# Casarett and Doull's
# TOXICOLOGY
## The Basic Science of Poisons

What is there that is not poison?
All things are poison and nothing (is)
without poison. Solely the dose
determines that a thing is not a poison.
*Paracelsus*
*(1493–1541)*

EDITOR

Curtis D. Klaassen, Ph.D.

Professor of Pharmacology and Toxicology
Department of Pharmacology, Toxicology, and Therapeutics
University of Kansas Medical Center
Kansas City, Kansas

EDITORS EMERITI

Mary O. Amdur, Ph.D.

Research Professor Emeritus
Institute of Environmental Medicine
New York University Medical Center
Tuxedo, New York

John Doull, Ph.D., M.D.

Professor Emeritus
Department of Pharmacology, Toxicology, and Therapeutics
University of Kansas Medical Center
Kansas City, Kansas

# Casarett and Doull's TOXICOLOGY
## The Basic Science of Poisons

Fifth Edition

McGraw-Hill
Health Professions Division

New York St. Louis San Francisco Auckland Bogotá Caracas Lisbon London Madrid
Mexico City Milan Montreal New Delhi San Juan Singapore Sydney Tokyo Toronto

*McGraw-Hill*
*A Division of The* ***McGraw-Hill*** *Companies*

**CASARETT AND DOULL'S TOXICOLOGY: THE BASIC SCIENCE OF POISONS**



34567890 DOW DOW 9876

ISBN 0-07-105476-6

This book was set in Times Roman by Northeastern Graphic Services, Inc.
The editors were Martin J. Wonsiewicz and Lester A. Sheinis.
The production supervisor was Richard C. Ruzycka.
The cover designer was Marsha Cohen/Parallelogram.
The indexer was Barbara Littlewood.
R.R. Donnelly & Sons Company was printer and binder.

This book is printed on acid-free paper.

**Library of Congress Cataloging-in-Publication Data**

Casarett and Doull's toxicology : the basic science of poisons /
editor, Curtis D. Klaassen, editors emeriti, Mary O. Amdur, John
Doull.—5th ed.
p. cm.
Includes bibliographical references and index.
ISBN 0-07-105476-6
1. Toxicology. I. Casarett, Louis J. II. Klaassen, Curtis D.
III. Amdur, Mary O. IV. Doull, John, date.
[DNLM: 1. Poisoning. 2. Poisons. QV 600 C335 1995]
RA 1211.C296 1995
615.9—dc20
DNLM/DLC
for Library of Congress 95-22362

# CONTENTS

# CONTRIBUTORS

**Daniel Acosta, Jr., Ph.D.**
Director, Toxicology Training Program
Department of Pharmacology and Toxicology
University of Texas
Austin, Texas
(Chapter 17)

**Mary O. Amdur, Ph.D.**
Research Professor Emeritus
Institute of Environmental Medicine
New York University Medical Center
Tuxedo, New York
(Chapter 28)

**Larry S. Andrews, Ph.D.**
Manager, Health Sciences and Regulatory Program
ARCO Chemical Company
Newtown Square, Pennsylvania
(Chapter 24)

**Douglas C. Anthony, Ph.D.**
Director, Neuropathology
Department of Pathology
Children's Hospital, Brigham and Women's Hospital, and Harvard Medical School
Boston, Massachusetts
(Chapter 16)

**Catherine M. Bens, M.S.**
The Institute of Wildlife and Environmental Toxicology (TIWET)
Lecturer
Department of Environmental Toxicology (ENTOX)
Clemson University
Pendleton, South Carolina
(Chapter 29)

**George A. Burdock, Ph.D., D.A.B.T.**
Burdock Associates
Reston, Virginia
(Chapter 30)

**Leigh Ann Burns, Ph.D.**
Toxicology Specialist, Immunotoxicology
Dow Corning Corporation
Midland, Michigan
(Chapter 12)

**Charles C. Capen, D.V.M., Ph.D.**
Professor and Chairperson
Department of Veterinary Biosciences
Ohio State University
Columbus, Ohio
(Chapter 21)

**Enrique Chacon, Ph.D.**
Senior Scientist
Cedra Corporation
Austin, Texas
(Chapter 17)

**George P. Cobb III, Ph.D.**
The Institute of Wildlife and Environmental Toxicology (TIWET)
Department of Environmental Toxicology (ENTOX)
Clemson University
Pendleton, South Carolina
(Chapter 29)

**David E. Cohen, M.D., M.P.H.**
Assistant Professor of Dermatology
Director of Occupational and Environmental Dermatology
New York University Medical Center
New York, New York
(Chapter 18)

**Daniel L. Costa, Sc.D.**
Chief, Pulmonary Toxicology Branch
Experimental Toxicology Division, NHEERL
US EPA
Research Triangle Park, North Carolina
(Chapter 28)

**Richard L. Dickerson, Ph.D.**
The Institute of Wildlife and Environmental Toxicology (TIWET)
Department of Environmental Toxicology (ENTOX)
Clemson University
Pendleton, South Carolina
(Chapter 29)

**Kenneth R. Dixon, Ph.D.**
The Institute of Wildlife and Environmental Toxicology (TIWET)
Department of Environmental Toxicology (ENTOX)
Clemson University
Pendleton, South Carolina
(Chapter 29)

**John Doull, Ph.D., M.D.**
Professor Emeritus
Department of Pharmacology, Toxicology, and Therapeutics
University of Kansas Medical Center
Kansas City, Kansas
(Appendix)

**Yvonne P. Dragan, Ph.D.**
Assistant Scientist
McArdle Laboratory for Cancer Research
University of Wisconsin Medical School
Madison, Wisconsin
(Chapter 8)

**David L. Eaton, Ph.D.**
Director
Center for Ecogenetics and Environmental Health
Department of Environmental Health
School of Public Health and Community Medicine
University of Washington
Seattle, Washington
(Chapter 2)

**Donald J. Ecobichon, Ph.D.**
Professor
Department of Pharmacology and Therapeutics
McGill University
Montreal, Canada
(Chapter 22)

**Elaine M. Faustman, Ph.D.**
Professor and Associate Chair
Department of Environmental Health
School of Public Health and Community Medicine
University of Washington
Seattle, Washington
(Chapter 4)

**W. Gary Flamm, Ph.D., F.A.C.T.**
Flamm Associates
Vero Beach, Florida
(Chapter 30)

**Michael A. Gallo, Ph.D.**
Professor
Director, NIEHS Center of Excellence
Department of Environmental and Community Medicine
UMDNJ-Robert Wood Johnson Medical School
Piscataway, New Jersey
(Chapter 1)

**Robin S. Goldstein, Ph.D.**
Director, Experimental Toxicology
Department of Toxicology/Pathology
Sandoz Pharmaceuticals Corporation
East Hanover, New Jersey
(Chapter 14)

**Robert A. Goyer, M.D.**
Professor Emeritus
University of Western Ontario
London, Ontario, Canada
(Chapter 23)

**Doyle G. Graham, M.D., Ph.D.**
Professor and Chair
Department of Pathology
Vanderbilt University Medical Center
Nashville, Tennessee
(Chapter 16)

**Zoltán Gregus, M.D., Ph.D.**
Professor
Department of Pharmacology
University Medical School of Pécs
Pécs, Hungary
(Chapter 3)

**Naomi H. Harley, Ph.D.**
Research Professor
The Nelson Institute of Environmental Medicine
New York University School of Medicine
New York, New York
(Chapter 25)

**George R. Hoffmann, Ph.D.**
Professor and Chair
Department of Biology
College of the Holy Cross
Worcester, Massachusetts
(Chapter 9)

**Robert J. Kavlock, Ph.D.**
Director
Reproductive Toxicology Division
National Health and Environmental Effects Research Laboratory
US EPA
Research Triangle Park, North Carolina
Adjunct Associate Professor of Pharmacology
Duke University
Durham, North Carolina
(Chapter 10)

**Ronald J. Kendall, Ph.D.**
Director
The Institute of Wildlife and Environmental Toxicology (TIWET)
Professor
Department of Environmental Toxicology (ENTOX)
Clemson University
Pendleton, South Carolina
(Chapter 29)

**Curtis D. Klaassen, Ph.D.**
Professor of Pharmacology and Toxicology
Department of Pharmacology, Toxicology, and Therapeutics
University of Kansas Medical Center
Kansas City, Kansas
(Chapters 2, 3, 5, 7)

**Stephen J. Klaine, Ph.D.**
The Institute of Wildlife and Environmental Toxicology (TIWET)
Departmental Chair and Professor
Department of Environmental Toxicology (ENTOX)
Clemson University
Pendleton, South Carolina
(Chapter 29)

**Frank N. Kotsonis, Ph.D., D.A.B.T.**
Corporate Vice President
Worldwide Regulatory Sciences
Monsanto
Deerfield, Illinois
(Chapter 30)

**Thomas E. Lacher, Jr., Ph.D.**
The Institute of Wildlife and Environmental Toxicology (TIWET)
Department of Environmental Toxicology (ENTOX)
Clemson University
Pendleton, South Carolina
(Chapter 29)

**Thomas W. La Point, Ph.D.**
The Institute of Wildlife and Environmental Toxicology (TIWET)
Department of Environmental Toxicology (ENTOX)
Clemson University
Pendleton, South Carolina
(Chapter 29)

**Jerold A. Last, Ph.D.**
Professor
Pulmonary/Critical Care Medicine
School of Medicine
University of California, Davis
Davis, California
(Chapter 15)

**Robert R. Lauwerys, M.D., D.Sc.**
Professor of Industrial Toxicology and Occupational Medicine
Faculty of Medicine
Catholic University of Louvain
Brussels, Belgium
(Chapter 33)

**Scott T. McMurry, Ph.D.**
The Institute of Wildlife and Environmental Toxicology (TIWET)
Department of Environmental Toxicology (ENTOX)
Clemson University
Pendleton, South Carolina
(Chapter 29)

**B. Jean Meade, DVM, Ph.D.**
Assistant Professor
Department of Pharmacology and Toxicology
Medical College of Virginia/Virginia Commonwealth University
Richmond, Virginia
(Chapter 12)

**Michele A. Medinsky, Ph.D.**
Senior Scientist
Chemical Industry Institute of Toxicology
Research Triangle Park, North Carolina
(Chapter 7)

**Richard A. Merrill, L.L.B., M.A.**
Daniel Caplin Professor of Law
University of Virginia
Charlottesville, Virginia
Special Counsel
Covington & Burling
Washington, DC
(Chapter 34)

**Thomas J. Montine, M.D., Ph.D.**
Assistant Professor
Department of Pathology
Vanderbilt University Medical Center
Nashville, Tennessee
(Chapter 16)

**Mary Treinen Moslen, Ph.D.**
Professor and Director
Toxicology Training Program
Department of Pathology
University of Texas Medical Branch
Galveston, Texas
(Chapter 13)

**Albert E. Munson, Ph.D.**
Professor
Department of Pharmacology and Toxicology
Medical College of Virginia/Virginia Commonwealth University
Richmond, Virginia
(Chapter 12)

**Raymond Noblet, Ph.D.**
The Institute of Wildlife and Environmental Toxicology (TIWET)
Department of Environmental Toxicology (ENTOX)
Clemson University
Pendleton, South Carolina
(Chapter 29)

**Stata Norton, Ph.D.**
Professor Emeritus
Department of Pharmacology, Toxicology, and Therapeutics
University of Kansas Medical Center
Kansas City, Kansas
(Chapter 27)

**Gilbert S. Omenn, M.D., Ph.D.**
Professor of Environmental Health and of Medicine
Dean, School of Public Health and Community Medicine
University of Washington
Seattle, Washington
(Chapter 4)

**Andrew Parkinson, Ph.D.**
Professor
Department of Pharmacology, Toxicology, and Therapeutics
University of Kansas Medical Center
Kansas City, Kansas
(Chapter 6)

**Henry C. Pitot III, M.D., Ph.D.**
Professor of Oncology and Pathology
McArdle Laboratory for Cancer Research and Center for Environmental Toxicology
University of Wisconsin
Madison, Wisconsin
(Chapter 8)

**Alphonse Poklis, Ph.D.**
Professor
Department of Pathology
Medical College of Virginia/Virginia Commonwealth University
Richmond, Virginia
(Chapter 31)

**Albert M. Potts, Ph.D., M.D.**
Distinguished Professor Emeritus
Department of Ophthalmology
University of Louisville
Louisville, Kentucky
(Chapter 20)

**Kenneth S. Ramos**
Professor
Department of Physiology and Pharmacology
College of Veterinary Medicine
Texas A&M University
College Station, Texas
(Chapter 17)

**Robert H. Rice, Ph.D.**
Professor and Chair
Department of Environmental Toxicology
University of California, Davis
Davis, California
(Chapter 18)

**John M. Rogers, Ph.D.**
Chief
Developmental Biology Branch
Reproductive Toxicology Division
National Health and Environmental Effects Research Laboratory
US EPA
Research Triangle Park, North Carolina
Adjunct Associate Professor
Curriculum in Toxicology
School of Medicine
University of North Carolina
Chapel Hill, North Carolina
(Chapter 10)

**Karl K. Rozman, Ph.D.**
Professor of Pharmacology and Toxicology
Department of Pharmacology, Toxicology, and Therapeutics
University of Kansas Medical Center
Kansas City, Kansas
(Chapter 5)

**Findlay E. Russell, M.D., Ph.D.**
Professor of Pharmacology and Toxicology
University of Arizona
Tucson, Arizona
Adjunct Professor of Neurology
University of Southern California
Los Angeles, California
(Chapter 26)

**Rick G. Schnellmann, Ph.D.**
Professor, Pharmacology and Toxicology
Department of Pharmacology and Toxicology
University of Arkansas for Medical Sciences
Little Rock, Arkansas
(Chapter 14)

**Ernest E. Smith, Ph.D.**
The Institute of Wildlife and Environmental Toxicology (TIWET)
Department of Environmental Toxicology (ENTOX)
Clemson University
Pendleton, South Carolina
(Chapter 29)

**Roger P. Smith, Ph.D.**
Irene Heinz Given Professor of Pharmacology and Toxicology
Department of Pharmacology and Toxicology
Dartmouth Medical School
Hanover, New Hampshire
(Chapter 11)

**Wayne R. Snodgrass, M.D., Ph.D.**
Professor
Pediatrics and Pharmacology–Toxicology
Head
Clinical Pharmacology–Toxicology Unit
Medical Director
Texas Poison Center
University of Texas Medical Branch
Galveston, Texas
(Chapter 32)

**Robert Snyder, Ph.D.**
Professor and Chair
Department of Pharmacology and Toxicology
Rutgers University College of Pharmacy
Environmental and Occupational
Health Science Institute
Piscataway, New Jersey
(Chapter 24)

**John A. Thomas, Ph.D.**
Professor of Pharmacology
The University of Texas Health Science Center at San Antonio
San Antonio, Texas
(Chapter 19)

**Hanspeter R. Witschi, M.D.**
Professor of Toxicology
School of Veterinary Medicine and ITEH
University of California, Davis
Davis, California
(Chapter 15)

# PREFACE

The fifth edition of *Casarett and Doull's Toxicology: The Basic Science of Poisons* marks its twentieth anniversary. The fifth edition, as the previous four, is meant to serve primarily as a text for, or an adjunct to, graduate courses in toxicology. Because the four previous editions have been widely used in courses in environmental health and related areas, an attempt has been made to maintain those characteristics that make it useful to scientists from other disciplines. This edition will again provide information on the many facets of toxicology and especially on the principles, concepts, and modes of thought that are the foundation of the discipline. Mechanisms of toxicity are emphasized. Research toxicologists will find this book an excellent reference source to find updated material in areas of their special or peripheral interests.

While the overall framework of the fifth edition is similar to the previous four, it has undergone some significant changes. Previously there were five sections, but the present edition has seven sections plus an appendix. The seven sections are "General Principles of Toxicology" (Unit 1), "Disposition of Toxicants" (Unit 2), "Nonorgan-Directed Toxicity" (carcinogenicity, mutagenicity, and teratogenicity) (Unit 3), "Target Organ Toxicity" (Unit 4), "Toxic Agents" (Unit 5), "Environmental Toxicology" (Unit 6), and "Applications of Toxicology" (Unit 7).

Without permitting the fifth edition to become unwieldy in size and prohibitive in cost, we have added three new chapters: "Toxicokinetics," "Mechanisms of Toxicity," and "Toxic Responses of the Endocrine System," as well as an Appendix on "Recommended Limits for Exposure to Chemicals." Half of the thirty-four chapters of the fifth edition have been written by authors not associated with the fourth edition.

The fifth edition reflects the marked progress made in toxicology this decade. For example, the importance of apoptosis, cytokines, growth factors, oncogenes, cell cycling, receptors, gene regulation, transcription factors, transgenic animals, polymorphisms, etc., in understanding the mechanisms of toxicity are included in this edition. More information on risk assessment is also included. The book has many more figures than previously to make it more "user-friendly."

The editor is grateful to our colleagues in academia, industry, and government who have made useful suggestions for improving this fifth edition both as a book and as a reference source. The editor is especially grateful to all the contributors, whose combined expertise has made possible a volume of this breadth. I dedicate this edition to John Doull and Mary Amdur, who have edited previous editions of this book and remain as Editors Emeriti to advise and help me on this fifth edition.

# PREFACE TO THE FIRST EDITION

This volume has been designed primarily as a textbook for, or adjunct to, courses in toxicology. However, it should also be of interest to those not directly involved in toxicologic education. For example, the research scientist in toxicology will find sections containing current reports on the status of circumscribed areas of special interest. Those concerned with community health, agriculture, food technology, pharmacy, veterinary medicine, and related disciplines will discover the contents to be most useful as a source of concepts and modes of thought that are applicable to other types of investigative and applied sciences. For those further removed from the field of toxicology or for those who have not entered a specific field of endeavor, this book attempts to present a selectively representative view of the many facets of the subject.

*Toxicology: The Basic Science of Poisons* has been organized to facilitate its use by these different types of users. The first section (Unit I) describes the elements of method and approach that identify toxicology. It includes those principles most frequently invoked in a full understanding of toxicologic events, such as dose-response, and is primarily mechanistically oriented. Mechanisms are also stressed in the subsequent sections of the book, particularly when these are well identified and extend across classic forms of chemicals and systems. However, the major focus in the second section (Unit II) is on the systemic site of action of toxins. The intent therein is to provide answers to two questions: What kinds of injury are produced in specific organs or systems by toxic agents? What are the agents that produce these effects?

A more conventional approach to toxicology has been utilized in the third section (Unit III), in which the toxic agents are grouped by chemical or use characteristics. In the final section (Unit IV) an attempt has been made to illustrate the ramifications of toxicology into all areas of the health sciences and even beyond. This unit is intended to provide perspective for the nontoxicologist in the application of the results of toxicologic studies and a better understanding of the activities of those engaged in the various aspects of the discipline of toxicology.

It will be obvious to the reader that the contents of this book represent a compromise between the basic, fundamental, mechanistic approach to toxicology and the desire to give a view of the broad horizons presented by the subject. While it is certain that the editors' selectivity might have been more severe, it is equally certain that it could have been less so, and we hope that the balance struck will prove to be appropriate for both toxicologic training and the scientific interest of our colleagues.

L.J.C.
J.D.

Although the philosophy and design of this book evolved over a long period of friendship and mutual respect between the editors, the effort needed to convert ideas into reality was undertaken primarily by Louis J. Casarett. Thus, his death at a time when completion of the manuscript was in sight was particularly tragic. With the help and encouragement of his wife, Margaret G. Casarett, and the other contributors, we have finished Lou's task. This volume is a fitting embodiment of Louis J. Casarett's dedication to toxicology and to toxicologic education.

J.D.

## NOTICE

# UNIT 1

# GENERAL PRINCIPLES OF TOXICOLOGY

CHAPTER 1

# HISTORY AND SCOPE OF TOXICOLOGY

*Michael A. Gallo*

Toxicology has been defined as the study of the adverse effects of xenobiotics and thus is a borrowing science that has evolved from ancient poisoners. Modern toxicology goes beyond the study of the adverse effects of exogenous agents to the study of molecular biology, using toxicants as tools. Historically, toxicology formed the basis of therapeutics and experimental medicine. Toxicology in this century (1900 to the present) continues to develop and expand by assimilating knowledge and techniques from most branches of biology, chemistry, mathematics, and physics. A recent addition to the field of toxicology (1975 to the present) is the application of the discipline to safety evaluation and risk assessment.

The contributions and activities of toxicologists are diverse and widespread. In the biomedical area, toxicologists are concerned with mechanisms of action and exposure to chemical agents as a cause of acute and chronic illness. Toxicologists contribute to physiology and pharmacology by using toxic agents to understand physiological phenomena. They are involved in the recognition, identification, and quantification of hazards resulting from occupational exposure to chemicals and the public health aspects of chemicals in air, water, other parts of the environment, foods and drugs. Traditionally, toxicologists have been intimately involved in the discovery and development of new drugs and pesticides. Toxicologists also participate in the development of standards and regulations designed to protect human health and the environment from the adverse effects of chemicals. Environmental toxicologists (a relatively new subset of the discipline) have expanded toxicology to study the effects of chemicals in flora and fauna. Molecular toxicologists are studying the mechanisms by which toxicants modulate cell growth and differentiation and cells respond to toxicants at the level of the gene. In all branches of toxicology, scientists explore the mechanisms by which chemicals produce adverse effects in biological systems. Clinical toxicologists develop antidotes and treatment regimes to ameliorate poisonings and xenobiotic injury. Toxicologists carry out some or all of these activities as members of academic, industrial, and governmental organizations. In doing so, they share methodologies for obtaining data about the toxicity of materials and the responsibility for using this information to make reasonable predictions regarding the hazards of the material to people and the environment. These different but complementary activities characterize the discipline of toxicology.

Toxicology, like medicine, is both a science and an art. The science of toxicology is defined as the observational and data-gathering phase, whereas the art of toxicology consists of the utilization of the data to predict outcomes of exposure in human and animal populations. In most cases, these phases are linked because the facts generated by the science of toxicology are used to develop extrapolations and hypotheses to explain the adverse effects of chemical agents in situations where there is little or no information. For example, the observation that the administration of TCDD (2,3,7,8-tetrachlorodibenzo-*p*-dioxin) to female Sprague-Dawley rats induces hepatocellular carcinoma is a fact. However, the conclusion that it will also do so in humans is a prediction or hypothesis. It is important to distinguish facts from predictions. When we fail to distinguish the science from the art, we confuse facts with predictions and argue that they have equal validity, which they clearly do not. In toxicology, as in all sciences, theories have a higher level of certainty than do hypotheses, which in turn are more certain than speculations, opinions, conjectures, and guesses. An insight into modern toxicology and the roles, points of view, and activities of toxicologists can be obtained by examining the historical evolution of the discipline.

## HISTORY OF TOXICOLOGY

### Antiquity

Toxicology dates back to the earliest humans, who used animal venoms and plant extracts for hunting, warfare, and assassination. The knowledge of these poisons must have predated recorded history. It is safe to assume that prehistoric humans categorized some plants as harmful and others as safe. The same is probably true for the classification of snakes and other animals. The Ebers papyrus (circa 1500 B.C.) contains information pertaining to many recognized poisons, including hemlock (the state poison of the Greeks), aconite (a Chinese arrow poison), opium (used as both a poison and an antidote), and metals such as lead, copper, and antimony. There is also an indication that plants containing substances similar to digitalis and belladonna alkaloids were known. Hippocrates (circa 400 B.C.) added a number of poisons and clinical toxicology principles pertaining to bioavailability in therapy and overdosage, while the Book of Job (circa 400 B.C.) speaks of poison arrows (Job 6:4). In the literature of ancient Greece, there are several references to poisons and their use. Some interpretations of Homer have Odysseus obtaining poisons for his arrows (Homer, circa 600 B.C.). Theophrastus (370–286 B.C.), a student of Aristotle, included numerous references to poisonous plants in *De Historia Plantarum*. Dioscorides, a Greek physician in the court of the Roman emperor Nero, made the first attempt at a classification of poisons, which was accompanied by descriptions and drawings. His classifiction into plant, animal, and mineral poisons not only remained a standard for 16 centuries but is still a convenient classification (Gunther, 1934). Dioscorides also dabbled in therapy, recognizing the use of emetics in poisoning and the use of caustic agents and cupping glasses in snakebite. Poisoning with plant and animal toxins was quite common. Perhaps the best known recipient of poison used as a state method of execution was Socrates (470–399 B.C.), whose cup of hemlock extract was apparently estimated to be the proper dose. Expeditious suicide on a voluntary basis also made use of toxicological knowledge. Demosthenes (385–322 B.C.), who took poison hidden in his pen, was one of many examples. The mode of suicide calling for one to fall on his sword, although manly and noble, carried little appeal and less significance for the women of the day. Cleopatra's (69–30 B.C.) knowledge of natural primitive toxicology permitted her to use the more genteel method of falling on her asp.

The Romans too made considerable use of poisons in politics. One legend tells of King Mithridates VI of Pontus, whose numerous acute toxicity experiments on unfortunate criminals led to his eventual claim that he had discovered an antidote for every venomous reptile and poisonous substance (Guthrie, 1946). Mithridates was so fearful of poisons that he regularly ingested a mixture of 36 ingredients (Galen reports 54) as protection against assassination. On the occasion of his imminent capture by enemies, his attempts to kill himself with poison failed because of his successful antidote concoction, and he was forced to use a sword held by a servant. From this tale comes the term "mithridatic," referring to an antidotal or protective mixture. The term "theriac" also has become synonymous with "antidote," although the word comes from the poetic treatise *Theriaca* by Nicander of Colophon (204–135 B.C.), which dealt with poisonous animals; his poem "Alexipharmaca" was about antidotes.

Poisonings in Rome reached epidemic proportions during the fourth century B.C. (Livy). It was during this period that a conspiracy of women to remove men from whose death they might profit was uncovered. Similar large-scale poisoning continued until Sulla issued the *Lex Cornelia* (circa 82 B.C.). This appears to be the first law against poisoning, and it later became a regulatory statute directed at careless dispensers of drugs. Nero (A.D. 37–68) used poisons to do away with his stepbrother Brittanicus and employed his slaves as food tasters to differentiate edible mushrooms from their more poisonous kin.

## Middle Ages

Come bitter pilot, now at once run on
The dashing rocks thy seasick weary bark!
Here's to my love! O true apothecary!
Thy drugs are quick. Thus with a kiss I die.
*Romeo and Juliet,* act 5, scene 3

Before the Renaissance, the writings of Maimonides (Moses ben Maimon, A.D. 1135–1204) included a treatise on the treatment of poisonings from insects, snakes, and mad dogs (*Poisons and Their Antidotes*, 1198). Maimonides, like Hippocrates before him, wrote on the subject of bioavailability, noting that milk, butter, and cream could delay intestinal absorption. Maimonides also refuted many of the popular remedies of the day and stated his doubts about others. It is rumored that alchemists of this period (circa A.D. 1200), in search of the universal antidote, learned to distill fermented products and made a 60% ethanol beverage that had many interesting powers.

In the early Renaissance, the Italians, with characteristic pragmatism, brought the art of poisoning to its zenith. The poisoner became an integral part of the political scene. The records of the city councils of Florence, particularly those of the infamous Council of Ten of Venice, contain ample testimony about the political use of poisons. Victims were named, prices set, and contracts recorded; when the deed was accomplished, payment was made.

An infamous figure of the time was a lady named Toffana who peddled specially prepared arsenic-containing cosmetics (*Agua Toffana*). Accompanying the product were appropriate instructions for its use. Toffana was succeeded by an imitator with organizational genius, Hieronyma Spara, who provided a new fillip by directing her activities toward specific marital and monetary objectives. A local club was formed of young, wealthy married women, which soon became a club of eligible young wealthy widows, reminiscent of the matronly conspiracy of Rome centuries earlier. Incidentally, arsenic-containing cosmetics were reported to be responsible for deaths well into the twentieth century (Kallett and Schlink, 1933).

Among the prominent families engaged in poisoning, the Borgias were the most notorious. However, many deaths that were attributed to poisoning are now recognized as having resulted from infectious diseases such as malaria. It appears true, however, that Alexander VI, his son Cesare, and Lucrezia Borgia were quite active. The deft application of poisons to men of stature in the Catholic Church swelled the holdings of the papacy, which was their prime heir.

In this period Catherine de Medici exported her skills from Italy to France, where the prime targets of women were their husbands. However, unlike poisoners of an earlier period, the circle represented by Catherine and epitomized by the notorious Marchioness de Brinvillers depended on developing direct evidence to arrive at the most effective compounds for their purposes. Under the guise of delivering provender to the sick and the poor, Catherine tested toxic concoctions, carefully noting the rapidity of the toxic response (onset of action), the effectiveness of the compound (potency), the degree of response of the parts of the body (specificity, site of action), and the complaints of the victim (clinical signs and symptoms).

The culmination of the practice in France is represented by the commercialization of the service by Catherine Deshayes, who earned the title "La Voisine." Her business was dissolved by her execution. Her trial was one of the most famous of those held by the Chambre Ardente, a special judicial commission established by Louis XIV to try such cases without regard to age, sex, or national origin. La Voisine was convicted of many poisonings, with over 2000 infants among her victims.

## Age of Enlightenment

All substances are poisons; there is none which is not a poison. The right dose differentiates a poison from a remedy.
*Paracelsus*

A significant figure in the history of science and medicine in the late Middle Ages was the renaissance man Philippus Aureolus Theophrastus Bombastus von Hohenheim-Paracelsus (1493–1541). Between the time of Aristotle and the age of Paracelsus, there was little substantial change in the biomedical sciences. In the sixteenth century, the revolt against the authority of the Catholic Church was accompanied by a parallel attack on the godlike authority exercised by the followers of Hippocrates and Galen. Paracelsus personally and professionally embodied the qualities that forced numerous changes in this period. He and his age were pivotal, standing between the philosophy and magic of classical antiquity and the philosophy and science willed to us by figures of the seventeenth and eighteenth centuries. Clearly, one can identify in Paracelsus's approach, point of view, and breadth of interest numerous similarities to the discipline that is now called toxicology.

Paracelsus, a physician-alchemist and the son of a physician, formulated many revolutionary views that remain an integral part of the structure of toxicology, pharmacology, and therapeutics today (Pagel, 1958). He promoted a focus on the "toxicon," the primary toxic agent, as a chemical entity, as opposed to the Grecian concept of the mixture or blend. A view initiated by Paracelsus that became a lasting contribution held as corollaries that (1) experimentation is essential in the examination of responses to chemicals, (2) one should make a distinction between the therapeutic and toxic properties of chemicals, (3) these properties are sometimes but not always indistinguishable except by dose, and (4) one can ascertain a degree of specificity of chemicals and their therapeutic or toxic effects. These principles led Paracelsus to introduce mercury as the drug of choice for the treatment of syphilis, a practice that survived 300 years but led to his famous trial. This viewpoint presaged the "magic bullet" (arsphenamine) of Paul Ehrlich and the introduction of the therapeutic index. Further, in a very real sense, this was the first sound articulation of the dose-response relation, a bulwark of toxicology (Pachter, 1961).

The tradition of the poisoners spread throughout Europe, and their deeds played a major role in the distribution of political power throughout the Middle Ages. Pharmacology as it is known today had its beginnings during the Middle Ages and early Renaissance. Concurrently, the study of the toxicity and the dose-response relationship of therapeutic agents was commencing.

The occupational hazards associated with metalworking were recognized during the fifteenth century. Early publications by Ellenbog (circa 1480) warned of the toxicity of the mercury and lead exposures involved in goldsmithing. Agricola published a short treatise on mining diseases in 1556. However, the major work on the subject, *On the Miners' Sickness and Other Diseases of Miners* (1567), was published by Paracelsus. This treatise addressed the etiology of miners' disease, along with treatment and prevention strategies. Occupational toxicology was further advanced by the work of Bernardino Ramazzini. His classic, published in 1700 and entitled *Discourse on the Diseases of Workers*, set the standard for occupational medicine well into the nineteenth century. Ramazzini's work broadened the field by discussing occupations ranging from miners to midwives and including printers, weavers, and potters.

The developments of the industrial revolution stimulated a rise in many occupational diseases. Percival Pott's (1775) recognition of the role of soot in scrotal cancer among chimney sweeps was the first reported example of polyaromatic hydrocarbon carcinogenicity, a problem that still plagues toxicologists as the year 2000 approaches. These findings led to improved medical practices, particularly in prevention. It should be noted that Paracelsus and Ramazzini also pointed out the toxicity of smoke and soot.

The nineteenth century dawned in a climate of industrial and political revolution. Organic chemistry was in its infancy in 1800, but by 1825 phosgene ($COCl_2$) and mustard gas (bis[B-chloroethyl]sulfide) had been synthesized. These two agents were used in World War I as war gases. By 1880 over 10,000 organic compounds had been synthesized including chloroform, carbon tetrachloride, diethyl ether, and carbonic acid, and petroleum and coal gasification by-products were used in trade (Zapp, 1982). Determination of the toxicological potential of these newly created chemicals became the underpinning of the science of toxicology as it is practiced today. However, there was little interest during the mid-nineteenth century in hampering industrial development. Hence, the impact of industrial toxicology discoveries was not felt until the passage of worker's insurance laws, first in Germany (1883), then in England (1897), and later in the United States (1910).

Experimental toxicology accompanied the growth of organic chemistry and developed rapidly during the nineteenth century. Magendie (1783–1885), Orfila (1787–1853), and Bernard (1813–1878) carried out truly seminal research in experimental toxicology and laid the groundwork for pharmacology and experimental therapeutics as well as occupational toxicology.

Orfila, a Spanish physician in the French court, was the first toxicologist to use autopsy material and chemical analysis systematically as legal proof of poisoning. His introduction of this detailed type of analysis survives as the underpinning of forensic toxicology (Orfila, 1818). Orfila published the first major work devoted expressly to the toxicity of natural agents (1815). Magendie, a physician and experimental physiologist, studied the mechanisms of action of emetine, strychnine, and "arrow poisons" (Olmsted, 1944). His research into the absorption and distribution of these compounds in the body remains a classic in toxicology and pharmacology. One of Magendie's more famous students, Claude Bernard, continued the study of arrow poisons (Bernard, 1850) but also added works on the mechanism of action of carbon monoxide. Bernard's treatise, *An Introduction to the Study of Experimental Medicine* (translated by Greene in 1949), is a classic in the development of toxicology.

Many German scientists contributed greatly to the growth of toxicology in the late nineteenth and early twentieth centuries. Among the giants of the field are Oswald Schmeideberg (1838–1921) and Louis Lewin (1850–1929). Schmiedeberg made many contributions to the science of toxicology, not the least of which was the training of approximately 120 students who later populated the most important laboratories of pharmacology and toxicology throughout the world. His research focused on the synthesis of hippuric acid in the liver and the detoxification mechanisms of the liver in several animal species (Schmiedeberg and Koppe, 1869). Lewin, who was educated originally in medicine and the natural sciences, trained in toxicology under Liebreich at the Pharmacological Institute of Berlin (1881). His contributions on the chronic toxicity of narcotics and other alkaloids remain a classic. Lewin also published much of the early work on the toxicity of methanol, glycerol, acrolein, and chloroform (Lewin, 1920, 1929).

## Modern Toxicology

Toxicology has evolved rapidly during this century. The exponential growth of the discipline can be traced to the World War II era with its marked increase in the production of drugs, pesticides, munitions, synthetic fibers, and industrial chemicals. The history of many sciences represents an orderly transition based on theory, hypothesis testing, and synthesis of new ideas. Toxicology, as a gathering and an applied science, has, by contrast, developed in fits and starts. Toxicology calls on almost all the basic sciences to test its hypotheses. This fact, coupled with the health and occupational regulations that have driven toxicology research since 1900, has made this discipline exceptional in the history of science. The differentiation of toxicology as an art and a science, though arbitrary, permits the presentation of historical highlights along two major lines.

Modern toxicology can be viewed as a continuation of the development of the biological and physical sciences in the late nineteenth and twentieth centuries (Table 1-1). During the second half of the nineteenth century, the world witnessed an explosion in science that produced the beginning of the modern era of medicine, synthetic chemistry, physics, and biology. Toxicology has drawn its strength and diversity from its proclivity to borrowing. With the advent of anesthetics and disinfectants and the advancement of experimental pharmacology

**Table 1-1**
**Selection of Developments in Toxicology**

*Development of early advances in analytic methods*
- Marsh, 1836: development of method for arsenic analysis
- Reinsh, 1841: combined method for separation and analysis of As and Hg
- Fresenius, 1845, and von Babo, 1847: development of screening method for general poisons
- Stas-Otto, 1851: extraction and separation of alkaloids
- Mitscherlich, 1855: detection and identification of phosphorus

*Early mechanistic studies*
- F. Magendie, 1809: study of "arrow poisons," mechanism of action of emetine and strychnine
- C. Bernard, 1850: carbon monoxide combination with hemoglobin, study of mechanism of action of strychnine, site of action of curare
- R. Bohm, ca. 1890: active anthelmintics from fern, action of croton oil catharsis, poisonous mushrooms

*Introduction of new toxicants and antidotes*
- R. A. Peters, L. A. Stocken, and R. H. S. Thompson, 1945: development of British Anti Lewisite (BAL) as a relatively specific antidote for arsenic, toxicity of monofluorocarbon compounds
- K. K. Chen, 1934: introduction of modern antidotes (nitrite and thiosulfate) for cyanide toxicity
- C. Voegtlin, 1923: mechanism of action of As and other metals on the SH groups
- P. Müller, 1944–1946: introduction and study of DDT (dichlorodiphenyltrichloroethane) and related insecticide compounds
- G. Schrader, 1952: introduction and study of organophosphorus compounds
- R. N. Chopra, 1933: indigenous drugs of India

*Miscellaneous toxicological studies*
- R. T. Williams: study of detoxication mechanisms and species variation
- A. Rothstein: effects of uranium ion on cell membrane transport
- R. A. Kehoe: investigation of acute and chronic effects of lead
- A. Vorwald: studies of chronic respiratory disease (beryllium)
- H. Hardy: community and industrial poisoning (beryllium)
- A. Hamilton: introduction of modern industrial toxicology
- H. C. Hodge: toxicology of uranium, fluorides; standards of toxicity
- A. Hoffman: introduction of lysergic acid and derivatives; psychotomimetics
- R. A. Peters: biochemical lesions, lethal synthesis
- A. E. Garrod: inborn errors of metabolism
- T. T. Litchfield and F. Wilcoxon: simplified dose-response evaluation
- C. J. Bliss: method of probits, calculation of dosage-mortality curves

in the late 1850s, toxicology as it is currently understood got its start. The introduction of ether, chloroform, and carbonic acid led to several iatrogenic deaths. These unfortunate outcomes spurred research into the causes of the deaths and early experiments on the physiological mechanisms by which these compounds caused both beneficial and adverse effects. By the late nineteenth century the use of organic chemicals was becoming more widespread, and benzene, toluene, and the xylenes went into larger-scale commercial production.

During this period, the use of "patent" medicines was prevalent, and there were several incidents of poisonings from these medicaments. The adverse reactions to patent medicines, coupled with the response to Upton Sinclair's exposé of the meat-packing industry in *The Jungle*, culminated in the passage of the Wiley Bill (1906), the first of many U.S. pure food and drug laws (see Hutt and Hutt, 1984, for regulatory history).

A working hypothesis about the development of toxicology is that the discipline expands in response to legislation, which itself is a response to a real or perceived tragedy. The Wiley Bill was the first such reaction in the area of food and drugs, and the worker's compensation laws cited above were a response to occupational toxicities. In addition, the National Safety Council was established in 1911, and the Division of Industrial Hygiene was established by the U. S. Public Health Service in 1914. A corollary to this hypothesis might be that the founding of scientific journals and/or societies is sparked by the development of a new field. The *Journal of Industrial Hygiene* began in 1918. The major chemical manufacturers in the United States (Dow, Union Carbide, and Du Pont) established internal toxicology research laboratories to help guide decisions on worker health and product safety.

During the 1890s and early 1900s, the French scientists Becquerel and the Curies reported the discovery of "radioactivity." This opened up for exploration a very large area in physics, biology, and medicine, but it would not actively affect the science of toxicology for another 40 years. However, another discovery, that of vitamins, or "vital amines," was to lead to the use of the first large-scale bioassays (multiple animal studies) to determine whether these "new" chemicals were beneficial or harmful to laboratory animals. The initial work in this area took place at around the time of World War I in several laboratories, including the laboratory of Philip B. Hawk in Philadelphia. Hawk and a young associate, Bernard L. Oser, were responsible for the development and verification of many early toxicological assays that are still used in a slightly amended form. Oser's contributions to food and regulatory toxicology were extraordinary. These early bioassays were made possible by a major advance in toxicology: the availability of developed and refined strains of inbred laboratory rodents (Donaldson, 1912).

The 1920s saw many events that began to mold the fledgling field of toxicology. The use of arsenicals for the treatment of diseases such as syphilis (arsenicals had been used in agriculture since the mid-nineteenth century) resulted in acute and chronic toxicity. Prohibition of alcoholic beverages in the United States opened the door for early studies of neurotoxicology, with the discovery that triorthocresyl phosphate (TOCP), methanol, and lead (all products of "bootleg" liquor) are neurotoxicants. TOCP, which is a modern gasoline additive, caused a syndrome that became known as "Ginger-Jake" walk, a spastic gait resulting from drinking adulterated ginger beer. Mueller's discovery of DDT (dichlorodiphenyltrichloroethane) and several other organohalides, such as hexachlorobenzene and hexachlorocyclohexane, during the late 1920s resulted in wider use of insecticidal agents. Other scientists were hard at work attempting to elucidate the structures and activity of the estrogens and androgens. Work on the steroid hormones led to the use of several assays for the determination of the biological activity of organ extracts and synthetic compounds. Efforts to synthesize steroidal-like chemicals were spearheaded by E. C. Dodds and his coworkers, one of whom was a young organic chemist, Leon Golberg. Dodds's work on the bioactivity of the estrogenic compounds resulted in the synthesis of diethylstilbestrol (DES), hexestrol, and other stilbenes and the discovery of the strong estrogenic activity of substituted stilbenes. Golberg's intimate involvement in this work stimulated his interest in biology, leading to degrees in biochemistry and medicine and a career in toxicology in which he oversaw the creation of the laboratories of the British Industrial Biological Research Association (BIBRA) and the Chemical Industry Institute of Toxicology (CIIT). Interestingly, the initial observations that led to the discovery of DES were the findings of feminization of animals treated with the experimental carcinogen 7,12-dimethylbenz[*a*]anthracene (DMBA)

The 1930s saw the world preparing for World War II and a major effort by the pharmaceutical industry in Germany and the United States to manufacture the first mass-produced antibiotics. One of the first journals expressly dedicated to experimental toxicology, *Archiv für Toxikologie*, began publication in Europe in 1930, the same year that Herbert Hoover signed the act that established the National Institutes of Health (NIH) in theUnited States.

The discovery of sulfanilamide was heralded as a major event in combating bacterial diseases. However, for a drug to be effective, there must be a reasonable delivery system, and sulfanilamide is highly insoluble in an aqueous medium. Therefore, it was originally prepared in ethanol (elixir). However, it was soon discovered that the drug was more soluble in ethylene glycol, which is a dihydroxy rather than a monohydroxy ethane. The drug was sold in glycol solutions but was labeled as an elixir, and several patients died of acute kidney failure resulting from the metabolism of the glycol to oxalic acid and glycolic acid, with the acids, along with the active drug, crystallizing in the kidney tubules. This tragic event led to the passage of the Copeland Bill in 1938, the second major bill involving the formation of the U.S. Food and Drug Administration (FDA). The sulfanilamide disaster played a critical role in the further development of toxicology, resulting in work by Eugene Maximillian Geiling in the Pharmacology Department of the University of Chicago that elucidated the mechanism of toxicity of both sulfanilamide and ethylene glycol. Studies of the glycols were simultaneously carried out at the U.S. FDA by a group led by Arnold Lehman. The scientists associated with Lehman and Geiling were to become the leaders of toxicology over the next 40 years. With few exceptions, toxicology in the United States owes its heritage to Geiling's innovativeness and ability to stimulate and direct young scientists and Lehman's vision of the use of experimental toxicology in public health decision making. Because of Geiling's reputation, the U.S. government turned to this group for help in the war effort. There were three main areas in which the Chicago group took part during World War II: the toxicology and pharmacology of organophosphate chemicals, antimalarial drugs, and radionuclides. Each of these areas produced teams of toxicologists who became academic, governmental, and industrial leaders in the field.

It was also during this time that DDT and the phenoxy herbicides were developed for increased food production and, in the case of DDT, control of insect-borne diseases. These efforts between 1940 and 1946 led to an explosion in toxicology. Thus, in line with the hypothesis advanced above, the crisis of World War II caused the next major leap in the development of toxicology.

If one traces the history of the toxicology of metals over the past 45 years, the role of the Chicago group is quite visible. This story commences with the use of uranium for the "bomb" and continues today with research on the role of metals in their interactions with DNA, RNA, and growth factors. Indeed, the Manhattan Project created a fertile environment that resulted in the initiation of quantitative biology, radiotracer technology, and inhalation toxicology. These innovations have revolutionized modern biology, chemistry, therapeutics, and toxicology.

Inhalation toxicology began at the University of Rochester under the direction of Stafford Warren, who headed the Department of Radiology. He developed a program with colleagues such as Harold Hodge (pharmacologist), Herb Stokinger (chemist), Sid Laskin (inhalation toxicologist), and Lou and George Casarett (toxicologists). These young scientists were to go on to become giants in the field. The other sites for the study of radionuclides were Chicago for the "internal" effects of radioactivity and Oak Ridge, Tennessee, for the effects of "external" radiation. The work of the scientists on these teams gave the scientific community data that contributed to the early understanding of macromolecular binding of xenobiotics, cellular mutational events, methods for inhalation toxicology and therapy, and toxicological properties of trace metals, along with a better appreciation of the complexities of the dose-response curve.

Another seminal event in toxicology that occurred during the World War II era was the discovery of organophosphate cholinesterase inhibitors. This class of chemicals, which was discovered by Willy Lange and Gerhard Schrader, was destined to become a driving force in the study of neurophysiology and toxicology for several decades. Again, the scientists in Chicago played major roles in elucidating the mechanisms of action of this new class of compounds. Geiling's group, Kenneth Dubois in particular, were leaders in this area of toxicology and pharmacology. Dubois's students, particularly Sheldon Murphy, continued to be in the forefront of this special area. The importance of the early research on the organophosphates has taken on special meaning in the years since 1960, when these nonbioaccumulating insecticides were destined to replace DDT and other organochlorine insectides.

Early in the twentieth century, it was demonstrated experimentally that quinine has a marked effect on the malaria parasite [it had been known for centuries that chincona bark extract is efficacious for "Jesuit fever" (malaria)]. This discovery led to the development of quinine derivatives for the treatment of the disease and the formulation of the early principles of chemotherapy. The pharmacology department at Chicago was charged with the development of antimalarials for the war effort. The original protocols called for testing of efficacy and toxicity in rodents and perhaps dogs and then the testing of efficacy in human volunteers. One of the investigators charged with generating the data needed to move a candidate drug from animals to humans was Fredrick Coulston. This young parasitologist and his colleagues, working under Geiling, were to evaluate potential drugs in animal models and then establish human clinical trials. It was during these experiments that the use of nonhuman primates came into vogue for toxicology testing. It had been noted by Russian scientists that some antimalarial compounds caused retinopathies in humans but did not apparently have the same adverse effect in rodents and dogs. This finding led the Chicago team to add one more step in the development process: toxicity testing in rhesus monkeys just before efficacy studies in people. This resulted in the prevention of blindness in untold numbers of volunteers and perhaps some of the troops in the field. It also led to the school of thought that nonhuman primates may be one of the better models for humans and the establishment of primate colonies for the study of toxicity. Coulston pioneered this area of toxicology and remains committed to it.

Another area not traditionally thought of as toxicology but one that evolved during the 1940s as an exciting and innovative field is experimental pathology. This branch of experimental biology developed from bioassays of estrogens and early experiments in chemical- and radiation-induced carcinogenesis. It is from these early studies that hypotheses on tumor promotion and cancer progression have evolved.

Toxicologists today owe a great deal to the researchers of chemical carcinogenesis of the 1940s. Much of today's work can be traced to Elizabeth and James Miller at Wisconsin. This husband and wife team started under the mentorship of Professor Rusch, the director of the newly formed McArdle Laboratory for Cancer Research, and Professor Baumann. The seminal research of the Millers led to the discovery of the role of reactive intermediates in carcinogenicity and that of mixed-function oxidases in the endoplasmic reticulum. These findings, which initiated the great works on the cytochrome P-450 family of proteins, were aided by two other major discoveries for which toxicologists (and all other biological scientists) are deeply indebted: paper chromatography in 1944 and the use of radiolabeled dibenzanthracene in 1948. Other major events of note in drug metabolism included the work of Bernard Brodie on the metabolism of methyl orange in 1947. This piece of seminal research led to the examination of blood and urine for chemical and drug metabolites. It became the tool with which one could study the relationship between blood levels and biological action. The classic treatise of R. T. Williams, *Detoxication Mechanisms*, was published in 1947. This text described the many pathways and possible mechanisms of detoxication and opened the field to several new areas of study.

The decade after World War II was not as boisterous as the period from 1935 to 1945. The first major U.S. pesticide act was signed into law in 1947. The significance of the initial Federal Insecticide, Fungicide, and Rodenticide Act was that for the first time in U.S. history a substance that was neither a drug nor a food had to be shown to be safe and efficacious. This decade, which coincided with the Eisenhower years, saw the dispersion of the groups from Chicago, Rochester, and

Oak Ridge and the establishment of new centers of research. Adrian Albert's classic *Selective Toxicity* was published in 1951. This treatise, which has appeared in several editions, presented a concise documentation of the principles of the site-specific action of chemicals.

## After World War II

You too can be a toxicologist in two easy lessons, each of ten years.
*Arnold Lehman* (circa 1955)

The mid-1950s witnessed the strengthening of the U.S. Food and Drug Administration's commitment to toxicology under the guidance of Arnold Lehman. Lehman's tutelage and influence are still felt today. The adage "You too can be a toxicologist" is as important a summation of toxicology as the often quoted statement of Paracelsus: "The dose makes the poison." The period from 1955 to 1958 produced two major events that would have a long-lasting impact on toxicology as a science and a professional discipline. Lehman, Fitzhugh, and their coworkers formalized the experimental program for the appraisal of food, drug, and cosmetic safety in 1955, updated by the U.S. FDA in 1982, and the Gordon Research Conferences established a conference on toxicology and safety evaluation, with Bernard L. Oser as its initial chairman. These two events led to close relationships among toxicologists from several groups and brought toxicology into a new phase. At about the same time, the U.S. Congress passed and the President signed the additives amendments to the Food, Drug, and Cosmetic Act. The Delaney clause (1958) of these amendments stated broadly that any chemical found to be carcinogenic in laboratory animals or humans could not be added to the U.S. food supply. The impact of this legislation cannot be overstated. Delaney became a battle cry for many groups and resulted in the inclusion at a new level of biostatisticians and mathematical modelers in the field of toxicology. It fostered the expansion of quantitative methods in toxicology and led to innumerable arguments about the "one-hit" theory of carcinogenesis. Regardless of one's view of Delaney, it has served as an excellent starting point for understanding the complexity of the biological phenomenon of carcinogenicity and the development of risk assessment models. One must remember that at the time of Delaney, the analytic detection level for most chemicals was 20 to 100 ppm (today, parts per quadrillion). Interestingly, the Delaney clause has been invoked only on a few occasions, and it has been stated that Congress added little to the food and drug law with this clause (Hutt and Hutt, 1984).

Shortly after the Delaney amendment and after three successful Gordon Conferences, the first American journal dedicated to toxicology was launched by Coulston, Lehman, and Hayes. *Toxicology and Applied Pharmacology* has been the flagship journal of toxicology ever since. The founding of the Society of Toxicology followed shortly afterward, and this journal became its official publication. The society's founding members were Fredrick Coulston, William Deichmann, Kenneth DuBois, Victor Drill, Harry Hayes, Harold Hodge, Paul Larson, Arnold Lehman, and C. Boyd Shaffer. These researchers deserve a great deal of credit for the growth of toxicology. DuBois and Geiling published their *Textbook of Toxicology* in 1959.

The 1960s were a tumultuous time for society, and toxicology was swept up in the tide. Starting with the tragic thalidomide incident, in which several thousand children were born with serious birth defects, and the publishing of Rachel Carson's *Silent Spring* (1962), the field of toxicology developed at a feverish pitch. Attempts to understand the effects of chemicals on the embryo and fetus and on the environment as a whole gained momentum. New legislation was passed, and new journals were founded. The education of toxicologists spread from the deep traditions at Chicago and Rochester to Harvard, Miami, Albany, Iowa, Jefferson, and beyond. Geiling's fledglings spread as Schmiedeberg's had a half century before. Many new fields were influencing and being assimilated into the broad scope of toxicology, including environmental sciences, aquatic and avian biology, cell biology, analytic chemistry, and genetics.

During the 1960s, particularly the latter half of the decade, the analytic tools used in toxicology were developed to a level of sophistication that allowed the detection of chemicals in tissues and other substrates at part per billion concentrations (today parts per quadrillion may be detected). Pioneering work in the development of point mutation assays that were replicable, quick, and inexpensive led to a better understanding of the genetic mechanisms of carcinogenicity (Ames, 1983). The combined work of Ames and the Millers (Elizabeth C. and James A.) at McArdle Laboratory allowed the toxicology community to make major contributions to the understanding of the carcinogenic process.

The low levels of detection of chemicals and the ability to detect point mutations rapidly created several problems and opportunities for toxicologists and risk assessors that stemmed from interpretation of the Delaney amendment. Cellular and molecular toxicology developed as a subdiscipline, and risk assessment became a major product of toxicological investigations.

The establishment of the National Center for Toxicologic Research (NCTR), the expansion of the role of the U.S. FDA, and the establishment of the U.S. Environmental Protection Agency (EPA) and the National Institute of Environmental Health Sciences (NIEHS) were considered clear messages that the government had taken a strong interest in toxicology. Several new journals appeared during the 1960s, and new legislation was written quickly after *Silent Spring* and the thalidomide disaster.

The end of the 1960s witnessed the "discovery" of TCDD as a contaminant in the herbicide Agent Orange (the original discovery of TCDD toxicity was reported in 1957). The research on the toxicity of this compound has produced some very good and some very poor research in the field of toxicology. The discovery of a high-affinity cellular binding protein designated the "Ah" receptor (see Poland and Knutsen, 1982, for a review) at the McArdle Laboratory and work on the genetics of the receptor at NIH (Nebert and Gonzalez, 1987) have revolutionized the field of toxicology. The importance of TCDD to toxicology lies in the fact that it forced researchers, regulators, and the legal community to look at the role of mechanisms of toxic action in a different fashion.

At least one other event precipitated a great deal of legislation during the 1970s: Love Canal. The "discovery" of Love Canal led to major concerns regarding hazardous wastes, chemical dump sites, and disclosure of information about those sites. Soon after Love Canal, the EPA listed several equally contaminated sites in the United States. The agency was given the responsibility to develop risk assessment methodology to determine health risks from exposure to effluents and to attempt to remediate these sites. These combined efforts led to broad-based support for research into the mechanisms of action of individual chemicals and complex mixtures. Love Canal and similar issues created the legislative environment that led to the Toxic Substances Control Act and eventually to the Superfund bill. These omnibus bills were created to cover the toxicology of chemicals from initial synthesis to disposal (cradle to grave).

The expansion of legislation, journals, and new societies involved with toxicology was exponential during the 1970s and 1980s and shows no signs of slowing down. Currently, in the United States there are dozens of professional, governmental, and other scientific organizations with thousands of members and over 120 journals dedicated to toxicology and related disciplines.

In addition, toxicology continues to expand in stature and in the number of programs worldwide. The International Congress of Toxicology is made up of toxicology societies from Europe, South America, Asia, Africa, and Australia and brings together the broadest representation of toxicologists.

The original Gordon Conference series has changed to Mechanisms of Toxicity, and several other conferences related to special areas of toxicology are now in existence. The American Society of Toxicology has formed specialty sections and regional chapters to accommodate the over 4000 scientists involved in toxicology today. Texts and reference books for toxicology students and scientists abound. Toxicology has evolved from a borrowing science to a seminal discipline seeding the growth and development of several related fields of science and science policy.

The history of toxicology has been interesting and varied but never dull. Perhaps as a science that has grown and prospered by borrowing from many disciplines, it has suffered from the absence of a single goal, but its diversification has allowed for the interspersion of ideas and concepts from higher education, industry, and government. As an example of this diversification, one now finds toxicology graduate programs in medical schools, schools of public health, and schools of pharmacy as well as programs in environmental science and engineering and undergraduate programs in toxicology at several institutions. Surprisingly, courses in toxicology are now being offered in several liberal arts undergraduate schools as part of their biology and chemistry curricula. This has resulted in an exciting, innovative, and diversified field that is serving science and the community at large.

Few disciplines can point to both basic sciences and direct applications at the same time. Toxicology—the study of the adverse effects of xenobiotics—may be unique in this regard.

# REFERENCES


Albert A: *Selective Toxicity*. London: Methuen, 1951.

Ames BN: Dietary carcinogens and anticarcinogens. *Science* 221:1249–1264, 1983.

Bernard C: Action du curare et de la nicotine sur le systeme nerveux et sur le systme musculaire. *CR Soc Biol* 2:195, 1850.

Bernard C: *Introduction to the Study of Experimental Medicine*, trans. Greene HC, Schuman H. New York: Dover, 1949.

Carson R: *Silent Spring*. Boston: Houghton Mifflin, 1962.

Christison R: *A Treatise on Poisons*, 4th ed. Philadelphia: Barrington & Howell, 1845.

Doll R, Peto R: *The Causes of Cancer*. New York: Oxford University Press, 1981.

Donaldson HH: The history and zoological position of the albino rat. *Natl Acad Sci* 15:365–369, 1912.

DuBois K, Geiling EMK: *Textbook of Toxicology*. New York: Oxford University Press, 1959.

Gunther RT: *The Greek Herbal of Dioscorides*. New York: Oxford University Press, 1934.

Guthrie DA: *A History of Medicine*. Philadelphia: Lippincott, 1946.

Handler P: Some comments on risk assessment, in *The National Research Council in 1979: Current Issues and Studies*. Washington, DC: NAS, 1979.

Hutt PB, Hutt PB II: A history of government regulation of adulteration and misbranding of food. *Food Drug Cosmet J* 39:2–73, 1984.

Kallet A, Schlink FJ: *100,000,000 Guinea Pigs: Dangers in Everyday Foods, Drugs and Cosmetics*. New York: Vanguard, 1933.

Levey M: Medieval arabic toxicology: The book on poisons of Ibn Wahshiya and its relation to early Indian and Greek texts. *Trans Am Philos Soc* 56(7): 1966.

Lewin L: *Die Gifte in der Weltgeschichte: Toxikologische, allgemeinverstandliche Untersuchungen der historischen Quellen*. Berlin: Springer, 1920.

Lewin L: *Gifte und Vergiftungen*. Berlin: Stilke, 1929.

Loomis TA: *Essentials of Toxicology*, 3d ed. Philadelphia: Lea & Febiger, 1978.

Macht DJ: Louis Lewin: Pharmacologist, toxicologist, medical historian. *Ann Med Hist* 3:179–194, 1931.

Meek WJ: *The Gentle Art of Poisoning*. Medico-Historical Papers. Madision: University of Wisconsin, 1954; reprinted from *Phi Beta Pi Quarterly*, May 1928.

Muller P: Uber zusammenhange zwischen Konstitution und insektizider Wirkung. I. *Helv Chim Acta* 29:1560–1580, 1946.

Munter S (ed).: *Treatise on Poisons and Their Antidotes. Vol. II of the Medical Writings of Moses Maimonides*. Philadelphia: Lippincott, 1966.

Nebert D, Gonzalez FJ: P450 genes: Structure, evolution and regulation. *Annu Rev Biochem* 56:945–993, 1987.

Olmsted JMD: *François Magendie: Pioneer in Experimental Physiology and Scientific Medicine in XIX Century France*. New York: Schuman, 1944.

Orfila MJB: *Traite des Poisons Tires des Regnes Mineral, Vegetal et Animal, ou, Toxicologie Generale Consideree sous les Rapports de la Physiologie, de la Pathologie et de la Medecine Legale.* Paris: Crochard, 1814–1815.

Orfila MJB: *Secours a Donner aux Personnes Empoisonees et Asphyxiees*. Paris: Feugeroy, 1818.

Pachter HM: *Paracelsus: Magic into Science*. New York: Collier, 1961.

Pagel W: *Paracelsus: An Introduction to Philosophical Medicine in the Era of the Renaissance*. New York: Karger, 1958.

Paracelsus (Theophrastus ex Hohenheim Eremita): *Von der Besucht*. Dillingen, 1567.

Poland A, Knutson JC: 2,3,7,8-Tetrachlorodibenzo-*p*-dioxin and related halogenated aromatic hydrocarbons, examination of the mechanism of toxicity. *Annu Rev Pharmacol Toxicol* 22:517–554, 1982.

Ramazzini B: *De Morbis Artificum Diatriba*. Modena: Typis Antonii Capponi, 1700.
Robert R: *Lehrbuch der Intoxikationen*. Stuttgart: Enke, 1893.
Schmiedeberg O, Koppe R: *Das Muscarin das giftige Alkaloid des Fliegenpilzes*. Leipzig: Vogel, 1869.
Thompson CJS: *Poisons and Poisoners: With Historical Accounts of Some Famous Mysteries in Ancient and Modern Times*. London: Shaylor, 1931.
U.S. FDA: *Toxicologic Principles for the Safety Assessment of Direct Food Additives and Color Additives Used in Food*. Washington, DC: U.S. Food and Drug Administration, Bureau of Foods, 1982.
Voegtlin C, Dyer HA, Leonard CS: On the mechanism of the action of arsenic upon protoplasm. *Public Health Rep* 38:1882–1912, 1923.
Williams RT: *Detoxication Mechanisms*, 2d ed. New York: Wiley, 1959.
Zapp JA Jr, Doull J: Industrial toxicology: Retrospect and prospect, in Clayton GD, Clayton FE (eds): *Patty's Industrial Hygiene and Toxicology*, 4th ed. New York: Wiley Interscience, 1993, pp 1–23.

# SUPPLEMENTAL READING

Adams F (trans.): *The Genuine Works of Hippocrates*. Baltimore: Williams & Wilkins, 1939.
Beeson BB: Orfila—pioneer toxicologist. *Ann Med Hist* 2:68–70, 1930.
Bernard C: Analyse physiologique des proprietes des systemes musculaire et nerveux au moyen du curare. *CR Acad Sci* (*Paris*) 43:325–329, 1856.
Bryan CP: *The Papyrus Ebers*. London: Geoffrey Bales, 1930.
Clendening L: *Source Book of Medical History*. New York: Dover, 1942.
Gaddum JH: *Pharmacology*, 5th ed. New York: Oxford University Press, 1959.
Garrison FH: *An Introduction to the History of Medicine*, 4th ed. Philadelphia: Saunders, 1929.
Hamilton A: *Exploring the Dangerous Trades*. Boston: Little, Brown, 1943. (Reprinted by Northeastern University Press, Boston, 1985.)
Hays HW: *Society of Toxicology History, 1961–1986*. Washington, DC: Society of Toxicology, 1986.
Holmstedt B, Liljestrand G: *Readings in Pharmacology*. New York: Raven Press, 1981.

# CHAPTER 2

# PRINCIPLES OF TOXICOLOGY

*David L. Eaton and Curtis D. Klaassen*

## INTRODUCTION TO TOXICOLOGY

*Toxicology* is the study of the adverse effects of chemicals on living organisms. A *toxicologist* is trained to examine the nature of those effects (including their cellular, biochemical, and molecular mechanisms of action) and assess the probability of their occurrence. Thus, the principles of toxicology are integral to the proper use of science in the process commonly called "risk assessment," where quantitative estimates are made of the potential effects on human health and environmental significance of various types of chemical exposures (e.g., pesticide residues on food, contaminants in drinking water). The variety of potential adverse effects and the diversity of chemicals in the environment make toxicology a very broad science. Therefore, toxicologists are usually specialized to work in one area of toxicology.

### Different Areas of Toxicology

The professional activities of toxicologists fall into three main categories: descriptive, mechanistic, and regulatory. A *descriptive toxicologist* is concerned directly with toxicity testing, which provides information for safety evaluation and regulatory requirements. The appropriate toxicity tests (as described later in this chapter) in experimental animals are designed to yield information that can be used to evaluate the risk posed to humans and the environment by exposure to specific chemicals. The concern may be limited to effects on humans, as in the case of drugs and food additives. Toxicologists in the chemical industry, however, must be concerned not only with the risk posed by a company's chemicals (insecticides, herbicides, solvents, etc.) to humans but also with potential effects on fish, birds, and plants, as well as other factors that might disturb the balance of the ecosystem.

A *mechanistic toxicologist* is concerned with identifying and understanding the mechanisms by which chemicals exert toxic effects on living organisms. The results of mechanistic studies are very important in many areas of applied toxicology. In risk assessment, mechanistic data may be very useful in demonstrating that an adverse outcome (e.g., cancer, birth defects) observed in laboratory animals is directly relevant to humans. For example, the relative toxic potential of organophosphate insecticides in humans, rodents, and insects can be accurately predicted on the basis of an understanding of common mechanisms (inhibition of acetylcholinesterase) and differences in biotransformation for these insecticides among the different species. Similarly, mechanistic data may be very useful in identifying adverse responses in experimental animals that may not be relevant to humans. For example, the bladder cancer–causing effects of the widely used artificial sweetener saccharin may not be relevant to humans at normal dietary intake rates because mechanistic studies have demonstrated that bladder cancer is induced only under conditions where saccharin is at such a high concentration in the urine that it forms a crystalline precipitate. Dose-response studies suggest that such high concentrations would not be achieved in the human bladder even after extensive dietary consumption. Mechanistic data also are useful in the design and production of safer alternative chemicals and in rational therapy for chemical poisoning and treatment of disease. For example, a highly effective antidote to organophosphate poisoning, pralidoxime, was designed on the basis of a complete understanding of the interaction between organophosphate insecticides and the active site of their target enzyme, acetylcholinesterase. In addition to aiding directly in the identification, treatment, and prevention of chemical toxicity, an understanding of the mechanisms of toxic action contributes to the knowledge of basic physiology, pharmacology, cell biology, and biochemistry. For example, studies on the toxicity of fluoroorganic alcohols and acids contributed to the knowledge of basic carbohydrate and lipid metabolism, and knowledge of regulation of ion gradients in nerve axonal membranes has been greatly aided by studies of natural and synthetic toxins such as tetrodotoxin and DDT (dichlorodiphenyltrichloroethane). Mechanistic toxicologists are active in universities, research institutes supported by the government or private sources, and the pharmaceutical and chemical industries.

A *regulatory toxicologist* has the responsibility for deciding, on the basis of data provided by descriptive and mechanistic toxicologists, whether a drug or another chemical poses a sufficiently low risk to be marketed for a stated purpose. The Food and Drug Administration (FDA) is responsible for allowing drugs, cosmetics, and food additives to be sold in the market according to the Federal Food, Drug and Cosmetic Act (FDCA). The U.S. Environmental Protection Agency (EPA) is responsible for regulating most other chemicals according to the Federal Insecticide, Fungicide and Rodenticide Act (FIFRA), the Toxic Substances Control Act (TSCA), the Resource Conservation and Recovery Act (RCRA), the Safe Drinking Water Act, and the Clean Air Act. The EPA is also responsible for enforcing the Comprehensive Environmental Response, Compensation and Liability Act [CERCLA, later revised as the Superfund Amendments Reauthorization Act (SARA)], more commonly called the Superfund. These regulations provide direction and financial support for the cleanup of waste sites that contain toxic chemicals and may present a risk to human health or the environment. The Occupational Safety and Health Administration (OSHA) of the Department of Labor was established to ensure that safe and healthful conditions exist in the workplace. The Consumer Product Safety Commission is responsible for protecting consumers from hazardous household substances, whereas the Department of Transportation (DOT) ensures that materials shipped in interstate commerce are labeled and packaged in a manner consistent with the degree of hazard they present. Regulatory toxicologists are also involved in the establishment of standards for the amount of chemicals permitted in ambient air, industrial atmospheres, and drinking water, often integrating scientific information from basic descriptive and mechanistic toxicology studies with the principles and approaches used for risk assessment (Chap. 4). Some of the philosophic and legal aspects of regulatory toxicology are discussed in Chap. 34.

There are three specialized areas of toxicology: forensic, clinical, and environmental toxicology. *Forensic toxicology* is a hybrid of analytic chemistry and fundamental toxicological principles. It is concerned primarily with the medicolegal aspects of the harmful effects of chemicals on humans and animals. The expertise of forensic toxicologists is invoked primarily to aid in establishing the cause of death and determining its circumstances in a postmortem investigation (Chap. 31). *Clinical toxicology* designates an area of professional emphasis in the realm of medical science that is concerned with disease caused by or uniquely associated with toxic substances (see Chap. 32). Generally, clinical toxicologists are physicians who receive specialized training in emergency medicine and poison management. Efforts are directed at treating patients poisoned with drugs or other chemicals and at the development of new techniques to treat those intoxications. *Environmental toxicology* focuses on the impacts of chemical pollutants in the environment on biological organisms. Although toxicologists concerned with the effects of environmental pollutants on human health fit into this definition, it is most commonly associated with studies on the impacts of chemicals on nonhuman organisms such as fish, birds, and terrestrial animals. *Ecotoxicology* is a specialized area within environmental toxicology that focuses more specifically on the impacts of toxic substances on population dynamics in an ecosystem. The transport, fate, and interactions of chemicals in the environment constitute a critical component of both environmental toxicology and ecotoxicology.

## Spectrum of Toxic Dose

One could define a *poison* as any agent capable of producing a deleterious response in a biological system, seriously injuring function or producing death. This is not, however, a useful working definition for the very simple reason that virtually every known chemical has the potential to produce injury or death if it is present in a sufficient amount. Paracelsus (1493–1541) phrased this well when he noted, "What is there that is not poison? All things are poison and nothing [is] without poison. Solely the dose determines that a thing is not a poison."

Among chemicals there is a wide spectrum of doses needed to produce deleterious effects, serious injury, or death. This is demonstrated in Table 2-1, which shows the dosage of chemicals needed to produce death in 50 percent of treated animals ($LD_{50}$). Some chemicals produce death in microgram doses and are commonly thought of as being extremely poisonous. Other chemicals may be relatively harmless after doses in excess of several grams. It should be noted, however, that measures of acute lethality such as $LD_{50}$ may not accurately reflect the full spectrum of toxicity, or hazard, associated

**Table 2–1**
**Approximate Acute $LD_{50}$s of Some Representative Chemical Agents**

| AGENT | $LD_{50}$, mg/kg* |
|---|---|
| Ethyl alcohol | 10,000 |
| Sodium chloride | 4,000 |
| Ferrous sulfate | 1,500 |
| Morphine sulfate | 900 |
| Phenobarbital sodium | 150 |
| Picrotoxin | 5 |
| Strychnine sulfate | 2 |
| Nicotine | 1 |
| *d*-Tubocurarine | 0.5 |
| Hemicholinium-3 | 0.2 |
| Tetrodotoxin | 0.10 |
| Dioxin (TCDD) | 0.001 |
| Botulinum toxin | 0.00001 |

* $LD_{50}$ is the dosage (mg/kg body weight) causing death in 50 percent of exposed animals.

with exposure to a chemical. For example, some chemicals with low acute toxicity may have carcinogenic or teratogenic effects at doses that produce no evidence of acute toxicity.

# CLASSIFICATION OF TOXIC AGENTS

Toxic agents are classified in a variety of ways, depending on the interests and needs of the classifier. In this textbook, for example, toxic agents are discussed in terms of their target organs (liver, kidney, hematopoietic system, etc.), use (pesticide, solvent, food additive, etc.), source (animal and plant toxins), and effects (cancer, mutation, liver injury, etc.). The term "toxin" generally refers to toxic substances which are produced naturally. The term "toxicant" is used in speaking of toxic substances that are produced by or are a by-product of anthropogenic (human-made) activities. Thus, zeralanone, produced by a mold, is a toxin, whereas "dioxin" [2,3-7,8-tetrachlorodibenzo-*p*-dioxin (TCDD)], produced during the combustion of certain chlorinated organic chemicals, is a toxicant. However, the distinction is not always clear; polyaromatic hydrocarbons are produced by the combustion of organic matter, which may occur both through natural processes (e.g., forest fires) and through anthropogenic activities (e.g., combustion of coal for energy production). Arsenic, a toxic metalloid, may occur as a natural contaminant of groundwater or may contaminate groundwater secondary to industrial activities. Generally, such toxic substances are referred to as toxicants, rather than toxins.

Toxic agents also may be classified in terms of their physical state (gas, dust, liquid), their labeling requirements (explosive, flammable, oxidizer), chemistry (aromatic amine, halogenated hydrocarbon, etc.), or poisoning potential (extremely toxic, very toxic, slightly toxic, etc.). Classification of toxic agents on the basis of their biochemical mechanisms of action (sulfhydryl inhibitor, methemoglobin producer) is usually more informative than classification by general terms such as irritants and corrosives, but more general classifications such as air pollutants, occupation-related agents, and acute and chronic poisons can provide a useful focus on a specific problem. It is evident from this discussion that no single classification is applicable to the entire spectrum of toxic agents and that combinations of classification systems or a classification based on other factors may be needed to provide the best rating system for a special purpose. Nevertheless, classification systems that take into consideration both the chemical and the biological properties of an agent and the exposure characteristics are most likely to be useful for legislative or control purposes and for toxicology in general.

## CHARACTERISTICS OF EXPOSURE

Adverse or toxic effects in a biological system are not produced by a chemical agent unless that agent or its metabolic breakdown (biotransformation) products reach appropriate sites in the body at a concentration and for a length of time sufficient to produce a toxic manifestation. Many chemicals are of relatively low toxicity in the "native" form but, when acted on by enzymes in the body, are converted to intermediate forms that interfere with normal cellular biochemistry and physiology. Thus, whether a toxic response occurs is dependent on the chemical and physical properties of the agent, the exposure situation, how the agent is metabolized by the system, and the overall susceptibility of the biological system or subject. Thus, to characterize fully the potential hazard of a specific chemical agent, we need to know not only what type of effect it produces and the dose required to produce that effect but also information about the agent, the exposure, and its disposition by the subject. The major factors that influence toxicity as it relates to the exposure situation for a specific chemical are the route of administration and the duration and frequency of exposure.

### Route and Site of Exposure

The major routes (pathways) by which toxic agents gain access to the body are the gastrointestinal tract (ingestion), lungs (inhalation), skin (topical, percutaneous, or dermal), and other parenteral (other than intestinal canal) routes. Toxic agents generally produce the greatest effect and the most rapid response when given directly into the bloodstream (the intravenous route). An approximate descending order of effectiveness for the other routes would be inhalation, intraperitoneal, subcutaneous, intramuscular, intradermal, oral, and dermal. The "vehicle" (the material in which the chemical is dissolved) and other formulation factors can markedly alter absorption after ingestion, inhalation, or topical exposure. In addition, the route of administration can influence the toxicity of agents. For example, an agent that is detoxified in the liver would be expected to be less toxic when given via the portal circulation (oral) than when given via the systemic circulation (inhalation).

Occupational exposure to toxic agents most frequently results from breathing contaminated air (inhalation) and/or direct and prolonged contact of the skin with the substance (dermal exposure), whereas accidental and suicidal poisoning occurs most frequently by oral ingestion. Comparison of the lethal dose of a toxic substance by different routes of exposure often provides useful information about its extent of absorption. In instances when the lethal dose after oral or dermal administration is similar to the lethal dose after intravenous administration, the assumption is that the toxic agent is absorbed readily and rapidly. Conversely, in cases where the lethal dose by the dermal route is several orders of magnitude higher than the oral lethal dose, it is likely that the skin provides an effective barrier to absorption of the agent. Toxic effects by any route of exposure also can be influenced by the concentration of the agent in its vehicle, the total volume of the vehicle and the properties of the vehicle to which the biological system is exposed, and the rate at which exposure occurs. Studies in which the concentration of a chemical in the blood is determined at various times after exposure are often needed to clarify the role of these and other factors in the toxicity of a compound. For more details on the absorption of toxicants, see Chap. 5.

### Duration and Frequency of Exposure

Toxicologists usually divide the exposure of animals to chemicals into four categories: acute, subacute, subchronic, and chronic. Acute exposure is defined as exposure to a chemical for less than 24 h, and examples of exposure routes are intraperitoneal, intravenous, and subcutaneous injection; oral intubation; and dermal application. While acute exposure usually refers to a single administration, repeated exposures may be given within a 24-h period for some slightly toxic or practically nontoxic chemicals. Acute exposure by inhalation refers to continuous exposure for less than 24 h, most frequently for 4 h. Repeated exposure is divided into three categories: subacute, subchronic, and chronic. Subacute exposure refers to repeated exposure to a chemical for 1 month or less, subchronic for 1 to 3 months, and chronic for more than 3 months. These three categories of repeated exposure can be by any route, but most often this occurs by the oral route, with the chemical added directly to the diet.

For many agents, the toxic effects that follow a single exposure are quite different from those produced by repeated exposure. For example, the primary acute toxic manifestation of benzene is central nervous system (CNS) depression, but repeated exposures can result in leukemia. Acute exposure to agents that are rapidly absorbed is likely to produce immediate toxic effects but also can produce delayed toxicity that may or may not be similar to the toxic effects of chronic exposure. Conversely, chronic exposure to a toxic agent may produce some immediate (acute) effects after each administration in addition to the long-term, low-level, or chronic effects of the toxic substance. In characterizing the toxicity of a specific chemical, it is evident that information is needed not only for the single-dose (acute) and long-term (chronic) effects but also for exposures of intermediate duration.

The other time-related factor that is important in the temporal characterization of exposure is the frequency of administration. The relationship between elimination rate and frequency of exposure is shown in Fig. 2-1. A chemical that produces severe effects with a single dose may have no effect if the same total dose is given in several intervals. For the chemical depicted by line B in Fig. 2-1, in which the half-life for elimination (time necessary for 50 percent of the chemical to be removed from the bloodstream) is approximately equal to the dosing frequency, a theoretical toxic concentration of

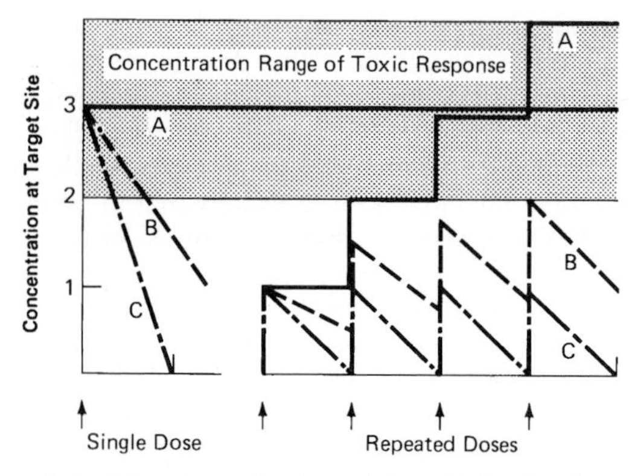


***Figure 2–1. Diagrammatic view of the relationship between dose and concentration at the target site under different conditions of dose frequency and elimination rate.***

Line A, a chemical with very slow elimination (e.g., half-life of one year); B, a chemical with a rate of elimination equal to frequency of dosing (e.g., 1 day); C, rate of elimination faster than the dosing frequency (e.g., 5 h). Shaded area is representative of the concentration of chemical at the target site necessary to elicit a toxic response.

2 units is not reached until the fourth dose of administration, whereas that concentration is reached with two dosing intervals for chemical A, which has an elimination rate much slower than the dosing frequency. Conversely, for chemical C, where the elimination rate is much shorter than the dosing interval, a toxic concentration at the site of toxic effect will never be reached regardless of how many doses are administered. Of course, it is possible that residual cell or tissue damage occurs with each dose even though the chemical itself is not accumulating. The important consideration, then, is whether the interval between doses is sufficient to allow for complete repair of tissue damage. It is evident that with any type of multiple dose the production of a toxic effect not only is influenced by the frequency of administration but may in fact be totally dependent on the frequency rather than duration of exposure. Chronic toxic effects may occur, therefore, if the chemical accumulates in the biological system (absorption exceeds biotransformation and/or excretion), if it produces irreversible toxic effects, or if there is insufficient time for the system to recover from the toxic damage within the exposure frequency interval. For additional discussion of these relationships, consult Chaps. 5 and 7.

## SPECTRUM OF UNDESIRED EFFECTS

The spectrum of undesired effects of chemicals is broad. Some effects are deleterious, and others are not. In therapeutics, for example, each drug produces a number of effects, but usually only one effect is associated with the primary objective of the therapy; all the other effects are referred to as undesirable or side effects of that drug for that therapeutic indication. However, some of these side effects may be desired for another therapeutic indication. For example, dryness of the mouth is a side effect of atropine used to decrease gastric secretion in the treatment of peptic ulcer but is the desired effect when atropine is for preanesthetic medication. Some side effects of drugs are never desirable and are always deleterious to the well-being of humans. These are referred to as the *adverse, deleterious,* or *toxic* effects of the drug.

### Allergic Reactions

*Chemical allergy* is an immunologically mediated adverse reaction to a chemical resulting from previous sensitization to that chemical or to a structurally similar one. The term "hypersensitivity" is most often used to describe this allergic state, but "allergic reaction" and "sensitization reaction" are also used to describe this situation when preexposure of the chemical is required to produce the toxic effect (Goldstein et al., 1974; Loomis, 1978). Once sensitization has occurred, allergic reactions may result from exposure to relatively very low doses of chemicals, and therefore population-based dose-response curves for allergic reactions have seldom been obtained. Because of this omission, some people assumed that allergic reactions are not dose-related. Thus, they do not consider the allergic reaction to be a true toxic response. However, for a given allergic individual, allergic reactions are dose-related. For example, it is well known that the allergic response to pollen in sensitized individuals is related to the concentration of pollen in the air. In addition, because the allergic response is an undesirable, adverse, deleterious effect, it obviously is also a toxic response. Sensitization reactions are sometimes very severe and may be fatal.

Most chemicals and their metabolic products are not sufficiently large to be recognized by the immune system as a foreign substance and thus must first combine with an endogenous protein to form an antigen (or immunogen). A molecule that must combine with an endogenous protein to elicit an allergic reaction is called a hapten. The hapten-protein complex (antigen) is then capable of eliciting the formation of antibodies, and usually at least 1 or 2 weeks is required for the synthesis of significant amounts of antibodies. Subsequent exposure to the chemical results in an antigen-antibody interaction, which provokes the typical manifestations of allergy. The manifestations of allergy are numerous. They may involve various organ systems and range in severity from minor skin disturbance to fatal anaphylactic shock. The pattern of allergic response differs in various species. In humans, involvement of the skin (e.g., dermatitis, urticaria, and itching) and involvement of the eyes (e.g., conjunctivitis) are most common, whereas in guinea pigs bronchiolar constriction leading to asphyxia is the most common. However, chemically induced asthma (characterized by bronchiolar constriction) certainly does occur in some humans, and the incidence of allergic asthma has increased substantially in recent years. Hypersensitivity reactions are discussed in more detail in Chap. 12.

### Idiosyncratic Reactions

*Chemical idiosyncrasy* refers to a genetically determined abnormal reactivity to a chemical (Goldstein et al., 1974; Levine, 1978). The response observed is usually qualitatively similar to that observed in all individuals but may take the form of extreme sensitivity to low doses or extreme insensitivity to high doses of the chemical. However, while some people use the term "idiosyncratic" as a catchall to refer to all reactions that occur with low frequency, it should not be used in that manner (Goldstein et al., 1974).

An example of an idiosyncratic reaction is provided by patients who exhibit prolonged muscular relaxation and apnea (inability to breathe) lasting several hours after a standard dose of succinylcholine. Succinylcholine usually produces skeletal muscle relaxation of only a short duration because of its very rapid metabolic degradation by an enzyme that is present normally in the bloodstream called plasma pseudocholinesterase. Patients exhibiting this idiosyncratic reaction have an unusual form of pseudocholinesterase which is less active in breaking down succinylcholine. Family pedigree studies have demonstrated that the presence of this atypical cholinesterase is a genetically determined characteristic. Similarly, there is a group of people who are abnormally sensitive to nitrites and certain other chemicals that have in common the ability to oxidize the iron in hemoglobin to produce "methemoglobin" that is incapable of carrying oxygen to the tissues. These individuals have a deficiency in NADH-methemoglobin reductase, which is inherited as an autosomal recessive trait. The consequence of this genetic deficiency is that these individuals may suffer from a serious lack of oxygen delivery to tissues after exposure to doses of methemoglobin-producing chemicals that would be harmless to individuals with normal NADH-methemoglobin reductase activity.

### Immediate versus Delayed Toxicity

Immediate toxic effects can be defined as those that occur or develop rapidly after a single administration of a substance, whereas delayed toxic effects are those that occur after the lapse of some time. Carcinogenic effects of chemicals usually have a long latency period, often 20 to 30 years after the initial exposure, before tumors are observed in humans. For example, the vaginal cancer produced by diethylstilbestrol in young women was due to their exposure *in utero* to diethylstilbestrol taken by their mothers to prevent miscarriage. Also, delayed neurotoxicity is observed after exposure to some organophosphorus insecticides that act by inhibiting the enzyme acetyl cholinesterase. The most notorious of the compounds that produce this type of neurotoxic effect is triorthocresylphosphate (TOCP). The effect is not observed until at least several days after exposure to the toxic compound. In contrast, most substances produce immediate toxic effects but do not produce delayed effects.

### Reversible versus Irreversible Toxic Effects

Some toxic effects of chemicals are reversible, and others are irreversible. If a chemical produces pathological injury to a tissue, the ability of that tissue to regenerate largely determines whether the effect is reversible or irreversible. Thus, for a tissue such as liver, which has a high ability to regenerate, most injuries are reversible, whereas injury to the CNS is largely irreversible because differentiated cells of the CNS cannot divide and be replaced. Carcinogenic and teratogenic effects of chemicals, once they occur, are usually considered irreversible toxic effects.

### Local versus Systemic Toxicity

Another distinction between types of effects is made on the basis of the general site of action. Local effects refer to those that occur at the site of first contact between the biological system and the toxicant. Local effects are produced by the ingestion of caustic substances or the inhalation of irritant materials. For example, chlorine gas reacts with lung tissue at the site of contact, causing damage and swelling of the tissue, with possibly fatal consequences, even though very little of the chemical is absorbed into the bloodstream. The alternative to local effects is systemic effects. Systemic effects require absorption and distribution of a toxicant from its entry point to a distant site at which deleterious effects are produced. Most substances, except highly reactive materials, produce systemic effects. For some materials, both effects can be demonstrated. For example, tetraethyl lead produces effects on skin at the site of absorption and then is transported systemically to produce its typical effects on the CNS and other organs. If the local effect is marked, there also may be indirect systemic effects. For example, kidney damage after a severe acid burn is an indirect systemic effect because the toxicant does not reach the kidney.

Most chemicals that produce systemic toxicity do not cause a similar degree of toxicity in all organs; instead, they usually elicit their major toxicity in only one or two organs. These sites are referred to as the *target organs* of toxicity of a particular chemical. The target organ of toxicity is often not the site of the highest concentration of the chemical. For example, lead is concentrated in bone, but its toxicity is due to its effects in soft tissues. DDT is concentrated in adipose tissue but produces no known toxic effects in that tissue.

The target organ of toxicity most frequently involved in systemic toxicity is the CNS. Even with many compounds having a prominent effect elsewhere, damage to the CNS, particularly the brain, can be demonstrated by the use of appropriate and sensitive methods. Next in order of frequency of involvement in systemic toxicity are the circulatory system; the blood and hematopoietic system; visceral organs such as the liver, kidney, and lung; and the skin. Muscle and bone are least often the target tissues for systemic effects. With substances that have a predominantly local effect, the frequency with which tissues react depends largely on the portal of entry (skin, gastrointestinal tract, or respiratory tract).

## INTERACTION OF CHEMICALS

Because of the large number of different chemicals an individual may come in contact with at any given time (workplace, drugs, diet, hobbies, etc), in assessing the spectrum of responses, it is necessary to consider how different chemicals may interact with each other. Interactions can occur in a variety of ways. Chemical interactions are known to occur by a number of mechanisms, such as alterations in absorption, protein binding, and the biotransformation and excretion of one or both of the interacting toxicants. In addition to these modes of interaction, the response of the organism to combinations of toxicants may be increased or decreased because of toxicological responses at the site of action.

The effects of two chemicals given simultaneously produce a response that may simply be additive of their individual responses or may be greater or less than that expected by addition of their individual responses. The study of these interactions often leads to a better understanding of the mechanism of toxicity of the chemicals involved. A number of terms have been used to describe pharmacological and toxicological interactions. An *additive* effect occurs when the combined effect of two chemicals is equal to the sum of the effects of each agent given alone (example: 2 + 3 = 5). The effect most commonly observed when two chemicals are given together is an additive effect. For example, when two organophosphate insecticides are given together, the cholinesterase inhibition is usually additive. A *synergistic* effect ocurs when the combined effects of two chemicals are much greater than the sum of the effects of each agent given alone (example: 2 + 2 = 20). For example, both carbon tetrachloride and ethanol are hepatotoxic compounds, but together they produce much more liver injury than the mathematical sum of their individual effects on liver would suggest. *Potentiation* occurs when one substance does not have a toxic effect on a certain organ or system but when added to another chemical makes that chemical much more toxic (example: 0 + 2 = 10). Isopropanol, for example, is not hepatotoxic, but when it is administered in addition to carbon tetrachloride, the hepatotoxicity of carbon tetrachloride is much greater than that when it is given alone. *Antagonism* occurs when two chemicals administered together interfere with each other's actions or one interferes with the action of the other (example: 4 + 6 = 8; 4 + (−4) = 0; 4 + 0 = 1). Antagonistic effects of chemicals are often very desirable in toxicology and are the basis of many antidotes. There are four major types of antagonism: functional, chemical, dispositional, and receptor. *Functional antagonism* occurs when two chemicals counterbalance each other by producing opposite effects on the same physiological function. Advantage is taken of this principle in that the blood pressure can markedly fall during severe barbiturate intoxication, which can be effectively antagonized by the intravenous administration of a vasopressor agent such as norepinephrine or metaraminol. Similarly, many chemicals, when given at toxic dose levels, produce convulsions, and the convulsions often can be controlled by giving anticonvulsants such as the benzodiazepines (e.g., diazepam). *Chemical antagonism* or *inactivation* is simply a chemical reaction between two compounds that produces a less toxic product. For example, dimercaprol (BAL) chelates with metal ions such as arsenic, mercury, and lead and decreases their toxicity. The use of antitoxins in the treatment of various animal toxins is also an example of chemical antagonism. The use of the strongly basic low-molecular-weight protein protamine sulfate to form a stable complex with heparin, which abolishes its anticoagulant activity, is another example.

*Dispositional antagonism* occurs when the disposition, that is, the absorption, biotransformation, distribution, or excretion of a chemical, is altered so that the concentration and/or duration of the chemical at the target organ are diminished. Thus, the prevention of absorption of a toxicant by ipecac or charcoal and the increased excretion of a chemical by administration of an osmotic diuretic or alteration of the pH of the urine are examples of dispositional antagonism. If the parent compound is responsible for the toxicity of the chemical (such as the organophosphate insecticide paraoxon) and its metabolic breakdown products are less toxic than the parent compound, increasing the compound's metabolism (biotransformation) by administering a drug which increases the activity of the metabolizing enzymes (e.g., a "microsomal enzyme inducer" such as phenobarbital) will decrease its toxicity. However, if the chemical's toxicity is largely due to a metabolic product (as in the case of the organophosphate insecticide parathion), inhibiting its biotransformation by an inhibitor of microsomal enzyme activity (SKF-525A or piperonyl butoxide) will decrease its toxicity. *Receptor antagonism* occurs when two chemicals that bind to the same receptor produce less of an effect when given together than the addition of their separate effects (example: 4 + 6 = 8) or when one chemical antagonizes the effect of the second chemical (example: 0 + 4 = 1). Receptor antagonists are often termed *blockers*. This concept is used to advantage in the clinical treatment of poisoning. For example, the receptor antagonist naloxone is used to treat the respiratory depressive effects of morphine and other morphinelike narcotics by competitive binding to the same receptor. The effect of oxygen in carbon monoxide poisoning is also an example of receptor antagonism. Treatment of organophosphate insecticide poisoning with atropine is an example not of the antidote competing with the poison for the receptor (cholinesterase) but involves blocking the receptor (cholinergic receptor) for the excess acetylcholine that accumulates by poisoning of the cholinesterase by the organophosphate.

## TOLERANCE

Tolerance is a state of decreased responsiveness to a toxic effect of a chemical resulting from prior exposure to that chemical or to a structurally related chemical. Two major mechanisms are responsible for tolerance: One is due to a decreased amount of toxicant reaching the site where the toxic effect is produced (*dispositional tolerance*), and the other is due to a reduced responsiveness of a tissue to the chemical. Comparatively less is known about the cellular mechanisms responsible for altering the responsiveness of a tissue to a toxic chemical than is known about dispositional tolerance. Two chemicals known to produce dispositional tolerance are carbon tetrachloride and cadmium. Carbon tetrachloride produces tolerance to itself by decreasing the formation of the reactive metabolite (trichloromethyl radical) that produces liver injury (Chap. 13). The mechanism of cadmium tolerance is explained by induction of a metal-binding protein, metallothionein. Subsequent binding of cadmium to metallothionein rather than to critical macromolecules thus decreases its toxicity (Goering and Klaassen, 1983).

## DOSE RESPONSE

The characteristics of exposure and the spectrum of effects come together in a correlative relationship customarily referred to as the *dose-response relationship.* This relationship is the most fundamental and pervasive concept in toxicology. Indeed, an understanding of this relationship is essential for the study of toxic materials.

From a practical perspective, there are two types of dose-response relationships: (1) that which describes the response of an *individual* to varying doses of a chemical, often referred to as "graded" responses because the measured effect is continuous over a range of doses, and (2) that which characterizes the distribution of responses to different doses in a *population* of individuals. Individual dose-response relationships are characterized by a dose-related increase in the severity of the response. The dose relatedness of the response often results from an alteration of a specific biochemical process. For example, Fig. 2-2 shows the dose-response relationship between different dietary doses of an organophosphate insecticide and the extent of inhibition of two different enzymes: cholinesterase and carboxylesterase. The degree of inhibition of both enzymes is clearly dose-related and spans a wide range, although the slopes of the curves are different. The toxicological response that results is directly related to the degree of cholinesterase enzyme inhibition, although the clinical expression (e.g., signs and symptoms) of the adverse response may vary with different doses because some organ systems are relatively more sensitive to cholinesterase inhibition than are others. In general, the observed response to varying doses of a chemical in the whole organism is often complicated by the fact that most toxic substances have multiple sites or mechanisms of toxicity, each with its own "dose-response" relationship and subsequent adverse effect.

In the example shown in Fig. 2-2, the dose expressed on an arithmetic scale yields the best fit for cholinesterase inhibition, whereas the data for inhibition of carboxylesterase fit best when the dose is expressed on a logarithmic scale. Dose-response relationships are most often expressed as log-normal distributions, although the basis for this is largely empirical.

The dose-response relationships in a population are by definition quantal in nature; for example, a specific endpoint is identified, and the dose required to produce that endpoint for each individual in the population is determined. Although these distinctions of "quantal population" and "graded individual" dose-response relationships are useful, the two types of responses are conceptually identical. The ordinate in both cases is simply labeled the response, which may be the degree of response in an individual or system or the fraction of a population responding, and the abscissa is the range in administered doses.

## Shape of the Dose-Response Curve

The shape of the dose-response relationship has many important implications in toxicity assessment. For example, for substances that are required for normal physiological function and survivial (e.g., vitamins and essential trace elements such as chromium, cobalt, and selenium), the shape of the "graded" dose-response relationship in an individual over the entire dose range is actually U-shaped (Fig. 2-3). That is, at very low doses, there is a high level of adverse effect, which decreases with an increasing dose. This region of the dose-response relationship for essential nutrients is commonly referred to as a deficiency. As the dose is increased to a point where the deficiency no longer exists, no adverse response is detected and the organism is in a state of homeostasis. However, as the dose is increased to abnormally high levels, an adverse response (usually qualitatively different from that observed at deficient doses) appears and increases in magnitude with increasing dose, just as with other toxic substances. Thus, it is recognized that high doses of vitamin A can cause liver toxicity and birth defects, high doses of selenium can affect the brain, and high doses of estrogens may increase the risk of breast cancer even though low doses of all these substances are essential for life.

Another important aspect of the dose-response relationship at low doses is the concept of the threshold. It has long been recognized that acute toxicological responses are associated with thresholds; that is, there is some dose below which the probability of an individual responding is zero. Obviously, the identification of a threshold depends on the particular response that is measured, the sensitivity of the measurement, and the number of subjects studied. For the individual dose-response relationship, thresholds for most toxic effects certainly exist, although interindividual variability in response and qualitative

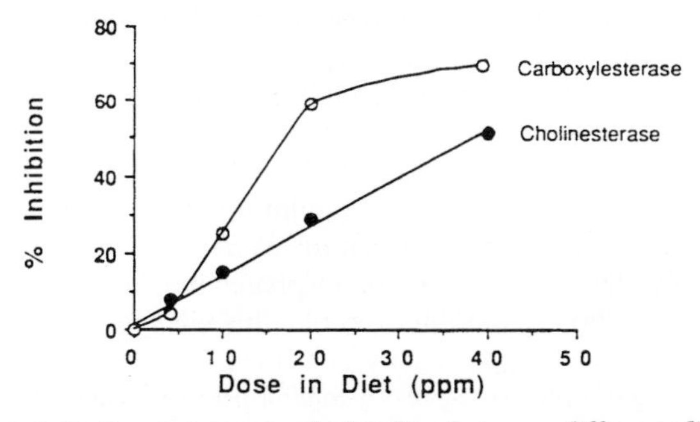


***Figure 2–2. Dose-response relationship between different dietary doses of the organophosphate insecticide dioxathion given for 7 days and enzyme inhibition.***

(From Murphy SD, Cheever KL: Effects of feeding insecticides: Inhibition of carboxylesterase and cholinesterase activities in rats. *Arch Environ Health* 17:749–756, 1968.)

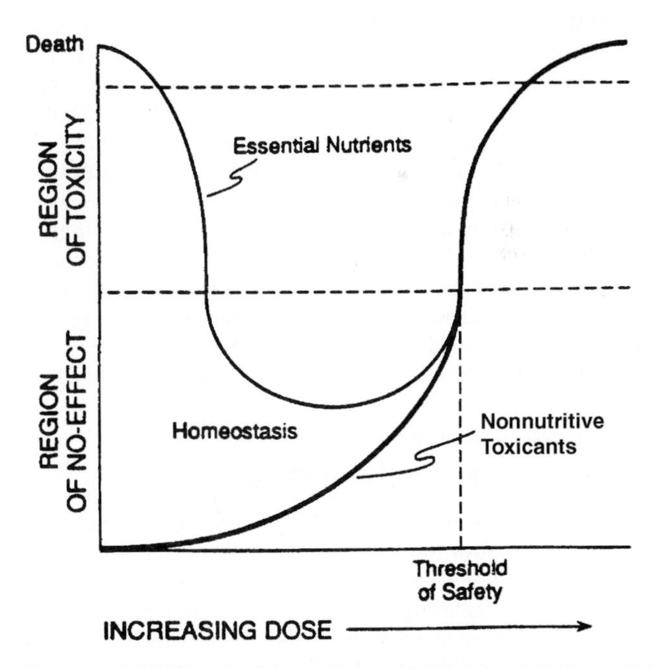


***Figure 2–3. Individual dose-response relationship. Dose-response curve for an individual exposed to either an essential substance or a nonnutritive substance.***

It is generally recognized that, for most types of toxic responses, a threshold exists such that at doses below the threshold, no toxicity is evident. For essential substances, doses below the minimum daily requirement, as well as those above the threshold for safety, may be associated with toxic effects. [From Eaton and Robertson, in Rosenstock L, Cullen MR (eds): *Textbook of Clinical Occupational and Environmental Medicine*. Philadelphia: Saunders, 1994, p 117.]

changes in response pattern with dose make it difficult to establish a true "no effects" threshold for any chemical. The biological basis of thresholds for acute responses is well established and frequently can be demonstrated on the basis of mechanistic information (Aldridge, 1986). The traditional approaches to establishing acceptable levels of exposure to chemicals are inherently different for threshold versus nonthreshold responses. The existence of thresholds for chronic responses is less well defined, especially in the area of chemical carcinogenesis. It is, of course, impossible to scientifically prove the absence of a threshold, as one can never prove a negative. Nevertheless, for the identification of "safe" levels of exposure to a substance, the absence or presence of a threshold is important for practical reasons (Chap. 4).

In evaluating the shape of the dose-response relationship in populations, it is realistic to consider inflections in the shape of the dose-response curve rather than absolute thresholds. That is, the slope of the dose-response relationship at high doses may be substantially different from the slope at low doses, usually because of dispositional differences in the chemical. Saturation of biotransformation pathways, protein-binding sites, or receptors and depletion of intracellular cofactors represent some reasons why sharp inflections in the dose-response relationship may occur. For example, the widely used analgesic acetaminophen has a very low rate of liver toxicity at normal therapeutic doses. Even though a toxic metabolite [*N*-acetyl-*p*-benzoquinoneimine (NAPQI)] is produced in the liver at therapeutic doses, it is rapidly detoxified through conjugation with the intracellular antioxidant glutathione. However, at very high doses, the level of intracellular glutathione in the liver is depleted and NAPQI accumulates, causing serious and potentially fatal liver toxicity. This effect is analogous to the rapid change in pH of a buffered solution that occurs when the buffer capacity is exceeded. Some toxic responses, most notably the development of cancer after the administration of genotoxic carcinogens, are often considered to be linear at low doses and thus do not exhibit a threshold. In such circumstances, there is no dose with "zero" risk, although the risk decreases proportionately with a decrease in the dose. The existence or lack of existence of a threshold dose for carcinogens has many regulatory implications and is a point of considerable controversy and research in the field of quantitative risk assessment (Chap. 4).

## Assumptions in Deriving the Dose-Response Relationship

A number of assumptions must be considered before dose-response relationships can be used appropriately. The first is that the response is due to the chemical administered. To describe the relationship between a toxic material and an observed effect or response, one must know with reasonable certainty that the relationship is indeed a causal one. For some data, it is not always apparent that the response is a result of chemical exposure. For example, an epidemiological study might result in the discovery of an "association" between a response (e.g., disease) and one or more variables. Frequently, the data are presented similarly to the presentation of "dose response" in pharmacology and toxicology. Use of the dose response in this context is suspect unless other convincing evidence supports a causal connection between the estimated dose and the measured endpoint (response). Unfortunately, in nearly all retrospective and case-control studies and even in many prospective studies, the dose, duration, frequency, and routes of exposure are seldom quantified, and other potential etiologic factors are frequently present. In its most strict usage, then, the dose-response relationship is based on the knowledge that the effect is a result of a known toxic agent or agents.

A second assumption seems simple and obvious: The magnitude of the response is in fact related to the dose. Perhaps because of its apparent simplicity, this assumption is often a source of misunderstanding. It is really a composite of three other assumptions that recur frequently:

1. There is a molecular or receptor site (or sites) with which the chemical interacts to produce the response.
2. The production of a response and the degree of response are related to the concentration of the agent at the receptor site.
3. The concentration at the site is, in turn, related to the dose administered.

The third assumption in using the dose-response relationship is that there exists both a quantifiable method of measuring and a precise means of expressing the toxicity. For any given dose-response relationship, a great variety of criteria or endpoints of toxicity could be used. The ideal criterion would be one closely associated with the molecular events resulting from exposure to the toxicant. It follows from this that a given chemical may have a family of dose-response relationships, one for each toxic endpoint. For example, a chemical that produces cancer through genotoxic effects, liver damage through inhibition of a specific enzyme, and CNS effects via a different mechanism may have three distinct dose-response relationships, one for each endpoint.

Early in the assessment of toxicity, little mechanistic information is usually available, and thus establishing a dose-response relationship based on the molecular mechanism of action is usually impossible; indeed, it might not be approachable even for well-known toxicants. In the absence of a mechanistic, molecular ideal criterion of toxicity, one looks to a measure of toxicity that is unequivocal and clearly relevant to the toxic effect. For example, with a new compound chemically related to the class of organophosphate insecticides, one might approach the measurement of toxicity by measuring the inhibition of cholinesterase in blood. In this way, one would be measuring, in a readily accessible system and using a technique that is convenient and reasonably precise, a prominent effect of the chemical and one that is usually pertinent to the mechanism by which toxicity is produced.

The selection of a toxic endpoint for measurement is not always so straightforward. Even the example cited above may be misleading, as an organophosphate may produce a decrease in blood cholinesterase, but this change may not be directly related to its toxicity (DuBois, 1961). As additional data are gathered to suggest a mechanism of toxicity for any substance, other measures of toxicity may be selected. Although many endpoints are quantitative and precise, they are often indirect measures of toxicity. Changes in enzyme levels in blood can be indicative of tissue damage. For example, alanine aminotransferase (ALT or SGPT) and aspartate aminotransferase (AST or SGOT) are used to detect liver damage. Patterns of isozymes and their alteration may provide insight into the organ or system that is the site of toxic effects. These measures may not be directly related to the mechanism of the toxic action.

Many direct measures of effects also are not necessarily related to the mechanism by which a substance produces harm to an organism but have the advantage of permitting a causal relation to be drawn between the agent and its action. For example, measurement of the alteration of the tone of smooth or skeletal muscle for substances acting on muscles represents a fundamental approach to toxicological assessment. Similarly, measures of heart rate, blood pressure, and electrical activity of heart muscle, nerve, and brain are examples of the use of physiological functions as indexes of toxicity. Measurement can also take the form of a still higher level of integration, such as the degree of motor activity or behavioral change.

The measurements used as examples in the preceding discussion all assume prior information about the toxicant, such as its target organ or site of action or a fundamental effect. However, such information is usually available only after toxicological screening and testing based on other measures of toxicity. With a new substance, the customary starting point in toxicological evaluation utilizes lethality as an index. Determination of lethality is precise, quantal, and unequivocal and is therefore useful in its own right, if only to suggest the level and magnitude of the potency of a substance. Lethality provides a measure of comparison among many substances whose mechanisms and sites of action may be markedly different. Furthermore, from these studies, clues to the direction of further studies are obtained. This comes about in two important ways. First, simply recording a death is not an adequate means of conducting a lethality study with a new substance. A key element must be a careful, disciplined, detailed observation of the intact animal extending from the time of administration of the toxicant to the death of the animal. From properly conducted observations, immensely informative data can be gathered by a trained toxicologist. Second, a lethality study ordinarily is supported by histological examination of major tissues and organs for abnormalities. From these observations, one can usually obtain more specific information about the events leading to the lethal effect, the target organs involved, and often a suggestion about the possible mechanism of toxicity at a relatively fundamental level.

## Evaluating the Dose-Response Relationship

Whatever response is selected for measurement, the relationship between the degree of response of the biological system and the amount of toxicant administered assumes a form that occurs so consistently as to be considered classic and fundamental and is referred to as the dose-response relationship.

In toxicology the quantal dose response is used extensively. Determination of the median lethal dose ($LD_{50}$) is usually the first experiment performed with a new chemical. The $LD_{50}$ is the statistically derived single dose of a substance that can be expected to cause death in 50 percent of the animals tested. If a large number of doses is used with a large number of animals per dose, a sigmoid dose-response curve is observed, as depicted in the top panel of Fig. 2-4. With the lowest dose (6 mg/kg), 1 percent of the animals die. A normally distributed sigmoid curve such as this one approaches a response of 0 percent as the dose is decreased and approaches 100 percent as the dose is increased but theoretically never passes through 0 and 100 percent. However, the minimally effective dose of any chemical that evokes a stated all-or-none response is called the *threshold dose* even though it cannot be determined experimentally.

The sigmoid curve has a relatively linear portion between 16 and 84 percent. These values represent the limits of 1 standard deviation (SD) of the mean (and the median) in a population with truly normal or gaussian distribution. However, it is usually not practical to describe the dose-response curve from this type of plot because one does not usually have large enough sample sizes to define the sigmoid curve adequately.

The middle panel of Fig. 2-4 shows that quantal dose responses such as lethality exhibit a normal or gaussian distri-

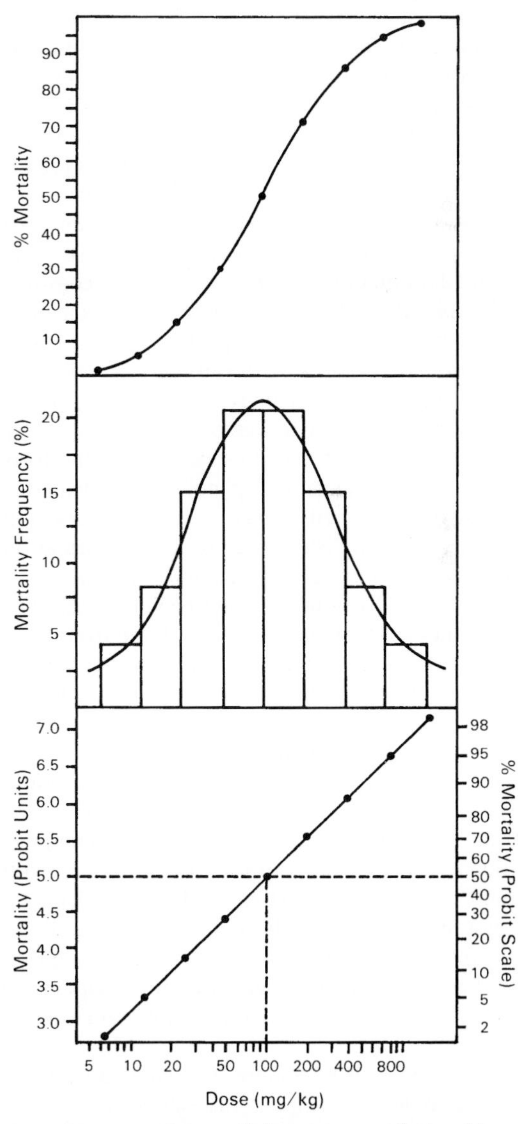


***Figure 2–4. Diagram of quantal dose-reponse relationship.***

The abscissa is a log dosage of the chemical. In the top panel the ordinate is percent mortality, in the middle panel the ordinate is mortality frequency, and in the bottom panel the mortality is in probit units (see text).

bution. The frequency histogram in this panel also shows the relationship between dose and effect. The data used to construct this histogram are the same as those used in the top panel. The bars represent the percentage of animals that died at each dose minus the percentage that died at the immediately lower dose. One can clearly see that only a few animals responded to the lowest dose and the highest dose. Larger numbers of animals responded to doses intermediate between these two extremes, and the maximum frequency of response occurred in the middle portion of the dose range. Thus, we have a bell-shaped curve known as a *normal frequency distribution*. The reason for this normal distribution is that there are differences in susceptibility to chemicals among individuals; this is known as biologic variation. Animals responding at the left end of the curve are referred to as *hypersusceptible*, and those at the right end of the curve are called *resistant*.

In a normally distributed population, the mean ±1 SD represents 68.3 percent of the population, the mean ±2 SD represents 95.5 percent of the population, and the mean ±3 SD equals 99.7 percent of the population. Since quantal dose-response phenomena are usually normally distributed, one can convert the percent response to units of deviation from the mean or normal equivalent deviations (NEDs). Thus, the NED for a 50 percent response is 0; an NED of +1 is equated with an 84.1 percent response. Later, it was suggested (Bliss, 1957) that units of NED be converted by the addition of 5 to the value to avoid negative numbers and that these converted units be called probit units. The probit (from the contraction of *prob*ability un*it*), then, is an NED plus 5. In this transformation, a 50 percent response becomes a probit of 5, a +1 deviation becomes a probit of 6, and a −1 deviation is a probit of 4.

The data given in the top two panels of Fig. 2-4 are replotted in the bottom panel with the mortality plotted in probit units. The data in the top panel (which was in the form of a sigmoid curve) and the middle panel (a bell-shaped curve) form a straight line when transformed into probit units. In essence, what is accomplished in a probit transformation is an adjustment of mortality or other quantal data to an assumed normal population distribution, resulting in a straight line. The $LD_{50}$ is obtained by drawing a horizontal line from the probit unit 5, which is the 50 percent mortality point, to the dose-effect line. At the point of intersection, a vertical line is drawn, and this line intersects the abscissa at the $LD_{50}$ point. It is evident from the line that information with respect to the lethal dose for 90 percent or for 10 percent of the population also may be derived by a similar procedure. Mathematically, it can be demonstrated that the range of values encompassed by the confidence limits is narrowest at the midpoint of the line ($LD_{50}$) and widest at both extremes ($LD_{10}$ and $LD_{90}$) of the dose-response curve (dotted lines in Fig. 2-5). In addition to the $LD_{50}$, the slope of the dose-response curve can also be obtained. Figure 2-5 demonstrates the dose-response curves for the mortality of two compounds. Compound A exhibits a "flat" dose-response curve, showing that a large change in dosage is required before a significant change in response will be observed. However, compound B exhibits a "steep" dose-response curve where a relatively small change in dosage will cause a large change in response. It is evident that the $LD_{50}$ for both compounds is the same (8 mg/kg). However, the slopes of the dose-response curves are quite different. At one-half of $LD_{50}$ of the compounds (4 mg/kg), less than 1 percent of the

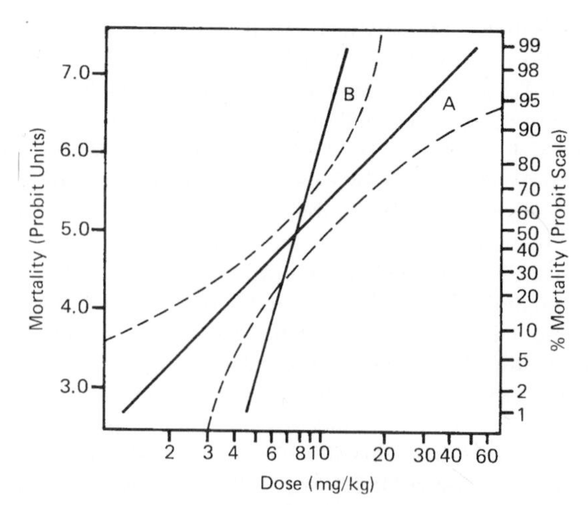


***Figure 2–5. Diagram of dose-response relationships.***

Dose-response relationship is steeper for chemical B than for chemical A. Dotted lines show the confidence limits for chemical A.

animals exposed to compound B would die but 20 percent of the animals given compound A would die.

Determination of the $LD_{50}$ has become a public issue because of increasing concern for the welfare and protection of laboratory animals. The $LD_{50}$ is not a biological constant. Many factors influence toxicity and thus may alter the estimation of the $LD_{50}$ in any particular study. Factors such as animal strain, age and weight, type of feed, caging, pretrial fasting time, method of administration, volume and type of suspension medium, and duration of observation have all been shown to influence adverse responses to toxic substances. These and other factors have been discussed in detail in earlier editions of this textbook (Doull, 1980). Because of this inherent variability in $LD_{50}$ estimates, it is now recognized that for most purposes it is only necessary to characterize the $LD_{50}$ within an order of magnitude range such as 5 to 50 mg/kg, 50 to 500 mg/kg, and so on.

There are several traditional approaches to determining the $LD_{50}$ and its 95 percent confidence limit as well as the slope of the probit line. The reader is referred to the classic works of Litchfield and Wilcoxon (1949), Bliss (1957), and Finney (1971) for a description of the mechanics of these procedures. A computer program in BASIC for determining probit and log-probit or logit correlations has been published (Abou-Setta et al., 1986). These traditional methods for determining $LD_{50}$s require a relatively large number of animals (40 to 50). Other statistical techniques that require fewer animals, such as the "moving averages" method of Thompson and Weill (1952; Weill, 1952), are available but do not provide confidence limits for the $LD_{50}$ and the slope of the probit line. Finney (1985) has succintly summarized the advantages and deficiencies of many of the traditional methods. For most circumstances, an adequate estimate of the $LD_{50}$ and an approximation of the 95 percent confidence intervals can be obtained with as few as six to nine animals, using the "up-and-down" method as modified by Bruce (1985). When this method was compared with traditional methods that typically utilize 40 to 50 animals, excellent agreement was obtained for all 10 compounds tested (Bruce, 1987).

When animals are exposed to chemicals in the air they breathe or the water they (fish) live in, the dose the animals receive is usually not known. For these situations, the lethal concentration 50 ($LC_{50}$) is usually determined, that is, the concentration of chemical in the air or water that causes death to 50 percent of the animals. In reporting an $LC_{50}$, it is imperative that the time of exposure be indicated.

Although by themselves $LD_{50}$ and $LC_{50}$ values are of limited significances, acute lethality studies are essential for characterizing the toxic effects of chemicals and their hazard to humans. The most meaningful scientific information derived from acute lethality tests comes from clinical observations and postmortem examination of animals rather than from the specific $LD_{50}$ value.

The *quantal all-or-none response* is not limited to lethality. Similar dose-effect curves can be constructed for cancer, liver injury, and other types of toxic responses as well as for beneficial therapeutic responses such as anesthesia. Figure 2-6 indicates the dose-response for three different chemical carcinogens. When higher doses were administered, higher percentages of the animals developed sarcomas. While some toxic and therapeutic responses, such as anesthesia, are all or none, other graded responses, such as blood pressure, can be transformed into quantal responses. This is usually performed by quantitating a particular parameter (e.g., blood pressure) in a large number of control animals and determining its standard deviation, which is a measure of its variability. Because the mean $\pm 3$ SD represents 99.7 percent of the population, one can assign all animals that lie outside this range after treatment with a chemical as being affected and those lying within this range as not being affected by the chemical. Using a series of doses of the chemical, one thus can construct a quantal dose-response curve similar to that described above for lethality.

In Figs. 2-4 and 2-5, the dosage has been given on a log basis. Although the use of the log of the dosage is empirical, log-dosage plots usually provide a more nearly linear representation of the data. It must be remembered, however, that this is not universally the case. Some radiation effects, for example, give a better probit fit when the dose is expressed arithmetically rather than logarithmically. There are other situations in which other functions (e.g., exponentials) of dosage provide a better fit to the data than does the log function. It is also conventional to express the dosage in milligrams per kilogram. It might be argued that expression of dosage on a mole per kilogram basis would be better, particularly for making comparisons among a series of compounds. Although such an argument has considerable merit, dosage is usually expressed in milligrams per kilogram.

One might also view dosage on the basis of body weight as being less appropriate than other bases, such as surface area, which is approximately proportional to (body weight)$^{2/3}$. In Table 2-2 selected values are given to compare the differences in dosage by the two alternatives. Given a dose of 100 mg/kg, it can be seen that the dose (milligrams per animal), of course, is proportional to the dose administered by body weight. Surface area is not proportional to weight: While the weight of a human is 3500 times greater than that of a mouse, the surface area of humans is only about 390 times greater than that of mice. Chemicals are usually administered in toxicological studies as mg/kg. The same dose given to humans and mice on a weight basis (mg/kg) would be approximately 10 times greater in humans than mice if that dosage were expressed per surface area (mg/cm$^2$). Cancer chemotherapeutic agents are usually administered on a surface area basis.

## Comparison of Dose Responses

Figure 2-7 illustrates the quantal dose-response curve for a desirable effect of a chemical (ED) such as anesthesia, a toxic effect (TD) such as liver injury, and the lethal dose (LD). As depicted in Fig. 2-7, a parallelism is apparent between the effective dose curve (ED) and the curve depicting mortality (LD). It

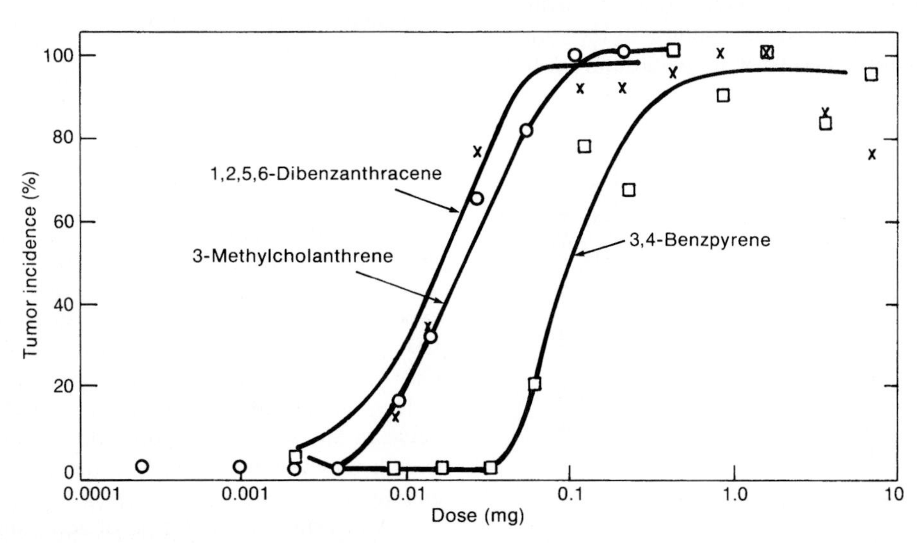


***Figure 2–6. Dose-response relationship for carcinogens.***

Three carcinogenic polycylic aromatic hydrocarbons were administered subcutaneously in a single dose, each to a group of 20 mice. The incidence of sarcomas at the site of injection was noted. (Modified from Bryan WR, Shimkin MB: Quantitave analysis of dose-response data obtained with three carcinogenic hydrocarbons in strain C3H male mice. *JNCI* 3:503–531. 1943.)

**Table 2–2**
**Comparison of Dosage by Weight and Surface Area**

| | WEIGHT g | DOSAGE mg/kg | DOSE mg/animal | SURFACE AREA $cm^2$ | DOSAGE $mg/cm^2$ |
|---|---|---|---|---|---|
| Mouse | 20 | 100 | 2 | 46 | 0.043 |
| Rat | 200 | 100 | 20 | 325 | 0.061 |
| Guinea pig | 400 | 100 | 40 | 565 | 0.071 |
| Rabbit | 1500 | 100 | 150 | 1270 | 0.118 |
| Cat | 2000 | 100 | 200 | 1380 | 0.145 |
| Monkey | 4000 | 100 | 400 | 2980 | 0.134 |
| Dog | 12000 | 100 | 1200 | 5770 | 0.207 |
| Human | 70000 | 100 | 7000 | 18000 | 0.388 |

is tempting to view the parallel dose-response curves as indicative of identity of mechanism, that is, to conclude that the lethality is a simple extension of the therapeutic effect. While this conclusion may ultimately prove to be correct in any particular case, it is not warranted solely on the basis of the two parallel lines. The same admonition applies to any pair of parallel "effect" curves or any other pair of toxicity or lethality curves.

**Therapeutic Index.** The hypothetical curves in Fig. 2-7 illustrate two other interrelated points: the importance of the selection of the toxic criterion and the interpretation of comparative effect. The concept of the "therapeutic index," which was introduced by Paul Ehrlich in 1913, can be used to illustrate this relationship. Although the therapeutic index is directed toward a comparison of the therapeutically effective dose to the toxic dose of a chemical, it is equally applicable to considerations of comparative toxicity. The *therapeutic index* (TI) in its broadest sense is defined as the ratio of the dose required to produce a toxic effect and the dose needed to elicit the desired therapeutic response. Similarly, an index of comparative toxicity is obtained by the ratio of doses of two different materials to produce an identical response or the ratio of doses of the same material necessary to yield different toxic effects.

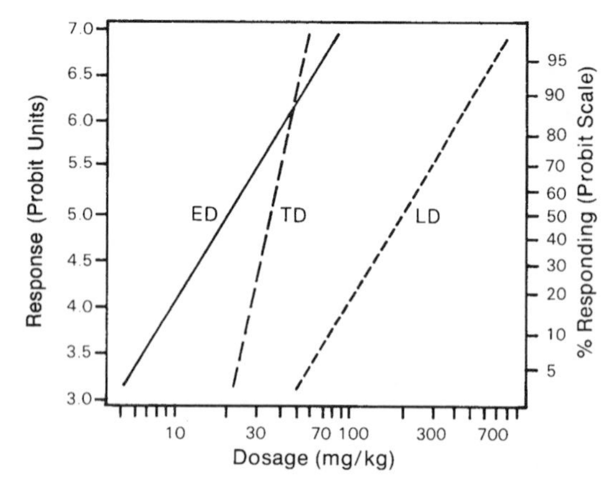


***Figure 2–7. Comparison of effective dose (ED), toxic dose (TD), and lethal dose (LD).***

The plot is of log dosage versus percentage of population responding in probit units.

The most commonly used index of effect, whether beneficial or toxic, is the median dose, that is, the dose required to result in a response in 50 percent of a population (or to produce 50 percent of a maximal response). The therapeutic index of a drug is an approximate statement about the relative safety of a drug expressed as the ratio of the lethal or toxic dose to the therapeutic dose:

$$TI = \frac{LD_{50}}{ED_{50}}$$

From Fig. 2-7 one can approximate a "therapeutic index" by using these median doses. The larger the ratio, the greater the relative safety. The $ED_{50}$ is approximately 20, and the $LD_{50}$ is about 200; thus, the therapeutic index is 10, a number indicative of a relatively safe drug. However, the use of the median effective and median lethal doses is not without disadvantages, because median doses tell nothing about the slopes of the dose-response curves for therapeutic and toxic effects.

**Margin of Safety.** One way to overcome this deficiency is to use the $ED_{99}$ for the desired effect and the $LD_1$ for the undesired effect. These parameters are used in the calculation of the margin of safety:

$$\text{Margin of safety} = \frac{LD_1}{ED_{99}}$$

The quantitative comparisons described above have been used mainly after a single administration of chemicals. However, for chemicals for which there is no beneficial or effective dose and exposures are likely to occur repeatedly, the ratio of $LD_1$ to $ED_{99}$ has little relevance. Thus, for nondrug chemicals, the term "margin of safety" has found use in risk assessment procedures as an indicator of the magnitude of the difference between an estimated exposed dose to a human population and the highest nontoxic dose determined in experimental animals.

A measure of the degree of accumulation of a chemical and/or its toxic effects also can be estimated from quantal toxicity data. The *chronicity index* (Hayes, 1975) of a chemical is a unitless value obtained by dividing its 1-dose $LD_{50}$ by its 90-dose (90-day) $LD_{50}$, with both expressed in milligrams per kilogram per day. Theoretically, if no cumulative effect occurs over the doses, the chronicity index will be 1. If a compound were absolutely cumulative, the chronicity index would be 90.

Similar statistical procedures that are used to calculate the $LD_{50}$ also can be used to determine the lethal time 50 ($LT_{50}$), or the time required for half the animals to die (Litchfield, 1949). The $LT_{50}$ value for a chemical indicates the time course of the toxic effects but does not indicate whether one chemical is more toxic than another.

**Potency versus Efficacy.** To compare the toxic effects of two or more chemicals, the dose response to the toxic effects of each chemical must be established. One can then compare the potency and maximal efficacy of the two chemicals to produce a toxic effect. These two important terms can be explained by reference to Fig. 2-8, which depicts dose-response curves to four different chemicals for the frequency of a particular toxic effect, such as the production of tumors. Chemical A is said to be more potent than chemical B because of their relative positions along the dosage axis. Potency thus refers to the range of doses over which a chemical produces increasing responses. Thus, A is more potent than B and C is more potent than D. Maximal efficacy reflects the limit of the dose-response relationship on the response axis to a certain chemical. Chemicals A and B have equal maximal efficacy, whereas the maximal efficacy of C is less than that of D.

# VARIATION IN TOXIC RESPONSES

## Selective Toxicity

*Selective toxicity* means that a chemical produces injury to one kind of living matter without harming another form of life even though the two may exist in intimate contact (Albert, 1965, 1973). The living matter that is injured is termed the *uneconomic form* (or undesirable), and the matter protected is called the *economic form* (or desirable). They may be related to each other as parasite and host or may be two tissues in one organism. This biological diversity interferes with the ability of toxicologists to predict the toxic effects of a chemical in one species (humans) from experiments performed in another species (laboratory animals). However, by taking advantage of the biological diversity, it is possible to develop agents that are lethal for an undesired species and harmless for other species. In agriculture, for example, there are fungi, insects, and even competitive plant life that injure the crop, and thus selective pesticides are needed. Similarly, animal husbandry and human medicine require agents, such as antibiotics, that are selectively toxic to the undesirable form but do not produce damage to the desirable form.

Drugs and other chemical agents used for selective toxic purposes are selective for one of two reasons. Either (1) the chemical is equitoxic to both economic and uneconomic cells but is accumulated mainly by uneconomic cells or (2) it reacts fairly specifically with a cytological or a biochemical feature that is absent from or does not play an important role in the economic form (Albert, 1965, 1973). Selectivity resulting from differences in distribution usually is caused by differences in the absorption, biotransformation, or excretion of the toxicant. The selective toxicity of an insecticide spray may be partly due to a larger surface area per unit weight that causes the insect to absorb a proportionally larger dose than does the mammal being sprayed. The effectiveness of radioactive iodine in the treatment of hyperthyroidism (as well as its thyroid carcinogenicity) is due to the selective ability of the thyroid gland to accumulate iodine. A major reason why chemicals are toxic to one but not to another type of tissue is that there are differences in accumulation of the ultimate toxic compound in various tissues. This in turn may be due to differences in the ability of various tissues to biotransform the chemical into the ultimate toxic product.

Selective toxicity caused by differences in comparative cytology is exemplified by a comparison of plant and animal cells. Plants differ from animals in many ways, for example, absence of a nervous system, an efficient circulatory system, and muscles and the presence of a photosynthetic mechanism and cell walls. The fact that bacteria contain cell walls and humans do not has been utilized in developing selective toxic chemotherapeutic agents, such as penicillin and cephalosporins, that kill bacteria but are relatively nontoxic to mammalian cells.

Selective toxicity also can be a result of a difference in biochemistry in the two types of cells. For example, bacteria do

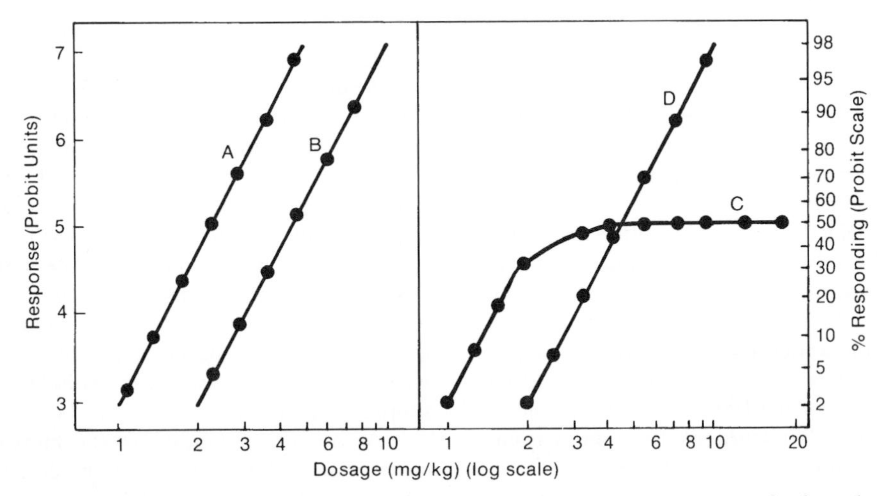


*Figure 2–8. Schematic representation of the difference in the dose-response curves for four chemicals (A–D), illustrating the difference between potency and efficacy (see text).*

not absorb folic acid but synthesize it from *p*-aminobenzoic acid, glutamic acid, and pteridine, whereas mammals cannot synthesize folic acid but have to absorb it from the diet. Thus, sulfonamide drugs are selectively toxic to bacteria because the sulfonamides, which resemble *p*-aminobenzoic acid in both charge and dimensions, antagonize the incorporation of *p*-aminobenzoic acid into the folic acid molecule, a reaction that humans do not carry out.

## Species Differences

Although a basic tenet of toxicology is that "experimental results in animals, when properly qualified, are applicable to humans," it is important to recognize that both quantitative and qualitative differences in response to toxic substances may occur among different species. As was discussed above, there are many reasons for selective toxicity among different species. Even among phylogenetically similar species (e.g., rats, mice, guinea pigs, and hamsters), large differences in response may occur. For example, the $LD_{50}$ for the highly toxic dioxin (TCDD) 2,3,7,8-tetrachlorodibenzo-*p*-dioxin differs by more than 1000-fold between guinea pigs and hamsters. Not only does the lethal dose for TCDD vary widely among species, so do the particular target organs affected.

Species differences in response to carcinogenic chemicals represent an important issue in regulatory risk assessment. As discussed in Chap. 4, extrapolation of laboratory animal data to infer human cancer risk is currently a key component of regulatory decision making. The validity of this approach of course depends on the relevance of the experimental animal model to humans. Large differences in carcinogenic response between experimental animal species are not unusal. For example, mice are highly resistent to the hepatocarcinogenic effects of the fungal toxin aflatoxin $B_1$. Dietary doses as high as 10,000 parts per billion (ppb) failed to produce liver cancer in mice, whereas in rats dietary doses as low as 15 ppb produced a significant increase in liver tumors (Wogan, 1973). The mechanistic basis for this dramatic difference in response appears to be entirely related to species differences in the expression of a particular form of glutathione S-transferase (mYc) that has unusually high catalytic activity toward the carcinogenic epoxide of aflatoxin (Eaton and Gallagher, 1994). Mice express this enzyme constitutively, whereas rats normally express a closely related form with much less detoxifying activity toward aflatoxin epoxide. Interestingly, rats do possess the gene for a form of glutathione S-transferase with high catalytic activity toward aflatoxin epoxide (*GST rYc2*) that is inducible by certain dietary antioxidants and drugs. Thus, dietary treatment can dramatically change the sensitivity of a species to a carcinogen.

Other examples in which large species differences in response to carcinogens have been observed include the development of renal tumors from 2,3,5-trimethylpentane and *d*-limonene in male rats (Lehman-McKeeman and Caudill, 1992), the production of liver tumors from "peroxisomal proliferators" such as the antilipidemic drug clofibrate and the common solvent trichloroethylene (Green, 1990), and the induction of nasal carcinomas in rats after inhalation exposure to formaldehyde (Monticello and Morgan, 1994).

Identifying the mechanistic basis for species differences in response to chemicals is an important part of toxicology because only through a thorough understanding of these differences can the relevance of animal data to human response be verified.

## Individual Differences in Response

Even within a species, large interindividual differences in response to a chemical can occur because of subtle genetic differences. Hereditary differences in a single gene are referred to as genetic polymorphism and may be responsible for idiosyncratic reactions to chemicals, as was discussed earlier in this chapter. However, genetic polymorphism may have other important but less dramatic effects than those described for acute idiosyncratic responses (such as that occuring in pseudocholinesterase-deficient individuals after succinylcholine exposure). For example, it is recognized that approximately 50 percent of the Caucasian population has a gene deletion for the enzyme glutathione S-transferase M1. This enzyme has no apparent significant physiological function, and thus homozygotes for the gene deletion (e.g., those who lack both copies of the normal gene) are functionally and physiologically normal. However, epidemiological studies have indicated that smokers who are homozygous for the null allele may be at increased risk (approximately three-fold) for developing lung cancer compared with smokers who have one or both copies of the normal gene (Sediegard et al., 1986; Nazar-Stewart et al., 1993). Chapter 6 provides additional examples of genetic differences in biotransformation enzymes that may be important determinants of variability in individual susceptibility to chemical exposures.

Genetic polymorphism in physiologically important genes may also be responsible for interindividual differences in toxic responses. For example, studies in transgenic mice have shown that mice possessing one copy of a mutated p53 gene (a so-called tumor suppressor gene; see Chap. 8) are much more susceptible to some chemical carcinogens than are wild-type mice with two normal copies of the gene (Lee et al., 1994). In humans, there is evidence that possessing one mutated copy of a tumor suppressor gene greatly increases the risk of developing certain cancers. For example, retinoblastoma is a largely inherited form of cancer that arises because of the presence of two copies of a defective tumor suppressor gene (the Rb gene) (Wieman, 1993). Individuals with one mutated copy of the Rb gene and one normal copy are not destined to acquire the disease (as are those with two copies of the mutated gene), although their chance of acquiring it is much greater than that of persons with two normal Rb genes. This is the case because both copies of the gene must be nonfunctional for the disease to develop. With one mutated copy present genetically, the probability of acquiring a mutation of the second gene (potentially from exposure to environmental mutagens) is much greater than the probability of acquiring independent mutations in both copies of the gene as would be necessary in people with two normal Rb alleles. (See Chap. 8 for additional discussion of onco-suppressor genes.)

As our understanding of the human genome increases, more "susceptibility" genes will be discovered, and it is likely that the etiology of many chronic diseases will be shown to be related to a combination of genetics and environment. Simple blood tests may ultimately be developed that allow an individual to learn whether he or she may be particularly susceptible to specific drugs or environmental pollutants. Although the public health significance of this type of information could be immense, the disclosure of such information raises many important ethical and legal issues that must be addressed before wide use of such tests.

## DESCRIPTIVE ANIMAL TOXICITY TESTS

Two main principles underlie all descriptive animal toxicity testing. The first is that the effects produced by a compound in laboratory animals, when properly qualified, are applicable to humans. This premise applies to all of experimental biology and medicine. On the basis of dose per unit of body surface, toxic effects in humans are usually in the same range as those in experimental animals. On a body weight basis, humans are generally more vulnerable than are experimental animals, probably by a factor of about 10. When one has an awareness of these quantitative differences, appropriate safety factors can be applied to calculate relatively safe doses for humans. All known chemical carcinogens in humans, with the possible exception of arsenic, are carcinogenic in some species but not in all laboratory animals. Whether the converse is true—that all chemicals carcinogenic in animals are also carcinogenic in humans—is not known with certainty, but this assumption serves as the basis for carcinogenicity testing in animals. This species variation in carcinogenic response appears to be due in many instances to differences in biotransformation of the procarcinogen to the ultimate carcinogen.

The second principle is that exposure of experimental animals to toxic agents in high doses is a necessary and valid method of discovering possible hazards in humans. This principle is based on the quantal dose-response concept that the incidence of an effect in a population is greater as the dose or exposure increases. Practical considerations in the design of experimental model systems require that the number animals used in toxicology experiments always be small compared with the size of human populations at risk. Obtaining statistically valid results from such small groups of animals requires the use of relatively large doses so that the effect will occur frequently enough to be detected. For example, an incidence of a serious toxic effect, such as cancer, as low as 0.01 percent would represent 20,000 people in a population of 200 million and would be considered unacceptably high. Detecting such a low incidence in experimental animals directly would require a minimum of about 30,000 animals. For this reason, there is no choice but to give large doses to relatively small groups and then use toxicological principles in extrapolating the results to estimate the risk at low doses.

Toxicity tests are not designed to demonstrate that a chemical is safe but to characterize the toxic effects a chemical can produce. There are no set toxicology tests that have to be performed on every chemical intended for commerce. Depending on the eventual use of the chemical, the toxic effects produced by structural analogues of the chemical, as well as the toxic effects produced by the chemical itself, contribute to the determination of the toxicology tests that should be performed. However, the FDA, EPA, and Organization for Economic Cooperation and Development (OECD) have written good laboratory practice (GLP) standards. These guidelines are expected to be followed when toxicity tests are conducted in support of the introduction of a chemical to the market.

### Acute Lethality

The first toxicity test performed on a new chemical is acute toxicity. The $LD_{50}$ and other acute toxic effects are determined after one or more routes of administration (one route being oral or the intended route of exposure) in one or more species. The species most often used are the mouse and rat, but sometimes the rabbit and dog are employed. In mice and rats the $LD_{50}$ is usually determined as described earlier in this chapter, but in the larger species only an approximation of the $LD_{50}$ is obtained by increasing the dose in the same animal until serious toxic effects are demonstrated. Studies are performed in both adult male and female animals. Food is often withheld the night before dosing. The number of animals that die in a 14-day period after a single dosage is tabulated. In addition to mortality and weight, daily examination of test animals should be conducted for signs of intoxication, lethargy, behavioral modifications, morbidity, food consumption, and so on. Acute toxicity tests (1) give a quantitative estimate of acute toxicity ($LD_{50}$) for comparison with other substances, (2) identify target organs and other clinical manifestations of acute toxicity, (3) establish the reversibility of the toxic response, and (4) provide dose-ranging guidance for other studies.

If there is a reasonable likelihood of substantial exposure to the material by dermal or inhalation exposure, acute dermal and acute inhalation studies are performed. The acute dermal toxicity test is usually performed in rabbits. The site of application is shaved. The test substance is kept in contact with the skin for 24 h by wrapping the skin with an impervious plastic material. At the end of the exposure period, the wrapping is removed and the skin is wiped to remove any test substance still remaining. Animals are observed at various intervals for 14 days, and the $LD_{50}$ is calculated. If no toxicity is evident at 2 g/kg, further acute dermal toxicity testing is usually not performed. Acute inhalation studies are performed that are similar to other acute toxicity studies except that the route of exposure is inhalation. Most often, the length of exposure is 4 h.

### Skin and Eye Irritations

The ability of a chemical to irritate the skin and eye after an acute exposure is usually determined in rabbits. For the dermal irritation test (Draize test), rabbits are prepared by removal of fur on a section of the back by electric clippers. The chemical is applied to the skin (0.5 ml of liquid or 0.5 g of solid) under four covered gauze patches (1 in. square; one intact and two abraded skin sites on each animal) and usually kept in contact for 4 h. The nature of the covering patches depends on whether occlusive, semiocclusive, or nonocclusive tests are desired. For occlusive testing the test material is covered with an impervious plastic sheet, whereas for semiocclusive tests a gauze dressing may be used. Occasionally, studies may require that the material be applied to abraded skin. The degree of skin irritation is scored for erythema, eschar and edema formation, and corrosive action. These dermal irritation observations are repeated at various intervals after the covered patch has been removed. To determine the degree of ocular irritation, the chemical is instilled into one eye (0.1 ml of liquid or 100 mg of solid) of each test rabbit. The contralateral eye is used as the control. The eyes of the rabbits are then examined at various times after application.

Controversy over this test has led to a reevaluation of the procedure. On the basis of reviews of this procedure and additional experimental data, a panel on eye irritancy of the National Academy of Sciences (NAS) recommended lowering the dose volume (National Academy of Sciences, 1977). More recent studies suggest that a volume of 0.01 ml is as sensitive a method for eye irritancy testing as the 0.1 ml test but causes less pain to the animals (Chan and Hayes, 1989).

## Sensitization

Information about the potential of a chemical to sensitize skin is needed in addition to irritation testing for all materials that may repeatedly come into contact with the skin. Numerous procedures have been developed to determine the potential of substances to induce a sensitization reaction in humans (delayed hypersensitivity reaction), including the Draize test, the open epicutaneous test, the Buehler test, Freund's complete adjuvant test, the optimization test, the split adjuvant test, and the guinea pig maximization test (Patrick and Maibach, 1989). Although they differ in regard to route and frequency of duration, they all utilize the guinea pig as the preferred test species. In general, the test chemical is administered to the shaved skin topically, intradermally, or both and may include the use of adjuvants to enhance the sensitivity of the assay. Multiple administrations of the test substance are generally given over a period of 2 to 4 weeks. Depending on the specific protocol, the treated area may be occluded. Two to 3 weeks after the last treatment, the animals are challenged with a nonirritating concentration of the test substance and the development of erythematous responses is evaluated.

## Subacute (Repeated-Dose Study)

Subacute toxicity tests are performed to obtain information on the toxicity of a chemical after repeated administration and as an aid to establish doses for subchronic studies. A typical protocol is to give three to four different dosages of the chemicals to the animals by mixing it in their feed. For rats 10 animals per sex per dose are often used, whereas for dogs three dosages and 3 to 4 animals per sex are used. Clinical chemistry and histopathology are performed after 14 days of exposure, as described below in the section on subchronic toxicity testing.

## Subchronic

The toxicity of a chemical after subchronic exposure is then determined. Subchronic exposure can last for different periods of time, but 90 days is the most common test duration. The principal goals of the subchronic study are to establish a no observed adverse effect level [NOAEL, referred to also as the no observed effect level (NOEL)], and to further identify and characterize the specific organ or organs affected by the test compound after repeated administration. One may also obtain a "lowest observed adverse effect level" (LOAEL) as well as the NOAEL for the species tested. The numbers obtained for NOAEL and LOAEL will depend on how closely the dosages are spaced and the number of animals examined. Determinations of NOAELs and LOAELs have numerous regulatory implications. For example, the EPA utilizes the NOAEL to calculate the *reference dose* (RfD), which may used to establish regulatory values for "acceptable" pollutant levels (Barnes and Dourson, 1988) (Chap. 4). An alternative to the NOAEL approach referred to as the *benchmark dose* uses all the experimental data to fit one or more dose-response curves (Crump, 1984). These curves are then used to estimate a benchmark dose that is defined as "the statistical lower bound on a dose corresponding to a specified level of risk" (Allen et al., 1994a). Although subchronic studies are frequently the primary or sole source of experimental data to determine both the NOAEL and the benchmark dose, these concepts can be applied to other types of toxicity testing protocols, such as that for chronic toxicity or developmental toxicity (Faustman et al., 1994; Allen et al., 1994a and b) (see also Chap. 4 for a complete discussion of the derivation and use of NOAELs, RfDs, and benchmark doses). If chronic studies have been completed, these data are generally used for NOAEL and LOAEL estimates in preference to data from subchronic studies.

A subchronic study is usually conducted in two species (rat and dog) by the route of intended exposure (usually oral). At least three doses are employed (a high dose that produces toxicity but does not cause more than 10 percent fatalities, a low dose that produces no apparent toxic effects, and an intermediate dose) with 10 to 20 rats and 4 to 6 dogs of each sex per dose. Each animal should be uniquely identified with permanent markings such as ear tags, tattoos, or electronically coded microchip implants. Only healthy animals should be used, and each animal should be housed individually in an adequately controlled environment. Animals should be observed once or twice daily for signs of toxicity, including changes in body weight, diet consumption, changes in fur color or texture, respiratory or cardiovascular distress, motor and behavioral abnormalities, and palpable masses. All premature deaths should be recorded and necropsied as soon as possible. Severely moribund animals should be terminated immediately to preserve tissues and reduce unnecessary suffering. At the end of the 90-day study, all the remaining animals should be terminated and blood and tissues should be collected for further analysis. The gross and microscopic condition of the organs and tissues (about 15 to 20) and the weight of the major organs (about 12) are recorded and evaluated. Hematology and blood chemistry measurements are usually done before, in the middle of, and at the termination of exposure. Hematology measurements usually include hemoglobin concentration, hematocrit, erythrocyte counts, total and differential leukocyte counts, platelet count, clotting time, and prothrombin time. Clinical chemistry determinations commonly made include glucose, calcium, potassium, urea nitrogen, alanine aminotransferase (ALT, formerly SGPT), serum aspartate aminotransferase (AST, formerly SGOT), gamma-glutamyltranspeptidase (GGT), sorbitol dehydrogenase, lactic dehydrogenase, alkaline phosphatase, creatinine, bilirubin, triglycerides, cholesterol, albumin, globulin, and total protein. Urinalysis is usually performed in the middle of and at the termination of the testing period and often includes determination of specific gravity or osmolarity, pH, glucose, ketones, bilirubin, and urobilinogen as well as microscopic examination of formed elements. If humans are likely to have significant exposure to the chemical by dermal contact or inhalation, subchronic dermal and/or inhalation experiments may also be required. Subchronic toxicity studies not only characterize the dose-response relationship of a test substance after repeated administration but also provide data for a more reasonable prediction of appropriate doses for chronic exposure studies.

For chemicals that are to be registered as drugs, acute and subchronic studies (and potentially additional special tests if a chemical has unusual toxic effects or therapeutic purposes) must be completed before the company can file an IND (Investigative New Drug) application with the FDA. If the application is approved, clinical trials can commence. At the same time phase I, phase II, and phase III clinical trials are performed, chronic exposure of the animals to the test compound can be carried out in laboratory animals, along with additional specialized tests.

## Chronic

Long-term or chronic exposure studies are performed similarly to subchronic studies except that the period of exposure is longer than 3 months. In rodents, chronic exposures are usually for 6 months to 2 years. Chronic studies in nonrodent species are usually for 1 year but may be longer. The length of exposure is somewhat dependent on the intended period of exposure in humans. If the agent is a drug planned to be used for short periods, such as an antimicrobial agent, a chronic exposure of 6 months may be sufficient, whereas if the agent is a food additive with the potential for lifetime exposure in humans, a chronic study up to 2 years in duration is likely to be required.

Chronic toxicity tests are performed to assess the cumulative toxicity of chemicals, but the study design and evaluation often include a consideration of the carcinogenic potential of chemicals so that a separate lifetime feeding study that addresses carcinogenicity does not have to be performed. These studies usually are performed in rats and mice and extend over the average lifetime of the species (18 months to 2 years for mice; 2 to 2.5 years for rats). To ensure that 30 rats per dose survive the 2-year study, 60 rats per group per sex are often started in the study. Both gross and microscopic pathological examinations are made not only on animals that survive the chronic exposure but also on those which die prematurely.

Dose selection is critical in these studies to ensure that premature mortality from chronic toxicity does not limit the number of animals that survive to a normal life expectancy. Most regulatory guidelines require that the highest dose administered be the estimated maximum tolerable dose (MTD). This is generally derived from subchronic studies, but additional longer studies (e.g., 6 months) may be necessary if delayed effects or extensive cumulative toxicity are indicated in the 90-day subchronic study. The MTD has had various definitions (Haseman, 1985). The National Toxicology Program's (NTP) Bioassay Program currently defines the MTD as the dose that suppresses body weight gain slightly (i.e., 10 percent) in a 90-day subchronic study, although the NTP and other testing programs are critically evaluating the use of parameters other than weight gain, such as physiological and pharmacokinetic considerations and urinary metabolite profiles, as indicators of an appropriate MTD. Generally, one or two additional doses, usually fractions of the MTD (e.g., 1/2 and 1/4 MTD), and a control group are tested.

The use of the MTD in carcinogenicity has been the subject of controversy. The premise that high doses are necessary for testing the carcinogenic potential of chemicals is derived from the statistical and experimental design limitations of chronic bioassays.

Consider that a 0.5 percent increase in cancer incidence in the United States would result in over 1 million additional cancer deaths each year—clearly an unacceptably high risk. However, identifying with statistical confidence a 0.5 percent incidence of cancer in a group of experimental animals would require a minimum of 1000 test animals, and this assumes that no tumors were present in the absence of exposure (zero background incidence).

Figure 2-9 shows the statistical relationship between minimum detectable tumor incidence and the number of test animals per group. This curve shows that in a chronic bioassay with 50 animals per test group, a tumor incidence of about 8 percent could exist even though no animals in the test group had tumors. This example assumes that there are no tumors in the control group. These statistical considerations illustrate why animals are tested at doses higher than those which occur in human exposure. Because it is impractical to use the large number of animals that would be required to test the potential carcinogenicity of a chemical at the doses usually encountered by people, the alternative is to assume that there is a relationship between the administered dose and the tumorigenic response and give animals doses of the chemical that are high enough to produce a measurable tumor response in a reasonable size test group, such as 40 to 50 animals per dose. The limitations of this approach are discussed in Chap. 4.

Recently, a new approach for establishing maximum doses for use in chronic animal toxicity testing of drugs has been proposed for substances for which basic human pharmacokinetic data are available (for example, new pharmaceutical agents which have completed phase I clinical trials). For chronic animal studies performed on drugs where single-dose human pharmacokinetic data are available, it has been suggested that a daily dose be used that would provide an area under the curve (AUC) in laboratory animals equivalent to 25 times the AUC in humans given the highest (single) daily dose to be used therapeutically. This value would then be used in place of the traditional MTD for chronic bioassays.

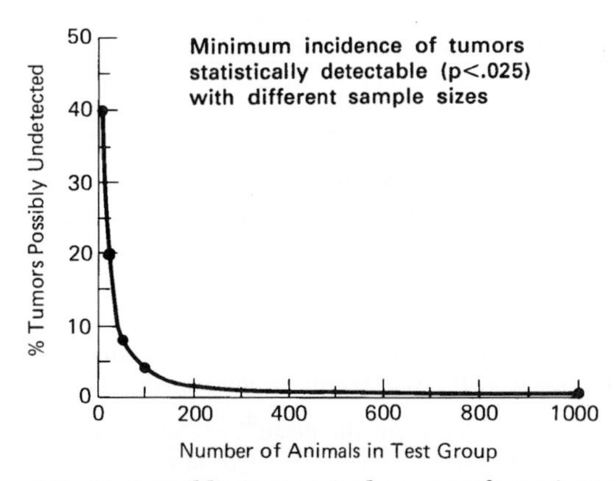


***Figure 2–9. Statistical limitations in the power of experimental animal studies to detect tumorigenic effects.***

Chronic toxicity assays are commonly used to evaluate the potential oncogenicity of test substances. Most regulatory guidelines require that both benign and malignant tumors be reported in the evaluation. Statistical increases above the control incidence of tumors (either all tumors or specific tumor types) in the treatment groups are considered indicative of carcinogenic potential of the chemical unless there are qualifying factors that suggest otherwise (lack of a dose response, unusually low incidence of tumors in the control group compared with "historical" controls, etc.). Thus, the conclusion as to whether a given chronic bioassay is positive or negative for carcinogenic potential of the test substance requires careful consideration of background tumor incidence. Properly designed chronic oncogenicity studies require that a concurrent control group matched for age, diet, housing conditions, and the like be used. For some tumor types, the "background" incidence of tumors is surprisingly high. Figure 2-10 shows the "background" tumor incidence for various tumors in male and female F-344 rats used in 27 recent National Toxicology Program 2-year rodent carcinogenicity studies. The data shown represent the percent of animals in control (nonexposed) groups that developed the specified tumor type by the end of the 2-year study. These studies involved more than 1300 rats of each sex. Figure 2-11 shows similar data for control (nonexposed) male and female B6C3F1 mice from 30 recent NTP 2-year carcinogenicity studies and includes data from over 1400 mice of each sex. There are several key points that can be derived from these summary data:

1. Tumors, both benign and malignant, are not uncommon events in animals even in the absence of exposure to any known carcinogen.
2. There are numerous different tumor types that develop "spontaneously" in both sexes of both rats and mice, but at different rates.
3. Background tumors that are common in one species may be uncommon in another (for example, testicular interstitial cell adenomas are very common in male rats but rare in male mice; liver adenomas/carcinomas are about 10 times more prevalent in male mice than in male rats).
4. Even within the same species and strain, large gender differences in background tumor incidence are sometimes observed (for example, adrenal gland pheochromocytomas are about seven times more prevalent in male F344

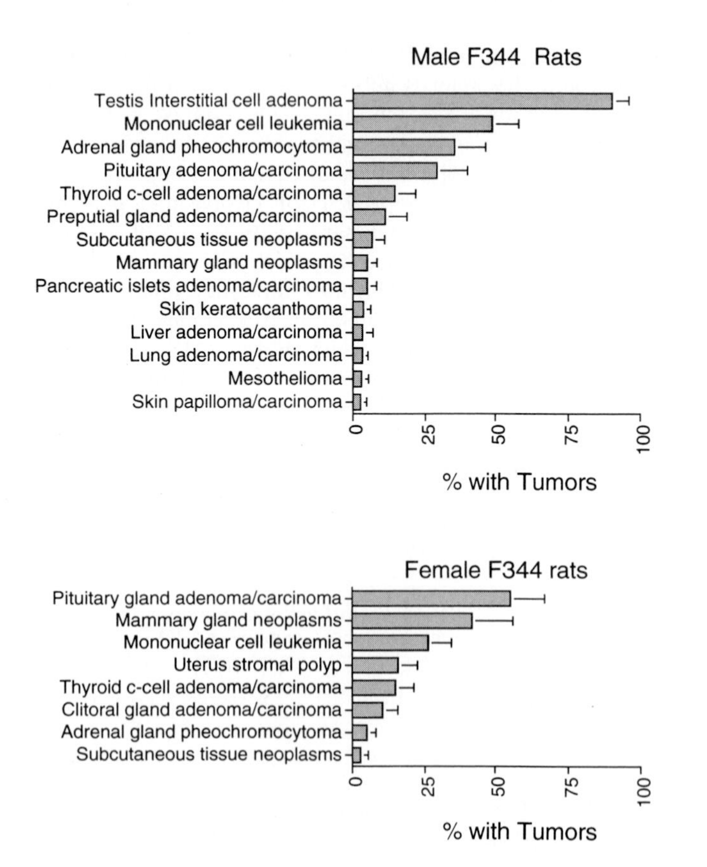


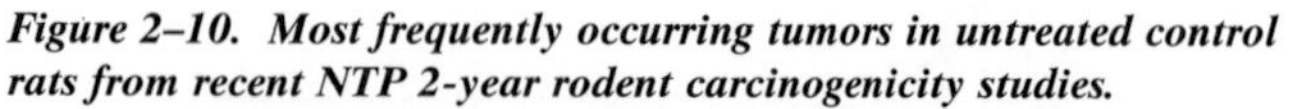


*Figure 2–10. Most frequently occurring tumors in untreated control rats from recent NTP 2-year rodent carcinogenicity studies.*

The values shown represent the mean ±SD of the percentage of animals developing the specified tumor type at the end of the 2-year study. The values were obtained from 27 different studies involving a combined total of between 1319 and 1353 animals per tumor type.

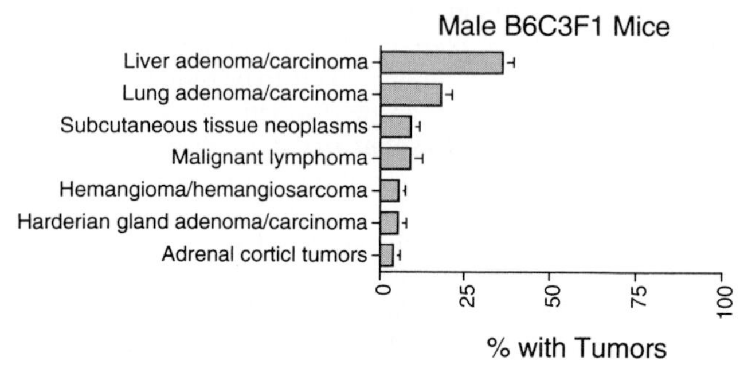


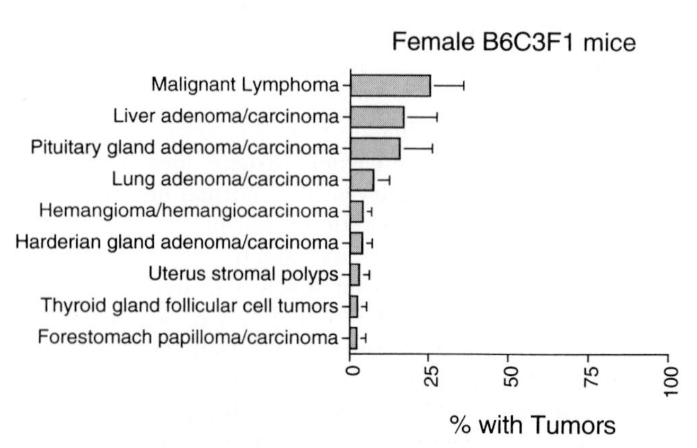


*Figure 2–11. Most frequently occurring tumors in untreated control mice from recent NTP 2-year rodent carcinogenicity studies.*

The values shown represent the mean ±SD of the percentage of animals developing the specified tumor type at the end of the 2-year study. The values were obtained from 30 different studies involving a total of between 1447 and 1474 animals per tumor type.

rats than in female F344 rats; lung and liver tumors are twice as prevalent in male B6C3F1 mice as in female B6C3F1 mice).

5. Even when the general protocols, diets, environment, strain and source of animals, and other variables are relatively constant, background tumor incidence can vary widely, as shown by the relatively large standard deviations for some tumor types in the NTP bioassay program. For example, the range in liver adenoma/carcinoma incidence in 30 different groups of unexposed (control) male B6C3F1 mice went from a low of 10 percent to a high of 68 percent. Pituitary gland adenomas/carcinomas ranged from 12 to 60 percent and 30 to 76 percent in unexposed male and female F344 rats, respectively, and from 0 to 36 percent in unexposed female B6C3F1 mice.

Taken together, these data demonstrate the importance of including concurrent control animals in such studies. In addition, comparisons of the concurrent control results to "historical" controls accumulated over years of study may be important in identifying potentially spurious "false-positive" results. The relatively high variability in background tumor incidence among groups of healthy, highly inbred strains of animals maintained on nutritionally balanced and consistent diets in rather sterile environments highlights the dilemma in interpreting the significance of both positive and negative results in regard to the human population, which is genetically diverse, has tremendous variability in diet, nutritional status and overall health; and lives in an environment full of potentially carcinogenic substances, both natural and human-made.

## Developmental and Reproductive Toxicity

The effects of chemicals on reproduction and development also need to be determined. *Developmental toxicology* is the study of adverse effects on the developing organism occurring anytime during the life span of the organism that may result from exposure to chemical or physical agents before conception (either parent), during prenatal development, or postnatally until the time of puberty. *Teratology* is the study of defects induced during development between conception and birth (see Chap. 10). *Reproductive toxicology* is the study of the occurrence of adverse effects on the male or female reproductive system that may result from exposure to chemical or physical agents (see Chap. 19).

Four types of animal tests are utilized to examine the potential of an agent to alter development and reproduction. General fertility and reproductive performance (segment I or phase I) tests are usually performed in rats with two or three doses (20 rats per sex per dose) of the test chemical (neither produces maternal toxicity). Males are given the chemical 60 days and females 14 days before mating. The animals are given the chemical throughout gestation and lactation. Typical observations made include the percentage of the females that become pregnant, the number of stillborn and live offspring, and the weight, growth, survival, and general condition of the offspring during the first 3 weeks of life.

The teratogenic potential of chemicals is also determined in laboratory animals (segment II). Teratogens are most effective when administered during the first trimester, the period of organogenesis. Thus, the animals (12 rabbits and 20 rats or mice per group) usually are exposed to one of three dosages during organogenesis (day 6 to 15 in rats and days 6 to 18 in rabbits), and the fetuses are removed by cesarean section a day before the estimated time of delivery (rabbit: day 31; rat: day 21). The uterus is excised and weighed and then examined for the number of live, dead, and resorbed fetuses. Live fetuses are weighed; half of each litter is examined for skeletal abnormalities, and the remaining half for soft tissue anomalies.

The perinatal and postnatal toxicities of chemicals also are often examined (segment III). This test is performed by administering the test compound to rats from the fifteenth day of gestation throughout delivery and lactation and determining its effect on the birthweight, survival, and growth of the offspring during the first 3 weeks of life.

A multigenerational study often is carried out to determine the effects of chemicals on the reproductive system. At least three dosage levels are given to groups of 25 female and 25 male rats shortly after weaning (30 to 40 days of age). These rats are referred to as the $F_0$ generation. Dosing continues throughout breeding (about 140 days of age), gestation, and lactation. The offspring ($F_1$ generation) thus have been exposed to the chemical *in utero*, via lactation, and in the feed thereafter. When the $F_1$ generation is about 140 days old, about 25 females and 25 males are bred to produce the $F_2$ generation, and administration of the chemical is continued. The $F_2$ generation is thus also exposed to the chemical *in utero* and via lactation. The $F_1$ and $F_2$ litters are examined as soon as possible after delivery. The percentage of $F_0$ and $F_1$ females that get pregnant, the number of pregnancies that go to full term, the litter size, the number of stillborn, and the number of live births are recorded. Viability counts and pup weights are recorded at birth and at 4, 7, 14, and 21 days of age. The fertility index (percentage of mating resulting in pregnancy), gestation index (percentage of pregnancies resulting in live litters), viability index (percentage of animals that survive 4 days or longer), and lactation index (percentage of animals alive at 4 days that survived the 21-day lactation period) are then calculated. Gross necropsy and histopathology are performed on some of the parents ($F_0$ and $F_1$), with the greatest attention being paid to the reproductive organs, and gross necropsy is performed on all weanlings.

Numerous short-term tests for teratogenicity have been developed (Faustman, 1988). These tests utilize whole embryo culture, organ culture, and primary and established cell cultures to examine developmental processes and estimate the potential teratogenic risks of chemicals. Many of these *in utero* test systems are under evaluation for use in screening new chemicals for teratogenic effects. These systems vary in their ability to identify specific teratogenic events and alterations in cell growth and differentiation. In general, the available assays cannot identify functional or behavioral teratogens (Faustman, 1988).

## Mutagenicity

Mutagenesis is the ability of chemicals to cause changes in the genetic material in the nucleus of cells in ways that allow the changes to be transmitted during cell division. Mutations can occur in either of two cell types, with substantially different consequences. Germinal mutations damage DNA in sperm and ova, which can undergo meiotic division and therefore have the potential for transmission of the mutations to future generations. If mutations are present at the time of fertilization in either the egg or the sperm, the resulting combination of genetic material may not be viable, and the death may occur in the early stages of embryonic cell division. Alternatively, the mutation in the genetic material may not affect early embryogenesis but may result in the death of the fetus at a later developmental period, resulting in abortion. Congenital abnormalities also may result from mutations. Somatic mutations refer to mutations in all other cell types and are not heritable but may result in cell death or transmission of a genetic defect to other cells in the same tissue through mitotic division. Because the initiation event of chemical carcinogenesis is thought to be a mutagenic event, mutagenic tests are often used to screen for potential carcinogens.

Several in vivo and in vitro procedures have been devised to test chemicals for their ability to cause mutations. Some genetic alterations are visible with the light microscope. In this case, cytogenetic analysis of bone marrow smears is used after the animals have been exposed to the test agent. Because some mutations are incompatible with normal development, the mutagenic potential of a chemical can also be measured by the dominant lethal test. This test is usually performed in rodents. The male is exposed to a single dose of the test compound and then is mated with two untreated females weekly for 8 weeks. The females are killed before term, and the number of live embryos and the number of corpora lutea are determined. The test for mutagens that has received the widest attention is the *Salmonella*/microsome test developed by Ames and colleagues (Ames et al., 1975). This test uses several mutant strains of *Salmonella typhimurium* that lack the enzyme phosphoribosyl ATP synthetase, which is required for histidine synthesis.

These strains are unable to grow in a histidine-deficient medium unless a reverse or back mutation to the wild type has occurred. Other mutations in these bacteria have been introduced to enhance the sensitivity of the strains to mutagenesis. The two most significant additional mutations enhance penetration of substances into the bacteria and decrease the ability of the bacteria to repair DNA damage. Since many chemicals are not mutagenic or carcinogenic unless they are biotransformed to a toxic product by the endoplasmic reticulum (microsomes), rat liver microsomes usually are added to the medium containing the mutant strain and the test chemical. The number of reverse mutations is then quantitated by the number of bacterial colonies that grow in a histidine-deficient medium. Mutagenicity is discussed in detail in Chap. 9.

## Other Tests

Most of the tests described above will be included in a "standard" toxicity testing protocol because they are required by the various regulatory agencies. Additional tests also may be required or included in the protocol to provide information relating a special route of exposure (inhalation) or a special effect (behavior). Inhalation toxicity tests in animals usually are carried out in a dynamic (flowing) chamber rather than in static chambers to avoid particulate settling and exhaled gas complications. Such studies usually require special dispersing and analytic methodologies, depending on whether the agent to be tested is a gas, vapor, or aerosol; additional information on methods, concepts, and problems associated with inhalation toxicology is provided in Chaps. 15 and 28. A discussion of behavioral toxicology can be found in Chap. 16. The duration of exposure for both inhalation and behavioral toxicity tests can be acute, subchronic, or chronic, but acute studies are more common with inhalation toxicology and chronic studies are more common with behavioral toxicology. Other special types of animal toxicity tests include immunotoxicology, toxicokinetics (absorption, distribution, biotransformation, and excretion), the development of appropriate antidotes and treatment regimes for poisoning, and the development of analytic techniques to detect residues of chemicals in tissues and other biological materials. The approximate costs of some descriptive toxicity tests are given in Table 2-3.

**Table 2–3**
**Typical Costs of Descriptive Toxicity Tests**

| TEST | COST, $ |
|---|---|
| *General acute toxicity* | |
| Acute toxicity (rat; two routes) | 6,500 |
| Acute dermal toxicity (rabbit) | 3,000 |
| Acute inhalation toxicity (rat) | 6,500 |
| Acute dermal irritation (rabbit) | 900 |
| Acute eye irritation (rabbit) | 500 |
| Skin sensitization (guinea pig) | 700 |
| *Repeated dose toxicity* | |
| 14-day exposure (rat) | 40,000 |
| 90-day exposure (rat) | 100,000 |
| 1-year (diet; rat) | 225,000 |
| 1-year (oral gavage; rat) | 275,000 |
| 2-year (diet; rat) | 625,000 |
| 2-year (oral gavage; rat) | 800,000 |
| *Genetic toxicology tests* | |
| Bacterial reverse mutation | 1,850*–13,650† |
| Mammalian cell forward mutation | 8,400*–13,650† |
| In vitro cytogenetics (CHO cells) | 8,000*–19,000† |
| In vivo micronucleus (mouse) | 10,775 |
| In vivo chromosome aberration (rat) | 26,500 |
| Dominant lethal (mouse) | 55,000 |
| *Drosophila* sex-linked recessive lethal | 35,000 |
| Mammalian bone marrow cytogenctics (in vivo; rat) | 26,500 |
| *Reproduction* | |
| Segment I (rat) | 95,000 |
| Segment II (rat) | 61,500 |
| Segment II (rabbit) | 66,500 |
| Segment III (rat) | 62,000 |
| Acute toxicity in fish ($LC_{50}$) | 1,750 |
| *Daphnia* reproduction study | 1,750 |
| Algae growth inhibition | 1,750 |

* Minimum cost for U.S. registration.
† Worldwide registration.

# REFERENCES


Abou-Setta MM, Sorrell RW, Childers CC: A computer program in BASIC for determining probit and log-probit or Logit correlation for toxicology and biology. *Bull Environ Contam Toxicol* 36:242–249, 1986.

Albert A: Fundamental aspects of selective toxicity. *Ann NY Acad Sci* 123:5–18, 1965

Albert A: *Selective Toxicity*. London: Chapman and Hall, 1973.

Aldridge WN: The biological basis and measurement of thresholds. *Annu Rev Pharmacol Toxicol* 26:39–58, 1986.

Allen BC, Kavlock RJ, Kimmel CA, Faustman EM: Dose-response assessment for developmental toxicity: II. Comparison of generic Benchmark Dose estimates with no observed adverse effect levels. *Fundam Appl Toxicol* 23:487–495, 1994a.

Allen BC, Kavlock RJ, Kimmel CA, Faustman EM: Dose-response assessment for developmental toxicity: III. Statistical models. *Fundam Appl Toxicol* 23:496–509, 1994b.

Ames B, McCann J, Yamasaki E: Methods for detecting carcinogens and mutagens with the *Salmonella*/mammalian microsome mutagenicity test. *Mutat Res* 31: 347–364, 1975.

Ames BN, Magaw R, Gold LW: Ranking possible carcinogenic hazards. *Science* 236:271–280, 1987.

Ariens EJ, Wius EW, Veringa EJ: Stereoselectivity of bioactive xenobiotics. *Biochem Pharmacol* 37:9–18, 1988.

Barnes DG, Dourson M: Reference dose (RfD): Description and use in health risk assessments. *Reg Toxicol Pharmacol* 8:471–486, 1988.

Bliss CL: Some principles of bioassay. *Am Sci* 45:449–466, 1957.

Boobis AR, Fawthrop DJ, Davis DS: Mechanisms of cell death. *TiPS* 10:275–280, 1989.

Bruce RD: An up-and-down procedure for acute toxicity testing. *Fundam Appl Toxicol* 5:15–157, 1985.

Bruce RD: A confirmatory study of the up-and-down method of acute oral toxicity testing. *Fundam Appl Toxicol* 8:97–100, 1987.

Bryan WR, Shimkin MB: Quantitative analysis of dose-response data obtained with three carcinogenic hydrocarbons in strain C3H male mice. *JNCI* 3:503–531, 1943.

Chan PK, Hayes, AW: Principles and methods for acute toxicity and eye irritancy, in Hayes AW (ed): *Principles and Methods of Toxicology*, 2d ed. New York: Raven Press, 1988, pp 169–220.

Crump KS: An improved procedure for low-doxe carcinogenic risk assessment from animal data. *J Environ Pathol Toxicol* 5:339–348, 1984.

Doull J: Factors influencing toxicity, in Doull J, Klaassen CD, Amdur MO (eds): *Casarett and Doull's Toxicology: The Basic Science of Poisons,* 2d ed. New York: Macmillan, 1980, pp 70–83.

DuBois KP: Potentiation of the toxicity or organophosphorus compounds. *Adv Pest Control Res* 4:117–151, 1961.

Eaton DL, Gallagher EP: Mechanisms of aflatoxin carcinogenesis. *Annu Rev Pharmacol Toxicol* 34:1325–1372, 1994.

Faustman EM: Short-term tests for teratogens. *Mutat Res* 205:355–384, 1988.

Faustman EM, Allen BC, Kavlock RJ, Kimmel CA: Dose-response assessment for developmental toxicity: I. Characterization of database and determination of no observed adverse effect levels. *Fundam Appl Toxicol* 23:478–486, 1994.

Finney DJ: *Probit Analysis*. Cambridge: Cambridge University Press, 1971.

Finney DJ: The median lethal dose and its estimation. *Arch Toxicol* 56:215–218, 1985.

Goering PL, Klaassen CD: Altered subcellular distribution of cadmium following cadmium pretreatment: Possible mechanism of tolerance to cadmium-induced lethality. *Toxicol Appl Pharmacol* 70:195–203, 1983.

Goldstein A, Aronow L, Kalman SM: *Principles of Drug Action*. New York: Wiley, 1974.

Green T: Species differences in carcinogenicity: The role of metabolism in human risk evaluation. *Teratogenesis Carcinog Mutagen* 10:103–119, 1990.

Haseman JD: Issues in carcinogenicity testing: Dose selection. *Fundam Appl Toxicol* 5:66–78, 1985.

Hayes WJ Jr: *Toxicology of Pesticides.* Baltimore: Williams & Wilkins, 1975.

Lee JM, Abhramson JL, Bernstein A: DNA damage, oncogenesis and the p53 tumour-suppressor gene. *Mutat Res* 307: 573–581, 1994.

Lehman-McKeeman LD, Caudill D: Biochemical basis for mouse resistance to hyaline droplet nephropathy: Lack of relevance of the alpha 2u-globulin protein superfamily in this male rat-specific syndrome. *Toxicol Appl Pharmacol* 112:214–221, 1992.

Levine RR: *Pharmacology: Drug Actions and Reactions*, 2d ed. Boston: Little, Brown, 1978.

Litchfield JT Jr: A method for rapid graphic solution of time-percent effective curve. *J Pharmacol Exp Ther* 97:399–408, 1949.

Litchfield JT, Wilcoxon F: Simplified method of evaluating dose-effect experiments. *J Pharmacol Exp Ther* 96:99–113, 1949.

Loomis TA: *Essentials of Toxicology*, 3d ed. Philidelphia: Lea & Febiger, 1978.

Lutz WK, Maier P: Genotoxic and epigenetic chemical carcinogenesis: One process, different mechanisms. *TiPS* 9:322–326, 1988.

Monticello TM, Morgan KT: Cell proliferation and formaldehyde-induced respiratory carcinogenesis. *Risk Anal* 14:313–319, 1994.

Murphy SD, Cheever KL: Effects of feeding insecticides: Inhibition of carboxylesterase and cholinesterase activities in rats. *Arch Environ Health* 17:749–756, 1968.

National Academy of Sciences: Committee for Revision of NAS Publication 1138: Dermal and eye toxicity tests, in *Principles and Procedures for Evaluating the Toxicity of Household Substances.* Washington, DC: National Academy of Sciences, 1977, pp 41–54.

Nazar-Stewart V, Motulsky AG, Eaton DL, et al: The glutathione S-transferase $\mu$ polymorphism as a marker for susceptibility to lung carcinoma. *Cancer Res* 53:2313–18, 1993.

Orrenius S, McConkey DJ, Bellomo G, Nicotera P: Role of $Ca^{2+}$ in toxic cell killing. *TiPS* 10:281–285, 1989.

Seidegard J, Voracheck WR, Pero RW, Pearson WR: Hereditary differences in the expression of the human glutathione transferase active on trans-stilbene oxide are due to a gene deletion. *Proc Natl Acad Sci* 85:7293–7297, 1988.

Thompson WR, Weil CS: On the construction of tables for moving average interpolation *Biometrics* 8:51–54, 1952.

Weil CS: Tables for convenient calculation of median-effective dose ($LD_{50}$ or $ED_{50}$) and instruction in their use. *Biometrics* 8:249–263, 1952.

Wieman KG: The retinoblastoma gene: Role in cell cycle control and cell differentiation. *FASEB J* 7:841–845, 1993.

# CHAPTER 3

# MECHANISMS OF TOXICITY

*Zoltán Gregus and Curtis D. Klaassen*

Depending primarily on the degree and route of exposure, chemicals may adversely affect the function and/or structure of living organisms. The qualitative and quantitative characterization of these harmful or toxic effects is essential for an evaluation of the potential hazard posed by a particular chemical. It is also valuable to understand the mechanisms responsible for the manifestation of toxicity, that is, how a toxicant enters an organism, how it interacts with target molecules, how it exerts its deleterious effects, and how the organism deals with the insult.

An understanding of the mechanisms of toxicity is of both practical and theoretical importance. Such information provides a rational basis for interpreting descriptive toxicity data, estimating the probability that a chemical will cause harmful effects, establishing procedures to prevent or antagonize the toxic effects, designing drugs and industrial chemicals that are less hazardous, and developing pesticides that are more selectively toxic for their target organisms. Elucidation of the mechanisms of chemical toxicity has led to a better understanding of fundamental physiological and biochemical processes ranging from neurotransmission (e.g., curare-type arrow poisons) to deoxyribonucleic acid (DNA) repair (e.g., alkylating agents). Pathological conditions such as cancer and Parkinson's disease are better understood because of studies on the mechanism of toxicity of chemical carcinogens and 1,2,3,6-tetrahydro-1-methyl-4-phenylpyridine (MPTP), respectively. Continued research on mechanisms of toxicity will undoubtedly continue to provide such insights.

This chapter reviews the cellular mechanisms that contribute to the manifestation of toxicities. Although such mechanisms are dealt with elsewhere in this volume, they are discussed in this chapter in an integrated and comprehensive manner. We provide an overview of the mechanisms of chemical toxicity by relating a series of events that begins with exposure, involves a multitude of interactions between the invading toxicant and the organism, and culminates in a toxic effect. This chapter focuses on mechanisms that have been identified definitively or tentatively in humans or animals.

As a result of the huge number of potential toxicants and the multitude of biological structures and processes that can be impaired, there are a tremendous number of possible toxic effects. Correspondingly, there are various pathways that may lead to toxicity (Fig. 3-1). The most direct pathway occurs when the chemical causes toxicity by its mere presence at critical sites in the body without interacting with a target molecule (path A). This pathway is followed, for example, when agents precipitate in renal tubules and block urine formation. With this type of toxicity, delivery (step 1) is the most important consideration.

An example of a more complex route (path B) to toxicity is that taken by the fugu fish poison, tetrodotoxin. After ingestion, this poison reaches the $Na^+$ channels of motoneurons (step 1). Interaction of tetrodotoxin with this target (step 2) results in blockade of $Na^+$ channels, inhibition of the activity of motor neurons (step 3), and ultimately skeletal muscle paralysis. No repair mechanisms can prevent the onset of such toxicity.

The most complex path to toxicity (path C) involves even more steps (Fig. 3-1). First, the toxicant is delivered to its target or targets (step 1), after which the ultimate toxicant interacts with endogenous target molecules (step 2), triggering perturbations in cell function and/or structure (step 3), which initiate repair mechanisms at the molecular, cellular, and/or tissue levels (step 4). When the perturbations induced by the toxicant exceed the repair capacity or when repair becomes malfunctional, toxicity occurs. Tissue necrosis, cancer, and fibrosis are examples of chemically induced toxicities whose development follow this four-step course.

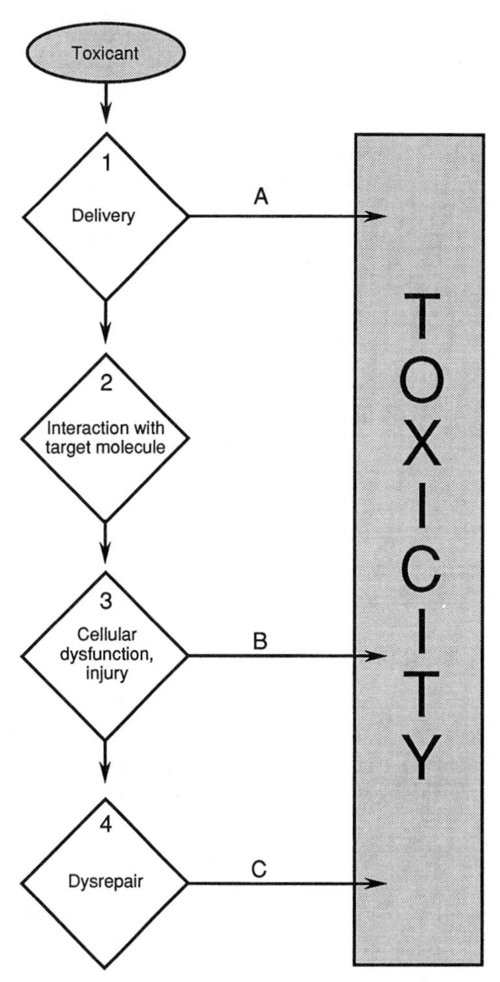


***Figure 3–1. Potential stages in the development of toxicity after chemical exposure.***

## DELIVERY: FROM THE SITE OF EXPOSURE TO THE TARGET

Theoretically, the intensity of a toxic effect depends primarily on the concentration and persistence of the ultimate toxicant at its site of action. The ultimate toxicant is the chemical species that reacts with the endogenous target molecule (e.g., receptor, enzyme, DNA, microfilamental protein, lipid), initiating structural and/or functional alterations that result in toxicity. Often the ultimate toxicant is the original chemical to which the organism is exposed (parent compound). In other cases, the ultimate toxicant is a metabolite of the parent compound or a reactive oxygen species generated during the biotransformation of the toxicant. Occasionally, the ultimate toxicant is an endogenous molecule (Table 3-1).

The concentration of the ultimate toxicant at the target molecule depends on the relative effectiveness of the processes that increase or decrease its concentration at the target site. The accumulation of the ultimate toxicant at its target is facilitated by its absorption, distribution to the site of action, reabsorption, and toxication (metabolic activation). Presystemic elimination, distribution away from the site of action, excretion, and detoxication oppose these processes and work against the accumulation of the ultimate toxicant at the target molecule (Fig. 3-2).

### Absorption versus Presystemic Elimination

**Absorption.** Absorption is the transfer of a chemical from the site of exposure, usually an external or internal body surface (e.g., skin, mucosa of the alimentary and respiratory tracts), into the systemic circulation. The vast majority of toxicants traverse epithelial barriers and reach the blood capillaries by diffusing through cells. The rate of absorption is related to the concentration of the chemical at the absorbing surface, which depends on the rate of exposure and the dissolution of the chemical. It is also related to the area of the exposed site, the characteristics of the epithelial layer through which absorption takes place (e.g., the thickness of the stratum corneum in the skin), the intensity of the subepithelial microcirculation, and the physicochemical properties of the toxicant. Lipid solubility is usually the most important physicochemical property influencing absorption. In general, lipid-soluble chemicals are absorbed more readily than are water-soluble substances.

**Presystemic Elimination.** During transfer from the site of exposure to the systemic circulation, toxicants may be eliminated. This is not unusual for chemicals absorbed from the gastrointestinal (GI) tract because they must first pass through

**Table 3–1**
**Types of Ultimate Toxicants and Their Sources**

| | | |
|---|---|---|
| Parent compounds as ultimate toxicants | | |
| Pb ions | | |
| Tetrodotoxin | | |
| TCDD | | |
| Methylisocyanate | | |
| HCN | | |
| CO | | |
| Metabolites as ultimate toxicants | | |
| Amygdalin | → | HCN |
| Arsenate | → | Arsenite |
| Fluoroacetate | → | Fluorocitrate |
| Ethylene glycol | → | Oxalic acid |
| Hexane | → | 2,5-Hexane dione |
| Acetaminophen | → | *N*-Acetyl-*p*-benzoquinoneimine |
| $CCl_4$ | → | $CCl_3OO^•$ |
| Benzo[*a*]pyrene (BP) | → | BP-7,8-diol-9,10-epoxide |
| Benzo[*a*]pyrene (BP) | → | BP-Radical cation |
| Reactive oxygen species as ultimate toxicants | | |
| Hydrogen peroxide | | |
| Diquat, doxorubicin, nitrofurantoin | → | Hydroxyl radical ($HO^•$) |
| Cr(V), Fe(II), Mn(II), Ni(II) | | |
| Endogenous compounds as ultimate toxicants | | |
| Sulfonamides → albumin-bound bilirubin | → | Bilirubin |
| $CCl_3OO^•$ → unsaturated fatty acids | → | Lipid peroxyl radicals |
| $CCl_3OO^•$ → unsaturated fatty acids | → | Lipid alkoxyl radicals |
| $CCl_3OO^•$ → unsaturated fatty acids | → | 4-Hydroxynonenal |
| $HO^•$ → proteins | → | Protein carbonyls |

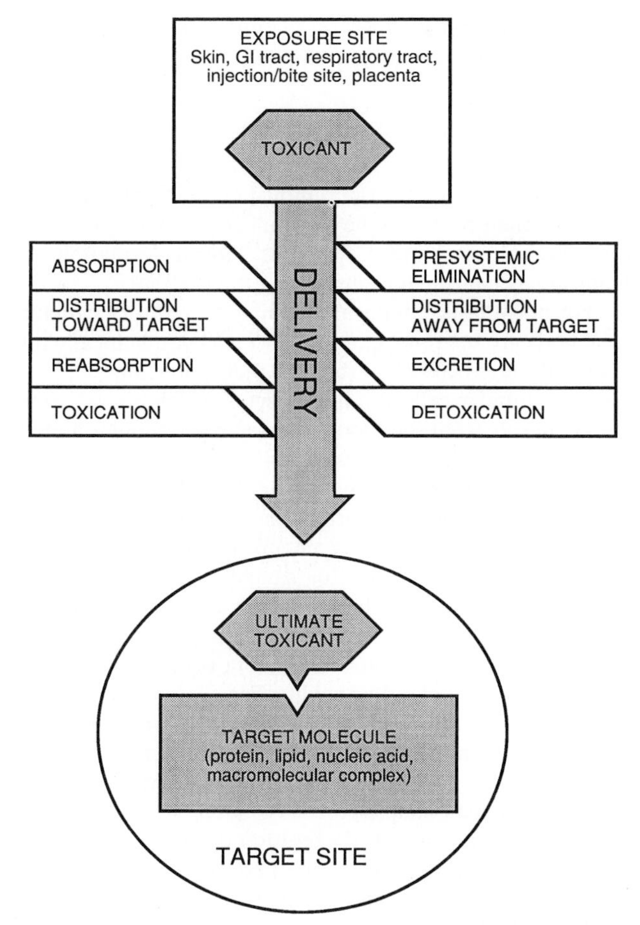


***Figure 3-2. The process of toxicant delivery is the first step in the development of toxicity.***

Delivery, that is, movement of the toxicant from the site of exposure to the site of its action in an active form, is promoted and opposed by the events indicated.

the GI mucosal cells, liver, and lung before being distributed to the rest of the body by the systemic circulation. The GI mucosa and the liver may eliminate a significant fraction of a toxicant during its passage through these tissues, decreasing its systemic availability. For example, ethanol is oxidized by alcohol dehydrogenase in the gastric mucosa (Lim et al., 1993), morphine is glucuronidated in the intestinal mucosa and liver, and the hepatic uptake of manganese and then its biliary excretion prevent a considerable amount of these chemicals from reaching the systemic blood. Thus, presystemic, or first-pass, elimination reduces the toxic effects of chemicals that reach their target sites by way of the systemic circulation. In contrast, presystemic elimination may contribute to injury of the digestive mucosa, the liver, and the lungs by chemicals such as ethanol, iron salts, $\alpha$-amanitin, and paraquat because it favors their delivery to those sites.

## Distribution To and Away from the Target

Toxicants exit the blood during the distribution phase, enter the extracellular space, and may penetrate into cells. Chemicals dissolved in plasma water may diffuse through the capillary endothelium via aqueous intercellular spaces and transcellular pores called fenestrae and/or across the cell membrane. Lipid-soluble compounds move readily into cells by diffusion. In contrast, highly ionized and hydrophilic xenobiotics (e.g., tubocurarine, aminoglycosides) are largely restricted to the extracellular space unless specialized membrane carrier systems are available to transport them.

During distribution, toxicants reach their site or sites of action, usually a macromolecule on either the surface or the interior of a particular type of cell. Chemicals also may be distributed to the site or sites of toxication, usually an intracellular enzyme, where the ultimate toxicant is formed. Some mechanisms facilitate, whereas others delay, the distribution of toxicants to their targets.

**Mechanisms Facilitating Distribution to a Target.** Distribution of toxicants to specific target sites may be enhanced by (1) the porosity of the capillary endothelium, (2) specialized membrane transport, and (3) reversible intracellular binding.

***Porosity of the Capillary Endothelium.*** Endothelial cells in the hepatic sinusoids and in the renal peritubular capillaries have large fenestrae (50 to 150 nm in diameter) that permit passage of even protein-bound xenobiotics. This favors the accumulation of chemicals in the liver and kidneys.

***Specialized Membrane Transport.*** A number of specialized membrane transport processes can contribute to the delivery of toxicants to the target. Included are voltage-gated $Ca^{2+}$ channels that permit the entry of cations such as lead or barium ions into excitable cells. Paraquat enteres into pneumocytes, $\alpha$-amanitin enters into hepatocytes (Kröncke et al., 1986), and an MPTP metabolite enters into extrapyramidal dopaminergic neurons by means of carrier-mediated uptake. Endocytosis of some toxicant-protein complexes, such as Cd-metallothionein or hydrocarbons bound to the male rat–specific $\alpha_{2u}$-globulin, by renal proximal tubular cells also can occur. In addition, lipoprotein receptor–mediated endocytosis leads to the accumulation of lipoprotein-bound toxicants. Membrane recycling can internalize cationic aminoglycosides associated with anionic phospholipids in the brush border membrane of renal tubular cells (Laurent et al., 1990). This process also may contribute to cellular uptake of heavy metal ions. Such uptake mechanisms facilitate the entry of toxicants into specific cells, rendering those cells targets. Thus, carrier-mediated uptake of paraquat by pneumocytes and internalization of aminoglycosides by renal proximal tubular cells expose those cells to toxic concentrations of those chemicals.

***Reversible Intracellular Binding.*** Binding to the pigment melanin, an intracellular polyanionic aromatic polymer, is a mechanism by which chemicals such as organic and inorganic cations and polycyclic aromatic hydrocarbons can accumulate in melanin-containing cells (Larsson, 1993). The release of melanin-bound toxicants is thought to contribute to the retinal toxicity associated with chlorpromazine and chloroquine, injury to substantia nigra neurons by MPTP and manganese, and the induction of melanoma by polycyclic aromatics.

**Mechanisms Opposing Distribution to a Target.** Distribution of toxicants to specific target sites may be hindered by several processes. These processes include (1) binding to plasma proteins, (2) specialized barriers, (3) distribution to storage sites such as adipose tissue, (4) association with intracellular binding proteins, and (5) export from cells.

***Binding to Plasma Proteins.*** As long as xenobiotics such as DDT and TCDD are bound to high-molecular-weight proteins or lipoproteins in plasma, they cannot leave the capillaries by diffusion. Even if they exit the bloodstream through fenestrae, they have difficulty permeating cell membranes. Dissociation from proteins is required for most xenobiotics to leave the blood and enter cells. Therefore, strong binding to plasma proteins delays and prolongs the effects and elimination of toxicants.

***Specialized Barriers.*** Brain capillaries have very low aqueous porosity because their endothelial cells lack fenestrae and are joined by extremely tight junctions. This blood-brain barrier prevents the access of hydrophilic chemicals to the brain except for those that can be actively transported. Water-soluble toxicants also have restricted access to reproductive cells, which are separated from capillaries by multiple layers of cells. The oocyte is surrounded by the granulosa cells, and the spermatogenic cells are surrounded by Sertoli's cells and other elements of the blood-testis barrier (Chap. 19). Transfer of hydrophilic toxicants across the placenta is also restricted. However, none of these barriers are effective against lipophilic substances.

***Distribution to Storage Sites.*** Some chemicals accumulate in tissues (i.e., storage sites) where they do not exert significant effects. For example, highly lipophilic substances such as chlorinated hydrocarbon insecticides concentrate in adipocytes, whereas lead is deposited in bone by substituting for $Ca^{2+}$ in hydroxyapatite. Such storage decreases the availability of these toxicants for their target sites and acts as a temporary protective mechanism. Lead is not readily mobilized from bone. However, insecticides may return to the circulation and be distributed to their target site, the nervous tissue, when there is a rapid lipid loss as a result of fasting. This is thought to contribute to the lethality to pesticide-exposed birds during migration or during the winter months, when food is restricted.

***Association with Intracelleular Binding Proteins.*** Binding to nontarget intracellular sites also reduces the concentration of toxicants at the target site, at least temporarily. Metallothionein, a cysteine-rich cytoplasmic protein, serves such a function in acute cadmium intoxication (Goering et al., 1995).

***Export from Cells.*** Intracellular toxicants may be transported back into the extracellular space. This occurs in brain capillary endothelial cells. These cells contain an ATP-dependent membrane transporter known as the multidrug-resistance (MDR) protein, or P-glycoprotein, which extrudes chemicals such as the neurotoxic pesticide ivermectin and contributes to the blood-brain barrier. Mice with a disrupted MDR gene have higher brain levels of and sensitivity to ivermectin (Schinkel et al., 1994). The oocyte is also equipped with the P-glycoprotein that provides protection against chemicals that are substrates for this efflux pump (Elbling et al., 1993).

## Excretion versus Reabsorption

**Excretion.** Excretion is the removal of xenobiotics from the blood and their return to the external environment. Excretion is a physical mechanism, whereas biotransformation is a chemical mechanism, for eliminating the toxicant.

For nonvolatile chemicals, the major excretory structures in the body are the renal glomeruli, which hydrostatically filter small molecules (<60 kDa) through their pores, and the proximal renal tubular cells and hepatocytes, which actively transport chemicals from the blood into the renal tubules and bile canaliculi, respectively. These cells are readily exposed to bloodborne chemicals through the large endothelial fenestrae and have membrane transporters that mediate the uptake and lumenal extrusion of certain chemicals. Renal transporters have a preferential affinity for smaller (<300 daltons), and hepatic transporters for larger (>400 daltons), amphiphilic molecules. A less common "excretory" mechanism consists of diffusion and partition into the excreta on the basis of their lipid content (see below) or acidity. For example, morphine is transferred into milk and amphetamine is transferred into gastric juice by nonionic diffusion. This is facilitated by pH trapping of those organic bases in those fluids, which are acidic relative to plasma (Chap. 5).

The route and speed of excretion depend largely on the physicochemical properties of the toxicant. The major excretory organs—the kidney and the liver—can efficiently remove only highly hydrophilic, usually ionized chemicals such as organic acids and bases. The reasons for this are as follows: (1) In the renal glomeruli, only compounds dissolved in the plasma water can be filtered, (2) transporters in hepatocytes and renal proximal tubular cells are specialized for the secretion of highly hydrophilic organic acids and bases, (3) only hydrophilic chemicals are freely soluble in the aqueous urine and bile, and (4) lipid-soluble compounds are readily reabsorbed by transcellular diffusion.

There are no efficient elimination mechanisms for nonvolatile, highly lipophilic chemicals such as polyhalogenated biphenyls and chlorinated hydrocarbon insecticides. If they are resistant to biotransformation, such chemicals are eliminated very slowly and tend to accumulate in the body upon repeated exposure. Three rather inefficient processes are available for the elimination of such chemicals: (1) excretion by the mammary gland after the chemical is dissolved in the milk lipids, (2) excretion in bile in association with biliary micelles and/or phospholipid vesicles, and (3) intestinal excretion, an incompletely understood transport from the blood into the intestinal lumen. Volatile, nonreactive toxicants such as gases and volatile liquids diffuse from pulmonary capillaries into the alveoli and are exhaled.

**Reabsorption.** Toxicants delivered into the renal tubules may diffuse back across the tubular cells into the peritubular capillaries. This process is facilitated by tubular fluid reabsorption, which increases the intratubular concentration as well as the residence time of the chemical by slowing urine flow. Reabsorption by diffusion is dependent on the lipid solubility of the chemical. For organic acids and bases, diffusion is inversely related to the extent of ionization, because the nonionized molecule is more lipid-soluble. The ionization of weak organic acids such as salicylic acid and phenobarbital and bases such as amphetamine, procainamide, and quinidine is strongly pH-dependent in the physiological range. Therefore, their reabsorption is influenced significantly by the pH of the tubular fluid. Acidification of urine favors the excretion of weak organic bases, while alkalinization favors the elimination of weak organic acids. In addition, some toxic metal oxyanions, such as chromate and molybdate, are reabsorbed in the kidney by the carrier-mediated sulfate transport system.

Toxicants delivered to the GI tract by biliary, gastric, and intestinal excretion and secretion by salivary glands and the exocrine pancreas may be reabsorbed by diffusion across the intestinal mucosa. Because compounds secreted into bile are usually organic acids, their reabsorption is possible only if they are sufficiently lipophilic or are converted to more lipid-soluble forms in the intestinal lumen. For example, glucuronides of toxicants such as diethylstilbestrol and glucuronides of the hydroxylated metabolites of polycyclic aromatic hydrocarbons, chlordecone, and halogenated biphenyls are hydrolyzed by $\beta$-glucuronidase in intestinal microorganisms, and the released aglycones are reabsorbed (Gregus and Klaassen, 1986). Glutathione conjugates of hexachlorobutadiene and trichloroethylene are hydrolyzed by intestinal and pancreatic peptidases, yielding the cysteine conjugates, which are reabsorbed and serve as precursors of additional metabolites with nephrotoxic properties (Dekant et al., 1989).

## Toxication versus Detoxication

**Toxication.** A number of xenobiotics (e.g., strong acids and bases, nicotine, aminoglycosides, ethylene oxide, methylisocyanate, heavy metal ions, HCN, CO) are directly toxic, whereas the toxicity of others is due largely to metabolites. Biotransformation to harmful products is called toxication or activation. With some xenobiotics, toxication confers physicochemical properties that adversely alter the microenvironment of biological processes or structures. For example, oxalic acid formed from ethylene glycol may cause acidosis and hypocalcemia as well as obstruction of renal tubules by precipitation as calcium oxalate. Occasionally, chemicals acquire structural features and reactivity by biotransformation that allows for a more efficient interaction with receptors or enzymes. For example the organophosphate insecticide parathion is biotransformed to an active cholinesterase inhibitor, paraoxon, and the rodenticide fluoroacetate is converted in the citric acid cycle to fluorocitrate, a false substrate that inhibits aconitase. Most often, however, toxication of xenobiotics renders them and occasionally other molecules in the body, such as oxygen, indiscriminately reactive toward endogenous compounds with susceptible functional groups. This increased reactivity may be due to conversion into (1) electrophiles, (2) free radicals, (3) nucleophiles, or (4) redox-active reactants.

***Formation of Electrophiles.*** Electrophiles are molecules containing an electron-deficient atom with a partial or full positive charge that allows it to react by sharing electron pairs with electron-rich atoms in nucleophiles. The formation of electrophiles is involved in the toxication of numerous chemicals (Table 3-2) (Chap. 6). Such reactants often are produced when xenobiotics are oxidized by cytochrome P-450 or other enzymes to ketones, epoxides and arene oxides, $\alpha,\beta$-unsaturated ketones and aldehydes, quinones or quinoneimines, and acyl halides. Thionoacyl halides and thioketenes are formed from halogenated alkenes in successive reactions catalyzed by glutathione *S*-transferase, $\gamma$-glutamyl transferase, dipeptidase, and cysteine conjugate $\beta$-lyase (Monks and Lau, 1994).

Cationic electrophiles are produced as a result of heterolytic bond cleavage. For example, methyl-substituted aromatics such as 7,12-dimethylbenzanthracene and aromatic amines (amides) such as 2-acetylaminofluorene are hydroxylated to form benzylic alcohols and *N*-hydroxy arylamines (amides), respectively (Miller and Surh, 1994). These substances are esterified, typically by sulfotransferases. Heterolytic cleavage of the C-O or N-O bonds of these esters results in a hydrosulfate anion and the concomitant formation of a benzylic carbonium ion or arylnitrenium ion, respectively. The oxidation of metallic mercury to $Hg^{2+}$ and the reduction of $CrO_4^{2-}$ to $Cr^{3+}$ as well as that of $AsO_4^{3-}$ to $AsO_3^{2-}/As^{3+}$ are examples of the formation of electrophilic toxicants from inorganic chemicals.

***Formation of Free Radicals.*** A free radical is a molecule or molecular fragment that contains one or more unpaired electrons in its outer orbital. Radicals are formed by accepting or losing an electron or by homolytic fission of a covalent bond.

Xenobiotics such as paraquat, doxorubicin, and nitrofurantoin can accept an electron from reductases to give rise to radicals (Fig. 3-3). These radicals typically transfer the extra electron to molecular oxygen, forming a superoxide anion radical ($O_2^{\bar{\bullet}}$) and regenerating the parent xenobiotic, which is ready to gain a new electron (Kappus, 1986). Through this "redox cycling," one electron acceptor xenobiotic molecule can generate many $O_2^{\bar{\bullet}}$ molecules. Alternatively, the xenobiotic radical with an excess electron can reduce and consequently release iron from ferritin, producing free Fe(II) ions, which are toxic (see below).

In contrast to these chemicals, nucleophilic xenobiotics such as phenols, hydroquinones, aminophenols, amines, hydrazines, phenothiazines, and thiols are prone to lose an electron in a reaction catalysed by peroxidases and form free radicals (Aust et al., 1993). Some of these chemicals, such as catechols and hydroquinones, may undergo two sequential one-electron oxidations, producing first semiquinone radicals and then quinones. Quinones are not only reactive electrophiles (Table 3-2) but also electron acceptors with the capacity to initiate redox cycling or oxidation of thiols and NAD(P)H. Polycyclic aromatic hydrocarbons with sufficiently low ionization potential such as benzo[*a*]pyrene and 7,12-dimethylbenzanthracene can be converted by one-electron oxidation by peroxidases or cytochrome P-450 to radical cations, which may be the ultimate toxicants for these carcinogens (Cavalieri and Rogan, 1992). Like peroxidases, oxyhemoglobin (Hb-FeII-$O_2$) can catalyze the oxidation of aminophenols to semiquinone radicals and quinoneimines. This is another example of toxication, because these products in turn oxidize ferrohemoglobin (Hb-FeII) to methemoglobin (Hb-FeIII), which cannot carry oxygen.

Free radicals also are formed by homolytic bond fission, which can be induced by electron transfer to the molecule (reductive fission). This mechanism is involved in the conver-

**Table 3–2**
**Toxication by Formation of Electrophilic Metabolites**

| ELECTROPHILIC METABOLITE | PARENT TOXICANT | ENZYMES CATALYZING TOXICATION | TOXIC EFFECT |
|---|---|---|---|
| **Nonionic electrophiles** | | | |
| Aldehydes, ketones | | | |
| Acetaldehyde | Ethanol | ADH | Hepatic fibrosis(?) |
| Zomepirac glucuronide (aldose form) | Zomepirac | GT→isomerization | Immune reaction(?) |
| 2,5-Hexane dione | Hexane | P450 | Axonopathy |
| *α,β*-Unsaturated aldehydes, ketones | | | |
| Acrolein | Allyl alcohol | ADH | Hepatic necrosis |
| Acrolein | Allyl amine | MAO | Vascular injury |
| Muconic aldehyde | Benzene | Multiple | Bone marrow injury |
| 4-Hydroxynonenal | Fatty acids | Lipid peroxidation | Cellular injury(?) |
| Quinones, quinoneimines | | | |
| DES-4,4′-quinone | DES | Peroxidases | Carcinogenesis(?) |
| *N*-Acetyl-*p*-benzoquinoneimine | Acetaminophen | P450, peroxidases | Hepatic necrosis |
| Epoxides, arene oxides | | | |
| Aflatoxin $B_1$ 8,9-epoxide | Aflatoxin $B_1$ | P450 | Carcinogenesis |
| 2-Chlorooxirane | Vinyl chloride | P450 | Carcinogenesis |
| Bromobenzene 3,4-oxide | Bromobenzene | P450 | Hepatic necrosis |
| Benzo[*a*]pyrene 7,8-diol 9,10-oxide | Benzo[*a*]pyrene | P450 | Carcinogenesis |
| Sulfoxides | | | |
| Thioacetamide *S*-oxide | Thioacetamide | FMO | Hepatic necrosis |
| Acyl halides | | | |
| Phosgene | Chloroform | P450 | Hepatic necrosis |
| Trifluoroacetyl chloride | Halothane | P450 | Immune reaction |
| Thionoacyl halides | | | |
| 2,3,4,4-Tetrachlorothiobut-3-enoic acid chloride | HCBD | GST→GGT →DP→CCL | Renal tubular necrosis |
| Thioketenes | | | |
| Chloro-1,2,2-trichlorovinyl-thioketene | HCBD | GST→GGT →DP→CC*β*L | Renal tubular necrosis |
| **Cationic Electrophiles** | | | |
| Carbonium ions | | | |
| Benzylic carbocation | 7,12-DMBA | P450→ST | Carcinogenesis |
| Carbonium cation | DENA | P450 →s.r. | |
| Nitrenium ions | | | |
| Arylnitrenium ion | AAF, DMAB<br>HCAAPP | P450→ST<br>P450→ST | Carcinogenesis |
| Sulfonium ions | | | |
| Episulfonium ion | Vicinal dihaloalkanes (e.g., DBE) | GST | Renal tubular necrosis |
| Metal ions | | | |
| Mercury(II) ion | Elemental Hg | Catalase | Brain injury |
| Diaquo-diamino platinate(II) | Cisplatinum | s.r. | Renal tubular necrosis |

AAF = 2-acetylaminofluorene, ADH = alcohol dehydrogenase, CC*β*L = cysteine conjugate *β*-lyase; DENA = diethylnitrosamine; DMAB = *N,N*-dimethyl-4-aminoazobenzene; 7,12-DMBA = 7,12-dimethylbenzanthracene; DBE = 1,2-dibromoethane; DES = diethylstilbestrol; DP = dipeptidase; FMO = flavin-containing monooxygenase; GT = UDP-glucuronosyltransferase; GGT = gamma-glutamyltransferase; GST = glutathione *S*-transferase; HCAAPP = heterocyclic arylamine pyrolysis products; HCBD = hexachlorobutadiene; MAO = monoamine oxidase; P450 = cytochrome P-450; ST = sulfotransferase; s.r. = spontaneous rearrangement.

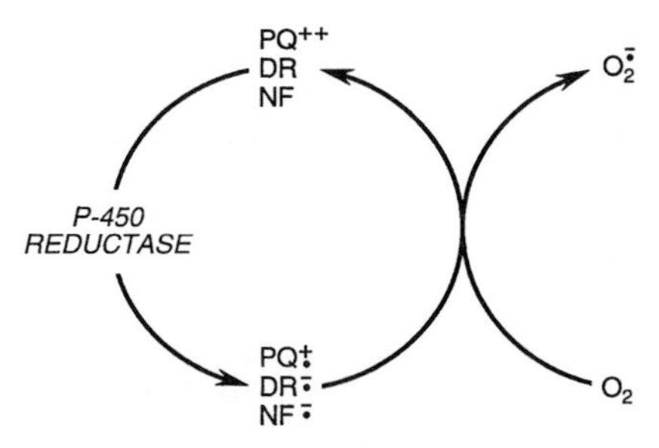


*Figure 3–3. Production of superoxide anion radical ($O_2^{\bar{\bullet}}$) by paraquat ($PQ^{++}$), doxorubicin (DR), and nitrofurantoin (NF).*

Note, that formation of ($O_2^{\bar{\bullet}}$) is not the final step in the toxication of these xenobiotics, because $O_2^{\bar{\bullet}}$ can yield the much more reactive hydroxyl radical, as depicted in Fig. 3-4.

sion of $CCl_4$ to the trichloromethyl free radical ($Cl_3C^{\bullet}$) by an electron transfer from cytochrome P-450 or the mitochondrial electron transport chain (reductive dehalogenation) (Recknagel et al., 1989). The $Cl_3C^{\bullet}$ reacts with $O_2$ to form the even more reactive trichloromethylperoxy radical ($Cl_3COO^{\bullet}$). The hydroxyl radical ($HO^{\bullet}$), a free radical of paramount toxicological significance, also is generated by homolytic (reductive) fission from hydrogen peroxide (HOOH) (Southorn and Powis, 1988). The Fenton reaction (Fig. 3-4), which is catalyzed by transition metal ions, typically Fe(II) or, Cu(I), Cr(V), Ni(II), or Mn(II), is a major toxication mechanism for HOOH and its precursor $O_2^{\bar{\bullet}}$ as well as for transition metals. Moreover, the toxicity of chemicals, such as nitrilotriacetic acid and bleomycin, that chelate transition metal ions is also based on Fenton chemistry because chelation increases the catalytic efficiency of some transition metal ions. The pulmonary toxicity of inhaled mineral particles such as asbestos and silica is caused, at least in part, by the formation of $HO^{\bullet}$ triggered by Fe ions on the particle surface (Guilianelli et al., 1993). Hydrogen peroxide is a direct or indirect by-product of several enzymatic reactions, including monoamine oxidase, xanthine oxidase, and acyl-coenzyme A oxidase. It is produced in large

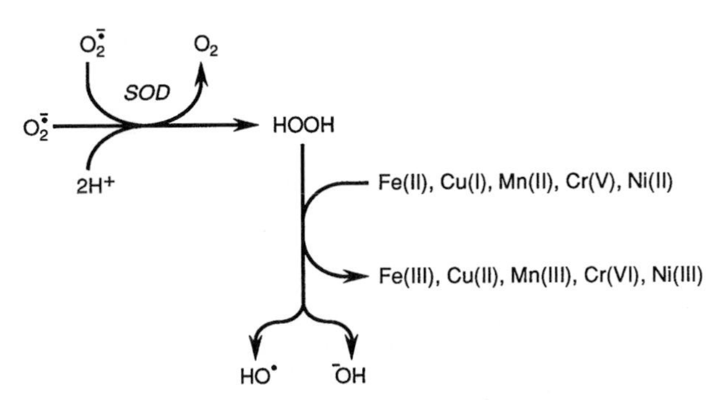


*Figure 3–4. Formation of hydroxyl radical ($HO^{\bullet}$), from superoxide anion radical ($O_2^{\bar{\bullet}}$) and hydrogen peroxide (HOOH).*

Conversion of ($O_2^{\bar{\bullet}}$) to HOOH is spontaneous or is catalyzed by superoxide dismutase (SOD). Homolytic cleavage of HOOH to hydroxyl radical and hydroxyl ion is called the Fenton reaction and is catalyzed by the transition metal ions shown. Hydroxyl radical formation is the ultimate toxication for xenobiotics that form $O_2^{\bar{\bullet}}$ (see Fig. 3-3) or HOOH, the transition metal ions listed, and some chemicals that form complexes with these transition metal ions.

quantities by spontaneous or superoxide dismutase-catalyzed dismutation of $O_2^{\bar{\bullet}}$ when this oxygen species is generated by redox cycling toxicants or by NAD(P)H oxidase in activated macrophages and granulocytes during a "respiratory burst."

***Formation of Nucleophiles.*** The formation of nucleophiles is a relatively uncommon mechanism for activating toxicants. Examples include the formation of cyanide from amygdalin, which is catalyzed by bacterial $\beta$-glucosidase in the gut; from acrylonitrile after epoxidation and subsequent glutathione conjugation; and from sodium nitroprusside by thiol-induced decomposition. Carbon monoxide is a toxic metabolite of dihalomethanes that undergo oxidative dehalogenation. Some nucleophilic metabolites formed in the liver by hydroxylation, such as dapsone hydroxylamine and 5-hydroxy primaquine, can produce methemoglobin by cooxidation (Fletcher et al., 1988).

***Formation of Redox-Active Reactants.*** There are specific mechanisms for the creation of redox-active reactants other than those already discussed. Examples include the formation of the methemoglobin-producing nitrite from nitrate by bacterial reduction in the intestine or from esters of nitrous or nitric acids in reaction with glutathione. Reductants such as ascorbic acid and reductases such as NADPH-dependent flavoenzymes reduce Cr(VI) to Cr(V) (Shi and Dalal, 1990). Cr(V) in turn catalyses $HO^{\bullet}$ formation (Fig. 3-4).

In summary, the most reactive metabolites are electron-deficient molecules and molecular fragments such as electrophiles and neutral or cationic free radicals. Although some nucleophiles are reactive (e.g., HCN, CO), many are activated by conversion to electrophiles. Similarly, free radicals with an extra electron cause damage by giving rise to the neutral $HO^{\bullet}$ radical after the formation and subsequent homolytic cleavage of HOOH.

**Detoxication.** Biotransformations which eliminate the ultimate toxicant or prevent its formation are called detoxications. In some cases, detoxication may compete with toxication for a chemical. Detoxication can take several pathways, depending on the chemical nature of the toxic substance.

***Detoxication of Toxicants with No Functional Groups.*** In general, chemicals without functional groups, such as benzene and toluene, are detoxicated in two phases. Initially, a functional group such as hydroxyl or carboxyl is introduced into the molecule, most often by cytochrome P-450 enzymes. Subsequently, an endogenous acid such as glucuronic acid, sulfuric acid, or an amino acid is added to the functional group by a transferase. With some exceptions, the final products are inactive, highly hydrophilic organic acids that are readily excreted.

***Detoxication of Nucleophiles.*** Nucleophiles generally are detoxicated by conjugation at the nucleophilic functional group. Hydroxylated compounds are conjugated by sulfation or glucuronidation, whereas thiols are glucuronidated and amines and hydrazines are acetylated. These reactions prevent peroxidase-catalyzed conversion of the nucleophiles to free radicals and biotransformation of phenols, aminophenols, catechols, and hydroquinones to electrophilic quinones and quinoneimines. An alternative mechanism for the elimination

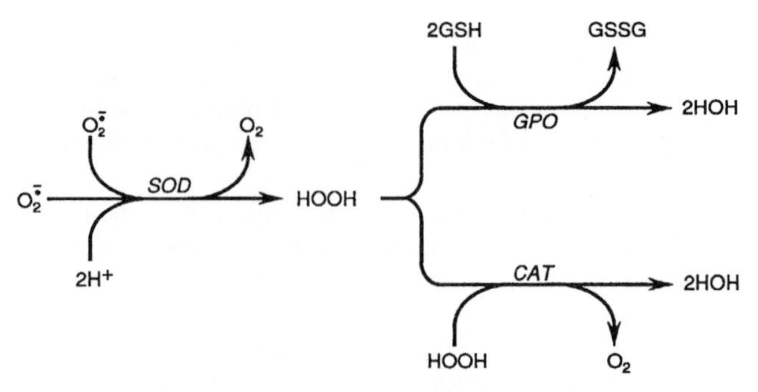


***Figure 3–5. Detoxication of superoxide anion radical ($O_2^{\bar{\bullet}}$) by superoxide dismutase (SOD), glutathione peroxidase (GPO), and catalase (CAT).***

GSH = glutathione; GSSG = glutathione disulfide.

of thiols, amines, and hydrazines is oxidation by flavin-containing monooxygenases (Jakoby and Ziegler, 1990). Some alcohols, such as ethanol, are detoxicated by oxidation to carboxylic acids by alcohol and aldehyde dehydrogenases. A specific detoxication mechanism is the biotransformation of cyanide to thiocyanate by rhodanese.

***Detoxication of Electrophiles.*** A general mechanism for the detoxication of electrophilic toxicants is conjugation with the thiol nucleophile glutathione (Ketterer, 1988). This reaction may occur spontaneously or can be facilitated by glutathione *S*-transferases. Metal ions such as $Ag^+$, $Cd^{2+}$, $Hg^{2+}$, and $CH_3Hg^+$ ions readily react with and are detoxicated by glutathione. Specific mechanisms for the detoxication of electrophilic substances include epoxide hydrolase–catalyzed biotransformation of epoxides and arene oxides to diols and dihydrodiols, respectively. Others are two-electron reduction of hydroquinones by DT-diaphorase, reduction of $\alpha,\beta$-unsaturated aldehydes to alcohols by alcohol dehydrogenase or oxidation to acids by aldehyde dehydrogenase, and complex formation of thiol-reactive metal ions by metallothionein and the redox-active ferrous iron by ferritin.

***Detoxication of Free Radicals.*** The ultimate toxicant produced by reductase-catalyzed redox cycling of xenobiotics is $HO^\bullet$ (Fig. 3-4). No enzyme eliminates $HO^\bullet$. While some relatively stable radicals, such as peroxyl radicals, can readily abstract a hydrogen atom from glutathione, $\alpha$-tocopherol (vitamin E), or ascorbic acid (vitamin C), thus becoming nonradicals, these antioxidants are generally ineffective in detoxifying $HO^\bullet$ (Sies, 1993). This is due to its extremely short half-life ($10^{-9}$ s), which provides little time for the $HO^\bullet$ to reach and react with antioxidants. Therefore, the only effective protection against $HO^\bullet$ is to prevent its formation. This can be done by coupling the conversion of $O_2^{\bar{\bullet}}$ to HOOH and the conversion of HOOH to water (Fig. 3-5). The first of these reactions is catalyzed by superoxide dismutases (SODs), high-capacity enzymes located in both the cytosol (Cu,Zn-SOD) and the mitochondria (Mn-SOD). The second reaction may be catalyzed by the selenoenzyme glutathione peroxidase in the cytosol or by catalase in the peroxisomes (Cotgreave et al., 1988).

Peroxidase-generated free radicals are eliminated by electron transfer from glutathione. This results in the oxidation of glutathione, which is reversed by NADPH-dependent glutathione reductase (Fig. 3-6). Thus, glutathione plays an important role in the detoxication of both electrophiles and free radicals.

***Detoxication of Protein Toxins.*** Presumably, extra- and intracellular proteases are involved in the inactivation of toxic polypeptides. Several toxins found in venoms, such as $\alpha$- and $\beta$-bungarotoxin, erabutoxin, and phospholipase, contain intramolecular disulfide bonds that are required for their activity. These proteins are inactivated by thioredoxin, an endogenous dithiol protein that reduces the essential disulfide bond (Lozano et al., 1994).

***When Detoxication Fails.*** Detoxication may be insufficient for several reasons:

1. Toxicants may overwhelm detoxification processes, leading to exhaustion of the detoxication enzymes, consumption of their cosubstrates, or depletion of cellular antioxidants such as glutathione, ascorbic acid, and $\alpha$-tocopherol. This results in the accumulation of the ultimate toxicant.
2. Some conjugation reactions can be reversed. For example, 2-naphthylamine, a bladder carcinogen, is *N*-hydroxylated and glucuronidated in liver, with the glucuronide excreted

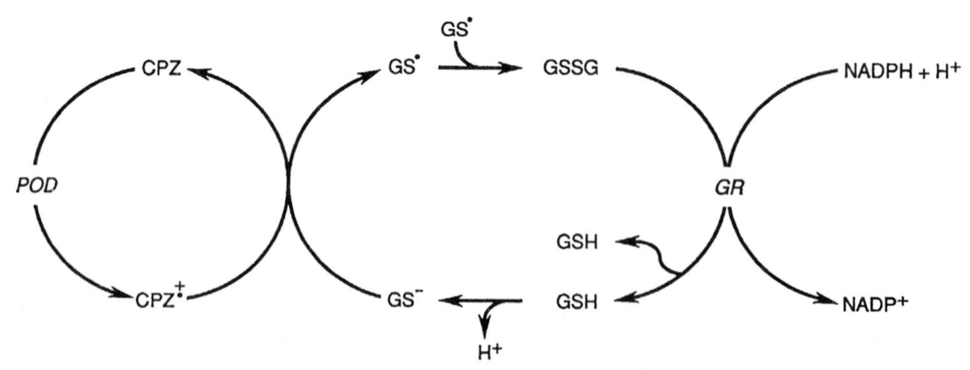


***Figure 3–6. Detoxication of peroxidase (POD)-generated free radicals such as chlorpromazine free radical (CPZ$^{+\bullet}$) by glutathione (GSH).***

The by-products are glutathione thiyl radical (GS) and glutathione disulfide (GSSG), from which GSH is regenerated by glutathione reductase (GR).

into urine. While in the bladder, the glucuronide is hydrolyzed, and the released arylhydroxylamine is converted by protonation and dehydration to the reactive electrophilic arylnitrenium ion (Bock and Lilienblum, 1994). Isocyanates and isothiocyanates form labile glutathione conjugates from which they can be released. Thus, methylisocyanate readily forms a glutathione conjugate in the lung after inhalation. From there, the conjugate is distributed to other tissues, where the reactive electrophilic parent compound may be regenerated (Baillie and Kassahun, 1994). Such conjugates are considered transport forms of toxicants.

3. Sometimes detoxication generates potentially harmful byproducts such as the glutathione thiyl radical and glutathione disulfide, which are produced during the detoxication of free radicals (Fig. 3-6). Glutathione disulfide can form mixed disulfides with protein thiols, whereas the thiyl radical ($GS^{\bullet}$), after reacting with thiolate ($GS^{-}$), forms a glutathione disulfide radical anion ($GSSG^{\overline{\bullet}}$) which can reduce $O_2$ to $O_2^{\overline{\bullet}}$.

## Toxicity Resulting from Delivery

Some xenobiotics do not or do not only interact with a specific endogenous target molecule to induce toxicity but instead alter the biological microenvironment (see path A in Fig. 3-1). Included here are (1) agents that alter ion concentrations in the aqueous biophase, such as acids and substances biotransformed to acids, such as methanol and ethylene glycol, as well as phenolic uncouplers such as 2,4-dinitrophenol and pentachlorophenol, which dissociate their phenolic protons in the mitochondrial matrix, thus dissipating the proton gradient that drives ATP synthesis, (2) solvents and detergents that physiochemically alter the lipid phase of cell membranes and destroy transmembrane solute gradients that are essential to cell functions, and (3) other xenobiotics that cause harm merely by occupying a site or space. For example, some chemicals (e.g., ethylene glycol) form water-insoluble precipitates in the renal tubules. By occupying bilirubin binding sites on albumin, compounds such as the sulfonamides induce bilirubin toxicity (kernicterus) in neonates. Carbon dioxide displaces oxygen in the pulmonary alveolar space and causes asphyxiation.

# REACTION OF THE ULTIMATE TOXICANT WITH THE TARGET MOLECULE

Toxicity is typically mediated by a reaction of the ultimate toxicant with a target molecule. Subsequently, a series of secondary biochemical events occur, leading to dysfunction or injury that is manifested at various levels of biological organization, such as at the target molecule itself, cell organelles, cells, tissues and organs, and even the whole organism. Because interactions of the ultimate toxicant with the target molecule trigger the toxic effect, consideration is given to (1) the types of reactions between ultimate toxicants and target molecules, (2) the attributes of target molecules, and (3) the effects of toxicants on the target molecules (Fig. 3-7).

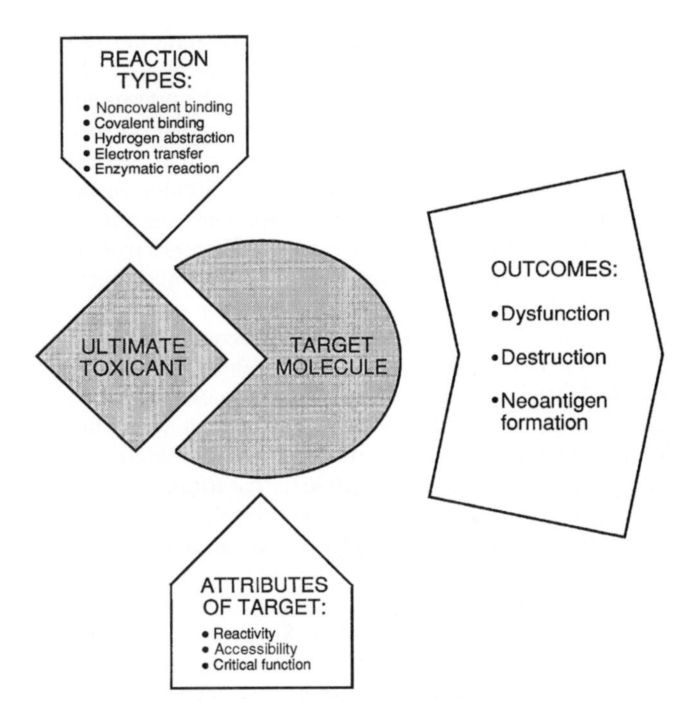


*Figure 3-7. Reaction of the ultimate toxicant with the target molecule: the second step in the development of toxicity.*

## Types of Reactions

The ultimate toxicant may bind to the target molecule noncovalently or covalently and may alter it by hydrogen abstraction, electron transfer, or enzymatically.

**Noncovalent Binding.** This type of binding can be due to apolar interactions (the formation of hydrogen and ionic bonds) and is typically involved in the interaction of toxicants with membrane receptors, intracellular receptors, ion channels, and some enzymes. For example, such interactions are responsible for the binding of strychnine to the glycine receptor on motor neurons in the spinal cord, TCDD to the aryl hydrocarbon receptor, saxitoxin to sodium channels, phorbol esters to protein kinase C, and warfarin to vitamin K 2,3-epoxide reductase. Such forces also are responsible for the intercalation of chemicals such as acridine yellow and doxorubicin into the double helix of DNA. These chemicals are toxic because the steric arrangement of their atoms allows them to combine with complementary sites on the endogenous molecule more or less as a key fits into a lock. Noncovalent binding usually is reversible because of the comparatively low bonding energy.

**Covalent Binding.** Being practically irreversible, covalent binding is of great toxicological importance because it permanently alters endogenous molecules (Boelsterli, 1993). Covalent adduct formation is common with electrophilic toxicants such as nonionic and cationic electrophiles and radical cations. These toxicants react with nucleophilic atoms that are abundant in biological macromolecules, such as proteins and nucleic acids. Electrophilic atoms exhibit some selectivity toward nucleophilic atoms, depending on their charge-to-radius ratio. In general, soft electrophiles prefer to react with soft nucleophiles (low charge-to-radius ratio in both), whereas hard electrophiles react more readily with hard nucleophiles (high charge-to-radius ratio in both). Examples are presented in Table 3-3. Metal ions such as silver and mercury also are classified as soft electrophiles which prefer to react with soft nucleophiles and hard electrophiles, such as lithium, calcium, and barium, which react preferentially with hard nucleophiles. Metals falling between these two extremes, such as chromium, zinc, and lead, exhibit universal reactivity with nucleophiles. The reactivity of an electrophile determines which endogenous nucleophiles can react with it and become a target.

Neutral free radicals such as $HO^{\bullet}$ and $CCl_3^{\bullet}$ also can bind covalently to biomolecules. The addition of $CCl_3^{\bullet}$ to double-bonded carbons in lipids or to lipid radicals yields lipids containing chloromethylated fatty acids. The addition of hydroxyl radicals to DNA bases results in the formation of numerous products, including 8-hydroxypurines, 5-hydroxymethylpyrimidines, and thymine and cytosine glycols (Breimer, 1990).

Nucleophilic toxicants are in principle reactive toward electrophilic endogenous compounds. Such reactions occur infrequently because electrophiles are rare among biomolecules. Examples include the covalent reaction of amines and hydrazides with the aldehyde pyridoxal, a cosubstrate for decarboxylases. Carbon monoxide, cyanide, hydrogen sulfide, and azide form coordinate covalent bonds with iron in various hemeproteins. Other nucleophiles react with hemoglobin in an electron-transfer reaction (see below).

**Hydrogen Abstraction.** Neutral free radicals can readily abstract H atoms from endogenous compounds, converting those compounds into radicals. Abstraction of hydrogen from thiols (R-SH) creates thiyl radicals ($R\text{-}S^{\bullet}$), which are precursors of other thiol oxidation products, such as sulfenic acids (R-SOH) and disulfides (R-S-S-R). Hydroxyl radicals can remove hydrogen from $CH_2$ groups of free amino acids or from amino acid residues in proteins and convert them to carbonyls. These carbonyls react with amines, forming cross-links with DNA or other proteins. Hydrogen abstraction from deoxyribose in DNA yields the C-4′-radical, which undergoes hydrolysis, yielding strand breaks. Abstraction of hydrogens from fatty acids produces lipid radicals and initiates lipid peroxidation.

**Electron Transfer.** Chemicals can oxidize Fe(II) in hemoglobin to Fe(III), producing methemoglobinemia. Nitrite can oxidize hemoglobin, whereas *N*-hydroxy arylamines (such as dapsone hydroxylamine), phenolic compounds (such as 5-hydroxy primaquine), and hydrazines (such as phenylhydrazine) are cooxidized with oxyhemoglobin, forming methemoglobin and hydrogen peroxide (Coleman and Jacobus, 1993).

**Enzymatic Reactions.** A few toxins act enzymatically on specific target proteins. For example, ricin induces hydrolytic fragmentation of ribosomes, blocking protein synthesis. Several bacterial toxins catalyze the transfer of ADP-ribose from NAD to specific proteins. For example, diphtheria toxin blocks the function of elongation factor 2 in protein synthesis and cholera toxin activates a G protein through such a mechanism. Snake venoms contain hydrolytic enzymes that destroy biomolecules.

In summary, most ultimate toxicants act on endogenous molecules on the basis of their chemical reactivity. Those with more than one type of reactivity may react by different mechanisms with various target molecules. For example, quinones may act as electrophiles and form covalent adducts but also may act as electron acceptors and initiate thiol oxidation or free radical reactions that lead to lipid peroxidation. The lead ion acts as a soft electrophile when it forms coordinate covalent bonds with critical thiol groups in $\delta$-aminolevulinic acid dehydratase, its major target enzyme in heme synthesis (Goering, 1993). However, it behaves like a hard electrophile or an ion when it binds to protein kinase C or blocks calcium channels, substituting for the natural ligand $Ca^{2+}$ at those target sites.

## Attributes of Target Molecules

Practically all endogenous compounds are potential targets for toxicants. The identification and characterization of the target molecules involved in toxicity constitute a major research priority, but a comprehensive inventory of potential target molecules is impossible. Nevertheless, the most prevalent and toxicologically relevant targets are macromolecules such as nucleic acids, especially DNA and proteins. Among the small molecules, membrane lipids are frequently involved, whereas

**Table 3-3**
**Examples of Soft and Hard Electrophiles and Nucleophiles**

| ELECTROPHILES | | NUCLEOPHILES |
|---|---|---|
| Carbon in polarized double bonds (e.g., quinones, $\alpha,\beta$-unsaturated ketones) | Soft ↑ | Sulfur in thiols (e.g., cysteinyl residues in proteins and glutathione) |
| Carbon in epoxides, strained-ring lactones, aryl halides | | Sulfur in methionine |
| Aryl carbonium ions | | Nitrogen in primary and secondary amino groups of proteins |
| Benzylic carbonium ions, nitrenium ions | | Nitrogen in amino groups in purine bases in nucleic acids |
| Alkyl carbonium ions | ↓ | Oxygen of purines and pyrimidines in nucleic acids |
| | Hard | Phosphate oxygen in nucleic acids |

SOURCE: Based on Coles (1984).

high-energy compounds such as ATP and cofactors such as coenzyme A and pyridoxal rarely are involved.

To be a target, an endogenous molecule must possess the appropriate reactivity and/or steric configuration to allow the ultimate toxicant to enter into covalent or noncovalent reactions. For these reactions to occur, the endogenous molecule must be accessible to a sufficiently high concentration of the ultimate toxicant. Thus, endogenous molecules that are in the vicinity of reactive chemicals or are adjacent to sites where they are formed are frequently targets. The first target for reactive metabolites is often the enzyme responsible for their production or the adjacent intracellular structures. For example, thyroperoxidase, the enzyme responsible for thyroid hormone synthesis, forms reactive free radical metabolites from some nucleophilic xenobiotics (such as methimazole, amitrole, and resorcinol) that inactivate it (Engler et al., 1982). This is the basis for the antithyroid as well as the thyroid tumor–inducing effect of these chemicals. Carbon tetrachloride, which is activated by cytochrome P-450, destroys this enzyme as well as the neighboring microsomal membranes (Osawa et al., 1995). Several mitochondrial enzymes, including pyruvate dehydrogenase, succinate dehydrogenase, and cytochrome c oxidase, are convenient targets for nephrotoxic cysteine conjugates such as dichlorovinyl cysteine, because these conjugates are converted to electrophiles in the same organelle by mitochondrial cysteine conjugate $\beta$-lyase (Dekant et al., 1989). Reactive metabolites that are unable to find appropriate endogenous molecules in close proximity to their site of formation may diffuse until they encounter such reactants. For example, hard electrophiles such as the arylnitrenium ion metabolite of *N*-methyl-4-aminoazobenzene react readily with hard nucleophilic atoms in nucleic acids and thus target DNA in the nucleus even though the electrophiles are produced in the cytoplasm.

Not all targets for chemicals contribute to the harmful effects. Thus, while carbon monoxide causes toxicity by binding to ferrohemoglobin, it also associates with the iron in cytochrome P-450 with little or no consequence. Binding of the ultimate toxicant of acetaminophen to several hepatic proteins does not appear to play a role in its acute hepatotoxic effect because a nonhepatotoxic regioisomer also binds covalently to those proteins (Nelson and Pearson, 1990). Thus, to conclusively identify a target molecule as being responsible for toxicity, it should be demonstrated that the ultimate toxicant (1) reacts with the target and adversely affects its function, (2) reaches an effective concentration at the target site, and (3) alters the target in a way that is mechanistically related to the observed toxicity.

## Effects of Toxicants on Target Molecules

Reaction of the ultimate toxicant with endogenous molecules may cause dysfunction or destruction; in the case of proteins, it may render them foreign (i.e., an antigen) to the immune system.

**Dysfunction of Target Molecules.** Some toxicants activate protein target molecules, mimicking endogenous ligands. For example, morphine activates opiate receptors, clofibrate is an agonist on the peroxisome proliferator–activated receptor, and phorbol esters and lead ions stimulate protein kinase C.

More commonly, chemicals inhibit the function of target molecules. Several xenobiotics, such as atropine, curare, and strychnine, block neurotransmitter receptors by attaching to the ligand binding sites or by interfering with the function of ion channels. Tetrodotoxin and saxitoxin, for example, inhibit channel opening, whereas DDT and the pyrethroid insecticides inhibit closure of the voltage-activated sodium channels in the neuronal membrane. Some toxicants block ion transporters, others inhibit mitochondrial electron transport complexes, and many inhibit enzymes. Chemicals that bind to tubulin (e.g., vinblastine, colchicine, taxol) or actin (e.g., cytochalasin B, phalloidin) impair the assembly (polymerization) and/or disassembly (depolymerization) of these cytoskeletal proteins.

Protein function is impaired when conformation or structure is altered by interaction with the toxicant. Many proteins possess critical moities, especially thiol groups, that are essential for catalytic activity or assembly into macromolecular complexes. The reaction of chemicals with such groups disrupts their function. For this reason, the activity of numerous proteins is impaired nonselectively by thiol-reactive chemicals.

Toxicants may interfere with the template function of DNA. The covalent binding of chemicals to DNA causes nucleotide mispairing during replication. For example, covalent binding of aflatoxin 8,9-oxide to *N*-7 of guanine results in pairing of the adducted guanine with adenine rather than cytosine, leading to the formation of an incorrect codon and the insertion of an incorrect amino acid into the protein. Such events are involved in the aflatoxin-induced mutation of the *ras* proto-oncogene and the *p53* tumor suppressor gene (Eaton and Gallagher, 1994). 8-Hydroxyguanine and 8-hydroxyadenine are mutagenic bases produced by $HO^\bullet$ that can cause mispairing with themselves as well as with neighboring pyrimidines, producing multiple amino acid substitutions (Breimer, 1990). Chemicals, such as doxorubicin, that intercalate between stacked bases in the double helical DNA push adjacent base pairs apart, causing an even greater error in the template function of DNA by shifting the reading frame.

**Destruction of Target Molecules.** In addition to adduct formation, toxicants alter the primary structure of endogenous molecules by means of cross-linking and fragmentation. Bifunctional electrophiles such as 2,5-hexane dione, carbon disulfide, acrolein, and nitrogen mustard alkylating agents cross-link cytoskeletal proteins, DNA, or DNA with proteins. Hydroxyl radicals also can induce cross-linking by converting these macromolecules into either reactive electrophiles (e.g., protein carbonyls), which react with a nucleophilic site in another macromolecule, or radicals, which react with each other. Cross-linking imposes both structural and functional constraints on the linked molecules.

Some target molecules are susceptible to spontaneous degradation after chemical attack. Free radicals such as $Cl_3COO^\bullet$ and $HO^\bullet$ can initiate peroxidative degradation of lipids by hydrogen abstraction from fatty acids (Recknagel et al., 1989). The lipid radical ($L^\bullet$) formed is converted successively to lipid peroxyl radical ($LOO^\bullet$) by oxygen fixation, lipid hydroperoxide (LOOH) by hydrogen abstraction, and lipid alkoxyl radical ($LO^\bullet$) by the Fe(II)-catalyzed Fenton reaction. Subsequent fragmentation gives rise to hydrocarbons such as ethane and reactive aldehydes such as 4-hydroxynonenal and malondialdehyde (Fig. 3-8). Thus, lipid peroxidation not only destroys lipids in cellular membranes but also generates endogenous toxicants, both free radicals (e.g., LOO•, LO•) and electrophiles (e.g., 4-hydroxynonenal). These substances can readily react with adjacent molecules such as membrane proteins or diffuse to more distant molecules such as DNA.

Apart from hydrolytic degradation by toxins, toxicant-induced fragmentation of proteins is not well documented. One example is the destruction of cytochrome P-450 by a reactive metabolite of allyl isopropyl acetamide produced by this enzyme (De Matteis, 1987). In this case, the heme prosthetic group of cytochrome P-450 is alkylated, leading to the loss of the altered heme and resulting in porphyria.

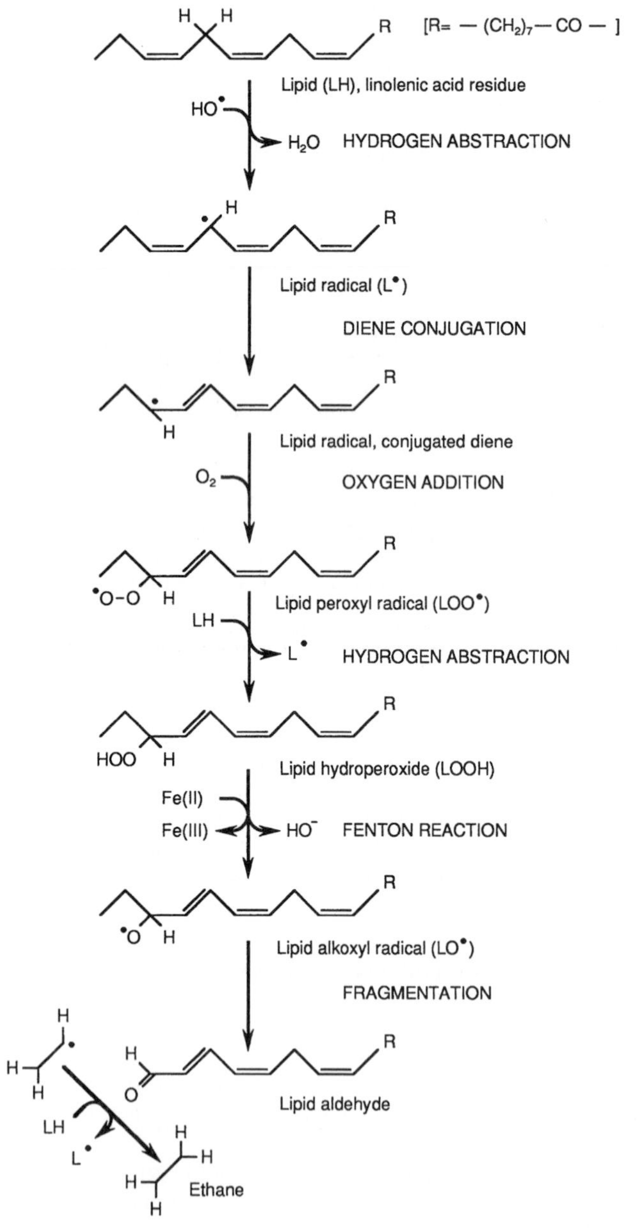

Several forms of DNA fragmentation are caused by toxicants. For instance, attack of DNA bases by HO• can result in the formation of imidazole ring–opened purines or ring-contracted pyrimidines, which block DNA replication (Breimer, 1990). Formation of a bulky adduct at guanine *N*-7 destabilizes the *N*-glycosylic bond, inducing depurination. Depurination results in apurinic sites that are mutagenic. Strand breaks typically are caused by hydroxyl radicals that attack the phosphodiester bonds.

***Figure 3–8. Lipid peroxidation initiated by the hydroxyl radical (HO•).***

Many of the products, such as the radicals and the $\alpha,\beta$-unsaturated aldehydes, are reactive, whereas others, such as ethane, are nonreactive but are indicators of lipid peroxidation.

**Neoantigen Formation.** While the covalent binding of xenobiotics or their metabolites is usually inconsequential with respect to the function of the immune system, in some individuals these altered proteins evoke an immune response. For example, cytochrome P-450 biotransforms halothane to an electrophile, trifluoroacetyl chloride, which binds as a hapten to various microsomal and cell surface proteins in the liver, inducing antibody production (Gut et al., 1993). The immune reaction is thought to be responsible for the hepatitislike syndrome in halothane-sensitive patients. Drug-induced lupus and possibly many cases of drug-induced agranulocytosis are mediated by immune reactions triggered by drug-protein adducts. The causative chemicals are typically nucleophiles, such as aromatic amines (e.g., procainamide and sulfonamides), hydrazines (e.g., hydralazine and isoniazid), and thiols (e.g., propylthiouracyl, methimazole, and captopril). These substances can be oxidized by myeloperoxidase discharged from activated granulocytes to reactive metabolites that bind to the surface proteins of these cells, making them antigens (Uetrecht, 1992). Unfortunately, some proteins that bear an adduct can mimic some normal proteins, which thus also can be attacked by the antibodies.

## CELLULAR DYSFUNCTION AND RESULTANT TOXICITIES

The reaction of toxicants with a target molecule may result in impaired cellular function as the third step in the development of toxicity (Fig. 3-1). The coordinated activity of multicellular organisms is achieved because each cell carries out defined programs. Long-term programs determine the destiny of cells, that is, whether they undergo division, differentiation (i.e., express proteins for specialized functions), or apoptosis. Short-term programs control the ongoing activity of differentiated cells, determining whether they secrete more or less of a substance, whether they contract or relax, and whether they transport or metabolize nutrients at higher or lower rates.

For coordination of these cellular programs, cells possess regulatory networks that can be activated and inactivated by external signaling molecules. To execute the programs, cells are equipped with synthetic, metabolic, kinetic, transport, and energy-producing systems organized into macromolecular complexes, cell membranes, and organelles, by which they maintain their own integrity (internal functions) and support the maintenance of other cells (external functions).

The type of cellular dysfunction caused by toxicants depends on the role of the target molecule affected (Fig. 3-9). If the target molecule is involved in cellular regulation, dysregulation of gene expression and/or dysregulation of momentary cellular activity occurs primarily. However, if the target molecule is involved predominantly in the cell's internal maintenance, the resultant dysfunction can compromise the survival of the cell. The reaction of a toxicant with targets serving external functions can influence the operation of other cells and integrated organ systems. The following discussion deals with these consequences.

## Toxicant-Induced Cellular Dysregulation

Cells are regulated by signaling molecules that activate specific cellular receptors linked to signal transducing networks that transmit the signals to the regulatory regions of genes and/or to functional proteins. Receptor activation may lead to (1) altered gene expression and/or (2) a chemical modification of specific proteins, typically by phosphorylation, to activate or inhibit those proteins. Programs controlling the destiny of cells primarily affect gene expression, whereas those regulating the ongoing activities primarily influence functional proteins; however, one signal may evoke both responses because of branching and interconnection of signaling networks.

**Dysregulation of Gene Expression.** Dysregulation of gene expression may occur at elements that are directly responsible for transcription, at components of the signal transduction pathway, and at the synthesis, storage, or release of the signaling molecules.

***Dysregulation of Transcription.*** Transcription of genetic information from DNA to mRNA is controlled largely by an interplay between transcription factors (TFs) and the regulatory or promoter region of genes. By binding to nucleotide sequences in this region, activated TFs facilitate the formation of the preinitiation complex, promoting transcription of the adjacent gene. Xenobiotics may interact with the promoter region of the gene, the TFs, or other components of the preinitiation complex. However, altered activation of TFs appears to be the most common modality. Functionally, two types of TFs are known: ligand-activated and signal-activated.

Many natural compounds, such as hormones (e.g., steroids, thyroid hormones) and vitamins (retinoids and vitamin D), influence gene expression by binding to and activating TFs (Table 3-4). Xenobiotics may mimic the natural ligands. For example, fibric acid–type lipid-lowering drugs and phthalate esters substitute for polyunsaturated fatty acids as ligands for the peroxisome proliferator–activated receptor (Poellinger et

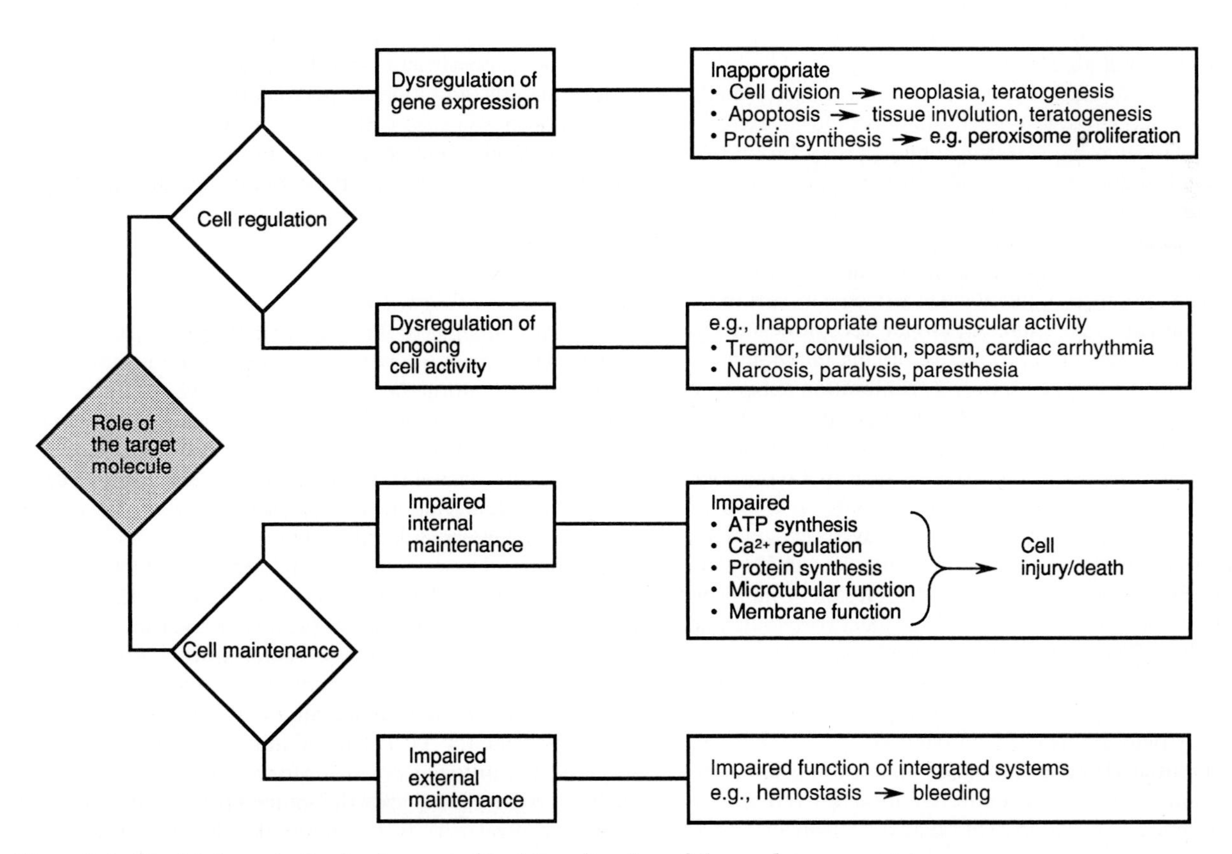


*Figure 3–9. The third step in the development of toxicity: alteration of the regulatory or maintenance function of the cell.*

**Table 3-4**
**Toxicants Acting on Ligand-Activated Transcription Factors**

| LIGAND-ACTIVATED TRANSCRIPTION FACTOR | ENDOGENOUS LIGAND | EXOGENOUS LIGAND | TOXIC EFFECT |
|---|---|---|---|
| Estrogen receptor | Estradiol | Ethynylestradiol<br>Diethylstilbestrol<br>DDT<br>Zeralenone | Mammary and hepatic carcinogenesis<br><br><br>Porcine vulval prolapse |
| Glucocorticoid receptor | Cortisol | Dexamethasone | Apoptosis of lymphocytes<br>Teratogenesis (cleft palate) |
| Retinoic acid receptor | All-*trans*-retinoic acid | A metabolite of 13-*cis* retinoic acid (?) | Teratogenesis (craniofacial, cardiac, thymic malformations) |
| Ah receptor | Unknown | TCDD | Apoptosis of thymocytes<br>Teratogenesis (cleft palate)<br>Hepatocarcinogenesis in rats<br>Altered protein synthesis (e.g., ↑ CYP1A1) |
| Peroxisome proliferator–activated receptor | Polyunsaturated fatty acids | Fibrate esters (e.g., clofibrate)<br>Phthalate esters (e.g., DEHP) | Hepatocarcinogenesis in rats<br>Peroxisome proliferation<br>Altered protein synthesis (e.g., ↑ CYP4A1, ↑ acyl-CoA oxidase) |
| Metal-responsive element-binding transcription factor (MTF-1) | $Zn^{2+}$ | $Cd^{2+}$ | ↑ synthesis of metallothionein |

al., 1992), and $Cd^{2+}$ substitutes for $Zn^{2+}$, the endogenous ligand of metal-responsive element-binding transcription factor (MTF-1) (Heuchel et al., 1994).

Natural or xenobiotic ligands may cause toxicity mediated by ligand-activated TFs when administered at extreme doses or at critical periods during ontogenesis (Table 3-4). Glucocorticoids induce apoptosis of lymphoid cells. While desirable in the treatment of lymphoid malignancies, this is an unwanted response in many other conditions. TCDD, a ligand of the aryl hydrocarbon (Ah) receptor, produces thymic atrophy by causing apoptosis of thymocytes. Estrogens exert mitogenic effects in cells that express estrogen receptors, such as those found in the female reproductive organs, the mammary gland, and the liver. Estrogen-induced proliferation appears to be responsible for tumor formation in these organs during prolonged estrogen exposure (Green, 1992). It has been speculated that environmental xenoestrogens such as DDT, polychlorinated biphenyls, and atrazine contribute to an increased incidence of breast cancer. Zearalenone, a mycoestrogen feed contaminant, causes vulval prolapse in swine, an example of an estrogen receptor–mediated proliferative lesion. Chemicals that act on ligand-activated TFs, such as glucocorticoids and retinoids, induce fetal malformations which may be regarded as inappropriate gene expression (Armstrong et al., 1992). Candidate target genes are the homeobox genes that determine the body plan during early ontogenesis.

In differentiated cells, compounds that act on ligand-activated TFs change the pattern of differentation by overexpressing various genes. For example, fibric acid derivatives stimulate genes that encode peroxisomal enzymes and induce proliferation of peroxisomes in rodent liver (Green, 1992). Likewise, TCDD increases the expression of genes for xenobiotic metabolizing enzymes such as cytochrome P-450 1A1, UDP-glucuronosyltransferase-1, and several subunits of mouse and rat glutathione *S*-transferase. In rats, a common feature of these genes is that the promoter region contains a dioxin response element with a consensus sequence of TCACGC that is recognized by the TCDD-activated Ah receptor complexed with its nuclear translocator protein (Poellinger et al., 1992).

***Dysregulation of Signal Transduction.*** A number of extracellular signaling molecules, such as cytokines, hormones, and growth factors, ultimately activate TFs. Phosphorylation is a common activation mechanism for TFs, which in turn stimulate gene transcription. Phosphorylation of signal-activated TFs is controlled by protein kinases and phosphatases. Any perturbation of signal transduction to TFs, including effects on protein phosphorylation or dephosphorylation, alters the expression of genes regulated by TFs.

Among the numerous signal-activated TFs, activation protein-1 (AP-1) plays a prominent role in toxicant-induced alterations in gene expression (Angel and Karin, 1991). AP-1 represents a family of dimeric proteins, with subunits of the Jun and Fos families, that promote transcription of genes with the tetradecanoylphorbol acetate (TPA) response element as the binding site for AP-1. This TF initiates the gene expression required for mitogenesis in response to signaling molecules such as cytokines and growth factors. Protein kinase C (PKC) plays a central role in the networks that transmit a signal toward AP-1. Therefore, direct stimulation of PKC activates AP-1. Phorbol esters (e.g., TPA) and lead ions are more effective activators of PKC than are the physiological regulators diacylglycerol and $Ca^{2+}$ (Goldstein, 1993). The mitogenic and carcinogenic effects of phorbol esters are most likely mediated by the PKC–AP-1 axis, although PKC-catalyzed phosphorylation of other regulatory proteins also could be involved and PKC-independent activation of AP-1 has been noted.

Toxicant-induced perturbation of signal transduction probably is responsible for altered gene expression after the exposure of cells to heat, oxidative stress, heavy metals, and chemicals forming covalent adducts. Oxidants can activate PKC and some TFs, such as AP-1 and NFκB (Colburn, 1992; Meyer et al., 1993). Genes with responsive elements for these TFs, such as the metallothionein gene and the heme oxygenase gene will be activated by the aforementioned stresses. The significance of such reprogramming of gene expression in toxicity and cellular defense is largely unknown.

It is likely that perturbation of signaling pathways and altered regulation of gene expression are involved in the apoptosis caused by various toxicants. Examples include the apoptosis of thymocytes after alkyltin exposure, that of enterocytes after treatment with antitumor agents, and that of hepatocytes after the administration of some hepatotoxins.

***Dysregulation of Signal Production.*** Hormones of the anterior pituitary exert mitogenic effects on endocrine glands in the periphery by acting on cell surface receptors. Pituitary hormone production is under negative feedback control by hormones of the peripheral glands. Perturbation of this circuit adversely affects pituitary hormone secretion and in turn the peripheral gland. For example, xenobiotics that inhibit thyroid hormone production (e.g., the herbicide amitrole and the fungicide metabolite ethylenethiourea) or enhance thyroid hormone elimination (e.g., phenobarbital) reduce thyroid hormone levels and increase thyroid stimulating hormone (TSH) secretion because of the reduced feedback inhibition. The increased TSH secretion stimulates cell division in the thyroid gland, which is responsible for the goiters or thyroid tumors caused by such toxicants (Chap. 21). Decreased secretion of pituitary hormone produces the opposite adverse affect, with apoptosis followed by involution of the peripheral target gland. For example, estrogens produce testicular atrophy in males by means of feedback inhibition of gonadotropin secretion. The low sperm count in workers intoxicated with the xenoestrogen chlordecone probably results from such a mechanism.

**Dysregulation of Ongoing Cellular Activity.** Ongoing control of specialized cells is exerted by signaling molecules that act on membrane receptors which transduce the signal by regulating $Ca^{2+}$ entry into the cytoplasm or stimulating the enzymatic formation of intracellular second messengers. The $Ca^{2+}$ or other second messengers ultimately alter the phosphorylation of functional proteins, altering their activity and in turn cellular functions almost instantly. Toxicants can adversely affect ongoing cellular activity by disrupting any step in signal coupling.

***Dysregulation of Electrically Excitable Cells.*** Many xenobiotics influence cellular activity in excitable cells, such as neurons, skeletal, cardiac, and smooth muscle cells. Cellular functions such as the release of neurotransmitters and muscle contraction are controlled by transmitters and modulators synthesized and released by adjacent neurons. The major mechanisms that control such cells are shown schematically in Fig. 3-10, and agents that interfere with these mechanisms are listed in Table 3-5.

Altered regulation of neural and/or muscle activity is the basic mechanism of action of many drugs and is responsible for toxicities associated with drug overdosage, pesticides, and microbial, plant, and animal toxins (Gilman et al., 1990; Herken and Hucho, 1992). As neurons are signal-transducing cells, the influence of chemicals on neurons is seen not only on the neuron affected by the toxicant but also on downstream cells influenced by the primary target. Thus, tetrodotoxin, which blocks voltage-gated $Na^{+}$ channels (item 7 in Fig. 3-10) in motor neurons, causes skeletal muscle paralysis. In contrast, cyclodiene insecticides, which block GABA receptors (item 3 in Fig. 3-10) in the central nervous system, induce neuronal excitation and convulsions (Narahashi, 1991).

Perturbation of ongoing cellular activity by chemicals may be due to an alteration in (1) the concentration of neurotransmitters, (2) receptor function, (3) intracellular signal transduction, or (4) the signal-terminating processes.

*Alteration in Neurotransmitter Levels.* Chemicals may alter synaptic levels of neurotransmitters by interfering with their synthesis, storage, release, or removal from the vicinity of the receptor. The convulsive effect of hydrazides is due to their ability to decrease the synthesis of GABA (Gale, 1992). Depletion of norepinephrine, 5-hydroxytryptamine, and dopamine by reserpine accounts for its many adverse effects. Skeletal muscle paralysis caused by botulinum toxin is due to inhibition of acetylcholine release from motor neurons. In contrast, inhibition of acetylcholinesterase by organophosphate or carbamate insecticides or chemical warfare agents (e.g., soman) prevents the hydrolysis of acetylcholine, resulting in massive stimulation of cholinergic receptors (receptors 1, 5, and 11 in Fig. 3-10) and a cholinergic crisis (Table 3-5). Inhibition of the neuronal reuptake of norepinephrine by cocaine or tricyclic antidepressants is responsible for overexcitation of $alpha_1$-adrenergic receptors on vascular smooth muscles, resulting in nasal mucosal ulceration and myocardial infarction in heavy cocaine abusers, whereas overstimulation of $beta_1$-adrenergic receptors contributes to life-threatening arryhthmias. Similar cardiac complications may result from amphetamine abuse, because amphetamine enhances the release of norepinephrine from adrenergic neurons and competitively inhibits neuronal reuptake of this transmitter. A hypertensive crisis can occur with the combined use of tricyclic antidepressants and monoamine oxidase inhibitors, drugs which block different mechanisms of norepinephrine elimination (Gilman et al., 1990).

*Toxicant–Neurotransmitter Receptor Interactions.* Some chemicals interact directly with neurotransmitter receptors, including (1) agonists that associate with the ligand binding site on the receptor and mimic the natural ligand, (2) antagonists that occupy the ligand binding site but cannot activate the receptor, (3) activators, and (4) inhibitors that bind to a site on the receptor that is not directly involved in ligand binding. In the absence of other actions, agonists and activators mimic, whereas antagonists and inhibitors block, the physiological responses characteristic of endogenous ligands. For example, muscimol, a mushroom poison, is an agonist at the inhibitory $GABA_A$ receptor (item 3 in Fig. 3-10), whereas barbiturates,

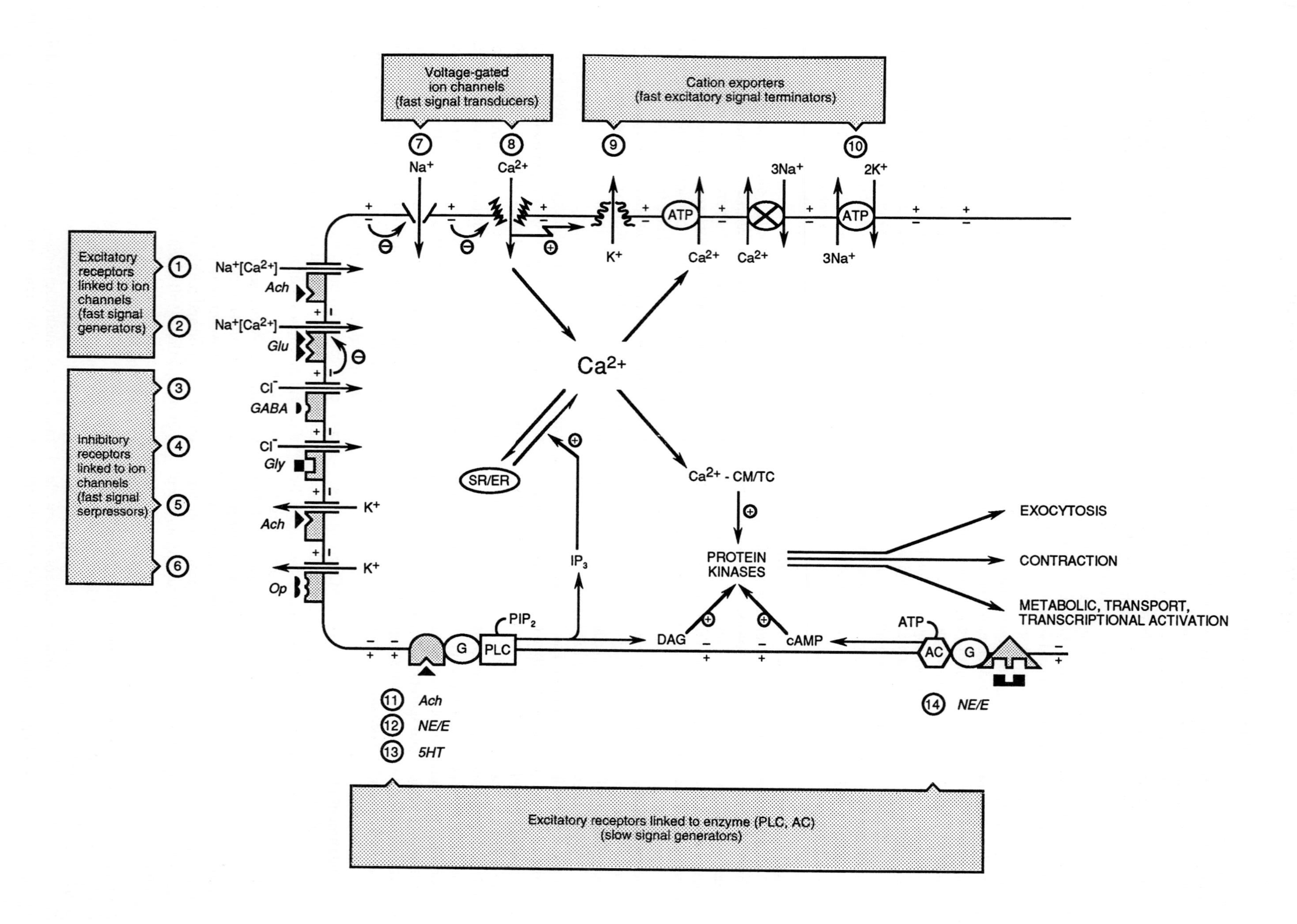
Voltage-gated ion channels (fast signal transducers)
Cation exporters (fast excitatory signal terminators)
Excitatory receptors linked to ion channels (fast signal generators)
Inhibitory receptors linked to ion channels (fast signal serpressors)
Excitatory receptors linked to enzyme (PLC, AC) (slow signal generators)
Na+
Ca2+
K+
ATP
3Na+
2K+
Na+[Ca2+]
Ach
Glu
Cl-
GABA
Gly
Op
Ca2+
SR/ER
IP3
Ca2+ - CM/TC
PROTEIN KINASES
EXOCYTOSIS
CONTRACTION
METABOLIC, TRANSPORT, TRANSCRIPTIONAL ACTIVATION
PIP2
G
PLC
DAG
cAMP
AC
Ach
NE/E
5HT
NE/E

benzodiazepines, general anaesthetics, and alcohols are activators (Narahashi, 1991). Thus, all these agents cause inhibition of central nervous system activity, resulting in sedation, general anesthesia, coma, and ultimately blockade of the medullary respiratory center, depending on the dose administered. There are also similarities in the responses evoked by agonist/activators on excitatory receptors and those elicited by antagonists/inhibitors on inhibitory sites. Thus, glutamate receptor agonists and muscarinic receptor agonists cause neuronal hyperactivity in the brain and ultimately convulsions, as do inhibitors of $GABA_A$ receptors. Because there are multiple types of receptors for each neurotransmitter, these receptors may be affected differentially by toxicants. For example, the neuronal nicotinic acetylcholine receptor is extremely sensitive to inhibition by lead ions, whereas the muscular nicotine receptor subtype is not (Oortgiesen et al., 1993). Other chemicals that produce neurotransmitter receptor–mediated toxicity are listed in Table 3-5.

Some sensory neurons have receptors that are stimulated by chemicals, such as the vanilloid or capsaicin receptor, which is a ligand-gated cation channel (Herken and Hucho, 1992). This receptor mediates the burning sensation of the tongue and reflex stimulation of the lacrimal gland associated with exposure to red pepper and other irritants. Lacrimators in tear gas, which are typically thiol-reactive chemicals, also stimulate these neurons, though their precise mode of action is unclear.

*Toxicant–Signal Transducer Interactions.* Many chemicals alter neuronal and/or muscle activity by acting on signal transduction processes. Voltage-gated $Na^+$ channels (item 7 in Fig. 3-10), which transduce and amplify excitatory signals generated by ligand-gated cation channels (receptors 1 and 2 in Fig. 3-10), are activated by a number of toxins derived from plants and animals (Table 3-5) as well as by synthetic chemicals such as DDT, resulting in overexcitation (Narahashi, 1992). In contrast, agents that block voltage-gated $Na^+$ channels (such as tetrodotoxin and saxitoxin) cause paralysis. The $Na^+$ channels are also important in signal transduction in sensory neurons; therefore, $Na^+$-channel activators evoke sensations and reflexes, whereas $Na^+$-channel inhibitors induce anesthesia. This explains the reflex bradycardia and burning sensation in the mouth that follow the ingestion of monkshood, which contains the $Na^+$-channel activator aconitine, as well as the use of $Na^+$-channel inhibitors such as procaine and lidocaine for local anesthesia.

*Toxicant–Signal Terminator Interactions.* The cellular signal generated by cation influx is terminated by removal of the cations through channels or by transporters (Fig. 3-10). Inhibition of cation export may prolong excitation, as occurs with the inhibition of $Ca^{2+}$-activated $K^+$ channels (item 9 in Fig. 3-10) by $Ba^{2+}$, which is accompanied by potentially lethal neuroexcitatory and spasmogenic effects. Glycosides from digitalis and other plants inhibit $Na^+,K^+$-ATPase (item 10 in Fig. 3-10) and thus increase the intracellular $Na^+$ concentration, which in turn decreases $Ca^{2+}$ export by $Ca^{2+}/Na^+$ exchange (Fig. 3-10). The resultant rise in the intracellular concentration of $Ca^{2+}$ enhances the contractility and excitability of cardiac muscle. Inhibition of brain $Na^+,K^+$-ATPase by chlordecone may be responsible for the tremor observed in chlordecone-exposed workers (Desaiah, 1982). Lithium salts, although used therapeutically, have the potential to produce hyperreflexia, tremor, convulsions, diarrhea, and cardiac arythmias (Gilman et al., 1990). Lithium also markedly potentiates cholinergically mediated seizures. A possible reason for these toxic effects is inefficient repolarization of neurons and muscle cells in the presence of $Li^+$. Whereas $Li^+$ readily enters these cells through $Na^+$ channels, contributing to the signal-induced depolarization, it is not a substrate for the $Na^+,K^+$ pump. Therefore, the cells fail to repolarize properly if a fraction of intracellular $Na^+$ is replaced by $Li^+$.

Failure of the $Na^+,K^+$ pump also is believed to contribute to the neuronal damage resulting from hypoxia, hypoglycemia, and cyanide intoxication. Inasmuch as 70 percent of the ATP produced in neurons is used to drive the $Na^+,K^+$ pump, cessation of ATP synthesis causes a cell to become or remain depolarized. The depolarization-induced release of neurotransmitters such as glutamate from such neurons is thought to be responsible for the hypoxic seizures and further amplification of neuronal injury by the neurotoxic actions of glutamate (Patel et al., 1993).

***Dysregulation of the Activity of Other Cells.*** While many signaling mechanisms also operate in nonexcitable cells, disturbance of these processes is usually less consequential. For example, rat liver cells possess $alpha_1$-adrenergic receptors (item 12 in Fig. 3-10) whose activation evokes metabolic changes, such as increased glycogenolysis and glutathione export, through elevation of intracellular $Ca^{2+}$, which may have toxicological significance.

Many exocrine secretory cells are controlled by muscarinic acetylcholine receptors (item 11 in Fig. 3-10). Salivation, lacrimation, and bronchial hypersecretion after organophosphate

← ***Figure 3–10. Signaling mechanisms for neurotransmitters.***

This simplified scheme depicts major cellular signaling mechanisms that are operational in many neurons and muscle and exocrine cells. Chemicals acting on the numbered elements are listed in Table 3-5. Fast signaling is initiated by the opening of ligand-gated $Na^+/Ca^{2+}$ channels (1,2). The resultant cation influx decreases the inside negative potential (i.e., evokes depolarization) and thus triggers the opening of the voltage-gated $Na^+$ and $Ca^{2+}$ channels (7,8). As a second messenger, the influxed $Ca^{2+}$ activates intracellular $Ca^{2+}$-binding proteins such as calmodulin (CM) and troponin C (TC), which in turn enhance the phosphorylation of specific proteins, causing activation of specific cellular functions. The signal is terminated by channels and transporters (e.g., 9,10) that remove cations from the cells and thus reestablish the inside negative resting potential (i.e., cause repolarization) and restore the resting $Ca^{2+}$ level. Fast signaling can be suppressed by opening the ligand-activated $Cl^-$ or $K^+$ channels (3–6), which increases the inside negativity (i.e., induces hyperpolarization) and thus counteracts opening of the voltage-gated $Na^+$ and $Ca^{2+}$ channels (7,8). Signal transduction from other receptors (11–14) is slower because it involves enzymatic generation of second messengers: inositol 1,4,5-triphosphate ($IP_3$) and diacylglycerol (DAG) by phospholipase C (PLC) and cyclic AMP (cAMP) by adenylyl cyclase (AC). These messengers influence cellular activities by activating protein kinases directly or by mobilizing $Ca^{2+}$ from the sarcoplasmic or endoplasmic reticulum (SR and ER), as $IP_3$ does. Ach = acetylcholine; Glu = glutamate; GABA = $\gamma$-aminobutyric acid; Gly = glycine; Op = opioid peptides; NE = norepinephrine; E = epinephrine; 5HT = 5-hydroxytryptamine; G = G protein; $PIP_2$ = phosphatidylinositol 4,5-bisphosphate. Encircled positive and negative signs indicate activation and inhibition, respectively.

**Table 3–5**
**Agents Acting on Signaling Systems for Neurotransmitters and Causing Deregulation of the Momentary Activity of Electrically Excitable Cells Such as Neurons and Muscle Cells.**

| RECEPTOR/CHANNEL/PUMP | | AGONIST/ACTIVATOR | | ANTAGONIST/INHIBITOR | |
|---|---|---|---|---|---|
| NAME | LOCATION | AGENT | EFFECT | AGENT | EFFECT |
| 1. Acetylcholine nicotinic receptor | Skeletal muscle | Nicotine<br>Anatoxin-a<br>Cytisine<br>*Ind*: ChE inhibitors | Muscle fibrillation, then paralysis | Tubocurarine, lophotoxin<br>α-Bungarotoxin<br>α-Cobrotoxin<br>α-Conotoxin<br>Erabutoxin b<br>*Ind*: botulinum toxin | Muscle paralysis |
| | Neurons | See above | Neuronal activation | $Pb^{2+}$ | Neuronal inhibition |
| 2. Glutamate receptor | CNS neurons | *N*-Methyl-*D*-aspartate<br>Kainate, domoate<br>Quinolinate<br>Quisqualate<br>*Ind*: hypoxia, HCN<br>→ glutamate release | Neuronal activation<br>→ convulsion, neuronal injury<br>("excitotoxicity") | Phencyclidine<br>Ketamine | Neuronal inhibition<br>→ "dissociative anesthesia"<br><br>Protection against "excitotoxicity" |
| 3. $GABA_A$ receptor | CNS neurons | Muscimol, avermectins<br>sedatives (barbiturates, benzodiazepines)<br>General anaesthetics (halothane)<br>Alcohols (ethanol) | Neuronal inhibition<br>→ sedation, general anaesthesia, coma, depression of vital centers | Bicuculline<br>Picrotoxin<br>Pentylenetetrazole<br>Cyclodiene insecticides<br>Lindane<br>*Ind*: isoniazid | Neuronal activation<br>→ tremor, convulsion |
| 4. Glycine receptor | CNS motor neurons | Avermectins (?) | Inhibition of motor neurons<br>→ paralysis | Strychnine<br>*Ind*: tetanus toxin | Disinhibition of motor neurons<br>→ tetanic convulsion |
| 5. Acetylcholine $M_2$ muscarinic receptor | Cardiac muscle | *Ind*: ChE inhibitors | Decreased heart rate and contractility | Belladonna alkaloids (e.g., atropine)<br>atropinelike drugs (e.g., TCAD) | Increased heart rate |
| 6. Opioid receptor | CNS neurons, visceral neurons | Morphine and congeners (e.g., heroin, meperidine) | Neuronal inhibition<br>→ analgesia, central respiratory depression, constipation, urine retention | Naloxone | Antidotal effects in opiate intoxication |

| | | | | | |
|---|---|---|---|---|---|
| 7. Voltage-gated $Na^+$ channel | Neurons, muscle cells, etc. | Aconitine, veratridine<br>Grayanotoxin<br>Batrachotoxin<br>Scorpion toxins<br>Ciguatoxin<br>DDT, pyrethroids | Neuronal activation → convulsion | Tetrodotoxin, saxitoxin<br>$\mu$-Conotoxin<br>Local anaesthetics<br>Phenytoin<br>Quinidine | Neuronal inhibition → paralysis, anesthesia<br>Anticonvulsive action |
| 8. Voltage-gated $Ca^+$ channel | Neurons, muscle cell, etc. | Maitotoxin (?)<br>Atrotoxin (?)<br>Latrotoxin (?) | Neuronal/muscular activation, cell injury | $\omega$-Conotoxin<br>$Pb^{2+}$ | Neuronal inhibition → paralysis |
| 9. Voltage/$Ca^{2+}$-activated $K^+$ Channel | Neurons, muscle cells | $Pb^{2+}$ | Neuronal/muscular inhibition | $Ba^{2+}$<br>Apamin (bee venom)<br>Dendrotoxin | Neuronal/muscular activation → convulsion/spasm |
| 10. $Na^+$,$K^+$-ATPase | Universal | | | Digitalis glycosides<br>Oleandrin<br>Chlordecone | Increased cardiac contractility, excitability<br>Increased neuronal excitability → tremor |
| 11. Acetylcholine $M_3$ muscarinic receptor | Smooth muscle glands | *Ind*: ChE inhibitors | Smooth muscle spasm<br>Salivation, lacrimation | Belladonna alkaloids (e.g., atropine)<br>Atropinelike drugs (e.g., TCAD) | Smooth muscle relaxation → intestinal paralysis, decreased salivation, decreased perspiration |
| Acetylcholine $M_1$ muscarinic receptor | CNS neurons | Oxotremorine<br>*Ind*: ChE inhibitors | Neuronal activation → convulsion | See above | |
| 12. Adrenergic $alpha_1$ receptor | Vascular smooth muscle | (Nor)epinephrine<br>*Ind*: cocaine, tyramine amphetamine, TCAD | Vasoconstriction → ischemia, hypertension | Prazosin | Antidotal effects in intoxication with $alpha_1$-receptor agonists |
| 13. 5-$HT_2$ receptor | Smooth muscle | Ergot alkaloids (ergotamine, ergonovine) | Vasoconstriction → ischemia, hypertension | Ketanserine | Antidotal effects in ergot intoxication |
| 14. Adrenergic $beta_1$ receptor | Cardiac muscle | (Nor)epinephrine<br>*Ind*: cocaine, tyramine amphetamine, TCAD | Increased cardiac contractility and excitability | Atenolol, metoprolol | Antidotal effects in intoxication with $beta_1$-receptor agonists |

Numbering of the signaling elements in this table corresponds to the numbering of their symbols in Fig. 3-10. This tabulation is simplified and incomplete. Virtually all receptors and channels listed occur in multiple forms with different sensitivity to the agents. The reader should consult the pertinent literature for more detailed information. CNS = central nervous system; ChE = cholinesterase; *Ind* = indirectly acting (i.e., by altering neurotransmitter level); TCAD = tricyclic antidepressants.

insecticide poisoning are due to stimulation of these receptors. In contrast, blockade of these receptors contributes to the hyperthermia characteristic of atropine poisoning.

The discovery that some sulfonamides produce hypoglycemia in experimental animals led to the development of oral hypoglycemic agents for diabetic patients. These drugs inhibit $K^+$ channels in pancreatic beta cells, inducing sequentially depolarization, $Ca^{2+}$ influx through voltage-gated $Ca^{2+}$ channels, and exocytosis of insulin (Gilman et al., 1990). The antihypertensive diazoxide acts in the opposite fashion on $K^+$ channels and impairs insulin secretion. While this effect is generally undesirable, it is exploited in the treatment of inoperable insulin-secreting pancreatic tumors.

## Toxic Alteration of Cellular Maintenance

Numerous toxicants interfere with cellular maintenance functions. In a multicellular organism, cells must maintain their own structural and functional integrity as well as provide supportive functions for other cells. Execution of these functions may be disrupted by chemicals, resulting in a toxic response.

**Impairment of Internal Cellular Maintenance: Mechanisms of Toxic Cell Death.** For survival, all cells must synthesize endogenous molecules; assemble macromolecular complexes, membranes, and cell organelles; maintain the intracellular environment; and produce energy for operation. Agents that disrupt these functions jeopardize survival. The following discussion focuses on major mechanisms that contribute to toxic cell death.

***Impaired ATP Synthesis.*** ATP plays a central role in cellular maintenance both as a chemical for biosynthesis and as the major source of energy. It is utilized in numerous biosynthetic reactions, activating endogenous compounds by phosphorylation and adenylation, and is incorporated into cofactors as well as nucleic acids. It is required for muscle contraction and polymerization of the cytoskeleton, fueling cellular motility, cell division, vesicular transport, and the maintenance of cell morphology. ATP drives ion transporters such as the $Na^+$,$K^+$-ATPase in the plasma membrane, the $Ca^{2+}$-ATPase in the plasma and the endoplasmic reticulum membranes, and $H^+$-ATPase in the lysosomal membrane. These pumps maintain conditions essential for various cell functions. For example, the $Na^+$ concentration gradient across the plasma membrane generated by the $Na^+$,$K^+$ pump drives $Na^+$-glucose and $Na^+$-amino acid cotransporters as well as the $Na^+/Ca^{2+}$ antiporter, facilitating the entry of these nutrients and the removal of $Ca^{2+}$.

Chemical energy is released by hydrolysis of ATP to ADP or AMP. The ADP is rephosphorylated in the mitochondria by ATP synthase (Fig. 3-11). Coupled to oxidation of hydrogen to water, this process is termed *oxidative phosphorylation*. In addition to ATP synthase, oxidative phosphorylation requires the (1) delivery of hydrogen in the form of reduced cofactors to the initial electron transport complex, (2) delivery of oxygen to the terminal electron transport complex, (3) delivery of ADP and inorganic phosphate to ATP synthase, (4) flux of electrons along the electron transport chain to $O_2$, accompanied by ejection of protons from the matrix space across the inner membrane, and (5) return of protons across the inner membrane into the matrix space down an electrochemical gradient to drive ATP synthase (Fig. 3-11).

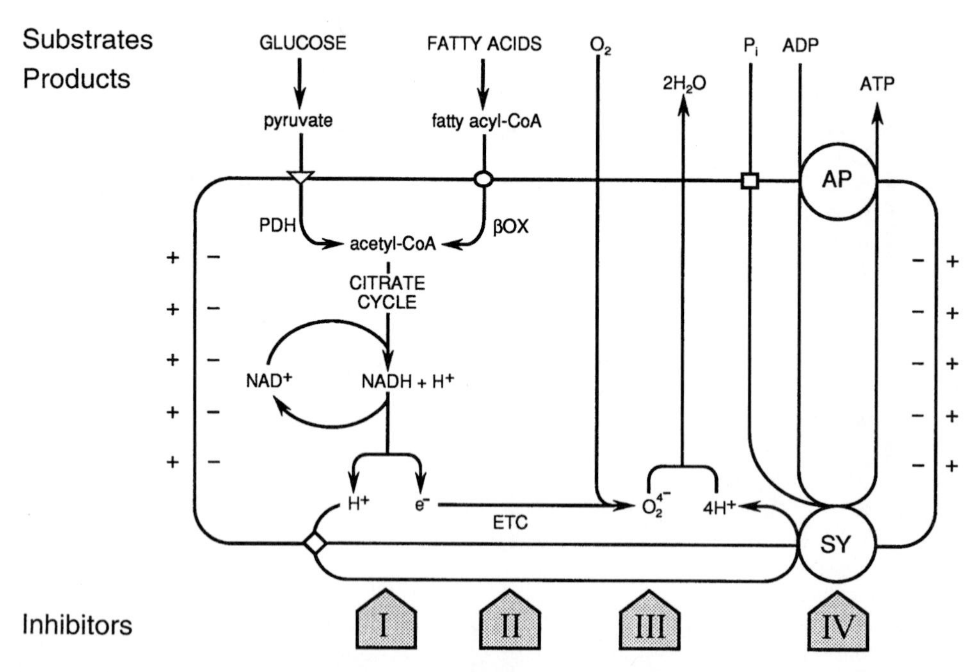


***Figure 3–11. ATP synthesis (oxidative phosphorylation) in mitochondria.***

Arrows with roman numerals point to the ultimate sites of action of four categories of agents that interfere with oxidative phosphorylation (Table 3-6). For simplicity, this scheme does not indicate that protons are extruded from the matrix space along the electron transport chain at three sites. AP = ADP/ATP antiporter; βOX = beta-oxidation of fatty acids; $e^-$ = electron; ETC = electron transport chain (respiratory chain); $P_i$ = inorganic phosphate; SY = ATP synthase ($F_oF_1$ATPase).

Several chemicals impede these processes, interfering with mitochondrial ATP synthesis (Commandeur and Vermeulen, 1990; Moreland, 1994). These chemicals are divided into four groups (Table 3-6). Substances in class I interfere with the delivery of hydrogen to the electron transport chain. For example, fluoroacetate inhibits the citric acid cycle and the production of reduced cofactors. Class II chemicals such as rotenone and cyanide inhibit the transfer of electrons along the electron transport chain to oxygen. Class III agents interfere with oxygen delivery to the terminal electron transporter, cytochrome oxidase. All chemicals that cause hypoxia ultimately act at this site. Finally, chemicals in class IV inhibit the activity of ATP synthase, the key enzyme for oxidative phosphorylation. At this site, the synthesis of ATP may be inhibited in one of four ways: (1) direct inhibition of ATP synthase, (2) interference with ADP delivery, (3) interference with inorganic phosphate delivery, and (4) deprivation of ATP synthase from its driving force, the controlled influx of protons into the matrix space. Protonophoric chemicals (uncouplers) such as 2,4-dinitrophenol and pentachlorophenol import protons into the mitochondrial matrix, dissipating the proton gradient that drives the controlled influx of protons into the matrix, which in turn drives ATP synthase. Table 3-6 lists other chemicals that impair ATP synthesis.

Impairment of oxidative phosphorylation is detrimental to cells because failure of ADP rephosphorylation results in the accumulation of ADP and its breakdown products as well as depletion of ATP. Accordingly, cultured hepatocytes exposed to KCN and iodoacetate exhibit a rapid rise in cytosolic $H^+$ and $Mg^{2+}$ as a result of the hydrolysis of adenosine di- and triphosphates (that exist as Mg salts) and the release of phosphoric acid and $Mg^{2+}$ (Herman et al., 1990). The increased conversion of pyruvate to lactate also may contribute to the acidosis. The lack of ATP compromises the operation of ATP-requiring ion pumps, leading to the loss of ionic and volume regulatory controls (Buja et al., 1993). Shortly after intracellular acidosis and hypermagnesemia, liver cells exposed to KCN and iodoacetate exhibit a rise in intracellular $Na^+$, probably as a result of failure of the $Na^+$ pump, after which plasma membrane blebs appear. The intracellular

**Table 3–6**
**Agents Impairing Mitochondrial ATP Synthesis**

I. By inhibition of hydrogen delivery to the electron transport chain and acting on/as
  1. Glycolysis (critical in neurons): hypoglycemia, iodoacetate
  2. Gluconeogenesis (critical in renal tubular cells): coenzyme A depletors (see below)
  3. Fatty acid oxidation (critical in cardiac muscle): hypoglycin, 4-pentenoic acid
  4. Pyruvate dehydrogenase: arsenite, DCVC, *p*-benzoquinone
  5. Citrate cycle
    (a) Aconitase: fluoroacetate, $NO^{\bullet}$
    (b) Isocitrate dehydrogenase: DCVC
    (c) Succinate dehydrogenase: malonate, DCVC, PCBD-cys, 2-bromohydroquinone, *cis*-crotonalide fungicides
  6. Depletors of TPP (inhibit TPP-dependent PDH and $\alpha$-KGDH): ethanol
  7. Depletors of coenzyme A: 4-(dimethylamino)phenol, *p*-benzoquinone
  8. Depletors of NADH
    (a) See group D in Table 3-7
    (b) Activators of poly(ADP-ribose) polymerase (e.g., MNNG, hydrogen peroxide): agents causing DNA damage
II. By inhibition of electron transport and acting on/as
  1. Inhibitors of electron transport complexes
    (a) NADH–coenzyme Q reductase (complex I): rotenone, amytal, $MPP^+$
    (b) Cycotochrome Q–cytochrome c reductase (complex III): antimycin-A, myxothiazole
    (c) Cytochrome oxidase (complex IV): cyanide, hydrogen sulfide, azide, formate
    (d) Multisite inhibitors: dinitroaniline and diphenylether herbicides, $NO^{\bullet}$
  2. Electron acceptors: $CCl_4$, doxorubicin, menadione, $MPP^+$
III. By inhibition of oxygen delivery to the electron transport chain
  1. Agents causing respiratory paralysis: CNS depressants, convulsants
  2. Agents causing ischemia: ergot alkaloids, cocaine
  3. Agents inhibiting oxygenation of Hb: carbon monoxide, methemoglobin-forming agents
IV. By inhibition of ADP phosphorylation and acting on/as
  1. ATP synthase: oligomycin, cyhexatin, DDT, chlordecone
  2. ADP/ATP antiporter: atractyloside, DDT, free fatty acids, lysophospholipids
  3. Phosphate transporter: *N*-ethylmaleimide, mersalyl, *p*-benzoquinone
  4. Agents dissipating the mitochondrial membrane potential (uncouplers)
    (a) Cationophores: pentachlorophenol, dinitrophenol-, benzonitrile-, thiadiazole herbicides, salicylate, valinomycin, gramicidin, calcimycin (A23187)
    (b) Agents permeabilizing the mitochondrial inner membrane: PCBD-cys, chlordecone

The ultimate sites of action of these agents are indicated in Fig. 3-11. DCVC = dichlorovinyl-cysteine; $\alpha$-KGDH = $\alpha$-ketoglutarate dehydrogenase; MNNG = *N*-methyl-*N*′-nitro-*N*-nitrosoguanidine; $MPP^+$ = 1-methyl-4-phenylpyridinium; PCBD-cys = pentachlorobutadienyl-cysteine; PDH = pyruvate dehydrogenase; TPP = thyamine pyrophosphate.

phosphoric acidosis is beneficial for the cells presumably because the released phosphoric acid forms insoluble calcium phosphate, preventing the rise of cytosolic $Ca^{2+}$ and the resultant $Ca^{2+}$-dependent activation of hydrolytic enzymes. Indeed, the increase in cytoplasmic $Ca^{2+}$ in cyanide- and iodoacetate-poisoned liver cells is not an early event (Herman et al., 1990). In addition, a low pH also directly decreases the activity of phospholipases. Terminally, the intracellular pH rises, increasing phospholipase activity, and this contributes to irreversible membrane damage (i.e., rupture of the blebs) not only by degrading phospholipids but also by generating endogenous detergents such as lysophospholipids and free fatty acids. The lack of ATP aggravates this condition because the reacylation of lysophospholipids with fatty acids is impaired. This chain of events is somewhat cell-specific. For example, cyanide toxicity in neurons is associated with depolarization and glutamate release (Patel et al., 1993) followed by $Ca^{2+}$ influx through voltage-gated as well as glutamate-gated channels (see items 8 and 2, respectively, in Fig. 3-10).

***Sustained Rise of Intracellular $Ca^{2+}$.*** Intracellular $Ca^{2+}$ levels are highly regulated (Fig. 3-12). The 10,000-fold difference between extracellular and cytosolic $Ca^{2+}$ concentration is maintained by the impermeability of the plasma membrane to $Ca^{2+}$ and by transport mechanisms that remove $Ca^{2+}$ from the cytoplasm (Richter and Kass, 1991). $Ca^{2+}$ is actively pumped from the cytosol across the plasma membrane and is sequestered in the endoplasmic reticulum and mitochondria (Fig. 3-12). Because they are equipped with a low-affinity transporter, the mitochondria play a significant role in $Ca^{2+}$ sequestration only when the cytoplasmic levels rise into the micromolar range. Under such conditions, a large amount of $Ca^{2+}$ accumulates in the mitochondria, where it is deposited as calcium phosphate.

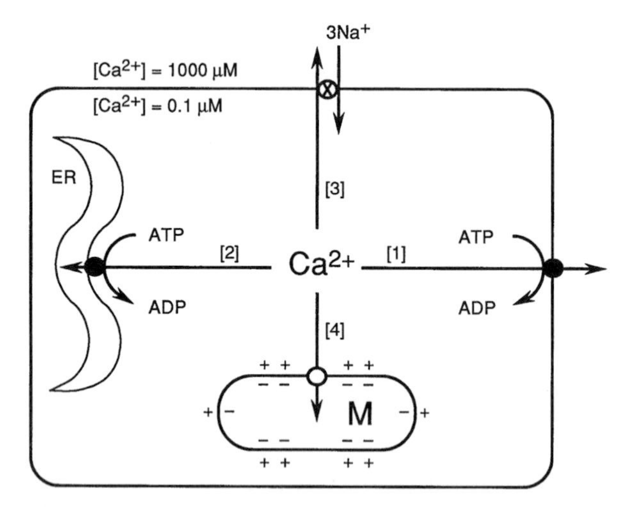


***Figure 3–12. Four mechanisms for the elimination of $Ca^{2+}$ from the cytoplasm: $Ca^{2+}$-ATPase–mediated pumping into (1) the extracellular space as well as (2) the endoplasmic reticulum (ER) and ion-gradient-driven transport into (3) the extracellular space (by the $Ca^{2+}/Na^{+}$ exhanger) as well as (4) the mitochondria (M; by the $Ca^{2+}$ uniporter).***

Some agents that inhibit these mechanisms are listed in Table 3-7, group B.

Toxicants induce elevation of cytoplasmic $Ca^{2+}$ levels by promoting $Ca^{2+}$ influx into or inhibiting $Ca^{2+}$ efflux from the cytoplasm. Opening of the ligand- or voltage-gated $Ca^{2+}$ channels or damage to the plasma membrane causes $Ca^{2+}$ to move down its concentration gradient from extracellular fluid to the cytoplasm. Toxicants also may increase cytosolic $Ca^{2+}$ by inducing its leakage from the mitochondria. They also may diminish $Ca^{2+}$ efflux through inhibition of $Ca^{2+}$ transporters or depletion of their driving forces. Several agents that can cause a sustained rise in cytoplasmic $Ca^{2+}$ levels are listed in Table 3-7. Sustained elevation of intracellular $Ca^{2+}$ is harmful because it can result in (1) depletion of energy reserves, (2) dysfunction of microfilaments, and (3) activation of hydrolytic enzymes.

There are at least three mechanisms by which sustained elevations in intracellular $Ca^{2+}$ unfavorably influence the cellular energy balance. First, high cytoplasmic $Ca^{2+}$ levels cause increased mitochondrial $Ca^{2+}$ uptake (step 1 in Fig. 3-13) by the $Ca^{2+}$ "uniporter," which, like ATP synthase, utilizes the inside negative mitochondrial membrane potential as the driving force. Consequently, mitochondrial $Ca^{2+}$ uptake inhibits the synthesis of ATP (step 2 in Fig. 3-13). A specific case of $Ca^{2+}$-induced deenergization is the so-called $Ca^{2+}$-cycling, which involves continuous mitochondrial release and reuptake of $Ca^{2+}$. The cycle is initiated by an increased export of $Ca^{2+}$ from the mitochondria, commonly in response to agents that oxidize mitochondrial NADH (group D in Table 3-7) (Richter and Kass, 1991). This ultimately results in activation of the transporter that extrudes $Ca^{2+}$ from the matrix space (see events starting at step 5 in Fig. 3-13). Second, $Ca^{2+}$ may deplete energy reserves by causing oxidative injury to the inner membrane as a consequence of the activation of mitochondrial dehydrogenases. The resultant increase of hydrogen output from the citrate cycle stimulates electron flux along the electron transport chain, increasing the formation of partially reduced oxygen species (steps 3 and 6 in Fig. 3-13), which damage the mitochondrial inner membrane. This injury further compromises oxidative phosphorylation. Third, a sustained rise in cytoplasmic $Ca^{2+}$ not only impairs ATP synthesis but also increases ATP consumption by the $Ca^{2+}$-ATPases working to eliminate the excess $Ca^{2+}$. Depletion of cellular ATP reserves, which may originate from intracellular hypercalcemia, can in turn increase cytoplasmic $Ca^{2+}$ levels further (see events starting with step 4 in Fig. 3-13), because extrusion of $Ca^{2+}$ from the cytoplasm is ATP-dependent. Thus, depletion of ATP and elevation of cytoplasmic $Ca^{2+}$ are interrelated events and may form a vicious cycle, as illustrated in Fig. 3-13.

A second mechanism by which an uncontrolled rise in cytoplasmic $Ca^{2+}$ causes cell injury is microfilamental dissociation (Nicotera et al., 1992). The cellwide network of actin filaments maintains cellular morphology by attachment of the filaments to actin-binding proteins in the plasma membrane. An increase of cytoplasmic $Ca^{2+}$ causes dissociation of actin filaments from $\alpha$-actinin and fodrin, proteins that promote anchoring of the filament to the plasma membrane. This represents a mechanism leading to plasma membrane blebbing, a condition that predisposes the membrane to rupture.

A third event in which $Ca^{2+}$ levels are deleterious to cells is activation of hydrolytic enzymes that degrade proteins, phospholipids, and nucleic acids (Nicotera et al., 1992). Many

**Table 3–7**
**Agents Causing Sustained Elevation of Cytosolic $Ca^{2+}$ and/or Impaired Synthesis of ATP**

A. Agents inducing $Ca^{2+}$ influx into the cytoplasm
  I. Via ligand-gated channels in neurons:
    1. Glutamate receptor agonists (“excitotoxins”): glutamate, kainate, domoate
    2. “Capsaicin receptor” agonists: capsaicin, resiniferatoxin
  II. Via voltage-gated channels: maitotoxin (?) $HO^{\bullet}$
  III. Via “newly formed pores”: maitotoxin, amphotericin B, chlordecone, methylmercury, alkyltins
  IV. Across disrupted cell membrane:
    1. Detergents: exogenous detergents, lysophospholipids, free fatty acids
    2. Hydrolytic enzymes: phospholipases in snake venoms, endogenous phospholipase $A_2$
    3. Lipid peroxidants: carbon tetrachloride
    4. Cytoskeletal toxins (by inducing membrane blebbing): cytochalasins, phalloidin
  V. From mitochondria: see D
B. Agents inhibiting $Ca^{2+}$ export from the cytoplasm (inhibitors of $Ca^{2+}$-ATPase in cell membrane and/or endoplasmic reticulum)
  I. Covalent binders: acetaminophen, bromobenzene, $CCl_4$, chloroform, DCE
  II. Thiol oxidants: cystamine (mixed disulfide formation), diamide, *t*-BHP, menadione, diquat
  III. Others: vanadate
C. Agents impairing mitochondrial ATP synthesis (see Table 3-6)
D. Agents causing hydrolysis of $NAD(P)^+$ in mitochondria
  I. By increasing $NAD(P)^+$ availability via oxidation of NAD(P)H
    1. Directly: alloxan
    2. Enzymatically: *t*-BHP, NAPBQI, divicine, fatty acid hydroperoxides, menadione, $MPP^+$
  II. By activation of “NAD-glycohydrolase”: phenylarsine oxide, gliotoxin, $NO^{\bullet}$

Sites of action of all agents are indicated in Fig. 3-13. DCE = 1,1-dichloroethylene; *t*-BHP = *t*-butyl hydroperoxide; $MPP^+$ = 1-methyl-4-phenylpyridinium; NAPBQI = *N*-acetyl-*p*-benzoquinoneimine.

integral membrane proteins are targets for $Ca^{2+}$-activated neutral proteases, or calpains (Saido et al., 1994). Calpain-mediated hydrolysis of actin-binding proteins also may cause membrane blebbing. It is assumed that $Ca^{2+}$-activated proteases proteolytically convert xanthine dehydrogenase to xanthine oxidase, whose by-products, $O_2^{\bar{\bullet}}$ and HOOH, contribute to cell injury. Calpains also activate protein kinase C proteolytically. Indiscriminate activation of phospholipases by $Ca^{2+}$ causes membrane breakdown directly and by the generation of detergents. Activation of a $Ca^{2+}$-$Mg^{2+}$-dependent endonuclease causes fragmentation of chromatin into oligonucleosomes when the internucleosomal DNA region is accessible to the enzyme after chromatin decondensation. Topoisomerases, which unwind supercoiled DNA, also are influenced by $Ca^{2+}$. Elevated levels of $Ca^{2+}$ can lock topoisomerase II in a form that cleaves but does not religate DNA. The $Ca^{2+}$-dependent chromatin fragmentation is observed in apoptotic cell death induced by toxicants such as TCDD. In summary, intracellular hypercalcemia activates several processes that interfere with the ability of cells to maintain their structural and functional integrity. The relative importance of these processes in vivo requires further definition.

***Other Mechanisms.*** Because both impaired oxidative phosphorylation and a sustained rise of cytoplasmic $Ca^{2+}$ have multiple consequences that are detrimental to cell vitality, these events may be regarded as common ultimate mechanisms for mediating lethal cellular toxicity. In addition to chemicals that disrupt oxidative phosphorylation and/or control of intracellular $Ca^{2+}$, there are toxicants that cause cell death by affecting other functions or structures primarily. Included here are (1) agents that directly damage the plasma membrane, such as lipid solvents, detergents, and venom-derived hydrolytic enzymes, (2) xenobiotics that damage the lysosomal membrane, such as aminoglycoside antibiotics and hydrocarbons binding to $\alpha_{2u}$-globulin, (3) toxins that destroy the cytoskeleton, such as the microfilamental toxin phalloidin and cytochalasins, the microtubular toxin colchicine, and the neurofilamental toxin 2,5-hexanedione, and (4) agents that disrupt protein synthesis, such as $\alpha$-amanitin and ricin, which inhibit cytoplasmic protein synthesis, and ethanol, which impairs mitochondrial protein synthesis (Cunningham et al., 1990).

The events leading to cell death after exposure to these agents is generally unknown. It is likely that cell death caused by these chemicals is ultimately mediated by impairment of oxidative phosphorylation and/or sustained elevation of intracellular $Ca^{2+}$. For example, direct plasma membrane injury would lead to increased intracellular $Ca^{2+}$ levels. Neurofilamental toxins that block axonal transport cause energy depletion in the distal axonal segment. Energy depletion also could be involved in ethanol-induced liver injury because ethanol impairs the synthesis of mitochondrial proteins that participate in oxidative phosphorylation.

**Impairment of External Cellular Maintenance.** Toxicants also may interfere with cells that are specialized to provide support to other cells, tissues, or the whole organism. Agents

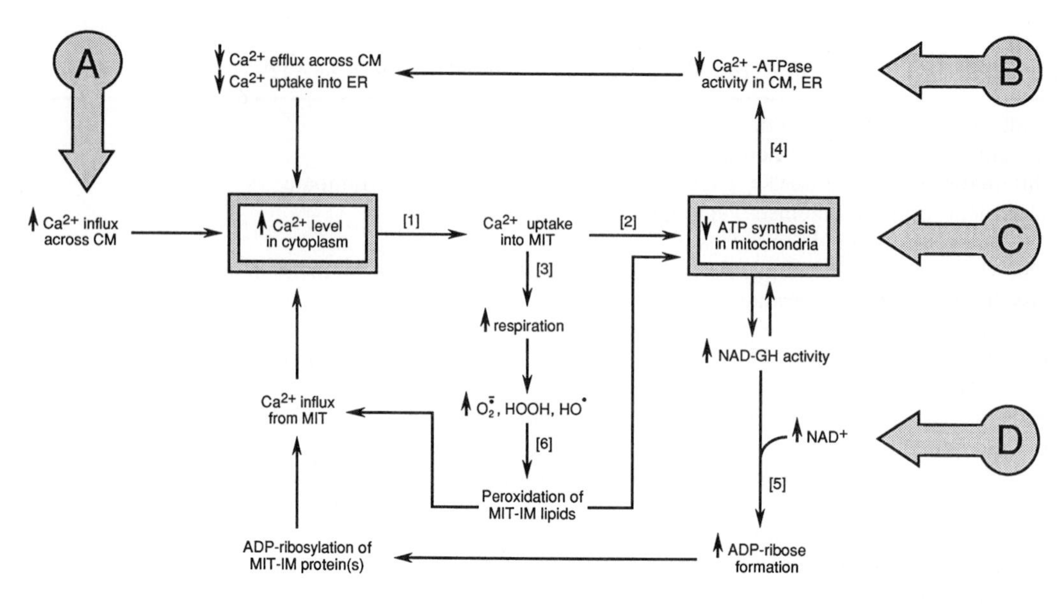


***Figure 3–13. Interrelationship between sustained increase in cytoplasmic $Ca^{2+}$ level and impaired mitochondrial ATP synthesis.***

This scheme represents a synopsis of processes definitively or tentatively identified in isolated cells and cell organelles. Circled letters indicate sites where toxicants and experimental chemicals are assumed to initiate alterations in $Ca^{2+}$ and ATP homeostasis. Such agents are listed in Table 3-7. Numbers in brackets point to events that are discussed below. They do not necessarily indicate the sequence of events. (1) Rise in cytoplasmic $Ca^{2+}$ level leads to $Ca^{2+}$ uptake by mitochondria (MIT) via a "uniporter" driven by the inside negative membrane potential. (2) $Ca^{2+}$ accumulation in the matrix space diminishes the mitochondrial membrane potential, the driving force for ATP synthase, and thus impairs ATP synthesis. (3) A second consequence of $Ca^{2+}$ uptake is acceleration of mitochondrial respiration (electron transport) with increased formation of oxygen radicals that can peroxidize lipids in the mitochondrial inner membrane (MIT-IM). (4) Impairment of mitochondrial ATP production compromises ATP supply for $Ca^{2+}$-ATPases ("$Ca^{2+}$ pumps") in the cell membrane (CM) and the endoplasmic reticulum (ER) as well as for the $Na^+$,$K^+$-ATPase in the CM, which drives the $Ca^{2+}/Na^+$ exchanger (see Fig. 3-12). Decreased pumping of cytoplasmic $Ca^{2+}$ out of the cell and into vesicles of the ER further elevates the concentration of $Ca^{2+}$ in the cytoplasm. (5) Increased formation of ADP-ribose from oxidized nicotinamide adenine dinucleotide ($NAD^+$) by NAD-glycohydrolase (NAD-GH) can lead to mono(ADP-ribosyl)ation of MIT-IM protein(s) (the $Ca^{2+}/H^+$-antiporter?), which purportedly enhances the $Ca^{2+}/H^+$-antiporter-mediated efflux of $Ca^{2+}$ from the mitochondria into the cytoplasm. Enhanced production of ADP-ribose may result from either increased formation of $NAD^+$ or increased activity of NAD-GH (e.g., in consequence of depletion of intramitochondrial ATP, which is an inhibitor of NAD-GH). (6) Continuous mitochondrial $Ca^{2+}$ uptake and release (i.e., "$Ca^{2+}$ cycling") ultimately can lead to peroxidative and possibly hydrolytic MIT-IM injury (the latter being evoked by $Ca^{2+}$-activated phospholipases). This results in further deterioration of ATP synthesis and flooding of the cytoplasm with $Ca^{2+}$ that had accumulated in the mitochondria as a result of high-capacity uptake but low-capacity efflux mechanisms. Further deleterious consequences of sustained elevation of cytoplasmic $Ca^{2+}$ and depletion of ATP are discussed in the text.

acting on the liver illustrate this type of toxicity. Hepatocytes produce and release into the circulation a number of proteins and nutrients. They remove cholesterol and bilirubin from the circulation, converting them into bile acids and bilirubin glucuronides, respectively, for subsequent excretion into bile. Interruption of these processes may be harmful to the organism, the liver, or both. For example, inhibition of the hepatic synthesis of coagulation factors by coumarins does not harm the liver but may cause death by hemorrhage (Gilman et al., 1990). This is the mechanism of the rodenticidal action of warfarin. In the fasting state, inhibitors of hepatic gluconeogenesis such as hypoglycin may be lethal by limiting the supply of glucose to the brain. Interference with the synthesis, assembly, and secretion of lipoproteins overloads the hepatocytes with lipids, causing hepatic dysfunction. $\alpha$-Naphthylisothiocyanate causes separation of extracellular tight junctions that seal bile canaliculi (Krell et al., 1987), impairing biliary secretion and leading to the retention of bile acids and bilirubin; this adversely affects the liver as well as the entire organism.

## REPAIR OR DYSREPAIR

The fourth step in the development of toxicity is inappropriate repair (Fig. 3-1). As was noted previously, many toxicants alter macromolecules which, if not repaired, cause damage at higher levels of the biological hierarchy in the organism. Because repair influences the progression of toxic lesions, mechanisms

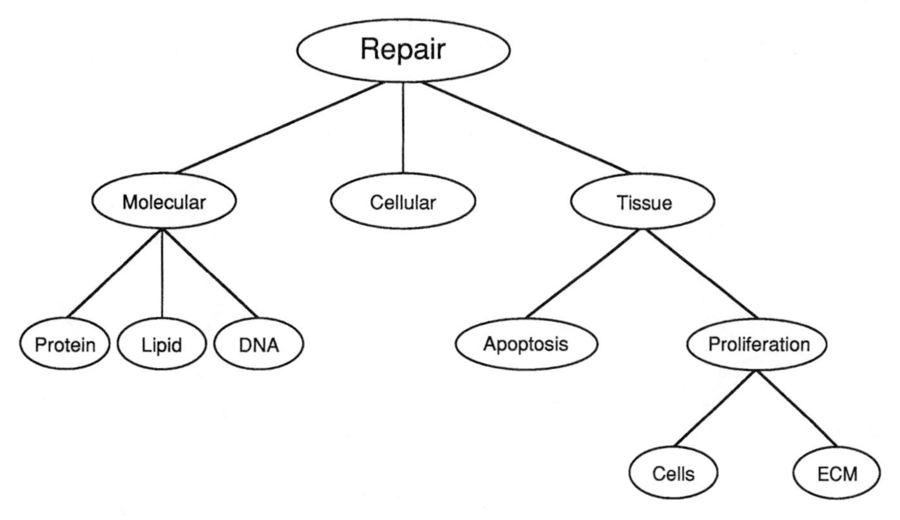


***Figure 3–14. Repair mechanisms.***

Dysfunction of these mechanisms results in dysrepair, the fourth step in the development of numerous toxic injuries. ECM = extracellular matrix.

of repair are categorized in Fig. 3-14 and discussed below in detail.

## Molecular Repair

Damaged molecules may be repaired in different ways. Some chemical alterations, such as oxidation of protein thiols and methylation of DNA, are simply reversed. Hydrolytic removal of the molecule's damaged unit or units and insertion of a newly synthesized unit or units often occur with chemically altered DNA and peroxidized lipids. In some instances, the damaged molecule is totally degraded and resynthesized. This process is time-consuming but unavoidable in cases such as the regeneration of cholinesterases after organophosphate intoxication.

**Repair of Proteins.** Thiol groups are essential for the function of numerous proteins, such as receptors, enzymes, cytoskeletal proteins, and TFs. Oxidation of protein thiols (Prot-SHs) to protein disulfides (Prot-SS, $Prot_1$-SS-$Prot_2$), protein-glutathione mixed disulfides, and protein sulfenic acids (Prot-SOH) can be reversed by enzymatic reduction (Fernando et al., 1992; Gravina and Mieyal, 1993) (Fig. 3-15). The endogenous reductants are thioredoxin and glutaredoxin, small ubiquitous proteins with two redox-active cysteines in their active centers. Because the catalytic thiol groups in these proteins are oxidized, they are recycled by reduction with NADPH generated by glucose-6-phosphate dehydrogenase and 6-phosphogluconate dehydrogenase in the pentose phosphate pathway.

Repair of oxidized hemoglobin (methemoglobin) occurs by means of electron transfer from cytochrome $b_5$, which is then regenerated by a NADH-dependent cytochrome $b_5$ reductase (also called methemoglobin reductase).

Soluble intracellular proteins are susceptible to denaturation by physical or chemical insults. Molecular chaperones such as the heat shock proteins are synthesized in large quantities in response to protein denaturation and are important in the refolding of altered proteins (Morimoto, 1993). The ATP/ubiquitin-dependent proteolytic enzymes are specialized for eliminating damaged intracellular proteins. These proteins are first conjugated with ubiquitin, allowing their recognition by proteasomes, large protease complexes in the cytosol that proteolytically degrade them. Removal of damaged and aggregated proteins is especially critical in the eye lens for maintenance of its transparency. Erythrocytes have ATP-independent, nonlysosomal proteolytic enzymes that rapidly and selectively degrade proteins denatured by $HO^•$ (Davies, 1987).

**Repair of Lipids.** Peroxidized lipids are repaired by a complex process that operates in concert with a series of reductants as well as with glutathione peroxidase and reductase (Fig. 3-16). Phospholipids containing fatty acid hydroperoxides are preferentially hydrolysed by phospholipase $A_2$, with the peroxidized fatty acids replaced with normal fatty acids (van Kuijk et al., 1987). Again, NADPH is needed to "repair" the reductants that are oxidized in the process.

**Repair of DNA.** Despite its high reactivity with electrophiles and free radicals, nuclear DNA is remarkably stable, in part because it is packaged in chromatin and because several repair mechanisms are available to correct alterations (Sancar and Sancar, 1988).

***Direct Repair.*** Certain covalent DNA modifications are directly reversed by enzymes such as DNA photolyase, which cleaves adjacent pyrimidines dimerized by ultraviolet (UV) light. Inasmuch as this chromophore-equipped enzyme uses the energy of visible light to correct damage, its use is restricted to light-exposed cells. Minor adducts, such as methyl groups, attached to the $O^6$ position of guanine are removed by $O^6$-alkylguanine-DNA-alkyltransferase (Pegg and Byers, 1992). While repairing the DNA, this alkyltransferase destroys itself, transferring the adduct onto one of its cysteine residues. This results in its inactivation and eventual degradation. Thus, similar to glutathione, which is depleted during detoxication of

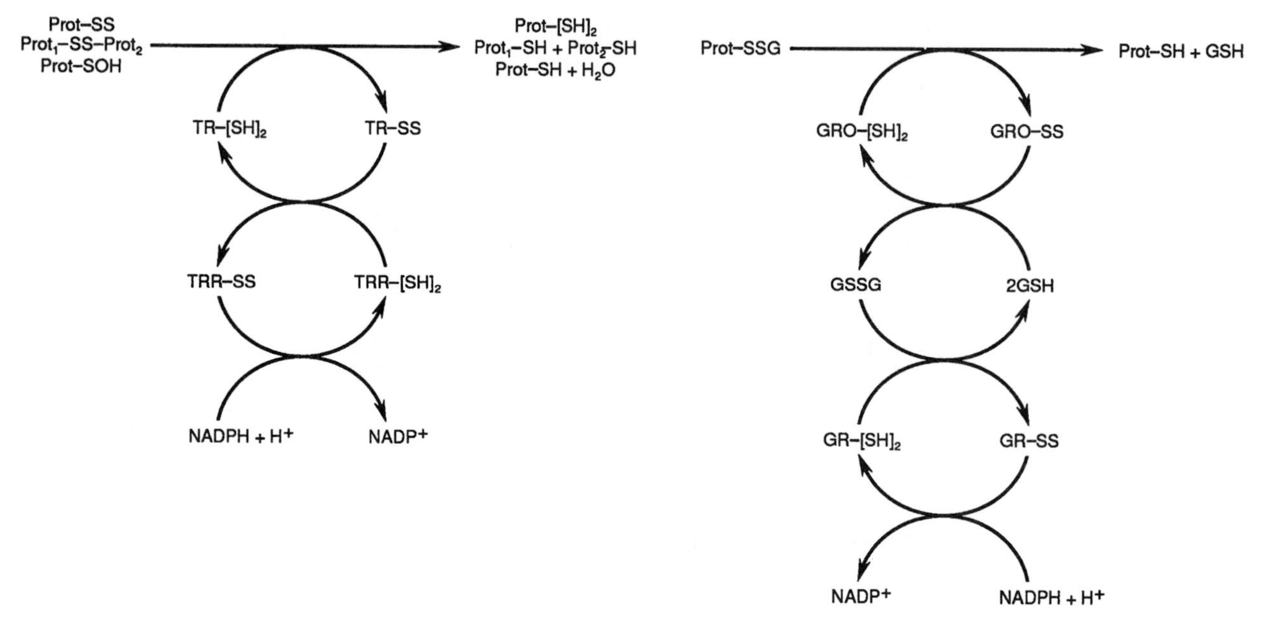


***Figure 3–15. Repair of proteins oxidized at their thiol groups.***

Protein disulfides (Prot-SS, $Prot_1$-SS-$Prot_2$) and protein sulfenic acids (Prot-SOH) are reduced by thioredoxin (TR-$[SH]_2$), whereas protein-glutathione mixed disulfides (Prot-SSG) are reduced by glutaredoxin (GRO-$[SH]_2$), which is also called thioltransferase. The figure also indicates how TR-$[SH]_2$ and GRO-$[SH]_2$ are regenerated from their disulfides (TR-SS and GRO-SS, respectively). In the mitochondria, TR-SS also can be regenerated by the dithiol dihydrolipoic acid, a component of the pyruvate- and $\alpha$-ketoglutarate dehydrogenase complexes. GSH = glutathione; GSSG = glutathione disulfide; GR-$[SH]_2$ and GR-SS = glutathione reductase (dithiol and disulfide forms, respectively); TRR-$[SH]_2$ and TRR-SS = thioredoxin reductase (dithiol and disulfide forms, respectively).

electrophiles, $O^6$-alkylguanine-DNA-alkyltransferase is consumed during the repair of DNA.

***Excision Repair.*** Base excision and nucleotide excision are two mechanisms for removing damaged bases from DNA (Fig. 8-13). Lesions that do not cause major distortion of the helix typically are removed by base excision, in which the altered base is recognized by a relatively substrate-specific DNA-glycosylase that hydrolyses the *N*-glycosidic bond, releasing the modified base and creating an apurinic or apyrimidinic (AP) site in the DNA. This site is recognized by the AP endonuclease that hydrolyses the phosphodiester bond adjacent to the abasic site. After its removal, the abasic sugar is replaced with the correct nucleotide by a DNA polymerase and is sealed in place by a DNA ligase.

Bulky lesions such as adducts produced by aflatoxins or aminofluorene derivatives and dimers caused by UV radiation are removed by nucleotide-excision repair. An ATP-dependent nuclease recognizes the distorted double helix and excises a number of intact nucleotides on both sides of the lesion, together with the one containing the adduct. The excised section of the strand is restored by insertion of nucleotides into the gap by DNA polymerase and ligase, using the complementary strand as a template. This phenomenon, designated "unscheduled DNA synthesis," can be detected by the appearance of altered deoxynucleosides in urine. Excision repair has a remarkably low error rate of less than 1 mistake in $10^9$ bases repaired.

Surveillance for damage by repair systems is not equally vigilant on the two DNA strands, and repair rates are not uniform for all genes (Scicchitano and Hanawalt, 1992). Actively transcribed genes are more rapidly repaired than are nontranscribed genes, and lesions in the transcribed strand that block RNA polymerase are more rapidly repaired than are lesions in the nontranscribed or coding strand. A protein termed transcription-repair coupling factor in *Escherichia coli* recognizes and displaces the RNA polymerase that has stalled at a DNA lesion, allowing access by the excision repair enzymes to the damage (Selby and Sancar, 1993).

***Recombinational (or Postreplication) Repair.*** Recombinational repair occurs when the excision of a bulky adduct or an intrastrand pyrimidine dimer fails to occur before DNA replication begins (Sancar and Sancar, 1988). At replication, such a lesion prevents DNA polymerase from polymerizing a daughter strand along a sizable stretch of the parent strand that carries the damage. The replication results in two homologous ("sister") yet dissimilar DNA duplexes: one that has a large postreplication gap in its daughter strand and an intact duplex synthesized at the opposite leg of the replication fork. This intact sister duplex is utilized to complete the postreplication gap in the damaged sister duplex. This is accomplished by recombination ("crossover") of the appropriate strands of the two homologous duplexes. After separation, the sister duplex that originally contained the gap carries in its daughter strand a section originating from the parent strand

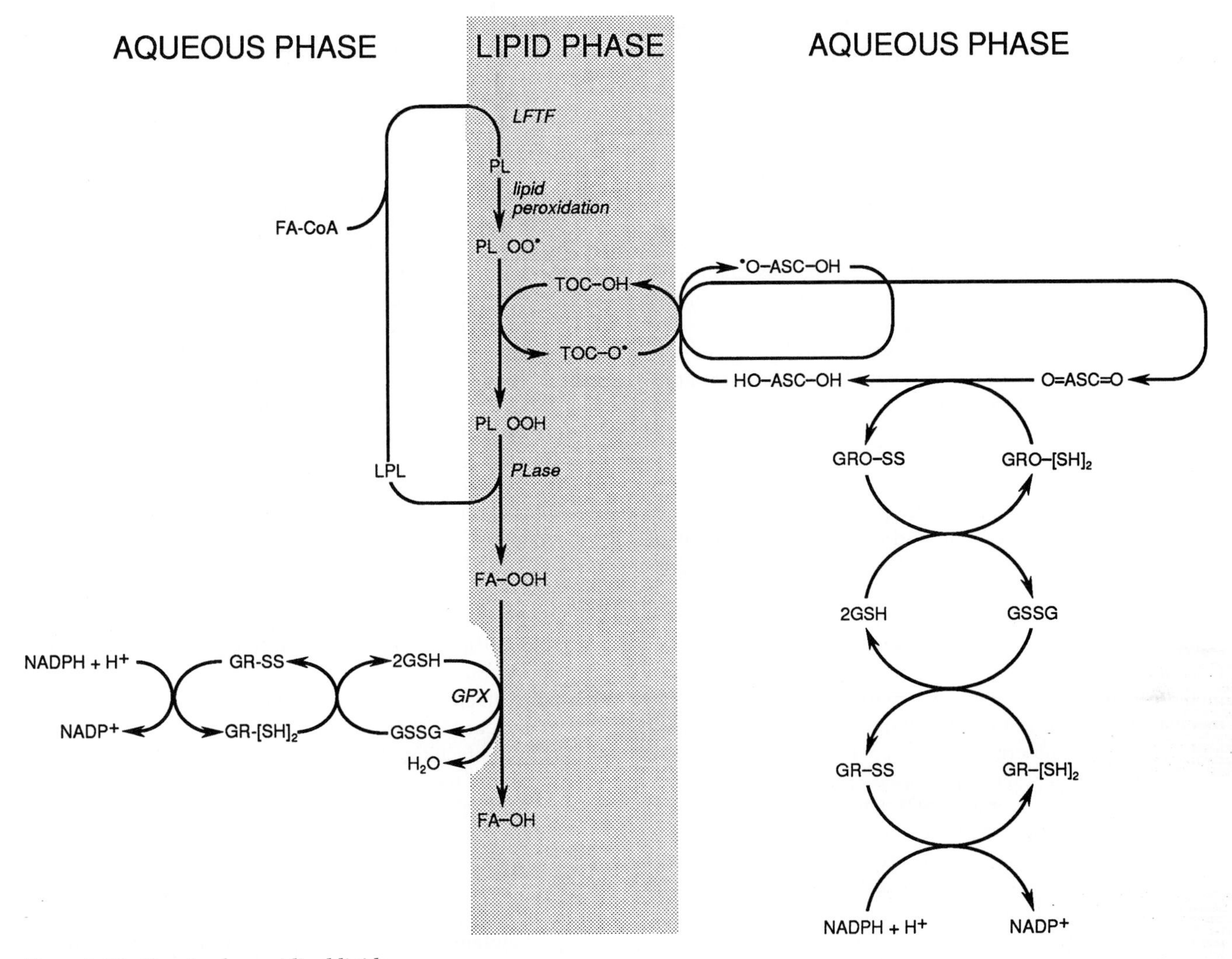


***Figure 3–16. Repair of peroxidized lipids.***

Phospholipid peroxyl radicals (PL-OO•) formed as a result of lipid peroxidation may abstract hydrogen from alpha-tocopherol (TOC-OH) and yield phospholipid hydroperoxide (PL-OOH). From the latter, the fatty acid carrying the hydroperoxide group is eliminated via hydrolysis catalyzed by phospholipase (PLase), yielding a fatty acid hydroperoxide (FA-OOH) and a lysophospholipid (LPL). The former is reduced to a hydroxy-fatty acid (FA-OH) by glutathione peroxidase (GPX), utilizing glutathione (GSH), whereas the latter is reacylated to phospholipid (PL) by lysophosphatide fatty acyl-coenzyme A transferase (LFTF), utilizing long-chain fatty acid–coenzyme A (FA-CoA). The figure also indicates regeneration of TOC-OH by ascorbic acid (HO-ASC-OH), regeneration of ascorbic acid from dehydroascorbic acid (O=ASC=O) by glutaredoxin (GRO-$[SH]_2$), and reduction of the oxidized glutaredoxin (GRO-SS) by GSH. Oxidized glutathione (GSSG) is reduced by glutathione reductase (GR-$[SH]_2$), which is regenerated from its oxidized form (GR-SS) by NADPH, the ultimate reductant. Most NADPH is produced during metabolism of glucose via the pentose phosphate shunt. TOC-O• = tocopheroxyl radical; •O-ASC-OH = ascorbyl radical.

of the intact sister, which in turn carries in its parent strand a section originating from the daughter strand of the damaged sister. This strand recombination explains the phenomenon of "sister chromatid exchange," which is indicative of DNA damage corrected by recombinational repair. This process also repairs double-strand breaks. A combination of excision and recombinational repairs occurs in restoration of DNA with interstrand cross-links. The process of recombinational repair at the molecular level has been partially characterized in *E. coli*. Much less is known about this process in eukaryotes.

## Cellular Repair: A Strategy in Peripheral Neurons

Repair of damaged cells is not a widely applied strategy in overcoming cellular injuries. In most tissues, injured cells die, with the survivors dividing to replace the lost cells. A notable exception is nerve tissue, because mature neurons have lost their ability to multiply. In peripheral neurons with axonal damage, repair does occur and requires macrophages and Schwann cells (Hall, 1989). Macrophages remove debris by phagocytosis and produce cytokines which activate Schwann cells to proliferate and produce nerve growth factor (NGF), express NGF receptors on their surface, and secrete neural cell adhesion molecules and extracellular matrix molecules. While comigrating with the regrowing axon, Schwann cells physically guide as well as chemically lure the axon to reinnervate the target cell.

In the mammalian central nervous system, axonal regrowth is prevented by growth inhibitory glycoproteins (e.g., NI-35, NI-250) produced by the oligodendrocytes and by the scar produced by astrocytes (Johnson, 1993). Thus, damage to central neurons is irreversible but is compensated for in part by the large number of reserve nerve cells that can take over the functions of lost neurons. For example, in Parkinson's disease, symptoms are not observed until there is at least an 80 percent loss of nigrostriatal neurons.

## Tissue Repair

In tissues with cells capable of multiplying, damage is reversed by deletion of the injured cells and regeneration of the tissue by proliferation. The damaged cells are eliminated by apoptosis or necrosis.

**Apoptosis: An Active Deletion of Damaged Cells.** Apoptosis and necrosis are two forms of cell death that are fundamentally different in terms of morphology, function, and mechanism. A cell destined for apoptosis shrinks; its nuclear and cytoplasmic materials condense, and then it breaks into membrane-bound fragments (apoptotic bodies) that are phagocytosed (Bursch et al., 1992). During necrosis, cells and intracellular organelles swell and desintegrate with membrane lysis. While apoptosis is orderly, necrosis is a disorderly process that ends with cell debris in the extracellular environment. The constituents of the necrotic cells attract aggressive inflammatory cells, and the ensuing inflammation amplifies cell injury. With apoptosis, dead cells are removed without inflammation.

While necrosis is passive, apoptosis is an active process, with gene activation necessary to direct the synthesis of proteins that aid in preparing the cell for programmed death. Apoptosis may be initiated by external signals or cell injury. Signal-induced apoptosis may be triggered by molecules that initiate the death program, such as glucocorticoids in thymocytes, or by the withdrawal of molecules that suppress apoptosis, such as uterotrophic placental hormones after birth (Bursch et al., 1992). Signal-induced apoptosis is a means for tissue remodeling and is of particular physiological importance during fetal development. It may also be exploited therapeutically to destroy malignant cells (Thompson, 1995). However, this mode of therapy may lead to toxicity by inducing involution in normal tissues as well.

While signal-induced apoptosis aids in tissue remodeling, apoptosis initiated by cell injury contributes to tissue repair. Damage to DNA appears to be a central event in triggering apoptosis in injured cells (Corcoran et al., 1994). Indeed, several agents that are known to react with DNA induce apoptosis. Included are ionizing radiation and drugs, such as alkylating agents, nucleoside analogues, and other drugs used in antitumor therapy. These substances exert both their desirable toxic effect against tumor cells and an undesirable cytotoxic effect against rapidly dividing normal cells such as hematopoetic and spermatogenic cells by inducing apoptosis. DNA-reactive toxicants and oxidative stress also induce apoptosis in cell culture. Moreover, necrogenic xenobiotics such as the hepatotoxin acetaminophen, 1,1-dichloroethylene, and thioacetamide, as well as the nephrotoxin ochratoxin, cause apoptosis early after exposure (Corcoran et al., 1994). Toxicants evoking apoptosis at low exposure levels or early after a high-dose exposure cause necrosis later at high exposure levels. Therefore, dysrepair of DNA, apoptosis, and necrosis appear to represent different stages of toxicity. When DNA repair mechanisms fail to cope with the damage, the cell initiates apoptosis. If cellular injury becomes so severe that it blocks the execution of this program, the apoptotic program is aborted and the cells are destroyed by necrosis. The significance of apoptosis after toxic cell injury is twofold: Apoptosis deletes injured cells without an aggressive inflammatory reaction, and deletion of cells with DNA damage prevents their malignant transformation.

While the mechanisms of apoptotic control are still being delineated, some important biochemical events have been characterized (Corcoran et al., 1994). These include the following:

1. The detachment of chromatin from the nuclear scaffold, leading to chromatin condensation.
2. Endonuclease-catalyzed hydrolysis of DNA at the internucleosomal linker regions into multimers of 180 base pairs which are visualized by electrophoresis as a "ladder" of nuclear DNA fragments. Access of the endonuclease to DNA is facilitated by depletion of polyamines, and the activity of the enzyme is increased by $Ca^{2+}$ and decreased by ADP-ribosylation. Thus, agents that increase intracellular $Ca^{2+}$ or inhibit poly(ADP-ribose) polymerase can induce apoptosis (Corcoran and Ray, 1992).
3. Apoptosis also is characterized by the induction of transglutaminase, an enzyme that cross-links proteins through $\varepsilon$-($\gamma$-glutamyl)lysine bonds and presumably contributes to the formation of membrane-bound apoptotic bodies.
4. Protein kinase A activation usually promotes, whereas protein kinase C activation retards, apoptosis.
5. Apoptotic cells increase synthesis of transforming growth factor-beta1, which blocks cell division and promotes apoptosis by interacting with its own membrane receptor (Bursch et al., 1992).
6. Cytotoxic T lymphocytes induce apoptosis of target cells by producing the Fas ligand, a signaling protein that activates Fas, a membrane receptor on potential target cells, including those of the liver, the heart, and the lungs (Nagata and Golstein, 1995).

Genetic control of apoptosis involves activation of the *c-myc* gene, which triggers passage of the differentiated resting cells from the $G_0$ to the $G_1$ phase of the cell cycle (Martin et al., 1994). The progression to S phase is blocked by activation of *p53*, a tumor-supressor gene. This blockade allocates time for DNA repair, but if the repair fails, the cell is diverted to the apoptotic pathway, presumably as a result of *bax* gene activation (Oltvai et al., 1993). In contrast, the *bcl-2* gene (a B-cell leukemia oncogene) blocks apoptosis, purportedly because the bcl-2 protein binds to the bax protein and inhibits its apoptogenic action (Oltvai et al., 1993). The molecular mechanisms of action of the proteins encoded by these genes are still unclear.

**Proliferation: Regeneration of Tissue.** Tissues are composed of various cells and the extracellular matrix. Tissue elements are anchored to each other by transmembrane proteins. Cadherins allow adjacent cells to adhere to one other, whereas connexins connect neighboring cells internally by association of these proteins into tubular structures (gap junctions). Integrins link cells to the extracellular matrix. Therefore, repair of injured tissues involves not only regeneration of lost cells and the extracellular matrix but also reintegration of the newly formed elements. In parenchymal organs such as liver, kidney, and lung, various types of cells are involved in the process of tissue restoration. Nonparenchymal cells of mesenchymal origin residing in the tissue, such as resident macrophages and endothelial cells, and those migrating to the site of injury, such as blood monocytes, produce factors that stimulate parenchymal cells to divide and stimulate some specialized cells (e.g., the perisinusoidal cells in the liver) to synthesize extracellular matrix molecules.

***Replacement of Lost Cells by Mitosis.*** Soon after injury, cells adjacent to the damaged area enter the cell division cycle (Fig. 3-17). Enhanced DNA synthesis is detected as an increase in the labeling index, which is the proportion of cells that incorporate $^{3}$H-thymidine or bromodeoxyuridine into their nuclear DNA during the S phase of the cycle. Also, mitotic cells can be observed microscopically. As early as 2 to 4 h after the administration of a low dose of carbon tetrachloride to rats, the mitotic index increases dramatically, indicating that cells already in the $G_2$ phase progress rapidly to the M phase (Calabrese et al., 1993). The mitotic activity of the hepatocytes culminates at 36 to 48 h, after a full transit through the cycle, indicating that quiescent cells residing in $G_0$ enter and progress to mitosis (M). Peak mitosis of nonparenchymal cells occurs later, after activation and replication of parenchymal cells (Burt, 1993). In some tissues, such as intestinal mucosa and bone marrow, stem cells first divide to provide self-renewal and then differentiate to replace more mature cells lost through injury. In an ozone-exposed lung, the damaged ciliated bronchial epithelial cells and type I pneumocytes are replaced by the nonciliated Clara cells and type II pneumocytes, respectively, which undergo mitosis and terminal differentiation (Mustafa, 1990).

Significant genetic alterations occur in cells that are destined to divide. Within minutes after injury, there is an increased expression of numerous genes. Among the so-called immediate-early growth response genes are those which code for TFs such as c-fos, c-jun and c-myc as well as cytokinelike secreted proteins (Mohn et al., 1991; Zawaski et al., 1993). These primary gene products amplify the initial gene activation process by stimulating other genes directly or through cell surface receptors and the coupled transducing networks (Fausto and Webber, 1993). Thus, the genetic expression is reprogrammed so that DNA synthesis and mitosis gain priority over specialized cellular activities. For example, as a result of dedifferentiation, regenerating hepatocytes underexpress cytochrome P-450 and hepatic perisinusoidal cells cease to accumulate fat and vitamin A.

It has been speculated that the regenerative process is initiated by the release of chemical mediators from damaged cells. The nonparenchymal cells, such as resident macrophages and endothelial cells, are receptive to these chemical signals and produce a host of secondary signaling molecules that promote and propagate the regenerative process (Fig. 3-18). One group of signaling molecules induces cell division. These mitogens, such as hepatocyte growth factor (HGF), or scatter factor, are especially important in tissue repair (Fausto, 1991). Despite its name, neither the formation nor the action of HGF is restricted to the liver. It is produced by resident macrophages and endothelial cells of various organs, including liver, lung, and kidney, and in a paracrine manner activates receptors on parenchymal cells. In rats intoxicated with carbon tetrachloride, the synthesis of HGF in hepatic and renal nonparenchymal cells increases markedly (Noji et al., 1990) and HGF levels in blood rise rapidly (Lindroos et al., 1991). The communication between parenchymal and nonparenchymal cells during tissue repair is mutual. For example, transforming growth factor-alpha (TGF-alpha), a potent mitogen produced by regenerating hepatocytes, acts both as an autocrine and a paracrine mediator on liver cells as well as on adjacent nonparenchymal cells.

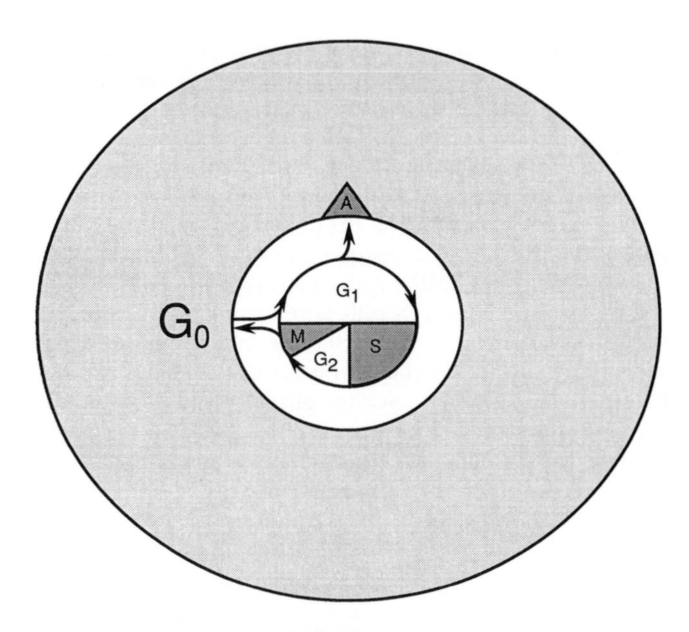


***Figure 3–17. The cell division cycle.***

Areas representing phases of the cycle are meant to be proportional to the number of cells in each phase. Normally, most cells are in $G_0$ phase, a differentiated and quiescent state. After receiving signals to divide, they progress into the $G_1$ phase of the cell division cycle. $G_0/G_1$ transition involves activation of immediate early genes so that cells acquire replicative competence. Now increasingly responsive to growth factors, these cells progress to the phase of DNA synthesis (S). If this progression is blocked (e.g., by expression of the tumor suppressor gene p53), the cells undergo apoptosis (A). After DNA replication, the cells prepare further for mitosis in the $G_2$ phase. During this phase there is a surge in the level of cyclins, proteins that activate cyclin-dependent kinases, which in turn activate proteins involved in mitosis (e.g., microtubular proteins of the mitotic apparatus). Mitosis (M) is the shortest phase of the cell cycle (approximately 40 min out of the 40-h-long cycle of hepatocytes) and most likely requires the largest energy expenditure per unit of time. The daughter cells produced may differentiate and enter into the pool of quiescent cells ($G_0$), substituting for those which had been lost. After tissue necrosis, the number of cells entering the cell division cycle markedly increases at areas adjacent to the injury. The proportion of cells that are in S phase in a given period is reflected by the labeling index, whereas the percentage of cells undergoing mitosis is the mitotic index (see text).

***Replacement of the Extracellular Matrix.*** The extracellular matrix is composed of proteins, glycosaminoglycans, and the glycoprotein and proteoglycan glycoconjugates (Gressner, 1992). In the liver, these molecules are synthesized by the perisinusoidal cells located in the space of Disse (Fig. 3-18). These cells are activated during liver regeneration by transforming growth factor-beta (TGF-beta) produced by the neighboring tissue macrophages residing in the hepatic sinusoids (Gressner, 1992). A dramatic increase in TGF-beta mRNA levels in Kupffer's cells is observed with in situ hybridization after carbon tetrachloride–induced hepatic necrosis (Burt, 1993). Another source of this mediator are the platelets that accumulate at sites of injury and degranulate, releasing stored TGF-beta. The TGF-beta acts on the perisinusoidal cells to stimulate the synthesis of extracellular matrix components, including collagens, fibronectin, tenascin, and proteoglycans. In addition, TGF-beta increases the synthesis of integrins, thus promoting reintegration of cells and the extracellular matrix into tissues. TGF-beta also plays a central role in extracellular matrix formation in the kidney and the lung, where its targets are the mesangial cells and the septal fibroblasts, respectively (Border and Ruoslahti, 1992).

The way in which tissue regeneration is terminated after repair is unclear, but the gradual dominance of TGF-beta, which is a potent antimitogen and apoptogen, over mitogens is a contributing factor in the termination of cell proliferation. Extracellular matrix production may be halted by products of the proliferative response that bind and inactivate TGF-beta. The proteoglycan decorin and the positive acute phase protein

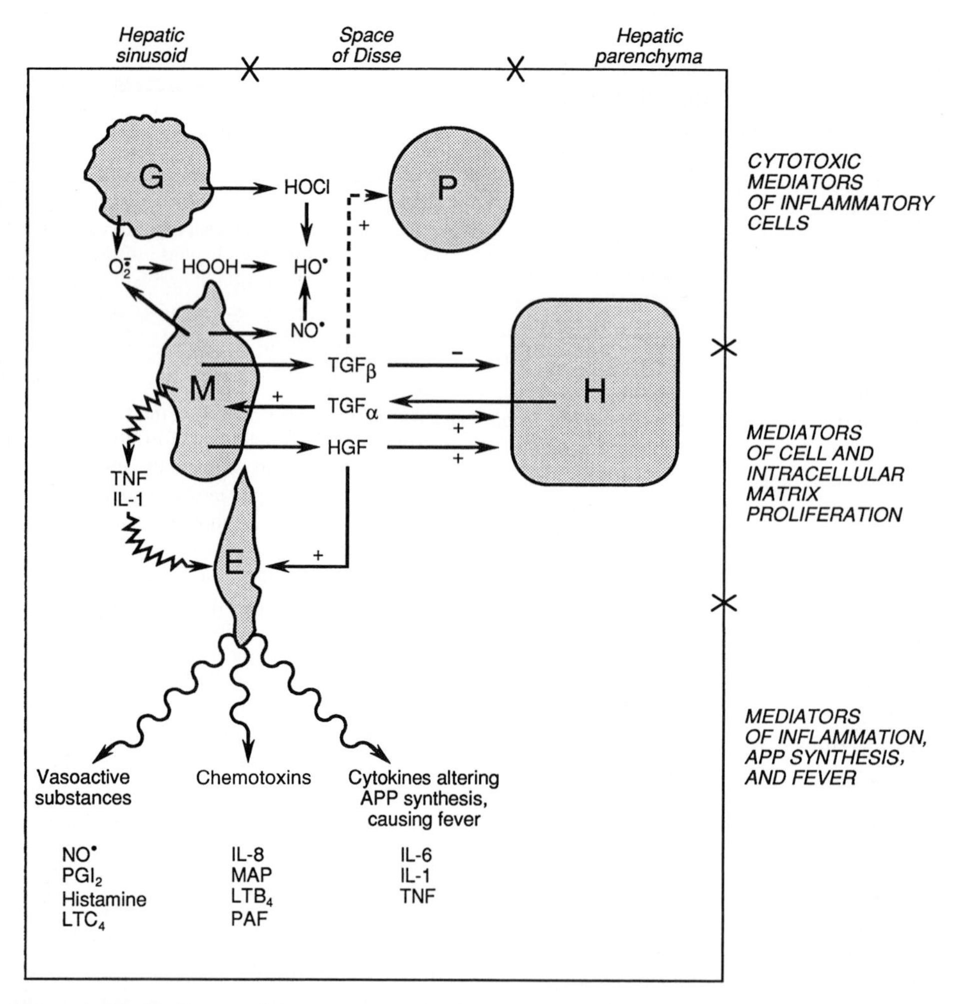


***Figure 3–18. Mediators of tissue repair and side reactions to tissue injury in liver: (1) growth factors promoting cell and extracellular matrix replacement, (2) mediators of inflammation, acute-phase protein (APP) synthesis, and fever, and (3) cytotoxic mediators of inflammatory cells.***

HGF = hepatocyte growth factor; TGF$\alpha$ = transforming growth factor-alpha, TGF$\beta$ = transforming growth factor-beta; NO• = nitric oxide; $PGI_2$ = prostacyclin; $LTC_4$ = leukotriene $C_4$; IL = interleukin; MAP = monocyte attractant protein; $LTB_4$ = leukotriene $B_4$; PAF = platelet-activating factor; TNF = tumor necrosis factor. Cells represented are E = endothelial cells; G = granulocyte; H = hepatocyte; M = macrophage (Kupffer's cell); P = perisinusoidal cell (also called Ito or fat-storing cell). Solid arrows represent effects of growth factors on cell division, whereas the dashed arrow shows the effect on extracellular matrix formation. Positive and negative signs indicate stimulation and inhibition, respectively. See text for further details.

alpha$_2$-macroglobulin are examples of such products (Gressner, 1992).

**Side Reactions to Tissue Injury.** In addition to mediators that aid in the replacement of lost cells and the extracellular matrix, resident macrophages and endothelial cells activated by cell injury also produce other mediators that induce ancillary reactions with uncertain benefit or harm to tissues (Fig. 3-18). Such reactions include inflammation, altered production of acute-phase proteins, and generalized reactions such as fever.

***Inflammation.*** Alteration of the microcirculation and accumulation of inflammatory cells are the hallmarks of inflammation. These processes are largely initiated by resident macrophages that secrete cytokines such as tumor necrosis factor (TNF) and interleukin-1 (IL-1) in response to tissue damage (Baumann and Gauldie, 1994) (Fig. 3-18). These cytokines in turn stimulate neighboring stromal cells, such as the endothelial cells and fibroblasts, to release mediators that induce dilation of the local microvasculature and cause permeabilization of capillaries. Activated endothelial cells also facilitate the egress of circulating leukocytes into the injured tissue by releasing chemotactic cytokines and lipid products as well as by expressing on their surface adhesion molecules, such as the intercellular adhesion molecule (ICAM). The invading leukocytes also synthesize mediators, propagating the inflammatory response.

Macrophages, as well as leukocytes, recruited to the site of injury undergo a respiratory burst, producing free radicals and hydrolytic enzymes (Weiss and LoBuglio, 1982) (Fig. 3-18). Free radicals, including the highly reactive hydroxyl radical ($HO^\bullet$), are produced in the inflammed tissue in three ways, each of which involves a specific enzyme: NAD(P)H oxidase, nitric oxide synthase, or myeloperoxidase.

During the respiratory burst, membrane-bound NAD(P)H oxidase is activated in both macrophages and granulocytes and produces superoxide anion radical ($O_2^{\bar{\bullet}}$) from molecular oxygen:

$$NAD(P)H + 2O_2 \rightarrow NAD(P)^+ + H^+ + 2\,O_2^{\bar{\bullet}}$$

The $O_2^{\bar{\bullet}}$ can give rise to the hydroxyl radical ($HO^\bullet$) in two sequential steps: The first is spontaneous or is catalyzed by superoxide dismutase, and the second, the Fenton reaction, is catalyzed by transition metal ions:

$$2O_2^{\bar{\bullet}} + 2H^+ \rightarrow O_2 + HOOH$$
$$HOOH + Fe^{2+} \rightarrow Fe^{3+} + HO^- + HO^\bullet$$

Macrophages, but not granulocytes, generate another cytotoxic free radical, nitric oxide ($NO^\bullet$). This radical is produced from arginine by nitric oxide synthase (Wang et al., 1993) that is inducible in macrophages by bacterial endotoxin and the cytokines IL-1 and TNF:

$$\text{L-arginine} + O_2 \rightarrow \text{L-citrulline} + NO^\bullet$$

Subsequently, $O_2^{\bar{\bullet}}$ and $NO^\bullet$, both of which are products of activated macrophages, can react with each other, yielding peroxynitrite anion, which upon protonation decays to nitrogen dioxide and hydroxyl radical:

$$O_2^{\bar{\bullet}} + NO^\bullet \rightarrow ONOO^-$$
$$ONOO^- + H^+ \rightleftarrows ONOOH$$
$$ONOOH \rightarrow NO_2^\bullet + HO^\bullet$$

Granulocytes, but not macrophages, discharge the lysosomal enzyme myeloperoxidase into engulfed extracellular spaces, the phagocytic vacuoles (Wang et al., 1993). Myeloperoxidase catalyzes the formation of hypochlorous acid (HOCl), a powerful oxidizing agent, from hydrogen peroxide (HOOH) and chloride ion:

$$HOOH + H^+ + Cl^- \rightarrow HOH + HOCl$$

Like HOOH, HOCl can form $HO^\bullet$ as a result of electron transfer from $Fe^{2+}$ or from $O_2^{\bar{\bullet}}$ to HOCl:

$$HOCl + O_2^{\bar{\bullet}} \rightarrow O_2 + Cl^- + HO^\bullet$$

All these reactive chemicals, as well as the discharged lysosomal proteases, are destructive products of inflammatory cells. Although these chemicals are responsible for antimicrobial activity at the site of injury, they also can damage the adjacent healthy tissue.

***Altered Protein Synthesis: Acute-Phase Proteins.*** Cytokines released from macrophages and endothelial cells of injured tissues also alter protein synthesis, predominantly in the liver (Baumann and Gauldie, 1994) (Fig. 3-18). Mainly interleukin-6 (IL-6) but also IL-1 and TNF act on cell surface receptors and increase or decrease the transcriptional activity of genes encoding certain proteins called positive and negative acute-phase proteins, respectively. Many of the hepatic acute-phase proteins, such as C-reactive protein, are secreted into the circulation, and their elevated levels in serum are diagnostic of tissue injury, inflammation, or neoplasm. Increased sedimentation of red blood cells, which is also indicative of these conditions, is due to enrichment of blood plasma with positive acute-phase proteins such as fibrinogen.

Apart from their diagnostic value, positive acute-phase proteins may play roles in minimizing tissue injury and facilitating repair. For example, many of them, such as alpha$_2$-macroglobulin and alpha$_1$-antiprotease, inhibit lysosomal proteases released from the injured cells and recruited leukocytes. Haptoglobin binds hemoglobin in blood, metallothionein complexes metals in the cells, heme oxygenase oxidizes heme to biliverdin, and opsonins facilitate phagocytosis. Thus, these positive acute-phase proteins may be involved in the clearance of substances released upon tissue injury.

Negative acute-phase proteins include some plasma proteins, such as albumin, transthyretin, and transferrin, as well as several forms of cytochrome P-450 and glutathione *S*-transferases. Because the latter enzymes play important roles in the toxication and detoxication of xenobiotics, the disposition and toxicity of chemicals may be altered markedly during the acute phase of tissue injury.

Although the acute-phase response is phylogenetically preserved, some of the acute-phase proteins are somewhat species-specific. For example, during the acute phase of tissue injury or inflammation, C-reactive protein and serum amyloid A levels dramatically increase in humans but not in rats, whereas the concentrations of alpha$_1$-acid glycoprotein and alpha$_2$-macroglobulin increase markedly in rats but only moderately in humans.

***Generalized Reactions.*** Cytokines released from activated macrophages and endothelial cells at the site of injury also may evoke neurohormonal responses. Thus IL-1, TNF, and IL-6 alter the temperature set point of the hypothalamus, triggering fever. IL-1 possibly also mediates other generalized reactions to tissue injury, such as hypophagia, sleep, and "sickness behavior" (Rothwell, 1991). In addition, IL-1 and IL-6 act on the pituitary to induce the release of ACTH, which in turn stimulates the secretion of cortisol from the adrenals. This represents a negative feedback loop because corticosteroids inhibit cytokine gene expression.

## When Repair Fails

Although repair mechanisms operate at molecular, cellular, and tissue levels, for various reasons they often fail to provide protection against injury. First, the fidelity of the repair mechanisms is not absolute, making it possible for some lesions to be overlooked. However, repair fails most typically when the damage overwhelms the repair mechanisms, such as when protein thiols are oxidized faster than they can be reduced. In other instances, the capacity of repair may become exhausted when necessary enzymes or cofactors are consumed. For example, alkylation of DNA may lead to consumption of $O^6$-alkylguanine-DNA-alkyltransferase (Pegg and Byers, 1992), and lipid peroxidation can deplete alpha-tocopherol. Sometimes the toxicant-induced injury adversely affects the repair process itself. Thus, after exposure to necrogenic chemicals, mitosis of surviving cells may be blocked and restoration of the tissue becomes impossible (Calabrese et al., 1993). Finally, some types of toxic injuries cannot be repaired effectively, as occurs when xenobiotics are covalently bound to proteins. Thus, toxicity is manifested when repair of the initial injury fails because the repair mechanisms become overwhelmed, exhausted, or impaired or are genuinely inefficient.

It is also possible that repair contributes to toxicity. This may occur in a passive manner, for example, if excessive amounts of NAD(P)H are consumed for the repair of oxidized proteins and endogenous reductants. This compromises oxidative phosphorylation, which is also dependent on the supply of reduced cofactors (see Fig. 3-11), thus causing or aggravating ATP depletion, an event that contributes to cell injury. Excision repair of DNA, degradation of damaged proteins by the ATP/ubiquitin-dependent proteases, and reacylation of lipids also contribute to cellular deenergization and injury by consuming significant amounts of ATP. However, repair also may play an active role in toxicity. This is observed after chronic tissue injury, when the repair process goes astray and leads to uncontrolled proliferation instead of tissue remodeling. Such proliferation may yield neoplasia or fibrosis.

## Toxicity Resulting from Dysrepair

Like repair, dysrepair occurs at the molecular, cellular, and tissue levels. Some toxicities involve dysrepair at an isolated level. For example, hypoxemia develops after exposure to methemoglobin-forming chemicals if the amount of methemoglobin produced overwhelms the capacity of methemoglobin reductase. Because this repair enzyme is deficient at early ages, neonates are especially sensitive to chemicals that cause methemoglobinemia. Formation of cataracts purportedly involves inefficiency or impairment of lenticular repair enzymes which normally reduce oxidized crystallins and hydrolyze damaged proteins to their constituent amino acids such as the endo- and exopeptidases. Dysrepair also is thought to contribute to the formation of Heinz bodies, which also are protein aggregates, in oxidatively stressed and aged red blood cells.

Several types of toxicity involve multiple failed and/or derailed repairs at different levels before they become apparent. This is true for the most severe toxic injuries, such as tissue necrosis, fibrosis, and chemical carcinogenesis.

**Tissue Necrosis.** As was discussed above, several mechanisms may lead to cell death. Most, if not all, involve molecular damage that is potentially reversible by repair mechanisms. If repair mechanisms operate effectively, they may prevent cell injury or at least retard its progression. For example, prooxidant toxicants cause no lipid fragmentation in microsomal membranes until alpha-tocopherol is depleted in those membranes. Membrane damage ensues when this endogenous antioxidant, which can repair lipids with peroxyl radical groups, becomes unavailable (Scheschonka et al., 1990). This suggests that cell injury progresses toward cell necrosis if molecular repair mechanisms are inefficient or the molecular damage is not readily reversible.

Progression of cell injury to tissue necrosis can be intercepted by two repair mechanisms working in concert: apoptosis and cell proliferation. As was discussed above, injured cells can initiate apoptosis, which counteracts the progression of the toxic injury. Apoptosis does this by preventing necrosis of injured cells and consequently the inflammatory response, which may cause injury by releasing cytotoxic mediators. Indeed, activation of the Kupffer's cells, the source of such mediators in the liver, by the administration of bacterial lipopolysaccharide (endotoxin) greatly aggravates the hepatotoxicity of galactosamine. In contrast, when the Kupffer's cells are selectively eliminated by pretreatment of rats with gadolinium chloride, the necrotic effect of carbon tetrachloride is markedly alleviated (Edwards et al., 1993).

Another important repair process that can halt the propagation of toxic injury is proliferation of cells adjacent to the injured cells. This response is initiated soon after cellular injury. A surge in mitosis in the liver of rats administered a low (nonnecrogenic) dose of carbon tetrachloride is detectable within a few hours. This early cell division is thought to be instrumental in the rapid and complete restoration of the injured tissue and the prevention of necrosis. This hypothesis is corroborated by the finding that in rats pretreated with chlordecone, which blocks the early cell proliferation in response to carbon tetrachloride, a normally nonnecrogenic dose of carbon tetrachloride causes hepatic necrosis (Calabrese et al., 1993).

It appears that the efficiency of repair is an important determinant of the dose-response relationship for toxicants that cause tissue necrosis. That is, tissue necrosis is caused by a certain dose of a toxicant not only because that dose ensures sufficient concentration of the ultimate toxicant at the target site but also because that quantity of toxicant causes a degree of damage sufficient to compromise repair, allowing for progression of the injury. Experimental observations with hepatotoxicants indicate that apoptosis and cell proliferation are operative with latent tissue injury caused by low (nonnecrogenic) doses of toxicants but are inhibited with severe injury induced by high (necrogenic) doses. For example, 1,1-dichloroethylene, carbon tetrachloride, and thioacetamide all induce apoptosis in the liver at low doses but cause hepatic necrosis after high-dose exposure (Corcoran and Ray, 1992). Similarly, there is an early mitotic response in the liver to low-dose carbon tetrachloride, but this response is absent after administration of the solvent at necrogenic doses (Calabrese et al., 1993). This suggests that tissue necrosis occurs because the injury overwhelms and disables the repair mechanisms, including (1) repair of damaged molecules, (2) elimination of damaged cells by apoptosis, and (3) replacement of lost cells by cell division.

**Fibrosis.** Fibrosis is a pathological condition characterized by excessive deposition of an extracellular matrix of abnormal composition. Hepatic fibrosis, or cirrhosis, results from chronic consumption of ethanol or intoxication with hepatic necrogens such as carbon tetrachloride and iron. Pulmonary fibrosis is induced by drugs such as bleomycin and amiodarone and prolonged inhalation of oxygen or mineral particles. Adriamycin may cause cardiac fibrosis, whereas exposure to ionizing radiation induces fibrosis in many organs. Most of these agents generate free radicals and cause chronic cell injury.

Dysrepair is a major contributing factor to fibrosis. As was discussed previously, cellular injury initiates a surge in cellular proliferation and extracellular matrix production which normally ceases when the injured tissue is remodeled. If increased production of extracellular matrix is not halted, fibrosis develops.

Overproduction of the extracellular matrix is controlled by cytokines produced by nonparenchymal cells. TGF-beta appears to be the major mediator of fibrogenesis, although other factors, such as TNF and platelet-derived growth factor, also may be involved (Border and Ruoslahti, 1992). Indeed, subcutaneous injection of TGF-beta induces local fibrosis, whereas TGF-beta antagonists such as anti-TGF-beta immunoglobulin and decorin ameliorate experimental fibrogenesis. In several types of experimental fibrosis and in patients with active liver cirrhosis, overexpression of TGF-beta in affected tissues has been demonstrated. The increased expression of TGF-beta is a common response mediating regeneration of the extracellular matrix after an acute injury. However, while TGF-beta production ceases when repair is complete, this does not occur when tissue injury leads to fibrosis. Failure to halt TGF-beta overproduction could be caused by continuous injury or a defect in the regulation of TGF-beta.

The fibrotic action of TGF-beta is due to (1) stimulation of the synthesis of individual matrix components by specific target cells and (2) inhibition of matrix degradation by decreasing the synthesis of metalloproteinases and increasing the level of tissue inhibitors of metalloproteinases (Burt, 1993). Interestingly, TGF-beta induces transcription of its own gene in target cells, suggesting that the TGF-beta produced by these cells can amplify in an autocrine manner the production of the extracellular matrix. This positive feedback may facilitate fibrogenesis (Border and Ruoslahti, 1992).

Fibrosis involves not only excessive accumulation of the extracellular matrix but also changes in its composition. The basement membrane components, such as collagen IV and laminin, as well as collagen I, which confers rigidity to tissues, increase disproportionately during fibrogenesis (Gressner, 1992).

Fibrosis is detrimental in a number of ways:

1. The scar compresses and may ultimately obliterate the parenchymal cells and blood vessels.
2. Deposition of basement membrane components between the capillary endothelial cells and the parenchymal cells presents a diffusional barrier which contributes to the malnutrition of the tissue cells.
3. An increased amount and rigidity of the extracellular matrix unfavorably affect the elasticity and flexibility of the whole tissue, compromising the mechanical function of organs such as the heart and lungs.
4. Furthermore, the altered extracellular environment is sensed by integrins. Through these transmembrane proteins, fibrosis may modulate several aspects of cell behavior, including polarity, motility, and gene expression (Burt, 1993; Raghow, 1994).

**Carcinogenesis.** Chemical carcinogenesis involves multiple failures and the malfunction of various repair mechanisms, including (1) failure of DNA repair, (2) failure of apoptosis, and (3) failure to terminate cell proliferation.

***Failure of DNA Repair: Mutation, the Initiating Event in Carcinogenesis.*** Chemical and physical insults may induce neoplastic transformation of cells by genotoxic and nongenotoxic mechanisms. Chemicals that react with DNA may cause damage such as adduct formation, oxidative alteration, and strand breakage (Fig. 3-19). In most cases, these lesions are repaired or injured cells are eliminated. If neither event occurs, a lesion in the parental DNA strand may induce a heritable alteration, or mutation, in the daughter strand during replication. The mutation may remain silent if it does not alter the protein encoded by the mutant gene or if the mutation causes an amino acid substitution that does not affect the function of the protein. Alternatively, the genetic alteration may be incompatible with cell survival. The most unfortunate scenario for the organism occurs when the altered genes express mutant proteins that reprogram cells for growth and multiplication. When such cells survive and undergo mitosis, their descendants also have a similar propensity for proliferation. Moreover, because enhanced cell division increases the likelihood of mutations, these cells eventually acquire additional mutations that may further increase their growth advantage over their normal counterparts. The final outcome of this process is a nodule, followed by a tumor consisting of transformed rapidly proliferating cells (Fig. 3-19).

The critical role of DNA repair in preventing carcinogenesis is examplified by the human heritable disease xeroderma pigmentosum. Affected individuals exhibit deficient excision repair and a greatly increased incidence of sunlight-induced squamous cell carcinomas and other skin cancers. Cells from these patients are also hypersensitive to DNA-reactive chemicals, including aflatoxin $B_1$, aromatic amines, polycyclic hydrocarbons, and 4-nitroquinoline-1-oxide (Lehmann and Dean, 1990).

A small set of cellular genes are the targets for genetic alterations that initiate neoplastic transformations. Included are proto-oncogenes and tumor suppressor genes (Barrett, 1992).

*Mutation of Proto-Oncogenes.* Proto-oncogenes are highly conserved genes encoding proteins that stimulate the

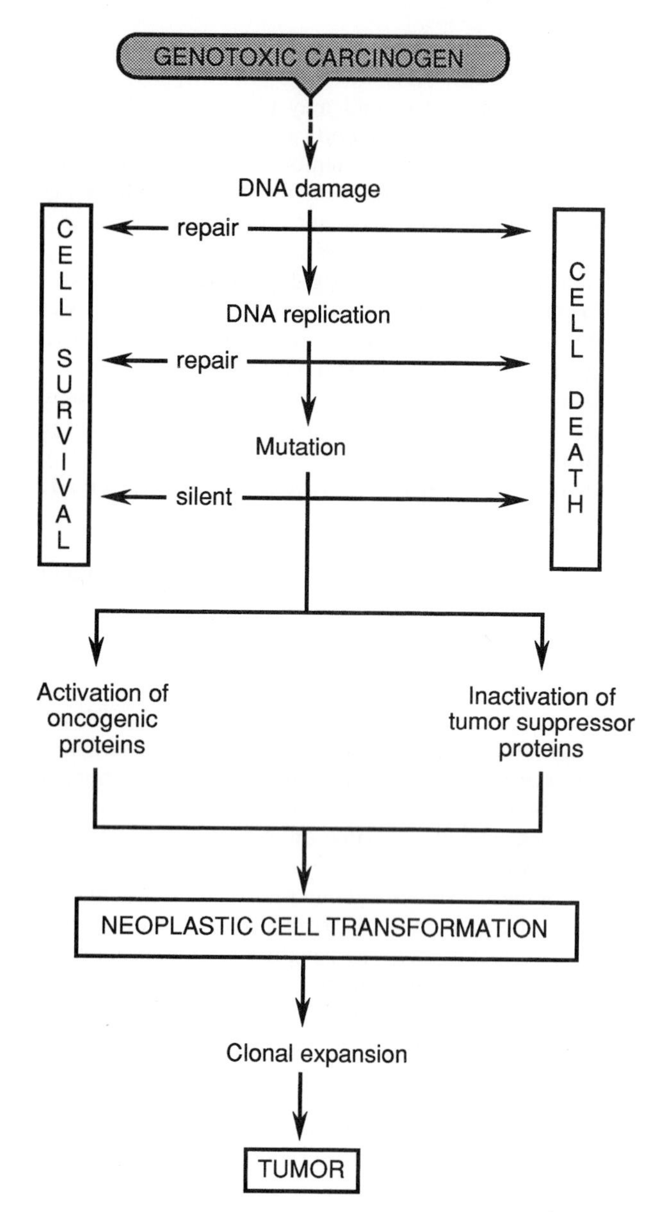


***Figure 3–19. The process of carcinogenesis initiated by genotoxic carcinogens (see text for explanation).***

progression of cells through the cell cycle (Smith et al., 1993). The products of proto-oncogenes include (1) growth factors, (2) growth factor receptors, (3) intracellular signal transducers such as G proteins and protein kinases, and (4) nuclear transcription factors. Transient increases in the production or activity of proto-oncogene proteins are required for regulated growth such as what occurs during embryogenesis, tissue regeneration, and stimulation of cells by growth factors or hormones. In contrast, permanent activation and/or overexpression of these proteins favors neoplastic transformation. Genotoxic carcinogens typically induce mutation of proto-oncogenes, with the mutant gene, then termed an oncogene, encoding a mutant protein. If this protein gains increased activity, it can initiate neoplastic transformation of the cell. An example of mutational activation of an oncogene protein is that of the Ras proteins.

Ras proteins represent a family of 21,000-dalton proteins (p21) with GTP/GDP binding capacity as well as GTPase activity (Anderson et al., 1992). They are localized on the inner surface of the plasma membrane and function as crucial mediators in responses initiated by growth factors. Ras is located downstream from growth factor receptors and nonreceptor protein tyrosine kinases and upstream from the cascade of kinases that includes Raf, mitogen-activated protein kinase kinase (MAPKK), and mitogen-activated protein kinase (MAPK). In this pathway, Ras serves as a molecular switch, being active in the GTP-bound form and inactive in the GDP-bound form. Mutation of a *ras* gene activates its product. For example, a point mutation in codon 12 of the gene changes amino acid 12 in the protein, resulting in dramatically lowered GTPase activity. This in turn locks Ras in the permanently active GTP-bound form. Continual rather than signal-dependent activation of Ras can lead eventually to uncontrolled proliferation and transformation. Indeed, microinjection of Ras-neutralizing monoclonal antibodies into cells blocks the mitogenic action of growth factors as well as cell transformation by several oncogenes. Numerous carcinogenic agents induce mutations of *ras* proto-oncogenes that lead to constitutive activation of Ras proteins (Anderson et al., 1992). These include *N*-methyl-*N*-nitrosourea, polycyclic aromatic hydrocarbons, benzidine, aflatoxin $B_1$, and ionizing radiation. Most of these agents induce point mutations by transversion of $G_{35}$ to T in codon 12.

While mutation-induced constitutive activation of oncogene proteins is a common mechanism in chemical carcinogenesis, overexpression of such proteins also can contribute to neoplastic cell transformation. This may result from (1) an alteration of the regulatory region of proto-oncogenes (e.g., by hypomethylation or translocation) and (2) amplification of the proto-oncogene (Anderson et al., 1992). Gene amplification (i.e., the formation of more than one copy) may be initiated by DNA strand breaks and therefore commonly results from exposure to ionizing radiation.

*Mutations of Tumor Suppressor Genes.* Tumor suppressor genes encode proteins which inhibit the progression of cells in the division cycle. Uncontrolled proliferation can occur when the mutant tumor suppressor gene encodes a protein which cannot suppress cell division. Inactivating mutations of specific tumor suppressor genes in germ cells are responsible for the inherited predisposition to cancer, as in familial retinoblastoma, Wilms' tumor, familial polyposis, and Li-Fraumeni syndrome (Levine et al., 1994). Mutations of tumor suppressor genes in somatic cells contribute to nonhereditary cancers. The best known tumor suppressor gene involved in both spontaneous and chemically induced carcinogenesis is *p53*.

The *p53* tumor suppressor gene encodes a 53,000-dalton protein with dual functions (Levine et al., 1994). First, it is a transcription factor increasing the rate of transcription of genes which possess p53 response elements in their regulatory regions, such as the growth arrest and DNA damage-inducible *gadd45* gene, as well as the apoptogenic *bax* gene (Zhan et al., 1994; Miyashita and Reed, 1995). Second, p53 protein binds to the TATA-binding protein, inhibiting the transcriptional activity of many genes that do not contain the p53 response element. Through unknown mechanisms, p53 arrests cell growth in the $G_1$ phase, allowing time for DNA repair. In addition, p53 promotes apoptosis. In this way, p53 counteracts the accumulation of genetic errors and inhibits the process leading to neoplastic transformation (Fig. 3-19). Indeed, cells that have no p53 are a million times more likely to permit DNA amplification than are cells with a normal level of the suppressor gene. Furthermore, transgenic mice missing the *p53* gene develop cancer by 6 to 9 months of age. These observations attest to the crucial role of the *p53* tumor suppressor gene in preventing carcinogenesis.

Mutations in the *p53* gene are found in a variety of induced cancers. The majority are "missense mutations" that change an amino acid and result in a faulty or altered protein (Harris, 1993). The faulty p53 protein forms a complex with endogenous wild-type p53 protein and inactivates it. Thus, the mutant p53 not only is unable to function as a tumor suppressor protein but also prevents tumor suppression by the wild-type p53. Moreover, some observations suggest that the mutant p53 can actively promote cell proliferation, much as an oncogene protein does.

Different carcinogens cause different mutations in the *p53* tumor suppressor gene. An example is the point mutation in codon 249 from AGG to AGT that changes amino acid 249 in the p53 protein from arginine to serine. This mutation predominates in hepatocellular carcinomas in individuals in regions where food is contaminated with aflatoxin $B_1$ (Harris, 1993). Because aflatoxin $B_1$ induces the transversion of G to T in codon 249 of the *p53* tumor suppressor gene in human hepatocytes (Aguilar et al., 1993), it appears likely that this mutation is indeed induced by this mycotoxin. Although the detected mutation in patients presumably contributes to the hepatocarcinogenecity of aflatoxin $B_1$ in humans, it is not required for aflatoxin $B_1$–induced hepatocarcinogenesis in rats, as rats do not show this aberration in the transformed liver cells.

*Cooperation of Proto-Oncogenes and Tumor Suppressor Genes in Carcinogenesis.* The accumulation of genetic damage in the form of (1) mutant proto-oncogenes (which encode activated proteins) and (2) mutant tumor suppressor genes (which encode inactivated proteins) is the main driving force in the transformation of normal cells with controlled proliferative activity to malignant cells with uncontrolled proliferative activity. Because the number of cells in a tissue is regulated by a balance between mitosis and apoptosis, the uncontrolled proliferation results from perturbation of this balance (Fig. 3-20).

***Failure of Apoptosis: Promotion of Mutation and Clonal Growth.*** In response to DNA damage caused by UV or gamma irradiation or genotoxic chemicals, the levels of p53 protein in cells are increased dramatically (fivefold to 60-fold) (Levine et al., 1994). The high p53 protein levels block the progression of cells in the $G_1$ phase and allow DNA repair to occur before replication or induce cell death by apoptosis. Consequently, apoptosis eliminates cells with DNA damage, preventing mutation, the initiating event in carcinogenesis.

Preneoplastic cells, or cells with mutations, have much higher apoptotic activity than do normal cells (Bursch et al., 1992). Therefore, apoptosis counteracts clonal expansion of the initiated cells and tumor cells. In fact, facilitation of apoptosis can induce tumor regression. This occurs when hormone-dependent tumors are deprived of the hormone that promotes growth and suppresses apoptosis. This is the rationale for the use of tamoxifen, an antiestrogen, and gonadotrophin-releasing-hormone analogues to combat hormone-dependent tumors of the mammary gland and the prostate gland, respectively (Bursch et al., 1992).

Thus, the inhibition of apoptosis is detrimental because it facilitates both mutations and clonal expansion of preneoplastic cells. Indeed, inhibition of apoptosis plays a role in the pathogenesis of human B-cell lymphomas. In this malignancy, a chromosomal translocation brings together the *bcl-2* gene and the immunoglobulin heavy-chain locus, resulting in aberrantly increased *bcl-2* gene expression. Overexpression of the *bcl-2* gene is oncogenic because its product overrides programmed cell death (McDonnell et al., 1993).

Inhibition of apoptosis is one mechanism by which phenobarbital, a tumor promoter, promotes clonal expansion of preneoplastic cells. This has been demonstrated in rats given a single dose of *N*-nitrosomorpholine followed by daily treatments with phenobarbital for 12 months to initiate and promote, respectively, neoplastic transformation in liver (Schulte-Hermann et al., 1990). From 6 months onward, phenobarbital did not increase DNA synthesis and cell division in the preneoplastic foci, yet it accelerated foci enlargement. The foci grow because phenobarbital lowers apoptotic activity, allowing the high cell replicative activity to manifest itself. The peroxysome proliferator nafenopin, a nongenotoxic hepatocarginogen, also suppresses apoptosis in primary rat hepatocyte cultures (Bayley et al., 1994), supporting the hypothesis that this mechanism may play a role in the hepatocarcinogenicity of peroxisome proliferators in rodents.

***Failure to Terminate Proliferation: Promotion of Mutation, Proto-Oncogene Expression, and Clonal Growth.*** Enhanced mitotic activity, whether it is induced by oncogenes inside the cell or by external factors such as xenobiotic or endogenous mitogens, promotes carcinogenesis for a number of reasons.

1. First, the enhanced mitotic activity increases the probability of mutations. This is due to activation of the cell division cycle which invokes a substantial shortening of the $G_1$ phase. Thus, less time is available for the repair of injured DNA before replication, increasing the chance that the damage will yield a mutation. Although repair still may be feasible after replication, postreplication repair is error-prone. In addition, activation of the cell division cycle increases the proportion of cells that replicate their DNA at any given time. During replication, the amount of DNA doubles and the DNA becomes unpacked, greatly increasing the effective target size for DNA-reactive mutagenic agents.
2. During increased proliferation, proto-oncogenes are overexpressed. These overproduced proto-oncogene proteins may cooperate with oncogene proteins to facilitate the neoplastic transformation of cells. In addition, enhanced mitotic activity indirectly enhances the transcriptional activity of proto-oncogenes and oncogenes by allowing less time for DNA methylation, which occurs in the early postreplication period. Methylation takes place at $C_5$ of specific cytosine residues in the regulatory region of genes and decreases the transcriptional activity of genes by inhibiting the interaction of transcription factors with the regulatory (promoter) region. Nonexpressed genes are

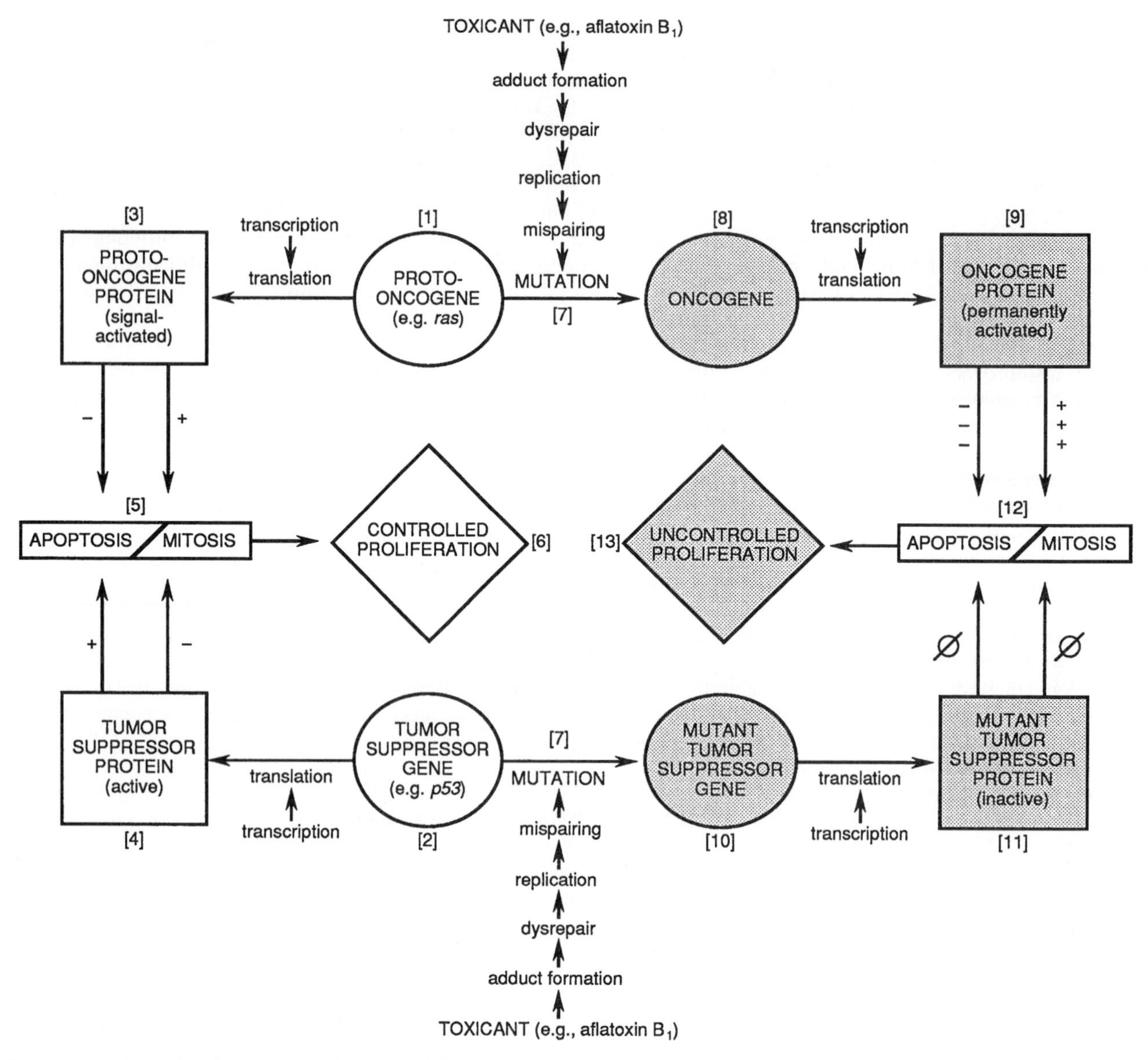


***Figure 3–20. A model of cooperation between a proto-oncogene (1) and a tumor suppressor gene (2) before and after mutation.***

The model shows that the normal proteins encoded by the cellular proto-oncogenes and the tumor suppressor genes [(3) and (4), respectively] reciprocally influence mitosis and apoptosis (5) and thus ensure controlled cell proliferation (6). However, the balance between the effects of these two types of proteins is offset by a toxicant-induced mutation of their genes (7) if the mutant proto-oncogene (oncogene) (8) encodes a constitutively (i.e., permanently) active oncogene protein (9) and the mutant tumor suppressor gene (10) encodes an inactive tumor suppressor protein (11). Under this condition, the effect of the oncogene protein on mitosis and apoptosis is unopposed (12), resulting in uncontrolled proliferation. Such a scenario may underlie the carcinogenicity of aflatoxin $B_1$, which can induce mutations in *ras* proto-oncogenes, and the *p53* tumor suppressor gene (see text for details). Positive and negative signs represent stimulation and inhibition, respectively; Ø means "no effect."

fully methylated. Hypomethylation of DNA, in contrast, enhances gene expression and may result in overexpression of proto-oncogenes and oncogenes. A "methyl-deficient diet" and ethionine, which deplete *S*-adenosylmethionine, induce hypomethylation of DNA and cancer, confirming the role of DNA hypomethylation in carcinogenesis (Poirier, 1994).

3. Another mechanism by which proliferation promotes the carcinogenic process is through clonal expansion of the initiated cells to form nodules (foci) and tumors.
4. Finally, cell-to-cell communication through gap junctions and intercellular adhesion through cadherins are temporarily disrupted during proliferation (Yamasaki et al., 1993). Lack of these junctions contributes to the invasive-

ness of tumor cells. Several tumor promoters, such as phenobarbital, phorbol esters, and peroxisome proliferators, decrease gap junctional intercellular communication. It has been hypothesized that this contributes to neoplastic transformation. It is unclear, however, whether diminished gap junctional communication plays a significant causative role in carcinogenesis or is merely a symptom of cell proliferation.

***Nongenotoxic Carcinogens: Promoters of Mitosis and Inhibitors of Apoptosis.*** A number of chemicals cause cancer by altering DNA and inducing a mutation. However, other chemicals do not alter DNA or induce mutations yet induce cancer after chronic administration (Barrett, 1992). These chemicals are designated nongenotoxic or epigenetic carcinogens and include (1) xenobiotic mitogens (e.g., phenobarbital, phorbol esters, DDT, peroxisomal proliferators), (2) endogenous mitogens such as growth factors (e.g., TGF-alpha) and hormones with mitogenic action on specific cells [e.g., estrogens on mammary gland or liver cells, TSH on the follicular cells of the thyroid gland, and luteinizing hormone (LH) on Leydig cells in testes], and (3) chemicals which when given chronically cause sustained cell injury (such as chloroform and *d*-limonene). Because several of these agents promote the development of tumors after neoplastic transformation has been initiated by a genotoxic carcinogen, they are referred to as tumor promoters. Despite the initial belief that promoters are unable to induce tumors by themselves, studies suggest that they can after prolonged exposure.

Nongenotoxic carcinogens cause cancer by promoting carcinogenesis initiated by genotoxic agents or spontaneous DNA damage (Fig. 3-21). Spontaneous DNA damage, some of which give rise to mutation, commonly occurs in normal cells (Barrett, 1992). The spontaneous mutation frequency per base pair in human cells is estimated to be in the range of $10^{-8}$ to $10^{-10}$. Genotoxic carcinogens increase the frequency tenfold to 1000-fold. Nongenotoxic carcinogens also increase the frequency of spontaneous mutations through a mitogenic effect and by the mechanisms discussed earlier. In addition, nongenotoxic carcinogens, by inhibiting apoptosis, increase the number of cells with DNA damage and mutations. Both enhanced mitotic activity and decreased apoptotic activity brought about by nongenotoxic carcinogens expand the population of transformed cells, promoting cancer development. In summary, nongenotoxic carcinogens appear to act by enhancing cell division and/or blocking apoptosis.

It is easy to recognize that even epigenetic carcinogens of the cytotoxic type act in this manner. As was discussed in the section on tissue repair, cell injury evokes the release of mitogenic growth factors such as HGF and TGF-alpha from tissue macrophages and endothelial cells. Thus, cells in chronically injured tissues are exposed continuously to endogenous mitogens. Although these growth factors are instrumental in tissue repair after acute cell injury, their continuous presence is potentially harmful because they may ultimately transform the affected cells into neoplastic cells. This view is supported by findings with transgenic mice that overexpress TGF-alpha. These animals exhibit hepatomegaly at a young age, and 80 percent develop tumors by 12 months (Fausto and Webber, 1993).

It is important to realize that even epigenetic carcinogens can exert a genotoxic effect, although indirectly. For example, chemicals causing chronic cell injury evoke a prolonged inflammatory response, with the free radicals produced by the inflammatory cells causing DNA injury in adjacent cells. Similarly, phorbol esters are not only potent mitogens but also activators of leukocytes, which release DNA-reactive free radicals during their respiratory burst (Weiss and LoBuglio, 1982).

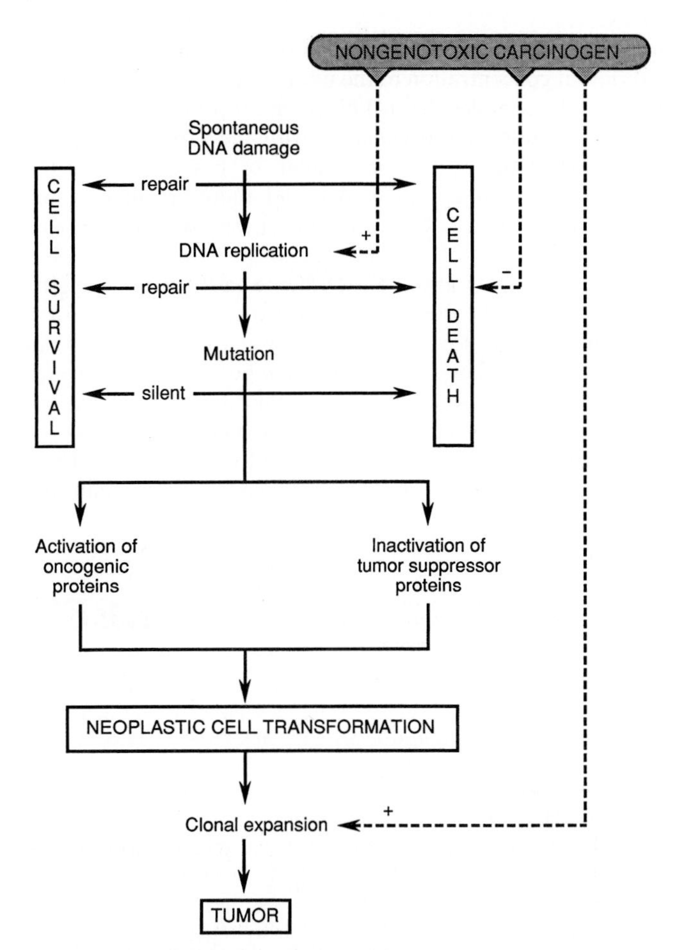


***Figure 3–21. The process of carcinogenesis promoted by nongenotoxic carcinogens.***

Positive and negative signs represent stimulation and inhibition, respectively. See text for explanation.

## CONCLUSIONS

This overview systematically surveys the mechanisms of the potential events that follow toxicant exposure and contribute to toxicity. This approach is also useful in the search for mechanisms responsible for (1) selective toxicity, that is, differences in the sensitivity to toxicants of various organisms, such as different species and strains of animals, organs, and cells, and (2) alteration of toxicity by exogenous factors such as chemicals and food and physiological or pathological conditions such as aging and disease. To identify the mechanisms that underlie selective toxicity or alterations in toxicity, all steps where variations might occur must be considered systematically. Selective or altered toxicity may be due to different or altered (1) exposure, (2) delivery, thus resulting in a different concentration of the ultimate toxicant at the target site, (3) target molecules, (4) biochemical processes triggered by the reaction of the chemical with the target molecules, (5) repair at the molecular, cellular, or tissue level, or (6) mechanisms, such as circulatory and thermoregulatory reflexes, by which the affected organism can adapt to some of the toxic effects.

In this chapter, a simplified scheme has been used to give an overview of the development of toxicity (Fig. 3-1). In reality, the route to toxicity can be considerably more diverse and complicated. For example, one chemical may yield several ultimate toxicants, one ultimate toxicant may react with several types of target molecules, and reaction with one type of target molecule may have a number of consequences. Thus, the toxicity of one chemical may involve several mechanisms which can interact with and influence each other in an intricate manner.

This chapter has emphasized the significance of the chemistry of a toxicant in governing its delivery to and reaction with the target molecule as well as the importance of the biochemistry, molecular and cell biology, immunology, and physiology of the affected organism in its response to the action of the toxicant. An organism has mechanisms that (1) counteract the delivery of toxicants, such as detoxication, (2) reverse the toxic injury, such as repair mechanisms, and (3) offset some dysfunctions, such as adaptive responses. Thus, toxicity is not an inevitable consequence of toxicant exposure, because it may be prevented, reversed, or compensated for by such mechanisms. Toxicity develops if the toxicant exhausts or impairs the protective mechanisms and/or overrides the adaptability of biological systems.

# REFERENCES


Aguilar F, Hussain SP, Cerutti P: Aflatoxin B1 induces the transversion of G → T in codon 249 of the *p53* tumor suppressor gene in human hepatocytes. *Proc Natl Acad Sci USA* 90:8586–8590, 1993.

Anderson MW, Reynolds SH, You M, Maronpot RM: Role of proto-oncogene activation in carcinogenesis. *Environ Health Perspect* 98:13–24, 1992.

Angel P, Karin M: The role of Jun, Fos and the AP-1 complex in cell-proliferation and transformation. *Biochim Biophys Acta* 1072:129–157, 1991.

Armstrong RB, Kim HJ, Grippo JF, Levin AA: Retinoids for the future: Investigational approaches for the identification of new compounds. *J Am Acad Dermatol* 27:S38–42, 1992.

Aust SD, Chignell CF, Bray TM, et al: Free radicals in toxicology. *Toxicol Appl Pharmacol* 120:168–178, 1993.

Baillie TA, Kassahun K: Reversibility in glutathione-conjugate formation. *Adv Pharmacol* 27:163–181, 1994.

Barrett JC: Mechanisms of action of known human carcinogens, in Vainio H, Magee PN, McGregor DB, McMichael AJ (eds): *Mechanisms of Carcinogenesis in Risk Identification*. Lyons: International Agency for Research on Cancer, 1992, pp 115–134.

Baumann H, Gauldie J: The acute phase response. *Immunol Today* 15:74–80, 1994.

Bayly AC, Roberts RA, Dive C: Suppression of liver cell apoptosis in vitro by the nongenotoxic hepatocarcinogen and peroxisome proliferator nafenopin. *J Cell Biol* 125:197–203, 1994.

Bock KW, Lilienblum W: Roles of uridine diphosphate glucuronosyltransferases in chemical carcinogenesis, in Kauffman FC (ed): *Conjugation-Deconjugation Reactions in Drug Metabolism and Toxicity*. Berlin: Springer-Verlag, 1994, pp 391–428.

Boelsterli UA: Specific targets of covalent drug-protein interactions in hepatocytes and their toxicological significance in drug-induced liver injury. *Drug Metab Rev* 25:395–451, 1993.

Border WA, Ruoslahti E: Transforming growth factor-$\beta$ in disease: The dark side of tissue repair. *J Clin Invest* 90:1–7, 1992.

Breimer LH: Molecular mechanisms of oxygen radical carcinogenesis and mutagenesis: The role of DNA base damage. *Mol Carcinog* 3:188–197, 1990.

Buja LM, Eigenbrodt ML, Eigenbrodt EH: Apoptosis and necrosis: Basic types and mechanisms of cell death. *Arch Pathol Lab Med* 117:1208–1214, 1993.

Bursch W, Oberhammer F, Schulte-Hermann R: Cell death by apoptosis and its protective role against disease. *Trends Pharmacol Sci* 13:245–251, 1992.

Burt AD: C. L. Oakley Lecture (1993): Cellular and molecular aspects of hepatic fibrosis. *J Pathol* 170:105–114, 1993.

Calabrese EJ, Baldwin LA, Mehendale HM: G2 subpopulation in rat liver induced into mitosis by low-level exposure to carbon tetrachloride: An adaptive response. *Toxicol Appl Pharmacol* 121:1–7, 1993.

Cavalieri EL, Rogan EG: The approach to understanding aromatic hydrocarbon carcinogenesis: The central role of radical cations in metabolic activation. *Pharmacol Ther* 55:183–199, 1992.

Colburn NH: Gene regulation by active oxygen and other stress inducers: Role in tumor promotion and progression, in Spatz L, Bloom AD (eds): *Biological Consequences of Oxidative Stress: Implications for Cardiovascular Disease and Carcinogenesis*. New York: Oxford University Press, 1992, pp 121–137.

Coleman MD, Jacobus DP: Reduction of dapsone hydroxylamine to dapsone during methaemoglobin formation in human erythrocytes in vitro. *Biochem Pharmacol* 45:1027–1033, 1993.

Coles B: Effects of modifying structure on electrophilic reactions with biological nucleophiles. *Drug Metab Rev* 15:1307–1334, 1984.

Commandeur JNM, Vermeulen NPE: Molecular and biochemical mechanisms of chemically induced nephrotoxicity: A review. *Chem Res Toxicol* 3:171–194, 1990.

Corcoran GB, Fix L, Jones DP, et al: Apoptosis: Molecular control point in toxicity. *Toxicol Appl Pharmacol* 128:169–181, 1994.

Corcoran GB, Ray SD: The role of the nucleus and other compartments in toxic cell death produced by alkylating hepatotoxicants. *Toxicol Appl Pharmacol* 113:167–183, 1992.

Cotgreave IA, Moldeus P, Orrenius S: Host biochemical defense mechanisms against prooxidants. *Annu Rev Pharmacol Toxicol* 28:189–212, 1988.

Cunningham CC, Coleman WB, Spach PI: The effects of chronic ethanol consumption on hepatic mitochondrial energy metabolism. *Alcohol Alcohol* 25:127–136, 1990.

Davies KJ: Protein damage and degradation by oxygen radicals: I. General aspects. *J Biol Chem* 262:9895–9901, 1987.

De Matteis F: Drugs as suicide substrates of cytochrome P-450, in De Matteis F, Lock EA (eds): *Selectivity and Molecular Mechanisms of Toxicity*. Houndmills, England: Macmillan, 1987, pp 183–210.

Dekant W, Vamvakas S, Anders MW: Bioactivation of nephrotoxic haloalkenes by glutathione conjugation: Formation of toxic and mutagenic intermediates by cysteine conjugate $\beta$-lyase. *Drug Metab Rev* 20:43–83, 1989.

Desaiah D: Biochemical mechanisms of chlordecone neurotoxicity: A review. *Neurotoxicology* 3:103–110, 1982.

Eaton DL, Gallagher EP: Mechanisms of aflatoxin carcinogenesis. *Annu Rev Pharmacol Toxicol* 34:135–172, 1994.

Edwards MJ, Keller BJ, Kauffman FC, Thurman RG: The involvement of Kupffer cells in carbon tetrachloride toxicity. *Toxicol Appl Pharmacol* 119:275–279, 1993.

Elbling L, Berger W, Rehberger A, et al: P-Glycoprotein regulates chemosensitivity in early developmental stages of the mouse. *FASEB J* 7:1499–1506, 1993.

Engler H, Taurog A, Nakashima T: Mechanism of inactivation of thyroid peroxidase by thioureylene drugs. *Biochem Pharmacol* 31:3801–3806, 1982.

Fausto N: Growth factors in liver development, regeneration and carcinogenesis. *Prog Growth Factor Res* 3:219–234, 1991.

Fausto N, Webber EM: Control of liver growth. *Crit Rev Eukaryot Gene Expr* 3:117–135, 1993.

Fernando MR, Nanri H, Yoshitake S, et al: Thioredoxin regenerates proteins inactivated by oxidative stress in endothelial cells. *Eur J Biochem* 209:917–922, 1992.

Fletcher KA, Barton PF, Kelly JA: Studies on the mechanisms of oxidation in the erythrocyte by metabolites of primaquine. *Biochem Pharmacol* 37:2683–2690, 1988.

Gale K: Role of GABA in the genesis of chemoconvulsant seizures. *Toxicol Lett* 64-65 (spec no):417–428, 1992.

Gilman AG, Rall TW, Nies AS, Taylor P (eds): *The Pharmacological Basis of Therapeutics*: New York: Pergamon, 1990.

Goering PL: Lead-protein interactions as a basis for lead toxicity. *Neurotoxicology* 14:45–60, 1993.

Goering PL, Waalkes MP, Klaassen CD: Toxicology of cadmium, in Goyer RA, Cherian MG (eds):*Toxicology of Metals: Biochemical Aspects*. Berlin: Springer-Verlag, 1995, pp 189–214.

Goldstein GW: Evidence that lead acts as a calcium substitute in second messenger metabolism. *Neurotoxicology* 14:97–101, 1993.

Gravina SA, Mieyal JJ: Thioltransferase is a specific glutathionyl mixed disulfide oxidoreductase. *Biochemistry* 32:3368–3376, 1993.

Green S: Nuclear receptors and chemical carcinogenesis. *Trends Pharmacol Sci* 13:251–255, 1992.

Gregus Z, Klaassen CD: Enterohepatic circulation of toxicants, in Rozman K, Hanninien O (eds): *Gastrointestinal Toxicology*. Amsterdam: Elsevier/North Holland, 1986, pp 57–118.

Gressner AM: Hepatic fibrogenesis: The puzzle of interacting cells, fibrogenic cytokines, regulatory loops, and extracellular matrix molecules. *Z Gastroenterol* 30(Suppl 1):5–16, 1992.

Guilianelli C, Baeza-Squiban A, Boisvieux-Ulrich E, et al: Effect of mineral particles containing iron on primary cultures of rabbit tracheal epithelial cells: Possible implication of oxidative stress. *Environ Health Perspect* 101:436–442, 1993.

Gut J, Christen U, Huwyler J: Mechanisms of halothane toxicity: Novel insights. *Pharmacol Ther* 58:133–155, 1993.

Hall SM: Regeneration in the peripheral nervous system. *Neuropathol Appl Neurobiol* 15:513–529, 1989.

Harris CC: *p53*: At the crossroads of molecular carcinogenesis and risk assessment. *Science* 262:1980–1981, 1993.

Herken H, Hucho F (eds): *Selective Neurotoxicity*. Berlin: Springer-Verlag, 1992.

Herman B, Gores GJ, Nieminen AL, et al: Calcium and pH in anoxic and toxic injury. *Crit Rev Toxicol* 21:127–148, 1990.

Heuchel R, Radtke F, Georgiev O, et al: The transcription factor MTF-1 is essential for basal and heavy metal-induced metallothionein gene expression. *EMBO J* 13:2870–2875, 1994.

Jakoby WB, Ziegler DM: The enzymes of detoxication. *J Biol Chem* 265:20715–20718, 1990.

Johnson AR: Contact inhibition in the failure of mammalian CNS axonal regeneration. *Bioessays* 15:807–813, 1993.

Kappus H: Overview of enzyme systems involved in bio-reduction of drugs and in redox cycling. *Biochem Pharmacol* 35:1–6, 1986.

Ketterer B: Protective role of glutathione and glutathione transferases in mutagenesis and carcinogenesis. *Mutat Res* 202:343–361, 1988.

Krell H, Metz J, Jaeschke H, et al: Drug-induced intrahepatic cholestasis: Characterization of different pathomechanisms. *Arch Toxicol* 60:124–130, 1987.

Kröncke KD, Fricker G, Meier PJ, et al: $\alpha$-Amanitin uptake into hepatocytes: Identification of hepatic membrane transport systems used by amatoxins. *J Biol Chem* 261:12562–12567, 1986.

Larsson BS: Interaction between chemicals and melanin. *Pigment Cell Res* 6:127–133, 1993.

Laurent G, Kishore BK, Tulkens PM: Aminoglycoside-induced renal phospholipidosis and nephrotoxicity. *Biochem Pharmacol* 40:2383–2392, 1990.

Lehmann AR, Dean SW: Cancer-prone human disorders with defects in DNA repair, in Cooper CS, Grover PL (eds): *Chemical Carcinogenesis and Mutagenesis II*. Berlin: Springer-Verlag, 1990, pp 71–101.

Levine AJ, Perry ME, Chang A, et al: The 1993 Walter Hubert Lecture: The role of the p53 tumour-suppressor gene in tumorigenesis. *Br J Cancer* 69:409–416, 1994.

Lim RT Jr, Gentry RT, Ito D, et al: First-pass metabolism of ethanol is predominantly gastric. *Alcohol Clin Exp Res* 17:1337–1344, 1993.

Lindroos PM, Zarnegar R, Michalopoulos GK: Hepatocyte growth factor (hepatopoietin A) rapidly increases in plasma before DNA synthesis and liver regeneration stimulated by partial hepatectomy and carbon tetrachloride administration. *Hepatology* 13:743–750, 1991.

Lozano RM, Yee BC, Buchanan BB: Thioredoxin-linked reductive inactivation of venom neurotoxins. *Arch Biochem Biophys* 309:356–362, 1994.

Martin SJ, Green DR, Cotter TG: Dicing with death: Dissecting the components of the apoptosis machinery. *Trends Biochem Sci* 19:26–30, 1994.

McDonnell TJ, Marin MC, Hsu B, et al: The *bcl-2* oncogene: Apoptosis and neoplasia. *Radiat Res* 136:307–312, 1993.

Meyer M, Schreck R, Baeuerle PA: $H_2O_2$ and antioxidants have opposite effects on activation of NF-KB and AP-1 in intact cells: AP-1 as secondary antioxidant-responsive factor. *EMBO J* 12:2005–2015, 1993.

Miller JA, Surh Y-J: Sulfonation in chemical carcinogenesis, in Kauffman FC (ed): *Conjugation-Deconjugation Reactions in Drug Metabolism and Toxicity*. Berlin: Springer-Verlag, 1994, pp 429–457.

Miyashita T, Reed JC: Tumor suppressor p53 is a direct transcriptional activator of the human *bax* gene. *Cell* 80:293–299, 1995.

Mohn KL, Laz TM, Hsu JC, et al: The immediate-early growth response in regenerating liver and insulin-stimulated H-35 cells: Comparison with serum-stimulated 3T3 cells and identification of 41 novel immediate-early genes. *Mol Cell Biol* 11:381–390, 1991.

Monks TJ, Lau SS: Glutathione conjugate mediated toxicities, in Kauffman FC (ed): *Conjugation-Deconjugation Reactionsin Drug Metabolism and Toxicity*. Berlin: Springer-Verlag, 1994, pp 459–509.

Moreland DE: Effects of toxicants on oxidative phosphorylation and photophosphorylation, in Hodgson E, Levi PE (eds): *Introduction to Biochemical Toxicology*, 2d ed. Norwalk, CT: Appleton, 1994, pp 345–366.

Morimoto RI: Cells in stress: Transcriptional activation of heat shock genes. *Science* 259:1409–1410, 1993.

Mustafa MG: Biochemical basis of ozone toxicity. *Free Radic Biol Med* 9:245–265, 1990.

Nagata S, Golstein P: The fas death factor. *Science* 267:1449–1456, 1995.

Narahashi T: Transmitter-activated ion channels as the target of chemical agents, in Kito S et al (eds): *Neuroreceptor Mechanisms in the Brain*. New York: Plenum, 1991, pp 61–73.

Narahashi T: Nerve membrane $Na^+$ channels as targets of insecticides. *Trends Pharmacol Sci* 13:236–241, 1992.

Nelson SD, Pearson PG: Covalent and noncovalent interactions in acute lethal cell injury caused by chemicals. *Annu Rev Pharmacol Toxicol* 30:169–195, 1990.

Nicotera P, Bellomo G, Orrenius S: Calcium-mediated mechanisms in chemically induced cell death. *Annu Rev Pharmacol Toxicol* 32:449–470, 1992.

Noji S, Tashiro K, Koyama E, et al: Expression of hepatocyte growth factor gene in endothelial and Kupffer cells of damaged rat livers, as revealed by in situ hybridization. *Biochem Biophys Res Commun* 173:42–47, 1990.

Oltvai ZN, Milliman CL, Korsmeyer SJ: Bcl-2 heterodimerizes in vivo with a conserved homolog, bax, that accelerates programed cell death. *Cell* 74:609–619, 1993.

Oortgiesen M, Leinders T, van Kleef RG, Vijverberg HP: Differential neurotoxicological effects of lead on voltage-dependent and receptor-operated ion channels. *Neurotoxicology* 14:87–96, 1993.

Osawa Y, Davila JC, Nakatsuka M, et al: Inhibition of P450 cytochromes by reactive intermediates. *Drug Metab Rev* 27:61–72, 1995.

Patel MN, Yim GK, Isom GE: N-methyl-D-aspartate receptors mediate cyanide-induced cytotoxicity in hippocampal cultures. *Neurotoxicology* 14:35–40, 1993.

Pegg AE, Byers TL: Repair of DNA containing $O^6$-alkylguanine. *FASEB J* 6:2302–2310, 1992.

Poellinger L, Göttlicher M, Gustafsson JA: The dioxin and peroxisome proliferator-activated receptors: Nuclear receptors in search of endogenous ligands. *Trends Pharmacol Sci* 13:241–245, 1992.

Poirier LA: Methyl group deficiency in hepatocarcinogenesis. *Drug Metab Rev* 26:185–199, 1994.

Raghow R: The role of extracellular matrix in postinflammatory wound healing and fibrosis. *FASEB J* 8:823–831, 1994.

Recknagel RO, Glende EA Jr, Dolak JA, Waller RL: Mechanisms of carbon tetrachloride toxicity. *Pharmacol Ther* 43:139–154, 1989.

Richter C, Kass GE: Oxidative stress in mitochondria: Its relationship to cellular $Ca^{2+}$ homeostasis, cell death, proliferation, and differentiation. *Chem Biol Interact* 77:1–23, 1991.

Rothwell NJ: Functions and mechanisms of interleukin 1 in the brain. *Trends Pharmacol Sci* 12:430–436, 1991.

Saido TC, Sorimachi H, Suzuki K: Calpain: New perspectives in molecular diversity and physiological-pathological involvement. *FASEB J* 8:814–822, 1994.

Sancar A, Sancar GB: DNA repair enzymes. *Annu Rev Biochem* 57:29–67, 1988.

Scheschonka A, Murphy ME, Sies H: Temporal relationships between the loss of vitamin E, protein sulfhydryls and lipid peroxidation in microsomes challenged with different prooxidants. *Chem Biol Interact* 74:233–252, 1990.

Schinkel AH, Smit JJ, van Tellingen O, et al: Disruption of the mouse *mdr1a* P-glycoprotein gene leads to a deficiency in the blood-brain barrier and to increased sensitivity to drugs. *Cell* 77:491–502, 1994.

Schulte-Hermann R, Timmermann-Trosiener I, Barthel G, Bursch W: DNA synthesis, apoptosis, and phenotypic expression as determinants of growth of altered foci in rat liver during phenobarbital promotion. *Cancer Res* 50:5127–5135, 1990.

Scicchitano DA, Hanawalt PC: Intragenomic repair heterogeneity of DNA damage. *Environ Health Perspect* 98:45–51, 1992.

Selby CP, Sancar A: Molecular mechanism of transcription-repair coupling. *Science* 260:53–58, 1993.

Shi X, Dalal NS: NADPH-dependent flavoenzymes catalyze one electron reduction of metal ions and molecular oxygen and generate hydroxyl radicals. *FEBS Lett* 276:189–191, 1990.

Sies H: Strategies of antioxidant defense. *Eur J Biochem* 215:213–219, 1993.

Smith MR, Matthews NT, Jones KA, Kung HF: Biological actions of oncogenes. *Pharmacol Ther* 58:211–236, 1993.

Southorn PA, Powis G: Free radicals in medicine: I. Chemical nature and biologic reactions. *Mayo Clin Proc* 63:381–389, 1988.

Thompson CB: Apoptosis in the pathogenesis and treatment of disease. *Science* 267:1456–1460, 1995.

Uetrecht JP: The role of leukocyte-generated reactive metabolites in the pathogenesis of idiosyncratic drug reactions. *Drug Metab Rev* 24:299–366, 1992.

Van Kuijk FJGM, Sevanian A, Handelman GJ, Dratz EA: A new role for phospholipase A2: Protection of membranes from lipid peroxidation damage. *TIBS* 12:31–34, 1987.

Wang JF, Komarov P, de Groot H: Luminol chemiluminescence in rat macrophages and granulocytes: The role of NO, $O_2^{\bullet-}$/$H_2O_2$, and HOCl. *Arch Biochem Biophys* 304:189–196, 1993.

Weiss SJ, LoBuglio AF: Phagocyte-generated oxygen metabolites and cellular injury. *Lab Invest* 47:5–18, 1982.

Yamasaki H, Krutovskikh V, Mesnil M, et al: Gap junctional intercellular communication and cell proliferation during rat liver carcinogenesis. *Environ Health Perspect* 101(Suppl 5):191–197, 1993.

Zawaski K, Gruebele A, Kaplan D, et al: Evidence for enhanced expression of c-fos, c-jun, and the $Ca^{2+}$-activated neutral protease in rat liver following carbon tetrachloride administration. *Biochem Biophys Res Commun* 197:585–590, 1993.

Zhan Q, Fan S, Bae I, et al: Induction of *bax* by genotoxic stress in human cells correlates with normal p53 status and apoptosis. *Oncogene* 9:3743–3751, 1994.

# CHAPTER 4

# RISK ASSESSMENT

*Elaine M. Faustman and Gilbert S. Omenn*

Risk assessment as an organized activity performed by federal agencies began in the 1970s. Earlier, the American Conference of Governmental Industrial Hygienists (ACGIH) had set threshold limit values for workers and the U.S. Food and Drug Administration (FDA) had established acceptable daily intakes for dietary pesticide residues and food additives. In 1958, Congress instructed the FDA in the Delaney clause to prohibit the addition to the food supply of all substances that cause cancer in animals or humans. Pragmatically, this policy allowed food sources that had nondetectable levels of these additives to be declared "safe." When advances in analytic chemistry revealed that "nondetects" were not equivalent to "not present" or "zero risk," regulatory agencies were forced to develop "tolerance levels" and "acceptable risk levels"; soon risk assessment methodologies blossomed (Albert, 1994). In response to these developments, the Office of Science and Technology Policy developed a framework for regulatory decision making (Fig. 4-1) and the National Research Council (NRC), in *Risk Assessment in the Federal Government: Managing the Process* (widely known as "the Red Book"), detailed the steps of hazard identification, dose-response assessment, exposure analysis, and characterization of risks to provide a consistent framework for risk assessment across agencies (Fig. 4-2) (NRC, 1983). This framework has been applied most frequently for the assessment of cancer risks; however, noncancer endpoints are receiving the same type of evaluation using such framework approaches. Recent advances in toxicology, epidemiology, exposure assessment, and the biologically based modeling of various adverse responses have led to improvements in risk assessment. Nevertheless, public policy objectives require extrapolations that go far beyond the observation of actual effects, causing uncertainty and controversy.

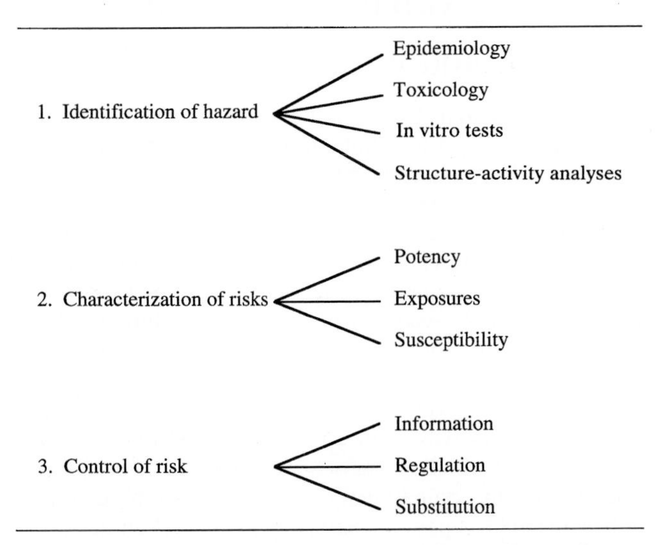


***Figure 4–1. Framework for regulatory decision making: risk assessment and risk management. [Based on Calkins et al. (1980).]***

## DEFINITIONS

*Risk assessment* is the systematic scientific characterization of potential adverse health effects resulting from human exposures to hazardous agents or situations (NRC, 1983). This type of assessment includes qualitative information on the strength of the evidence and the nature of the outcomes, quantitative assessment of the exposure and the potential magnitude of the risks, and a description of the uncertainties in the conclusions and estimates. *Risk* is defined as the probability of an adverse outcome. The term "hazard" is used by North Americans to refer to intrinsic toxic properties; internationally, this term is defined as the probability of an adverse outcome. This chapter presents risk assessment approaches for both cancer and noncancer hazards. Analogous approaches can be applied to ecological risks (NRC, 1993a). The objectives of risk assessment are outlined in Table 4-1.

*Risk management* refers to the process by which policy actions to deal with the hazards identified in the risk assessment process are chosen. Risk managers consider scientific evidence and risk estimates, along with statutory, engineering, economic, social, and political factors, in evaluating alternative regulatory options and choosing among those options (NRC, 1983). Chapter 34 discusses approaches to regulatory options.

*Risk communication* is the process of making risk assessment and risk management information comprehensible to lawyers, politicians, judges, business and labor, environmentalists, and community groups. These groups and individuals often want to know whether something is safe, not whether its risks are uncertain and complicated.

## RISK PERCEPTION

Individuals respond differently to hazardous situations, as do societies. An event that is accepted by one individual may be unacceptable to another (Fischhoff et al., 1981, 1993). Understanding these behavioral responses is critical in developing risk management options. Experts and laypersons commonly disagree. In a classic study, students, League of Women Voters members, active club members, and scientific experts were asked to rank 30 activities or agents in order of their annual contribution to deaths (Slovic et al., 1979). The lay groups all ranked motorcycles and handguns as highly risky and vaccinations, home appliances, power mowers, and football as relatively safe. Club members viewed pesticides, spray cans, and nuclear power as safer than did other laypersons. Students ranked contraceptives and food preservatives as riskier and mountain climbing as safer than did the others. The experts, however, ranked electric power, surgery, swimming, and x-rays

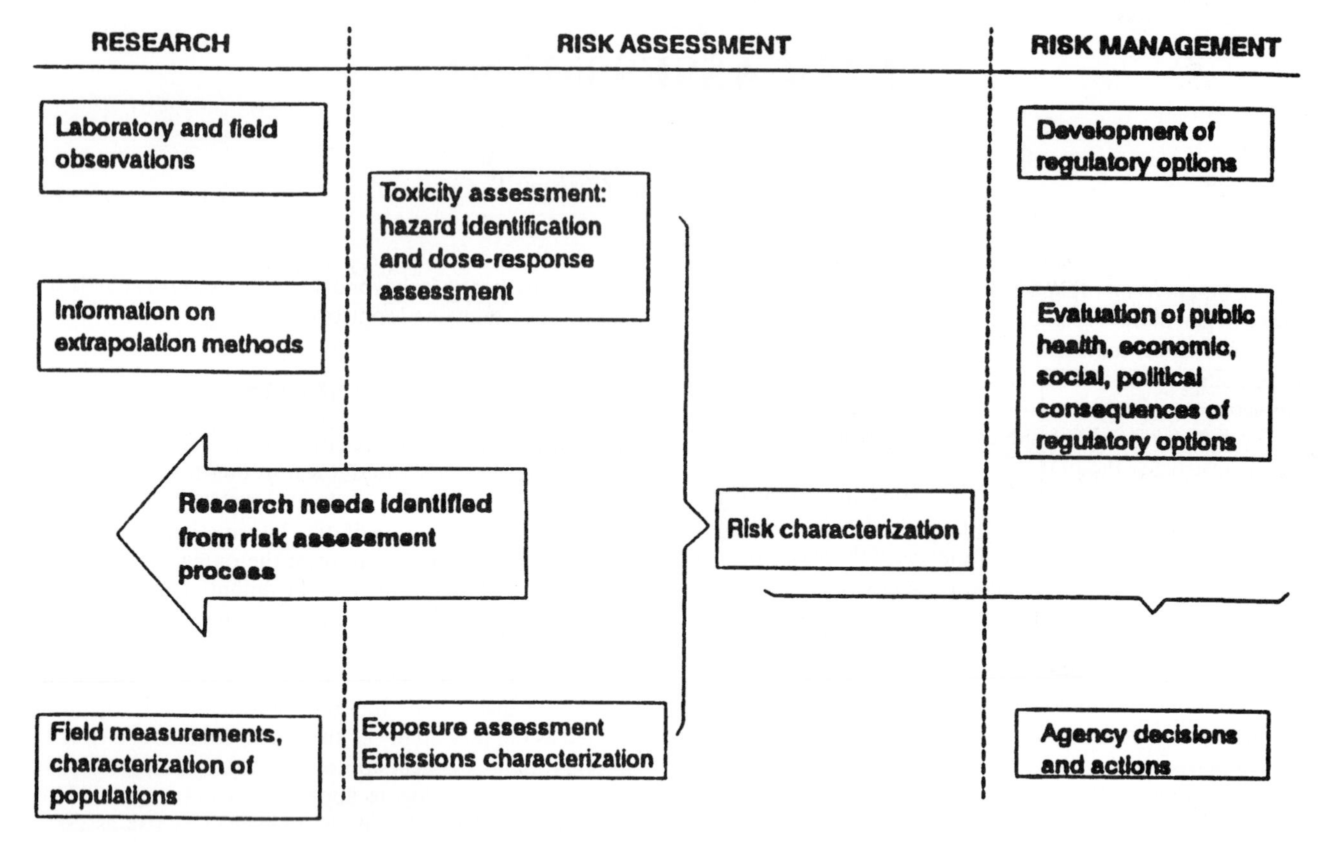


***Figure 4–2.** Elements of risk assessment and risk management.*

This risk assessment/management paradigm was adapted from the original from the National Research Council, 1983, and now emphasizes even more the importance of research and the interative nature of the risk-assessment process. (Reprinted from *Science and Judgement in Risk Assessment*, 1994, with permission from the National Academy Press, Washington, DC.)

as more risky and nuclear power and police work as less risky than did laypersons. Perceptions of risk by toxicologists in academia, industry, and government also have been studied (Neil et al., 1994); there were group differences in responses involving chemical hazards.

Figure 4-3 illustrates the relationship of psychological factors such as dread, perceived uncontrollability, and involuntary exposure (horizontal axis) to factors that represent the extent to which a hazard is familiar, observable, and "essential" (vertical axis) (Morgan, 1993). For example, the upper right sector of risk space includes pesticide use, radioactive waste, DNA technology, electromagnetic fields, asbestos insulation, and mercury. Risks that have these features are good candidates for public demand for government regulations and are less likely to be "acceptable" (Lowrance, 1976).

**Table 4–1**
**Objectives of Risk Assessment**

1. Balance risks and benefits
   - Drugs
   - Pesticides
2. Set target levels of risk
   - Food contaminants
   - Water pollutants
3. Set priorities for program activities
   - Regulatory agencies
   - Manufacturers
   - Environmental and consumer organizations
4. Estimate residual risks and extent of risk reduction after steps are taken to reduce risks

## HAZARD IDENTIFICATION

### Structure-Activity Relationships

In many cases, toxicity information on chemicals is limited. Given the 1 million to 2 million dollars in cost and the 3 to 5 years required to test a single chemical in a lifetime rodent carcinogenicity bioassay, initial decisions on whether to continue the development of a chemical, submit a premanufacturing notice (PMN), or require additional testing may be based largely on structure-activity relationships (SARs) and limited short-term assays. A test agent's structure, solubility, stability, pH sensitivity, electrophilicity, and chemical reactivity can represent important information for hazard identification. Historically, certain key molecular structures have provided regulators with some of the most readily available information on which to assess hazard potential. For example, 8 of the first 14 occupational carcinogens were regulated together by the Occupational Safety and Health Administration (OSHA) as belonging to the aromatic amine chemical class. The EPA Office of Toxic Substances relies on structure-activ-

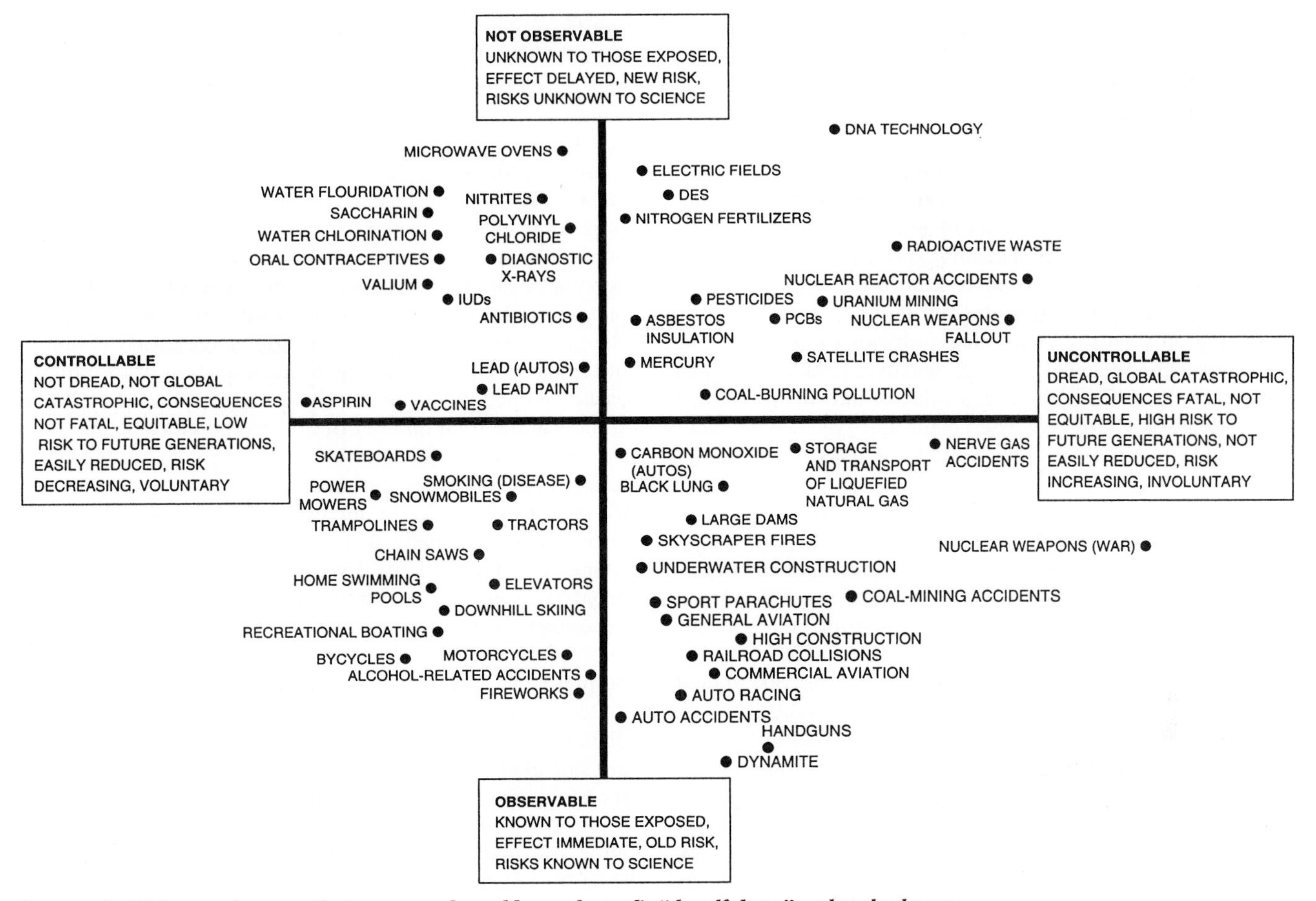


***Figure 4–3. Risk space has axes that correspond roughly to a hazard's "dreadfulness" and to the degree to which it is understood.***

Risks in the upper right quadrant of this space are most likely to provoke calls for government regulation. [From Morgan (1993) and Slovic (1988).]

ity relationships to meet deadlines for responding to premanufacturing notice for new chemical manufacture under the Toxic Substances Control Act (TSCA). Structural alerts such as *n*-nitroso or aromatic amine groups, amino azo dye structures, and phenanthrene nuclei are clues to prioritizing agents for additional evaluation as potential carcinogens. The limited database of known developmental toxicants limits structure-activity relationships to only a few chemical classes, including chemicals with structures related to those of valproic acid and retinoic acid.

SARs are useful in assessing the relative toxicity of chemically related compounds. The EPA's 1994 reassessment of the risks of 2,3,7,8 tetrachlorodibenzo-*p*-dioxin and related chlorinated and brominated dibenzo-*p*-dioxins, dibenzofurans, and planar biphenyls might have relied too heavily on toxicity equivalence factors (TEFs) based on induction of the Ah receptor (EPA, 1994c). The estimated toxicity of environmental mixtures containing those chemicals is a product of the concentration of each chemical times its TEF value. However, it is difficult to predict activity across chemical classes and especially across multiple toxic endpoints by using a single biological response. Many complex chemical-physical interactions are not easily understood and may be oversimplified by researchers. Several computerized SAR methods gave disappointing results in the National Toxicology Program's (NTP) 44-chemical rodent carcinogenicity prediction challenge (Omenn et al., 1995; Ashby and Tennant, 1994; Tennant et al., 1990).

## In Vitro and Short-Term Tests

The next approach to hazard identification includes in vitro or short-term tests ranging from bacterial mutation assays performed entirely in vitro to more elaborate short-term tests such as skin-painting studies in mice and altered rat liver foci assays conducted in vivo. Chapter 9 describes various assays of genetic and mutagenic endpoints, and Chap. 8 discusses the uses of these assays for identifying chemical carcinogens. Other assays assess developmental toxicity (Faustman, 1988; Whittaker and Faustman, 1994), reproductive toxicity (Shelby et al., 1993; Harris et al., 1992; Gray, 1988), neurotoxicity (Atterwill et al., 1992), and immunotoxicity (Chap. 12). Less information is available on the extrapolation of these tests for risk assessment than on the mutagenicity and carcinogenicity endpoints; however, the mechanistic information obtained in these systems has been applied to risk assessment (Abbott et al., 1992; EPA, 1994c; Leroux et al., in press).

The validation and application of short-term assays are particularly important in risk assessment, because these assays can be designed to provide information about mechanisms of effects and are fast and inexpensive compared with lifetime bioassays. The NTP rodent carcinogenicity prediction challenge gave promising results for the prediction of genotoxic carcinogens; a second round with the next 30 chemicals entering NTP rodent bioassays has been announced (Ashby and Tennant, 1994; Tennant et al., 1990). As with other kinds of tests, to validate in vitro assays, it is necessary to determine their sensitivity (ability to identify true carcinogens), specificity (ability to recognize noncarcinogens as noncarcinogens), and predictive value for the toxic endpoint under evaluation. The societal costs of relying on such tests, with false positives (noncarcinogens classified as carcinogens) and false negatives (true carcinogens not detected), are the subject of a value-of-information model for testing aspects of risk assessment and risk management (Lave and Omenn, 1986; Omenn and Lave, 1988).

## Animal Bioassays

The use of animal bioassay data is a key component of the hazard identification process. Chemicals that cause tumors in animals are presumed to be likely to cause tumors in humans. All the human carcinogens that have been adequately tested in animals have produced positive results in at least one animal model. Thus, "although this association cannot establish that all agents and mixtures that cause cancer in experimental animals also cause cancer in humans, nevertheless, in the absence of adequate data on humans, it is biologically plausible and prudent to regard agents and mixtures for which there is sufficient evidence of carcinogenicity in experimental animals as if they presented a carcinogenic risk to humans" (IARC, 1994). In general, the most appropriate rodent bioassays are those which test the exposure pathways of most relevance to predicted or known human exposure pathways. Bioassays for reproductive and developmental toxicity and other noncancer endpoints have a similar rationale (see Chaps. 10 and 19 for details).

Consistent features in the design of standard cancer bioassays include testing in two species, testing both sexes, using 50 animals per dose group, and using near-lifetime exposure. Important choices include the strains of rats and mice, the number of doses and dose levels [typically 90, 50, and 10 to 25 percent of the maximal tolerated dose (MTD)], and the complexity of the required histopathology. Positive evidence of chemical carcinogenicity can include increases in the number of tumors at a particular organ site, induction of rare tumors, earlier induction of commonly observed tumors, and/or increases in the total number of observed tumors.

There are serious problems in using the rodent bioassay as a gold standard for the prediction of human carcinogenicity risk. Tumors may be increased only at the highest dose tested, which is usually at or near a dose that causes toxicity (Ames and Gold, 1990). Even without toxicity, a high dose may trigger events different from those triggered by low-dose exposures. Table 4-2 presents some mechanistic details about two rodent tumor responses that are no longer thought to be predictive of cancer risk for humans: thyroid tumors mediated by hyperstimulation and male rat kidney tumors mediated by $\alpha_{2u}$-globulin induction. Other rodent responses that are not likely to be predictive for humans include localized forestomach tumors after gavage, bladder tumors in response to supersaturating concentrations of salts, and lung tumors after overloading of clearance mechanisms with particles (McClain, 1994; Omenn, in press). Nevertheless, tumors in unusual sites, such as the pituitary gland, the eighth cranial

**Table 4–2**
**Two Examples of Mechanistic Considerations for Nongenotoxic Carcinogens: Explanation for Lack of Relevancy of Rodent Bioassay Data for Human Risk Evaluation**

| SYSTEM | TARGET ORGAN | MECHANISM FOR SUSCEPTIBLE SPECIES | SPECIES DIFFERENCES | ILLUSTRATIVE CHEMICAL AGENTS |
|---|---|---|---|---|
| Endocrine | Thyroid gland tumors in rodents | Alteration in thyroid homeostasis<br>Decrease thyroid hormone production<br>Sustain increase in thyroid stimulating hormone (TSH)<br>Thyroid tumors | Lack of thyroid-binding protein in rodents versus humans<br>Decreased $t_{1/2}$ for $T_4$; increased TSH levels in rodents | Ethylene bisdithiocarbamate, fungicides, amitrol, goitrogens, sulfamethazine |
| Urinary tract | Renal tumors in male rats | Chemicals bind to $\alpha_{2u}$-globulin<br>Accumulation in target kidney cells<br>Increased necrosis<br>Increased regenerative hyperplasia<br>Renal tubular calcification, neoplasia | $\alpha_{2u}$-globulin male rat specific low-molecular weight protein not found in female rats, humans, or other resistant species/mice, monkeys | Unleaded gasoline<br>1,4-Dichlorobenzene<br>D-Limonene<br>Isophorons<br>Dimethyl-methylphosphonate<br>Perchloroethylene<br>Pentachloroethane<br>Hexachloroethane |

nerve, and the Zymbal gland should not be dismissed as irrelevant, because organ-organ correlation is often lacking (NRC, 1994). It is desirable to use the same route of administration as the likely exposure pathway in humans.

Rats and mice give concordant positive or negative results in only 70 percent of these bioassays, and so it is unlikely that rodent-human concordance would be higher (Lave et al., 1988). Even when concordant positive results are observed, there can be great differences in potency, as is observed in aflatoxin-induced tumors in rats and mice. In this example, an almost 100,000-fold difference in susceptibility to $AFB_1$-induced liver tumors is seen between the sensitive rat and trout species versus the more resistant mouse strains. Genetic differences in the expression of cytochrome P-450 and glutathione-S-transferase isoenzymes explain most of these species differences and suggest that humans may be as sensitive to $AFB_1$-induced liver tumors as are rats (Eaton and Gallagher, 1994).

Haseman and Lockhart (1993) concluded that most target sites in cancer bioassays showed a strong correlation (65 percent) between males and females, especially for stomach, liver, and thyroid tumors, and suggested that bioassays could rely on a combination of male rats and female mice for efficiency. In any case, results must be extrapolated from a dose-response curve in the 10 to 100 percent tumor response range down to $10^{-6}$ risk estimates at the upper confidence limit or to a benchmark or reference dose–related risk. The addition of investigations of mechanisms and assessment of multiple noncancer endpoints in the same study represents an important enhancement of lifetime bioassays. It is feasible and desirable to tie these bioassays together with mechanistically oriented short-term tests and biomarker and genetic studies of epidemiology (Perera et al., 1991). In the example of $AFB_1$-induced liver tumors, $AFB_1$-DNA adducts have proved to be an extremely useful biomarker. A highly linear relationship was observed between liver tumor incidence in rats and trout and $AFB_1$-DNA adduct formation over a dose range of 5 orders of magnitude (Bechtel, 1989). Such approaches extend biologically observable phenomena to doses lower than those causing frank tumor development.

### Use of Epidemiological Data in Risk Assessment

The most convincing evidence for human risk is a well-conducted epidemiological study in which a positive association between exposure and disease has been observed (NRC, 1983). Epidemiological studies are essentially opportunistic. These studies begin with known or presumed exposures, comparing exposed versus nonexposed individuals, or with known cases compared with persons lacking the particular diagnosis. There are important limitations. When the study is exploratory, the hypotheses are often weak. Exposures are often crude and retrospective, especially for conditions with a long latency before clinical manifestations appear. Generally, there are multiple exposures, especially when a full week or a lifetime is considered. There is always a trade-off between detailed information on relatively few persons and very limited information on large numbers of persons. Contributions from lifestyle factors such as smoking and diet represent a challenge. Humans are highly outbred, and so the method must consider variation in susceptibility among those who are exposed. The expression of results in terms of odds ratios, relative risks, and confidence intervals may be unfamiliar to nonepidemiologists. Finally, the caveats self-effacing epidemiologists often cite may discourage risk managers and toxicologists (Omenn, 1993).

Nevertheless, human epidemiology studies provide very useful information for hazard identification and sometimes quantitative information for data characterization. Three major types of epidemiology studies are available: cross-sectional studies, cohort studies, and case-control studies. Cross-sectional studies survey groups of humans to identify risk factors (exposure) and disease but are not useful for establishing cause-and-effect relationships. Cohort studies evaluate individuals selected on the basis of their exposure to the agent under study. Thus, on the basis of exposure status, these individuals are monitored for development of disease. Prospective studies monitor individuals who initially are disease-free to determine if they develop the disease over time. In case-control studies, subjects are selected on the basis of disease status: disease cases and matched cases of disease-free individuals. The exposure histories of the two groups are compared to determine key consistent features. All case-control studies are retrospective studies.

Epidemiological findings are judged by the following criteria: strength of association, consistency of observations (i.e., reproducibility in time and space), specificity (uniqueness in quality or quantity of response), appropriateness of temporal relationship (i.e., did the exposure precede the responses?), dose responsiveness, biological plausibility and coherence, verification, and analogy (biological extrapolation) (Hill, 1965). In addition, epidemiological studies should be evaluated for power of detection, appropriateness of outcomes, verification of exposure assessments, completeness of assessing confounders, and general applicability of the outcomes to other populations at risk. Power of detection is calculated by using study size, variability, accepted detection limits for the endpoints under study, and a specified significance level. [See Healey (1987) for calculation formulas or computer programs such as EPI-INFO (Dean et al., 1990) or EGRET (SERC, 1994) for determination of the experimental power of detection.] The biological plausibility of epidemiological associations will be increased remarkably by the use of biomarkers of exposure, effects, and susceptibility (Perera et al., 1991).

## CHARACTERIZATION OF RISK

### Quantitative Risk Assessment

Quantitative considerations in risk assessment under the rubric of the Red Book, include dose-response assessment, exposure assessment, and characterization of uncertainty. With dose-response assessment, varying approaches have been proposed for threshold and nonthreshold endpoints. Traditionally, threshold approaches have been applied for the assessment of noncancer endpoints and nonthreshold approaches have been used for the assessment of cancer endpoints. Each approach and its inherent assumptions will be discussed below.

**Dose-Response Assessment.** The fundamental basis of the quantitative relationships between exposure to an agent and the incidence of an adverse response is the dose-response assessment. As described extensively in Chapter 2, approaches to characterizing dose-response relationships include effect levels such as $LD_{50}$, $LC_{50}$, $ED_{10}$, and no observed adverse effect levels (NOAELs); margins of safety; therapeutic indexes; and models for extrapolation to very low doses far below the observed range.

For risk assessment purposes, human exposure data for the prediction of human response are usually limited. Thus, animal bioassay data are generally used for dose-response assessment; however, the risk assessor is normally interested in low environmental exposures of humans, which are way below the experimentally observable range of responses in animal assays. Thus, low-dose extrapolation and animal-to-human risk extrapolation methods are required and constitute major aspects of dose-response assessment.

Figure 4-4 shows an observed effect at 10 percent incidence and five hypothetical options for the extrapolated dose-response curve below the 10 percent response dose. The first curve on the right represents a threshold and by definition represents a dose below which no response is observed (8.0 $\mu$g/wk).

Figure 4-5 expands this concept of a threshold and shows that, depending on the response that is modeled, each response to an agent can have a separate threshold dose. In this example, progressively adverse responses are modeled from changes in body weight to reduced fertility and liver pathology. Increased body weight (defined in the example as an increase of 5 percent) would probably be identified not as an adverse effect but only as an effect level, hence the use of the no observed effect level (NOEL) and the lowest observed effect level (LOEL) to describe this first curve. As doses increase and reduced fertility is observed, no observed adverse effect levels (NOAELs) and lowest observed adverse effect levels (LOAELs) are observed. At higher doses, signs of liver necrosis are observed and a frank effect level (FEL) is shown.

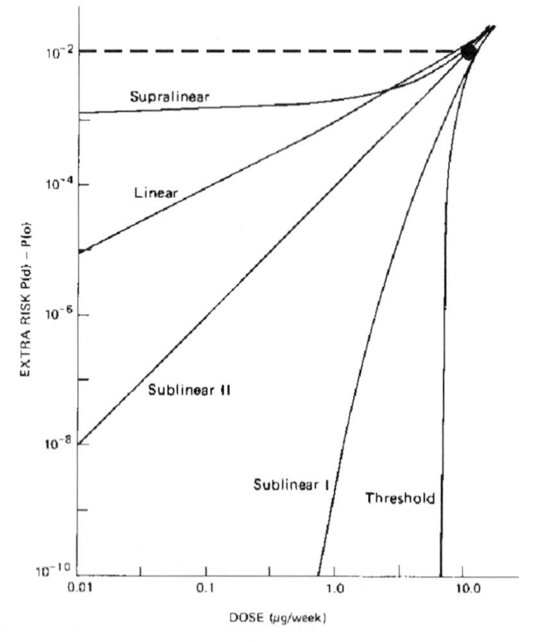


*Figure 4–4. Results of alternative extrapolation models for the same experimental data. [From NRC (1983).]*

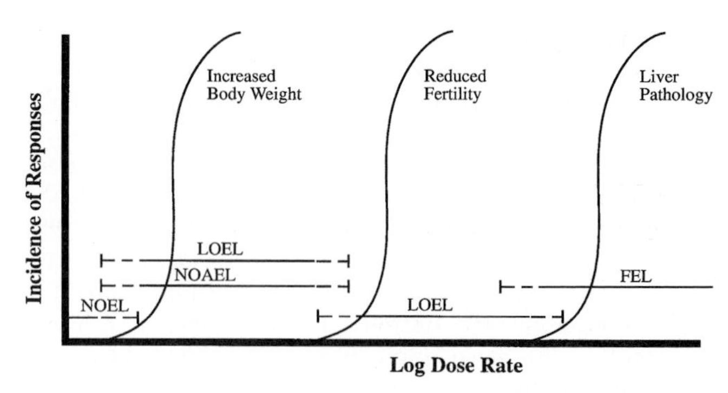


*Figure 4–5. The "threshold" region for chronic dose-response curves.*

The illustrated dose-response curves represent idealized "true" dose-response curves; the brackets illustrate the ranges for individual experimental results that might be categorized according to this scheme. NOEL = no observed effect level; NOAEL = no observed adverse effect level; LOEL = lowest observed effect level; LOAEL = lowest observed adverse effect level; FEL = frank effect level. Depending on the quality of the data, some of these categories (e.g., NOAEL and LOEL) may overlap. [From Hartung (1987).]

The highest dose level that does not produce a significantly elevated increase in an adverse response is the NOAEL. Significance usually refers to both biological and statistical criteria (Faustman et al., 1994) and is dependent on the number of dose levels tested, the number of animals tested at each dose, and the background incidence of the adverse response in nonexposed control groups. The NOAEL should not be perceived as risk-free, as several reports have shown that the response of NOAELs for continuous endpoints averages 5 percent risk, and NOAELs based on quantal endpoints can be associated with a risk of greater than 10 percent (Faustman et al., 1994; Allen et al., 1994a and b).

NOAELs can be used as a basis for risk assessment calculations such as reference doses and acceptable daily intake values. References doses (RfDs) and concentrations (RfCs) are estimates of a daily exposure to an agent that is assumed to be without an adverse health impact on the human population. The acceptable daily intake (ADI) values are used by the World Health Organization (WHO) for pesticides and food additives to define "the daily intake of chemical, which during an entire lifetime appears to be without appreciable risk on the basis of all known facts at that time" (WHO, 1962). Reference doses (introduced in Chap. 2) and ADI values typically are calculated from NOAEL values by dividing by uncertainty (UF) and/or modifying factors (MFs) (EPA, 1991b):

$$\text{RfD} = \text{NOAEL}/(\text{UF} * \text{MF})$$
$$\text{ADI} = \text{NOAEL}/(\text{UF} * \text{MF})$$

In principle, these safety factors allow for intraspecies and interspecies (animal to human) variation with default values of 10. An additional uncertainty factor is used to extrapolate from short-exposure-duration studies to a situation more relevant for chronic study or to account for inadequate numbers of animals or other experimental limitations. Modifying factors can be used to adjust the uncertainty factors if data on mechanisms, pharmacokinetics, and the relevance of the animal response to human risk justify such modifications. If only a LOAEL value is available, an additional 10-fold factor commonly is used to arrive at a value more comparable to a NOAEL.

Allen and associates (1994a) have shown that for developmental toxicity endpoints, the 10-fold factor for conversion from LOAEL to NOAEL is too large. Reference doses for developmental toxicity are usually reported as $RfD_{DT}$ or $RfC_{DT}$ to distinguish these results from oral or dermal RfD and inhalation RfC values.

Another way in which NOAEL values have been utilized for risk assessment is in evaluating a "margin of exposure" (MOE) or "margin of safety" (MOS), where the ratio of the NOAEL determined in animals and expressed as mg/kg/day is compared with the level to which a human may be exposed. For example, if human exposures are calculated to occur via drinking water and the water supply in the equation contains 1 ppm, the exposure per day is 1 mg/liter × 2 liters/day ÷ 50 kg = 0.04 mg/kg/day for a 50-kg woman. If the NOAEL for neurotoxicity is 100 mg/kg/day, the MOE is 2500 for the oral exposure route for neurotoxicity. Such a large value is reassuring for public health officials. Low values of MOE indicate that human levels of exposure are close to levels for the NOAEL in animals. No factor is included in this calculation for differences in human and animal susceptibility or animal-to-human extrapolation; thus, MOE values below 100 have been used by regulatory agencies as flags for further evaluation.

The NOAEL approach has been criticized in several areas, including the following: (1) The NOAEL must by definition be one of the experimental doses tested, (2) once it is identified, the rest of the dose-response curve is ignored, (3) experiments that test fewer animals result in larger NOAELs and thus larger reference doses, rewarding testing procedures that produce less certain rather than more certain NOAEL values, and (4) the NOAEL approach does not identify the actual responses at the NOAEL and will vary based on experimental design, resulting in regulatory limits set at varying levels of risk. Because of these limitations, an alternative to the NOAEL approach, the benchmark dose (BMD) method, was proposed by Crump (1984) and then extended by Kimmel and Gaylor (1988). In this approach, the dose response is modeled and the lower confidence bound for a dose at a specified response level [benchmark response (BMR)] is calculated. The benchmark response is usually specified as a 1 to 10 percent response. Figure 4-6 shows how a benchmark dose is calculated by using a 10 percent benchmark response and a 95 percent lower confidence bound on the dose. The $BMD_x$ (with x representing the x percent benchmark response) is used as an alternative to the NOAEL value for reference dose calculations. Thus, the RfD would be

$$RfD = BMD_x / UF * MF$$

The proposed values used for the UFs and MFs for benchmark doses can range from the same factors used for the NOAEL to lower values because of increased confidence in the response level and increased recognition of experimental variability caused by the use of a lower confidence bound on the dose (Barnes et al., 1995).

The benchmark dose approach has been applied to study several noncancer endpoints, including developmental (Allen et al., 1994a and b) and reproductive toxicity (Auton et al., 1994). The most extensive studies with developmental toxicity

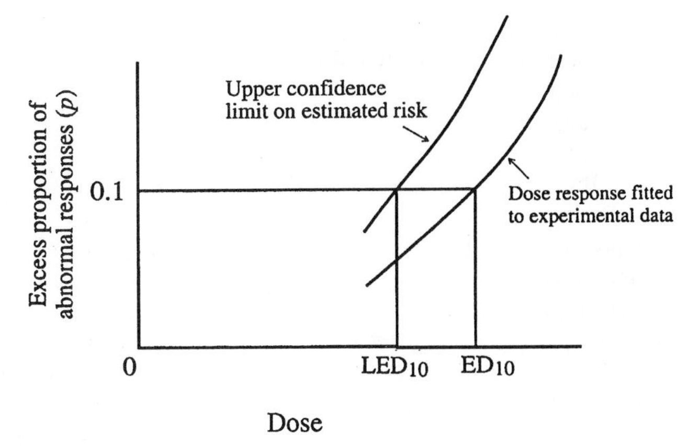


*Figure 4–6. Benchmark dose.*

have shown that $BMD_5$ were similar to a statistically derived NOAEL for a wide range of developmental toxicity endpoints and that the results from using generalized dose-response models were similar to those from statistical models designed specifically to incorporate unique features of developmental toxicity testing. A generalized log logistic dose-response model did offer other advantages in dealing with litter size and intralitter correlations (Allen et al., 1994b). Examples of how the benchmark dose approach can be used with continuous endpoints such as body weight changes have also been evaluated (Kavlock et al., 1995).

Clear advantages of the BMD approach include (1) the ability to take into account the full dose-response curve as opposed to focusing on a single test dose as is done in the NOAEL approach, (2) the inclusion of a measure of variability (confidence limit), (3) the use of responses within the experimental range versus extrapolation of responses to low doses not tested experimentally, and (4) the use of a consistent benchmark response level for RfD calculations across studies.

Some common exposures, such as lead and criteria air pollutants, are so close to LOAELs that regulatory agencies use an informal margin of safety approach that is heavily weighted with a consideration of technical feasibility.

**Nonthreshold Approaches.** As Fig. 4-4 shows, numerous dose-response curves can be proposed in the low-dose region of the dose-response curve if a threshold assumption is not made. Because the risk assessor generally needs to extrapolate beyond the region of the dose-response curve for which experimentally observed data are available, the choice of models to generate curves in this region of the dose-response curve has received much attention. Two general types of dose-response models exist: statistical (or probability distribution) models and mechanistic models (Krewski and Van Ryzin, 1981). Table 4-3 shows common models that have been used in risk extrapolation.

The distribution models are based on the assumption that each individual has a tolerance level for a test agent and that this response level is a variable that follows a specific probability distribution function. These responses can be modeled by using a cumulative-dose response function. Chapter 2 discusses the common normal distribution pattern (see Fig. 4-3). A log-probit model estimates the probability of response at a specified dose (d); thus, $P(d) = \Phi[\alpha + \beta \log d]$, where $\Phi$ is the

**Table 4–3**
**Models Used in Risk Extrapolation**

| |
|---|
| *Statistical or distribution models* |
| Log-probit |
| Logit |
| Weibull |
| *Mechanistic models* |
| One-hit |
| Multihit |
| Multistage |
| Linearized multistage |
| Stochastic two-stage model (Moolgavkar-Venson-Knudson) |
| *Model enhancement* |
| Time to tumor response |
| Physiologically based toxicokinetic models |
| Biologically based dose-response models |

cumulative function for a standard normal distribution of the log tolerances with standard deviations $\sigma$ and mean $\mu$, $a$ equals $\mu/\sigma$, and $\beta$ equals the slope of the probit line $(-1/\sigma)$. The probit curve at low doses usually assumes an S shape. Chapter 2 discusses the determination of the $LD_{50}$ value from such a curve. However, extrapolation of the experimental data from 50 percent response levels to a "safe" or "acceptable" level of exposure such as one in a million risk above background illustrates the huge gap between scientific observations and highly protective risk limits (sometimes called "virtually safe doses," with the dose corresponding to a 95 percent upper confidence limit on adverse response rates).

The log logistic model was derived from chemical kinetic theory. The probability of a response at dose d is defined as $P(d) = [1 - \exp(a + \beta \log d)]^{-1}$. Like the probit model, this model defines sigmoidal curves that are symmetrical around the 50 percent response level; however, the log logistic curves approach the 0 and 100 percent response levels with a more shallow curve shape (Fig. 4-4). The logit and probit curves are indistinguishable in fitting the data in the region of the response curve where experimentally derived data are present (Brown, 1984; Hartung, 1987).

**Models Derived from Mechanistic Assumptions.** This modeling approach involves the use of a mathematical equation to describe dose-response relationships that are consistent with postulated biological mechanisms of response. These models are based on the idea that a response (toxic effect) in a particular biological unit (animal, human, pup, etc.) results from the random occurrence of one or more biological events (stochastic events).

Radiation research has spawned a series of such "hit models" for cancer modeling, where a "hit" is defined as a critical cellular event that must occur before a toxic effect is produced. These models assume that (1) an infinitely large number of targets exists, for example, in the DNA, (2) the organism responds with a toxic response only after a minimum number of targets has been modified, (3) a critical target is altered if a sufficient number of hits occurs, and (4) the probability of a hit in the low-dose range of the dose-response curve is proportional to the dose of the toxicant (Brown, 1984).

The simplest mechanistic model is the one-hit (one-stage) linear model in which only one hit or critical cellular interaction is required for a cell to be altered. For example, based on somatic mutation theory, a single mutational change would be sufficient for a cell to become cancerous through a transformational event and dose-independent clonal expansion. The probability statement for these models is $(d) = 1 - \exp^{(-\lambda d)}$, where $\lambda d$ equals the number of hits occurring during a time period. A single molecule of a genotoxic carcinogen will have a minute but finite chance of causing a mutational event.

As theories of cancer have grown in complexity, so too have these "hit-based" mechanistic models. Multihit models have been developed that can describe hypothesized single-target multihit events as well as multitarget, multihit events in carcinogenesis. The probability statement for these models is $P(d) = \int^{\lambda d} X^{k-1} \exp^{-x} / \Gamma(k)\, dx$, where $\Gamma(k)$ denotes the gamma function and k denotes the critical number of hits for the adverse response. The Weibull model has a dose-response function with characteristics similar to those in the multihit models where the response equation is $P(d) = 1 - \exp[-\lambda d^k]$, where again k denotes the critical number of hits for the toxic cellular response.

Armitage and Doll (1957) developed a multistage model for carcinogenesis that was based on these equations and on the hypothesis that a series of ordered stages is required before a cell can undergo mutation, initiation, transformation, and progression to form a tumor. This relationship was generalized by Crump (1980) by maximizing the likelihood function over polynomials so that the probability statement is

$$P(d) = 1 - \exp[-\lambda_0 + \lambda d_1 + \lambda d_2 + \ldots \lambda_1 d^k]$$

If the true value of $\lambda_1$ is replaced with $\lambda_1^*$ (the upper confidence limit of $\lambda_1$), a linearized multistage model can be derived in which the expression is dominated by $(\lambda d^*)d$ at low doses. The slope of this confidence interval, $q_1^*$, is used by EPA for quantitative cancer assessment. To obtain an upper 95 percent confidence interval on risk, the $q_1^*$ value ($\Delta$ risk/$\Delta$ dose in mg/kg/day) is multiplied by the amount of exposure (mg/kg/day). Thus, the upper bound estimate on risk (R) is calculated as

$$R = q_1^* \text{ [risk (mg/kg/day)}^{-1}] \times \text{exposure (mg/kg/day)}$$

This relationship has been used to calculate a "virtually safe dose" (VSD) which represents the lower 95 percent confidence limit on a dose that gives an "acceptable level" of risk (e.g., upper confidence limit for $10^{-6}$ excess risk). Since both the $q_1^*$ and VSD values are calculated by using 95 percent confidence intervals, the values are believed to represent conservative estimates. The use of the maximum likelihood estimate (MLE) values from the linearized multistage models has not been accepted because of problems with the stability of a MLE estimate at a low dose using the linearized multistage (LMS) model.

The EPA utilizes the LMS model to calculate "unit risk estimates" in which the increased individual lifetime risk of cancer for a 70-kg human breathing 1 $\mu g/m^3$ of contaminated air or drinking 2 liters per day of water containing 1 ppm (1 mg/liter) is estimated over a 70-year life span.

**Toxicologic Enhancements of the Models.** Table 4-3 lists three areas of research that have improved the application of models used in risk extrapolation. Interim sacrifice data from animal bioassays had provided useful time to tumor information that allowed researchers to identify and model the early onset of some carcinogen-induced tumors. Other model enhancements include physiologically based toxicokinetic modeling (PBTK), and Chapter 7 discusses in detail these improvements in our estimation of exposure and offers approaches to modeling the "target internal effective dose" in risk assessment rather than just using single-value "external exposure doses."

Biologically based dose-response (BBDR) modeling is intended to make the generalized mechanistic models discussed in the previous section more clearly reflect specific biological processes. Measured rates are incorporated into the mechanistic equations to replace default or computer-generated values. For example, the Moolgavkar-Venson-Knudson (MVK) model (Moolgavkar, 1986, 1990) is based on a two-stage model for carcinogenesis where two mutations are required for carcinogenesis and the birth and death rates of cells are modeled through clonal expansion and tumor formation. This model has been applied effectively to human epidemiological data on retinoblastoma and to animal data on kidney and liver tumors in the 2-acetylaminofluorene (2-AAF) "megamouse" study, bladder cancer in saccharin-exposed rats, rat lung tumors after radiation exposure, rat liver tumors after *N*-nitroso-morpholine exposure, respiratory tract tumors after benzo[*a*]pyrene exposure, and mouse liver tumors after chlordane exposure (NRC, 1993a; Cohen and Ellwein, 1990; Moolgavkar and Luebeck, 1990). Additional exploratory applications are needed to continue validation of the model (NRC, 1993a). EPA discusses receptor binding theory in its dioxin risk reassessment (EPA, 1994c). Kohn and colleagues (1993) and Andersen and coworkers (1993) used PBTK and BBDR information to improve dioxin risk assessment.

The development of biologically based dose-response models for endpoints other than cancer are limited; however, several approaches are being explored in developmental toxicity, utilizing cell cycle kinetics, enzyme activity, litter effects, and cytotoxicity as critical endpoints (Shuey et al., 1994; Leroux et al., in press; Rai and Van Ryzin, 1985; Faustman et al., 1989). Unfortunately, there is a lack of specific quantitative biological information for most toxicants and endpoints.

## Exposure Assessment

The primary objectives of exposure assessment are to determine the source, type, magnitude, and duration of contact with the agent of interest. Obviously, this is a key element of the risk assessment process, as hazard does not occur in the absence of exposure. However, it is also frequently identified as the key area of uncertainty in overall risk determination. Chapter 5 discusses the basic principles of the absorption and excretion of toxicants, and Chap. 7 discusses toxicokinetics. Here the primary focus is on the uses of exposure information in quantitative risk assessment. Chapters 15 and 28 discuss exposure considerations that are important in risk assessment for inhalation toxicology.

A key step in making an exposure assessment is determining which exposure pathways are relevant for the risk scenario under development. The subsequent steps entail quantitating each pathway identified as a potentially relevant exposure and then summarizing these pathway-specific exposures for the calculation of overall exposure. The EPA has published numerous documents which provide guidelines for determining such exposures (EPA, 1992, 1989a and b). Such calculations can include an estimation of total exposures for a specified population as well as calculation of exposure for highly exposed individuals. The use of a hypothetical maximally exposed individual (MEI) is no longer favored in exposure assessment because of its extremely conservative assumptions at each step of the estimation. High-end exposure estimates (HEEEs) and theoretical upper-bound estimates (TUBEs) are now recommended.

Conceptually, HEEE calculations are designed to represent a "plausible estimate" of the exposure of the individuals in the upper ninetieth percentile of the exposure distribution. TUBEs are "bounding calculations" designed to represent exposures at a level that exceeds the exposures experienced by all individuals in the exposure distribution and are calculated by assuming limits for all exposure variables. A calculation for individuals exposed at levels near the middle of the exposure distribution is a central estimate. A lifetime average daily dose (LADD) is calculated as follows:

$$\text{LADD} = \frac{\begin{array}{c}\text{concentration}\\ \text{of the}\\ \text{toxicant in the}\\ \text{exposure media}\end{array} \times \begin{array}{c}\text{contact}\\ \text{rate}\end{array} \times \begin{array}{c}\text{contact}\\ \text{fraction}\end{array} \times \begin{array}{c}\text{exposure}\\ \text{duration}\end{array}}{(\text{body weight})\ (\text{lifetime})}$$

Table 4-4 illustrates an application of this exposure calculation. This table provides an HEEE and a central estimate for a potential dioxin exposure in recreational fish (EPA, 1994d). These estimates differ in the estimates for the amount of fish ingested, the contamination level in the fish, and the frequency of eating meals of recreationally captured fish. Obviously, such estimates would differ even more if the full range of potential toxicant containment levels were used. Utilizing better estimates for the distribution of containment levels is a major focus of recent risk assessment research. To obtain such estimates, several techniques, such as generating subjective uncertainty distributions and Monte Carlo composite analyses of parameter uncertainty, have been applied (NRC, 1994). The recent health assessment documents of EPA on TCDD and related compounds (EPA, 1994c) provide detailed examples of how to approach exposure uncertainties. These are approaches that can provide a reality check that is useful in generating more realistic exposure estimates.

Several endpoint-specific exposure considerations need to be discussed. In general, estimates for cancer risk use averages over a lifetime. In a few cases, short-term exposure limits (STELs) are required (for example, ethylene oxide), along with characterization of short but high levels of exposure. In these cases, exposures are not averaged over the lifetime. Another example of endpoint-specific considerations is the assumption with developmental toxicity that a single exposure can be sufficient to produce an adverse developmental effect; thus, daily doses rather than lifetime weighted averages are used. This is also important because of the time-dependent

**Table 4–4**
**Exposure Scenario for Dioxin via Ingestion of Contaminated Recreational Fish**

Central exposure estimate*

$$\text{LADD} = \frac{\dfrac{3 \times 10^{-9}\ \text{mg dioxin}}{\text{g fish}} \times \dfrac{150\ \text{g fish}}{\text{meal}} \times \dfrac{3\ \text{meals}}{\text{year}} \times \dfrac{1.0\ \text{contact}}{\text{fraction}}}{70\ \text{kg body weight} \times \dfrac{70\ \text{years}}{\text{lifetime}} \times \dfrac{365\ \text{days}}{\text{year}}}$$

$\text{LADD} = 5.3 \times 10^{-11}$ mg/kg/day

High-end exposure estimate†

$\text{LADD} = 1.2 \times 10^{-9}$ mg/kg/day

* Daily ingestion is calculated using 150 g of fish consumed per meal for three meals per year of recreationally caught fish and averaged over 365 days/year. Rate of ingestion for central estimates is 1.2 g of fish per day. Estimated fish contaminant levels are $3 \times 10^{-9}$ mg/g fish.

† The high-end exposure estimate uses 200 g fish per meal for 10 meals per year of recreationally caught fish and 15 ppt for dioxin contaminant level in the fish tissue based on a study downstream from 104 pulp mills. The rate of ingestion for this high-end exposure estimate is 4.1 g fish per day.

SOURCE: EPA(1994d).

specificity of many adverse developmental outcomes (EPA 1991b). Table 4-5 provides useful reference values for calculating exposure doses.

**Variation in Susceptibility.** Toxicologists have been slow to recognize the marked variation that occurs among humans. Generally, assay results and toxicokinetic modeling utilize means and standard deviations or even standard errors of the mean to make the range as small as possible. Outliers are seldom investigated. However, in occupational and environmental medicine, physicians are often asked, Why me, Doc? when they inform a patient that exposures on the job might explain a clinical problem. The patient insists that he or she is "no less careful than the next person." Thus, it is important to know whether and how the patient might be at higher risk. Furthermore, EPA and OSHA are expected under the Clean Air Act and the Occupational Safety and Health Act to promulgate standards that protect the most susceptible subgroups and individuals in the population. When investigators focus on the most susceptible individuals, there also may be a better chance to recognize and elucidate the underlying mechanisms (Omenn et al., 1990).

Host factors that influence susceptibility to environmental exposures include genetic traits, sex, and age; preexisting diseases; behavioral traits (most importantly smoking); coexisting exposures; medications; vitamins; and protective measures. Genetic studies are of two kinds: (1) investigations of the effects of chemicals and radiation on the genes and chromosomes, which are termed "genetic toxicology" (Chap. 9) (these tests measure evidence of mutations, adduct formation, chromosomal aberrations, sister chromatid exchange, DNA repair, and oncogene activation); and (2) ecogenetics studies identifying inherited variation in susceptibility (predisposition and resistance) to specific exposures ranging across pharmaceuticals ("pharmacogenetics"), pesticides, inhaled pollutants, foods, food additives, sensory stimuli, allergic and sensitizing agents, and infectious agents. Inherited variation in susceptibility has been demonstrated for all these kinds of external agents. In turn, ecogenetic variation may affect either the biotransformation systems that activate and detoxify chemicals or the sites of action in target tissues. Ecogenetics is still in its infancy; the development of new methods and specific biomarkers for biotransformation and sites of action of chemicals may soon permit rapid advances.

## Information Resources

There has been a virtual explosion of toxicology information that is now available on-line. Haz Dat can be accessed through the World Wide Web by using the address http://atsdr1.atsdr.cdc.gov:8080/atsdrhome.html. This database contains information on hazardous substance releases and contaminants as well as over 160 public health statements from the ATSDR's chemical-specific toxicology profiles. EXTOXNET (http://www.oes.orst.edu:70/l/ext) provides information

**Table 4–5**
**Reference Values for Dose Calculations: Life Span, Body Weight, Food and Water Intake, and Nominal Air Intake for Adults**

| SPECIES | SEX | LIFE SPAN, YEARS | BODY WEIGHT, kg | FOOD INTAKE (WET WEIGHT), g/day | WATER INTAKE, ml/day | AIR INTAKE, $m^3$/day |
|---|---|---|---|---|---|---|
| Human | M | 70 | 75 | 1500 | 2500 | 20 |
| | F | 78 | 60 | 1500 | 2500 | 20 |
| Mouse | M | 2 | 0.03 | 5 | 5 | 0.04* |
| | F | 2 | 0.025 | 5 | 5 | 0.04* |
| Rat | M | 2 | 0.5 | 20 | 25 | 0.2† |
| | F | 2 | 0.35 | 18 | 20 | 0.2† |
| Hamster | M | 2 | 0.125 | 12 | 15 | 0.09 |
| | F | 2 | 0.110 | 12 | 15 | 0.09 |

* For more exact values, use $m^3$/day (mouse) $= 0.0345\ (W/0.025)^{2/3}$, where W = body weight in kg (EPA, 1980).

† For more exact values, use $m^3$/day (rat) $= 0.105\ (W/0.113)^{2/3}$, where W = body weight in kg (EPA, 1980).

SOURCE: Hallenbeck (1993).

on the environmental chemistry and toxicology of pesticides, food additives, natural toxicants, and environmental contaminants. It is the product of an ad hoc consortium of university toxicologists and environmental chemists and specialists.

Other key sources of information for toxicologists are available through large databases such as RTECS, Toxline, and Medline. Scientific publications from the International Agency for Research on Cancer (IARC) have also been useful. The EPA provides health hazard information on over 500 chemicals and includes the most current oral reference doses, inhalation reference concentrations, and carcinogen unit risk estimates on the integrated risk information system (IRIS). To access IRIS, call the IRIS Risk Information Hotline at (513) 569-7254.

## Integrating the Qualitative and Quantitative Aspects of Risk Assessment

Qualitative assessment of hazard information should include a consideration of the consistency and concordance of the findings. Such an assessment should include a determination of the consistency of the toxicological findings across species and target organs, an evaluation of consistency across duplicate experimental conditions, and the adequacy of the experiments to detect the adverse endpoints of interest.

The National Toxicology Program (NPT) uses several categories to classify bioassay results, with the category "clear evidence of carcinogenicity" describing bioassays in which dose-related increases in malignant or combined malignant and benign neoplasms are seen across all doses or at least significant increases in two of the four species/sex test groups are noted. The NTP's evaluation guidelines allow for categories of some, equivocal, no evidence, and inadequate study.

Qualitative assessment of animal or human evidence is done by many agencies, including the EPA and IARC. Similar evidence classifications are used for both animal and human evidence categories by both agencies. These evidence classifications include levels of sufficient, limited, inadequate, no evidence (EPA, 1994b), and "evidence suggesting lack of carcinogenicity" (IARC, 1994). EPA also includes a specific no data category.

These evidence classifications are used for overall weight of evidence carcinogenicity classification schemes. Although differing group number or letter categories are used, striking similarities exist between these approaches. EPA's newly proposed changes to its risk assessment guidelines for carcinogenic substances include changes in how likelihood categories are used, with new references to categories described as "known," "likely," or "not likely" to be carcinogenic to humans. A category representing a "cannot evaluate" level includes inadequate data, incomplete or inconclusive data, and "no data" categories.

This section has presented approaches to evaluating cancer endpoints. Similar weight of evidence approaches have been proposed for reproductive risk assessment [refer to sufficient and insufficient evidence categories in EPA proposed guidelines for reproductive risk (EPA, 1994d)]. The Institute for Evaluating Health Risks has recently defined an "evaluative process" by which reproductive and developmental toxicity data can be evaluated consistently and integrated to ascertain its relevance for human health risk assessment (Moore et al., 1995). Application of such carefully deliberated approaches for assessing noncancer endpoints should help researchers avoid the tendency to list chemicals as yes or no (or positive or negative) without human relevancy information.

For many years there has been an information-sharing process aimed at harmonizing chemical testing regimes and clinical trial methodologies so that data might be accepted in the multiple countries that are members of the Organization for Economic Cooperation and Development (OECD). The United Nations Conference on the Environment in Rio de Janeiro in 1992 established harmonization of risk assessment as one of its goals, with a coordinating role for the International Programme on Chemical Safety. The negotiation in 1994 of the General Agreement on Trade and Tariffs (GATT) and the establishment of a World Trade Organization make harmonization of various aspects of testing, risk assessment, labeling, registration, and standards important elements in trade, not just in regulatory science. Moolenaar (1994) has summarized the carcinogen risk assessment methodologies used by various countries as a basis for regulatory actions. He tabulated the risk characterization, carcinogen identification, risk extrapolation, and chemical classification schemes of EPA, US Public Health Service, IARC, ACGIH, Australia, the European Economic Community (EEC), Germany, Netherlands, Norway, and Sweden. The approach of the EPA in estimating an upper bound to human risk is unique; all other countries estimate human risk values on the basis of the expected incidence of cancer from the exposures under review. The United Kingdom follows a case-by-case approach to risk evaluations for both genotoxic and nongenotoxic carcinogens, using no generic procedures. Denmark, the EEC, the United Kingdom, and the Netherlands all divide carcinogens into genotoxic and nongenotoxic agents and use different extrapolation procedures for each. Norway does not extrapolate data to low doses, using instead the $TD_{50}$ to divide category I carcinogens into tertiles by potency. The United Kingdom, the EEC, and the Netherlands all treat nongenotoxic chemical carcinogens as threshold toxicants. A NOAEL and a safety factor are used to set ADIs. It may be time for the United States to consider applying the BMD method to nongenotoxic carcinogens.

A politically controversial matter in recent years has been the introduction of organized comparative risk analysis projects. Comparative risk analysis is a planning and decision-making tool that ranks various kinds of environmental problems to establish their relative significance and priority for action. Many states have mounted explicit programs, as did EPA for itself, leading to its reports *Unfinished Business* (1987) and *Reducing Risks* (1990). After the 1994 national elections, the campaign of local officials to resist "unfunded mandates" was merged with the comparative risk method in an attempt to figure out which actions would be affordable and which would have priority both for federal assistance and for local spending. Typical problems compared in local projects are indoor air pollution, outdoor air pollution, alteration and/or destruction of terrestrial ecosystems, drinking water contamination, aesthetic degradation of the landscape, changes in land use patterns, and non-point-source pollution from everyday activities. The community participants express their preferences in a mostly qualitative process that leads to ranking and prioritization. There is also an effort to identify cultural and social aspects of living circumstances that might put certain population groups at higher risk through subsistence fishing, poor nutrition, or coexisting exposures; this element is called environmental justice. An even broader analysis might be called social justice, or the general public health approach of attending to all the modifiable determinants of poor health in a community. Increasingly, toxicologists and other regulatory scientists are being drawn in to these value-laden and sometimes emotionally charged community-based risk assessment and risk management processes.

## SUMMARY

The NRC framework for risk assessment has provided us with a consistent databased tool for evaluating risks. As listed in Table 4-1, the objectives of risk assessment can vary with risk management needs. However, the framework has been flexible enough to address these varying objectives and has provided guidance for priority setting in industrial research and development processes, resource allocation in environmental organizations, and government regulatory and public health agencies in setting public health priorities.

One of the strengths of this framework approach to risk assessment is the ability to organize the processes and allow new scientific findings to be substituted for default assumptions. Although the public, Congress, and regulatory agencies have long been preoccupied with cancer as the primary health risk, recent efforts to expand the application of framework approaches reflect a clear consensus to pay as much attention to noncancer endpoints as to ecological risks. Evidence of the commitment of scientists to a steadily increasing scientific basis for risk assessment can be seen in recent NRC publications such as *Science and Judgment in Risk Assessment* (NRC, 1994), which deals with the appropriateness of the default assumption and provides guidance on approaches for dealing with uncertainty. It is important to realize that risk assessment is an interactive process that is constantly being refined as a delicate balance of science and judgment that should improve with time and knowledge.

# REFERENCES

Abbott BD, Harris MW, Birnbaum LS: Comparisons of the effects of TCDD and hydrocortisone on growth factor expression provide insight into their interaction in the embryonic mouse palate. *Teratology* 45:35–53, 1992.

Albert RE: Carcinogen risk assessment in the US Environmental Protection Agency. *CRC Crit Rev Toxicol* 24:75–85, 1994.

Allen BC, Kavlock RJ, Kimmel CA, Faustman EM: Dose response assessments for developmental toxicity: II. Comparison of generic benchmark dose estimates with NOAELs. *Fundam Appl Toxicol* 23:487–495, 1994a.

Allen BC, Kavlock RJ, Kimmel CA, Faustman EM: Dose-response assessment for developmental toxicity: III. Statistical models. *Fundam Appl Toxicol* 23:496–509, 1994b.

Ames BN, Gold LS: Too many rodent carcinogens: Mitogenesis increases mutagenesis. *Science* 249:970–971, 1990.

Andersen ME, Mills JJ, Gargas ML, et al: Modeling receptor-mediated processes with dioxin: Implications for pharmacokinetics and risk assessment. *Risk Anal* 13(1):25–36, 1993.

Anderson EL: Quantitative approaches in use to assess cancer risk. *Risk Anal* 3:277–295, 1983.

Armitage P, Doll R: A two-stage theory of carcinogenesis in relation to the age distribution of human cancer. *Br J Cancer* 11:161–169, 1957.

Ashby J, Tennant RW: Prediction of rodent carcinogenicity of 44 chemicals: Results. *Mutagenesis* 9:7–15, 1994.

Atterwill CK, Johnston H, Thomas SM: Models for the *in vitro* assessment of neurotoxicity in the nervous system in relation to xenobiotic and neurotrophic factor-mediated events. *Neurotoxicology* 13:39–54, 1992.

Auton TR: Calculation of benchmark doses from teratology data. *Regul Toxicol Pharmacol* 19(2):152–167, 1994.

Barnes DG, Daston JS, Evans JS, et al: Benchmarks dose workshop: Criteria for use of a benchmark dose to estimate a reference dose. *Regul Toxicol Pharmacol* 21(2):296–306, 1995.

Bechtel DH: Molecular dosimetry of hepatic aflatoxin $B_1$-DNA adducts: Linear correlation with hepatic cancer risk. *Reg Toxicol Pharmacol* 10:74–81, 1989.

Brown CC: High- to low-dose extrapolation in animals, in Rodricks JV, Tardiff RG (eds.): *Assessment and Management of Chemical Risks*. Washington, DC: American Chemical Society, 1984, pp 57–79.

Calkins DR, Dixon RL, Gerber CR, et al: Identification, characterization, and control of potential human carcinogens: A framework for federal decision-making. *JNCI* 61:169–175, 1980.

Cohen SM, Ellwein LB: Proliferative and genotoxic cellular effects in 2-acetylaminofluorene bladder and liver carcinogenesis: Biological modeling of the EDO1 study. *Toxicol Appl Pharmacol* 104:79–93, 1990.

Crump KS: An improved procedure for low-dose carcinogenic risk assessment from animal data. *J Environ Pathol Toxicol* 5:675–684, 1980.

Crump KS: A new method for determining allowable daily intakes. *Fundam Appl Toxicol* 4:854–871, 1984.

Dean AG, Dean JA, Burton AH, Dicker RC: Epi Info, Version 5: A word processing, database, and statistics program for epidemiology on microcomputers. Stone Mountain, Ga.: USD, 1990.

Eaton DL, Gallagher EP: Mechanisms of aflatoxin carcinogenesis. *Annu Rev Pharmacol Toxicol* 34:135–172, 1994.

EPA: *Guidelines and Methodology Used in the Preparation of Health Effect Assessment Chapters of the Consent Decree Water Criteria Documents*. Federal Register 45:79347–79357, 1980.

EPA: *Unfinished Business: A Comparative Assessment of Environmental Problems*, vol 1. Overview Report. Washington, DC: Office of Policy Analysis, Office of Policy Planning and Evaluation, *Human Health Evaluation Manual*: Part A. *Risk Assessment Guidance for Superfund*. Interim Final. 6.1– 6.53, 1989a.

EPA: *Human Health Evaluation Manual*: Part A. Risk *Assessment Guidance for Superfund*, vol 1. Interim Final. Washington, DC: The Office of Emergency and Remedial Response, 1989a, pp 6.1–6.53.

EPA: *Exposure Factors Handbook*. Final Report. Washington, DC: Exposure Assessment Group. Office of Health and Evironmental Assessment, 1989b.

EPA: *Reducing Risk*. Washington, DC: Relative Risk Reduction Strategies Committee. Report No. SAB-EC-90-021, 1990.

EPA: *Exposure Factors Handbook* Final Report. Washington, DC: Exposure Assessment Group. Office of Health and Environmental Assessment, 1989b.

EPA: *Alpha2μ-Globulin: Association with Chemically-Induced Renal Toxicity and Neoplasia in the Male Rat.* EPA/625/3-91/0-19F. Washington, DC: EPA, 1991a.

EPA: Guidelines for developmental toxicity risk assessment. *Federal Register* 56:63798–63826, 1991b. Washington, DC: Office of the Federal Register, National Archives and Records Administration.

EPA: Guidelines for exposure assessment. *Federal Register* 57:22888–22938, 1992.

EPA: Guidelines for reproductive toxicity risk assessment, external review draft. EPA/600/AP94001. Washington, DC: Office of Research and Development, Office of Health and Environmental Assessment, 1994a.

EPA: Draft revisions to the guidelines for carcinogen risk assessment. Washington, DC: Office of Health and Environmental Assessment, Office of Research and Development, 1994b.

EPA: Health assessment document for 2,3,7,8-tetrachlorodibenzo-p-dioxin (TCDD) and related compounds. External Review Draft. EPA/600/BP-92/001b. Washington, DC: Office of Health and Environmental Assessment, Office of Research and Development, 1994c.

EPA: Estimating exposure to dioxin-like compounds. Washington, DC: Office of Health and Environmental Assessment, Exposure Assessment Group, 1994d.

Faustman EM: Short-term test for teratogens. *Muta Res* 205:355–384, 1988.

Faustman EM, Allen BC, Kavlock RJ, Kimmel CA: Quantitative dose-response assessment of developmental toxicity: I. Characterization of data base and determination of NOAELs. *Fundam Appl Toxicol* 23:478–486, 1994.

Faustman EM, Wellington DG, Smith WP, Kimmel CS: Characterization of a developmental toxicity dose response model. *Environ Health Perspect* 79:229–241, 1989.

Fischhoff B, Bostrom A, Quandrel MJ: Risk perception and communication. *Annu Rev Public Health* 14:183–203, 1993.

Fischhoff B, Lichtenstein S, Slovic P: *Acceptable Risk.* New York: Cambridge University Press, 1981.

Gray TJB: Application of *in vitro* systems in male reproductive toxicology, in Lamb JC IV, Foster PMD (eds): *Physiology and Toxicology of Male Reproduction.* San Diego: Academic Press, 1988, pp 225–257.

Hallenbeck, WH: *Quantitative Risk Assessment for Environmental and Occupational Health*, 2d ed. Boca Raton, Fla: Lewis, 1993.

Harris MW, Chapin RE, Lockhart AC, et al: Assessment of a short-term reproductive and developmental toxicity screen. *Fundam Appl Toxicol* 19:186–196, 1992.

Hartung R: Dose-response relationships, in Tardiff RG, Rodricks JV (eds): *Toxic Substances and Human Risk: Principles of Data Interpretation.* New York: Plenum Press, 1987, pp 29–46.

Haseman JK, Lockhart AM: Correlations between chemically related site-specific carcinogenic effects in long-term studies in rats and mice. *Environ Health Perspect* 101:50–54, 1993.

Healey GF: Power calculations in toxicology. *ATLA* 15:132–139, 1987.

Hill AB: The environment and disease: Association or causation. *Proc R Soc Lond Med* 58:295–300, 1965.

IARC: *IARC Monographs on the Evaluation of Carcinogenic Risks to Humans.* Lyon: World Health Organization, 1994.

Kavlock RJ, Allen BC, Faustman EM, Kimmel CA: Dose response assessments for developmental toxicity: IV. Benchmark doses for fetal weight changes. *Fundam Appl Toxicol* 26:211–222, 1995.

Kimmel CA, Gaylor DW: Issues in qualitative and quantitative risk analysis for developmental toxicology. *Risk Anal* 8:15–20, 1988.

Kohn MC, Lucier GW, Clark GC, et al: A mechanistic model of effects of dioxin on gene expression in the rat liver. *Toxical Appl Pharmcol* 120:138–154, 1993.

Krewski D, Van Ryzin J: Dose response models for quantal response toxicity data, in Csörgö M, Dawson DA, Rao JNK, Seleh AK (eds): *Statistics and Related Topics: Proceedings of the International Symposium on Statistics and Related Topics.* North-Holland, 1981, pp 201–229.

Lave LB, Ennever F, Rosenkranz HS, Omenn GS: Information value of the rodent bioassay. *Nature* 336:631–633, 1988.

Lave LB, Omenn GS: Cost-effectiveness of short-term tests for carcinogenicity. *Nature* 334:29–34, 1986.

Leroux BG, Leisenring WM, Moolgavkar SH, Faustman EM: A biologically based dose-response model for development. *Risk Anal*, (in press).

Lowrance WW: *Of Acceptable Risk.* Los Altos, Calif: William Kaufmann, 1976.

McClain RM: Mechanistic considerations in the regulation and classification of chemical carcinogens, in Kotsonis FN, Mackey M, Hijele J (eds): *Nutritional Toxicology.* New York: Raven Press, 1994, pp 273–304.

Moolenaar RJ: Carcinogen risk assessment: International comparison. *Reg Toxicol Pharmacol* 20:302–336, 1994.

Moolgavkar SH: Carcinogenesis modeling: From molecular biology to epidemiology. *Annu Rev Public Health* 7:151–169, 1986.

Moolgavkar SH, Luebeck G: Two-event model for carcinogenesis: Biological, mathematical, and statistical considerations. *Risk Anal* 10:323–341, 1990.

Moore JA, Daston GP, Faustman EM, et al: An evaluative process for assessing human reproductive and developmental toxicity of agents. *Reprod Toxicol* 9:61–95, 1995.

Morgan GM: Risk analysis and management. *Sci Am* 269:32–35, 38–41, 1993.

Neil N, Malmfors T, Slovic P: Intuitive toxicology: Expert and lay judgments of chemical risks. *Toxicol Pathol* 22(2):198–201, 1994.

NRC: *Risk Assessment in the Federal Government: Managing the Process.* Washington, DC: National Academy Press, 1983.

NRC: *Issues in Risk Assessment.* Washington, DC: National Academy Press, 1993a.

NRC: *Pesticides in the Diets of Infants and Children.* Washington, DC: National Academy Press, 1993b.

NRC: *Science and Judgment in Risk Assessment.* Washington, DC: National Academy Press, 1994.

Omenn GS: The role of epidemiology in public policy. *Ann Epidemiol* 3:319–322, 1993.

Omenn GS: The risk assessment paradigm. *Toxicology* 102:23–28, 1995.

Omenn GS, Lave LB: Scientific and cost-effectiveness criteria in selecting batteries of short-term tests. *Mutat Res* 205:41–49, 1988.

Omenn GS, Omiecinski CJ, Eaton DL: Eco-genetics of chemical carcinogens, in Cantor C, Caskey C, Hood L, et al (eds): *Biotechnology and Human Genetic Predispostion to Disease.* New York: Wiley-Liss, 1990, pp 81–93.

Omenn GS, Steubbe S, Lave LB: Predictions of rodent carcinogenicity testing results: Interpretation in light of the Lave-Omenn value-of-information model. *Mol Carcinogen* 14:37–45, 1995.

Perera F, Mayer J, Santella RM, et al: Biologic markers in risk assessment for environmental carcinogens. *Environ Health Perspect* 90:247–254, 1991.

Rai K, Van Ryzin J: A dose response model for teratological experiments involving quantal responses. *Biometrics* 41:1–10, 1985.

Shelby MD, Bishop JB, Mason JM, Tindall KR: Fertility, reproduction and genetic disease: Studies on the mutagenic effects of environmental agents on mammalian germ cells. *Environ Health Perspect* 100:283–291, 1993.

Shuey DL, Lau C, Logsdon TR, et al: Biologically based dose-response modeling in developmental toxicology: Biochemical and cellular sequelae of 5-fluorouracil exposure in the developing rat. *Toxicol Appl Pharmacol* 126:129–144, 1994.

Slovic P: Risk perception, in Travis CC (ed): *Carcinogen Risk Assessment*. New York: Plenum Press, 1988, pp 171–192.

Slovic P, Fischhoff B, Lichtenstein S: Rating the risks. *Environ* 21:1–20, 36–39, 1979.

Statistics and Epidemiology Research Corporation (SERC): EGRET. Seattle: Statistics and Epidemiology Research Corporation, 1994.

Tennant RW, Spalding JW, Stasiewicz S, Ashby J: Prediction of the outcome of rodent carcinogenicity bioassays currently being conducted on 44 chemicals by the US NTP. *Mutagenesis* 5:3–14, 1990.

Whittaker SG, Faustman EM: *In vitro* assays for developmental toxicity, in Gad SC (ed): *In Vitro Toxicology. New York: Raven Press, 1994, pp. 97–122.*

WHO: Principles governing consumer safety in relation to pesticide residues. *WHO Tech Rep Ser* 240, Geneva, 1962.

# UNIT 2

# DISPOSITION OF TOXICANTS

CHAPTER 5

# ABSORPTION, DISTRIBUTION, AND EXCRETION OF TOXICANTS

*Karl K. Rozman and Curtis D. Klaassen*

## INTRODUCTION

As was noted in Chaps. 2 and 3, the toxicity of a substance depends on the dose; that is, the greater the amount of a chemical taken up by an organism, the greater the toxic response. This concept, which is known as *dose-response,* requires elaboration, because ultimately it is not the dose but the concentration of a toxicant at the site or sites of action (target organ or tissue) that determines toxicity. It should be noted that the words "toxicant," "drug," "xenobiotic" (foreign compound), and "chemical" are used interchangeably throughout this chapter, since all chemical entities, whether endogenous or exogenous in origin, can cause toxicity at some dose. The concentration of a chemical at the site of action is proportional to the dose, but the same dose of two or more chemicals may lead to vastly different concentrations in a particular target organ of toxicity. This differential pattern is due to differences in the disposition of chemicals. Disposition may be conceptualized as consisting of absorption, distribution, biotransformation, and excretion. It should be noted, however, that these processes may occur simultaneously. The various factors affecting disposition are depicted in Fig. 5-1. They are discussed in detail in this chapter and Chap. 6. Any or all of these factors may have a minor or major impact on the concentration and thus the toxicity of a chemical in a target organ. For example, (1) if the fraction absorbed or the rate of absorption is low, a chemical may never attain a sufficiently high concentration at a potential site of action to cause toxicity, (2) the distribution of a toxicant may be such that it is concentrated in a tissue other than the target organ, thus decreasing the toxicity, (3) biotransformation of a chemical may result in the formation of less toxic or more toxic metabolites at a fast or slow rate with obvious consequences for the concentration and thus the toxicity at the target site, and (4) the more rapidly a chemical is eliminated from an organism, the lower

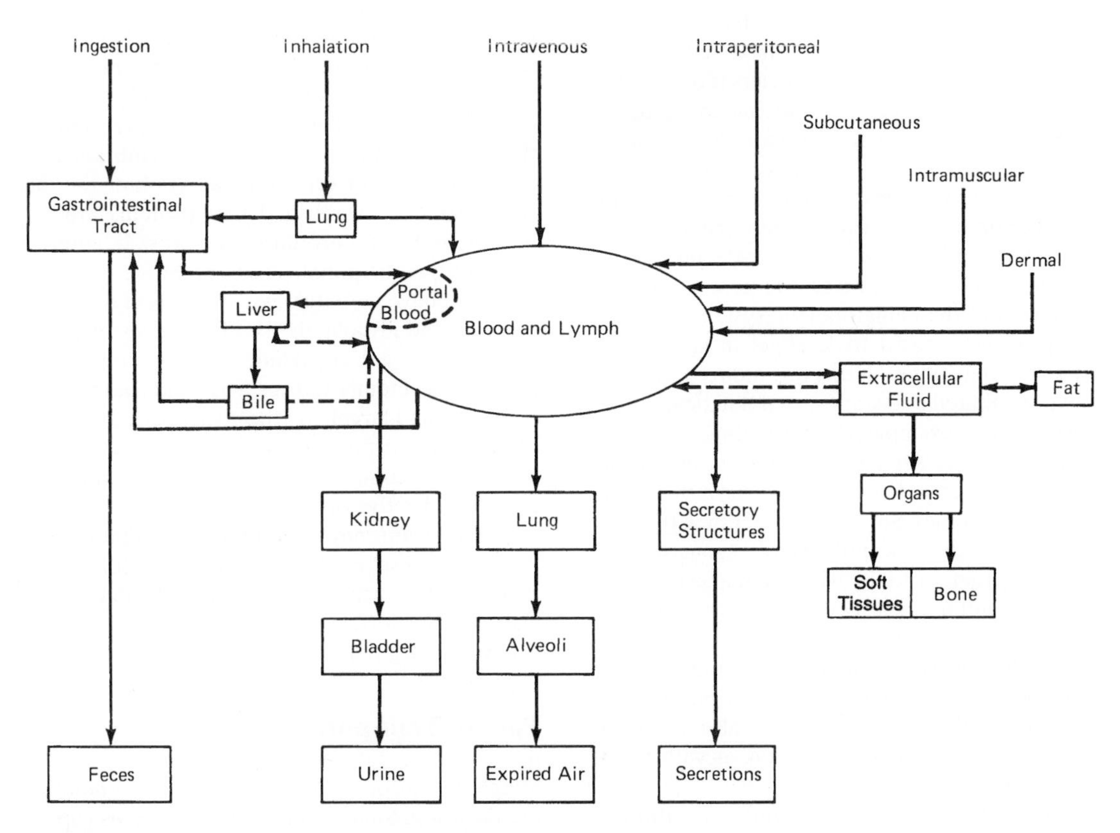


***Figure 5-1.** Routes of absorption, distribution, and excretion of toxicants in the body.*

will be its concentration and hence its toxicity in a target tissue or tissues. Furthermore, all these processes are interrelated and thus influence each other. For example, the rate of excretion of a chemical may depend to a large extent on its distribution and/or biotransformation. If a chemical is distributed to and stored in fat, its elimination is likely to be slow because very low plasma levels preclude rapid renal clearance or other clearances. Some lipid-soluble chemicals are very resistant to biotran<sup>c</sup>formation. Their rate of excretion depends on biotransformation to water-soluble products and/or slow intestinal excretion of the parent compounds. As this brief introduction illustrates, the disposition of xenobiotics is very important in determining the concentration and thus the toxicity of chemicals in organisms.

The quantitation and determination of the time course of absorption, distribution, biotransformation, and excretion of chemicals are referred to as *pharmacokinetics* or *toxicokinetics* (see Chap. 7). Mathematical models are used to describe parts or the whole process of the disposition of a chemical. Calculations based on these models allow a numerical characterization of disposition (half-life, elimination rate constants, tissue profiles, etc.), which is essential for the assessment of the toxicity of a compound. Examination of species differences combined with knowledge of species-specific pathways of handling chemicals often provides the tools that allow toxicologists to predict disposition and its role in the toxicity of a compound for human exposure.

The skin, lungs, and alimentary canal are the main barriers that separate higher organisms from an environment that contains a high number of chemicals. Toxicants have to cross one or several of these incomplete barriers to exert their deleterious effects at one site or several sites in the body. Exceptions are caustic and corrosive agents (acids, bases, salts, oxidizers), which act topically. A chemical absorbed into the bloodstream through any of these three barriers is distributed, at least to some extent, throughout the body, including the site where it produces damage. This site is often called the *target organ* or *target tissue*. A chemical may have one or several target organs, and in turn, several chemicals may have the same target organ or organs. For example, benzene affects the hematopoietic system and carbon tetrachloride injures the liver. Lead and mercury both damage the central nervous system, the kidneys, and the hematopoietic system. It is self-evident that to produce a direct toxic effect in an organ, a chemical must reach that organ. However, indirect toxic responses may be precipitated at distant sites if a toxicant alters regulatory functions. For example, cholestyramine, a nonabsorbable resin, may trap certain acidic vitamins in the intestinal lumen and cause systemic toxicity in the form of various vitamin deficiency syndromes. Several factors other than the concentration influence the susceptibility of organs to toxicants. Therefore, the organ or tissue with the highest concentration of a toxicant is not necessarily the site where toxicity is exerted. For example, chlorinated hydrocarbon insecticides such as dichlorodiphenyltrichloroethane (DDT) attain their highest concentrations in fat depots of the body but produce no known toxic effect in that tissue. A toxicant also may exert its adverse effect directly on the bloodstream, as with arsine gas, which causes hemolysis.

Toxicants are removed from the systemic circulation by biotransformation, excretion, and storage at various sites in the body. The relative contribution of these processes to total elimination depends on the physical and chemical properties of the chemical. The kidney plays a major role in the elimination of most toxicants, but other organs may be of critical importance with some toxic agents. Examples include the elimination of a volatile agent such as carbon monoxide by the lungs and that of lead in the bile. Although the liver is the most active organ in the biotransformation of toxicants, other organs or tissues (enzymes in plasma, kidney, lungs, GI tract, etc.) also may contribute to overall biotransformation. Biotransformation often is a prerequisite for renal excretion, because many toxicants are lipid-soluble and are therefore reabsorbed from the renal tubules after glomerular filtration. After a toxicant is biotransformed, its metabolites may be excreted preferentially into bile, as are the metabolites of DDT, or may be excreted into urine, as are the metabolites of organophosphate insecticides.

In this chapter, the qualitative aspects of absorption, distribution, and excretion are outlined, whereas their quantitative aspects will be treated in Chap. 7. The fourth aspect of disposition—the biotransformation of chemicals—is dealt with in Chap. 6 As most toxic agents have to pass several membranes before exerting toxicity, we will start with a discussion of some general characteristics of this ubiquitous barrier in the body.

## CELL MEMBRANES

Toxicants usually pass through a number of cells, such as the stratified epithelium of the skin, the thin cell layers of the lungs or the gastrointestinal tract, the capillary endothelium, and the cells of the target organ or tissue. The plasma membranes surrounding all these cells are remarkably similar. The thickness of the cell membrane is about 7 to 9 nm. Biochemical, physiological, and morphological (electron microscopy) studies have provided strong evidence that membranes consist of a phospholipid bilayer with polar head groups (phosphatidylcholine, phosphatidylethanolamine) predominating on both the outer and inner surfaces of the membrane and more or less perpendicularly directed fatty acids filling out the inner space. It is also well established that proteins are inserted in the bilayer, and some proteins even cross it, allowing the formation of aqueous pores (Fig. 5-2). Some cell membranes (eukaryotic) have an outer coat or glycocalyx consisting of glycoproteins and glycolipids. The fatty acids of the membrane do not have a rigid crystalline structure but are quasi-fluid at physiological temperatures. The fluid character of membranes is determined largely by the structure and relative abundance of unsaturated fatty acids. The more unsaturated fatty acids membranes contain, the more fluidlike they are, facilitating more rapid active or passive transport.

A toxicant may pass through a membrane by one of two general processes: (1) passive transport (diffusion according to Fick's law), in which the cell expends no energy, and (2) specialized transport, in which the cell provides energy to translocate the toxicant across its membrane.

### Passive Transport

**Simple Diffusion.** Most toxicants cross membranes by simple diffusion. Small hydrophilic molecules (up to a molecular weight of about 600) presumably permeate membranes

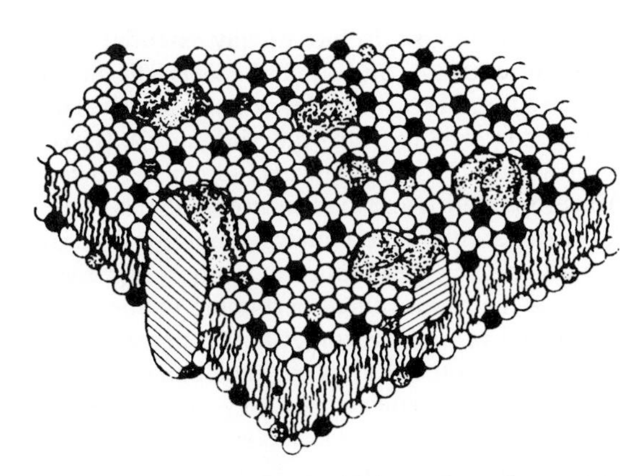

***Figure 5-2. Schematic model of a biological membrane.***

Spheres represent the ionic and polar head groups of the phospholipid molecules, with different types represented as black, white, or stippled. Zigzag lines represent the fatty acid chains. Proteins associated with the membrane are represented by the large bodies with cross-hatching.

through aqueous pores (Benz et al., 1980), whereas hydrophobic molecules diffuse across the lipid domain of membranes. The smaller a hydrophilic molecule is, the more readily it traverses membranes by simple diffusion through aqueous pores. Consequently, ethanol is absorbed rapidly from the stomach and intestine and is distributed equally rapidly throughout the body by simple diffusion from blood into all tissues. The majority of toxicants consist of larger organic molecules with differing degrees of lipid solubility. Their rate of transport across membranes correlates with their lipid solubility, which is frequently expressed as hexane/water or chloroform/water partition coefficients.

Many chemicals are weak organic acids or bases. In solution, they are ionized according to Arrhenius' theory. The ionized form usually has low lipid solubility and thus does not permeate readily through the lipid domain of a membrane. Some transport of organic anions and cations (depending on their molecular weight) may occur through the aqueous pores, but this is a slow process (except for very low molecular weight compounds), as the total surface area of aqueous pores is small compared with the total surface area of the lipid domain of a membrane. In general, the nonionized form of weak organic acids and bases is to some extent lipid-soluble, resulting in diffusion across the lipid domain of a membrane. The rate of transport of the nonionized form is proportional to its lipid solubility. The molar ratio of ionized to nonionized molecules of a weak organic acid or base in solution depends on the ionization constant. The ionization constant provides a measure for the weakness of organic acids and bases. The pH at which a weak organic acid or base is 50 percent ionized is called its p*K*a or p*K*b. Like pH, p*K*a and p*K*b are defined as the negative logarithm of the ionization constant of a weak organic acid or base. With the equation p*K*a = 14 − p*K*b, p*K*as can also be calculated for weak organic bases. An organic acid with a low p*K*a is a relatively strong acid, and one with a high p*K*a is a weak acid. The opposite is true for bases. The numerical value of p*K*a does not indicate whether a chemical is an organic acid or a base. Knowledge of the chemical structure is required to distinguish between organic acids and bases.

The degree of ionization of a chemical depends on its p*K*a and on the pH of the solution. The relationship between p*K*a and pH is described by the Henderson-Hasselbalch equations:

$$\text{For acids: } pK_a - pH = \log \frac{[\text{nonionized}]}{[\text{ionized}]}$$

$$\text{For bases: } pK_a - pH = \log \frac{[\text{ionized}]}{[\text{nonionized}]}$$

The effect of pH on the degree of ionization of an organic acid (benzoic acid) and an organic base (aniline) is shown in Fig. 5-3. According to the Brönsted-Lowry acid-base theory, an acid is a proton ($H^+$) donor and a base is a proton acceptor. Thus, the ionized and nonionized forms of an organic acid represent an acid-base pair, with the nonionized moiety being the acid and the ionized moiety being the base. At a low pH, a weak organic acid such as benzoic acid is largely nonionized. At pH 4, exactly 50 percent of benzoic acid is ionized and 50 percent is nonionized, because this is the p*K*a of the compound. As the pH increases, more and more protons are neutralized by hydroxyl groups, and benzoic acid continues to dissociate until almost all of it is in the ionized form. For an organic base such as aniline, the obverse is true. At a low pH, when protons are abundant, almost all of aniline is protonated, that is, ionized. This form of aniline is an acid because it can donate protons. As the pH increases, anilinium ions continue to dissociate until almost all the aniline is in the nonionized form, which is the aniline base. As transmembrane passage is largely restricted to the nonionized form, benzoic acid is more readily translocated through a membrane from an acidic environment, whereas more aniline is transferred from an alkaline environment.

**Filtration.** When water flows in bulk across a porous membrane, any solute small enough to pass through the pores flows with it. Passage through these channels is called *filtration,* as it involves bulk flow of water caused by hydrostatic or osmotic force. One of the main differences between various membranes is the size of these channels. In the kidney glomeruli these pores are relatively large (about 70 nm), allowing molecules smaller than albumin (molecular weight 60,000) to pass through. The channels in most cells are much smaller (<4 nm), permitting substantial passage of molecules with molecular weights of no more than a few hundred (Schanker, 1961, 1962).

## Special Transport

There are numerous compounds whose movement across membranes cannot be explained by simple diffusion or filtration. Some compounds are too large to pass through aqueous

| pH | Benzoic Acid | % Nonionized | Aniline | % Nonionized |
|---|---|---|---|---|
| 1 | COOH | 99.9 | $NH_3^+$ | |
| 2 | | 99 | | 0.1 |
| 3 | | 90 | | 1 |
| 4 | | 50 | | 10 |
| 5 | ↕ | 10 | ↕ | 50 |
| 6 | $COO^-$ | 1 | $NH_2$ | 90 |
| 7 | | 0.1 | | 99 |

***Figure 5–3. Effect of pH on the ionization of benzoic acid (pKa = 4) and aniline (pKa = 5).***

pores or too insoluble in lipids to diffuse across the lipid domains of membranes. Nevertheless, they often are transported very rapidly across membranes, even against concentration gradients. To explain these phenomena, the existence of specialized transport systems has been postulated. These systems are responsible for the transport across cell membranes of many nutrients, such as sugars and amino and nucleic acids, and also that of some foreign compounds.

**Active Transport.** The following properties characterize an active transport system: (1) Chemicals are moved against electrochemical or concentration gradients, (2) the transport system is saturated at high substrate concentrations and thus exhibits a transport maximum ($T_m$), (3) the transport system is selective for certain structural features of chemicals and has the potential for competitive inhibition between compounds that are transported by the same transporter, and (4) the system requires expenditure of energy so that metabolic inhibitors block the transport process.

Substances actively transported across cell membranes presumably form a complex with a membrane-bound macromolecular carrier on one side of the membrane. The complex subsequently traverses to the other side of the membrane, where the substance is released. Afterward, the carrier returns to the original surface to repeat the transport cycle.

Active transport is particularly important in regard to eliminating xenobiotics from an organism. The central nervous system (CNS) has two transport systems at the choroid plexus to transport compounds out of the cerebrospinal fluid (CSF): one for organic acids and one for organic bases. The kidney also has two active transport systems, whereas the liver has at least four, two of which transport organic acids, one organic bases, and one neutral organic compounds.

**Facilitated Diffusion.** Facilitated diffusion applies to carrier-mediated transport that exhibits the properties of active transport, except that the substrate is not moved against an electrochemical or concentration gradient and the transport process does not require the input of energy; that is, metabolic poisons do not interfere with this transport. The transport of glucose from the gastrointestinal (GI) tract across the basolateral membrane of the intestinal epithelium, from plasma into red blood cells and from blood into the CNS, occurs by facilitated diffusion.

**Additional Transport Processes.** Other forms of specialized transport have been proposed, but their overall importance is not as well established as that of active transport and facilitated diffusion. Phagocytosis and pinocytosis are proposed mechanisms for cell membranes flowing around and engulfing particles. This type of transfer has been shown to be important for the removal of particulate matter from the alveoli by phagocytes and from blood by the reticuloendothelial system of the liver and spleen.

## ABSORPTION

The process by which toxicants cross body membranes and enter the bloodstream is referred to as *absorption*. There are no specific systems or pathways for the sole purpose of absorbing toxicants. Xenobiotics penetrate membranes during absorption by the same processes as do biologically essential substances such as oxygen, foodstuffs, and other nutrients. The main sites of absorption are the GI tract, the lungs, and the skin. However, absorption also may occur from other sites, such as the subcutis, peritoneum, or muscle, if a chemical is administered by special routes. Experimentalists and medical professionals often distinguish between parenteral and enteral administration of drugs and other xenobiotics. It is important to know that enteral administration includes all routes pertaining to the alimentary canal (sublingual, oral, and rectal), whereas parenteral administration involves all other routes (intravenous, intraperitoneal, intramuscular, subcutaneous, etc.).

### Absorption of Toxicants by the Gastrointestinal Tract

The GI tract is one of the most important sites where toxicants are absorbed. Many environmental toxicants enter the food chain and are absorbed together with food from the GI tract. This site of absorption is of particular interest to toxicologists because suicide attempts frequently involve an overdose of an orally ingested drug. Oral intake is also the most common route by which children are accidentally exposed to poisons.

The GI tract may be viewed as a tube traversing the body. Although it is within the body, its contents can be considered exterior to the body. Therefore, poisons in the GI tract usually do not produce systemic injury to an individual until they are absorbed unless a noxious agent has caustic or irritating properties.

Absorption of toxicants can take place along the entire GI tract, even in the mouth and rectum. Therefore, drugs such as nitroglycerin are administered sublingually and others are administered rectally, whereas the majority of drugs are given orally. If a toxicant is an organic acid or base, it tends to be absorbed by simple diffusion in the part of the GI tract in which it exists in the most lipid-soluble (nonionized) form. Because gastric juice is acidic and the intestinal contents are nearly neutral, the lipid solubility of weak organic acids or bases can differ markedly in these two areas of the GI tract. One can determine by the Henderson-Hasselbalch equations the fraction of a toxicant that is in the nonionized (lipid-soluble) form and estimate the rate of absorption from the stomach or intestine. According to this equation, a weak organic acid is present mainly in the nonionized (lipid-soluble) form in the stomach and predominantly in the ionized form in the intestine. Therefore, one would expect that weak organic acids are absorbed more readily from the stomach than from the intestine. In contrast, organic bases (except very weak organic bases) are not in the lipid-soluble form in the stomach but are in that form in the intestine, suggesting that the absorption of such compounds occurs predominantly in the intestine rather than in the stomach. However, the Henderson-Hasselbalch equations have to be interpreted with some qualifications because other factors, such as the mass action law, surface area, and blood flow rate, have to be taken into consideration in examining the absorption of weak organic acids or bases. For example, only 1 percent of benzoic acid is present in the lipid-soluble form in the intestine. Therefore, one might conclude that the intestine has little capacity to absorb this organic acid. However, absorption is a dynamic process. The blood keeps removing benzoic acid from the lamina propria of the intes-

*For Weak Acids*

$$pK_a - pH = \log \frac{[nonionized]}{[ionized]}$$

Benzoic acid pKa ≈ 4

Stomach pH ≈ 2

$$4 - 2 = \log \frac{[nonionized]}{[ionized]}$$

$$2 = \log \frac{[nonionized]}{[ionized]}$$

$$10^2 = \log \frac{[nonionized]}{[ionized]}$$

$$100 = \log \frac{[nonionized]}{[ionized]}$$

Ratio favors absorption

Intestine pH ≈ 6

$$4 - 6 = \log \frac{[nonionized]}{[ionized]}$$

$$-2 = \log \frac{[nonionized]}{[ionized]}$$

$$10^{-2} = \frac{[nonionized]}{[ionized]}$$

$$\frac{1}{100} = \frac{[nonionized]}{[ionized]}$$

*For Weak Bases*

$$pKa - pH = \log \frac{[ionized]}{[nonionized]}$$

Aniline p*K*a ≈ 5

Stomach pH ≈ 2

$$5 - 2 = \log \frac{[ionized]}{[nonionized]}$$

$$3 = \log \frac{[ionized]}{[nonionized]}$$

$$10^3 = \log \frac{[ionized]}{[nonionized]}$$

$$1000 = \log \frac{[ionized]}{[nonionized]}$$

Intestine pH ≈ 6

$$5 - 6 = \log \frac{[ionized]}{[nonionized]}$$

$$-1 = \log \frac{[ionized]}{[nonionized]}$$

$$10^{-1} = \frac{[ionized]}{[nonionized]}$$

$$\frac{1}{10} = \frac{[ionized]}{[nonionized]}$$

Ratio favors absorption

tine, and according to the mass action law, the equilibrium will always be maintained at 1 percent in the nonionized form, providing continuous availability of benzoic acid for absorption. Moreover, absorption by simple diffusion also is proportional to the surface area. Because the small intestine has a very large surface (the villi and microvilli increase the surface area approximately 600-fold), the overall capacity of the intestine for absorption of benzoic acid is quite large. Similar considerations are valid for the absorption of all weak organic acids from the intestine.

The mammalian GI tract has specialized transport systems (carrier-mediated) for the absorption of nutrients and electrolytes (Table 5-1). The absorption of some of these substances is complex and depends on a number of factors. The absorption of iron, for example, depends on the need for iron and takes place in two steps: Iron first enters the mucosal cells and then moves into the blood. The first step is relatively rapid, whereas the second is slow. Consequently, iron accumulates within the mucosal cells as a protein-iron complex termed *ferritin*. When the concentration of iron in blood drops below normal values, some iron is liberated from the mucosal stores of ferritin and transported into the blood. As a consequence, the absorption of more iron from the intestine is triggered to replenish these stores. Calcium also is absorbed by a two-step process: first absorption from the lumen and then exudation into the interstitial fluid. The first step is faster than the second, and therefore intracellular calcium rises in mucosal cells during absorption. Vitamin D is required for both steps of calcium transport.

Some xenobiotics can be absorbed by the same specialized transport systems. For example, 5-fluorouracil is absorbed by the pyrimidine transport system (Schanker and Jeffrey, 1961), thallium by the system that normally absorbs iron (Leopold et al., 1969), and lead by the calcium transporter (Sobel et al., 1938). Cobalt and manganese compete for the iron transport system (Schade et al., 1970; Thomson et al., 1971a, 1971b). Some dipeptide and oligopeptide transporters have been well characterized and have been shown to play an important role in the active absorption of drugs containing a $\beta$-lactam structure (Tsuji et al., 1993; Dantzig et al., 1994). Transepithelial absorption of dipeptides (e.g., glycylsarcosine) and $\beta$-lactam antibiotics at low concentrations occurs predominantly by active carrier-mediated mechanisms at both apical and basolateral membranes (Thwaites et al., 1993).

The number of toxicants actively absorbed by the GI tract is low; most enter the body by simple diffusion. Although lipid-soluble substances are absorbed by this process more rapidly and extensively than are water-soluble substances, the latter also may be absorbed to some degree. After oral ingestion, about 10 percent of lead, 4 percent of manganese, 1.5 percent of cadmium, and 1 percent of chromium salts are absorbed. If a compound is very toxic, even small amounts of absorbed material produce serious systemic effects. An organic compound that would not be expected to be absorbed on the basis of the pH-partition hypothesis is the fully ionized quaternary ammonium compound pralidoxime chloride (2-PAM; molecular weight 137), yet it is absorbed almost entirely from the GI tract (Levine and Steinberg, 1966). The mechanism by which some lipid-insoluble compounds are absorbed is not entirely clear. It appears that organic ions of low molecular weight (122 to 188) can be transported across the mucosal barrier by paracellular transport, that is, passive penetration

**Table 5–1**
**Site Distribution of Specialized Transport Systems in the Intestine of Man and Animals**

| | LOCATION OF ABSORPTIVE CAPACITY | | | |
|---|---|---|---|---|
| | *Small Intestine* | | | |
| SUBSTRATES | *Upper* | *Middle* | *Lower* | *Colon* |
| Sugar (glucose, galactose, etc.) | + + | + + + | + + | 0 |
| Neutral amino acids | + + | + + + | + + | 0 |
| Basic amino acids | + + | + + | + + | ? |
| Gamma globulin (newborn animals) | + | + + | + + + | ? |
| Pyrimidines (thymine and uracil) | + | + | ? | ? |
| Triglycerides | + + | + + | + | ? |
| Fatty acid absorption and conversion to triglyceride | + + + | + + | + | 0 |
| Bile salts | 0 | + | + + + | |
| Vitamin $B_{12}$ | 0 | + | + + + | 0 |
| $Na^+$ | + + + | + + | + + + | + + + |
| $H^+$ (and/or $HCO_3^-$ secretion) | 0 | + | + + | + + |
| $Ca^{2+}$ | + + + | + + | + | ? |
| $Fe^{2+}$ | + + + | + + | + | ? |
| $Cl^-$ | + + + | + + | + | 0 |

SOURCE: Adapted from Wilson TH: *Mechanisms of Absorption.* Saunders, Philadelphia, 1962, pp 40–68.

through aqueous pores at the tight junctions (Aungst and Shen, 1986), or by active transport as discussed above.

It is interesting that even particulate matter can be absorbed by the GI epithelium. Particles of an azo dye, variable in size but averaging several thousand nanometers in diameter, have been shown to be taken up by the duodenum (Barnett, 1959). Emulsions of polystyrene latex particles of 22 $\mu$m in diameter have been demonstrated to be carried through the cytoplasm of the intestinal epithelium in intact vesicles and discharged into the interstices of the lamina propria, followed by absorption into the lymphatics of the mucosa (Sanders and Ashworth, 1961). Particles appear to enter intestinal cells by pinocytosis, a process that is much more prominent in newborns than in adults (Williams and Beck, 1969). These examples demonstrate some of the principles and the variety of toxicants that can be absorbed at least to some extent by the GI tract.

The resistance or the lack of resistance of chemicals to alteration by the acidic pH of the stomach, enzymes of the stomach or intestine, or the intestinal flora is of extreme importance. A toxicant may be hydrolyzed by stomach acid or biotransformed by enzymes of the microflora of the intestine to new compounds with a toxicity greatly different from that of the parent compound. For example, snake venom is much less toxic when administered orally rather than intravenously because it is broken down by digestive enzymes of the GI tract. Ingestion of well water with a high nitrate content produces methemoglobinemia much more frequently in infants than in adults. This is due to the higher pH of the GI tract in newborns, with the consequence of greater abundance of certain bacteria, especially *Escherichia coli (E. coli),* which convert nitrate to nitrite. Nitrite formed by bacterial action produces methemoglobinemia (Rosenfield and Huston, 1950). Nitrite also is used as a food additive in meats and smoked fish. Some fish, vegetables, and fruit juices contain secondary amines. The acidic environment of the stomach facilitates a chemical reaction between nitrite and secondary amines, leading to the formation of carcinogenic nitrosamines (Chap. 8). Also, the intestinal flora can reduce aromatic nitro groups to aromatic amines that may be goitrogenic or carcinogenic (Thompson et al., 1954). Intestinal bacteria, specifically *Aerobacter aerogenes,* have been shown to degrade DDT to DDE (Mendel and Walton, 1966).

Many factors alter the GI absorption of toxicants. For example, editic acid [ethylenediaminetetraacetic acid (EDTA)] increases the absorption of some toxicants by increasing intestinal permeability. Simple diffusion is proportional not only to surface area and permeability but also to residency time in various segments of the alimentary canal. Therefore, the rate of absorption of a toxicant remaining for longer periods in the intestine increases, whereas that with a shorter residency time decreases. The residency time of a chemical in the intestine depends on intestinal motility. Some agents used as laxatives are known to exert such effects on the absorption of xenobiotics by altering intestinal motility (Levine, 1970).

Experiments have shown that the oral toxicity of some chemicals is increased by diluting the dose (Ferguson, 1962; Borowitz et al., 1971). This phenomenon may be explained by more rapid stomach emptying induced by increased dosage volume, which in turn leads to more rapid absorption in the duodenum because of the larger surface area there.

The absorption of a toxicant from the GI tract also depends on the physical properties of a compound, such as lipid solubility, and the dissolution rate. Although it is often generalized that an increase in lipid solubility increases the absorption of chemicals, an extremely lipid-soluble chemical does not dissolve in the GI fluids, and absorption is low (Houston et al., 1974). If the toxicant is a solid and is relatively insoluble in GI fluids, it will have limited contact with the GI mucosa, and therefore its rate of absorption will be low. Also, the larger the particle size is, the less will be absorbed, as the dissolution rate is inversely proportional to particle size (Gorringe and Sproston, 1964; Bates and Gibaldi, 1970). This explains why metallic mercury is relatively nontoxic when ingested orally and why finely powdered arsenic is significantly more toxic than its coarse, granular form (Schwartze, 1923).

The amount of a chemical entering the systemic circulation after oral administration depends on several factors. First, it depends on the amount absorbed into the GI cells. Further, before a chemical enters the systemic circulation, it can be biotransformed by the GI cells or extracted by the liver and excreted into bile with or without prior biotransformation. The lung can also contribute to the biotransformation or elimination of chemicals before their entrance into the systemic circulation, although its role is less well defined than that of the intestine and liver. This phenomenon of the removal of chemicals before entrance to the systemic circulation is referred to as *presystemic elimination,* or *first-pass effect.*

A number of other factors have been shown to alter absorption. For example, one ion can alter the absorption of another: Cadmium decreases the absorption of zinc and copper, and calcium that of cadmium; zinc decreases the absorption of copper, and magnesium that of fluoride (Pfeiffer, 1977). Milk has been found to increase lead absorption (Kelly and Kostial, 1973), and starvation enhances the absorption of dieldrin (Heath and Vandekar, 1964). The age of animals also appears to affect absorption: Newborn rats absorbed 12 percent of a dose of cadmium, whereas adult rats absorbed only 0.5 percent (Sasser and Jarboe, 1977). While lead and many other heavy metal ions are not absorbed readily from the GI tract, EDTA and other chelators increase the lipid solubility and thus the absorption of complexed ions. Thus, it is important not to give a chelator orally when excess metal is still present in the GI tract after oral ingestion.

The principles of GI absorption may be summarized in the following way. Penetration of amphophilic (having both lipophilic and hydrophilic molecular characteristics) substances across the GI wall occurs according to the basic principles of physicochemistry, with the unstirred water layer representing the rate-determining barrier for the more lipophilic molecules and the epithelial cell membrance representing that for the more hydrophilic compounds. Unlike the skin, which is virtually impenetrable to molecules at the extreme ends of the lipophilicity/hydrophilicity scale, the GI tract can also absorb such compounds. Some extremely hydrophilic compounds are absorbed by active processes, whereas extremely lipophilic compounds [2, 3, 7, 8-tetrachlorodibenzo-*p*-dioxin (TCDD), DDT, polychlorinated biphenyls (PCBs), etc.] ride in on the "coattails" of lipids via the micelles and subsequent biological processes related to lipid metabolism.

## Absorption of Toxicants by the Lungs

It is well known that toxic responses to chemicals can result from their absorption after inhalation. The most frequent cause of death from poisoning—carbon monoxide—and probably the most important occupational disease—silicosis—are both due to the absorption or deposition of airborne poisons in the lungs. This site of absorption has been employed in chemical warfare (chlorine and phosgene gas, lewisite, mustard gas) and in the execution of criminals in the gas chamber (hydrogen cyanide).

Toxicants absorbed by the lungs are usually gases (e.g., carbon monoxide, nitrogen dioxide, and sulfur dioxide), vapors of volatile or volatilizable liquids (e.g., benzene and carbon tetrachloride), and aerosols. Because the absorption of inhaled gases and vapor differs from that of aerosols, aerosols will be discussed separately below. However, the absorption of gases and vapors is governed by the same principles, and therefore the word "gas" will represent both in this section.

**Gases and Vapors.** The absorption of inhaled gases takes place mainly in the lungs. However, before a gas reaches the lungs, it passes through the nose with its turbinates, which increase the surface area. Because the mucosa of the nose is covered by a film of fluid, gas molecules can be retained by the nose and not reach the lungs if they are very water soluble or react with cell surface components. Therefore, the nose acts as a "scrubber" for water-soluble gases and highly reactive gases, partially protecting the lungs from potentially injurious insults. A case in point is formaldehyde. The drawback of this protective mechanism for the lungs is that a typical nose breather such as a rat develops tumors of the nasal turbinates when chronically exposed to high levels of formaldehyde by inhalation.

Absorption of gases in the lungs differs from intestinal and percutaneous absorption of compounds in that the dissociation of acids and bases and the lipid solubility of molecules are less important factors in pulmonary absorption because diffusion through cell membranes is not rate-limiting in the pulmonary absorption of gases. There are at least three reasons for this. First, ionized molecules are of very low volatility, and consequently, their concentration in normal ambient air is insignificant. Second, the epithelial cells lining the alveoli—that is, type I pneumocytes—are very thin and the capillaries are in close contact with the pneumocytes, so that the distance for a chemical to diffuse is very short. Third, chemicals absorbed by the lungs are removed rapidly by the blood, as it takes only about three-fourths of a second for the blood to go through the extensive capillary network in the lungs.

When a gas is inhaled into the lungs, gas molecules diffuse from the alveolar space into the blood and then dissolve. Except for some gases with a special affinity for certain body components (e.g., the binding of carbon monoxide to hemoglobin), the uptake of a gas by a tissue usually involves a simple physical process of dissolving. The end result is that gas molecules partition between the two media: air and blood during the absorptive phase and blood and other tissues during the distribution phase. As the contact of the inspired gas with blood continues in the alveoli, more molecules dissolve in blood until gas molecules in blood are in equilibrium with gas molecules in the alveolar space. At equilibrium, the ratio of the concentration of chemical in the blood and chemical in the gas phase is constant. This solubility ratio is called the *blood-to-gas partition coefficient.* This constant is unique for each gas. Note that only the ratio is constant, not the concentrations, as, according to Henry's law, the amount of gas dissolved in a liquid is proportional to the partial pressure of the gas in the gas phase at any given concentration before or at saturation. Thus, the higher the inhaled concentration of a gas (i.e., the higher the partial pressure), the higher the gas concentration in blood, but the ratio does not change unless saturation has occurred. When equilibrium is reached, the rate of transfer of gas molecules from the alveolar space to blood equals the rate of removal by blood from the alveolar space. For example, chloroform has a high (15) and ethylene a low (0.14) blood/gas phase solubility ratio. For a substance with a low solubility ratio such as ethylene, only a small percentage of the total gas in the lungs is removed by blood during each circulation because blood is soon saturated with the gas. Therefore, an increase in the respiratory rate or minute volume does not change the transfer of such a gas to blood. In contrast, an increase in the rate of blood flow markedly increases the rate of uptake of a compound with a low solubility ratio because of more rapid removal from the site of equilibrium, that is, the alveolar membranes. It has been calculated that the time to equilibrate between the blood and the gas phase for a relatively insoluble gas is about 8 to 21 min.

Most of a gas with a high solubility ratio, such as chloroform, is transferred to blood during each respiratory cycle so that little, if any, remains in the alveoli just before the next inhalation. The more soluble a toxic agent is in blood, the more of it will be dissolved in blood by the time equilibrium is reached. Consequently, the time required to equilibrate with blood is very much longer for a gas with a high solubility ratio than for a gas with a low ratio. This has been calculated to take a minimum of 1 h for compounds with a high solubility ratio, although it may take even longer if the gas also has high tissue affinity (i.e., high fat solubility). With these highly soluble gases, the principal factor limiting the rate of absorption is respiration. Because the blood is already removing virtually all of a gas with a high solubility ratio from the lungs, increasing the blood flow rate does not substantially increase the rate of absorption. However, the rate can be accelerated greatly by increasing the rate of respiration, or the minute volume.

Thus, the rate of absorption of gases in the lungs is variable and depends on a toxicant's solubility ratio (concentration in blood/concentration in gas phase before or at saturation) at equilibrium. For gases with a very low solubility ratio, the rate of transfer depends mainly on blood flow through the lungs (perfusion-limited), whereas for gases with a high solubility ratio, it is primarily a function of the rate and depth of respiration (ventilation-limited). Of course, there is a wide spectrum of intermediate behavior between the two extremes, with the median being a blood/gas concentration ratio of about 1.20.

The blood carries the dissolved gas molecules to the rest of the body. In each tissue, the gas molecules are transferred from the blood to the tissue until equilibrium is reached at a tissue concentration dictated by the tissue-to-blood partition coefficient. After releasing part of the gas to tissues, blood returns to the lungs to take up more of the gas. The process continues until a gas reaches equilibrium between blood and each tissue according to the tissue-to-blood partition coefficients characteristic of each tissue. At this time, no net absorption of gas takes place as long as the exposure concentration remains constant, because a steady state has been reached. Of course, if biotransformation and excretion occur, alveolar absorption will continue until a corresponding steady state is established.

**Aerosols and Particles.** The degree of ionization and the lipid solubility of chemicals are very important for oral and percutaneous exposures, whereas water solubility, tissue reactivity, and blood-to-gas phase partition coefficients are important after exposure to gases and vapors. The important characteristics that affect absorption after exposure to aerosols are the aerosol size and water solubility of a chemical present in the aerosol.

The site of deposition of aerosols depends largely on the size of the particles. This relationship is discussed in detail in Chap. 15. Particles 5 μm or larger usually are deposited in the nasopharyngeal region (Fig. 5-4). Those deposited on the unciliated anterior portion of the nose tend to remain at the site of deposition until they are removed by nose wiping, blowing, or sneezing. The mucous blanket of the ciliated nasal surface propels insoluble particles by the movement of the cilia. These particles and particles inhaled through the mouth are swallowed within minutes. Soluble particles may dissolve in the mucus and be carried to the pharynx or may be absorbed through the nasal epithelium into blood.

Particles of 2 to 5 μm are deposited mainly in the tracheobronchiolar regions of the lungs, from which they are cleared by retrograde movement of the mucus layer in the ciliated portions of the respiratory tract. The rate of cilia-propelled movement of mucus varies in different parts of the respiratory tract, although in general it is a rapid and efficient transport mechanism. Measurements have shown transport rates between 0.1 and 1 mm per minute, resulting in removal half-lives between 30 and 300 min. Coughing and sneezing greatly increase the movement of mucus and particulate matter toward the mouth. Particles eventually may be swallowed and absorbed from the GI tract.

Particles 1 μm and smaller penetrate to the alveolar sacs of the lungs. They may be absorbed into blood or cleared through the lymphatics after being scavenged by alveolar macrophages.

In addition to gases, liquid aerosols and particles can be absorbed in the alveoli. The mechanisms responsible for the removal or absorption of particulate matter from the alveoli

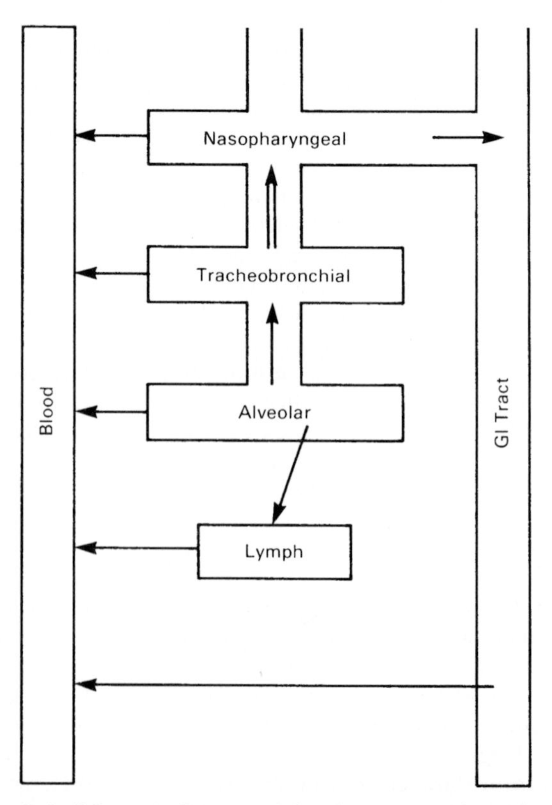


***Figure 5–4. Schematic diagram of the absorption and translocation of chemicals by lungs.***

(usually less than 1 μm in diameter) are less clear than those responsible for the removal of particles deposited in the tracheobronchial tree. Removal appears to occur by three major mechanisms. First, particles may be removed from the alveoli by a physical process. It is thought that particles deposited on the fluid layer of the alveoli are aspirated onto the mucociliary escalator of the tracheobronchial region. From there, they are transported to the mouth and may be swallowed, as was mentioned previously. The origin of the thin fluid layer in the alveoli is probably a transudation of lymph and secretions of lipids and other components by the alveolar epithelium. The alveolar fluid flows by an unknown mechanism to the terminal bronchioles. This flow seems to depend on lymph flow, capillary action, the respiratory motion of the alveolar walls, the cohesive nature of the respiratory tract fluid blanket, and the propelling power of the ciliated bronchioles. Second, particles from the alveoli may be removed by phagocytosis. The principal cells responsible for engulfing alveolar debris are the mononuclear phagocytes, the macrophages. These cells are found in large numbers in normal lungs and contain many phagocytized particles of both exogenous and endogenous origin. They apparently migrate to the distal end of the mucociliary escalator and are cleared and eventually swallowed. Third, removal may occur via the lymphatics. The endothelial cells lining lymphatic capillaries are permeable for very large molecules (molecular weight $> 10^6$) and for particles, although the rate of penetration is low above a molecular weight of 10,000 (Renkin, 1968). Nevertheless, the lymphatic system plays a prominent role in collecting high-molecular-weight proteins leaked from cells or blood capillaries and particulate matter from the interstitium and the alveolar spaces. Particulate matter may remain in lymphatic tissue for long periods, and this explains the name "dust store of the lungs."

For the reasons discussed above, the overall removal of particles from the alveoli is relatively inefficient; on the first day only about 20 percent of particles are cleared, and the portion remaining longer than 24 h is cleared very slowly. The rate of clearance by the lungs can be predicted by a compound's solubility in lung fluids. The lower the solubility, the lower the removal rate. Thus, it appears that removal of particles from the lungs is largely due to dissolution and vascular transport. Some particles may remain in the alveoli indefinitely. This may occur when proliferating, instead of desquamating, alveolar cells ingest dust particles and, in association with a developing network of reticulin fibers, form an alveolar dust plaque or nodule.

## Absorption of Toxicants through the Skin

Human skin comes into contact with many toxic agents. Fortunately, the skin is not very permeable and therefore is a relatively good barrier for separating organisms from their environment. However, some chemicals can be absorbed by the skin in sufficient quantities to produce systemic effects. For example, nerve gases such as sarin are readily absorbed by intact skin. Also, carbon tetrachloride can be absorbed through the skin in sufficient quantities to cause liver injury. Various insecticides have caused death in agricultural workers after absorption through intact skin (Chaps. 18 and 22).

To be absorbed through the skin, a toxicant must pass through the epidermis or the appendages (sweat and sebaceous glands and hair follicles). Sweat glands and hair follicles are scattered in varying densities on the skin. Their total cross-sectional area is probably between 0.1 and 1.0 percent of the total skin surface. Although the entry of small amounts of toxicants through the appendages may be rapid, chemicals are absorbed mainly through the epidermis, which constitutes the major surface area of the skin. Chemicals that are absorbed through the skin have to pass through several cell layers (a total of seven) before entering the small blood and lymph capillaries in the dermis (Fig. 5-5). The rate-determining barrier in the dermal absorption of chemicals is the epidermis. More accurately, it is the stratum corneum (horny layer), the uppermost layer of the epidermis (Dugard, 1983). This is the outer horny layer of the skin, consisting of densely packed keratinized cells that have lost their nuclei and thus are biologically inactive. Passage through the six other cell layers is much more rapid than is passage through the stratum corneum. Therefore, the most important considerations regarding the dermal absorption of xenobiotics relate to the stratum corneum.

The first phase of percutaneous absorption is diffusion of xenobiotics through the rate-limiting barrier, the stratum corneum. Studies have shown that the stratum corneum is replenished about every 3 to 4 weeks in adults. This complex process includes a gross dehydration and polymerization of intracellular matrix that results in keratin-filled dried cell layers. In the course of keratinization, the cell walls apparently double in thickness owing to the inclusion or deposition of chemically resistant materials. This change in the physical state of the tissue causes a commensurate change in its diffusion barrier property. The transformation is from an aqueous fluid medium that is characterized by liquid state to a dry, keratinous semisolid state with much lower permeability for toxicants by diffusion (permeability by diffusion = diffusivity).

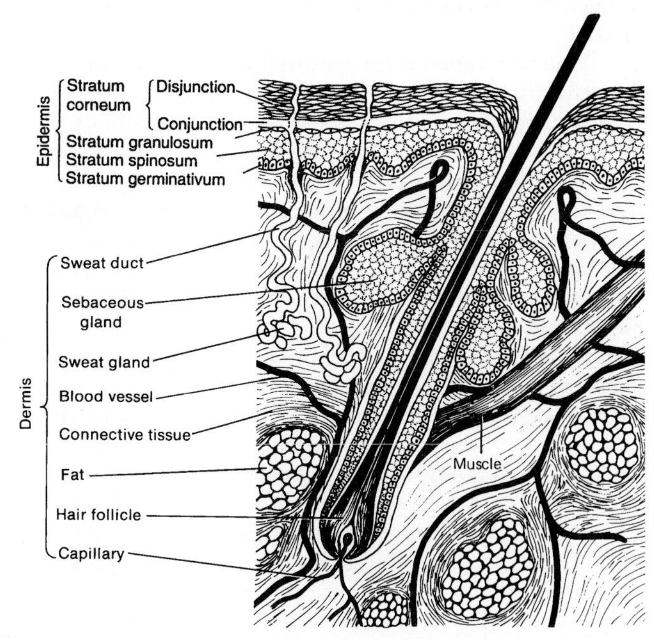


*Figure 5–5. Diagram of a cross section of human skin.*

In contrast to the complexity of the GI tract, the skin is a simpler penetration barrier for chemicals because passage through dead cell layers is the rate-determining step. It is clear that all toxicants move across the stratum corneum by passive diffusion. Kinetic measurements suggest that polar and nonpolar toxicants may diffuse through the stratum corneum by different mechanisms. Polar substances appear to diffuse through the outer surface of protein filaments of the hydrated stratum corneum, whereas nonpolar molecules dissolve in and diffuse through the lipid matrix between the protein filaments (Blank and Scheuplein, 1969). The rate of diffusion of nonpolar toxicants is proportional to their lipid solubility and is inversely related to their molecular weight (Marzulli et al., 1965). However, there are limits to the generalization of this theory. The rate of dermal penetration of highly lipophilic chemicals such as TCDD is very limited (Weber et al., 1991). Their solubility in triglycerides is relatively good, but not in phospholipids and other lipids with polar head groups. Because the stratum corneum contains very little triglycerides (2.8 percent in pigs, 0 percent in humans) and much cholesterol (26.0 percent in pigs, 26.9 percent in humans), some cholesterol esters (4.1 percent in pigs, 10 percent in humans), and various ceramides (44.2 percent in pigs, 41.1 percent in humans), it is not surprising that the absorption of highly lipophilic toxicants through the skin remains quite limited (Wertz and Downing, 1991). Ceramides are moderately lipophilic, as they are amides and/or esters of saturated and unsaturated fatty acids. Thus, the stratum corneum consists of about 75 to 80 percent moderately lipophilic materials. The simple physicochemical fact of *similis similibus solvontur* ("similar dissolves similar") explains the validity of the lipophilicity theory for molecules of moderate lipophilicity which also possess some hydrophilic regions. However, for both extreme ends of the lipophilicity/hydrophilicity spectrum, the stratum corneum represents a nearly impenetrable barrier unless those compounds damage the upper layer of the skin. A slow rate of penetration is possible for such substances via the appendages, provided that they remain in contact with a large skin surface area for prolonged periods.

Human stratum corneum displays significant differences in structure and chemistry from one region of the body to another, and these differences affect the permeability of the skin to chemicals. Skin from the plantar and palmar regions is much different from skin from other areas of the body in that the stratum corneum of the palms and soles is adapted for weight bearing and friction. The stratum corneum of the rest of the body surface is adapted for flexibility and fine sensory discrimination. The permeability of the skin depends on both the diffusivity and the thickness of the stratum corneum. While the stratum corneum is much thicker on the palms and soles (400 to 600 $\mu$m in callous areas) than on the arms, back, legs, and abdomen (8 to 15 $\mu$m), it has much higher diffusivity per unit thickness. Consequently, toxicants readily cross scrotum skin, since it is extremely thin and has high diffusivity; cross the abdominal skin less rapidly, as it is thicker and exhibits less diffusivity; and cross the sole with the greatest difficulty because the distance to traverse is great even though diffusivity there is highest.

The second phase of percutaneous absorption consists of diffusion of the toxicant through the lower layers of the epidermis (stratum granulosum, spinosum, and germinativum) and the dermis. These cell layers are far inferior to the stratum corneum as diffusion barriers. In contrast to the stratum corneum, they contain a porous, nonselective, aqueous diffusion medium. Toxicants pass through this area by diffusion and enter the systemic circulation through the numerous venous and lymphatic capillaries in the dermis. The rate of diffusion depends on blood flow, interstitial fluid movement, and perhaps other factors, including interactions with dermal constituents.

The absorption of toxicants through the skin varies, depending on the condition of the skin. Because the stratum corneum plays a critical role in determining cutaneous permeability, removal of this layer causes a dramatic increase in the permeability of the epidermis for a variety of large or small molecules, both lipid-soluble and water-soluble (Malkinson, 1964). Agents such as acids, alkalis, and mustard gases that injure the stratum corneum increase its permeability. The most frequently encountered penetration enhancing damage to the skin results from burns and various skin diseases. Water plays an extremely important role in skin permeability. Under normal conditions, the stratum corneum is partially hydrated, containing about 7 percent water by weight. This amount of water increases the permeability of the stratum corneum approximately 10-fold over the permeability that exists when it is completely dry. On additional contact with water, the stratum corneum can increase its weight of tightly bound water up to three- to fivefold, and this results in an additional two- to threefold increase in permeability. Studies of the dermal absorption of toxicants often utilize the method of Draize and associates (1944), wrapping plastic around animals and placing the chemical between the plastic and the skin (occlusive application). This hydrates the stratum corneum and enhances the absorption of some toxicants.

Solvents such as dimethyl sulfoxide (DMSO) also can facilitate the penetration of toxicants through the skin. DMSO increases the permeability of the barrier layer of the skin, that is, the stratum corneum. Little information is available about the mechanism by which DMSO enhances skin permeability. However, it has been suggested that DMSO (1) removes much of the lipid matrix of the stratum corneum, making holes or artificial shunts in the penetration barrier, (2) produces reversible configurational changes in protein structure brought about by the substitution of integral water molecules, and (3) functions as a swelling agent (Allenby et al., 1969; Dugard and Embery, 1969).

Various species have been employed in studying the dermal absorption of toxicants. Considerable species variation has been observed in cutaneous permeability. For many chemicals the skin of rats and rabbits is more permeable whereas the skin of cats is usually less permeable, while the cutaneous permeability characteristics of guinea pigs, pigs, and monkeys are often similar to those observed in humans (Scala et al., 1968; Coulston and Serrone, 1969; Wester and Maibach, 1977). Species differences in percutaneous absorption account for the differential toxicity of insecticides in insects and humans. For example, the $LD_{50}$ of injected DDT is approximately equal in insects and mammals, but DDT is much less toxic to mammals than to insects when it is applied to the skin. This appears to be due to the fact that DDT is poorly absorbed through the skin of mammals but passes readily through the chitinous exoskeleton of insects. Furthermore, insects have a much greater body surface area relative to weight than do mammals (Winteringham, 1957; Albert, 1965; Hayes, 1965).

### Absorption of Toxicants after Special Routes of Administration

Toxicants usually enter the bloodstream after absorption through the skin, lungs, or GI tract. However, in studying chemical agents, toxicologists frequently administer them to laboratory animals by special routes. The most common routes are (1) intraperitoneal, (2) subcutaneous, (3) intramuscular, and (4) intravenous. The intravenous route introduces the toxicant directly into the bloodstream, eliminating the process of absorption. Intraperitoneal injection of toxicants into laboratory animals is also a common procedure. It results in rapid absorption of xenobiotics because of the rich blood supply and the relatively large surface area of the peritoneal cavity. In addition, this route of administration circumvents the delay and variability of gastric emptying. Intraperitoneally administered compounds are absorbed primarily through the portal circulation and therefore must pass through the liver before reaching other organs (Lukas et al., 1971). Subcutaneously and intramuscularly administered toxicants are usually absorbed at slower rates but enter directly into the general circulation. The rate of absorption by these two routes can be altered by changing the blood flow to the injection site. For example, epinephrine causes vasoconstriction and will decrease the rate of absorption if it is coinjected intramuscularly with a toxicant. The formulation of a xenobiotic also may affect the rate of absorption; toxicants are absorbed more slowly from suspensions than from solutions.

The toxicity of a chemical may or may not depend on the route of administration. If a toxicant is injected intraperitoneally, most of the chemical enters the liver via the portal circulation before reaching the general circulation. Therefore, an intraperitoneally administered compound may be completely extracted and biotransformed by the liver with subsequent excretion into the bile without gaining access to the systemic circulation. Propranolol (Shand and Rangno, 1972) and lidocaine (Boyes et al., 1970) are two drugs with efficient extraction during the first pass through the liver. Any toxicant displaying the first-pass effect with selective toxicity for an organ other than the liver and GI tract is expected to be much less toxic when administered intraperitoneally than when injected intravenously, intramuscularly, or subcutaneously. For compounds with no appreciable biotransformation in the liver, toxicity ought to be independent of the route of administration if the rates of absorption are equal. This discussion indicates that it is possible to obtain some preliminary information on the biotransformation and excretion of xenobiotics by comparing their toxicity after administration by different routes.

## DISTRIBUTION

After entering the blood by absorption or intravenous administration, a toxicant is available for distribution (translocation) throughout the body. Distribution usually occurs rapidly. The rate of distribution to organs or tissues is determined primarily by blood flow and the rate of diffusion out of the capillary bed into the cells of a particular organ or tissue. The final distribution depends largely on the affinity of a xenobiotic for various tissues. In general, the initial phase of distribution is dominated by blood flow, whereas the eventual distribution is determined largely by affinity. The penetration of toxicants into cells occurs by passive diffusion or special transport processes, as was discussed previously. Small water-soluble molecules and ions apparently diffuse through aqueous channels or pores in the cell membrane. Lipid-soluble molecules readily permeate the membrane itself. Very polar molecules and ions of even moderate size (molecular weight of 50 or more) cannot enter cells easily except by special transport mechanisms because they are surrounded by a hydration shell, making their actual size much larger.

### Volume of Distribution

Total body water may be divided into three distinct compartments: (1) plasma water, (2) interstitial water, and (3) intracellular water. Extracellular water is made up of plasma water plus interstitial water. The concentration of a toxicant in blood depends largely on its volume of distribution. For example, if 1 g of each of several chemicals were injected directly into the bloodstream of 70-kg humans, marked differences in their plasma concentrations would be observed depending on the distribution: A high concentration would be observed in the plasma if the chemcial was distributed into plasma water only, and a much lower concentration would be reached if it was distributed into a large pool, such as total body water (see below).

The distribution of toxicants is usually complex and cannot be equated with distribution into one of the water compartments of the body. Binding to and/or dissolution in various storage sites of the body, such as fat, liver, and bone, are usually more important factors in determining the distribution of chemicals.

Some toxicants do not readily cross cell membranes and therefore have restricted distribution, whereas other toxicants rapidly pass through cell membranes and are distributed throughout the body. Some toxicants accumulate in certain parts of the body as a result of protein binding, active transport,

| COMPARTMENT | % OF TOTAL | LITERS IN 70-kg HUMAN | PLASMA CONCENTRATION AFTER 1 g OF CHEMICAL |
|---|---|---|---|
| Plasma water | 4.5 | 3 | 333 mg/liter |
| Total extracellular water | 20 | 14 | 71 mg/liter |
| Total body water | 55 | 38 | 26 mg/liter |
| Tissue binding | — | — | 0–25 mg/liter |

or high solubility in fat. The site of accumulation of a toxicant also may be its site of major toxic action, but more often it is not. If a toxicant accumulates at a site other than the target organ or tissue, the accumulation may be viewed as a protective process in that plasma levels and, consequently, the concentration of a toxicant at the site of action are diminished. In this case, it is assumed that the chemical in the storage depot is toxicologically inactive. However, because any chemical in a storage depot is in equilibrium with the free fraction of toxicant in plasma, it is released into the circulation as the unbound fraction of toxicant is eliminated, for example, by biotransformation.

## Storage of Toxicants in Tissues

Since only the free fraction of a chemical is in equilibrium throughout the body, binding to or dissolving in certain body constituents greatly alters the distribution of a xenobiotic. Toxicants often are concentrated in a specific tissue. Some xenobiotics attain their highest concentrations at the site of toxic action, such as carbon monoxide, which has a very high affinity for hemoglobin, and paraquat, which accumulates in the lungs. Other agents concentrate at sites other than the target organ. For example, lead is stored in bone, but manifestations of lead poisoning appear in soft tissues. The compartment where a toxicant is concentrated can be thought of as a storage depot. Toxicants in these depots are always in equilibrium with the free fraction in plasma. As a chemical is biotransformed or excreted from the body, more is released from the storage site. As a result, the biological half-life of stored compounds can be very long. The following discussion deals with the major storage sites for xenobiotics in the body.

**Plasma Proteins as Storage Depot.** Several plasma proteins bind xenobiotics as well as some physiological constituents of the body. As depicted in Fig. 5-6, albumin can bind a large number of different compounds. Transferrin, a beta$_1$ globulin, is important for the transport of iron in the body. The other main metal-binding protein in plasma is ceruloplasmin, which carries most of the copper. The alpha- and beta-lipoproteins are very important in the transport of lipid-soluble compounds such as vitamins, cholesterol, and steroid hormones as well as xenobiotics. The gamma globulins are antibodies that interact specifically with antigens. Compounds possessing basic characteristics often bind to $\alpha_1$-acid glycoprotein (Wilkinson, 1983).

Many therapeutic agents have been examined with respect to plasma protein binding. The extent of plasma protein binding varies considerably among xenobiotics. Some, such as antipyrine, are not bound; others, such as secobarbital, are bound to about 50 percent; and some, like warfarin, are 99 percent bound. Plasma proteins can bind acidic compounds such as phenylbutazone, basic compounds such as imipramine, and neutral compounds such as digitoxin.

The binding of toxicants to plasma proteins usually is determined by equilibrium dialysis or ultrafiltration. The fraction that passes through the dialysis membrane or appears in the ultrafiltrate is the unbound, or free, fraction. The total concentration is the sum of the bound and free fractions. The bound fraction thus can be determined from the difference between the total and free fractions. The binding of toxicants to plasma proteins can be analyzed through the use of Scatchard plots (Scatchard, 1949). In this analysis, the ratio of bound to free ligand (toxicant) is plotted on the ordinate and the concentration of bound ligand is plotted on the abscissa, as depicted in Fig. 5-7. From this analysis, the number of ligand binding sites (N) per molecule of protein and the affinity constant of the protein-ligand complex can be determined. The Scatchard plot frequently exhibits nonlinearity, indicating the presence of two or more classes of binding sites with different affinities and capacity characteristics.

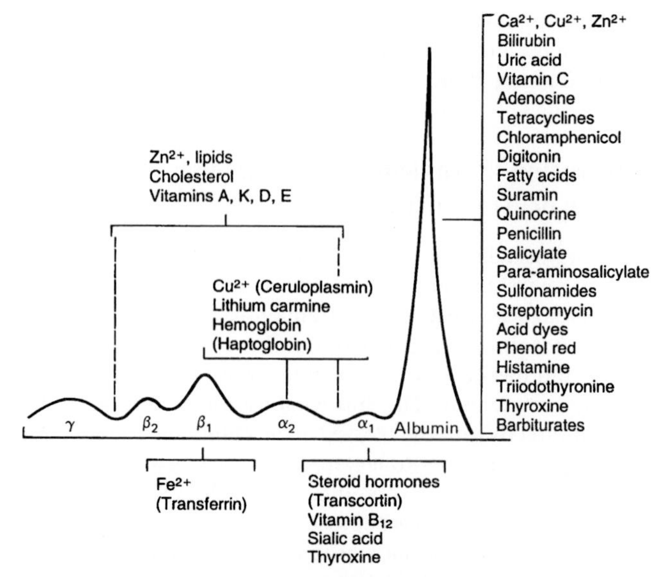


*Figure 5–6. Ligand interactions with plasma proteins.*

Plasma proteins are depicted according to their relative amounts (y axis) and electrophoretic mobilities (x axis). Some representative interactions are listed. [From Goldstein A, Aronow L, Kalman SM: *Principles of Drug Action* (copyright © 1968, by Harper and Row; reprinted by permission of John Wiley & Sons, Inc., copyright proprietor). Modified from Putman FW: Structure and function of the plasma proteins, in Neurath H (ed): *The Proteins*, 2d ed. Academic Press, Inc., New York, 1965, vol III.]

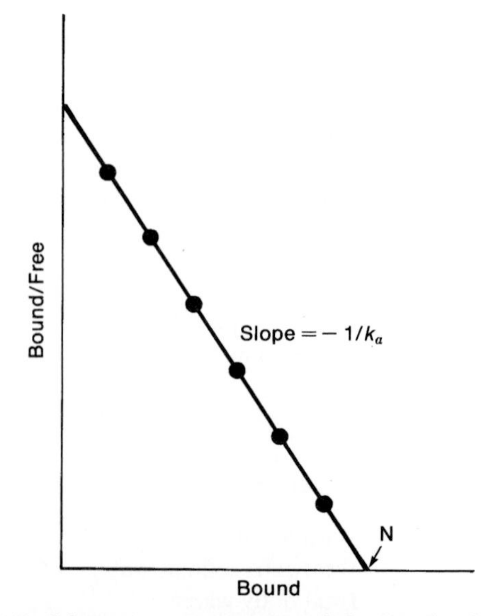


*Figure 5–7. Schematic representation of the Scatchard plot for the analysis of the binding of toxicants to proteins.*

Most xenobiotics that are bound to plasma proteins bind to albumin. Albumin is the most abundant protein in plasma and serves as a depot and transport protein for many endogenous and exogenous compounds. Long-chain fatty acids and bilirubin are endogenous ligands with affinity for albumin. There appear to be six binding regions on the protein (Kragh-Hansen, 1981). Protein-ligand interactions occur primarily as a result of hydrophobic forces, hydrogen bonding, and Van der Waals forces. Because of their high molecular weight, plasma proteins and the toxicants bound to them cannot cross capillary walls. Consequently, the fraction of toxicant bound to plasma proteins is not immediately available for distribution into the extravascular space or filtration by the kidneys. However, the interaction of a chemical with plasma proteins is a reversible process. As unbound chemical diffuses out of capillaries, bound chemical dissociates from the protein until the free fraction reaches equilibrium between the vascular space and the extravascular space. In turn, diffusion in the extravascular space to sites more distant from the capillaries continues, and the resulting concentration gradient provides the thermodynamic force for continued dissociation of the bound fraction in plasma. Active transport processes are not limited by the binding of chemicals to plasma proteins.

The binding of chemicals to plasma proteins is of special importance to toxicologists because severe toxic reactions can occur if a toxicant is displaced from plasma proteins by another agent, increasing the free fraction of the toxicant in plasma. This will result in an increased equilibrium concentration of the toxicant in the target organ, with the potential for toxicity. For example, if a strongly bound sulfonamide is given concurrently with an antidiabetic drug, the sulfonamide may displace the antidiabetic drug and induce a hypoglycemic coma. Xenobiotics can also compete with and displace endogenous compounds that are bound to plasma proteins. The importance of this phenomenon was demonstrated in a clinical trial comparing the efficacy of tetracycline with that of a penicillin-sulfonamide mixture in the management of bacterial infections in premature infants (Silverman et al., 1956). The penicillin-sulfonamide mixture led to much higher mortality than did the tetracycline because the sulfonamide displaced a considerable amount of bilirubin from albumin. The bilirubin then diffused into the brain through the not fully developed blood-brain barrier of the newborn, causing a severe form of brain damage termed *kernicterus*.

Most research on the binding of xenobiotics to plasma proteins has been conducted with drugs. However, other chemicals, such as the insecticide dieldrin, also bind avidly to plasma proteins (99 percent). Therefore, it is to be expected that chemical-chemical interactions that alter plasma protein binding occur with many different xenobiotics.

**Liver and Kidney as Storage Depots.** The liver and kidney have a high capacity for binding a multitude of chemicals. These two organs probably concentrate more toxicants than do all the other organs combined. Although the mechanisms by which the liver and kidney remove toxicants from the blood have not been established, active transport or binding to tissue components seems to be involved in most cases.

A protein in the cytoplasm of the liver (ligandin) has been identified as having a high affinity for many organic acids. It has been suggested that this protein may be important in the transfer of organic anions from plasma into liver (Levi et al., 1969). This protein also binds azo dye carcinogens and corticosteroids (Litwack et al., 1971). Another protein—metallothionein—has been found to bind cadmium and zinc with high affinities in the kidney and liver. Hepatic uptake of lead illustrates how rapidly liver binds foreign compounds: Just 30 min after a single dose, the concentration of lead in liver is 50 times higher than the concentration in plasma (Klaassen and Shoeman, 1974).

**Fat as Storage Depot.** Many organic compounds in the environment are highly lipophilic. This characteristic permits rapid penetration of cell membranes and uptake by tissues. Therefore, it is not surprising that highly lipophilic toxicants are distributed and concentrated in body fat. Such accumulation in adipose tissue has been demonstrated for a number of chemicals, including chlordane, DDT, and polychlorinated and polybrominated biphenyls.

Toxicants appear to accumulate in fat by dissolution in neutral fats, which constitute about 50 percent and 20 percent of the body weight of obese individuals and lean athletic individuals, respectively. Thus, large amounts of toxicants with a high lipid/water partition coefficient may be stored in body fat. Storage lowers the concentration of the toxicant in the target organ; therefore, the toxicity of such a compound can be expected to be less severe in an obese person than in a lean individual. However, of more practical concern is the possibility of a sudden increase in the concentration of a chemical in the blood and thus in the target organ of toxicity when rapid mobilization of fat occurs. Several studies have shown that signs of intoxication can be produced by short-term starvation of experimental animals that previously were exposed to persistent organochlorine insecticides.

**Bone as Storage Depot.** Compounds such as fluoride, lead, and strontium may be incorporated and stored in bone matrix. For example, 90 percent of the lead in the body is eventually found in the skeleton.

Skeletal uptake of xenobiotics is essentially a surface chemistry phenomenon, with exchange taking place between the bone surface and the fluid in contact with it. The fluid is the extracellular fluid, and the surface is that of the hydroxyapatite crystals of bone mineral. Many of those crystals are very small so that the surface is large in proportion to the mass. The extracellular fluid brings the toxicant into contact with the hydration shell of the hydroxyapatite, allowing diffusion through it and penetration of the crystal surface. As a result of similarities in size and charge, $F^-$ may readily displace $OH^-$, whereas lead or strontium may substitute for calcium in the hydroxyapatite lattice matrix through an exchange-absorption reaction.

Deposition and storage of toxicants in bone may or may not be detrimental. Lead is not toxic to bone, but the chronic effects of fluoride deposition (skeletal fluorosis) and radioactive strontium (osteosarcoma and other neoplasms) are well documented.

Foreign compounds deposited in bone are not sequestered irreversibly by that tissue. Toxicants can be released from the bone by ionic exchange at the crystal surface and dissolution of bone crystals through osteoclastic activity. An increase in osteolytic activity such as that seen after parathyroid hormone administration leads to enhanced mobilization of hydroxyapatite lattice, which can be reflected in an increased plasma concentration of toxicants.

## Blood-Brain Barrier

The blood-brain barrier is not an absolute barrier to the passage of toxic agents into the CNS. Instead, it represents a site that is less permeable than are most other areas of the body. Nevertheless, many poisons do not enter the brain in appreciable quantities because of this barrier.

There are four major anatomic and physiological reasons why some toxicants do not readily enter the CNS. First, the capillary endothelial cells of the CNS are tightly joined, leaving few or no pores between the cells. Second, the brain capillary endothelial cells contain an ATP-dependent transporter, the multidrug-resistant (MDR) protein that transports some chemicals into the blood. Third, the capillaries in the CNS are to a large extent surrounded by glial cell processes (astrocytes). Fourth, the protein concentration in the interstitial fluid of the CNS is much lower than that in other body fluids. For small- to medium-size water-soluble molecules, the tighter junctions of the capillary endothelium and the lipid membranes of the glial cell processes represent the major barrier. Lipid-soluble compounds have to traverse not only the membranes of the endothelial cells but also those of glial cell processes. More important, perhaps, the low protein content of the interstitial fluid in the brain greatly limits the movement of water-insoluble compounds by paracellular transport, which is possible in a largely aqueous medium only when they are bound to proteins. These features provide some protection against the distribution of toxicants to the CNS and thus against toxicity.

The effectiveness of the blood-brain barrier varies from one area of the brain to another. For example, the cortex, the lateral nuclei of the hypothalamus, the area postrema, the pineal body, and the posterior lobe of the hypophysis are more permeable than are other areas of the brain. It is not clear whether this is due to the increased blood supply to those areas, a more permeable barrier, or both.

In general, the entrance of toxicants into the brain follows the same principle that applies to transfer across other cells in the body. Only the free fraction of a toxicant (i.e., not bound to plasma proteins) equilibrates rapidly with the brain. Lipid solubility plays an important role in determining the rate of entry of a compound into the CNS, as does the degree of ionization, as was discussed earlier. In general, increased lipid solubility enhances the rate of penetration of toxicants into the CNS, whereas ionization greatly diminishes it. Pralidoxime (2-PAM), a quaternary nitrogen derivative, does not readily penetrate the brain and is ineffective in reversing the inhibition of brain cholinesterase caused by organophosphate insecticides. It is not clear why some very lipophilic chemicals such as TCDD, are not readily distributed into the brain, which in fact displays the lowest concentration among all tissues and body fluids (Weber et al., 1993). It is likely, though, that strong binding to plasma proteins or lipoproteins, as well as the composition of the brain (mainly phospholipids), limits the entry of very lipophilic compounds into the brain. Some xenobiotics, although very few, appear to enter the brain by carrier-mediated processes. For example, methylmercury combines with cysteine, forming a structure similar to methionine (see below), and the

$$CH_3Hg^+ + {}^-S-CH_2-\underset{NH_3^+}{\underset{|}{CH}}-COO^- \quad \text{Cysteine}$$

$$CH_3-Hg-S-CH_2-\underset{NH_3^+}{\underset{|}{CH}}-COO^- \quad \text{Methylmercury-Cysteine (complex)}$$

$$CH_3-S-CH_2-CH_2-\underset{NH_3^+}{\underset{|}{CH}}-COO^- \quad \text{Methionine}$$

complex is then accepted by the large neutral amino acid carrier of the capillary endothelial cells (Clarkson, 1987).

The blood-brain barrier is not fully developed at birth, and this is one reason why some chemicals are more toxic to newborns than to adults. Morphine, for example, is 3 to 10 times more toxic to newborn than to adult rats because of the higher permeability of the brain of a newborn to morphine (Kupferberg and Way, 1963). Lead produces encephalomyelopathy in newborn rats but not in adults, also apparently because of differences in the stages of development of the blood-brain barrier (Pentschew and Garro, 1966).

## Passage of Toxicants across the Placenta

For years the term "placental barrier" was associated with the concept that the main function of the placenta is to protect the fetus against the passage of noxious substances from the mother. However, the placenta has many functions: It provides nutrition for the conceptus, exchanges maternal and fetal blood gases, disposes of fetal excretory material, and maintains pregnancy through complex hormonal regulation. Most of the vital nutrients necessary for the development of the fetus are transported by active transport systems. For example, vitamins, amino acids, essential sugars, and ions such as calcium and iron are transported from mother to fetus against a concentration gradient (Young, 1969; Ginsburg, 1971). In contrast, most toxic agents pass the placenta by simple diffusion. The only exceptions are a few antimetabolites that are structurally similar to endogenous purines and pyrimidines, which are the physiological substrates for active transport from the maternal to the fetal circulation.

Many foreign substances can cross the placenta. In addition to chemicals, viruses (e.g., rubella virus), cellular pathogens (e.g., syphilis spirochetes), globulin antibodies, and even erythrocytes (Goldstein et al., 1974) can traverse the placenta.

Anatomically, the placental barrier consists of a number of cell layers interposed between the fetal and maternal circulations. The number of layers varies with the species and the state of gestation. Placentas in which the maximum number of cell layers are present (all six layers) are called *epitheliochorial* (Table 5-2). Those in which the maternal epithelium is absent are referred to as *syndesmochorial.* When only the endothelial layer of the maternal tissue remains, the tissue is termed *endotheliochorial;* when even the endothe-

**Table 5–2**
**Tissues Separating Fetal and Maternal Blood**

| | MATERNAL TISSUE | | | FETAL TISSUE | | | |
|---|---|---|---|---|---|---|---|
| | *Endothelium* | *Connective Tissue* | *Epithelium* | *Trophoblast* | *Connective Tissue* | *Endothelium* | *Species* |
| Epitheliochorial | + | + | + | + | + | + | Pig, horse, donkey |
| Syndesmochorial | + | + | — | + | + | + | Sheep, goat, cow |
| Endotheliochorial | + | — | — | + | + | + | Cat, dog |
| Hemochorial | — | — | — | + | + | + | Human, monkey |
| Hemoendothelial | — | — | — | — | — | + | Rat, rabbit, guinea pig |

SOURCE: Modified from Amaroso EC: Placentation, in Parkes AS (ed): *Marshall's Physiology of Reproduction,* Longmans, Green, London, vol. 2, 1952.

lium is gone, so that the chorionic villi bathe in the maternal blood, the tissue is called *hemochorial.* In some species, some of the fetal layers are absent and are called *hemoendothelial* (Dames, 1968). Within the same species, the placenta also may change its histological classification during gestation (Amaroso, 1952). For example, at the beginning of gestation the placenta of a rabbit has six major layers (epitheliochorial), and at the end it has only one (hemoendothelial). One might suspect that a relatively thin placenta such as that of a rat would be more permeable to toxic agents than is the placenta of humans, whereas a thicker placenta such as that of a goat would be less permeable. The exact relationship of the number of layers of the placenta to its permeability has not been investigated. Currently, it is not considered to be of primary importance in determining the distribution of chemicals to the fetus.

The same factors are important determinants of the placental transfer of xenobiotics by passive diffusion (particularly lipid/water solubility), as was discussed above for the passage of molecules across body membranes. It is uncertain whether the placenta plays an active role in preventing the transfer of noxious substances from mother to fetus. However, the placenta has biotransformation capabilities that may prevent some toxic substances from reaching the fetus (Juchau, 1972). Among the substances that cross the placenta by passive diffusion, more lipid-soluble substances more rapidly attain a maternal-fetal equilibrium. Under steady-state conditions, the concentrations of a toxic compound in the plasma of the mother and fetus are usually the same. The concentration in the various tissues of the fetus depends on the ability of fetal tissue to concentrate a toxicant. For example, the concentration of diphenylhydantoin in the plasma of the fetal goat was about half of that found in the mother. This was due to differences in plasma protein concentration and the binding affinity of diphenylhydantoin to plasma proteins (Shoeman et al., 1972). Also, some organs, such as the liver of the newborn (Klaassen, 1972) and the fetus, do not concentrate some xenobiotics, and therefore lower levels are found in the liver of the fetus. In contrast, higher concentrations of some chemicals, such as lead and dimethylmercury, are encountered in the brain of the fetus because of the fetus's not fully developed blood-brain barrier. Differential body composition between mother and fetus may be another reason for an apparent placental barrier. For example, fetuses have very little fat. Accordingly, and in contrast to the mothers, they do not accumulate highly lipophilic chemicals such as TCDD (Li et al., 1995).

## Redistribution of Toxicants

As was mentioned earlier, blood flow to and the affinity of an organ or tissue are the most critical factors that affect the distribution of xenobiotics. Chemicals can have an affinity to a binding site (e.g., intracellular protein or bone matrix) or to a cellular constituent (e.g., fat). The initial phase of distribution is determined primarily by blood flow to the various parts of the body. Therefore, a well-perfused organ such as the liver may attain high initial concentrations of a xenobiotic. However, the affinity of less well perfused organs or tissues may be higher for a particular xenobiotic, causing redistribution with time. For example, 2 h after administration, 50 percent of a dose of lead is found in the liver (Klaassen and Shoeman, 1974). However, 1 month after dosing, 90 percent of the dose remaining in the body is associated with the crystal lattice of bone. Similarly, 5 min after an intravenous dose of a lipophilic chemical such as TCDD, about 15 percent of the dose is localized in the lungs, but only about 1 percent in adipose tissue. However, 24 h later, only 0.3 percent of the remaining dose is found in the lungs but about 20 percent in adipose tissue (Weber et al., 1993).

# EXCRETION

Toxicants are eliminated from the body by several routes. The kidney is perhaps the most important organ for the excretion of xenobiotics, as more chemicals are eliminated from the body by this route than by any other (Chap. 14). Many xenobiotics, though, have to be biotransformed to more water-soluble products before they can be excreted into urine (Chap. 6). The second important route of elimination of many xenobiotics is via feces, and the third, primarily for gases, is via the lungs. Biliary excretion of xenobiotics and/or their metabolites is most often the major source of fecal excretion, but a number of other sources can be significant for some compounds. All body secretions appear to have the ability to excrete chemicals; toxicants have been found in sweat, saliva, tears, and milk (Stowe and Plaa, 1968).

## Urinary Excretion

The kidney is a very efficient organ for the elimination of toxicants from the body. Toxic compounds are excreted with urine by the same mechanisms the kidney uses to remove the end products of intermediary metabolism from the body: glomerular filtration, tubular excretion by passive diffusion, and active tubular secretion.

The kidney receives about 25 percent of the cardiac output, about 20 percent of which is filtered at the glomeruli. The glomerular capillaries have large pores (70 nm). Therefore, compounds up to a molecular weight of about 60,000 (proteins smaller than albumin) are filtered at the glomeruli. The degree of plasma protein binding affects the rate of filtration because protein-xenobiotic complexes are too large to pass through the pores of the glomeruli.

A toxicant filtered at the glomeruli may remain in the tubular lumen and be excreted with urine. Depending on the physicochemical properties of a compound, it may be reabsorbed across the tubular cells of the nephron back into the bloodstream. The principles governing the reabsorption of toxicants across the kidney tubules are the same as those discussed earlier in this chapter for passive diffusion across cell membranes. Thus, toxicants with a high lipid/water partition coefficient are reabsorbed efficiently, whereas polar compounds and ions are excreted with urine. As can be deduced from the Henderson-Hasselbalch equations, bases are excreted (i.e., not reabsorbed) to a greater extent at lower and acids at higher urinary pH values. A practical application of this knowledge is illustrated by the treatment of phenobarbital poisoning with sodium bicarbonate. The percentage of ionization can be increased markedly within physiologically attainable pH ranges for a weak organic acid such as phenobarbital (p*K*a 7.2). Consequently, alkalinization of urine by the administration of sodium bicarbonate results in a significant increase in the excretion of phenobarbital (Weiner and Mudge, 1964). Similarly, acceleration of salicylate loss via the kidney can be achieved through the administration of sodium bicarbonate.

Toxic agents also can be excreted from plasma into urine by passive diffusion through the tubule. This process is probably of minor significance because filtration is much faster than excretion by passive diffusion through the tubules, providing a favorable concentration gradient for reabsorption rather than excretion. Exceptions to this generalization may be some organic acids (p*K*a $\approx$ 3 to 5) and bases (p*K*a $\approx$ 7 to 9) that would be largely ionized and thus trapped at the pH of urine (pH $\approx$ 6). For renal excretion of such compounds, the flow of urine is likely to be important for the maintenance of a concentration gradient, favoring excretion. Thus, diurectics can hasten the elimination of weak organic acids and bases.

Toxic agents can also be excreted into urine by active secretion. Two tubular secretory processes are known: one for organic anions (acids) and the other for organic cations (bases). *p*-Aminohippurate is the prototype for the organic acid transport system, and *N*-methylnicotinamide is the prototype for the organic base transporter. Specialized renal transport systems are located in the proximal tubules. The organic anion transport process is thought to be localized primarily at the basolateral membrane of the proximal tubule. The transport of organic anions across this membrane appears to occur through a three-step process (Fig. 5-8). In the first step, ATP is hydrolyzed to drive the sodium pump. The resulting sodium gradient drives sodium $\alpha$-ketoglutarate cotransport, which is the second step. The third step appears to be cotransport of $\alpha$-ketoglutarate with the organic anion, as $\alpha$-ketoglutarate markedly stimulates the transport of organic anions (Pritchard and Miller, 1993). Once inside the proximal tubule cell, the organic acid appears to be eliminated on the luminal side of the cell by a carrier-mediated transport system; however, this process is less well understood than are the processes on the basolateral side. Some less polar xenobiotics may diffuse into the lumen. In contrast to filtration, protein-bound toxicants are available for active transport. As in all active transport systems, renal secretion of xenobiotics also reveals competition. This fact was put to use during World War II, when penicillin was in short supply. Penicillin is actively secreted by the organic acid system of the kidney. To lengthen its half-life and duration of action, another acid was sought to compete with penicillin for renal secretion; probenecid was successfully introduced for this purpose. Uric acid also is secreted actively by renal tubules. It is of clinical relevance that toxicants transported by the organic acid transport system can increase the plasma uric acid concentration and precipitate an attack of gout.

Because many functions of the kidney are incompletely developed at birth, some xenobiotics are eliminated more slowly in newborns than in adults and therefore may be more toxic to newborns. For example, the clearance of penicillin by premature infants is only about 20 percent of that observed in older children (Barnett et al., 1949). It has been demonstrated that the development of this organic acid transport system in newborns can be stimulated by the administration of substances normally excreted by this system (Hirsch and Hook, 1970). Some compounds, such as cephaloridine, are known to be nephrotoxic in adult animals but not in newborns. Because active uptake of cephaloridine by the kidneys is not well de-

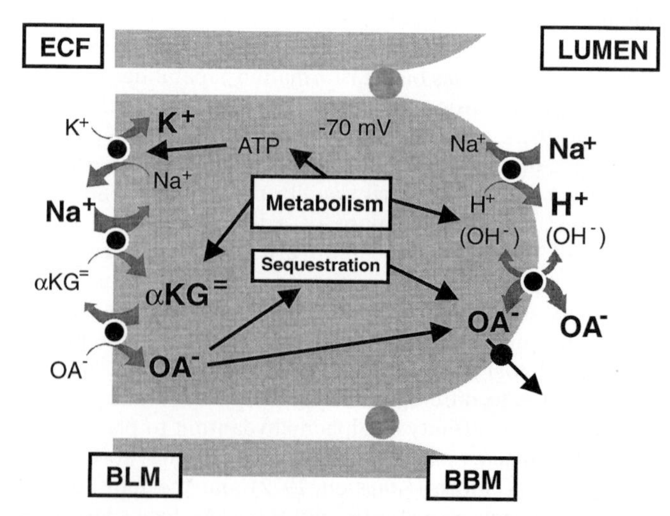


*Figure 5–8. Schematic model showing the processes involved in basolateral and luminal organic anion (OA⁻) transport. ECF = extracellular fluid; BLM = basolateral membrane; BBM = brush border or luminal membrane; αKG⁻ = a-ketoglutarate. (Based on Pritchard and Miller, 1993.)*

veloped in newborns, this agent is not concentrated in the tubules and consequently is not nephrotoxic. If the development of active transport in newborns is stimulated, the kidneys take up cephaloridine more readily and nephrotoxicity is observed (Wold et al., 1977). Also, nephrotoxicity can be blocked by probenecid, which competitively inhibits the uptake of cephaloridine into the kidneys (Tune et al., 1977).

Species differences in regard to the urinary excretion of weak organic acids and bases are observed frequently, as the pH of urine varies widely among species. Differences in renal clearance also can occur for compounds filtered at the glomeruli because of differences in plasma protein binding. Interestingly, species variations also can arise as a result of differences in active renal secretion, as has been shown for captopril (Migdalof et al., 1984).

The renal proximal tubule reabsorbs small plasma proteins that are filtered at the glomerulus. Thus, if a toxicant binds to those small proteins, it can be carried into the proximal tubule cells and exert toxicity. For example, cadmium bound to metallothionein, a small metal-binding protein, is readily taken up by the kidney leading to kidney injury (Dorian et al., 1992). Similarly, chemicals such as limonene (present in orange juice) and trimethyl pentane (present in gasoline) bind to a $\alpha_{2U}$-globulin and are taken up by the proximal tubule to produce hyaline droplet nephropathy and eventually renal tumors in male rats (Lehman-McKeeman and Caudill, 1992). Fortunately, a $\alpha_{2U}$-globulin is expressed only by male rats.

## Fecal Excretion

Fecal excretion is the other major pathway for the elimination of xenobiotics from the body. Fecal excretion of chemicals is a complex process that is not as well understood as urinary excretion is. Several important sources and many more minor sources contribute to the excretion of toxicants via the feces.

**Nonabsorbed Ingesta.** In addition to indigestible material, varying proportions of nutrients and xenobiotics that are present in food or are ingested voluntarily (drugs) pass through the alimentary canal unabsorbed, contributing to fecal excretion. The physicochemical properties of xenobiotics and the biological characteristics that facilitate absorption were discussed earlier in this chapter. In general, most human-made chemicals are at least to some extent lipophilic and thus are available for absorption. Exceptions include some macromolecules and some essentially completely ionized compounds of higher molecular weight. For example, the absorption of polymers or quaternary ammonium bases is quite limited in the intestine. Consequently, most of a dose of orally administered sucrose polyester, cholestyramine, or paraquat can be found in feces. It is rare for 100 percent of a compound to be absorbed. Therefore, the nonabsorbed portion of xenobiotics contributes to the fecal excretion of most chemicals to some extent.

**Biliary Excretion.** The biliary route of elimination is perhaps the most important contributing source to the fecal excretion of xenobiotics and is even more important for the excretion of their metabolites. The liver is in a very advantageous position for removing toxic agents from blood after absorption from the GI tract, because blood from the GI tract passes through the liver before reaching the general circulation. Thus, the liver can extract compounds from blood and prevent their distribution to other parts of the body. Furthermore, the liver is the main site of biotransformation of toxicants, and the metabolites thus formed may be excreted directly into bile. Xenobiotics and/or their metabolites entering the intestine with bile may be excreted with feces; when the physicochemical properties favor reabsorption, an enterohepatic circulation may ensue.

Foreign compounds excreted into bile are often divided into three classes on the basis of ratio of their concentration in bile versus that in plasma. Class A substances have a ratio of nearly 1 and include sodium, potassium, glucose, mercury, thallium, cesium, and cobalt. Class B substances have a ratio of bile to plasma greater than 1 (usually between 10 and 1000). Class B substances include bile acids, bilirubin, sulfobromophthalein, lead, arsenic, manganese, and many other xenobiotics. Class C substances have a ratio below 1 (e.g., inulin, albumin, zinc, iron, gold, and chromium). Compounds rapidly excreted into bile are most likely to be found among class B substances. However, a compound does not have to be highly concentrated in bile for biliary excretion to be of quantitative importance. For example, mercury is not concentrated in bile, yet bile is the main route of excretion for this slowly eliminated substance.

The mechanism of transport of foreign substances from plasma into liver and from liver into bile is not known with certainty. Especially little is known about the mechanism of the transfer of class A and class C compounds. However, it is thought that most class B compounds are actively transported across both sides of the hepatocyte. Liver has at least four transport systems for active excretion of organic compounds into bile. Two of those systems specifically transport organic acids; one, organic bases; and one, neutral compounds. The biliary excretion of two organic acids—sulfobromophthalein (BSP) and indocyanine green (ICG)—has been particularly well examined. The rate of removal of these two dyes has long been used in liver function tests. The test is performed by injecting the dye intravenously and determining its plasma disappearance profile. A lack of proper plasma clearance of BSP or ICG indicates reduced biliary excretion, suggesting liver injury. Bilirubin is also actively transported from plasma into bile. Therefore, jaundice is often observed after a liver injury.

Like the kidneys, the liver has an active transport system for the excretion of bases; procainamide ethyl bromide is the prototype for this transport system. There is an additional transport system in the liver for the excretion of neutral compounds such as ouabain. It appears that the liver has at least one more active transport system for the excretion of metals (Klaassen, 1976). For example, lead is excreted into the bile against a large bile/plasma concentration ratio (100) with an apparent transport maximum. It is not known whether other metals are excreted into bile by the same or similar mechanisms.

As with renal tubular secretion, toxic agents bound to plasma proteins are fully available for active biliary excretion. The relative importance of biliary excretion depends on the substance and species concerned. It is not known which factors determine whether a chemical will be excreted into bile or into urine. However, low-molecular-weight compounds are poorly excreted into bile while compounds or their conjugates with molecular weights exceeding about 325 can be excreted in appreciable quantities. Glutathione and glucuronide conjugates have a high predilection for excretion into bile. The percentages of a large number of compounds excreted into bile have been tabulated (Klaassen et al., 1981). Marked species variation in the biliary excretion of foreign compounds exists and can result in species differences in the biological half-life of a compound and its toxicity. This species variation in biliary excretion is compound-specific. It is therefore difficult to categorize species into "good" or "poor" biliary excretors. However, in general, rats and mice tend to be better biliary excretors than are other species (Klaassen and Watkins, 1984).

Once a compound is excreted into bile and enters the intestine, it can be reabsorbed or eliminated with feces. Many organic compounds are conjugated before excretion into bile. Such polar metabolites are not sufficiently lipid-soluble to be reabsorbed. However, intestinal microflora may hydrolyze glucuronide and sulfate conjugates, making them sufficiently lipophilic for reabsorption. Reabsorption of a xenobiotic completes an enterohepatic cycle. Repeated enterohepatic cycling may lead to very long half-lives of xenobiotics in the body. Therefore, it is often desirable to interrupt this cycle to hasten the elimination of a toxicant from the body. This principle has been utilized in the treatment of dimethylmercury poisoning; ingestion of a polythiol resin binds the mercurial and thus prevents its reabsorption (Magos and Clarkson, 1976).

An increase in hepatic excretory function also has been observed after pretreatment with some drugs (Klaassen and Watkins, 1984). For example, it has been demonstrated that phenobarbital increases plasma disappearance by enhancing the biliary excretion of BSP and a number of other compounds. The increase in bile flow caused by phenobarbital appears to be an important factor in increasing the biliary excretion of BSP. However, other factors, such as the induction of some phase II enzymes, also can increase the conjugating capacity of the liver and thus enhance the plasma disappearance and biliary excretion of some compounds. Not all microsomal enzyme inducers increase bile flow and excretion; 3-methylcholanthrene and benzo[*a*]pyrene are relatively ineffective in this regard.

An increase in biliary excretion can decrease the toxicity of xenobiotics. Phenobarbital treatment of laboratory animals has been shown to enhance the biliary excretion and elimination of methylmercury from the body (Klaassen, 1975a; Magos and Clarkson, 1976). Two steroids known to induce microsomal enzymes—spironolactone and pregnenolone-16$\alpha$-carbonitrile—have also been demonstrated to increase bile production and enhance biliary excretion of BSP (Zsigmond and Solymoss, 1972). These two steroids have also been shown to decrease the toxicity of several chemicals (Selye, 1971), including cardiac glycosides (Selye, 1969), by increasing their biliary excretion. This in turn decreases the concentration of cardiac glycosides in the heart, their target organ of toxicity (Castle and Lage, 1972, 1973; Klaassen, 1974a).

The toxicity of some compounds can be directly related to their biliary excretion. For example, indomethacin can cause intestinal lesions. The sensitivity of various species to this toxic response is directly related to the amount of indomethacin excreted into bile. The formation of intestinal lesions can be abolished by means of bile duct ligation (Duggan et al., 1975).

The hepatic excretory system is not fully developed in newborns, and this is another reason why some compounds are more toxic to newborns than to adults (Klaassen, 1972, 1973a). For example, ouabain is about 40 times more toxic in newborn than in adult rats. This is due to an almost complete inability of the newborn rat liver to remove ouabain from plasma. A decreased excretory function of newborn liver also has been demonstrated for other xenobiotics (Klaassen, 1973b). The development of hepatic excretory function can be promoted in newborns by administering microsomal enzyme inducers (Klaassen, 1974b).

**Intestinal Excretion.** It has been shown for a fairly large number of diverse chemicals (e.g., digitoxin, dinitrobenzamide, hexachlorobenzene, ochratoxin A) that their excretion into feces can be explained neither by the unabsorbed portion of an oral dosage nor by excretion into bile (Rozman, 1986). Experiments in bile duct–ligated animals and animals provided with bile fistulas have revealed that the source of many chemicals in feces is a direct transfer from blood into the intestinal contents. This transfer is thought to occur by passive diffusion for most xenobiotics. In some instances, rapid exfoliation of intestinal cells also may contribute to the fecal excretion of some compounds. Intestinal excretion is a relatively slow process. Therefore, it is a major pathway of elimination only for compounds that have low rates of biotransformation and/or low renal or biliary clearance. The rate of intestinal excretion of some lipid-soluble compounds can be substantially enhanced by increasing the lipophilicity of the GI contents, for example by adding mineral oil to the diet (Rozman, 1986). Active secretion of organic acids and bases also has been demonstrated in the large intestine (Lauterbach, 1977). The importance of active intestinal secretion for fecal elimination has been established only for a few chemicals.

**Intestinal Wall and Flora.** No systematic attempts have been undertaken to assess the role of biotransformation in the intestinal wall in the fecal excretion of xenobiotics. Nevertheless, in recent years evidence has accumulated that mucosal biotransformation and reexcretion into the intestinal lumen occur with many compounds. The significance of these findings for fecal excretion is difficult to judge because further interaction with the intestinal flora may alter these compounds, making them more or less suitable for reabsorption or excretion (Rozman, 1986). More is known about the contribution of the intestinal flora to fecal excretion. It has been estimated that 30 to 42 percent of fecal dry matter originates from bacteria. Chemicals originating from the nonabsorbed portion of an oral dose, the bile, or the intestinal wall are taken up by these microorganisms according to the principles of membrane permeability. Therefore, a considerable proportion of fecally excreted xenobiotics is associated with the excreted bacteria. However, chemicals may be profoundly altered by bacteria before excretion with feces, particularly in the large intestine, where intestinal flora are most abundant, and intestinal contents remain for 24 h or longer. It seems that biotransformation by intestinal flora favors reabsorption rather than excretion. Nevertheless, there is evidence that in many instances xenobiotics found in feces derive from bacterial biotransformation. The importance of microbial biotransformation for fecal excretion can be studied by performing experiments in normal versus gnotobiotic animals (animals with no microflora).

## Exhalation

Substances that exist predominantly in the gas phase at body temperature are eliminated mainly by the lungs. Because volatile liquids are in equilibrium with their gas phase in the alveoli, they also may be excreted via the lungs. The amount of a liquid eliminated via the lungs is proportional to its vapor pressure. A practical application of this principle is seen in the breath analyzer test for determining the amount of ethanol in the body. Highly volatile liquids such as diethyl ether are excreted almost exclusively by the lungs.

No specialized transport systems have been described for the excretion of toxic substances by the lungs. These substances seem to be eliminated by simple diffusion. Elimination of gases is roughly inversely proportional to the rate of their absorption. Therefore, gases with low solubility in blood, such as ethylene, are rapidly excreted, whereas chloroform, which has a much higher solubility in blood, is eliminated very slowly by the lungs. Trace concentrations of highly lipid-soluble anesthetic gases such as halothane and methoxyflurane may be present in expired air for as long as 2 to 3 weeks after a few hours of anesthesia. Undoubtedly, this prolonged retention is due to deposition in and slow mobilization from adipose tissue of these highly lipid-soluble agents. The rate of elimination of a gas with low solubility in blood is perfusion-limited, whereas that of a gas with high solubility in blood is ventilation-limited.

## Other Routes of Elimination

**Cerebrospinal Fluid.** A specialized route of removal of toxic agents from a specific organ is represented by the CSF. All compounds can leave the CNS with the bulk flow of CSF through the arachnoid villi. In addition, lipid-soluble toxicants also can exit at the site of the blood-brain barrier. It is noteworthy that toxicants also can be removed from the CSF by active transport, similar to the transport systems of the kidneys for the excretion of organic ions.

**Milk.** The secretion of toxic compounds into milk is extremely important because (1) a toxic material may be passed with milk from the mother to the nursing offspring and (2) compounds can be passed from cows to people via dairy products. Toxic agents are excreted into milk by simple diffusion. Because milk is more acidic (pH $\approx$ 6.5) than plasma, basic compounds may be concentrated in milk, whereas acidic compounds may attain lower concentrations in milk than in plasma (Findlay, 1983; Wilson, 1983). More important, about 3 to 4 percent of milk consists of lipids, and the lipid content of colostrum after parturition is even higher. Lipid-soluble xenobiotics diffuse along with fats from plasma into the mammary gland and are excreted with milk during lactation. Compounds such as DDT and polychlorinated and polybrominated biphenyls, dibenzo-*p*-dioxins, and furans (Van den Berg et al., 1987; Li et al., 1995) are known to occur in milk, and milk can be a major route of their excretion. Species differences in the excretion of xenobiotics with milk are to be expected, as the proportion of milk fat derived from the circulation versus that synthesized de novo in the mammary gland differs widely among species. Metals chemically similar to calcium, such as lead, and chelating agents that form complexes with calcium also can be excreted into milk to a considerable extent.

**Sweat and Saliva.** The excretion of toxic agents in sweat and saliva is quantitatively of minor importance. Again, excretion depends on the diffusion of the nonionized, lipid-soluble form of an agent. Toxic compounds excreted into sweat may produce dermatitis. Substances excreted in saliva enter the mouth, where they are usually swallowed and thus are available for GI absorption.

# CONCLUSION

Humans are in continuous contact with toxic agents. Toxicants are in the food we eat, the water we drink, and the air we breathe. Depending on their physical and chemical properties, toxic agents may be absorbed by the GI tract, lungs, and/or skin. Fortunately, the body has the ability to biotransform and excrete these compounds into urine, feces, and air. However, when the rate of absorption exceeds the rate of elimination, toxic compounds may accumulate and reach a critical concentration at a certain target site, and toxicity may ensue (Fig. 5-9). Whether a chemical elicits toxicity depends not only on its inherent potency and site specificity but also on how an organism can handle—that is, dispose of—a particular toxicant. Therefore, knowledge of the disposition of chemicals is of great importance in judging the toxicity of xenobiotics. For example, for a potent CNS suppressant that displays a strong hepatic first-pass effect, oral exposure is of less concern than is exposure by inhalation. Also, two equipotent gases—with the absorption of one being perfusion rate–limited and that of the other being ventilation rate–limited—will exhibit completely different toxicity profiles at a distant site because of differences in the concentrations attained in the target organ.

Many chemicals have very low inherent toxicity but have to be activated by biotransformation into toxic metabolites; the toxic response then depends on the rate of production of toxic metabolites. Alternatively, a very potent toxicant may be detoxified rapidly by biotransformation. Toxic effects are related to the concentration of the "toxic chemical" at the site of action (in the target organ) whether a chemical is administered or generated by biotransformation in the target tissue or at a distant site. Thus, the toxic response exerted by chemicals is critically influenced by the rates of absorption, distribution, biotransformation, and excretion.

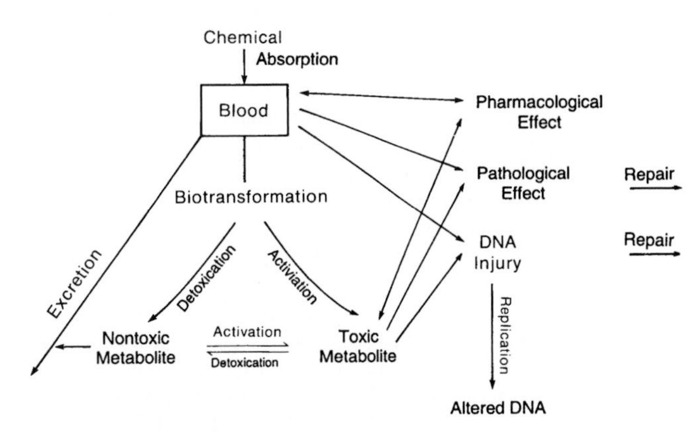


***Figure 5-9. Schematic representation of the disposition and toxic effects of chemicals.***

# REFERENCES


Albert A: *Selective Toxicity,* 3d ed. London: Methuen, 1965.

Allenby AC, Creasey NH, Edginton JAG, et al: Mechanism of action of accelerants on skin penetration. *Br J Dermatol* 81 (Suppl 4):47–55, 1969.

Amaroso EC: Placentation, in Parks AS (ed): *Marshall's Physiology of Reproduction,* 3d ed. London: Longmans, Green, 1952, vol 2, 127–311.

Aungst B, Shen DD: Gastrointestinal absorption of toxic agents, in Rozman K, Hänninen O (eds): *Gastrointestinal Toxicology.* Amsterdam/New York/Oxford: Elsevier, 1986, pp 29–56.

Barnett HL, McNamara H, Schultz S, Tomposett R: Renal clearances of sodium penicillin G, procaine penicillin G, and inulin in infants and children. *Pediatrics* 3:418–422, 1949.

Barnett RJ: The demonstration with the electron microscope of the end-products of histochemical reactions in relation to the fine structure of cells. *Exp Cell Res* (Suppl 7):65–89, 1959.

Bates TR, Gibaldi M: Gastrointestinal absorption of drugs, in Swarbrick J (ed): *Current Concepts in the Pharmaceutical Sciences: Biopharmaceutics*. Philadelphia: Lea & Febiger, 1970, pp 57–100.

Benz R, Janko K, Länger P: Pore formation by the matrix protein (porin) to *Escherichia coli* in planar bilayer membranes. *Ann NY Acad Sci* 358:13–24, 1980.

Blank IH, Scheuplein RJ: Transport into and within the skin. *Br J Dermatol* 81 (Suppl 4):4–10, 1969.

Borowitz JL, Moore PF, Him GKW, Miya TS: Mechanism of enhanced drug effects produced by dilution of the oral dose. *Toxicol Appl Pharmacol* 19:164–168, 1971.

Boyes RN, Adams HJ, Duce BR: Oral absorption and disposition kinetics of lidocaine hydrochloride in dogs. *J Pharmacol Exp Ther* 174:1–8, 1970.

Castle MC, Lage GL: Effect of pretreatment with spironolactone, phenobarbital or *β*-diethylaminoethyl diphenylpropylacetate (SKF 525-A) on tritium levels in blood, heart and liver of rats at various times after administration of [$^3$H]digitoxin. *Biochem Pharmacol* 21:1149–1155, 1972. *Biochem. Pharmacol* 21:1149–1155, 1972.

Castle MC, Lage GL: Enhanced biliary excretion of digitoxin following spironolactone as it relates to the prevention of digitoxin toxicity. *Res Commun Chem Pathol Pharmacol* 5:99–108, 1973.

Clarkson, TW: Metal toxicity in the central nervous system. *Environ Health Perspect* 75:59–64, 1987.

Coulston F, Serrone DM: The comparative approach to the role of nonhuman primates in evaluation of drug toxicity in man: A review. *Ann NY Acad Sci* 162:681–704, 1969.

Dames, GS: *Foetal and Neonatal Physiology: A Comparative Study of the Changes at Birth.* Chicago: Year Book, 1968.

Dantzig AH, Duckworth DC, Tabas LB: Transport mechanisms responsible for the absorption of loracarbef, cefixime, and cefuroxime axetil into human intestinal Caco-2 cells. *Biochem Biophys Acta* 1191:7–13, 1994.

Dorian C, Gattone VH II, Klaassen CD: Renal cadmium deposition and injury as a result of accumulation of cadmium-metallothionein (CdMT) by proximal convoluted tubules—a light microscope autoradiographic study with $^{109}$CdMT. *Toxicol Appl Pharmacol* 114:173–181, 1992.

Dowling, RH: Compensatory changes in intestinal absorption. *Br Med Bull* 23:275–278, 1967.

Draize JH, Woodard G, Calvery HO: Methods for the study of irritation and toxicity of substances applied topically to the skin and mucous membranes. *J Pharmacol Exp Ther* 82:377–390, 1944.

Dugard PH: Skin permeability theory in relation to measurements of percutaneous absorption in toxicology, in Marzulli FN, Maibach HI (eds): *Dermatotoxicology,* 2d ed. Washington/New York/London: Hemisphere, 1983, pp 91–116.

Dugard PH, Embery G: The influence of dimethylsulphoxide on the percutaneous migration of potassium butyl [$^{35}$S]sulphate, potassium methyl [$^{35}$S]sulphate and sodium [$^{35}$S]sulphate. *Br J Dermatol* 81 (Suppl 4):69–74, 1969.

Duggan DE, Hooke KF, Noll RM, Kwan KC: Enterohepatic circulation of indomethacin and its role in intestinal irritation. *Biochem Pharmacol* 24:1749–1754, 1975.

Ferguson HC: Dilution of dose and acute oral toxicity. *Toxicol Appl Pharmacol* 4:759–762, 1962.

Findlay JWA: The distribution of some commonly used drugs in human breast milk. *Drug Metab Rev* 14:653–686, 1983.

Ginsburg J: Placental drug transfer. *Annu Rev Pharmacol* 11:387–408, 1971.

Goldstein A, Aronow L, Kalman SM (eds): *Principles of Drug Action: The Basis of Pharmacology,* 2d ed. New York: Wiley, 1974.

Gorringe JAL, Sproston EM: The influence of particle size upon the absorption of drugs from the gastrointestinal tract, in Binn TB (ed): *Absorption and Distribution of Drugs*. Baltimore: Williams & Wilkins, 1964, pp 128–139.

Hayes WJ Jr: Review of the metabolism of chlorinated hydrocarbon insecticides especially in mammals. *Annu Rev Pharmacol* 5:27–52, 1965.

Heath DF, Vandekar M: Toxicity and metabolism of dieldrin in rats. *Br J Ind Med* 21:269–279, 1964.

Hirsch GH, Hook JB: Maturation of renal organic acid transport: Substrate stimulation by penicillin and *p*-aminohippurate (PAH). *J Pharmacol Exp Ther* 171:103–108, 1970.

Houston JB, Upshall DG, Bridges JW: A re-evaluation of the importance of partition coefficients in the gastrointestinal absorption of nutrients. *J Pharmacol Exp Ther* 189:244–254, 1974.

Juchau MR: Mechanisms of drug biotransformation reactions in the placenta. *Fed Proc* 31:48–51, 1972.

Kelly D, Kostial K: The effect of milk diet on lead metabolism in rats. *Environ Res,* 6:355–360, 1973.

Klaassen CD: Immaturity of the newborn rat's hepatic excretory function for ouabain. *J Pharmacol Exp Ther,* 183:520–526, 1972.

Klaassen CD: Comparison of the toxicity of chemicals in newborn rats to bile duct-ligated and sham-operated rats and mice. *Toxicol Appl Pharmacol* 24:37–44, 1973a.

Klaassen CD: Hepatic excretory function in the newborn rat. *J Pharmacol Exp Ther* 184:721–728, 1973b.

Klaassen CD: Effect of microsomal enzyme inducers on the biliary excretion of cardiac glycosides. *J Pharmacol Exp Ther* 191:201–211, 1974a.

Klaassen CD: Stimulation of the development of the hepatic excretory mechanism for ouabain in newborn rats with microsomal enzyme inducers. *J Pharmacol Exp Ther* 191:212–218, 1974b.

Klaassen CD: Biliary excretion of mercury compounds. *Toxicol Appl Pharmacol* 33:356–365, 1975a.

Klaassen CD: Biliary excretion of metals. *Drug Metab Rev* 5:165–196, 1976.

Klaassen CD, Eaton DL,Cagen SZ: Hepatobiliary disposition of xenobiotics, in Bridges JW, Chasseaud LF (eds): *Progress in Drug Metabolism*. New York: Wiley, 1981, pp 1–75.

Klaassen CD, Shoeman DW: Biliary excretion of lead in rats, rabbits and dogs. *Toxicol Appl Pharmacol* 29:434–446, 1974.

Klaassen CD, Watkins JB: Mechanisms of bile formation, hepatic uptake, and biliary excretion. *Pharmacol Rev* 36:1–67, 1984.

Kragh-Hansen U: Molecular aspects of ligand binding to serum albumin. *Pharmacol Rev* 33:17–53, 1981.

Kupferberg HJ, Way EL: Pharmacologic basis for the increased sensitivity of the newborne rat to morphine. *J Pharmacol Exp Ther* 141:105–112, 1963.

Lauterbach F: Intestinal secretion of organic ions and drugs, in Kramer M, Lauterbach F (eds): *Intestinal Permeation. Amsterdam/Oxford: Excerpta Medica, 1977, pp 173–195.*

Lehman-McKeeman LD, Caudill D: α2U-Globulin is the only member of the lipocalin protein superfamily that binds to hyaline droplet inducing agents. *Toxicol Appl Pharmacol* 116:170–176, 1992.

Leopold G, Furukawa E, Forth W, Rummel W: Comparative studies of absorption of heavy metals in vivo and in vitro. *Arch Pharmacol Exp Pathol* 263:275–276, 1969.

Levi AJ, Gatmaitan Z, Arias IM: Two hepatic cytoplasmic protein fractions, Y and Z, and their possible role in the hepatic uptake of bilirubin, sulfobromophthalein, and other anions. *J Clin Invest* 48:2156–2167, 1969.

Levine RR: Factors affecting gastrointestinal absorption of drugs. *Am J Dig Dis* 15:171–188, 1970.

Levine RR, Steinberg GM: Intestinal absorption of pralidoxime and other aldoximes. *Nature* 209:269–271, 1966.

Li X, Weber LWD, Rozman KK: Toxicokinetics of 2,3,7,8-tetrachlorodibenzo-*p*-dioxin (TCDD) in female Sprague-Dawley rats including placental and lactational transfer to fetuses and neonates. *Fundam Appl Toxicol* 27: 70–76, 1995.

Litwack G, Ketterer B, Arias IM: Ligandin: A hepatic protein which binds steroids, bilirubin, carcinogens and a number of exogenous organic anions. *Nature* 234:466–467, 1971.

Lukas G, Brindle SD, Greengard P: The route of absorption of intraperitoneally administered compounds. *J Pharmacol Exp Ther* 178:562–566, 1971.

Magos L, Clarkson TW: The effect of oral doses of a polythiol resin on the excretion of methylmercury in mice treated with cystein, d-penicillamine or phenobarbitone. *Chem Biol Interact* 14:325–335, 1976.

Malkinson FD: Permeability of the stratus corneum, in Montagna W, Lobitz WC Jr (eds): *The Epidermis*. New York: Academic Press, 1964, pp 435–452.

Marzulli FN, Callahan JF, Brown DWC: Chemical structure and skin penetrating capacity of a short series of organic phosphates and phosphoric acid. *J Invest Dermatol* 44:339–344, 1965.

Mendel JL, Walton MS: Conversion of *p,p*-DDT to *p,p*-DDD by intestinal flora of the rat. *Science* 151:1527–1528, 1966.

Migdalof BH, Antonaccio MJ, McKinstry DN, et al: Captopril: Pharmacology, metabolism, and disposition. *Drug Metab Rev* 15:841–869, 1984.

Pentschew A, Garro F: Lead encephalomyelopathy of the suckling rat and its implication on the porphyrinopathic nervous diseases. *Acta Neuropathol (Berl)* 6:266–278, 1966.

Pfeiffer CJ: Gastroenterologic response to environmental agents—absorption and interactions, in Lee DHK (ed): *Handbook of Physiology. Section 9: Reactions to Environmental Agents*. Bethesda, MD: American Physiological Society, 1977, pp 349–374.

Pritchard JB, Miller DS: Mechanisms mediating renal secretion of organic anions and cations. *Physiol Rev* 73:765–796, 1993.

Renkin EM: Capillary permeability, in Mayerson HS (ed): *Lymph and the Lymphatic System*. Springfield, IL: Thomas, 1968, pp 76–88.

Rosenfield AB, Huston R: Infant methemoglobinemia in Minnesota due to nitrates in well water. *Minn Med* 33:787–796, 1950.

Rozman K: Fecal excretion of toxic substances, in Rozman K, Hänninen O (eds): *Gastrointestinal Toxicology*. Amsterdam/New York/Oxford: Elsevier, 1986, pp 119–145.

Sanders E, Ashworth CT: A study of particulate intestinal absorption of hepatocellular uptake: Use of polystyrene latex particles. *Exp Cell Res* 22:137–145, 1961.

Sasser LB, Jarboe GE: Intestinal absorption and retention of cadmium in neonatal rat. *Toxicol Appl Pharmacol* 41:423–431, 1977.

Scala J, McOsker DE, Reller HH: The percutaneous absorption of ionic surfactants. *J Invest Dermatol* 50:371–379, 1968.

Scatchard G: The attraction of proteins for small molecules and ions. *Ann NY Acad Sci* 51:660–672, 1949.

Schade SG, Felsher BF, Glader BE, Conrad ME: Effect of cobalt upon iron absorption. *Proc Soc Exp Biol Med* 134:741–743, 1970.

Schanker LS: Mechanisms of drug absorption and distribution. *Annu Rev Pharmacol* 1:29–44, 1961.

Schanker LS: Passage of drugs across body membranes. *Pharmacol Rev* 14:501–530, 1962.

Schanker LS, Jeffrey J: Active transport of foreign pyrimidines across the intestinal epithelium. *Nature* 190:727–728, 1961.

Schwartze EW: The so-called habituation to arsenic: Variation in the toxicity of arsenious oxide. *J Pharmacol Exp Ther* 20:181–203, 1923.

Selye H: Mercury poisoning: Prevention by spironolactone. *Science* 169:775–776, 1970.

Selye H: Hormones and resistance. *J Pharm Sci* 60:1–28, 1971.

Selye H, Krajny M, Savoie L: Digitoxin poisoning: Prevention by spironolactone. *Science* 164:842–843, 1969.

Shand DG, Rangno RE: The deposition of propranolol: I. Elimination during oral absorption in man. *Pharmacology* 7:159–168, 1972.

Shoeman DW, Kauffman RE, Azarnoff DL, Boulos BM: Placental transfer of diphenylhydantoin in the goat. *Biochem Pharmacol* 21:1237–1243, 1972.

Silverman WA, Andersen DH, Blanc WA, Crozier DN: A difference in mortality rate and incidence of kernicterus among premature infants allotted to two prophylactic antibacterial regimens. *Pediatrics* 18:614–625, 1956.

Sobel AE, Gawron O, Kramer B: Influence of vitamin D in experimental lead poisoning. *Proc Soc Exp Biol Med* 38:433–435, 1938.

Stowe CM, Plaa GL: Extrarenal excretion of drugs and chemicals. *Annu Rev Pharmacol* 8:337–356, 1968.

Thompson RQ, Sturtevant M, Bird OD, Glazko AJ: The effect of metabolites of chloramphenicol (Chloromycetin) on the thyroid of the rat. *Endocrinology* 55:665–681, 1954.

Thomson ABR, Olatunbosun D, Valberg LS: Interrelation of intestinal transport system for manganese and iron. *J Lab Clin Med* 78:642–655, 1971a.

Thomson ABR, Valberg LS, Sinclair DG: Competitive nature of the intestinal transport mechanism for cobalt and iron in the rat. *J Clin Invest* 50:2384–2394, 1971b.

Thwaites DT, Brown CD, Hirst BH, Simmons NL: $H^+$-coupled dipeptide (glycylsarcosine) transport across apical and basal borders of human intestinal Caco-2 cell monolayers display distinctive characteristics. *Biochem Biophys Acta* 1151:237–245, 1993.

Tsuji A, Tamai I, Nakanishi M, et al: Intestinal brush-border transport of the oral cephalosporin antibiotic, cefdinir, mediated by dipeptide and monocarboxylic acid transport systems in rabbits. *J Pharm Pharmacol* 45:996–998, 1993.

Tune BM, Wu KY, Kempson RL: Inhibition of transport and prevention of toxicity of cephaloridine in the kidney: Dose-responsiveness of the rabbit and the guinea pig to probenecid. *J Pharmacol Exp Ther* 202:466–471, 1977.

Van den Berg M, Heeremans C, Veerhoven E, Oliek: Transfer of polychlorinated dibenzo-*p*-dioxins and dibenzofurans to fetal and neonatal rats. *Fundam Appl Toxicol* 9:635–644, 1987.

Weber LWD, Ernst SW, Stahl BU, Rozman KK: Tissue distribution and toxicokinetics of 2,3,7,8-tetrachloro-dibenzo-*p*-dioxin in rats after intravenous injection. *Fundam Appl Toxicol* 21:523–534, 1993.

Weber LWD, Zesch A, Rozman KK: Penetration, distribution and kinetics of 2,3,7,8-tetrachlorodibenzo-*p*-dioxin in human skin in vitro. *Arch Toxicol* 65:421–428, 1991.

Weiner IM, Mudge GH: Renal tubular mechanisms for excretion of organic acids and bases. *Am J Med* 36:743–762, 1964.

Wertz PhW, Downing DT: Epidermal lipids, in Goldsmith LA (ed): *Physiology, Biochemistry and Molecular Biology of the Skin.* NewYork/Oxford: Oxford University Press, 1991, pp 206–236.

Wester RC, Maibach HI: Percutaneous absorption in man and animal: A perspective, in Drill VA, Lazar P (eds): *Cutaneous Toxicity*. New York: Academic Press, 1977, pp 111–126.

Wilkinson GR: Plasma and tissue binding considerations in drug disposition. *Drug Metab Rev* 14:427–465, 1983.

Williams RM, Beck F: A histochemical study of gut maturation. *J Anat* 105:487–501, 1969.

Wilson JT: Determinants and consequences of drug excretion in breast milk. *Drug Metab Rev* 14:619–652, 1983.

Winteringham FPW: Comparative biochemical aspects of insecticidal action. *Chem Ind (Lond)* 1195–1202, 1957.

Wold JS, Joost RR, Owen NV: Nephrotoxicity of cephaloridine in newborn rabbits: Role of the renal anionic transport system. *J Pharmacol Exp Ther* 201:778–785, 1977.

Young M: Three topics in placental transport: Amino transport; oxygen transfer; placental function during labour, in Klopper A, Diczfalusy E (eds): *Foetus and Placenta*. Oxford: Blackwell Scientific Publications, 1969, pp 139–189.

Zsigmond G, Solymoss B: Effect of spironolactone, pregnenolone-16α-carbonitrile and cortisol on the metabolism and biliary excretion of sulfobromophthalein and phenol-3,6-dibromophthalein disulfonate in rats. *J Pharmacol Exp Ther* 183:499–507, 1972.

# CHAPTER 6

# BIOTRANSFORMATION OF XENOBIOTICS

*Andrew Parkinson*

All organisms are exposed constantly and unavoidably to foreign chemicals, or *xenobiotics*, which include both man-made and natural chemicals such as drugs, industrial chemicals, pesticides, pollutants, pyrolysis products in cooked food, alkaloids, secondary plant metabolites, and toxins produced by molds, plants, and animals. Unfortunately, the physical property that enables many xenobiotics to be absorbed through the skin, lungs, or gastrointestinal tract, namely their lipophilicity, is an obstacle to their elimination because lipophilic compounds can be readily reabsorbed. Consequently, the elimination of xenobiotics often depends on their conversion to water-soluble chemicals by a process known as *biotransformation*, which is catalyzed by enzymes in the liver and other tissues. An important consequence of biotransformation is that the physical properties of a xenobiotic are generally changed from those favoring absorption (lipophilicity) to those favoring excretion in urine or feces (hydrophilicity). An exception to this general rule is the elimination of volatile compounds by exhalation, in which case biotransformation to nonvolatile, water-soluble chemicals can retard their rate of elimination.

Without biotransformation, lipophilic xenobiotics would be excreted from the body so slowly that they would eventually overwhelm and kill an organism. This principle is illustrated by comparing the theoretical and observed rates of elimination of barbital and hexobarbital. The theoretical half-life of barbital, which is water soluble, closely matches the observed elimination half-life of this drug ($t_{1/2}$55–75 h), which is eliminated largely unchanged. In contrast, the observed elimination half-life of hexobarbital ($t_{1/2}$5–6 h) is considerably shorter than the theoretical rate of elimination of this highly lipophilic drug ($t_{1/2}$2–5 months), the difference being that hexobarbital is biotransformed to water-soluble metabolites that are readily excreted.

A change in pharmacokinetic behavior is not the only consequence of xenobiotic biotransformation nor, in some cases, is it the most important outcome. Xenobiotics exert a variety of effects on biological systems. These may be beneficial, in the case of drugs, or deleterious, in the case of poisons. These effects are dependent on the physicochemical properties of the xenobiotic. In many instances, chemical modification of a xenobiotic by biotransformation alters its biological effects. The importance of this principle to pharmacology is that some drugs must undergo biotransformation to exert their pharmacodynamic effect (i.e., it is the metabolite of the drug, and not the drug itself, that exerts the pharmacological effect). The importance of this principle to toxicology is that many xenobiotics must undergo biotransformation to exert their characteristic toxic or tumorigenic effect (i.e., many chemicals would be considerably less toxic or tumorigenic if they were not converted to reactive metabolites by xenobiotic-biotransforming enzymes). In most cases, however, biotransformation terminates the pharmacological effects of a drug and lessens the toxicity of xenobiotics. Enzymes catalyzing biotransformation reactions often determine the intensity and duration of action of drugs and play a key role in chemical toxicity and chemical tumorigenesis (Anders, 1985; Jakoby, 1980; Jakoby et al., 1982; Kato et al., 1989).

To a limited extent, the degree to which organisms are exposed to xenobiotics determines their biotransformation capacity. For example, insects that feed on a variety of plants have a greater capacity to biotransform xenobiotics than insects that feed on a limited number of plants, which in turn have a greater capacity to biotransform xenobiotics than insects that feed on a single species of plant. Compared with mammals, fish have a low capacity to metabolize xenobiotics, ostensibly because they can eliminate xenobiotics unchanged across their gills. Species differences in the capacity of mammals to biotransform xenobiotics do not simply reflect differences in exposure. However, some chemicals stimulate the synthesis of enzymes involved in xenobiotic biotransformation. This process, known as enzyme induction, is an adaptive and reversible response to xenobiotic exposure. Enzyme induction enables some xenobiotics to accelerate their own biotransformation and elimination (Conney, 1967). The mechanism and consequences of enzyme induction are discussed in "Induction of Cytochrome P450."

## Xenobiotic Biotransformation versus the Immune System

Xenobiotic biotransformation is the principal mechanism for maintaining homeostasis during exposure of organisms to small foreign molecules, such as drugs. For large foreign molecules, including invading organisms (such as viruses and bacteria), homeostasis is achieved by the immune system. It is instructive to compare how these two homeostatic mechanisms evolved to cope with exposure to a limitless variety of small and large foreign molecules. The immune system produces a seemingly infinite number of highly specific antibodies. Antibody production is triggered by the foreign agent, which ensures the specificity of the immune response. In contrast, xenobiotic biotransformation is accomplished by a limited number of enzymes with broad substrate specificities. The synthesis of some of these enzymes is triggered by the xenobiotic (by the process of enzyme induction), but in most cases the enzymes are expressed constitutively (i.e., they are synthesized in the absence of a discernible, external stimulus).

Both homeostatic systems have beneficial and detrimental effects. Neutralization of foreign antigens and killing of invading pathogens and cancerous cells are benefits of the immune system, whereas autoimmune disease due to recognition of host antigens is a detriment. Detoxication and enhanced elimination of foreign chemicals are benefits of xenobiotic biotransformation, but conversion of chemicals to toxic metabolites is a detriment. The specificity of xenobiotic-biotransforming enzymes is so broad that they metabolize a large variety of endogenous chemicals, such as ethanol, acetone, steroid hormones, vitamins A and D, bilirubin, bile acids, fatty acids, and eicosanoids.

Indeed, xenobiotic-biotransforming enzymes, or enzymes that are closely related, play an important role in the synthesis of many of these same molecules. For example, several steps in the synthesis of steroid hormones are catalyzed by cytochrome P450 enzymes in steroidogenic tissues. In general, these steroidogenic enzymes play little or no role in the biotransformation of xenobiotics. In the liver, however, other cytochrome P450 enzymes convert steroid hormones to water-soluble metabolites that are excreted in urine or bile, in an analogous manner to the biotransformation and elimination of xenobiotics.

## Biotransformation versus Metabolism

The terms *biotransformation* and *metabolism* are often used synonymously, particularly when applied to drugs. For example, xenobiotic-biotransforming enzymes are often called drug-metabolizing enzymes. The term *xenobiotic-biotransforming enzymes* is more encompassing, although this term conceals the fact that steroids and several other endogenous chemicals are substrates for these enzymes. The term *metabolism* is often used to describe the total fate of a xenobiotic, which includes absorption, distribution, biotransformation, and elimination. However, metabolism is commonly used to mean biotransformation, which is understandable from the standpoint that the products of xenobiotic biotransformation are known as *metabolites*. Furthermore, individuals with a genetic enzyme deficiency resulting in impaired xenobiotic biotransformation are described as *poor metabolizers* rather than poor biotransformers. (Individuals with the normal phenotype are called *extensive metabolizers*).

## Phase I and Phase II Biotransformation

The reactions catalyzed by xenobiotic-biotransforming enzymes are generally divided into two groups, called phase I and phase II, as shown in Table 6-1 (Williams, 1971). Phase I reactions involve hydrolysis, reduction, and oxidation. These reactions expose or introduce a functional group (-OH, $-NH_2$, -SH or -COOH), and usually result in only a small increase in hydrophilicity. Phase II biotransformation reactions include glucuronidation, sulfation, acetylation, methylation, conjugation with glutathione (mercapturic acid synthesis) and conjugation with amino acids (such as glycine, taurine, and glutamic acid). The cofactors for these reactions (discussed later) react with functional groups that are either present on the xenobiotic or are introduced/exposed during phase I biotransformation. Most phase II biotransformation reactions result in a large increase in xenobiotic hydrophilicity, hence they greatly promote the excretion of foreign chemicals.

Phase II biotransformation of xenobiotics may or may not be preceded by phase I biotransformation. For example, morphine, heroine, and codeine are all converted to morphine-3-glucuronide. In the case of morphine, this metabolite forms by direct conjugation with glucuronic acid. In the other two cases, however, conjugation with glucuronic acid is preceded by phase I biotransformation: hydrolysis (deacetylation) in the case of heroine, and *O*-demethylation (involving oxidation by cytochrome P450) in the case of codeine. Similarly, acetaminophen can be glucuronidated and sulfated directly, whereas phenacetin must undergo phase I metabolism (involving *O*-deethylation to acetaminophen) prior to undergoing phase II biotransformation. These examples illustrate how phase I biotransformation is often required for subsequent phase II biotransformation. In general, phase II biotransformation does not precede phase I biotransformation, although there are exceptions to this rule. For example, some sulfated steroids (including some steroid disulfates) are hydroxylated by cytochrome P450.

**Table 6–1**
**General Pathways of Xenobiotic Biotransformation and Their Major Subcellular Location**

| REACTION | ENZYME | LOCALIZATION |
|---|---|---|
| | Phase I | |
| *Hydrolysis* | Carboxylesterase | Microsomes, cytosol |
| | Peptidase | Blood, lysosomes |
| | Epoxide hydrolase | Microsomes, cytosol |
| *Reduction* | Azo- and nitro-reduction | Microflora, microsomes, cytosol |
| | Carbonyl reduction | Cytosol |
| | Disulfide reduction | Cytosol |
| | Sulfoxide reduction | Cytosol |
| | Quinone reduction | Cytosol, microsomes |
| | Reductive dehalogenation | Microsomes |
| *Oxidation* | Alcohol dehydrogenase | Cytosol |
| | Aldehyde dehydrogenase | Mitochondria, cytosol |
| | Aldehyde oxidase | Cytosol |
| | Xanthine oxidase | Cytosol |
| | Monoamine oxidase | Mitochondria |
| | Diamine oxidase | Cytosol |
| | Prostaglandin H synthase | Microsomes |
| | Flavin-mono-oxygenases | Microsomes |
| | Cytochrome P450 | Microsomes |
| | Phase II | |
| | Glucuronide conjugation | Microsomes |
| | Sulfate conjugation | Cytosol |
| | Glutathione conjugation | Cytosol, microsomes |
| | Amino acid conjugation | Mitochondria, microsomes |
| | Acylation | Mitochondria, cytosol |
| | Methylation | Cytosol |

### Nomenclature of Xenobiotic-Biotransforming Enzymes

The enzymes involved in xenobiotic biotransformation tend to have broad and overlapping substrate specificities, which precludes the possibility of naming the individual enzymes after the reactions they catalyze (which is how most other enzymes are named). Many of the enzymes involved in xenobiotic biotransformation have been cloned and sequenced, and in several cases arbitrary nomenclature systems have been developed based on the primary amino acid sequence of the individual enzymes.

### Distribution of Xenobiotic-Biotransforming Enzymes

Xenobiotic-biotransforming enzymes are widely distributed throughout the body, and are present in several subcellular compartments. In vertebrates, the liver is the richest source of enzymes catalyzing biotransformation reactions. These enzymes are also located in the skin, lung, nasal mucosa, eye, and gastrointestinal tract, which can be rationalized on the basis that these are major routes of exposure to xenobiotics, as well as numerous other tissues, including the kidney, adrenal, pancreas, spleen, heart, brain, testis, ovary, placenta, plasma, erythrocytes, platelets, lymphocytes, and aorta (Gram, 1980; Farrell, 1987; Krishna and Klotz, 1994). Intestinal microflora play an important role in the biotransformation of certain xenobiotics. Within the liver (and most other organs), the enzymes catalyzing xenobiotic biotransformation reactions are located primarily in the endoplasmic reticulum (microsomes) or the soluble fraction of the cytoplasm (cytosol), with lesser amounts in mitochondria, nuclei, and lysosomes (see Table 6-1). Their presence in the endoplasmic reticulum can be rationalized on the basis that those xenobiotics requiring biotransformation for urinary or biliary excretion will likely be lipophilic and, hence, soluble in the lipid bilayer of the endoplasmic reticulum.

By extracting and biotransforming xenobiotics absorbed from the gastrointestinal tract, the liver limits the systemic bioavailability of orally ingested xenobiotics, a process known as *first pass elimination*. In some cases, xenobiotic biotransformation in the intestine contributes significantly to the first pass elimination of foreign chemicals. For example, the oxidation of cyclosporin by cytochrome P450 and the conjugation of morphine with glucuronic acid in the small intestine limit the systemic bioavailability of these drugs. Under certain circumstances, oxidation of ethanol to acetaldehyde in the gastric mucosa reduces the systemic bioavailability of alcohol.

Some extrahepatic sites contain high levels of xenobiotic-biotransforming enzymes, but their small size minimizes their overall contribution to the biotransformation of xenobiotics. For example, certain xenobiotic-biotransforming enzymes (such as cytochrome P450 enzymes, flavin-containing monooxygenases, glutathione *S*-transferases and carboxylesterases) are present in nasal epithelium at levels that rival those found in the liver. The nasal epithelium plays an important role in the biotransformation of inhaled xenobiotics, including odorants, but is quantitatively unimportant in the biotransformation of orally ingested xenobiotics (Brittebo, 1993).

The fact that tissues differ enormously in their capacity to biotransform xenobiotics has important toxicological implications in terms of tissue-specific chemical injury. Several xenobiotics, such as acetaminophen and carbon tetrachloride, are hepatotoxic due to their activation to reactive metabolites in the liver (Anders, 1985). Cells within an organ also differ in their capacity to biotransform xenobiotics, and this heterogeneity also has toxicological implications. For example, the cytochrome P450 enzymes that activate acetaminophen and carbon tetrachloride to their reactive metabolites are localized in the centrilobular region of the liver (zone 3), which is why these xenobiotics cause centrilobular necrosis. Species differences in xenobiotic-biotransforming enzymes have both toxicological and pharmacological consequences, as do factors that influence the activity of xenobiotic-biotransforming enzymes (Kato, 1979). For example, the duration of action of hexobarbital (i.e., narcosis) in mice (~10 min), rabbits (~50 min), rats (~100 min) and dogs (~300 min) is inversely related to the rate of hexobarbital biotransformation (i.e., 3-hydroxylation) by liver microsomal cytochrome P450, which follows the rank order: mouse > rabbit > rat > dog. The duration of action of hexobarbital in rats can be shortened from ~100 min to ~30 min by prior treatment with phenobarbital, which induces cytochrome P450 and thereby increases the rate of hexobarbital 3-hydroxylation. By inducing cytochrome P450, treatment of rats with phenobarbital also increases the hepatotoxic effects of acetaminophen and carbon tetrachloride. Species differences in xenobiotic-biotransforming enzymes and factors that affect the pharmacological or toxicological effects of xenobiotics will be discussed throughout this chapter as each of the major xenobiotic-biotransforming enzyme systems is described.

## XENOBIOTIC BIOTRANSFORMATION BY PHASE I ENZYMES

Phase I reactions involve hydrolysis, reduction and oxidation of xenobiotics, as shown in Table 6-1. These reactions expose or introduce a functional group (-OH, $-NH_2$, -SH, or -COOH), and usually result in only a small increase in the hydrophilicity of xenobiotics. The functional groups exposed or introduced during phase I biotransformation are often sites of phase II biotransformation.

### Hydrolysis

**Carboxylesterases.** Mammals contain a variety of carboxylesterases that hydrolyze xenobiotics containing such functional groups as a carboxylic acid ester (procaine), amide (procainamide), thioester (spironolactone), phosphoric acid ester (paraoxon), and acid anhydride (diisopropylfluorophosphate), as shown in Fig. 6-1 (Satoh, 1987). In the presence of an alcohol, carboxylesterases can catalyze the transesterification of xenobiotics, which accounts for the conversion of cocaine (a methyl ester) to ethylcocaine (the corresponding ethyl ester) (Fig. 6-1). Carboxylesterases are not the only enzymes capable of cleaving esters. Examples are given later in this chapter in which the cleavage of xenobiotics containing a carboxylic or phosphoric acid ester is catalyzed by cytochrome P450.

Carboxylesterases determine the duration and site of action of certain drugs. For example, procaine, a carboxylic acid

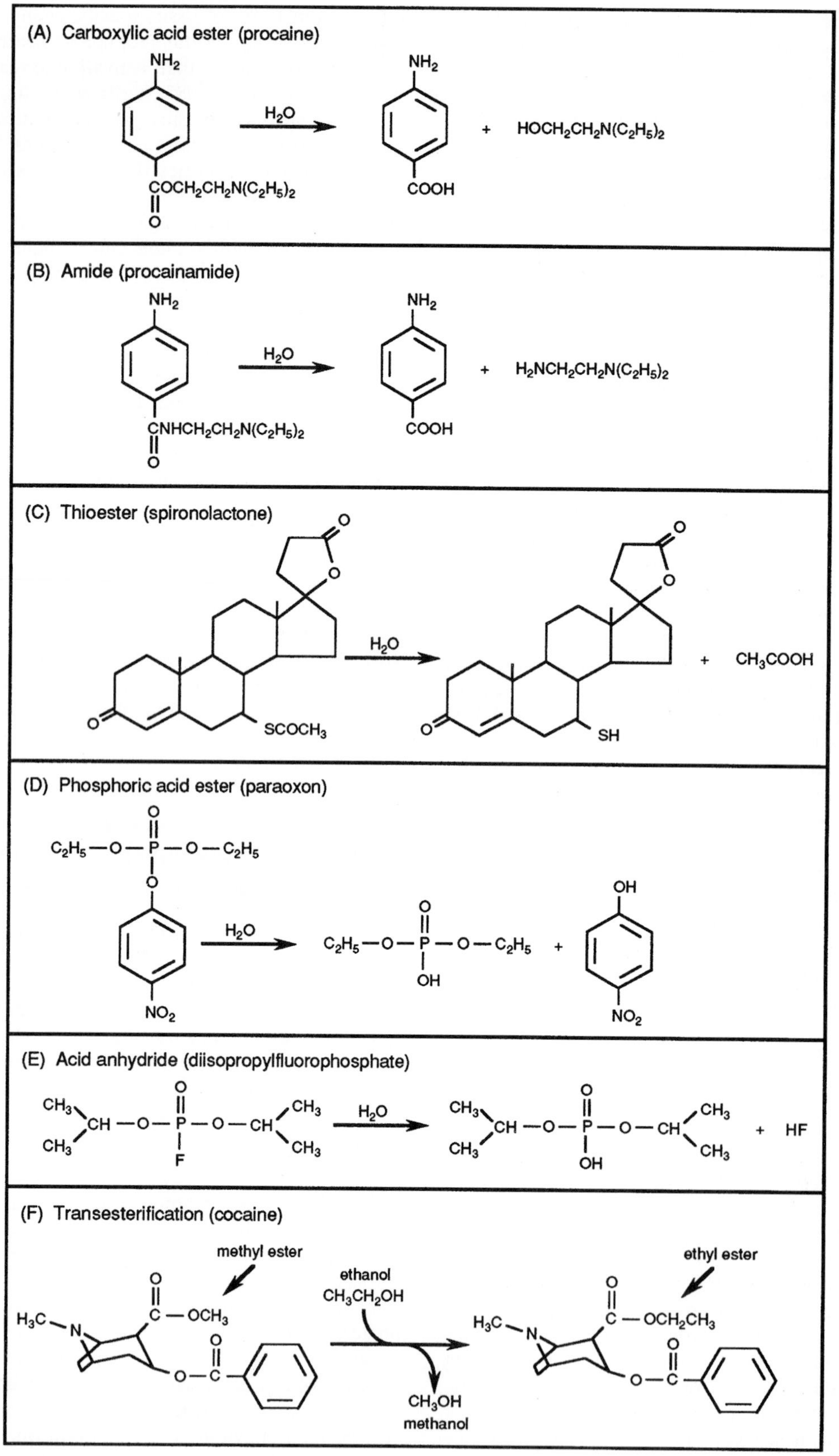

(A) Carboxylic acid ester (procaine)

$NH_2$ … $COCH_2CH_2N(C_2H_5)_2$ $\xrightarrow{H_2O}$ $NH_2$ … $COOH$ + $HOCH_2CH_2N(C_2H_5)_2$

(B) Amide (procainamide)

$NH_2$ … $CNHCH_2CH_2N(C_2H_5)_2$ $\xrightarrow{H_2O}$ $NH_2$ … $COOH$ + $H_2NCH_2CH_2N(C_2H_5)_2$

(C) Thioester (spironolactone)

$SCOCH_3$ $\xrightarrow{H_2O}$ $SH$ + $CH_3COOH$

(D) Phosphoric acid ester (paraoxon)

$C_2H_5—O—P—O—C_2H_5$ … $NO_2$ $\xrightarrow{H_2O}$ $C_2H_5—O—P—O—C_2H_5$ (OH) + OH … $NO_2$

(E) Acid anhydride (diisopropylfluorophosphate)

$(CH_3)_2CH—O—P(O)(F)—O—CH(CH_3)_2$ $\xrightarrow{H_2O}$ $(CH_3)_2CH—O—P(O)(OH)—O—CH(CH_3)_2$ + HF

(F) Transesterification (cocaine)

methyl ester

$H_3C—N$ … $C—OCH_3$ … $O—C$

ethanol
$CH_3CH_2OH$

$CH_3OH$
methanol

ethyl ester

$H_3C—N$ … $C—OCH_2CH_3$ … $O—C$

*Figure 6–1. Examples of reactions catalyzed by carboxylesterases.*

ester, is rapidly hydrolyzed by serum carboxylesterase, which is why this drug is used mainly as a local anesthetic. In contrast, procainamide, the amide analog of procaine, is hydrolyzed much more slowly; hence, this drug reaches the systematic circulation, where it is useful in the treatment of cardiac arrhythmia. In general, enzymatic hydrolysis of amides occurs more slowly than esters, although electronic factors can influence the rate of hydrolysis. The presence of electron-withdrawing substituents weakens an amide bond, making it more susceptible to enzymatic hydrolysis. The duration of action of the muscle relaxant, succinylcholine, is determined by serum carboxylesterase (also known as pseudocholinesterase). In individuals who are genetically deficient in the normal enzyme (~2 percent of Caucasians), succinylcholine causes prolonged muscular relaxation and apnea (La Du, 1992; Lockridge, 1992).

In addition to hydrolyzing numerous drugs and other xenobiotics, carboxylesterases can hydrolyze or bind stoichiometrically to organophosphorus pesticides. Both types of interactions (i.e., hydrolysis and covalent binding) play an important role in the detoxication of these compounds. Numerous studies have shown an inverse relationship between carboxylesterase activity and susceptibility to the toxic effect of organophosphates. Factors that decrease carboxylesterase activity potentiate the toxic effects of organophosphates, whereas factors that increase carboxylesterase activity have a protective effect. For example, the susceptibility of animals to the toxicity of parathion, malathion, and diisopropylfluorophosphate is inversely related to the level of serum carboxylesterase activity. Differences in the susceptibility of several mammalian species to organophosphate toxicity can be abolished by pretreatment with selective inhibitors of carboxylesterases such as cresylbenzodioxaphosphorin oxide, the active metabolite of tri-*ortho*-tolylphosphate (which is also known as tri-*ortho*-cresylphosphate or TOCP). Carboxylesterases are not the only enzymes involved in the detoxication of organophosphorus pesticides. Certain organophosphorus compounds are detoxified by cytochrome P450, flavin-containing monooxygenases, and glutathione *S*-transferases. In addition to xenobiotics, carboxylesterases hydrolyze numerous endogenous compounds, such as palmitoyl-CoA, monoacylglycerol, diacylglycerol, retinyl ester, and other esterified lipids.

Metabolism of xenobiotics by carboxylesterases is not always a detoxication process. Figure 6-2 shows some examples in which carboxylesterases convert xenobiotics to toxic and tumorigenic metabolites. The transesterification of cocaine to ethylcocaine can also be considered an example of xenobiotic activation by carboxylesterases (Fig. 6-1). Normally, hydrolysis of cocaine by carboxylesterases is a detoxication reaction. In the presence of ethanol, however, carboxylesterases catalyze the transesterification of cocaine and some of its metabolites to the corresponding ethyl esters. The ethylated metabolites of cocaine are pharmacologically active and slightly more lipophilic than the parent methyl esters. It has been proposed, therefore, that the increased mortality and hepatotoxicity seen with acute combined consumption of cocaine and ethanol may be due, in part, to the formation of toxic ethylated metabolites of cocaine.

Carboxylesterases are widely distributed throughout the body, with high levels in the centrilobular region of the liver, the proximal tubules of the kidney, the interstitial

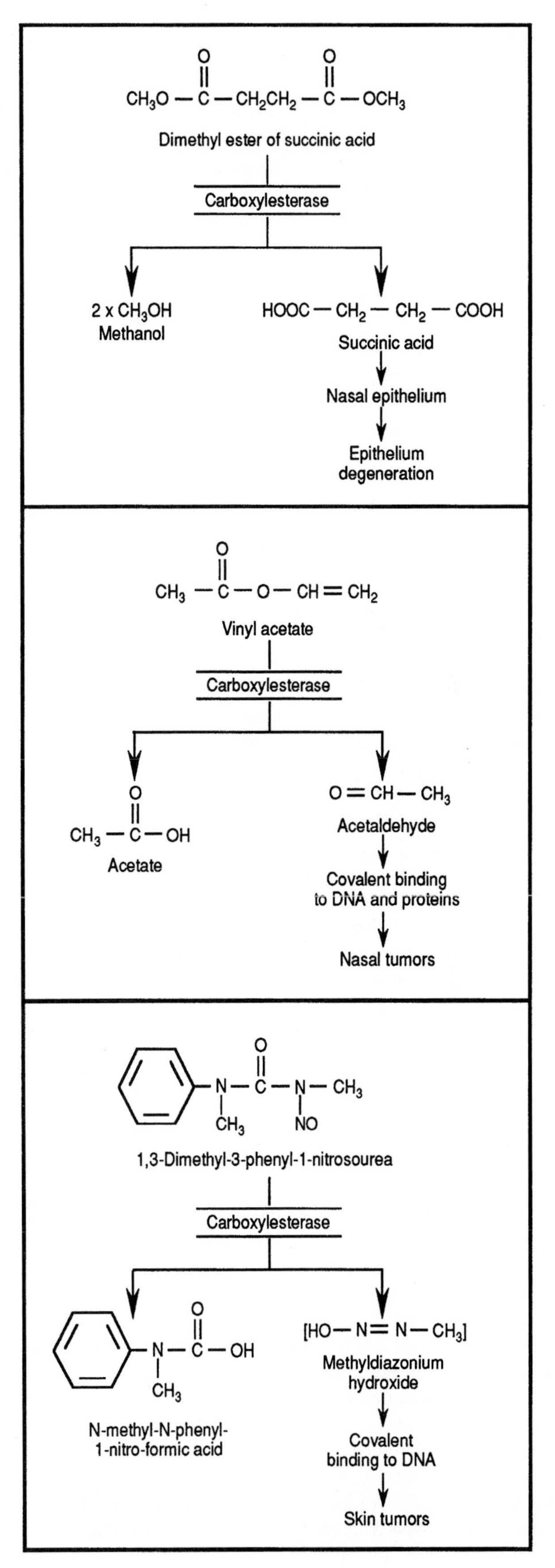


***Figure 6–2.** Activation of xenobiotics to toxic and tumorigenic metabolites by carboxylesterases.*

(Leydig) cells of the testis, the Clara cells of the lung, and the red blood cells and plasma of the blood. Carboxylesterases are present in several subcellular organelles, with high levels in the endoplasmic reticulum (microsomes) and cytosol. Carboxylesterases are abundant cellular components, and they appear to have certain structural roles. For example, egasyn, a liver microsomal carboxylesterase identified in both rat and mouse, binds $\beta$-glucuronidase via its active site, which results in sequestration of the protein within the endoplasmic reticulum.

A systematic nomenclature system for classifying carboxylesterases remains to be established. The broad substrate specificity of these enzymes precludes the possibility of naming them for the reactions they catalyze. Even the term *carboxylesterases* is misleading because these enzymes can also function as amidases and phosphatases, as shown in Fig. 6-1. Several carboxylesterases have been cloned and sequenced, and a nomenclature system based on the structure of these enzymes may soon be developed. Although it is unsatisfactory for naming individual enzymes, the classification system developed in 1953 by Aldridge is still widely used because it has practical value in toxicology (La Du, 1992). Aldridge (1953) classified carboxylesterases based on the nature of their interaction with organophosphates. Carboxylesterases that hydrolyze organophosphates are classified as A-esterases; carboxylesterases that are inhibited by organophosphates are classified as B-esterases, whereas carboxylesterases that do not interact with organophosphates are classified as C-esterases.

Although they are not inhibited by organophosphates, A-esterases are inhibited by *para*-chloromercurobenzoate (PCMB), whereas the opposite is true of B-esterases (i.e., they are inhibited by organophosphates but not by PCMB). It has been postulated that the major difference between A- and B-esterases is that the former contain a cysteine residue at their active site, whereas the latter contain a serine residue. In A-esterases, organophosphates ostensibly interact with the functional SH-group on cysteine and form a phosphorus-sulfur bond, which is readily cleaved by water. In B-esterases, however, organophosphates interact with the functional OH-group on serine and form a phosphorus-oxygen bond, which is not readily cleaved by water. Therefore, organophosphates bind stoichiometrically to B-esterases and inhibit their enzymatic activity. Most of the carboxylesterases that have been purified or cloned from mammalian sources are B-esterases with a serine residue at the active site. The mechanism of catalysis by carboxylesterases containing a serine residue at their active site is analogous to the mechanism of catalysis by serine-proteases. It involves charge relay among a catalytic triad comprised of an acidic amino acid residue (aspartate or glutamate), a basic residue (histidine), and a nucleophilic residue (serine) (Yan et al., 1994).

The mechanism of toxicity of organophosphorus pesticides (and carbamate insecticides) involves inhibition of acetylcholinesterase, which is a serine-containing esterase that terminates the action of the neurotransmitter, acetylcholine. The symptoms of organophosphate toxicity resemble those caused by excessive stimulation of cholinergic nerves. The covalent interaction between organophosphates and acetylcholinesterase is analogous to their binding to the active site serine residue in B-esterases. It should be noted, however, that acetylcholinesterase is structurally distinct from the B-esterases involved in xenobiotic biotransformation.

Liver microsomes from all mammalian species, including humans, contain at least one carboxylesterase, but the exact number of carboxylesterases expressed in any one tissue or species is not known. Because carboxylesterases are glycoproteins, variations in carbohydrate content can give rise to multiple forms of the same enzyme. Consequently, the large number of carboxylesterases that have been identified by isoelectric focussing and nondenaturing gel electrophoresis probably overestimates the number of genes encoding these enzymes.

**Peptidases.** With the advent of recombinant DNA technology, numerous human peptides have been mass-produced for use as drugs, and several recombinant peptide hormones, growth factors, and cytokines currently are used therapeutically. To avoid acid-precipitation and proteolytic degradation in the gastrointestinal tract, peptides are administered parenterally. Nevertheless, peptides are hydrolyzed in the blood and tissues by a variety of peptidases, including aminopeptidases and carboxypeptidases, which hydrolyze amino acids at the *N*- and *C*-terminus, respectively, and endopeptidases, which cleave peptides at specific internal sites (trypsin, for example, cleaves peptides on the *C*-terminal side of arginine or lysine residues) (Humphrey and Ringrose, 1986). Peptidases cleave the amide linkage between adjacent amino acids, hence, they function as amidases. As in the case of carboxylesterases, the active site of peptidases contains either a serine or cysteine residue, which initiates a nucleophilic attack on the carbonyl moiety of the amide bond. As previously noted, the mechanism of catalysis by serine proteases, such as chymotrypsin, is similar to that by serine carboxylesterases (B-esterases).

**Epoxide Hydrolase.** Epoxide hydrolase catalyzes the *trans*-addition of water to alkene epoxides and arene oxides (oxiranes), which can form during the cytochrome P450-dependent oxidation of aliphatic alkenes and aromatic hydrocarbons, respectively. The products of this hydrolyation are *trans*-1,2-dihydrodiols, as shown in Fig. 6-3. Epoxide hydrolase plays an important role in detoxifying electrophilic epoxides that might otherwise bind to proteins and nucleic acids and cause cellular toxicity and genetic mutations. Although the levels vary from

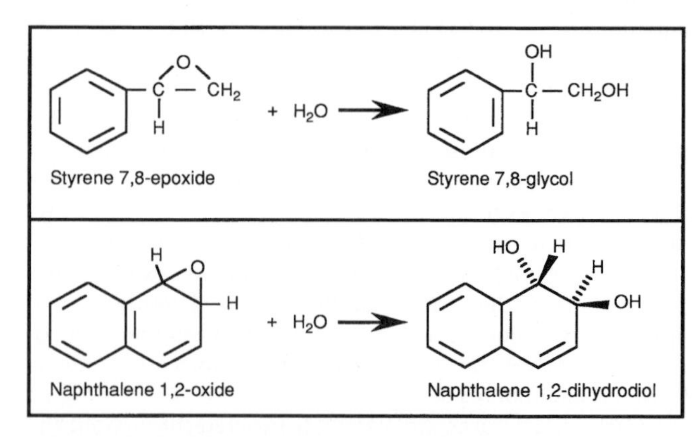


***Figure 6–3. Examples of the hydrolyation of an alkene epoxide (top) and an arene oxide (bottom) by epoxide hydrolase.***

one tissue to the next, epoxide hydrolase has been found in the microsomal fraction of virtually all tissues, including the liver, testis, ovary, lung, kidney, skin, intestine, colon, spleen, thymus, brain, and heart. Within certain tissues, such as liver and lung, the distribution of epoxide hydrolase parallels that of cytochrome P450. In other words, both enzymes are located in the centrilobular region of the liver (zone 3), and in Clara and type II cells in the lung. The cellular distribution and microsomal location of epoxide hydrolase ensure the rapid detoxication of alkene epoxides and arene oxides generated by cytochrome P450.

There are three immunologically distinct forms of epoxide hydrolase in the liver; two in the endoplasmic reticulum, and one in cytosol. One of the microsomal enzymes hydrates cholesterol 5,6$\alpha$-oxide but has virtually no capacity to detoxify xenobiotic oxides. The other microsomal epoxide hydrolase and the cytosolic epoxide hydrolase can hydrate a wide variety of alkene epoxides and arene oxides, as described above. These two forms of epoxide hydrolase are distinct gene products and have different substrate specificities. In rat and mouse, the two enzymes can be distinguished by their stereoselective hydration of stilbene-oxide; microsomal epoxide hydrolase preferentially hydrates the *cis*-isomer at pH 9.0, whereas cytosolic epoxide hydrolase preferentially hydrates the *trans*-isomer at pH 7.4, as shown in Fig. 6-4.

The mechanism of catalysis by epoxide hydrolase is distinct from that of carboxylesterases and peptidases. In contrast to these latter enzymes, epoxide hydrolase does not form a covalent intermediate with its substrates, but hydrolyses epoxides by increasing the nucleophilicity of water. The active site of epoxide hydrolase contains a basic histidine residue ($His^{431}$ in the rat microsomal enzyme), which abstracts a proton ($H^+$) from water to generate a hydroxide ion ($OH^-$) (Bell and Kasper, 1993). This nucleophile hydroxylates the least hindered carbon atom on the opposite side of the oxirane ring. Ring opening produces an alkoxide anion, which is converted to a hydroxyl group by transfer of a proton from a general acid, such as the protonated form ($^-NH_3^+$) of lysine. The initial hydroxylation event and ring opening occur on opposite sides of the molecule, so that the resulting dihydrodiols have a *trans* configuration.

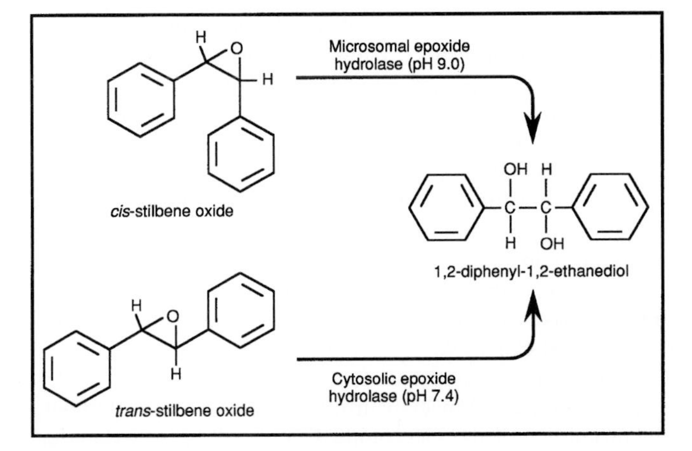


***Figure 6–4. Stereoselective hydrolyation of stilbene oxide by microsomal and cytosolic epoxide hydrolase.***

Some xenobiotic oxides are not hydrated by epoxide hydrolase because the oxirane ring is protected by bulky substituents that sterically hinder interaction with the enzyme. This point proved to be extremely important in elucidating the mechanism by which polycyclic aromatic hydrocarbons cause tumors in laboratory animals (Conney, 1982). Tumorigenic polycyclic aromatic hydrocarbons, such as benzo[a]pyrene, are converted by cytochrome P450 to a variety of arene oxides that bind covalently to DNA, making them highly mutagenic to bacteria. One of the major arene oxides formed from benzo[a]pyrene, namely the 4,5-oxide, is highly mutagenic to bacteria but weakly mutagenic to mammalian cells. This discrepancy reflects the rapid inactivation of benzo[a]pyrene 4,5-oxide by epoxide hydrolase in mammalian cells. However, one of the arene oxides formed from benzo[a]pyrene, namely benzo[a]pyrene 7,8-dihydrodiol-9,10-oxide, is not a substrate for epoxide hydrolase and is highly mutagenic to mammalian cells and considerably more potent than benzo[a]pyrene as a lung tumorigen in mice.

Benzo[a]pyrene 7,8-dihydrodiol-9,10-oxide is known as a bay-region diolepoxide, and analogous bay-region diolepoxides are now recognized as tumorigenic metabolites of numerous polycyclic aromatic hydrocarbons. A feature common to all bay-region epoxides is their resistance to hydrolyation by epoxide hydrolase, which results from steric hindrance from the nearby dihydrodiol group. As shown in Fig. 6-5, benzo[a]-pyrene 7,8-dihydrodiol-9,10-oxide is formed in three steps: Benzo[a]pyrene is converted to the 7,8-oxide, which is converted to the 7,8-dihydrodiol, which is converted to the corresponding 9,10-epoxide. The first and third steps are epoxidation reactions catalyzed by cytochrome P450 or prostaglandin H synthase, but the second step is catalyzed by epoxide hydrolase. Consequently, even though epoxide hydrolase plays a major role in detoxifying several benzo[a]pyrene oxides, such as the 4,5-oxide, it nevertheless plays a role in converting benzo[a]pyrene to its ultimate tumorigenic metabolite, benzo[a]pyrene 7,8-dihydrodiol-9,10-oxide.

Not all epoxides are highly reactive and toxic. The major metabolite of carbamazepine is an epoxide, which is so stable that carbamazepine 10,11-epoxide is a major circulating metabolite in patients treated with this antiepileptic drug. Vitamin K epoxide is also a nontoxic epoxide, which is formed and consumed during the vitamin K-dependent $\gamma$-carboxylation of prothrombin and other clotting factors in the liver. Vitamin K epoxide is not hydrated by epoxide hydrolase but is reduced by vitamin K epoxide reductase. This enzyme is inhibited by warfarin and related coumarin anticoagulants, which interrupts the synthesis of several clotting factors.

Epoxide hydrolase is one of several inducible enzymes in liver microsomes. Induction of epoxide hydrolase is invariably associated with the induction of cytochrome P450, and several cytochrome P450 inducers, such as phenobarbital and *trans*-stilbene oxide, increase the levels of microsomal epoxide hydrolase by twofold or threefold. In mice, the levels of epoxide hydrolase in liver microsomes can be increased by almost an order of magnitude by antioxidants such as butylated hydroxytoluene (BHT), butylated hydroxyanisole (BHA), and ethoxyquin. Epoxide hydrolase is one of several preneoplastic antigens that are overexpressed in chemically-induced foci and nodules that eventually develop into liver tumors. Several alcohols, ketones, and imidazoles stimulate microsomal epox-

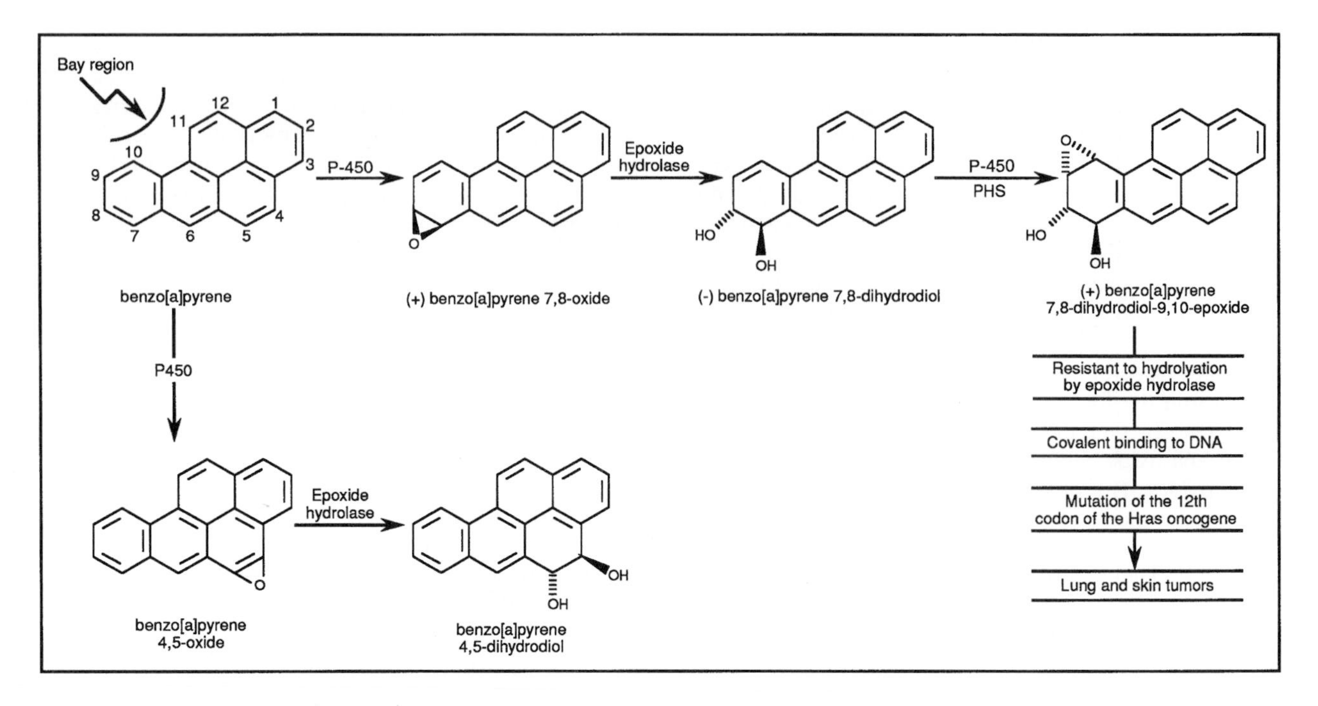


***Figure 6–5.** Role of epoxide hydrolase in the inactivation of benzo[a]pyrene 4,5-oxide and in the conversion of benzo[a]pyrene to its tumorigenic bay-region diolepoxide.*

ide hydrolase activity in vitro. Epoxide hydrolase cannot be inhibited by antibodies raised against the purified enzyme, but it can be inhibited by certain epoxides, such as 1,1,1-trichloropropene oxide and cyclohexene oxide, and certain drugs, such as valpromide (the amide analog of valproic acid) and progabide, a $\gamma$-aminobutyric acid (GABA) agonist. These latter two drugs potentiate the neurotoxicity of carbamazepine by inhibiting epoxide hydrolase, leading to increased plasma levels of carbamazepine 10,11-epoxide (Kroetz et al., 1993).

## Reduction

Certain metals (e.g., pentavalent arsenic) and xenobiotics containing an aldehyde, ketone, disulfide, sulfoxide, quinone, *N*-oxide, alkene, azo, or nitro group are often reduced in vivo, although it is sometimes difficult to ascertain whether the reaction proceeds enzymatically or nonenzymatically by interaction with reducing agents (such as the reduced forms of glutathione, FAD, FMN and NAD[P]). Some of these functional groups can be either reduced or oxidized. For example, aldehydes (RCHO) can be reduced to an alcohol ($RCH_2OH$) or oxidized to a carboxylic acid (RCOOH), whereas sulfoxides ($R_1SOR_2$) can be reduced to a sulfide ($R_1SR_2$) or oxidized to a sulfone ($R_1SO_2R_2$). In the case of halogenated hydrocarbons, such as halothane, dehalogenation can proceed by an oxidative or reductive pathway, both of which are catalyzed by the same enzyme (namely cytochrome P450). In some cases, such as azo-reduction, nitro-reduction, and the reduction of some alkenes (e.g., cinnamic acid, $C_6H_5CH{=}CHCOOH$), the reaction is largely catalyzed by intestinal microflora.

**Azo- and Nitro-Reduction.** Prontosil and chloramphenicol are examples of drugs that undergo azo- and nitro-reduction, respectively, as shown in Fig. 6-6 (Herwick, 1980). Reduction of prontosil is of historical interest. Treatment of streptococcal and pneumococcal infections with prontosil marked the beginning of specific antibacterial chemotherapy. Subsequently, it was discovered that the active drug was not prontosil but its metabolite, sulfanilamide (*para*-aminobenzene sulfonamide), a product of azo-reduction. During azo-reduction, the nitrogen-nitrogen double bond is sequentially reduced and cleaved to produce two primary amines, a reaction requiring four reducing equivalents. Nitro-reduction requires six reducing equivalents, which are consumed in three sequential reactions, as shown in Fig. 6-6 for the conversion of nitrobenzene to aniline.

Azo- and nitro-reduction are catalyzed by intestinal microflora and by two liver enzymes: cytochrome P450 and NAD(P)H-quinone oxidoreductase (a cytosolic flavoprotein, also known as DT-diaphorase). The reactions require NAD(P)H and are inhibited by oxygen. The anaerobic environment of the lower gastrointestinal tract is well suited for azo- and nitro-reduction, which is why intestinal microflora contribute significantly to these reactions. Most of the reactions catalyzed by cytochrome P450 involve oxidation of xenobiotics. Azo- and nitro-reduction are examples in which, under conditions of low oxygen tension, cytochrome P450 can catalyze the reduction of xenobiotics.

Nitro-reduction by intestinal microflora is thought to play an important role in the toxicity of several nitroaromatic compounds including 2,6-dinitrotoluene, which is hepatotumorigenic to male rats. The role of nitro-reduction in the metabolic activation of 2,6-dinitrotoluene is shown in Fig. 6-7 (Long and Rickert, 1982; Mirsalis and Butterworth, 1982). The biotransformation of 2,6-dinitrotoluene begins in the liver, where it is oxidized by cytochrome P450 and conjugated with glucuronic acid. This glucuronide is excreted in bile and undergoes biotransformation by intestinal microflora. One or both of the nitro groups are reduced to amines by nitroreductase,

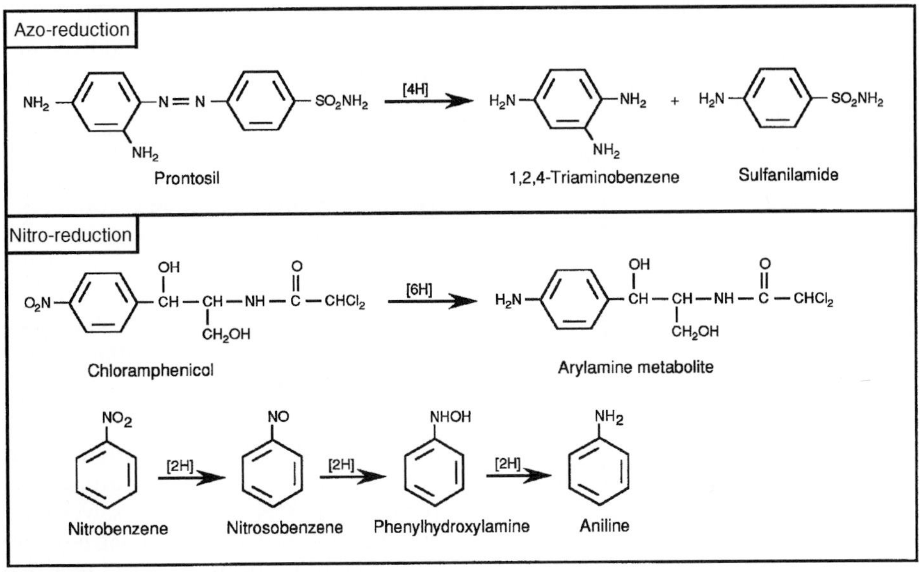

Azo-reduction

Prontosil $\xrightarrow{[4H]}$ 1,2,4-Triaminobenzene + Sulfanilamide

Nitro-reduction

Chloramphenicol $\xrightarrow{[6H]}$ Arylamine metabolite

Nitrobenzene $\xrightarrow{[2H]}$ Nitrosobenzene $\xrightarrow{[2H]}$ Phenylhydroxylamine $\xrightarrow{[2H]}$ Aniline

*Figure 6–6. Examples of drugs that undergo azo reduction (prontosil) and nitro reduction (chloramphenicol and nitrobenzene).*

and the glucuronide is hydrolyzed by $\beta$-glucuronidase. The deconjugated metabolites are absorbed and transported to the liver, where the newly formed amine group is *N*-hydroxylated by cytochrome P450 and conjugated with acetate or sulfate. These conjugates form good leaving groups, which renders the nitrogen highly susceptible to nucleophilic attack from proteins and DNA; this ostensibly leads to mutations and the formation of liver tumors. The complexity of the metabolic scheme shown in Fig. 6-7 underscores an important principle, namely that the activation of some chemical tumorigens to DNA-reactive metabolites involves several different biotransforming enzymes and may take place in more than one tissue. Consequently, the ability of 2,6-dinitrotoluene to bind to DNA and cause mutations is not revealed in most of the short-term assays for assessing the genotoxic potential of chemical agents. These in vitro assays for genotoxicity do not make allowance for biotransformation by intestinal microflora or, in some cases, the phase II (conjugating) enzymes.

**Carbonyl Reduction.** The reduction of certain aldehydes to primary alcohols and of ketones to secondary alcohols is catalyzed by alcohol dehydrogenase and by a family of carbonyl

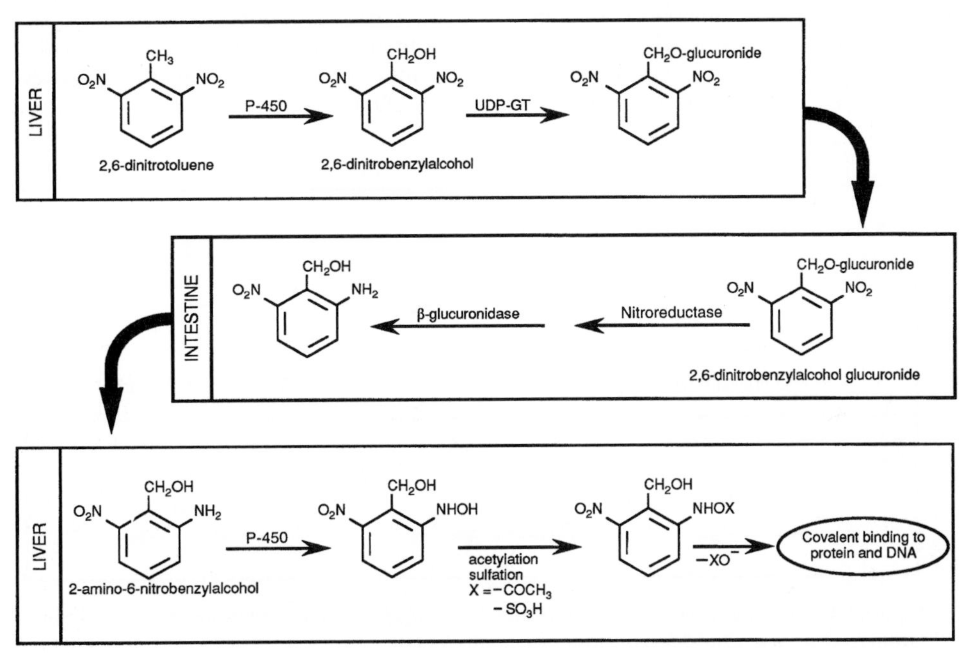


*Figure 6–7. Role of nitro reduction by intestinal microflora in the activation of the rat liver tumorigen, 2,6-dinitrotoluene.*

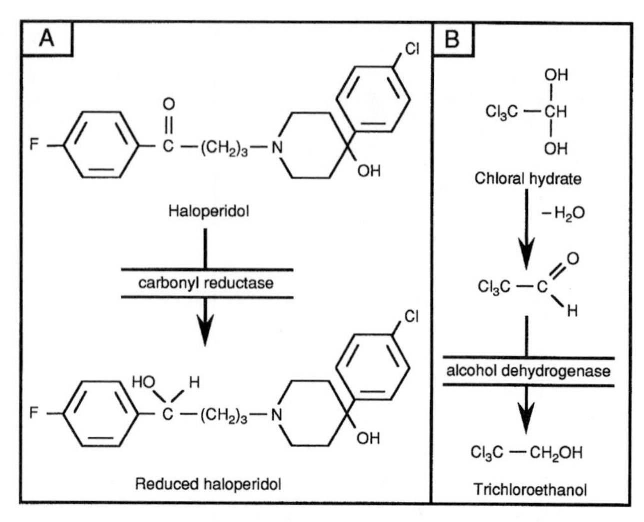


*Figure 6–8.* ***Reduction of xenobiotics by carbonyl reductase (A) and alcohol dehydrogenase (B).***

reductases (Weiner and Flynn, 1989). Carbonyl reductases are NADPH-dependent enzymes present in blood and the cytosolic fraction of the liver, kidney, brain, and other tissues. The major circulating metabolite of the antipsychotic drug, haloperidol, is a secondary alcohol formed by carbonyl reductases in the blood and liver, as shown in Fig. 6-8 (Inaba and Kovacs, 1989). Other xenobiotics that are reduced by carbonyl reductases include acetohexamide, daunorubicin, ethacrynic acid, warfarin, menadione and *para*nitroacetophenone. Prostaglandins are physiological substrates for carbonyl reductases. The activity of low- and high-affinity carbonyl reductases in human liver cytosol varies about tenfold among individuals (Wong et al., 1993).

In rat liver cytosol, the reduction of quinones is primarily catalyzed by DT-diaphorase (see "Quinone Reduction," below), whereas in human liver cytosol, quinone reduction is catalyzed by both DT-diaphorase and carbonyl reductases. In certain cases, the reduction of aldehydes to alcohols can be catalyzed by alcohol dehydrogenase, as shown in Fig. 6-8 for the conversion of the sedative-hypnotic, chloral hydrate, to trichloroethanol. Alcohol dehydrogenase typically converts alcohols to aldehydes. In the case of chloral hydrate, the reverse reaction is favored by the presence of the trichloromethyl group, which is a strong electron-withdrawing group.

**Disulfide Reduction.** Some disulfides are reduced and cleaved to their sulfhydryl components, as shown in Fig. 6-9 for the alcohol deterrent, disulfiram (Antabuse). As shown in Fig. 6-9, disulfide reduction by glutathione is a three-step process, the last of which is catalyzed by glutathione reductase. The first steps can be catalyzed by glutathione *S*-transferase, or they can occur nonenzymatically.

**Sulfoxide and N-Oxide Reduction.** Thioredoxin-dependent enzymes in liver and kidney cytosol have been reported to reduce sulfoxides, which themselves may be formed by cytochrome P450 or flavin-containing monooxygenases (Anders et al., 1981). It has been suggested that recycling through these counteracting enzyme systems may prolong the half-life of certain xenobiotics. Sulindac is a sulfoxide that undergoes reduction to a sulfide, which is excreted in bile and reabsorbed from the intestine (Ratnayake et al., 1981). This enterohepatic cycling prolongs the duration of action of the drug such that this nonsteroidal anti-inflammatory drug (NSAID) need only be taken twice daily. Diethyldithiocarbamate methyl ester, a metabolite of disulfiram, is oxidized to a sulfine, which is reduced to the parent methyl ester by glutathione. In the latter reaction, two molecules of glutathione (GSH) are oxidized with reduction of the sulfine oxygen to water ($R_1R_2C = S^+—O^- + 2\ GSH \rightarrow R_1R_2C = S + GSSG + H_2O$) (Madan et al., 1994).

Just as sulfoxide reduction can reverse the effect of sulfoxidation, so the reduction of *N*-oxides can reverse the *N*-oxygenation of amines, which are formed by flavin-containing monooxygenases and possibly cytochrome P450. Under reduced oxygen tension, reduction of the *N*-oxides of imipramine, tiaramide, indicine, and *N,N*-dimethylaniline can be catalyzed by mitochondrial and/or microsomal enzymes in the presence of NADH or NADPH (Sugiura and Kato, 1977). The NADPH-

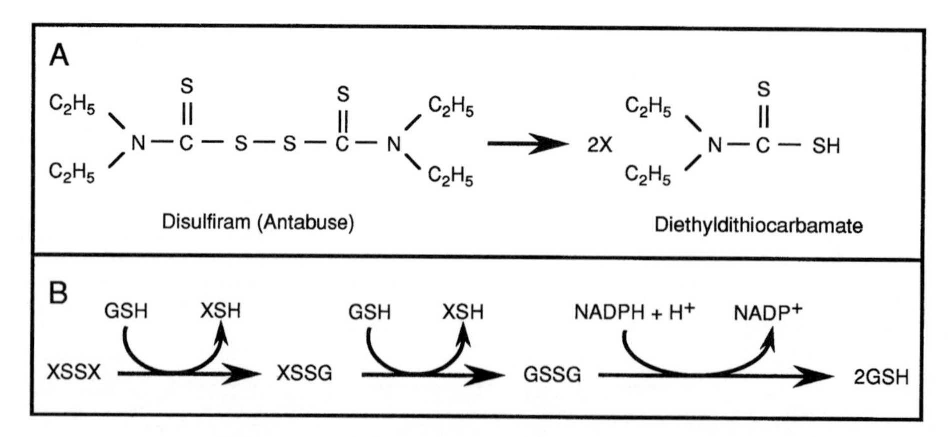


*Figure 6–9.* ***Biotransformation of disulfiram by disulfide reduction (A) and the mechanism of glutathione-dependent disulfide reduction of xenobiotics (B).***

Abbreviations: GSH, glutathione; XSSX, xenobiotic disulfide; GSSG, reduced glutathione. The last reaction is catalyzed by glutathione reductase.

dependent reduction of *N*-oxides in liver microsomes appears to be catalyzed by cytochrome P450 (Sugiura et al., 1976). Most *N*-oxides are reduced slowly, but SR 4233 is an exception (Walton et al., 1992). This benzotriazine di-*N*-oxide is preferentially toxic to hypoxic cells, such as those present in solid tumors, apparently due to its activation by one-electron reduction of the *N*-oxide to an oxidizing nitroxide radical, as shown in Fig. 6-10. This reaction is catalyzed by cytochrome P450 and/or NADPH-cytochrome P450 reductase. Two-electron reduction of the di-*N*-oxide, SR 4233, produces a mono-*N*-oxide, SR 4317, which undergoes a second *N*-oxide reduction to SR 4330. Like SR 4233, the antibacterial agent, quindoxin, is a di-*N*-oxide whose cytotoxicity is dependent on reductive activation, which is favored by anaerobic conditions.

**Quinone Reduction.** Quinones can be reduced to hydroquinones by NAD(P)H-quinone oxidoreductase, a cytosolic flavoprotein also known as DT-diaphorase (Ernster, 1987; Riley and Workman, 1992). An example of this reaction is shown in Fig. 6-11. Formation of the relatively stable hydroquinone involves a two-electron reduction of the quinone with stoichiometric oxidation of NAD[P]H *without* oxygen consumption. The two-electron reduction of quinones also can be catalyzed by carbonyl reductase. Although there are exceptions (see below, this section), this pathway of quinone reduction is essentially nontoxic, that is, it is not associated with oxidative stress, unlike the one-electron reduction of quinones by NADPH-cytochrome P450 reductase (Fig. 6-11). In addition to quinones, substrates for DT-diaphorase include a variety of potentially toxic compounds, including quinone epoxides, quinoneimines, azo dyes and *C*-nitroso derivatives of arylamines.

The second pathway of quinone reduction is catalyzed by NADPH-cytochrome P450 reductase (a microsomal flavoprotein) and results in the formation of a semiquinone free radical by a one-electron reduction of the quinone. Semiquinones are readily autooxidizable, which leads to nonstoichiometric oxidation of NADPH and oxygen consumption. The oxidative stress associated with autooxidation of a semiquinone free radical, which produces a superoxide anion, hydrogen peroxide, and other active oxygen species, can be extremely cytotoxic, as illustrated in Fig. 6-11 for menadione. Oxidative stress appears to be an important component to the mechanism of toxicity of several xenobiotics that either contain a quinone or can be biotransformed to a quinone (Anders, 1985). The production of superoxide anion radicals and oxidative stress are responsible, at least in part, for the cardiotoxic effects of doxorubicin (adriamycin) and daunorubicin (daunomycin), the pulmonary toxicity of paraquat and nitrofurantoin, and the neurotoxic effects of 6-hydroxydopamine. Oxidative stress also plays an important role in the destruction of pancreatic beta cells by alloxan and dialuric acid. Tissues low in superoxide dismutase activity, such as the heart, are especially susceptible to the oxidative stress associated with the redox cycling of quinones. This accounts, at least in part, for the cardiotoxic effects of adriamycin and related anticancer agents.

DT-diaphorase levels are often elevated in tumor cells, which has implications for cancer chemotherapy with agents that are biotransformed by DT-diaphorase (Riley and Workman, 1992). Some cancer chemotherapeutic agents are inactivated by DT-diaphorase, such as SR 4233 (Fig. 6-10), whereas others are activated to cytotoxic metabolites, as in the case of diaziquone. High levels of DT-diaphorase predispose tumor cells to the cytotoxic effects of diaziquone, which is converted by DT-diaphorase to a hydroquinone that readily autooxidizes to a semiquinone with production of reactive oxygen species. It is now apparent that the structure of the hydroquinones produced by DT-diaphorase determines whether the two-elec-

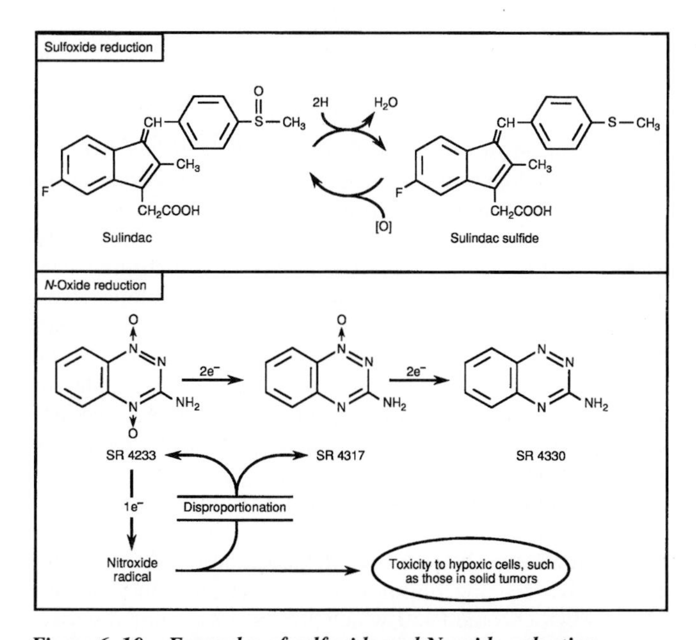


*Figure 6–10. Examples of sulfoxide and N-oxide reduction.*

Note that SR 4233 (3-amino-1,2,4-benzotriazine-1,4-dioxide) is a representative of a class of agents that are activated by reduction, which may be clinically useful in the treatment of certain tumors.

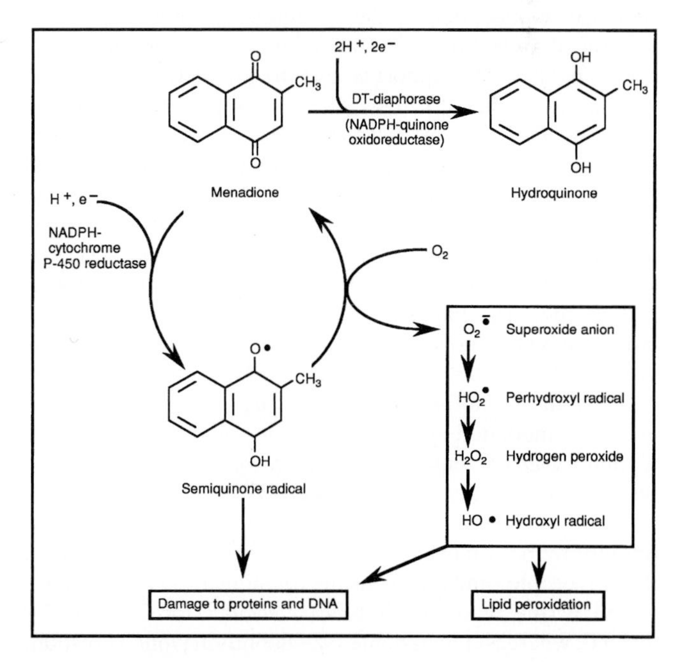


*Figure 6–11. Two-electron reduction of menadione to a hydroquinone, and production of reactive oxygen species during the one-electron reduction to a semiquinone radical.*

tron reduction of quinones results in xenobiotic detoxication or activation. Hydroquinones formed by two-electron reduction of unsubstituted or methyl-substituted 1,4-naphthoquinones (such as menadione) or the corresponding quinone epoxides are relatively stable to autooxidation, whereas the methoxyl, glutathionyl, and hydroxyl derivatives of these compounds undergo autooxidation with production of semiquinones and reactive oxygen species. The ability of glutathionyl derivatives to undergo redox cycling indicates that conjugation with glutathione does not prevent quinones from serving as substrates for DT-diaphorase. The glutathione conjugates of quinones can also be reduced to hydroquinones by carbonyl reductases, which actually have a binding site for glutathione.

DT-diaphorase is a dimer of two equal subunits (*Mr* ~27 kDa) each containing FAD. Mouse, rat, and human appear to possess two, three, and four forms of DT-diaphorase, respectively (Riley and Workman, 1992). The human enzymes are encoded by four distinct gene loci (*DIA 1* through *DIA 4*). The fourth gene locus encodes the form of DT-diaphorase known as NADPH-quinone oxidoreductase-1 ($NQO_1$), which accounts for the majority of DT-diaphorase activity in most human tissues. This enzyme is inducible (see below, this section), and is the orthologue of rat $NQO_1$. A second, noninducible form of DT-diaphorase, $NQO_2$, is polymorphically expressed in humans (Jaiswal et al., 1990).

DT-diaphorase is inducible up to tenfold by two classes of agents, which have been categorized as *bifunctional* and *monofunctional* inducers (Prochaska and Talalay, 1992). The bifunctional agents include compounds like 3-methylcholanthrene and 2,3,7,8-tetrachlorodibenzo-*p*-dioxin (TCDD or dioxin), which induce both phase I enzymes (such as the cytochrome P450 enzyme known as CYP1A1) and phase II enzymes (such as glutathione *S*-transferase and uridine diphosphate [UDP]-glucuronosyltransferase). The induction of CYP1A1, DT-diaphorase, and phase II enzymes by these chemicals is mediated by the *Ah* receptor (discussed in "Induction of Cytochrome P450," below.). The monofunctional agents induce DT-diaphorase and the phase II enzymes, but they do not induce CYP1A1. The monofunctional agents can be subdivided into two classes: those that cause oxidative stress through redox cycling (e.g., the quinone, menadione, and the phenolic antioxidants *tert*-butylhydroquinone and 3,5-di-*tert*-butylcatechol), and those that cause oxidative stress by depleting glutathione (e.g., fumarates, maleates, acrylates, isothiocyanates, and other Michael acceptors that react with glutathione). The *trans*-acting factor responsible for enzyme induction by the monofunctional agents is not known, but it is not the *Ah* receptor. These effects of bifunctional agents (e.g., TCDD) and monofunctional agents (e.g., *tert*-butylhydroquinone) are mediated by two different responsive elements (i.e., regulatory DNA sequences) in the 5′-region of the DT-diaphorase gene (Favreau and Pickett, 1991; Rushmore et al., 1991). The flavonoid, $\beta$-naphthoflavone, induces DT-diaphorase by both mechanisms; the parent compound binds to the *Ah* receptor and is responsible for inducing DT-diaphorase via XRE (the *xenobiotic-responsive element* for CYP1A1 inducers), whereas a metabolite of $\beta$-naphthoflavone is responsible for inducing DT-diaphorase via ARE (the *antioxidant responsive element*). Among the monofunctional agents that apparently induce DT-diaphorase via ARE is sulforaphane, an ingredient of broccoli that may be responsible for its anticarcinogenic effects (Zhang et al., 1992).

**Dehalogenation.** There are three major mechanisms for removing halogens (F, Cl, Br, and I) from aliphatic xenobiotics (Anders, 1985). The first, known as *reductive dehalogenation*, involves replacement of a halogen with hydrogen, as shown below.

$$X_3C{-}CHX_2 \xrightarrow[-HX]{+2H} X_2HC{-}CHX_2$$

Pentahaloethane → Tetrahaloethane

In the second mechanism, known as *oxidative dehalogenation*, a halogen and hydrogen on the same carbon atom are replaced with oxygen. Depending on the structure of the haloalkane, oxidative dehalogenation leads to the formation of an acylhalide or aldehyde, as shown below.

$$X_3C{-}CHX_2 \xrightarrow[-HX]{+[O]} X_3C{-}C(X){=}O$$

Pentahaloethane → Tetrahaloacetylhalide

$$X_3C{-}CH_2X \xrightarrow[-HX]{+[O]} X_3C{-}C(H){=}O$$

Tetrahaloethane → Trihaloacetaldehyde

A third mechanism of dehalogenation involves the elimination of two halogens on adjacent carbon atoms to form a carbon-carbon double bond, as shown below:

$$X_3C{-}CHX_2 \xrightarrow[-2HX]{+2H} X_2C{=}CXH$$

Pentahaloethane → Trihaloacetylene

A variation on this third mechanism is *dehydrohalogenation*, in which a halogen and hydrogen on adjacent carbon atoms are eliminated to form a carbon-carbon double bond.

Reductive and oxidative dehalogenation are both catalyzed by cytochrome P450. (The ability of cytochrome P450 to catalyze both reductive and oxidative reactions is explained later in this chapter.) Dehalogenation reactions leading to double bond formation are catalyzed by cytochrome P450 and glutathione *S*-transferase. These reactions play an important role in the biotransformation and metabolic activation of several halogenated alkanes, as the following examples illustrate.

The hepatotoxicity of carbon tetrachloride ($CCl_4$) and several related halogenated alkanes is dependent on their biotransformation by reductive dehalogenation. The first step in reductive dehalogenation is a one-electron reduction catalyzed by cytochrome P450, which produces a potentially toxic, carbon-centered radical and inorganic halide. In the case of $CCl_4$, reductive dechlorination produces a trichloromethyl radical ($\cdot CCl_3$), which initiates lipid peroxidation and produces a variety of other metabolites, as shown in Fig. 6-12.

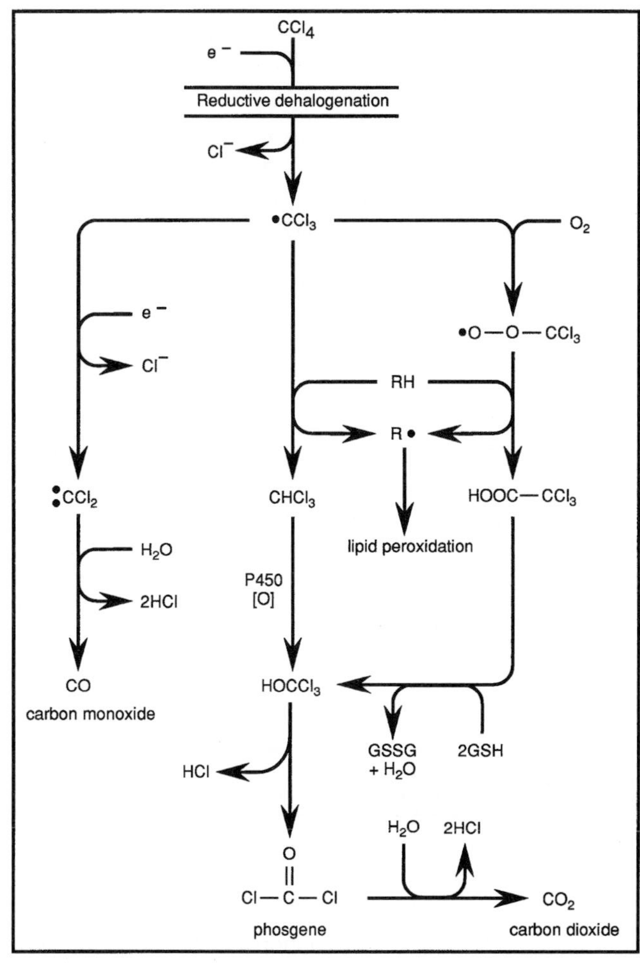


***Figure 6–12. Reductive dehalogenation of carbon tetrachloride to a trichloromethyl free radical that initiates lipid peroxidation.***

Abbreviations: RH, unsaturated lipid; R˙, lipid dienyl radical; GSH, reduced glutathione; GSSG, oxidized glutathione.

Halothane can also be converted by reductive dehalogenation to a carbon-centered radical, as shown in Fig. 6-13. The mechanism is identical to that described for carbon tetrachloride, although in the case of halothane the radical is generated through loss of bromine, which is a better leaving group than chlorine. Figure 6-13 also shows that halothane can undergo oxidative dehalogenation, which involves oxygen insertion at the C-H bond to generate an unstable halohydrin ($CF_3COHClBr$) that decomposes to a reactive acylhalide ($CF_3COCl$), which can bind to cellular proteins (particularly to amine groups) or further decompose to trifluoroacetic acid ($CF_3COOH$).

Both the oxidative and reductive pathways of halothane metabolism generate reactive intermediates capable of binding to proteins and other cellular macromolecules. The relative importance of these two pathways to halothane-induced hepatotoxicity appears to be species dependent. In rats, halothane-induced hepatotoxicity is promoted by those conditions favoring the reductive dehalogenation of halothane, such as moderate hypoxia (10–14% oxygen) plus treatment with the cytochrome P450 inducers, phenobarbital and pregnenolone-16$\alpha$-carbonitrile. In contrast to the situation in rats, halothane-induced hepatotoxicity in guinea pigs is largely the result of oxidative dehalogenation of halothane (Lunam et al., 1989). In guinea pigs, halothane hepatotoxicity is not enhanced by moderate hypoxia and is diminished by the use of deuterated halothane, which impedes the oxidative dehalogenation of halothane because the P450-dependent insertion of oxygen into a carbon-deuterium bond is energetically less favorable (and therefore slower) than inserting oxygen into a carbon-hydrogen bond.

Halothane hepatitis in humans is a rare but severe form of liver necrosis associated with repeated exposure to this volatile anesthetic. In humans, as in guinea pigs, halothane hepatotoxicity appears to result from the oxidative dehalogenation of halothane, as shown in Fig. 6-13. Serum samples from patients suffering from halothane hepatitis contain antibodies directed against neoantigens formed by the trifluoroacetylation of proteins. These antibodies have been used to identify which specific proteins in the endoplasmic reticulum are targets for trifluoroacetylation during the oxidative dehalogenation of halothane (Pohl et al., 1989).

The concept that halothane is activated by cytochrome P450 to trifluoroacetylhalide, which binds covalently to proteins and elicits an immune response, has been extended to other volatile anesthetics, such as enflurane, methoxyflurane, and isoflurane. In other words, these halogenated aliphatic hydrocarbons, like halothane, may be converted to acylhalides that form immunogens by binding covalently to proteins. In addition to accounting for rare instances of enflurane hepatitis, this mechanism of hepatotoxicity can also account for reports of a *cross-sensitization* between enflurane and halothane, in which enflurane causes liver damage in patients previously exposed to halothane.

One of the metabolites generated from the reductive dehalogenation of halothane is 2-chloro-1,1-difluoroethylene (Fig. 6-13). The formation of this metabolite involves the loss of two halogens from adjacent carbon atoms with formation of a carbon-carbon double bond. This type of dehalogenation reaction can also be catalyzed by glutathione *S*-transferases. Glutathione initiates the reaction with a nucleophilic attack either on the electrophilic carbon to which the halogen is attached (mechanism A) or on the halide itself (mechanism B), as shown in Fig. 6-14 for the dehalogenation of 1,2-dihaloethane to ethylene. The insecticide DDT is detoxified by dehydrochlorination to DDE by DDT-dehydrochlorinase, as shown in Fig. 6-15. The activity of this glutathione-dependent reaction correlates well with resistance to DDT in houseflies.

## Oxidation

**Alcohol, Aldehyde, Ketone Oxidation-Reduction Systems.** Alcohols, aldehydes and ketones are oxidized or reduced by a number of enzymes, including alcohol dehydrogenase, aldehyde dehydrogenase, aldehyde oxidase, and carbonyl reductase. For example, simple alcohols (such as methanol and ethanol) are oxidized to aldehydes (namely formaldehyde and acetaldehyde) by alcohol dehydrogenase. These aldehydes are further oxidized to carboxylic acids (formic acid and acetic acid) by aldehyde dehydrogenase, as shown in Fig. 6-16. $NAD^+$ is the preferred cofactor for both alcohol and aldehyde dehydrogenase.

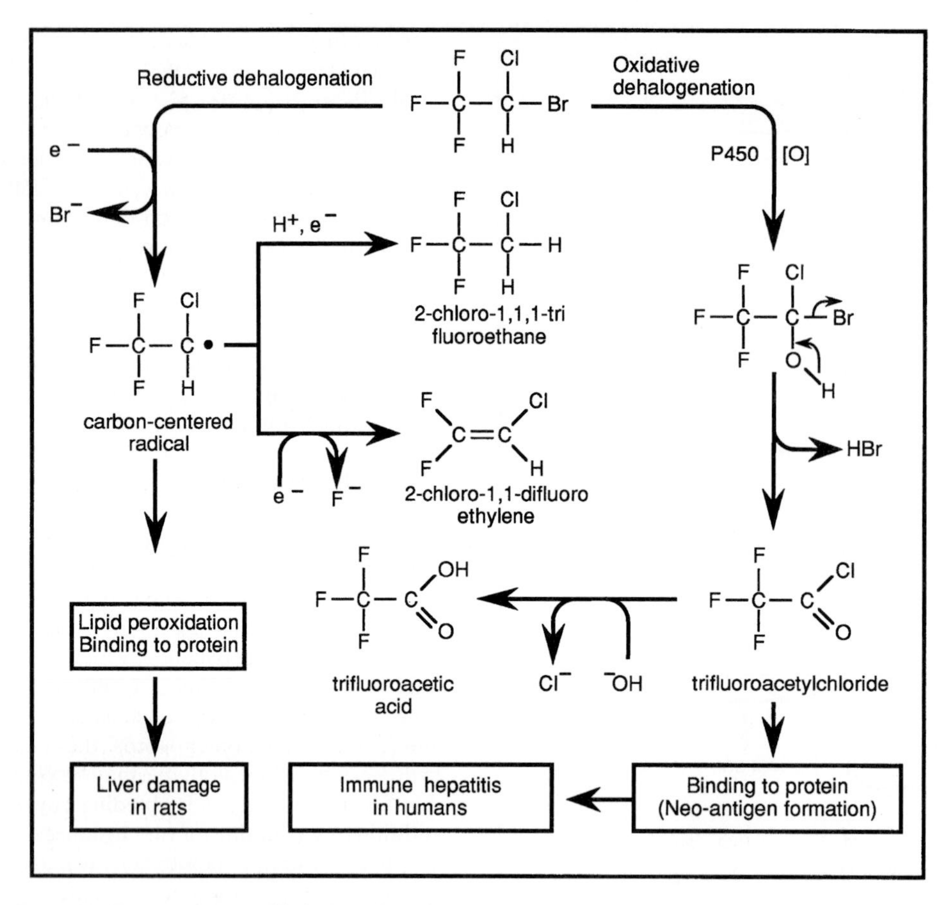


*Figure 6–13. Activation of halothane by reductive and oxidative dehalogenation and their role in liver toxicity in rats and humans.*

Alcohol dehydrogenase (ADH) is a zinc-containing, cytosolic enzyme present in several tissues including the liver, which has the highest levels, the kidney, the lung, and the gastric mucosa (Agarwal and Goedde, 1992). Human ADH is a dimeric protein consisting of two 40-kDa subunits. The subunits ($\alpha$, $\beta$, $\gamma$, $\pi$, and $\chi$) are encoded by five different gene loci ($ADH_1$ through $ADH_5$). However, because there are three allelic variants of the beta subunit ($\beta_1$, $\beta_2$, and $\beta_3$) and two allelic variants of the gamma subunit ($\gamma_1$ and $\gamma_2$), the human ADH enzymes are comprised of eight subunits, which can combine as heterodimers or homodimers. The different molecular forms of ADH are divided into three major classes. Class I contains $ADH_1$, $ADH_2$, and $ADH_3$. $ADH_1$ contains either two alpha subunits or one alpha subunit plus a beta or gamma subunit. $ADH_2$ contains either two beta subunits (which could be $\beta_1$, $\beta_2$, or $\beta_3$) or a beta subunit plus a gamma subunit (which could be $\gamma_1$ or $\gamma_2$). $ADH_3$ contains two gamma subunits (which could be $\gamma_1$ or $\gamma_2$). Class II contains $ADH_4$,

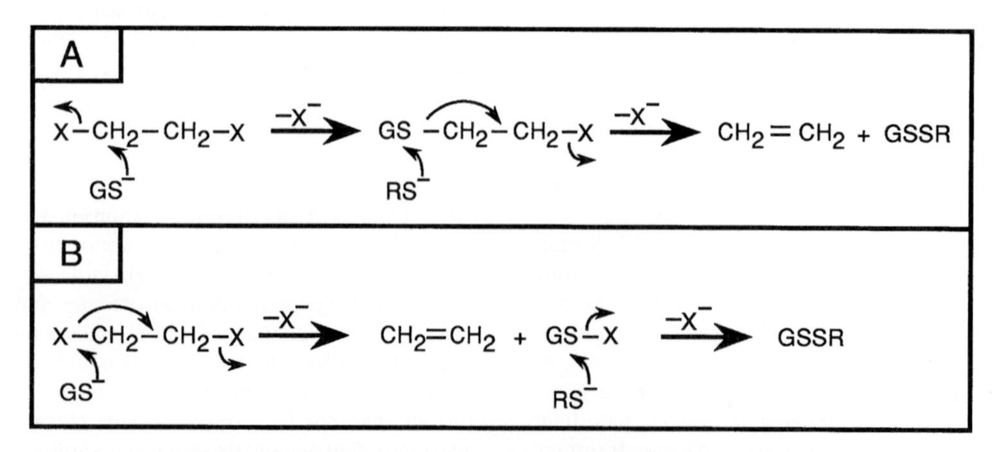


*Figure 6–14. Glutathione-dependent dehalogenation of 1,2-dihaloethane to ethylene.*

(*A*) Nucleophilic attack on carbon. (*B*) Nucleophilic attack on halide.

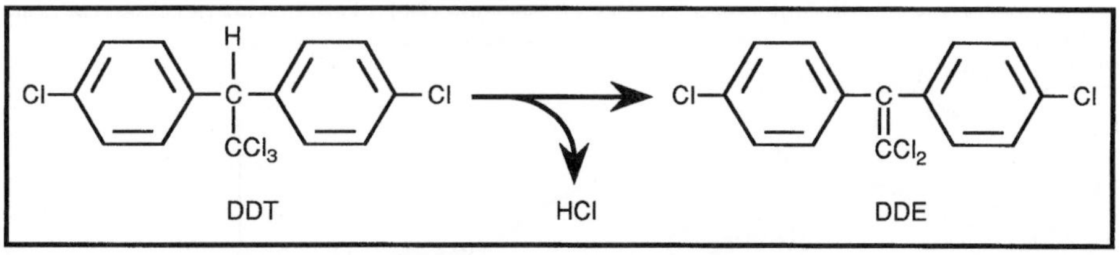

*Figure 6–15. Dehydrochlorination of the pesticide DDT to DDe, a glutathione-dependent reaction.*

which is made up of two pi subunits (named pi because this form of ADH is not inhibited by pyrazole). Class III contains $ADH_5$, which is made up of two chi subunits (for which reason it is also known as chi-ADH) (Agarwal and Goedde, 1992).

The class I ADH isozymes are responsible for the oxidation of ethanol and other small, aliphatic alcohols, and they are strongly inhibited by pyrazole and its 4-alkyl derivatives (e.g., 4-methylpyrazole). Class II isozymes preferentially oxidize larger aliphatic and aromatic alcohols and play little role in ethanol oxidation. Class II isozymes do not oxidize methanol and are not inhibited by pyrazole. Long-chain alcohols (pentanol and larger) and aromatic alcohols (such as cinnamyl alcohol) are preferred substrates for the class III isozymes, which also are not inhibited by pyrazole. Class III ADH and formaldehyde dehydrogenase are identical enzymes (Koivusalo et al., 1989).

The class I isozymes of ADH differ in their capacity to oxidize ethanol. The homodimer, $\beta_2\beta_2$, and heterodimers containing at least one $\beta_2$ subunit are especially active in oxidizing ethanol at physiological pH. These isozymes, known as *atypical* ADH, are responsible for the unusually rapid conversion of ethanol to acetaldehyde in 85 percent of the Japanese and Chinese population. The atypical ADH is expressed to a much lesser degree in Caucasians (<5 percent of Americans, ~8 percent of English, ~12 percent of Germans and ~20 percent of Swiss), African Americans (<10 percent), Native Americans (0 percent) and Asian Indians (0 percent) (Agarwal and Goedde, 1992).

Class I isozymes of $ADH_1$, $ADH_2$, and $ADH_3$ are expressed mainly in the liver, with lesser amounts in kidney, gastrointestinal tract and lung. Gastric ADH is mainly $ADH_3$ (composed of gamma subunits); hence, ethanol oxidation in the stomach differs somewhat from that in the liver. Compared with hepatic ADH, gastric ADH has a lower affinity (higher $K_m$) for alcohol, but gastric ADH nevertheless can limit the systemic bioavailability of alcohol. This first-pass elimination of alcohol by gastric ADH can be significant depending on the manner in which the alcohol is consumed; large doses over a short time produce high ethanol concentrations in the stomach, which compensate for the high $K_m$ of gastric ADH. Women have lower gastric ADH activity than do men, and gastric ADH activity tends to be lower in alcoholics (Frezza et al., 1990). Some alcoholic women have no detectable gastric ADH, and blood levels of ethanol after oral consumption of alcohol are the same as those that are obtained after intravenous administration. Gastric ADH activity decreases during fasting, which is one reason alcohol is more intoxicating when consumed on an empty stomach. Several commonly used drugs (cimetidine, ranitidine, aspirin) are noncompetitive inhibitors of gastric ADH. Under certain circumstances these drugs increase the systemic availability of alcohol, although the effect is too small to have serious medical, social, or legal consequences (Levitt, 1993).

Alcohols can be oxidized to aldehydes by non-ADH enzymes in microsomes and peroxisomes, although these are quantitatively less important than ADH for ethanol oxidation (Lieber, 1990). The microsomal ethanol oxidizing system (formerly known as MEOS) is the cytochrome P450 enzyme, CYP2E1. The corresponding peroxisomal enzyme is catalase. The oxidation of ethanol to acetaldehyde by these three enzyme systems is shown in Fig. 6-17.

Aldehyde dehydrogenase (ALDH) oxidizes aldehydes to carboxylic acids with $NAD^+$ as the cofactor. Several ALDH enzymes are involved in the oxidation of xenobiotic aldehydes (Goedde and Agarwal, 1992). Formaldehyde dehydrogenase, which specifically oxidizes formaldehyde that is complexed with glutathione, is not a member of the ALDH family but is a class III ADH (Koivusalo et al., 1989).

The ALDH enzymes are divided into three classes. Members of class 1 (ALDH1) are cytosolic enzymes that oxidize a wide variety of xenobiotic aldehydes. Members of class 2 (ALDH2) are mitochondrial enzymes that, by virtue of their low $K_m$ (high affinity) are primarily responsible for oxidizing simple aldehydes, such as acetaldehyde, as shown in Fig. 6-17. Members of class 3 (ALDH3) are cytosolic enzymes present

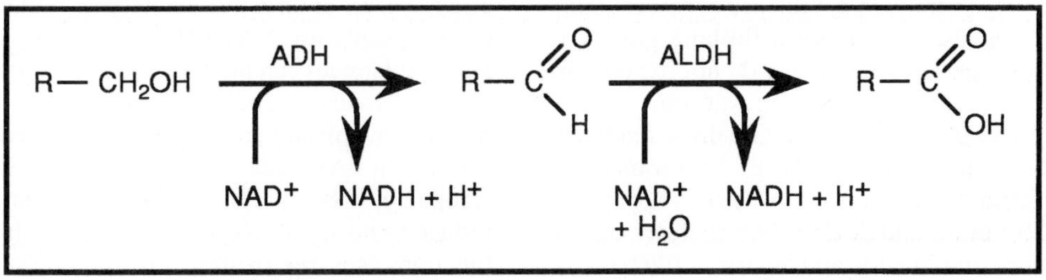

*Figure 6–16. Oxidation of alcohols to aldehydes and carboxylic acids by alcohol dehydrogenase (ADH) and aldehyde dehydrogenase (ALDH).*

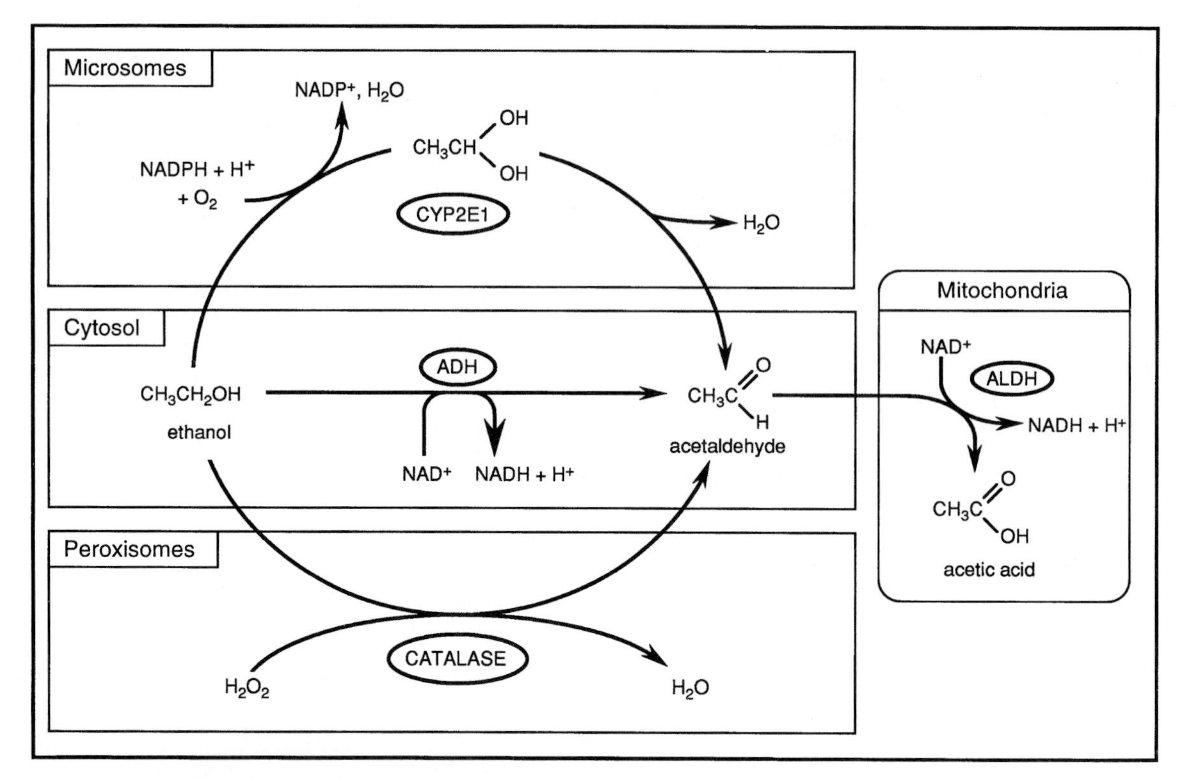


***Figure 6–17. Oxidation of alcohol to acetaldehyde by alcohol dehydrogenase (ADH), cytochrome P450 (CYP2E1), and catalase.***

Note the oxidation of alcohol to acetic acid involves multiple organelles.

in the stomach and certain other extrahepatic tissues. ALDH3 would seem well placed to detoxify acetaldehyde produced by the oxidation of ethanol by gastric ADH. However, acetaldehyde is not a substrate for ALDH3. In contrast to ALDH1 and ALDH2, which specifically reduce $NAD^+$, ALDH3 reduces both $NAD^+$ and $NADP^+$ due to its low affinity for these cofactors. ALDH3 appears to be a dimer of two 85-kDa subunits, whereas ALDH1 and ALDH2 appear to be homotetramers of 54-kDa subunits (Goedde and Agarwal, 1992).

A genetic polymorphism for ALDH2 has been documented in humans. A high percentage (45 to 53 percent) of Japanese, Chinese, and Vietnamese populations are deficient in ALDH2 activity due to a point mutation ($Glu^{487} \rightarrow Lys^{487}$). These same ethnic groups also have a high incidence of the atypical form of ADH, which means that they rapidly convert ethanol to acetaldehyde but only slowly convert acetaldehyde to acetic acid. For this reason, many Japanese and Chinese subjects experience a flushing syndrome after consuming alcohol due to a build-up of acetaldehyde, which triggers the dilation of facial blood vessels through the release of catecholamines. Native Americans also experience a flushing syndrome after consuming alcohol, even though they do not express the atypical ADH or lack ALDH2. The flushing syndrome in these individuals may be caused by impaired acetaldehyde oxidation in blood erythrocytes. Inhibition of ALDH by disulfiram (Antabuse) causes an accumulation of acetaldehyde in alcoholics. The nauseating effect of acetaldehyde serves to deter continued ethanol consumption (Goedde and Agarwal, 1992).

The toxicological consequences of an inherited or acquired deficiency of ALDH illustrate that aldehydes are more cytotoxic than the corresponding alcohol. This is especially true of allyl alcohol ($CH_2 = CHCH_2OH$), which is converted by ADH to the hepatotoxic aldehyde, acrolein ($CH_2 = CHCHO$).

The oxidation of ethanol by ADH and ALDH leads to the formation of acetic acid, which is rapidly oxidized to carbon dioxide and water. However, in certain cases, alcohols are converted to toxic carboxylic acids, as in the case of methanol and ethylene glycol, which are converted via aldehyde intermediates to formic acid and oxalic acid, respectively. Formic and oxalic acids are considerably more toxic than acetic acid. For this reason methanol and ethylene glycol poisoning are commonly treated with ethanol, which competitively inhibits the oxidation of methanol and ethylene glycol by ADH and ALDH. The potent inhibitor of ADH, 4-methylpyrazole (fomepizole), is also used to treat methanol and ethylene glycol poisoning.

The reduction of aldehydes and ketones to primary and secondary alcohols by carbonyl reductases has already been discussed. In contrast to ADH and ALDH, carbonyl reductases typically use NADPH as the source of reducing equivalents. Aldehydes can also be oxidized by aldehyde oxidase and xanthine oxidase. The aldehyde oxidase in liver cytosol is a metalloflavoprotein composed of two identical subunits each containing FAD, molybdenum, and iron in a 1:1:4 ratio (Rajagopalan, 1980). During substrate oxidation, the enzyme is reduced and then reoxidized by molecular oxygen; hence, it functions as a true oxidase. The oxygen incorporated into the xenobiotic is derived from water rather than oxygen, which distinguishes the oxidases from oxygenases. Aldehyde oxidase is something of a misnomer because the enzyme can oxidize a number of substituted pyrroles, pyridines, pyrimidines, purines, and pteridines. Substrates for human aldehyde oxidase include $N^1$-methylnicotinamide, benzaldehyde and 6-methylpurine (Rodrigues, 1994). Aldehyde oxidase is the second of two enzymes involved in the formation of cotinine, a major metabolite of nicotine excreted in the urine of cigarette smokers. The initial step in this reaction is the formation of a double bond (C = N) in the pyrrole ring, which produces nicotine $\Delta^{1',5'}$-iminium ion. Like nicotine, several other drugs are oxidized either sequentially or concomitantly by cytochrome P450 and aldehyde oxidase, including quinidine, azapetine, cyclophosphamide, carbazeran, and prolintane. Aldehydes generated by cytochrome P450 can also be further oxidized by cytochrome P450 to carboxylic acids. In contrast to aldehyde oxidase, the cytochrome P450-dependent oxidation of alcohols and aldehydes occurs in microsomes and proceeds by oxygenation, such that the oxygen incorporated into the substrate is derived from molecular oxygen, not water. Some of the substrates oxidized by aldehyde oxidase are also oxidized by xanthine oxidase.

Several purine derivatives (e.g., allopurinol, 6-mercaptopurine) can be oxidized by xanthine oxidase, which normally catalyzes the sequential oxidation of hypoxanthine to xanthine and uric acid, as shown in Fig. 6-18 (Rajagopalan, 1980). By competing with hypoxanthine and xanthine for oxidation by xanthine oxidase, allopurinol inhibits the formation of uric acid, making allopurinol a useful drug in the treatment of gout. Monomethylated xanthines can also be oxidized to the corresponding uric acid derivatives by xanthine oxidase. In contrast, dimethylated and trimethylated xanthines, such as theophylline (1,3-dimethylxanthine) and caffeine (1,3,7-trimethylxanthine), are oxidized to the corresponding uric acid derivatives primarily by cytochrome P450. Substrates for xanthine oxidase are not limited to purine derivatives, as illustrated by the oxidation of phthalazine to phthalazinone (see Fig. 6-18). This same reaction is also catalyzed by aldehyde oxidase.

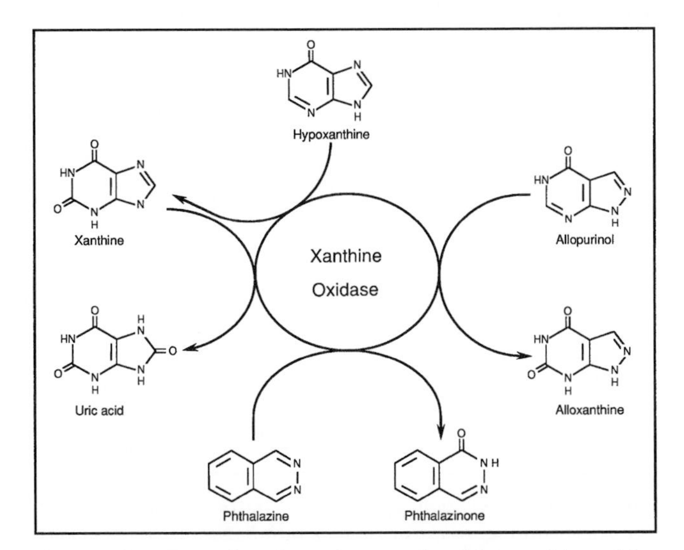


***Figure 6–18. Examples of reactions catalyzed by xanthine oxidase.***

Note that the conversion of hypoxanthine and xanthine to uric acid is a normal part of purine catabolism.

**Monoamine Oxidase, Diamine Oxidase and Polyamine Oxidase.** Monoamine oxidase (MAO), diamine oxidase (DAO), and polyamine oxidase (PAO) are all involved in the oxidative deamination of primary, secondary, and tertiary amines (Weyler et al., 1992; Benedetti and Dostert, 1994). Substrates for these enzymes include several naturally occurring amines, such as the monoamine, serotonin (5-hydroxytryptamine), the diamine, putrescine, and monoacetylated derivatives of the polyamines, spermine and spermidine. A number of xenobiotics are substrates for these enzymes, particularly MAO. Oxidative deamination of primary amines produces ammonia and an aldehyde, whereas oxidative deamination of secondary amines produces a primary amine and an aldehyde. The aldehydes are usually oxidized further by other enzymes to the corresponding carboxylic acids, although in some cases they are reduced to alcohols. Examples of reactions catalyzed by MAO, DAO, and PAO are shown in Fig. 6-19.

Monoamine oxidase is a mitochondrial flavoprotein present in the liver, kidney, intestine, blood platelets, and neuronal tissue. Its substrates include primaquine, haloperidol, milacemide, a dealkylated metabolite of propranolol, $\beta$-phenylethylamine, tyramine, catecholamines (dopamine, norepinephrine, epinephrine), and tryptophan derivatives (tryptamine, serotonin). At least two forms of monoamine oxidase, called MAO-A and MAO-B, are present in liver and other tissues. MAO-A preferentially oxidizes serotonin (5-hydroxytryptamine) and the dealkylated metabolite of propranolol and is preferentially inhibited by clorgyline, whereas MAO-B preferentially oxidizes $\beta$-phenylethylamine and is preferentially inhibited by *l*-deprenyl. Most tissues contain both forms of the enzyme, each encoded by a distinct gene, although some tissues express only one MAO. In humans, for example, only MAO-A is expressed in the placenta, whereas only MAO-B is expressed in blood platelets and lymphocytes.

The mechanism of catalysis by monoamine oxidase is illustrated below:

$$\begin{aligned} RCH_2NH_2 + FAD &\rightarrow RCH = NH + FADH_2 \\ RCH = NH + H_2O &\rightarrow RCHO + NH_3 \\ FADH_2 + O_2 &\rightarrow FAD + H_2O_2 \end{aligned}$$

The substrate is oxidized by the enzyme, which itself is reduced ($FAD \rightarrow FADH_2$). The oxygen incorporated into the substrate is derived from water, not molecular oxygen. The catalytic cycle is completed by reoxidation of the reduced enzyme ($FADH_2 \rightarrow FAD$) by oxygen, which generates hydrogen peroxide. The initial step appears to be abstraction of hydrogen from the $\alpha$-carbon adjacent to the nitrogen atom, hence, the oxidative deamination of xenobiotics by MAO is generally blocked by substitution of the $\alpha$-carbon. For example, amphetamine and other phenylethylamine derivatives carrying a methyl group on the $\alpha$-carbon atom are not oxidized well by MAO. (Amphetamines can undergo oxidative deamination, but the reaction is catalyzed by cytochrome P450). The abstraction of hydrogen from the $\alpha$-carbon adjacent to the nitrogen atom can occur stereospecifically; therefore, one enantiomer of an $\alpha$-substituted compound may be the substrate for MAO. For example, whereas MAO-B catalyzes the oxidative deamination of both *R*- and *S*-$\beta$-phenylethylamine, only the *R*-enantiomer is a substrate for MAO-A. The oxidative deamination of the dealkylated metabolite of propranolol is cata-

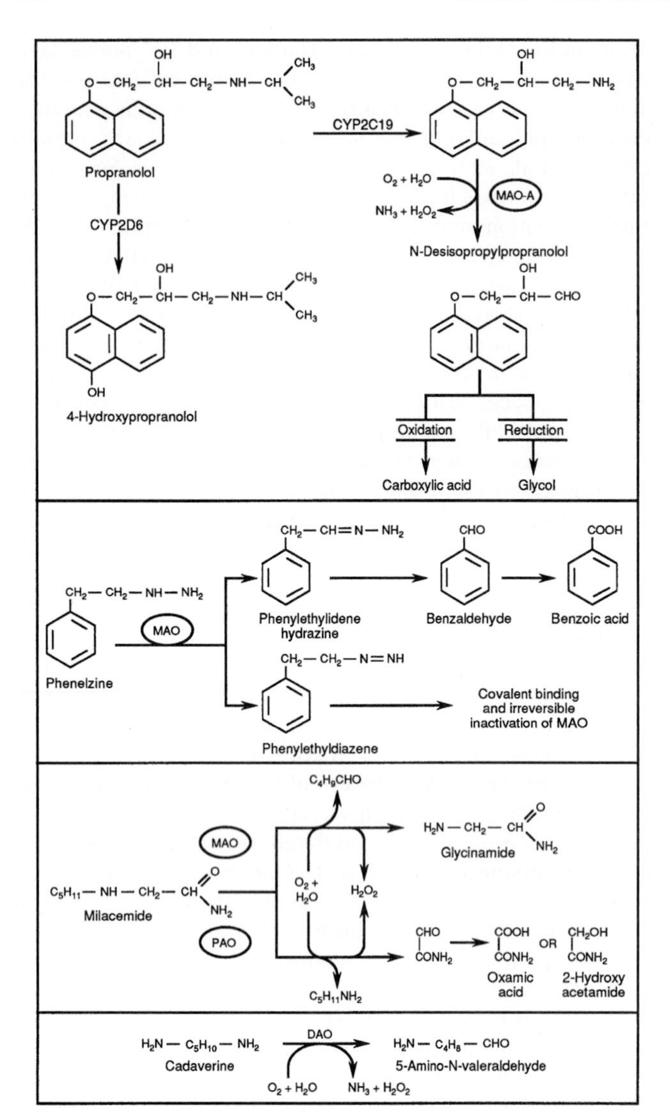


***Figure 6–19. Examples of reactions catalyzed by monoamine oxidase (MAO), diamine oxidase (DAO), and polyamine oxidase (PAO).***

Note that pheneizine is a mechanism-based inhibitor of MAO-A and MAO-B.

lyzed stereoselectively by MAO-A, although in this case the preferred substrate is the *S*-enantiomer (which has the same absolute configuration as the *R*-enantiomer of $\beta$-phenylethylamine) (Benedetti and Dostert, 1994).

Clorgyline and *l*-deprenyl are mechanism-based inhibitors (suicide inactivators) of MAO-A and MAO-B, respectively. Both enzymes are irreversibly inhibited by phenelzine, a hydrazine that can be oxidized either by abstraction of hydrogen from the $\alpha$-carbon atom, which leads to oxidative deamination with formation of benzaldehyde and benzoic acid, or by abstraction of hydrogen from the nitrogen atom, which leads to formation of phenylethyldiazene and covalent modification of the enzyme, as shown in Fig. 6-19.

Monoamine oxidase has received considerable attention for its role in the activation of MPTP (1-methyl-4-phenyl-1,2,5,6-tetrahydropyridine) to a neurotoxic metabolite that causes symptoms characteristic of Parkinson's disease in humans and monkeys but not rodents (Gerlach et al., 1991). In 1983, Parkinsonism was observed in young individuals who, in attempting to synthesize and use a narcotic drug related to meperidine (demerol), instead synthesized and self-administered MPTP, which causes selective destruction of dopaminergic neurones in the substantia nigra. MPTP crosses the blood–brain barrier, where is it oxidized by MAO in the astrocytes (a type of glial cell) to 1-methyl-4-phenyl-2,3-dihydropyridine ($MPDP^+$), which in turn autooxidizes to the neurotoxic metabolite, 1-methyl-4-phenylpyridine $MPP^+$, as shown in Fig. 6-20. Because it is transported by the dopamine transporter, $MPP^+$ concentrates in dopaminergic neurones, where it impairs mitochondrial respiration. The neurotoxic effects of MPTP can be blocked with pargyline (an inhibitor of both MAO-A and MAO-B), by *l*-deprenyl (a selective inhibitor of MAO-B) but not by clorgyline (a selective inhibitor of MAO-A). This suggests that the activation of MPTP to its neurotoxic metabolite is catalyzed predominantly by MAO-B. Species differences in the neurotoxic effects of MPTP are due in part to the low levels of MAO-B in rodents compared with the high levels in humans and primates. These studies with MPTP are significant because they have provided an animal model to study Parkinson's disease, and they suggest Parkinson's disease may be caused by xenobiotics. It is interesting that the bipyridyl herbicide, paraquat, is similar in structure to the toxic metabolite of MPTP, as shown in Fig. 6-20. Some epidemiological studies have shown a positive correlation between herbicide exposure and the incidence of Parkinsonism in some but not all rural communities. Haloperidol can also be converted to a potentially neurotoxic pyridinium metabolite (Subramanyam et al., 1991).

Although not present in mitochondria, PAO resembles MAO in its cofactor requirement and basic mechanism of action. Both enzymes use oxygen as an electron acceptor, which results in the production of hydrogen peroxide. The MAO inhibitor, pargyline, also inhibits PAO. The anticonvulsant, milacemide, is one of the few xenobiotic substrates for PAO, although it is also a substrate for MAO (Fig. 6-19). By converting milacemide to glycine (via glycinamide), MAO

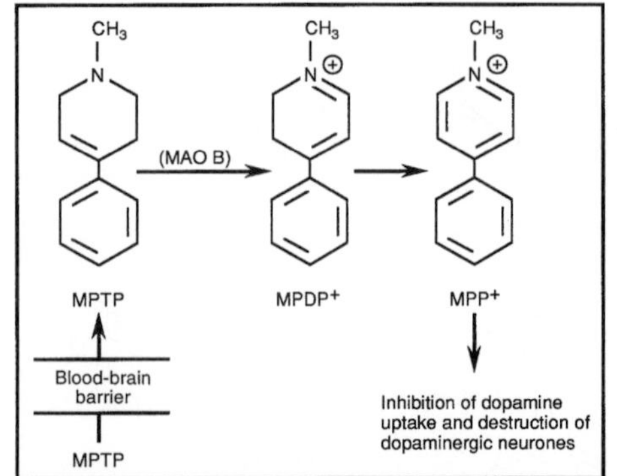


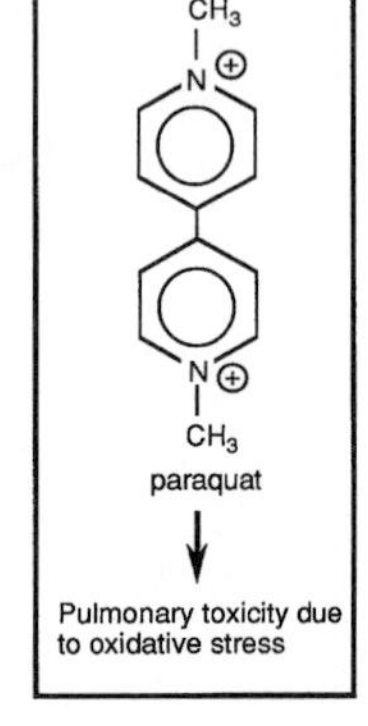


***Figure 6–20. Activation of MPTP (1-methyl-4-phenyl-1,2,5,6,-tetrahydropyridine) to the neurotoxic metabolite, $MPP^+$ (1-methyl-4-phenylpyridine), by monoamine oxidase B.***

The toxic pyridinium metabolite, $MPP^+$, is structurally similar to the herbicide paraquat. $MPDP^+$, 1-methyl-4-phenyl-2,3-dihydropyridine.

plays an important role the anticonvulsant therapy with milacemide (Benedetti and Dostert, 1994).

Diamine oxidase is a cytosolic, copper-containing, pyridoxal phosphate-dependent enzyme present in liver, kidney, intestine, and placenta. Its preferred substrates include histamine and simple alkyl diamines with a chain length of 4 (putrescine) or 5 (cadaverine) carbon atoms. Diamines with carbon chains longer than 9 are not substrates for DAO, although they can be oxidized by MAO. DAO or a similar enzyme is present in cardiovascular tissue and appears to be responsible for the cardiotoxic effects of allylamine, which is converted by oxidative deamination to acrolein.

**Aromatization.** The conversion of MPTP to $MPP^+$ (Fig. 6-20) is an example of a xenobiotic whose oxidation involves the introduction of multiple double bonds to achieve some semblance of aromaticity (in this case, formation of a pyridinium ion). Aromatization of xenobiotics is an unusual reaction, but some examples have been documented. A mitochondrial enzyme in guinea pig and rabbit liver can oxidize several cyclohexane derivatives to the corresponding aromatic hydrocarbon, as shown in Fig. 6-21 for the aromatization of cyclohexane carboxylic acid (hexahydrobenzoic acid) to benzoic acid. Mitochondria from rat liver are less active, and those from cat, mouse, dog, monkey, and human are completely inactive. The reaction requires magnesium, coenzyme A, oxygen, and ATP. The first step appears to be the formation of hexahydrobenzoyl-CoA, which is then dehydrogenated to the aromatic product. Glycine stimulates the reaction, probably by removing benzoic acid through conjugation to form hippuric acid (a phase II reaction). The conversion of androgens to estrogens involves aromatization of the A-ring of the steroid nucleus. This reaction is catalyzed by CYP19, one of the cytochrome P450 enzymes involved in steroidogenesis.

**Peroxidase-Dependent Cooxidation.** The oxidative biotransformation of xenobiotics generally requires the reduced pyridine nucleotide cofactors, NADPH and NADH. An exception is xenobiotic biotransformation by peroxidases, which couple the reduction of hydrogen peroxide and lipid hydroperoxides to the oxidation of other substrates, a process known as *cooxidation* (Eling et al., 1990). Several different peroxidases catalyze the biotransformation of xenobiotics, and these enzymes occur in a variety of tissues and cell types. For example, kidney medulla, platelets, vascular endothelial cells, the gastrointestinal tract, brain, lung, and urinary bladder epithelium contain prostaglandin H synthase (PHS); mammary gland epithelium contains lactoperoxidase, and leukocytes contain myeloperoxidase. PHS is the most extensively studied peroxidase involved in the xenobiotic biotransformation. This enzyme possesses two catalytic activities: a *cyclooxygenase* that converts arachidonic acid to the cyclic endoperoxide-hydroperoxide $PGG_2$ (which involves the addition of two molecules of oxygen to each molecule of arachidonic acid), and a *peroxidase* that converts the hydroperoxide to the corresponding alcohol $PGH_2$ (which can be accompanied by the oxidation of xenobiotics). The conversion of arachidonic acid to $PGH_2$, which is subsequently converted to a variety of eicosanoids (prostaglandins, thromboxane, and prostacyclin), is shown in Fig. 6-22. PHS and other peroxidases play an important role in the activation of xenobiotics to toxic or tumorigenic metabolites, particularly in extrahepatic tissues that contain low levels of cytochrome P450 (Eling et al., 1990).

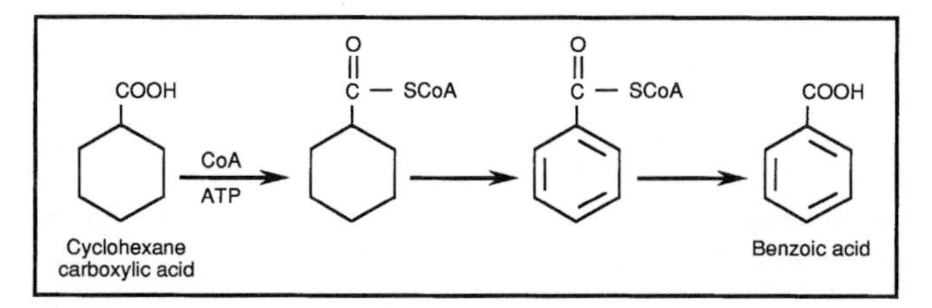


*Figure 6–21. Aromatization of cyclohexane carboxylic acid, a reaction catalyzed by rabbit and guinea pig liver mitochondria.*

In certain cases, the oxidation of xenobiotics by peroxidases involves direct transfer of the peroxide oxygen to the xenobiotic, as shown in Fig. 6-22 for the conversion of substrate X to product XO. An example of this type of reaction is the PHS-catalyzed epoxidation of benzo[a]pyrene 7,8-dihydrodiol to the corresponding 9,10-epoxide (see Fig. 6-5). Although PHS can catalyze the final step (i.e., 9,10-epoxidation) in the formation of this tumorigenic metabolite of benzo[a]pyrene, it cannot catalyze the initial step (i.e., 7,8-epoxidation), which is catalyzed by cytochrome P450. The 9,10-epoxidation of benzo[a]pyrene 7,8-dihydrodiol can also be catalyzed by 15-lipoxygenase, which is present at high concentrations in human pulmonary epithelial cells, and by peroxyl radicals formed during lipid peroxidation in skin. Cytochrome P450 and peroxyl radicals formed by PHS, lipoxygenase, and/or lipid peroxidation may all play a role in activating benzo[a]pyrene to metabolites that cause lung and skin tumors. These same enzymes can also catalyze the 8,9-epoxidation of aflatoxin $B_1$, which is one of the most potent hepatotumorigens known. Epoxidation by cytochrome P450 is thought to be primarily responsible for the hepatotumorigenic effects of aflatoxin $B_1$. However, aflatoxin $B_1$ also causes neoplasia of rat renal papilla. This tissue has very low levels of cytochrome P450, but contains relatively high levels of PHS, which is suspected, therefore, of mediating the nephrotumorigenic effects of aflatoxin (Fig. 6-23).

The direct transfer of the peroxide oxygen from a hydroperoxide to a xenobiotic is not the only mechanism of xenobiotic oxidation by peroxidases, nor is it the most common. As shown in Fig. 6-22, xenobiotics that can serve as electron donors, such as amines and phenols, can be oxidized to free radicals during the reduction of a hydroperoxide. In this case, the hydroperoxide is still converted to the corresponding alcohol, but the peroxide oxygen is reduced to water instead of being incorporated into the xenobiotic. For each molecule of hydroperoxide reduced (which is a two-electron process), two molecules of xenobiotic can be oxidized (each by a one-electron process). Important classes of compounds that undergo one-electron oxidations by peroxidase include aromatic amines, phenols, hydroquinones and polycyclic hydrocarbons. Many of the metabolites produced are reactive electrophiles. For example, polycyclic aromatic hydrocarbons, phenols, and hydroquinones are oxidized to electrophilic quinones. Acetaminophen is similarly converted to a quinoneimine, namely *N*-acetyl-benzoquinoneimine, a cytotoxic electrophile that binds to cellular proteins, as shown in Fig. 6-24. The formation of this toxic metabolite by cytochrome P450 causes

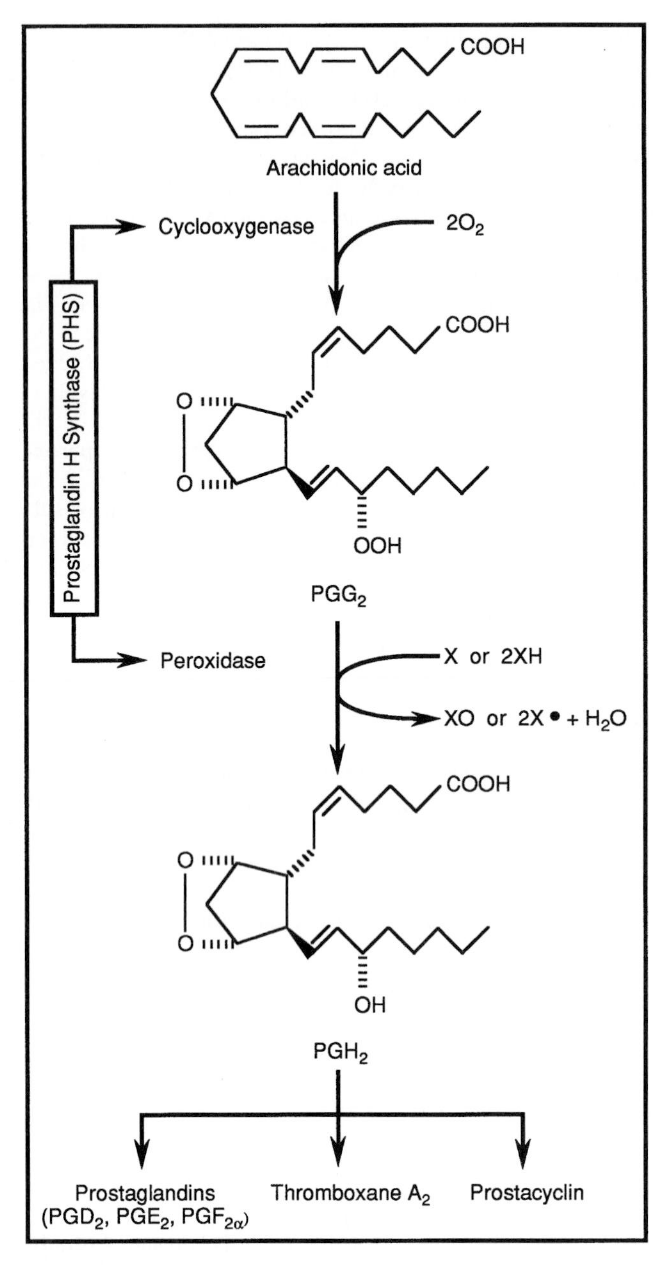


*Figure 6–22. Cooxidation of xenobiotics (X) during the conversion of arachidonic acid to $PGH_2$ by prostaglandin H synthase.*

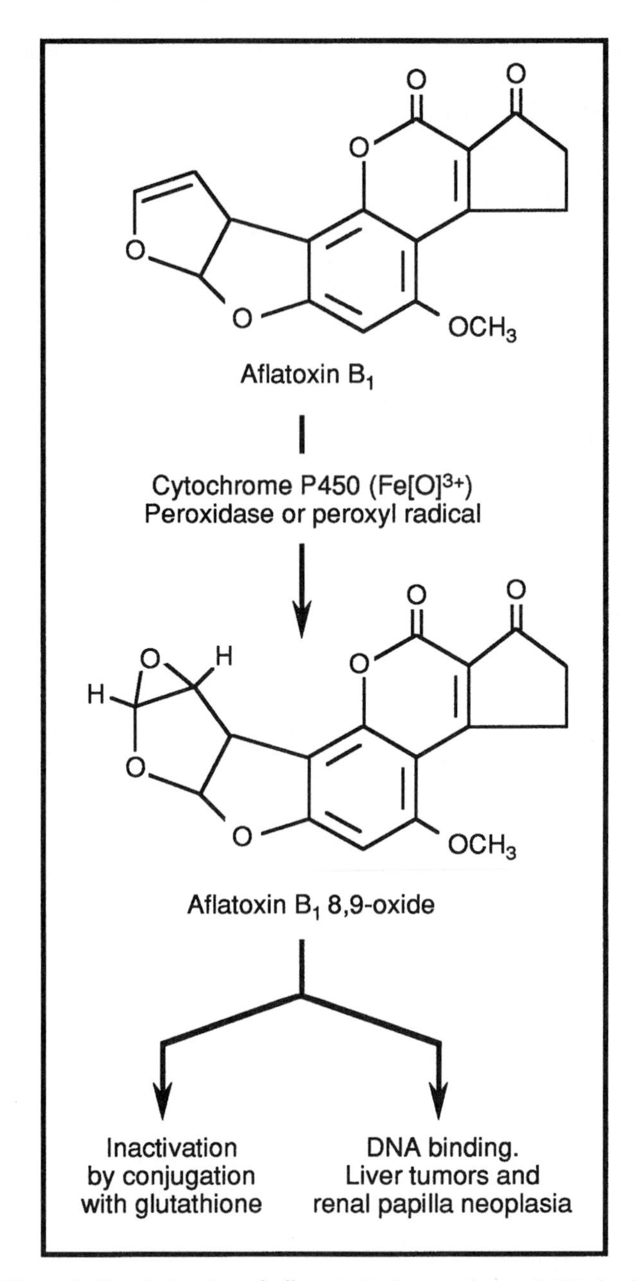


*Figure 6–23. Activation of aflatoxin $B_1$ by cytochrome P450, leading to liver tumor formation, and peroxidases, leading to renal papilla neoplasia.*

centrilobular necrosis of the liver. However, acetaminophen can also damage the kidney medulla, which contains low levels of cytochrome P450 but relatively high levels of PHS; hence, PHS may play a significant role in the nephrotoxicity of acetaminophen. The two-electron oxidation of acetaminophen to *N*-acetyl-benzoquinoneimine by PHS likely involves the formation of a one-electron oxidation product, namely *N*-acetyl-benzosemiquinoneimine radical. Formation of this semiquinoneimine radical by PHS likely contributes to the nephrotoxicity of acetaminophen and related compounds, such as phenacetin and *p*-aminophenol.

Like the kidney medulla, urinary bladder epithelium also contains low levels of cytochrome P450 but relatively high levels of PHS. Just as PHS in kidney medulla can activate aflatoxin and acetaminophen to nephrotoxic metabolites, so PHS in urinary bladder epithelium can activate certain aromatic amines, such as benzidine, 4-aminobiphenyl, and 2-aminonaphthalene, to DNA-reactive metabolites that cause bladder cancer in certain species, including humans and dogs. As illustrated in Fig. 6-25, PHS can convert aromatic amines to reactive radicals, which can undergo nitrogen-nitrogen or nitrogen-carbon coupling reactions, or they can undergo a second one-electron oxidation to reactive diimines. Binding of these reactive metabolites to DNA is presumed to be the underlying mechanism by which several aromatic amines cause bladder cancer in humans and dogs. In some cases the one-electron oxidation of an amine leads to *N*-dealkylation. For example, PHS catalyzes the *N*-demethylation of ami-

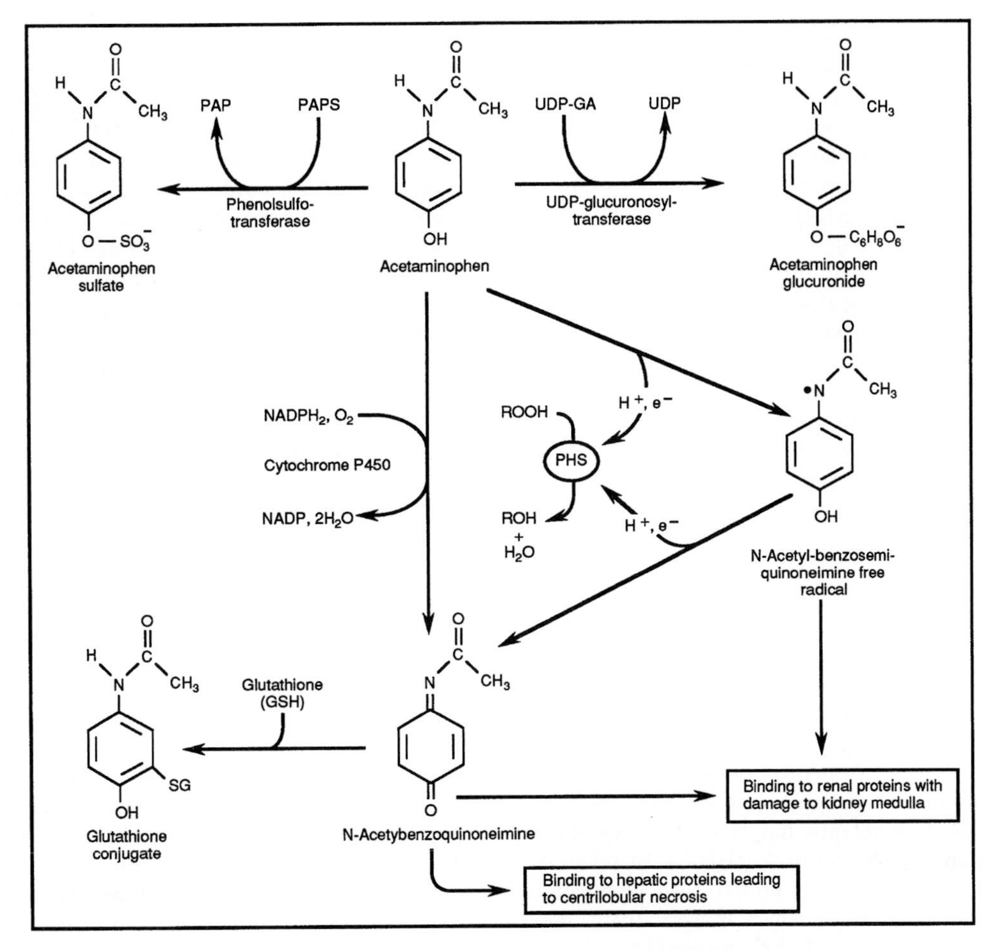


***Figure 6–24. Activation of acetaminophen by cytochrome P450, leading to hepatotoxicity, and prostaglandin H synthase (PHS), leading to nephrotoxicity.***

Conjugation with sulfate, glucuronic acid, or glutathione represent detoxication reactions.

nopyrine, although in vivo this reaction is mainly catalyzed by cytochrome P450. In contrast to cytochrome P450, PHS does not catalyze the *N*-hydroxylation of aromatic amines.

Many of the aromatic amines known or suspected of causing bladder cancer in humans have been shown to cause bladder tumors in dogs. In rats, however, aromatic amines cause liver tumors by a process that involves *N*-hydroxylation by cytochrome P450, followed by conjugation with acetate or sulfate, as shown in Fig. 6-7. This species difference has complicated an assessment of the role of PHS in aromatic amine-induced bladder cancer, because such experiments must be carried out in dogs. However, another class of compounds, the 5-nitrofurans, such as *N*-[4-(5-nitro-2-furyl)-2-thiazole]formamide (FANFT) and its deformylated analog 2-amino-4-(5-nitro-2-furyl)thiazole (ANFT), are substrates for PHS and are potent bladder tumorigens in rats. The tumorigenicity of FANFT is thought to involve deformylation to ANFT, which is oxidized to DNA-reactive metabolites by PHS. The ability of FANFT to cause bladder tumors in rats is blocked by the PHS cyclooxygenase inhibitor, aspirin, which suggests that PHS plays an important role in the metabolic activation and tumorigenicity of this nitrofuran. Unexpectedly, combined treatment of rats with FANFT and aspirin causes forestomach tumors, which are not observed when either compound is administered alone. This example underscores the complexity of chemically induced tumor formation.

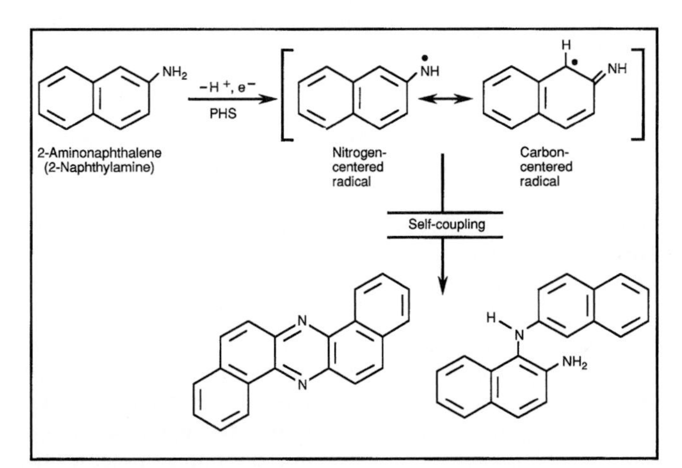


***Figure 6–25. Products of the one-electron oxidation of 2-aminoaphthalene by the peroxidase, prostaglandin H synthase (PHS).***

Many phenolic compounds can serve as reducing substrates for PHS peroxidase. The phenoxyl radicals produced by one-electron oxidation reactions can undergo a variety of reactions, including binding to critical nucleophiles, such as protein and DNA, reduction by antioxidants such as glutathione, and self-coupling. The reactions of phenoxyl radicals are analogous to those of the nitrogen-centered free radicals produced during the one-electron oxidation of aromatic amines by PHS (see Fig. 6-25). Peroxidases appear to play an important role in the bone marrow suppression produced by chronic exposure to benzene. Liver cytochrome P450 converts benzene to phenol, which in turn is oxidized to hydroquinone, which can be converted to DNA-reactive metabolites by PHS in bone marrow and by myeloperoxidase in bone marrow leukocytes. The myelosuppressive effect of benzene can be blocked by the PHS inhibitor, indomethacin, which suggests an important role for peroxidase-dependent activation in the myelotoxicity of benzene. The formation of phenol and hydroquinone in the liver is also important for myelosuppression by benzene. However, such bone marrow suppression cannot be achieved simply by administering phenol or hydroquinone to mice, although it can be achieved by coadministering hydroquinone with phenol. Phenol stimulates the PHS-dependent activation of hydroquinone. Therefore, bone marrow suppression by benzene involves the cytochrome P450-dependent oxidation of benzene to phenol and hydroquinone in the liver, followed by phenol-enhanced peroxidative oxidation of hydroquinone to reactive intermediates that bind to protein and DNA in the bone marrow (Fig. 6-26).

The ability of phenol to enhance the peroxidative metabolism of hydroquinone is analogous to the interaction between the phenolic antioxidants, butylated hydroxytoluene (BHT), and butylated hydroxyanisole (BHA). In mice, the pulmonary toxicity of BHT, which is a relatively poor substrate for PHS, is enhanced by BHA, which is a relatively good substrate for PHS. The mechanism by which BHA enhances the pulmonary toxicity of BHT appears to involve the peroxidase-dependent conversion of BHA to a phenoxyl radical that interacts with BHT, converting it to a phenoxyl radical (by one-electron oxidation) or a quinone methide (by two-electron oxidation), as shown in Fig. 6-27. Formation of the toxic quinone methide of BHT can also be catalyzed by cytochrome P450, which is largely responsible for activating BHT in the absence of BHA.

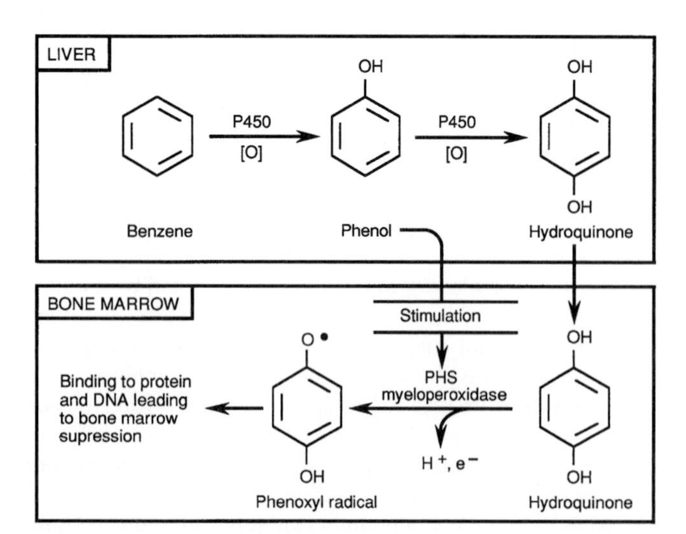


***Figure 6–26. Role of cytochrome P450 and peroxidases in the activation of benzene to myelotoxic metabolites.***

PHS, prostaglandin H synthase.

Several reducing substrates, such phenylbutazone, retinoic acid, 3-methylindole, sulfite, and bisulfite, are oxidized by PHS to carbon-or sulfur-centered free radicals that can trap oxygen to form a peroxyl radical, as shown in Fig. 6-28 for phenylbutazone. The peroxyl radical can oxidize xenobiotics in a peroxidative manner. For example, the peroxyl radical of phenylbutazone can convert benzo[a]pyrene 7,8-dihydrodiol to the corresponding 9,10-epoxide.

PHS is unique among peroxidases because it can both generate hydroperoxides and catalyze peroxidase-dependent reactions, as shown in Fig. 6-22. Xenobiotic biotransformation by PHS is controlled by the availability of arachidonic acid. The biotransformation of xenobiotics by other peroxidases is controlled by the availability of hydroperoxide substrates. Hydrogen peroxide is a normal product of cellular respiration, and lipid peroxides can form during lipid peroxidation. The levels of these peroxides and their availability for peroxidase reactions depends on the efficiency of hydroperoxide scavenging by glutathione peroxidase and catalase.

**Flavin-Containing Monooxygenases.** Liver, kidney, and lung contain one or more FAD-containing monooxygenases (FMO) that oxidize the nucleophilic nitrogen, sulfur and phosphorus heteroatom of a variety of xenobiotics (Ziegler, 1993; Lawton et al., 1994; Cashman, 1995). Like cytochrome P450, the FMOs are microsomal enzymes that require NADPH and $O_2$, and many of the reactions catalyzed by FMO also can be catalyzed by cytochrome P450. Several in vitro techniques have been developed to distinguish reactions catalyzed by FMO from those catalyzed by cytochrome P450. In contrast to cytochrome P450, FMO is heat labile and can be inactivated in the absence of NADPH by warming microsomes to 50°C for 1 min. By comparison, cytochrome P450 can be inactivated with nonionic detergent, such as 1% Emulgen 911, which has a minimal effect on FMO activity. Antibodies raised against purified P450 enzymes can be used not only to establish the role of cytochrome P450 in a microsomal reaction but also to identify which particular P450 enzyme catalyzes the reaction. In contrast, antibodies raised against purified FMO do not inhibit the enzyme. The use of chemical inhibitors to ascertain the relative contribution of FMO and cytochrome P450 to microsomal reactions is often complicated by a lack of specificity. For example, cimetidine and SKF 525A, which are well-recognized cytochrome P450 inhibitors, are both substrates for FMO. The situation is further complicated by the observation that the various forms of FMO differ in their thermal stability and sensitivity to detergents and other chemical modulators.

FMO catalyzes the oxidation of nucleophilic tertiary amines to *N*-oxides, secondary amines to hydroxylamines and nitrones, and primary amines to hydroxylamines and oximes. FMO also oxidizes several sulfur-containing xenobiotics (such as thiols, thioethers, thiones, and thiocarbamates) and phosphines to *S*- and *P*-oxides, respectively. Hydrazines, iodides, selenides, and boron-containing compounds and selenides are also substrates for FMO. Examples of these reactions are shown in Fig. 6-29a and b. In general, the metabolites produced by FMO are the products of a chemical reaction between a xenobiotic and a peracid or peroxide. In general, the reactions catalyzed by FMO are detoxication reactions, al-

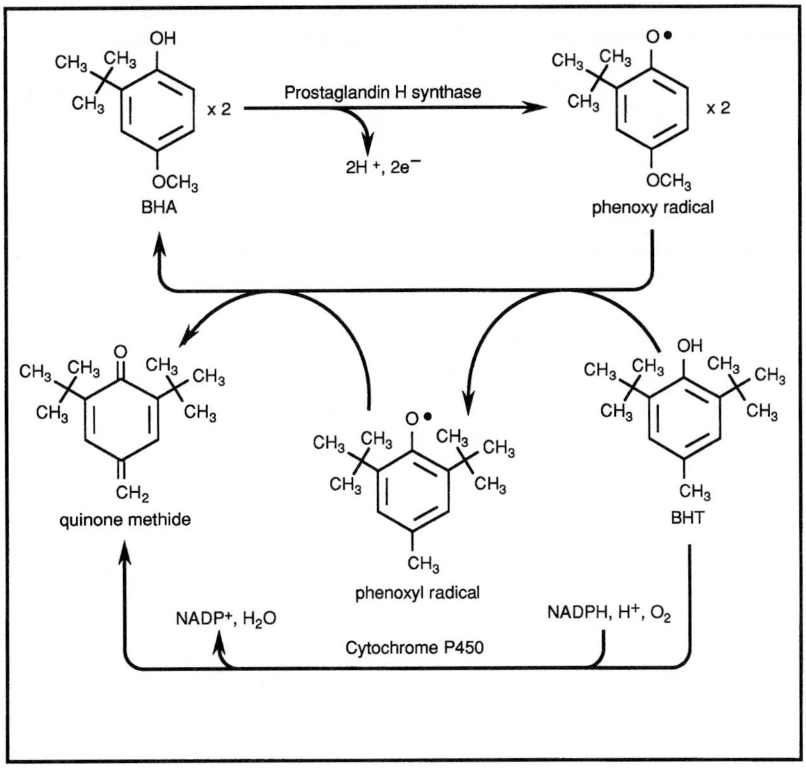

***Figure 6–27. Metabolic interaction between the phenolic antioxidants, butylated hydroxytoluene (BHT) and butylated hydroxyanisole (BHA).***

Note that activation of BHT to a toxic quinone methide can be catalyzed by cytochrome P450 or, in the presence of BHA, by prostaglandin H synthase.

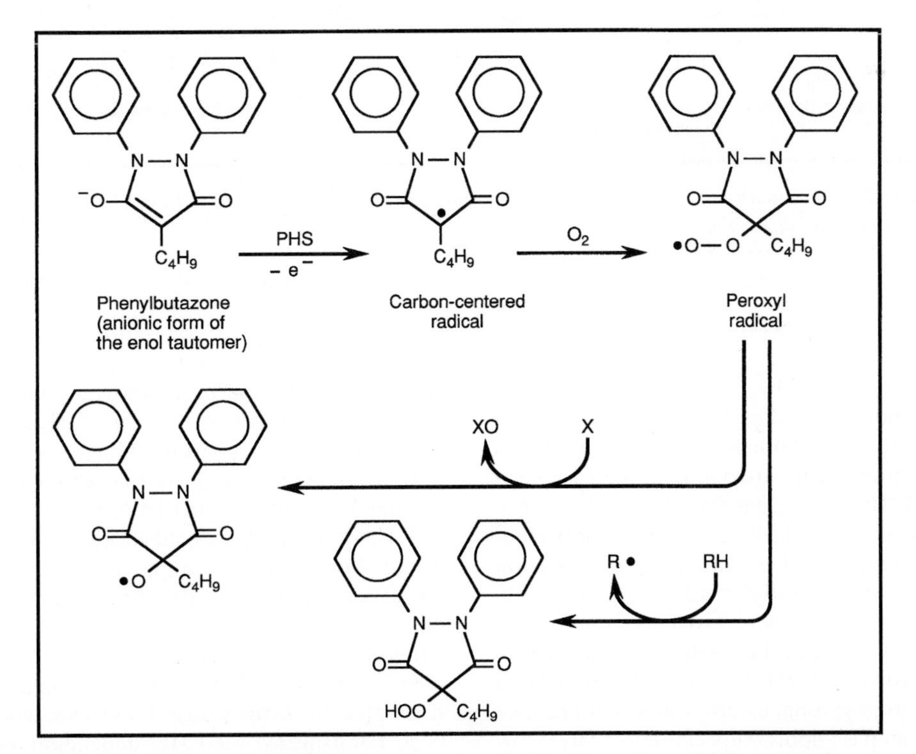


***Figure 6–28. Oxidation of phenylbutazone by prostaglandin H synthase (PHS) to a carbon-centered radical and peroxyl radical.***

Note that the peroxyl radical can oxidize xenobiotics (X) in a peroxidative manner.

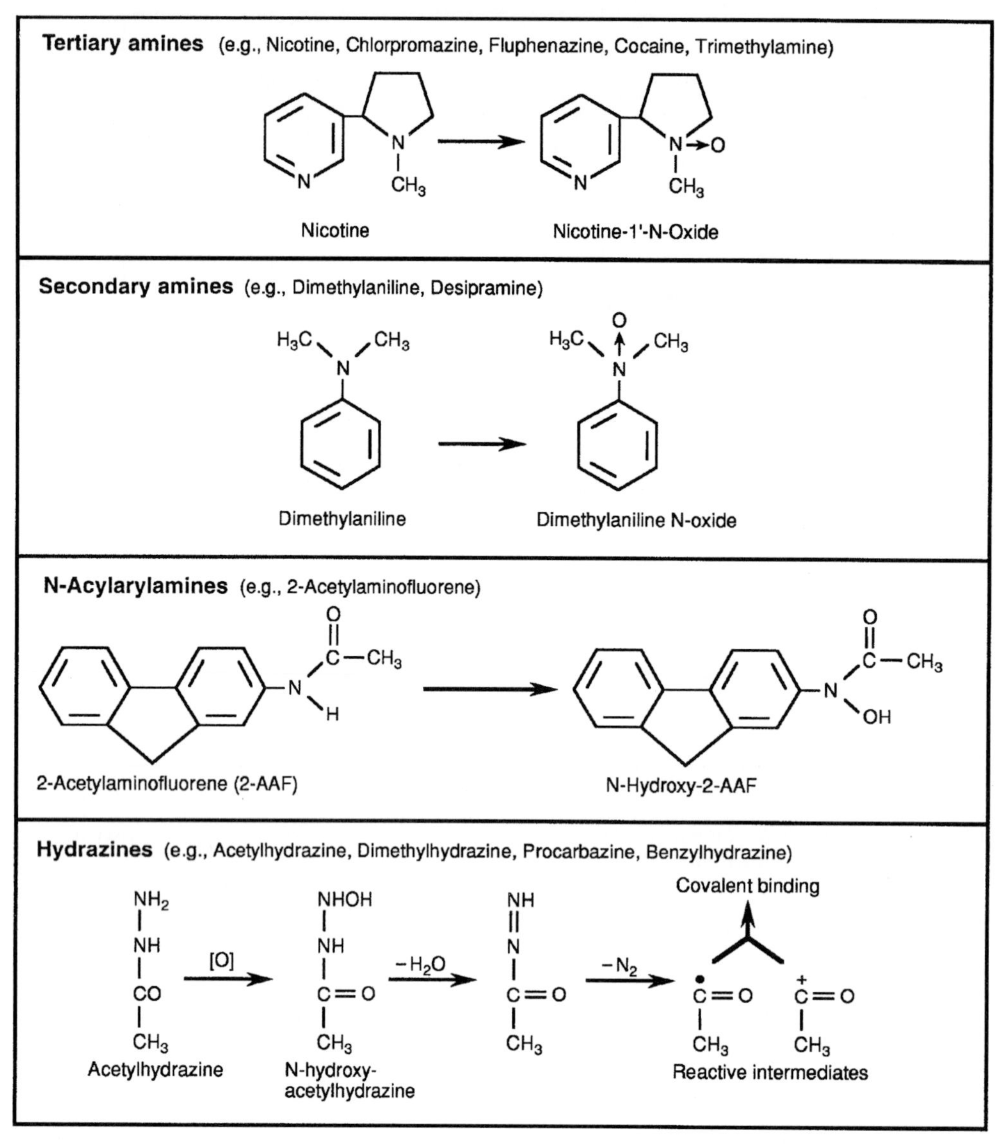


*Figure 6–29A. Examples of reactions catalyzed by flavin-containing monooxygenases (FMO): Nitrogen-containing xenobiotics.*

though there are exceptions to this rule, which are described below (this section).

The mechanism of catalysis by FMO is depicted in Fig. 6-30. After the FAD moiety is reduced by NADPH, the oxidized cofactor, $NADP^+$, remains bound to the enzyme, which then binds oxygen to produce a peroxide (i.e., the 4a-hydroperoxyflavin of FAD). The peroxide is relatively stable, probably because the active site of FMO comprises nonnucleophilic, lipophilic amino acid residues. During the oxygenation of xenobiotics, the 4a-hydroperoxyflavin is converted to 4a-hydroxyflavin with transfer of the flavin peroxide oxygen to the substrate (depicted as X → XO in Fig. 6-30). The final step in the catalytic cycle involves dehydration of 4a-hydroxyflavin (which restores FAD to its resting, oxidized state) and release of $NADP^+$. This final step is important because it is rate limiting, and it occurs after substrate oxygenation. Consequently, this step determines the upper limit of the rate of substrate oxidation. Therefore all good substrates for FMO are converted to products at the same maximum rate (i.e., $V_{max}$ is determined by the final step in the catalytic cycle). Binding of $NADP^+$ to FMO during catalysis is important because it prevents the reduction of oxygen to $H_2O_2$. In the absence of bound $NADP^+$, FMO would function as an NADPH-oxidase that would consume NADPH and cause oxidative stress through excessive production of $H_2O_2$.

The oxygenation of substrates by FMO does not lead to inactivation of the enzyme, even though some of the products are strong electrophiles capable of binding covalently to critical and noncritical nucleophiles such as protein and glutathione, respectively. The products of the oxygenation reactions catalyzed by FMO and/or the oxygenation of the same substrates by cytochrome P450 can inactivate cytochrome P450. For example, the FMO-dependent *S*-oxygenation of spironolactone thiol (which is formed by the deacetylation of spironolactone by carboxylesterases, as shown in Fig. 6-1) leads to the formation of an electrophilic sulfenic acid (R-SH

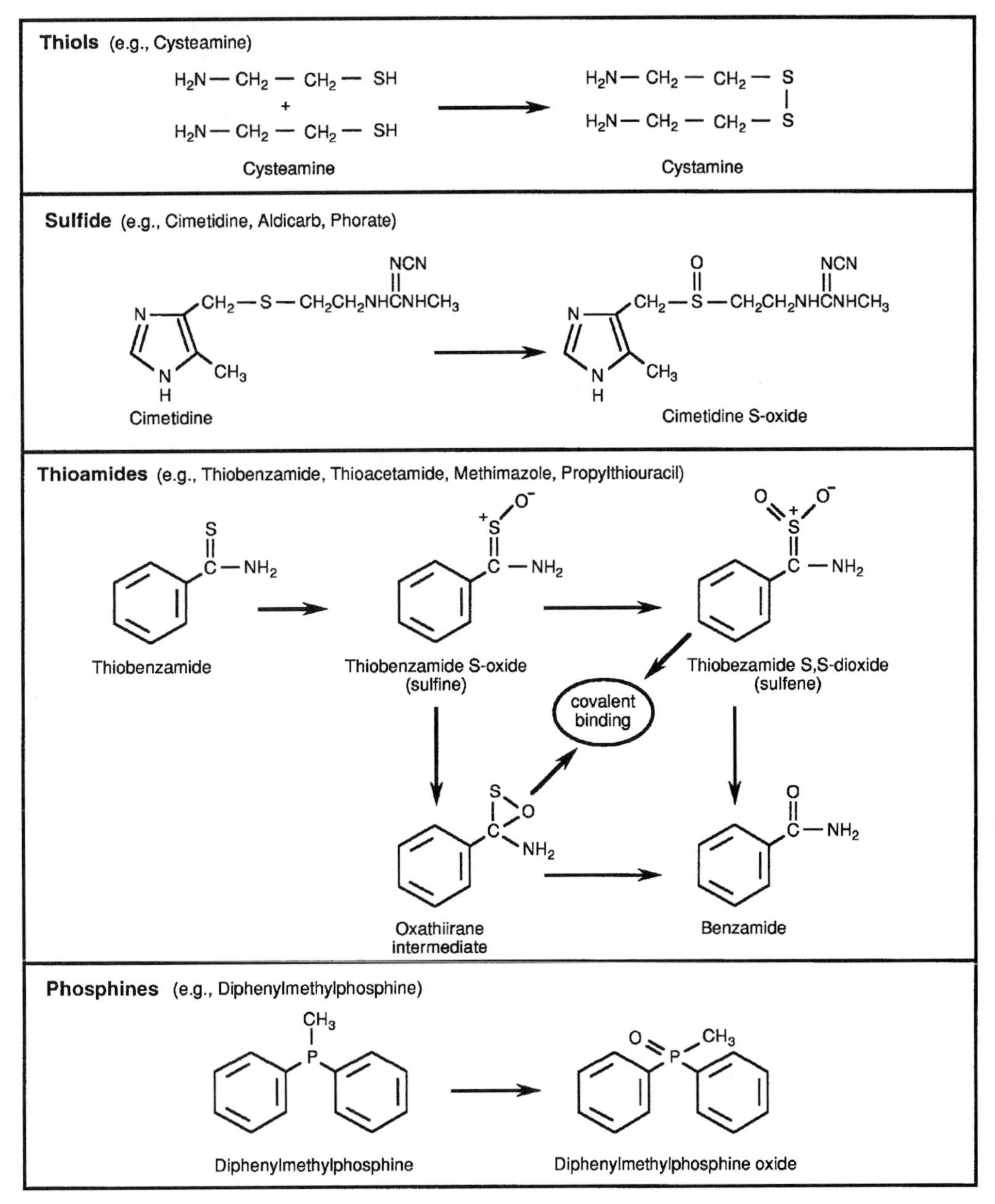


*Figure 6–29B. Examples of reactions catalyzed by flavin-containing monooxygenases (FMO): Sulfur- and phosphorus-containing xenobiotics.*

→ R-SOH) that inactivates cytochrome P450 and binds covalently to other proteins.

FMO plays an important role in the biotransformation of several drugs and xenobiotics in humans. The major flavin-containing monooxygenase in human liver microsomes, FMO3, is predominantly if not solely responsible for converting (*S*)-nicotine to (*S*)-nicotine *N*-1′-oxide (which is one of the reactions shown in Fig. 6-29A). The reaction proceeds stereospecifically; only the *trans* isomer is produced by FMO3, and this is the only isomer of (*S*)-nicotine *N*-1′-oxide excreted in the urine of cigarette smokers or individuals wearing a nicotine patch. Therefore, the urinary excretion of *trans*-(*S*)-nicotine *N*-1′-oxide can be used as an in vivo probe of FMO3 activity in humans. FMO3 is also the principal enzyme involved in the *S*-oxygenation of cimetidine, an $H_2$-antagonist widely used in the treatment of gastric ulcers and other acid-related disorders (this reaction is shown in Fig. 6-29B). Cimetidine is stereoselectively sulfoxidated by FMO3 to an 84:16 mixture of (+) and (−) enantiomers, which closely matches the 75:25 enantiomeric composition of cimetidine *S*-oxide in human urine. Therefore, the urinary excretion of cimetidine *S*-oxide, like that of (*S*)-nicotine *N*-1′-oxide, is an in vivo indicator of FMO3 activity in humans. It should be noted, however, that in some species (such as pig, rat, and rabbit) FMO1 is the major flavin-containing monooxygenase expressed in the liver and that FMO1 converts (*S*)-nicotine and cimetidine to 1:1 mixtures of *cis*- and *trans*-(*S*)-nicotine *N*-1′-oxide and (+) and (−) cimetidine *S*-oxide, respectively. There-

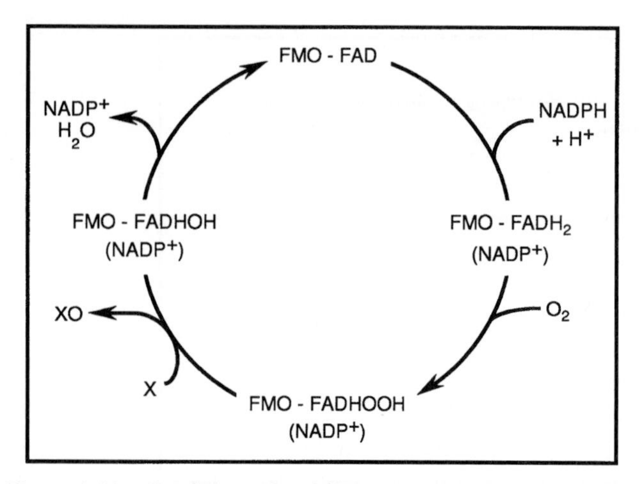


***Figure 6–30.** Catalytic cycle of flavin-containing monooxygenase (FMO).*

X and XO are the xenobiotic substrate and oxygenated product, respectively. The 4a-hydroperoxyflavin and 4a-hydroxyflavin of FAD are depicted as FADHOOH and FADHOH, respectively.

fore, statements concerning the role of FMO in the disposition of xenobiotics in humans may not apply to other species, or vice versa.

Several sulfur-containing xenobiotics are oxygenated by FMO to electrophilic reactive intermediates. Such xenobiotics include various thiols, thioamides, 2-mercaptoimidazoles, thiocarbamates, and thiocarbamides. The electrophilic metabolites of these xenobiotics do not inactivate FMO, but they can covalently modify and inactivate neighboring proteins, including cytochrome P450. Some of these same xenobiotics are substrates for cytochrome P450, and their oxygenation to electrophilic metabolites leads to inactivation of cytochrome P450, a process known as mechanism-based inhibition (suicide inactivation). 2-Mercaptoimidazoles undergo sequential *S*-oxygenation reactions by FMO, first to sulfenic acids and then to sulfinic acids (R-SH $\rightarrow$ R-SOH $\rightarrow$ R-$SO_2$H). These electrophilic metabolites, like the sulfenic acid metabolite produced from spironolactone thiol (see above), bind to critical nucleophiles (such as proteins) or interact with glutathione to form disulfides. The thiocarbamate functionality present in numerous agricultural chemicals is converted by FMO to *S*-oxides (sulfoxides), which can be further oxygenated to sulfones. These reactions involve *S*-oxygenation adjacent to a ketone, which produces strong electrophilic acylating agents, which may be responsible for the toxicity of many thiocarbamate herbicides and fungicides. The hepatotoxicity of thiobenzamide is dependent on *S*-oxidation by FMO and/or cytochrome P450. As shown in Fig. 6-29B, the *S*-oxidation of thiobenzamide can lead to the formation of an oxathiirane (a three-membered ring of carbon, sulfur, and oxygen) that can bind covalently to protein (which leads to hepatocellular necrosis) or rearrange to benzamide, a reaction known as *oxidative group transfer*.

Endogenous FMO substrates include cysteamine, which is oxidized to the disulfide, cystamine, and trimethylamine (TMA), which is converted to TMA *N*-oxide (Fig. 6-29B). By converting cysteamine to cystamine, FMO may serve to produce a low molecular weight disulfide-exchange agent, which may participate in the formation of disulfide bridges during peptide synthesis or the renaturation of proteins. By converting TMA to TMA *N*-oxide, FMO converts a malodorous and volatile dietary product of choline catabolism to an inoffensive metabolite. TMA smells of rotting fish, and people who lack FMO (presumably FMO3, the major FMO expressed in human liver microsomes) suffer from *fish-odor syndrome*, which is caused by the excretion of TMA in urine, sweat, and breath (Ayesh and Smith, 1992).

Humans and other mammals express five different flavin-containing monooxygenases (FMO1, FMO2, FMO3, FMO4, and FMO5) in a species- and tissue-specific manner, as shown in Table 6-2 (adapted from Cashman, 1995). For example, the

**Table 6–2**
**Putative Tissue Levels of FMO Forms Present in Animals and Humans**

| | FMO1 | FMO2 | FMO3 | FMO4 | FMO5 |
|---|---|---|---|---|---|
| Liver | | | | | |
| Mouse | Low | NP* | High | ? | Low |
| Rat | High | ?* | Low | ? | Low |
| Rabbit | High | NP | Low | ? | Low |
| Human | Very low | Low | High | Very low | Low |
| Kidney | | | | | |
| Mouse | High | ? | High | ? | Low |
| Rat | High | ? | High | High | Low |
| Rabbit | Low | Low | Very low | High | Low |
| Human | High | Low | ? | ? | ? |
| Lung | | | | | |
| Mouse | ? | High | Very low | NP | Low |
| Rat | ? | ? | ? | NP | Low |
| Rabbit | ? | Very high | ? | NP | NP |
| Human | ? | Low | ? | NP | ? |

*NP, apparently not present. A question mark indicates that no data are available or the presence of an FMO form is in doubt.
From Cashman (1995).

major FMO expressed in human and mouse liver microsomes is FMO3, whereas FMO1 is the major FMO expressed in rat, rabbit, and pig liver. In humans, high levels of FMO1 are expressed in the kidney, and low levels of FMO2 are expressed in the lung. However, lung microsomes from other species, particularly rabbit and mouse, contain high levels of FMO2.

The various forms of FMO are distinct gene products with different physical properties and substrate specificities. For example, FMO2 *N*-oxygenates *n*-octylamine, whereas such long aliphatic primary amines are not substrates for FMO1, although they stimulate its activity toward other substrates (in some cases causing a change in stereospecificity). Conversely, short-chain tertiary amines, such as chlorpromazine and imipramine, are substrates for FMO1 but not FMO2. Certain substrates are oxygenated stereospecifically by one FMO enzyme but not another. For example, FMO2 and FMO3 convert (*S*)-nicotine exclusively to *trans*-(*S*)-nicotine *N*-1′-oxide, whereas the *N*-oxides of (*S*)-nicotine produced by FMO1 are a 1:1 mixture of *cis* and *trans* isomers. FMO2 is heat stable under conditions that completely inactivate FMO1, and FMO2 is resistant to anionic detergents that inactivate FMO1. Low concentrations of bile salts, such as cholate, stimulate FMO activity in rat and mouse liver microsomes but inhibit FMO activity in rabbit and pig liver.

The FMO enzymes expressed in liver microsomes are not under the same regulatory control as cytochrome P450. In rats, the expression of FMO1 is repressed rather than induced by phenobarbital or 3-methylcholanthrene treatment. The levels of FMO3 in mouse liver microsomes are sexually differentiated (female > male) due to suppression of expression by testosterone. The opposite is true of FMO1 levels in rat liver microsomes, the expression of which is positively regulated by testosterone and negatively regulated by estradiol. In pregnant rabbits, lung FMO2 is positively regulated by progesterone and/or corticosteroids.

Species differences in the relative expression of FMO and cytochrome P450 appear to determine species differences in the toxicity of the pyrrolizidine alkaloids, senecionine, retrorsine and monocrotaline. These compounds are detoxified by FMO, which catalyzes the formation of tertiary amine *N*-oxides, but are activated by cytochrome P450, which oxidizes these alkaloids to pyrroles that generate toxic electrophiles through the loss of substituents on the pyrrolizidine nucleus. Rats have a high pyrrole-forming cytochrome P450 activity and a low *N*-oxide forming FMO activity, whereas the opposite is true of guinea pigs. This likely explains why pyrrolizidine alkaloids are highly toxic to rats but not to guinea pigs. Many of the reactions catalyzed by FMO are also catalyzed by cytochrome P450, but differences in the oxidation of pyrrolizidine alkaloids by FMO and cytochrome P450 illustrate that this is not always the case.

**Cytochrome P450.** Among the phase I biotransforming enzymes, the cytochrome P450 system ranks first in terms of catalytic versatility and the sheer number of xenobiotics it detoxifies or activates to reactive intermediates (Guengerich, 1987; Waterman and Johnson, 1991). The highest concentration of P450 enzymes involved in xenobiotic biotransformation are found in liver endoplasmic reticulum (microsomes), but P450 enzymes are present in virtually all tissues. The liver microsomal P450 enzymes play a very important role in determining the intensity and duration of action of drugs, and they also play a key role in the detoxication of xenobiotics. P450 enzymes in liver and extrahepatic tissues play important roles in the activation of xenobiotics to toxic and/or tumorigenic metabolites. Microsomal and mitochondrial P450 enzymes play key roles in the biosynthesis or catabolism of steroid hormones, bile acids, fat-soluble vitamins, fatty acids and eicosanoids, which underscores the catalytic versatility of cytochrome P450.

All P450 enzymes are heme-containing proteins. The heme iron in cytochrome P450 is usually in the ferric ($Fe^{3+}$) state. When reduced to the ferrous ($Fe^{2+}$) state, cytochrome P450 can bind ligands such as $O_2$ and carbon monoxide (CO). The complex between ferrous cytochrome P450 and CO absorbs light maximally at 450 nm, from which cytochrome P450 derives its name. The absorbance maximum of the CO complex differs slightly among different P450 enzymes and ranges from 447 nm to 452 nm. All other hemoproteins that bind CO absorb light maximally at ~420 nm. The unusual absorbance maximum of cytochrome P450 is due to an unusual fifth ligand to the heme (a cysteine-thiolate). The amino acid sequence around the cysteine residue that forms the thiolate bond with the heme moiety is highly conserved in all P450 enzymes. When this thiolate bond is disrupted, cytochrome P450 is converted to a catalytically inactive form called cytochrome P420. By competing with oxygen, CO inhibits cytochrome P450. The inhibitory effect of carbon monoxide can be reversed by irradiation with light at 450 nm, which photodissociates the cytochrome P450-CO complex. These properties of cytochrome P450 are of historical importance. The observation that treatment of rats with certain chemicals, such as 3-methylcholanthrene, causes a shift in the peak absorbance of cytochrome P450 (from 450 nm to 448 nm) provided some of the earliest evidence for the existence of multiple forms of cytochrome P450 in liver microsomes. The conversion of cytochrome P450 to cytochrome P420 by detergents and phospholipases helped to establish the hemoprotein nature of cytochrome P450. The inhibition of cytochrome P450 by CO and the reversal of this inhibition by photo-dissociation of the cytochrome P450-CO complex established cytochrome P450 as the microsomal and mitochondrial enzyme involved in drug biotransformation and steroid biosynthesis.

The basic reaction catalyzed by cytochrome P450 is monooxygenation in which one atom of oxygen is incorporated into a substrate, designated RH, and the other is reduced to water with reducing equivalents derived from NADPH, as follows:

$$\text{Substrate (RH)} + O_2 + \text{NADPH} + H^+ \rightarrow \text{Product (ROH)} + H_2O + \text{NADP}^+$$

Although cytochrome P450 functions as a monooxygenase, the products are not limited to alcohols and phenols due to rearrangement reactions (Guengerich, 1991). During catalysis, cytochrome P450 binds directly to the substrate and molecular oxygen, but it does not interact directly with NADPH or NADH. The mechanism by which cytochrome P450 receives electrons from NAD(P)H depends on the subcellular localization of cytochrome P450. In the endoplasmic reticulum, which is where most of the P450 enzymes involved in xenobiotic biotransformation are localized, electrons are relayed from

NADPH to cytochrome P450 via a flavoprotein called NADPH-cytochrome P450 reductase. Within this flavoprotein, electrons are transferred from NADPH to cytochrome P450 via FMN and FAD. In mitochondria, which house many of the P450 enzymes involved in steroid hormone biosynthesis and vitamin D metabolism, electrons are transferred from NAD(P)H to cytochrome P450 via two proteins; an iron-sulfur protein called ferredoxin, and an FMN-containing flavoprotein called ferredoxin reductase (these proteins are also known as adrenodoxin and adrenodoxin reductase). In bacteria such as *Pseudomonas putida* electron flow is similar to that in mitochondria (NADH → flavoprotein → putidaredoxin → P450).

There are some notable exceptions to the general rule that cytochrome P450 requires a second enzyme (i.e., a flavoprotein) for catalytic activity. One exception applies to two P450 enzymes involved in the conversion of arachidonic acid to eicosanoids, namely thromboxane synthase and prostacyclin synthase. These two P450 enzymes convert the endoperoxide, $PGH_2$, to thromboxane ($TXA_2$) and prostacyclin ($PGI_2$) in platelets and the endothelial lining of blood vessels, respectively. In both cases, cytochrome P450 functions as an isomerase and catalyzes a rearrangement of the oxygen atoms introduced into arachidonic acid by cyclooxygenase. The plant cytochrome P450, allene oxide synthase, and certain invertebrate P450 enzymes also catalyze the rearrangement of oxidized chemicals.

The second exception are two cytochrome P450 enzymes expressed in the bacterium *Bacillus megaterium*, which are known as BM-1 and BM-3 (or CYP106 and CYP102, respectively). These P450 enzymes are considerably larger than most P450 enzymes because they are linked directly to a flavoprotein. In other words, the P450 moiety and flavoprotein are expressed in a single protein encoded by a single gene. Through recombinant DNA techniques, mammalian P450 enzymes have been linked directly to NADPH-cytochrome P450 reductase and, like the bacterial enzyme, the resultant fusion protein is catalytically active. Most mammalian P450 enzymes are not synthesized as a single enzyme containing both the hemoprotein and flavoprotein moieties, but this arrangement is found in nitric oxide (NO) synthase. In addition to its atypical structure, the P450 enzyme expressed in *Bacillus megaterium*, CYP102, is unusual for another reason: It is inducible by phenobarbital, which has provided insight into the mechanism of cytochrome P450 induction.

Phospholipids and cytochrome $b_5$ also play an important role in cytochrome P450 reactions. Cytochrome P450 and NADPH-cytochrome P450 reductase are embedded in the phospholipid bilayer of the endoplasmic reticulum, which facilitates their interaction. When the *C*-terminal region that anchors NADPH-cytochrome P450 reductase in the membrane is cleaved with trypsin, the truncated flavoprotein can no longer support cytochrome P450 reactions, although it is still capable of reducing cytochrome c and other soluble electron acceptors. The ability of phospholipids to facilitate the interaction between NADPH-cytochrome P450 reductase and cytochrome P450 does not appear to depend on the nature of the polar head group (serine, choline, inositol, ethanolamine), although certain P450 enzymes (those in the CYP3A subfamily) have a requirement for phospholipids containing unsaturated fatty acids.

Cytochrome $b_5$ can donate the second of two electrons required by cytochrome P450. Although this would be expected simply to increase the rate of catalysis of cytochrome P450, cytochrome $b_5$ can also increase the apparent affinity with which certain P450 enzymes bind their substrates, hence, cytochrome $b_5$ can increase $V_{max}$ and/or decrease the apparent $K_m$ of cytochrome P450 reactions. Liver microsomes contain numerous forms of cytochrome P450 but contain a single form of NADPH-cytochrome P450 reductase and cytochrome $b_5$. For each molecule of NADPH-cytochrome P450 reductase in rat liver microsomes, there are 5–10 molecules of cytochrome $b_5$ and 10–20 molecules of cytochrome P450. NADPH-cytochrome P450 reductase will reduce electron acceptors other than cytochrome P450, which enables this enzyme to be measured based on its ability to reduce cytochrome c (which is why NADPH-cytochrome P450 reductase is often called NADPH-cytochrome c reductase). NADPH-cytochrome P450 reductase can transfer electrons much faster than cytochrome P450 can use them, which more than likely accounts for the low ratio of NADPH-cytochrome P450 reductase to cytochrome P450 in liver microsomes. Low levels of NADPH-cytochrome P450 reductase may also be a safeguard to protect cells from the often deleterious one-electron reduction reactions catalyzed by this flavoprotein (see Fig. 6-11).

The catalytic cycle of cytochrome P450 is shown in Fig. 6-31 (Dawson, 1988). The first part of the cycle involves the activation of oxygen, and the final part of the cycle involves substrate oxidation, which entails the abstraction of a hydrogen atom or an electron from the substrate followed by oxygen rebound (radical recombination). Following the binding of substrate to the P450 enzyme, the heme iron is reduced from the ferric ($Fe^{3+}$) to the ferrous ($Fe^{2+}$) state by the addition of a single electron from NADPH-cytochrome P450 reductase. The reduction of cytochrome P450 is facilitated by substrate binding, possibly because binding of the substrate in the vicinity of the heme moiety converts the heme iron from a low-spin to a high-spin state. Oxygen binds to cytochrome P450 in its ferrous state, and the $Fe^{2+}O_2$ complex is converted to an $Fe^{2+}OOH$ complex by the addition of a proton ($H^+$) and a second electron, which is derived from NADPH-cytochrome P450 reductase or cytochrome $b_5$. Introduction of a second proton cleaves the $Fe^{2+}OOH$ complex to produce water and an $(FeO)^{3+}$ complex, which transfers its oxygen atom to the substrate. Release of the oxidized substrate returns cytochrome P450 to its initial state. If the catalytic cycle is interrupted (uncoupled) following introduction of the first electron, oxygen is released as superoxide anion ($O_2^{\bar{\cdot}}$). If the cycle is interrupted after introduction of the second electron, oxygen is released as hydrogen peroxide ($H_2O_2$). The final oxygenating species, $(FeO)^{3+}$, can be generated directly by the transfer of an oxygen atom from hydrogen peroxide and certain other hydroperoxides, a process known as the peroxide shunt. For this reason certain P450 reactions can be supported by hydroperoxides in the absence of NADPH-cytochrome P450 reductase and NADPH.

Cytochrome P450 catalyzes several types of oxidation reactions, including:

1. Hydroxylation of an aliphatic or aromatic carbon;
2. Epoxidation of a double bond;

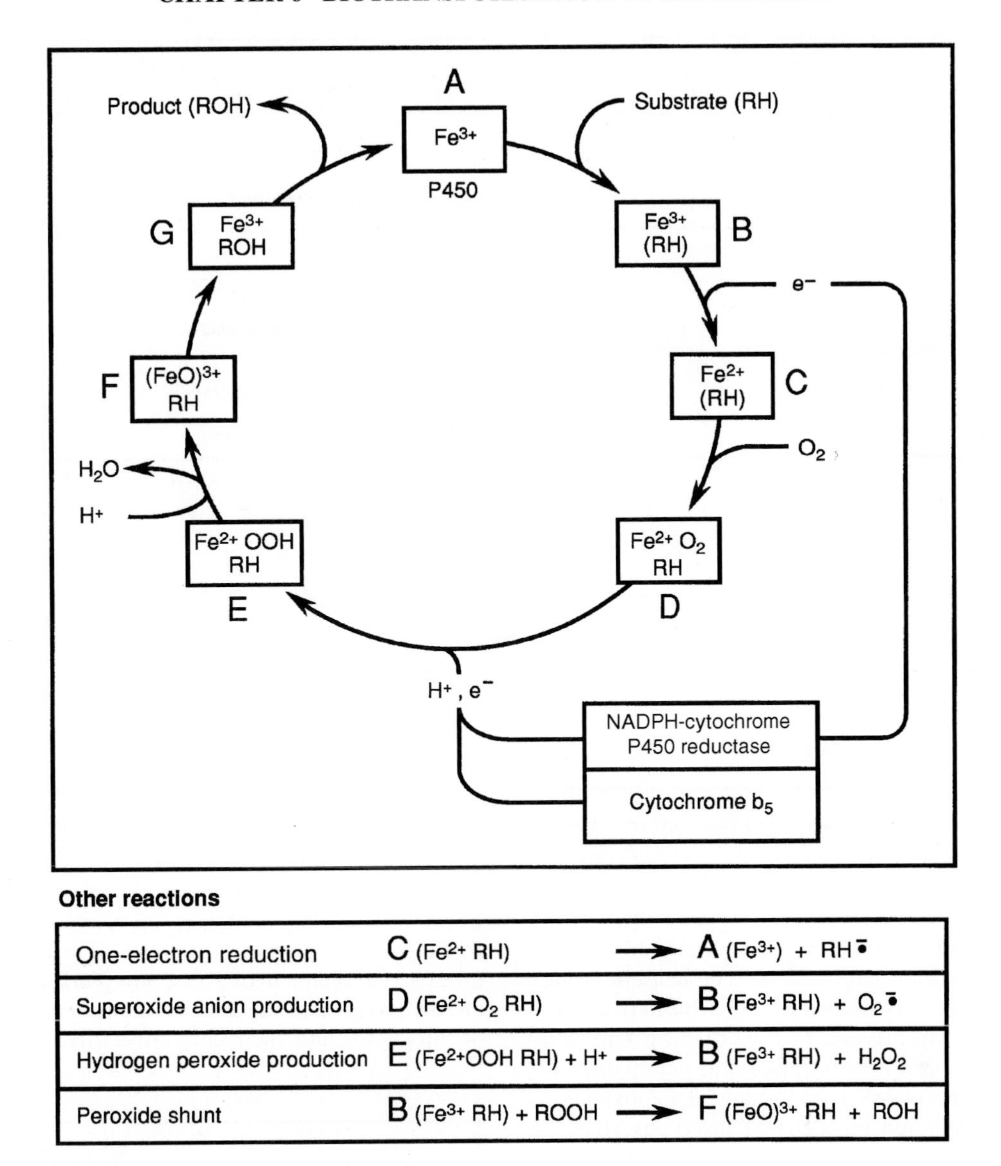


| | | | |
|---|---|---|---|
| One-electron reduction | C ($Fe^{2+}$ RH) | → | A ($Fe^{3+}$) + $RH^{\bar{\bullet}}$ |
| Superoxide anion production | D ($Fe^{2+}$ $O_2$ RH) | → | B ($Fe^{3+}$ RH) + $O_2^{\bar{\bullet}}$ |
| Hydrogen peroxide production | E ($Fe^{2+}$OOH RH) + $H^+$ | → | B ($Fe^{3+}$ RH) + $H_2O_2$ |
| Peroxide shunt | B ($Fe^{3+}$ RH) + ROOH | → | F $(FeO)^{3+}$ RH + ROH |

*Figure 6–31. Catalytic cycle of cytochrome P450.*

3. Heteroatom (*S*-, *N*-, and *I*-) oxygenation and *N*-hydroxylation;
4. Heteroatom (*O*-, *S*-, and *N*-) dealkylation;
5. Oxidative group transfer;
6. Cleavage of esters;
7. Dehydrogenation.

In the first three cases, oxygen from the $(FeO)^{3+}$ complex is incorporated into the substrate, which otherwise remains intact. In the fourth case, oxygenation of the substrate is followed by a rearrangement reaction leading to cleavage of an amine (*N*-dealkylation) or an ether (*O*- and *S*-dealkylation). Oxygen from the $(FeO)^{3+}$ complex is incorporated into the alkyl-leaving group, producing an aldehyde or ketone. In the fifth case, oxygenation of the substrate is followed by a rearrangement reaction leading to loss of a heteroatom (oxidative group transfer). The sixth case, the cleavage of esters, resembles heteroatom dealkylation in that the functional group is cleaved with incorporation of oxygen from the $(FeO)^{3+}$ complex into the leaving group, producing an aldehyde. In the seventh case, two hydrogens are abstracted from the substrate with the formation of a double bond (C=C, C=O, or C=N), with the reduction of oxygen from the $(FeO)^{3+}$ complex to water. It should be noted that this long list of reactions does not encompass all of the reactions catalyzed by cytochrome P450. As noted above (this section), cytochrome P450 can catalyze reductive reactions (such as azo reduction, nitro reduction, and reductive dehalogenation) and isomerization reactions (such as the conversion of $PGH_2$ to thromboxane and prostacyclin). During the synthesis of steroid hormones, cytochrome P450 catalyzes the cleavage of carbon-carbon bonds, which occurs during the conversion of cholesterol to pregnenolone by side-chain cleavage enzyme (also known as $P450_{scc}$ and CYP11A1) and the aromatization of a substituted cyclohexane, which occurs during the conversion of androgens to estrogens by aromatase (also known as $P450_{aro}$ and CYP19).

Examples of aliphatic and aromatic hydroxylation reactions catalyzed by cytochrome P450 are shown in Figs. 6-32 and

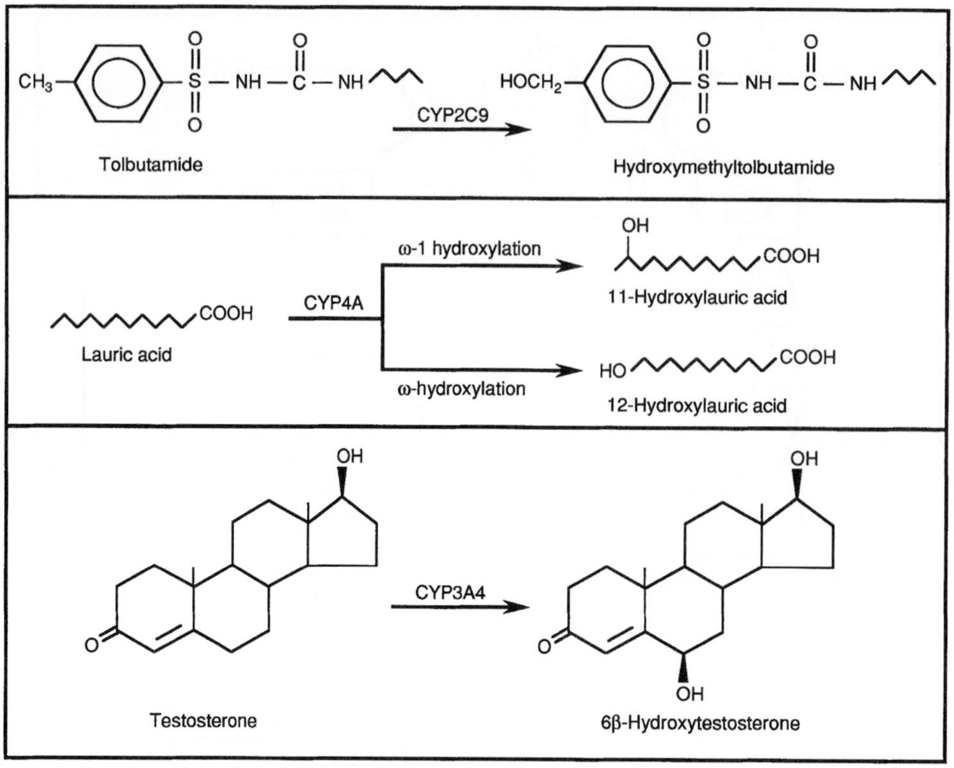

Figure 6–32. *Examples of reactions catalyzed by cytochrome P450: Hydroxylation of aliphatic carbon.*

6-33, respectively. The hydroxylation of aromatic hydrocarbons may proceed via an oxirane intermediate (i.e., an arene oxide) that isomerizes to the corresponding phenol. Alternatively aromatic hydroxylation can proceed by a mechanism known as direct insertion. The *ortho*hydroxylation and *para*hydroxylation of chlorobenzene proceed via 2,3-and 3,4-epoxidation, whereas *meta*hydroxylation proceeds by direct insertion, as shown in Fig. 6-34. When aromatic hydroxylation involves direct insertion, hydrogen abstraction (i.e., cleavage of the C-H bond) is the rate-limiting step, so that substitution of hydrogen with deuterium or tritium considerably slows the hydroxylation reaction. This *isotope effect* is less marked when aromatic hydroxylation proceeds via an arene oxide intermediate. Arene oxides are electrophilic and, therefore, potentially toxic metabolites that are detoxified by such enzymes as epoxide hydrolase (see Fig. 6-8) and glutathione *S*-transferase. Depending on the ring substituents, the rearrangement of arene oxides to the corresponding phenol can lead to an intramolecular migration of a substituent (such as hydrogen or a halogen) from one carbon to the next. This intramolecular migration occurs at the site of oxidation and is known as the NIH shift; so named for its discovery at the National Institutes of Health.

Aliphatic hydroxylation involves insertion of oxygen into a C-H bond. As in the case of aromatic hydroxylation by direct insertion, cleavage of the C-H bond by hydrogen abstraction is the rate-limiting step, as shown below:

$$(FeO)^{3+} \quad HC\!- \rightarrow Fe(OH)^{3+} \quad \bullet C\!- \rightarrow Fe^{3+} \quad HO\!-\!C\!-$$

In the case of simple, straight chain hydrocarbons, such as n-hexane, aliphatic hydroxylation occurs at both the terminal methyl groups and the internal methylene groups. In the case of fatty acids and their derivatives (i.e., eicosanoids such as

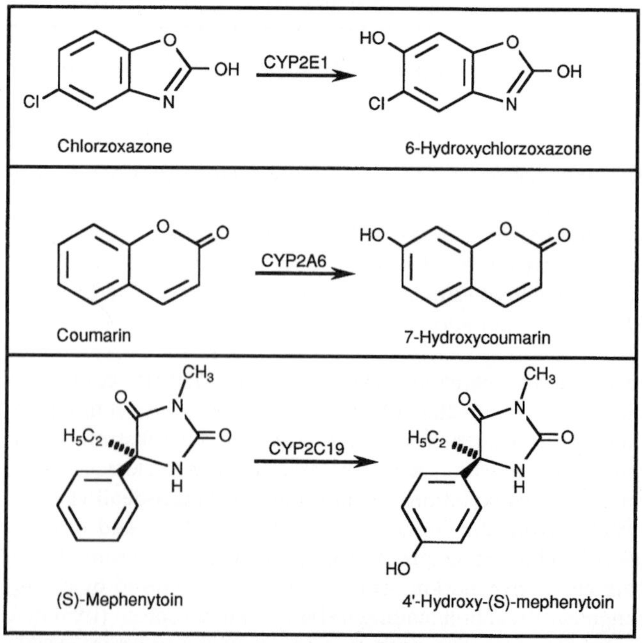

Figure 6–33. *Examples of reactions catalyzed by cytochrome P450: Hydroxylation of aromatic carbon.*

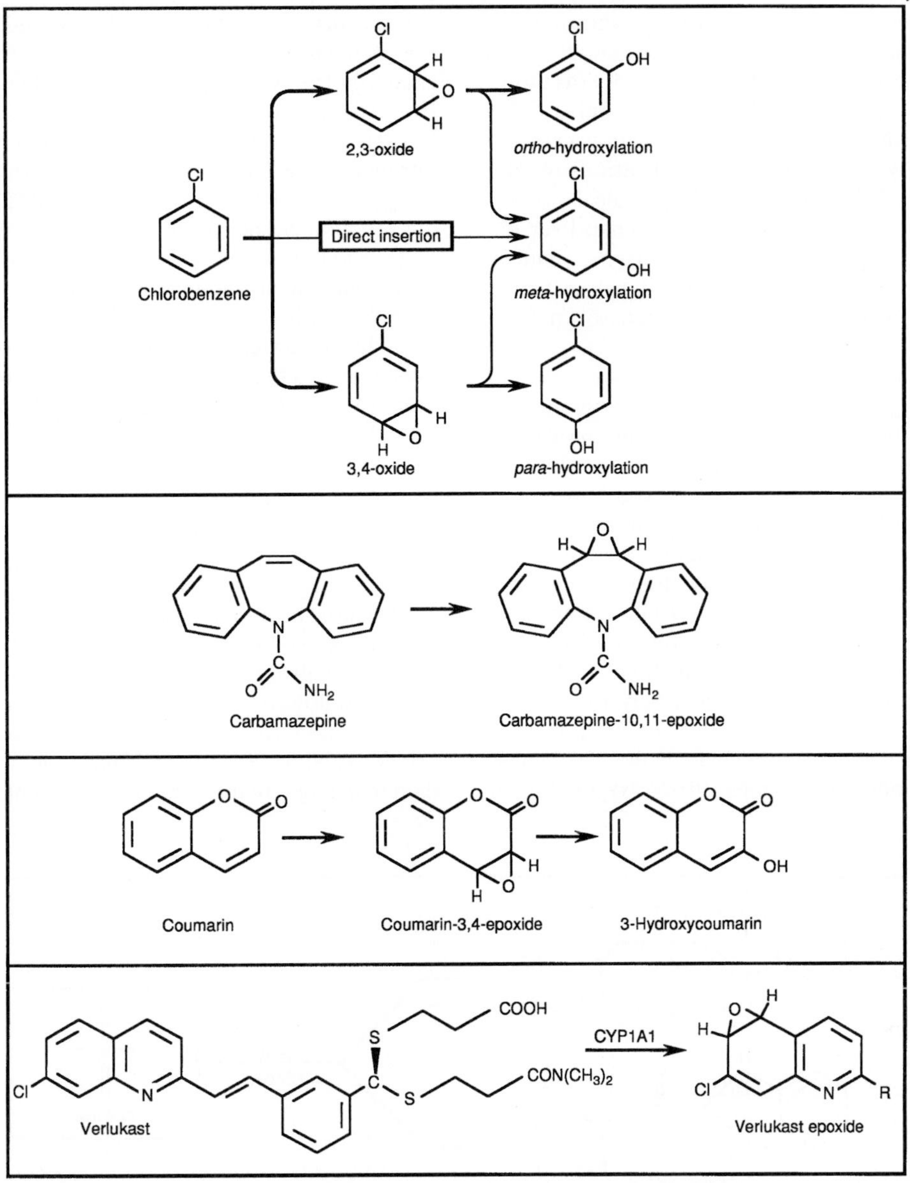

***Figure 6–34. Examples of reactions catalyzed by cytochrome P450: Epoxidation.***

prostaglandins and leukotrienes), aliphatic hydroxylation occurs at the $\omega$-carbon (terminal methyl group) and the $\omega$-1carbon (penultimate carbon), as shown for lauric acid in Fig. 6-32. Most P450 enzymes preferentially catalyze the $\omega$-1 hydroxylation of fatty acids and their derivatives, but one group of P450 enzymes (those encoded by the *CYP4A* genes) preferentially catalyzes the $\omega$-hydroxylation of fatty acids, which can be further oxidized to dicarboxylic acids.

Xenobiotics containing a carbon-carbon double bond (i.e., alkenes) can be epoxidated (i.e., converted to an oxirane) in an analogous manner to the oxidation of aromatic compounds to arene oxides. Just as arene oxides can isomerize to phenols, so aliphatic epoxides can isomerize to the corresponding ene-ol, the formation of which may involve an intramolecular migration (NIH shift) of a substituent at the site of oxidation. Like arene oxides, aliphatic epoxides are also potentially toxic metabolites that are inactivated by other xenobiotic-metabolizing enzymes. Oxidation of some aliphatic alkenes and alkynes produces metabolites that are sufficiently reactive to bind covalently to the heme moiety of cytochrome P450, a process known as suicide inactivation or mechanism-based inhibition. As previously discussed in the section on epoxide hydrolase, not all epoxides are highly reactive electrophiles. Although the 3,4-epoxidation of coumarin produces an hepatotoxic metabolite, the 10,11-epoxidation of carbamazepine produces a stable, relatively nontoxic metabolite (Fig. 6-34).

In the presence of NADPH and $O_2$, liver microsomes catalyze the oxygenation of several *S*-containing xenobiotics, including chlorpromazine, cimetidine, lansoprazole and omeprazole. Sulfur-containing xenobiotics can potentially undergo two consecutive sulfoxidation reactions: one that converts the sulfide (S) to the sulfoxide (SO), which occurs during the sulfoxidation of chlorpromazine and cimetidine, and one that converts the sulfoxide (SO) to the sulfone ($SO_2$), which occurs during the sulfoxidation of omeprazole and lansoprazole, as shown in Fig. 6-35. Albendazole is converted first to a sulfoxide and then to a sulfone. All of these reactions are catalyzed by FMO (as shown in Fig. 6-29B) and/or cytochrome P450 (as shown in Fig. 6-35). Both enzymes are efficient catalysts of *S*-oxygenation, and both contribute significantly to the sulfoxidation of various xenobiotics. For example, the sulfoxidation of omeprazole, lansoprazole, chlorpromazine, and phenothiazine by human liver microsomes is primarily catalyzed by a P450 enzyme (namely CYP3A4), whereas the sulfoxidation of cimetidine is primarily catalyzed by a flavin-containing monooxygenase (namely FMO3).

In the presence of NADPH and $O_2$, liver microsomes catalyze the oxygenation of several *N*-containing xenobiotics, including chlorpromazine, doxylamine, oflaxacin, morphine, nicotine, MPTP, methapyrilene, methaqualone, metronidazole, pargyline, pyridine, senecionine, strychnine, trimethylamine, trimipramine, and verapamil, all of which are converted to stable *N*-oxides. Whereas *S*-oxygenation might be catalyzed by both cytochrome P450 and FMO, *N*-oxygenation is more likely to be catalyzed by just one of these enzymes. For example, the conversion of (*S*)-nicotine to *trans*-(*S*)-nicotine *N*-1′-oxide by human liver microsomes is catalyzed by FMO3, with little or no contribution from cytochrome P450. Conversely, the conversion of pyridine to its *N*-oxide is primarily catalyzed by cytochrome P450. Both enzymes can participate in the *N*-oxygenation of certain xenobiotics. For example, the *N*-oxygenation of chlorpromazine is catalyzed by FMO3 and, to a lesser extent, by two P450 enzymes (CYP2D6 and CYP1A2). In general, FMO catalyzes the *N*-oxygenation of xenobiotics containing electron-deficient nitrogen atoms, whereas cytochrome P450 catalyzes the *N*-oxygenation of xenobiotics containing electron-rich nitrogen atoms. Therefore, substrates primarily *N*-oxygenated by cytochrome P450 are somewhat limited to pyridine-containing xenobiotics, such as the tobacco-specific nitrosamine NNK and the antihistamine temelastine, and to xenobiotics containing a quinoline or isoquinoline group, such as the muscle relaxant 6,7-dimethoxy-4-(4′-chlorobenzyl)isoquinoline.

The initial step in heteroatom oxygenation by cytochrome P450 involves the abstraction of an electron from the heteroatom (*N, S* or *I*) by the $(FeO)^{3+}$ complex, as shown below for sulfoxidation.

$$(FeO)^{3+}\ :\!\overset{|}{\underset{|}{S}} \rightarrow (FeO)^{2+}\ +\bullet\overset{|}{\underset{|}{S}}- \rightarrow Fe^{3+}\ \ O^{-}-\overset{|}{\underset{|}{^{+}S}}$$

Abstraction of an electron from *N, O*, or *S* by the $(FeO)^{3+}$ complex is also the initial step in heteroatom dealkylation, but in this case abstraction of the electron from the heteroatom is quickly followed by abstraction of a proton ($H^+$) from the $\alpha$-carbon atom (the carbon atom attached to the heteroatom). Oxygen rebound leads to hydroxylation of the $\alpha$-carbon, which then rearranges to form the corresponding aldehyde or ketone

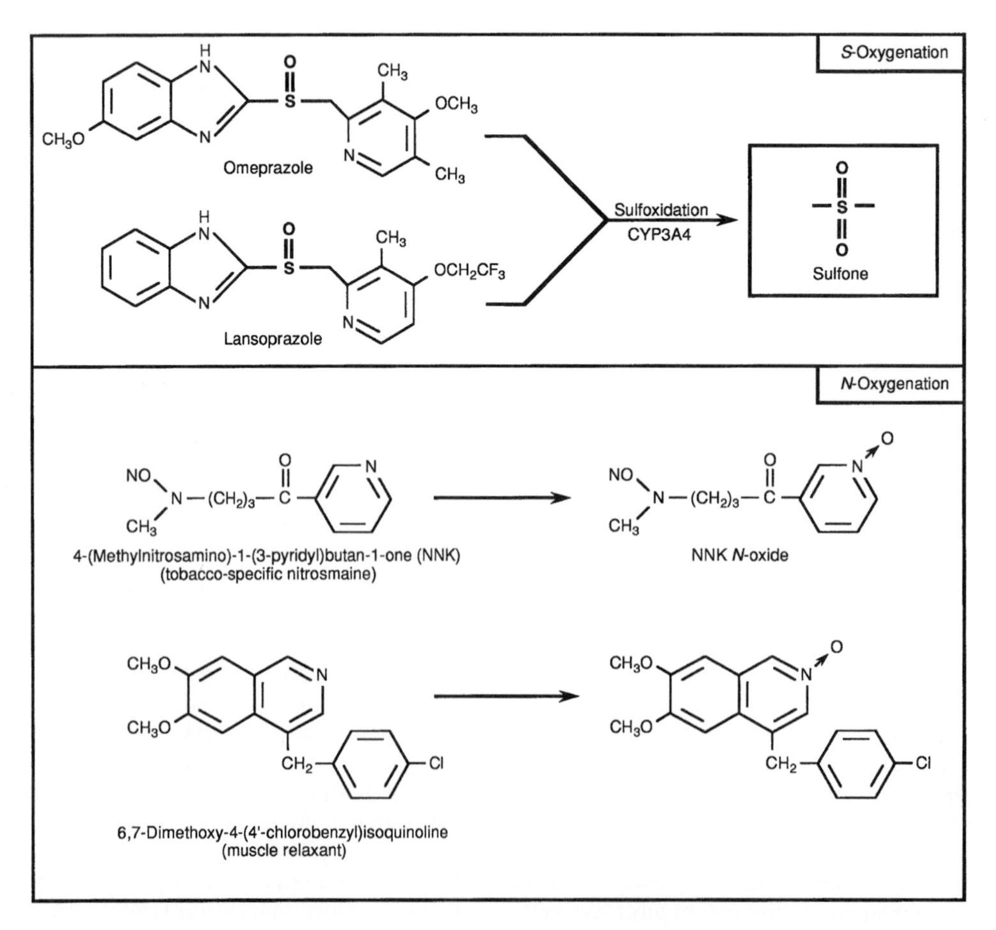


*Figure 6–35. Examples of reactions catalyzed by cytochrome P450: Heteroatom oxygenation.*

with cleavage of the $\alpha$-carbon from the heteroatom, as shown below for the *N*-dealkylation of an *N*-alkylamine:

$$(FeO)^{3+}\ :\!N(CH_2R) \rightarrow (FeO)^{2+} + \bullet N(CH_2R) \rightarrow Fe(OH)^{3+}\ :\!N(\bullet CHR) \rightarrow$$

$$Fe^{3+}\ :\!N(HOCHR) \rightarrow\ :\!N(H) + O{=}CHR$$

Although the initial steps in heteroatom oxygenation and heteroatom dealkylation are the same (abstraction of an electron from the heteroatom to produce a radical cation), the nature of the radical cation determines whether the xenobiotic will undergo oxygenation or dealkylation. The sulfur radical cations of numerous xenobiotics are sufficiently stable to allow oxygen rebound with the heteroatom itself, which results in *S*-oxygenation. However, this is not generally the case with nitrogen radical cations, which undergo rapid deprotonation at the $\alpha$-carbon, which in turn results in *N*-dealkylation. In general, therefore, cytochrome P450 catalyzes the *N*-dealkylation, not the *N*-oxygenation, of amines. *N*-oxygenation by cytochrome P450 can occur if the nitrogen radical cation is stabilized by a nearby electron-donating group (making the nitrogen electron rich) or if $\alpha$-protons are either absent (e.g., aromatic amines) or inaccessible (e.g., quinidine). In the case of primary and secondary aromatic amines, *N*-oxygenation by cytochrome P450 usually results in the formation of hydroxylamines, as illustrated in Fig. 6-7. *N*-Hydroxylation of aromatic amines with subsequent conjugation with sulfate or acetate is one mechanism by which tumorigenic aromatic amines, such as 2-acetylaminofluorene, are converted to electrophilic reactive intermediates that bind covalently to DNA (Anders, 1985).

In contrast to cytochrome P450, which oxidizes nitrogen-containing xenobiotics by a radicaloid mechanism involving an initial one-electron oxidation of the heteroatom, the flavin-containing monooxygenases oxidize nitrogen-containing xenobiotics by a heterolytic mechanism involving a two-electron oxidation by the 4a-hydroperoxide of FAD (see Fig. 6-30). These different mechanisms explain why the *N*-oxygenation of xenobiotics by cytochrome P450 generally results in *N*-dealkylation, whereas *N*-oxygenation by the flavin-containing monooxygenases results in *N*-oxide formation. In contrast to cytochrome P450, the flavin-containing monooxygenases do not catalyze *N*-, *O*-, or *S*-dealkylation reactions.

Numerous xenobiotics are *N*-, *O*-, or *S*-dealkylated by cytochrome P450, and some examples of these heteroatom dealkylation reactions are shown in Fig. 6-36. The dealkylation of xenobiotics containing an *N*-, *O*-, or *S*-methyl group results in the formation of formaldehyde, which can easily be measured by a simple colorimetric assay to monitor the demethylation of substrates in vitro. The expiration of $^{13}C$- or $^{14}C$-labelled carbon dioxide following the demethylation of drugs containing a $^{13}C$- or $^{14}C$-labelled methyl group has been used to probe cytochrome P450 activity in vivo (Watkins, 1994). The activity of the human P450 enzymes involved in the *N*-demethylation of aminopyrine, erythromycin, and caffeine can be assessed by this technique. Although caffeine has three *N*-methyl groups, all of which can be removed by cytochrome P450, the major pathway in humans involves *N3*-demethylation of caffeine to paraxanthine (see Fig. 6-36).

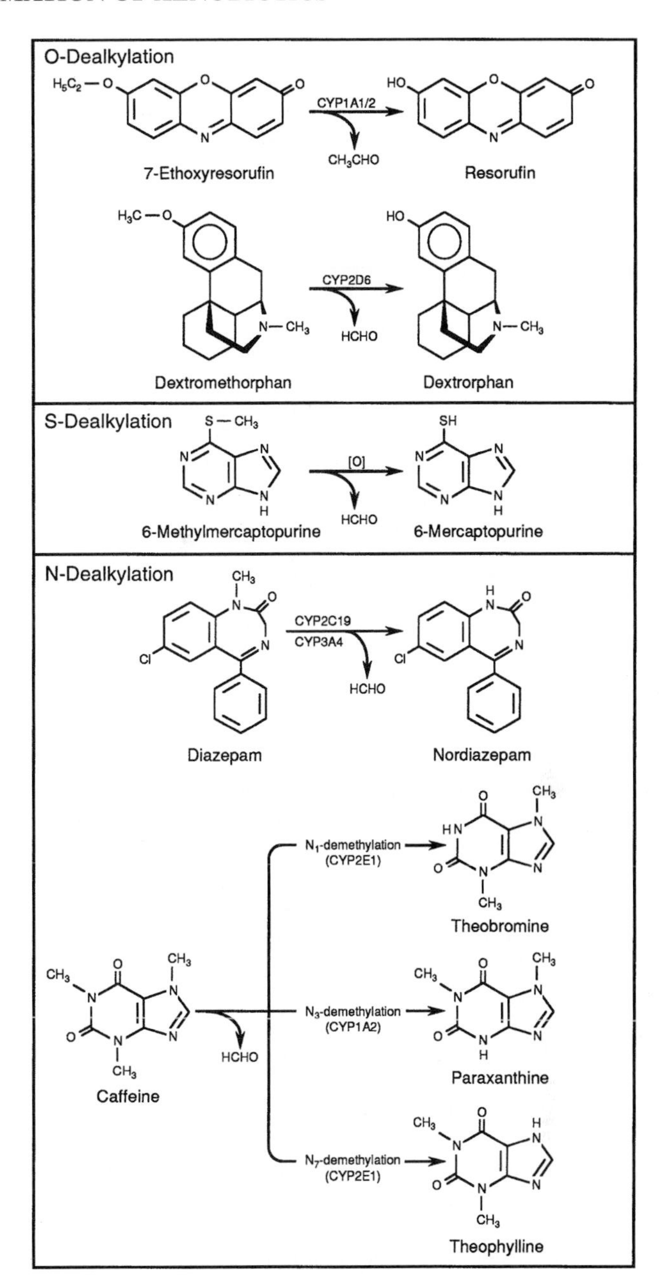


***Figure 6–36. Examples of reactions catalyzed by cytochrome P450: Hetroatom dealkylation.***

In addition to *N*-dealkylation, primary amines can also undergo oxidative deamination by cytochrome P450, which is an example of oxidative group transfer. The mechanism is similar to that of *N*-dealkylation: The $\alpha$-carbon adjacent to the primary amine is hydroxylated, which produces an unstable intermediate that rearranges to eliminate ammonia with the formation of an aldehyde or ketone. The conversion of amphetamine to phenylacetone is an example of oxidative deamination, as shown in Fig. 6-37. Oxidative deamination is also catalyzed by monoamine oxidase (MAO). In the example given above, however, the substrate, amphetamine, contains an $\alpha$-methyl group which renders it a poor substrate for MAO (as described in "Monoamine Oxidase, Diamine Oxidase, and Polyamine Oxidase," above).

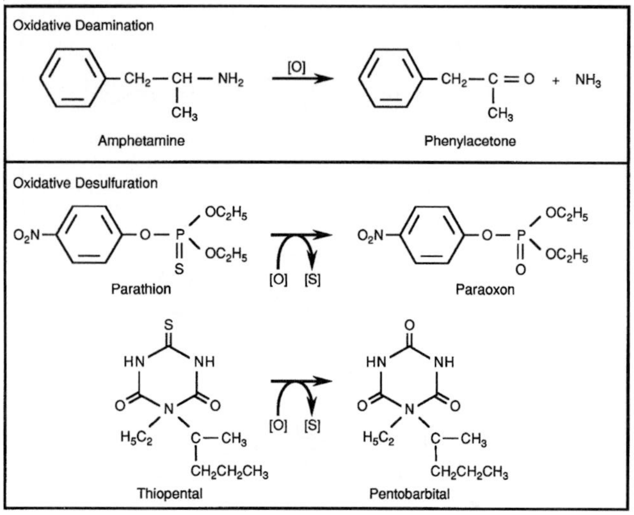

***Figure 6–37. Examples of reactions catalyzed by cytochrome P450: Oxidative group transfer.***

In addition to oxidative deamination, cytochrome P450 catalyzes two other types of oxidative group transfer, namely oxidative desulfuration and oxidative dehalogenation. In all cases the heteroatom (*N, S,* or halogen) is replaced with oxygen. As shown in Fig. 6-37, oxidative desulfuration converts parathion, which has little insecticidal activity, to paraoxon, which is a potent insecticide. The same reaction converts thiopental to pentobarbital. Diethyldithiocarbamate methyl ester, a metabolite of disulfiram, also undergoes oxidative desulfuration. The initial reaction involves *S*-oxidation by cytochrome P450 or FMO to a sulfine ($R_1R_2C = S \rightarrow R_1R_2C = S^+—O^-$). In the presence of glutathione (GSH) and glutathione *S*-transferase, this sulfine is either converted back to the parent compound ($R_1R_2C = S^+—O^- + 2\ GSH \rightarrow R_1R_2C = S + GSSG + H_2O$) or it undergoes desulfuration ($R_1R_2C = S^+—O^- + 2\ GSH \rightarrow R_1R_2C = O + GSSG + H_2S$) (Madan et al., 1994).

Cytochrome P450 catalyzes both reductive and oxidative dehalogenation reactions (Guengerich, 1991). During oxidative dehalogenation, a halogen and hydrogen from the same carbon atom are replaced with oxygen ($R_1R_2CHX \rightarrow R_1R_2CO$) to produce an aldehyde or acylhalide, as shown in Fig. 6-13 for the conversion of halothane ($CF_3CHClBr$) to trifluoroacetylchloride ($CF_3COCl$). Oxidative dehalogenation does not involve a direct attack on the carbon-halogen bond, but it involves the formation of an unstable halohydrin by oxidation of the carbon atom bearing the halogen substituent. The carbon-halogen bond is broken during the rearrangement of the unstable halohydrin. When the carbon atom contains a single halogen, the resulting product is an aldehyde, which can be further oxidized to a carboxylic acid or reduced to a primary alcohol. When the carbon atom contains two halogens, the dihalohydrin intermediate rearranges to an acylhalide, which can be converted to the corresponding carboxylic acid (see Fig. 6-13). As discussed previously, aldehydes and, in particular, acylhalides are reactive compounds that can bind covalently to protein and other critical cellular molecules. The immune hepatitis caused by repeated exposure of humans to halothane and related volatile anesthetics is dependent on oxidative dehalogenation by cytochrome P450, with neoantigens produced by the trifluoroacetylation of proteins, as shown in Fig. 6-13.

As shown in Figs. 6-12 and 6-13 above, cytochrome P450 also can catalyze the reductive dehalogenation of halogenated alkanes and the reduction of certain azo- and nitro-containing xenobiotics (Fig. 6-6). The ability of cytochrome P450 to reduce xenobiotics can be understood from the catalytic cycle shown in Fig. 6-31. Binding of a substrate to cytochrome P450 is followed by a one-electron reduction by NADPH-cytochrome P450 reductase. Under aerobic conditions, reduction of the heme iron to the ferrous state permits binding of oxygen. Anaerobic conditions, in contrast, interrupt the cycle at this point, which allows cytochrome P450 to reduce those substrates capable of accepting an electron. Therefore, cytochrome P450 can catalyze reduction reactions, such as azo-reduction, nitro-reduction, and reductive dehalogenation, particularly under conditions of low oxygen tension. In effect, the substrate rather than molecular oxygen accepts electrons and is reduced. In fact, oxygen acts as an inhibitor of these reactions because it competes with the substrate for the reducing equivalents. The toxicity of many halogenated alkanes is dependent on their biotransformation by reductive dehalogenation. The first step in reductive dehalogenation is a one-electron reduction catalyzed by cytochrome P450, which produces a potentially toxic, carbon-centered radical and inorganic halide. The conversion of $CCl_4$ to a trichloromethyl radical and other toxic metabolites is shown in Fig. 6-12.

The oxidative desulfuration of parathion involves the production of an intermediate that rearranges to paraoxon (see Fig. 6-37). This same intermediate can decompose to *para*-nitrophenol and diethylphosphorothioic acid, which are the same products formed by the hydrolysis of parathion (Fig. 6-38). In addition to facilitating the hydrolysis of phosphoric acid esters, cytochrome P450 also catalyzes the cleavage of carboxylic acid esters, as shown in Fig. 6-38. Carboxylic acid esters typically are cleaved by carboxylesterases, which results in the formation of an acid and an alcohol ($R_1COOCH_2R_2 + H_2O \rightarrow R_1COOH + R_2CH_2OH$). In contrast, cytochrome P450 converts carboxylic acid esters to an acid plus aldehyde ($R_1COOCH_2\ R_2 + [O] \rightarrow R_1COOH + R_2CHO$), as shown in Fig. 6-38. The deacylation of loratadine is the major route of biotransformation of this nonsedating antihistamine. The reaction is catalyzed predominantly by cytochrome P450 (namely CYP3A4 with a minor contribution from CYP2D6), with little contribution from carboxylesterases.

Cytochrome P450 can also catalyze the dehydrogenation of a number of compounds, including acetaminophen, nifedipine, and related dihydropyridine calcium-channel blockers, sparteine, nicotine, digitoxin and testosterone, as shown in Fig. 6-39. Dehydrogenation by cytochrome P450 converts acetaminophen to its hepatotoxic metabolite, *N*-acetylbenzoquinoneimine, as shown in Fig. 6-24. Dehydrogenation of digitoxin ($dt_3$) to 15′-dehydro-$dt_3$ leads to cleavage of the terminal sugar residue to produce digitoxigenin bisdigitoxoside ($dt_2$), which can similarly be converted to 9′-dehydro-$dt_2$, which undergoes digitoxosyl cleavage to digitoxigenin monodigitoxoside ($dt_1$). In contrast to digitoxin, this latter metabolite is an excellent substrate for glucuronidation. In rats, the P450 enzymes responsible for converting digitoxin to $dt_1$ (namely the CYP3A enzymes) and the UDP-glucuronosyltransferase responsible for glucuronidating $dt_1$ are inducible by dexamethasone, pregnenolone-16$\alpha$-carbonitrile and spironolactone, all of which protect rats from the toxic effects of digitoxin. The dehydrogena-

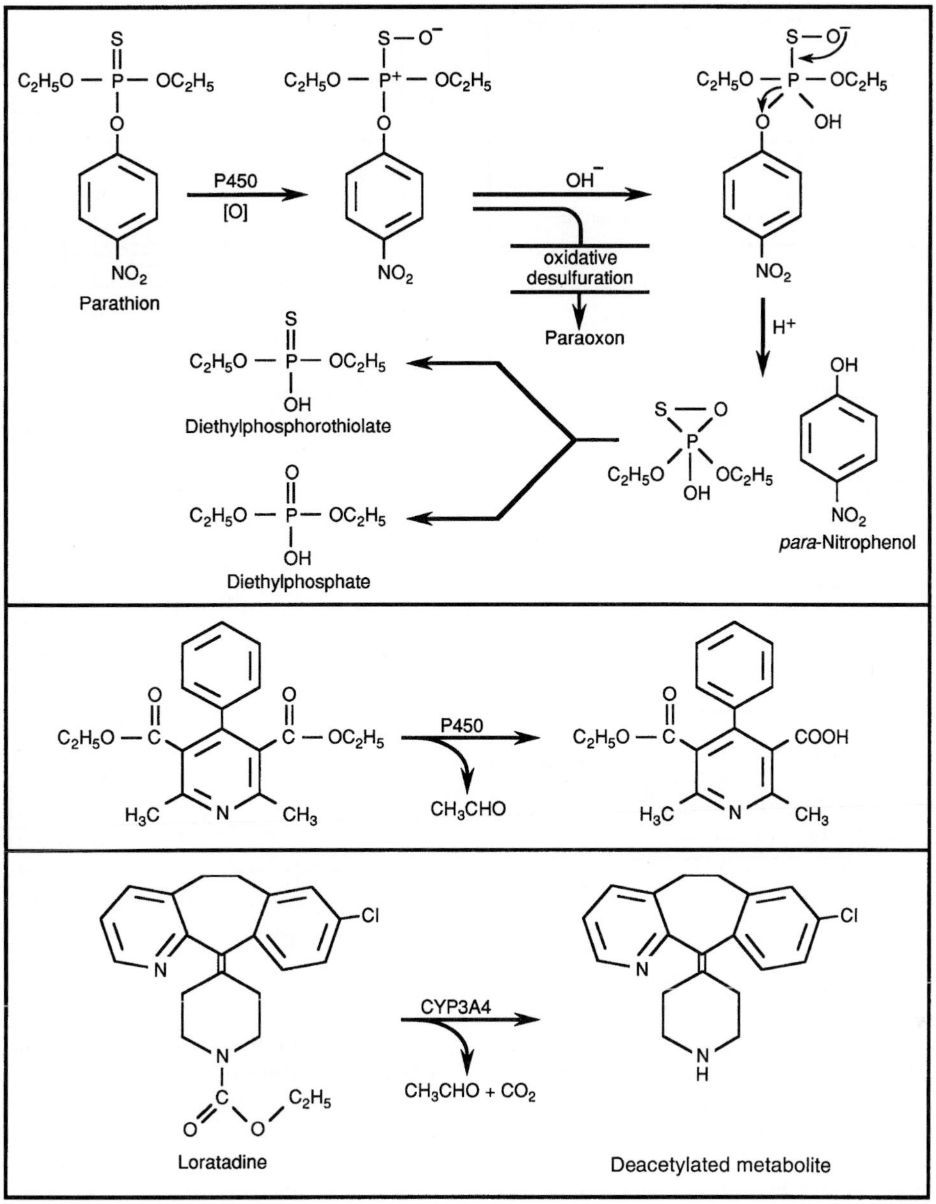

***Figure 6–38. Examples of reactions catalyzed by cytochrome P450: Cleavage of esters.***

tion of nicotine produces nicotine $\Delta^{1',5'}$-iminium ion, which is oxidized by cytosolic aldehyde oxidase to cotinine, a major metabolite of nicotine excreted in the urine of cigarette smokers.

Testosterone is dehydrogenated by cytochrome P450 to two metabolites: 6-dehydrotestosterone, which involves formation of a carbon-carbon double bond, and androstenedione, which involves formation of a carbon-oxygen double bond. The conversion of testosterone to androstenedione is one of several cases where cytochrome P450 converts a primary or secondary alcohol to an aldehyde or ketone, respectively. The reaction can proceed by formation of a *gem*-diol (two hydroxyl groups on the same carbon atom), with subsequent dehydration to a keto group, as shown in Fig. 6-17 for the conversion of ethanol to acetaldehyde. However, *gem*-diols are not obligatory intermediates in the oxidation of alcohols by cytochrome P450, and in fact the conversion of testosterone to androstenedione by CYP2B1 (the major phenobarbital-inducible P450 enzyme in rats) does not involve the intermediacy of a *gem*-diol but proceeds by direct dehydrogenation (Fig. 6-39). In contrast, a *gem*-diol is involved in the formation of androstenedione from *epi*-testosterone (which is identical to testosterone except the hydroxyl group at C17 is in the $\alpha$-configuration, not the $\beta$-configuration). The fact that formation of androstenedione from *epi*-testosterone involves formation of a *gem*-diol, whereas its formation from testosterone does not, makes it difficult to generalize the mechanism by which cytochrome P450 converts alcohols to aldehydes and ketones.

Liver microsomes from all mammalian species contain numerous P450 enzymes, each with the potential to catalyze the various types of reactions shown in Figs. 6-32 through 6-39. In other words, all of the P450 enzymes expressed in liver microsomes have the potential to catalyze xenobiotic hydroxy-

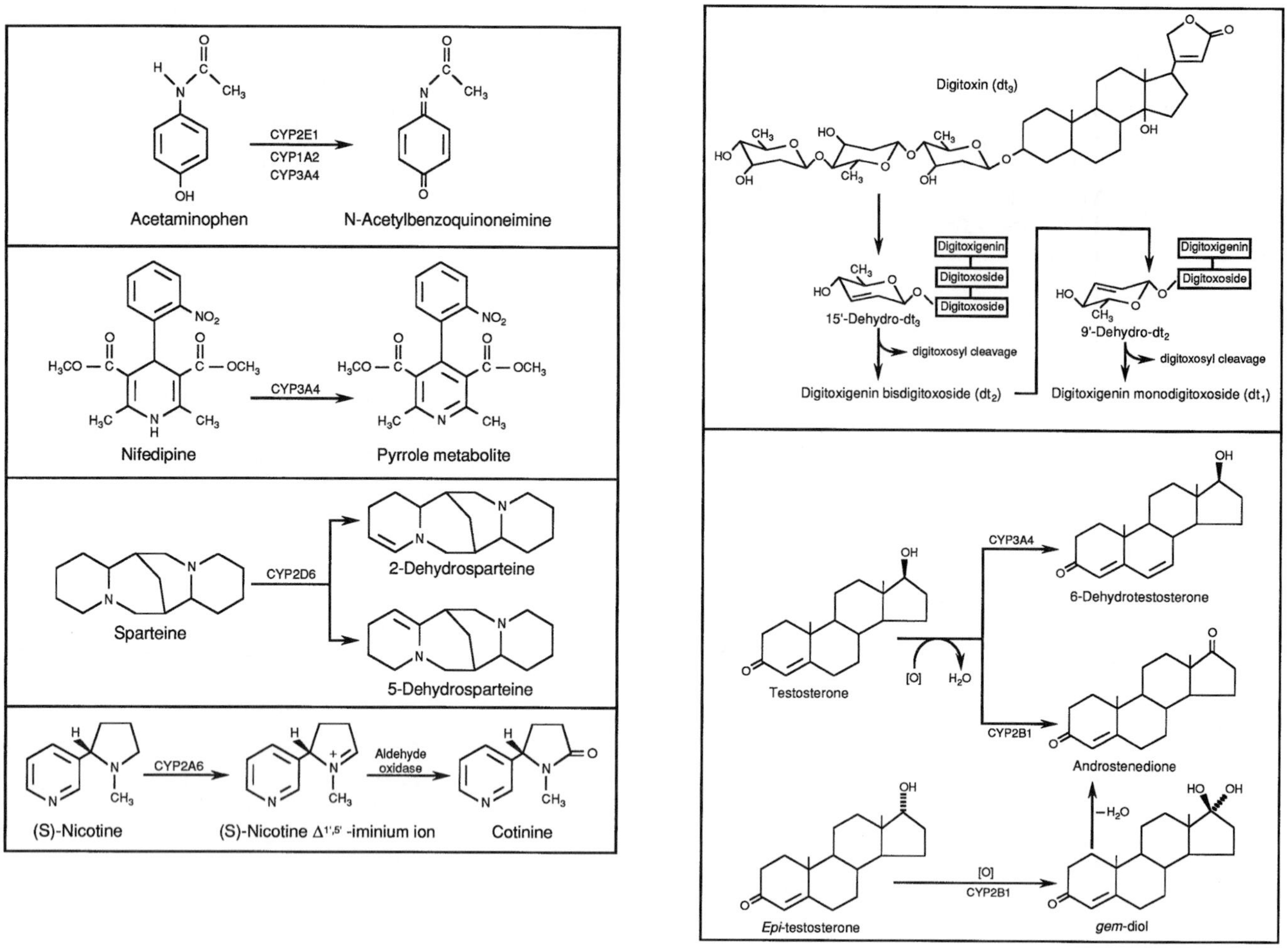

*Figure 6–39. Examples of reactions catalyzed by cytochrome P450: Dehydrogenation.*

lation, epoxidation, dealkylation, oxygenation, dehydrogenation, and so forth. The broad and often overlapping substrate specificity of liver microsomal P450 enzymes precludes the possibility of naming these enzymes for the reactions they catalyze. The amino acid sequence of numerous P450 enzymes has been determined, largely by recombinant DNA techniques, and such sequences now form the basis for classifying and naming P450 enzymes (Gonzalez, 1989; Nelson et al., 1993). In general, P450 enzymes with less than 40 percent amino acid sequence identity are assigned to different gene families (gene families 1, 2, 3, 4 etc.). P450 enzymes that are 40 to 55 percent identical are assigned to different subfamilies (e.g., 2A, 2B, 2C, 2D, 2E, etc.). P450 enzymes that are more than 55 percent identical are classified as members of the same subfamily (e.g., 2A1, 2A2, 2A3, etc.). The liver microsomal P450 enzymes involved in xenobiotic biotransformation belong to three main P450 gene families, namely CYP1, CYP2, and CYP3. Liver microsomes also contain P450 enzymes encoded by the CYP4 gene family, substrates for which include several fatty acids and eicosanoids but relatively few xenobiotics. The liver microsomal P450 enzymes in each of these gene families generally belong to a single subfamily (i.e., CYP1A, CYP3A and CYP4A). A notable exception is the CYP2 gene family, which contains five subfamilies (i.e., CYP2A, CYP2B, CYP2C, CYP2D and CYP2E). The number of P450 enzymes in each subfamily differs from one species to the next.

Human liver microsomes can contain 15 or more different P450 enzymes (CYP1A1, 1A2, 2A6, 2B6, 2C8, 2C9, 2C18, 2C19, 2D6, 2E1, 3A4, 3A5, 3A7, 4A9, and 4A11) that biotransform xenobiotics and/or endogenous substrates (Guengerich, 1994; Wrighton and Stevens, 1992). Other P450 enzymes in human liver microsomes have been described but they appear to be allelic variants of the aforementioned enzymes rather than distinct gene products. For example, CYP2C10 and CYP3A3 appear to be allelic variants of CYP2C9 and CYP3A4, respectively. Unfortunately, a nomenclature system based on structure does not guarantee that structurally related proteins in different species will perform the same function (examples of such functional differences are given later). Some P450 enzymes have the same name in all mammalian species, whereas others are named in a species-specific manner. For example, all mammalian species contain two P450 enzymes belonging to the CYP1A subfamily, and in all cases these are known as CYP1A1 and CYP1A2 because the function and regulation of these enzymes are highly conserved among mammalian species. The same is true of CYP2E1. In other words, CYP1A1, CYP1A2, and CYP2E1 are not species-specific names, but rather they are names given to proteins in all mammalian species. In all other cases, functional or evolutionary relationships are not immediately apparent, hence, the P450 enzymes are named in a species-specific manner, and the names are assigned in chronological order regardless of the species of origin. For example, human liver microsomes express CYP2A6, but this is the only functional member of the CYP2A subfamily found in the human liver. The other members of this subfamily (i.e., CYP2A1–CYP2A5) are the names given to rat and mouse proteins, which were sequenced before the human enzyme. With the exception of CYP1A1, CYP1A2, and CYP2E1, the names of all of the other P450 enzymes in human liver microsomes refer specifically to human P450 enzymes.

Without exception, the levels and activity of each P450 enzyme have been shown to vary from one individual to the next, due to environmental and/or genetic factors (Meyer, 1994; Shimada et al., 1994). Decreased P450 enzyme activity can result from (1) a genetic mutation that either blocks the synthesis of a P450 enzyme or leads to the synthesis of a catalytically compromised or inactive enzyme, (2) exposure to an environmental factor (such as an infectious disease or a xenobiotic) that suppresses P450 enzyme expression, or (3) exposure to a xenobiotic that inhibits or inactivates a preexisting P450 enzyme. By inhibiting cytochrome P450, one drug can impair the biotransformation of another, which may lead to an exaggerated pharmacological or toxicological response to the second drug. In this regard, inhibition of cytochrome P450 mimics the effects of a genetic deficiency in P450 enzyme expression. Increased P450 enzyme activity can result from (1) gene duplication leading to overexpression of a P450 enzyme, (2) exposure to environmental factors, such as xenobiotics, that induce the synthesis of cytochrome P450, or (3) stimulation of pre-existing enzyme by a xenobiotic.

Although activation of cytochrome P450 has been documented in vitro, it appears to occur in vivo only under special circumstances. Although duplication of functional P450 genes has been documented, induction of cytochrome P450 by xenobiotics is the most common mechanism by which P450 enzyme activity is increased. By inducing cytochrome P450, one drug can stimulate the metabolism of a second drug and thereby decrease or ameliorate its therapeutic effect. A dramatic effect of this type of drug interaction is the induction of ethinylestradiol metabolism by phenobarbital and rifampin, which can ameliorate the contraceptive effect of the former drug and lead to unplanned pregnancy. Allelic variants, which arise by point mutations in the wild-type gene, are another source of interindividual variation in P450 activity. Amino acid substitutions can increase or, more commonly, decrease P450 enzyme activity, although the effect may be substrate-dependent. Examples of genetic factors that influence P450 activity are given below, this section. The environmental factors known to affect P450 levels include medications (e.g., barbiturates, rifampin, isoniazid), foods (e.g., cruciferous vegetables, charcoal-broiled beef), social habits (e.g., alcohol consumption, cigarette smoking), and disease status (diabetes, inflammation, hyperthyroidism, and hypothyroidism). When environmental factors influence P450 enzyme levels, considerable variation may be observed during repeated measures of xenobiotic biotransformation (e.g., drug metabolism) in the same individual. Such variation is not observed when alterations in P450 activity are determined genetically.

Due to their broad substrate specificity, it is possible that two or more P450 enzymes can contribute to the metabolism of a single compound. For example, two P450 enzymes, designated CYP2D6 and CYP2C19, both contribute significantly to the metabolism of propranolol in humans: CYP2D6 oxidizes the aromatic ring to give 4-hydroxypropranolol, whereas CYP2C19 oxidizes the isopropanolamine side chain to give naphthoxylactic acid (see Fig. 6-19). Consequently, changes in either CYP2D6 or CYP2C19 do not markedly affect the disposition of propranolol. Three human P450 enzymes, CYP1A2, CYP2E1, and CYP3A4, can convert the commonly used analgesic, acetaminophen, to its hepatotoxic metabolite, *N*-acetylbenzoquinoneimine (Fig. 6-39). It is also possible for a single P450 enzyme to catalyze two or more metabolic pathways for the same drug. For example, CYP2D6 catalyzes both the *O*-demethylation and 5-hydroxylation (aromatic ring hydroxylation) of methoxyphenamine, and CYP3A4 catalyzes the 3-hydroxylation and *N*-oxygenation of quinidine, the M1-, M17-, and M21-oxidation of cyclosporin, the 1-and 4-hydroxylation of midazolam, the *tert*-butyl-hydroxylation and *N*-dealkylation of terfenadine, and several pathways of testosterone oxidation, including 1$\beta$-, 2$\beta$-, 6$\beta$-, and 15$\beta$-hydroxylation and dehydrogenation to 6-dehydrotestosterone (Figs. 6-32 and 6-39).

The pharmacological or toxic effects of certain drugs are exaggerated in a significant percentage of the population due to a heritable deficiency in a P450 enzyme (Tucker, 1994; Meyer, 1994). The cytochrome P450 deficiencies identified to date include CYP2D6 and CYP2C19, which appear to be inherited as autosomal recessive traits (which in the case of CYP2D6 have been shown to result from a variety of mutations in the *CYP2D6* gene). Individuals lacking CYP2D6 or CYP2C19 were initially identified as poor metabolizers of debrisoquine and *S*-mephenytoin, respectively. However, because each P450 enzyme has a broad substrate specificity, each genetic defect affects the metabolism of several drugs. The incidence of the poor-metabolizer phenotype varies among different ethnic groups. For example, 5 to 10 percent of Caucasians are poor metabolizers of debrisoquine (an antihypertensive drug metabolized by CYP2D6), whereas less than 1 percent of Japanese subjects are defective in CYP2D6 activity. In contrast, ~20 percent of Japanese subjects are poor metabolizers of *S*-mephenytoin (an anticonvulsant metabolized by CYP2C19), whereas less than 5 percent of Caucasians are so affected. Some individuals have been identified as poor metabolizers of tolbutamide and phenytoin, both of which are metabolized by CYP2C9, or as poor metabolizers of phenacetin, which is metabolized by CYP1A2. However, the incidence of each of these phenotypes is apparently less than 1 percent.

The observation that individuals who are genetically deficient in a particular P450 enzyme are poor metabolizers of one or more drugs illustrates a very important principle; namely that the rate of elimination of drugs can be largely determined by a single P450 enzyme. This observation seems to contradict the fact that P450 enzymes have broad and overlapping substrate specificities. The resolution to this apparent paradox lies in the fact that although more than one human P450 enzyme can catalyze the biotransformation of a xenobiotic, they may do so with markedly different affinities. Consequently, xenobiotic biotransformation in vivo, where only low substrate concentrations are usually achieved, is often determined by the P450 enzyme with the highest affinity (lowest apparent $K_m$) for the xenobiotic. For example, the *N*-demethylation of diazepam (shown in Fig. 6-36) and the 5-hydroxylation of omeprazole are both catalyzed by two human P450 enzymes, namely CYP2C19 and CYP3A4. However, these reactions are catalyzed by CYP3A4 with such low affinity that the *N*-demethylation of diazepam and the 5-hydroxylation of omeprazole in vivo appear to be dominated by CYP2C19 (Kato and Yamazoe, 1994a). When several P450 enzymes catalyze the same reaction, their relative contribution to xenobiotic biotransformation is determined by the kinetic parameter, $V_{max}/K_m$, which is a measure of in vitro intrinsic clearance at low substrate concentrations (<10 percent of $K_m$) (Houston, 1994).

Inasmuch as the biotransformation of a xenobiotic in humans is frequently dominated by a single P450 enzyme, considerable attention has been paid to defining the substrate specificity of the P450 enzymes expressed in human liver microsomes (a process commonly referred to as *reaction phenotyping*). Four in vitro approaches have been developed for reaction phenotyping. Each has its advantages and disadvantages, and a combination of approaches is usually required to identify which human P450 enzyme is responsible for metabolizing a xenobiotic (Wrighton et al., 1993). The four approaches to reaction phenotyping are:

1. *Correlation analysis*, which involves measuring the rate of xenobiotic metabolism by several samples of human liver microsomes and correlating reaction rates with the variation in the level or activity of the individual P450 enzymes in the same microsomal samples. This approach is successful because the levels of the P450 enzymes in human liver microsomes vary enormously from sample to sample (up to 100-fold) but vary independently from each other.
2. *Chemical inhibition*, which involves an evaluation of the effects of known P450 enzyme inhibitors on the metabolism of a xenobiotic by human liver microsomes. Chemical inhibitors of cytochrome P450, which are discussed later, must be used cautiously because most of them can inhibit more than one P450 enzyme. Some chemical inhibitors are mechanism-based inhibitors that require biotransformation to a metabolite that inactivates or noncompetitively inhibits cytochrome P450.
3. *Antibody inhibition*, which involves an evaluation of the effects of inhibitory antibodies against selected P450 enzymes on the biotransformation of a xenobiotic by human liver microsomes. Due to the ability of antibodies to inhibit selectively and noncompetitively, this method alone can establish which human P450 enzyme is responsible for biotransforming a xenobiotic. Unfortunately, the utility of this method is limited by the availability of inhibitory antibodies.
4. *Biotransformation by purified or cDNA-expressed human P450 enzymes*, which can establish whether a particular P450 enzyme can or cannot biotransform a xenobiotic, but it does not address whether that P450 enzyme contributes substantially to reactions catalyzed by human liver microsomes. The information obtained with purified or cDNA-expressed human P450 enzymes can be improved by taking into account large differences in the extent to which the individual P450 enzymes are expressed in human liver microsomes, which is summarized in Table 6-3 (adapted from Shimada et al., 1994). Some P450 enzymes, such as CYP1A1 and CYP2B6, are expressed at such low levels in human liver microsomes that they seldom contribute significantly to the biotransformation of xenobiotics that are excellent substrates for these enzymes. Other P450 enzymes are expressed in some but not all livers. For example, CYP3A5 is expressed in ~25 percent of human livers. By definition, allelic variants, such as CYP2C10 and CYP3A3, are not expressed in all human livers.

**Table 6–3**
**Concentration of Individual P450 Enzymes in Human Liver Microsomes**

| | CONCENTRATION IN LIVER MICROSOMES (n = 60) | |
|---|---|---|
| P450 ENZYME | SPECIFIC CONTENT (PMOL/MG PROTEIN) | PERCENTAGE OF TOTAL SPECTRAL P450 |
| Total P450 (Determined spectrally) | 344 ± 167 | |
| Total P450 (Sum of individual enzymes determined immunochemically) | 240 ± 100 | 72.0 ± 15.3 |
| CYP1A2 | 42 ± 23 | 12.7 ± 6.2 |
| CYP2A6 | 14 ± 13 | 4.0 ± 3.2 |
| CYP2B6 | 1 ± 2 | 0.2 ± 0.3 |
| CYP2C* | 60 ± 27 | 18.2 ± 6.7 |
| CYP2D6 | 5 ± 4 | 1.5 ± 1.3 |
| CYP2E1 | 22 ± 12 | 6.6 ± 2.9 |
| CYP3A† | 96 ± 51 | 28.8 ± 10.4 |

*Sum of CYP2C8, 2C9, 2C18, and 2C19 and allelic variants (e.g., CYP2C10).
†Sum of CYP3A4, 3A5, and 3A7 and allelic variants (e.g., CYP3A3).
From Shimada et al. (1994).

These in vitro approaches have been used to characterize the substrate specificity of several of the P450 enzymes expressed in human liver microsomes. Examples of reactions catalyzed by human P450 enzymes are shown in Figs. 6-32 through 6-39, and lists of substrates, inhibitors and inducers for each P450 enzyme are given in Table 6-4. It should be emphasized that reaction phenotyping in vitro is not always carried out with pharmacologically or toxicologically relevant substrate concentrations. As a result, the P450 enzyme that appears responsible for biotransforming the drug in vitro may not be the P450 enzyme responsible for biotransforming the drug in vivo. This may be particularly true of CYP3A4, which metabolizes several drugs with high capacity but low affinity. The salient features of the major P450 enzymes in human liver microsomes are summarized below (subsequent sections, this chapter).

***CYP1A1/2.*** All mammalian species apparently possess two inducible CYP1A enzymes, namely CYP1A1 and CYP1A2 (see Table 6-3). Human liver microsomes contain relatively high levels of CYP1A2, but not CYP1A1, even though this enzyme is readily detectable in the human lung, intestine, skin, lymphocytes, and placenta, particularly from cigarette smokers. In addition to cigarette smoke, inducers of the CYP1A enzymes include charcoal-broiled meat (a source of polycyclic aromatic hydrocarbons), cruciferous vegetables (a source of various indoles), and omeprazole, a proton-pump inhibitor used to suppress gastric acid secretion. In contrast to CYP1A1, CYP1A2 is not expressed in extrahepatic tissues. CYP1A1 and CYP1A2 both catalyze the *O*-dealkylation of 7-methoxyresorufin and 7-ethoxyresorufin (see Fig. 6-36). Reactions preferentially catalyzed by CYP1A1 include the hydroxylation and epoxidation of benzo[a]pyrene (see Fig. 6-5) and the epoxidation of the leukotriene $D_4$ receptor antagonist, verlukast (Fig. 6-34). CYP1A2 catalyzes the *N*-hydroxylation of aromatic amines, such as 4-aminobiphenyl and 2-aminonaphthalene, which in many cases represents the initial step in the conversion of aromatic amines to tumorigenic metabolites (see Fig. 6-7). CYP1A2 also catalyzes the *O*-dealkylation of phenacetin and the 4-hydroxylation of acetanilide, both of which produce acetaminophen, which can be converted by CYP1A2 and other P450 enzymes to a toxic benzoquinoneimine (Fig. 6-24). As shown in Fig. 6-36, CYP1A2 catalyzes the *N3*-demethylation of caffeine to paraxanthine. By measuring rates of formation of paraxanthine in blood, urine, or saliva or by measuring the exhalation of isotopically labelled $CO_2$ from $^{13}C$- or $^{14}C$-labeled caffeine, the *N3*-demethylation of caffeine can be used as an in vivo probe of CYP1A2 activity, which varies enormously from one individual to the next. CYP1A1 and CYP1A2 are both inhibited by $\alpha$-naphthoflavone. Ellipticine preferentially inhibits CYP1A1, whereas the mechanism-based inhibitor furafylline is a specific inhibitor of CYP1A2.

Although CYP1A1 and CYP1A2 are expressed in all mammals, there are species differences in their function and regulation. For example, although CYP1A1 is not expressed in human liver (or in the liver of most other mammalian species), it appears to be constitutively expressed in Rhesus monkey and guinea pig liver. Conversely, although CYP1A2 is expressed in human liver (and in most other mammalian species), it does not appear to be constitutively expressed in Cynomolgus monkey liver. Polycyclic and polyhalogenated aromatic hydrocarbons appear to induce CYP1A enzymes in all mammalian species. In contrast, omeprazole is an inducer of CYP1A enzymes in humans, but not in mice or rabbits (Diaz et al., 1990). The function of the CYP1A enzymes is fairly well conserved across species, although there are subtle differences. For example, in some species, such as the rat, CYP1A1 is considerably more effective than CYP1A2 as a catalyst of 7-ethoxyresorufin *O*-dealkylation, whereas the opposite is true in other species, such as rabbit. In mice, CYP1A1 and CYP1A2 catalyze the *O*-dealkylation of 7-ethoxyresorufin at comparable rates. In the rat, CYP1A1 preferentially catalyzes the *O*-dealkylation of 7-ethoxyresorufin whereas CYP1A2 preferentially catalyzes the *O*-dealkylation of 7-methoxyresorufin. However, in other species, such as the mouse and the human, CYP1A2 catalyzes the *O*-dealkylation of 7-ethoxyresorufin and 7-methoxyresorufin at about the same rate. There are also species differences in the affinity with which CYP1A2 interacts with xenobiotics. For example, furafylline is a potent, mechanism-based inhibitor of human CYP1A2, but it is a weak inhibitor of rat CYP1A2. Although the levels of CYP1A2 vary enormously from one individual to the next, genetic defects in CYP1A2 are rare (<1 percent).

***CYP2B6.*** Human liver microsomes generally contain little or no CYP2B6 (see Table 6-5); therefore, this P450 enzyme does not appear to play an important role in xenobiotic biotransformation. By analogy with the rodent CYP2B enzymes, CYP2B6 would be expected to be inducible by barbiturates and other drugs (discussed below, in "Induction of Cytochrome P450"). However, the levels of CYP2B6 are extremely low even in individuals treated with phenobarbital. It would appear that the ability of phenobarbital to stimulate the biotransformation of xenobiotics in humans largely stems from its ability to induce the CYP2C and CYP3A enzymes.

***CYP2A6.*** Enzymes belonging to the *CYP2A* gene family show marked species differences in catalytic function. For example, the two CYP2A enzymes expressed in rat liver, namely CYP2A1 and CYP2A2, primarily catalyze the $7\alpha$- and $15\alpha$-hydroxylation of testosterone, respectively. In contrast, the CYP2A enzyme expressed in human liver, namely CYP2A6, catalyzes the 7-hydroxylation of coumarin, as shown in Fig. 6-33. Just as rat CYP2A1 and CYP2A2 have little or no capacity to 7-hydroxylate coumarin, human CYP2A6 has little or no capacity to hydroxylate testosterone. Mouse liver microsomes contain three CYP2A enzymes; a testosterone $7\alpha$-hydroxylase (CYP2A1), a testosterone $15\alpha$-hydroxylase (CYP2A4), and a coumarin 7-hydroxylase (CYP2A5). Functionally, CYP2A5 can be converted to CYP2A4 by a single amino acid substitution ($Phe^{209} \rightarrow Leu^{209}$). In other words, this single amino substitution converts CYP2A5 from a coumarin 7-hydroxylating to a testosterone $15\alpha$-hydroxylating enzyme (Lindberg and Negishi, 1989). The fact that a small change in primary structure can have a dramatic effect on substrate specificity makes it difficult to predict whether orthologous proteins in different species (which are structurally similar but never identical) will catalyze the same reactions.

Differences in CYP2A function have important implications for the adverse effects of coumarin, which is hepatotoxic to rats but not humans. Whereas coumarin is detoxified in humans by conversion to 7-hydroxycoumarin, which is sub-

**Table 6–4**
**Examples of Substrates, Inhibitors, and Inducers of the Major Human Liver Microsomal P450 Enzymes Involved in Xenobiotic Biotransformation**

| CYP1A2 | CYP2A6 | CYP2B6 | CYP2C8 | CYP2C9 | CYP2C19 | CYP2D6 | CYP2E1 | CYP3A4 |
|---|---|---|---|---|---|---|---|---|
| | | | | *Substrates* | | | | |
| Acetaminophen | Coumarin | Cyclophosphamide | Carbamazepine | Diclofenac | Citalopram | Amiflamine | Acetaminophen | Acetaminophen |
| Acetanilide | Butadiene | Ifosphamide | Taxol | Phenytoin | Diazepam | Amitriptyline | Alcohols | Aldrin |
| Aromatic amines | Nicotine | | | Piroxicam | Diphenylhydantoin | Aprindine | Aniline | Alfentanil |
| Caffeine | | | | Tenoxicam | Hexobarbital | Brofaromine | Benzene | Amiodarone |
| Estradiol | | | | Tetrahydrocannabinol | Imipramine | Bufurolol | Caffeine | Astemizole |
| Ethoxyresorufin | | | | Tienilic acid | Lansoprazole | Captopril | Chlorzoxazone | Benzphetamine |
| Imipramine | | | | Tolbutamide | *S*-Mephenytoin | Cinnarizine | Dapsone | Budesonide |
| Methoxyresorufin | | | | Torsemide | Mephobarbital | Citalopram | Enflurane | Carbemaze- |
| Phenacetin | | | | Warfarin | Omeprazole | Clonipramine | Halogenated | pine |
| Theophylline | | | | | Pentamidine | Clozapine | aklanes | Cyclophospha- |
| Warfarin | | | | | Proguanil | Codeine | Isoflurane | mide |
| | | | | | Propranolol | Debrisoquine | Methylformamide | Cyclosporin |
| | | | | | | Deprenyl | p-Nitrophenol | Dapsone |
| | | | | | | Desmethylcita- | Nitrosamines | Digitoxin |
| | | | | | | lopram | Styrene | Diltiazem |
| | | | | | | Despiramine | Theophylline | Diazepam |
| | | | | | | Dextro- | | Erythromycin |
| | | | | | | methorphan | | Ethinylestradiol |
| | | | | | | Encainide | | Etoposide |
| | | | | | | Flecainide | | Flutamide |
| | | | | | | Fluoxetine | | Hydroxyarginine |
| | | | | | | Flunarizine | | Ifosphamide |
| | | | | | | Fluphenazine | | Imipramine |
| | | | | | | Guanoxan | | Lansoprazole |
| | | | | | | Haloperidol (reduced) | | Lidocaine |
| | | | | | | Hydrocodone | | Loratadine |
| | | | | | | Imipramine | | Losartan |
| | | | | | | Indoramin | | Lovastatin |
| | | | | | | Methoxyampheta- | | Midazolam |
| | | | | | | mine | | Nifedipine |
| | | | | | | Methoxyphenamine | | Omeprazole |
| | | | | | | Metoprolol | | Quinidine |
| | | | | | | Mexiletene | | Rapamycin |
| | | | | | | Mianserin | | Retinoic Acid |
| | | | | | | Miniaprine | | Steroids |
| | | | | | | Nortriptyline | | (e.g., cortisol) |
| | | | | | | Ondansetron | | Tacrolimus (FK 506) |
| | | | | | | Paroxetine | | Tamoxifen |
| | | | | | | Perhexiline | | Taxol |
| | | | | | | Perphenazine | | Teniposide |
| | | | | | | Propafenone | | Terfenadine |

| | | | | | | | | |
|---|---|---|---|---|---|---|---|---|
| | | | | | | Propranolol<br>*N*-Propylajmaline<br>Remoxipride<br>Sparteine<br>Thioridazine<br>Timolol<br>Tomoxetine<br>Trifluperidol<br>Tropisetron | | Tetrahydrocan-<br>nabinol<br>Theophylline<br>Toremifene<br>Triazolam<br>Troleandomycin<br>Verapamil<br>Warfarin<br>Zatosetron<br>Zonisamide |
| *Inhibitors* | | | | | | | | |
| Furafylline*<br>α-Naphthoflavone<br><I> | Diethyldithio-<br>carbamate<br>8-Metho-<br>xypsoralen*<br>Tranylcypromine | Orphenadrine* | Quercetin | Sulfaphenazole<br>Sulfinpyrazone | Tranylcypromine | Ajmalicine<br>Chinidin<br>Corynanthine<br>Fluoxetine<br>Lobelin<br>Propidin<br>Quinidine<br>Trifluperidol<br>Yohimbine | 3-Amino-1,2,4-<br>triazole*<br>Diethyldithio-<br>carbamate<br>Dihydrocapsaicin<br>Dimethyl sulfoxide<br>Disulfiram<br>4-Methylpyrazole<br>Phenethyl<br>isothiocyanate* | Clotrimazole<br>Ethinylestradiol*<br>Gestodene*<br>Itraconazole<br>Ketoconazole<br>Miconazole<br>Naringenin<br>Troleandomycin*<br>Activator:<br>α-Naphthoflavone |
| *Inducers* | | | | | | | | |
| Charcoal-broiled beef<br>Cigarette smoke<br>Cruciferous vegetables<br>Omeprazole | Barbiturates | Not known | Not known | Rifampin | Rifampin | None<br>known | Ethanol<br>Isoniazid | Carbamazepine<br>Dexamethasone<br>Phenobarbital<br>Phenytoin<br>Rifampin<br>Sulfadimidine<br>Sulfinpyrazone<br>Troleandomycin |

*Mechanism-based inhibitor.

**Table 6–5**
**Examples of Xenobiotics Activated by Human P450**

CYP1A1
- Benzo[a]pyrene and other polycyclic aromatic hydrocarbons

CYP1A2
- Acetaminophen
- 2-Acetylaminofluorene
- 4-Aminobiphenyl
- 2-Aminofluorene
- 2-Naphthylamine
- NNK*
- Amino acid pyrrolysis products (DiMeQx, MelQ, MelQx, Glu P-1, Glu P-2, IQ, PhIP, Trp P-1, Trp P-2)

CYP2A6
- *N*-nitrosodiethylamine
- NNK*

CYP2B6
- 6-Aminochrysene
- Cyclophosphamide
- Ifosphamine

CYP2C8, 9, 18, 19
- None known

CYP2D6
- NNK*

CYP2E1
- Acetaminophen
- Acrylonitrile
- Benzene
- Carbon tetrachloride
- Chloroform
- Dichloromethane
- 1,2-Dichloropropane
- Ethylene dibromide
- Ethylene dichloride
- Ethyl carbamate
- *N*-Nitrosodimethylamine
- Styrene
- Trichlorothylene
- Vinyl chloride

CYP3A4
- Acetaminophen
- Aflatoxin $B_1$ and $G_1$
- 6-Aminochrysene
- Benzo[a]pyrene 7,8-dihydrodiol
- Cyclophosphamide
- Ifosphamide
- 1-Nitropyrene
- Sterigmatocystin
- Senecionine
- *Tris*(2,3-dibromopropyl) phosphate

CYP4A9/11
- None known

*NNK, 4-(methylnitrosamino)-1-(3-pyridyl)-1-butanone, a tobacco-specific nitrosamine.
Adapted from Guengerich (1991).

sequently conjugated with glucuronic acid and excreted, a major pathway of coumarin biotransformation in rats involves formation of the hepatotoxic metabolite, coumarin 3,4-epoxide, as shown in Fig. 6-34. In addition to catalyzing the 7-hydroxylation of coumarin, CYP2A6 converts 1,3-butadiene to butadiene monoxide and nicotine to nicotine $\Delta^{1',5'}$-iminium ion, which is further oxidized by aldehyde oxidase to cotinine, as shown in Fig. 6-39. 8-Methoxypsoralen, a structural analog of coumarin, is a potent, mechanism-based inhibitor of CYP2A6. Although the levels of CYP2A6 vary enormously from one individual to the next, genetic defects in this enzyme are rare (<1 percent).

***CYP2C9.*** A genetic polymorphism for tolbutamide metabolism was first described in 1978–1979, although its incidence is still unknown (Back and Orme, 1992). Poor metabolizers are presumably defective in CYP2C9, which catalyzes the methylhydroxylation of this hypoglycemic agent. Poor metabolizers of tolbutamide are also poor metabolizers of phenytoin, which is consistent with in vitro data suggesting that CYP2C9 catalyzes both the methylhydroxylation of tolbutamide and the 4-hydroxylation of phenytoin. CYP2C9 is responsible for the biotransformation of several nonsteroidal anti-inflammatory drugs (NSAIDs), including the 4′-hydroxylation of diclofenac and the 5′-hydroxylation of piroxicam and tenoxicam. Tienilic acid is also metabolized by CYP2C9, but with potentially deleterious effects. CYP2C9 converts tienilic acid to an electrophilic thiophene sulfoxide that can react either with water to give 5-hydroxytienilic acid or with a nucleophilic amino acid in CYP2C9 to form a covalent adduct, which inactivates the enzyme (Lecoeur et al., 1994). Antibodies directed against the adduct between CYP2C9 and tienilic acid are thought to be responsible for the immunoallergic hepatitis that develops in about 1 out of every 10,000 patients treated with this uricosuric diuretic drug. Sulfaphenazole is a potent inhibitor of CYP2C9, both in vitro and in vivo.

CYP2C10 ($Cys^{358}$ and $Asp^{417}$) and CYP2C9 ($Tyr^{358}$ and $Gly^{417}$) differ by only two amino acids and are probably allelic variants rather than distinct gene products. A number of other allelic variants of CYP2C9 have been described, which are generated by one or more amino acid substitutions at positions 144, 358, 359, and 417. These amino acid substitutions can influence catalytic activity in substrate-dependent manner. For example, although the wild-type CYP2C9 ($Arg^{144}$, $Tyr^{358}$, $Ile^{359}$, $Gly^{417}$) and its allelic variant CYP2C9($Arg^{144} \rightarrow Cys^{144}$) both catalyze the methylhydroxylation of tolbutamide (the former being twice as active as the latter), the latter enzyme is virtually devoid of *S*-warfarin 6- and 7-hydroxylase activity (Rettie et al., 1994). This raises the intriguing possibility that individuals who express only the allelic variant CYP2C9 ($Arg^{144} \rightarrow Cys^{144}$) could be poor metabolizers of warfarin but extensive metabolizers of tolbutamide.

***CYP2C19.*** A genetic polymorphism for the metabolism of *S*-mephenytoin was first described in 1984 (reviewed in Wilkinson et al., 1989). The deficiency affects the 4′-hydroxylation (aromatic ring hydroxylation) of this anticonvulsant drug. The other major pathway of *S*-mephenytoin metabolism, namely *N*-demethylation to *S*-nirvanol, is not affected. Consequently, poor metabolizers excrete little or no 4′-hydroxymephenytoin in their urine, but they do excrete increased amounts of the *N*-demethylated metabolite, *S*-nirvanol (*S*-phenylethylhydantoin). Interestingly, the P450 enzyme responsible for this genetic polymorphism, namely CYP2C19, is highly stereoselective for the *S*-enantiomer of mephenytoin. In contrast to the *S*-enantiomer, the *R*-enantiomer is not converted to 4′-hydroxymephenytoin, but it is *N*-demethylated to *R*-nirvanol (*R*-phenylethylhydantoin). The formulation of mephenytoin used clinically is mesantoin, which is a racemic mixture of *S*- and *R*-enantiomers. An exaggerated central response has been observed in poor metabolizers administered mephenytoin at doses that were without effect in extensive metabolizers of mephenytoin. There is considerable interethnic variation in the incidence of the poor metabolizer phenotype for *S*-mephenytoin. In Caucasians, CYP2C19 is defective in as few as 2 to 5 percent of the population, but it is defective in as many as 12 to 23 percent of Japanese, Chinese, and Korean subjects. Other substrates for CYP2C19 are listed in Table 6-4. Based on clinical observations, CYP2C19 appears to determine the in vivo rate of diazepam *N*-demethylation and omeprazole 5-hydroxylation. CYP2C19 also converts proguanil to its active antimalarial metabolite, cycloguanil. The monoamine oxidase inhibitor, tranylcypromine, is a potent but not specific inhibitor of CYP2C19.

***CYP2C8 and CYP2C18.*** The 6$\alpha$-hydroxylation of the taxane ring of taxol (which generates a metabolite known variously as M5, VIII′, and HM3) is catalyzed primarily by CYP2C8 (Rahman et al., 1994). The minor pathway of taxol metabolism, aromatic hydroxylation to M4 (also known as VII′), is catalyzed by CYP3A enzymes. Like CYP2C9, CYP2C8 catalyzes the methylhydroxylation of tolbutamide. However, because of its higher $K_m$ and lower $V_{max}$, CYP2C8 probably contributes negligibly to the methylhydroxylation of tolbutamide in vivo. CYP2C8 catalyzes the 10,11-epoxidation of carbamazepine, although this reaction in human liver microsomes is dominated by CYP3A4. The functions of CYP2C18 are largely unknown. The levels of CYP2C18 mRNA vary independently of the mRNAs encoding CYP2C8 and CYP2C9, which tend to be coregulated.

The multiplicity, function, and regulation of the CYP2C enzymes vary enormously from one species to the next. For example, whereas the 4′-hydroxylation of *S*-mephenytoin in humans is catalyzed by CYP2C19, this same reaction in rats is catalyzed by a CYP3A enzyme, not a CYP2C enzyme. Conversely, one of the reactions catalyzed by rat CYP2C11, namely the 2$\alpha$-hydroxylation of testosterone, is not catalyzed by the human CYP2C enzymes (or any of the other P450 enzymes in human liver microsomes).

***CYP2D6.*** In the late 1950s, clinical trials in the United States established that sparteine was as potent as oxytocin for inducing labor at term. However, the duration and intensity of action of sparteine was dramatically increased in ~7 percent of all patients tested. The exaggerated response to sparteine included prolonged (tetanic) uterine contraction and abnormally rapid labor. In some cases, sparteine caused the death of the fetus. The drug was not recommended for clinical use because these side effects were unpredictable and occurred at doses of 100–200 mg/kg, which were well tolerated by other patients. The antihypertensive drug, debrisoquine, was subsequently found to cause a marked and prolonged hypotension in 5 to 10 percent of patients, and a genetic polymorphism for the metabolism of debrisoquine and sparteine was discovered in 1977–1979 (Gonzalez, 1989; Meyer, 1994). Poor metabolizers lack CYP2D6, which catalyzes the 4-hydroxylation of debrisoquine and the $\Delta^2$- and $\Delta^5$-oxidation of sparteine (see Fig. 6-39).

In addition to debrisoquine and sparteine, CYP2D6 biotransforms a large number of drugs, as shown in Table 6-4. Individuals lacking CYP2D6 have an exaggerated response to most but not all of these drugs. For example, even though debrisoquine and propranolol are both biotransformed by CYP2D6, the effects of propranolol are not exaggerated in poor metabolizers of debrisoquine, for two reasons. First, 4-hydroxypropranolol is a $\beta$-adrenoceptor antagonist, so the 4-hydroxylation of propranolol by CYP2D6 does not terminate the pharmacological effects of the drug. Second, CYP2D6 is not the only P450 enzyme to biotransform propranolol. As mentioned above, CYP2C19 catalyzes the side-chain oxidation of propranolol to naphthoxylactic acid (see Fig. 6-19). Because CYP2D6 and CYP2C19 both contribute significantly to the biotransformation of propranolol, a deficiency in either one of these enzymes does not markedly alter the pharmacokinetics of this beta blocker. However, in one individual who lacked both enzymes, the total oral clearance of propranolol was markedly reduced (Wilkinson et al., 1989). CYP2D6 catalyzes the *O*-demethylation of codeine to the potent analgesic, morphine. Pain control with codeine is reduced in individuals lacking CYP2D6.

The biotransformation of substrates for CYP2D6 occurs 5 to 7.5Å from a basic nitrogen, which interacts with an anionic residue ($Glu^{301}$) in the enzyme's substrate-binding site (Strobl et al., 1993). Quinidine is a potent inhibitor of CYP2D6 because it interacts favorably with the anionic site on CYP2D6 but it cannot be oxidized at a site 5 to 7.5Å from its basic nitrogen atoms. Fluoxetine (and several other serotonin-uptake inhibitors), ajmalicine, and yohimbine are also potent competitive inhibitors of CYP2D6. A poor metabolizer phenotype can be induced pharmacologically with these potent inhibitors of CYP2D6. Quinine, the levorotatory diasteriomer of quinidine, is not a potent inhibitor of CYP2D6, and neither drug is a potent inhibitor of the CYP2D enzymes expressed in rats. CYP2D6 is one of the few P450 enzymes that efficiently use the peroxide shunt, so that reactions catalyzed by CYP2D6 can be supported by cumene hydroperoxide.

As shown in Fig. 6-36, CYP2D6 catalyzes the *O*-demethylation of dextromethorphan to dextrorphan, which is glucuronidated and excreted in urine. Dextromethorphan can also be *N*-demethylated, a reaction catalyzed predominantly by CYP3A4, but this metabolite is not glucuronidated and excreted in urine. Because the urinary excretion of dextromethorphan is dependent on *O*-demethylation, this over-the-counter antitussive drug can be used to identify individuals lacking CYP2D6, although most poor metabolizers can be identified by DNA analysis. There is considerable interethnic variation in the incidence of the poor metabolizer phenotype for debrisoquine/sparteine. In caucasians, CYP2D6 is defective in 5 to 10 percent of the population, but it is defective in less than 2 percent of African Americans, Africans, Thai, Chinese, and Japanese subjects. Individuals lacking CYP2D6 have an unusually low incidence of some chemically induced neoplastic diseases, such as lung cancer, bladder cancer, hepatocellular carcinoma, and endemic Balkan nephropathy (Idle, 1991). It has been hypothesized that CYP2D6 may play a role in the metabolic activation of chemical carcinogens, such as those present in the environment, in the diet, and/or in cigarette smoke. According to this hypothesis, individuals lacking CYP2D6 have a low incidence of cancer because they fail to activate chemical carcinogens. However, CYP2D6 appears to play little or no role in the activation of known chemical carcinogens to DNA-reactive or mutagenic metabolites, with the possible exception of the tobacco-smoke specific nitrosamine, 4-(methylnitrosamino)-1-(3-pyridyl)-1-butanone (NNK), which is also activated by other P450 enzymes. Therefore, it remains to be determined whether a deficiency of CYP2D6 is causally or coincidentally related to a low incidence of certain cancers.

***CYP2E1.*** As shown in Fig. 6-17, CYP2E1 was first identified as MEOS, the microsomal ethanol oxidizing system (Lieber, 1990). In addition to ethanol, CYP2E1 catalyzes the biotransformation of a large number halogenated alkanes (Guengerich et al., 1991). CYP2E1 is expressed constitutively in human liver and possibly in extrahepatic tissues, such as the kidney, lung, and lymphocytes, and the enzyme is inducible by ethanol and isoniazid. CYP2E1 catalyzes the *N1*- and *N7*-demethylation of caffeine to theobromine and theophylline, as shown in Fig. 6-36, and it can activate acetaminophen to the hepatotoxic metabolite, *N*-acetylbenzoquinoneimine, as shown in Figs. 6-24 and 6-39. The mechanism by which alcohol potentiates the hepatotoxic effects of acetaminophen (Tylenol) is thought to involve increased activation of acetaminophen, due to the induction of CYP2E1, and decreased inactivation, due to a lowering of glutathione levels. Induction of CYP2E1 by isoniazid stimulates the dehalogenation of the volatile anesthetics, enflurane and isoflurane. In human liver microsomes, CYP2E1 activity can be conveniently measured by the 6-hydroxylation of chlorzoxazone and the hydroxylation of *para*-nitrophenol. The 6-hydroxylation of chlorzoxazone can also be catalyzed by CYP1A1, but this enzyme is rarely expressed in human liver. Chlorzoxazone is an FDA-approved muscle relaxant (Paraflex), and the urinary excretion of 6-hydroxychlorzoxazone and the plasma ratio of 6-hydroxychlorzoxazone to chlorzoxazone have been used as noninvasive in vivo probes of CYP2E1. The levels of CYP2E1 are by no means constant among individuals, but they do not exhibit the marked interindividual variation characteristic of other P450 enzymes. CYP2E1 is one of the P450 enzymes that requires cytochrome $b_5$, which lowers the $K_m$ for several substrates biotransformed by CYP2E1. The function and regulation of CYP2E1 are well conserved among mammalian species.

***CYP3A.*** The most abundant P450 enzymes in human liver microsomes belong to the CYP3A gene subfamily, which includes CYP3A4 (or its allelic variant CYP3A3), CYP3A5, and CYP3A7. CYP3A7 is considered a fetal enzyme, whereas the others are considered to be adult forms, although livers from some adults contain CYP3A7 and some fetal livers contain CYP3A5. All human livers appear to contain CYP3A4, although the levels vary enormously (>10-fold) among individuals (Wrighton and Stevens, 1992; Shimada et al., 1994). CYP3A5 is expressed in relatively few livers (10–30 percent). One or more of these enzymes is expressed in extrahepatic tissues. For example, CYP3A4 is expressed in the small intestine, whereas CYP3A5 is expressed in 80 percent of all human kidneys. The CYP3A enzymes biotransform an extraordinary array of xenobiotics and steroids, as shown in Table 6-4. CYP3A enzymes also catalyze the oxidation of hydroxyarginine to citrulline and nitric oxide. Factors that influence the levels and/or activity of the CYP3A enzymes influence the biotransformation of many of the drugs listed in Table 6-4, and many of these drugs have been shown to inhibit each other's metabolism (Pichard et al., 1990).

In humans, CYP3A enzymes are inducible by numerous drugs, such as rifampin, dexamethasone, phenobarbital, and phenytoin (Pichard et al., 1990). Inhibitors of human CYP3A include imidazole-type antimycotics (e.g., ketoconazole and clotrimazole), macrolide antibiotics (e.g., erythromycin and troleandomycin), the ethynylprogesterone analog, gestodene, and certain flavones or other component(s) present in grapefruit juice. Although inhibited by naringenin (a grapefruit-derived flavone), CYP3A enzymes can also be stimulated by flavones in vitro, such as 7,8-benzoflavone ($\alpha$-naphthoflavone). Several noninvasive, clinical tests of CYP3A activity have been proposed, including the [$^{14}$C-*N*-methyl]-erythromycin breath test, the plasma clearance of midazolam and nifedipine, and the urinary excretion of 6$\beta$-hydroxycortisol and *N*-hydroxydapsone (Watkins, 1994). However, for reasons that are not yet understood, there can be marked differences in the results obtained with different tests in the same individuals. Nevertheless, the various noninvasive tests suggest that CYP3A activity varies widely among individuals (>10-fold), but there appear to be no individuals who are completely devoid of CYP3A activity, possibly due to the multiplicity of enzymes in the human CYP3A subfamily.

The function and regulation of the CYP3A enzymes is fairly well conserved among mammalian species, with some notable exceptions. For example, rifampin is an inducer of the CYP3A enzymes in humans and rabbits but not rats or mice, whereas the opposite appears to be true of pregnenolone-16$\alpha$-carbonitrile (Pichard et al., 1990). In adult rats, the levels of CYP3A2 in males are much greater (>10-fold) than in females, whereas no marked sex difference in CYP3A levels is observed in humans (if anything, the levels of CYP3A enzymes are higher in females than in males).

***CYP4A9/11.*** The CYP4A enzymes in humans and other mammalian species catalyze the $\omega$- and $\omega$-1 hydroxylation of fatty acids and their derivatives, including prostaglandins, thromboxane, prostacyclin, and leukotrienes. With lauric acid as substrate, the CYP4A enzymes preferentially catalyze the $\omega$-hydroxylation to 12-hydroxylauric acid (see Fig. 6-32), which can be further oxidized to form a dicarboxylic acid. Although CYP4A enzymes also catalyze the $\omega$-1 hydroxylation of lauric acid, other P450 enzymes, including CYP2E1, can contribute significantly to the formation of 11-hydroxylauric acid. The CYP4A enzymes are unusual for ability to preferentially catalyze the $\omega$-hydroxylation of fatty acids over the thermodynamically more favorable reaction leading to $\omega$-1 hydroxylation. Despite their physiological importance, the CYP4A enzymes appear to play a very limited role in the metabolism of drugs.

**Activation of Xenobiotics by Cytochrome P450.** Biotransformation by cytochrome P450 does not always lead to detoxication, and several examples have been given previously where the toxicity or tumorigenicity of a chemical depends on its activation by cytochrome P450. The role of individual human P450 enzymes in the activation of procarcinogens and protoxicants is summarized in Table 6-5 (adapted from Guengerich and Shimada, 1991). A variety of cytochrome P450-dependent reactions are involved in the activation of the chemicals listed in Table 6-5. The conversion of polycyclic aromatic hydrocarbons to tumor-forming metabolites involves the formation of bay-region diolepoxides, as shown in Fig. 6-5, for the conversion of benzo[a]pyrene to benzo[a]pyrene 7,8-dihydrodiol-9,10, epoxide. Epoxidation generates hepatotoxic metabolites of chlorobenzene and coumarin (Fig. 6-34), and generates an hepatotumorigenic metabolite of aflatoxin $B_1$ (Fig. 6-23).

The initial step in the conversion of aromatic amines to tumor-forming metabolites involves *N*-hydroxylation, as shown for 2-amino-6-nitrobenzylalcohol (Fig. 6-7) and 2-acetylaminofluorene (Fig. 6-29*A*). In the case of acetaminophen, activation to an hepatotoxic metabolite involves dehydrogenation to *N*-acetylbenzoquinoneimine, as shown in Fig. 6-24. A similar reaction converts butylated hydroxytoluene to a toxic quinone methide, as shown in Fig. 6-27. The myelotoxicity of benzene depends on its conversion to phenol and hydroquinone (Fig. 6-26). The toxicity of several organophosphorus insecticides involves oxidative group transfer to the corresponding organophosphate, as shown for the conversion of parathion to paraoxon in Figs. 6-37 and 6-38. The hepatotoxicity of carbon tetrachloride involves reductive dechlorination to a trichloromethyl free radical, which binds to protein and initiates lipid peroxidation, as shown in Fig. 6-12. The hepatotoxicity and nephrotoxicity of chloroform involves oxidative dechlorination to phosgene (Fig. 6-12). Oxidative and reductive dehalogenation both play a role in the activation of halothane, although hepatotoxicity in rats is more dependent on reductive dehalogenation, whereas the immune hepatitis in humans is largely a consequence of oxidative dehalogenation, which leads to the formation of neoantigens (Pohl et al., 1989). Formation of neoantigens (by covalent binding to CYP2C9) is also the mechanism by which the uricosuric diuretic drug, tienilic acid, causes immune hepatitis (Lecoeur et al., 1994).

Some of the chemicals listed in Table 6-5 are activated to toxic or tumorigenic metabolites by mechanisms not mentioned previously. For example, *N*-nitrosodimethylamine, which is representative of a large class of tumorigenic nitrosamines, is activated to an alkylating electrophile by *N*-demethylation, as shown in Fig. 6-40. The activation of ethyl carbamate (urethan) involves two sequential reactions catalyzed by cytochrome P450 (CYP2E1): dehydrogenation to vinyl carbamate followed by epoxidation, as shown in Fig. 6-40. CYP2E1 is one of several P450 enzymes that can catalyze the epoxidation of tetrachloroethylene. The rearrangement of this epoxide to a carbonyl is accompanied by migration of chlorine, which produces the highly reactive metabolite, trichloroacetylchloride, as shown in Fig. 6-40. The toxic pyrrolizidine alkaloids, such as senecionine, are cyclic arylamines that are dehydrogenated by cytochrome P450 (CYP3A4) to the corresponding pyrroles. Pyrroles themselves are nucleophiles, but electrophiles are generated through the loss of substituents on the pyrrolizidine nucleus, as shown in Fig. 6-40. Cyclophosphamide and ifosphamide are examples of chemicals designed to be activated to toxic electrophiles for the treatment of malignant tumors and other proliferative diseases. These drugs are nitrogen mustards, which have a tendency to undergo intramolecular nucleophilic displacement to form an electrophilic aziridinium species. In the case of cyclophosphamide and ifosphamide, the nitrogen mustard is stabilized by the presence of a phosphoryl oxygen, which delocalizes the lone pair of nitrogen electrons required for intramolecular nucleophilic displacement. For this reason, formation of an electrophilic aziridinium species requires hydroxylation by cytochrome P450, as shown in Fig. 6-40 for cyclophosphamide. Hydroxylation of the carbon atom next to the ring nitrogen leads spontaneously to ring opening and elimination of acrolein. In the resultant phosphoramide mustard, delocalization of the lone pair of nitrogen electrons to the phosphoryl oxygen is now disfavored by the presence of the lone pair of electrons on the oxygen anion, hence, the phosphoramide undergoes an intramolecular nucleophilic elimination to generate an electrophilic aziridinium species. This reaction is catalyzed by CYP3A4 and CYP2B6. In liver, the activation of cyclophosphamide by CYP2B6 may be negligible because relatively few human livers express this P450 enzyme (see Table 6-3). Cyclophosphamide is also activated by CYP2B enzymes in rats, one of which (CYP2B12) is expressed in the skin (Friedberg et al., 1992). Activation of cyclophosphamide by P450 enzymes in the skin would generate a cytotoxic metabolite at the base of hair follicles, which may be the reason why hair loss is one of the side effects of cyclophosphamide treatment.

Many of the chemicals listed in Table 6-5 are also detoxified by cytochrome P450 by biotransformation to less toxic metabolites. In some cases, the same P450 enzyme catalyzes both activation and detoxication reactions. For example, CYP3A4 activates aflatoxin $B_1$ to the hepatotoxic and tumorigenic 8,9-epoxide, but it also detoxifies aflatoxin $B_1$ by 3-hydroxylation to aflatoxin $Q_1$. Similarly, CYP3A4 activates senecionine by converting this pyrrolizidine alkaloid to the corresponding pyrrole, but it also detoxifies senecionine through formation of an *N*-oxide (a reaction mainly catalyzed by FMO3). Epoxidation of trichloroethylene by CYP2E1 appears to be both an activation and detoxication pathway, as shown in Fig. 6-40. Rearrangement of trichloroethylene epoxide can be accompanied by migration of chlorine, which produces chloral (trichloroacetaldehyde), or hydrogen, which produces dichloroacetylchloride. Chloral is much less toxic than dichloroacetylchloride, hence, migration of the chlorine during epoxide rearrangement is a detoxication reaction, whereas migration of the hydrogen is an activation reaction. These few examples serve to underscore the complexity of factors that determine the balance between xenobiotic activation and detoxication.

**Inhibition of Cytochrome P450.** In addition to predicting the likelihood of some individuals being poor metabolizers due to a genetic deficiency in P450 expression, information on which human P450 enzyme metabolizes a drug can help predict or explain drug interactions (Peck et al., 1993). For example, when administered with azole antifungals (e.g., ketoconazole and itraconazole) or macrolide antibiotics (e.g., erythromycin and troleandomycin), the antihistamine terfenadine (Seldane) can cause *Torsades de Pointes*, which in some individuals has apparently led to lethal ventricular arrhythmias

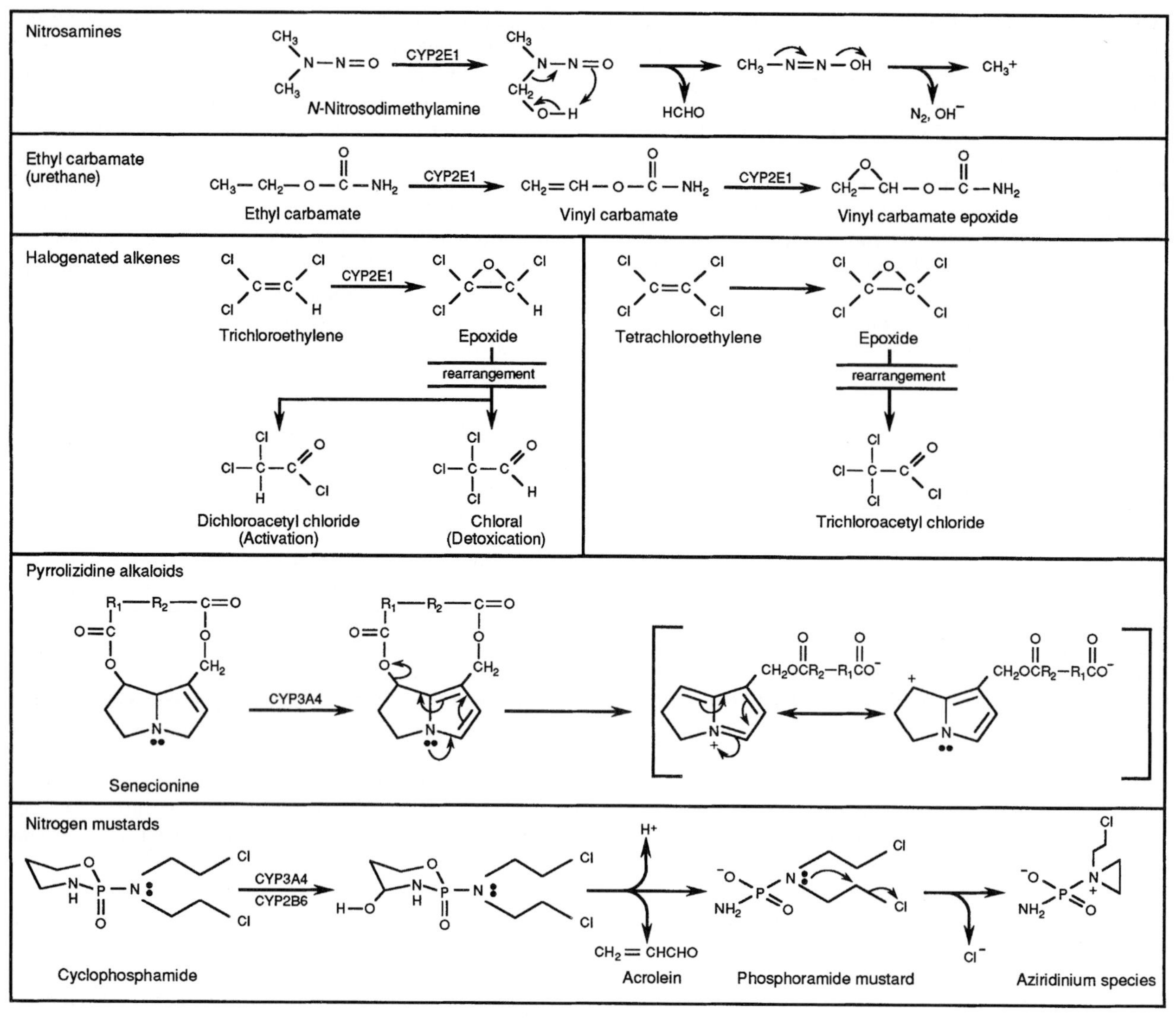


***Figure 6–40. Additional mechanisms of cytochrome P450-dependent activation of xenobiotics to electrophilic metabolites.***

(Kivsito et al., 1994). This drug interaction can be rationalized on the basis that terfenadine is normally converted by intestinal and liver CYP3A4 to a *tertiary*-butyl alcohol, which is further oxidized to a carboxylic acid metabolite. This latter metabolite blocks $H_1$-receptors and does not cross the blood–brain barrier, which is why terfenadine is a nonsedating antihistamine. When formation of the carboxylic acid metabolite is blocked by CYP3A4 inhibitors, such as ketoconazole, itraconazole, erythromycin, or troleandomycin, the plasma levels of the parent drug, terfenadine, become sufficiently elevated to block cardiac potassium channels, which can lead to arrhythmias. In some cases, inhibition of cytochrome P450 is advantageous. For example, ketoconazole and erythromycin inhibit the biotransformation of cyclosporin by intestinal and liver CYP3A4 and consequently increase the bioavailability of cyclosporin and decrease the rate of elimination of this expensive immunosuppressant. However, much higher doses of cyclosporin must be given to patients taking the CYP3A4 inducer, rifampin, in order to achieve therapeutic levels and immune suppression.

Inhibitory drug interactions generally fall into three categories. The first involves competition between two drugs that are metabolized by the same P450 enzyme. For example, omeprazole and diazepam are both metabolized by CYP2C19. When the two drugs are administered simultaneously, omeprazole decreases the plasma clearance of diazepam and prolongs its plasma half-life. The inhibition of diazepam metabolism by omeprazole is presumed to involve competition for metabolism by CYP2C19 because no such inhibition occurs in individuals who, for genetic reasons, lack this polymorphically expressed P450 enzyme. The second inhibitory drug interaction is also competitive in nature, but the inhibitor is not a substrate for the affected P450 enzyme. The inhibition of dextromethorphan biotransformation by quinidine is a good example of this type of drug interaction. Dextromethorphan is *O*-demethylated by CYP2D6, and the clearance of dextromethorphan is impaired in individuals lacking this polymorphically expressed enzyme. The clearance of dextromethorphan is similarly impaired when this antitussive agent is taken with quinidine, a potent inhibitor of CYP2D6. However, quinidine is not biotransformed by CYP2D6, even though it binds to this enzyme with high affinity ($K_i$ ~100 nM). Quinidine is actually biotransformed by CYP3A4, and is a weak competitive inhibitor of this enzyme ($K_i > 100\ \mu M$).

The third type of drug interaction results from noncompetitive inhibition of cytochrome P450, and it often involves mechanism-based inhibition or suicide inactivation of cytochrome P450 (Halpert et al., 1994). The inhibition of terfenadine metabolism by macrolide antibiotics appears to be an example of this type of drug interaction. CYP3A4 converts macrolide antibiotics to a metabolite that binds so tightly (but noncovalently) to the heme moiety of CYP3A4 that it is not released from the enzyme's active site. The noncompetitive inhibition of a P450 enzyme by a mechanism-based inhibitor can completely block the metabolism of a drug. As the fatal interactions between macrolide antibiotics and terfenadine indicate, noncompetitive inhibition of cytochrome P450 can have profound consequences. Numerous compounds are activated by cytochrome P450 to metabolites that bind covalently to the heme moiety or surrounding protein. These compounds, known as suicide inactivators, include various halogenated alkanes ($CCl_4$), halogenated alkenes (vinyl chloride, trichloroethylene), allylic compounds (allylisopropylacetamide and secobarbital), and acetylenic compounds (ethinylestradiol and the ethynylprogesterone, gestodene). Ethinyl derivatives of various P450 substrates have been synthesized as potential selective mechanism-based inhibitors of individual P450 enzymes. For example, polycyclic aromatic hydrocarbons are preferred substrates for CYP1A1, and this enzyme can be inactivated by various ethinyl derivatives of naphthalene and pyrene. Furafylline is a mechanism-based inhibitor of CYP1A2, for which the structurally related xanthine, caffeine, is a substrate. Similarly, 8-methoxypsoralen, which is a derivative of coumarin, is a mechanism-based inhibitor of CYP2A6 (Table 6-4).

**Induction of Cytochrome P450.** In contrast to inhibitors, inducers of cytochrome P450 increase the rate of xenobiotic biotransformation (Conney, 1967,1982; Batt et al., 1992). Some of the P450 enzymes in human liver microsomes are inducible, as summarized in Table 6-4 (Pichard et al., 1990). Clinically important consequences of P450 enzyme induction include the enhanced biotransformation of cyclosporin, warfarin, and contraceptive steroids, by inducers of the CYP3A and CYP2C enzymes, and enhanced activation of acetaminophen to its hepatotoxic metabolite, *N*-acetylbenzoquinoneimine, by the CYP2E1 inducers, ethanol and isoniazid, and possibly by CYP3A enzyme inducers. As an underlying cause of serious adverse effects, P450 induction is generally less important than P450 inhibition, because the latter can cause a rapid and profound increase in blood levels of a drug, which can cause toxic effects and symptoms of drug overdose. In contrast, cytochrome P450 induction lowers blood levels, which compromises the therapeutic goal of drug therapy but does not cause an exaggerated response to the drug. An exception to this rule is the potentiating effect of alcohol and isoniazid on acetaminophen hepatotoxicity, which is in part because of cytochrome P450 induction.

However, even this drug interaction is complicated by the fact that ethanol and isoniazid are inhibitors as well as inducers of CYP2E1 (Zand et al., 1993). Consequently, increased activation of acetaminophen by ethanol and isoniazid is a delayed response, due to the time required for increased synthesis of CYP2E1 and the time required for the inducers to be cleared to the point where they no longer cause an overall inhibition of CYP2E1 activity. CYP3A4 and CYP1A2 are also inducible enzymes capable of activating acetaminophen to a reactive quinoneimine. By inducing CYP3A4, rifampin and barbiturates would be expected to enhance the hepatotoxicity of acetaminophen, and there is some clinical evidence that this does occur. In contrast, induction of CYP1A2 by cigarette smoking or dietary exposure to polycyclic aromatic hydrocarbons (in charcoal-broiled beef) or indole-3-carbinol derivatives (in cruciferous vegetables) has been reported to have no effect on the hepatotoxicity of acetaminophen, even though CYP1A2 induction in rodents potentiates the hepatocellular necrosis caused by acetaminophen.

Induction of cytochrome P450 would be expected to increase the activation of procarcinogens to DNA-reactive metabolites, leading to increased tumor formation. Contrary to expectation, there is little evidence from either human epidemiological studies or animal experimentation that P450 induction enhances the incidence or multiplicity of tumors caused by known chemical carcinogens. In fact, most evidence points to a protective role of enzyme induction against chemical-induced neoplasia (Parkinson and Hurwitz, 1991). P450 induction can cause pharmacokinetic tolerance, as in the case of barbiturates and glutethimide, in which case larger doses of drug must be administered to achieve therapeutic blood levels due to increased drug biotransformation. In many cases, however, P450 induction does not necessarily enhance the biotransformation of the inducer, in which case the induction is said to be gratuitous. Drugs are also known to induce enzymes that play no role in their biotransformation. For example, omeprazole induces CYP1A2, even though the disposition of this acid-suppressing drug is largely determined by CYP2C19. Some of the most effective inducers of cytochrome P450 are polyhalogenated aromatic hydrocarbons, such as polychlorinated derivatives of dibenzo-*p*-dioxin (PCDDs), dibenzofurans (PCDFs), azobenzenes and azoxybenzenes, biphenyl (PCBs), and naphthalene. In general, highly chlorinated compounds are resistant to biotransformation and cause a prolonged induction of cytochrome P450 and other enzymes.

Due to the increased demand for heme, persistent induction of cytochrome P450 can lead to porphyria, a disorder characterized by excessive accumulation of intermediates in the heme biosynthetic pathway. In 1956, widespread consumption of wheat contaminated with the fungicide hexachlorobenzene caused an epidemic of porphyria cutanea tarda in Turkey. Another outbreak occurred in 1964 among workers at a factory in the United States manufacturing 2,4,5-trichlorophenoxyacetic acid (the active ingredient in several herbicides and in the defoliant, Agent Orange). The outbreak of porphyria cutanea tarda was caused not by the herbicide itself but by a contaminant, 2,3,7,8-tetrachlorodibenzo-*p*-dioxin, also known as dioxin and TCDD. Drugs that cause P450 induction have not been shown to cause porphyria cutanea tarda under normal circumstances, but phenobarbital, phenytoin, and alcohol are recognized as *precipitating factors* because they cause episodes of porphyria cutanea tarda in individuals with an inherited deficiency in the heme-biosynthetic enzyme, uroporphyrinogen decarboxylase.

The mechanism of P450 induction has been studied extensively in rats and other laboratory animals (Gonzalez, 1989; Okey, 1990; Ryan and Levin, 1990; Porter and Coon, 1991). Currently, five classes of P450 enzyme inducers are recognized, which are represented by 3-methylcholanthrene, phenobarbital, isoniazid, pregnenolone-16$\alpha$-carbonitrile (PCN) and clofibric acid. Treatment of rats with 3-methylcholanthrene causes a marked (>20-fold) induction of CYP1A1 and CYP1A2, which are structurally related enzymes (69 percent identical), but which catalyze different reactions. Liver microsomes from untreated rats contain low levels of CYP1A2 and virtually undetectable levels of CYP1A1. In addition to polycyclic aromatic hydrocarbons, such as 3-methylcholanthrene and benzo[a]pyrene, inducers of the CYP1A enzymes include flavones (e.g., $\beta$-naphthoflavone), polyhalogenated aromatic hydrocarbons (e.g., TCDD, 3,3′,4,4′,5,5′-hexachlorobiphenyl), acid condensation products of indole-3-carbinol, and certain drugs and food additives (e.g., chlorpromazine, phenothiazine, clotrimazole, ketoconazole, miconazole, isosafrole). Induction of CYP1A1 involves transcriptional activation of the *CYP1A1* gene, which, together with message stabilization, results in an increase in the levels of mRNA and newly synthesized protein.

In the absence of an inducer, transcription of the *CYP1A1* gene is suppressed by a repressor protein, which accounts for the low constitutive levels of CYP1A1 in most species. (Guinea pig and Rhesus monkey appear to express CYP1A1 constitutively and, hence, are exceptions to this general rule). Induction of CYP1A1 involves both derepression and activation of transcription by the *Ah* receptor. Although this cytosolic receptor binds several *a*romatic *h*ydrocarbons, such as 3-methylcholanthrene and benzo[a]pyrene, the ligand with the highest binding affinity is TCDD, which is why the *Ah* receptor is also known as the dioxin receptor (Whitlock, 1993). The *Ah* receptor is normally complexed in a 1:2 ratio with heat-shock protein (hsp90), which dissociate upon binding of ligand to the *Ah* receptor, enabling the receptor to be phosphorylated by tyrosine kinase. The activated *Ah* receptor then enters the nucleus and forms a heterodimer complex with the *Ah*-receptor-nuclear translocator, *Arnt*. Inside the nucleus, the *Ah* receptor-*Arnt* complex binds to regulatory sequences (known as *dioxin-responsive elements, DRE*, or *xenobiotic responsive elements, XRE*) and enhances the transcription of the *CYP1A1* gene and other genes with an XRE or XRE-like sequence in their upstream enhancer region (namely CYP1A2, DT-diaphorase, glutathione *S*-transferase, UDP-glucuronosyltransferase, and aldehyde dehydrogenase). The XRE is only a small segment of DNA (the consensus sequence is 5′-TXGCGTG-3′, where X is normally T or A), which can be located more than one thousand bases from the initiation site for transcription. The enhancer region of the *CYP1A1* gene contains multiple XREs, which accounts for the marked (<100-fold) increase in CYP1A1 mRNA and protein levels following exposure to ligands for the *Ah* receptor.

*Arnt* was initially thought to be a cytosolic protein that simply facilitates the translocation of the ligand-bound *Ah* receptor into the nucleus. It is now recognized as an important component of the receptor complex that binds to DNA and activates transcription of genes under the control of the *Ah* receptor. For heterodimer formation, the *Ah* receptor must be bound to ligand and possibly phosphorylated, and *Arnt* must be phosphorylated, apparently by protein kinase C. The *Ah* receptor is often compared with the steroid/thyroid/retinoid family of receptors, which also bind ligands in the cytoplasm and are translocated to the nucleus where they bind to DNA and enhance gene transcription. However, the *Ah* receptor is a novel ligand-activated transcription factor, very distinct from these other receptors. Whereas the steroid/thyroid/retinoid receptors have "zinc-finger" DNA-binding domains and form homodimers, the *Ah* receptor forms a heterodimer with *Arnt*; both of these contain a basic helix-loop-helix (bHLH) domain near their *N*-terminus. The basic region binds DNA and the helix-loop-helix is involved in protein-protein interactions. The XRE recognized by the *Ah* receptor-*Arnt* complex contains a sequence of four base pairs (5′-GCGT-3′) that is part of the recognition motif for other bHLH proteins (Whitlock, 1993).

In mice, the *Ah* receptor is encoded by a single gene, but there are four allelic variants: a low-affinity form known as $Ah^{d}$ (an ~104 kDa protein expressed in strains DBA/2, AKR, and 129) and three high-affinity forms known as $Ah^{b-1}$ (an ~95 kDa protein expressed in C57 mice), $Ah^{b-2}$ (an ~104 kDa protein expressed in BALB/c, C3H, and A mice), and $Ah^{b-3}$ (an ~105 kDa protein expressed in MOLF/Ei mice) (Poland et al., 1994). Mice that express the low affinity form of the receptor ($Ah^{d}$) require higher doses (~10 times) of TCDD to induce CYP1A1. Even though they respond to high doses of TCDD, $Ah^{d}$ mice are called *nonresponsive* because it is not possible to administer sufficient amounts of polycyclic aromatic hydrocarbons to cause induction of CYP1A1. Although several genetic alterations give rise to the four allelic variants of the *Ah* receptor, the low-affinity binding of ligands to the $Ah^{d}$ receptor from nonresponsive mice is attributable to a single amino acid substitution ($Ala^{375} \rightarrow Val^{375}$). In vivo, the $Ah^{d}$ and $Ah^{b}$ genotypes can be distinguished by phenotypic differences in the effects of 3-methylcholanthrene treatment on the duration of action of the muscle relaxant, zoxazolamine. Treatment of nonresponsive ($Ah^{d}$) mice with 3-methylcholanthrene results in no change in zoxazolamine-induced paralysis time. In contrast, such treatment of responsive ($Ah^{b}$) mice causes an induction of CYP1A1, which accelerates the 6-hydroxylation of zoxazolamine and reduces paralysis time from about 1 h to several minutes.

Some of the genes regulated by the *Ah* receptor contain other responsive elements and their expression is controlled by other transcription factors (Nebert, 1994). To a limited extent, the induction of CYP1A1 by polycyclic aromatic hydrocarbons can also be mediated by another cytosolic receptor known as the 4S-binding protein, which has recently been identified as the enzyme, glycine *N*-methyltransferase. The first intron of the CYP1A1 gene contains a glucocorticoid responsive element (GRE), hence, the induction of CYP1A1 by TCDD can be augmented by glucocorticoids. DT-diaphorase is inducible up to tenfold by two classes of agents: chemicals like 3-methylcholanthrene and TCDD that bind to the *Ah* receptor, and chemicals that cause oxidative stress, such as menadione, *tert*-butylhydroquinone and 3,5-di-*tert*-butylcatechol, which produce reactive oxygen species through redox cycling reactions. These latter effects are mediated by the antioxidant responsive elements (ARE); therefore these enzymes are inducible by so-called *monofunctional* agents that do not induce CYP1A1 (see this section on DT-diaphorase above). The flavonoid $\beta$-naphthoflavone induces DT-diaphorase by both mechanisms; the parent compound binds to the *Ah* receptor and is responsible for inducing DT-diaphorase via XRE (the XRE for CYP1A1 inducers), whereas a metabolite of $\beta$-naphthoflavone is responsible for inducing DT-diaphorase via ARE. The ARE core sequence for enzyme induction (5′-**GTGAC**AAA**GC**-3′) is similar to the AP-1 DNA-binding site (5′-TGACTCA-3′), which is regulated by redox status. However, ARE is not regulated by known AP-1 transcription factors (i.e., dimerized Jun/Fos protein). The *trans*-acting factor(s) that bind(s) to ARE and activates transcription of DT-diaphorase in response to oxidative stress is(are) yet to be identified. In addition to DT-diaphorase (which is encoded by the *Nmo1* gene), the ARE regulates the expression of three other genes: *Ugt1.6*, a UDP-glucuronosyltransferase, *Ahd4*, a class 3 aldehyde dehydrogenase, and *Gsta1 (Ya)*, a glutathione *S*-transferase (Nguyen et al., 1994).

The enhancer region of *CYP1A2* also contains an XRE (or XRE-like sequences), so inducers of CYP1A1 are also inducers of CYP1A2. However, the induction of CYP1A2 differs from that of CYP1A1 in several respects: It occurs at lower doses of inducer; it often involves stabilization of mRNA or enzyme from degradation, and it requires liver-specific factors. The first of these differences (dose-response) may explain why low-level exposure of humans to CYP1A inducers results in an increase in hepatic levels of CYP1A2 but not CYP1A1. The second of these differences (namely stabilization of mRNA and/or enzyme) apparently explains why compounds that form stable complexes with CYP1A2, such as isosafrole, can induce CYP1A2 even in nonresponsive ($Ah^d$) mice. The third difference (the requirement for hepatic factors) explains why CYP1A2 is not expressed or inducible in extrahepatic tissues, hepatoma-derived cell lines, or isolated hepatocytes cultured under conditions that do not restore liver-specific gene expression.

Liver microsomes from untreated rats contain low levels of CYP2B2 and extremely low or undetectable levels of CYP2B1, which are structurally related enzymes (97 percent identical) with very similar substrate specificities. Treatment of rats with phenobarbital causes a marked (>20-fold) induction of cytochromes CYP2B1 and CYP2B2. In addition to barbiturates, such as phenobarbital and glutethimide, inducers of the CYP2B enzymes include drugs (e.g., phenytoin, loratadine, doxylamine, griseofulvin, chlorpromazine, phenothiazine, clotrimazole, ketoconazole, miconazole), pesticides (e.g., DDT, chlordane, dieldrin), food additives (e.g., butylated hydroxytoluene and butylated hydroxyanisole), and certain polyhalogenated aromatic hydrocarbons [e.g., 2,2′,4,4′,5,5′-hexachlorobiphenyl and 1,4-bis[2]-(3,5-chloropyridyloxy)benzene or TCPOBOP]. Treatment of rats with phenobarbital also results in a 2- to 4-fold increase in the levels of CYP2A1, CYP2C6, and CYP3A2, as well as a 50 to 75 percent decrease in the levels of CYP2C11, which is present only in adult male rats. In addition, treatment of rats with phenobarbital generally causes an increase (50 to 300 percent) in the concentration of cytochrome $b_5$, NADPH-cytochrome P450 (*c*) reductase, epoxide hydrolase, aldehyde dehydrogenase, glutathione *S*-transferase and UDP-glucuronosyltransferase. Indeed treatment of rodents with phenobarbital and related inducers causes hepatocellular hyperplasia and/or hypertrophy, which is accompanied by a proliferation of the endoplasmic reticulum.

The mechanism of induction of CYP2B1 by phenobarbital has not been elucidated in as much detail as the induction of CYP1A1 by TCDD. In the latter case, progress was facilitated by the early identification of a sensitive and fairly specific marker for CYP1A1, namely benzo[a]pyrene 3-hydroxylation (which is the basis of the aryl hydrocarbon hydroxylase or AHH assay), and the identification of *Ah* responsive ($Ah^b$) and nonresponsive ($Ah^d$) mouse strains. More importantly, CYP1A1 is inducible by TCDD in numerous cell lines, whereas CYP2B1 is not. As in the case of CYP1A1, induction of CYP2B1 involves transcriptional activation of the *CYP2B1* gene, which, together with message stabilization, results in an increase in the levels of mRNA and newly synthesized protein. However, a cytosolic *phenobarbital receptor* equivalent to the *Ah* receptor has not been identified. In contrast to CYP1A1 inducers, the CYP2B1 inducers are so structurally diverse that no structure-activity relationship is apparent.

Considerable progress in our understanding of the mechanism of induction by phenobarbital followed the discovery that the bacterium *Bacillus megaterium* contains two cytochrome P450 enzymes, known as P450BM-1 and P450BM-3, that are inducible by phenobarbital and other compounds that induce rat CYP2B1 (Liang et al., 1995). The 5′-enhancer regions of these bacterial genes contain a 15-base pair DNA sequence that, when deleted or mutated, results in P450BM-1 or P450BM-2 expression. A similar 15-base pair DNA sequence, which is known as the *Barbie box* (after *barbiturate*), is present in the 5′-enhancer region of CYP2B1, CYP2B2, and numerous other mammalian genes that are transcriptionally activated by phenobarbital. All Barbie boxes contain a four base pair sequence (5′-AAAG-3′), making this the likely site of DNA-protein interactions. In the absence of inducer, a repressor protein binds to the Barbie box and impedes or prevents transcription of the structural gene. Binding of the inducer to this repressor causes its dissociation from the Barbie box, which results in increased transcription. In the presence of an inducer, a second transcription factor may bind to the Barbie box and enhance transcription of the structural gene. Therefore, induction of CYP2B1, like that of CYP1A1, may result from a combination of inducer-dependent derepression and inducer-dependant activation of gene expression. The proteins that bind phenobarbital and the Barbie box and either repress or promote gene transcription have not yet been characterized, but it is now apparent that the mechanism of regulating gene expression by phenobarbital and related chemicals has been highly conserved during the evolution of bacteria, plants, and mammals.

Treatment of rodents with PCN causes an induction of CYP3A1 and CYP3A2, which are two independently regulated CYP3A enzymes with very similar structures (87 percent similar) and substrate specificities. In contrast to CYP3A1, CYP3A2 is present in liver microsomes from untreated rats, although the levels of this enzyme decline markedly after puberty in female rats. Consequently, CYP3A2 is a male-specific protein in mature rats, and it is inducible in mature male but not mature female rats (whereas CYP3A1 is inducible in mature male and female rats). In addition to PCN, inducers of CYP3A enzymes include steroids (e.g., dexamethasone and spironolactone), macrolide antibiotics (e.g., troleandomycin and erythromycin estolate), and imidazole antifungals (e.g., clotrimazole, ketoconazole, and miconazole). Although it primarily induces the CYP2B enzymes (see above), phenobarbital is also an inducer of CYP3A2, which contains three Barbie boxes located 48, 1007, and 1166 base pairs upstream from the translation start site.

The induction of CYP3A1, like that of CYP1A1 and CYP2B1, involves transcriptional activation of the structural gene, which, together with message stabilization, results in an increase in the levels of CYP3A1 mRNA and newly synthesized protein. The mechanism of induction of CYP3A1 by PCN and related steroids has not yet been fully elucidated. PCN is a glucocorticoid receptor antagonist, and dexamethasone induces CYP3A1 only at doses that far exceed those required to induce tyrosine aminotransferase (TAT), which is regulated by the glucocorticoid receptor. Therefore, induction of CYP3A1 is not simply mediated by the glucocorticoid receptor. In the case of macrolide antibiotics, such as troleandomycin and erythromycin, induction of CYP3A1 involves both transcriptional activation and stabilization of the newly synthesized enzyme against protein degradation. This latter effect involves biotransformation of the macrolide antibiotic to a metabolite that binds tightly to the heme moiety. The induction of CYP3A1 by macrolide antibiotics is often masked by their ability to function as mechanism-based inhibitors. The enzyme-inducing effects of clotrimazole, ketoconazole, and miconazole are similarly masked by the ability of these imidazole antimycotics to bind to and inhibit cytochrome P450 enzymes (including CYP3A1). Substrates and ligands stabilize CYP3A1 by inhibiting its cAMP-dependent-phosphorylation on $Ser^{393}$, which otherwise denatures the protein and targets it for degradation in the endoplasmic reticulum.

Treatment of rats with isoniazid causes a 2- to 5-fold induction of CYP2E1. In sexually mature rats, the levels of liver microsomal CYP2E1 are slightly greater in female than in male rats. In addition to isoniazid, inducers of CYP2E1 include ethanol, acetone, pyrazole, pyridine, ketoconazole, fasting, and uncontrolled diabetes. A common feature of CYP2E1 inducers is their ability to inhibit or be biotransformed by CYP2E1 and/or their ability to increase serum ketone bodies. Like CYP3A1, CYP2E1 is induced both by transcriptional activation of the gene and stabilization of the protein against degradation (Koop and Tierney, 1990). Induction of CYP2E1 can also involve mRNA stabilization and/or increased efficiency of mRNA translation. The mechanism of CYP2E1 induction varies even among closely related inducers. For example, although diabetes and fasting both increase the levels of CYP2E1 mRNA by ~10-fold, the increase with diabetes results from mRNA stabilization, whereas the increase with fasting results from increased gene transcription. Acetone and other substrates stabilize CYP2E1 by blocking its cAMP-dependent-phosphorylation on $Ser^{129}$, which otherwise causes the denaturation and degradation of this enzyme. The enzyme-inducing effects of ethanol, acetone, pyrazole, pyridine, and isoniazid are often masked in vivo by the binding of these substrates to CYP2E1.

Treatment of male rats with clofibric acid causes a marked induction (up to 40-fold) of CYP4A1, CYP4A2, and CYP4A3, which are three independently regulated CYP4A enzymes with similar substrate specificities (Sundseth and Waxman, 1991). CYP4A1 is expressed in the liver, whereas CYP4A3 is expressed in the liver and kidney. CYP4A2 is expressed in the liver and kidney of male rats, but it is neither expressed nor inducible in female rats. In addition to clofibric acid, inducers of CYP4A enzymes include perfluorodecanoic acid, phthalate ester plasticizers, 2,4-dichlorophenoxyacetic acid (2,4-D), ciprofibrate and other hypolipidemic drugs, aspirin and other NSAIDs, nicotinic acid, dehydroepiandrosterone sulfate, and leukotriene receptor antagonists (MK-0571 and RG 7512). A feature common to all these CYP4A enzyme inducers is their ability to cause proliferation of hepatic peroxisomes.

As in the case of CYP1A1, CYP2B1, and CYP3A1, the induction of CYP4A enymes by clofibric acid involves activation of the structural gene which results in an increase in the levels of mRNA and newly synthesized protein. The transcription factor that activates the *CYP4A* genes is the peroxisome proliferator-activated receptor (PPAR), a member of the steroid/thyroid/retinoid superfamily of nuclear receptors that regulates transcription of the genes for fatty acyl-CoA oxidase, bifunctional enzyme (enoyl-CoA hydratase/3-hydroxyacyl-CoA dehydrogenase) and fatty acid binding protein (Muerhoff et al., 1992; Demoz et al., 1994). Binding of a peroxisome proliferator to PPAR results in the formation of a heterodimer with another nuclear receptor, the retinoid X receptor (RXR), which is activated by 9-*cis*-retinoic acid. The ligand-bound heterodimer of PPAR and RXR binds to a regulatory DNA sequence known as the peroxisome proliferator response element. Three PPREs have been identified in the 5′-enhancer region of the rabbit *CYP4A6* gene. Each of these elements contains a sequence known as DR1, an imperfect repeat of the nuclear receptor binding consensus sequence separated by one nucleotide (PuGGTCA N PuGGTCA). Peroxisome proliferators can bind to PPAR stereoselectively; therefore, the enantiomers of certain drugs differ in their ability to induce CYP4A and cause a proliferation of peroxisomes. Androsterone sulfate and arachidonic acid are physiological ligands for PPAR.

In mature rats, the levels of certain P450 enzymes are sexually differentiated; that is, they are higher in either male or female rats. Male-specific enzymes include CYP2A2, CYP2C11, CYP2C13, CYP3A2, and CYP4A2. The only known female-specific P450 enzyme is CYP2C12, although the levels of several other P450 enzymes are greater in female than male rats, including CYP2A1, CYP2C7, and CYP2E1. These gender-related differences in P450 enzyme expression are due in large part to sex differences in the pattern of secretion of growth hormone, which is pulsatile in male rats and more or less continuous in females (Waxman et al., 1991). Treatment of mature male rats with various xenobiotics perturbs the pattern of growth hormone secretion and causes a partial "feminization" of P450 enzyme expression, which includes decreased expression of CYP 2C11. Sex differences in the expression of P450 enzymes occur to a limited extent in mice, but no marked sex differences in P450 expression have been observed in dogs, monkeys, or humans.

Enzymatic assays have been developed to monitor the induction of the aforementioned P450 enzymes. A series of 7-alkoxyresorufin analogs has proven very useful for monitoring the induction of rat and mouse CYP1A and CYP2B enzymes. CYP1A enzymes preferentially catalyze the *O*-dealkylation of 7-methoxyresorufin and 7-ethoxyresorufin, whereas CYP2B enzymes preferentially catalyze the *O*-dealkylation of

7-pentoxyresorufin and 7-benzyloxyresorufin. The effects of treating rats with phenobarbital on the levels of liver CYP2A1, CYP2B1/2, CYP2C11, and CYP3A1/2 can be monitored by changes in specific pathways of testosterone oxidation. For all practical purposes, the rates of testosterone $2\alpha$-, $7\alpha$- and $16\beta$-hydroxylation accurately reflect the levels of CYP2C11, CYP2A1, and CYP2B1/2, respectively. The $2\beta$-, $6\beta$-, and $15\beta$-hydroxylation of testosterone collectively reflect the levels of CYP3A1 and/or CYP3A2. Induction of CYP2E1 can be monitored by increases in *para*-nitrophenol hydroxylase, aniline 4-hydroxylase, and chlorzoxazone 6-hydroxylase activity, although none of these reactions is specifically catalyzed by CYP2E1. The 12-hydroxylation of lauric acid appears to be catalyzed specifically by CYP4A enzymes. Indeed the $\omega$-hydroxylation of fatty acids and their derivatives (such as eicosanoids) appears to be a physiological function of these enzymes. CYP4A enzymes also catalyze the 11-hydroxylation of lauric acid, but this reaction is also catalyzed by other P450 enzymes, including the CYP2B and CYP2E enzymes. Induction of CYP4A enzymes by clofibric acid increases the ratio 12- to 11-hydroxylauric acid, whereas induction of CYP2B enzymes by phenobarbital or CYP2E1 by isoniazid has the opposite effect.

In addition to measuring certain enzyme activities, changes in the levels of specific P450 enzymes can also be monitored by immunochemical techniques, such as Western immunoblotting. When P450 induction involves increased gene transcription and/or mRNA stabilization, the increase in mRNA levels can be measured by Northern blotting. These techniques are particularly useful for detecting P450 induction by chemicals that bind tightly to the active site of cytochrome P450 enzymes and thus mask their detection by enzymatic assays. Such chemicals include macrolide antibiotics (e.g., erythromycin and troleandomycin), methylenedioxy-containing compounds (e.g., safrole and isosafrole) and imidazole antimycotics (e.g., clotrimazole, ketoconazole, and miconazole).

Numerous phenobarbital-type inducers and peroxisome proliferators are epigenetic tumorigens (Grasso et al., 1991). Rodents treated chronically with these chemicals develop liver and/or thyroid tumors. The liver tumors seem to be a consequence of hepatocellular hyperplasia/hypertrophy and the sustained proliferation of either the endoplasmic reticulum (in the case of CYP2B inducers) or peroxisomes (in the case of CYP4A inducers). The thyroid tumors are the result of UDP-glucuronosyltransferase induction, which accelerates the glucuronidation of thyroid hormones, leading to a compensatory increase in thyroid-stimulating hormone (TSH). Sustained stimulation of the thyroid gland by TSH leads to the development of thyroid follicular tumors. These epigenetic mechanisms of chemical-induced tumor formation do not appear to operate in humans. Prolonged treatment with anticonvulsants, such as phenobarbital or phenytoin, does not lead to liver or thyroid tumor formation in humans. Prolonged elevation of TSH in humans does not lead to tumor formation but causes goiter, a reversible enlargement of the thyroid gland associated with iodide deficiency and treatment with drugs that block thyroid hormone synthesis. Chemicals that cause peroxisome proliferation in rodents do not do so in humans and other primates, possibly because of low levels of PPAR in primate liver.

## PHASE II ENZYME REACTIONS

Phase II biotransformation reactions include glucuronidation, sulfation, acetylation, methylation, conjugation with glutathione (mercapturic acid synthesis) and conjugation with amino acids (such as glycine, taurine, and glutamic acid) (Paulson et al., 1986). The cofactors for these reactions, which are shown in Fig. 6-41, react with functional groups that are either present on the xenobiotic or are introduced/exposed during phase I biotransformation. With the exception of methylation and acetylation, phase II biotransformation reactions result in a large increase in xenobiotic hydrophilicity, so they greatly promote the excretion of foreign chemicals. Glucuronidation, sulfation, acetylation, and methylation involve reactions with activated or "high-energy" cofactors, whereas conjugation with amino acids or glutathione involves reactions with activated xenobiotics. Most phase II biotransforming enzymes are located in the cytosol; a notable exception is the UDP-glucuronosyltransferases, which are microsomal enzymes (Table 6-1). Phase II reactions generally proceed much faster than phase I reactions, such as those catalyzed by cytochrome P450. Therefore, the rate of elimination of xenobiotics whose excretion depends on biotransformation by cytochrome P450 followed by phase II conjugation is generally determined by the first reaction.

### Glucuronidation

Glucuronidation is a major pathway of xenobiotic biotransformation in mammalian species except for members of the cat family (lions, lynxes, civets, and domestic cats) (Miners and Mackenzie, 1992; Mackenzie et al., 1992; Burchell and Coughtrie, 1992). Glucuronidation requires the cofactor uridine diphosphate-glucuronic acid (UDP-glucuronic acid), and the reaction is catalyzed by UDP-glucuronosyltransferases, which are located in the endoplasmic reticulum of liver and other tissues, such as the kidney, intestine, skin, brain, spleen and nasal mucosa (Fig. 6-42). Examples of xenobiotics that are glucuronidated are shown in Fig. 6-43. The site of glucuronidation is generally an electron-rich nucleophilic heteroatom (O, N, or S). Therefore, substrates for glucuronidation contain such functional groups as aliphatic alcohols and phenols (which form *O*-glucuronide ethers), carboxylic acids (which form *O*-glucuronide esters), primary and secondary aromatic and aliphatic amines (which form *N*-glucuronides), and free sulfhydryl groups (which form *S*-glucuronides). In humans, the tertiary amine tripelennamine is also a substrate for *N*-glucuronidation. Certain xenobiotics, such as phenylbutazone and sulfinpyrazone, contain carbon atoms that are sufficiently nucleophilic to form *C*-glucuronides. In addition to numerous xenobiotics, substrates for glucuronidation include several endogenous compounds, such as bilirubin, steroid hormones and thyroid hormones. Glucuronide conjugates of xenobiotics and endogenous compounds are polar, water-soluble conjugates that are eliminated from the body in urine or bile.

Whether glucuronides are excreted from the body in bile or urine depends on the size of the aglycone (parent compound or phase I metabolite). In rat, glucuronides are preferentially excreted in urine if the molecular weight of the aglycone is less than 250, whereas glucuronides of larger molecules (aglycones with molecular weight $> 350$) are preferentially

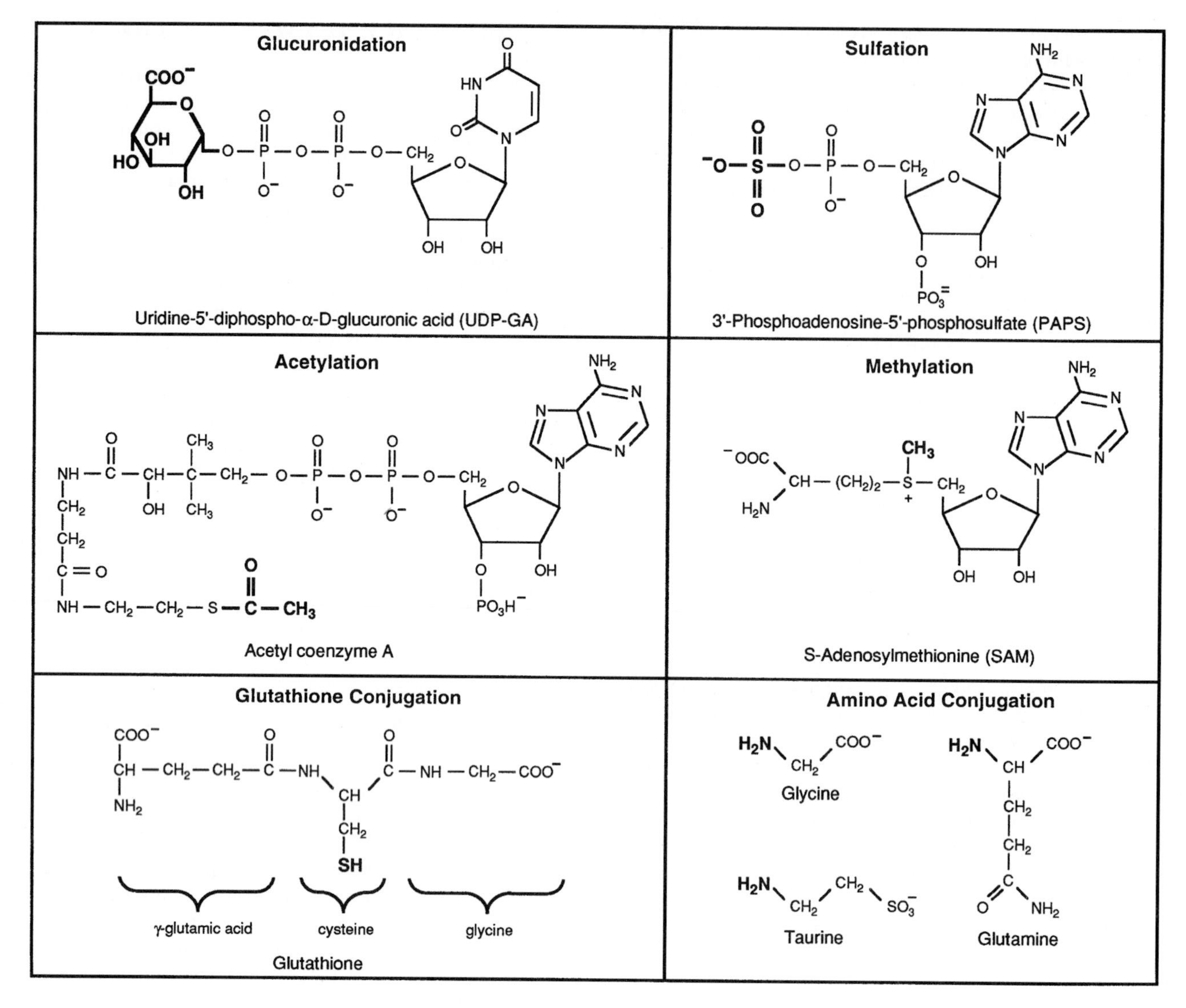


***Figure 6–41. Structures of cofactors for phase II biotransformation.***

The functional group that reacts with or is transferred to the xenobiotics is shown in bold.

excreted in bile. Molecular weight cutoffs for the preferred route of excretion vary among mammalian species. The carboxylic acid moiety of glucuronic acid, which is ionized at physiological pH, promotes excretion because (1) it increases the aqueous solubility of the xenobiotic and (2) it is recognized by the biliary and renal organic anion transport systems, which enables glucuronides to be secreted into urine and bile.

The cofactor for glucuronidation is synthesized from glucose-1-phosphate, and the linkage between glucuronic acid and UDP has an $\alpha$-configuration, as shown in Fig. 6-42. This configuration protects the cofactor from hydrolysis by $\beta$-glucuronidase. However, glucuronides of xenobiotics have a $\beta$-configuration. This inversion of configuration occurs because glucuronides are formed by nucleophilic attack by an electron-rich atom (usually O, N, or S) on UDP-glucuronic acid, and this attack occurs on the opposite side of the linkage between glucuronic acid and UDP, as shown in Fig. 6-42. In contrast to the UDP-glucuronic acid cofactor, xenobiotics conjugated with glucuronic acid are substrates for $\beta$-glucuronidase. Although present in the lysosomes of some mammalian tissues, considerable $\beta$-glucuronidase activity is present in the intestinal microflora. The intestinal enzyme can release the aglycone, which can be reabsorbed and enter a cycle called *enterohepatic circulation*, which delays the elimination of xenobiotics. Nitrogen-glucuronides are more slowly hydrolyzed by $\beta$-glucuronidase than *O*- or *S*-glucuronides, whereas *O*-glucuronides tend to be more stable to acid-catalyzed hydrolysis than *N*- or *S*-glucuronides. The potential for glucuronides to be hydrolyzed in the presence of acid or base complicates the analysis of conjugates in urine or feces.

The *C*-terminus of all UDP-glucuronosyltransferases contains a membrane-spanning domain that anchors the enzyme in the endoplasmic reticulum. The enzyme faces the lumen of the endoplasmic reticulum, where it is ideally placed to conju-

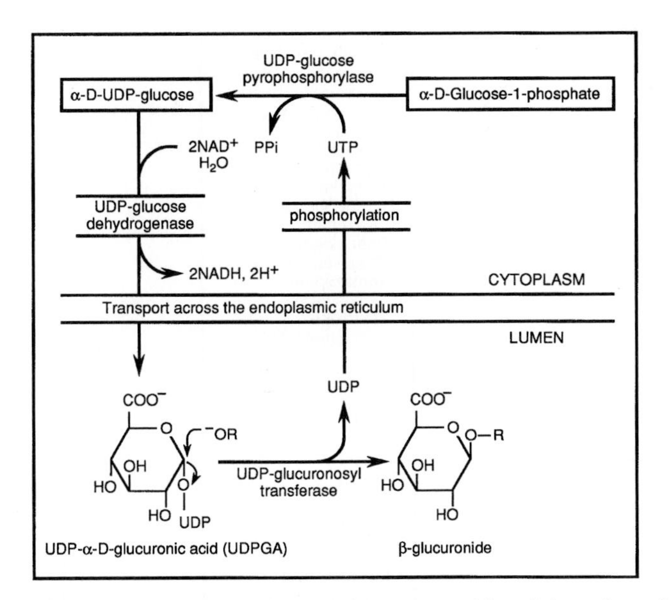


***Figure 6–42. Synthesis of UDP-glucuronic acid and inversion of configuration ($\alpha \rightarrow \beta$) during glucuronidation of a phenolic xenobiotic (designated $RO^-$).***

gate lipophilic xenobiotics and their metabolites generated by cytochrome P450 and other microsomal phase I enzymes. The lumenal orientation of UDP-glucuronosyltransferases poses a problem because UDP-glucuronic acid is a water-soluble cofactor synthesized in the cytoplasm. A transporter has been postulated to shuttle this cofactor into the lumen of the endoplasmic reticulum, and it may also shuttle UDP (the byproduct of glucuronidation) back into the cytoplasm for synthesis of UDP-glucuronic acid, as shown in Fig. 6-42. In vitro, the glucuronidation of xenobiotics by liver microsomes can be stimulated by detergents, which disrupt the lipid bilayer of the endoplasmic reticulum and allow UDP-glucuronosyltransferases free access to UDP-glucuronic acid. High concentrations of detergent can inhibit UDP-glucuronosyltransferases, presumably by disrupting their interaction with phospholipids, which are important for catalytic activity. Cofactor availability can limit the rate of glucuronidation of drugs that are administered in high doses and are conjugated extensively, such as aspirin and acetaminophen. In experimental animals, the glucuronidation of xenobiotics can be impaired in vivo by factors that reduce or deplete UDP-glucuronic acid levels, such as diethyl ether, borneol, and galactosamine.

The existence of multiple forms of UDP-glucuronosyltransferase was first suggested by the observation that in rats developmental changes in glucuronidation rates were substrate dependent, and the glucuronidation of xenobiotics could be differentially affected by treatment of rats with chemicals known to induce cytochrome P450. Based on their ontogeny and inducibility, the UDP-glucuronosyltransferase activities in rat liver microsomes were categorized into four groups. The activity of enzyme(s) in the first group peaks 1 to 5 days *before* birth, and it is inducible by 3-methylcholanthrene and other CYP1A enzyme inducers. Substrates for the group 1 enzyme(s) tend to be planar chemicals, such as 1-naphthol, 4-nitrophenol, and 4-methylumbelliferone. The activity of enzyme(s) in the second group peaks ~5 days *after* birth and is inducible by phenobarbital and other CYP2B enzyme inducers. Substrates for the group 2 enzyme(s) tend to be bulky chemicals, such as chloramphenicol, morphine, 4-hydroxybiphenyl, and monoterpenoid alcohols. The activity of enzyme(s) in the third group peaks around the time of puberty (~1 month) and is inducible by PCN and other CYP3A enzyme inducers. Substrates for the group 3 enzyme(s) include digitoxigenin monodigitoxoside ($dt_1$), a metabolite of digitoxin formed by CYP3A (see Fig. 6-39), and possibly bilirubin. The activity of enzyme(s) in the fourth group also peak around the time of puberty (~1 month) and is inducible by clofibrate and other CYP4A enzyme inducers. Substrates for the group 4 enzyme(s) include bilirubin but not $dt_1$, which distinguishes group 3 from group 4 UDP-glucuronosyltransferases.

Although this classification system still has some practical value, it has become evident that the four groups of UDP-glucuronosyltransferases do not simply represent four independently regulated enzymes with different substrate specificities. This realization stems from various studies, including those conducted with Gunn rats, which are hyperbilirubinemic due to a genetic defect in bilirubin conjugation. The glucuronidation defect in Gunn rats is substrate-dependent in a manner that does not match the categorization of UDP-glucuronosyltransferases into the four aforementioned groups. For example, in Gunn rats the glucuronidation of the group 2 substrates, morphine and chloramphenicol, is not impaired, whereas the glucuronidation of 1-naphthol, $dt_1$ and bilirubin (group 1, 3, and 4 substrates) is low or undetectable. The induction of UDP-glucuronosyltransferase activity by 3-methylcholanthrene, PCN, and clofibric acid is impaired in Gunn rats, whereas the induction by phenobarbital is normal. (Although phenobarbital does not induce the conjugation of bilirubin in Gunn rats, it does so in normal Wistar rats.)

Only when the UDP-glucuronosyltransferases were cloned did it become apparent why the genetic defect in Gunn rats affects three of the four groups of UDP-glucuronosyltransferases that are otherwise independently regulated as a function of age and xenobiotic treatment (Owens and Ritter, 1992). It is now apparent that the UDP-glucuronosyltransferases expressed in rat liver microsomes belong to two gene families (UGT1 and UGT2), each containing at least four members. Members of family 1 are formed by alternate splicing of a single gene, whereas members of family 2 are all distinct gene products. As shown in Fig. 6-44, the multiple enzymes encoded by the UGT1 locus are constructed by linking different substrate binding sites (encoded by multiple copies of exon 1) to a constant portion of the enzyme (encoded by exons 2–5). This constant region is involved in cofactor binding and membrane insertion. This method of generating multiple forms of an enzyme from a single gene locus is economical, but it is also the genetic equivalent of putting all of one's eggs in the same basket. Whereas a mutation in any one of the UGT2 enzymes affects a single enzyme, a mutation in the constant region of the UGT1 gene affects all enzymes encoded by this locus. In the Gunn rat, a mutation at codon 415 introduces a premature stop signal, so that all forms of UDP-glucuronosyltransferase encoded by the UGT1 locus are truncated and functionally inactive. The UDP-glucuronosyltransferases known to be encoded by the rat UGT1 locus include the 3-methylcholanthrene-inducible enzyme that conjugates planar molecules like 1-naphthol (UGT1.6), the phenobarbital- and clofibric acid-inducible enzyme that conjugates bilirubin

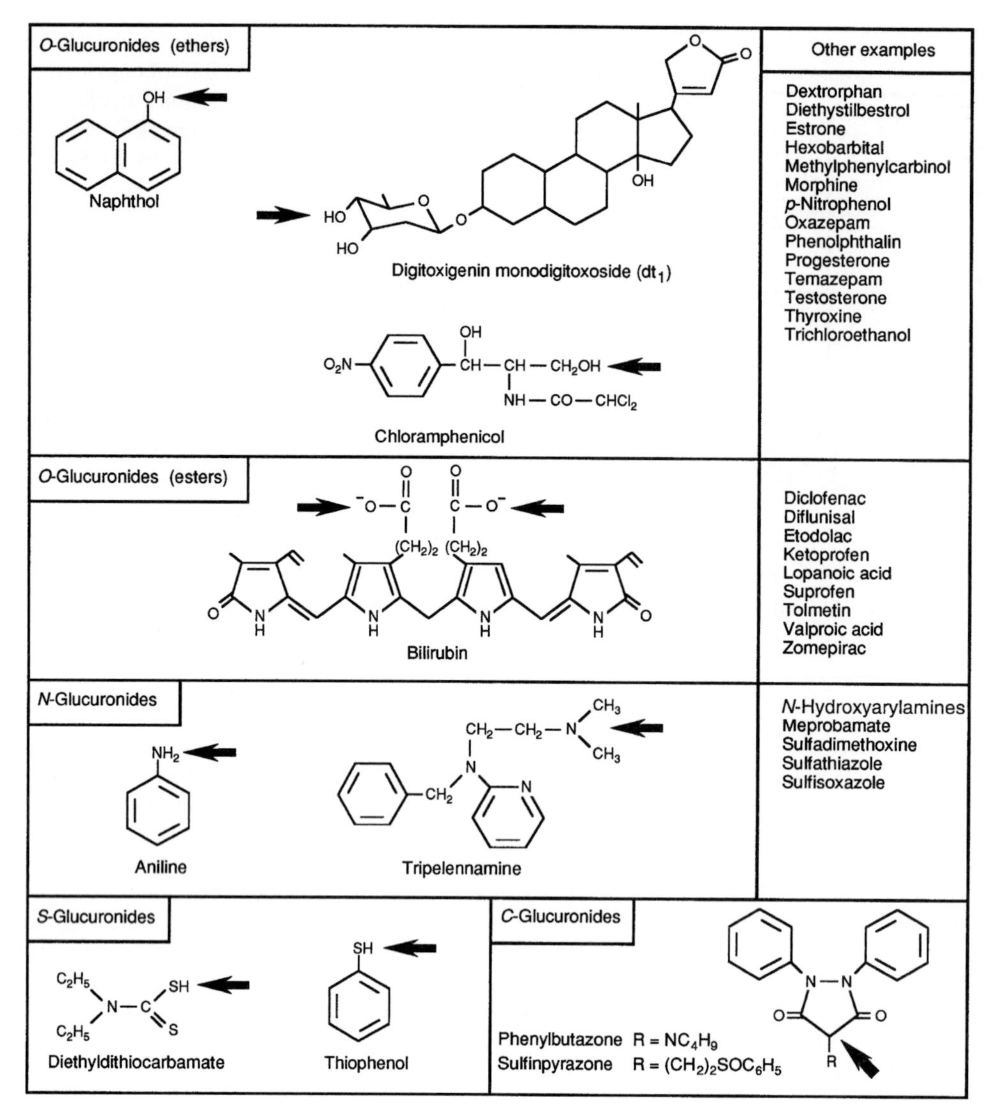


***Figure 6–43. Examples of xenobiotics and endogenous substrates that are glucuronidated.***

The arrow indicates the site of glucuronidation.

(UGT1.1 and UGT1.4), and the PCN-inducible enzyme that conjugates $dt_1$ (which will be named when the first exon for this enzyme is cloned and localized within the UGT1 locus). All of these UGT1 enzymes are defective in Gunn rats.

The second family of UDP-glucuronosyltransferase, which share less than 50 percent of amino acid sequence identity with the first family, are divided into two subfamilies (UGT2A and UGT2B), and its members are distinct gene products. Members of the 2A subfamily are expressed specifically in olfactory epithelium whereas members of the 2B subfamily (UGT2B1, 2, 3, 6, and 12) are expressed in liver microsomes. Members of the UGT2B subfamily are named in the order they are cloned, regardless of the species of origin (much like the nomenclature system for most of the P450 enzymes). UGT2B enzymes have been cloned from rat (forms 1, 2, 3, and 12), humans (forms 4, 7, 8, 9, 10, and 11), mouse (form 5), and rabbits (forms 13 and 14). In rats, two of the four UGT2B enzymes (forms 2 and 12) are inducible by phenobarbital. The genes encoding these enzymes are not defective in Gunn rats; therefore, treatment of Gunn rats with phenobarbital induces the glucuronidation of bulky group 2 substrates. However, these enzymes do not conjugate bilirubin (a reaction mainly catalyzed by UGT1.1 and/or UGT1.4), which is why phenobarbital cannot induce the conjugation of bilirubin in Gunn rats.

The multiple forms of UDP-glucuronosyltransferase in human liver microsomes are also products of either a single UGT1 gene locus (which generate at least six enzymes through alternative splicing of exon 1, as shown in Fig. 6-44) or multiple UGT2B genes (namely UGT2B4, 7, 8, 9, 10, 11). In humans, Crigler-Najjar syndrome is a congenital defect in bilirubin conjugation analogous to that seen in Gunn rats. The UGT1 locus in humans encodes two bilirubin conjugation enzymes, namely UGT1.1 and UGT1.4, although the latter enzyme is quantitatively less important (Bosma et al., 1994). Mutations in exons 2-5, which affect all enzymes encoded by the UGT1 locus, have been identified in patients with type I Crigler-Najjar syndrome, a severe form of the disease charac-

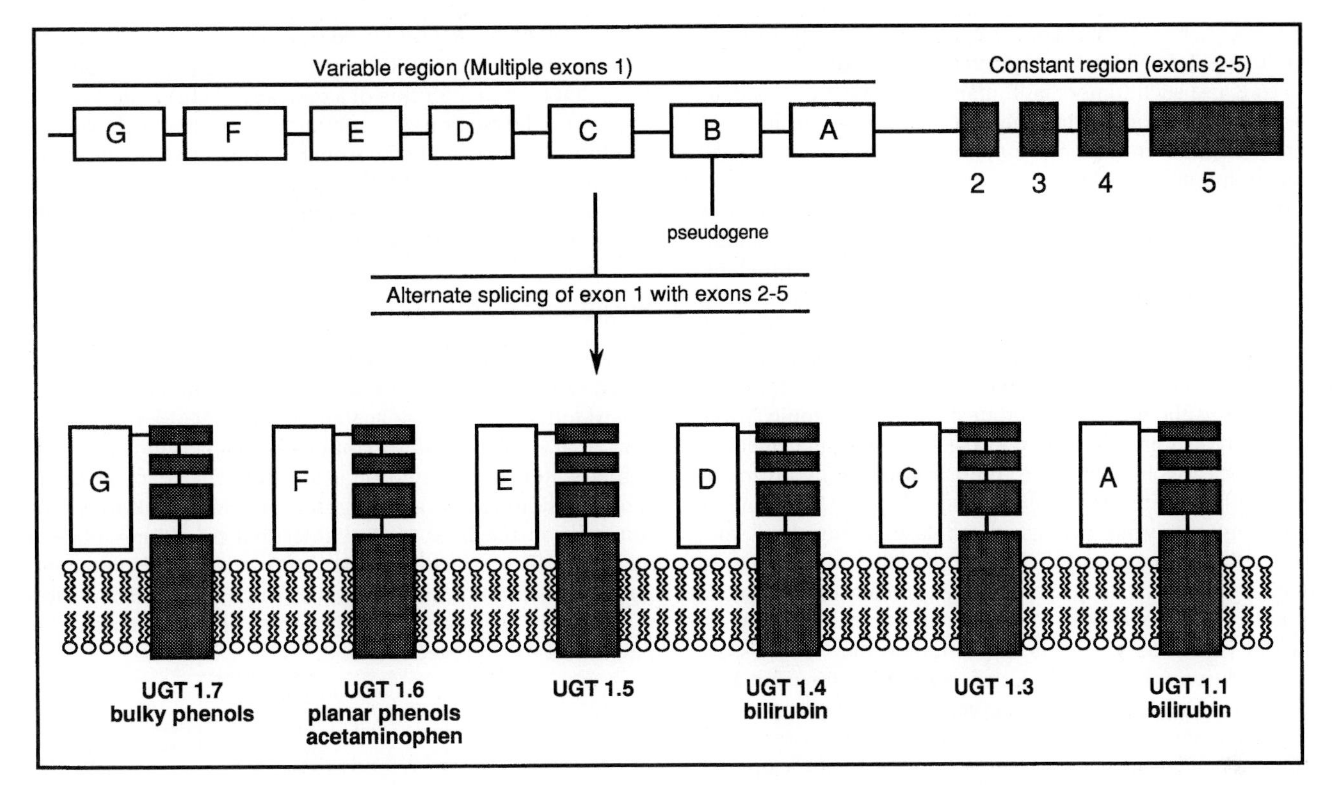


***Figure 6–44.*** ***Structure of the human UGT 1 locus which encodes multiple forms of UDP-glucuronosyl-transferase.***

Note that these microsomal enzymes face the lumen of the endoplasmic reticulum.

terized by a complete loss of bilirubin-conjugating activity and marked hyperbilirubinemia. Type I Crigler-Najjar syndrome can also be caused by mutations in exon 1 of UGT1.1 that specifically inactivate the major bilirubin-conjugating enzyme. Other mutations in exon 1 of UGT1.1 reduce but do not abolish enzyme activity and give rise to the less severe form of Crigler-Najjar syndrome (type II) or the even milder form of hyperbilirubinemia known as Gilbert's disease (which affects 5–7 percent of the population). Gilbert's syndrome can also be caused by "soft" mutations in exons 2–5, which reduce but do not abolish the activity of all UDP-glucuronosyltransferases encoded by the UGT1 locus. The milder forms of hyperbilirubinemia respond to phenobarbital, which stimulates bilirubin conjugation by inducing UGT1.1 and UGT1.4.

In rats, UGT1.6 is the major 3-methylcholanthrene-inducible form of UDP-glucuronosyltransferase. The corresponding enzyme in humans has been shown to glucuronidate acetaminophen. The glucuronidation of acetaminophen in humans is enhanced by cigarette smoking and dietary cabbage and brussels sprouts, which suggests that human UGT1.6, like the rat enzyme, is inducible by polycyclic aromatic hydrocarbons and derivatives of indole 3-carbinol (Bock et al., 1994). These ligands for the *Ah* receptor also induce CYP1A2, which would be expected to enhance the hepatotoxicity of acetaminophen. Increased glucuronidation due to induction of UGT1.6 may explain why cigarette smoking does not enhance the hepatotoxicity of acetaminophen. Conversely, decreased glucuronidation may explain why some individuals with Gilbert's syndrome are predisposed to the hepatotoxic effects of acetaminophen (De Morais et al., 1992). Low rates of glucuronidation also predispose humans to the adverse gastrointestinal effects of irinotecan, a derivative of camptothecin (Gupta et al., 1994). Low rates of glucuronidation predispose newborns to jaundice and to the toxic effects of chloramphenicol; the latter was once used prophylactically to prevent opportunistic infections in newborns until it was found to cause severe cyanosis and even death (gray baby syndrome).

Glucuronidation generally detoxifies xenobiotics and potentially toxic endobiotics, such as bilirubin, for which reason glucuronidation is generally considered a beneficial process. However, steroid hormones glucuronidated on the D-ring (but not the A-ring) cause cholestasis, and induction of UDP-glucuronosyltransferase activity has been implicated as an epigenetic mechanism of thyroid tumor formation in rodents (Curran and DeGroot, 1991; McClain, 1989). Inducers of UDP-glucuronosyltransferases cause a decrease in serum thyroid hormone levels, which triggers a compensatory increase in thyroid stimulating hormone (TSH). During sustained exposure to the enzyme-inducing agent, prolonged stimulation of the thyroid gland by TSH (>6 months) results in the development of thyroid follicular cell neoplasia. Glucuronidation followed by biliary excretion is a major pathway of thyroxine biotransformation in rodents whereas deiodination is the major pathway (up to 85 percent) of thyroxine metabolism in humans. In contrast to the situation in rodents, prolonged stimulation of the thyroid gland by TSH in humans will result in malignant tumors only in exceptional circumstances and possibly only in conjunction with some thyroid abnormality.

Therefore, chemicals that cause thyroid tumors in rats or mice by inducing UDP-glucuronosyltransferase activity are unlikely to cause such tumors in humans. In support of this conclusion, epidemiological data suggest that phenobarbital and other anticonvulsants do not function as thyroid tumor promoters in humans.

In some cases, glucuronidation represents an important event in the toxicity of xenobiotics. For example, the aromatic amines that cause bladder cancer, such as 2-aminonaphthalene and 4-aminobiphenyl, undergo *N*-hydroxylation in the liver followed by *N*-glucuronidation of the resultant *N*-hydroxyaromatic amine. The *N*-glucuronides, which accumulate in the urine of the bladder, are unstable in acidic pH and thus are hydrolyzed to the corresponding unstable, tumorigenic *N*-hydroxyaromatic amine, as shown in Fig. 6-45. A similar mechanism may be involved in colon tumor formation by aromatic amines, although in this case hydrolysis of the *N*-glucuronide is probably catalyzed by $\beta$-glucuronidase in intestinal microflora. Some acylglucuronides are reactive intermediates that bind covalently to protein by mechanisms that may or may not result in cleavage of the glucuronic acid moiety, as shown in Fig. 6-45. Several drugs, including the NSAIDs diclofenac, diflunisal, etodolac, ketoprofen, suprofen, and tolmetin, contain a carboxylic acid moiety that is glucuronidated to form a reactive acylglucuronide. Neoantigens formed by binding of acylglucuronides to protein might be the cause of rare cases of NSAID-induced immune hepatitis. Binding of acylglucuronides to protein can involve isomerization reactions that lead to retention of a rearranged glucuronide moiety (Fig. 6-45). Formation of a common neoantigen (i.e., one that contains a rearranged glucuronic acid moiety) might explain the allergic cross-reactivities (cross-sensitization) observed among different NSAIDs (Spahn-Langguth and Benet, 1992; Kretz-Rommel and Boesterli, 1994).

## Sulfation

Many of the xenobiotics and endogenous substrates that undergo *O*-glucuronidation also undergo sulfate conjugation, as illustrated in Fig. 6-24 for acetaminophen (Mulder, 1981; Paulson et al., 1986). Sulfate conjugation generally produces a highly water-soluble sulfuric acid ester. The reaction is catalyzed by sulfotransferases, a group of soluble enzymes found primarily in the liver, kidney, intestinal tract, lung, platelets, and brain. The cofactor for the reaction is 3′-phosphoadenosine-5′-phosphosulfate (PAPS), the structure of which is shown in Fig. 6-41. The sulfate conjugation of aliphatic alcohols and phenols, R-OH, proceeds as follows:

$$\text{R—OH} + \text{phosphoadenosine}\text{—O—}\overset{\overset{\displaystyle O^-}{|}}{\underset{\underset{\displaystyle O}{\|}}{P}}\text{—O—}\overset{\overset{\displaystyle O}{\|}}{\underset{\underset{\displaystyle O}{\|}}{S}}\text{—O}^- \longrightarrow \text{R—O—}\overset{\overset{\displaystyle O}{\|}}{\underset{\underset{\displaystyle O}{\|}}{S}}\text{—O}^- + \text{phosphoadenosine}\text{—O—}\overset{\overset{\displaystyle O^-}{|}}{\underset{\underset{\displaystyle O}{\|}}{P}}\text{—O}^- + H^+$$

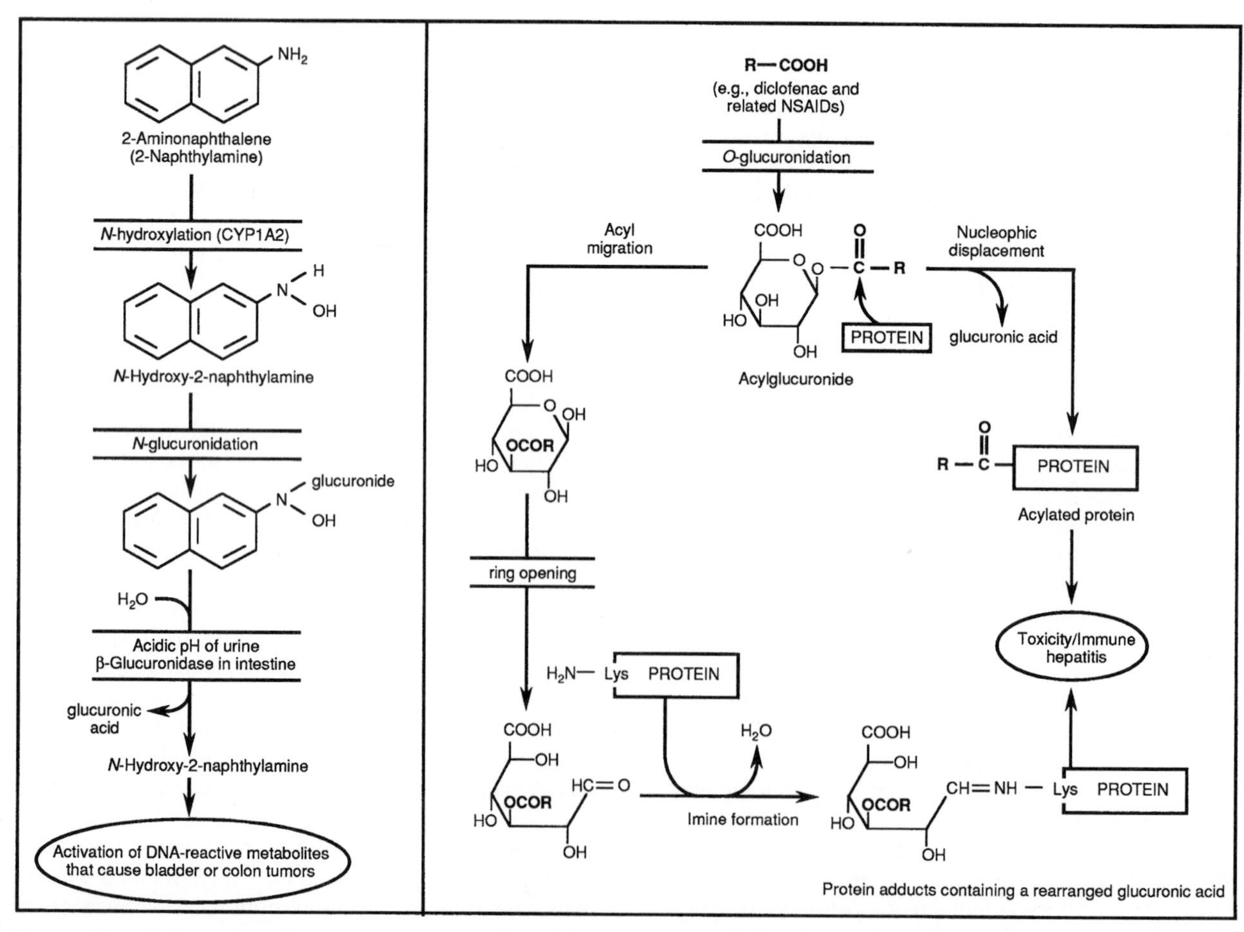


*Figure 6–45. Role of glucuronidation in the activation of xenobiotics to toxic metabolites.*

Sulfate conjugation involves the transfer of $SO_3^-$ (not $SO_4^-$) from PAPS to the xenobiotic. Sulfation is not limited to phenols and aliphatic alcohols (which are often the products of phase I biotransformation), although these represent the largest groups of substrates for sulfotransferases. Certain aromatic amines, such as aniline and 2-aminonaphthalene, can undergo sulfate conjugation to the corresponding sulfamates. The *N*-oxide group in minoxidil and the *N*-hydroxy group in *N*-hydroxy-2-aminonaphthalene and *N*-hydroxy-2-acetylaminofluorene can also be sulfated. In all cases, the conjugation reaction involves nucleophilic attack of oxygen or nitrogen on the electrophilic sulfur atom in PAPS with cleavage of the phosphosulfate bond. Table 6-6 lists some examples of xenobiotics and endogenous compounds that are sulfated without prior biotransformation by phase I enzymes. An even greater number of xenobiotics are sulfated after a hydroxyl group is exposed or introduced during phase I biotransformation. Carboxylic acids can be conjugated with glucuronic acid but not with sulfate. However, a number of carboxylic acids, such as benzoic acid, naphthoic acid, naphthylacetic acid, salicylic acid, and naproxen, are competitive inhibitors of sulfotransferases (Rao and Duffel, 1991). Pentachlorophenol and 2,6-dichloro-4-nitrophenol are potent sulfotransferase inhibitors because they bind to the enzyme but cannot initiate a nucleophilic attack on PAPS due to the presence of electron-withdrawing substituents in the *ortho*- and *para*-positions on the aromatic ring.

Sulfate conjugates of xenobiotics are excreted mainly in urine. Those excreted in bile may be hydrolyzed by aryl sulfatases present in gut microflora, which contributes to the enterohepatic circulation of certain xenobiotics. Sulfatases are also present in the endoplasmic reticulum and lysosomes, where they primarily hydrolyze sulfates of endogenous compounds. Their role in the disposition of sulfate conjugates is poorly understood. Some sulfate conjugates are substrates for further biotransformation. For example, dehydroepiandrosterone-3-sulfate is 16$\alpha$-hydroxylated by CYP3A7, the major P450 enzyme expressed in human fetal liver, whereas androstane-3,17-diol-3,17-disulfate is 15$\beta$-hydroxylated by CYP2C12, a female-specific P450 enzyme in rats. Sulfation facilitates the deiodination of thyroxine and triiodothyronine and can determine the rate of elimination of thyroid hormones.

The sulfate donor PAPS is synthesized from inorganic sulfate ($SO_4^{2-}$) and ATP in a two step reaction: The first reaction is catalyzed by ATP sulfurylase, which converts ATP and $SO_4^{2-}$ to adenosine-5′-phosphosulfate (APS) and pyrophosphate. The second reaction is catalyzed by APS kinase, which transfers a phosphate group from ATP to the 3′-position of APS. The major source of sulfate required for the synthesis of PAPS appears to be derived from cysteine through a complex oxidation sequence. Because the concentration of free cysteine is limited, the cellular concentrations of PAPS (~75 $\mu$M) are considerably lower than those of UDP-glucuronic acid (~350 $\mu$M) and glutathione (~10 mM). The relatively low concentration of PAPS limits the capacity for xenobiotic sulfation. In general, sulfation is a high-affinity but low-capacity pathway of xenobiotic conjugation, whereas glucuronidation is a low-affinity but high-capacity pathway. Acetaminophen is one of several xenobiotics that are substrates for both sulfotransferases and UDP-glucuronosyltransferases (see Fig. 6-24). The relative amount of sulfate and glucuronide conjugates of acetaminophen is dependent on dose. At low doses, acetaminophen sulfate is the main conjugate formed due the high affinity of sulfotransferases. As the dose increases, the proportion of acetaminophen conjugated with sulfate decreases, whereas the proportion conjugated with glucuronic acid increases. In some cases, even the absolute amount of xenobiotic conjugated with sulfate can decrease at high doses apparently because of substrate inhibition of sulfotransferase.

More than a dozen forms of sulfotransferase have been identified in rat liver cytosol, which have been categorized into five classes: *Arylsulfotransferase*, which sulfates numerous phenolic xenobiotics; *alcohol sulfotransferase*, which sulfates primary and secondary alcohols including nonaromatic hydroxysteroids (for which reason these enzymes are also known as hydroxysteroid sulfotransferases); *estrogen sulfotransferase*, which sulfates estrone and other aromatic hydroxysteroids; *tyrosine ester sulfotransferase*, which sulfates tyrosine methyl ester and 2-cyanoethyl-*N*-hydroxythioacetamide, and *bile salt sulfotransferase*, which sulfates conjugated and unconjugated

**Table 6–6**
**Examples of Xenobiotics and Endogenous Compounds That Undergo Sulfate Conjugation**

| FUNCTIONAL GROUP | EXAMPLE |
|---|---|
| Primary alcohol | Chloramphenicol, ethanol, hydroxymethyl polycyclic aromatic hydrocarbons, polyethylene glycols |
| Secondary alcohol | Bile acids, 2-butanol, cholesterol, dehydroepiandrosterone, doxaminol |
| Phenol | Acetaminophen, estrone, ethinylestradiol, naphthol, pentachlorophenol, phenol, picenadol, salicylamide, trimetrexate |
| Catechol | Dopamine, ellagic acid, $\alpha$-methyl-DOPA |
| *N*-oxide | Minoxidil |
| Aliphatic amine | 2-Amino-3,8-dimethylimidazo[4,5,-f]-quinoxaline (MeIQx)* 2-Amino-3-methylinidazo [4,5-f]-quinoline (IQ)* 2-Cyanoethyl-*N*-hydroxythioacetamide, despramine |
| Aromatic amine | 2-Aminonaphthalene, aniline |
| Aromatic hydroxylamine | *N*-hydroxy-2-aminonaphthalene |
| Aromatic hydroxyamide | *N*-hydroxy-2-acetylaminofluorene |

*Amino acid pyrolysis products.

bile acids. The activity of these enzymes is known to vary considerably with the sex and age of rats. In mature rats, arylsulfotransferase activity is higher in males, whereas alcohol sulfotransferase and bile salt sulfotransferase activities are higher in females. Sex differences in the developmental expression of individual sulfotransferase are the result of a complex interplay between gonadal, thyroidal, and pituitary hormones, which similarly determine sex differences in P450 enzyme expression. However, compared with P450 enzymes, the sulfotransferases are refractory or only marginally responsive to the enzyme-inducing effects of 3-methylcholanthrene and phenobarbital, although one or more forms of the alcohol and bile acid sulfotransferases are inducible by PCN. In general, sulfotransferase activity is low in pigs but high in cats. The high sulfotransferase activity in cats offsets their low capacity to conjugate xenobiotics with glucuronic acid.

Three sulfotransferases have been purified from human liver cytosol and extensively characterized (Weinshilboum, 1992). Two of the enzymes are phenol sulfotransferases (PST) that can be distinguished by their thermal stability; hence, they are known as TS-PST (*thermally stable*) and TL-PST (*thermally labile*). Because of differences in their substrate specificity, TS-PST and TL-PST are also known as phenol-PST and monoamine-PST, respectively. TL-PST preferentially catalyzes the sulfation of dopamine, epinephrine, and levadopa, whereas TS-PST preferentially catalyzes the sulfation of simple phenols, such as phenol, *para*-nitrophenol, minoxidil, and acetaminophen. TS-PST also catalyzes the *N*-sulfation of 2-aminonaphthalene. TS-PST (sensitive) and TL-PST (insensitive) can also be distinguished by differences in their sensitivity to the inhibitory effects of 2,6-dichloro-4-nitrophenol. The third enzyme is an alcohol sulfotransferase known as DHEA-ST. In addition to dehydroepiandrosterone (DHEA), substrates for DHEA-ST include several steroid hormones, bile acids, and cholesterol. The thermal stability of DHEA-ST is intermediate between that of the two phenol sulfotransferases, and the enzyme is resistant to the inhibitory effects of 2,6-dichloro-4-nitrophenol. These enzymes have been cloned from human liver. A fourth enzyme cloned from human liver is an estrogen sulfotransferase. It is distinct from the other three human sulfotransferases and from an estrogen sulfotransferase expressed in human placenta, breast, and uterine tissue.

The expression of PSTs in human liver is largely determined by genetic factors, which also determine the level of these sulfotransferases in blood platelets. Inherited variation in platelet TS-PST is correlated with interindividual variation in the sulfation of acetaminophen. Low TS-PST predisposes individuals to diet-induced migraine headaches, possibly due to impaired sulfation of unidentified phenolic compounds in the diet that cause such headaches. DHEA-ST is not expressed in blood platelets, but the activity of this enzyme has been measured in human liver cytosol. DHEA-ST is bimodally distributed, possibly due to a genetic polymorphism, with a high activity group comprised of ~25 percent of the population.

In general, sulfation is an effective means of decreasing the pharmacological and toxicological activity of xenobiotics. There are cases, however, in which sulfation increases the toxicity of foreign chemicals because certain sulfate conjugates are chemically unstable and degrade to form potent electrophilic species. As shown in Fig. 6-46, sulfation plays an important role in the activation of aromatic amines, methyl-substituted polycyclic aromatic hydrocarbons, and safrole to tumorigenic metabolites. To exert its tumorigenic effect in rodents, safrole must be hydroxylated by cytochrome P450 to 1′-hydroxysafrole, which is then sulfated to the electrophilic and tumor-initiating metabolite, 1′-sulfooxysafrole (Boberg et al., 1983). 1′-Hydroxysafrole is a more potent hepatotumorigen than safrole. Two lines of evidence support a major role for sulfation in the hepatotumorigenic effect of 1′-hydroxysafrole. First, the hepatotumorigenic effect of 1′-hydroxysafrole can be inhibited by treating mice with the sulfotransferase inhibitor, pentachlorophenol. Second, the hepatotumorigenic effect of 1′-hydroxysafrole is markedly reduced in brachymorphic mice, which have a diminished capacity to sulfate xenobiotics because of a genetic defect in PAPS synthesis. Brachymorphic mice are undersized because the defect in PAPS synthesis prevents the normal sulfation of glycosaminoglycans and proteoglycans such as heparin and chondroitin, which are important components of cartilage.

## Methylation

Methylation is a common but generally minor pathway of xenobiotic biotransformation. Methylation differs from most other phase II reactions because it generally decreases the water solubility of xenobiotics and masks functional groups that might otherwise be conjugated by other phase II enzymes. An exception to this rule is the *N*-methylation of pyridine-containing xenobiotics, such as nicotine, which produces quaternary ammonium ions that are water soluble and readily excreted. The cofactor for methylation is *S*-adenosylmethionine (SAM), the structure of which is shown in Fig. 6-41. The methyl group bound to the sulfonium ion in SAM has the characteristics of a carbonium ion and is transferred to xenobiotics and endogenous substrates by nucleophilic attack from an electron-rich heteroatom (*O, N*, or *S*). Consequently, the functional groups involved in methylation reactions are phenols, catechols, aliphatic and aromatic amines, *N*-heterocyclics, and sulfhydryl-containing compounds. The conversion of benzo[a]-pyrene to 6-methylbenzo[a]pyrene is a rare example of *C*-methylation. Another reaction that appears to involve *C*-methylation, the conversion of cocaine to ethylcocaine, is actually a transesterification reaction, as shown in Fig. 6-1. Metals can also be methylated. Inorganic mercury and arsenic can both be dimethylated, and inorganic selenium can be trimethylated. The selenium atom in ebselen is methylated following the ring opening of this anti-inflammatory drug. Some examples of xenobiotics and endogenous substrates that undergo *O*-, *N*-, or *S*-methylation are shown in Fig. 6-47. During these methylation reactions, SAM is converted to *S*-adenosylhomocysteine.

The *O*-methylation of phenols and catechols is catalyzed by two different enzymes known as phenol *O*-methyltransferase (POMT) and catechol-*O*-methyltransferase (COMT) (Weinshilboum, 1989, 1992b). POMT is a microsomal enzyme that methylates phenols but not catechols, and COMT is a cytosolic enzyme with the converse substrate specificity. COMT plays a greater role in the biotransformation of catechols than POMT plays in the biotransformation of phenols. COMT is present in virtually all tissues, including erythrocytes, but the highest concentrations are found in liver and kidney. Substrates for COMT include several catecholamine

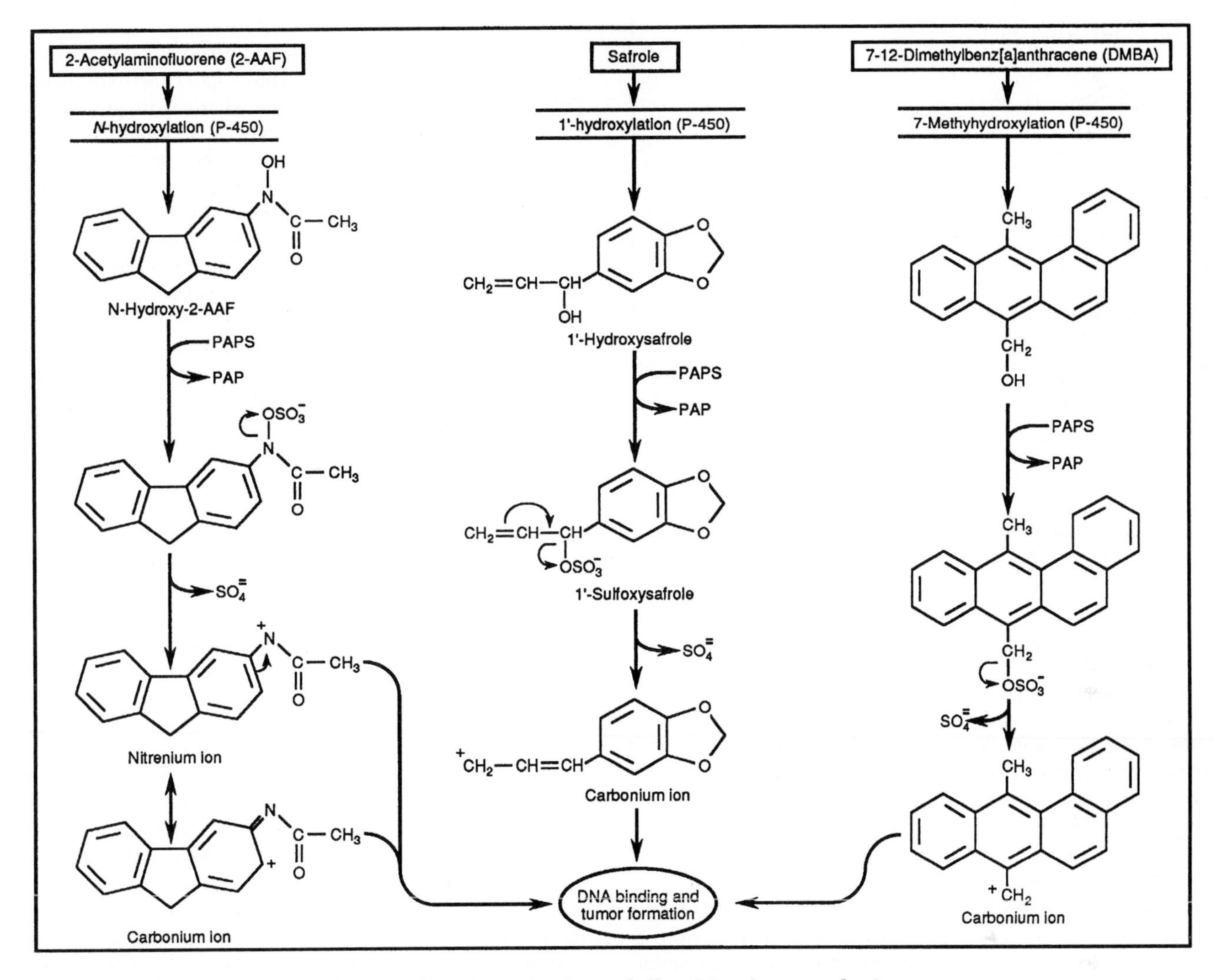


*Figure 6–46. Role of sulfation in the generation of tumorigenic metabolites (nitrenium or carbonium ions) of 2-acetylaminofluorene, safrole, and 7-12-dimethylbenz[a]anthracene.*

neurotransmitters, such as epinephrine, norepinephrine, and dopamine, and catechol drugs, such as the anti-Parkinson's disease agent L-dopa (3,4-dihydroxyphenylalanine) and the antihypertensive drug methyldopa ($\alpha$-methyl-3,4-dihydroxyphenylalanine). Catechol estrogens, which are formed by 2- or 4-hydroxylation of the steroid A-ring, are substrates for COMT, as are drugs that are converted to catechols either by two consecutive hydroxylation reactions (as in the case of phenobarbital and diclofenac), by ring opening of a methylenedioxy group (as in the case of stiripentol and 3,4-methylenedioxymethamphetamine), or by hydrolysis of vicinal esters (as in the case of ibopamine). Formation of catechol estrogens, particularly 4-hydroxyestradiol, has been suggested to play an important role in estrogen-induced tumor formation in hamster kidney, rat pituitary, and mouse uterus (Zhu and Liehr, 1993). These tissues contain high levels of epinephrine or dopamine, which inhibit the *O*-methylation of 4-hydroxyestradiol by COMT. Nontarget tissues do not contain high levels of catecholamines, which suggests that 4-hydroxyestradiol induces tumor formation in those tissues that fail to methylate and detoxify this catechol estrogen.

In humans, COMT is encoded by a single gene with alleles for a low activity form ($COMT^{L}$) and high activity form ($COMT^{H}$) (Weinshilboum, 1989, 1992b). In Caucasians, these allelic variants are expressed with equal frequency, so that 25 percent of the population is homozygous for either the low or high activity enzyme, and 50 percent is heterozygous and have intermediate COMT activity. COMT activity is generally higher in African Americans due to a higher frequency of the $COMT^{H}$ allele (~0.75 for blacks vs. ~0.5 for whites) (McLeod et al., 1994). The genetically determined levels of COMT in erythrocytes correlates with individual differences in the proportion of L-dopa converted to 3-*O*-methyldopa and the proportion of methyldopa converted to its 3-*O*-methyl metabolite. *O*-Methylation is normally a minor pathway of L-dopa biotransformation, but 3-*O*-methyldopa is the major metabolite when L-dopa is administered with a dopa decarboxylase inhibitor, such as carbidopa or benserazide, which is common practice. High COMT activity, resulting in extensive *O*-methylation of L-dopa to 3-*O*-methyldopa, has been associated with poor therapeutic management of Parkinson's disease and an increased incidence of drug-induced toxicity (dyskinesia).

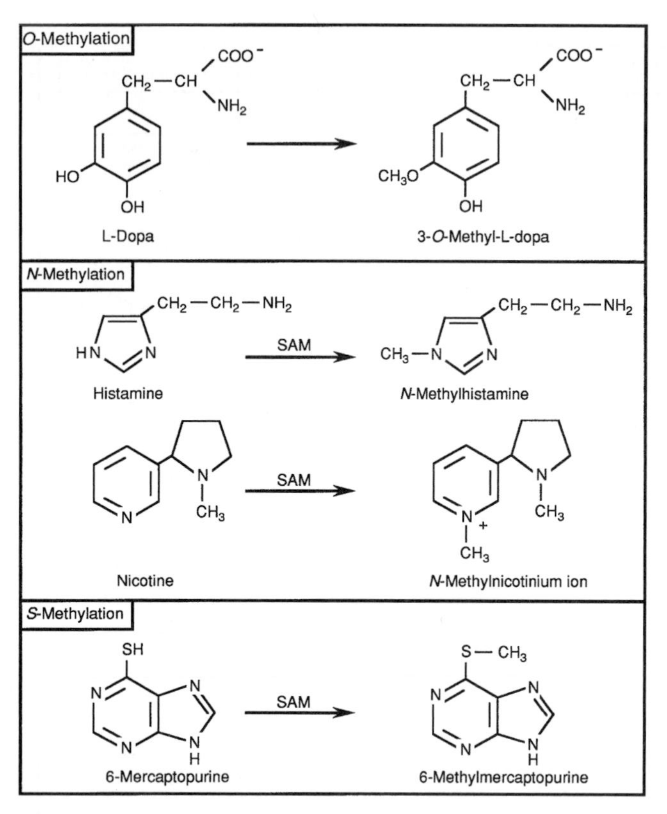


***Figure 6–47. Examples of compounds that undergo O-, N-, or S-methylation.***

SAM, S-adenosylmethionine.

Two *N*-methyltransferases have been described in humans. The first is known as histamine *N*-methyltransferase, which specifically methylates the imidazole ring of histamine and closely related compounds (Weinshilboum, 1989, 1992b). The second enzyme is known as nicotinamide *N*-methyltransferase, which methylates compounds containing a pyridine ring, such as nicotinamide and nicotine, or an indole ring, such as tryptophan and serotonin. Like COMT, histamine *N*-methyltransferase is a cytoplasmic enzyme expressed in numerous tissues including erythrocytes. The activity of histamine *N*-methyltransferase in erythrocytes is largely under genetic control and varies sixfold among individuals. It is not known whether inheritance is similarly involved in the regulation of nicotinamide *N*-methyltransferase. The system that is used to classify human *N*-methyltransferases may not be appropriate for other species. In guinea pigs, for example, nicotine and histamine are both methylated by a common *N*-methyltransferase. Guinea pigs have an unusually high capacity to methylate histamine and xenobiotics. The major route of nicotine biotransformation in the guinea pig is methylation, although *R*-(+)-nicotine is preferentially methylated over its *S*-(−)-enantiomer (Cundy et al., 1985). Guinea pigs also methylate the imidazole ring of cimetidine.

*S*-Methylation is an important pathway in the biotransformation of sulfhydryl-containing xenobiotics, such as the antihypertensive drug captopril, the antirheumatic agent D-penicillamine, the antineoplastic drug 6-mercaptopurine, metabolites of the alcohol deterrent disulfiram, and the deacetylated metabolite of the antidiuretic, spironolactone. In humans, *S*-methylation is catalyzed by two enzymes, thiopurine methyltransferase (TPMT) and thiol methyltransferase (TMT). TPMT is cytoplasmic enzyme that preferentially methylates aromatic and heterocyclic compounds such as the thiopurine drugs 6-mercaptopurine and azathioprine. TMT is a microsomal enzyme that preferentially methylates aliphatic sulfhydryl compounds such as captopril, D-penicillamine, and disulfiram derivatives. Both enzymes are present in erythrocytes at levels that reflect the expression of TPMT and TMT in liver and other tissues. Although TPMT and TMT are independently regulated, their expression in erythrocytes is largely determined by genetic factors. TPMT is encoded by a single gene with alleles for a low activity form ($TPMT^L$) and for a high activity form ($TPMT^H$). The gene frequency of $TPMT^L$ and $TPMT^H$ are 6 and 94 percent, respectively, which produces a trimodal distribution of TPMT activity with low, intermediate and high activity expressed in 0.3, 11.1, and 88.6 percent of the population, respectively. Cancer patients with low TPMT activity are at increased risk for thiopurine-induced myelotoxicity, in contrast to the potential need for higher-than-normal doses to achieve therapeutic levels of thiopurines in patients with TPMT high activity (Weinshilboum, 1989, 1992b). A genetic polymorphism for TMT also has been described, but its pharmacological and toxicological significance remain to be determined.

The hydrogen sulfide produced by anaerobic bacteria in the intestinal tract is converted by *S*-methyltransferases to methane thiol and then to dimethylsulfide. Another source of substrates for *S*-methyltransferase are the thioethers of glutathione conjugates. Glutathione conjugates are hydrolyzed to cysteine conjugates, which can either be acetylated to form mercapturic acids or cleaved by beta lyase. This beta lyase pathway converts the cysteine conjugate to pyruvate, ammonia and a sulfhydryl-containing xenobiotic, which is a potential substrate for *S*-methylation.

## Acetylation

*N*-Acetylation is a major route of biotransformation for xenobiotics containing an aromatic amine ($R\text{-}NH_2$) or a hydrazine group ($R\text{-}NH\text{-}NH_2$), which are converted to aromatic amides ($R\text{-}NH\text{-}COCH_3$) and hydrazides ($R\text{-}NH\text{-}NH\text{-}COCH_3$), respectively (Evans, 1992). Xenobiotics containing primary aliphatic amines are rarely substrates for *N*-acetylation, a notable exception being cysteine conjugates, which are formed from glutathione conjugates and converted to mercapturic acids by *N*-acetylation in the kidney (see "Glutathione Conjugation"). Like methylation, *N*-acetylation masks an amine with a nonionizable group, so that many *N*-acetylated metabolites are less water soluble than the parent compound. Nevertheless, *N*-acetylation of certain xenobiotics, such as isoniazid, facilitates their urinary excretion.

The *N*-acetylation of xenobiotics is catalyzed by *N*-acetyltransferases and requires the cofactor acetyl-coenzyme A (acetyl-CoA), the structure of which is shown in Fig. 6-41. The reaction occurs in two sequential steps according to a *ping-pong Bi-Bi* mechanism (Hein, 1988). In the first step, the acetyl group from acetyl-CoA is transferred to an active site cysteine residue within an *N*-acetyltransferase with release of coenzyme A ($E\text{-}SH + CoA\text{-}S\text{-}COCH_3 \rightarrow E\text{-}S\text{-}COCH_3 + CoA\text{-}$

SH). In the second step, the acetyl group is transferred from the acylated enzyme to the amino group of the substrate with regeneration of the enzyme. For strongly basic amines, the rate of *N*-acetylation is determined by the first step (acetylation of the enzyme), whereas the rate of *N*-acetylation of weakly basic amines is determined by the second step (transfer of the acetyl group from the acylated enzyme to the acceptor amine). In certain cases (discussed below), *N*-acetyltransferases can catalyze the *O*-acetylation of xenobiotics.

*N*-Acetyltransferases are cytosolic enzymes found in liver and many other tissues of most mammalian species, with the notable exception of the dog and fox, which are unable to acetylate xenobiotics. In contrast to other xenobiotic-biotransforming enzymes, the number of *N*-acetyltransferases is limited (Vatsis et al., 1995). Humans, rabbits and hamsters express only two *N*-acetyltransferases, known as NAT1 and NAT2, whereas mice express three distinct forms of the enzymes, namely NAT1, NAT2 and NAT3. In each species examined, NAT1 and NAT2 are closely related proteins (79-95% identical in amino acid sequence) with an active site cysteine residue ($Cys^{68}$) in the *N*-terminal region (Grant et al., 1992, Vatsis et al., 1995). Although they are encoded by intronless genes on the same chromosome, NAT1 and NAT2 are independently regulated proteins: NAT1 is expressed in most tissues of the body whereas NAT2 appears to be expressed only in liver and gut. NAT1 and NAT2 also have different but overlapping substrate specificities, although no substrate is exclusively *N*-acetylated by one enzyme or the other. Substrates preferentially *N*-acetylated by human NAT1 include *para*-aminosalicylic acid, *para*-aminobenzoic acid, sulfamethoxazole, and sulfanilamide, while substrates preferentially *N*-acetylated by human NAT2 include isoniazid, hydralazine, procainamide, dapsone, aminoglutethimide, and sulfamethazine. Some xenobiotics, such as the carcinogenic aromatic amine, 2-aminofluorene, are *N*-acetylated equally well by NAT1 and NAT2.

Several drugs are *N*-acetylated following their biotransformation by phase I enzymes. For example, caffeine is *N3*-demethylated by CYP1A2 to paraxanthine (Fig. 6-36), which is then *N*-demethylated to 1-methylxanthine and *N*-acetylated to 5-acetylamino-6-formylamino-3-methyluracil (AFMU) by NAT2. Other drugs converted to metabolites that are *N*-acetylated by NAT2 include sulfasalazine, nitrazepam, and clonazepam. Examples of drugs that are *N*-acetylated by NAT1 and NAT2 are shown in Fig. 6-48. It should be noted, however, that there are species differences in the substrate specificity of *N*-acetyltransferases. For example, *para*-aminobenzoic acid is preferentially *N*-acetylated by NAT1 in humans and rabbits but by NAT2 in mice and hamsters.

Genetic polymorphisms for *N*-acetylation have been documented in humans, hamsters, rabbits, and mice (Heim, 1988; Evans, 1992; Grant et al., 1992; Vatsis et al., 1995). A series of clinical observations in the 1950s established the existence of *slow* and *fast acetylators* of the antituberculosis drug isoniazid. The incidence of the slow acetylator phenotype is high in Middle Eastern populations (e.g., ~70 percent in Egyptians, Saudi Arabians, and Moroccans), intermediate in Caucasian populations (~50 percent in Americans, Australians, and Europeans), and low in Asian populations (e.g., <25 percent of Chinese, Japanese, and Koreans). The slow acetylator phenotype is caused by various mutations in the NAT2 gene that either decrease NAT2 activity or enzyme stability. For example, a point mutation in nucleotide 341 (which causes the amino acid substitution $Ile^{114} \rightarrow Thr$) decreases $V_{max}$ for *N*-acetylation without altering the $K_m$ for substrate binding or the stability of the enzyme. This mutation is the most common cause of the slow acetylator phenotype in Caucasians but is rarely observed in Asians. In contrast, a point mutation in nucleotide 857, which decreases the stability of NAT2, is more prevalent in Asians than Caucasians. Within the slow acetylator phenotype there is considerable variation in rates of xenobiotic *N*-acetylation. This is because different mutations in *NAT2* have different effects on NAT2 activity and/or enzyme stability, and because the *N*-acetylation of "NAT2-substrates" by NAT1 becomes significant in slow acetylators.

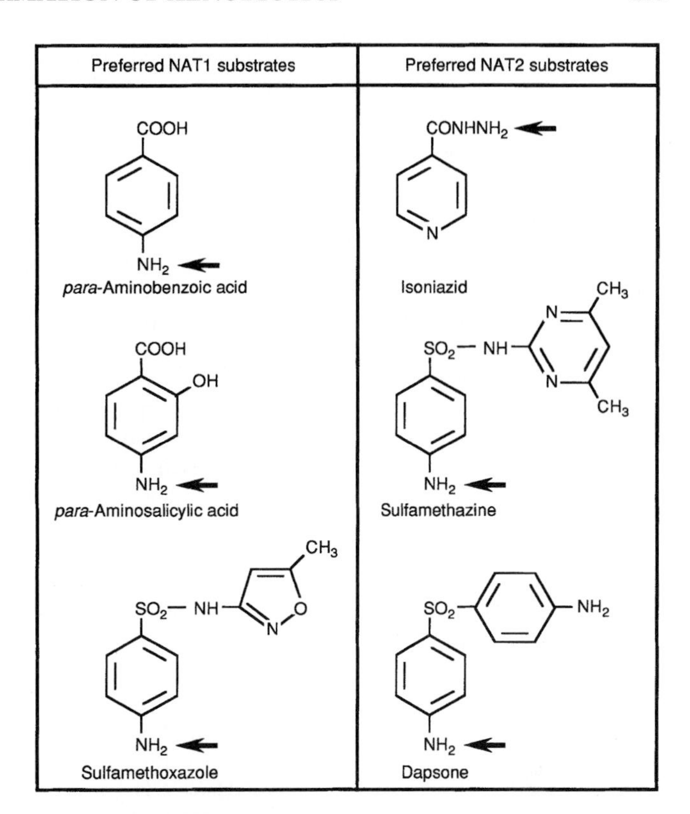


***Figure 6–48. Examples of substrates for the human N-acetyltransferases, NAT1, and the highly polymorphic NAT2.***

Arrows indicate the site of acetylation.

NAT1 and NAT2 are often referred to as *monomorphic* and *polymorphic* *N*-acetyltransferases because only the latter enzyme was thought to be genetically polymorphic. However, recent evidence suggests that phenotypic differences in the *N*-acetylation of *para*-aminosalicylic acid are distributed bimodally, suggesting the existence of low and high activity forms of NAT1. Furthermore, an extremely slow acetylator of *para*-aminosalicylic acid has been identified with mutations in both NAT1 alleles; one that decreases NAT1 activity and stability and one that encodes a truncated and catalytically inactive form of the enzyme. The incidence and pharmacological/toxicological significance of genetic polymorphisms in *NAT1* that produce phenotypically discernible alterations in NAT1 activity remain to be determined.

Genetic polymorphisms in NAT2 have a number of pharmacological and toxicological consequences for drugs that are

*N*-acetylated by this enzyme. The pharmacological effects of the antihypertensive drug hydralazine are more pronounced in slow acetylators. Slow acetylators are predisposed to several drug toxicities, including nerve damage (peripheral neuropathy) from isoniazid and dapsone, systemic lupus erythematosus from hydralazine and procainamide, and the toxic effects of coadministration of the anticonvulsant phenytoin with isoniazid. Slow acetylators that are deficient in glucose-6-phosphate dehydrogenase are particularly prone to hemolysis from certain sulfonamides. Fast acetylators are predisposed to the myelotoxic effects of amonafide because *N*-acetylation retards the clearance of this antineoplastic drug.

Some epidemiological studies suggest that rapid acetylators are at increased risk for the development of isoniazid-induced liver toxicity, although several other studies contradict these findings. Indeed, some studies have demonstrated convincingly that slow acetylation is a risk factor for isoniazid-induced hepatotoxicity. Following its acetylation by NAT2, isoniazid can be hydrolyzed to isonicotinic acid and acetylhydrazine ($CH_3CO$-$NHNH_2$). This latter metabolite can be *N*-hydroxylated by FMO or cytochrome P450 to a reactive intermediate, as shown in Fig. 6-29a. The generation of a reactive metabolite from acetylhydrazine would seem to provide a mechanistic basis for enhanced isoniazid hepatotoxicity in fast acetylators. However, acetylhydrazine can be further acetylated to diacetlyhydrazine ($CH_3CO$-NHNH-$COCH_3$), and this detoxication reaction is also catalyzed by NAT2. Therefore, acetylhydrazine is both produced and detoxified by NAT2, hence slow acetylation, not fast acetylation, is a possible risk factor for isoniazid-induced hepatotoxicity, just as it is for isoniazid-induced peripheral neuropathy. Rifampin and alcohol have been reported to enhance the hepatotoxicity of isoniazid. These drug interactions are probably the result of increased *N*-hydroxylation of acetylhydrazine due to cytochrome P450 induction rather than to an alteration in NAT2 activity.

Aromatic amines can be both activated and deactivated by *N*-acetyltransferases (Kato and Yamazoe, 1994b). The *N*-acetyltransferases detoxify aromatic amines by converting them to the corresponding amides because aromatic amides are less likely than aromatic amines to be activated to DNA-reactive metabolites by cytochrome P450, PHS, and UDP-glucuronosyltransferase. However, *N*-acetyltransferases can activate aromatic amines if they are first *N*-hydroxylated by cytochrome P450 because *N*-acetyltransferases can also function as *O*-acetyltransferases and convert *N*-hydroxyaromatic amines (hydroxylamines) to acetoxy esters. As shown in Fig. 6-7, the acetoxy esters of *N*-hydroxyaromatic amines, like the corresponding sulfate esters (Fig. 6-46), can break down to form highly reactive nitrenium and carbonium ions that bind to DNA. *N*-acetyltransferases catalyze the *O*-acetylation of *N*-hydroxyaromatic amines by two distinct mechanisms. The first reaction, which is exemplified by the conversion of *N*-hydroxyaminofluorene to *N*-acetoxyaminofluorene, requires acetyl-CoA and proceeds by the same mechanism previously described for *N*-acetylation. The second reaction is exemplified by the conversion of 2-acetylaminofluorene to *N*-acetoxyaminofluorene, which does not require acetyl-CoA but involves an intramolecular transfer of the *N*-acetyl group from nitrogen to oxygen. These reactions are shown in Fig. 6-49.

Genetic polymorphisms in NAT2 have been reported to influence susceptibility to aromatic amine-induced bladder and colon cancer (Heim, 1988; Evans, 1992; Kadlubar, 1994). Bladder cancer is thought to be caused by bicyclic aromatic amines (benzidine, 2-aminonaphthalene, and 4-aminobiphenyl), whereas colon cancer is thought to be caused by heterocyclic aromatic amines, such as the products of amino acid pyrolysis (e.g., 2-amino-6-methylimidazo[4,5-*b*]pyridine or PhIP, and others listed in Table 6-5). Epidemiological studies suggest that slow acetylators are more likely than fast acetylators to develop bladder cancer from cigarette smoking and from occupational exposure to bicyclic aromatic amines. The possibility that slow acetylators are at increased risk for aromatic amine-induced cancer is supported by the finding that dogs, which are poor acetylators, are highly prone to aromatic amine-induced bladder cancer. By comparison, fast acetylators appear to be at increased risk for colon cancer from heterocyclic aromatic amines.

The influence of acetylator phenotype on susceptibility to aromatic amine-induced cancer can be rationalized on the ability of *N*-acetyltransferases to activate and detoxify aromatic amines and by differences in the substrate specificity and tissues distribution of NAT1 and NAT2 (recall that NAT1 is expressed in virtually all tissues, whereas NAT2 is expressed only in the liver and gut). Both NAT1 and NAT2 catalyze the *O*-acetylation (activation) of *N*-hydroxy bicyclic aromatic amines, whereas the *O*-acetylation of *N*-hydroxy heterocyclic aromatic amines is preferentially catalyzed by NAT2. Bicyclic aromatic amines can also be *N*-acetylated (detoxified) by NAT1 and NAT2, but heterocyclic aromatic amines are poor substrates for both enzymes. Therefore, the fast acetylator phenotype protects against aromatic amine-induced bladder cancer because NAT2 (as well as NAT1) catalyzes the *N*-acetylation (detoxication) of bicyclic aromatic amines in the liver. In slow acetylators, a greater proportion of the bicyclic aromatic amines are activated through *N*-hydroxylation by CYP1A2. These *N*-hydroxylated aromatic amines can be activated by *O*-acetylation, which can be catalyzed in the bladder itself by NAT1. Recent evidence suggests that a high level of NAT1 in the bladder is a risk factor for aromatic amine-induced bladder cancer. In addition, the fast acetylator phenotype potentiates the colon cancer-inducing effects of heterocyclic aromatic amines. These aromatic amines are poor substrates for NAT1 and NAT2, so that high levels of NAT2 in the liver do little to prevent their *N*-hydroxylation by CYP1A2. The *N*-hydroxylated metabolites of heterocyclic aromatic amines can be activated by *O*-acetylation, which can be catalyzed in the colon itself by NAT2. The presence of NAT2 (and NAT1) in the colons of fast acetylators probably explains why this phenotype is a risk factor for the development of colon cancer.

Whether fast acetylators are protected from or predisposed to the cancer-causing effects of aromatic amines depends on the nature of the aromatic amine (bicyclic vs. heterocyclic) and on other important risk factors. For example, CYP1A2 plays an important role in the *N*-hydroxylation of both bicyclic and heterocyclic amines, and high CYP1A2 activity has been shown or is strongly suspected of being a risk factor for aromatic amine-induced bladder and colon cancer. It remains to be determined whether the activation of aromatic amines by *N*-glucuronidation and the activation of *N*-

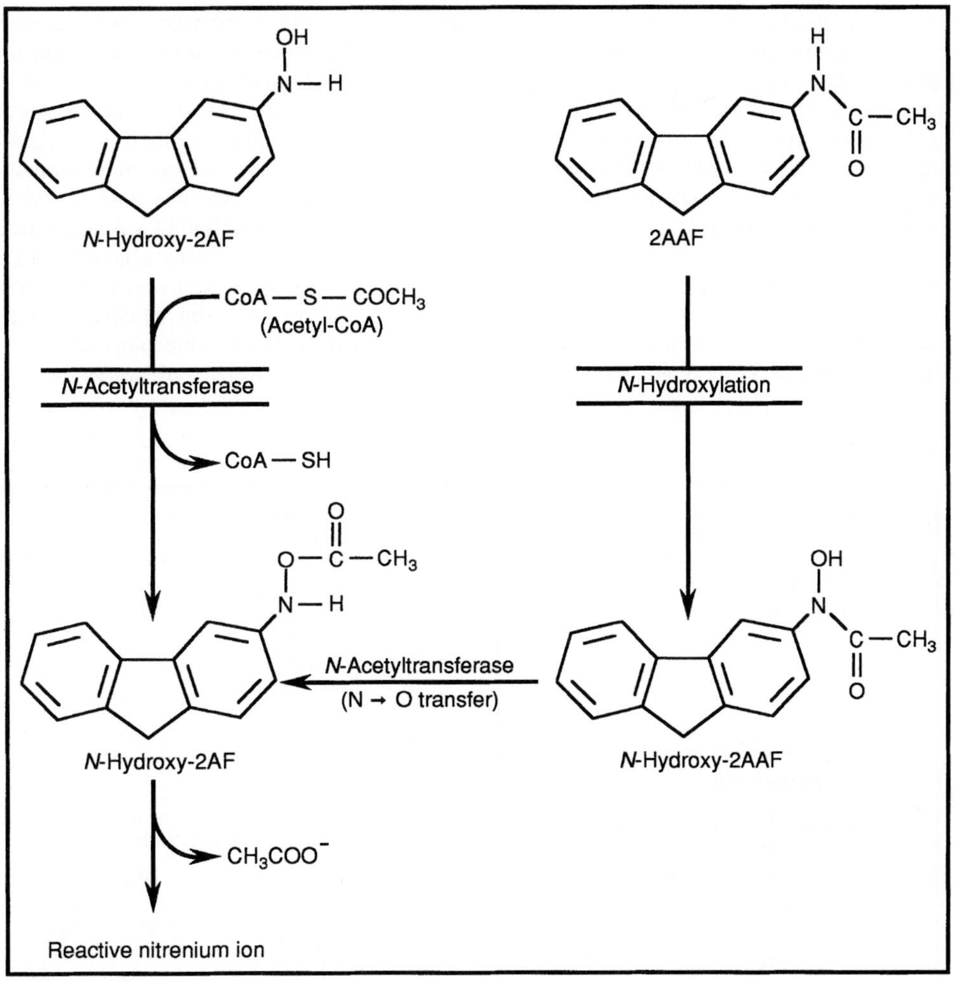

*Figure 6–49. Role of N-acetyltransferase in the O-acetylation of N-hydroxy-2-aminofluorene (N-hydroxy-2AF) and the intramolecular rearrangement of N-hydroxy-2-acetylaminofluorene (N-hydroxy-2-AAF).*

hydroxy aromatic amines by sulfation have a significant impact on the incidence of bladder and colon cancer. These and other risk factors may explain why some epidemiological studies, contrary to expectation, have shown that slow acetylators are at increased risk for aromatic amine-induced bladder cancer, as was demonstrated recently for benzidine manufacturers in China (Hayes et al., 1993).

The *N*-acetylation of aromatic amines (a detoxication reaction) and the *O*-acetylation of *N*-hydroxy aromatic amines (an activation reaction) can be reversed by a microsomal enzyme called arylacetamide deacetylase (Probst et al., 1994). This enzyme is similar to but distinct from the microsomal carboxylesterases that hydrolyze esters and amides. Whether arylacetamide deacetylase alters the overall balance between detoxication and activation of aromatic amines remains to be determined.

## Amino Acid Conjugation

There are two principal pathways by which xenobiotics are conjugated with amino acids, as illustrated in Fig. 6-50. The first involves conjugation of xenobiotics containing a carboxylic acid group with the amino group of amino acids such as glycine, glutamine and taurine (see Fig. 6-41). This pathway involves activation of the xenobiotic by conjugation with CoA, which produces an acyl-CoA thioether that reacts with the *amino group* of an amino acid to form an amide linkage. The second pathway involves conjugation of xenobiotics containing an aromatic hydroxylamine (*N*-hydroxy aromatic amine) with the *carboxylic acid group* of such amino acids as serine and proline. This pathway involves activation of an amino acid by aminoacyl-tRNA-synthetase, which reacts with an aromatic hydroxylamine to form a reactive *N*-ester (Kato and Yamazoe, 1994b).

The conjugation of benzoic acid with glycine to form hippuric acid was discovered in 1842, making it the first biotransformation reaction discovered (Paulson et al., 1985). The first step in this conjugation reaction involves activation of benzoic acid to an acyl-CoA thioester. This reaction requires ATP and is catalyzed by acyl-CoA synthetase (ATP-dependent acid:CoA ligase). The second step is catalyzed by acyl-CoA:amino acid *N*-acyltransferase, which transfers the acyl moiety of the xenobiotic to the amino group of the acceptor amino acid. The reaction proceeds by a *ping-pong Bi-Bi* mechanism, and involves transfer of the xenobiotic to a cysteine residue in the enzyme with release of coenzyme A, followed by transfer of the xenobiotic to the acceptor amino acid with regeneration of the enzyme. The second step in amino acid conjugation is analogous to amide formation during the acetylation of aromatic amines by *N*-acetyltransferase. Substrates for amino acid conjugation are restricted to certain aliphatic, aromatic, heteroaromatic, cinnamic, and arylacetic acids.

The ability of xenobiotics to undergo amino acid conjugation depends on steric hindrance around the carboxyl acid group, and by substituents on the aromatic ring or aliphatic side chain. In rats, ferrets, and monkeys, the major pathway of phenylacetic acid biotransformation is amino acid conjugation. However, due to steric hindrance, diphenylacetic acid cannot be conjugated with an amino acid, so the major pathway of diphenylacetic acid biotransformation in these same three species is acylglucuronidation. Bile acids are endogenous substrates for glycine and taurine conjugation. However, the activation of bile acids to an acyl-CoA thioester is catalyzed by a microsomal enzyme, cholyl-CoA synthetase, and conjugation with glycine or taurine is catalyzed by a single cytosolic enzyme, bile acid-CoA:amino acid *N*-acyltransferase (Falany et al., 1994). In contrast, the activation of xenobiotics occurs mainly in mitochondria, which appear to contain multiple acyl-CoA synthetases. The second step in the conjugation of xeno-

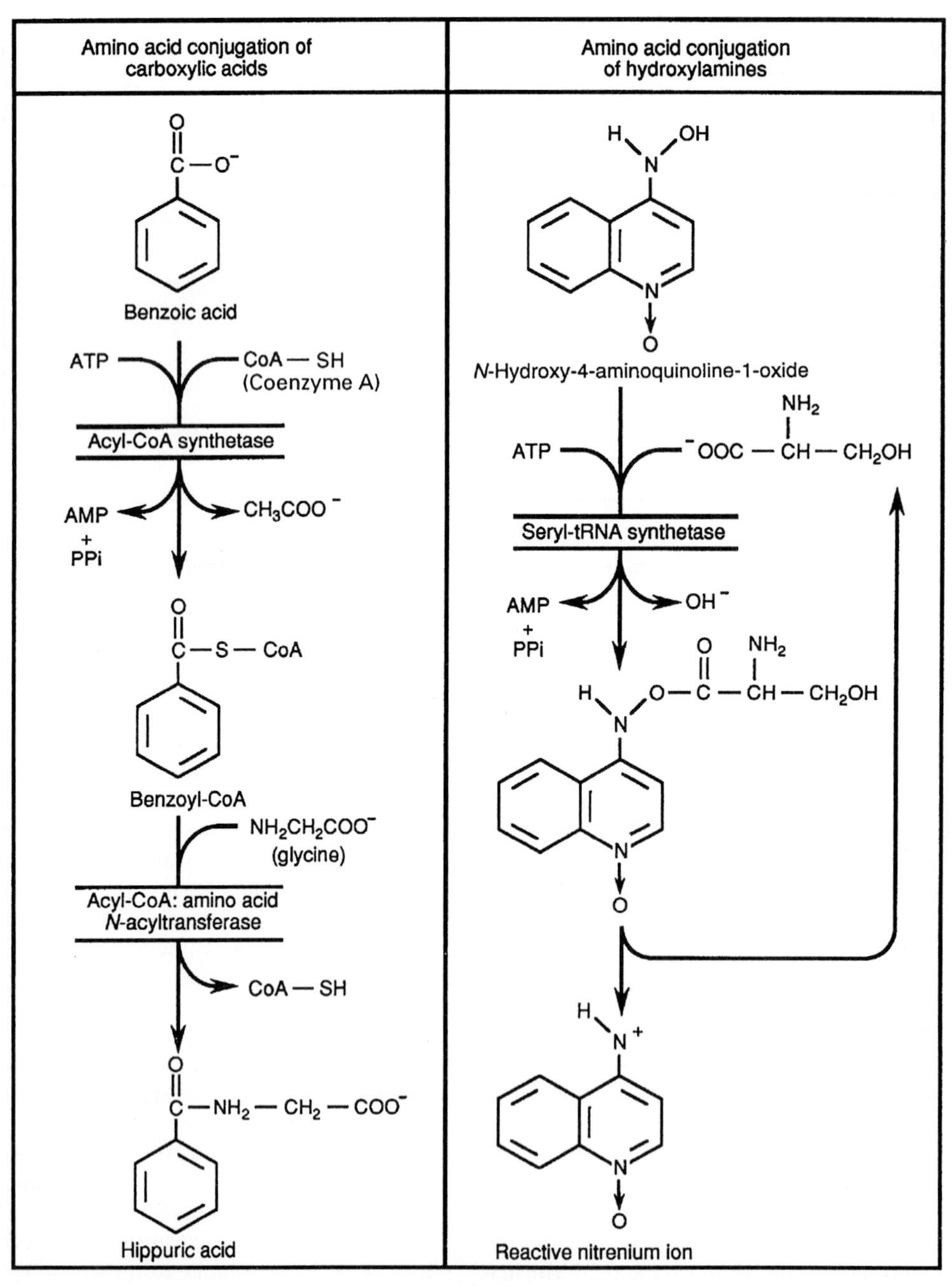


*Figure 6–50. Conjugation of xenobiotics with amino acids.*

biotics with amino acid is catalyzed by cytosolic and/or mitochondrial forms of *N*-acyltransferase. Two different types of *N*-acyltransferases have been purified from mammalian hepatic mitochondria. One prefers benzoyl-CoA as substrate, whereas the other prefers arylacetyl-CoA. Another important difference between the amino acid conjugates of xenobiotics and bile acids is their route of elimination: Bile acids are secreted into bile whereas amino acid conjugates of xenobiotics are eliminated primarily in urine. The addition of an endogenous amino acid to xenobiotics may facilitate this elimination by increasing their ability to interact with the tubular organic anion transport system in the kidney.

In addition to glycine, glutamine, and taurine, acceptor amino acids for xenobiotic conjugation include ornithine, arginine, histidine, serine, aspartic acid, and several dipeptides, such as glycylglycine, glycyltaurine, and glycylvaline. The acceptor amino acid used for conjugation is both species- and xenobiotic-dependent. For benzoic, heterocyclic, and cinnamic acids, the acceptor amino acid is glycine, except in birds and reptiles, which use ornithine. Arylacetic acids are also conjugated with glycine except in primates, which use glutamine. In mammals, taurine is generally an alternative acceptor to glycine. Taurine conjugation is well developed in nonmammalian species and carnivores. Whereas most species conjugate bile acids with both glycine and taurine, cats and dogs conjugated bile acids only with taurine.

Conjugation of carboxylic acid-containing xenobiotics is an alternative to glucuronidation. Conjugation with amino acids is a detoxication reaction, whereas the glucuronidation of carboxylic acid-containing xenobiotic produces potentially toxic acylglucuronides (see Fig. 6-45). Amino acid conjugation of ibuprofen and related *profens* (2-substituted propionic acid NSAIDs) is significant for two reasons: It limits the formation of potentially toxic acylglucuronides, and it leads to chiral inversion (the interconversion of *R*- and *S*-enantiomers) (Shirley et al., 1994). This latter reaction requires conversion of the profen to its acyl-CoA thioester, which undergoes chiral inversion by 2-arylpropionyl-CoA epimerase (this involves the intermediacy of a symmetrical, conjugated enolate anion). Chiral inversion explains why the *R*- and *S*-enantiomers of several profen NSAIDs have comparable anti-inflammatory effects in vivo, even though the *S*-enantiomers are considerably more potent than their antipodes as inhibitors of cyclooxygenase (the target of NSAID therapy).

In contrast to amino acid conjugation of carboxylic acid-containing xenobiotics, which is a detoxication reaction, amino acid conjugation of *N*-hydroxy aromatic amines (hydroxylamines) is an activation reaction because it produces *N*-esters that can degrade to form electrophilic nitrenium and carbonium ions (Anders, 1985; Kato and Yamazoe, 1994b). Conjugation of hydroxylamines with amino acids is catalyzed by cytosolic aminoacyl-tRNA synthetases and requires ATP (Fig. 6-50). Hydroxylamines activated by aminoacyl-tRNA synthetases include *N*-hydroxy-4-aminoquinoline 1-oxide, which is conjugated with serine, and *N*-hydroxy-Trp-P-2, which is conjugated with proline. (*N*-hydroxy-Trp-P-2 is the *N*-hydroxylated metabolite of Trp-P-2, a pyrolysis product of tryptophan [see Table 6-5]). It is now apparent that the hydroxylamines formed by the cytochrome P450-dependent *N*-hydroxylation of aromatic amines can potentially be activated by numerous reactions, including *N*-glucuronidation by UDP-glucuronosyltransferase (Fig. 6-45), *O*-acetylation by *N*-acetyltransferase (Fig. 6-7), *O*-sulfation by sulfotransferase (Fig. 6-46), and conjugation with amino acids by seryl- or prolyl-tRNA synthetase (Fig. 6-50).

## Glutathione Conjugation

The preceding section described the conjugation of xenobiotics with certain amino acids, including some simple dipeptides, such as glycyltaurine. This section describes the conjugation of xenobiotics with the tripeptide glutathione, which is comprised of glycine, cysteine, and glutamic acid (the latter being linked to cysteine via the $\gamma$-carboxyl group, not the usual $\alpha$-carboxyl group, as shown in Fig. 6-41). Conjugation of xenobiotics with glutathione is fundamentally different from their conjugation with other amino acids and dipeptides (Sies and Ketterer, 1988; Mantle et al., 1987). Substrates for glutathione conjugation include an enormous array of electrophilic xenobiotics, or xenobiotics that can be biotransformed to electrophiles. In contrast to the amides formed by conjugation of xenobiotics to other amino acids, glutathione conjugates are thioethers, which form by nucleophilic attack of glutathione thiolate anion ($GS^-$) with an electrophilic carbon atom in the xenobiotic. Glutathione can also conjugate xenobiotics containing electrophilic heteroatoms (*O*, *N*, and *S*).

The synthesis of glutathione involves formation of the peptide bond between cysteine and glutamic acid, followed by peptide bond formation with glycine. The first reaction is catalyzed by $\gamma$-glutamylcysteine synthetase; the second by glutathione synthetase. At each step, ATP is hydrolyzed to ADP and inorganic phosphate. The first reaction is inhibited by buthionine-*S*-sulfoximine, which can be used in vivo to decrease glutathione levels in experimental animals. The conjugation of xenobiotics with glutathione is catalyzed by a family of glutathione *S*-transferases. These enzymes are present in most tissues, with high concentrations in the liver, intestine, kidney, testis, adrenal, and lung, where they are localized in the cytoplasm (>95 percent) and endoplasmic reticulum (<5 percent).

Substrates for glutathione *S*-transferase share three common features: They are hydrophobic, they contain an electrophilic atom, and they react nonenzymatically with glutathione at some measurable rate. The mechanism by which glutathione *S*-transferase increases the rate of glutathione conjugation involves deprotonation of GSH to $GS^-$ by an active site tyrosinate (Tyr-$O^-$), which functions as a general base catalyst (Atkins et al., 1993; Dirr et al., 1994). The concentration of glutathione in liver is extremely high (~10 mM); hence, the nonenzymatic conjugation of certain xenobiotics with glutathione can be significant. However, some xenobiotics are conjugated with glutathione stereoselectively, indicating that the reaction is largely catalyzed by glutathione *S*-transferase. Like glutathione, the glutathione *S*-transferases are themselves abundant cellular components, accounting for up to 10 percent of the total cellular protein. These enzymes bind, store, and/or transport a number of compounds that are not substrates for glutathione conjugation. The cytoplasmic protein formerly known as ligandin, which binds heme, bilirubin, steroids, azo-dyes and polycyclic aromatic hydrocarbons, is glutathione *S*-transferase.

As shown in Fig. 6-51, substrates for glutathione conjugation can be divided into two groups: Those that are sufficiently

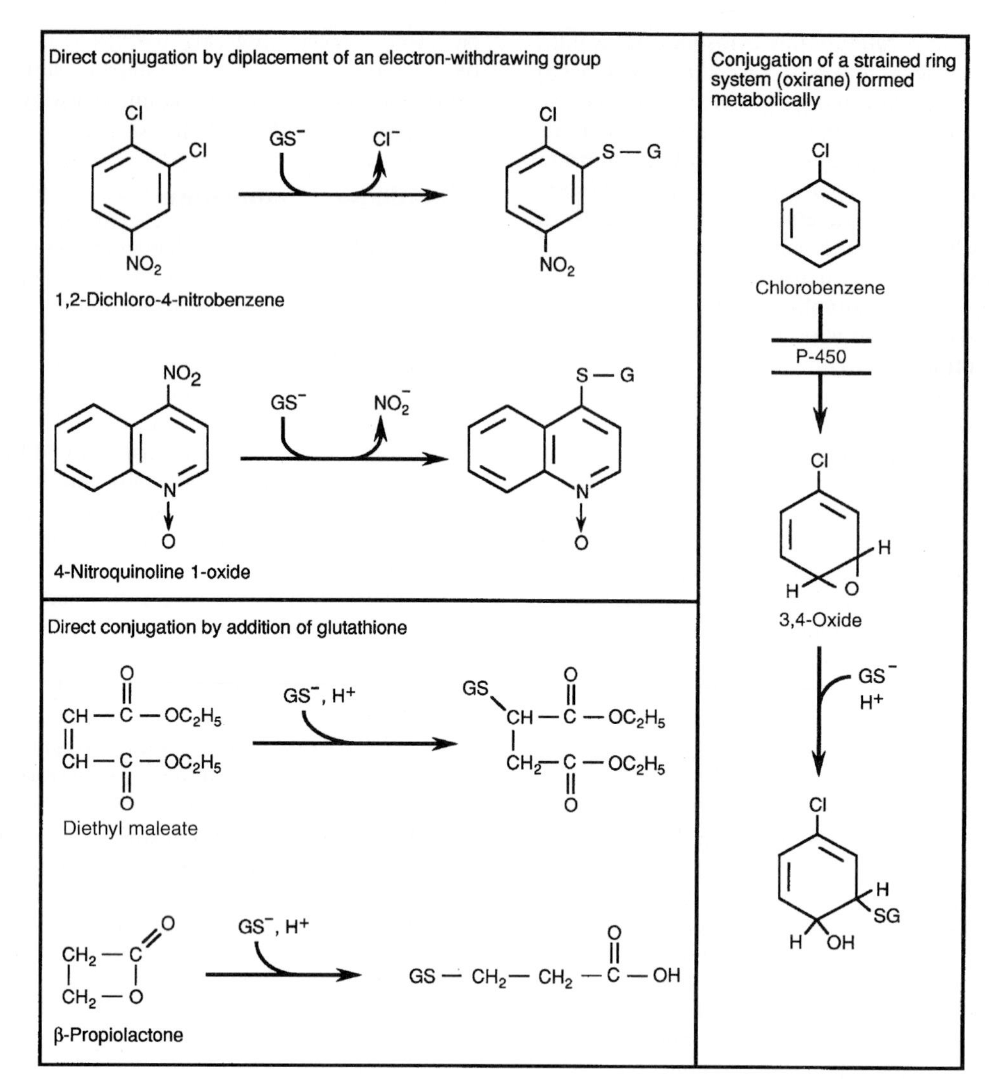


***Figure 6–51.*** ***Examples of glutathione conjugation of xenobiotics with an electrophilic carbon.*** $GS^-$ represents the anionic form of glutathione.

electrophilic to be conjugated directly, and those that must first be biotransformed to an electrophilic metabolite prior to conjugation. The second group of substrates for glutathione conjugation includes reactive intermediates produced during phase I or phase II biotransformation, and include oxiranes (arene oxides and alkene epoxides), nitrenium ions, carbonium ions, and free radicals. The conjugation reactions themselves can be divided into two types: *displacement reactions*, in which glutathione displaces an electron-withdrawing group, and *addition reactions*, in which glutathione is added to an activated double bond or strained ring system.

The displacement of an electron-withdrawing group by glutathione typically occurs when the substrate contains halide, sulfate, sulfonate, phosphate, or a nitro group (i.e., good *leaving groups*) attached to an allylic or benzylic carbon atom. Displacement of an electron-withdrawing group from aromatic xenobiotics is decreased by the presence of other substituents that donate electrons to the aromatic ring (-$NH_2$, -OH, -OR, and -R). Conversely, such displacement reactions are increased by the presence of other electron-withdrawing groups (-F, -Cl, -Br, -I, -$NO_2$, -CN, -CHO, and -COOR). This explains why 1,2-dichloro-4-nitrobenzene and 1-chloro-2,4-dinitrobenzene, each of which contains three electron-withdrawing groups, are commonly used as substrates for measuring glutathione *S*-transferase activity in vitro. Glutathione *S*-transferase can catalyze the *O*-demethylation of dimethylvinphos and other methylated organophosphorus compounds. The reaction is analogous to the interaction between methyliodide and glutathione, which produces methylglutathione and iodide ion ($GS^- + CH_3I \rightarrow GS\text{-}CH_3 + I^-$). In this case, iodide is the leaving group. In the case of dimethylvinphos, the entire organophosphate molecule (minus the methyl group) functions as the leaving group.

The addition of glutathione to a carbon-carbon double bond is also facilitated by the presence of a nearby electron-withdrawing group, hence, substrates for this reaction typically contain a double bond attached to -CN, -CHO, -COOR, or -COR. The double bond in diethyl maleate is attached to two electron-withdrawing groups and readily undergoes a Michael addition reaction with glutathione, as shown in Fig. 6-51. Diethyl maleate reacts so well with glutathione that it is often used in vivo to decrease glutathione levels in experimental animals. The loop diuretic, ethacrynic acid, contains an $\alpha,\beta$-unsaturated ketone that readily reacts with glutathione and other sulfhydryls by Michael addition. The conversion of acetaminophen to a glutathione conjugate involves addition of glutathione to an activated double bond, which is formed during the cytochrome P450-dependent dehydrogenation of acetaminophen to *N*-acetylbenzoquinoneimine, as shown in Fig. 6-24.

Arene oxides and alkene epoxides, which are often formed by cytochrome P450-dependent oxidation of aromatic hydrocarbons and alkenes, are examples of strained ring systems that open during the addition of glutathione (Fig. 6-51). In many cases, conjugation of arene oxides with glutathione proceeds stereoselectively, as shown in Fig. 6-52 for the 1,2-oxides of naphthalene. The glutathione conjugates of arene oxides may undergo rearrangement reactions, which restore aromaticity and possibly lead to migration of the conjugate to the adjacent carbon atom (through formation of an episulfonium ion), as shown in Fig. 6-52. Conjugation of quinones and quinoneimines with glutathione also restores aromaticity, as shown in Fig. 6-24 for *N*-acetylbenzoquinoneimine, the reactive metabolite of acetaminophen. Compared with glucuronidation and sulfation, conjugation with glutathione is a minor pathway of acetaminophen biotransformation, even though liver contains high levels of both glutathione and glutathione *S*-transferases. The relatively low rate of glutathione conjugation reflects the slow rate of formation of *N*-acetylbenzoquinoneimine, which is catalyzed by cytochrome P450 (Fig. 6-24).

Glutathione can also conjugate xenobiotics with an electrophilic heteroatom (*O*, *N*, and *S*), as shown in Fig. 6-53. In each of the examples shown in Fig. 6-53, the initial conjugate formed between glutathione and the heteroatom is cleaved by a second molecule of glutathione to form oxidized glutathione (GSSG). The initial reactions shown in Fig. 6-53 are catalyzed by glutathione *S*-transferase, whereas the second reaction (which leads to GSSG formation) generally occurs nonenzymatically. Analogous reactions leading to the reduction and cleavage of disulfides have been described previously (see Fig. 6-9). Some of the reactions shown in Fig. 6-53, such as the reduction of hydroperoxides to alcohols, can also be catalyzed by glutathione peroxidase, which is a selenium-dependent enzyme. (For their role in the reduction of hydroperoxides, the glutathione *S*-transferases are sometimes called nonselenium-requiring glutathione peroxidases.) Cleavage of the nitrate esters of nitroglycerin releases nitrite, which can be converted to the potent vasodilator, nitric oxide. The ability of sulfhydryl-generating agents to partially prevent or reverse tolerance to nitroglycerin suggests that glutathione-dependent denitration may play a role in nitroglycerin-induced vasodilation.

Glutathione *S*-transferases catalyze two important isomerization reactions, namely the conversion of the endoperoxide, $PGH_2$, to the prostaglandins $PGD_2$ and $PGE_2$, and the conversion of $\Delta^5$ steroids to $\Delta^4$ steroids, such as the formation of androstenedione from androst-5-ene-3,17-dione. Another physiological function of glutathione *S*-transferase is the synthesis of leukotriene $C_4$, which is catalyzed by a microsomal form of the enzyme.

Glutathione conjugates formed in the liver can be excreted intact in bile, or they can be converted to mercapturic acids in the kidney and excreted in urine. As shown in Fig. 6-54, the conversion of glutathione conjugates to mercapturic acids involves the sequential cleavage of glutamic acid and glycine

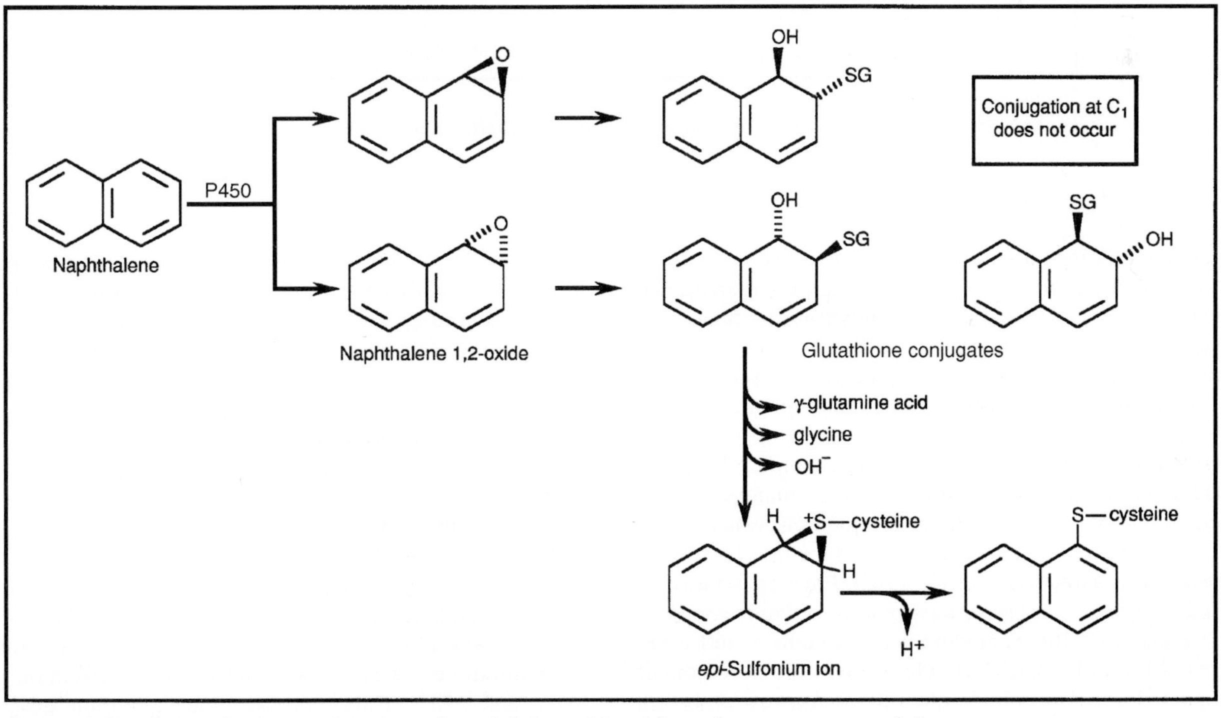

***Figure 6–52.** Stereoselective conjugation of naphthalene 1,2-oxide and rearrangement of 2-naphthyl to 1-naphthyl conjugates.*

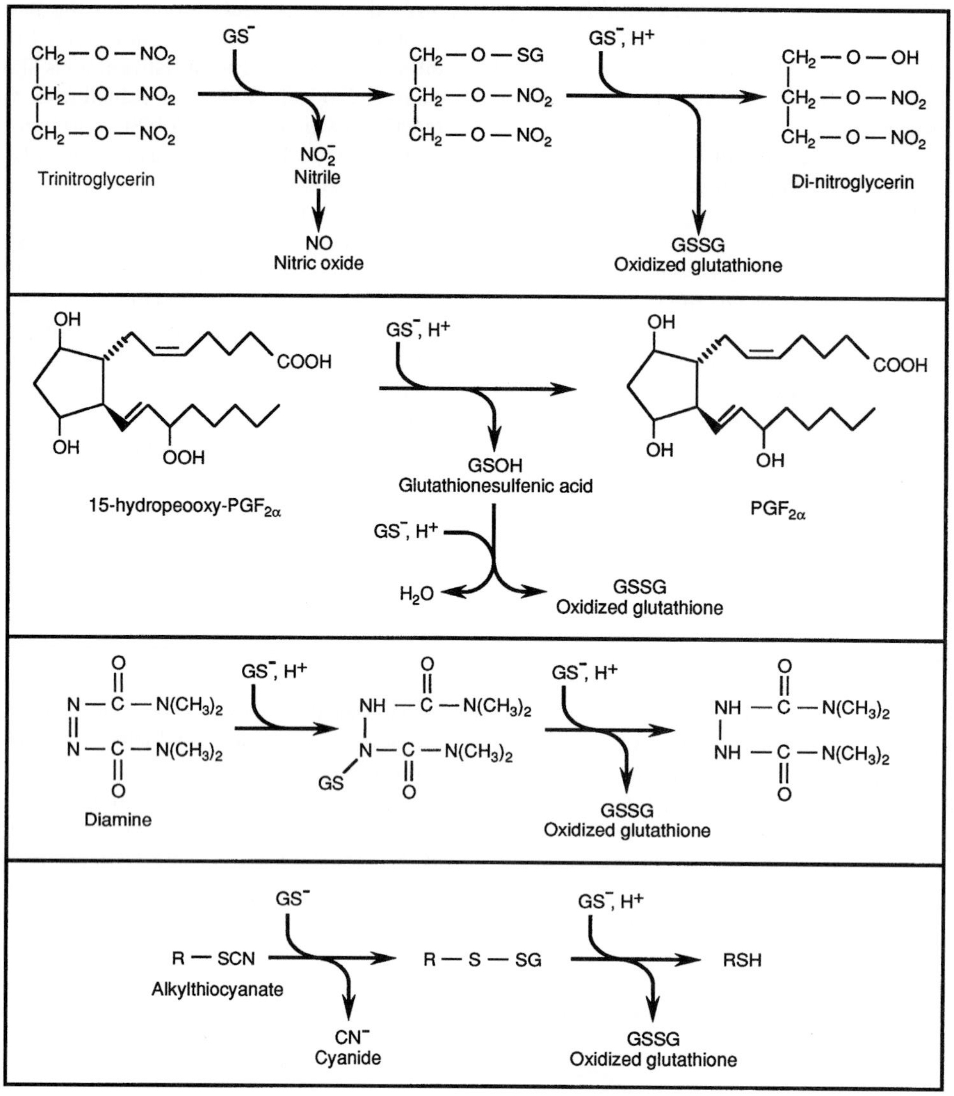

*Figure 6–53. Examples of glutathione conjugation of electrophilic heteroatoms.*

from the glutathione moiety, followed by *N*-acetylation of the resulting cysteine conjugate. The first two steps in mercapturic acid synthesis are catalyzed by $\gamma$-glutamyltranspeptidase and aminopeptidase M. The glutathione conjugate, leukotriene $C_4$, is similarly hydrolyzed by $\gamma$-glutamyltranspeptidase to form leukotriene $D_4$, which is hydrolyzed by aminopeptidase M to form leukotriene $E_4$.

Glutathione *S*-transferases are dimers composed of identical subunits, although some forms are heterodimers. Numerous subunits have been cloned and sequenced, which forms the basis of a nomenclature system for naming the glutathione *S*-transferases (Mannervick et al., 1992). Each enzyme is assigned a two-digit number to designate its subunit composition. For example, the homodimers of subunits 1 and 2 are designated 1-1 and 2-2, respectively, whereas the heterodimer is designated 1-2. The soluble glutathione *S*-transferases are arranged into four classes designated A, M, P, and T (which refer to alpha, mu, pi, and theta or $\alpha, \mu, \pi$, and $\theta$). By definition, the subunits in different classes share less than 50 percent amino acid identity. Generally, the subunits within a class are ~70 percent identical and can form heterodimers, whereas the subunits in different classes are only ~30 percent identical, which appears to prevent dimerization of two subunits from different classes.

Humans express two subunits belonging to the alpha class of glutathione *S*-transferases, designated hGSTA1 and hGSTA2, which are also known as $B_1$ and $B_2$. Rats express four GSTA subunits, which are also known as $Ya_1$, $Ya_2$, $Yc_1$, and $Yc_2$. Rat GSTA1 is also known as ligandin. The alpha class of glutathione *S*-transferases has basic isoelectric points. They are the major glutathione *S*-transferases in liver and kidney.

Humans express four subunits belonging to the mu class of glutathione *S*-transferases, designated hGSTM1a, -M1b, -M2, and -M3. Rats express five subunits, designated rGSTM1–rGSTM5. Rat M1, M2, and M3 are also known as $Yb_1$, $Yb_2$, and $Yb_3$. The mu class of glutathione *S*-transferases

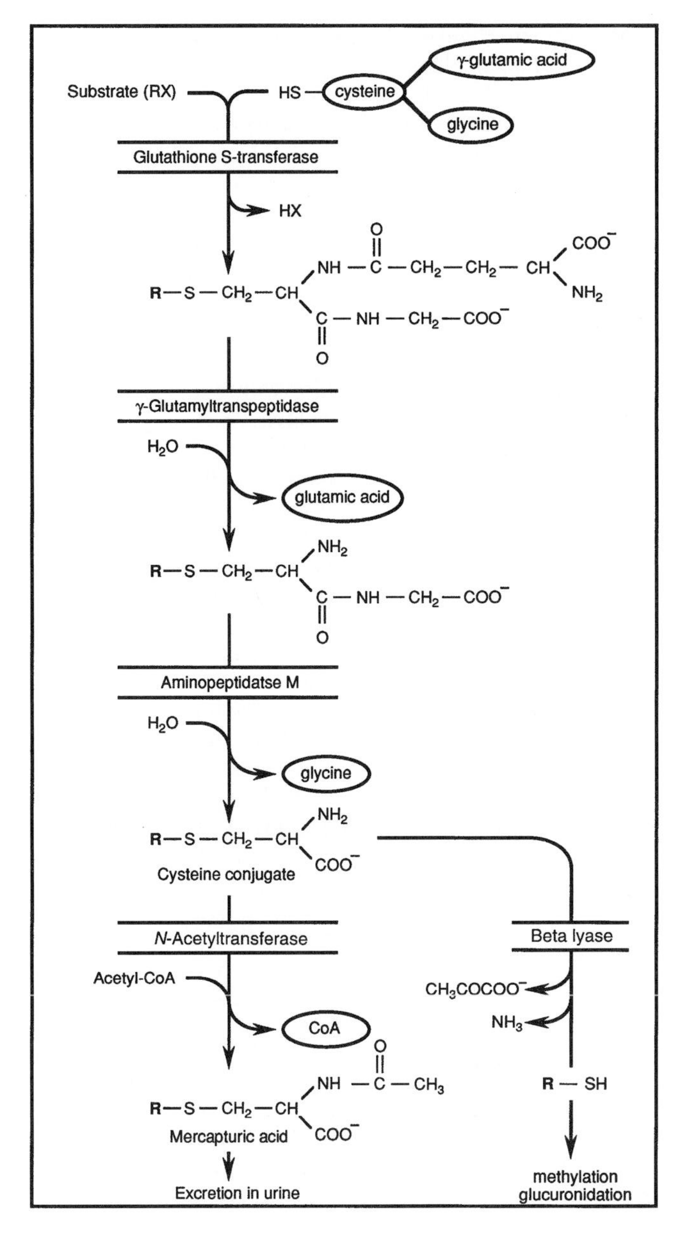


*Figure 6–54. Glutathione conjugation and mercapturic acid biosynthesis.*

has neutral isoelectric points. Human GSTM2 and M3 are expressed in muscle and brain, respectively.

Humans express two subunits belonging to the pi class of glutathione *S*-transferases (hGSTP1a and hGSTP1b), whereas rats express only one subunit (rGSTP1). The pi class of glutathione *S*-transferases have acidic isoelectric points. They are expressed in the placenta, lung, gut, and other extrahepatic tissues. In rats, GSTP1 is one of several preneoplastic antigens that are overexpressed in chemical-induced tumors. Humans and rats appear to express a single subunit of the theta class of glutathione *S*-transferases, which appears to be an ancestral form of the enzyme.

The microsomal glutathione *S*-transferases are distinct from the soluble enzymes. Two microsomal glutathione *S*-transferases have been identified: one is a trimeric enzyme that conjugates xenobiotics with glutathione, the other is a distinct enzyme that conjugates leukotriene $A_4$ (a lipid epoxide derived of arachidonic acid) with glutathione to form leukotriene $C_4$. This latter enzyme is known as leukotriene $C_4$ synthase.

The conjugation of certain xenobiotics with glutathione is catalyzed by all classes of glutathione *S*-transferase. For example, the alpha, mu, and pi classes of human glutathione *S*-transferase all catalyze the conjugation of 1-chloro-2,4-dinitrobenzene. Other reactions are fairly specific for one class of enzymes. For example, the alpha glutathione *S*-transferases preferentially isomerize $\Delta^5$ steroids to $\Delta^4$ steroids and reduce linoleate and cumene hydroperoxide to their corresponding alcohols. The mu glutathione *S*-transferases preferentially conjugate certain arene oxides and alkene epoxides, such as styrene-7,8-epoxide. The pi glutathione *S*-transferases preferentially conjugate ethacrynic acid. However, individual members within a class of glutathione *S*-transferases can differ markedly in their substrate specificity. In rodents, for example, the alpha glutathione *S*-transferases comprised of Yc subunits rapidly conjugate aflatoxin $B_1$ 8,9-oxide, whereas those comprised of Ya subunits are virtually incapable of catalyzing this reaction (Eaton and Gallagher, 1994).

In rodents, individual members of the alpha and mu class of glutathione *S*-transferases are inducible (generally 2- to 3-fold) by 3-methylcholanthrene, phenobarbital, corticosteroids, anti-oxidants and Michael acceptors (i.e., substrates for glutathione conjugation) (Rushmore et al., 1991; Daniel, 1993; Nguyen et al., 1994). Induction is usually associated with increased levels of mRNA due to transcriptional activation of the gene encoding a subunit of glutathione *S*-transferase. The enhancer regions of the genes encoding some of the rodent glutathione *S*-transferases have been shown to contain a xenobiotic (dioxin)-responsive element (XRE), a Barbie box, a glucocorticoid responsive element (GRE), and/or an antioxidant responsive element (ARE). In rodents, certain glutathione *S*-transferase subunits, such as rGSTA1 (Ya), are regulated by both *monofunctional* and *bifunctional* agents, as described previously for DT-diaphorase (see also the section on CYP1A1 induction). Induction of glutathione *S*-transferases by sulforaphane is thought to be responsible, at least in part, for the anti-cancer effects of broccoli (Zhang et al., 1992). It remains to be determined whether factors that regulate the expression of glutathione *S*-transferases in rodents have similar effects in humans.

Conjugation with glutathione represents an important detoxication reaction because electrophiles are potentially toxic species that can bind to critical nucleophiles, such as proteins and nucleic acids, and cause cellular damage and genetic mutations. All of the enzymes involved in xenobiotic biotransformation have the potential to generate reactive intermediates, most of which are detoxified to some extent by conjugation with glutathione. Glutathione is also a cofactor for glutathione peroxidase, which plays an important role in protecting cells against lipid peroxidation. Resistance to toxic compounds is often associated with an over-expression of glutathione *S*-transferase. Examples include the resistance of insects to DDT (see Fig. 6-15), of corn to atrazine, and of cancer cells to chemotherapeutic agents. Glutathione *S*-transferase is the major determinant of certain species differences in chemical-induced toxicity. For example, low doses of aflatoxin

$B_1$ cause liver toxicity and tumor formation in rats but not mice, even though rats and mice convert aflatoxin $B_1$ to the highly reactive 8,9-oxide at similar rates (this reaction is shown in Fig. 6-23). This species difference arises because mice express high levels of an alpha class glutathione *S*-transferase (Yc) enabling them to conjugate aflatoxin $B_1$ 8,9-epoxide with glutathione up to 50 times faster than rats (or humans, which are also considered a susceptible species) (Eaton and Gallagher, 1994). Mice become sensitive to the adverse effects of aflatoxin $B_1$ following treatment with agents that decrease glutathione levels, such as diethyl maleate (which depletes glutathione) or buthionine-*S*-sulfoximine (which inhibits glutathione synthesis). Conversely, treatment of rats with inducers of glutathione *S*-transferase ($Yc_1Yc_2$), such as ethoxyquin, BHA, oltipraz, and phenobarbital, protects them from the hepatotoxic/tumorigenic action of aflatoxin $B_1$ (Hayes et al., 1994). These studies in experimental animals suggest that individual differences in glutathione *S*-transferase may determine susceptibility to the toxic effects of certain chemicals. In support of this interpretation, a genetic polymorphism for hGSTM1 has been identified, and individuals with the null allele (i.e., those with low glutathione *S*-transferase activity) appear to be at increased risk for cigarette smoking-induced lung cancer.

In some cases, conjugation with glutathione enhances the toxicity of a xenobiotic (Monks et al., 1990; Dekant and Vamvakas, 1993). Four mechanisms of glutathione-dependent activation of xenobiotics have been identified, as shown in Fig. 6-55. These mechanisms are (1) formation of glutathione conjugates of haloalkanes, organic thiocyanates, and nitrosoguanides that release a toxic metabolite; (2) formation of glutathione conjugates of vicinal dihaloalkanes that are inherently toxic because they can form electrophilic sulfur mustards; (3) formation of glutathione conjugates of halogenated alkenes that are degraded to toxic metabolites by beta lyase in the kidney, and (4) formation of glutathione conjugates of quinones, quinoneimines, and isothiocyanates that are degraded to toxic metabolites by $\gamma$-glutamyltranspeptidase and endopeptidase M in the kidney.

The first mechanism is illustrated by dichloromethane, conjugated with glutathione to form chloromethyl-glutathione, which then breaks down to formaldehyde. Both formaldehyde and the glutathione conjugate are reactive metabolites, and either or both may be responsible for dichloromethane-induced tumorigenesis in sensitive species. The rate of conjugation of dichloromethane with glutathione is considerably faster in mice, which are susceptible to dichloromethane-induced tumorigenesis, than rats or hamsters, which are resistant species.

The second mechanism accounts for the toxicity of dichloroethane and dibromoethane. These vicinal dihaloalkanes are converted to glutathione conjugates that can rearrange to form mutagenic and nephrotoxic episulfonium ions (sulfur half-mustards) (Fig. 6-55). Dichloroethane and dibromoethane can also be oxidized by cytochrome P450 to chloroacetaldehyde and bromoacetaldehyde (by reactions analogous to those shown in Fig. 6-40). Either pathway can

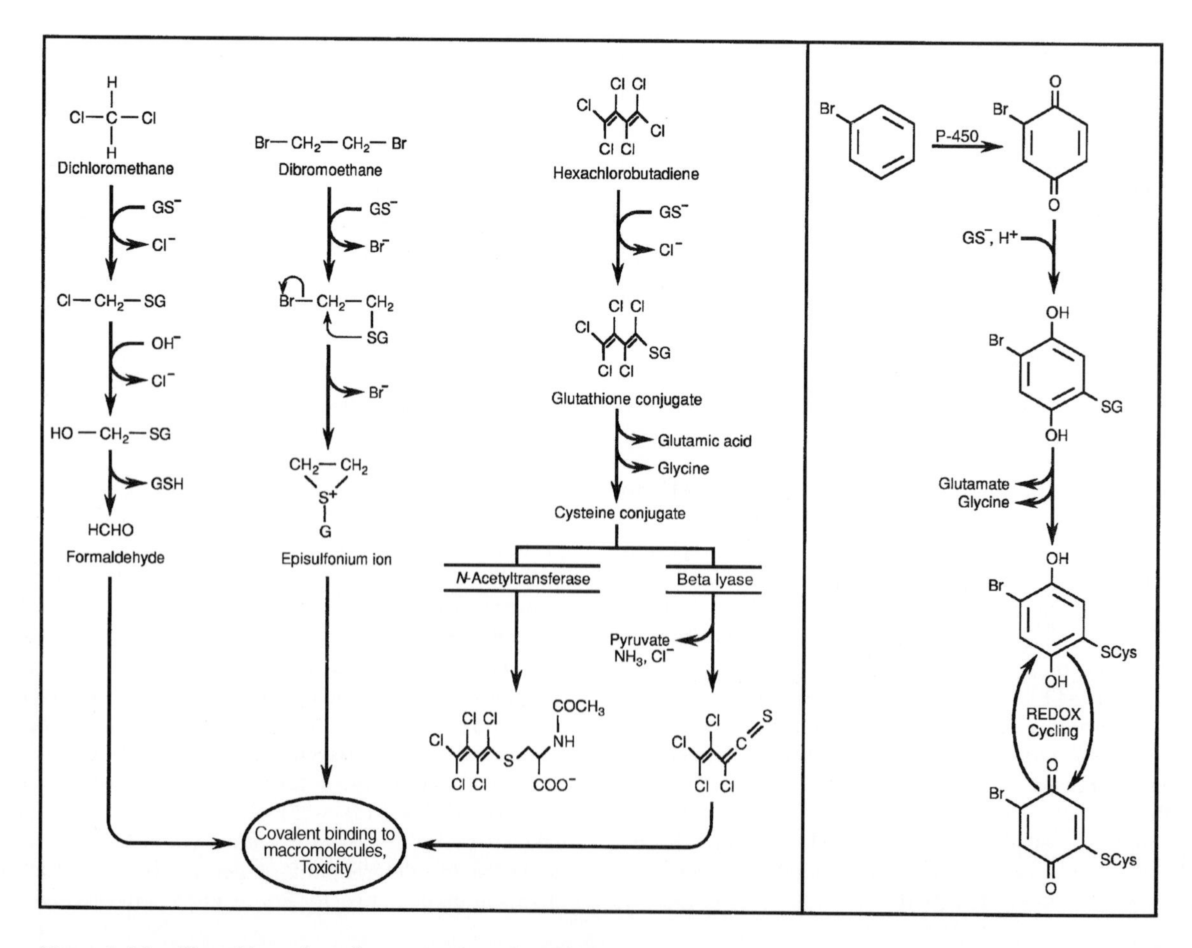


*Figure 6–55. Glutathione-dependent activation of xenobiotics.*

potentially account for the toxic and tumorigenic effects of these dihaloalkanes. However, the toxicity and DNA-binding of dihaloalkanes are increased by factors that decrease their oxidation by cytochrome P450 and increase their conjugation with glutathione.

The third mechanism accounts for the nephrotoxicity of several halogenated alkenes. Several halogenated alkenes, such as hexachlorobutadiene, cause damage to the kidney tubules in rats, which leads to carcinoma of the proximal tubules. These nephrotoxic halogenated alkenes are conjugated with glutathione and transported to the kidney for processing to mercapturic acids. The cysteine conjugates, which form by removal of glutamic acid and glycine, are substrates for *N*-acetyltransferase, which completes the synthesis of mercapturic acids, and $\beta$-lyase, which removes pyruvate and ammonia from the cysteine conjugate to produce thionylacyl halides and thioketenes. The early damage to renal mitochondria caused by halogenated alkenes is probably because cysteine conjugate beta lyase is a mitochondrial enzyme.

The fourth mechanism accounts for the nephrotoxicity of bromobenzene, which causes damage to the proximal tubules in rats. Bromobenzene is oxidized by cytochrome P450 in the liver to bromohydroquinone, which is conjugated with glutathione and transported to the kidney (Fig. 6-55). The glutathione conjugate is converted to the cysteine derivative by $\gamma$-glutamyltranspeptidase and aminopeptidase M. Substitution of bromohydroquinones with cysteine lowers their redox potential and thereby facilitates their oxidation to toxic quinones. The cysteine conjugates of bromohydroquinone are thought to undergo redox cycling and cause kidney damage through the generation of reactive oxygen species. *para*-Aminophenol is thought to cause kidney damage by a similar mechanism, except a benzoquinoneimine is involved in conjugation with glutathione and subsequent damage to proximal tubules of the kidney. Treatment of rats with the glutathione depletor, buthionine-*S*-sulfoximine, protects them against the nephrotoxic effects of *para*-aminophenol, which implicates glutathione conjugation in the activation of this compound.

## Rhodanese

Rhodanese is a mitochondrial enzyme that converts cyanide to the far less toxic metabolite, thiocyanate. The reaction involves transfer of sulfur from thiosulfate (or another sulfur donor) as follows:

$$\underset{\text{cyanide}}{CN^-} + \underset{\text{thiosulfate}}{S_2O_3^{2-}} \longrightarrow \underset{\text{thiocyanate}}{SCN^-} + \underset{\text{sulfite}}{SO_3^{2-}}$$

*para*-Dimethylaminophenol is used to induce methemoglobinemia as an antidote to cyanide poisoning because methemoglobin competes with cytochrome oxidase for the cyanide ion. *para*-Dimethylaminophenol is nephrotoxic to rats, presumably by a mechanism similar to that described above for the structural analog, *para*-aminophenol.

# REFERENCES


Agarwal DP, Goedde HW: Pharmacogenetics of alcohol dehydrogenase, in Kalow W (ed): *Pharmacogenetics of Drug Metabolism*. New York: Pergamon, 1992, pp 263–280.

Aldridge WN: Serum esterases: Two types of esterases (A and B) hydrolyzing para-nitrophenylacetate, propionate, and a method for their determination. *Biochem J* 53:110–119, 1953.

Anders MW, Ratnayake JH, Hanna PE, Fuchs JA: Thioredoxin-dependent sulfoxide reduction by rat renal cytosol. *Drug Metab Dispos* 9:307–310, 1981.

Anders MW (ed): *Bioactivation of Foreign Compounds*. New York: Academic, 1985.

Atkins WM, Wang RW, Bird AW, et al: The catalytic mechanism of glutathione *S*-transferase (GST): Spectroscopic determination of the pKa of Tyr-9 in rat a1-1 GST. *J Biol Chem* 268:19188–19191, 1993.

Ayesh R, Smith RL: Genetic polymorphism of trimethylamine *N*-oxidation, in Kalow W (ed): *Pharmacogenetics of Drug Metabolism*. New York: Pergamon, 1992, pp 315–332.

Back DJ, Orme LE: Genetic factors influencing the metabolism of tolbutamide, in Kalow W (ed): *Pharmacogenetics of Drug Metabolism*. New York: Pergamon, 1992, pp 737–746.

Batt AM, Siest G, Magdalou J, Galteau M-M: Enzyme induction by drugs and toxins. *Clin Chem Acta* 209:109–121, 1992.

Bell PA, Kasper CB: Expression of rat microsomal epoxide hydrolase in *Escherichia coli*: Identification of a histidyl residue essential for catalysis. *J Biol Chem* 268:14011–14017, 1993.

Benedetti MS, Dostert P: Contribution of amine oxidases to the metabolism of xenobiotics. *Drug Metab Rev* 26:507–535, 1994.

Boberg EW, Miller EC, Miller JA, et al: Strong evidence from studies with brachymorphic mice and pentachlorophenol that 1′-sulfoöxysafrole is the major ultimate electrophilic and carcinogenic metabolite of 1′-hydroxysafrole in mouse liver. *Cancer Res* 43:5163–5173, 1983.

Bock KW, Schrenk D, Forster A, et al: The influence of environmental and genetic factors on CYP2D6, CYP1A2, and UDP-glucuronosyltransferases in man using sparteine, caffeine, and paracetamol as probes. *Pharmacogenetics* 4:209–218, 1994.

Bosma PJ, Seppen J, Goldhoorn B, et al: Bilirubin UDP-glucuronosyltransferase 1 is the only relevant bilirubin glucuronidating isoform in man. *J Biol Chem* 269:17960–17964, 1994.

Brittebo EB: Metabolism of xenobiotics in the nasa olfactory mucosa: Implications for local toxicity. *Pharmacol and Toxicol* 72(suppl III):50–52, 1993.

Burchell B, Coughtrie MWH: UDP-glucuronosyltransferases, in Kalow W (ed): *Pharmacogenetics of Drug Metabolism*. New York: Pergamon, 1992, pp 195–225.

Cashman JR: Structural and catalytic properties of the mammalian flavin-containing monooxygenase. *Chem Res Toxicol* 8:165–181, 1995.

Conney AH: Pharmacological implications of microsomal enzyme induction. *Pharmacol Rev* 19:317–366, 1967.

Conney A: Induction of microsomal enzymes by foreign chemicals and carcinogenesis by polycyclic aromatic hydrocarbons: G. H. A. Clowes Memorial Lecture. *Cancer Res* 42:4875–4917, 1982.

Cundy KC, Sato M, Crooks PA: Stereospecific in vivo *N*-methylation of nicotine in the guinea pig. *Drug Metab* 13:175–185, 1985.

Curran PG, DeGroot LJ: The effect of hepatic enzyme-inducing drugs on thyroid hormones and the thyroid gland. *Endocrin Rev* 12:135–150, 1991.

Daniel V: Glutathione *S*-transferases: Gene structure and regulation of expression. *Crit Rev Biochem Mol Biol* 28:173–207, 1993.

Dawson JH: Probing structure-function relations in heme-containing oxygenases and peroxidases. *Science* 240:433–439, 1988.

Dekant W, Vamvakas S: Glutathione-dependent bioactivation of xenobiotics. *Xenobiotica* 23:873–887, 1993.

DeMorais SMF, Uetrecht JP, Wells PG: Decreased glucuronidation and increased bioactivation of acetaminophen in Gilbert's syndrome. *Gastroenterology* 102:577–586, 1992.

Demoz A, Vaagenes H, Aarsaether N, et al: Coordinate induction of hepatic fatty acyl-CoA oxidase and P4504A1 in rat after activation of the peroxisome proliferator-activated receptor (PPAR) by sulphur-substituted fatty acid analogues. *Xenobiotica* 24:943–956, 1994.

Diaz D, Fabre I, Daujat M, et al: Omeprazole is an aryl hydrocarbon-like inducer of human hepatic cytochrome P450. *Gastroenterology* 99:737–747, 1990.

Dirr H, Reinemer P, Huber R: X-ray crystal structures of cytosolic glutathione *S*-transferases: Implications for protein architecture, substrate recognition and catalytic function. *Eur J Biochem* 220:645–661, 1994.

Eaton DL, Gallagher EP: Mechanisms of aflatoxin carcinogenesis. *Annu Rev Pharmacol Toxicol* 34:135–172, 1994.

Eling TE, Thompson DC, Foureman GL, et al: Prostaglandin H synthase and xenobiotic oxidation. *Annu Rev Pharmacol Toxicol* 30:1–45, 1990.

Ernster L: DT-diaphorase: A historical review. *Chem Scripta* 27A:1–17, 1987.

Evans DAP: *N*-Acetyltransferase, in Kalow W (ed): *Pharmacogenetics of Drug Metabolism*. New York: Pergamon, 1992, pp 95–178.

Falany CN, Johnson MR, Barnes S, Diasio RB: Glycine and taurine conjugation of bile acids by a single enzyme: Molecular cloning and expression of human liver bile acid CoA:amino acid *N*-acetyltransferase. *J Biol Chem* 269:19375–19379, 1994.

Farrell GC: Drug metabolism in extrahepatic diseases. *Pharmacol Ther* 35:375–404, 1987.

Favreau LV, Pickett CB: Transcriptional regulation of the rat NAD(P)H:quinone reductase gene. Identification of regulatory elements controlling basal level expression and inducible expression by planar aromatic compounds and phenolic antioxidants. *J Biol Chem* 266:4556–4561, 1991.

Frezza C, DiPadova G, Pozzato M, et al: High blood alcohol levels in women. The role of decreased gastric alcohol dehydrogenase activity and blood ethanol levels. *N Engl J Med* 322:95–99, 1990.

Friedberg T, Grassow MA, Bartlomowiczoesch B, et al: Sequence of a novel CYP2B cDNA coding for a protein which is expressed in a sebaceous gland but not in the liver. *Biochem J* 297:775–783, 1992.

Gerlach M, Riederer P, Przuntek H, Youdim MBH: MPTP mechanisms of neurotoxicity and their implications for Parkinson's disease. *Eur J Pharmacol* 208:273–286, 1991.

Goedde HW, Agarwal DP: Pharmacogenetics of aldehyde dehydrogenase, in Kalow W (ed): *Pharmacogenetics of Drug Metabolism*. New York: Pergamon, 1992, pp 281–311.

Gonzalez FJ: The molecular biology of cytochrome P450s. *Pharmacol Rev* 40:243–288, 1989.

Gram TE (ed): *Extrahepatic Metabolism of Drugs and Other Foreign Compounds*. New York: Spectrum, 1980, pp 1–601.

Grant DM, Blum M, Meyers UA: Polymorphisms of *N*-acetyltransferase genes. *Xenobiotica* 22:1073–1081, 1992.

Grasso P, Sharratt M, Cohen AJ: Role of persistent, non-genotoxic tissue damage in rodent cancer and relevance to humans. *Annu Rev Pharmacol Toxicol* 31:253–287, 1991.

Guengerich FP: Catalytic selectivity of human cytochrome P450 enzymes: Relevance to drug metabolism and toxicity. *Toxicol Letters* 70:133–138, 1994.

Guengerich FP: Reactions and significance of cytochrome P450 enzymes. *J Biol Chem* 266:10019–10022, 1991.

Guengerich FP: *Mammalian Cytochrome P450*. Boca Raton, FL: CRC, 1987.

Guengerich FP, Kim D-H, Iwasaki M: Role of human cytochrome P450 IIE1 in the oxidation of many low molecular weight cancer suspects. *Chem Res Toxicol* 4:168–179, 1991.

Guengerich FP, Shimada T: Oxidation of toxic and carcinogenic chemicals by human cytochrome P450 enzymes. *Chem Res Toxicol* 4:391–407, 1991.

Gupta E, Lestingi TM, Mick R, et al: Metabolic fate of irinotecan in humans: Correlation of glucuronidation with diarrhea. *Cancer Res* 54:3723–3725, 1994.

Halpert JR, Guengerich FP, Bend JR, Correia MA: Contemporary issues in toxicology: Selective inhibitors of cytochromes P450. *Toxicol App Pharmacol* 125:163–175, 1994.

Hayes JD, Nguyen T, Judah DJ, et al: Cloning of cDNAs from fetal rat liver encoding glutathione *S*-transferase Yc polypeptides. *J Biol Chem* 269:20707–20717, 1994.

Hayes RB, Bi W, Rothman N, et al: *N*-Acetylation phenotype and genotype and risk of bladder cancer in benzidine-exposed workers. *Carcinogenesis* 14:675–678, 1993.

Hein DW: Acetylator genotype and arylamine-induced carcinogenesis. *Biochem Biophys Acta* 948:37–66, 1988.

Herwick DS: Reductive metabolism of nitrogen-containing functional groups, in Jakoby WB, Bend JR, Caldwell J (eds): *Metabolic Basis of Detoxication*. New York: Academic, 1980, pp 151–170.

Houston JB: Utility of in vitro drug metabolism data in predicting in vivo metabolic clearance. *Biochem Pharmacol* 47:1469–1479, 1994.

Humphrey MJ, Ringrose PS: Peptides and related drugs: A review of their adsorption, metabolism, and excretion. *Drug Metab Rev* 17:283–310, 1986.

Idle JR: Is environmental carcinogenesis modulated by host polymorphism? *Mutat Res* 247:259–266, 1991.

Inaba T, Kovacs J: Haloperidol reductase in human and guinea pig livers. *Drug Metab Dispos* 17:330–333, 1989.

Jaiswal AK, Burnett P, Adesnik M, McBride OW: Nucleotide and deduced amino acid sequence of a human cDNA ($NQO_2$) corresponding to a second member of the NAD(P)H: Quinone oxidoreductase gene family. Extensive polymorphism at the $NQO_2$ gene locus on chromosome 6. *Biochemistry* 29:1899–1906, 1990.

Jakoby WB (ed): *Enzymatic Basis of Detoxication*. New York: Academic, 1980, vols 1 and 2.

Jakoby WB, Bend JR, Caldwell J: *Metabolic Basis of Detoxification: Metabolism of Functional Groups*. New York: Academic, 1982, pp 1–375.

Kadlubar FF: Biochemical individuality and its implications for drug and carcinogen metabolism: Recent insights from acetyltransferase and cytochrome P4501A2 phenotyping and genotyping in humans. *Drug Metab Rev* 26:37–46, 1994.

Kato R: Characteristics and differences in the hepatic mixed function oxidases of different species. *Pharmacol Ther* 6:41–98, 1979.

Kato R, Estabrook RW, Cayen MN (eds): *Xenobiotic Metabolism and Disposition*. London: Taylor and Francis, 1989, pp 1–538.

Kato R, Yamazoe Y: The importance of substrate concentration in determining cytochromes P450 therapeutically relevant in vivo. *Pharmacogenetics* 4:359–362, 1994a.

Kato R, Yamazoe Y: Metabolic activation of *N*-hydroxylated metabolites of carcinogenic and mutagenic arylamines and arylamides by esterification. *Drug Metab Rev* 26:413–430, 1994b.

Kivsito KT, Neuvonen PJ, Klotz U: Inhibition of terfenadine metabolism: Pharmacokinetic and pharmacodynamic consequences. *Clin Pharmacokin* 27:1–5, 1994.

Koivusalo M, Baumann M, Uotila L: Evidence for the identity of glutathione-dependent formaldehyde dehydrogenase and class III alcohol dehydrogenase. *FEBS Lett* 257:105–109, 1989.

Koop DR, Tierney DJ: Multiple mechanisms in the regulation of ethanol-inducible cytochrome P450IIE1. *BioEssays* 12:429–435, 1990.

Kretz-Rommel A, Boesterli UA: Mechanism of covalent adduct formation of diclofenac to rat hepatic microsomal proteins: Retention of the glucuronic acid moiety in the adduct. *Drug Metab Dispos* 22:956–961, 1994.

Krishna DR, Klotz U: Extrahepatic metabolism of drugs in humans. *Clin Pharmacokinet* 26:144–160, 1994.

Kroetz DL, Loiseau P, Guyot M, Levy RH: In vivo and in vitro correlation of microsomal epoxide hydrolase inhibition by progabide. *Clin Pharmacol Ther* 54:485–497, 1993.

La Du BN: Human serum paraoxonase/arylesterase, in Kalow W (ed): *Pharmacogenetics of Drug Metabolism*. New York: Pergamon, 1992, pp 51–91.

Lawton MP, Cashman JR, Cresteil T, et al: A nomenclature for the mammalian flavin-containing monooxygenase gene family based on amino acid sequence identities. *Arch Biochem Biophys* 308:254–257, 1994.

Lecoeur S, Bonierbale E, Challine D, et al: Specificity of in vitro covalent binding of tienilic acid metabolites to human liver microsomes in relationship to the type of hepatotoxicity: Comparison with two directly hepatotoxic drugs. *Chem Res Toxicol* 7:434–442, 1994.

Levitt MD: Review article: Lack of clinical significance of the interaction between H2-receptor antagonists and ethanol. *Aliment Pharmacol Ther* 7:131–138, 1993.

Liang Q, He J-S, Fulco A: The role of barbie box sequences as cis-acting elements involved in the barbiturate-mediated induction of cytochromes P450 BM-1 and P450 BM-3 in Bacillus megaterium. *J Biol Chem* 270:4438–4450, 1995.

Lieber CS: Mechanism of ethanol induced hepatic injury. *Pharmacol Ther* 46:1–41, 1990.

Lindberg R, Negishi M: Alteration of mouse cytochrome P459coh substrate specificity by mutation of a single amino acid residue. *Nature* 336:632–634, 1989.

Lockridge O: Genetic variants of human serum butyrylcholinesterase influence the metabolism of the muscle relaxant succinylcholine, in Kalow W (ed): *Pharmacogenetics of Drug Metabolism*. New York: Pergamon, 1992, pp 15–50.

Long RM, Rickert DE: Metabolism and excretion of 2,6-dinitro-[14C]toluene in vivo and in isolated perfused rat livers. *Drug Metab Dispos* 10:455–458, 1982.

Lunam CA, Hall PM, Cousins MJ: The pathology of halothane hepatotoxicity in a guinea pig model: A comparison with human halothane hepatitis. *Brit J Exp Pathol* 70:533–541, 1989.

Mackenzie PI, Rodbourne L, Stranks S: Steroid UDP glucuronosyltransferases. *J Steroid Biochem* 43:1099–1105, 1992.

Madan A, Williams TD, Faiman MD: Glutathione- and glutathione-*S*-transferase-dependent oxidative desulfuration of the thione xenobiotic diethyldithiocarbamate methyl ester. *Mol Pharmacol* 46:1217–1225, 1994.

Mannervik B, Awasthi YC, Board PG, et al: Nomenclature for human glutathione transferases. *Biochem J* 282:305–308, 1992.

Mantle TJ, Pickett CB, Hayes JD (eds): *Glutathione S-Transferases and Carcinogenesis*. London: Taylor and Francis, 1987, pp 1–267.

McClain RM: The significance of hepatic microsomal enzyme induction and altered thyroid function in rats: Implications for thyroid gland neoplasia. *Toxicol Pathol* 17:294–306, 1989.

McLeod HL, Fang L, Luo X, et al: Ethnic differences in erythrocyte catechol-*O*-methyltransferase activity in black and white americans. *J Pharmacol Exp Ther* 270:26–29, 1994.

Meyer UA: The molecular basis of genetic polymorphisms of drug metabolism. *J Pharm Pharmacol* 46(suppl 1):409–415, 1994.

Miners JO, Mackenzie PI: Drug glucuronidation in humans. *Pharmacol Ther* 51:347–369, 1992.

Mirsalis JC, Butterworth BE: Induction of unscheduled DNA synthesis in rat hepatocytes following in vivo treatment with dinitrotoluene. *Carcinogenesis* 3:241–245, 1982.

Monks TJ, Anders MW, Dekant W, et al: Contemporary issues in toxicology: Glutathione conjugate mediated toxicities. *Toxicol and Pharmacol* 106:1–19, 1990.

Muerhoff AS, Griffin KJ, Johnson EF: The peroxisome proliferator-activated receptor mediates the induction of CYP4A6, a cytochrome P450 fatty acid $\chi$-hydroxylase, by clofibric acid. *J Biol Chem* 267:10951–19053, 1992.

Mulder GJ (ed): *Sulfation of Drugs and Related Compounds*. Boca Raton, FL: CRC, 1981.

Nebert D: Drug-metabolizing enzymes in ligand-modulated transcription. *Biochem Pharmacol* 47:25–37, 1994.

Nelson DR, Kamataki T, Waxman DJ, et al: The P450 superfamily: Update on new sequences, gene mapping, accession numbers, early trivial names, and nomenclature. *DNA Cell Biol* 12:1–51, 1993.

Nguyen T, Rushmore TH, Pickett CB: Transcriptional regulation of a rat liver glutathione *S*-transferase Ya subunit gene. *J Biol Chem* 269:13656–13663, 1994.

Okey AB: Enzyme induction in the cytochrome P450 system. *Pharmacol Ther* 45:241–298, 1990.

Owens IS, Ritter JK: The novel bilirubin/phenol UDP-glucuronosyltransferase *UGT1* gene locus: Implications for multiple nonhemolytic familial hyperbilirubinemia phenotypes. *Pharmacogenetics* 2:93–108, 1992.

Parkinson A, Hurwitz A: Omeprazole and the induction of human cytochrome P450: A response to concerns about potential adverse effects. *Gastroenterology* 100:1157–1164, 1991.

Paulson GD, Caldwell J, Hutson DH, Menn JJ (eds): *Xenobiotic Conjugation Chemistry*. Washington, DC: American Chemical Society, 1986, pp 1–358.

Peck CC, Temple R, Collins JM: Understanding consequences of concurrent therapies. *J Am Med Assoc* 269:1550–1552, 1993.

Pichard L, Fabre I, Fabre G, et al: Cyclosporin A drug interactions: Screening for inducers and inhibitors of cytochrome P450 (cyclosporin A oxidase) in primary cultures of human hepatocytes and in liver microsomes. *Drug Metab Dispos* 18:595–606, 1990.

Pohl LR, Kenna JG, Satoh H, et al: Neoantigens associated with halothane hepatitis. *Drug Metab Rev* 20:203–217, 1989.

Poland A, Palen D, Glover E: Analysis of the four alleles of the murine aryl hydrocarbon receptor. *Mol Pharmacol* 46:915–921, 1994.

Porter TD, Coon MJ: Multiplicity of isoforms, substrates, and catalytic and regulatory mechanisms. *J Biol Chem* 266:13469–13472, 1991.

Probst MR, Beer M, Beer D, et al: Molecular cloning of a novel esterase involved in the metabolic activation of arylamine carcinogens with high sequence similarity to hormone-sensitive lipase. *J Biol Chem* 269:21650–21656, 1994.

Prochaska HJ, Talalay P: Regulatory mechanisms of monofunctional and bifunctional anticarcinogenic enzyme inducers in murine liver. *Cancer Res* 48:4776–4782, 1992.

Rahman A, Korzekwa KR, Grogan J, et al: Selective biotransformation of taxol to 6$\alpha$-hydroxytaxol by human cytochrome P450 2C8. *Cancer Res* 54:5543–5546, 1994.

Rajagopalan KV: Xanthine oxidase and aldehyde oxidase, in Jakoby WB (ed): *Enzymatic Basis of Detoxication*. New York: Academic, 1980, vol 1, pp 295–306.

Rao SI, Duffel MW: Inhibition of aryl sulfotransferase by carboxylic acids. *Drug Metab Disp* 19:543–545, 1991.

Ratnayake JH, Hanna PE, Anders MW, Duggan DE: Sulfoxide reduction in vitro reduction of sulindac by rat hepatic cytosolic enzymes. *Drug Metab Dispos* 9:85–87, 1981.

Rettie A, Wienkers L, Gonzalez FJ, et al: Impaired (*S*)-warfarin metabolism catalyzed by the R144C allelic variant of CYP2C9. *Pharmacogenetics* 4:39–42, 1994.

Riley RJ, Workman P: DT-diaphorase and cancer chemotherapy. *Biochem Pharmacol* 43:1657–1669, 1992.

Rodrigues AD: Comparison of levels of aldehyde oxidase with cytochrome P450 activities in human liver in vitro. *Biochem Pharmacol* 48:197–200, 1994.

Rushmore TH, Morton MR, Pickett CB: The antioxidant responsive element. Activation by oxidative stress and identification of the DNA consensus sequence required for functional activity. *J Biol Chem* 266:11632–11639, 1991.

Ryan DE, Levin W: Purification and characterization of hepatic microsomal cytochrome P450. *Pharmacol Ther* 45:153–239, 1990.

Satoh T: Role of carboxylesterases in xenobiotic metabolism. *Rev Biochem Toxicol* 8:155–181, 1987.

Shimada T, Yamazaki H, Mimura M, et al: Interindividual variations in human liver cytochrome P450 enzymes involved in the oxidation of drugs, carcinogens and toxic chemicals: Studies with liver microsomes of 30 Japanese and 30 Caucasians. *J Pharmacol Exp Ther* 270:414–423, 1994.

Shirley MA, Guan X, Kaiser DG, et al: Taurine conjugation of ibuprofen in humans and in rat liver in vitro. Relationship to metabolic chiral inversion. *J Pharmacol Exp Ther* 269:1166–1175, 1994.

Sies H, Ketterer B (eds): *Glutathione Conjugation Mechanisms and Biological Significance*. London: Academic, 1988, pp 1–480.

Spahn-Langguth H, Benet LZ: Acyl glucuronides revisited: Is the glucuronidation process a toxification as well as a detoxification mechanism? *Drug Metab Rev* 24:5–48, 1992.

Strobl GR, von Kruedener S, Stockigt J, et al: Development of a pharmacophore for inhibition of human liver cytochrome P450 -6: Molecular modeling and inhibition studies. *J Med Chem* 36:1136–1145, 1993.

Subramanyam B, Woolf T, Castagnoli N: Studies on the in vitro conversion of haloperidol to a potentially neurotoxic pyridinium metabolite. *Chem Res Toxicol* 4:123–128, 1991.

Sugiura M, Iwasaki K, Kato R: Reduction of tertiary amine *N*-oxides by microsomal cytochrome P450. *Mol Pharmacol* 12:322–334, 1976.

Sugiura M, Kato R: Reduction of tertiary amine N-oxides by rat liver mitochondria. *J Pharmacol Exp Ther* 200:25–32, 1977.

Sundseth SS, Waxman DJ: Sex-dependent expression and clofibrate inducibility of cytochrome P450 4A fatty acid $\chi$-hydroxylases. *J Biol Chem* 267:3915–3921, 1991.

Tucker GT: Clinical implications of genetic polymorphism in drug metabolism. *J Pharm Pharmacol* 46(suppl 1):417–424, 1994.

Vatsis KP, Weber WW, Bell DA, et al: Nomenclature for *N*-acetyltransferases. *Pharmacogenetics* 5:1–17, 1995.

Walton MI, Wolf CR, Workman P: The role of cytochrome P450 and cytochrome P450 reductase in the reductive bioactivation of the novel benzotriazine di-*N*-oxide hypoxic cytotoxin 3-amino-1,2,4-benzotriazine-1,4-dioxide (SR 4233, WIN 59075) by mouse liver. *Biochem Pharmacol* 44:251–259, 1992.

Waterman MR, Johnson EF (eds): *Cytochrome P450. Methods in Enzymology*, New York: Academic, 1991, vol 206.

Watkins PB: Noninvasive tests of CYP3A enzymes. *Pharmacogenetics* 4:171–184, 1994.

Waxman DJ, Pampori NA, Ram PA, et al: Interpulse interval in circulating growth hormone patterns regulates sexually dimorphic expression of hepatic cytochrome P450. *Biochemistry* 88:6868–6872, 1991.

Weiner H, Flynn TG (eds): *Enzymology and Molecular Biology of Carbonyl Metabolism 2: Aldehyde Dehydrogenase, Alcohol Dehydrogenase, and Aldo-Keto Reductase*. New York: Alan R. Liss, 1989.

Weinshilboum R: Methyltransferase pharmacogenetics. *Pharmacol Ther* 43:77–90, 1989.

Weinshilboum R: Sulfotransferase pharmacogenetics, in Kalow W (ed): *Pharmacogenetics of Drug Metabolism*. New York: Pergamon, 1992a, pp 227–242.

Weinshilboum RM: Methylation pharmacogenetics: Thiopurine methyltransferase as a model system. *Xenobiotica* 22:1055–1071, 1992b.

Weyler W, Hsu YP, Breakefield XO: Biochemistry and genetics of monoamine oxidase, in Kalow W (ed): *Pharmacogenetics of Drug Metabolism*. New York: Pergamon, 1992, pp 333–366.

Whitlock JP: Mechanistic aspects of dioxin action. *Chem Res Toxicol* 6:754–763, 1993.

Wilkinson GR, Guengerich FP, Branch RA: Genetic polymorphism of *S*-mephenytoin hydroxylation. *Pharmacol Ther* 43:53–76, 1989.

Williams RT: *Detoxification Mechanisms*, 2d ed. New York: Wiley, 1971.

Wong JMY, Kalow W, Kadar D, et al: Carbonyl (phenone) reductase in human liver: Inter-individual variability. *Pharmacogenetics* 3:110–115, 1993.

Wrighton SA, Stevens JC: The human hepatic cytochromes P450 involved in drug metabolism. *Crit Rev Toxicol* 22:1–21, 1992.

Wrighton SA, Vandenbranden M, Stevens JC, et al: In vitro methods for assessing human hepatic drug metabolism: Their use in drug development. *Drug Metab Rev* 25:453–484, 1993.

Yan B, Yang D, Brady M, Parkinson A: Rat kidney carboxylesterase: Cloning, sequencing, cellular localization, and relationship to rat liver hydrolase. *J Biol Chem* 269:29688–29696, 1994.

Zand R, Sidney N, Slattery J, et al: Inhibition and induction of cytochrome P4502E1-catalyzed oxidation by isoniazid in humans. *Clin Pharmacol Ther* 54:142–149, 1993.

Zhang Y, Talalay P, Cho C-G, Posner GH: A major inducer of anticarcinogenic protective enzymes from broccoli: Isolation and elucidation of structure. *Proc Natl Acad Sci USA* 89:2399–2403, 1992.

Zhu BT, Liehr JG: Inhibition of the catechol-*O*methyltransferase-catalyzed *O*-methylation of 2- and 4-hydroxyestradiol by catecholamines: Implications for the mechanism of estrogen-induced carcinogenesis. *Arch Biochem Biophys* 304:248–256, 1993.

Ziegler DM: Recent studies on the structure and function of multisubstrate flavin-containing monooxygenases. *Annu Rev Pharmacol Toxicol* 33:179–199, 1993.

# CHAPTER 7

# TOXICOKINETICS

*Michele A. Medinsky and Curtis D. Klaassen*

The study of the kinetics of chemicals was oringinally initiated for drugs and consequently was termed *pharmacokinetics*. However, toxicology is not limited to the study of adverse drug effects but entails an investigation of the deleterious effects of all chemicals. Therefore, the study of the kinetics of xenobiotics is more properly called *toxicokinetics*. Toxicokinetics refers to the modeling and mathematical description of the time course of disposition (absorption, distribution, biotransformation, and excretion) of xenobiotics in the whole organism. In the past, the most common way to characterize the kinetics of drugs was to represent the body as consisting of one or two compartments even if those compartments had no apparent physiological or anatomic reality. More recently, physiologically based pharmacokinetic models have been developed in which mass balance equations allow the modeling of each organ or tissue on the basis of physiological considerations. It should be emphasized that there is no inherent contradiction between the classical and physiologically based approaches. Classical pharmacokinetics, as will be shown, requires certain assumptions that the physiologically based models do not require. Under ideal conditions, physiological pharmacokinetic models can predict tissue concentrations, whereas classical models cannot. However, the appropriate physiological (e.g., blood flow rate, tissue volume) and biochemical (e.g., rate of biotransformation in a particular tissue) parameters are often unknown or inexact, hampering meaningful physiologically based pharmacokinetic modeling.

## CLASSICAL TOXICOKINETICS

### One-Compartment Model

The simplest toxicokinetic analysis entails measurement of the plasma concentrations of a xenobiotic at several time points after the administration of a bolus intravenous injection. If the data obtained yield a straight line when they are plotted as the logarithms of plasma concentrations versus time, the kinetics of the xenobiotic can be described with a one-compartment model (Fig. 7-1). Compounds whose toxicokinetics can be described with a one-compartment model rapidly equilibrate, or mix uniformly, between blood and the various tissues relative to the rate of elimination. The one-compartment model depicts the body as a homogeneous unit. This does not mean that the concentration of a compound is the same throughout the body, but it does assume that the changes that occurr in the plasma concentration reflect changes in tissue concentrations.

The elimination from the body of a chemical whose disposition is described by a one-compartment model usually occurs through a first-order process; that is, the rate of elimination at any time is proportional to the amount of the chemical in the body at that time. Elimination includes biotransformation, exhalation, and excretion. The first-order elimination rate constant $k_{el}$ has units of reciprocal time (e.g., $min^{-1}$ and $h^{-1}$). Thus, if the elimination rate constant is, for example, 0.3 $h^{-1}$, the percentage of the dose excreted after 1 h is the same regardless of the administered dose (Table 7-1). In this case, the percentage of the dose excreted after 1 h is 26 percent, even though the rate constant is 0.3/h (or 30 percent/h), because the remaining dose ($C$) continuously decreases with time. The rate of elimination, or $k_{el} \cdot C$, decreases as $C$ decreases. The mathematical expression of this first-order process is a monoexponential equation, $C = C_o \cdot e^{-k_{el}t}$, where $C$ is the plasma concentration, $k_{el}$ is the first-order elimination rate constant, and $t$ is the time of blood sampling. The logarithmic equation for this exponen-

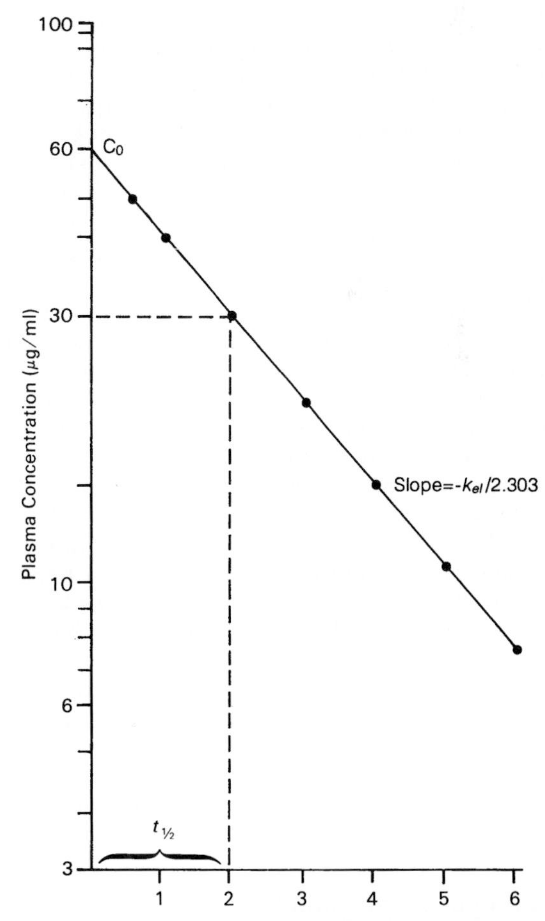


***Figure 7–1.*** ***Schematic representation of the concentration of a chemical in the plasma as a function of time after an intravenous injection if the body acts as a one-compartment system and elimination of the chemical obeys first-order kinetics with a rate constant ($k_{el}$).***

**Table 7–1**
**Elimination of Four Different Doses of a Chemical Described by a One Compartment Open Model and First-Order Kinetics**

| DOSE, mg | CHEMICAL REMAINING, mg | CHEMICAL ELIMINATED, mg | CHEMICAL ELIMINATED, % of dose |
|---|---|---|---|
| 10 | 7.4 | 2.6 | 26 |
| 30 | 22 | 8 | 26 |
| 90 | 67 | 23 | 26 |
| 250 | 185 | 65 | 26 |

tial function has the general form of an equation describing a straight line:

$$\log C = \log C_0 - \frac{k_{el} \cdot t}{2.303}$$

where log $C_0$ represents the intercept and $-k_{el} / 2.303$ represents the slope of the line. Thus, the first-order elimination rate constant can be determined from the slope of the log $C$ versus time plot.

Another important and frequently used parameter to characterize the time course of xenobiotics in an organism is the half-life ($t_{1/2}$). The half-life or elimination $t_{1/2}$ is the time required for the plasma concentration of a chemical to decrease by one-half. Because of the relationship $t_{1/2} = 0.693/k_{el}$, the half-life of a compound can be calculated after $k_{el}$ has been determined from the slope of the line. The $t_{1/2}$ also can be determined by means of visual inspection of the log $C$ versus time plot, as shown in Fig. 7-1. For compounds eliminated by first-order kinetics, the time required for the plasma concentration to decrease by one-half is constant. Therefore, xenobiotics eliminated from the body by first-order processes are theoretically never completely eliminated. However, during seven half-lives, 99.2 percent of a chemical is eliminated, and for practical purposes this can be viewed as complete elimination. The half-life of a chemical obeying first-order elimination kinetics is independent of the dose. This means that plotting the logarithm of concentration divided by dose as a function of time yields a single straight line independent of the dose (Fig. 7-2). This is known as the *principle of superposition*.

In summary, the important characteristics of first-order elimination according to a one-compartment model are as follows: (1) The rate at which a chemical is eliminated at any time is directly proportional to the amount of that chemical in the body at that time, (2) a semilogarithmic plot of plasma concentration versus time yields a single straight line, (3) the half-life ($t_{1/2}$) is independent of dose, and (4) the concentration of the chemical in plasma and other tissues decreases by some constant fraction per unit of time, the elimination rate constant ($k_{el}$).

## Two-Compartment Model

After the rapid intravenous administration of some chemicals, the semilogarithmic plot of plasma concentration versus time does not yield a straight line but a curve. In these cases, a multicompartmental analysis of the results is necessary. As was

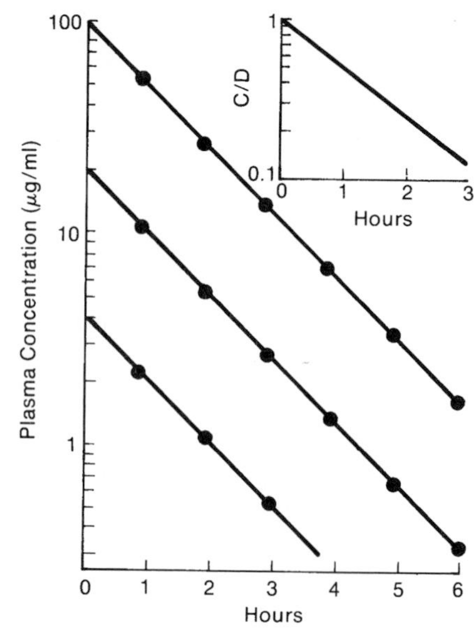


***Figure 7–2. Schematic representation of the time course of elimination of three different doses of a chemical after intravenous injection, assuming that the body acts as a one-compartment system and elimination obeys first-order kinetics.***

The inset is a semilogarithmic plot of plasma concentrations ($C$) divided by dose ($D$) as a function of time. Note that the separate curves in the main figure collapse into the single line in the inset.

noted earlier, a chemical whose toxicokinetics can be described by a one-compartment model is rapidly distributed between the plasma and various tissues. However, some chemicals require a longer time for their concentration in tissues to reach equilibrium with the concentration in plasma, as depicted in the bottom panel of Fig. 7-3. This results in a multiexponential elimination of the xenobiotic from the plasma. The disposition of such a chemical is said to obey a multicompartment model.

In the simplest case, a curve of this type can be resolved into two monoexponential terms (a two-compartment model) and is described by $C = Ae^{-\alpha t} + Be^{-\beta t}$, where $A$ and $B$ are proportionality constants and $\alpha$ and $\beta$ are rate constants with dimensions of reciprocal time (Fig. 7-3). During the distribution ($\alpha$) phase, concentrations of the chemical in the plasma decrease more rapidly than they do in the postdistribution ($\beta$) phase (also referred to as equilibrium or the elimination phase) (Fig. 7-3). The distribution phase may last for only a few minutes or for hours or days. Whether the distribution phase becomes apparent depends on the time when the first plasma samples are obtained.

The equivalent of $k_{el}$ in a one-compartment model is $\beta$ in a two-compartment model. Thus, the termimal half-time for the elimination of a compound that displays the characteristics of a two-compartment model can be calculated by using the equation, $\beta = 0.693 / t_{1/2}$.

The plasma concentration profile of many compounds cannot be described satisfactorily by an equation with two exponential terms. Sometimes three or four exponential terms are needed to fit a curve to the log $C$ versus time plot. Such compounds are viewed as displaying characteristics of three- or four-compartment open models. The principles for dealing

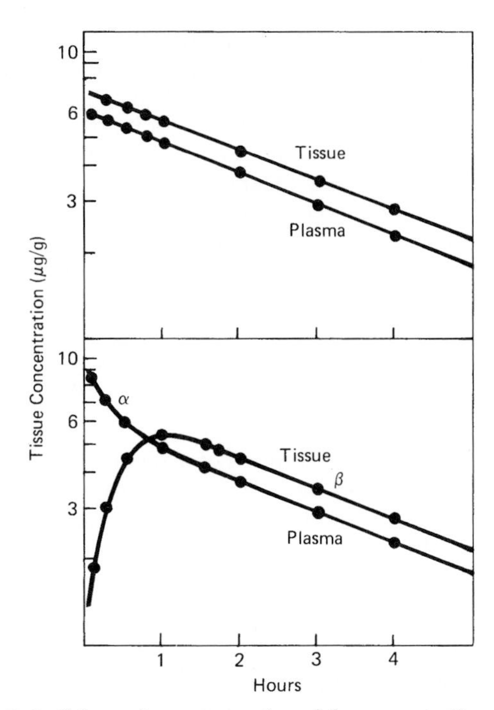


*Figure 7–3. Schematic representation of the concentration of a xenobiotic in plasma and tissue with time in a one-compartment open model (top panel) and a two-compartment open model (bottom panel).*

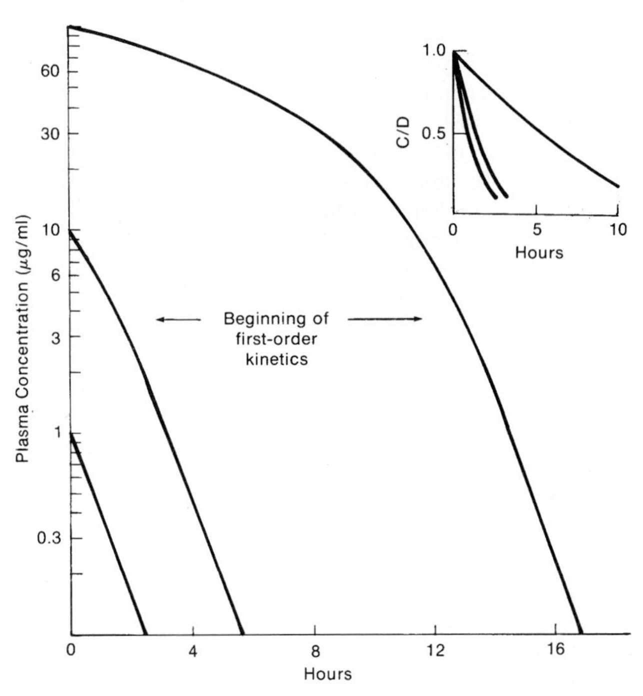


*Figure 7–4. Schematic representation of the time course of elimination of three different doses of a chemical after rapid intravenous administration, assuming that the body acts as a one-compartment system and elimination is easily saturated.*

The inset is a plot of the plasma concentrations (*C*) divided by dose (*D*).

with such models are the same as those used for the two-compartment open model, but the mathematics are more complex.

## Saturation of Elimination

The elimination of most chemicals occurs by first-order processes. However, as the dose of a compound increases, its rate of elimination may decrease, as shown in Fig. 7-4. This is usually referred to as saturation or Michaelis-Menten kinetics. Biotransformation, active transport processes, and protein binding have finite capacities and can be saturated. When the concentration of a chemical in the body is higher than the $K_M$ (chemical concentration at one-half the maximum capacity), the rate of elimination is no longer proportional to the dose. The transition from first-order to saturation kinetics is important in toxicology because it leads to prolonged residency time of a compound in the body, which can result in increased toxicity.

Some of the criteria that indicate nonlinear pharmacokinetics include the following: (1) The decline in the levels of the chemical in the body is not exponential, (2) $t_{1/2}$ increases with increasing dose, (3) the area under the plasma concentration versus time curve (AUC) is not proportional to the dose, (4) the composition of excretory products changes quantitatively or qualitatively with the dose, (5) competitive inhibition by other chemicals that are biotransformed or actively transported by the same enzyme system occurs, and (6) dose-response curves show a nonproportional change in response with an increasing dose, starting at the dose level at which saturation effects become evident.

The elimination of some chemicals from the body is readily saturated. These compounds follow zero-order kinetics. Ethanol is an example of a chemical whose elimination follows zero-order kinetics, with its biotransformation being the rate-limiting step in its elimination. As shown in Table 7-2, a constant amount is biotransformed per unit of time regardless of the amount of ethanol present in the body. Important characteristics of zero-order processes are as follows: (1) An arithmetic plot of plasma concentration versus time yields a straight line, (2) the rate or amount of chemical eliminated at any time is constant and is independent of amount of chemical in the body, and (3) a true $t_{1/2}$ or $k_{el}$ does not exist.

## Apparent Volume of Distribution

The apparent volume of distribution ($V_d$) is a proportionality constant that relates the concentration of a xenobiotic in plasma to the total amount of chemical in the body. $V_d$ is cor-

**Table 7–2**
**Elimination of a Chemical Which Follows Zero-Order Kinetics**

| TIME, h | ETHANOL REMAINING, ml | ETHANOL ELIMINATED, ml | ETHANOL ELIMINATED, % of that remaining |
|---|---|---|---|
| 0 | 50 | 0 | 0 |
| 1 | 40 | 10 | 20 |
| 2 | 30 | 10 | 25 |
| 3 | 20 | 10 | 33 |
| 4 | 10 | 10 | 50 |
| 5 | 0 | 10 | 100 |

rectly called the *apparent volume of distribution* because it has no direct physiological meaning and usually does not refer to a real volume. A chemical with high affinity for tissues will have a large volume of distribution. In fact, binding to tissues may be so avid that the $V_d$ of a chemical is much larger than the actual body volume. The apparent volume of distribution of a chemical displaying the characteristics of a one-compartment model is mathematically defined as the quotient between the amount of chemical in the body and its plasma concentration. Determination of $V_d$ is analogous to adding a known amount of dye to a container with an unknown volume of liquid. After the liquid has been well stirred, the volume of the liquid (i.e., the volume of distribution) can be determined by dividing the amount of dye added by the concentration measured in the container. Unlike the dye in the container, the concentration of a chemical in plasma declines as a result of excretion, distribution, and biotransformation in tissues. Therefore, to estimate $V_d$, it is necessary to extrapolate the plasma disappearance curve after intravenous injection to the zero time point. This extrapolation yields the plasma concentration $C_0$ at time zero, that is, before any elimination has taken place (Fig. 7-1). The apparent volume of distribution can be calculated by the equation $V_d = \text{Dose}_{iv} / C_0$, where $\text{Dose}_{iv}$ is the intravenous dose and $C_0$ is the extrapolated plasma concentration at time zero. This equation is appropriate for chemicals that display characteristics of a one-compartment model but is not valid for those which require two or more compartments for their modeling.

## Clearance

Clearance is an important toxicokinetic concept that is frequently used to characterize various compounds. Clearance is a ratio relating the *rate* of transfer or elimination of a chemical from an appropriate reference fluid, usually plasma (in milligrams per minute), to its *concentration* in that same fluid (in milligrams per milliliter). Thus, clearance has the units of flow rate (milliliters per minute). A clearance of 100 ml/min of a xenobiotic means that 100 ml of blood or plasma is completely cleared of the compound in each minute that passes. The overall efficiency of the removal of a chemical from the body can be characterized by clearance. High values of clearance indicate efficient and generally rapid removal, whereas low clearance values indicate slow and less efficient removal of a xenobiotic from the body. Chemicals are cleared from the body by various routes, for example, via the kidneys, liver, or intestine. *Total body clearance* is defined as the sum of clearances by individual organs:

$$\text{Cl} = \text{Cl}_r + \text{Cl}_h + \text{Cl}_i + \ldots$$

where $\text{Cl}_r$ depicts renal, $\text{Cl}_h$ hepatic, and $\text{Cl}_i$ intestinal clearance. Clearance of xenobiotics from the blood by a particular organ cannot be higher than blood flow to that organ. In the case of a xenobiotic that is being eliminated by hepatic biotransformation, clearance cannot exceed the hepatic blood flow rate. Total body clearance is defined as

$$\text{Cl} = \frac{\text{Dose}_{iv}}{\text{AUC}_{0\rightarrow x}}$$

where $AUC_{0 \rightarrow x}$ is the area under the plasma concentration versus time curve from time $= 0$ to time $= x$ and $\text{Dose}_{iv}$ is the amount of chemical given by intravenous injection. Clearance can also be defined as $\text{Cl} = V_d \cdot k_{el}$ for a one-compartment model and $\text{Cl} = V_d \cdot \beta$ for a two-compartment model. Clearance is an exceedingly important concept in toxicokinetics. It is the single most important index of the capacity of an organism to remove xenobiotics. Clearance is also the major determinant of the extent to which a xenobiotic accumulates during multiple dosing regimens. Often it is more useful to define specific organ clearances because they may provide important information about the proper functioning or diseased state of an organ.

## Bioavailability

The extent of systemic absorption of a xenobiotic can be determined experimentally by comparing the plasma AUC after intravenous and oral dosing. The resulting index is called *bioavailability*. Bioavailability can be determined by using different doses, provided that the compound does not display dose-dependent kinetics:

$$\text{Bioavailability} = \frac{\text{Dose}_{iv} \cdot \text{AUC}_{0\rightarrow \text{x oral}}}{\text{Dose}_{oral} \cdot \text{AUC}_{0\rightarrow \text{x iv}}}$$

where $\text{AUC}_{0\rightarrow x}$ is the area under the plasma concentration versus time curve from time $= 0$ to time $= x$ for oral or intravenous administration. Bioavailability is an exceedingly important concept in pharmacokinetics and toxicokinetics. As was discussed earlier, the most critical factor influencing toxicity is not necessarily the dose but rather the concentration of a xenobiotic at the site of action. Xenobiotics are delivered to most organs by the systemic circulation. Therefore, the fraction of a chemical that reaches the systemic circulation is of critical importance in determining toxicity. Several factors can greatly alter this systemic availability, including (1) limited absorption after oral dosing, (2) intestinal first-pass effect, (3) hepatic first-pass effect, and (4) mode of formulation, which affects, for example, dissolution rate or incorporation into micelles (for lipid-soluble compounds).

# PHYSIOLOGICAL TOXICOKINETICS

The primary difference between *physiological* compartmental models and *classical* compartmental models lies in the basis underlying the rate constants that describe the transport of chemicals into and out of the compartments (Andersen, 1991). In classical kinetics, the rate constants are defined by the data; thus, these models are often referred to as *data-based*. In physiological models, the rate constants represent known or hypothesized biological processes, and these models are commonly referred to as *physiologically based*. The concept of incorporating biological realism into the analysis of drug or xenobiotic distribution and elimination is not new. For example, one of the first physiological models was proposed by Teorell (1937). This model contained all the important determinants in chemical disposition that are considered valid today. Unfortunately, the computational tools required to solve the underlying equations were not available at that time. With advances in computer science, the software and hardware needed to implement physiological models are now well within the reach of toxicologists.

The advantages of physiologically based models compared with classical pharmacokinetics are that (1) these models can provide the time course of distribution of xenobiotics to any organ or tissue, (2) they allow estimation of the effects of changing physiological parameters on tissue concentrations, (3) the same model can predict the toxicokinetics of chemicals across species by allometric scaling, and (4) complex dosing regimes are easily accommodated (Gargas and Andersen, 1988). The disadvantages are that (1) more information is needed for these models compared with classical models, (2) the mathematics can be difficult for many toxicologists to handle, and (3) parameters are often ill defined in various species, strains, and disease states. Nevertheless, physiologically based toxicokinetic models are conceptually sound and are potentially useful tools for gaining insight into the kinetics of xenobiotics beyond what classical toxicokinetics can provide.

## Basic Model Structure

Physiological models often look like a number of classical one-compartmental models that are linked together. The actual model *structure*, or *how* the compartments are linked together, depends on both the chemical and the organism being studied. For example, a physiological model describing the disposition of a chemical in fish would require a description of the gills (Nichols et al., 1994), whereas a model for the same chemical in mammals would require a lung (Ramsey and Andersen, 1984). Model structures can also vary with the chemicals being studied. As shown in Figs. 7-5 and 7-6, a model for phenobarbital, which may be administered by intravenous injection, has a structure different from that for a model for benzene, a volatile chemical for which inhalation is the likely route of exposure. The route of administration is not the only difference between these two models: The phenobarbital model has compartments for the large intestine and bile, and the benzene model has a compartment for fat. However, the models are not *completely* different. Both contain a liver compartment because the hepatic metabolism of each chemical is an important element of its disposition. It is important to realize that there is no generic physiological model.

In view of the fact that physiological modeling requires more effort than does classical compartmental modeling, what accounts for the increase in the popularity of the kinetic approach among toxicologists? The answer lies in the potential predictive power of physiological models. Toxicologists are constantly faced with the issue of extrapolation from laboratory animals to humans, from high to low doses, from intermittent to continuous exposure, and from single chemicals to mixtures. Because the kinetic constants in physiological models represent measurable biological or chemical processes, the resultant physiological models have the potential for extrapolation from observed data to predicted situations.

One of the best illustrations of the predictive power of physiological models is their ability to extrapolate kinetic behavior from laboratory animals to humans. For example, Fig. 7-7 shows the results of physiological model simulations of the concentration of styrene in the blood of rats and humans. *Simulations* are the outcomes or results (such as a chemical's

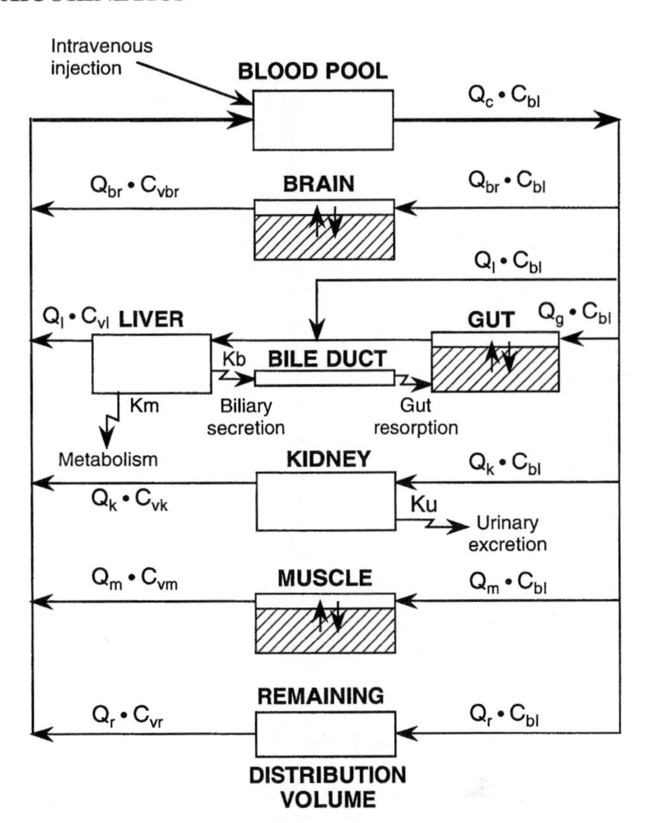


***Figure 7–5. Physiological model for phenobarbital.***

[Reproduced from Engasser et al. (1981), with permission of the American Pharmaceutical Association.]

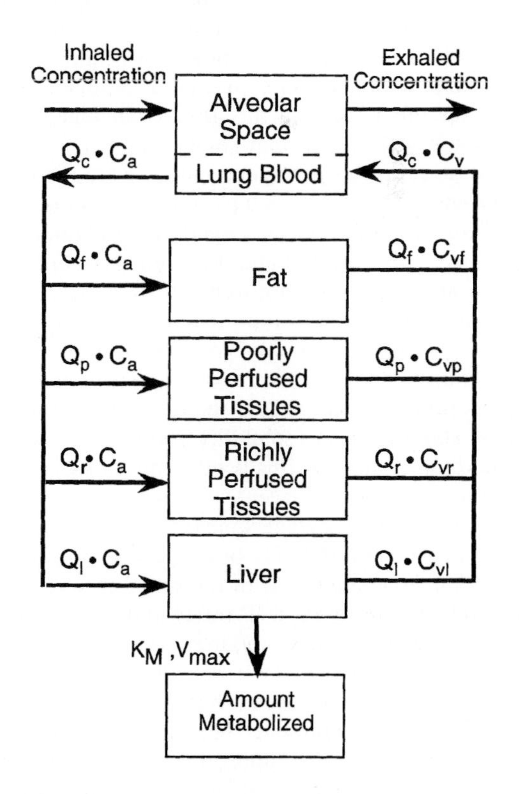


***Figure 7–6. Physiological model for the volatile organic chemical benzene***

[Redrawn from Medinsky et al. (1989), with permission.]

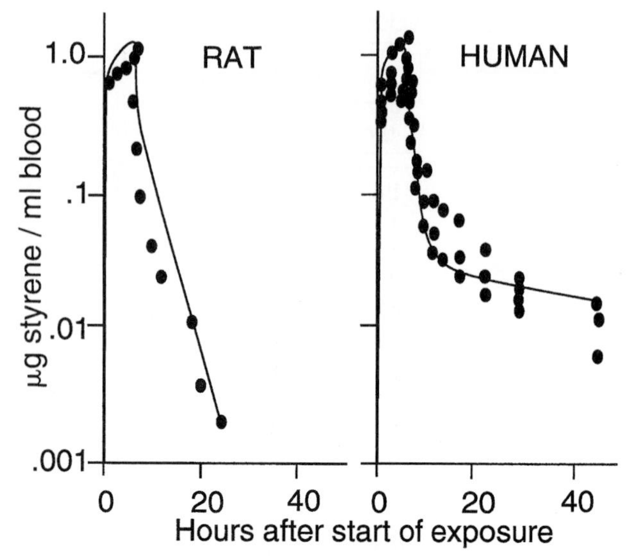


***Figure 7–7. Concentration of styrene in the venous blood of rats and humans exposed to 80 ppm styrene for 6 h.***

Data points represent individual measurements of styrene in blood. Lines are results of simulations using the physiological model of Ramsey and Andersen (1984). [From Michele A. Medinsky, Critical determinants in the systemic availability and dosimetry of volatile organic chemicals, in Gerrity and Henry (eds): Principles of Route-to-Route Extrapolation for Risk Assessment, © 1990, p 157. Reprinted by permission of Prentice-Hall, Inc., Englewood Cliffs, N.J.]

concentration in blood or tissue) of numerically integrating model equations over a simulated time period, using a set of initial conditions (such as intravenous dose) and parameter values (such as organ weights). Styrene is a volatile organic chemical; thus, the model structure for styrene kinetics in rats and humans is identical to that for benzene (Fig. 7-6). The exposure conditions for the rat and human were the same: 80 ppm of styrene inhaled over a 6-h period. Some of the parameter values for rats and humans were different. Humans have larger body weights than rats, and thus weights of organs such as the liver are larger. Because humans are larger, they also breathe more air per unit of time than do rats, and a human heart pumps a larger volume of blood per unit of time than does that of a rat, although the rat heart beats more times in the same period. The parameters that describe the chemical behavior of styrene, such as solubility in tissues, are similar in the rat and human models. This is often the case because the composition of tissues in different species is similar.

In the example of styrene kinetics in humans and rats, there are experimental data for both species and the model simulations can be compared with the actual data to see how well the model has performed (Ramsey and Andersen, 1984; Andersen et al., 1984). As is apparent in Fig. 7-7, the same model structure is capable of describing the kinetics of styrene in two different species. Because the parameters underlying the model structure represent measurable biological and chemical determinants, the appropriate values for those parameters can be chosen for each species, forming the basis for successful interspecies extrapolation.

In the example of styrene, even though the same model structure is used for both rats and humans, both the simulated and the observed kinetic behavior of styrene differs between rats and humans. As can be seen in Fig. 7-7, the terminal half-life of styrene is longer in the human compared with the rat. This longer half-life for humans is due to the fact that clearance rates for smaller species are faster than those for larger ones. Even though the larger species breathes more air or pumps more blood per unit of time than does the smaller species, blood flows and ventilation rates *per unit of body mass* are greater for the smaller species. The smaller species has more breaths per minute or heartbeats per minute than does the larger one even though each breath or stroke volume is smaller. These faster flows per unit mass bring more xenobiotic to organs responsible for elimination. Thus, a smaller species can eliminate a xenobiotic faster than a larger one can. Because the parameters in physiological models represent real, measurable values such as blood flows and ventilation rates, the same model structure can resolve such disparate kinetic behaviors among species.

## Compartments

The basic unit of the physiological model is the lumped compartment, which is often depicted as a box (Fig. 7-8). A *compartment* is a single region of the body with a *uniform* xenobiotic concentration (Rowland, 1984; Rowland, 1985). A compartment may be a particular functional or anatomical portion of an organ, a single blood vessel with surrounding tissue, an entire discrete organ such as the liver or kidney, or a widely distributed tissue type such as fat or skin. Compartments consist of three individual well-mixed phases, or *subcompartments*, that correspond to specific physiological portions of the organ or tissue. These subcompartments are (1) the *vascular* space through which the compartment is perfused with blood, (2) the *interstitial* space that forms the matrix for the cells, and (3) the *intracellular* space consisting of the cells in the tissue (Gerlowski and Jain, 1983).

In Fig. 7-8, the xenobiotic enters the vascular subcompartment at a certain rate in mass per unit of time (e.g., milligrams per hour). The rate of entry is a product of the blood flow rate to the tissue ($Q_t$, in liters per hour) and the concentration of the xenobiotic in the blood entering the tissue ($C_{in}$, in milligrams per liter). Within the compartment, the xenobiotic moves from the vascular space to the interstitial space at a certain net rate ($Flux_1$) and moves from the interstitial space

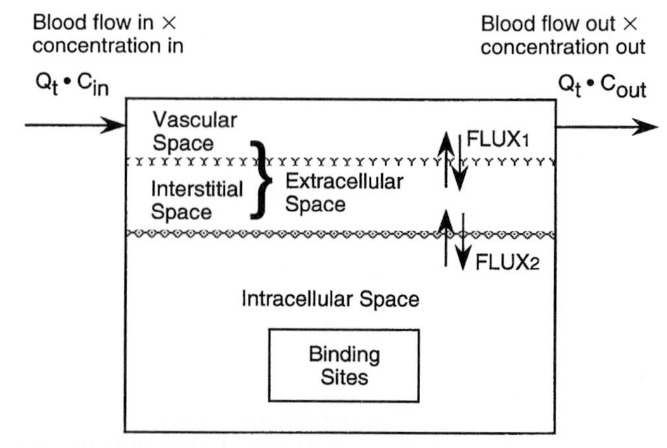


***Figure 7–8. Schematic representation of a lumped compartment in a physiological model.***

to the intracellular space at different net rate ($Flux_2$). Some xenobiotics can bind to cell components; thus, within a compartment there may be both free and bound xenobiotic. The xenobiotic leaves the vascular space at a certain venous concentration ($C_{out}$). $C_{out}$ is equal to the concentration of the xenobiotic in the vascular space.

## Parameters

The most common types of parameters, or information required, in physiological models are *anatomic, physiological, thermodynamic,* and *transport.*

**Anatomic.** The size of each of the compartments in the physiological model must be known. The size is generally specified as a volume (milliliters or liters) because a unit density is assumed even though weights are most frequently obtained experimentally. If a compartment contains subcompartments such as those in Fig. 7-8, those volumes also must be known. Volumes of compartments often can be obtained from the literature or from specific toxicokinetic experiments. For example, kidney, liver, brain, and lung can be weighed. Obtaining precise data for volumes of compartments representing widely distributed tissues such as fat or muscle is more difficult. If necessary, these tissues can be removed by dissection and weighed. Among the numerous sources of general information on organ and tissue volumes, Arms (1988) is a good starting point.

**Physiological.** The blood flow rate ($Q_t$, in volume per unit time, such as ml/min or liters/h) to individual compartments must be known. Additionally, information on the total blood flow rate or *cardiac output* ($Q_c$) is necessary. If inhalation is the route for exposure to the xenobiotic or is a route of elimination, the alveolar ventilation rate ($Q_p$) also must be known. Blood flow rates and ventilation rates can be taken from the literature or can be obtained experimentally. Renal clearance rates and parameters to describe rates of biotransformation, or metabolism, such as $V_{max}$ and $K_M$ also can be required physiological parameters if these processes are important in describing the elimination of a xenobiotic.

**Thermodynamic.** Thermodynamic parameters relate the *total* concentration of a xenobiotic in a tissue (C) to the concentration of *free* xenobiotic in that tissue ($C_f$). Two important assumptions are that (1) total and free concentrations are in equilibrium with each other and (2) only free xenobiotic can enter and leave the tissue (Lutz et al., 1980). Most often, total concentration is measured experimentally; however, it is the free concentration that is available for binding, metabolism, or removal from the tissue by blood. Various mathematical expressions describe the relationship between these two entities. In the simplest situation, the xenobiotic is a freely diffusible water-soluble chemical that does not bind to any molecules. In this case, the free concentration of the xenobiotic is exactly equal to the total concentration of the xenobiotic: total = free, or $C = C_f$.

The affinity of many xenobiotics for tissues of different composition varies. The extent to which a xenobiotic partitions into a tissue is directly dependent on the composition of the tissue and independent of the concentration of the xenobiotic. Thus, the relationship between free and total concentration becomes one of proportionality: total = free · partition coefficient, or $C = C_f \cdot P$. In this case, P is called a *partition* or *distribution* coefficient. Knowledge of the value of P permits an indirect calculation of the free concentration of xenobiotic or $C_f$. $C_f = C/P$.

Table 7-3 compares the partition coefficients for a number of toxic volatile organic chemicals. The larger values for the fat/blood partition coefficients compared with those for other tissues suggests that these chemicals distribute into fat to a greater extent than they distribute into other tissues. This has been observed experimentally. Fat and fatty tissue such as bone marrow contain higher concentrations of benzene than do tissues such as liver and blood. Similarly, styrene concentrations in fatty tissue are higher than styrene concentrations in other tissues.

A more complex relationship between the free concentration and the total concentration of a chemical in tissues is also possible. For example, the chemical may bind to saturable binding sites on tissue components. In these cases, nonlinear functions relating the free concentration in the tissue to the total concentration are necessary. An example in which more complex binding has been used is the physiological model for the chemical dioxin developed by Andersen and associates (1993).

**Transport.** The passage of a xenobiotic across a biological membrane is complex and may occur by passive diffusion, carrier-mediated transport, facilitated transport, or a combination of processes (Himmelstein and Lutz, 1979). The simplest of these processes—passive diffusion—is a first-order process described by Fick's law of diffusion. Diffusion of xenobiotics can occur across the blood capillary membrane ($Flux_1$ in Fig. 7-8) or across the cell membrane ($Flux_2$ in Fig. 7-8). *Flux* refers to the rate of transfer of a xenobiotic across a boundary. For simple diffusion, the net flux (milligrams per hour) from one side of a membrane to the other is described as Flux = permeability coefficient · driving force, or

$$\text{Flux} = [PA] \cdot (C_1 - C_2) = [PA] \cdot C_1 - [PA] \cdot C_2$$

The permeability coefficient [PA] is often called the *permeability-area cross-product* for the membrane (in units of liters per hour) and is a product of the cell membrane permeability constant (P, in micrometers per hour) for the xenobiotic and the total membrane area (A, in square micrometers). The cell membrane permeability constant takes into account the rate of diffusion of the specific xenobiotic and the thickness of the cell membrane. $C_1$ and $C_2$ are the *free* concentrations of

**Table 7–3**
**Partition Coefficients for Four Volatile Organic Chemicals**

| CHEMICAL | BLOOD/AIR | MUSCLE/BLOOD | FAT/BLOOD |
|---|---|---|---|
| Isoprene | 3 | 0.67 | 24 |
| Benzene | 18 | 0.61 | 28 |
| Styrene | 40 | 1 | 50 |
| Methanol | 1350 | 1.3 | 1.1 |

xenobiotic on each side of the membrane. For any given xenobiotic, thin membranes, large surface areas, and large concentration differences enhance diffusion.

There are two *limiting conditions* for the transport of a xenobiotic across membranes: *perfusion-limited* and *diffusion-limited*. An understanding of the asumptions underlying the limiting conditions is critical because the assumptions change the way in which the differential equations are written to describe the compartment.

## Perfusion-Limited Compartments

A perfusion-limited compartment is also referred to as *blood flow-limited*, or simply *flow-limited*. A flow-limited compartment can be developed if the cell membrane permeability coefficient [PA] for a particular xenobiotic is much greater than the blood flow rate to the tissue ($Q_t$) or $[PA] \gg Q_t$. In this case, the rate of xenobiotic uptake by tissue subcompartments is limited by the rate at which the blood containing a xenobiotic arrives at the tissue, not by the rate at which the xenobiotic crosses the cell membranes. In most tissues, the rate of entry of a xenobiotic into the interstitial space from the vascular space is not limited by the rate of xenobiotic transport across vascular cell membranes and is therefore perfusion rate–limited. In the generalized tissue compartment in Fig. 7-8, this means that transport of the xenobiotic through the loosely knit blood capillary walls of most tissues is rapid compared with delivery of the xenobiotic to the tissue by the blood. As a result, the vascular blood is in equilibrium with the interstitial subcompartment and the two subcompartments are usually lumped together as a single compartment that is often called the *extracellular space*. An important exception to this vascular-interstitial equilibrium relationship is the brain, where the tightly knit blood capillary walls form a barrier between the vascular space and the interstitial space.

As indicated in Fig. 7-8, the cell membrane separates the extracellular compartment from the intracellular compartment. The cell membrane is the most important diffusional barrier in a tissue. Nonetheless, for molecules that are very small (molecular weight <100) or lipophilic, cellular permeability generally does not limit the rate at which a molecule moves across cell membranes. For these molecules, flux across the cell membrane is fast compared with the tissue perfusion rate ($[PA] \gg Q_t$), and the molecules rapidly distribute through the subcompartments. In this case, the intracellular compartment is in equilibrium with the extracellular compartment, and these tissue subcompartments are usualy lumped as a single compartment. This flow-limited tissue compartment is shown in Fig. 7-9. Movement into and out of the entire tissue compartment can be described by a single equation:

$$V_t dC/dt = Q_t \cdot (C_{in} - C_{out})$$

where $V_t$ is the volume of the tissue compartment, C is the concentration of free xenobiotic in the compartment ($V_t \cdot C$ equals the amount of xenobiotic in the compartment), $V_t\, dC/dt$ is the change in the amount of xenobiotic in the compartment with time expressed as mass per unit of time, $Q_t$ is blood flow to the tissue, $C_{in}$ is xenobiotic concentration entering the compartment, and $C_{out}$ is xenobiotic concentration leaving the compartment. Equations of this type are called mass balance *differential* equations. Differential refers to the term d*x*/dt. Mass balance refers to the requirement that input into one equation must be balanced by outflow from another equation in the physiological model.

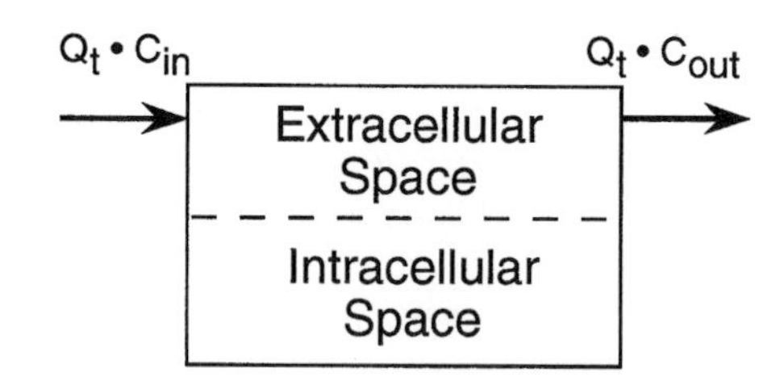


***Figure 7–9. Schematic representation of a compartment that is blood-flow–limited.***

Rapid exchange between the extracellular and intracellular spaces maintains the equilibrium between them.

In the perfusion-limited case, $C_{out}$, or the venous concentration of xenobiotic leaving the tissue, is equal to the free concentration of xenobiotic in the tissue, $C_f$. As was noted above, if $C_f$ (or $C_{out}$) can be related to the total concentration of xenobiotic in the tissue through a simple linear partition coefficient, $C_{out} = C_f = C/P$. In this case, the differential equation describing the rate of change in the amount of a xenobiotic in a tissue becomes

$$V_t\, dC/dt = Q_t \cdot (C_{in} - C/P)$$

The physiological model shown in Fig. 7-6, which was developed for volatile organic chemicals such as styrene and benzene, is a good example of a model in which all the compartments are described as flow-limited. Distribution of xenobiotic in all the compartments is described by using equations of the type noted above. In a flow-limited compartment, the assumption is that the concentrations of a xenobiotic in all parts of the tissue are in equilibrium. For this reason, the compartments are generally drawn as simple boxes (Fig. 7-6) or boxes with dashed lines that symbolize the equilibrium between the intracellular and extracellular subcompartments (Fig. 7-9). Additionally, with a flow-limited model, estimates of flux are not required to develop the mass balance differential equation for the compartment. Given the information required to estimate flux, this is a simplifying assumption that significantly reduces the number of parameters required in the physiological model.

## Diffusion-Limited Compartments

When uptake into a compartment is governed by cell membrane permeability and total membrane area, the model is said to be *diffusion-limited*, or *membrane-limited*. Diffusion-limited transport occurs when the flux, or the transport of a xenobiotic across cell membranes, is slow compared with blood flow to the tissue. In this case, the permeability-area cross-product [PA] is small compared with blood flow, $Q_t$, or $PA \ll Q_t$. The distribution of large polar molecules into tissue cells is likely to be limited by the rate at which the molecules pass through cell membranes. In contrast, entry into the interstitial space of the tissue through the leaky capillaries of the vascular space is usually flow-limited

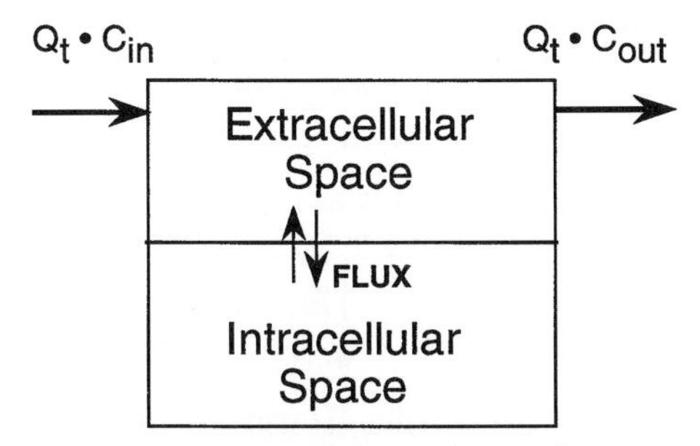


***Figure 7–10. Schematic representation of a compartment that is membrane-limited, showing perfusion of blood to the extracellular compartment and transmembrane transport from the extracellular to the intracellular subcompartment.***

even for large molecules. Figure 7-10 shows the structure of such a model. The xenobiotic concentrations in the interstitial and vascular spaces are in equilibrium and make up the extracellular subcompartment where uptake from the incoming blood is flow-limited. The rate of xenobiotic uptake across the cell membrane (into the intracellular space from the extracellular space) is limited by cell membrane permeability and is thus diffusion-limited. Two mass balance differential equations are necessary to describe this compartment:

Extracellular space: $V_{t1}\, dC_1/dt = Q_t \cdot (C_{in} - C_{out}) - [PA] \cdot C_1 + [PA] \cdot C_2$

Intracellular space: $V_{t2}\, dC_2/dt = [PA] \cdot C_1 - [PA] \cdot C_2$

$Q_t$ is blood flow, and C is *free* xenobiotic concentration in entering blood (in), exiting blood (out), extracellular space (1), or intracellular space (2). Both equations contain terms for flux, or transfer across the cell membrane, $[PA] \cdot (C_1 - C_2)$. The physiological model for phenobarbital in Fig. 7-5 is composed of several diffusion-limited compartments each of which contain two subcompartments—extracellular and intracellular space—and several perfusion-limited compartments.

## Specialized Compartments

**Lung.** The inclusion of a lung compartment in a physiological model is an important consideration because inhalation is a common route of exposure to many toxic chemicals. Additionally, the lung compartment serves as an instructive example of the assumptions and simplifications that can be incorporated into physiological models while maintaining the overall objective of describing processes and compartments in biologically relevant terms. For example, although lung physiology and anatomy are complex, Haggard (1924) developed a simple approximation that sufficiently describes the uptake of many volatile xenobiotics by the lungs. A diagram of this simplified lung compartment is shown in Fig. 7-11. The assumptions inherent in this compartment description are as follows: (1) Ventilation is continuous, not cyclic, (2) conducting airways (nasal passages, larynx, trachea, bronchi, and bronchioles) function as inert tubes, carrying the vapor to the pulmonary or gas exchange region, (3) diffusion of vapor across the lung cell and capillary walls is rapid compared with blood flow through the lung, (4) all xenobiotic disappearing from the inspired air

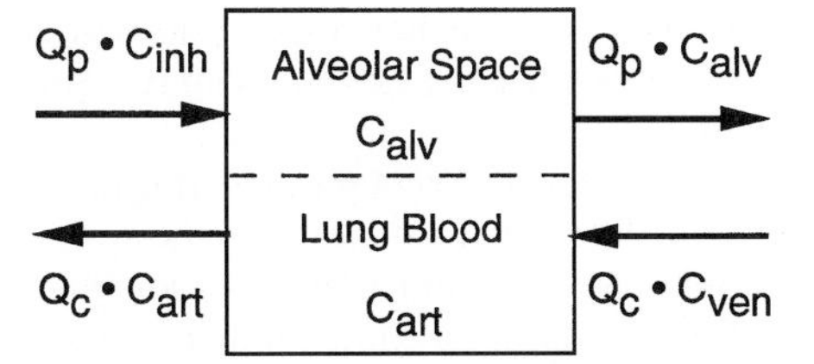


***Figure 7–11. Simple model of gas exchange in the alveolar region of the respiratory tract.***

$Q_p$ = alveolar ventialtion (L/h); $Q_c$ = cardiac output (L/h); $C_{inh}$ = inhaled concentration (mg/L); $C_{art}$ = concentration of vapor in the arterial blood; $C_{ven}$ = concentration of vapor in the mixed venous blood. The equilibrium relationship between the chemical in the alveolar air and the chemical in the arterial blood is determined by the blood/air partition coefficient $P_b$, eg, $C_{alv} = C_{art}/P_b$. [Adapted from Gargas et al. (1993) with permission.]

appears in the arterial blood (i.e., there is no storage of xenobiotic in the lung tissue and insignificant lung mass), (5) vapor in the alveolar air and arterial blood within the lung compartment are in rapid equilibrium and are related by $P_b$, the blood/air partition coefficient (e.g., $C_{alv} = C_{art}/P_b$). $P_b$ is a thermodynamic parameter that quantifies the distribution or partitioning of a xenobiotic into blood compared with air.

In the lung compartment depicted in Fig. 7-11, the rate of inhalation of xenobiotic is controlled by the ventilation rate ($Q_p$) and the inhaled concentration ($C_{inh}$). The rate of exhalation of a xenobiotic is a product of the ventilation rate and the xenobiotic concentration in the alveoli ($C_{alv}$). Xenobiotic also can enter the lung compartment via venous blood returning from the heart, represented by the product of cardiac output ($Q_c$) and the concentration of xenobiotic in venous blood ($C_{ven}$). Xenobiotic leaving the lungs via the blood is a function of both cardiac output and the concentration of xenobiotic in arterial blood ($C_{art}$). Putting these four processes together, a mass balance differential equation can be written for the rate of change in the amount of xenobiotic in the lung compartment (L):

$$dL/dt = Q_p \cdot (C_{inh} - C_{alv}) + Q_c \cdot (C_{ven} - C_{art})$$

Because of some of these assumptions, the rate of change in the amount of xenobiotic in the lung compartment becomes equal to zero ($dL/dt = 0$). $C_{alv}$ can be replaced by $C_{art}/P_b$, and the differential equation can be solved for the arterial blood concentration:

$$C_{art} = (Q_p \cdot C_{inh} + Q_c \cdot C_{ven}) / (Q_c + Q_p/P_b)$$

This algebraic equation is incorporated into physiological models for many volatile organics. Because the lung is viewed here as a portal of entry and not as a target organ, the concentration of a xenobiotic delivered to other organs by the blood, or the arterial concentration of that xenobiotic, is of primary interest. The assumptions of continuous ventilation, dead space, rapid equilibration with arterial blood, and no storage of vapor in the lung tissues have worked extremely well with many volatile organics, especially relatively lipophilic chemicals. Indeed, the use of these assumptions simplifies and speeds model calculations and may be entirely adequate for describing the chemical behavior of relatively inert vapors with low water solubility.

Inspection of the equation for calculating the arterial concentration of the inhaled organic vapor indicates that the term $P_b$, the xenobiotic-specific blood/air partition coefficient, becomes an important term for simulating the uptake of various volatile organic xenobiotics. As the value for $P_b$ increases, xenobiotic concentration in the arterial blood increases. Figure 7-12 demonstrates the relationship between $P_b$ and the blood concentration of a xenobiotic during and after inhalation of the same concentration of three volatile organic chemicals. The blood/air partition coefficients for the three vapors are shown in Table 7-3. As $P_b$ increases, the maximum concentration of the xenobiotic in the blood increases (Figure 7-12). Additionally, the time to reach the steady-state concentration and the time to clear the xenobiotic also increase with increasing $P_b$. Fortunately, $P_b$ is readily measured by using in vitro techniques in which a volatile chemical in air is equilibrated with blood in a closed system, such as a sealed vial (Gargas and Andersen, 1988).

**Liver.** The liver is often represented as a compartment in physiological models because hepatic biotransformation is an important aspect of the toxicokinetics of many xenobiotics. The effects of multiple factors such as concentration, dose rate, and species on the metabolism of xenobiotics are important in assessing risk. Because the liver is often the major organ for the biotransformation of xenobiotics, the task of metabolism is generally assigned to the liver compartment in physiological models. A simple compartmental structure for the liver is depicted in Fig. 7-13 where the liver compartment is assumed to be flow-limited and is similar to the general tissue compartment in Fig. 7-9, except that the liver compartment contains an additional process for metabolic elimination. One of the simplest expressions for this process is first-order elimination, which is written

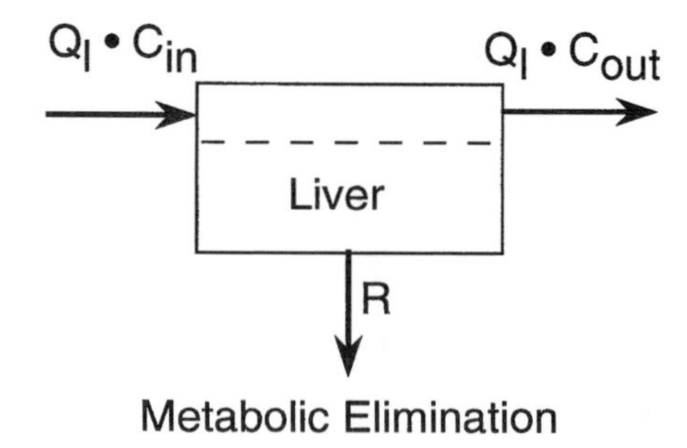


*Figure 7–13. Schematic representation of a flow-limited liver compartment in which metabolic elimination occurs. R, in milligrams per hour, is the rate of metabolism.*

$$R = C_f \cdot V_l \cdot K_f$$

R is the rate of metabolism (milligrams per hour), $C_f$ is the free concentration of xenobiotic in the liver (milligrams per liter), $V_l$ is the liver volume (liters), and $K_f$ is the first-order rate constant for metabolism in units of $h^{-1}$. Another widely used expression for metabolism in physiological models is the Michaelis-Menten expression for *saturable metabolism* (Andersen, 1981). Other, more complex expressions for metabolism also can be incorporated into physiological models. Bisubstrate second-order reactions, or reactions involving the destruction of enzymes, the inhibition of enzymes, and the depletion of cofactors, have been simulated using physiological models. Additionally, metabolism can be included in other compartments in much the same way.

The usefulness of physiological models for describing the complex toxicokinetic profiles resulting from saturable metabolism is responsible to a large extent for the popularity of these models. The ability of physiological models to extrapolate across a range of doses is illustrated in Fig. 7-14. The same parameters and model structure were used for each of the experiments. The model accounted for inhalation of xenobiotic, distribution to and uptake by tissues, and metabolism. The complex shapes of the curves in Fig. 7-14 are largely due to the transition from saturable metabolism at the high starting concentrations to apparent first-order metabolism at the low concentrations.

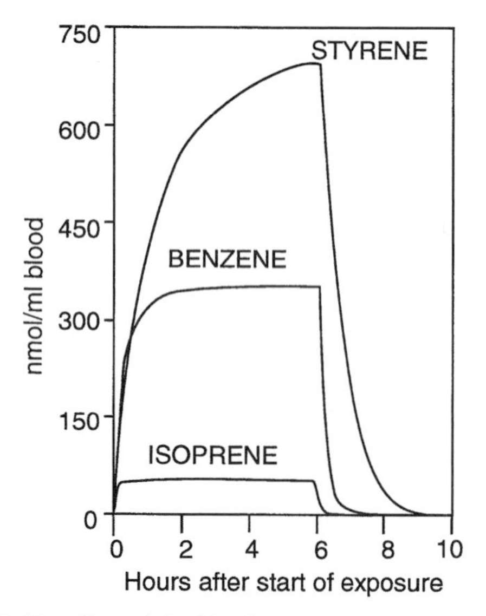


*Figure 7–12. Effect of the blood/air partition coefficient on venous blood concentrations in rats of three volatile organic chemicals during and after a 6-h exposure to 2000 mg/m³.*

Lines are physiological model simulations. [From Michele A. Medinsky, Critical determinants in the systemic availability and dosimetry of volatile organic chemicals, in Gerrity and Henry (eds): *Principles of Route-to-Route Extrapolation for Risk Assessment*, © 1990, p. 161. Reprinted by permission of Prentice-Hall, Inc., Englewood Cliffs, N.J.]

**Blood.** In a physiological model, as in a living organism, the tissue compartments are linked together by the blood. Figures 7-5 and 7-6 represent different approaches toward describing the blood in physiological models. In general, a tissue receives a xenobiotic in the systemic arterial blood. Exceptions are the liver, which receives arterial and portal blood, and the lungs, which receive mixed venous blood. In the body, the venous blood supplies draining from tissue compartments eventually merge in the large blood vessels and heart chambers to form mixed venous blood. In Fig. 7-5, a blood compartment is created in which the input is the sum of the xenobiotic efflux from

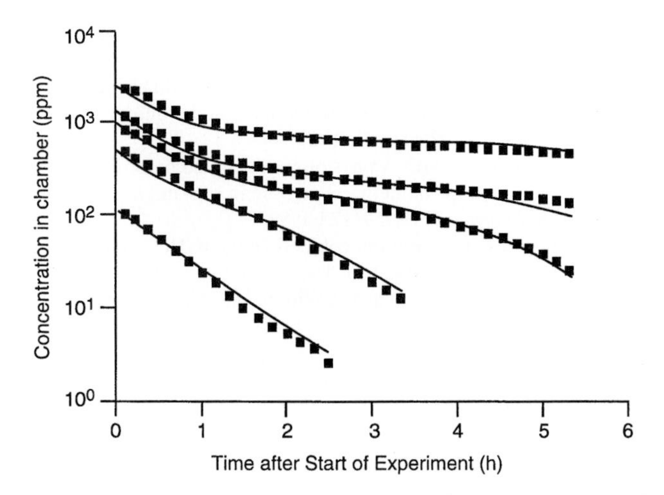


***Figure 7–14. Disappearance of chloroform after injection (at t = 0) into a closed chamber containing three rats.***

The experimental data (squares) are the results of measurements of air samples taken from the chamber. The lines are physiological model simulations of the experiments. After an initial period of equililbration, further decline in the chamber concentration is due to metabolism of chloroform by the rats. (From *Inhalation Toxicology*, volume 2, page 301, Gargas et al., Taylor and Francis, Inc., Wahsington, D.C. Reproduced with permission. All rights reserved.).

each compartment ($Q_t \cdot C_{vt}$). Efflux from the blood compartment is a product of the blood concentration in the compartment and the total cardiac output ($Q_c \cdot C_{bl}$). The differential equation for the blood compartment in Fig. 7-5 looks like this:

$$dV_{bl}C_{bl}/dt = Q_r \cdot C_{vr} + Q_m \cdot C_{vm} + Q_k \cdot C_{vk} + Q_l \cdot C_{vl} + Q_{br} \cdot C_{vbr} - Q_c \cdot C_{bl}$$

In contrast, the physiological model in Fig. 7-6 does not have a blood compartment. For simplicity, the blood volumes of the heart and the major blood vessels that are not within organs are assumed to be negligible. The venous concentration of xenobiotic returning to the lungs is simply the weighted average of the xenobiotic concentrations in the venous blood emerging from the tissues:

$$C_v = (Q_l \cdot C_{vl} + Q_r \cdot C_{vr} + Q_p \cdot C_{vp} + Q_f \cdot C_{vf}) / Q_c$$

The blood concentration going to the tissue compartments is the arterial concentration ($C_{art}$) that was calculated above for the lung compartment. The decision to use one formulation as oposed to another to describe blood in a physiological model depends on the role the blood plays in disposition. If the toxicokinetics after intravenous injection are to be simulated or if binding to or metabolism by blood components is suspected, a separate compartment for the blood that incorporates these additional processes is the best solution. If, as in the case of the volatile organics shown in Fig. 7-6, the blood is simply a conduit to the other compartments, the algebraic solution is acceptable.

## CONCLUSION

This chapter provides a basic overview of the simpler elements of physiological models and the important and often neglected assumptions that underlie model structures. Detailed descriptions of individual models of a wide variety of xenobiotics have been published. Several review articles describing how to construct a model step by step are included in the references. The field of physiological modeling is rapidly expanding and evolving as toxicologists and pharmacologists develop increasingly more sophisticated applications. Three-dimensional visualizations of xenobiotic transport in fish and vapor transport in the rodent nose, physiological models of a parent chemical linked in series with one or more active metabolites, models describing biochemical interactions among xenobiotics, and more biologically realistic descriptions of tissues previously viewed as simple lumped compartments are just a few of the exciting trends. Finally, physiologically based *toxicokinetic* models are beginning to be linked to biologically based *toxicodynamic* models to simulate the entire exposure→dose→response paradigm that is basic to the science of toxicology.

# REFERENCES

Andersen ME: A physiologically based toxicokinetic description of the metabolism of inhaled gases and vapors: Analysis at steady state. *Toxicol Appl Pharmacol* 60:509–526, 1981.

Andersen ME: Physiological modeling of organic compounds. *Ann Occup Hyg*. 35(3):309–321, 1991.

Andersen ME, Gargas ML, Ramsey JC: Inhalation pharmacokinetics: Evaluating systemic extraction, total *in vivo* metabolism, and the time course of enzyme induction for inhaled styrene in rats based on arterial blood:inhaled air concentration ratios. *Toxicol Appl Pharmacol* 73:176–187, 1984.

Andersen ME, Mills JJ, Gargas ML, et al: Modeling receptor-mediated processes with dioxin: Implications for pharmacokinetics and risk assessment. *Risk Anal* 13(1):25–36, 1993.

Arms AD: Reference Physiological Parameters in Pharmacokinetic Modeling. Washington, DC: U.S. Environmental Protection Agency (PB88-196019), 1988.

Engasser JM, Sarhan F, Falcoz C: Distribution, metabolism, and elimination of phenobarbital in rats: Physiologically based pharmacokinetic model. *J Pharmaceut Sci* 70(11):1233–1238, 1981.

Gargas ML, Andersen ME: Physiologically based approaches for examining the pharmacokinetics of inhaled vapors, in Gardner DE, Crapo JD, Massaro EJ (eds): *Toxicology of the Lung*. New York: Raven Press, 1988, pp 449–476.

Gargas ML, Andersen ME, Clewell HJ III: Gas uptake techniques and the rates of metabolism of chloromethanes, chloroethanes, and chloroethylenes in the rat. *Inhal Toxicol* 2:295–319, 1990.

Gargas ML, Medinsky MA, Andersen ME: Advances in physiological modeling approaches for understanding the disposition of inhaled vapors, in Gardner DE, Crapo JD, McClellan RO (eds): *Toxicology of the Lung*, 2d ed. New York: Raven Press, 1993, pp 461–483.

Gerlowski LE, Jain RK: Physiologically based pharmacokinetic modeling: Principles and applications. *J Pharm Sci* 72(10):1103–1127, 1983.

Haggard HW: The absorption, distribution, and elimination of ethyl ether: II. Analysis of the mechanism of the absorption and elimination of such a gas or vapor as ethyl ether. *J Biol Chem* 49:753–770, 1924.

Himmelstein KJ, Lutz RJ: A review of the applications of physiologically based pharmacokinetic modeling. *J Pharmacokinet Biopharm* 7(2):127–145, 1979.

Lutz RJ, Dedrick RL, Zaharko DS: Physiological pharmacokinetics: An *in vivo* approach to membrane transport. *Pharmac Ther* 11:559–592, 1980.

Medinsky MA: Critical determinants in the systemic availability and dosimetry of volatile organic chemicals, in Gerrity TR, Henry CJ (eds): *Principles of Route-to-Route Extrapolation for Risk Assessment.* New York: Elsevier, 1990, pp 155–172.

Medinsky MA, Sabourin PJ, Lucier G, et al: A physiological model for simulation of benzene metabolism by rats and mice. *Toxicol Appl Pharmacol* 99:193–206, 1989.

Nichols J, Rheingans P, Lothenbach D, et al: Three-dimensional visualization of physiologically based kinetic model outputs. *Environ Health Perspect* 102(11):952–956, 1994.

Ramsey JC, Andersen ME: A physiologically based description of the inhalation pharmacokinetics of styrene in rats and humans. *Toxicol Appl Pharmacol* 73:159–175, 1984.

Rowland M: Physiologic pharmacokinetic models: Relevance, experience, and future trends. *Drug Metab Rev* 15:55–74, 1984.

Rowland M: Physiologic pharmacokinetic models and interanimal species scaling. *Pharmac Ther* 29:49–68, 1985.

Teorell T: Kinetics of distribution of substances administered to the body: I. The extravascular modes of administration. *Arch Int Pharmacodyn Ther* 57:205–225, 1937.

# UNIT 3

# NONORGAN-DIRECTED TOXICITY

# CHAPTER 8

# CHEMICAL CARCINOGENESIS

*Henry C. Pitot III and Yvonne P. Dragan*

Cancer resulting from exposure to chemicals in the environment, though known for millennia, has taken on new importance in this century. With the advent of advanced technology, new chemical agents enter the environment, although at relatively low levels in most cases, at a prodigious rate. It has been estimated (Korte and Coulston, 1994) that the number of organic chemicals that are continually being brought into the environment (about 300 million tons per year) may include more than 100,000 compounds. Chemical contamination of waste (Landrigan, 1983), the food chain (Foran et al., 1989), and the occupational environment (Anttila et al., 1993) is reportedly substantial. However, other researchers (Ames and Gold, 1990) have noted numerous misconceptions about the relationship of exposure to industrially based environmental chemicals and the incidence of human cancer. Therefore, knowledge about the mechanisms and natural history of cancer development as well as the epidemiology of human cancer is critical to the control and prevention of human neoplastic disease.

## HISTORICAL FOUNDATION

The historical foundations for the induction of carcinogenesis by chemicals date back several thousand years to the description of breast cancer in the Edwin Smith Papyrus (Shimkin, 1977). In 1700, Ramazzini described the first example of occupational cancer. He noted the high incidence of breast cancer among nuns, which he attributed to their celibate life. A specific causal relationship between exposure to environmental mixtures and the induction of cancer was reported in 1775 by an eminent English physician and surgeon, Percivall Pott. Pott described the occurrence of cancer of the scrotum in a number of patients with a history of employment as chimney sweeps. With remarkable insight, Pott concluded that the occupation of those men was directly and causally related to their malignant disease. In addition, Pott suggested that the soot to which they were exposed was the causative agent of their condition. While Pott's publication soon led other observers to attribute cancer in various sites to soot exposure, his work had little impact on British public health practice during the succeeding century (Lawley, 1994). Thus, more than a century later, Butlin (1892) reported the relative rarity of scrotal cancer among chimney sweeps on the European continent compared with those in England. This difference was attributed to the relatively low standards of hygiene in Britain and the practice of exposing young "climbing boys" to the combustion products of coal. However, the lesson from Pott's findings has been a long time in the learning. A hundred years after the publication of Pott's monograph, the high incidence of skin cancer among certain German workers was traced to their exposure to coal tar, the chief constituent of the chimney sweeps' soot (Miller, 1978). Even today—more than 200 years after Pott's original scientific report on the association of soot and smoke products with cancer—a large percentage of the world's population is exposed to carcinogenic products that result from the combustion of tobacco and organic fuels.

During the nineteenth century, industrial chemicals, including cutting oils and dyes, were implicated as causative factors in the development of skin and bladder cancer, respectively (Lawley, 1994). Coal tar derivatives became the basis for the dye industry during the middle of the nineteenth century in Europe. Amine-containing aromatics such as 2-naphthylamine and benzidine were discovered and subsequently were synthesized and used to yield a variety of chemical species of pigments for coloring a variety of materials. In 1895 Rehn reported the occurrence of bladder cancer in workers in the aniline dye industry. This finding was rapidly supported by other reports (Miller, 1978). Epidemiological studies incriminated a number of aromatic amines, such as naphthylamines and benzidines, as the inciting agents (Hueper et al., 1938). Today, 2-naphthylamine is not used in the U.S. chemical industry and exposure to a variety of other aromatic amines is regulated by law. Thus, the reader may appreciate that the human being was the first experimental animal in which chemical carcinogenesis was studied. Later we will consider both the development and the data derived from studies of chemical carcinogenesis in animals.

## DEFINITIONS

Cancer describes a subset of lesions of the disease neoplasia. *Neoplasia* or the constituent lesion, a *neoplasm*, is defined as a heritably altered, relatively autonomous growth of tissue (Pitot, 1986a). The critical points of this definition are (1) the heritable aspects of neoplasia at the somatic or germ cell level and (2) the relative autonomy of neoplastic cells, reflecting their abnormal regulation of genetic expression, which is inherent in the neoplastic cell or occurs in response to environmental stimuli. Neoplasms may be either *benign* or *malignant*. The critical distinction between these classes is related to the characteristic of successful *metastatic* growth of malignant, but not benign, neoplasms. *Metastases* are secondary growths of cells from the primary neoplasm. Cancers are malignant neoplasms, whereas the term "tumor" describes space-occupying lesions that may or may not be neoplastic.

The nomenclature of neoplasia depends primarily on whether the neoplasm is benign or malignant and, in the latter case, whether it is derived from epithelial or mesenchymal tissue. For most benign neoplasms, the tissue of origin is followed by the suffix *-oma*: fibroma, lipoma, adenoma, and so on. For malignant neoplasms derived from tissues of mesenchymal origin, the term "sarcoma" is added to the tissue descriptor: fibrosarcoma, osteosarcoma, liposarcoma, and so on. Malignant neoplasms derived from tissues of ectodermal or endodermal (epithelial) origin are termed carcinomas with an antecedent tissue descriptor: epidermoid carcinoma (skin), hepatocellular carcinoma, gastric adenocarcinoma, and so on.

In general a *carcinogen* is an agent that causes or induces neoplasia. However, this definition is insufficient by current standards. The following definition may be more appropriate.

A *carcinogen* is an agent whose administration to previously untreated animals leads to a statistically significant increased incidence of neoplasms of one or more histogenetic types as compared with the incidence in appropriate untreated animals (Pitot, 1986a).

This definition includes the induction of neoplasms that usually are not observed, the earlier induction of neoplasms that usually are observed, and/or the induction of more neoplasms than usually are found. Although it is important to distinguish between agents that induce neoplasms through direct action on the cells that become neoplastic and those which produce neoplasia through indirect actions in the animal as a whole, this is not always possible. Some agents, such as immune suppressants, can increase the incidence of neoplasms in tissues that previously were exposed to carcinogens through indirect effects on the host. When the action of a chemical in causing an increase in neoplasms is known to be indirect—that is, mediated by its effect on cells other than those undergoing carcinogenesis—that agent should not be designated as a carcinogen. Later in this chapter the stages and modifying factors of the process of chemical carcinogenesis will be considered, necessitating a further refinement of the term "carcinogen" in relation to the action of specific chemicals in the carcinogenic process.

## CARCINOGENESIS BY CHEMICALS

At the turn of this century, studies in humans showed that environmental and possibly internal chemical agents are causative factors in the development of cancer (Shimkin, 1977; Lawley, 1994). However, a systematic study of the mechanisms of chemical carcinogenesis was not possible without defined experimental systems. In 1915, the Japanese pathologists Yamagawa and Ichikawa (1915) described the first production of skin tumors in animals by the application of coal tar to the skin. These investigators repeatedly applied crude coal tar to the ears of rabbits for a number of months, finally producing both benign and later malignant epidermal neoplasms. Later studies demonstrated that the skin of mice is also susceptible to the carcinogenic action of such organic tars. During the next 15 years, extensive attempts were made to determine the nature of the material in the crude tars that causes malignancy. In 1932, Kennaway and associates reported the production of carcinogenic tars by means of pyrolysis of organic compounds consisting only of carbon and hydrogen (Kennaway, 1955).

### Organic Chemical Carcinogens

In the early 1930s, several polycyclic aromatic hydrocarbons were isolated from active crude tar fractions. In 1930, the first synthetic carcinogenic polycyclic aromatic hydrocarbon was produced (Miller, 1978). This compound, dibenz(*a,h*)anthracene (Fig. 8-1), was demonstrated to be a potent carcinogen after repeated painting on the skin of mice. The isolation from coal tar and the synthesis of benzo(*a*)pyrene (3,4-benzpyrene) were achieved in 1932. The structures of several polycyclic aromatic hydrocarbons are shown in Fig. 8-1. Polycyclic hydrocarbons vary in their carcinogenic potencies; for example, the compound dibenz(*a,c*)anthracene has very little carcinogenic activity, while the *a,h* isomer is carcinogenic (Heidelberger, 1970). The more potent polycyclic aromatic hydrocarbon carcinogens are 3-methylcholanthrene and 7,12-dimethylbenz(*a*)-anthracene. The carcinogenic dibenzo(*c,q*)carbazole, which has a nitrogen in its central ring, also is considered to be in this class of compounds. Benzo(*e*)pyrene is reportedly inactive in inducing skin cancer in mice but can "initiate" the carcinogenic process. Perylene is inactive as a chemical carcinogen, whereas chrysene may have slight carcinogenic activity.

In 1935, Sasaki and Yoshida opened another field of chemical carcinogenesis by demonstrating that feeding of the azo dye *o*-aminoazotoluene (2′,3-dimethyl-4-aminoazobenzene) (Fig. 8-2) to rats can result in the development of liver neoplasms. Similarly, Kinosita (1936) demonstrated that the administration of 4-dimethylaminoazobenzene in the diet also causes neoplasms in the liver. A number of analogues of this compound were prepared and tested for carcinogenic potential. Unlike the polycyclic aromatic hydrocarbons, the azo dyes generally acted not at the site of first contact of the compound with the organism but instead at a remote site, the liver.

Another important carcinogen that acts at remote sites is 2-acetylaminofluorene (Fig. 8-2). This chemical induces neoplasms of the mammary gland, ear duct, and liver in rats (Miller et al., 1949) and neoplasms of the bladder in mice (Miller et al., 1964). The aromatic amine 2-naphthylamine and several other aromatic amines are carcinogenic for the urinary bladder in humans (Vainio et al., 1991). Benzidine (4,4′-diaminobiphenyl) is also a bladder carcinogen for humans and serves as an intermediate in the production of a number of dyes in the United States, several of which have been labeled as carcinogenic to humans (Radomski, 1979). The carcinogenic chemical ethyl carbamate appears to be a general "initiating agent" in the mouse. Ethyl carbamate was in use in Japan from 1950 to 1975 as a cosolvent for dissolving water-insoluble analgesic drugs (Miller, 1991), but this practice was stopped after 1975. No systematic study of the incidence of cancer in this cohort has been conducted. In addition, certain cytocidal alkylating agents, such as the nitrogen mustards (Fig. 8-2), have been used to treat cancer in humans and also are known to be potent carcinogens in both animals and humans (Vainio et al., 1991). The other three agents depicted on the bottom line of Fig. 8-2 are also alkylating agents that are used industrially. Bis(chloromethyl)ether, a popular intermediate in organic synthetic reactions, has been classified as carcinogenic to humans on the basis of epidemiological and animal studies (Vainio et al., 1991).

Dimethylnitrosamine is the smallest of the class of dialkylnitrosamines in which the alkyl substituents on the nitrogen linked to the nitroso group may vary widely, including fusion to yield a cyclic aliphatic substituent. Dimethylnitrosamine (Fig. 8-2) is highly carcinogenic for the liver and kidney in virtually all the mammalian species tested (Schmähl and Habs,

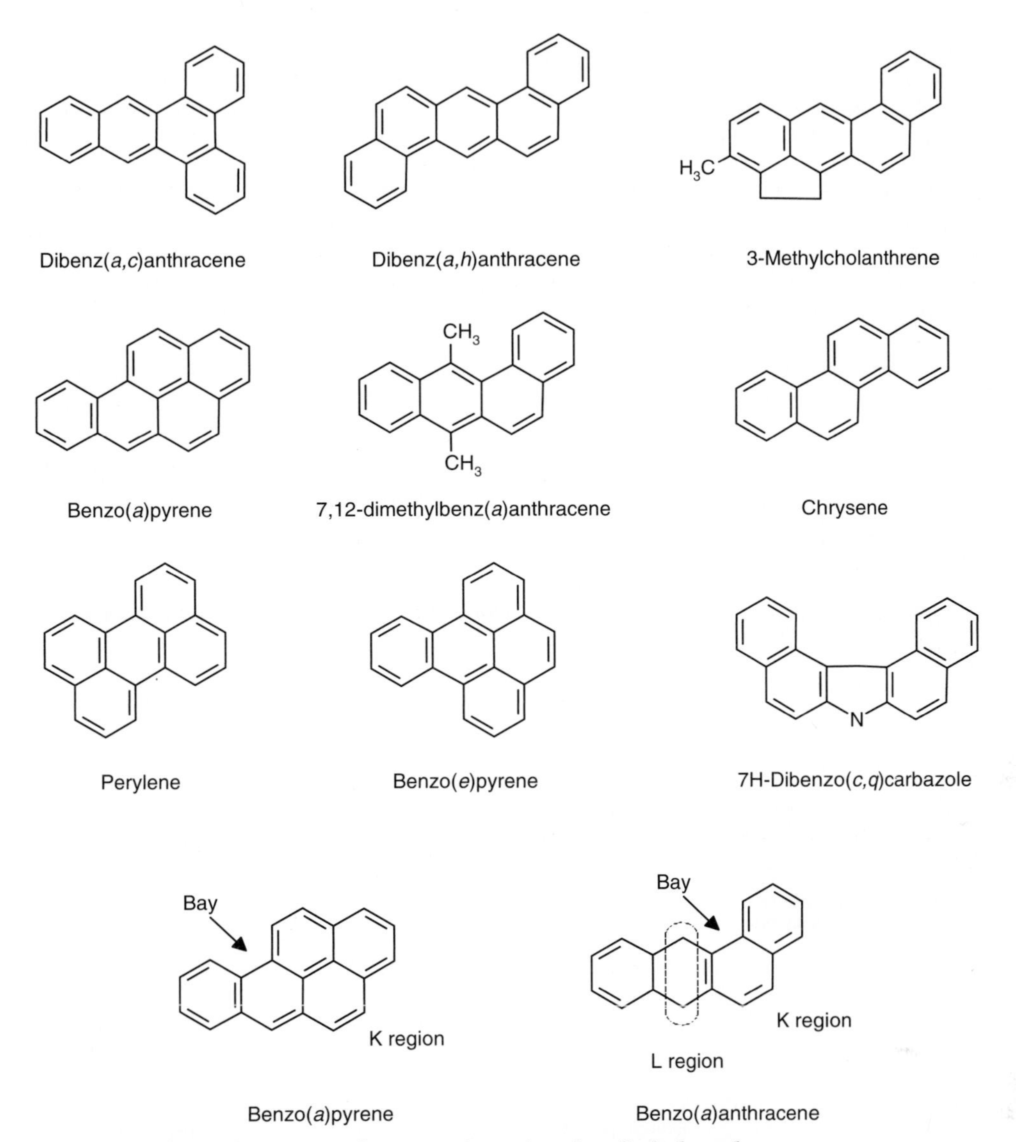


***Figure 8–1.*** ***Chemical structures of some carcinogenic polycyclic hydrocarbons.***

1980). There is substantial epidemiological evidence for a role of nitroso compounds in the induction of human cancer. The nitrosamine NNK (Fig. 8-2) is produced in tobacco smoke from nicotine, a tobacco alkaloid (Hecht, 1985). This is an extremely potent carcinogen that may play a role in the induction of tobacco-related cancers in humans. Methapyrilene was developed as an antihistamine but is a potent carcinogen in the rat (Mirsalis, 1987). Several investigators (Lijinsky, 1977; Magee and Swann, 1969; Mirvish et al., 1983) have shown that certain dietary components, especially in the presence of high levels of nitrite, may give rise to low levels of nitrosamines or nitrosamides and induce neoplasia of the gastrointestinal tract in experimental animals. The action of bacterial flora in the intestine may enhance the formation of these compounds. There is increasing evidence of an etiologic role for endogenously formed *N*-nitroso compounds in the development of certain human cancers (Bartsch et al., 1990).

Another important environmental and experimental hepatocarcinogenic agent is aflatoxin $B_1$. This toxic substance is produced by certain strains of the mold *Aspergillus flavus*. Aflatoxin $B_1$ is one of the most potent hepatocarcinogenic agents known and has produced neoplasms in rodents, fish, birds, and primates (Dragan and Pitot, 1994). This agent is a potential contaminant of many farm products (for example, grains and peanuts) that are stored under warm and humid conditions for some time. Aflatoxin $B_1$ and related compounds may cause some of the toxic hepatitis and hepatic neoplasia seen in various parts of Africa and the Far East (Wogan, 1992). Other products of molds and fungi are potentially carcinogenic in humans and animals (Schoental, 1985). A number of plants, some of which are edible, also contain chemical carcinogenic agents whose structures have been elucidated (Hirono, 1993).

Ethionine is an antimetabolite of the amino acid methionine. Farber (1963) was the first to show definitively that the administration of ethionine in the diet for extended periods can result in the development of liver cancer in rats. This was the first example of direct interference with the metabolism of a normal metabolic constituent, resulting in the development of cancer.

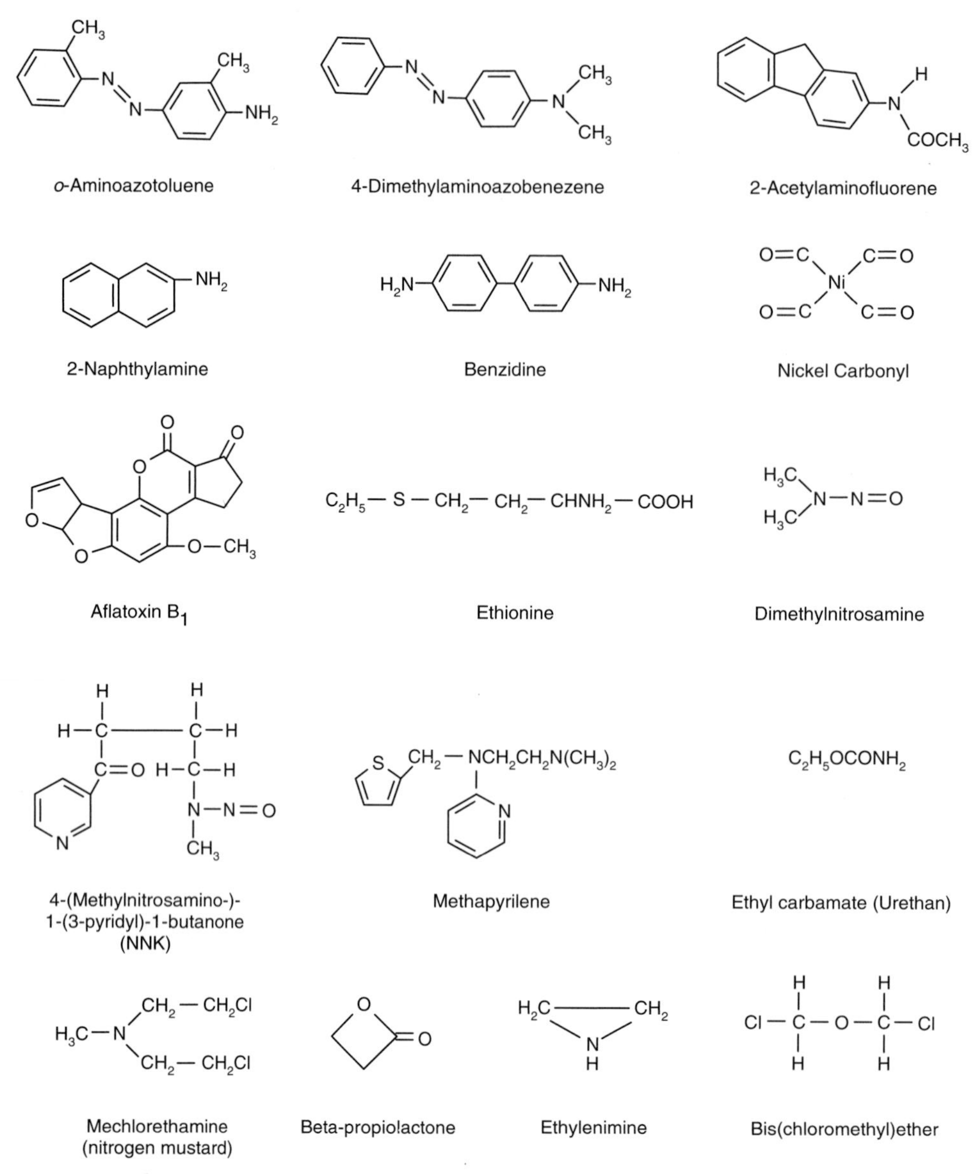


*Figure 8–2. Chemical structures of other representative chemical carcinogens.*

## Inorganic Chemical Carcinogenesis

In addition to organic compounds such as those illustrated in Figs. 8-1 and 8-2, a number of inorganic elements and their compounds have been shown to be carcinogenic in both animals and humans (Vainio and Wilbourn, 1993). Table 8-1 lists metals that are carcinogenic in some form to humans (part 1A) and experimental animals (part 1B) (Sky-Peck, 1986). Many elements and their compounds have not been adequately tested for carcinogenicity in animals, and at this time there is no evidence that such elements exhibit effects in humans on the basis of epidemiological studies. By contrast, compounds of cadmium, chromium, and nickel have induced malignant neoplasms in humans primarily in industrial and refining situations (Table 8-1A) (Magos, 1991). In the case of cadmium, the evidence for carcinogenicity in humans is somewhat limited (Waalkes et al., 1992) because of the variety of confounding factors that occur in situations of human exposure. However, its carcinogenic effect in animals is well documented. By contrast, organonickel compounds, especially nickel carbonyl (Fig. 8-2), are carcinogenic to humans in several tissues, as noted in Table 8–1. Exposures to several metals and their compounds, including lead (Verschaeve et al., 1979) and beryllium (Kuschner, 1981), have been implicated as causes of cancer in humans, but the data are not sufficient to demonstrate such an association unequivocally. In contrast, arsenic and its derivatives present an interesting paradox (Landrigan, 1981) in that there is essentially no experimental evidence to substantiate the carcinogenicity of this element and its compounds in lower animals, whereas the evidence for its carcinogenicity in humans is quite clear (Sky-Peck, 1986).

## Film and Fiber Carcinogenesis

A class of chemical carcinogens different from those described thus far is the group of inert plastic and metal films or similar forms that cause sarcomas at the implantation site in some rodents (Brand et al., 1975). The implantation site is usually

**Table 8–1**
**Induction of Cancer by Exposure to Specific Metals**

*A. Metals Causally Associated with Human Cancer*

| METAL AND SOURCE | MALIGNANCY |
|---|---|
| *Arsenic* | |
| Cu refinery | Pulmonary carcinoma |
| As pesticides | Lymphoma, leukemia |
| Chemical plants | Dermal carcinoma |
| Drinking water (oral) | Hepatic angiosarcoma |
| Cigarette smoke | |
| *Cadmium* | |
| Cd refinery | Pulmonary carcinoma |
| | Prostatic carcinoma |
| *Chromium* | |
| Cr refinery | Pulmonary carcinoma |
| Chrome plating | Gastrointestinal carcinoma |
| Chromate pigments | |
| *Nickel* | |
| Ni refinery | Pulmonary carcinoma |
| | Nasolaryngeal carcinoma |
| | Gastric and renal carcinoma |
| | Sarcoma (?) |

*B. Carcinogenicity of Metals in Experimental Animals*

| METALS | ANIMALS | TUMOR | SITE | ROUTE |
|---|---|---|---|---|
| Beryllium | Mice, rats, monkeys | Osteosarcoma | Bone | IV, INH |
| | | Carcinoma | Lung | |
| Cadmium | Mice, rats, chickens | Sarcoma | Injection site | IM, SC, ITS |
| | | Teratoma | Testes | |
| Cobalt | Rats, rabbits | Sarcoma | Injection site | IM, SC |
| Chromium | Mice, rats, rabbits | Sarcoma | Injection site | IM, SC, IP, |
| | | Carcinoma | Lung | INH |
| Iron | Hamsters, mice, rats, rabbits | Sarcoma | Injection site | IM, IP, SC |
| Nickel | Mice, rats, cats, hamsters, rabbits | Sarcoma | Injection site | IM, ITS, SC |
| | Guinea pigs, rats | Carcinoma | Lung | INH, IP, IR |
| | | Carcinoma | Kidney | |
| Lead | Mice, rats | Carcinoma | Kidney | IP, PO, SC |
| Titanium | Rats | Sarcoma | Injection site | IM |
| Zinc | Chickens, rats, hamsters | Carcinoma | Testes | ITS |
| | | Teratoma | Testes | |

IV = intravenous; INH = inhalation; IM = intramuscular; SC = subcutaneous; ITS = intratesticular; IP = intraperitoneal; IR = intrarenal; PO = per os.
SOURCE: From Sky-Peck (1986).

subcutaneous. Rats and mice are highly susceptible to this form of carcinogenesis, but guinea pigs appear to be resistant (Stinson, 1964). The carcinogenic properties of the implant are to a large extent dependent on its physical characteristics and surface area. Multiple perforations each greater than a certain diameter (for example, 0.4 $\mu$m), pulverization, and roughening of the surface of the implant (Ferguson, 1977) markedly reduced the incidence of neoplasms. Plastic sponge implants also may induce sarcomas subcutaneously, and in this instance the yield of tumors is dependent on the thickness of the sponge implant (Roe et al., 1967). The age of the animal at implantation also affects the time that elapses between implantation and tumor development (Paulini et al., 1975).

The chemical nature of the implant is not the critical factor in its ability to transform normal cells to neoplastic cells. Brand and associates (Johnson et al., 1970) studied this phenomenon intensively and demonstrated a variety of kinetic and morphological characteristics of the process of "foreign-body tumorigenesis" in mice. These investigations have shown that DNA synthesis occurs in the film-attached cell population throughout the preneoplastic phase and that preneoplastic cells may be identified well before neoplasms develop (Thomassen et al., 1978). Brand suggested that such "preneoplastic" cells may be present in normal tissue before implantation and that the implant appears to "create the conditions" required for carcinogenesis of these cells (Brand et al., 1975).

Other possible mechanisms for this unique type of carcinogenesis are discussed later in this chapter.

While the epidemiological evidence that implants of prostheses in humans, such as those used for the repair of hernias and joint replacements, induce the formation of sarcomas is not substantial, there have been a number of isolated reports of neoplasms arising in association with such foreign bodies (Sunderman, 1989). A study in the rat of the carcinogenic potential of a number of materials used in such prostheses demonstrated a small increase in sarcomas in animals with certain metal alloy implants that contained significant amounts of cobalt, chromium, or nickel (Memoli et al., 1986). Of greater significance is the induction of malignant mesothelioma and bronchogenic carcinoma in humans by exposure to asbestos fibers. In this case, the induction of the malignant mesothelioma appears to be dependent on the crystal structure rather than the composition of the asbestos both in experimental animals and in humans (Craighead, 1982). In experimental animals, fibers longer than 8 $\mu$m and with a diameter less than 1.5 $\mu$m induce mesothelioma fairly effectively. Similarly, certain types of asbestos, such as the crocidolite form, are most strongly associated with the occurrence of this neoplasm, whereas exposure to other forms, such as chrysotile, may not be as important a cause of malignant mesothelioma. Thus, in both humans and animals, film and fiber carcinogenesis is largely independent of the chemical nature of the inciting agent.

## Hormonal Carcinogenesis

Hormones consist of amines, steroids, and polypeptides. Beatson (1896) was the first to point out that hormones may be causally associated with the development of specific neoplasms. He suggested that a relationship exists between breast cancer and the ovary, the major site of production of female sex hormones.

Hormones play an important physiological role in maintaining the "internal milieu" (Bernard, 1878, 1879). Some cancers may result from abnormal internal production of specific hormones. Alternatively, excessive production or the derangement of the homeostatic mechanisms of an organism may result in neoplastic transformation (Clifton and Sridharan, 1975). Furth (1975) was emphatic in his propositions and demonstrations that disruption of the cybernetic relationship between peripheral endocrine glands and the anterior pituitary can result in neoplasia of one of the glands involved (Fig. 8-3). One of the classic examples is the experimental transplantation of normal ovaries into the spleen of castrated rodents (Biskind and Biskind, 1944). This results in a break in the pituitary-gonadal hormone feedback loop. The break occurs

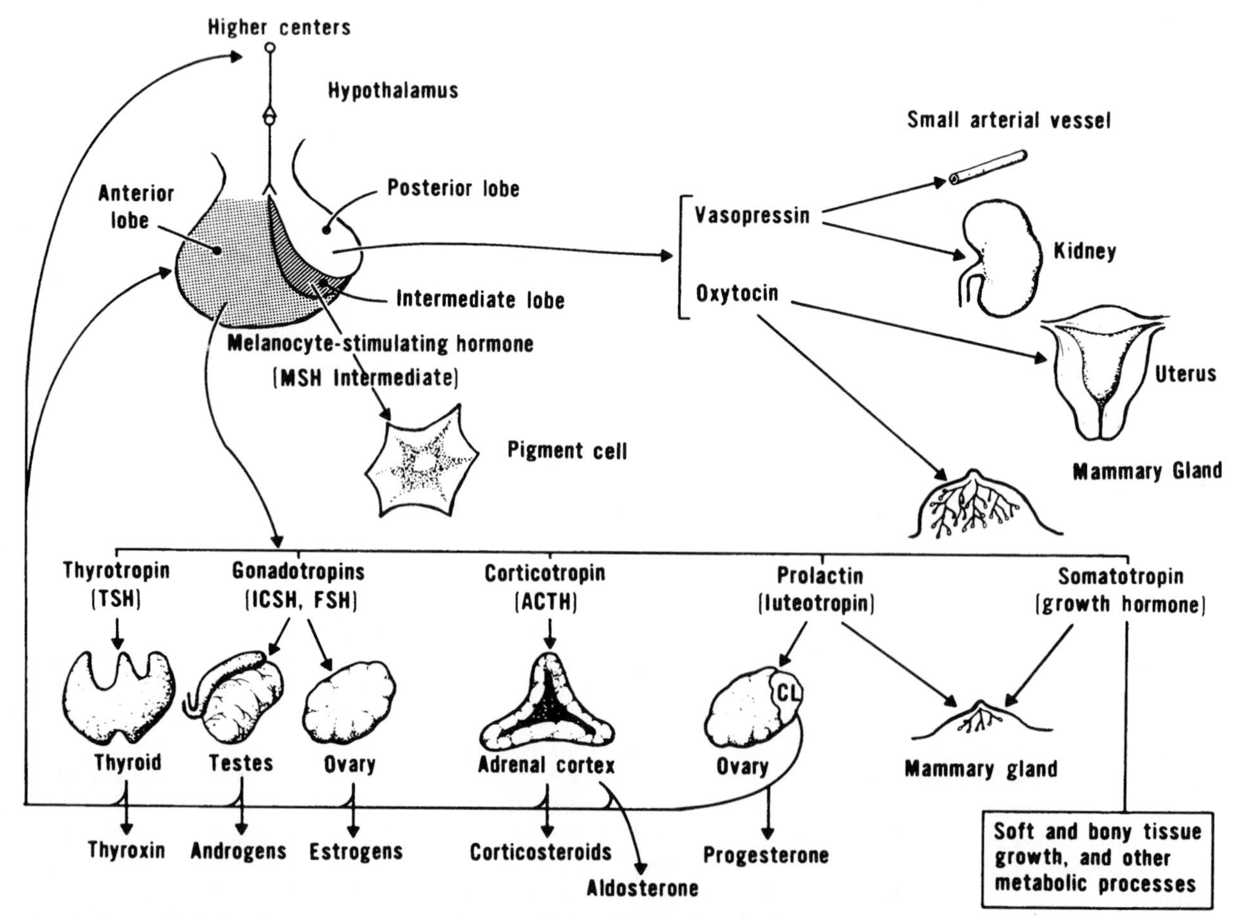


*Figure 8–3. Cybernetic relations of the pituitary gland (anterior, intermediate, and posterior lobes) with the hypothalamus, other endocrine organs, and tissues of the organism. [After Furth (1975), reproduced with the permission of the author and publisher.]*

because estrogens produced by the ovary are carried by the splenic venous system to the liver. In the liver, the estrogens are metabolized and thus are prevented from entering the general circulation to suppress the pituitary production of gonadotropins. The excessive production of gonadotropins and their constant stimulus of the ovarian fragment in the spleen result ultimately in neoplasia of the ovarian implant.

A similar mechanism is likely to be involved in the production of thyroid neoplasms either by the administration of goitrogens (chemicals that inhibit the synthesis and/or secretion of normal thyroid hormone) or by a marked increase in the circulating levels of thyrotropin secreted by thyrotropin-secreting pituitary neoplasms transplanted into the host. In the former instance, there is a break in the feedback loop and the pituitary gland produces high levels of thyrotropin in the absence of normal feedback regulation by the thyroid hormone (Furth, 1975). In fact, in humans there is substantial evidence that this may be the mechanism of the development of many thyroid cancers (Williams, 1989). In this case, high levels of circulating thyrotropin result from the unregulated production of this hormone by the transplanted neoplasm (Ueda and Furth, 1967). Thyroidectomy and neonatal gonadectomy result in the development of neoplasms of the pituitary, presumably because of the lack of inhibition by the hormone from the target end organ (Furth, 1975). Chronic administration of pituitary growth hormone also induces a variety of neoplasms in the rat (Moon et al., 1950a, b). Theoretically, then, neoplasms of any of the end organs shown in Fig. 8–3 may be produced by some manipulation that breaks the feedback loop between the pituitary and the target organ.

Some examples of carcinogenesis resulting from the interruption of the cybernetics of hormonal relationships shown in Fig. 8-3 are listed in Table 8-2. In addition to effecting carcinogenesis in the ovary (Biskind and Biskind, 1944), endogenous gonadotropins are involved in the development of adrenocortical and interstitial (Leydig's) cell neoplasms in mice and rats, respectively (Table 8-2). Unleaded gasoline acts like an antiestrogen, thus removing the estrogen protection usually provided against the development of liver neoplasms in the mouse (Standeven et al., 1994) and leading to an increased number of hepatic neoplasms in the female. Phenobarbital acts to decrease serum levels of thyroid hormone ($T_3$) by stimulating enzymes that metabolize and eliminate the hormone before it can be recycled to the hypothalamus (McClain, 1989). This mechanism is very similar to the effects of goitrogens, which prevent $T_3$ formation and release from the thyroid. The induction of pituitary adenomas, which themselves produce large amounts of prolactin, is due to an inhibition of the formation of dopamine in the hypothalamus. Dopamine acts like an inhibitor of prolactin synthesis and release by the pituitary. When this inhibition is eliminated by estrogen inhibition of dopamine formation, prolactin-producing pituitary cells replicate at a very high rate. Furthermore, they produce extensive amounts of prolactin, which in turn, in the presence of estrogens, leads to mammary neoplasia (Neumann, 1991).

Figure 8-4 shows some representative structures of hormones, both naturally occurring and synthetic, for which there is substantial evidence of carcinogenicity in lower animals and/or humans. In addition to the structure of growth hormone, two other growth factors expressed in adult tissues—transforming growth factor-$\alpha$ (TGF-$\alpha$), which is expressed in the small intestine (Barnard et al., 1991), the major salivary glands (Wu et al., 1993), and other tissues (Lee et al., 1993), and insulin-like growth factor-II (IGF-II), which is expressed in the forebrain, uterus, kidney, heart, skeletal muscle, and to a very small degree the liver (Murphy et al., 1987)—may be considered chemical carcinogens. The carcinogenic action of these two growth factor hormones in vivo has been demonstrated by the use of transgenic mice, among which animals overexpressing TGF-$\alpha$ developed liver neoplasms in dramatic excess of the number seen in controls (Lee et al., 1992), and animals expressing high levels of IGF-II developed excessive numbers of hepatocellular carcinomas and lymphomas (Rogler et al., 1994).

As noted in Table 8-2, neoplasms of the pituitary and the peripheral endocrine organs may be induced by the administration of steroid sex hormones. Although the kidney is not usually considered a peripheral endocrine organ, its cells produce erythropoietin. Synthetic or natural estrogen administration can induce renal cortical carcinomas in male hamsters (Li

**Table 8–2**
**Interrupted Cybernetics of Hormonal Carcinogenesis in Rodents**

| SPECIES/TISSUE | INDUCING AGENT | HORMONAL CARCINOGEN | INTERRUPTED PATHWAY | REFERENCE |
|---|---|---|---|---|
| Mouse/ovary | Ovary transplant to spleen | Gonadotropin | Estrogen → hypothalamus | Biskind and Biskind, 1944 |
| Rat/thyroid | Goitrogen or thyrotropin-secreting tumor | Thyrotropin | $T_3$ → hypothalamus | Furth, 1975 |
| Mouse/adrenal cortex | Ovariectomy | Gonadotropins | Estrogen → hypothalamus | Kawashima et al., 1980 |
| Female mouse/liver | Unleaded gasoline | Androgens | Estrogen synthesis | Standeven et al., 1994 |
| Rat/thyroid | Phenobarbital | Thyrotropin | $T_3$ → hypothalamus | McClain, 1989 |
| Rat/pituitary | Estrogens | ? | Dopamine → pituitary | Neumann, 1991 |
| Rat/Leydig's cells | Antiandrogens | Gonadotropins | Androgens → hypothalamus | Neumann, 1991 |
| Rat/mammary | Estrogens | Prolactin | Dopamine → pituitary | Neumann, 1991 |

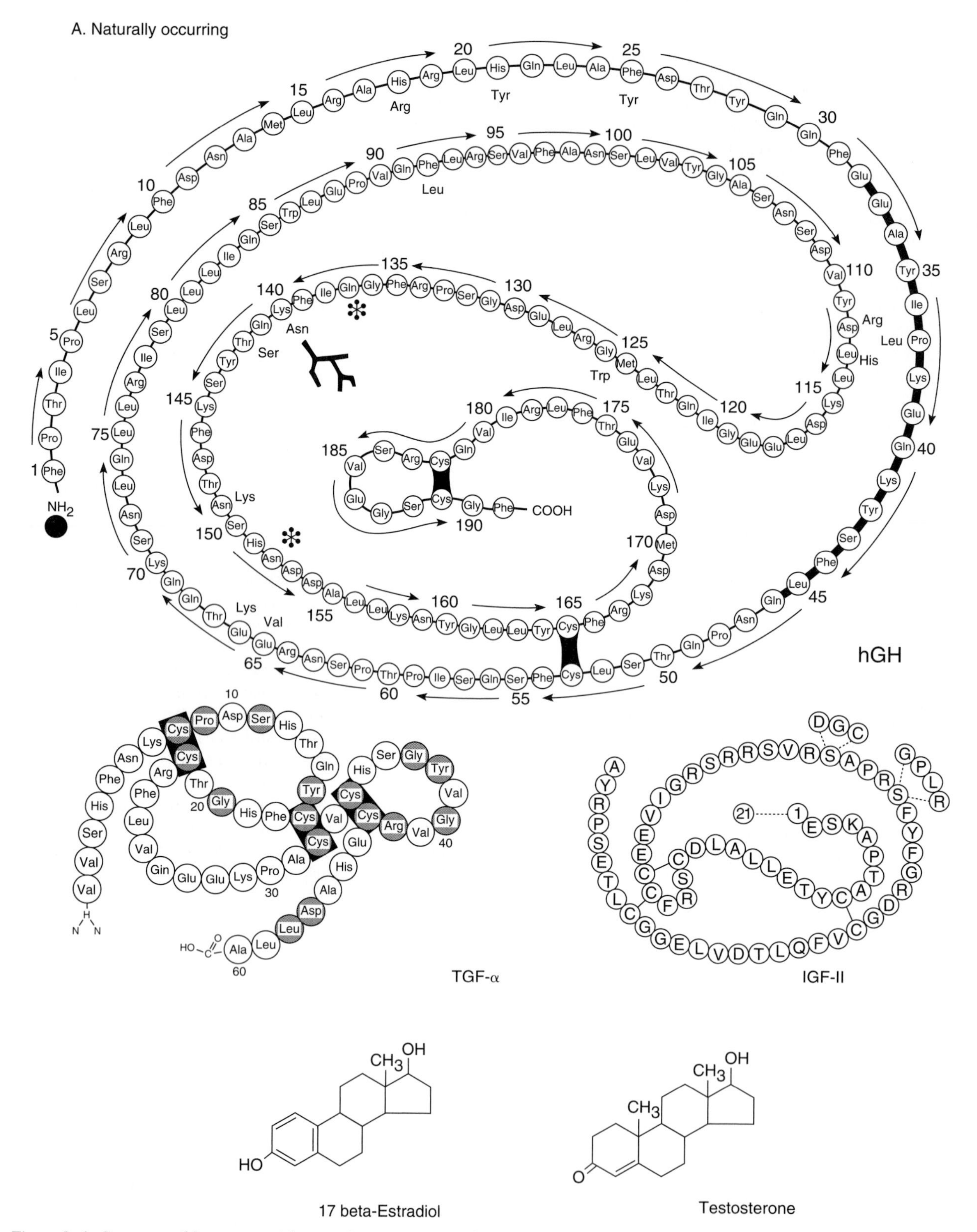


***Figure 8–4. Structure of hormones with a carcinogenic potential.***

A. Structures of polypeptide hormones. hGH-human growth hormone; TGF-$\alpha$-transforming growth factor alpha; IGF-II-insulin-like growth factor-II.

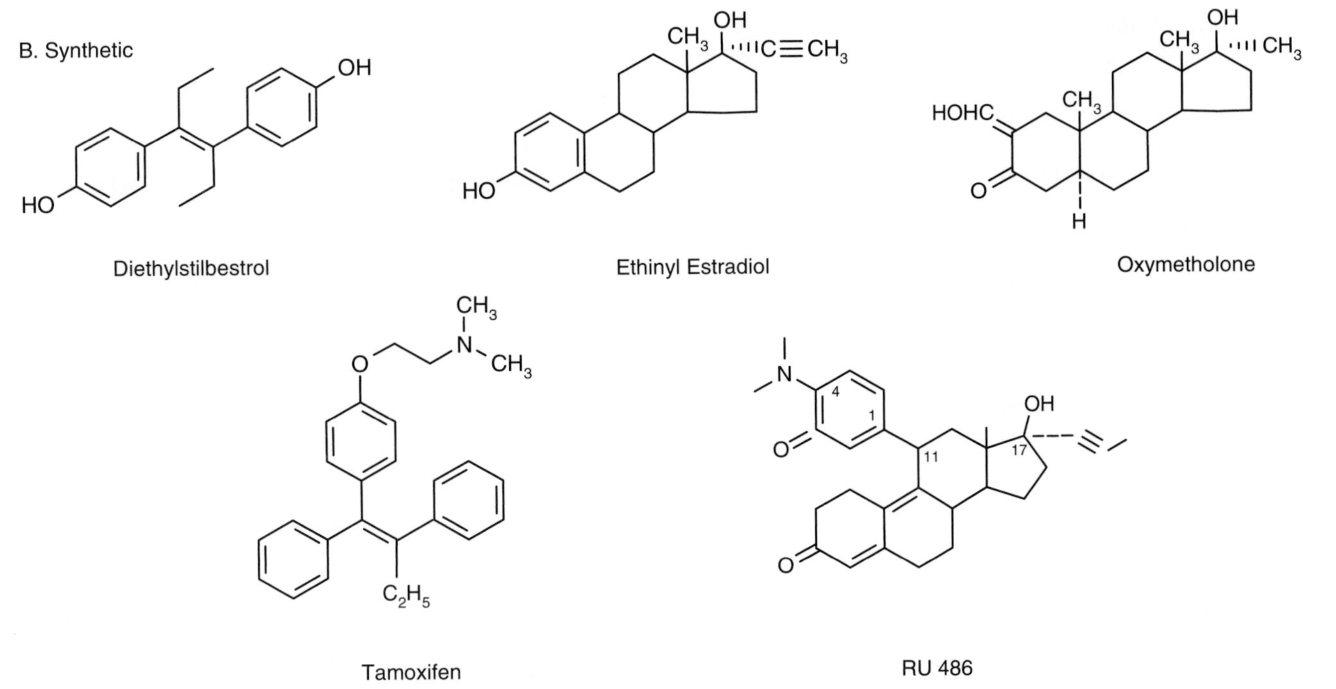

B. Synthetic

Diethylstilbestrol

Ethinyl Estradiol

Oxymetholone

Tamoxifen

RU 486

*Figure 8–4. (continued).*

B. Structures of some naturally occurring (beta-estradiol and testosterone) and synthetic steroid hormones and antihormones.

and Li, 1990), and estradiol induces Leydig's cell tumors of the testes in mice (Huseby, 1980). However, a closely related structural analogue, 2-fluoroestradiol, which exhibits significant estrogenic potency, did not induce renal carcinoma in the same sex and species (Liehr, 1983). Recently, the synthetic antiestrogen tamoxifen was found to induce carcinomas of the liver in the rat as well (Williams et al., 1993). Evidence that male hormones by themselves are carcinogenic is not as strong as the data for the carcinogenicity of female hormones. The natural male hormone testosterone does exhibit a weak ability to "transform" hamster embryo cells in culture into a neoplastic phenotype (Lasne et al., 1990). The evidence that synthetic androgens are carcinogenic is somewhat greater, especially in humans. In addition, elevated serum testosterone levels are associated with an increased risk of hepatocellular carcinoma in humans (Yu and Chen, 1993). A number of reports (Mays and Christopherson, 1984; Chandra et al., 1984) have indicated a causative relationship between the administration of synthetic androgens such as oxymetholone (Fig. 8-4B) for various clinical conditions and the appearance of hepatocellular neoplasms, predominantly benign.

In addition to apparently direct induction of neoplasia by hormonal stimuli, hormones act in concert with known carcinogenic agents to induce neoplasia. One of the better studied examples of this phenomenon is the induction of mammary adenocarcinomas in rodents. Bittner (1956) demonstrated that three factors are essential for the production of mammary carcinoma in mice: genetic susceptibility, hormonal influence, and a virus transmitted through the milk. The importance of the first two factors has been demonstrated repeatedly in a variety of species, including humans, but incontrovertible evidence for the participation of a virus in mammary carcinogenesis has been obtained only in mice. In the rat, high levels of endogenous prolactin enhance the induction of mammary carcinomas by dimethylbenz(*a*)anthracene (Ip et al., 1980). Chronic treatment with synthetic or natural estrogens alone may induce mammary carcinomas in rodents. Thus, mammary carcinogenesis in rodents is a complicated process that requires several components that may differ from species to species.

Both male and female sex steroid hormones also have been shown to act in concert with known carcinogenic agents to increase the incidence of neoplasia. Various synthetic estrogens administered chronically to animals that had been dosed with a known carcinogen markedly enhanced the development of hepatocellular carcinomas in the rat (Yager and Yager, 1980). Both testosterone and synthetic androgens given with or after chemical carcinogens enhance the induction of adenocarcinomas of the prostate and other accessory sex organs of the male (Hoover et al., 1990). A combination of testosterone and estradiol-17$\beta$ after treatment with methylnitrosourea also resulted in the development of adenocarcinomas of the prostate (Bosland et al., 1991).

## Chemical Carcinogenesis by Mixtures: Defined and Undefined

While most of this chapter is concerned with the carcinogenic action of specific chemicals, it is relatively unusual for an individual to be exposed to a single carcinogenic agent. Despite this, relatively few detailed studies on mixtures of carcinogenic chemicals have been carried out experimentally. The most common environmental mixtures are those seen in tobacco smoke and other combustion products, including engine exhaust and air pollution (Mauderly, 1993). Interactions between the chemicals in mixtures may be additive, greater, or inhibitory (Mumtaz et al., 1993). In the examples given above, however, the exact chemical nature of the components in tobacco smoke or air pollution is not always known and their amounts have not been determined. Thus, one may be forced to deal with a mixture as if it were a single entity or, if the constituents are known, treat the effects of the mixture in an empirical way that usually is related to the most potent component in the mixture.

Studies on the carcinogenic action of defined mixtures of chemicals are usually done with a knowledge of the carcinogenic effect of the chemicals involved. Warshawsky and coworkers (1993) demonstrated that extremely low levels of benzo[*a*]pyrene, which produced no skin tumors on repeated application, resulted in a significant yield of neoplasms when applied in the presence of five noncarcinogenic polycyclic aromatic hydrocarbons. In an earlier study, the administration of two noncarcinogenic aminoazo dyes in the diet of the rat for a year resulted in the appearance of a variety of neoplasms (Neish et al., 1967). More recently, the administration of three to five *N*-nitrosamines resulted in either an additive or a synergistic carcinogenic effect of the combinations of the compounds given at low dose rates (Berger et al., 1987; Lijinsky et al., 1983). In contrast, the administration of a mixture of 40 chemical carcinogens to rats for 2 years at 50 percent of the dose normally used to induce neoplasms in 50 percent of the animals resulted in significant tumor incidences only in the thyroid and liver (Takayama et al., 1989). In a more recent study, ingestion of a mixture of 20 pesticides given at "acceptable daily intake levels" was found to exert no effect on carcinogenesis in rat liver (Ito et al., in press). Thus, the toxicological study of complex mixtures, not only in the area of carcinogenesis, is a critical field in human health, as evidenced by disease resulting from tobacco smoke, engine exhaust, and other components of air pollution (Mauderly, 1993). One of the most important chemical mixtures associated with human neoplasia is diet.

**Chemical Carcinogenesis by Diet.** There is substantial evidence in humans to indicate that many dietary components, including excessive caloric intake (Osler, 1987; Lutz and Schlatter, 1992), excessive alcohol intake (IARC, 1987), and a variety of chemical contaminants of the diet including aflatoxin $B_1$ (Fig. 8-2) (Gorchev and Jelinek, 1985; Lutz and Schlatter, 1992), are carcinogenic. Other general and specific studies have supported these views (Jensen and Madsen, 1988; Habs and Schmähl, 1980; Miller et al., 1994), whereas others have been more controversial (Willett and MacMahon, 1984; Pariza, 1984). Evidence for the association of dietary factors with cancer incidence in animals is more substantial and supports much of the evidence relating environmental factors to increased cancer incidence in the human (Kritchevsky, 1988; Rogers et al., 1993).

Although a relative lack of "antioxidant micronutrients" such as carotenoids, selenium, and the vitamins A, C, and E has been implicated as a factor in the incidence of neoplastic development (Dorgan and Schatzkin, 1991), more studies are needed before the effectiveness of these agents in cancer prevention can be established. In contrast, experimental evidence that the lack of available sources of methyl groups can actually induce liver cancer in rats is well documented (Mikol et al., 1983; Ghoshal and Farber, 1984). This observation may be closely related to earlier studies by Farber (1963) on the induction of liver cancer in rats by the administration of ethionine, which indirectly may cause a lack of available methyl groups in this tissue.

## MECHANISMS INVOLVED IN CHEMICAL CARCINOGENESIS

Although the discovery that polycyclic hydrocarbons and other chemical compounds can induce cancer in experimental animals gave hope that the complete understanding of the nature of neoplasia might be forthcoming, more than 60 years has elapsed since those initial findings, and it appears that we are still a long way from such an understanding. The realization that chemical carcinogens are altered within a living organism by metabolic reactions paralleled our increased knowledge about metabolic mechanisms.

### Metabolism of Chemical Carcinogens in Relation to Carcinogenesis

When it became apparent from the studies of Yoshida and others that chemicals other than polycyclic hydrocarbons are carcinogenic by a variety of metabolic routes, the dilemma of understanding the mechanisms of action of this variety of agents appeared to be almost insurmountable. It was noted that the excretory metabolites of polycyclic hydrocarbons are hydroxylated derivatives, which usually have little or no carcinogenic activity. Similarly, hydroxylation of the rings of aromatic amine carcinogens such as 2-acetylaminofluorene (AAF) and 4-dimethyl-aminoazobenzene often resulted in a complete loss of activity. The enzymatic production of these more polar metabolites facilitated further metabolism and excretion of the parent compound. The beginning of our understanding of this dilemma was reported by Elizabeth and James Miller (1947), who first demonstrated that azo dyes become covalently bound to proteins of the liver but not to proteins of the resulting neoplasms (Miller, 1978). These initial studies of the Millers led them to suggest that the binding of carcinogens to proteins might lead to the loss or deletion of proteins critical for growth control.

As an extension of this work, Elizabeth Miller (1951) demonstrated the covalent binding of benzo(*a*)pyrene or some of its metabolites to proteins in the skin of mice treated with the hydrocarbon. Later, Abell and Heidelberger (1962) described the same phenomenon with another carcinogenic polycyclic hydrocarbon, 3-methylcholanthrene. These findings strongly suggested that a critical step in the induction of cancer by chemicals is the covalent interaction of some form of the chemical with macromolecules. Since the parent compound was incapable of covalent binding directly with macromolecules, the logical conclusion was that the interaction of the chemical with the macromolecule was a result of the metabolic activation of the parent compound.

Although a number of studies in the 1950s (Weisburger and Weisburger, 1958) demonstrated that ring hydroxylation is a major pathway in the metabolism of AAF, the Millers and Cramer (Miller et al., 1960) reported that hydroxylation of the nitrogen of the acetylamino group also occurred. They isolated *N*-hydroxy-AAF from the urine of AAF-treated rats and found this metabolite to be more carcinogenic than was the parent compound, AAF. Furthermore, *N*-hydroxy-AAF induced neoplasms that were not observed with the parent compound, such as subcutaneous sarcomas at the site of injection. In animals, such as the guinea pig, that convert little of the AAF to its *N*-hydroxy derivative, cancer of the liver was not produced by feeding the parent compound. These findings strongly supported the suggestion that the parent compound might not be the direct carcinogen; instead, certain metabolic derivatives were active in the induction of neoplasia. These studies paved the way for further investigations of the activation of carcinogens by means of their metabolism (Miller, 1970).

Figure 8-5 depicts a number of metabolic reactions involved in the "activation" of chemicals to their ultimate carcinogenic forms. One may divide such metabolic functions into two general classes (Goldstein and Faletto, 1993). Those involved in phase I metabolism (Fig. 8-5) occur within the endoplasmic reticulum. These reactions involve metabolism by cytochrome P-450 mixed-function oxidases and their reductase, as well as the mixed-function amine oxidase. Generally, these metabolic reactions induce biotransformation by converting a substrate to a more polar compound through the introduction of molecular oxygen. Phase II metabolic reactions (Fig. 8-6) are biosynthetic reactions that involve conjugation and occur primarily in the cytosol of the cell. A detailed consideration of xenobiotic metabolic pathways is beyond the scope of this text; the reader is referred to several pertinent reviews (Porter and Coon, 1991; Guengerich, 1992).

As noted in Fig. 8-5, the *N*-hydroxylation of AAF can be followed by esterification of the *N*-hydroxyl group to yield a highly reactive compound that is capable of nonenzymatic reaction with nucleophilic sites on proteins and nucleic acids. The demonstration of the metabolism of AAF to a highly reactive chemical led the Millers to propose that chemical carcinogens are or can be converted into electrophilic reactants (chemicals with electron-deficient sites). These electrophilic agents exert their carcinogenic effects by means of covalent interaction with cellular macromolecules (Miller, 1978). Furthermore, the Millers proposed that chemical carcinogens that require metabolism to exert their carcinogenic effect be termed procarcinogens, whereas their highly reactive metabolites were termed ultimate carcinogens. Metabolites intermediate between procarcinogens and ultimate carcinogens were called "proximate" carcinogens. The "ultimate" form of the carcinogen, that is, the form that actually interacts with cellular constituents and probably causes the neoplastic transformation, is the final product shown in the pathways in Fig. 8-5. In some instances the structure of the ultimate form of certain carcinogenic chemicals is still not known, while in other cases there may be more than one ultimate carcinogenic metabolite.

After the demonstration by the Millers of the critical significance of electrophilic metabolites in chemical carcinogenesis, the ultimate forms of a number of compounds, specifically the aromatic amines such as benzidine, naphthylamine, and 4-aminobiphenyl, were described. However, the carcinogenic polycyclic hydrocarbons still posed a problem. Pullman and Pullman (1955) had earlier proposed that the K region (Fig. 8-1) of polycyclic hydrocarbons is important in predicting their carcinogenicity. Boyland (1950) proposed the formation of epoxide intermediates in the metabolism of these chemicals. However, it was not until 1970 that Jerina and associates detected the formation of such an intermediate in a biological system (Jerina et al., 1970). Other investigations showed that epoxides of polycyclic hydrocarbons could react with nucleic acids and proteins in the absence of any metabolizing system. Surprisingly, K-region epoxides of a number of carcinogenic polycyclic hydrocarbons were weaker carcinogens than were the parent hydrocarbons. After this finding, scientific attention shifted to other reactive metabolites of these molecules. Benzo(*a*)pyrene has been used as a model compound in studies of carcinogenic polycyclic hydrocarbons, and some of the metabolic reactions observed in vivo are shown in Figs. 8-5 and 8-6. In 1974, Sims and associates proposed that a diol epoxide of benzo(*a*)pyrene is the ultimate form of this carcinogen (Dims et al., 1974). Subsequent studies by a number of investigators have demonstrated that the structure of this ultimate form is (+)anti-benzo(*a*)pyrene-7,8-dihydrodiol-9,10-epoxide (Yang et al., 1976; also see reviews by: Conney, 1982; Harvey, 1981; Lowe and Silverman, 1984).

One of the ramifications of these findings is the realization of the importance of oxidation of the carbons in the "bay region" of potentially carcinogenic polycyclic hydrocarbons. Figure 8-1 indicated the bay regions of benz(*a*)anthracene and benzo(*a*)pyrene. Analogous bay regions may be identified in other polycyclic aromatic hydrocarbons (Fig. 8-1). The bay region is the sterically hindered region formed by the angular benzo ring. Although the bay-region concept has not been tested with all known carcinogenic polycyclic hydrocarbons, it appears to be generally applicable. Several authors (Levin et al., 1978; Conney, 1982) have proposed that epoxidation of the dihydro, angular benzo ring that forms part of the bay region of a polycyclic hydrocarbon may form the ultimate carcinogenic form. In addition, Cavalieri and Rogan (1992) have proposed that radical cations of polycyclic aromatic hydrocarbons (PAHs) formed by oxidation of the parent compound via the cytochrome P-450 pathway are also important intermediates in the formation of the ultimate carcinogenic metabolites of these chemicals. Thus, oxidation can result in the metabolic activation of a number of procarcinogens, including the PAHs.

Although the administration of polypeptide hormones and growth factors can result in neoplasia, these compounds do not have "ultimate" carcinogenic forms. There is, however, evidence that synthetic steroid hormones, especially estrogens, are metabolized to more reactive intermediates. In the intensively studied estrogen-induced renal neoplasia in hamsters, Zhu and colleagues (1993) developed substantial evidence that synthetic estrogens are converted to catechol metabolites in significant amounts. These authors proposed that such metabolites may act as the ultimate carcinogenic forms of the synthetic estrogens.

Although conjugation reactions usually inactivate chemical carcinogens and permit rapid urinary excretion as a result of increased water solubility, an exception to this has been shown. Both haloalkanes and haloalkenes react with glutathione in a conjugation reaction catalyzed by glutathione *S*-transferase. Halogenated aliphatics may induce neoplasia in several organs, with the kidney as the predominant target site. The glutathione-dependent bioactivation of ethylene dibromide provides an example (Fig. 8-6). The proximate carcinogen of ethylene dibromide, glutathione *S*-ethylbromide, spontaneously forms an episulfonium ion as the ultimate carcinogenic form. This highly reactive chemical alkylates DNA at the $N^7$ position of guanine (Koga et al., 1986). In addition to glutathione conjugates, cysteine *S*-conjugates of several ha-

**Procarcinogen (Pr)→Proximate (Px) Carcinogen→Ultimate (Ut) Carcinogen**

*C*-Hydroxylation, *N*-hydroxylation, and epoxidation

a. Aromatic

Direct epoxidation

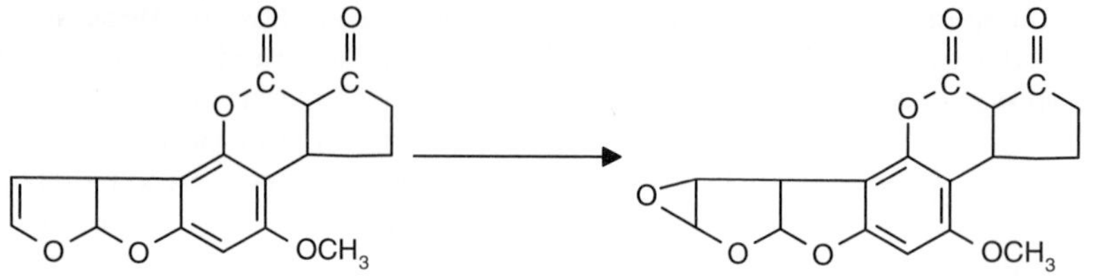

Aflatoxin $B_1$ (Pr) → Aflatoxin $B_1$, 2,3 epoxide (Ut)

*N*-Hydroxylation

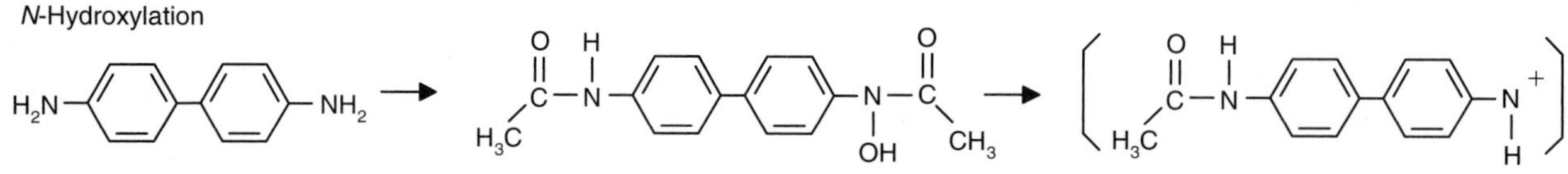

Benzidine (Pr) → *N* hydroxy dacetyl Benzidine (Px) → *N* Acetyl benzidine Nitrenium ion (Ut)

Two-step epoxidation

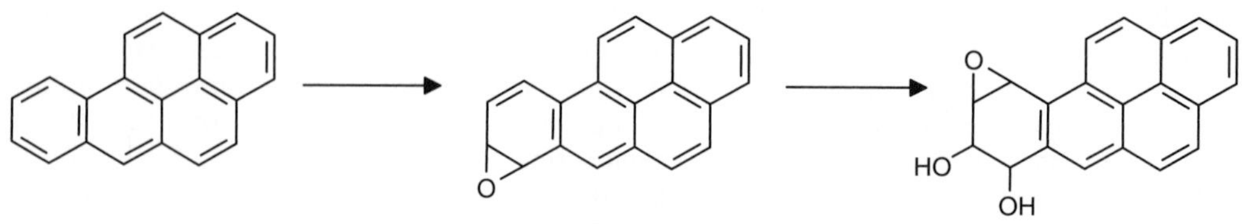

Benzo(*a*)pyrene (Pr) → Benzo(*a*)pyrene 7,8 epoxide (Px) → Benzo(*a*)pyrene 7,8 diol-9,10 epoxide (Ut)

b. Aliphatic

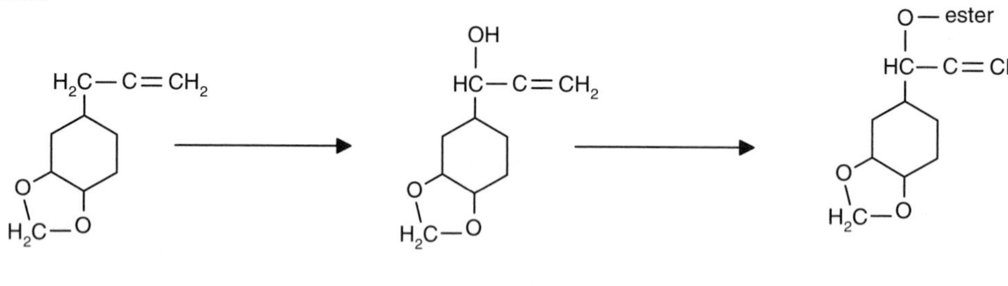

Safrole → I' hydroxy Safrole (Px) → Safrole I' O-ester (Ut)

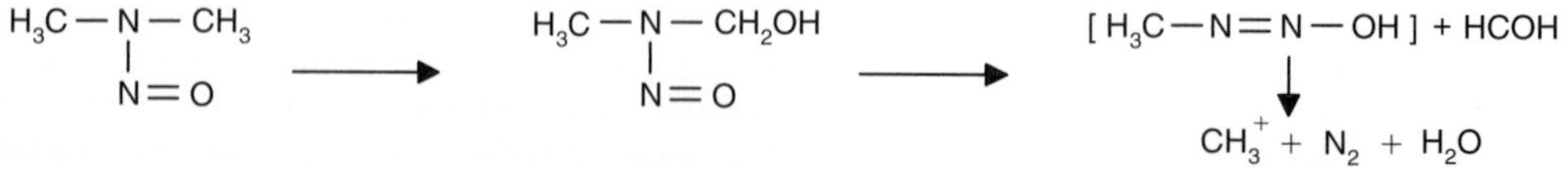

Dimethynitrosamine (Pr) → Hydroxymethyl, methyl nitrosamine (Px) → $[H_3C-N=N-OH]$ + HCOH → $CH_3^+ + N_2 + H_2O$ Methyl carbonium ion (Ut)

*Figure 8–5. Structures of representative chemical carcinogens and their metabolic derivatives, the proximate (Px) and ultimate (Ut) carcinogenic forms resulting from the action of phase I metabolism of procarcinogens (Pr).*

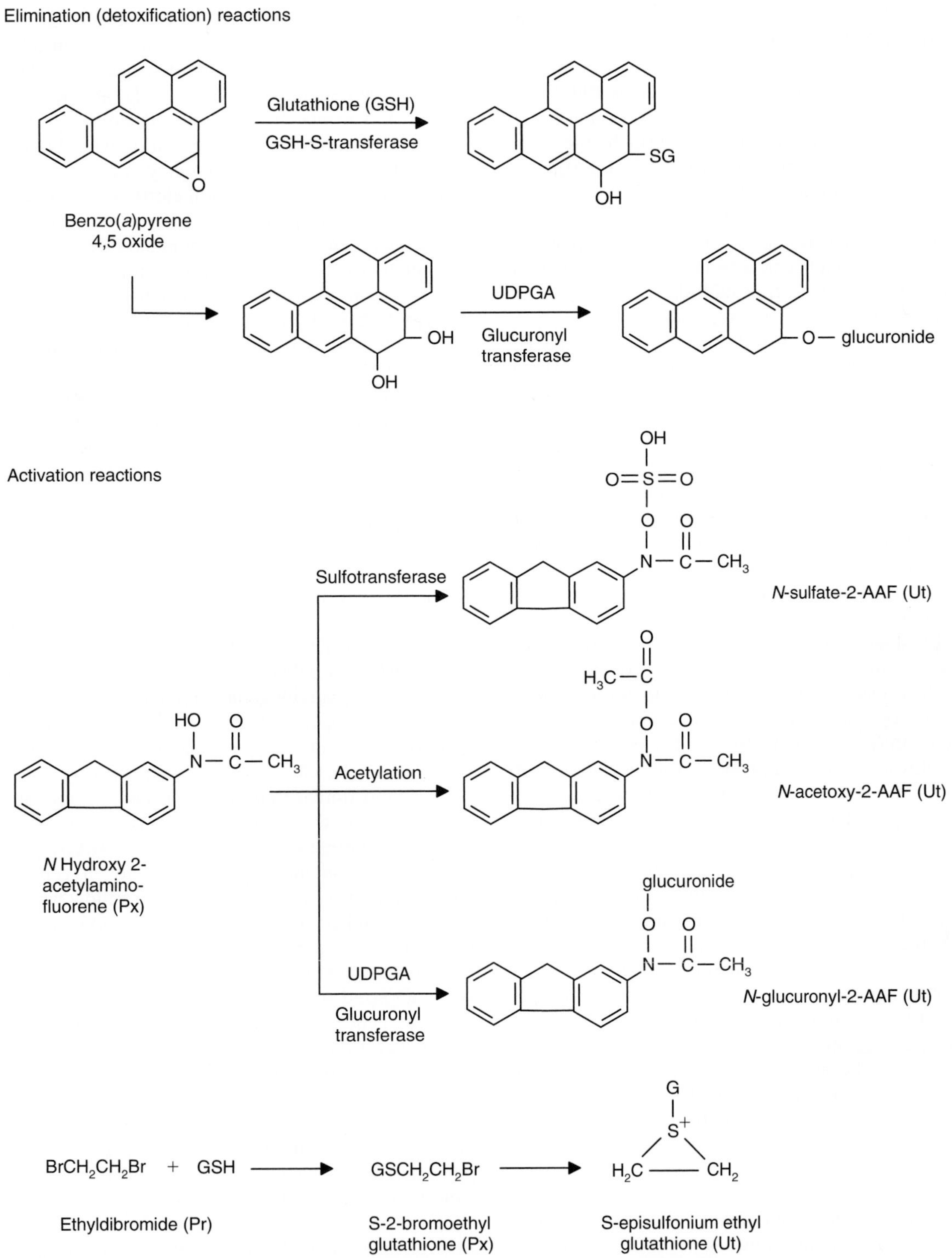

Elimination (detoxification) reactions

Benzo(*a*)pyrene 4,5 oxide

Glutathione (GSH)
GSH-S-transferase

SG
OH

OH
OH

UDPGA
Glucuronyl transferase

O— glucuronide

Activation reactions

*N* Hydroxy 2-acetylamino-fluorene (Px)

HO O
N— C— $CH_3$

Sulfotransferase

OH
O=S=O
O O
N— C— $CH_3$

*N*-sulfate-2-AAF (Ut)

Acetylation

O
$H_3C$—C
O O
N— C— $CH_3$

*N*-acetoxy-2-AAF (Ut)

UDPGA
Glucuronyl transferase

glucuronide
O O
N— C— $CH_3$

*N*-glucuronyl-2-AAF (Ut)

$BrCH_2CH_2Br$ + GSH → $GSCH_2CH_2Br$ → $H_2C$—$CH_2$ (G—$S^+$)

Ethyldibromide (Pr)

S-2-bromoethyl glutathione (Px)

S-episulfonium ethyl glutathione (Ut)

***Figure 8–6. Structures of representative chemical carcinogens and their metabolic derivatives resulting from the action of phase II metabolism of procarcinogens.***

loalkenes are nephrotoxic and mutagenic (Monks et al., 1990). The actual mechanism of the carcinogenic effect is not clear despite these observations (Monks et al., 1990).

In addition to the electrophilic intermediates that constitute many of the ultimate forms of chemical carcinogens, substantial evidence also implicates free radical derivatives of chemicals in their carcinogenic action (Nagata et al., 1982). Free radicals may be positively or negatively charged, or neutral, but all possess a single unpaired electron. Although a wide range of stabilities are known for different species, most radicals are extremely reactive. Two lines of evidence suggest that free radicals may be important in the induction of neoplastic transformation by chemicals. Several molecules that inhibit the formation of free radicals, including antioxidants, are capable of inhibiting the carcinogenic action of many chemical carcinogens (Ito and Hirose, 1987; Simic, 1988). In addition, free radical intermediates sometimes are formed during the metabolism of chemical carcinogens (Guengerich, 1992), and the metabolic reactions of a number of chemical carcinogens may proceed through free radical intermediates. Chemical carcinogens, including nitrosamines (Bartsch et al., 1989), nitro compounds (Conaway et al., 1991), and diethylstilbestrol (Wang and Liehr, 1994), may possess ultimate forms that are free radicals in nature. The formation of free radicals plays an important role in the carcinogenic effects of ionizing radiation (Biaglow, 1981). Furthermore, free radicals are important in the process of cancer development (see below).

Pathways other than the mixed-function oxidase may be involved in the bioactivation of compounds. Marnett (1981) described the cooxygenation of polyunsaturated fatty acids, especially arachidonic acid, and polycyclic aromatic hydrocarbons with bioactivation of the hydrocarbon. Such cooxygenation can occur during the synthesis of prostaglandins, a series of autocoids that are important in normal homeostasis. Prostaglandin H synthase has two catalytic activities. In the first reaction, the cyclooxygenase activity of prostaglandin H synthase catalyzes the oxygenation of arachidonic acid to the endoperoxide prostaglandin $G_2$ (Fig. 8-7). The associated peroxidase activity of prostaglandin H synthase reduces the hydroperoxide prostaglandin $G_2$ to the alcohol prostaglandin $H_2$. Many tissues that have a low expression of monooxygenases contain prostaglandin H synthase. In these tissues, compounds can be activated to reactive forms by prostaglandin H synthase, since oxidation by the peroxidase activity often yields a free radical product. The cooxidation of 2-aminofluorene is an example (Fig. 8-7). In the case of benzo(*a*)pyrene 7,8 diol, peroxidase-catalyzed transfer of the free radical from the hydroperoxide to the hydrocarbon results in the formation of the ultimate carcinogenic form of benzo(*a*)pyrene, the 7,8 diol 9,10 epoxide. This pathway of metabolic activation of carcinogens, while not ubiquitous, is important in some extrahepatic tissues. For example, Wise and colleagues (1984) demonstrated a marked metabolic activation of 2-naphthylamine via prostaglandin synthase in dog bladder without activation in the liver. Mattammal and associates (1981) have suggested that a number of renal and bladder carcinogens may be activated by this pathway. Several reviews on the role of prostaglandin synthase in the metabolism of compounds, including their bioactivation in extrahepatic tissues, can be consulted for additional information (Eling et al., 1990; Smith et al., 1991).

**Chemical Structure and Chemical Carcinogenesis.** Knowledge of the metabolic activation of chemicals has dramatically advanced our understanding of the carcinogenic mechanisms that underlie the extreme diversity of chemical structures involved in cancer development. The relationship of chemical structure to carcinogenic activity plays a significant role in the potential identification and mechanism of potential chemical carcinogens. Computerized databases of carcinogenic and noncarcinogenic chemicals have been developed to relate structure to carcinogenic activity in a variety of carcinogens (Enslein et al., 1994; Rosenkranz and Klopman, 1994).

Using the results of rodent bioassays of more than 500 chemicals, Ashby and Paton (1993) studied the influence of chemical structure on both the extent and the target tissue specificity of carcinogenesis for those chemicals. From an analysis of the presence of potential electrophilic sites (DNA-reactive), mutagenicity to *Salmonella*, and level of carcinogenicity to rodents, these authors developed a list of chemical structures that have a high correlation with the development of neoplasia in rodent tests (Ashby et al., 1989; Tennant and Ashby, 1991). These "structural alerts" signify that a chemical that has such structures should be examined closely for carcinogenic potential. These authors have developed a composite model structure indicating the various "structural alerts" that appear to be associated with DNA reactivity or carcinogenicity (Fig. 8-8). The substantial database used to generate these structural alerts indicates the utility of this information for the identification of potential carcinogens and the mechanisms of their action in specific tissues. In addition, investigation of the metabolic activation of such functional groups during the carcinogenic process should provide insight into their role in the induction of cancer.

## Mutagenesis and Carcinogenesis

Most chemical carcinogens must be metabolized in the cell before they exert their carcinogenic activity. In this respect, the metabolism of some chemicals results in bioactivation instead of elimination. Thus, metabolic capabilities may underlie the way in which a substance that is not carcinogenic for one species may be carcinogenic for another. This becomes important for carcinogen testing in whole animals for both hazard identification and risk assessment. Such considerations directly affect the choice of the most sensitive species or the species most similar to humans for these evaluations.

Studies on the induction of liver neoplasms by the food dye *N,N*-dimethyl-4-aminoazobenzene (DAB) provided the first evidence that metabolites of carcinogens can bind to macromolecules. This dye, known as butter yellow, was found to be covalently linked to proteins. Because DAB did not bind to purified protein in vitro and yet could not be extracted from protein after in vivo administration, it was deduced that DAB is metabolized in vivo to a reactive form which covalently binds to cellular macromolecules. The Millers (Miller and Miller, 1947) demonstrated a high degree of correlation between the extent of protein binding and carcinogenicity in different species. Because carcinogens are reactive per se or are activated by metabolism to reactive intermediates that bind to cellular components, including DNA, these electrophilic derivatives, which bind to a variety of nucleophilic (electron-dense) moieties in DNA, RNA, and protein, were considered the carcinogenic form of the compounds of interest. Several lines of evidence indicate that DNA is the critical target for carcinogenesis. The first hint that DNA is the target for heritable alterations caused by carcinogen administration came from the increased incidence of cancer in genetically prone individuals with a defective ability to repair DNA damage (xeroderma pigmentosum; Friedberg, 1992). The second major piece of evidence that DNA is the target of carcinogen action was the observation of carcinogen-induced mutations in specific target genes associated with neoplasia in a multitude of experimental systems. A comparison of DNA-adduct formation with biologically effective doses of carcinogens with different potencies demonstrated that the level of DNA dam-

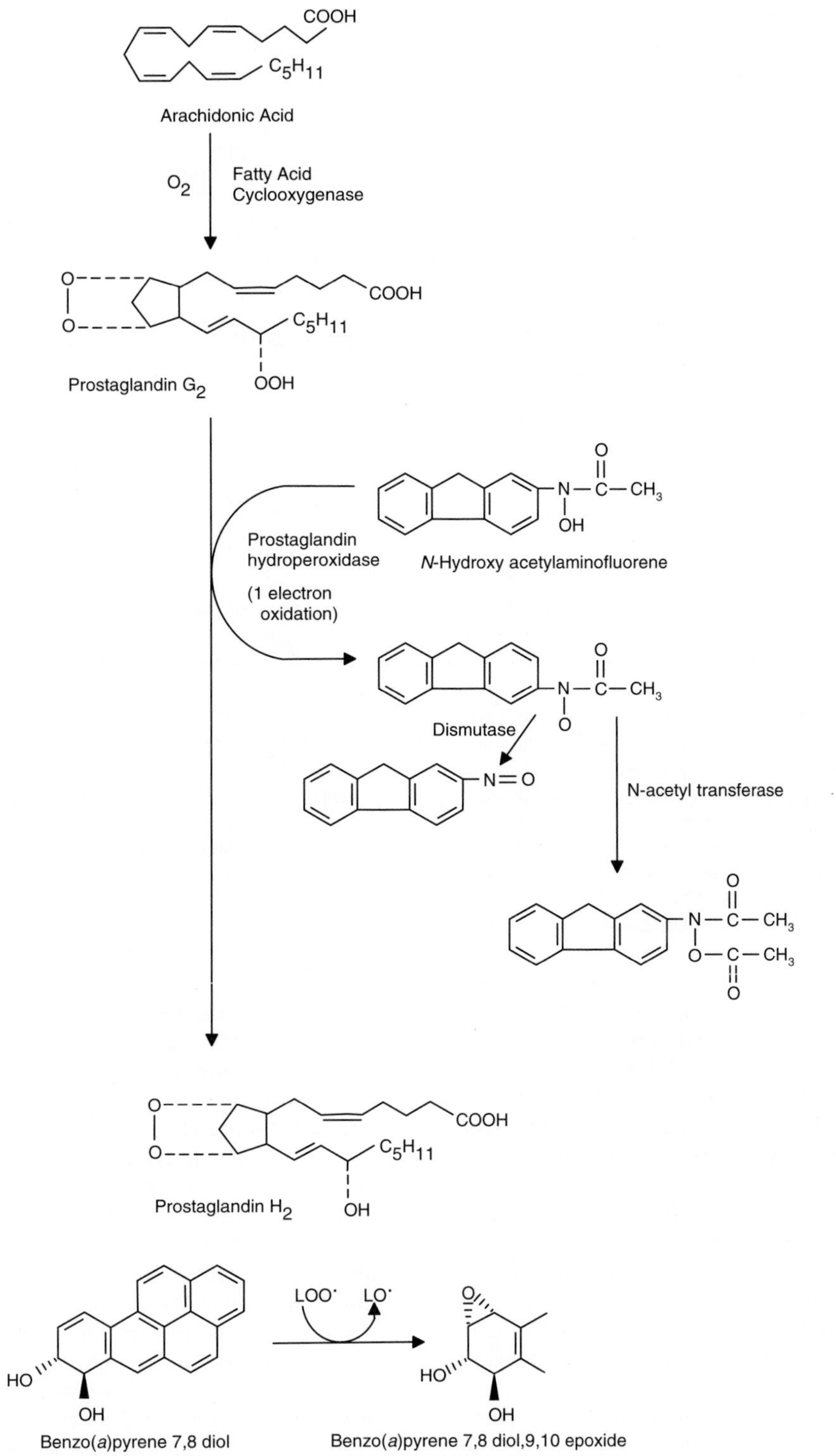

***Figure 8–7. The metabolic activation of benzo(a)pyrene 7,8 diol and N-hydroxy 2-acetylaminofluorene during the peroxidation of arachidonic acid.***

age was relatively similar. Since covalent adducts in DNA could be derived from carcinogenic compounds, the mechanism by which mutations arise and their relationship to carcinogenesis was the next area to be examined in the quest for an understanding of cancer development.

The induction of mutations is due primarily to chemical or physical alterations in the structure of DNA that result in inaccurate replication of a particular region of the genome. The process of mutagenesis consists of structural DNA alteration, cell proliferation that fixes the DNA damage, and DNA repair that either directly repairs the alkylated base or bases or results in the removal of larger segments of DNA. Electrophilic compounds can interact with the ring nitrogens, exocyclic amino groups, carbonyl oxygens, and the phosphodiester

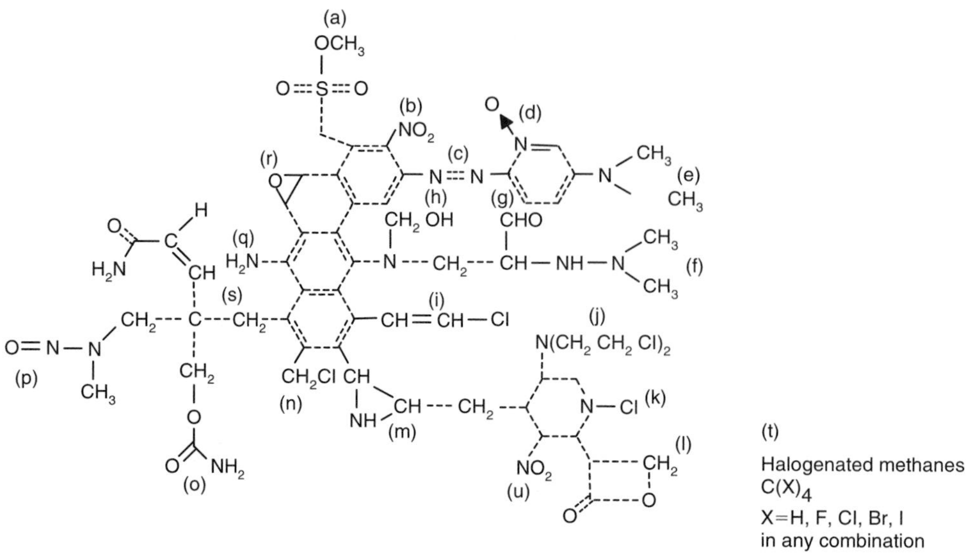

(t)
Halogenated methanes
$C(X)_4$
X=H, F, Cl, Br, I
in any combination

***Figure 8–8. Potential structural alerts for mutagenicity.***

The substituents are as follows: (a) alkyl esters of either phosphonic or sulfonic acids, (b) aromatic nitro groups, (c) aromatic azo groups, not per se but by virtue of their possible reduction to an aromatic amine, (d) aromatic ring *N*-oxides, (e) aromatic mono- and dialkylamino groups, (f) alkyl hydrazines, (g) alkyl aldehydes, (h) *N*-methylol derivatives, (i) monohaloalkenes, (j) a large family of *N* and *S* mustards (*β*-haloethyl), (k) *N*-chloramines (see below), (l) propiolactones and propiosultones, (m) aromatic and aliphatic aziridinyl derivatives, (n) both aromatic and aliphatic substituted primary alkyl halides, (o) derivatives of urethane (carbamates), (p) alkyl-*N*-nitrosamines, (q) aromatic amines, their *N*-hydroxy derivatives and the derived esters, and (r) aliphatic and aromatic epoxides. The *N*-chloramine substructure (k) has not been associated with carcinogenicity, but potent genotoxic activity has been reported for it (discussed in Ashby et al., 1989). Michael-reactive *α,β*-unsaturated esters, amides, and nitriles form a relatively new class of genotoxin (e.g., acrylamide). However, the structural requirements for genotoxicity have not been established, and this structural unit is not shown in the figure. [Adapted from Tennant and Ashby (1991) with permission of the author and publisher.]

backbone. The reaction of electrophiles with DNA results in alkylation products that are covalent derivatives of the reactive chemical species with DNA. Direct-acting alkylation agents induce preferential binding to highly nucleophilic centers such as the $N^7$ position of guanine. Less reactive species such as the active form of diethylnitrosamine also react with the nucleophilic oxygens in DNA. Carcinogenic agents that result in the formation of bulky adducts often specifically react with sites in the purine ring. For example, aromatic amines bind to the $C^8$ position of guanine, while the diol epoxide of polycyclic aromatic hydrocarbons binds to the $N^2$ and $N^6$ positions of guanine. The position of an adduct in DNA and its chemical and physical properties in that context dictate the types of mutations induced (Essigman and Wood, 1993). This indicates that different adducts can induce a distinct spectrum of mutations and that any given adduct can result in a multitude of different DNA lesions. Observations on the need for metabolic activation of compounds to the ultimate reactive form were rapidly extended to a number of other compounds, including 2-acetylaminofluorene. In tests of mutagenicity, it was demonstrated that whereas 2-acetylaminofluorene itself is not mutagenic, its sulfate metabolite is highly mutagenic for transforming DNA (Maher et al., 1968). These findings led to the development of mutagenesis assays for the detection of chemical carcinogens on the basis of the premise that one could detect carcinogens in highly mutable strains of bacteria given exogenous liver microsomal preparations for in vitro metabolism of the test agent (see below). Cultured mammalian cells also have been developed for the evaluation of the mutagenic action of potential carcinogenic agents. Compounds are evaluated in the presence (Michalopoulos et al., 1981) or absence (Li et al., 1991) of metabolic activation systems such as irradiated hepatic feeder layers and hepatic microsomes. The use of these in vitro screens of mutagenicity has permitted analysis of the mutational specificity of some carcinogens (Table 8-3). While the data shown in the table were derived from bacterial mutagenesis studies, several other systems have been utilized to determine the mutagenic specificity of various agents (Essigmann and Wood, 1993).

Point mutations, frameshift mutations, chromosomal aberrations, aneuploidy, and polyploidization can be induced by chemicals with varying degrees of specificity that are in part dose-dependent. Mutagenesis can result from several different alterations in the physical and chemical nature of DNA. While alkylation of DNA with small alkyl groups or large bulky adducts can result in mutation, other processes also may be involved. Conformation of the DNA has a major impact on the potential mutagenic activity of a compound. This is best demonstrated by the related compounds 2-acetylaminofluorene and 2-aminofluorene, which both form bulky DNA adducts at guanine residues in DNA. The AAF adduct distorts the double helix, while the AF adduct remains outside the helix and does not distort it. The AAF adduct induces frameshift mutations, whereas the AF adduct induces primarily transversions

**Table 8–3**
**A Comparison of the Mutagenic Spectrum of Aflatoxin $B_1$, Benzo[*a*]pyrene Diolepoxide, and 2-Acetylaminofluorene**

| MUTATION | AFLATOXIN $B_1$ | BENZO[A]PYRENE DIOLEPOXIDE | 2-ACETYLAMINOFLUORENE |
|---|---|---|---|
| GC to TA | 0.94 | 0.76 | 0.88 |
| GC to AT | 0.06 | 0.11 | 0.06 |
| GC to CG | 0.00 | 0.13 | 0.06 |

SOURCE: Modified from Loechler (1989).

(Bichara and Fuchs, 1985). Planar agents that can intercalate between the base pairs in DNA can effectively induce frameshift mutations by exacerbating slippage mispairing in repetitive sequences. In addition, agents that lie within the major or minor groove of DNA can perturb nucleosome formation and may alter DNA replication. Some of these agents are potential chemotherapeutic agents. Agents such as irradiation and topoisomerase inhibitors that induce double-strand breaks also can enhance mutagenesis (Eastman and Barry, 1992).

Several mechanisms of mutagenesis exist. The presence of certain alkylation products, such as *O*-6 alkyl deoxyguanosine and *O*-4 alkyl deoxythymidine, permits a degenerate base pairing that can base pair with the appropriate base as well as with an inappropriate base. This can be demonstrated in vitro and in vivo as the induction of transition mutations after treatment with certain alkylating agents (Singer, 1986). Thus, methylating and ethylating agents result in mutations as a result of base mispairing. The active metabolites of numerous compounds, such as PAHs and aromatic amines, can form bulky DNA adducts that block DNA synthesis, resulting in a noncoding lesion. The synthetic machinery employs bypass synthesis to avoid the lethal impact of these unrepaired lesions (Friedberg, 1994). In this condition, the most prevalent base, frequently deoxyadenosine (Shearman and Loeb, 1979), is inserted opposite the offending adducted nucleotide base. Thus, DNA binding and repair, induction of point mutations, and clastogenicity have proved useful as endpoints in the identification of potential carcinogens and biomarkers of carcinogen exposure. The role of DNA repair in the protection of the genome and the induction of mutations is an essential component in the process of mutagenesis process (see below).

Not all chemical carcinogens require intracellular metabolism to become ultimate carcinogens. Examples of direct-acting mutagens include alkylating agents such as *β*-propiolactone, nitrogen mustard, ethyleneimine, and bis(chloromethyl)ether (Fig. 8-3). Direct-acting carcinogens are typically carcinogenic at multiple sites and in all the species examined. A number of direct-acting alkylating agents, including some used in chemotherapy, are carcinogenic for humans (Vainio et al., 1991).

## Macromolecular Adducts Resulting from Reaction with Ultimate Carcinogens

One of the most intriguing problems in chemical carcinogenesis is the chemical characterization of covalent compounds derived from reactions between the ultimate metabolite of a chemical carcinogen and a macromolecule. The structures of several carcinogens covalently bound to protein and nucleic acids are shown in Fig. 8-9. As noted in the figure, the reaction of the ultimate form of *N*-methyl-4-aminoazobenzene with polypeptides involves a demethylation of methionine and a reaction of the electrophilic position ortho to the amino group of the azobenzene with the nucleophilic sulfur of methionine and subsequent loss of the methyl of methionine. The most nucleophilic site in DNA is the *N*-7 position of guanine, and many carcinogens form covalent adducts at that site. Adducts formed with DNA exhibit stereospecific configurations, as exemplified by the reaction of the epoxide of aflatoxin $B_1$ with the *N*-7 position of guanine. The ultimate carcinogenic form of AAF also reacts with guanine at two positions on the DNA base, as shown in the figure. In contrast, ethylene oxide directly alkylates the *N*-7 position of guanine in DNA (Bolt et al., 1988). An interesting adduction occurs during the metabolism of 2-nitropropane, which results in the formation of 8-aminoguanine possibly from the spontaneous reaction with the highly reactive intermediate ($NH_2^+$) formed during the metabolism of the nitro group (Sodum et al., 1993). The formation of an additional ring structure in adenine and cytosine occurs with the ultimate form of vinyl chloride and structurally similar carcinogens (Bolt, 1988). For the detailed chemistry of the reactions involved in the formation of such adducts, several reviews are suggested (Miller, 1970, 1978; Weisburger and Williams, 1982; Hathway and Kolar, 1980; Dipple et al., 1985).

Several carcinogens that adduct DNA by direct methylation, ethylation, or higher alkylations are of considerable experimental and environmental significance. The sites on DNA that are alkylated by ethylating and methylating chemicals are shown in Fig. 8-10 (Pegg, 1984). Pegg (1984) also described the relative proportions of the methylated bases present in DNA after reaction with carcinogen-methylating agents (Table 8-4). The predominant adduct seen with methylating agents such as methylmethane sulfonate is 7-methylguanine. In contrast, ethylation of DNA occurs predominantly in the phosphate backbone. Pegg argued that the principal carcinogenic adduct is the $O^6$-alkylguanine. In contrast, Swenberg and associates (1984) reported that $O^4$-alkylthymine may be a more important adduct for carcinogenesis because this DNA adduct is retained in the DNA for more extended periods than is the $O^6$-alkylguanine adduct. The importance of the persistence of DNA adducts of ultimate carcinogens will be discussed below.

Another common structural change in DNA is the hydroxylation of DNA bases. Such changes have been found in all four of the bases making up DNA (Marnett and Burcham, 1993), but the most commonly analyzed are 5-hydroxymethylthymine (Srinivasan and Glauert, 1990) and 8-hydroxyguanine (Floyd, 1990). These hydroxylated bases have been found in the DNA of target organs in animals that were

3-(homocyctein-S-yl) *N*-methyl-4-aminoazobenzene in peptide linkage

Aflatoxin $B_1$ $N$-$^7$ guanine-adduct

*N*-(deoxyguanosin-8-yl)-acetylaminofluorene in DNA

3-(deoxyguanosin $N^2$-yl)-acetylaminofluorene in DNA

1, $N^6$-ethenoadenine in DNA

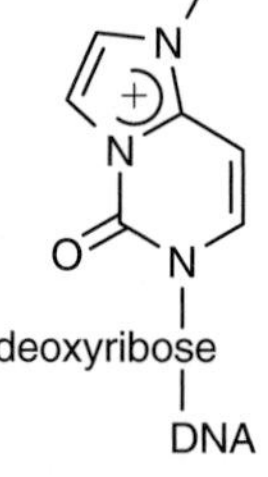


3, $N^4$-ethenocytosine in DNA

7,-(2-hydroxyethyl) guanosine in DNA

***Figure 8–9. Structures of some protein- and nucleic acid–bound forms of certain chemical carcinogens. The macromolecular linkages are shown schematically.***

Esters of 2-acetylaminofluorene react predominantly with the 8 position of guanine, whereas the epoxide of aflatoxin $B_1$ reacts primarily with the $N$-$^7$ position of guanine. The ethanoadenine and ethanocytosine adducts result from the reaction of DNA with halogenated acetaldehydes or ultimate forms of vinyl chloride and related structures. 7,-(2-Hydroxyethyl)guanosine is a product of the reaction of ethylene oxide with DNA.

administered chemical carcinogens but also are present in the DNA of organisms not subjected to any known carcinogenic agent (Marnett and Burcham, 1993). Estimates of a rate of endogenous depurination of DNA of 580 bases/h per cell and DNA strand breaks at a rate of 2300/h per cell have been reported (Shapiro, 1981). These estimates are not incompatible with the presence of oxidative DNA lesions at a level of $10^6$ per cell in young rats and almost twice that in old rats (Ames et al., 1993). The source of such oxidative damage is presumably free radical reactions occurring endogenously in the cell that are capable of producing activated oxygen radicals (Floyd, 1990; Ames et al., 1993). Such oxidative reactions,

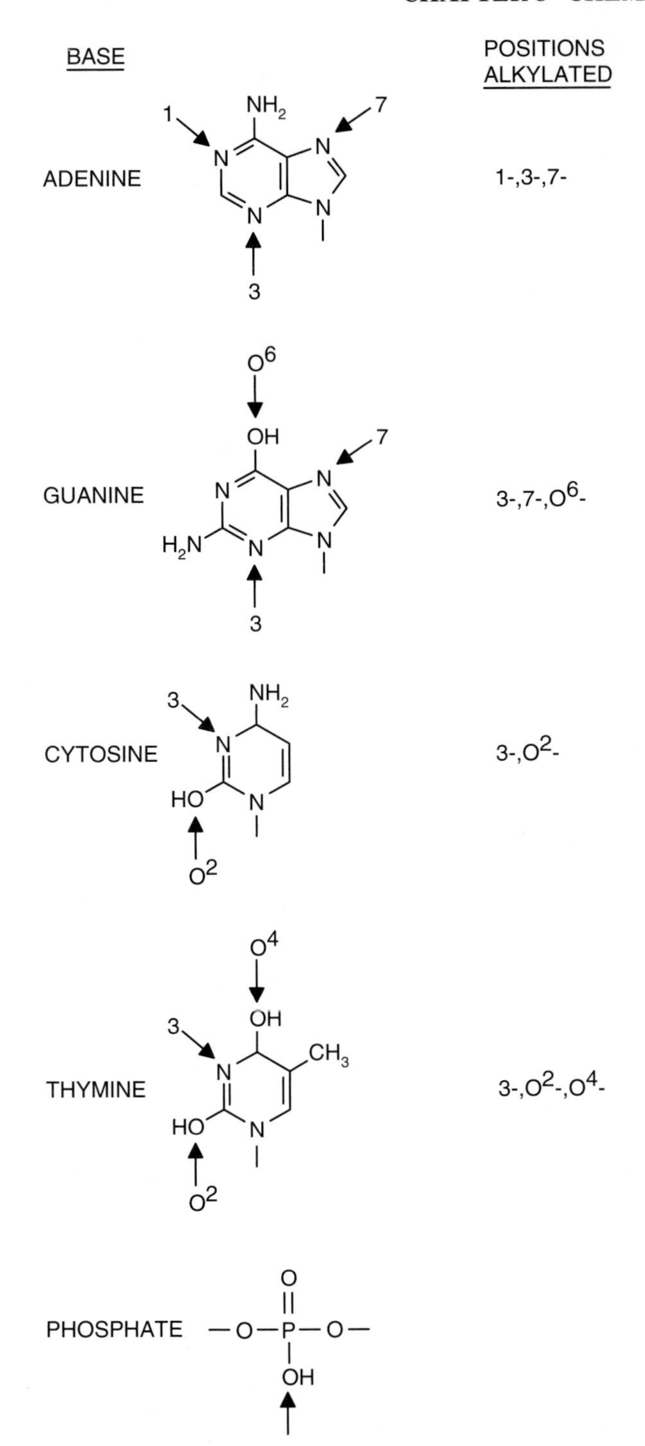


***Figure 8–10. Sites of alkylation of DNA under physiological conditions. [From Pegg (1984), with permission of the author and publisher.]***

which occur either as a result of an endogenous oxidative phenomenon or from the administration of exogenous chemical and radiation carcinogens, presumably are rapidly repaired by the mechanisms discussed below. Thus, endogenous mutations are kept to a minimum.

The best studied endogenous modification of DNA is the methylation of deoxycytidine residues by the transfer of a methyl group from *S*-adenosylmethionine by DNA methyl-

**Table 8–4**
**Relative Proportions of Methylated Bases Present in DNA after Reaction with Carcinogenic Alkylating Agents**

| | PERCENTAGE OF TOTAL ALKYLATION BY | |
|---|---|---|
| | DIMETHYL-NITROSAMINE, *N*-METHYL-*N* NITROSOUREA, or 1,2-DIMETHYL-HYDRAZINE | DIETHYL-NITROSAMINE or *N*-ETHYL-*N*-NITROSOUREA |
| 1-Alkyladenine | 0.7 | 0.3 |
| 3-Alkyladenine | 8 | 4 |
| 7-Alkyladenine | 1.5 | 0.4 |
| 3-Alkylguanine | 0.8 | 0.6 |
| 7-Alkylguanine | 68 | 12 |
| $O^6$-Alkylguanine | 7.5 | 8 |
| 3-Alkylcytosine | 0.5 | 0.2 |
| $O^2$-Alkylcytosine | 0.1 | 3 |
| 3-Alkylthymine | 0.3 | 0.8 |
| $O^2$-Alkylthymine | 0.1 | 7 |
| $O^4$-Alkylthymine | 0.1–0.7 | 1–4 |
| Alkylphosphates | 12 | 53 |

SOURCE: Adapted from Pegg (1984).

transferase (Holliday, 1989; Michalowsky and Jones, 1989). Such methylation results in the heritable expression or repression of specific genes in eukaryotic cells. Genes that are actively transcribed are hypomethylated, whereas those which are hypermethylated rarely tend to be transcribed. When such methylation occurs during development, the expression or repression of specific genes may be "imprinted" by DNA methylation at various stages during development (Barlow, 1993). Chemical carcinogens may inhibit DNA methylation by several mechanisms, including the formation of covalent adducts, single-strand breaks in the DNA, alteration in methionine pools, and the direct inactivation of the enzyme DNA *S*-adenosylmethionine methyltransferase, which is responsible for methylation (Riggs and Jones, 1983). Therefore, the inhibition of DNA methylation by chemical carcinogens may represent a further potential mechanism for carcinogenesis induced by chemicals. Mikol and colleagues (1983) demonstrated the importance of this mechanism in hepatocarcinogenesis; half the animals receiving a diet devoid of methionine and choline for 18 months developed hepatocellular carcinomas and cholangiomas. A methyl-deficient diet induces a drastic hypomethylation of hepatic nuclear DNA (Wilson et al., 1984), which may heritably alter the phenotype of the cell.

Finally, structural changes in DNA of largely unknown character have been reported with the $^{32}P$ postlabeling assay (Reddy and Randerath, 1987). This procedure is outlined in Fig. 8-11. After digestion of DNA to its constituent nucleotides, each nucleotide is labeled by using $\gamma^{32}P$-labeled ATP and a bacterial kinase, an enzyme that transfers the terminal phosphate of ATP to the available 5′ hydroxyl of the 3′ nucleotides to convert all the nucleotides to a radioactive biphosphorylated form. Nucleotides of the normal DNA bases are removed by appropriate

Carcinogen-adducted DNA

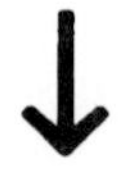

Cleavage into component nucleotides:
micrococcal endonuclease
+ spleen exonuclease

Ap + Gp + Tp + Cp + m$^5$Cp + Xp + Yp + . . .
(Normal nucleotides) (Adducts)

Phosphate transfer:
[γ-$^{32}$P] ATP + T4 polynucleotide kinase

*pAp + *pGp + *pTp + *pCp + *pm$^5$Cp + *pXp + *pYp + . . .

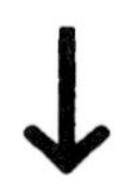

Removal of normal nucleotides:
PE1-cellulose or reversed-phase TLC
or reversed-phase HPLC

*pXp + *pYp + . . .

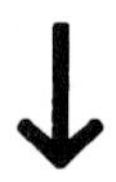

Separation and detection of adducts:
PEI-cellulose TLC
Autoradiography

Maps of $^{32}$P-labeled carcinogen-DNA adducts

***Figure 8–11. The basic features of $^{32}$P-postlabeling assay for carcinogen-adducted DNA.***

The $^{32}$P assay involves four steps: digestion of DNA, $^{32}$P labeling of the digestion products, removal of $^{32}$P-labeled nucleotides not containing adducts, and thin-layer chromatography mapping of the [$^{32}$P] nucleotides with adducts. Asterisks indicate the position of the $^{32}$P label. [Modified from Gupta et al. (1982)].

chromatographic procedures, leaving only the nucleotides that contain structural adducts. Although this technique has been used to demonstrate adduction of DNA by a variety of known chemical carcinogens, it is equally interesting that a number of adducts of unknown structure have been discovered in living cells. Some of these structurally unknown DNA adducts, termed I-compounds (Li and Randerath, 1992), change with dietary modifications or drug administration (Randerath et al., 1992) and exhibit species and tissue differences (Li et al., 1990). I-compounds occur in human fetal tissues (Hansen et al., 1993), increase with age and caloric restriction, but decrease during hepatocarcinogenesis (Randerath et al., 1991). Thus, the exact role, if any, of these DNA adducts of unknown structure in the process of carcinogenesis remains an open question.

Thus, the role of structural adducts of DNA in carcinogenesis is not a simple matter of adduct = mutation = carcinogenesis. Adducts of known carcinogens (Fig. 8-9) may play a significant role in the carcinogenesis induced by their procarcinogenic forms, but the function of structurally undefined, endogenously produced adducts such as I-compounds in the carcinogenic process is not clear. There is no substantial evidence that endogenously formed adducts lead to mutation. Whether a

DNA adduct results in the formation of mutations is a consequence of its persistence through a period of cell proliferation, which in turn is partially a function of the process of DNA repair.

## DNA REPAIR AND CHEMICAL CARCINOGENESIS

### Persistence of DNA Adducts and DNA Repair

The extent to which DNA adducts occur after the administration of chemical carcinogens depends on the overall metabolism of the chemical agent and the chemical reactivity of the ultimate metabolite. Once the adduct is formed, its continued presence in the DNA of the cell depends primarily on the ability of the cellular machinery to repair the structural alteration in the DNA.

It is from such considerations, as well as the presumed critical nature of the adduct in the carcinogenic process, that a working hypothesis on the relationship between mutagenesis and carcinogenesis has evolved. It has been postulated that the extent of DNA adduct formation and the persistence of adducts in the DNA should correlate with the biological effect of the agent (Neumann, 1983). In accordance with this hypothesis, several studies have correlated the persistence of DNA adducts during chemical carcinogenesis with the high incidence of neoplasms in specific tissues (Table 8-5). Among the earliest of those studies was that of Goth and Rajewsky (1974), who demonstrated the relative persistence of $O^6$-ethylguanine in DNA of brain but not liver of animals administered ethylnitrosourea at 10 days of age. The rapid loss of the adduct in liver DNA contrasted with the sevenfold slower loss in DNA of the brain. In this study, neoplastic lesions were observed in the brain but not in the liver later in life. Swenberg and associates (1985) demonstrated an analogous situation in the liver, in which the administration of dimethylhydrazine induced a high incidence of neoplasms in hepatic vascular endothelium, but a very low incidence in hepatocytes. Examination of the analogous adduct $O^6$-methylguanine demonstrated its rapid removal from the DNA of hepatocytes but much slower removal from the DNA of vascular endothelial cells. Similarly, Kadlubar and associates (1981) demonstrated that more 2-naphthylamine adducts of guanine persisted in bladder epithelium (urothelium) than in liver after the administration of the carcinogen to dogs. The bladder, but not the liver, is a target for this carcinogen in that species. When the susceptibility to carcinogenesis by diethylnitrosamine was investigated in the same tissue in two different species, significant alkylation and the development of neoplasia were observed in the hamster but not the mouse lung. Thus, the difference in the persistence of DNA adducts plays an important role in the target organ and species specificity of certain carcinogens.

Although the correlations noted in Table 8-4 support the working hypothesis for the importance of specific adducts during the carcinogenic process, the mere presence of DNA adducts is probably not sufficient for the carcinogenic process to proceed; equally or more important is the persistence of the adducts in the DNA of viable cells. For example, Swenberg and associates (1984) demonstrated that the $O^4$-ethylthymine adduct but not the $O^6$-ethylguanine adduct is stable in liver parenchymal cells after the continuous exposure of rats to diethylnitrosamine. Furthermore, Müller and Rajewsky (1983) found that the $O^4$-ethylthymine adduct persisted in all organs after the administration of ethylnitrosourea to neonatal or adult rats. By contrast, persistence of DNA adducts of the carcinogenic *trans*-4-aminostilbene does not correlate with tissue susceptibility. While the liver and kidney exhibited the greatest burden and persistence of the adduct and the ear duct glands of Zymbal showed the lowest adduct concentration, it is the latter tissue that is most susceptible to carcinogenesis by this agent (Neumann, 1983). Such differences in susceptibility to carcinogenesis are undoubtedly the result of a number of factors, including replication of the target cells and repair of the carcinogen-DNA adduct (see below).

Despite exceptions to the working hypothesis, our knowledge about the persistence of covalent adducts of DNA in tissues has been utilized to quantitate the exposure of humans to carcinogenic chemicals and relate the potential risk of neoplastic development to such exposure. The occurrence of ad-

**Table 8–5**
**Organ and Species Specificity of Chemical Carcinogenesis in Relation to Persistence of Adducts in DNA**

| SPECIES | CARCINOGEN | TISSUE | DNA ADDUCT ($T\frac{1}{2}$) | NEOPLASTIC DEVELOPMENT | REFERENCE |
|---|---|---|---|---|---|
| Rat (neonates) | ENU* | Liver | $O^6$EtG (30 h) | ±† | Goth and Rajewsky, 1974 |
| Rat (neonates) | ENU | Brain | $O^6$EtG (220 h) | +++ | |
| Rat | SDMH | Liver, hepatocytes | $O^6$MeG (~1.6 days) | ± | Swenberg et al., 1985 |
| Rat | SDMH | Liver, nonparenchymal cells | $O^6$MeG (>20 days) | +++ | |
| Dog | 2-NA | Liver | *N*-(dG-8-yl)-2-NA (~2 days) | 0 | Kadlubar et al., 1981 |
| Dog | 2-NA | Urothelium | *N*-(dG-8-yl)-2-NA (>20 days) | +++ | |
| Hamster | DEN | Lung | $O^6$EtG (91 hr) | 0 | Becker and Shank, 1985 |
| Rat | DEN | Lung | $O^6$EtG (undetectable) | +++ | |

* ENU = ethylnitrosourea; SDMH = symmetrical dimethylhydrazine; 2-NA = 2-naphthylamine; DEN = diethylnitrosamine; $O^6$EtG = $O^6$ ethylguanine; *N*-(dG-8-yl)-2-NA = *N*-(deoxyguanosin-8-yl)-2-naphthylamine.

† ± = occasional neoplasm; +++ = high incidence of neoplasms; 0 = no increased incidence of neoplasia above untreated controls.

ducts of benzo(*a*)pyrene throughout the tissues of exposed animals at unexpectedly similar levels (Stowers and Anderson, 1985) further supports the rationale for the investigation of persistent adducts of DNA and protein as biomarkers of human exposure. Immunologic and highly sensitive chromatographic technologies have been used to demonstrate the presence of adducts of several carcinogenic species (Perera et al., 1991; Shields and Harris, 1991). DNA adducts of carcinogenic PAHs have been demonstrated at relatively high levels in tissues, especially blood cells, of smokers and foundry workers compared with nonexposed individuals (Perera et al., 1991). Huh and coworkers (1989) demonstrated an increased level of $O^4$-ethylthymine in the DNA of liver from individuals with no known exposure to ethylating agents, and a statistically significant increased level of ethylation of this base was noted in cancer patients compared with controls. In a more recent study by Hsieh and Hsieh (1993), DNA adducts of aflatoxin $B_1$ were demonstrated in samples of human placenta and cord blood from patients in Taiwan, an area with a high incidence of liver cancer. In addition to detection of specific structural DNA adducts, the $^{32}P$-postlabeling assay has been exploited to determine the presence of DNA adducts in human tissues (Beach and Gupta, 1992). As expected, a variety of adducts are found in both normal individuals and those potentially exposed to specific carcinogenic agents. In addition to DNA adducts, specific carcinogens also bind covalently to serum proteins. For example, Bryant and colleagues (1987) showed a five- to sixfold greater level of hemoglobin adducts of 4-aminobiphenyl in smokers than in nonsmokers. While this adduct has a finite lifetime, chronic exposure to cigarette smoke maintains the dramatic increase in the adduct level between these two groups, suggesting a potential use of such determinations in estimating exposure to carcinogenic agents. Thus, the persistence of macromolecular adducts of the ultimate forms of chemical carcinogens may be very important in the carcinogenic mechanism of such agents. However, as was noted above, the presence and persistence of DNA adducts are only one factor in the complex process of cancer development.

## Mechanisms of DNA Repair

The persistence of DNA adducts results predominantly from failure of DNA repair. The types of structural alterations that may occur in the DNA molecule as a result of interaction with reactive chemical species or directly with radiation are considerable. A number of the more frequently seen structural changes in DNA are schematically represented in Fig. 8-12. The reaction of DNA with reactive chemical species produces

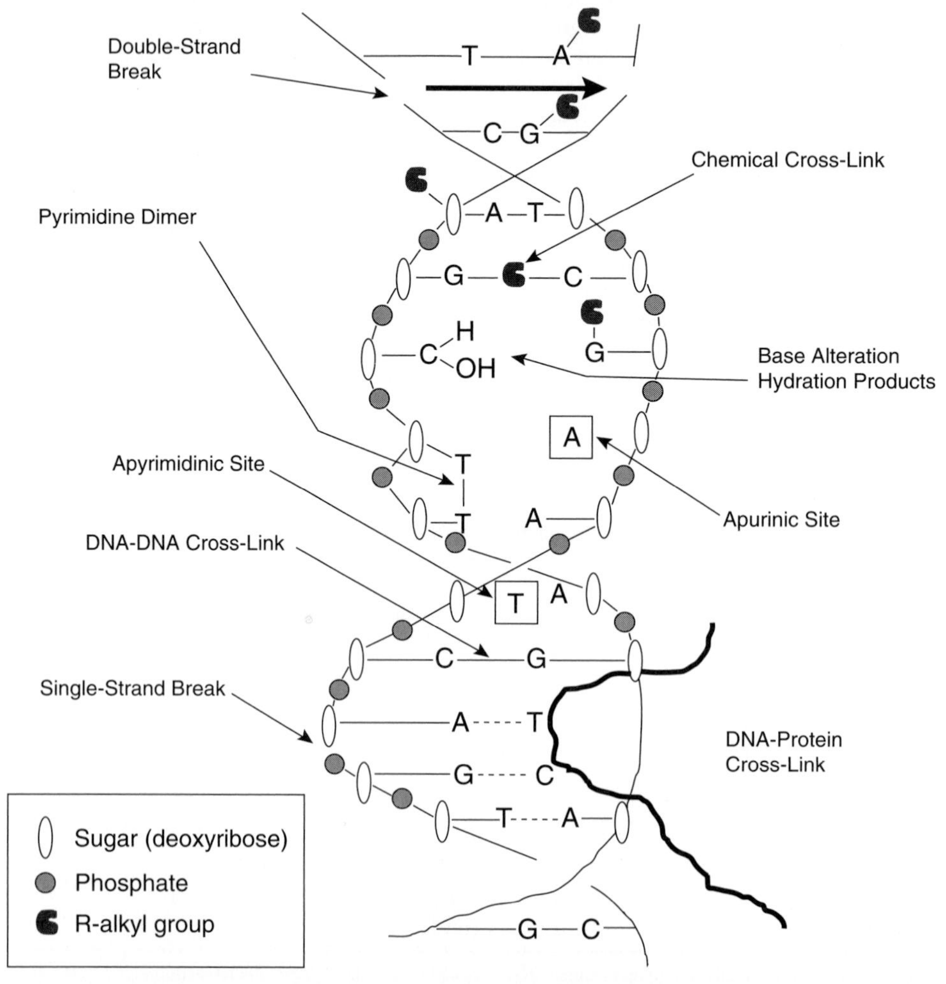


*Figure 8–12. Schematic representation of chemical and radiation-induced lesions in DNA. [Adapted from Fry et al. (1982), with permission of the authors and publisher.]*

adducts on bases, sugars, and the phosphate backbone. In addition, bifunctional reactive chemicals may cause the cross-linking of DNA strands through a reaction with two opposing bases. Other structural changes, such as pyrimidine dimer formation, are specific for ultraviolet radiation, while double-strand DNA breaks are most commonly seen with ionizing radiation (see below). Most of the other lesions depicted in Fig. 8-12 may occur as a result of either chemical or radiation effects on the DNA molecule. To cope with the many structurally distinct types of DNA damage, a variety of mechanisms have evolved to effectively repair each type of damage shown in Fig. 8-12. It has been estimated that over 100 genes are dedicated to DNA repair, emphasizing the essential nature of the genetic information. A summary of the types of DNA repair most commonly encountered in mammalian systems appears in Table 8-6.

Two types of damage response pathways exist: repair pathways and a tolerance mechanism (Friedberg, 1994). In repair mechanisms the DNA damage is removed, while tolerance mechanisms circumvent the damage without fixing it. Tolerance mechanisms are by definition error-prone. Certain repair mechanisms reverse the DNA damage, for example, removal of adducts from bases and insertion of bases into apurinic/apyrimidinic (AP) sites. An example of direct reversal is provided by the removal of small alkyl groups from the $O^6$ portion of guanine by alkyltransferases. Alkyltransferases directly transfer the alkyl (methyl or ethyl) group from the DNA base guanine to a cysteine acceptor site in the alkyltransferase protein (Pegg and Byers, 1992). In microorganisms, the intracellular concentration of the alkyltransferase protein is regulated by environmental factors, including the concentration of the alkylating agents. A similar adaptation may occur in certain mammalian tissues in response to DNA-damaging agents and treatments that cause an increase in cell proliferation. In mammalian tissues, the level of the alkyltransferase protein is a major factor in the resistance of some cancer cells to certain chemotherapeutic agents. At least for the alkyltransferase reaction, direct reversal of the premutational lesions restores normal base-pairing specificity.

The excisional repair of DNA may involve the removal of damaged bases, mispaired bases, or regions of DNA damage. Distinct pathways are involved in the removal of a single altered base with a relatively low molecular weight adduct (small patch) and the removal of a base with a very large bulky group adducted to it (large patch). Pyrimidines dimerized by ultraviolet light also may be removed by the latter pathway. These two pathways are represented diagrammatically in Fig. 8-13. In the instance of base excision or small-patch repair, enzymes specific for the different types of altered bases have been described in mammalian cells. Such base excisional repair is complemented by the alkyltransferase reaction noted above (Bronstein et al., 1992). In base excision repair, the altered or mispaired base is removed and then there is cleavage of the damaged DNA strand by an AP endonuclease. An exonuclease removes several of the neighboring bases in the cleaved strand with subsequent action of one or more of the DNA polymerases. Finally, the strand is filled in by a DNA ligase, yielding completed, nonadducted double-stranded DNA. However, since DNA polymerases are not absolutely faithful in their replication of the template strand, there is a potential for a mutation to occur in the form of a mispaired base. This possibility is even greater in the nucleotide excision (large patch) repair mechanism, in which a much longer base sequence of more than 20 nucleotides usually is removed after the recognition and demarcation of the DNA lesion (Hoeijmakers and Bootsma, 1994). In this pathway in mammals, the endonuclease step is complex and occurs as a result of the concerted action of a number of proteins (Sancar and Tang, 1993). The existence and characterization of several proteins involved in this step have resulted from studies of patients with mutations in the genes coding for proteins involved in the endonuclease action. This disease—xeroderma pigmentosum—is an autosomal recessive condition in which the patients are very sensitive to and have defects in the repair of DNA damage caused by ultraviolet light. If exposed to sunlight, such patients have a much greater risk of developing skin cancer than do unaffected individuals. This emphasizes the important role of altered DNA repair in the development of neoplasia. After removal of the altered base or dimer and the associated nucleotides, DNA polymerases synthesize the complementary DNA to close the strand gap and ligase completes the formation of the double-stranded DNA. The effectiveness of excisional repair is influenced both by the DNA sequences in immediate proximity to the DNA damage (sequence context) (Horsfall et al., 1990) and by the transcriptional activity of the gene in which the mutation occurs (Scicchitano and Hanawalt, 1992).

While the repair of adducts involves several possible pathways, the repair of either single or double DNA strand breaks is more difficult and as a result more prone to error than is either the excisional or the direct removal pathway. Single-strand breaks may result from a variety of agents and during the repair process itself. Double-strand breaks in DNA are largely the result of ionizing radiation, although even under normal conditions, transient double-strand DNA breaks occur as a result of the normal function of topoisomerases involved in the unwinding of DNA (Eastman and Barry, 1992). Double-strand breaks may occur at sites of single-strand DNA that result from attempts to repair adduction with bulky molecules. Bulky adducts can prevent further polymerase action with subsequent endonuclease cleavage, resulting in double-strand breaks and the potential for the induction of chromosomal aberrations (Kaufmann, 1989). Double-strand breaks and some single-strand breaks are repaired after DNA synthesis by a process termed postreplication repair. The exact mechanisms involved in such repair have not been fully clari-

**Table 8–6**
**Types of DNA Repair**

1. Direct reversal of DNA damage
   Alkyltransferases
2. Base excision repair
   Glycosylase and apurinic/apyrimidinic endonuclease
3. Nucleotide excision repair
   Pyrimidine dimer repair
   "Bulky" adduct repair
4. Recombination: postreplication repair
5. Mismatch repair
   Repair of deamination of 5-methylcytosine

SOURCE: Adapted from Myles and Sancar (1989), with permission.

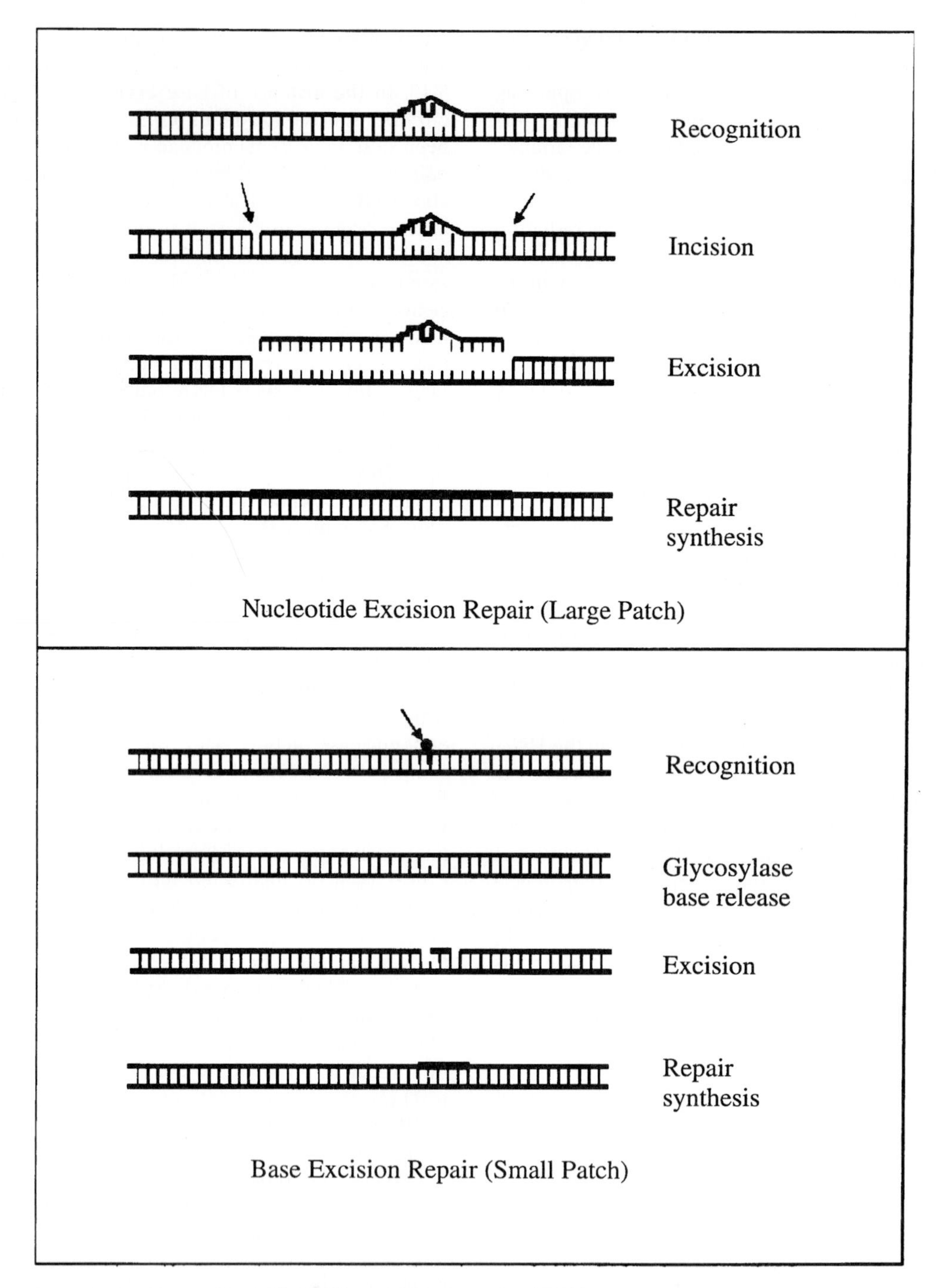


***Figure 8–13. Two major pathways for excisional repair of DNA.***

Both pathways may involve cofactors that make damaged sites accessible to repair enzymes or regulate the repair process. Nucleotide excision repair (acting on dimers, large carcinogen-DNA adducts, etc.) involves the actions of an endonuclease, an exonuclease, polymerase, and ligase for the last three steps, respectively. Base excision repair (action on uracil, alkylated bases, etc.) involves the actions of an *N*-glycosylase, apurinic/apyrimidinic endonuclease, exonuclease, polymerase, and ligase. Nucleotide and base excision pathways may correspond to large patch and small patch excision repair as described by Regan and Setlow (1974).

fied. Recombination and annealing of single strands are steps known to occur during this process (Price, 1993). By an annealing mechanism, the DNA termini at the break are digested by exonuclease until complementary sequences are exposed, at which time annealing and ligation occur. Although this method provides a rapid means of repairing double-strand breaks, deletions are inevitable. An alternative method involves recombination through homologous pairing between the damaged segment of DNA and the duplicate sequence from the second copy of this stretch of the genomic DNA (Figure 8-14). In this instance, DNA repair replication precedes strand exchange, and thus the resolution of the recombination intermediates is possible. Both of these events are quite prone to errors leading both to deletion mutations and to chromosomal abnormalities.

Several processes can induce base mismatches, including DNA polymerase infidelity, formation and/or repair of AP sites, and modification of bases. The deamination of 5-methylcytosine, which converts this base to thymine and therefore induces a G-T mispair or the misincorporation of nucleotides during DNA replication, can result in base pair mismatches. The mispaired thymine formed from the deamination of 5-methylcytosine is removed by a specific DNA glycosylase (Wiebauer et al., 1993), followed by repair via the short patch pathway noted in Fig. 8-13. Deamination of cytosine as well as adenine also can occur. Presumably glycosylases specific for uracil and hypoxanthine, the products of cytosine and adenine deamination, would effect the repair of those lesions. Recently, genes analogous to the bacterial "mutator" genes that repair mismatched bases that can result from DNA replication have been reported, these genes may be important in the hereditary development of colon cancer in humans (Fishel et al., 1993; Karran and Bignami, 1994).

The critical importance of the fidelity of DNA repair in the maintenance of cellular and organismal homeostasis is apparent from this brief discussion. Because induction of DNA repair processes occurs as a response to genetic damage, induction can be used as an endpoint for its detection indirectly. In addition, an increase in repair mechanisms above constitutive levels can increase the magnitude of the genotoxic insult. The relative importance of DNA repair in understanding the mechanisms of chemical carcinogenesis is most apparent in relating DNA damage and repair to DNA synthesis and cell replication. This is required to exceed the intrinsic capacity of a cell to repair this damage.

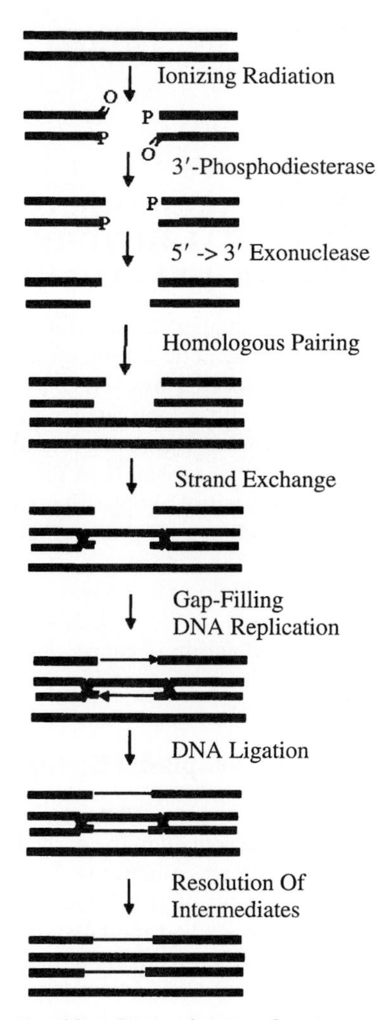


***Figure 8–14. Possible scheme of postreplication repair of double-strand breaks in DNA.***

The model shown is for stretches of DNA lacking direct repeats. This includes most of the sequences that encode proteins. Correction of the damage is carried out by the double-strand break repair pathway, as shown. After a double-strand break by ionizing radiation or some chemical action, the altered residues at the 3′ termini are first excised by a 3′-phosphodiesterase. Then the double-strand gap is extended on both strands by a magnesium-dependent 5′→3′ exonuclease. Homologous sequences from the two chromosomal copies of the gene are paired, and strand exchange, DNA replication, DNA ligation, and resolution of intermediates follow in sequence. [After Price (1993), with permission of the author and publisher.]

## DNA Repair, Cell Replication, and Chemical Carcinogenesis

The persistence of DNA adducts in relation to the development of neoplasia in specific tissues (Table 8-5) and differences in the repair of the adducts are critical factors in chemical carcinogenesis. The removal of methyl, ethyl, and similar small alkyl radicals from individual bases is to a great extent dependent on the presence of alkyltransferases (see above). While in some tissues, such as liver, it may be possible to increase the level of such enzymes in response to damage and hormonal or other influences, many tissues do not have inducible repair mechanisms. Furthermore, some adducts are extremely difficult, if not impossible, for a cell to repair. An example of such a lesion, the 3-(deoxyguanosine)-$N^2$-yl)-acetylaminofluorene adduct first described by Kriek and associates (Westra et al., 1976), is depicted in Fig. 8-9. This may in part account for the relatively wide spectrum of neoplasms inducible by this chemical carcinogen.

Of equal importance is the continuous damage to DNA that occurs in cells as a result of ambient mutagens, radiation, and endogenous processes including oxidation, methylation, deamination, and depurination. DNA damage induced by oxidative reactions (oxidative stress) is probably the source of most endogenous DNA damage. Ames and associates (1993) estimated that the individual reactive "hits" in DNA per cell per day are of the order of $10^5$ in rats and $10^4$ in humans as a result of endogenous oxidative reaction. Such reactions can produce alkylation through peroxidative reactions such as those described in Fig. 8-7 or hydroxylation of bases and single-strand breaks (Fig. 8-12). The end product of oxidative damage to DNA can also be interstrand cross-links and double-strand breaks (Demple and Harrison, 1994) with the potential for subsequent major genetic damage noted below. A more complete listing of the estimates of endogenous DNA

**Table 8–7**
**Estimates of Endogenous DNA Damage and Repair Processes in Human Cells in Vivo**

| TYPE OF DAMAGE | ESTIMATED OCCURRENCES OF DAMAGE PER HOUR PER CELL | MAXIMAL REPAIR RATE, BASE PAIRS PER HOUR PER CELL |
|---|---|---|
| Depurination | 1000 | $10^4$ |
| Depyrimidination | 55 | $10^4$ |
| Cytosine deamination | 15 | $10^4$ |
| Single-stranded breaks | 5000 | $2 \times 10^5$ |
| $N^7$-methylguanine | 3500 | Not reported |
| $O^6$-methylguanine | 130 | $10^4$ |
| Oxidation products | 120 | $10^5$ |

SOURCE: Modified from data from the National Academy of Science (1989).

damage and repair processes in humans is given in Table 8-7. The data in this table emphasize the considerable degree and significant variation in types of DNA damage and repair that occur in each cell of the organism at a molecular level.

Experimental studies in mammalian cells have demonstrated that active oxygen radicals may contribute to clastogenesis directly (Ochi and Kaneko, 1989) and indirectly through the production of lipid peroxides (Emerit et al., 1991). While methods for the repair of some types of oxidative damage, including base hydroxylation (Bessho et al., 1993) and single-strand breaks (Satoh and Lindahl, 1994), exist, such repair requires time and may be dependent on many other intracellular factors. Because the formation of a mutation occurs during the synthesis of a new DNA strand through the use of the damaged template, cell replication becomes an important factor in the "fixation" of a mutation. The importance of the rate of cell division and DNA synthesis in carcinogenesis has been emphasized by several authors (Ames et al., 1993; Butterworth, 1991; Cohen and Ellwein, 1991). Thus, while many DNA repair mechanisms may not be abnormal in neoplastic cells compared with their normal counterpart, a high rate of cell division tends to enhance both the spontaneous level and the induced level of mutation through the chance inability of a cell to repair damage before DNA synthesis. An important pathway of DNA repair that is genetically defective in a number of hereditary and spontaneous neoplasms in humans (Umar et al., 1994) is the mismatch repair mechanism that corrects spontaneous and post-replicative base alterations and thus is an important pathway for the avoidance of mutation in normal cells. Genetic defects in mismatch repair mechanisms lead to microsatellite DNA and instability with subsequent alteration in the stabilization of the genome (Modrich, 1994). Enhanced mitogenesis also may trigger more dramatic genetic alterations, including mitotic recombination, gene conversion, and nondisjunction. These genetic changes result in further progressive genetic alterations that have a high likelihood of resulting in cancer. The types of mutational events, the numbers of such mutations, and the cellular responses to them thus become important factors in our understanding of the mechanisms of chemical carcinogenesis.

## CHEMICAL CARCINOGENS AND THE NATURAL HISTORY OF NEOPLASTIC DEVELOPMENT

A number of chemicals can alter the structure of the genome and/or the expression of genetic information with the subsequent appearance of cancer. However, cancer as a disease usually develops slowly, with a long latency period between the first exposure to a chemical carcinogen and the ultimate development of malignant neoplasia. Thus, the process of carcinogenesis (the pathogenesis of neoplasia) involves a variety of biological changes which to a great extent reflect the structural and functional alterations in the genome of the affected cell. However, when the biological changes occurring during carcinogenesis are assessed at the molecular level, a better understanding of the mechanisms of cancer development may be generated.

### The Pathogenesis of Neoplasia: Biology

Although morphological changes occurring during the early stages of neoplasia were described in the early decades of this century, not until the 1940s was a better understanding of the biological changes that occur after carcinogen exposure obtained. The first and best studied model system was mouse skin carcinogenesis. The early investigations of Rous and Kidd (1941), Mottram (1944), and Berenblum and Shubik (1947) used the development of benign papillomas as an endpoint for studies of epidermal carcinogenesis in mouse skin induced by polycyclic hydrocarbons. These investigators coined the term "initiation" to designate the initial alteration in individual cells within the tissue resulting from a single subcarcinogenic dose of a chemical carcinogen. In these circumstances, papillomas were obtained only with subsequent chronic, multiple doses of a second agent that by itself was essentially noncarcinogenic. This latter "stage" was termed "promotion." Subsequent studies of a mammary adenocarcinoma model in the mouse led to the proposal that processes subsequent to initiation constitute a stage termed "progression" (Foulds, 1954). Foulds's description of this stage emphasized changes characteristic of malignant neoplasia and its evolution to higher degrees of autonomy.

During the last two decades, these investigations have been extended to a variety of tissue systems and to humans (Pitot, in press). At present the pathogenesis of neoplasia is felt to consist of at least three operationally defined stages beginning with initiation and followed by an intermediate stage of promotion, from which evolves the stage of progression. The third stage exhibits many of the characteristics described by Foulds. The biological characteristics of the stages of initiation, promotion, and progression are listed in Table 8-8 (Pitot and Dragan, 1994; Boyd and Barrett, 1990; Harris, 1991). It is in the first and last stages of neoplastic development—initiation and progression—that structural changes in the genome (DNA) can be observed. The structural changes discussed previously are most likely to be involved in the induction of these stages, especially the stage of initiation (Figs. 8-8 and 8-9). The intermediate stage of promotion does not appear to involve direct structural changes in the genome of the cell but instead depends on an altered expression of genes.

**Initiation.** Until recently, the stage of initiation had been characterized and quantitated well after the process of carcinogenesis had begun. As with mutational events (see above), initiation requires one or more rounds of cell division for the "fixation" of the process (Kakunaga, 1975; Columbano et al., 1981). The quantitative parameters of initiation noted in Table 8-8—dose response and relative potency—have been demonstrated in a variety of experimental systems (Pitot et al., 1987; Dragan et al., 1994); however, these parameters may be modulated by alteration of xenobiotic metabolism (Talalay et al., 1988) and by trophic hormones (Liao et al., 1993). The metabolism of initiating agents to nonreactive forms and the high efficiency of DNA repair of tissue can alter the process of initiation.

One of the characteristics of the stage of initiation is its irreversibility in the sense that the genotype and or phenotype of the initiated cell is established at the time of initiation; there is accumulating evidence that not all initiated cells survive over the life span of the organism or the period of an experiment. Their demise appears to be due to the normal process of programmed cell death, or apoptosis (Wyllie, 1987).

Spontaneous preneoplastic lesions have been described in a number of experimental systems (Maekawa and Mitsumori, 1990; Pretlow, 1994) as well as in humans (Dunham, 1972; Pretlow, 1994; Pretlow et al., 1993). Thus, it would appear that the spontaneous or fortuitous initiation of cells in a variety of tissues is a very common occurrence. If this is true, the development of neoplasia can be a function solely of the action of agents at the stages of promotion and/or progression.

**Promotion.** As in the stage of initiation, a variety of chemicals have been shown to induce promotion. However, unlike chemicals that induce the stage of initiation, there is no evidence that promoting agents or their metabolites directly interact with DNA or that metabolism is required for their effectiveness. Figure 8-15 shows some representative structures of various promoting agents. Tetradecanoyl phorbol acetate (TPA) is a naturally occurring alicyclic chemical that is the active ingredient of croton oil, a promoting agent used for the promotion of mouse skin tumors. Saccharin is an effective promoting agent for the bladder, and phenobarbital is an ef-

**Table 8–8**
**Morphological and Biological Characteristics of the Stages of Initiation, Promotion, and Progression During Carcinogenesis**

| INITIATION | PROMOTION | PROGRESSION |
|---|---|---|
| Irreversible | Operationally reversible both at the level of gene expression and at the cellular level | Irreversible |
| Initiated "stem cell" not morphologically identifiable | | Morphologically discernible alteration in cellular genomic structure resulting from karyotypic instability |
| Efficiency sensitive to xenobiotic and other chemical factors | Promoted cell population existence dependent on continued administration of promoting agent | |
| Spontaneous (endogenous) occurrence of initiated cells | Efficiency sensitive to aging and dietary and hormonal factors | Growth of altered cells sensitive to environmental factors during early phase of this stage |
| | Endogenous promoting agents may effect "spontaneous" promotion | |
| Requirement for cell division for "fixation" | | |
| Dose-response not exhibiting a readily measurable threshold | Dose response exhibits measurable threshold and maximal effect | Benign or malignant neoplasms observed in this stage |
| Relative potency of initiators dependent on quantitation of preneoplastic lesions after defined period of promotion | Relative potency of promoters measured by their effectiveness in causing an expansion of the initiated cell population | "Progressor" agents advance promoted cells into this stage |

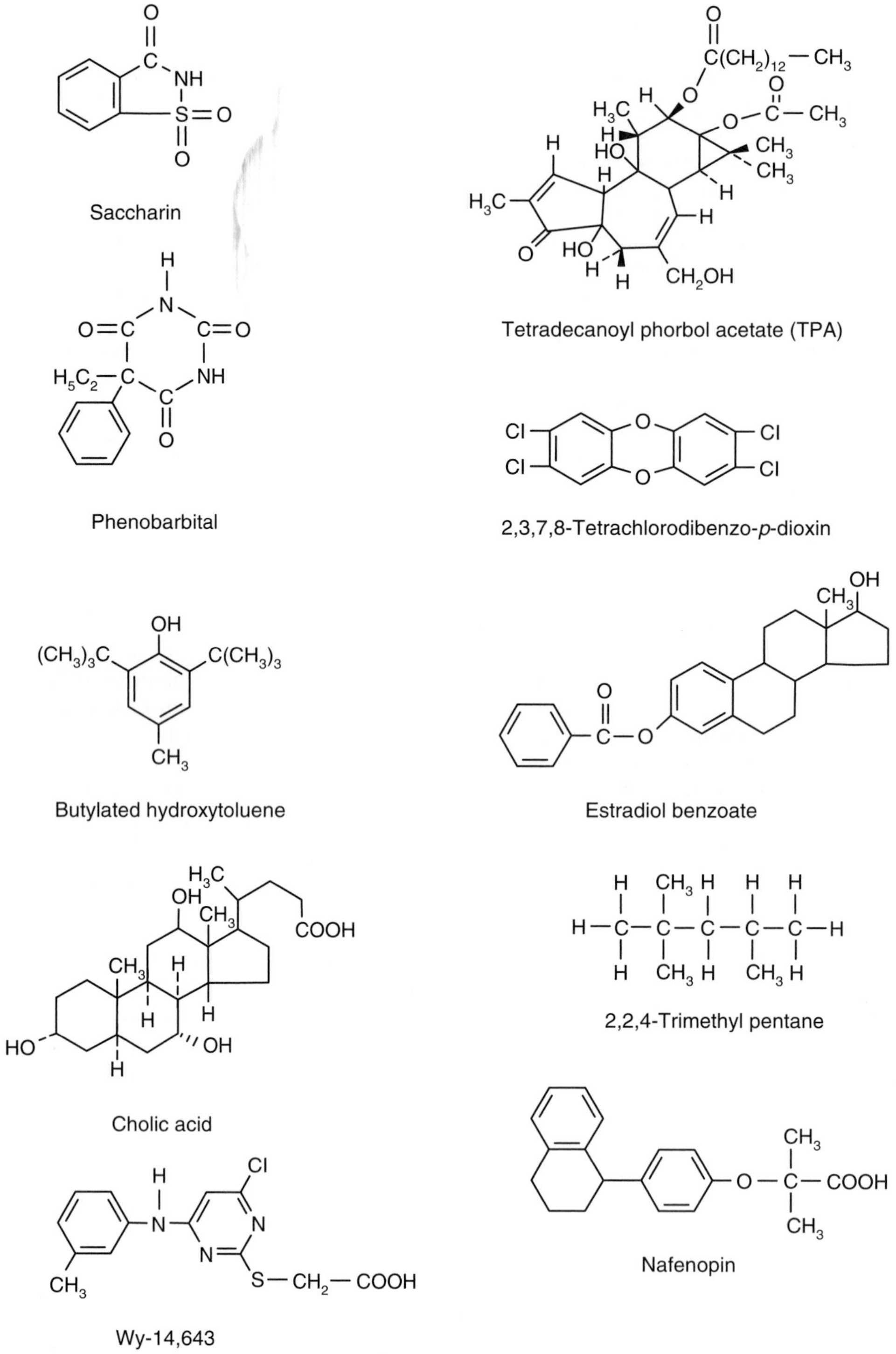

Saccharin

Tetradecanoyl phorbol acetate (TPA)

Phenobarbital

2,3,7,8-Tetrachlorodibenzo-*p*-dioxin

Butylated hydroxytoluene

Estradiol benzoate

Cholic acid

2,2,4-Trimethyl pentane

Nafenopin

Wy-14,643

***Figure 8–15. Structures of representative promoting agents.***

fective promoting agent for hepatocarcinogenesis. 2,3,7,8-Tetrachlorodibenzo-*p*-dioxin (TCDD) is probably the most effective promoting agent known for rat liver carcinogenesis but is also effective in the lung and skin. Estradiol is shown as a representative of endogenous hormones that are effective promoting agents. Both androgens and estrogens, natural and synthetic, are effective promoting agents in their target end organs as well as in the liver (Taper, 1978; Sumi et al., 1980; Kemp, 1989). Cholic acid enhances preneoplastic and neoplastic lesions in the rat colon (Magnuson et al., 1993), whereas 2,2,4-trimethylpentane and unleaded gasoline effectively promote renal tubular cell tumors in rats (Short et al., 1989). The final two structures noted—Wy-14,643 and Nafenopin—are two members of the large class of carcinogenic peroxisome proliferators that induce the synthesis of peroxisomes in liver, are effective promoting agents, and induce hepatic neoplasms on long-term administration at high doses to rodents (Reddy and Lalwani, 1983). Many other agents including polypeptide hormones (see above), dietary factors including total calories, many other halogenated hydrocarbons, and numerous other chemicals have been found to enhance the development of preneoplastic and neoplastic lesions in one or more systems of carcinogenesis, including the human system.

The distinctive characteristic of promotion as opposed to initiation or progression is the reversible nature of this stage (Pitot and Dragan, in press) (Table 8-6). Boutwell (1964) first demonstrated that when the frequency of application of the promoting agent was decreased after initiation in mouse skin there was a lower yield of papillomas in comparison with that obtained by a more frequent application of the promoting agent. Other investigators (Andrews, 1971; Burns et al., 1978) later demonstrated that papillomas developing during promotion in mouse epidermal carcinogenesis regress in large numbers both on removal of the promoting agent and during its continued application. The regression of preneoplastic lesions after withdrawal of the promoting agents may be due to apoptosis (Schulte-Hermann et al., 1990). This proposed mechanism is supported by the demonstration that many promoting agents inhibit apoptosis in preneoplastic lesions (Schulte-Hermann et al., 1993; Wright et al., 1994). Another potential pathway of this operational reversibility is "redifferentiation" or remodeling (Tatematsu et al., 1983). Thus, cells in the stage of promotion are dependent on continued administration of the promoting agent (Hanigan and Pitot, 1985), as was implied by the early studies of Furth (1959) on hormonally dependent neoplasia.

Another characteristic of the stage of promotion is its susceptibility to modulation by physiological factors. The stage of promotion may be modulated by the aging process (Van Duuren et al., 1975, and by dietary and hormonal factors (Sivak, 1979). Glauert and associates (1986) demonstrated that promotion of hepatocarcinogenesis was less effective in rats fed a semisynthetic diet than in those fed a crude, cereal-based diet. The promotion stage of chemically induced rat mammary cancer also is modulated by dietary (Cohen et al., 1991) and hormonal (Carter et al., 1988) factors. Many modulating factors are themselves promoting agents. Several hormones can be carcinogenic. These hormones are effective promoting agents and thus may serve as an exogenous or endogenous source for the modulation of cell proliferation during carcinogenesis (Pitot, 1991). Such physiological agents may be one component of the endogenous promotion of initiated cells.

The dose-response relationships of promoting agents exhibit sigmoidlike curves with an observable threshold and a maximal effect. Such relationships are depicted in Fig. 8-16, in which the dose-response curve for the binding of the phorbol TPA with its receptor is compared with a dose-response curve for the TPA promotion of dimethylbenzanthracene-initiated papillomas in mouse skin (Ashendel, 1985; Verma and Boutwell, 1980). The threshold effect of promoting agents may be considered a consequence of the reversible nature of their effects at the cellular level (see above). The maximal effect is due to a saturation of ligand binding in the former case and to the promotion of all initiated cells in the latter (Fig. 8-16). Although one may not directly equate the variables in the two processes, the similarity in the shapes of the curves is striking (Fig. 8-16). The relative potency of promoting agents may be

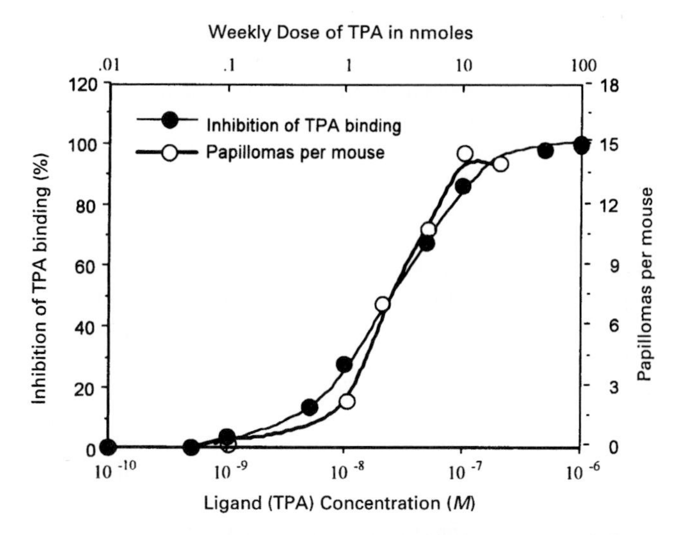


***Figure 8–16. Composite showing the specific interaction of the receptor for phorbol esters with its ligand determined as the inhibition of radioactive TPA binding (closed circles).***

The tumor response expressed as papillomas per mouse on mice initiated with dimethylbenzanthracene and promoted with various weekly doses of TPA is noted in the open circles. [Composite graph from data of Ashendel (1985) and Verma and Boutwell (1980) as published in Pitot (1986a).]

determined as a function of their ability to induce the clonal growth of initiated cells. Thus, the net rate of growth of preneoplastic lesions can be employed to determine the relative potencies of promoting agents (Pitot et al., 1987).

The format of an experimental protocol for the demonstration of initiation and promotion is shown in Fig. 8-17. As noted in the figure, the endpoint of the study, which usually takes from 3 to 6 months, depends on the tissue under investigation, the dose and nature of the initiating and promoting agents utilized, and factors, such as diet and hormonal status, that were mentioned above. The endpoint analyzed in such studies is properly a preneoplastic lesion (PNL) that develops clonally from initiated cells in the tissue under study. These are altered hepatic foci in the rat or mouse liver (Pitot, 1990), epidermal papillomas in mouse skin (Wigley, 1983), hyperplasia of terminal end buds in rat mammary carcinomas (Purnell, 1980; Russo et al., 1983), and aberrant crypts in rat colon carcinogenesis (Pretlow et al., 1993). Administration of

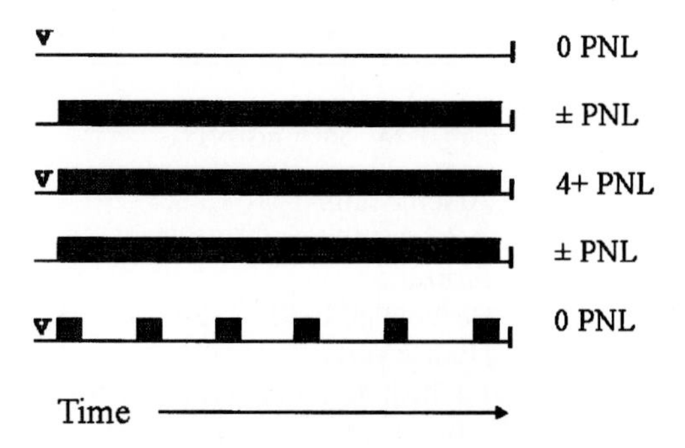


***Figure 8–17. General experimental format demonstrating initiation (v) and promotion (▬) for use in carcinogenesis studies of rodent tissues. PNL = preneoplastic lesions.***

the promoting agent for the entire period of the experiment after initiation results in many preneoplastic lesions, whereas alteration of the format of administration of the promoting agent results in the development of very few preneoplastic lesions. This reinforces the fact that the stage of promotion is operationally reversible (Boutwell, 1964) and indicates that a threshold dose effect level may exist.

**Progression.** The transition from the early progeny of initiated cells to the biologically malignant cell population constitutes the major part of the natural history of neoplastic development. Foulds recognized the importance of the development of neoplasia beyond the appearance of any initial identifiable lesions (Foulds, 1965). The characteristics of malignant progression that Foulds observed—growth rate, invasiveness, metastatic frequency, hormonal responsiveness, and morphological characteristics—vary independently as the disease develops. These characteristics have been ascribed to karyotypic instability during the irreversible progression stage. Environmental alterations can influence the stage of progression. For example, exposure to promoting agents can alter gene expression and induce cell proliferation. However, as the growth of the neoplasm continues and karyotypic instability evolves, responses to environmental factors may be altered or lost (Noble, 1977; Welch and Tomasovic, 1985). Agents that act only to effect the transition of a cell from the stage of promotion to that of progression may properly be termed *progressor agents*. Some examples are listed in Table 8-9. Such agents presumably have the characteristic of inducing chromosomal aberrations, may not necessarily be capable of initiation, and in some cases may enhance the clastogenesis associated with evolving karyotypic instability. Mechanisms during progression that may contribute to the evolving karyotypic instability include the inhibition of DNA repair (Fornace et al., 1980), including topoisomerase activity (Cortés et al., 1993), gene amplification (Ottaggio et al., 1993), and altered telomere integrity (Ledbetter, 1992). As with the two stages of initiation and promotion, spontaneous progression also may occur. In fact, spontaneous progression would be greatly fostered by increased cell replication (Ames et al., 1993).

The experimental demonstration of the stage of progression is somewhat more complex than that of initiation and promotion. Figure 8-18 shows a general experimental format designed to demonstrate the effect of the administration of a progressor agent after a course of initiation and promotion with all the appropriate controls. However, in this instance the endpoint that is quantitated is the number of neoplastic lesions (NL). In experimental systems, the most effective development of neoplasia involves the continued administration of the promoting agent even after the administration of the progressor agent. This might be expected because cells early in the stage of progression respond to promoting agents, increasing the yield of neoplastic lesions in the experimental system (Table 8-8). As was noted, a lower yield that usually is still significant may be obtained without additional administration of the promoting agent. Because of the duration of the experiments, preneoplastic lesions occur to varying degrees in each of the experimental groups. The difficulty in such studies is the quantitation of the neoplastic lesions, usually carried out by determining the number, incidence, and multiplicity of malignant tumors. However, premalignant lesions in the stage of progression occur stochastically (Henson and Albores-Saavedra, 1986), and thus the appropriate endpoint is the quantitation of such lesions. This has been extremely difficult to do, and thus quantitative analyses of the effects of progressor agents remain crude.

## Cellular and Molecular Mechanisms of the Stages of Carcinogenesis

Although the descriptive and morphological characteristics of the stages of carcinogenesis are critical to our initial understanding of the pathogenesis of neoplasia, a complete knowledge of the molecular mechanisms of carcinogenesis may be necessary to control the disease through rational therapy, earlier diagnosis, and reasonable methods of prevention. However, our understanding of the molecular mechanisms of carcinogenesis is incomplete. Nonetheless, there has been an exponential explosion of knowledge in this area during the past decade.

**Initiation.** While the morphological and biological characterization of the stage of initiation has been somewhat limited, mechanistic studies of this stage have been more extensively reported. This is strikingly true in relation to the metabolic activation of chemical carcinogens and the structure of their

**Table 8–9**
**Putative Progressor Agents in Carcinogenesis**

| AGENT | INITIATING ACTIVITY | CLASTOGENIC ACTIVITY | CARCINOGENIC ACTIVITY |
|---|---|---|---|
| Arsenic salts | — | + | + |
| Asbestos fibers | ? | + | + |
| Benzene | — | + | + |
| Benzoyl peroxide | — | + | ± |
| Hydroxyurea | — | + | ± |
| 1,4-Bis[2-(3,5-dichloropyridyloxy)]-benzene | — | + | + |
| 2,5,2′,5′-Tetrachlorobiphenyl | — | + | ± |

SOURCE: Modified from Pitot and Dragan (1994).

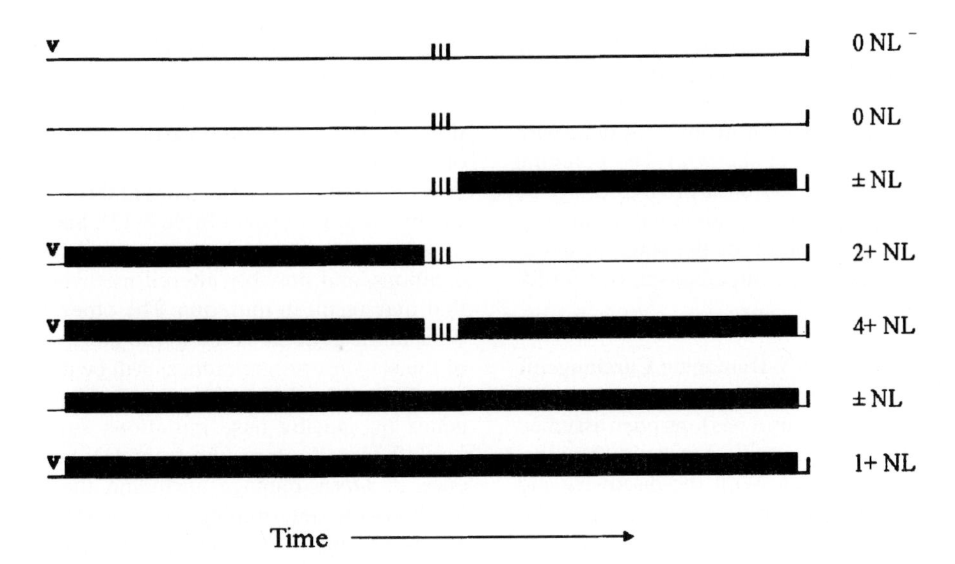


*Figure 8–18. General experimental format for demonstration of the stage of progression and the effect of progressor agents in experimental systems.*

NL = neoplastic lesions; ± = occasional or infrequent; 1+ = few; 2+ = some; 4+ = many; **III** = administration of progressor agent as single or several multiple doses; **v** = initiation; ▬ = promoting agent doses.

DNA adducts. As was indicated earlier, however, the molecular mechanisms of initiation must conform to the observable biological characteristics of this stage. At least three processes are important in initiation: metabolism, DNA repair, and cell proliferation. Perturbation of any of these pathways will have an impact on initiation. Initiated cells are difficult to distinguish morphologically and phenotypically from their normal counterparts, and the molecular alterations responsible for initiation may be equally subtle. Table 8-10 lists a number of the molecular mechanistic characteristics of the stages of initiation, promotion, and progression. As was already indicated, initiating agents or their metabolites are mutagenic to DNA. Thus, carcinogenic agents administered at doses that do not induce neoplasia (incomplete carcinogenesis) are capable of initiating cells in experimental models of multistage carcinogenesis (Boutwell, 1964; Dragan et al., 1994). Furthermore, such subcarcinogenic doses of initiating agents may induce substantial DNA alkylation (Pegg and Perry, 1981; Brambilla et al., 1983; Ward, 1987). The genetic changes necessary to induce the stage of initiation need not be those which cause obvious or gross structural chromosomal alterations. Sargent and colleagues (1989) demonstrated normal karyotypes in

**Table 8–10**
**Some Cellular and Molecular Mechanisms in Multistage Carcinogenesis**

| INITIATION | PROMOTION | PROGRESSION |
|---|---|---|
| Simple mutations (transitions, transversions, small deletions, etc.) involving the cellular genome | Reversible enhancement or repression of gene expression mediated via receptors specific for the individual promoting agent | Complex genetic alterations (chromosomal translocations, deletions, gene amplification, recombination, etc.) resulting from evolving karyotypic instability |
| In some species and tissues, point mutations in protooncogenes and/or potential cellular oncogenes | Inhibition of apoptosis by promoting agent | Irreversible changes in gene expression, including fetal gene expression, altered major histocompatibility complex (MHC) gene expression, and ectopic hormone production |
| Mutations in genes of signal transduction pathways that may result in an altered phenotype | No direct structural alteration in DNA from action or metabolism of promoting agent | Selection of neoplastic cells for optimal growth genotype/phenotype in response to the cellular environment and including the evolution of karyotypic instability |

SOURCE: After Pitot (1993a).

cells from altered hepatic foci in the stage of promotion in the rat. A number of investigations have demonstrated specific point mutations in genes that are compatible with those induced in vitro by the adducts resulting from treatment with carcinogenic chemicals (Anderson et al., 1992). The potential genetic targets for initiating agents as well as progressor agents have been elucidated to some extent. Individual variability, species differences, and organotropism of the stage of initiation involve a balance of carcinogen metabolism, cell proliferation, and DNA repair.

**Molecular Genetic Targets of DNA-Damaging Carcinogenic Agents.** Although many genes are affected by the mutagenic action of certain chemical carcinogens, it has long been assumed that mutations in a relatively few specific genes may be most critical to neoplastic transformation. With the discovery and elucidation of the function of viral oncogenes (Bishop, 1985) and their cellular counterparts, proto-oncogenes (Garrett, 1986), the original assumption moved closer to reality. Three different classes of genes have been described that play major roles in the neoplastic process (Table 8-11). Although a variety of other genes involved in DNA repair (Friedberg et al., 1985; Jass et al., 1994), carcinogen metabolism (Nebert, 1991), and abnormalities in the immune system (Müller, 1990) generate inherited predispositions to the development of neoplasia, it is the products of the proto-oncogenes and cellular oncogenes and the tumor suppressor genes that have been most closely associated with neoplastic transformation (Table 8-11).

Table 8-12 shows a listing of a number of functions of proto-oncogenes and cellular oncogenes and tumor suppressor genes, with specific examples and their localization in the cell where known. It is immediately obvious that the oncogenes are involved primarily in cellular growth, signal transduction, and nuclear transcription. Interestingly, similar functions are attributed to known tumor suppressor genes, but in addition, at least two tumor suppressor genes are involved in regulation of the cell cycle. This table is not meant to be all inclusive, and interested readers are referred to recent reviews and texts for a more detailed discussion of these genes and their products (Hunter, 1991; Levine, 1993).

Mutations in proto-oncogenes can result in their activation with subsequent neoplastic transformation similar to that observed after the altered expression of cellular oncogenes. Activation of proto-oncogenes and cellular oncogenes can occur by various means (Table 8-13). Scrutiny of these mechanisms suggests that only point mutations, small insertions and deletions, and possibly altered methylation status are events that may result in initiation. The other, more complex alterations in the genome listed in the table would be characteristic of the stage of progression, as will be discussed below.

The activation of proto-oncogenes and cellular oncogenes by specific base mutations, small deletions, and frameshift mutations results from DNA synthesis in the presence of DNA damage, including the presence of adducts. Methods for determining such alterations in specimens that consist of only a few hundred or a thousand cells have been available only during the last decade (Mies, 1994). The analysis of mutations in specific genes potentially involved in the neoplastic transformation is possible from very small samples by various molecular techniques.

The *ras* genes code for guanosine triphosphatases, which function as molecular switches for signal transduction pathways involved in the control of growth, differentiation, and other cellular functions (Hall, 1994). Table 8-14 lists a number of examples in rodent tissues of specific mutation in two of the *ras* genes, the Ha-*ras* proto-oncogene, and the Ki-*ras* cellular oncogene. With the exception of mouse skin, the frequency of such mutations in preneoplastic lesions in experimental animals in the stage of promotion is about 20 to 60 percent. In instances of multistage carcinogenesis in mouse skin, the frequency increases to nearly 100 percent (Bailleul et al., 1989). In general, the mutations noted are those which theoretically could result from DNA adducts formed by the particular carcinogen. Interestingly, spontaneously occurring neoplasms in mice also exhibit a significant incidence of point mutations in *ras* proto-oncogenes and cellular oncogenes (Rumsby et al.,

**Table 8–11**
**Characteristics of Proto-Oncogenes, Cellular Oncogenes, and Tumor Suppressor Genes**

| PROTO-ONCOGENES | CELLULAR ONCOGENES | TUMOR SUPPRESSOR GENES |
|---|---|---|
| Dominant | Dominant | Recessive |
| Broad tissue specificity for cancer development | Broad tissue specificity for cancer development | Considerable tissue specificity for cancer development |
| Germline inheritance rarely involved in cancer development | Germline inheritance rarely involved in cancer development | Germline inheritance frequently involved in cancer development |
| Analogous to certain viral oncogenes | No known analogues in oncogenic viruses | No known analogues in oncogenic viruses |
| Somatic mutations activated during all stages of neoplastic development | Somatic mutations activated during all stages of neoplastic development | Germline mutations may initiate, but mutation to neoplasia occurs only during stage of progression |

SOURCE: After Pitot (1993b).

**Table 8–12**
**Functions of Representative Oncogenes and Tumor Suppressor Genes**

| *A. Oncogenes* | | |
|---|---|---|
| FUNCTIONS OF GENE PRODUCT | GENES | CELL LOCALIZATION |
| Growth factors | *sis, fgf* | Extracellular |
| Receptor/protein tyrosine kinases | *met, neu* | Extra cell/cell membrane |
| Protein tyrosine kinases | *src, ret* | Cell membrane/cytoplasmic |
| Membrane-associated G proteins | *ras, gip-2* | Cell membrane/cytoplasmic |
| Cytoplasmic protein serine kinases | *raf, pim-1* | Cytoplasmic |
| Nuclear transcription factors | *myc, fos, jun* | Nuclear |
| Unknown, undetermined | *bcl-2, crk* | Mitochondrial, cytoplasmic |

| *B. Tumor suppressor genes* | | |
|---|---|---|
| FUNCTIONS OF GENE PRODUCT | GENES | CELL LOCALIZATION |
| GTPase activation | NF1 | Cell membrane/cytoplasmic |
| Cell cycle–regulated nuclear transcriptional repressor | RB-1 | Nuclear |
| Cell cycle–regulated nuclear transcription factor | p53 | Nuclear |
| Zinc finger transcription factor | WT1 | Nuclear |
| Mismatch DNA repair | hMLH1 | Nuclear |
| Zinc finger transcription factor (?) | BRCA1 | Unknown |

SOURCE: Part A was modified from Hunter (1991). Information for part B was obtained from Levine (1993) as well as Papadopoulos et al. (1994) and Bronner et al. (1994), while that for BRCA1 was obtained from Miki et al. (1994) and Futreal et al. (1994).

1991; Candrian et al., 1991), but neoplasms in corresponding tissues in other species do not necessarily exhibit activating mutations in proto-oncogenes or cellular oncogenes (Tokusashi et al., 1994; Kakiuchi et al., 1993; Schaeffer et al., 1990). In addition, mutated *ras* genes have been described in normal-appearing mouse skin after dimethylbenz(*a*)anthracene (DMBA) or urethane application (Nelson et al., 1992). By contrast, Cha and associates (1994) recently reported that a very high percentage of untreated rats contained detectable levels of Ha-*ras* mutations in normal mammary tissue. Thus,

**Table 8–13**
**Potential Mechanisms of Oncogene Activation**

| EVENT | CONSEQUENCE | EXAMPLES |
|---|---|---|
| Base mutation in coding sequences | New gene product with altered activity | v-*onc* genes, bladder carcinoma |
| Deletion in noncoding sequences | Altered regulation of normal gene product | Fibroblast transformation in vitro |
| Altered promoter for RNA polymerase | Increased transcription of mRNA (normal gene product) | Cell transformation in vitro, lymphoma in chickens |
| Insertion or substitution with repetitive DNA elements ("transposons") | Altered regulation of gene product (? normal) | Canine venereal tumor, mouse myeloma |
| Chromosomal translocation | Altered mRNA, new gene product (?), no altered regulation of gene expression | Burkitt's lymphoma in humans, mouse plasmacytoma |
| Gene amplification | Increased expression of normal gene | Human colon carcinoma, human bladder carcinoma |
| Hypomethylation of c-*onc* gene | Altered regulation of gene expression (?), normal gene product | Human colon and lung cancer |

SOURCE: Adapted from Pitot (1986b).

**Table 8–14**
**Mutational Activation of *ras* Oncogenes during the Stages of Initiation and Promotion**

| SPECIES/ TISSUE | CARCINOGEN | LESION | GENE/MUTATION* | FREQUENCY† | REFERENCE |
|---|---|---|---|---|---|
| Rat/colon | Azoxymethane | Aberrant crypt foci | K-*ras*/G→A/12 | 5/16 | Shivapurkar et al., 1994 |
| Mouse/liver | Diethylnitrosamine | G6Pase⁻ foci | Ha-*ras*/C→A/61 A→G | 12/127 | Bauer-Hofmann et al., 1992 |
| Mouse/lung | Urethane | Small adenomas | Ki-*ras*/A→G/61 A→T | 32/100 | Nuzum et al., 1990 |
| Rat/mammary gland | *N*-methyl-*N*-nitrosourea | Initiated cell clones | H-*ras*/G→A/12 | 17% | Zhang et al., 1991 |
| Hamster/ pancreas | *N*-nitroso-bis (2-oxopropyl)-amine | Papillary hyperplasia | K-*ras*/G→A/12 | 12/26 | Cerny et al., 1992 |
| Mouse/skin | DMBA/TPA | Papilloma | Ha-*ras*/A→T/61 | 12/14 | Quintanilla et al., 1986 |

*The numbers in this column refer to the codon position in the cDNA (mRNA) of the gene product.
†The numerator indicates the number of animals exhibiting the mutation; the denominator refers to the total number of animals studied.

the mutations seen in neoplasms in untreated animals may result from the selective proliferation of cells containing preexisting mutations.

Thus, while several classes of genes appear to be appropriate as targets for DNA-damaging carcinogens, the actual role of proto-oncogene and cellular oncogene mutations in establishing carcinogenesis is not entirely clear. Among the earliest preneoplastic lesions studied (Table 8-13), only about one-third exhibit mutations in the *ras* gene family, but it is quite possible that other proto-oncogenes and cellular oncogenes are targets. Evidence that tumor suppressor genes may be targets for the initiation of early malignant development come largely from studies of genetically inherited neoplasia. In these rare hereditary cancers, one of the alleles of a tumor suppressor gene contains a germline mutation in all the cells of the organism (Paraskeva and Williams, 1992; Knudson, 1993).

**Promotion.** Boutwell (1974) was the first to propose the theory that promoting agents may induce their effects through their ability to alter gene expression. During the past decade, our understanding of mechanisms involving the alteration of gene expression by environmental agents has increased exponentially (Morley and Thomas, 1991; Rosenthal, 1994). The regulation of genetic information is mediated through recognition of the environmental effector, hormone, promoting agent, drug, and so on, and their specific molecular interaction with either a surface or a cytosolic receptor. Several types of receptors exist in cells (Mayer, 1994; Pawson, 1993; Strader et al., 1994). Plasma membrane receptors may possess a tyrosine protein kinase domain on the intracellular region, while others have multiple transmembrane domains with the intracellular signal being transduced through G proteins and cyclic nucleotides (Mayer, 1994). The other general type of receptor mechanism involves a cytosolic receptor that interacts with the ligand (usually lipid-soluble) that has diffused through the plasma membrane. The ligand-receptor complex then travels to the nucleus before interacting directly with specific DNA sequences known as response elements.

Promoting agents exert their effects on gene expression primarily through perturbation of the signal transduction pathways, as indicated in Fig. 8-19. Table 8-15 lists some of the best studied promoting agents known to be effectors in signal transduction pathways. Thus, the mechanism of action of promoting agents in altering gene expression may be mediated through specific receptors. This hypothesis provides a partial explanation of the tissue specificity demonstrated by many promoting agents. The receptor-ligand concept of promoting agent action is based on dose-response relationships involving pharmacological agents. The basic assumptions of such interactions argue that the effect of the agent is directly proportional to the number of receptors occupied by the ligand. The intrinsic activity of the chemical and the signal transduction pathways available in the tissue are important factors in determining the type and degree of response observed.

The selective induction of the proliferation of initiated cell populations was first intimated by the work of Solt and Farber (1976), who used AAF administration as a "selection agent" for the enhancement of the proliferation of altered hepatic foci in a modified initiation-promotion protocol. A similar "selection" of certain initiated clones by TPA promotion also has been postulated as occurring during multistage carcinogenesis in mouse skin (DiGiovanni, 1992). Later studies demonstrated that AAF was in fact acting as a promoting agent in this protocol (Saeter et al., 1988). Farber and colleagues espoused the concept that the lowered xenobiotic metabolism of preneoplastic cell populations gives such cells a competitive advantage in toxic environments such as those provided by the chronic administration of carcinogens. Schulte-Hermann and associates (Schulte-Hermann et al., 1981) demonstrated that several hepatic promoting agents, including phenobarbital, certain steroids, and peroxisome proliferators, selectively enhance the proliferation of cells within preneoplastic lesions in rat liver. A similar effect was reported by Klaunig in preneoplastic and neoplastic hepatic lesions in mice that responded to promotion by phenobarbital (Klaunig, 1993). The response of preneoplastic hepatocytes in the rat to partial hepatectomy is also greater than that of normal hepatocytes (Laconi et al., 1994). Thus, the ability of promoting agents at the cellular and molecular levels to selectively increase cell proliferation of preneoplastic cell populations more than that of their normal

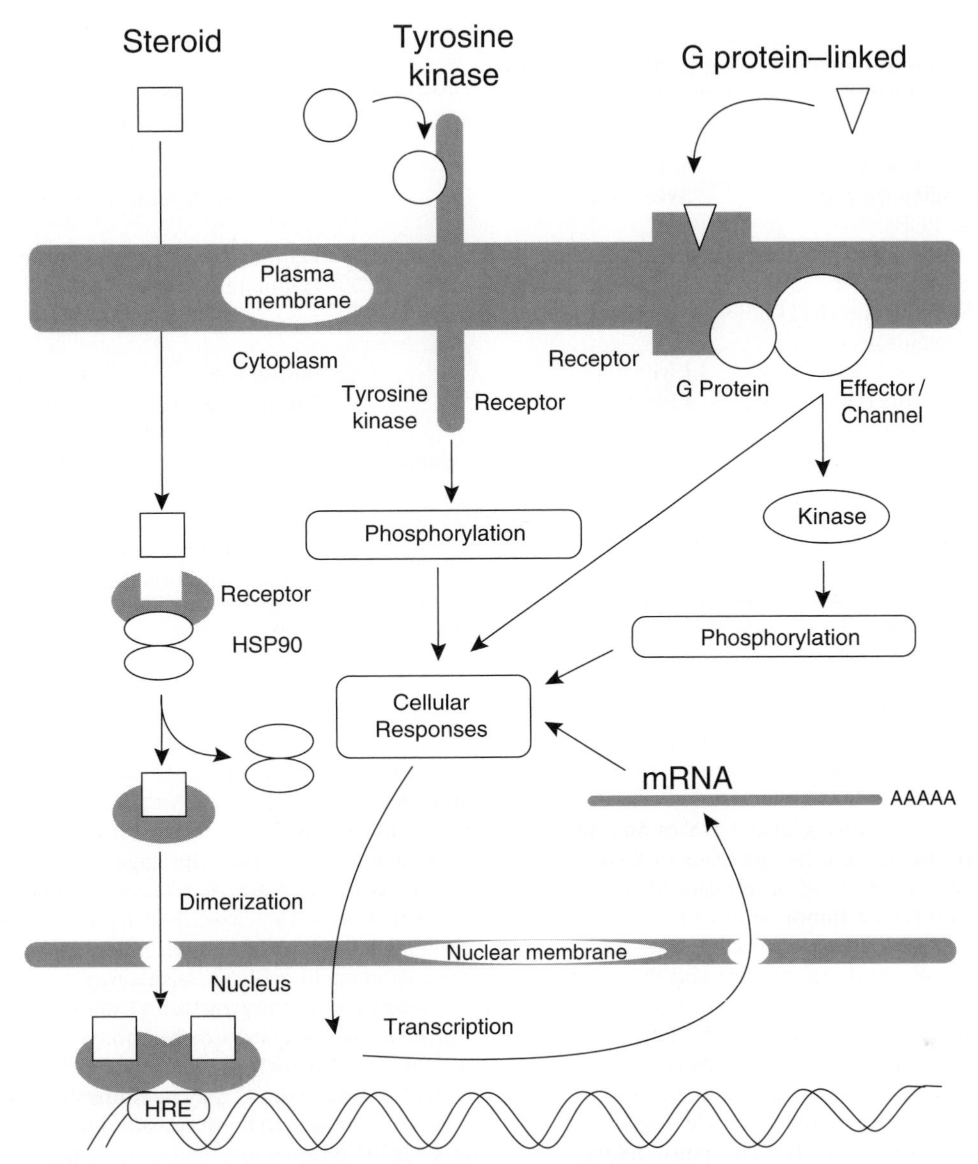


***Figure 8–19. Diagram of the principal mechanisms of intracellular signal transduction initiated either within the cytosol or at the plasma membrane. [From Mayer (1994), with permission of author and publisher.]***

counterparts may result from altered mechanisms of cell cycle control in the preneoplastic cell. The cell parameter opposed to mitosis is programmed cell death, or apoptosis (Majno and Joris, 1995). This process is dramatically inhibited by many promoting agents (Schulte-Hermann et al., 1993), but its mechanisms are not well understood. Several specific genes appear to be involved in this process (Corcoran et al., 1994; Wyllie, 1994), including the c-*myc* proto-oncogene, the *bcl-2* cellular oncogene, TGF-$\beta$, and the p53 tumor suppressor gene (Lowe et al., 1993).

***Cell Cycle Regulation.*** Although the exact mechanisms by which promoting agents selectively enhance cell replication and decrease apoptosis in preneoplastic cells are unknown, our understanding of the cell cycle and its regulation has increased dramatically in recent years. Figure 8-20 diagrams an integration of the cell cycle and apoptosis with the signal transduction pathways (Fig. 8-19). The connecting links between signal transduction and the cell cycle are still somewhat uncertain. In Fig. 8-20 it may be noted that a critical mechanism for the regulation of all phases of the cell cycle is protein phosphorylation. A variety of kinases with different amino acid and protein specificities control the activation and inactivation of cell cycle–dependent genes. The principal molecular mechanism relating signal transduction to the cell cycle is phosphorylation of various transcription factors. One pathway of cell proliferation is mediated by mitogen-activated protein kinases (MAPKs), which in turn are activated by phosphorylation mediated through the signal transduction pathways. The phosphorylation of cyclins—proteins that are critical in the passage of a cell through the cell cycle (Sherr, 1993)—by a variety of cyclin-dependent kinases (CDKs) results in different levels of phosphorylation during different parts of the cell cycle. This, coupled with the rapid synthesis and degradation of

**Table 8–15**
**Some Promoter-Receptor Interactions in Target Tissues**

| PROMOTING AGENT | TARGET TISSUE(S) | RECEPTOR STATUS |
|---|---|---|
| Tetradecanoylphorbol acetate (TPA) | Skin | Defined (protein kinase C) |
| 2,3,7,8-Tetrachlorodibenzo-*p*-dioxin (TCDD); planar PCBs | Skin, liver | Defined (Ah receptor) |
| Sex steroids (androgens and estrogens) | Liver, mammary tissue, kidney | Defined (estrogen and androgen receptors) |
| Synthetic antioxidants [butylated hydroxytoluene (BHT), butylated hydroxyanisole(BHA)] | Liver, lung, forestomach | Postulated |
| Phenobarbital | Liver | Postulated |
| Peroxisome proliferators (WY-14,643, nafenopin, clofibrate) | Liver | Defined peroxisome proliferator-activated receptor (PPAR) |
| Polypeptide trophic hormones and growth factors [prolactin, epidermal growth factor (EGF), glucagon] | Liver, skin, mammary gland | Defined or partially characterized |
| Okadaic acid | Skin | Defined (?) (protein phosphatase-2A) |
| Cyclosporin | Liver | Defined (cyclophilin) |

SOURCE: Most of the examples cited in this table are taken from Pitot (1993b). References to okadaic acid (Fujiki and Suganuma, 1993) and cyclosporin (Masuhara et al., 1993) were not cited in that reference.

cyclins and other cell cycle–dependent proteins during the cycle, allows the cycle to take place in a reproducible manner. From studies in yeast (Hartwell and Kastan, 1994), it is known that excessive production of any cyclin or CDK or an absence of the production of one of these factors leads to karyotypic instability, which is characteristic of progression (see below). The retinoblastoma protein, a tumor suppressor gene, alters the cell cycle at the level of cyclin E just before the important "checkpoint" at the $G_1$-S transition (Hunter and Pines, 1994). Phosphorylation of the retinoblastoma protein prevents its interaction with both cyclins and transcription factors, allowing the cycle to continue (Draetta, 1994). Another tumor suppressor gene, the p53 gene, also plays a role as a transcription factor, preventing continuance of the cell cycle when there is DNA damage (Wu and Levine, 1994). This pause allows the cells to repair such damage or, if the damage is excessive, to undergo apoptosis. If the p53 gene is mutated or absent, the pause does not occur and the cell cycle continues replication despite the presence of damage resulting in mutations and clastogenesis (Lane, 1992; Sander et al., 1993; Dulic et al., 1994). Obviously, the missing mechanistic link is a clear understanding of the selective enhancement of the cell cycle in preneoplastic cells by promoting agents. A variety of possibilities exist, including increased concentrations of receptors or any one or more of the components of the signal transduction pathway and mutations in transcription factors, cyclins, CDKs, or other components of the cell cycle. However, definitive studies to pinpoint such mechanisms have not been performed.

**Progression.** The stage of progression usually develops from cells in the stage of promotion but may develop directly from normal cells, usually as a result of the administration of relatively high, usually cytotoxic doses of complete carcinogenic agents that are capable of inducing both initiation and progression. In addition, the incorporation into the genome of genetic information such as oncogenic viruses, the stable transfection of genetic material, or spontaneous chromosomal alterations may induce the stage of progression. As noted in Tables 8-8 through 8-10 the major hallmark of the stage of progression is evolving karyotypic instability. It is this molecular characteristic of cells in the stage of progression that potentially leads to the multiple "stages" or changes in malignant cells which were first described by Foulds (1954) as "independent characteristics." Foulds noted that cells in the stage of progression might evolve in such a way that the characteristics of invasion, metastatic growth, and anaplasia as well as the rate of growth and responses to hormonal influences change toward higher and higher degrees of malignancy. Such "independent characteristics" may be understood as resulting from karyotypic changes that are constantly evolving in cells during the stage of progression. Included in these "characteristics" may be such things as fetal gene expression, the expression of the major histocompatibility complex (MHC) class I and II surface proteins, and the ectopic production of hormones by cells derived from non-hormone-producing tissues. Thus, in some tissues it may be possible to describe multiple "stages" that reflect the evolving karyotypic instability of neoplasms, such as in the evolution of colonic (Fearon and Vogelstein, 1992) and other neoplasms (Nowell, 1990). Simultaneous with these changes there may be the occurrence of mutated proto-oncogenes and cellular oncogenes (Liu et al., 1988; Burns et al., 1991) and tumor suppressor genes (Yokota and Sugimura, 1993). However, since karyotypic instability is unlikely to lead directly to point mutations in oncogenes and tumor suppressor genes, it is more likely that their appearance reflects the selection of cells that are better suited to the growth environment of a neoplasm.

The critical molecular characteristic of the stage of progression is karyotypic instability. As pointed out by Harris (1991), the genetic instability of this stage is primarily a reflection of the karyotypic changes seen rather than reflecting point mutations or gene amplification. Mechanisms that can lead to karyotypic instability are numerous and include disrup-

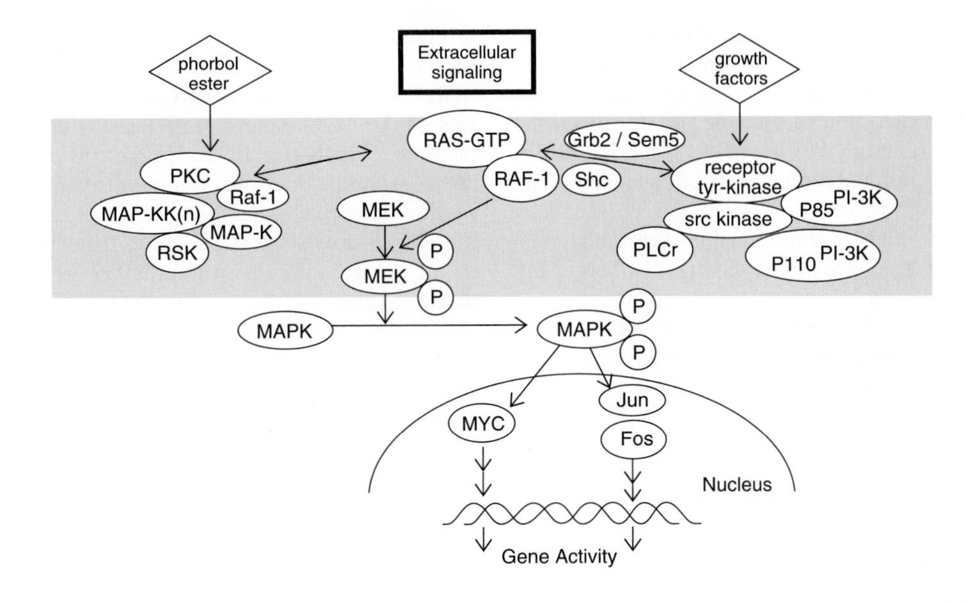


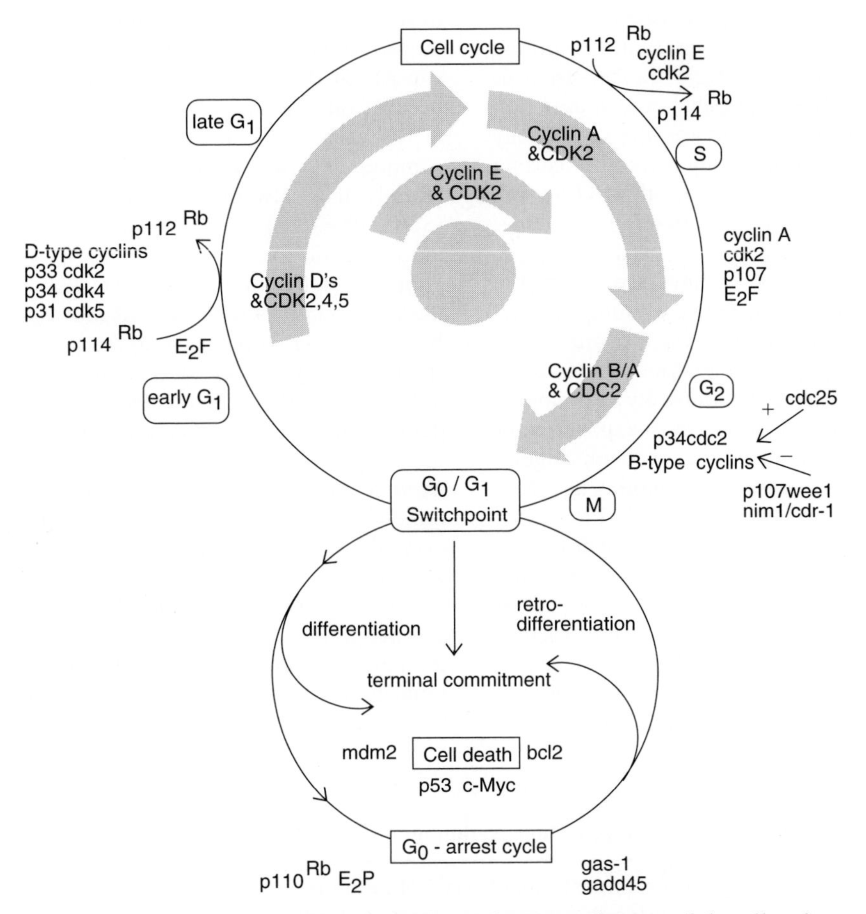


***Figure 8–20. Diagram of components of signal transduction pathways and the cell cycle.***

As indicated in the text and the figure, there is no known direct interaction between signal transduction pathways and regulation of the cell cycle, although numerous potential pathways primarily through protein phosphorylation are known. The lower portion of the figure indicates the extension of the cell into the $G_0$ phase from which apoptosis (cell death) occurs.

tion of the mitotic apparatus, alteration in telomere function (Blackburn, 1994), DNA hypomethylation, recombination, gene amplification, and gene transposition (Cheng and Loeb, 1993). The recent demonstration of the role of alterations in mismatch repair genes (see above) in some forms of cancer suggests a potential for both karyotypic and genetic instability. Many neoplasms exhibit one or more of these events, which very likely play a role in the evolution of the carcinogenic process. Numerical and structural genetic changes can occur in populations of cells without adequate repair, such as those with mutant p53 genes (see above). Histologically distinct neoplasms may exhibit different pathways during their evolution throughout the stage of progression (Heim et al., 1988; Fearon and Vogelstein, 1992).

## Genetic and Nongenetic Mechanisms of Chemical Carcinogenesis in Relation to the Natural History of Cancer Development

Chemical carcinogenesis is significantly more complex than the mere formation of DNA adducts which result from the reaction of ultimate carcinogens with DNA. In view of the multistage nature of carcinogenesis, including the occurrence of endogenous effectors in each stage, it is reasonable to classify chemical agents in regard to their primary action during one or more of the stages of carcinogenesis. Table 8-16 gives such a classification. Agents that are capable only of initiation and thus are true incomplete carcinogens are very rare, if they exist at all. Although the "pure" initiating activity of certain chemicals in specific tissues has been reported (DiGiovanni, 1992), in most instances, at higher doses or in different tissues, such agents can be shown to be carcinogenic, usually acting as complete carcinogens. However, as we have seen from the experimental basis for a distinction between initiation and promotion, very low doses of complete carcinogens act to initiate cells but cannot sustain the remainder of the carcinogenic process. This consideration is undoubtedly very important in carcinogenesis in humans, in whom most exposures are at extremely or relatively low levels of a carcinogenic agent. The list of promoting agents and putative promoting agents is, like that of complete carcinogens, growing steadily. Progressor agents in the strict sense of inducing the characteristics noted in Table 8-8 have not been identified. Some agents, specifically initiating and progressor agents, have as a primary aspect of their carcinogenic mechanism the ability to alter the structure of DNA and/or chromosomes. Such "genotoxic" effects of these agents have been linked directly to the induction of neoplasia. However, a number of chemicals, when administered chronically to animals, induce the development of neoplasia, although there is no evidence of their direct "genotoxic" action on target cells. Considering the effects of chemicals on the development of neoplasia via a multistage process, one may quickly classify such agents as promoting agents that act to expand clones of spontaneously initiated cells. The consequent selective enhancement of cell replication in these initiated cell clones sets the stage for the spontaneous transition of an occasional cell into the stage of progression, as was discussed above. However, this explanation of "nongenotoxic" carcinogenesis may be oversimplified. Table 8-17 lists a representative sample of chemicals that are nonmutagenic as assessed by induction of mutations in bacteria or mammalian cells but that on chronic administration are carcinogenic in experimental systems. As indicated in the table, a number of these chemicals have been shown to be promoting agents, but some are not. Several of those which are not promoting agents may be classified as putative progressor agents, as evidenced by their effectiveness as clastogens in experimental systems (see above). A number of other chemicals (Tennant, 1993) have not been tested for their action at specific stages of carcinogenesis and thus cannot be placed neatly in the classification in Table 8-17.

In addition to the potential progressor agents such as benzene noted in Table 8-17, other nongenotoxic mechanisms have been proposed to account for carcinogenesis by some of these chemicals (Grasso and Hinton, 1991). One such class consists of the so-called peroxisome proliferators, so named because on administration to rodents they induce an increase in the number of peroxisomes primarily in the liver. These compounds now constitute a relatively large list of chemicals (Reddy and Lalwani, 1983) that are generally nongenotoxic (Stott, 1988), but many are hepatocarcinogenic and are promoting agents for hepatocarcinogenesis in the rat (Cattley and Popp, 1989). Because of the peroxidative function of many of the enzymes in peroxisomes, Reddy and others (Reddy and Rao, 1989) have proposed that the carcinogenic action of these chemicals may be mediated by an increased oxidative potential for DNA damage in cells treated with such agents. The demonstration of such increased oxidative damage to DNA in the livers of peroxisome proliferator–treated rats has been variable (Kasai et al., 1989; Hegi et al., 1990). It should also be remembered (Table 8-15) that many peroxisome proliferators exert their effects through a specific receptor (Issemann and Green, 1990; Motojima, 1993).

Another series of chemical carcinogens that induce renal cell neoplasms in rodents also have been found to induce a dramatic increase in the accumulation of urinary proteins in renal tubular cells. This is observed only in the male rat, in which there is an accumulation of the male specific urinary

**Table 8–16**
**Classification of Chemical Carcinogens in Relation to Their Action on One or More Stages of Carcinogenesis**

Initiating agent (incomplete carcinogen): a chemical capable only of initiating cells
Promoting agent: a chemical capable of causing the expansion of initiated cell clones
Progressor agent: a chemical capable of converting an initiated cell or a cell in the stage of promotion to a potentially malignant cell
Complete carcinogen: a chemical possessing the ability to induce cancer from normal cells, usually with properties of initiating, promoting, and progressor agents

**Table 8–17**
**Some Nonmutagenic Chemical Carcinogens**

| COMPOUND | SPECIES/TARGET ORGAN | PROMOTING ACTION |
|---|---|---|
| Benzene | Rat, mouse/Zymbal gland | − |
| Butylated hydroxyanisole | Rat, hamster/forestomach | + |
| Chlorobenzilate | Rat/liver | + |
| Chloroform | Rat, mouse/liver | + |
| Clofibrate | Rat/liver | + |
| Dieldrin | Mouse/liver | + |
| Diethylhexyl phthalate | Rat/liver | ± |
| *p,p'*-Dichlorodiphenyl-dichloroethylene | Rat/liver | + |
| 1,4-Dioxane | Mouse, rat/liver, nasal turbinate | NT |
| Furfural | Mouse/liver | + |
| Lindane | Mouse/liver | + |
| Methapyrilene | Rat/liver | + |
| Polychlorinated biphenyls | Rat, mouse/liver | + |
| Reserpine | Mouse/mammary tissue | NT |
| Saccharin | Rat/bladder | + |
| 2,3,7,8-Tetrachlorodibenzo-*p*-dioxin | Rat/liver, lung | + |
| Trichloroethylene | Mouse/liver | + |

NT = not tested.
SOURCE: Modified from Lijinsky (1990) and Tennant (1993).

protein, $\alpha$2u-globulin, which is correlated with the production of renal neoplasms in male but not female rats. This has been found with *d*-limonene (Dietrich and Swenberg, 1991) and unleaded gasoline (Short et al., 1989). Several halogenated hydrocarbons induce $\alpha$2u-globulin and renal neoplasms in male rats (Konishi and Hiasa, 1994). Compounds that induce $\alpha$2u-globulin dramatically increase cell proliferation in the kidney as a result of the chronic accumulation of the protein with subsequent cell degeneration. However, this $\alpha$2u-globulin nephropathy is not itself carcinogenic (Dominick et al., 1991).

Agents that are not mutagenic or genotoxic may induce direct toxicity with sustained tissue damage and subsequent cell proliferation. Both direct DNA toxicity and increased cell proliferation may lead to clastogenesis (Scott et al., 1991) or damage genetic DNA indirectly through oxidative mechanisms. Finally, the cell proliferation resulting from toxicity may selectively induce enhanced replication of an already damaged genome in the initiated cell population. While cell toxicity does not directly induce carcinogenesis, it can enhance the process. Because many agents that are tested at chronic doses induce at least a mild degree of toxicity, it has been argued that the format of the testing system leads to the induction of neoplasia. Thus, neoplastic development observed with the administration of a test compound may occur as a result of the toxicity and cell proliferation associated with the chronic high doses utilized rather than from a direct carcinogenic effect of the agent (Ames and Gold, 1990). Thus, nongenotoxic or nonmutagenic mechanisms of carcinogenesis involve mechanisms that have been characterized. Several types of compounds appear to have primarily a promoting type of effect, including agents that induce P-450s, other mitogenic agents, cytotoxic agents, and many agents that act through receptor-mediated processes.

## CHEMICAL CARCINOGENESIS IN HUMANS

There is substantial evidence that chemical agents can cause cancer in humans. Ramazzini reported in 1700 that breast cancer had a very high incidence in celibate nuns (Wright, 1940). Ramazzini proposed that the development of this neoplasm in that occupational group was the result of the nun's lifestyle, a thesis compatible with current knowledge that endogenous hormone exposure plays a causal role in breast cancer development (Henderson et al., 1982). The initial evidence for an exogenous chemical cause of cancer in humans was related by Hill, who described the association of the use of tobacco snuff with the occurrence of nasal polyps (Hill, 1761). As discussed earlier in this chapter, Pott demonstrated the causal relationship of chimney soot to scrotal cancer in young individuals employed as chimney sweeps. During the last 150 years a number of specific chemicals or chemical mixtures, industrial processes, and lifestyles have been causally related to increased incidences of a variety of human cancers. The proportion of human cancer caused by a variety of environmental agents is provided in Fig. 8-21 (Doll and Peto, 1981). While this chart is more than two decades old, substantial evidence has accrued to support these proportional differences. How these proportions were determined and the specific chemicals associated with the segments related to chemical carcinogenesis are the subject of this section.

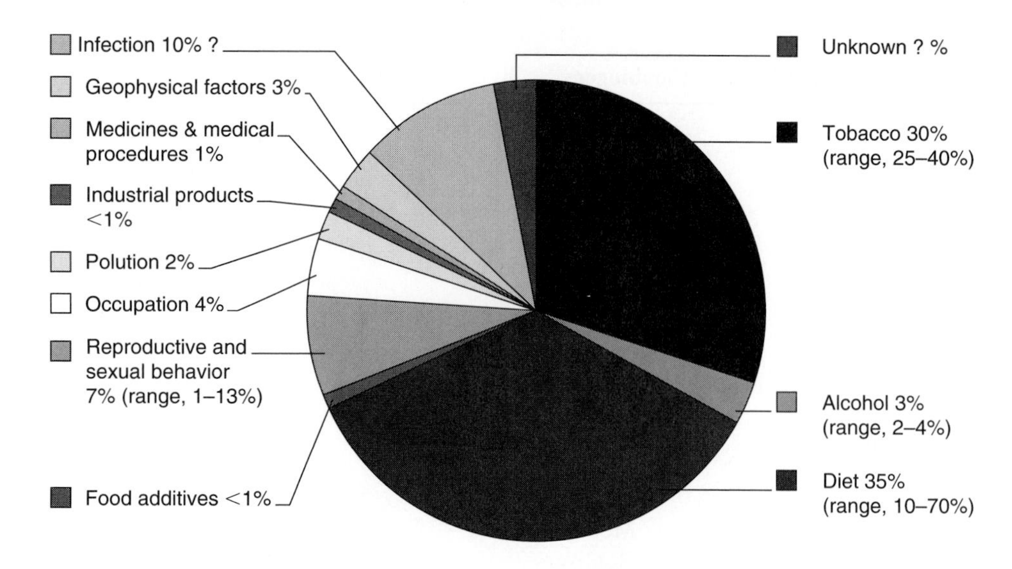


***Figure 8–21. Proportions of cancer deaths attributed to various environmental factors. [After Doll and Peto (1981).]***

## Epidemiological and Animal Studies as Bases for the Identification of Chemical Carcinogens in Humans

Epidemiology has been defined as the study of the distribution and determinants of disease (Stewart and Sarfaty, 1978). Epidemiological methodologies involve findings from observation rather than from controlled experimentation. Animal studies of carcinogenesis provide data from controlled experiments in vivo and in vitro. Because human beings cannot and should not be treated as experimental animals, epidemiological observations may take a number of forms (Rogan and Brown, 1979; Pitot, 1986a), including the following.

1. *Episodic observations.* Observations of isolated cases of cancer in relation to a specific environmental factor or factors have yielded information in the past on cause-and-effect relationships. However, deductions from these types of observations must be evaluated carefully in properly designed studies.
2. *Retrospective studies.* Retrospective studies, which are investigations of the histories and habits of groups of individuals who have developed a disease, have been frequent sources of epidemiological data. An important factor in such investigations is the use of case controls: individuals not exposed to the variable under study. In many instances, the suitable designation of such controls is the critical component in the study. This type of study usually represents the first step in attempting to identify factors that may be causative in the development of human cancer.
3. *Prospective studies.* Prospective investigations involve analyses of the continuing and future development of cancers in individuals with specific social habits, occupational exposures, and so on. Such investigations require large populations and long follow-up periods (usually 10 to 30 years), with a large percentage of both controls and test groups continuing for the duration of the study. Many of these investigations are under way in the United States and throughout the world.

Epidemiological studies may be concerned with a single factor or with multiple factors potentially causative of specific human cancers. However, it is rarely possible to identify a single chemical as the sole causative factor in the development of a specific type of human cancer because of the many other environmental variables to which the human population or cohort (group under study) is exposed. In addition, environmental factors in the causation of human cancer, including chemical exposure, infection with various parasites, ultraviolet and ionizing radiation, and individual genetic background, may be additive, synergistic, or antagonistic in relation to one another. As a confounding factor, an agent may act at the same stage or different stages in carcinogenesis.

Epidemiological studies can only identify factors that differ between two populations and are sufficiently important in the etiology of the condition under study to play a determining role under the conditions of exposure. Furthermore, on the basis of epidemiological studies alone, it usually is very difficult to determine whether a specific chemical is or is not carcinogenic to humans. The reasons for this difficulty are the extended period between first exposure and the clinical occurrence of the neoplasm, the high background incidence for many cancers in the general population, the relatively imprecise knowledge of the nature of the exposure in most instances, and other confounding variables. Thus, many negative epidemiological studies must be considered inconclusive for indicating the risk factor of relatively weak carcinogens or low doses of carcinogens for the induction of neoplastic disease in the human population (Pitot, 1986a). In view of the fact that epidemiological studies in themselves are often insufficient to establish the carcinogenicity of an agent for humans, laboratory studies with laboratory animals in vivo and cells in vitro have been employed to complement or in some cases supplant epidemiological observations where they exist.

(Heyne et al., 1992). In a similar vein, methoxypsoralen, which directly alkylates DNA, has been used in combination with ultraviolet light exposure for the treatment of the autoimmune skin condition psoriasis. Although this treatment is in many ways the treatment of choice, there is distinct evidence that squamous cell carcinoma of the skin is induced by this combination (Green et al., 1992).

Immunosuppression as a result of genetic abnormalities, therapeutic immunosuppression (such as for transplants), and immunosuppression resulting from diseases such as advanced cancer and the acquired immunodeficiency syndrome (AIDS) are associated with increased incidences of a variety of different cancers (Penn, 1989). In these instances, the development of neoplasia results from a loss of host resistance to the growth of neoplastic cells, especially those infected with viruses such as the Epstein-Barr virus or one of the herpes simplex viruses (Purtilo and Linder, 1983).

Besides the chemicals listed in Table 8-23, a number of other chemicals used as drugs in therapy for a variety of human diseases are carcinogenic in lower forms of life (Griffith, 1988). Thus, it is clear that some forms of medical therapy and diagnosis pose a carcinogenic risk to humans under certain circumstances. The decision about which is greater, the benefit to the patient or the risk of producing further pathology, must be made ultimately by the patient in consultation with the physician.

**Table 8–24**
**Modes of Prevention of Cancer Caused by Chemicals**

| MODE | STAGE |
|---|---|
| Passive | |
| Smoking cessation | Pr, Pg* |
| Dietary restriction | Pr |
| Moderation of alcohol intake | Pr |
| Modification of sexual and reproductive habits | I, Pr |
| Avoidance of excessive ultraviolet exposure | I, Pr |
| Active | |
| Dietary modification and supplements | Pr |
| Vaccination against oncogenic viruses | I, Pr |
| Application of ultraviolet blocking agents in appropriate situations | I, Pr |
| Selective screening for certain preneoplastic lesions | I, Pr |
| Determination of genetic background in relation to neoplastic disease | I, Pr |
| Administration of antihormones | Pr |

*I=initiation; Pr=promotion; Pg=progression.
SOURCE: After Pitot (1993c).

## THE PREVENTION OF HUMAN CANCER INDUCED BY CHEMICALS

More than two-thirds of human cancers are theoretically preventable through personal and societal decisions. Since the prevention of disease is by far the most effective and inexpensive mode of health care, it is appropriate that the prevention of this feared disease condition is of paramount importance.

Cancer prevention in humans may in general be grouped into two approaches: active prevention and passive prevention. Table 8-24 supplies an outline of various methods in cancer prevention with an indication of the stage of carcinogenesis toward which the preventive measure is directed. The passive prevention of cancer involves the cessation of habits such as smoking, dietary restrictions, and modification of other personal habits such as those of a sexual nature. Active prevention of cancer development signifies the administration of an agent to prevent infection by carcinogenic viruses and other organisms or the intake of chemicals, nutrients, or other factors that may modify or prevent the action of carcinogenic agents. Theoretically, passive cancer prevention or the alteration of one's "carcinogenic" habits can be the most effective and unintrusive method of cancer prevention. However, for many individuals, passive prevention requires external persuasion such as governmental regulation or peer pressure to force an alteration of their habits. Obviously, in many instances such methods are doomed to failure. Active cancer prevention, which many consider a form of preventive "therapy," is likely to be the most effective method in this area.

Most of the examples noted in Table 8-24 were discussed earlier in this chapter, with the exception of the consideration of ultraviolet light and oncogenic viruses as carcinogens. Individuals with hereditary conditions involving alterations in specific oncogenes or tumor suppressor genes constitute a relatively small part of the population. However, genes that may modify the susceptibility of an individual to the development of certain types of neoplasms probably represent significant factors in the development of an important fraction of human cancers (Spitz and Bondy, 1993). In reviewing the table, however, one may note that most methods of cancer prevention are linked to an action at the stage of promotion. Because this is the reversible stage of neoplastic development, such a finding is not surprising. However, since we still do not know all, or even most, of the causes of human cancer, the continued identification of agents, especially chemicals, that might induce human cancer is important. The final sections of this chapter will consider the identification of potential carcinogenic chemicals, evaluate the risk to humans of such agents, and describe methods that have been used, primarily by the government, to enforce cancer prevention through the passive mode.

### Identification of Potential Carcinogenic Agents

The primary factors involved in the determination of carcinogenic potential are hazard identification and risk estimation. These two components also form the basis of cancer risk assessment and much of the legislation concerning it. The trend in carcinogen identification has been to move away from the epidemiological detection of human cancer risks that provided the original evidence that chemicals can be carcinogenic to humans. At present, animals are used as surrogates for human exposure to identify agents that pose a potential risk for human cancer induction. Because the purpose of these studies is to detect agents that might under some conditions of exposure result in human cancer development, the trend has been toward the use of the most sensitive species and endpoints. In addition, the maximum tolerated dose (MTD) of a compound is administered for a majority of the life span of the animal to ensure that if any carcinogenic hazard exists, it will be detected (Carr and Kolbye, 1991). Since the primary interest lies in whether a given compound is carcinogenic under the likely exposure conditions that exist for humans, this assessment requires several additional factors, including a knowledge of exposure dose, duration, and frequency. In addition, the similarity of the biological responses to the compound in the surrogate organism and in humans is important, as is a knowledge of comparative physiology, pharmacokinetics, repair systems, and mechanisms of action (Boorman et al., 1994; Faccini et al., 1992). The basis for any risk assessment must be the comparative dose-response relationship for the cancer endpoint. Recently, endpoints for other related actions of the compound have been suggested. As with noncancer toxicology risk assessment, the concepts of dose response and exposure duration and frequency, in concert with the similarity of the responsiveness of the test system to human action to the underlying mechanism for the carcinogenic action of the test compound, are of paramount importance in the estimation of cancer risk.

Cancer is a complex process consisting of multiple stages and pathways. The natural history of the development of neoplasia should serve as the basis for determining the mechanism of action of a carcinogenic agent. Extrapolation of risk between species should be based on the similarity of response of the compared species, along with dose and pharmacokinetic and pharmacodynamic considerations. As was noted earlier, a chemical can have an impact on the course of each of the stages in a distinctive manner specific for the compound and for the stage. Clues about the mechanisms of action of an agent can come from structure-activity relationships and from the stage or stages during the carcinogenic process at which the compound is active.

## Classification Schemes for Compounds as Carcinogens

The original classification scheme for the designation of compounds as carcinogenic in humans was provided by the International Agency for Research on Cancer (Table 8-18). In this scheme, convincing epidemiological evidence of carcinogenicity is required to establish the fact that an agent has carcinogenic action in humans. While such studies examine the species of interest (human) at biologically relevant doses, epidemiological studies often are limited by the expense and long duration necessary for the detection of clinically relevant malignancy. In addition, numerous confounders exist (Peto et al., 1980; Weinberg, 1992). Because most epidemiological studies are performed after exposure to a compound has occurred, they are not protective of human health. Animal studies, primarily in rodents, coupled with short-term genotoxicity tests are thus used to provide weight to the argument for the potential risk from exposure to a compound, with the stipulation that the endpoint be primarily hazard identification. Many advantages result from the use of animal studies, including the ability to address multiple endpoints, host characteristics, and exposure conditions.

**The 2-Year Bioassay.** The primary factor used in risk assessment for the cancer endpoint is tumor incidence from 2-year bioassays in rodents. This test is used to define a carcinogen. As dictated by federal regulations and as performed by the National Cancer Institute/National Toxicology Program, the 2-year rodent bioassay is performed by chronically administering a compound and assessing the incidence of tumors at all sites. The dose of the compound is MTD and one-half the MTD. In addition, both a solvent-treated control and an untreated control usually are included. The compound generally is administered by the route through which human exposure is believed to occur or will occur. This is often an oral route through gavage or dietary administration. Animals with a low spontaneous tumor incidence result in the lowest background on which to detect an increased tumor incidence. The animals should be susceptible but not hypersensitive to the tested effect. However, the two strains typically used in these studies—the B6C3F1 mouse and the F344 rat—have high spontaneous rates of certain tumor types, limiting their predictive value and utility in risk estimation for these sites (Table 8-25). The number of animals is minimally set at 50 per dose per sex per species to approach statistical relevance for the dose-response data needed for use in risk assessment.

**Table 8–25**
**Spontaneous Tumor Incidence (Combined Benign and Malignant) in Selected Sites of the Two Species, B6C3F1 Mice and F344 Rats, Used in the NCI/NTP Bioassay**

| | B6C3F1 MICE | | F344 RATS | |
|---|---|---|---|---|
| *Site* | *Male* | *Female* | *Male* | *Female* |
| Liver | | | | |
| Adenoma | 10.3 | 4.0 | 3.4 | 3.0 |
| Carcinoma | 21.3 | 4.1 | 0.8 | 0.2 |
| Pituitary | 0.7 | 8.3 | 24.7 | 47.5 |
| Adrenal | 3.8 | 1.0 | 19.4 | 8.0 |
| Thyroid | 1.3 | 2.1 | 10.7 | 9.3 |
| Hematopoetic | 12.7 | 27.2 | 30.1 | 18.9 |
| Mammary gland | 0 | 1.9 | 2.5 | 26.1 |
| Lung | 17.1 | 7.5 | 2.4 | 1.2 |

SOURCE: From Goodman et al. (1979) and Chandra and Frith (1992).

Because so many research dollars go into carcinogenicity testing and because the data resulting from such studies are expected to be useful not only in hazard identification but also in risk estimation, an acceptable scientific protocol with quality assurance must be followed to produce scientifically and statistically valid data. Several factors are relevant to the acceptable outcome of a carcinogenicity study. These factors include parameters related to the compound to be studied and the animals to be used, including their husbandry. It is essential that the identity and purity of the test compound and any contaminants be known. The homogeneity and physical properties of the test compound should be uniform, and the chemical stability of the chemical under various storage conditions and in various matrices should be known. In addition, the formulation should be either that which is to be administered to humans or that which permits bioavailability in the test organism. The solubility, stability, and availability of the test compound in the solvent should be optimized. Appropriate mixing procedures should be detailed and ascertained, because, for example, the dilution method and volume can have effects on the final outcome. Various factors impinge on each of these parameters, and problems in the use of the data for risk estimation and submission to regulatory agencies as a result of inattention to each parameter have been noted. The environment of the rodent is also important, and care should be taken to control for sources of variability in the animals, their diet, and their housing. While the most appropriate comparison in animal studies is the concurrent control, for some situations, such as rare tumors, historical controls may be more appropriate.

The underlying basis for risk extrapolation from animals to human is that the animal is a good model for human cancer development. In fact, 2-year bioassay models have been used to detect the compounds listed by IARC (Vainio et al., 1991) as known human carcinogens. Also, most known human chemical carcinogens have a carcinogenic potential in animals that supports the results of epidemiological studies (Vainio et al., 1985). The only exceptions are arsenic and benzene. It should be recognized that under some conditions certain animal strains are not good models for the detection of potential human carcinogens. These conditions include differences in pharmacokinetics, susceptibility to the agent in question, and species-dependent responses such as thyroid neoplasia (McClain, 1989) and the induction of $\alpha_2$-microglobulin (Swenberg et al., 1985) or peroxisome proliferation (Ashby et al., 1994). In addition, animal strains that have a high spontaneous incidence of tumor formation at a particular site, such as liver tumors in mice, are poor models for the estimation of risk for the induction of human cancer. While only a limited number of compounds have been examined, the total dose per unit of body weight required to induce carcinogenicity is fairly similar (within an order or two of magnitude) across species. Perhaps the best examples of this are the antineoplastic agents for which there are both epidemiological and animal data (Crouch and Wilson, 1979). The use of extreme concentrations of a test compound, while useful under some conditions for the identification of a potential carcinogenic risk, may not be required or even useful for human risk estimation. In fact, the use of an MTD can result in a number of confounding results that create difficulty for extrapolation across species including extrapolation from high-dose to low-dose exposure scenarios. Specifically, overt toxicity may result from the administration of high doses of compounds that result in pathologies that are not hinted at with lower-dose administration. In addition, metabolic and repair pathways may be overwhelmed at higher compared with lower doses. These types of factors can lead to a loss in the continuity of the spectrum of toxicities likely to be observed at the lower doses of human exposures, thus hampering extrapolation from observations at the higher dose to possible risks at the human exposure level.

**Short-Term Tests for Mutagenicity in Vitro.** Numerous short-term tests are used to aid in the identification of potential carcinogens. In addition, several cell lines and animal strains have been genetically engineered to increase their sensitivity to specific classes of carcinogens. All these methodologies may be useful in carcinogen identification but pose problems for risk estimation. The first unifying mechanism for carcinogenesis was the somatic mutation theory suggested by Boveri and other genetic researchers. This concept was solidified by the observations of the Millers that the carcinogenic substances they studied are electrophilic. These concepts of carcinogenic agents were developed into short-term screens to aid in the identification of carcinogenic agents. The majority of the short-term tests are in vitro screens for mutagenicity and are dependent on the assumption that all carcinogens are mutagenic. While almost half the agents known to be carcinogenic in humans are also mutagenic, not all compounds that test positive in a 2-year bioassay are mutagenic either directly or after metabolic activation. Because our definition of a carcinogenic agent is an agent that increases the incidence of tumors, it is also important to understand the mechanism by which nonmutagenic agents induce neoplasia.

***Bacterial Mutagenicity Tests.*** A number of short-term tests are available for testing the potential carcinogenicity of an agent (Table 8-26). The common feature of these short-term assays is the use of genetic damage or a phenotype reflecting sustained genetic damage as the endpoint. The best studied assay is the mutagenicity assay originally developed in *Salmonella typhimurium* by Bruce Ames and associates (Ames et al., 1973). In this assay, bacterial cells that are deficient in DNA repair and lack the ability to grow in the absence of histidine are treated with several dose levels of the compound of interest, after which reversion to the histidine-positive phenotype is ascertained. Because bacteria differ in their metabolic capabilities compared with mammals, a drug-metabolizing system is added to these assays. Specifically, the 9000*g* supernate (S9) that results from centrifuging a liver homogenate prepared from a rat treated with an inducer of multiple P-450's, such as Aroclor 1254, is used in combination with an NADPH regenerating system. The method for performing the *Salmonella* assay (the Ames assay) is described in Fig. 8-22. Several different lines of *Salmonella* have been generated to permit the detection of point mutations (TA100, TA1535) and frameshift mutations (TA98, TA1537, TA1538), and the assay is continuously being refined. Typically, five dose levels of the test compound are used in addition to the solvent control. In addition, activation-dependent and activation-independent positive control mutagenic substances are tested concurrently. Certain types of carcinogens are not detected by these bacterial mutagenicity assays, including hormonal carcinogens, metals,

**Table 8–26**
**Short-Term Tests for Carcinogen Identification**

| |
|---|
| Gene mutation assay |
| Bacterial-Ames assay (histidine reversion assay in *Salmonella*) |
| Mammalian mouse lymphoma thymidine kinase assay |
| Chinese hamster ovary hypoxanthine-guanine phosphiphoribosyltransferase |
| Chromosome aberration |
| In vitro assay in cell lines |
| Mouse micronuclei |
| Rat bone marrow cytogenetics |
| Primary DNA damage |
| DNA adducts: $^{32}P$ postlabeling |
| Strand breakage |
| Induction of DNA repair |
| Bacteria: SOS response |
| Rat liver: unscheduled DNA synthesis (UDS) induction |
| Sister chromatid exchange (SCE) |
| Morphological transformation |
| Syrian hamster embryo (SHE) |
| Balb/c 3T3 |

agents that have a multiple-target-organ mode of action, and agents with a nongenotoxic mode of action. This bacterial reverse mutation system, when performed in the presence of a mammalian S9 activation system, is, however, a very sensitive screen for the detection of many mutagenic agents.

***Mammalian Mutation Assays.*** In addition to the bacterial mutational assay, several in vitro mammalian cell mutation assays exist, including the mouse lymphoma L5178Y (MOLY) assay, the Chinese hamster ovary (CHO) assay, and the V79 fibroblast assay. These mammalian mutagenicity assays use either the hypoxanthine-guanine phosphoribosyltransferase (HGPRT) or the thymidine kinase (TK) gene as the endpoint. The basis for these assays is provided in Fig. 8-23. They are similar to the Ames assay in that the phenotypic expression of a mutation in a single-copy gene is compared in treated and untreated cells. These assays are frequently performed in the presence of an exogenous metabolizing source such as an epithelial cell layer that has been irradiated. The mammalian mutation test systems are forward mutation assays in which the heterozygous state of a gene is used as a tool to detect genetic damage that might result in the loss of a phenotype: growth in the presence of a toxic compound. In CHO and V79 cells, the X-linked HPGRT locus is used as the target gene for analysis. This enzyme is important in purine salvage and allows the incorporation of toxic purine analogues such as 6-thioguanine and 8-azaguanine into DNA, resulting in inhibition of cell growth and/or cell death. Alternatively, a mutation in this gene that results in phenotype loss may permit colony formation in the presence of toxic analogues. Assays based on the forward mutation of TK are similar in that colony formation in the presence of a DNA-damaging agent is scored in the presence of a pyrimidine analogue. Because these short-term tests are based on the premise that carcinogens damage DNA, their concordance with the bioassay is between 30 and 80 percent. In addition, the results of tests are coincident with each other and tend to detect the same types of carcinogens without providing the battery approach that has been suggested. Among the short-term mutagenicity tests that use mutation as the endpoint, the Ames assay has been the best studied and has been applied to the greatest number of compounds.

**Genetically Engineered Cells and Animals for Carcinogen Identification.** The inherent problems of metabolism in cell lines have led to an interest in developing mutagenesis assays that employ engineered cells containing various human P-450s to more closely mimic the metabolic activation systems available for various potential target organs in humans (Gonzalez et al., 1991). In addition, the disruption of the internal cellular milieu associated with cell culture techniques and the lack of congruence between metabolic activation and conjugation systems has led to the development of in vivo mutagenesis assays, including transgenic mice (Cordaro, 1989), with some lines containing a shuttle vector with the *lacI* or *lacZ* gene (Mirsalis et al., 1994). In Mutamouse, the target *lacZ* gene is within a $\lambda$gt10 shuttle vector with *Eco*R1 linkers. The shuttle vector is found at a copy number of 80 in all cells of these mice. Genomic DNA can be isolated from target tissues of interest and with packaging extracts, the shuttle vector containing the target gene can be amplified and plated out with X-gal and isopropylthio-$\beta$-galactoside (IPTC) for the detection of white colonies, which may contain mutations compared with blue colonies. The DNA in the white colonies then can be sequenced to determine the mutational spectrum (specific base pair and frameshift mutations) resulting from background and chemically induced mutation. This is a versatile in vivo assay for mutagen identification, its ability to detect clastogenic agents has not been validated, and its ability to detect nonmutagenic carcinogens is doubtful. While useful for identification of mutagens and for developing a mechanistic understanding of members of certain classes of carcinogens that lack the dose-response data generated in a 2-year bioassay, this assay does not allow risk estimation. Such tests are very sensitive to genotoxic compounds that are readily detected by the in vitro mutagenicity assay, but information has not been forthcoming that other types of genetic and epigenetic changes are as readily detected.

**Endogenous Genes for Use in Mutation Detection.** In vivo mutagenesis assays can provide a more realistic mutation level than can many in vitro systems, and this has led to the development of several in vivo assays. In vitro systems are more sensitive, but in vivo systems more accurately reflect the human situation in which repair of genetic damage occurs and are an important homeostatic response to such damage. Other approaches to the problem of using genomic DNA to assess mutagenic potential with in vivo systems have involved endogenous genes as targets for carcinogenic alteration. Mutation in the HPGRT gene has been assessed after mutagen administration in vivo to compare the incidence and mutational spectrum with those obtained after in vitro administration. In addition, oncogenes including the *ras* genes and tumor suppressor genes such as p53 have been used as targets for mutational analysis. The use of endogenous genes, which are

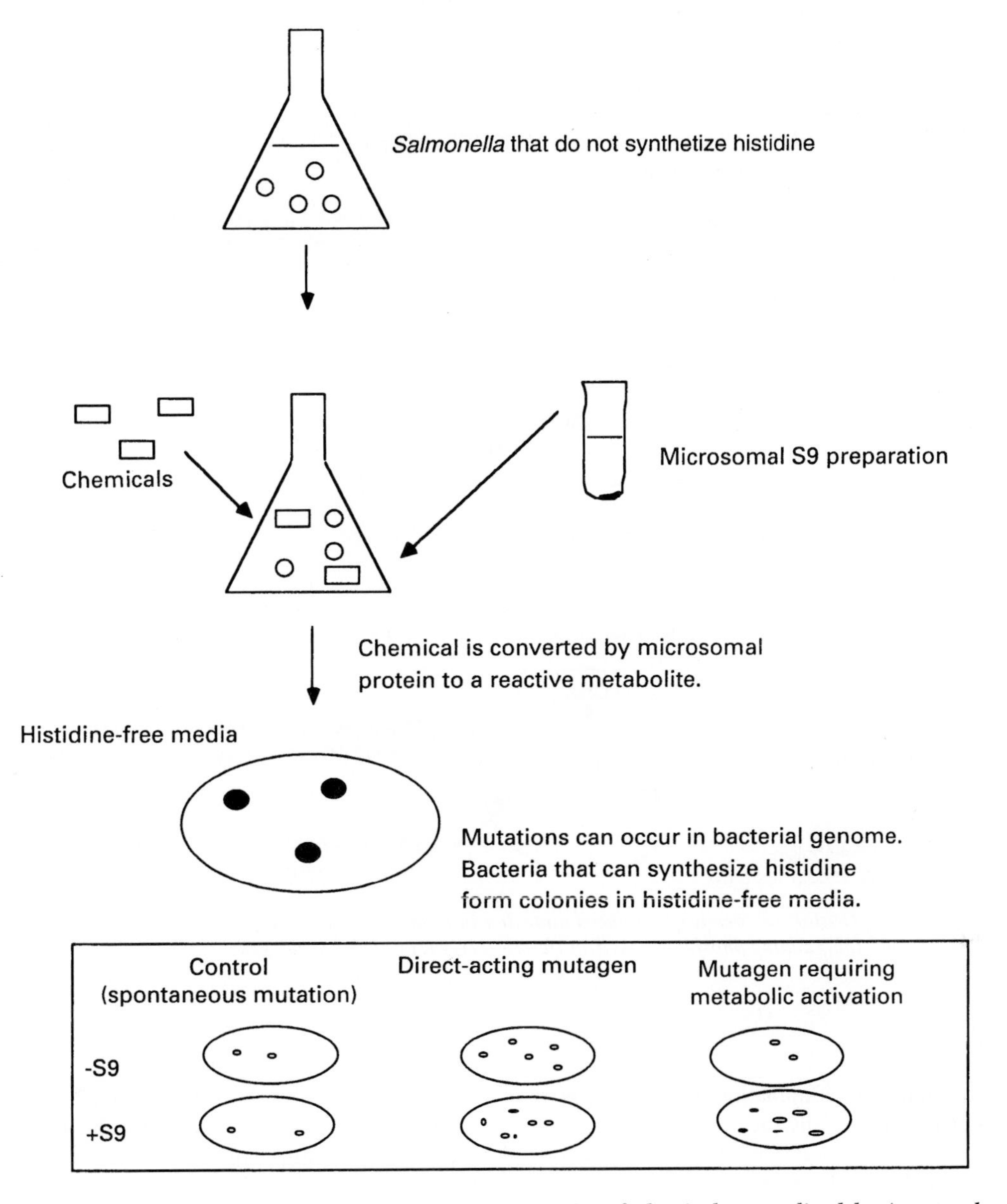


*Figure 8–22. Bacterial assay used to test the mutagenicity of chemicals as outlined by Ames and colleagues (1973).*

altered during the carcinogenesis process in some tissues and for which a large database exists from in vitro studies, provides a unique opportunity for molecular toxicologists.

**Indirect Tests for the Detection of Carcinogenicity.** Other short-term tests indirectly assess genetic damage or assess damage at the chromosomal level. For example, induction of SOS repair in bacteria and unscheduled DNA synthesis (UDS) in rat hepatocytes have been used to indicate DNA damage. Primary rat hepatocytes have been used to examine compound-based induction of DNA repair after both in vitro and in vivo compound administration. While the type of genetic damage is not determined in this assay, the assay is sufficient to induce the DNA repair system to incorporate radiolabeled thymidine into the DNA and can be quantified by the number of grains on an autoradiography film. DNA strand breakage in rat hepatocytes also has been used as an indirect measure of genetic damage. A very popular though poorly understood indirect measure of genetic damage is sister chromatid exchange (SCE).

The SCE assay is typically performed in CHO cells or peripheral lymphocytes. In this assay, an increase in SCE as a function of dose or an increase above background levels is determined for several doses of the compound of interest and for activation-dependent and activation-independent positive control compounds. The toxicity of the compound to the CHO

**Mammalian Cell Lines Used for Gene Mutation Studies**

| | |
|---|---|
| Mouse lymphoma L5178Y | TK, HGPRT |
| CHO | HGPRT |
| V79 hamster cells | HGPRT |

Selection of forward mutations by loss of HPGRT+ phenotype in V79 or chinese hamster ovary cells.

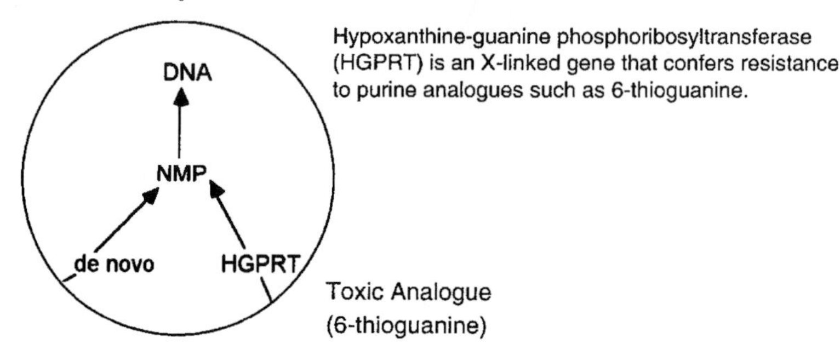


Performed in the presence of an activation system or hepatic feeder layer

Selection of mutagen-induced TK -/- phenotype in TK+/- in mouse lymphoma assay (MOLY) in L5178Y cells. This assay detects forward mutations at the TK locus.

Treat TK (+/-) cells with test compound. Fluoruracil is converted to a toxin, killing the cells. If mutation in TK occurs, FU is not metabolized to a toxin and colonies grow.

DNA

TMP

de novo

TK

Thymidine kinase (TK) confers resistance to pyrimidine analogues. It is a somatic gene.

Toxic analogue (bromodeoxyuridine)

*Figure 8–23. Outline of chemically induced mutation in mouse cell lines using thymidine kinase (TK) or hypoxanthine-guanine phosphoribosyltransferase (HGPRT) as the target gene.*

cells must be determined in conjunction with analysis of changes in SCE induction. Generally, the doses chosen bracket the highest dose that results in no overt toxicity, and one higher dose and three lower doses are used. The cells are incubated with the thymidine analogue bromodeoxyuridine (BrdU) to label the DNA in cells that are undergoing cell replication. Excess BrdU is washed from the cells, and the cells are permitted to grow in the dark through two cell cycles (the duration is dependent on whether the compounds induce mitotic delay). Colcemid is added for the last several hours of the culture to block cells in mitosis. Slides are prepared, and mitotic spreads are examined to determine whether two sister chromatids have exchanged material during mitosis. Many types of carcinogens, including some promoting agents, can be detected with this method.

**Cytogenetic Assessment of Chromosomal Aberration Induction.** Cytogenetics is assessed in vitro and in vivo after compound administration. Karyotypic analyses permit the detection of the number and integrity of the chromosomes. Analysis of chromosomal aberrations often is performed in CHO cells. Alternatively, rodent bone marrow cells are analyzed and evidence of clastogenicity, including the induction of chromosome breakage, and ploidy are scored. Gaps are noted but are not considered as damage unless the incidence is unusually high. Open breaks indicate that genetic damage has occurred. The number of cells with damage and the incidence of damage per cell are important parameters in such studies. Gross genetic changes, both numerical and structural, in cells that can survive more than one mitotic cycle may contribute to carcinogenesis. An in vivo version of this assay is performed in rat bone marrow; the structural integrity and number of chromosomes are assessed. The mouse micronucleus test permits detection of clastogenic agents and compounds that affect spindle formation and function. This test uses the polychromatic erythrocyte stem cells of the mouse as the in vivo target of potential carcinogens. The detected fragments are scored during interphase on a per animal basis. Recently, the comet assay has been proposed as a rapid screen for the induction of genetic damage. This assay is simple and rapid to perform but does not permit the detail on the type of genetic change provided by karyotypic analysis.

## Induction of Aneuploidy

An association between changes in the genetic material of a cell and neoplasia was first noted by von Hansemann (1890). This suggestion was extended by Boveri (1914) to include the observation that neoplasia was associated with the sequence of events that follow a chromosomal alteration. In neoplastic cells, chromosomal abnormalities were frequently present, and within a single tumor, most of the cells appeared to contain the same chromosomal change. It was not until the discovery of the Philadelphia chromosome that specific chromosomal changes began to be associated with one cancer type (Nowell and Hungerford, 1960). Several forms of hereditary chromosomal imbalances led to a heightened susceptibility for cancer development. The observation that children with Down syndrome or Klinefelter's syndrome had a significantly increased risk of cancer development (Harnden et al., 1971) increased awareness that aneuploidy plays a role in neoplasia. Other hereditary susceptibilities, especially those of childhood cancers, led to the development of the two-hit theory of carcinogenesis (Knudson, 1976). These hereditary cancers form the basis of our understanding of tumor suppressor genes, whose products are necessary for maintenance of the nonneoplastic state. Aneuploidy has been defined classically as a deviation of chromosome number from an exact multiple of the haploid state. Thus, the presence of an extra chromosome or the loss of one that normally is present was considered aneuploidy, while polyploidization was not. Both structural and numerical changes in chromosomes can have an adverse effect. Two mechanisms involved in the ordered distribution between daughter cells are the formation of a bipolar spindle and appropriate attachment of the chromosomes to the spindle. This is accomplished in part by elongation of microtubules from the centrosomes. Some sources of aneuploidy include failure to form a bipolar spindle, the absence of a functional kinetocore, and mistakes during cell cycle progression.

While the cellular mechanisms of aneuploidy induction are not known, multiple cellular targets other than DNA are clearly important (Oshimura and Barrett, 1986; Liang and Brinkley, 1985). These targets include tubulin, centromeres/kinetocores, centrioles/centrosomes, and microtubule-associated proteins and regulatory molecules. The factors that may result in aneuploidy include damage of chromosomes such as increased stickiness, altered chromosome condensation, pairing, and loss of telomeric region. Many compounds that alter tubulin polymerization or spindle movement can induce aneuploidy. Colchicine, benzimidazole derivatives, griseofulvin, sulfhydral reagents (mercurials and arsenicals), diethylstilbesterol, and *p*-fluorophenylalanine prevent tubulin polymerization, and their administration thus can result in aneuploidy. The Vinca alkaloids, which cause tubulin to crystallize, and taxol, which enhances tubulin polymerization, can induce aneuploidy in mammalian systems. Additionally, agents that affect spindle elongation (e.g., chloral hydrate) or movement of the kinetocore to the pole (taxol) can induce aneuploidy. Agents that can induce aneuploidy through an effect on centrioles or centrosomes include diazepam, diethylstilbesterol, ethidium bromide, and actinomycin D. Kinetocores and centromeres also can be a target for aneuploidy-inducing agents, including colchicine and mitomycin C. Compounds that alter microtubule assembly, including calmodulin, microtubule-associated proteins, and numerous enzymes (kinases and phosphatases), can induce aneuploidy. Membrane-active agents also may induce aneuploidy. Thus, unlike direct genotoxic agents whose target is DNA, agents that induce aneuploidy can react with a number of non-DNA targets.

A number of agents induce aneuploidy in at least two tests (Table 8-27), including pesticides, solvents, anesthetics, and anticancer, antianxiety, and antifungal drugs. Many are known to interact with microtubules. Another group consists of the alkylating agents, which may induce aneuploidy through their mutagenic and clastogenic action or through the adduction of proteins that are important in chromosome segregation. However, a number of compounds of clinical and environmental importance also may induce aneuploidy and have tested positive in at least one system. These compounds include fungicides such as benomyl and herbicides such as trifluralin and atrazine. In addition, a number of solvents, including benzene, chloroform, formaldehyde, and trichloroethylene, potentially induce aneuploidy. Several drugs, including diazepam, griseofulvin, vincristine, and taxol, may induce aneuploidy.

**Cell Transformation Assays.** A very interesting short-term test that holds promise for the detection of several classes of genotoxic compounds is called the cell transformation assay. These assays have been developed in mouse fibroblast cell lines that include 3T3 cells. Changes in the morphological appearance of these cells serve as an indication that transformation has occurred. Several caveats must be addressed, including differences in metabolism in vitro and in vivo, differences in biology when morphologically "transformed" cells are placed in vivo or malignant cells are placed in culture, and

**Table 8–27**
**Chemicals That Cause Aneuploidy in Two or More Test Systems**

| |
|---|
| Agents affecting microtubules |
| Benomyl |
| Chloral hydrate |
| Colcemid |
| Colchicine |
| Griseofulvin |
| Methyl 2-benzimidazolecarbamate |
| Trifluralin |
| Vinblastine |
| Alkylating agents |
| Cyclophosphamide |
| Ethyl methanesulfonate |
| Methyl methanesulfonate |
| *N*-Methyl-*N'*-nitro-*N*-nitrosoguanidine |
| Agents acting by other mechanisms |
| Actinomycin D |
| Atrazine |
| Methotrexate |
| *p*-Fluorophenylalanine |
| Pyrimethamine |
| 12-*O*-Tetradecanoyl-phorbol-13-acetate |

SOURCE: Adapted from Liang and Brinkley (1985); Oshimura and Barrett (1986).

the altered metabolic activation and detoxification pathways in cells in culture compared with cells in vivo. Because the majority of human neoplasms are epithelial in origin and because extraction of DNA from human tumors often does not transform the fibroblast test cells, other assays have been developed. Specifically, Syrian hamster embryo cells contain the three primary tissue types, and different histological cells theoretically can give rise to the morphological transformation. Besides questions involving in vitro metabolism, the use of hamster cells has a limited database compared with the mouse and rat. More recently, rat epithelial cell transformation assays have been described for epidermal and hepatic cells. The sensitivity of these assays may be enhanced by the integration of drug-metabolizing enzymes, an activated oncogene, or an inactivated tumor suppressor gene.

**Non-Genotoxic Carcinogens.** While most of the agents that test positive in one or more genotoxicity screens are carcinogenic in animal bioassays, as was noted earlier, many nongenotoxic carcinogens occur. Some agents may be mutagenic in vitro but fail to demonstrate carcinogenic action in vivo because of a short chemical half-life, rapid excretion of the test chemical in vivo, metabolic detoxification of the ultimate carcinogen, or enhanced detoxification relative to activation in vivo. Species specificity for the observed response also can occur. Tests for nongenotoxic compounds have been less well developed than have those for genotoxic agents. The effects of nongenotoxic compounds often are organ-specific and/or species-dependent, leading to difficulty in testing. Therefore, specific tests are used to assess mechanisms of toxicity indirectly. For example, an increase in liver weight is indicative of P-450 induction, including that of the peroxisome proliferators. Suggestions have been made that one could use the promoter sequences of various xenobiotic metabolizing enzymes in conjunction with a reporter construct to rapidly screen for these types of compounds.

Cell proliferation is another commonly used endpoint that can be detected by assessing the effect of compound administration on the incorporation of BrdU into DNA compared with that in appropriate controls that are not given the test compound. This method may be hindered by the need for treatment with a second chemical, BrdU, in addition to the one of interest. More recently, induction of proliferating cell nuclear antigen (PCNA) in chemically treated rodents has been assessed. This marker is expressed to varying degrees in all cycling cells, and care must be taken in determining S-phase synthesis versus growth fraction. The difficulty in scoring these slides compared with those labeled with BrdU and the smaller database are to some extent overruled by the lack of a need to treat the animals except with the test agent. Interest in cell proliferation has led to the development of assays to detect proteins expressed specifically during the S phase of the cell cycle, such as p34cdc2 kinase (Ma et al., 1992). In all cases, increases in the labeling index should be compared with changes in the mitotic index because the labeling index reflects polyploidization as well as cell proliferation (Styles, 1993). In addition, results indicate that mitogenesis should be correlated with pathology to determine whether cytotoxicity is the underlying cause.

Disruption of cell-cell communication also has been suggested as an important component in the progression toward frank neoplasia, and assays to assess this parameter in several organs, primarily rodent liver, are being developed. Structural alerts, which have proved so useful in the classification of potential genotoxic mechanisms, are useful only in receptor-based mechanisms, and even there the functional response of an organism is still difficult to predict. A number of organ-specific initiation-promotion studies have been established. The most extensively studied are the mouse epidermis, mouse liver, mouse lung, rat liver, rat mammary gland, and rat bladder (Pitot, 1986a).

## Evaluation and Regulation of Carcinogenic Potential

Regulatory toxicology has evolved from concern over overt toxicity resulting from high-dose acute exposure to examination of the more subtle effects of low-level chronic exposure. Controversy with respect to the differences between science and policy is most evident in this part of toxicology, especially as it applies to the regulation of carcinogens. Contributing to this controversy are differences in the underlying assumptions regarding the cancer development process and the meaning of extrapolation from data obtained with high doses in animals to the lower doses typical of human exposure. In addition, the original belief that a zero level risk for carcinogens is attainable has been challenged by improved analytic capabilities that result in ever lowered detection limits and the presence of natural carcinogens in the food supply (Ames and Gold, 1990).

Epidemiology provides the most definitive means of estimating the carcinogenicity to humans from exposure to an agent (IARC; see above). However, such studies can be performed only after an exposure has occurred and thus cannot be preventive. In addition, epidemiological studies can only detect differences between populations that are great enough to effect a twofold increase above the background tumor induction rate in the control population. Thus, animals are used as a surrogate for human exposure in order to make an estimate of risk. This entails that the biological responses observed in animals be relevant to humans and indicate the possibility of human hazard under some exposure format. Such scenarios assume that the physiological responses are similar between the test organism and humans and that exposure at the MTD in animals has some relevance to the actual exposure of humans.

For risk analysis, it is assumed that cancer induction differs from all other toxicological events in that the induction of cancer is a nonthreshold phenomenon or an accumulation of many such irreversible events. However, we know that compensatory methods exist for all homeostatic processes and that functional redundancy and repair processes limit the effects from exposure to potential carcinogens. At least one stage in the carcinogenesis process—promotion—is characterized by a dose-response curve with a threshold below which there is no discernible promoting effect. Thus, while for all other toxicological events a threshold approach that uses the acceptable daily intake approach of Lehman and Fitzhugh (1954) is used to approximate risk, a nonthreshold approach is applied to potential carcinogens. It has been argued on theoretical grounds that a single adduct can result in the initiation of the carcinogenesis process. The absence of a detectable threshold for radiation-induced DNA damage has been used to support this hypothesis. In addition, it has been argued that, inasmuch as individuals all have their own thresholds, assumptions of a single threshold for a population are unrealistic. The threshold approach has, however, proved applicable in regulating acceptable dietary levels of the known human carcinogen aflatoxin (Lu, 1988).

**Cancer Risk Assessment from Biomathematical Models.** Models of cancer risk assessment assume that all carcinogens are the same and that there is no threshold for their carcinogenic action. However, it is known that for most carcinogens, repair processes are available within the cell. In addition, most early changes are adaptive in nature, and functionally redundant pathways exist to compensate for those changes. While thresholds exist for each of the processes involved in the carcinogenesis process, the default assumption in the risk assessment process is that there is not a measurable threshold. This assumption predicts all further risk estimation, because most statistical and probabilistic models contain this concept as a central premise. Generally, it also is assumed that all individuals have the same risk of cancer development, which is known not to be true. Thus, given the same exposure, individuals vary with respect to their susceptibility to disease induction because of factors including genetic constitution, gender, age, and nutritional and disease status. This difference in susceptibility may also include differences in carcinogen metabolism, DNA repair, and the regulation of net cell growth (proliferation and apoptosis).

Numerous mathematical relationships have been devised to provide a statistical method for extrapolating whole-animal bioassay data to human exposure and, insofar as possible, quantitate the potential for human risk. Most of these mathematical models have as a basic tenet the assumption that carcinogenic agents lack a threshold, act irreversibly, and have effects that are additive. The lack of a threshold is assumed because no threshold has been demonstrated for radiation-induced carcinogenesis. As was indicated above, one molecule of a carcinogen could theoretically induce an initiated cell, thus allowing no margin for a threshold, since carcinogenic action (at least for some agents) is irreversible and potentially cumulative. The assumption that the effects of carcinogens are additive is based on the finding of the additive effects of radiation in carcinogenesis. The one-hit hypothesis or linear model of cancer development is based on the paradigm that a single molecule can induce a neoplasm through interaction with a cellular target. The multihit model assumes that more than one hit is required for the development of frank neoplasia (Hanes and Wedel, 1985). An extension of this model is the log-probit model, which made the assumption that every agent is carcinogenic but that a safe dose could be calculated where, for example, the acceptable risk was set at a very low level, for example 1 per 1 million. The linear multistage model incorporates the ideas of multiple steps into a statistical approach for risk analysis, as first suggested by Armitage and Doll (1954). This multistage model (Fig. 8-24) incorporates one aspect of the pathogenesis of cancer development, but cell-cycle-dependent processes and the dynamics of cell kinetics, including birth rate and death rate, are not considered. Furthermore, the transition from one stage to the next is considered irreversible. Despite these deficiencies, the linearized multistage model is the one that is most commonly used. At a low dose, the multistage model is used to fit the observed tumor incidence data to a polynomial of the dose where risk is approximated by dose as a function of the q1*, where this potency estimate is in inverse units of dose. The q1* defines the linear component of the excess tumor risk at these low doses to a 95 percent upper confidence bound on the q1 term. The q1* calculation is a characteristic of the species for which the calculation was determined and assumes a constant lifetime exposure.

The linear multistage model is not appropriate for estimating low-dose carcinogenic potency for many chemicals. In most cases, the dose response at high doses of testing differs substantially from the considerably lower doses for exposure. Pharmacokinetic and pharmacodynamic models provide information that can help bridge the gap between the high-dose and low-dose scenarios (Anderson et al., 1989). A second problem is associated with extrapolation of lifetime exposure of animals to the MTD of a compound to the less than lifetime exposure common for humans. This problem is addressed by EPA through the use of the Weibull model (Hanes and Wedel, 1985), which assumes that risk is greater when encountered at a younger age and that once exposure occurs, risk continues to accrue despite the cessation of exposure. However, observations in humans and experimental animals have demonstrated that in many cases risk decreases after exposure ceases.

More recently, biomathematical modeling of cancer risk assessment has been used in an attempted to relate such models more closely to the biological characteristics of the pathogenesis of neoplasia. The best known of these biologically based models is that described originally by Moolgavkar, Venzon, and Knudson, termed the MVK model (Moolgavkar, 1986). This model, which is depicted in Fig. 8-24, reproduces quite well the multistage characteristics of neoplastic development with $\mu_1$, the rate at which normal cells are converted to "intermediate" cells (initiated cells), and $\mu_2$, the rate at which intermediate cells are converted to neoplastic (N) cells. These rates model the rates of initiation and progression in multistage carcinogenesis, while the stage of promotion represents the expansion of the intermediate cell population, which is a function of $\alpha_2$, the rate of division of "intermediate cells," and $\beta_2$, the rate of differentiation and/or death of intermediate cells. Other factors in the model that are also true in biology are the rate of replication and cell death of normal or stem cells. While this model originally was developed to explain certain epidemiological characteristics of breast cancer incidence and mortality in humans (Moolgavkar, 1986), it has found potential application in a variety of multistage models, including that of rat liver (Luebeck et al., 1991). Application of the model to risk assessment problems has not found wide use, but this may change in the next few years (Anderson et al., 1992). In addition, integration of biological data, including pharmacokinetic and pharmacodynamic parameters, should aid in the development of a more biologically based risk assessment model.

**Practical Considerations in Risk Extrapolation from Animals to Humans.** Zeise and colleagues (1987) noted that a variety of dose-response curve shapes for carcinogen action are observed in both animals and humans. In addition, none of these response curves indicate doses that result in a lifetime risk of 1 in a 1 million. There are several classes of chemical carcinogens, each with a unique mechanism of action and thus a unique dose-response curve. The linearity of the dose-re-

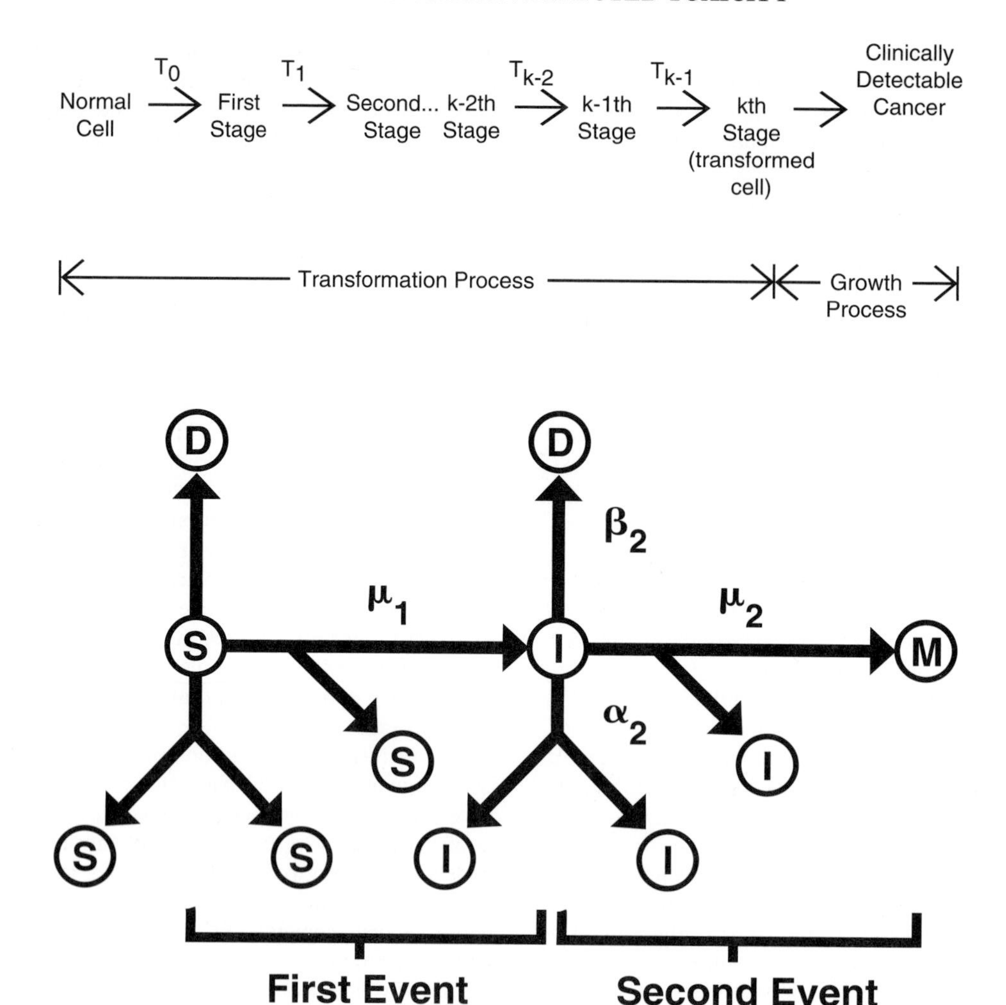


***Figure 8–24. The Armitage and Doll (upper) and MKV (lower) models of multistage carcinogenesis.***

In the former, the number of stages is unspecified ($T_k$) and the transition between them is irreversible. In the MKV model the fates of stem cells (S) and intermediate (I) cells are death (D) or proliferation. Rarely, I cells undergo $\mu_2$ to malignancy (M). The rates of replication ($\alpha_2$) and apoptosis ($\beta_2$) for I cells are indicated, and similar rates for S cells are implied. $\mu_1$ and $\mu_2$ are the rates of the first genetic event (initiation) and the second genetic event (progression).

sponse curve also may be affected by the background tumor incidence in the species and target organ of interest (Gaylor, 1992). In addition, the mechanism of action of a carcinogen and the pharmacokinetic and pharmacodynamic impact of the formulation tested can result in nonlinear kinetics with apparent threshold doses for carcinogenic action.

The acceptance of the presence of a threshold or at least a practical threshold permits the use of a safety factor approach (Lehman and Fitzhugh, 1954) such as that of the reference dose (RfD) or the benchmark dose (Barnes and Doursen, 1988). The RfD approach uses the no-effect or low-effect dose level as a function of a number of uncertainty factors. These uncertainty factors can be restricted in magnitude or defined by legislation and include factors for both variability and uncertainty. Commonly used uncertainty factors include ones that attempt to account for the heterogeneity in the human population (10X), animal-to-human extrapolation (10X), progression from subchronic to chronic (10X), use of a low-effect dose instead of a no-effect dose (10X), adequacy of the database (10X), and other modifying factors (10X). Some criticisms of the use of thresholds are based on the fact that uncertainty factors are not validated and may not include all sources of variability. In addition, the calculation may be wrong 5 percent of the time, and the assumption that there is a population threshold also may be wrong. The Weibull and log-logistic models are used to establish a threshold dose below which no increase in response is expected. This approach uses both the dose and the dose rate as parameters for the calculation.

Several issues are relevant to cross-species extrapolation, including differences in metabolism between species. Typically, metabolic schemes are qualitatively similar across species, although they can be markedly dissimilar quantitatively. There is a difference in the metabolic rate, which is partly due to elimination kinetics. Exposure estimation frequently is based on the daily dose administered or on plasma concentration as a surrogate for tissue concentration. Extrapolation across species through the use of the plasma concentration assumes that each species responds in the same manner to a given dose of a compound. However, allosteric scaling is appropriate only under conditions in which the process by which the toxicity occurs is scalable in a concentration- and time-dependent manner, the mechanism of toxicity is the same in the species being compared, and the difference in biological responses between species is dependent only upon the difference in size of the species and thus is independent of other susceptibility factors. Allometric scaling has been suggested as the best indicator of the toxicity of anticancer agents in humans compared with animals (Freireich et al., 1966). Perhaps milligrams per kilogram is the best basis for cross-species comparison because it better predicts tissue concentration–response effects after chronic administration (Allen et al., 1988; Monro, 1992).

The other point involves the use of the MTD, which is justified on the basis that if a compound is negative for carcinogenicity after exposure to the highest dose tolerated, it is doubtful that it is a human carcinogen. This provides a very conservative approach for hazard identification. Several factors can indicate that exposure has exceeded the MTD, including compensatory mitogenesis after tissue damage, which can be measured crudely by an increase in cell proliferation. The other crude measure indicating that the MTD has been exceeded is a change in excretion patterns with an increased dose (Melnick et al., 1984). Metabolic saturation can result in abnormal metabolism (Munro, 1977) or abnormal clearance (Morrow, 1992). Thus, use of the MTD can result in an inability of the animal to compensate for any adaptive changes that were induced by the treatment. This compromise is often detected by means of the induction of cytotoxicity and compensatory hyperplasia.

## Regulation of Carcinogenic Risk at the Federal Level

At least four federal agencies have as their primary responsibility the regulation of risk. These agencies include the Consumer Products Safety Commission (CPSC), the EPA, the U.S. Food and Drug Administration (FDA), and the Occupational Safety and Health Administration (OSHA). At least two types of regulations affect risk analysis; these include regulations similar to the Clean Water Act, which imposes technology-based standards that are dictated by the best available technology, and the Clean Air Act, which imposes health- or risk-based standards to protect human health by providing an ample margin of safety. A number of laws have been passed that control exposure to carcinogens in food, drugs, and the environment (Table 8-28). Perhaps the most controversial is the Food, Drug, and Cosmetic Act of 1938, including the 1958 amendment known as the Delaney amendment. The Delaney amendment was passed to curtail any possible use of additives in food and drugs that had been demonstrated to induce cancer in humans or animals. This law ignores the presence of endogenous or endogenously produced compounds that have carcinogenic action. For example, nitrites are effective bactericidal agents when used at low levels as food additives, but nitrites are produced extensively in vivo during normal metabolism of nitrogenous compounds, especially when nitrates are present in the diet (Rogers, 1982). High doses of nitrites given with secondary amines result in the formation of nitrosamines, which are carcinogenic in rodents (Rogers, 1982). Thus, a number of difficulties are encountered when food and additives are regulated with strict adherence to the Delaney amendment.

Besides science, a major driving force in legislative actions concerning the regulation of carcinogenic or potentially carcinogenic chemicals in the environment is the benefit obtained from such regulation. The saccharin-cyclamate debates were an interesting example of this (Kraybill, 1976). Saccharin is carcinogenic at very high doses in rat uroepithelium (Anderson et al., 1988). After considerable debate, the U.S. Congress passed a law permitting the use of this "carcinogenic" compound as an artificial sweetener because of its low cost and benefit to a variety of individuals, especially diabetics. Recently, the courts rejected the use of two food colorings

**Table 8–28**
**Selected Federal Laws for the Regulation of Toxic and Carcinogenic Agents**

| NAME OF ACT AND YEAR PASSED AND AMENDED | AREA OF CONCERN |
|---|---|
| Food Drug and Cosmetic Act (FDC): 1906, 1938, amended 1958 (Delaney), 1960, 1962, 1968, 1976, 1980, 1984, 1986, 1987, 1990, 1992 | Food, drugs, cosmetics, food additives, color additives, new drugs, animal feed additives, medical devices |
| Federal Insecticide, Fungicide, and Rodenticide Act (FIFRA): 1948, amended 1972, 1975, 1976 | Pesticides |
| Clean Air Act: 1970, amended 1974, 1977, 1978, 1980, 1981, 1982, 1983, 1990 | Air pollutants |
| Clean Water Act: 1972, amended 1977–1983, 1987, 1988, 1990, 1992; originally the Federal Water Control Act | Water pollutants |
| Occupational Safety and Health Act (OSHA): 1970, amended 1974, 1978, 1979, 1982, 1990, 1992 | Workplace exposure to toxicants |
| Toxic Substances Control Act (TOSCA): 1976, amended 1981, 1983, 1984, 1986, 1988, 1990, 1992 | Hazardous chemicals not covered elsewhere, including premarket review |

SOURCE: Adapted from Office of Science and Technology Policy (1986).

in drugs and cosmetics on the basis of an interpretation of the Delaney amendment as prohibitive of the use of additives even when only minimal risk can be demonstrated. The EPA faces a difficult situation in the regulation of pesticides when it attempts to balance the requirement of the Federal Insecticide, Fungicide, and Rodenticide Act (FIFRA), which requires a balance of risk and benefit in the application of pesticides to raw agricultural products, and the zero tolerance for carcinogens in processed foodstuffs mandated by the Delaney amendment. OSHA is responsible for regulating workers' exposure to potential toxins, including carcinogens. The statutes require that feasibility be considered in concert with lack of effect on workers' health. In the case of *Industrial Union Department v American Petroleum Institute*, the Supreme Court found that the allowable levels of a compound (i.e., benzene) could be powered only if a significant risk from exposure could be demonstrated and that this risk could be lessened by a change in practice. In the final analysis, a significant proportion of risk to the average citizen is based on the perception of risk.

# REFERENCES


Abell CW, Heidelberger C: Interaction of carcinogenic hydrocarbons with tissues: VIII. Binding of tritium-labeled hydrocarbons to the soluble proteins of mouse skin. *Cancer Res* 22:931–946, 1962.

Allen B, Crump K, Shipp A: Correlation between carcinogenic potency of chemicals in animals and humans. *Risk Anal* 8:531–561, 1988.

Ames BN, Durston WE, Yamasaki E, Lee FD: Carcinogens are mutagens: A simple test system combining liver homogenates for activation and bacteria for detection. *Proc Natl Acad Sci USA* 70:2281–2285, 1973.

Ames BN, Gold LS: Misconceptions on pollution and the causes of cancer. *Angew Chem Int Ed Engl.* 29:1197–1208, 1990a.

Ames B, Gold L: Dietary carcinogens, environmental pollution, and cancer: Some misconceptions. *Med Oncol Tumor Pharmacother* 7:69–85, 1990b.

Ames BN, Shigenaga MK, Gold LS: DNA lesions, inducible DNA repair, and cell division: Three key factors in mutagenesis and carcinogenesis. *Environ Health Perspect* 93:35–44, 1993.

Anderson ME: Tissue dosimetry, physiologically-based pharmacokinetic modeling, and cancer risk assessment. *Cell Biol Toxicol* 5:405–415, 1989.

Anderson ME, Krishnan K, Conolly RB, McClellan RO: Mechanistic toxicology research and biologically-based modeling: partners for improving quantitative risk assessments. *Chem Indust Inst Toxicol* 12:1–7, 1992.

Anderson MW, Reynolds SH, You M, Maronpot RM: Role of protooncogene activation in carcinogenesis. *Environ Health Perspect* 98:13–24, 1992.

Anderson R, Lefever F, Maurer J: Comparison of the responses of male rats to dietary sodium saccharin exposure initiated during nursing with responses to exposure initiated to weaning. *Food Chem Toxicol* 26:899–907, 1988.

Andrews EJ: Evidence of the nonimmune regression of chemically induced papillomas in mouse skin. *JNCI* 47:653–665, 1971.

Anttila A, Sallmén M, Hemminki K: Carcinogenic chemicals in the occupational environment. *Pharmacol Toxicol* 72:69–76, 1993.

Armitage P, Doll R: The age distribution of cancer and a multi-stage theory of carcinogenesis. *Br J Cancer* 8:1–12, 1954.

Ashby J, Brady A, Elcombe CR, Elliott BM, Ishmael J, Odum J, Tugwood JD, Kettle S, Purchase IFH: Mechanistically-based human hazard assessment of peroxisome proliferator-induced hepatocarcinogenesis. *Hum Exp Toxicol* 13:S1-S117, 1994.

Ashby J, Paton D: The influence of chemical structure on the extent and sites of carcinogenesis for 522 rodent carcinogens and 55 different human carcinogen exposures. *Mutat Res* 286:3–74, 1993.

Ashby J, Tennant RW, Zeiger E, Stasiewicz S: Classification according to chemical structure, mutagenicity to Salmonella and level of carcinogenicity of a further 42 chemicals tested for carcinogenicity by the U.S. National Toxicology Program. *Mutat Res* 223:73–103, 1989.

Ashendel CL: The phorbol ester receptor: A phospholipid-regulated protein kinase. *Biochim Biophys Acta,* 822:219–242, 1985.

Bailleul B, Brown K, Ramsden M, et al: Chemical induction of oncogene mutations and growth factor activity in mouse skin carcinogenesis. *Environ Health Perspect* 81:23–27, 1989.

Barlow DP: Methylation and imprinting: From host defense to gene regulation? *Science* 260:309–310, 1993.

Barnard JA, Polk WH, Moses HL, Coffey RJ: Production of transforming growth factor-*α* by normal rat small intestine. *Am J Physiol* 261:C994-C1000, 1991.

Barnes D, Doursen M: Reference dose (RFD): Description and use in health risk assessments. *Regul Toxicol Pharmacol* 8:471–486, 1988.

Barrows GH, Mays ET, Christopherson WM: Steroid related neoplasia in human liver, in Miller RW et al (eds): *Unusual Occurrences as Clues to Cancer Etiology.* Tokyo: Japan Science Society Press /Taylor & Francis, 1988, pp 47–59.

Bartsch H, Hietanen E, Malaveille C: Carcinogenic nitrosamines: Free radical aspects of their action. *Free Radic Biol Med* 7:637–644, 1989.

Bartsch H, Ohshima H: Endogenous *N*-nitroso compounds: How relevant are they to human cancer? in Rhoads JE, Fortner J (eds): *GMCRF.* Philadelphia: Lippincott, 1989, pp 304–317.

Bartsch H, Ohshima H, Shuker DEG, et al: Exposure of humans to endogenous *N*-nitroso compounds: Implications in cancer etiology. *Mutat Res* 238:255–267, 1990.

Bauer-Hofmann R, Klimek F, Buchmann A, et al: Role of mutations at codon 61 of the c-Ha-*ras* gene during diethylnitrosamine-induced hepatocarcinogenesis in C3H/He mice. *Mol Carcinog* 6:60–67, 1992.

Beach AC, Gupta RC: Human biomonitoring and the $^{32}$P-postlabeling assay. *Carcinogenesis* 13:1053–1074, 1992.

Beatson GT: On the treatment of inoperable cases of carcinoma of the mamma: Suggestions for a new method of treatment, with illustrative cases. *Lancet* 2:104–107, 1896.

Becker RA, Shank RC: Kinetics of formation and persistence of ethylguanines in DNA of rats and hamsters treated with diethylnitrosamine. *Cancer Res* 45:2076–2084, 1985.

Berenblum I, Shubik P: A new quantitative approach to the study of stages of chemical carcinogenesis in the mouse's skin. *Br J Cancer* 1:383, 1947.

Berger MR, Schmähl D, Zerban H: Combination experiments with very low doses of three genotoxic *N*-nitrosamines with similar organotropic carcinogenicity in rats. *Carcinogenesis* 8:1635–1643, 1987.

Bernard C: Leçons sur les phénomènes de la vie, 2 vols. Paris: J-B Bailliere et fils, 1878, 1879.

Bessho T, Roy R, Yamamoto K, et al: Repair of 8-hydroxyguanine in DNA by mammalian *N*-methylpurine-DNA glycosylase. *Proc Natl Acad Sci USA* 90:8901–8904, 1993.

Bhide SV, Shivapurkar NM, Gothoskar SV, Ranadive KJ: Carcinogenicity of betel quid ingredients: Feeding mice with aqueous extract and the polyphenol fraction of betel nut. *Br J Cancer* 40:922–926, 1979.

Biaglow JE: The effects of ionizing radiation on mammalian cells. *J Chem Educ* 58:144–156, 1981.

Bichara M, Fuchs RPP: DNA binding and mutation spectra of the carcinogen *N*-2-aminofluorene in *Escherichia coli*: A correlation between the conformation of the premutagenic lesion and the mutation specificity. *J Mol Biol* 183:341–351, 1985.

Bishop JM: Viral oncogenes. *Cell* 42:23–38, 1985.

Biskind MS, Biskind GR: Development of tumors in the rat ovary after transplantation into the spleen. *Proc Soc Exp Biol Med* 55:176–179, 1944.

Bittner JJ: Mammary cancer in C3H mice of different sublines and their hybrids. *JNCI* 16:1263–1286, 1956.

Blackburn EH: Telomeres: No end in sight. *Cell* 77:621–623, 1994.

Blayney DW, Longo DL, Young RC, et al: Decreasing risk of leukemia with prolonged follow-up after chemotherapy and radiotherapy for Hodgkin's disease. *N Engl J Med* 316:710–714, 1987.

Blot WJ: Alcohol and cancer. *Cancer Res* 52:2119s–2123s, 1992.

Bogen KT: Cancer potencies of heterocyclic amines found in cooked foods. *Food Chem Toxicol* 32:505–515, 1994.

Bolt HM: Roles of etheno-DNA adducts in tumorigenicity of olefins. *CRC Crit Rev Toxicol* 18:299–309, 1988.

Bolt HM, Peter H, Föst U: Analysis of macromolecular ethylene oxide adducts. *Int Arch Occup Environ Health* 60:141–144, 1988.

Bond GG, Rossbacher R: A review of potential human carcinogenicity of the chlorophenoxy herbicides MCPA, MCPP, and 2,4-DP. *Br J Ind Med* 50:340–348, 1993.

Boorman GA, Maronpot RR, Eustis SL: Rodent carcinogenicity bioassay: past, present, and future. *Toxicol Pathol* 22:105–111, 1994.

Bosland MC, Dreef-Van Der Meulen HC, Sukumar S, et al: Multistage prostate carcinogenesis: the role of hormones. *Int Symp Princess Takamatsu Cancer Res Fund* 22:109–123, 1991.

Boutwell RK: Some biological aspects of skin carcinogenesis. *Prog Exp Tumor Res* 4:207–250, 1964.

Boutwell RK: Function and mechanism of promoters of carcinogenesis. *CRC Crit Rev Toxicol* 2:419–443, 1974.

Boutwell RK: Caloric intake, dietary fat level, and experimental carcinogenesis, in Jacobs MN (eds): *Exercise, Calories, Fat, and Cancer*. New York: Plenum Press, 1992, pp 95–101.

Boveri T: *Zur frage der enstebung maligner tumorgen*. Jena: G. Fischer, 1914.

Boyd JA, Barrett JC: Genetic and cellular basis of multistep carcinogenesis. *Pharmacol Ther* 46:469–486, 1990.

Boyland E: The biological significance of metabolism of polycyclic compounds. *Biochem Soc Symp* 5:40–54, 1950.

Brambilla G, Carlo P, Finollo R, et al: Viscometric detection of liver DNA fragmentation in rats treated with minimal doses of chemical carcinogens. *Cancer Res* 43:202–209, 1983.

Brand KG, Buoen LC, Johnson KH, Brand I: Etiological factors, stages, and the role of the foreign body in foreign body tumorigenesis: A review. *Cancer Res* 35:279–286, 1975.

Bronner CE, Baker SM, Morrison PTet al: Mutation in the DNA mismatch repair gene homologue *hMLH 1* is associated with hereditary non-polyposis colon cancer. *Nature* 368:258–261, 1994.

Bronstein SM, Skopek TR, Swenberg JA: Efficient repair of $O^6$-ethylguanine, but not $O^4$-ethylthymine or $O^2$-ethylthymine, is dependent upon $O^6$-alkylguanine-DNA alkyltransferase and nucleotide excision repair activities in human cells. *Cancer Res* 52:2008–2011, 1992.

Bryant MS, Skipper PL, Tannenbaum SR, Maclure M: Hemoglobin adducts of 4-aminobiphenyl in smokers and nonsmokers. *Cancer Res* 47:602–608, 1987.

Burns FJ, Vanderlaan M, Snyder E, Albert RE: Induction and progression kinetics of mouse skin papillomas, in Slaga TJ, Sivak A, Boutwell RK (eds): *Carcinogenesis*, vol 2: *Mechanism of Tumor Promotion and Cocarcinogenesis*.New York: Raven Press, 1978, pp 91–96.

Burns P, Brown K, Bremner R, et al: Molecular alterations in oncogenes or tumor suppressor genes during chemical carcinogenesis. *Prog Histochem Cytochem* 23:100–106, 1991.

Butlin HJ: Three lectures on cancer of the scrotum in chimney-sweeps and others: I. Secondary cancer without primary cancer: II. Why foreign sweeps do not suffer from scrotal cancer. III. Tar and paraffin cancer. *Br Med J* 1:1341–1346, 1892; 2:1–6, 66–71, 1892.

Butterworth BE: Chemically induced cell proliferation as a predictive assay for potential carcinogenicity, in Butterworth BE et al. (eds): *Chemically Induced Cell Proliferation: Implications for Risk Assessment*. New York: Wiley-Liss, 1991, pp 457–467.

Candrian U, You M, Goodrow T, et al: Activation of protooncogenes in spontaneously occurring non-liver tumors from C57BL/6 x C3H $F_1$ mice. *Cancer Res* 51:1148–1153, 1991.

Carr CJ, Kolbye AC Jr: A critique of the use of the maximum tolerated dose in bioassays to assess cancer risks from chemicals. *Regul Toxicol Pharmacol* 14:78–87, 1991.

Carter JH, Carter HW, Meade J: Adrenal regulation of mammary tumorigenesis in female Sprague-Dawley rats: Incidence, latency, and yield of mammary tumors. *Cancer Res* 48:3801–3807, 1988.

Cattley RC, Popp JA: Differences between the promoting activities of the peroxisome proliferator WY-14,643 and phenobarbital in rat liver. *Cancer Res* 49:3246–3251, 1989.

Cavalieri EL, Rogan EG: The approach to understanding aromatic hydrocarbon carcinogenesis: The central role of radical cations in metabolic activation. *Pharmacol Ther* 55:183–199, 1992.

Cerny WL, Mangold KA, Scarpelli DG: K-*ras* mutation is an early event in pancreatic duct carcinogenesis in the Syrian golden hamster. *Cancer Res* 52:4507–4513, 1992.

Cha RS, Thilly WG, Zarbl H: *N*-Nitroso-*N*-methylurea-induced rat mammary tumors arise from cells with preexisting oncogenic *Hras1* gene mutations. *Proc Natl Acad Sci USA* 91:3749–3753, 1994.

Chandra M, Frith CH: Spontaneous neoplasms in B6C3F1 mice. *Toxicol Lett* 60:91–98, 1992.

Chandra RS, Kapur SP, Kelleher J, et al: Benign hepatocellular tumors in the young. *Arch Pathol Lab Med* 108:168–171, 1984.

Cheng KC, Loeb LA: Genomic instability and tumor progression: Mechanistic considerations. *Adv Cancer Res* 60:121–156, 1993.

Clifton KH, Sridharan BN: Endocrine factors and tumor growth, in Becker FF (ed): *Cancer—A Comprehensive Treatise*. New York: Plenum, 1975, vol 3, pp 249–285.

Cohen LA, Kendall ME, et al: Modulation of *N*-nitrosomethylurea-induced mammary tumor promotion by dietary fiber and fat. *JNCI* 83:496–501, 1991.

Cohen SM, Ellwein LB: Genetic errors, cell proliferation, and carcinogenesis. *Cancer Res* 51:6493–6505, 1991.

Columbano A, Rajalakshmi S, Sarma DSR: Requirement of cell proliferation for the initiation of liver carcinogenesis as assayed by three different procedures. *Cancer Res* 41:2079–2083, 1981.

Conaway CC, Nie G, Hussain NS, Fiala ES: Comparison of oxidative damage to rat liver DNA and RNA by primary nitroalkanes, secondary nitroalkanes, cyclopentanone oxime, and related compounds. *Cancer Res* 51:3143–3147, 1991.

Conney AH: Induction of microsomal enzymes by foreign chemicals and carcinogenesis by polycyclic aromatic hydrocarbons: G. H. A. Clowes Memorial Lecture. *Cancer Res* 42:4875–4917, 1982.

Connolly JG, White EP: Malignant cells in the urine of men exposed to beta-naphthylamine. *Can Med Assoc J* 100:879–882, 1969.

Cooper WC: Epidemiologic study of vinyl chloride workers: Mortality through December 31, 1972. *Environ Health Perspect* 41:101–106, 1981.

Corcoran GB, Fix L, Jones DP, et al: Apoptosis: Molecular control point in toxicity. *Toxicol Appl Pharmacol* 128:169–181, 1994.

Cordaro JC: Transgenic mice as future tools in risk assessment. *Risk Anal* 9:157–168, 1989.

Cortés F, Piñero J, Ortiz T: Importance of replication fork progression for the induction of chromosome damage and SCE by inhibitors of DNA topoisomerases. *Mutat Res* 303:71–76, 1993.

Craighead JE: Asbestos-associated diseases. *Arch Pathol Lab Med* 106:542–597, 1982.

Crouch E, Wilson R: Interspecies comparison of carcinogenic potency. *J Toxicol Environ Health* 5:1095–1118, 1979.

Cullen MR, Cherniack MG, Rosenstock L: Occupational medicine. *N Engl J Med* 322:675–682, 1990.

Demple B, Harrison L: Repair of oxidative damage to DNA: Enzymology and biology. *Annu Rev Biochem* 63:915–948, 1994.

Dietrich DR, Swenberg JA: The presence of $\alpha_{2u}$-globulin is necessary for d-limonene promotion of male rat kidney tumors. *Cancer Res* 51:3512–3521, 1991.

DiGiovanni J: Multistage carcinogenesis in mouse skin. *Pharmacol Ther* 54:63–128, 1992.

Dipple A, Michejda CJ, Weisburger EK: Metabolism of chemical carcinogens. *Pharmacol Ther* 27:265–296, 1985.

Doll R, Peto R: *The Causes of Cancer.* Oxford: Oxford University Press, 1981.

Dominick MA, Robertson DG, Bleavins MR, et al: $\alpha_{2u}$-Globulin nephropathy without nephrocarcinogenesis in male Wistar rats administered 1-(aminomethyl)cyclohexaneacetic acid. *Toxicol Appl Pharmacol* 111:375–387, 1991.

Dorgan JF, Schatzkin A: Antioxidant micronutrients in cancer prevention. *Nutr Cancer* 5:43–68, 1991.

Draetta GF: Mammalian $G_1$ cyclins. *Curr Opinion Cell Biol* 6:842–846, 1994.

Dragan YP, Hully JR, Nakamura J, et al: Biochemical events during initiation of rat hepatocarcinogenesis. *Carcinogenesis* 15:1451–1458, 1994.

Dragan YP, Pitot HC: Aflatoxin carcinogenesis in the context of the multistage nature of cancer, in Eaton DL, Groopman JD (eds): *The Toxicology of Aflatoxins: Human Health, Veterinary, and Agricultural Significance.* San Diego: Academic Press, 1994, pp 179–206.

Dulic V, Kaufmann WK, Wilson SJ, et al: p53-Dependent inhibition of cyclin-dependent kinase activities in human fibroblasts during radiation-induced G1 arrest. *Cell* 76:1013–1023, 1994.

Dunham LJ: Cancer in man at site of prior benign lesion of skin or mucous membrane: A review. *Cancer Res* 32:1359–1374, 1972.

Eastman A, Barry MA: The origins of DNA breaks: a consequence of DNA damage, DNA repair, or apoptosis? *Cancer Invest* 10:229–240, 1992.

Eaton DL, Groopman JD, eds: *The Toxicology of Aflatoxins—Human Health, Veterinary, and Agricultural Significance*. San Diego: Academic Press, 1994.

Eling TE, Thompson DC, Foureman GL, et al: Prostaglandin H synthase and xenobiotic oxidation. *Annu Rev Pharmacol Toxicol* 30:1–45, 1990.

Emerit I, Khan SH, Esterbauer H: Hydroxynonenal, a component of clastogenic factors? *Free Radic Biol Med* 10:371–377, 1991.

Enslein K, Gombar VK, Blake BW: Use of SAR in computer-assisted prediction of carcinogenicity and mutagenicity of chemicals by the *TOPKAT* program. *Mutat Res* 305:47–61, 1994.

Essigmann JM, Wood ML: The relationship between the chemical structures and mutagenic specificities of the DNA lesions formed by chemical and physical mutagens. *Toxicol Lett* 67:29–39, 1993.

Faccini JM, Butler WR, Friedmann J-C, et al: IFSTP guidelines for the design and interpretation of the chronic rodent carcinogenicity bioassay. *Exp Toxic Pathol* 44:443–456, 1992.

Farber E: Ethionine carcinogenesis. *Adv Cancer Res* 7:383–474, 1963.

Fearon ER, Vogelstein B: A genetic model for colorectal tumorigenesis. *Cell* 61:759–761, 1992.

Ferguson DJ: Cellular attachment to implanted foreign bodies in relation to tumorigenesis. *Cancer Res* 37:4367–4371, 1977.

Fingerhut MA, Halperin WE, Marlow DA, et al: Cancer mortality in workers exposed to 2,3,7,8-tetrachlorodibenzo-*p*-dioxin. *N Engl J Med* 324:212–218, 1991.

Fishel R, Lescoe MK, Rao MRS, et al: The human mutator gene homolog *MSH2* and its association with hereditary nonpolyposis colon cancer. *Cell* 75:1027–1038, 1993.

Fisher B, Costantino JP, Redmond CK, et al: Endometrial cancer in tamoxifen-treated breast cancer patients: Findings from the National Surgical Adjuvant Breast and Bowel Project (NSABP) B-14. *JNCI* 86:527–537, 1994.

Floyd RA: Role of oxygen free radicals in carcinogenesis and brain ischemia. *FASEB J* 4:2587–2597, 1990.

Foran JA, Cox M, Croxton D: Sport fish consumption advisories and projected cancer risks in the Great Lakes basin. *Am J Public Health* 79:322–325, 1989.

Fornace AJ Jr, Nagasawa H, Little JB: Relationship of DNA repair to chromosome aberrations, sister-chromatid exchanges and survival during liquid-holding recovery in X-irradiated mammalian cells. *Mutat Res* 70:323–336, 1980.

Foulds L: The experimental study of tumor progression: A review. *Cancer Res* 14:327–339, 1954.

Foulds L: Multiple etiologic factors in neoplastic development. *Cancer Res* 25:1339–1347, 1965.

Freedman LS, Clifford C, Messina M: Analysis of dietary fat, calories, body weight, and the development of mammary tumors in rats and mice: A review. *Cancer Res* 50:5710–5719, 1990.

Freireich E, Gehan E, Rall D, et al: Quantitative comparison of toxicity of anticancer agents in mouse, rat, hamster, dog, monkey, and man. *Cancer Chemother* 50:219–244, 1966.

Friedberg EC: Nucleotide excision repair of DNA in eucaryotes: Comparison between human cells and yeast. *Cancer Surv* 4:529–555, 1985.

Friedberg EC: Xeroderma pigmentosum, Cockayne's syndrome, helicases, and DNA repair: what's the relationship? *Cell* 71:887–889, 1992.

Friedberg EC: DNA repair: Looking back and peering forward. *Bioessays* 16:645–649, 1994.

Fry RJM, Ley RD, Grube D, Staffeldt E: Studies on the multistage nature of radiation carcinogenesis, in Hecker E, Fusenig NE, Kunz W, et al (eds): *Carcinogenesis—A Comprehensive Survey: Cocarcinogenesis and Biological Effects of Tumor Promoters.* New York: Raven Press, 1982, vol 7, pp 155–165.

Fujiki H, Suganuma M: Tumor promotion by inhibitors of protein phosphatases 1 and 2A: The okadaic acid class of compounds. *Adv Cancer Res* 61:143–194, 1993.

Furth J: A meeting of ways in cancer research: Thoughts on the evolution and nature of neoplasms. *Cancer Res* 19:241–256, 1959.

Furth J: Hormones as etiological agents in neoplasia, in Becker FF (ed): *Cancer—A Comprehensive Treatise.* New York: Plenum, 1975, vol 1, pp 75–120.

Futreal PA, Liu Q, Shattuck-Eidens D, et al: *BRCA1* mutations in primary breast and ovarian carcinomas. *Science* 266:120–122, 1994.

Gambrell RD Jr: Cancer and the use of estrogens. *Int J Fertil* 31:112–122, 1986.

Garrett CT: Oncogenes. *Clin Chim Acta* 156:1–40, 1986.

Garro AJ, Lieber CS: Alcohol and cancer. *Annu Rev Pharmacol Toxicol* 30:219–249, 1990.

Gaylor DW: Relationship between the shape of dose-response curves and background tumor rates. *Regul Toxicol Pharmacol* 16:2–9, 1992.

Ghoshal AK, Farber E: The induction of liver cancer by dietary deficiency of choline and methionine without added carcinogens. *Carcinogenesis* 5:1367–1370, 1984.

Glauert HP, Schwarz M, Pitot HC: The phenotypic stability of altered hepatic foci: Effect of the short-term withdrawal of phenobarbital and of the long-term feeding of purified diets after the withdrawal of phenobarbital. *Carcinogenesis* 7:117–121, 1986.

Gold LS, Slone TH, Manley NB, Ames BN: Heterocyclic amines formed by cooking food: Comparison of bioassay results with other chemicals in the Carcinogenic Potency Database. *Cancer Lett* 83:21–29, 1994.

Goldfarb S: Sex hormones and hepatic neoplasia. *Cancer Res* 36:2584–2588, 1976.

Goldstein JA, Faletto MB: Advances in mechanisms of activation and deactivation of environmental chemicals. *Environ Health Perspect* 100:169–176, 1993.

Gonzalez F, Crespi C, Gelboin H: cDNA-expressed human cytochrome P450s: A new age of molecular toxicology and human risk assessment. *Mutat Res* 247:113–127, 1991.

Goodman DG, Ward JM, Squire RA, et al: Neoplastic and nonneoplastic lesions in aging F344 rats. *Toxicol Appl Pharmacol* 48:237–248, 1979.

Gorchev HG, Jelinek CF: A review of the dietary intakes of chemical contaminants. Bull WHO 63:945–962, 1985.

Goth R, Rajewsky MF: Persistence of $O^6$-ethylguanine in rat-brain DNA: correlation with nervous system-specific carcinogenesis by ethylnitrosourea. *Proc Natl Acad Sci USA* 71:639–643, 1974.

Grasso P, Hinton RH: Evidence for and possible mechanisms of non-genotoxic carcinogenesis in rodent liver. *Mutat Res* 248:271–290, 1991.

Green C, Diffey BL, Hawk JLM: Ultraviolet radiation in the treatment of skin disease. *Phys Med Biol* 37:1–20, 1992.

Griffith RW: Carcinogenic potential of marketed drugs. *J Clin Res Drug Dev* 2:141–144, 1988.

Guengerich FP: Metabolic activation of carcinogens. *Pharmacol Ther* 54:17–61, 1992.

Gupta RC, Reddy MV, Randerath K: $^{32}$P-postlabeling analysis of non-radioactive aromatic carcinogen—DNA adducts. *Carcinogenesis* 3:1081–1092, 1982.

Habs M, Schmähl D: Diet and cancer. *J Cancer Res Clin Oncol* 96:1–10, 1980.

Hall A: A biochemical function for ras—at last. *Science* 264:1413–1414, 1994.

Hanes B, Wedel T: A selected review of risk models: one hit, multihit, multistage, probit, Weibull, and pharmacokinetic. *J Am Coll Toxicol* 4:271–278, 1985.

Hanigan MH, Pitot HC: Growth of carcinogen-altered rat hepatocytes in the liver of syngeneic recipients promoted with phenobarbital. *Cancer Res* 45:6063–6070, 1985.

Hansen C, Asmussen I, Autrup H: Detection of carcinogen-DNA adducts in human fetal tissues by the $^{32}$P-postlabeling procedure. *Environ Health Perspect* 99:229–231, 1993.

Hardell L, Eriksson M, Degerman A: Exposure to phenoxyacetic acids, chlorophenols, or organic solvents in relation to histopathology, stage, and anatomical localization of non-Hodgkin's lymphoma. *Cancer Res* 54:2386–2389, 1994.

Harnden D, Maclean N, Langlands A: Carcinoma of the breast and Klinefelter's syndrome. *J Med Genet* 8:460–461, 1971.

Harris CC: Chemical and physical carcinogenesis: Advances and perspectives for the 1990s. *Cancer Res* 51:5023s–5044s, 1991.

Hartwell LH, Kastan MB: Cell cycle control and cancer. *Science* 266:1821–1828, 1994.

Harvey RG: Activated metabolites of carcinogenic hydrocarbons. *Accid Chem Res* 14:218–226, 1981.

Hathway DE, Kolar GF: Mechanisms of reaction between ultimate chemical carcinogens and nucleic acid. *Chem Soc Rev* 9:241–253, 1980.

Hecht SS: Chemical carcinogenesis: An overview. *Clin Physiol Biochem* 3:89–97, 1985.

Hegi ME, Ulrich D, Sagelsdorff P, et al: No measurable increase in thymidine glycol or 8-hydroxydeoxyguanosine in liver DNA of rats treated with nafenopin or choline-devoid low-methionine diet. *Mutat Res* 238:325–329, 1990.

Heidelberger C: Chemical carcinogenesis, chemotherapy: cancer's continuing core challenges. G. H. A. Clowes Memorial Lecture. *Cancer Res* 30:1549–1569, 1970.

Heim S, Mandahl N, Mitelman F: Genetic convergence and divergence in tumor progression. *Cancer Res* 48:5911–5916, 1988.

Henderson BE, Ross R, Bernstein L: Estrogens as a cause of human cancer: The Richard and Hinda Rosenthal Foundation Award Lecture. *Cancer Res* 48:246–253, 1988.

Henderson BE, Ross RK, Pike MC, Casagrande JT: Endogenous hormones as a major factor in human cancer. *Cancer Res* 42:3232–3239, 1982.

Henson DE, Albores-Saavedra J: *The Pathology of Incipient Neoplasia.* Philadelphia: Saunders, 1986.

Herbst AL: Clear cell adenocarcinoma and the current status of DES-exposed females. *Cancer* 48:484–488, 1981.

Heyne KH, Lippman SM, Lee JJ, et al: The incidence of second primary tumors in long-term survivors of small-cell lung cancer. *J Clin Oncol* 10:1519–1524, 1992.

Hill J: *Cautions against the Immoderate Use of Snuff*, 2d ed. London, 1761.

Hirono I: Edible plants containing naturally occurring carcinogens in Japan. *Jpn J Cancer Res* 84:997–1006, 1993.

Hoeijmakers JHJ, Bootsma D: Incisions for excision. *Nature* 371:654–655, 1994.

Holliday R: A different kind of inheritance. *Sci Am* 260:60–73, 1989.

Hoover DM, Best KL, McKenney BK, et al: Experimental induction of neoplasia in the accessory sex organs of male Lobund-Wistar rats. *Cancer Res* 50:142–146, 1990.

Hoover R, Fraumeni JF Jr: Drug-induced cancer. *Cancer* 47:1071–1080, 1981.

Horsfall MJ, Gordon AJE, Burns PA, et al: Mutational specificity of alkylating agents and the influence of DNA repair. *Environ Mol Mutagen* 15:107–122, 1990.

Hsieh LL, Hsieh TT: Detection of aflatoxin B1-DNA adducts in human placenta and cord blood. *Cancer Res* 53:1278–1280, 1993.

Hueper WC, Wiley FH, Wolfe HD: Experimental production of bladder tumors in dogs by administration of beta-naphthylamine. *J Indust Hyg Toxicol* 20:46–84, 1938.

Huh, N.-H., Satoh MS, Shiga J, et al: Immunoanalytical detection of $O^4$-ethylthymine in liver DNA of individuals with or without malignant tumors. *Cancer Res* 49:93–97, 1989.

Hunter T: Cooperation between oncogenes. *Cell* 64:249–270, 1991.

Hunter T, Pines J: Cyclins and cancer II: Cyclin D and CDK inhibitors come of age. *Cell* 79:573–582, 1994.

Huseby RA: Demonstration of a direct carcinogenic effect of estradiol on Leydig cells of the mouse. *Cancer Res* 40:1006–1013, 1980.

IARC Monographs on the Evaluation of Carcinogenic Risks to Humans: *Alcohol Drinking*. Lyon, France: International Agency for Research on Cancer. 1987, vol 44, pp 101–105.

Ip C, Yip P, Bernardis LL: Role of prolactin in the promotion of dimethylbenz[*a*]anthracene-induced mammary tumors by dietary fat. *Cancer Res* 40:374–378, 1980.

Issemann I, Green S: Activation of a member of the steroid hormone receptor superfamily by peroxisome proliferators. *Nature* 347:645–650, 1990.

Ito N, Hasegawa R, Imaida K, et al: Ingestion of 20 pesticides in combination at acceptable daily intake levels exerts no effects on rat liver carcinogenesis. *Food Chem Toxicol* 33:159–163, 1995.

Ito N, Hirose M: The role of antioxidants in chemical carcinogenesis. *Jpn J Cancer Res (Gann)* 78:1011–1026, 1987.

Jass JR, Stewart SM, Stewart J, Lane MR: Hereditary non-polyposis colorectal cancer—morphologies, genes and mutations. *Mutat Res* 310:125–133, 1994.

Jensen H, Madsen JL: Diet and cancer. *Acta Med Scand* 223:293–304, 1988.

Jerina DM, Daly JW, Witkop B, et al: 1,2-Naphthalene oxide as an intermediate in the microsomal hydroxylation of naphthalene. *Biochemistry* 9:147–156, 1970.

Johnson ES: Human exposure to 2,3,7,8-TCDD and risk of cancer. *Crit Rev Toxicol* 21:451–462, 1992.

Johnson KH, Buoen LC, Brand I, Brand KG: Polymer tumorigenesis: Clonal determination of histopathological characteristics during early preneoplasia: Relationships to karyotype, mouse strain, and sex. *JNCI* 44:785–793, 1970.

Kadlubar FF, Anson JF, Dooley KL, Beland FA: Formation of urothelial and hepatic DNA adducts from the carcinogen 2-naphthylamine. *Carcinogenesis* 2:467–470, 1981.

Kakiuchi H, Ushijima T, Ochiai M, et al: Rare frequency of activation of the Ki-*ras* gene in rat colon tumors induced by heterocyclic amines: Possible alternative mechanisms of human colon carcinogenesis. *Mol Carcinog* 8:44–48, 1993.

Kakunaga T: The role of cell division in the malignant transformation of mouse cells treated with 3-methylcholanthrene. *Cancer Res* 35:1637–1642, 1975.

Karran P, Bignami M: DNA damage tolerance, mismatch repair and genome instability. *Bioessays* 16:833–839, 1994.

Kasai H, Okada Y, Nishimura S, et al: Formation of 8-hydroxydeoxyguanosine in liver DNA of rats following long-term exposure to a peroxisome proliferator. *Cancer Res* 49:2603–2605, 1989.

Kaufmann WK: Pathways of human cell post-replication repair. *Carcinogenesis* 10:1–11, 1989.

Kawashima S, Wakabayashi K, Nishizuka Y: Low incidence of nodular hyperplasia of the adrenal cortex after ovariectomy in neonatally estrogenized mice than in the controls. *Proc Jpn Acad* 56:350–354, 1980.

Kemp CJ, Leary CN, Drinkwater NR: Promotion of murine hepatocarcinogenesis by testosterone is androgen receptor-dependent but not cell autonomous. *Proc Natl Acad Sci USA* 86:7505–7509, 1989.

Kennaway E: The identification of a carcinogenic compound in coal-tar. *Br Med J* 2:749–752, 1955.

Kinosita R: Researches on the cancerogenesis of the various chemical substances. *Gann* 30:423–426, 1936.

Klaunig JE: Selection induction of DNA synthesis in mouse preneoplastic and neoplastic hepatic lesions after exposure to phenobarbital. *Environ Health Perspect* 101:235–240, 1993.

Knudson AG: Genetics and the etiology of childhood cancer. *Pediatr Res* 10:513–517, 1976.

Knudson AG: Antioncogenes and human cancer. *Proc Natl Acad Sci USA* 90:10914–10921, 1993.

Koga N, Inskeep PB, Harris TM, Guengerich FP: *S*-[2-*N*7-Guanyl)-ethyl]glutathione, the major DNA adduct formed from 1,2-dibromoethane. *Biochemistry*, 25:2192–2198, 1986.

Konishi N, Hiasa Y: Renal carcinogenesis, in Waalkes MP, Ward JM (eds): *Carcinogenesis*. New York: Raven Press, 1994, pp 123–159.

Korte F, Coulston F: Some consideration of the impact of energy and chemicals on the environment. *Regul Toxicol Pharmacol* 19:219–227, 1994.

Kraybill H: Food chemicals and food additives, in Newberne, P (ed): *Trace Substances and Health, A Handbook, Part I*. New York: Marcel Dekker, 1976, pp 245–318.

Kritchevsky D: Dietary effects in experimental carcinogenesis: Animal models, in Beynen AC, West CE (eds): *Use of Animal Models for Research in Human Nutrition*. Basel: Karger, 1988, vol 6, pp 174–185.

Kritchevsky D, Weber MM, Buck CL, Klurfeld DM: Calories, fat and cancer. *Lipids* 21:272–274, 1986.

Kuschner M: The carcinogenicity of beryllium. *Environ Health Perspect* 40:101–105, 1981.

Laconi E, Vasudevan S, Rao PM, et al: An earlier proliferative response of hepatocytes in $\gamma$-glutamyl transferase positive foci to partial hepatectomy. *Cancer Lett* 81:229–235, 1994.

Landrigan PJ: Arsenic—state of the art. *Am J Ind Med* 2:5–14, 1981.

Landrigan PJ: Epidemiologic approaches to persons with exposures to waste chemicals. *Environ Health Perspect* 48:93–97, 1983.

Lane DP: p53, guardian of the genome. *Cancer,* 358:15–16, 1992.

Lasne C, Lu YP, Orfila L, et al: Study of various transforming effects of the anabolic agents trenbolone and testosterone on Syrian hamster embryo cells. *Carcinogenesis* 11:541–547, 1990.

Lawley PD: Historical origins of current concepts of carcinogenesis. *Adv Cancer Res* 65:17–111, 1994.

Leaf CD, Wishnok JS, Tannenbaum SR: Mechanisms of endogenous nitrosation. *Cancer Surv* 8:323–334, 1989.

Ledbetter DH: Minireview: Cryptic translocations and telomere integrity. *Am J Hum Genet* 51:451–456, 1992.

Lee DC, Luetteke NC, Qiu TH, et al: Transforming growth factor alpha: Its expression, regulation, and role in transformation, in Tsang RC, Lemons JA, Balistren WF (eds): *Growth Factors in Perinatal Development*. New York: Raven Press, 1993, pp 21–38.

Lee G-H, Merlino G, Fasuto N: Development of liver tumors in transforming growth factor $\alpha$ transgenic mice. *Cancer Res* 52:5162–5170, 1992.

Lehman A, Fitzhugh O: 100-fold margin of safety. *Assoc Food Drug Off US Q Bull* 18:33–35, 1954.

Levin W, Thakker DR, Wood AW, et al: Evidence that benzo[*a*]anthracene 3,4-diol-1,2-epoxide is an ultimate carcinogen on mouse skin. *Cancer Res* 38:1705–1710, 1978.

Levine AJ: The tumor suppressor genes. *Annu Rev Biochem* 62:623–651, 1993.

Li AP, Aaron CS, Auletta AE, et al: An evaluation of the roles of mammalian cell mutation assays in the testing of chemical genotoxicity. *Regul Toxicol Pharmacol* 14:24–40, 1991.

Li D, Randerath K: Modulation of DNA modification (I-compound) levels in rat liver and kidney by dietary carbohydrate, protein, fat, vitamin, and mineral content. *Mutat Res* 275:47–56, 1992.

Li D, Xu D, Randerath K: Species and tissue specificities of I-compounds as contrasted with carcinogen adducts in liver, kidney and skin DNA of Sprague-Dawley rats, ICR mice and Syrian hamsters. *Carcinogenesis* 11:2227–2232, 1990.

Li JJ, Li SA: Estrogen carcinogenesis in hamster tissues: A critical review. *Endocr Rev* 11:524–531, 1990.

Liang JC, Brinkley BR: Chemical probes and possible targets for the induction of aneuploidy, in Dellarco V, Voytek P, Hollaender A (eds): *Aneuploidy, Etiology, and Mechanisms*. New York: Plenum Press, 1985, pp 491–505.

Liao D, Porsch-Hällström I, Gustafsson J-A, and Blanck A: Sex differences at the initiation stage of rat liver carcinogenesis—influence of growth hormone. *Carcinogenesis* 14:2045–2049, 1993.

Liehr JG: 2-Fluoroestradiol: Separation of estrogenicity from carcinogenicity. *Mol Pharmacol* 23:278–281, 1983.

Lijinsky W: Nitrosamines and nitrosamides in the etiology of gastrointestinal cancer. *Cancer* 40:2446–2449, 1977.

Lijinsky W: Non-genotoxic environmental carcinogens. *J Environ Sci Health* C8(1):45–87, 1990.

Lijinsky W, Reuber MD, Riggs CW: Carcinogenesis by combinations of *N*-nitroso compounds in rats. *Food Chem Toxicol* 21:601–605, 1983.

Liu E, Dollbaum C, Scott G, et al: Molecular lesions involved in the progression of a human breast cancer. *Oncogene* 3:323–327, 1988.

Loechler EL: Adduct-induced base-shifts: A mechanism by which the adducts of bulky carcinogens might induce mutations. *Biopolymers* 28:909–927, 1989.

Lowe JP, Silverman BD: Predicting carcinogenicity of polycyclic aromatic hydrocarbons. *Chem Res* 17:332–338, 1984.

Lowe SW, Ruley HW, Jacks T, Housman DE: p53-Dependent apoptosis modulates the cytotoxicity of anticancer agents. *Cell* 74:957–967, 1993.

Lu F: Acceptable daily intake: Inception, evolution, and application. *Reg Toxicol Pharmacol* 8:45–60, 1988.

Luebeck E, Moolgavkar S, Buchman A, Schwarz M: Effects of polychlorinated biphenyls in rat liver: Quantitative analysis of enzyme-altered foci. *Toxicol Appl Pharmacol* 111:469–484, 1991.

Lutz WK, Schlatter J: Chemical carcinogens and overnutrition in diet-related cancer. *Carcinogenesis* 13:2211–2216, 1992.

Lutz WK, Schlatter J: The relative importance of mutagens and carcinogens in the diet. *Pharmacol Toxicol* 72:s104-s107, 1993.

Ma X, Mufti N, Babish J: Protein tyrosine phosphorylation as an indicator of 2,3,7,8-tetrachloro-p-dioxin exposure in vivo and in vitro. *Biochem Biophys Res Commun* 189:59–65, 1992.

Mack TM, Pike MC, Henderson BE, et al: Estrogens and endometrial cancer in a retirement community. *N Engl J Med* 294:1262–1267, 1976.

Maekawa A, Mitsumori K: Spontaneous occurrence and chemical induction of neurogenic tumors in rats—influence of host factors and specificity of chemical structure. *Crit Rev Toxicol* 20:287–310, 1990.

Magee PN, Swann PF: Nitroso compounds. *Br Med Bull* 25:240–244, 1969.

Magnuson BA, Carr I, Bird RP: Ability of aberrant crypt foci characteristics to predict colonic tumor incidence in rats fed cholic acid. *Cancer Res* 53:4499–4504, 1993.

Magos L: Epidemiological and experimental aspects of metal carcinogenesis: Physicochemical properties, kinetics, and the active species. *Environ Health Perspect* 95:157–189, 1991.

Maher VM, Miller EC, Miller JA, Szybalski W: Mutations and decreases in density of transforming DNA produced by derivatives of the carcinogens 2-acetylaminofluorene and *N*-methyl-4-aminoazobenzene. *Mol Pharmacol* 4:411–426, 1968.

Majno G, Joris I: Apoptosis, oncosis, and necrosis: An overview of cell death. *Am J Pathol* 146: 3–15,1995.

Marnett LJ: Polycyclic aromatic hydrocarbon oxidation during prostaglandin biosynthesis. *Life Sci* 29:531–546, 1981.

Marnett LJ, Burcham PC: Endogenous DNA adducts: Potential and paradox. *Chem Res Toxicol* 6:771–785, 1993.

Masuhara M, Ogasawara H, Katyal SL, et al: Cyclosporine stimulates hepatocyte proliferation and accelerates development of hepatocellular carcinomas in rats. *Carcinogenesis* 14:1579–1584, 1993.

Mattammal MB, Zenser TV, Davis BB: Prostaglandin hydroperoxidase—mediated 2-amino-4-(5-nitro-furyl)[$^{14}$C]thiazole metabolism and nucleic acid binding. *Cancer Res* 41:4961–4966, 1981.

Mauderly JL: Toxicological approaches to complex mixtures. *Environ Health Perspect* 101:155–165, 1993.

Mayer EA: Signal transduction and intercellular communication, in Walsh JH, Dockray GJ (eds): *Gut Peptides: Biochemistry and Physiology*. New York: Raven Press, 1994, pp 33–73.

Mays ET, Christopherson W: Hepatic tumors induced by sex steroids. *Semin Liver Dis* 4:147–157, 1984.

McClain RM: The significance of hepatic microsomal enzyme induction and altered thyroid function in rats: Implications for thyroid gland neoplasia. *Toxicol Pathol* 17:294–306, 1989.

Melnick R, Boorman G, Haseman J, Huff J: Toxicity and carcinogenicity of melamine in F344 rats and B6C3F$_1$ mice. *Toxicol Appl Pharmacol* 72:292–303, 1984.

Memoli VA, Urban RM, Alroy J, Galante JO: Malignant neoplasms associated with orthopedic implant materials in rats. *J Orthop Res* 4:346–355, 1986.

Merchant JA: Human epidemiology: A review of fiber type and characteristics in the development of malignant and nonmalignant disease. *Environ Health Perspect* 88:287–293, 1990.

Michalopoulos G, Strom SC, Kligerman AD, et al: Mutagenesis induced by procarcinogens at the hypoxanthine-guanine phosphoribosyl transferase locus of human fibroblasts cocultured with rat hepatocytes. *Cancer Res* 41:1873–1878, 1981.

Michalowsky LA, Jones PA: DNA methylation and differentiation. *Environ Health Perspect* 80:189–197, 1989.

Mies C: Molecular biological analysis of paraffin-embedded tissues. *Hum Pathol* 25:555–560, 1994.

Miki Y, Swensen J, Shattuck-Eidens D, et al: A strong candidate for the breast and ovarian cancer susceptibility gene *BRCA1*. *Science* 266:66–71, 1994.

Mikol YB, Hoover KL, Creasia D, Poirier LA: Hepatocarcinogenesis in rats fed methyl-deficient, amino acid-defined diets. *Carcinogenesis* 4:1619–1629, 1983.

Miller AB, Berrino F, Hill M, et al: Diet in the aetiology of cancer: A review. *Eur J Cancer* 30A:207–220, 1994.

Miller EC: Studies on the formation of protein-bound derivatives of 3,4-benzopyrene in the epidermal fraction of mouse skin. *Cancer Res* 11:100–108, 1951.

Miller EC: Some current perspectives on chemical carcinogenesis in humans and experimental animals: Presidential address. *Cancer Res* 38:1479–1496, 1978.

Miller EC, Miller JA: The presence and significance of bound aminoazo dyes in the livers of rats fed p-dimethylaminoazobenzene. *Cancer Res* 7:468–480, 1947.

Miller EC, Miller JA, Enomoto M: The comparative carcinogenicities of 2-acetylaminofluorene and its *N*-hydroxy metabolite in mice, hamsters, and guinea pigs. *Cancer Res* 24:2018–2026, 1964.

Miller EC, Miller JA, Sandin RB, Brown RK: The carcinogenic activities of certain analogues of 2-acetylaminofluorene in the rat. *Cancer Res* 9:504–509, 1949.

Miller JA: Carcinogenesis by chemicals: An overview—G.H.A. Clowes Memorial Lecture. *Cancer Res* 30:559–576, 1970.

Miller JA: The need for epidemiological studies of the medical exposures of Japanese patients to the carcinogen ethyl carbamate (urethane) from 1950 to 1975. *Jpn J Cancer Res* 82:1323–1324, 1991.

Miller JA, Cramer JW, Miller EC: The *N*- and ring-hydroxylation of 2-acetylaminofluorene during carcinogenesis in the rat. *Cancer Res* 20:950–962, 1960.

Mirsalis JC: Genotoxicity, toxicity, and carcinogenicity of the antihistamine methapyrilene. *Mutat Res* 185:309–317, 1987.

Mirsalis JC, Monforte JA, Winegar RA: Transgenic animal models for measuring mutations in vivo. *Crit Rev Toxicol* 24:255–280, 1994.

Mirvish SS, Salmasi S, Cohen SM, et al: Liver and forestomach tumors and other forestomach lesions in rats treated with morpholine and sodium nitrite, with and without sodium ascorbate. *JNCI* 71:81–85, 1983.

Modrich P: Mismatch repair, genetic stability, and cancer. *Science* 266:1959–1960, 1994.

Monks TJ, Anders MW, Dekant W, et al: Contemporary issues in toxicology: Glutathione conjugate mediated toxicities. *Toxicol Appl Pharmacol* 106:1–19, 1990.

Monro A: What is an appropriate measure of exposure when testing drugs for carcinogenicity in rodents? *Toxicol Appl Pharmacol* 112:171–181, 1992.

Moolgavkar SH: Carcinogenesis modeling: From molecular biology to epidemiology. *Annu Rev Public Health* 7:151–169, 1986.

Moon HD, Simpson ME, Li CH, Evans HM: Neoplasms in rats treated with pituitary growth hormone: I. Pulmonary and lymphatic tissues. *Cancer Res* 10:297, 1950a.

Moon HD, Simpson ME, Li CH, Evans HM: Neoplasms in rats treated with pituitary growth hormone: III. Reproductive organs. *Cancer Res* 10:549, 1950b.

Morley SJ, Thomas G: Intracellular messengers and the control of protein synthesis. *Pharmacol Ther* 50:291–319, 1991.

Morrow PE: Dust overloading of the lungs: Update and appraisal. *Toxicol Appl Pharmacol* 113:1–12, 1992.

Motojima K: Peroxisome proliferator-activated receptor (PPAR): structure, mechanisms of activation and diverse functions. *Cell Struct Funct* 18:267–277, 1993.

Mottram JC: A developing factor in experimental blastogenesis. *J Pathol Bacteriol* 56:181–187, 1944.

Müller H: Recessively inherited deficiencies predisposing to cancer. *Anticancer Res* 10:513–518, 1990.

Müller R, Rajewsky MF: Enzymatic removal of O$^6$-ethylguanine *versus* stability of O$^4$-ethylthymine in the DNA of rat tissues exposed to the carcinogen ethylnitrosourea: Possible interference of guanine-O6 alkylation with 5-cytosine methylation in the DNA of replicating target cells. *Z Naturforsch [c]* 38:1023–1029, 1983.

Mumtaz MM, Sipes IG, Clewell HJ, Yang RSH: Risk assessment of chemical mixtures: Biologic and toxicologic issues. *Fundam Appl Toxicol* 21:258–269, 1993.

Munro IC: Considerations in chronic toxicity testing: the chemical, the dose, the design. *J Environ Pathol Toxicol* 1:183–197, 1977.

Murphy LJ, Bell GI, Friesen HG: Tissue distribution of insulin-like growth factor I and II messenger ribonucleic acid in the adult rat. *Endocrinology* 120:1279–1282, 1987.

Muscat JE, Wynder EL: Cigarette smoking, asbestos exposure, and malignant mesothelioma. *Cancer Res* 51:2263–2267, 1991.

Myles GM, Sancar A: DNA repair. *Chem Res Toxicol* 2:197–226, 1989.

Nagata C, Kodama M, Ioki Y, Kimura T: Free radicals produced from chemical carcinogens and their significance in carcinogenesis, in Floyd RA (ed): *Free Radicals and Cancer*. New York: Marcel Dekker, 1982, pp 1–62.

National Academy of Science: Biological significance of DNA adducts and protein adducts, in *Drinking Water and Health*. Washington, DC: National Academy Press, 1989, vol 9, pp 6–37.

Nebert DW: Role of genetics and drug metabolism in human cancer risk. *Mutat Res* 247:267–281, 1991.

Neish WJP, Parry EW, Ghadially FN: Tumour induction in the rat by a mixture of two non-carcinogenic aminoazo dyes. *Oncology* 21:229–240, 1967.

Nelson MA, Futscher BW, Kinsella T, et al: Detection of mutant Ha-*ras* genes in chemically initiated mouse skin epidermis before the development of benign tumors. *Proc Natl Acad Sci USA* 89:6398–6402, 1992.

Neumann F: Early indicators for carcinogenesis in sex-hormone-sensitive organs. *Mutat Res* 248:341–356, 1991.

Neumann H-G: Role of extent and persistence of DNA modifications in chemical carcinogenesis by aromatic amines. *Recent Results Cancer Res* 84:77–89, 1983.

Noble RL: Hormonal control of growth and progression in tumors of Nb rats and a theory of action. *Cancer Res* 37:82–94, 1977.

Nowell P, Hungerford D: A minute chromosome in human chronic granulocytic leukemia. *Science* 132:1497, 1960.

Nowell PC: Cytogenetics of tumor progression. *Cancer* 65:2172–2177, 1990.

Nuzum EO, Malkinson AM, Beer DG: Specific Ki-*ras* codon 61 mutations may determine the development of urethan-induced mouse lung adenomas or adenocarcinomas. *Mol Carcinog* 3:287–295, 1990.

Ochi T, Kaneko M: Active oxygen contributes to the major part of chromosomal aberrations in V79 Chinese hamster cells exposed to *N*-hydroxy-2-naphthylamine. *Free Radic Res Commun* 5:351–358, 1989.

Office of Science and Technology Policy: Chemical carcinogens: A review of the science and its associated principles. US Interagency Staff Group on Cacinogens. *Environ Health Perspec* 67:201–282.

Ohnishi K, Iida S, Iwama S, et al: The effect of chronic habitual alcohol intake on the development of liver cirrhosis and hepatocellular carcinoma: Relation to hepatitis B surface antigen carriers. *Cancer* 49:672–677, 1982.

Olsson H, Möller TR, Ranstam J: Early oral contraceptive use and breast cancer among premenopausal women: Final report from a study in southern Sweden. *JNCI* 81:1000–1004, 1989.

Oshimura M, Barrett JC: Chemically induced aneuploidy in mammalian cells: Mechanisms and biological significance in cancer. *Environ Mutagen* 8:129–159, 1986.

Oshimura M, Hesterberg TW, Tsutsui T, Barrett JC: Correlation of asbestos-induced cytogenetic effects with cell transformation of Syrian hamster embryo cells in culture. *Cancer Res* 44:5017–5022, 1984.

Osler M: Obesity and cancer. *Dan Med Bull* 34:267–274, 1987.

Ottaggio L, Bonatti S, Cavalieri Z, Abbondandolo A: Chromosomes bearing amplified genes are a preferential target of chemicals inducing chromosome breakage and aneuploidy. *Mutat Res* 301:149–155, 1993.

Papadopoulos N, Nicolaides N, Wei Y, et al: Mutation of a mutL homolog in hereditary colon cancer. *Science* 263:1559–1560.

Paraskeva C, Williams AC: Promotability and tissue specificity of hereditary cancer genes: Do hereditary cancer patients have a reduced requirement for tumor promotion because all their somatic cells are heterozygous at the predisposing locus? *Mol Carcinog* 5:4–8, 1992.

Pariza MW: A perspective on diet, nutrition, and cancer. *JAMA* 251:1455–1458, 1984.

Paulini K, Beneke G, Körner B, Enders R: The relationship between the latent period and animal age in the development of foreign body sarcomas. *Beitr Pathol* 154:161–169, 1975.

Pawson T: Signal transduction—a conserved pathway from the membrane to the nucleus. *Dev Genetics* 14:333–338, 1993.

Pegg AE: Methylation of the O6 position of guanine in DNA is the most likely initiating event in carcinogenesis by methylating agents. *Cancer Invest* 2:223–231, 1984.

Pegg AE, Byers TL: Repair of DNA containing *O*6-alkylguanine. *FASEB J* 6:2302–2310, 1992.

Pegg AE, Perry W: Alkylation of nucleic acids and metabolism of small doses of dimethylnitrosamine in the rat. *Cancer Res* 41:3128–3132, 1981.

Penn I: Why do immunosuppressed patients develop cancer? *Crit Rev Oncog* 1:27–52, 1989.

Perera F, Mayer J, Santella RM, et al: Biologic markers in risk assessment for environmental carcinogens. *Environ Health Perspect* 90:247–254, 1991.

Peto R, Pike M, Day N, et al: Guidelines for simple, sensitive significance tests for carcinogenic effects in long-term animal experiments. IARC Monogr (Suppl) 2:311–426, 1980.

Pike MC, Krailo MD, Henderson BE, et al: "Hormonal" risk factors, "breast tissue age" and the age-incidence of breast cancer. *Nature* 303:767–770, 1983.

Pirkle JL, Wolfe WH, Patterson DG: Estimates of the half-life of 2,3,7,8-tetrachlorodibenzo-*p*-dioxin in Vietnam veterans of operation ranch hand. *J Toxicol Environ Health* 27:165–171, 1989.

Pitot HC: *Fundamentals of Oncology*, 3d ed New York: Marcel Dekker, 1986a.

Pitot HC: Oncogenes and human neoplasia. *Clin Lab Med* 6:167–179, 1986b.

Pitot HC: Altered hepatic foci: Their role in murine hepatocarcinogenesis. *Annu Rev Pharmacol Toxicol* 30:465–500, 1990.

Pitot HC: Endogenous carcinogenesis: The role of tumor promotion. *Proc Soc Exp Biol Med* 198:661–666, 1991.

Pitot HC: The dynamics of carcinogenesis: Implications for human risk. *CIIT Activities* 13:1–6, 1993a.

Pitot HC: The molecular biology of carcinogenesis. *Cancer* 72:962–970, 1993b.

Pitot HC: Multistage carcinogenesis—genetic and epigenetic mechanisms in relation to cancer prevention. *Cancer Detect Prevent* 17:567–573, 1993c.

Pitot HC: The role of receptors in multistage carcinogenesis. *Mutat Res* (in press).

Pitot HC, Dragan YP: Chemical induction of hepatic neoplasia, in Arias IM, Boyer JL, Fausto N, et al (eds): *The Liver: Biology and Pathobiology,* 3d ed. New York: Raven Press, 1994, pp 1467–1495.

Pitot HC, Dragan YP: The instability of tumor promotion in relation to human cancer risk (in press).

Pitot HC, Goldsworthy TL, Moran S, et al: A method to quantitate the relative initiating and promoting potencies of hepatocarcinogenic agents in their dose-response relationship to altered hepatic foci. *Carcinogenesis* 8:1491–1499, 1987.

Porter TD, Coon MJ: Cytochrome P-450: Multiplicity of isoforms, substrates, and catalytic and regulatory mechanisms. *J Biol Chem* 266:13469–13472, 1991.

Pretlow TP: Alterations associated with early neoplasia in the colon, in Pretlow TG, Pretlow TP (eds): *Biochemical and Molecular Aspects of Selected Cancers*. San Diego: Academic Press, 1994, vol 2, pp 93–141.

Pretlow TP, O'Riordan MA, Spancake KM, Pretlow TG: Two types of putative preneoplastic lesions identified by hexosaminidase activity in whole-mounts of colons from F344 rats treated with carcinogen. *Am J Pathol* 142:1695–1700, 1993.

Price A: The repair of ionizing radiation-induced damage to DNA. *Cancer Biol* 4:61–71, 1993.

Pullman A, Pullman B: Electronic structure and carcinogenic activity of aromatic molecules: New developments. *Adv Cancer Res* 3:117–169, 1955.

Purnell DM: The relationship of terminal duct hyperplasia to mammary carcinoma in 7,12-dimethylbenzo($a$)anthracene-treated LEW/Mai rats. *Am J Pathol* 98:311–324, 1980.

Purtilo DT, Linder J: Oncological consequences of impaired immune surveillance against ubiquitous viruses. *J Clin Immunol* 3:197–206, 1983.

Quintanilla M, Brown K, Ramsden M, Balmain A: Carcinogen-specific mutation and amplification of Ha-*ras* during mouse skin carcinogenesis. *Nature* 322:78–80, 1986.

Radomski JL: The primary aromatic amines: Their biological properties and structure-activity relationships. *Annu Rev Pharmacol Toxicol* 19:129–157, 1979.

Randerath E, Hart RW, Turturro A, et al: Effects of aging and caloric restriction on I-compounds in liver, kidney and white blood cell DNA of male Brown-Norway rats. *Mech Ageing Dev* 58:279–296, 1991.

Randerath K, van Golen KL, Dragan YP, Pitot HC: Effects of phenobarbital on I-compounds in liver DNA as a function of age in male rats fed two different diets. *Carcinogenesis* 13:125–130, 1992.

Reddy JK, Lalwani ND: Carcinogenesis by hepatic peroxisome proliferators: Evaluation of the risk of hypolipidemic drugs and industrial plasticizers to humans. *CRC Crit Rev Toxicol* 12:1–58, 1983.

Reddy JK, Rao MS: Oxidative DNA damage caused by persistent peroxisome proliferation: its role in hepatocarcinogenesis. *Mutat Res* 214:63–68, 1989.

Reddy MV, Randerath K: $^{32}$P-Postlabeling assay for carcinogen-DNA adducts: nuclease $P_1$-mediated enhancement of its sensitivity and applications. *Environ Health Perspect* 76:41–47, 1987.

Regan JD, Setlow RB: Two forms of repair in the DNA of human cells damaged by chemical carcinogens and mutagens. *Cancer Res* 34:3318–3325, 1974.

Reif AE: Effect of cigarette smoking on susceptibility to lung cancer. *Oncology* 38:76–85, 1981.

Riggs AD, Jones PA: 5-Methylcytosine, gene regulation, and cancer. *Adv Cancer Res* 40:1–30, 1983.

Roe FJC, Dukes CE, Mitchley BCV: Sarcomas at the site of implantation of a polyvinyl plastic sponge: incidence reduced by use of thin implants. *Biochem Pharmacol* 16:647–650, 1967.

Rogan WJ, Brown SM: Some fundamental aspects of epidemiology: A guide for laboratory scientists. *Fed Proc* 38:1875–1879, 1979.

Rogers A: Nitrosamines, in Newberne P (ed): *Trace Substances and Health: A Handbook, Part 2*. New York: Marcel Dekker, 1982, pp 47–80.

Rogers AE, Zeisel SH, Groopman J: Diet and carcinogenesis. *Carcinogenesis* 14:2205–2217, 1993.

Rogler CE, Yang D, Rossetti L, et al: Altered body composition and increased frequency of diverse malignancies in insulin-like growth factor-II transgenic mice. *J Biol Chem* 269:13779–13784, 1994.

Rosenkranz HS, Klopman G: Structural implications of the ICPEMC method for quantifying genotoxicity data. *Mutat Res* 305:99–116, 1994.

Rosenthal N: Molecular medicine. Regulation of gene expression. *N Engl J Med* 331:931–933, 1994.

Rous P, Kidd JG: Conditional neoplasms and sub-threshold neoplastic states: A study of the tar tumors of rabbits. *J Exp Med* 73:369–390, 1941.

Rumsby PC, Barrass NC, Phillimore HE, Evans JG: Analysis of the Ha-*ras* oncogene in C3H/He mouse liver tumors derived spontaneously or induced with diethylnitrosamine or phenobarbitone. *Carcinogenesis* 12:2331–2336, 1991.

Russo J, Tait L, Russo IH: Susceptibility of the mammary gland to carcinogenesis: III. The cell of origin of rat mammary carcinoma. *Am J Pathol* 113:50–66, 1983.

Saeter G, Schwarze PE, Nesland JM, Seglen PO: 2-Acetylaminofluorene promotion of liver carcinogenesis by a non-cytotoxic mechanism. *Carcinogenesis* 9:581–587, 1988.

Sancar A, Tang M-S: Nucleotide excision repair. *Photochem Photobiol* 57:905–921, 1993.

Sandén A, Järvholm B, Larsson S, Thiringer G: The risk of lung cancer and mesothelioma after cessation of asbestos exposure: A prospective cohort study of shipyard workers. *Eur Respir J* 5:281–285, 1992.

Sander CA, Yano T, Clark HM, et al: p53 mutation is associated with progression in follicular lymphomas. *Blood* 82:1994–2004, 1993.

Sargent L, Xu Y-H Sattler GL, et al: Ploidy and karyotype of hepatocytes isolated from enzyme-altered foci in two different protocols of multistage hepatocarcinogenesis in the rat. *Carcinogenesis* 10:387–391, 1989.

Sasaki T, Yoshida T: Experimentelle Erzeugung des Lebercarcinoms durch Fütterung mit o-Amidoazotoluol. *Virchows Arch [A]* 295:175–200, 1935.

Satoh MS, Lindahl T: Enzymatic repair of oxidative DNA damage. *Cancer Res* 54:1899s–1901s, 1994.

Schaeffer BK, Zurlo J, Longnecker DS: Activation of c-Ki-*ras* not detectable in adenomas or adenocarcinomas arising in rat pancreas. *Mol Carcinog* 3:165–170, 1990.

Schlesselman JJ, Stadel BV, Murray P, Shenghan L: Breast cancer in relation to early use of oral contraceptives. *JAMA* 259:1828–1833, 1988.

Schmähl D, Habs M: Carcinogenicity of *N*-nitroso compounds: Species and route differences in regard to organotropism. *Oncology* 37:237–242, 1980.

Schoental R: Trichothecenes, zearalenone, and other carcinogenic metabolites of *Fusarium* and related microfungi. *Adv Cancer Res* 45:217–274, 1985.

Schulte-Hermann R, Bursch W, Kraupp-Grasl B, et al: Cell proliferation and apoptosis in normal liver and preneoplastic foci. *Environ Health Perspect* 101:87–90, 1993.

Schulte-Hermann R, Ohde G, Schuppler J, Timmermann-Trosiener I: Enhanced proliferation of putative preneoplastic cells in rat liver following treatment with the tumor promoters phenobarbital, hexachlorocyclohexane, steroid compounds, and nafenopin. *Cancer Res* 41:2556–2562, 1981.

Schulte-Hermann R, Timmermann-Trosiener I, Barthel G, Bursch W: DNA synthesis, apoptosis, and phenotypic expression as determinants of growth of altered foci in rat liver during phenobarbital promotion. *Cancer Res* 50:5127–5135, 1990.

Scicchitano DA, Hanawalt PC: Intragenomic repair heterogeneity of DNA damage. *Environ Health Perspect* 98:45–51, 1992.

Scott D, Galloway SM, Marshall RR, et al: Genotoxicity under extreme culture conditions. *Mutat Res* 257:147–204, 1991.

Seitz HK, Simanowski UA: Alcohol and carcinogenesis. *Annu Rev Nutr* 8:99–119, 1988.

Shapiro R: Damage to DNA caused by hydrolysis, in Seeberg E, Kleppe K (eds): *Chromosome Damage and Repair*. New York: Plenum Press, 1981, pp 3–18.

Shearman CW, Loeb LA: Effects of depurination on the fidelity of DNA synthesis. *J Mol Biol* 128:197–218, 1979.

Shephard SE, Schlatter, Ch.; and Lutz WK: Assessment of the risk of formation of carcinogenic *N*-nitroso compounds from dietary precursors in the stomach. *Food Chem Toxicol* 25:91–108, 1987.

Sherr CJ: Mammalian $G_1$ cyclins. *Cell* 73:1059–1065, 1993.

Shields PG, Harris CC: Molecular epidemiology and the genetics of environmental cancer. *JAMA* 266:681–687, 1991.

Shimkin MB: *Contrary to Nature*. Washington, DC: U.S. Department of Health, Education, and Welfare, Public Health Service, National Institutes of Health, 1977.

Shivapurkar N, Tang Z, Ferreira A, et al: Sequential analysis of K-*ras* mutations in aberrant crypt foci and colonic tumors induced by azoxymethane in Fischer-344 rats on high-risk diet. *Carcinogenesis* 15:775–778, 1994.

Shixin L, Mingxin L, Chuan J, et al: An *N*-nitroso compound, N-3-methylbutyl-N-1-methylacetonylnitrosamine, in cornbread inoculated with fungi. *Sci Sin* 22:601, 1979.

Short BG, Steinhagen WH, Swenberg JA: Promoting effects of unleaded gasoline and 2,2,4-trimethylpentane on the development of atypical cell foci and renal tubular cell tumors in rats exposed to *N*-ethyl-*N*-hydroxyethylnitrosamine. *Cancer Res* 49:6369–6378, 1989.

Simic MG: Mechanisms of inhibition of free-radical processes in mutagenesis and carcinogenesis. *Mutat Res* 202:377–386, 1988.

Sims P, Grover PL, Swaisland A, et al: Metabolic activation of benzo[a]pyrene proceeds by a diol-epoxide. *Nature* 252:326–328, 1974.

Singer B: *O*-Alkyl pyrimidines in mutagenesis and carcinogenesis: Occurrence and significance. *Cancer Res* 46:4879–4885, 1986.

Sivak A: Cocarcinogenesis. *Biochim Biophys Acta* 560:67–89, 1979.

Sky-Peck HH: Trace metals and neoplasia. *Clin Physiol Biochem* 4:99–111, 1986.

Smith BJ, Curtis JF, Eling TE: Bioactivation of xenobiotics by prostaglandin H synthase. *Chem Biol Interact* 79:245–264, 1991.

Snyder R, Kalf GF: A perspective on benzene leukemogenesis. *Crit Rev Toxicol* 24:177–209, 1994.

Sodum RS, Nie G, Fiala ES: 8-Aminoguanine: A base modification produced in rat liver nucleic acids by the hepatocarcinogen 2-nitropropane. *Chem Res Toxicol* 6:269–276, 1993.

Solt D, Farber E: New principle for the analysis of chemical carcinogenesis. *Nature* 263:701–703, 1976.

Spitz MR, Bondy ML: Genetic susceptibility to cancer. *Cancer* 72:991–995, 1993.

Srinivasan S, Glauert HP: Formation of 5-hydroxymethyl-2′-deoxyuridine in hepatic DNA of rats treated with $\gamma$-irradiation, diethylnitrosamine, 2-acetylaminofluorene or the peroxisome proliferator ciprofibrate. *Carcinogenesis* 11:2021–2024, 1990.

Standeven AM, Wolf DC, Goldsworthy TL: Investigation of antiestrogenicity as a mechanism of female mouse liver tumor induction by unleaded gasoline. *Chem Indust Inst Toxicol* 14:1–5, 1994.

Stanford JL, Brinton LA, Hoover RN: Oral contraceptives and breast cancer: Results from an expanded case-control study. *Br J Cancer* 60:375–381, 1989.

Stanton MF, Layard M, Tegeris A, et al: Carcinogenicity of fibrous glass: Pleural response in the rat in relation to fiber dimension. *JNCI* 58:387–603, 1977.

Stanton MF, Layard M, Tegeris A, et al: Relation of particle dimension to carcinogenicity in amphibole asbestoses and other fibrous minerals. *JNCI* 67:965–975, 1981.

Starr TB, Gibson JE: The mechanistic toxicology of formaldehyde and its implications for quantitative risk estimation. *Annu Rev Pharmacol Toxicol* 25:745–767, 1985.

Statland BE: Nutrition and cancer. *Clin Chem* 38:1587–1594, 1992.

Steinbrecher UP, Lisbona R, Huang SN, Mishkin S: Complete regression of hepatocellular adenoma after withdrawal of oral contraceptives. *Digest Dis Sci* 26:1045–1050, 1981.

Stewart BW, Sarfaty GA: Environmental chemical carcinogenesis. *Med J Aust* 1:92–95, 1978.

Stinson NE: The tissue reaction induced in rats and guinea-pigs by polymethylmethacrylate (acrylic) and stainless steel (18/8/Mo). *Br J Exp Pathol* 45:21–29, 1964.

Stott WT: Chemically induced proliferation of peroxisomes: Implications for risk assessment. *Regul Toxicol Pharmacol* 8:125–159, 1988.

Stowers SJ, Anderson MW: Formation and persistence of benzo(a)pyrene metabolite-DNA adducts. *Environ Health Perspect* 62:31–39, 1985.

Strader CD, Fong TM, Tota MR, et al: Structure and function of G protein-coupled receptors. *Annu Rev Biochem* 63:101–132, 1994.

Styles JA: Measurement of ploidy and cell proliferation in the rodent liver. *Environ Health Perspect* 101(suppl 5):67–71, 1993.

Sumi C, Yokoro K, Kajitani T, Ito A: Synergism of diethylstilbestrol and other carcinogens in concurrent development of hepatic, mammary, and pituitary tumors in castrated male rats. *JNCI* 65:169–175, 1980.

Sunderman FW Jr: Carcinogenicity of metal alloys in orthopedic prostheses: clinical and experimental studies. *Fundam Appl Toxicol* 13:205–216, 1989.

Swenberg JA, Dyroff MC, Bedell MA, et al: $O^4$-Ethyldeoxythymidine, but not $O^6$-ethyldeoxyguanosine, accumulates in hepatocyte DNA of rats exposed continuously to diethylnitrosamine. *Proc Natl Acad Sci USA* 81:1692–1695, 1984.

Swenberg JA, Richardson FC, Boucheron JA, Dyroff MC: Relationships between DNA adduct formation and carcinogenesis. *Environ Health Perspect* 62:177–183, 1985.

Swerdlow AJ, Douglas AJ, Hudson GV, et al: Risk of second primary cancers after Hodgkin's disease by type of treatment: Analysis of 2846 patients in the British National Lymphoma Investigation. *Br Med J* 304:1137–1143, 1992.

Takayama S, Hasegawa H, Ohgaki H: Combination effects of forty carcinogens administered at low doses to male rats. *Jpn J Cancer Res* 80:732–736, 1989.

Talalay P, De Long MJ, Prochaska HJ: Identification of a common chemical signal regulating the induction of enzymes that protect against chemical carcinogenesis. *Proc Natl Acad Sci USA* 85:8261–8265, 1988.

Taper HS: The effect of estradiol-17-phenylpropionate and estradiol benzoate on *N*-nitrosomorpholine-induced liver carcinogenesis in ovariectomized female rats. *Cancer* 42:462–467, 1978.

Tatematsu M, Nagamine Y, Farber E: Redifferentiation as a basis for remodeling of carcinogen-induced hepatocyte nodules to normal appearing liver. *Cancer Res* 43:5049–5058, 1983.

Tennant RW: A perspective on nonmutagenic mechanisms in carcinogenesis. *Environ Health Perspect* 101(suppl):231–236, 1993.

Tennant RW, Ashby J: Classification according to chemical structure, mutagenicity to Salmonella and level of carcinogenicity of a further 39 chemicals tested for carcinogenicity by the U.S. National Toxicology Program. *Mutat Res* 257:209–227, 1991.

Thomas DB: Oral contraceptives and breast cancer: Review of the epidemiologic literature. *Contraception* 43:597–642, 1991.

Thomassen MJ, Buoen LC, Brand I, Brand KG: Foreign-body tumorigenesis in mice: DNA synthesis in surface-attached cells during preneoplasia. *JNCI* 61:359–363, 1978.

Tokusashi Y, Fukuda I, Ogawa K: Absence of *p53* mutations and various frequencies of Ki-*ras* exon 1 mutations in rat hepatic tumors induced by different carcinogens. *Mol Carcinog* 10:45–51, 1994.

Ueda G, Furth J: Sacromatoid transformation of transplanted thyroid carcinoma. *Arch Pathol* 83:3, 1967.

Umar A, Boyer JC, Thomas DC, et al: Defective mismatch repair in extracts of colorectal and endometrial cancer cell lines exhibiting microsatellite instability. *J Biol Chem* 269:14367–14370, 1994.

Vainio H, Coleman M, Wilbourn J: Carcinogenicity evaluations and ongoing studies: The IARC databases. *Environ Health Perspect* 96:5–9, 1991.

Vainio H, Hemminki K, Wilbourn J: Data on the carcinogenicity of chemicals in the *IARC Monographs* programme. *Carcinogenesis* 6:1653–1665, 1985.

Vainio H, Wilbourn J: Cancer etiology: Agents causally associated with human cancer. *Pharmacol Toxicol* 72:4–11, 1993.

Van Duuren BL, Sivak A, Katz C, et al: The effect of aging and interval between primary and secondary treatment in two-stage carcinogenesis on mouse skin. *Cancer Res* 35:502–505, 1975.

Verma AK, Boutwell RK: Effects of dose and duration of treatment with the tumor-promoting agent, 12-O-tetradecanoylphorbol-13-acetate on mouse skin carcinogenesis. *Carcinogenesis* 1:271–276, 1980.

Verschaeve L, Driesen M, Kirsch-Volders M, et al: Chromosome distribution studies after inorganic lead exposure. *Hum Genet* 49:147–158 1979.

Von Hansemann D: Uber assymetrische Zellteilung im Epithelkrebsen und deren biologische Bedeutung. *Virchows Arch [A]* 119:299–326, 1890.

Waalkes MP, Coogan TP, Barter RA: Toxicological principles of metal carcinogenesis with special emphasis on cadmium. *Crit Rev Toxicol* 22:175–201, 1992.

Wallace LA: The exposure of the general population to benzene. *Cell Biol Toxicol* 5:297–314, 1989.

Wang M-Y, Liehr JG: Identification of fatty acid hydroperoxide cofactors in the cytochrome P450-mediated oxidation of estrogens to quinone metabolites. *J Biol Chem* 269:284–291, 1994.

Ward EJ: Persistent and heritable structural damage induced in heterochromatic DNA from rat liver by *N*-nitrosodimethylamine. *Biochemistry* 26:1709–1717, 1987.

Warshawsky D, Barkley W, Bingham E: Factors affecting carcinogenic potential of mixtures. *Fundam Appl Toxicol* 20:376–382, 1993.

Weinberg RA: The integration of molecular genetics into cancer management. *Cancer* 70(suppl 6):1653–1658, 1992.

Weisburger EK, Weisburger JH: Chemistry, carcinogenicity and metabolism of 2-fluorenamine and related compounds. *Adv Cancer Res* 5:331–431, 1958.

Weisburger JH, Williams GH: Metabolism of chemical carcinogens, in Becker FF (ed): *Cancer: A Comprehensive Treatise*. New York: Plenum, 1982, vol 1, pp 241–333.

Welch DR, Tomasovic SP: Implications of tumor progression on clinical oncology. *Clin Exp Metastasis* 3:151–188, 1985.

Westra JG, Kriek E, Hittenhausen H: Identification of the persistently bound form of the carcinogen *N*-acetyl-2-aminofluorene to rat liver DNA in vivo. *Chem.-Biol Interact* 15:149–164, 1976.

White E, Malone KE, Weiss NS, Daling JR: Breast cancer among young U.S. women in relation to oral contraceptive use. *JNCI* 86:505–514, 1994.

Wiebauer K, Neddermann P, Hughes M, Jiricny J: The repair of 5-methylcytosine deamination damage, in Jost JP, Saluz HP (eds): *DNA Methylation: Molecular Biology and Biological Significance*. Basel: Birkhäuser Verlag, 1993, pp 510–522.

Wigley CB: Experimental approaches to the analysis of precancer. *Cancer Surv* 2:495–515, 1983.

Willett WC, MacMahon B: Diet and cancer—an overview. *N Engl J Med* 310:633–638, 697–701, 1984.

Williams ED: TSH and thyroid cancer, in Pfeiffer EF, Reaven GM (eds): *Hormone and Metabolic Research*. New York: Theime, Inc., 1989, vol 23, pp 72–75.

Williams GM, Iatropoulos MJ, Djordjevic MV, Kaltenberg OP: The triphenylethylene drug tamoxifen is a strong liver carcinogen in the rat. *Carcinogenesis* 14:315–317, 1993.

Wilson MJ, Shivapurkar N, Poirier LA: Hypomethylation of hepatic nuclear DNA in rats fed with a carcinogenic methyl-deficient diet. *Biochem J* 218:987–990, 1984.

Winick NJ, McKenna RW, Shuster JJ, et al: Secondary acute myeloid leukemia in children with acute lymphoblastic leukemia treated with etoposide. *J Clin Oncol* 11:209–217, 1993.

Wise RW, Zenser TV, Kadlubar FF, Davis BB: Metabolic activation of carcinogenic aromatic amines by dog bladder and kidney prostaglandin H synthase. *Cancer Res* 44:1893–1897, 1984.

Wogan GN: Aflatoxins as risk factors for hepatocellular carcinoma in humans. *Cancer Res* 52:2114s-2118s, 1992.

Wright SC, Zhong J, Larrick JW: Inhibition of apoptosis as a mechanism of tumor promotion. *FASEB J* 8:654–660, 1994.

Wright WC: *De Morbis Artificum* by Bernardino Ramazzini: The Latin Text of 1713. Chicago: U of Chicago Press, 1940, p 191.

Wu HH, Kawamata H, Wang DD, Oyasu R: Immunohistochemical localization of transforming growth factor in the major salivary glands of male and female rats. *Histochem J* 25:613–618, 1993.

Wu X, Levine AJ: p53 and E2F-1 cooperate to mediate apoptosis. *Proc Natl Acad Sci USA* 91:3602–3606, 1994.

Wyllie AH: Apoptosis: Cell death in tissue regulation. *J Pathol* 153:313–316, 1987.

Wyllie AH: Death from inside out: An overview. *Philos Trans R Soc Lond [Biol]* 345:237–241, 1994.

Wynder EL, Weisburger JH, Horn C: On the importance and relevance of tumour promotion systems in the development of nutritionally linked cancers. *Cancer Surv* 2:557–576, 1983.

Yager JD, Yager R: Oral contraceptive steroids as promoters of hepatocarcinogenesis in female Sprague-Dawley rats. *Cancer Res* 40:3680–3685, 1980.

Yamagawa K, Ichikawa K: Experimentelle Studie über die Pathogenese der Epithelialgeschwülste. *Mitteilungen Med Fakultät Kaiserl Univ Tokyo* 15:295–344, 1915.

Yang SK, McCourt DW, Roller PP, Gelboin HV: Enzymatic conversion of benzo[*a*]pyrene leading predominantly to the diol-epoxide *r*-7, *t*-8-dihydroxy-*t*-9,10-oxy-7,8,9,10-tetrahydrobenzo[*a*]pyrene through a single enantiomer of *r*-7, *t*-8-dihydroxy-7,8-dihydrobenzo[*a*]pyrene. *Proc Natl Acad Sci USA* 73:2594–2598, 1976.

Yokota J, Sugimura T: Multiple steps in carcinogenesis involving alterations of multiple tumor suppressor genes. *FASEB J* 7:920–925, 1993.

Yu M-W, Chen C: Elevated serum testosterone levels and risk of hepatocellular carcinoma. *Cancer Res* 53:790–794, 1993.

Zatonski W, Becher H, Lissowska J: Smoking cessation: Intermediate nonsmoking periods and reduction of laryngeal cancer risk. *JNCI* 82:1427–1428, 1990.

Zeise L, Wilson R, Crouch E: Dose response relationships for carcinogens: A review. *Environ Health Perspect* 73:259–308, 1987.

Zhang R, Haag JD, Gould MN: Quantitating the frequency of initiation and cH-ras mutation in *in situ* *N*-methyl-*N*-nitrosourea-exposed rat mammary gland. *Cell Growth Differ* 2:1–6, 1991.

Zhu BT, Roy D, Liehr JG: The carcinogenic activity of ethinyl estrogens is determined by both their hormonal characteristics and their conversion to catechol metabolites. *Endocrinology* 132:577–583, 1993.

CHAPTER 9

# GENETIC TOXICOLOGY

*George R. Hoffmann*

## SCOPE OF GENETIC TOXICOLOGY

Genetic toxicology deals with the mutagenic effects of chemicals and radiation and the consequences for human health of exposure to mutagens. Genetic toxicologists conduct research on the mechanisms of mutagenesis, apply test systems to detect and characterize mutagens, and formulate means of assessing the health risks posed by mutagens. Defined broadly, mutagenesis includes the induction of DNA damage and genetic alterations that range from changes in one or a few DNA base pairs (gene mutations) to gross changes in chromosome structure (chromosome aberrations) or number (aneuploidy and polyploidy). Any agent that causes mutations is a mutagen. The more specialized terms "clastogen" and "aneugen" are used for agents that cause chromosome aberrations and aneuploidy, respectively.

There are two major reasons for concern about human exposure to mutagens. First, an increase in the mutation rate in human germ cells (eggs, sperm, and their precursors) may cause an increased incidence of genetic disease in future generations. Second, mutations in somatic cells may contribute to various disorders, most notably cancer, in exposed individuals. Gene mutations, chromosome aberrations, and aneuploidy all contribute to human genetic disease, and diverse genetic alterations have been implicated in carcinogenesis.

This chapter discusses the historical development of genetic toxicology, the nature of genetic damage, mechanisms of mutagenesis and DNA repair, assays used in mutagenicity testing, the implications of mutagenesis for human health, and assessment of mutational hazards. For brevity, reviews and other syntheses of information are often cited instead of original research papers. Further information can be found in the literature cited and in the three major journals in the field: *Mutation Research*, *Environmental and Molecular Mutagenesis*, and *Mutagenesis*.

## HISTORICAL DEVELOPMENT

The beginning of the modern era of mutation research was marked by H. J. Muller's discovery in 1927 that x-rays cause sex-linked recessive lethal mutations in the fruit fly *Drosophila melanogaster*. One year later, L. R. Stadler reported that x-rays are mutagenic in plants. The mutagenicity of ultraviolet light (UV) was demonstrated soon afterward. The first unequivocal evidence of chemical mutagenesis was obtained in Scotland in 1942 by Charlotte Auerbach and J. M. Robson, who found that mustard gas is mutagenic in *Drosophila*. The research of Auerbach and Robson was not reported until after World War II, when wartime censorship was lifted. In Germany during the war, Friedrich Oehlkers found that urethane causes chromosome aberrations. Shortly thereafter, I. A. Rapoport reported in the Soviet Union that ethylene oxide, ethylenimine, epichlorohydrin, diazomethane, diethyl sulfate, glycidol, and several other chemicals are mutagenic. By the end of the 1940s chemical mutagenesis was a well-established and growing area of interest in genetics.

Early interest in mutagens focused on the nature of mutation, the use of mutagens to obtain mutants for genetic studies, and the introduction of new genetic variations into organisms of agricultural or industrial importance. H. J. Muller suggested in his 1927 paper and during the 1930s that mutagenesis in somatic cells can cause cancer, but it was not until the late 1950s and early 1960s that the health hazard of mutagenesis was generally recognized. The primary focus was on germ cell mutagenesis and genetic disease. The idea that mutagenicity should be considered in the toxicological evaluation of chemicals became widespread during this period. A driving force in the newly evolving field of genetic toxicology in the 1960s was that of Alexander Hollaender, who led the founding of the Environmental Mutagen Society (EMS) in 1969. The EMS and related organizations now include hundreds of geneticists and toxicologists involved in research on mutation or public health policy related to mutagenesis.

The past two decades have given rise to an extensive literature on basic mutation research and mutagenicity testing, and mutagenesis has gradually been integrated into the broad field of toxicology. National and international agencies have become increasingly interested in mutagenesis, recognizing its importance not only for genetic disease but also for carcinogenesis. In the United States, agencies such as the National Institutes of Health and National Toxicology Program (NTP), Environmental Protection Agency (EPA), Food and Drug Administration (FDA), and Department of Energy have supported basic research on mutagenesis. Moreover, mutagenesis is among the biological effects considered in regulating chemicals to ensure public safety, and private industry has developed mutagenicity programs in an effort to develop safe chemical products. The historical development of mutation research and genetic toxicology has been reviewed by Auerbach (1976) and Wassom (1989).

## KINDS OF GENETIC DAMAGE

Genetic toxicologists are principally concerned with three categories of genetic alterations: gene mutations, chromosome aberrations, and changes in chromosome number.

### Gene Mutations

Gene mutations are changes in the DNA sequence in a gene. They are also called point mutations because they are restricted to a particular site. Gene mutations typically are detected on the basis of the changes they cause in the phenotype.

For example, they are detected in the mouse visible specific locus test by altered pigmentation or ear length (Ehling, 1991). Mutations have traditionally been characterized by subjecting mutants to genetic analysis, but they are also being characterized by direct analysis of DNA sequences. The two principal kinds of gene mutations are base-pair substitutions and frameshift mutations (Griffiths et al., 1993), which are illustrated in Fig. 9-1.

In a base-pair substitution, one base pair in DNA (e.g., G:C) is replaced by another (e.g., A:T). Base-pair substitutions are called transitions if the purine to pyrimidine orientation of the base pair remains the same. This is the same as saying that one purine (e.g., G) is replaced by another (e.g., A) in a transition. In contrast, a base-pair substitution in which a purine is replaced by a pyrimidine (and vice versa) is called a transversion. Because of the specific pairing of adenine with thymine and guanine with cytosine, there are several possible transitions (G:C → A:T and A:T → G:C) and transversions (G:C → T:A, G:C → C:G, A:T → C:G, and A:T → T:A). The consequences of a transition or transversion depend on whether it results in missense or nonsense in protein synthesis. In a missense mutation, there is a coding change in which one amino acid replaces another in the gene product. The mutation can inactivate the gene product, have only a slight effect on func-

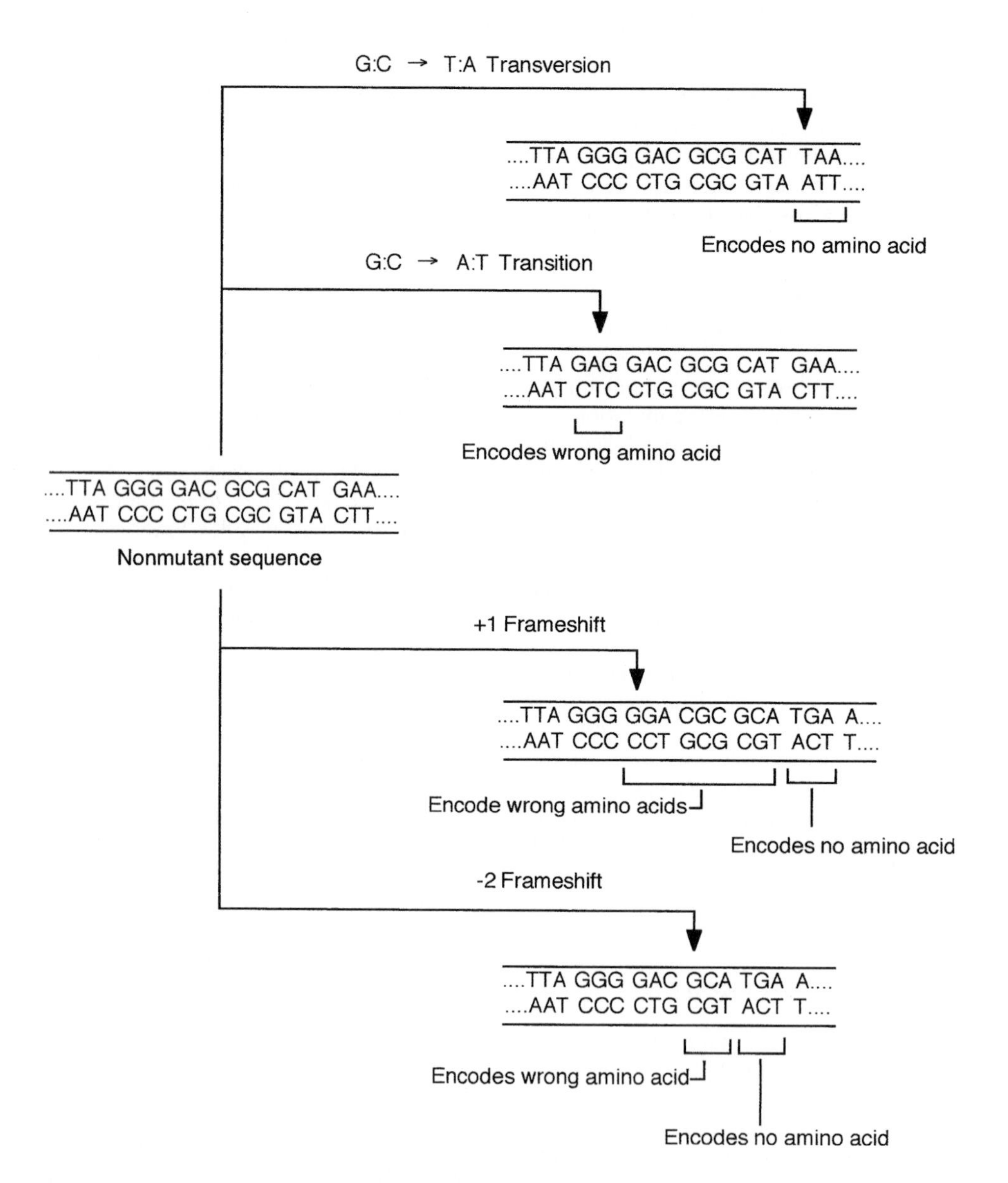


***Figure 9–1. Base-pair substitutions and frameshift mutations.***

The arrows indicate the sites of the mutations in a DNA sequence that is shown in units of three bases to denote the reading frame of the mRNA codons specified by the DNA. The base-pair substitutions are a transversion (G:C → T:A) and a transition (G:C → A:T). One of the base-pair substitutions (the transition) is a missense mutation, and the other is a nonsense mutation. The frameshift mutations are examples in which one base pair (G:C) has been added (+1 frameshift) or two base pairs (G:C and C:G) have been deleted (−2 frameshift). In frameshift mutations, the reading frame of the genetic code is altered for all codons after the point of the mutation.

tion (i.e., a "leaky" mutation), or be virtually without effect, depending on the specific amino acid substitution and its position in the protein. In a nonsense mutation, the gene product is incomplete and nonfunctional because of premature termination of protein synthesis. A mutation also can prevent the formation of a functional gene product by preventing transcription or normal splicing of RNA.

Mutations that alter the reading frame of the genetic code during the translation of RNA into protein are called frameshift mutations. Most commonly, frameshifts involve the gain or loss of one or two base pairs in a gene. In a frameshift mutation, the gene product is grossly altered because every triplet is changed in the messenger RNA after the point of the mutation. The gene product is also apt to be incomplete because the new reading frame is likely to include a nonsense codon (UAA, UAG, or UGA), which specifies no amino acid at all, somewhere in the altered message. Frameshift mutations therefore lead to nonfunctional gene products. The phenotypic effect of a frameshift mutation depends on how the lack of that specific gene function affects the viability and metabolism of the cell or organism.

An exciting development in the last few years has been the discovery in humans of a new class of mutations called triplet repeats (Martin, 1993a). Triplet repeats resemble gene mutations in that they are alterations at the level of DNA sequence in individual genes. In a triplet repeat mutation, a particular trinucleotide is amplified (e.g., CTG/CTG/CTG/CTG). Triplet repeats are involved in several genetic diseases, including myotonic dystrophy, Huntington's disease, and fragile X syndrome. For example, the CGG trinucleotide, which normally is repeated 6 to 54 times in the FMR-1 gene, expands to 50 to 1500 copies in a person with fragile X syndrome. The factors that modulate the expansion of these triplets are not clear.

## Chromosome Aberrations

Chromosome aberrations are changes in chromosome structure. They involve gross alteration of the genetic material and are generally detected by using light microscopy to examine metaphase chromosomes in appropriately prepared cells. Cytologically detected damage includes chromosome breakage and various chromosomal rearrangements that result from broken chromosomes. Aberrations that involve only one of the two chromatids in a replicated chromosome are called chromatid-type aberrations, whereas those which involve both chromatids are called chromosome-type aberrations. Ionizing radiation induces chromosome-type aberrations when cells are treated before DNA replication and chromatid-type aberrations after DNA replication. Unlike ionizing radiation, most chemical clastogens induce only chromatid aberrations, because the aberrations result from DNA synthesis on a damaged DNA template in the S period of the cell cycle (Bender et al., 1988; Sorsa et al., 1992). A few exceptions, such as bleomycin, are said to be radiomimetic because, like ionizing radiation, they are S-independent and induce chromosome-type aberrations in the $G_1$ period or in nondividing ($G_0$) cells (Littlefield and Hoffmann, 1993).

Some aberrations are stable in that they can be transmitted through repeated cell divisions and thus persist in the cell population. Deletions, duplications, inversions, and balanced translocations are chromosomal rearrangements that can be transmitted in populations of cells or organisms. Besides stable aberrations, chromosome breaks give rise to acentric fragments (i.e., broken pieces of chromosomes with no centromere), dicentric chromosomes, ring chromosomes, and various other asymmetrical rearrangements that are unstable in that they usually cause the death of the cell through the loss of vital genetic material or mechanical hindrance of mitosis. Stable rearrangements can be detected with staining techniques that reveal banding patterns on chromosomes but are not readily detected with routine cytogenetic analysis of unbanded chromosomes. The analysis of banded chromosomes, however, is more labor-intensive than is standard cytogenetic analysis. Metaphase analysis for chromosome damage therefore is usually performed by analyzing unbanded chromosomes for gross structural changes. Although many of the alterations detected in this manner are unstable, they provide direct evidence of chromosome breakage and are representative of aberrations as a whole in that clastogens induce both stable and unstable aberrations. Easily scored aberrations include chromatid breaks, chromosome breaks, acentric fragments, chromatid exchanges, dicentric chromosomes, ring chromosomes, and some reciprocal translocations (Bender et al., 1988; Kirkland et al., 1990).

While gene mutations and chromosome aberrations appear to be distinct categories, they may overlap. Small deletions within a gene resemble gene mutations in that they are confined to a localized site but may arise by the same mechanisms that cause gross chromosomal rearrangements. Such deletions are too small to detect by microscopy but may be detected by the loss of gene function that they impart. Thus, small deletions may be detected on the basis of phenotype, as are gene mutations. Many assays for gene mutations also detect small deletions that remove part or all of the target gene and sometimes some of the surrounding DNA.

## Aneuploidy and Polyploidy

Aneuploid and polyploid cells have chromosome numbers that differ from the normal number for the species. Aneuploidy involves the gain or loss of one or a few chromosomes, whereas polyploidy involves complete sets of chromosomes. For example, in humans, the normal diploid ($2n$) chromosome number is 46, and those cells or individuals with 45 or 47 chromosomes would be described as aneuploid, whereas those with 69 chromosomes would be described as polyploid, in this case triploid ($3n$). Aneuploids lacking a chromosome are said to be monosomic, whereas those with an extra chromosome are called trisomic (Griffiths et al., 1993). Down syndrome, for example, results when an individual has three copies of chromosome 21 (i.e., trisomy 21). Aneuploidy and polyploidy are sometimes referred to as numerical chromosome aberrations, as opposed to the structural chromosome aberrations discussed in the preceding section.

# HEALTH IMPACT OF MUTATIONS

The importance of mutations and chromosomal alterations for human health is evident from their roles in genetic disorders and cancer. Therefore, mutations in both germ cells and somatic cells must be considered here.

## Mutations in Germ Cells

The relevance of gene mutations to health is evident from the many disorders that are inherited as simple mendelian characteristics (Mohrenweiser, 1991). About 1.3 percent of newborns suffer from autosomal dominant (1 percent), autosomal recessive (0.25 percent), or sex-linked (0.05 percent) genetic diseases (National Research Council, 1990; Sankaranarayanan, 1993). Molecular analysis of the mutations responsible for mendelian diseases has revealed that almost half these mutations are base-pair substitutions; of the remainder, most are small deletions (Sankaranarayanan, 1993). Among base-pair substitutions, transitions at sites of adjacent cytosine and guanine nucleotides (i.e., at CpG dinucleotides) are especially prevalent, constituting about one-third of the total (Cooper and Krawczak, 1990). These transitions result primarily from the spontaneous deamination of the naturally occurring methylated base 5-methylcytosine. Transitions at CpG sites would not be expected to be as prevalent among induced mutations as they are among spontaneous mutations.

Many genetic disorders (e.g., cystic fibrosis, phenylketonuria, Tay-Sachs disease) are caused by the expression of recessive mutations. These mutations are mainly inherited from previous generations and are expressed when an individual inherits the mutant gene from both parents. New mutations make a larger contribution to the incidence of dominant diseases than to that of recessive diseases, because only a single dominant mutation is required for expression. Thus, new dominant mutations are expressed in the first generation. If a dominant disorder is severe, its transmission between generations is unlikely because of reduced fitness. For dominants with a mild effect, reduced penetrance, or a late age of onset, however, the contribution from previous generations is apt to be greater than that from new mutations. Estimating the proportion of all mendelian genetic disease that can be ascribed to new mutations is not straightforward; a rough estimate is 20 percent (Wyrobek, 1993; Shelby, 1994).

Besides causing diseases that exhibit mendelian inheritance, gene mutations undoubtedly contribute to human disease through the genetic component of disorders with a complex etiology. Some 3 percent (National Research Council, 1990) to 6 percent (Sankaranarayanan, 1993) of infants are affected by congenital abnormalities; if one includes multifactorial disorders that often have a late onset, such as heart disease, hypertension, and diabetes, the proportion of the population affected increases to more than 60 percent (National Research Council, 1990; Sankaranarayanan, 1993). Such frequencies are necessarily approximate because of differences among surveys in the reporting and classification of disorders. A higher prevalence would be found if less severe disorders were included in the tabulation. Nevertheless, such estimates provide a sense of the large impact of genetic disease.

Refined cytogenetic methods have led to the discovery of minor variations in chromosome structure that have no apparent effect. Nevertheless, other chromosome aberrations cause fetal death or serious abnormalities. Aneuploidy also contributes to fetal deaths and causes disorders such as Down syndrome. About 4 infants per 1000 have syndromes associated with chromosomal abnormalities, including translocations and aneuploidy. The majority of these syndromes (about 85 percent) are trisomic (National Research Council, 1990). Much of the effect of chromosomal abnormalities occurs prenatally. It has been estimated that 5 percent of all recognized pregnancies involve chromosomal abnormalities, as do about 6 percent of infant deaths and 30 percent of all spontaneous embryonic and fetal deaths (Mohrenweiser, 1991). Among the abnormalities, aneuploidy is the most common, followed by polyploidy. Structural aberrations constitute about 5 percent of the total. Unlike gene mutations, many of which are inherited from the previous generation, about 85 percent of the chromosomal anomalies detected in newborns arise de novo in the germ cells of the parents (Mohrenweiser, 1991).

## Mutations in Somatic Cells

An association between mutation and cancer has long been evident on indirect grounds, such as a correlation between the mutagenicity and carcinogenicity of chemicals, especially in biological systems that have the requisite metabolic activation capabilities. Moreover, human chromosome instability syndromes and DNA repair deficiencies are associated with increased cancer risk (Friedberg, 1985). Cancer cytogenetics has greatly strengthened the association in that specific chromosomal alterations, including deletions, translocations, and inversions, have been implicated in many human leukemias and lymphomas as well as in some solid tumors (Rabbitts, 1994).

Critical evidence that mutation plays a central role in cancer has come from molecular studies of oncogenes and tumor suppressor genes. Oncogenes are genes that stimulate the transformation of normal cells into cancer cells (Bishop, 1991). They originate when genes, called proto-oncogenes, that are involved in normal cellular growth and development are genetically altered. Normal regulation of cellular proliferation requires a balance between factors that promote growth and those that restrict it. Mutational alteration of proto-oncogenes can lead to overexpression of their growth-stimulating activity, while mutations that inactivate tumor suppressor genes, which normally restrain cellular proliferation, free cells from their inhibitory influence (Evans and Prosser, 1992).

The action of oncogenes is genetically dominant in that a single active oncogene is expressed even though its normal allele is present in the same cell. Proto-oncogenes can be converted into active oncogenes by point mutations or chromosomal alterations. Base-pair substitutions in *ras* proto-oncogenes are found in many human tumors (Bishop, 1991; Barrett, 1993). Among chromosomal alterations that activate proto-oncogenes, translocations are especially prevalent (Rabbitts, 1994). For example, Burkitt's lymphoma involves a translocation between the long arm of chromosome 8, which is the site of the *c-MYC* oncogene, and chromosome 14 (about 90 percent of cases), 22, or 2. A translocation can activate a proto-oncogene by moving it to a new chromosomal location, typically the site of a T-cell receptor or immunoglobulin gene, where its expression is enhanced. This mechanism applies to Burkitt's lymphoma and various other hematopoietic cancers. Alternatively, the translocation may join two genes, resulting in a protein fusion that contributes to cancer development. Fusions have been implicated in other hematopoietic cancers and some solid tumors (Rabbitts, 1994). Like translocations, other chromosomal alterations can activate proto-oncogenes, and genetic amplification of oncogenes can magnify their expression (Bishop, 1991).

Mutational inactivation or deletion of tumor suppressor genes has been implicated in many cancers. Unlike oncogenes, the cancer-causing alleles that arise from tumor suppressor genes are typically recessive in that they are not expressed when they are heterozygous (Evans and Prosser, 1992). However, several genetic mechanisms, including mutation, deletion, chromosome loss, and mitotic recombination, can inactivate or eliminate the normal dominant allele, leading to the expression of the recessive cancer gene in a formerly heterozygous cell (Bishop, 1991; Marshall, 1991). The inactivation of tumor suppressor genes has been associated with various cancers, including those of the eye, kidney, colon, brain, breast, lung, and bladder (Fearon and Vogelstein, 1990; Marshall, 1991). Gene mutations in a tumor suppressor gene on chromosome 17 called p53 occur in many different human cancers, and molecular characterization of p53 mutations has linked specific human cancers to mutagen exposures (Harris, 1993; Aguilar et al., 1994).

In the simplest model for the action of tumor suppressor genes, two events are required for the development of the cancer, as both normal alleles must be inactivated or lost (Evans and Prosser, 1992). In sporadic forms of the cancer (i.e., no family history), the two genetic events occur independently, but in familial forms (e.g., familial retinoblastoma), the first mutation is inherited, leaving the need for only a single additional event for expression. The strong predisposition to cancer in the inherited disease stems from the high likelihood that a loss of heterozygosity will occur by mutation, recombination, or aneuploidy in at least one or a few cells in the development of the affected organ. The simple model involving two events and a single pair of alleles cannot explain all observations concerning tumor suppressor genes, because many cancers involve more than one tumor suppressor gene. For example, the childhood kidney tumor called Wilms' tumor can be caused by damage in at least three different genes (Marshall, 1991), and colorectal carcinomas are often found to have lost not only the wild-type p53 tumor suppressor gene but also other tumor suppressor genes (Fearon and Vogelstein, 1990). Moreover, a single mutation in a tumor suppressor gene, even though not fully expressed, may contribute to carcinogenesis. For example, a single p53 mutation in a developing colorectal tumor may confer a growth advantage that contributes to the development of the disease. Subsequent loss of heterozygosity will increase the growth advantage as the tumor progresses from benign to malignant (Fearon and Vogelstein, 1990).

Many cancers involve both activation of oncogenes and inactivation of tumor suppressor genes (Fearon and Vogelstein, 1990; Bishop, 1991). The observation of multiple genetic changes supports the view that cancer results from an accumulation of genetic alterations and that carcinogenesis is a multistep process (Hollstein et al., 1991; Barrett, 1993). At least three stages can be recognized in carcinogenesis: initiation, promotion, and progression (Barrett, 1993). *Initiation* involves the induction of a genetic alteration, such as the mutational activation of a *ras* proto-oncogene, by a mutagen. It is an irreversible step that starts the process toward cancer. *Promotion* involves cellular proliferation in an initiated cell population. Promotion can lead to the development of benign tumors such as papillomas. Agents called promoters stimulate this process. Promoters may be mutagenic but are not necessarily so. *Progression* involves the continuation of cell proliferation and the accumulation of additional irreversible genetic changes; it is marked by increasing genetic instability and malignancy.

Gene mutations, chromosome aberrations, and aneuploidy are all implicated in the development of cancer. Mutagens and clastogens contribute to carcinogenesis as initiators. Their role does not have to be restricted to initiation, however, in that mutagens, clastogens, and aneugens may contribute to the multiple genetic alterations that characterize progression. Other agents that contribute to carcinogenesis, such as promoters, need not be mutagens. With the complexity of carcinogenesis, it is not surprising that chemicals can affect it in a multiplicity of ways and that some carcinogens have been found to be nonmutagenic (Butterworth and Slaga, 1987). However, the role of mutations is critical, and analyzing mutations and mutagenic effects is therefore essential for understanding and predicting chemical carcinogenesis.

## MUTAGENESIS AND DNA REPAIR

Gene mutations, chromosome aberrations, aneuploidy, and polyploidy are all subject to induction by chemicals in experimental organisms. Although some mutagens may induce all these effects, most show some degree of specificity. It is useful to separate the induction of gene mutations and chromosome aberrations from the induction of aneuploidy and polyploidy, because the cellular targets tend to be different. The principal target for the induction of gene mutations and chromosome aberrations is DNA, whereas the targets for the induction of aneuploidy and polyploidy are often components of the mitotic and meiotic apparatus, such as spindle fibers.

### DNA Alterations Causing Mutation

The underlying basis for mutagenesis is a chemical or physical alteration in the structure of DNA. For example, many electrophilic compounds react with DNA, forming covalent addition products called adducts. The positions on DNA bases at which adducts are formed can be specific for a given agent. Because mutagens differ with respect to the positions and properties of the chemical and physical alterations they cause in DNA, they also differ in the kinds of mutations they induce.

Monofunctional alkylating agents such as ethylnitrosourea (ENU) cause the addition of alkyl groups to DNA (Fig. 9-2). Alkylated bases may exhibit the same pairing specificity as normal bases or may exhibit altered pairing. For example, guanine alkylated on the nitrogen at its 7 position pairs normally, but guanine alkylated on the oxygen at its 6 position is apt to mispair with thymine (Laval et al., 1990). Mispairing of $O^6$-alkylguanine leads to G:C → A:T transitions. Although not as prevalent as $O^6$-alkylguanine, $O^4$-alkylthymine is also likely to mispair, giving rise to A:T → G:C transitions (Shevell et al., 1990). ENU, whose alkylation products include a relatively high proportion of $O^6$-ethylguanine, is a potent mutagen in microorganisms, *Drosophila*, and mammals, effectively inducing base-pair substitutions, especially G:C → A:T transitions (Pastink et al., 1990; Sierra et al., 1993).

Mispairing is not the only mechanism by which alkylating agents induce mutations. Some alkylated bases lead to secondary alterations in DNA. For example, the alkyl group in N7-alkylguanine, which is the major adduct formed by many alky-

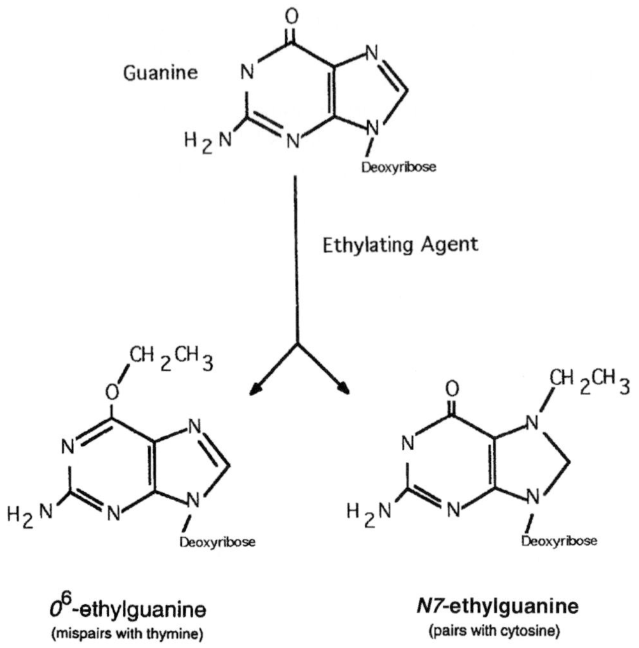

Guanine

Ethylating Agent

$O^6$-ethylguanine (mispairs with thymine)

*N7*-ethylguanine (pairs with cytosine)

***Figure 9–2. Formation of O⁶-ethylguanine and N7-ethylguanine by the reaction of a guanine residue with an alkylating agent.***

$O^6$-ethylguanine causes G:C → A:T transitions by mispairing with thymine. Although N7-ethylguanine does not mispair, it is more apt to be lost from DNA than is normal guanine, and mutations may arise at the sites of base loss.

lating agents, labilizes the bond that connects the base to deoxyribose and thus stimulates base loss. Base loss from DNA leaves an apurinic or apyrimidinic site commonly called an AP site, and the insertion of incorrect bases into AP sites causes mutations, especially transversions (Laval et al., 1990; Walker and Skopek, 1993). Alkylation of nitrogen sites in DNA also leads to chromosome aberrations (Sierra et al., 1993). In general, the induction of point mutations correlates best with the formation of $O^6$-alkylguanine, whereas the induction of chromosome aberrations correlates better with the alkylation of nitrogen sites (Sierra et al., 1993).

Most chemical mutagenesis requires covalent reaction of the mutagen with DNA. However, in the case of some planar molecules, such as 9-aminoacridine, mutagenesis results from the intercalation of the chemical between the base pairs of DNA. Such noncovalent interactions can stimulate the deletion of base pairs or the insertion of extra base pairs when the DNA is replicated. Consequently, 9-aminoacridine is a frameshift mutagen. A widely accepted model that can explain many frameshift mutations involves slippage, or localized pairing out of register, at sites of repetitive bases in DNA. Agents such as 9-aminoacridine preferentially induce mutations in repetitive sequences (e. g., GGGGG) and may operate by enhancing or stabilizing the slipped mispairing (Ferguson and Denny, 1990). Related compounds that both intercalate in DNA and bind to it covalently, such as the acridine mustard ICR-191, also induce frameshift mutations and tend to be more potent mutagens than are simple intercalators (Ferguson and Denny, 1991).

When cells or organisms are irradiated with UV, chemical alterations occur in DNA; major premutational lesions in UV-irradiated DNA are the cyclobutane pyrimidine dimer and the (6-4)-photoproduct (Friedberg, 1985). These bulky lesions can block replication and cause the death of the cell. Moreover, intracellular processing of damaged DNA leads to mutations. Bulky adducts of chemical mutagens such as that of the aromatic amide *N*-2-acetylaminofluorene (AAF) on the 8 position of guanine also impede replication, and mutations are produced as cellular processes bypass the lesions (Heflich and Neft, 1994). The mutagenicity of UV and many chemicals therefore shows the complexity of mutation as a cellular process that involves not only the pairing specificity of altered bases but also their interactions with cellular mechanisms of replication and repair.

## DNA Repair

DNA is subject to spontaneous chemical degradation that would interfere with its functioning as the genetic material if it were not corrected (Lindahl, 1993). It is therefore not surprising that organisms have evolved diverse mechanisms for coping with the spontaneous hydrolysis, oxidation, and nonenzymatic methylation of DNA as well as damage induced by naturally occurring chemical mutagens and radiation that have been present throughout the evolution of life. Mechanisms by which organisms cope with DNA damage fall into two broad categories: damage-tolerance mechanisms and repair mechanisms (Friedberg, 1985). Damage tolerance entails bypassing a lesion in DNA that could block replication. For example, in recombinational repair in bacteria, the replication mechanism bypasses an unrepaired pyrimidine dimer or bulky chemical adduct, leaving a gap in the new strand opposite the damage; the gap is then filled with the segment of DNA from the opposite parental strand by means of a recombinational process (Griffiths et al., 1993). The bypass of potentially lethal lesions promotes survival, and the damage can be removed later by DNA repair mechanisms.

DNA repair mechanisms may be classified into direct repair, in which the reaction that caused the DNA damage is reversed, and excision, in which damaged or incorrect bases are removed and replaced (Sancar and Tang, 1993). Examples of direct reversal include the photorepair of UV damage, the removal of adducts from DNA bases, the insertion of purines into sites of base loss, and the sealing of single-strand breaks by DNA ligase (Friedberg, 1985). Photorepair is a light-dependent process in which an enzyme cleaves pyrimidine dimers in DNA, returning the two adjacent pyrimidines to their original configuration. Direct reversal of methylation on the $O^6$-position of guanine occurs through the transfer of the methyl group to the protein $O^6$-methylguanine-DNA methyltransferase and restores the normal base-pairing specificity (Shevell et al., 1990). The *Escherichia coli* (*E. coli*) methyltransferase also removes methyl groups from the $O^4$ position of thymine, though less efficiently, and from phosphate groups in the DNA backbone. Although best characterized in *E. coli*, $O^6$-methylguanine-DNA methyltransferases occur in yeasts, rodents, and humans. Specific repair systems also exist for alkylated bases other than $O^6$-methylguanine (Shevell et al., 1990).

Processes that remove damaged bases, mispaired bases, or a segment of DNA containing damage are collectively called excision-repair mechanisms. Unlike photorepair and repair by a methyltransferase, excision mechanisms respond to a broad range of premutational lesions. Two major pathways of excision repair—nucleotide excision and base excision—are shown in Fig. 9-3. These general patterns of excision repair are applicable to both bacteria and eukaryotes, though there are variations in details.

Nucleotide excision (Fig. 9-3) is initiated by an endonuclease (e.g., the *uvrABC* excinuclease of *E. coli*) that nicks the DNA backbone on both sides of the damage (Hanawalt and Mellon, 1993; Sancar and Tang, 1993). Removal of the oligonucleotide that contains the damage requires a helicase and leaves a gap 27 to 29 nucleotides long in eukaryotes and 12 to 13 nucleotides long in bacteria. A repair polymerase (e.g., DNA polymerase I of *E. coli*) fills the gap with the correct bases, using the opposite strand as a template. The remaining break in the DNA strand is sealed by DNA ligase. The net result is restoration of the original DNA sequence.

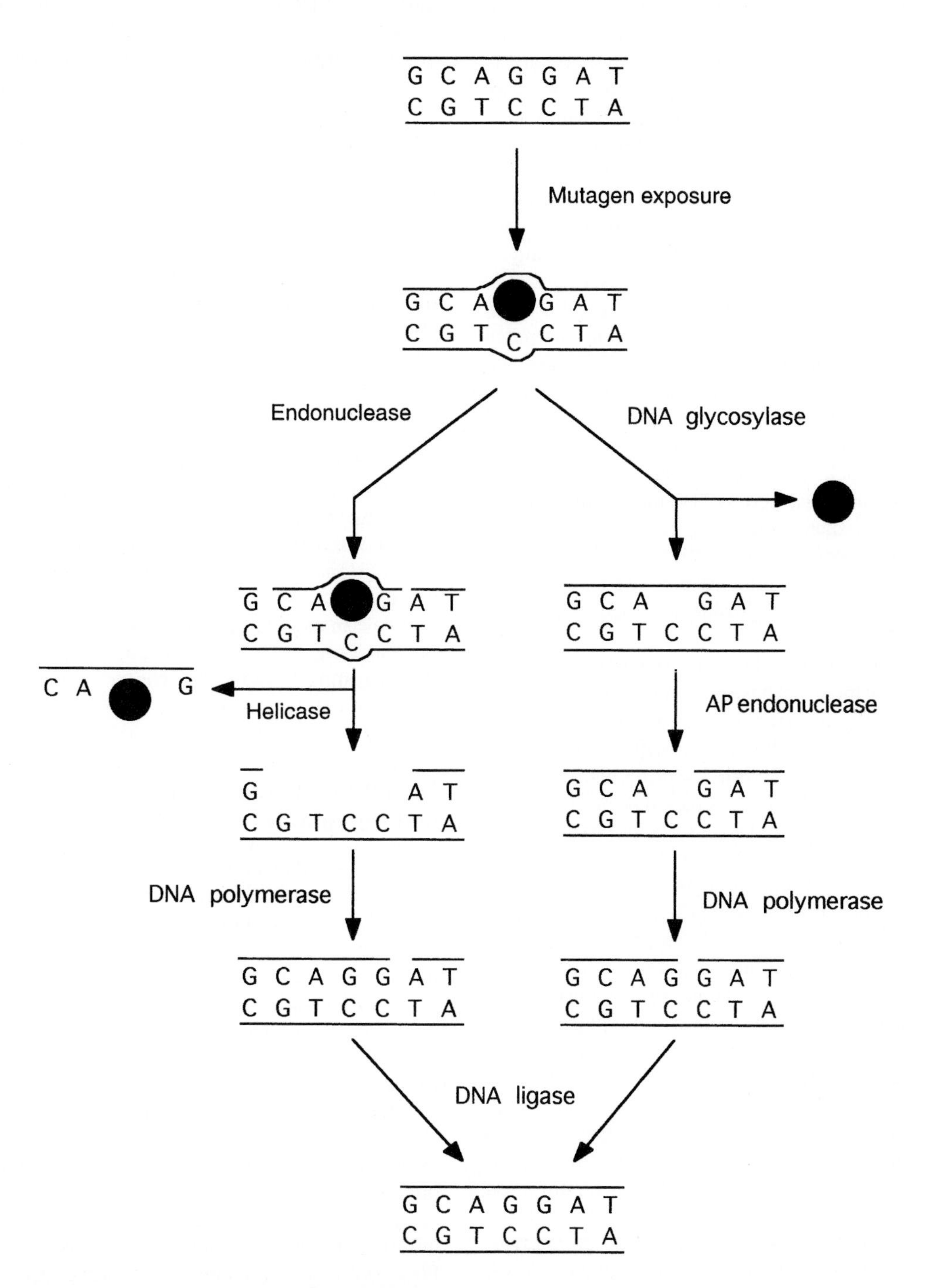


***Figure 9–3. Excision repair of DNA damage.***

Photoproducts or chemical adducts (●) are formed in DNA as a consequence of exposure to UV or a chemical mutagen. The repair pathways called nucleotide excision (*left*) and base excision (*right*) remove the damaged region and restore the intact DNA. The excised segments in nucleotide excision are longer than those shown in this generalized scheme.

Nucleotide excision repair is the most general repair mechanism in all organisms (Hanawalt and Mellon, 1993; Sancar and Tang, 1993). It repairs essentially all kinds of DNA damage, including UV photoproducts, bulky chemical adducts that are not removed by other mechanisms, and interstrand cross-links produced by chemicals such as cisplatin (Holbrook and Fornace, 1991). Pyrimidine dimers and some chemical adducts in actively transcribed strands of DNA are removed preferentially to those in the complementary nontranscribed strand or in inactive sequences (Sancar and Tang, 1993; Hanawalt and Mellon, 1993). Research on such heterogeneity in repair is revealing unforeseen relationships among transcription, repair, and mutagenesis, and these relationships may have implications for mutational risk assessment (Scicchitano and Hanawalt, 1992).

In base excision (Fig. 9-3), DNA damage is acted on by a DNA glycosylase. The glycosylase releases the damaged base by cleaving the bond that links it to deoxyribose, creating an AP site. An AP endonuclease then cleaves the DNA backbone and removes the deoxyribose to which the damaged base had been attached. Compared with nucleotide excision, the patch repaired is short, usually a single nucleotide. Polymerase and ligase steps complete the repair process as in nucleotide excision, though the particular enzymes may differ (Sancar and Tang, 1993). DNA glycosylases are much more specific than is the endonuclease of nucleotide excision, but collectively they remove pyrimidine dimers caused by UV; the nonbulky damage caused by agents such as ionizing radiation, alkylating agents, and hydrogen peroxide (Friedberg, 1985; Holbrook and Fornace, 1991); and spontaneous damage such as that caused by the deamination of cytosine to uracil (Friedberg, 1985; Lindahl, 1993).

Mismatch repair is a distinct kind of excision by which cells recognize and remove incorrect base pairs such as G:T and A:C. Such base pairs can arise by errors in replication, as intermediates in recombination, or by chemical modification of bases, such as the deamination of 5-methylcytosine, which occurs naturally in many species. Mismatch repair systems have been studied extensively in bacteria and are now being characterized in eukaryotes, including humans (Modrich, 1991).

Repair does not provide complete protection against mutagenesis, because repair processes may become saturated or may inefficiently repair some kinds of damage. Some lesions in DNA may be fixed as mutations before repair, and mutations may be generated during the cellular processing of DNA damage. The occurrence of mutations as a consequence of the repair or bypass of damage is sometimes called error-prone repair, and the best-characterized example is the dependence of the mutagenicity of UV on the SOS system in *E. coli* (Friedberg, 1985). UV mutagenesis had been studied for many years when the surprising discovery was made that UV is nonmutagenic in strains of *E. coli* that carry a *recA* or *lexA* mutation and are sensitive to killing by UV. This observation led to the proposal that these genes are somehow involved in an error-prone response to DNA damage. It turned out that DNA damage caused by UV stimulates the activation of a complex network of genetic functions called the SOS system in which the $recA^+$ and $lexA^+$ genes play a central role. This inducible system permits the bypass of bulky, potentially lethal lesions in replicating DNA. Since mutations arise during the process, the SOS system promotes survival at the expense of an elevated mutation frequency.

Genetic systems that are activated in response to DNA damage in bacteria include the SOS system, a response to oxidative stress (Holbrook and Fornace, 1991), and the adaptive response, in which methyl groups are removed from the $O^6$ position of guanine (Shevell et al., 1990). Inducible responses to DNA damage are not as well characterized in eukaryotes, but there is ample evidence for the activation of yeast genes that function in DNA repair, replication, and growth control (Holbrook and Fornace, 1991). The gene encoding the repair enzyme DNA polymerase $\beta$ is activated by DNA alkylation in mammalian cells, but most other mammalian genes activated by DNA damage have unknown functions or are involved in general host defenses or transcriptional regulation rather than having known functions in DNA repair (Holbrook and Fornace, 1991). The analysis of cellular responses to DNA damage indicates that mutations, repair, and metabolism cannot be considered in isolation, as mutagenesis is a complex cellular process involving many interactions among these elements.

Mutations that eliminate repair processes often confer heightened sensitivity to DNA damage. For example, bacteria carrying a *uvrA*, *uvrB*, or *uvrC* mutation are defective in excision repair and are therefore killed by smaller exposures to UV than are wild-type strains. In humans, the genetic disease xeroderma pigmentosum (XP), in which there is unusually high susceptibility to the induction of skin cancer by UV, involves a deficiency in an early step in nucleotide excision repair (Hanawalt and Mellon, 1993). Repair-deficient mutants in bacteria, yeast, and mammalian cells have played an important role in elucidating the mechanisms of DNA repair (Sancar and Tang, 1993). They have also found use in genetic toxicology testing, because they confer increased sensitivity to the effects of many mutagens.

## Induction of Aneuploidy and Polyploidy

Aneuploid cells can arise from a normal cell by nondisjunction: the failure of homologous chromosomes to separate properly in meiosis I or of sister chromatids to do so in meiosis II or mitosis (Griffiths et al., 1993). The result of nondisjunction is that one pole of the spindle receives both homologues or chromatids while the other receives neither. Assuming that only one chromosome or pair of chromosomes is involved, the daughter nuclei will have one chromosome too many or too few.

Unlike aneuploidy, polyploidy involves the entire set of chromosomes. The chromosome number may be doubled, for example, if the chromosomes duplicate normally in interphase but the chromatids do not separate to daughter cells when their centromeres divide in the subsequent mitotic division. Such a mitotic error in a diploid cell gives rise to a tetraploid cell. Polyploid cells are commonly observed in some tissues and organs (e.g., mammalian liver and bronchial epithelium). Just as mitotic errors can give rise to polyploid cells, meiotic errors can give rise to gametes that are diploid rather than being normal haploids. If diploid gametes are involved in fertilization, the result is a polyploid zygote. Another mechanism by which polyploid individuals can arise is the fertilization of an egg by more than one sperm.

The induction of aneuploidy and polyploidy is distinct from other aspects of mutagenesis because it involves different cellular targets (Dellarco et al., 1985; Natarajan, 1993). For example, colchicine blocks the polymerization of tubulin, the principal protein of spindle fibers. Treatment of dividing cells with colchicine disrupts spindle formation and causes polyploidy if there is complete blockage or aneuploidy if there is a lesser disruption. Agents that damage kinetochores, which are the structures by which chromosomes attach to a spindle, also can cause aneuploidy. Although some of the targets are common to mitosis and meiosis, others can be specific (Dellarco et al., 1985). Agents that damage the synaptonemal complex can disrupt the pairing or segregation of homologous chromosomes in meiosis I. Cyclophosphamide, for example, has been reported to cause fragmentation of the synaptonemal complex and synaptic failure in mammalian germ cells; it induces aneuploidy as well as other genetic effects by different mechanisms. In principle, an agent that causes any of the following events can induce meiotic aneuploidy: extra chromosome replication, premature centromere division, improper pairing of homologous chromosomes in prophase I, and nondisjunction or chromosome loss in anaphase I or II. Besides the structural components of the meiotic apparatus, the system of genetic recombination should be considered as a potential target for the induction of aneuploidy because crossing over and chiasma formation are involved in normal disjunction in meiosis.

Because of the difference in targets, aneugens do not have to be clastogens or inducers of point mutations. Known or suspected aneugens include diverse agents such as cadmium chloride, chloral hydrate, colchicine, diazepam, econazole, hydroquinone, pyrimethamine, thiabendazole, thimerosal, and vinblastine (Natarajan, 1993).

### Recombinagenic Effects

Genetic recombination between homologous DNA sequences is a normal part of meiosis and is integral to the genetic variation of populations. Recombination also occurs in mitosis, though at a much lower frequency. Many mutagens and carcinogens increase the frequency of mitotic recombination in organisms as diverse as fungi, plants, insects, and mammals (Hoffmann, 1994). Such agents are referred to as *recombinagens*, and their effects include the induction of reciprocal mitotic recombination, also called mitotic crossing over, and nonreciprocal mitotic recombination, also called mitotic gene conversion. The recombinagenic effects of mutagens have been used for many years as a general indicator of DNA damage. Mitotic recombination is also of interest because it has been linked to the etiology of some cancers and may play a role in other disorders (Morley, 1991; Hoffmann, 1994; Sengstag, 1994).

## STRUCTURE-ACTIVITY RELATIONSHIPS

The first indication that a chemical is a mutagen often lies in its chemical structure. Most mutagens contain substituent groups that can serve as "structural alerts" to their mutagenicity and possible carcinogenicity. Potential electrophilic sites in chemical structures suggest mutagenicity, because such sites indicate reactivity with nucleophilic sites in DNA. The following chemical groups have been identified as structural alerts for mutagenicity: alkyl esters of phosphonic or sulfonic acids, aliphatic or aromatic nitro groups, aromatic azo groups, aromatic ring *N*-oxides, aromatic alkylamino or dialkylamino groups, alkyl hydrazines, alkyl aldehydes, *N*-methylol derivatives, monohaloalkenes, nitrogen and sulfur mustards, *N*-chloramines, propiolactones, propiosultones, aliphatic and aromatic aziridines, aromatic and aliphatic substituted primary alkyl halides, carbamates, alkyl *N*-nitrosamines, aromatic amines, *N*-hydroxy and ester derivatives of aromatic amines, aliphatic epoxides, and aromatic oxides (Tennant and Ashby, 1991).

Though informative, structural alerts cannot eliminate the need for biological data and must be used with cognizance of other factors that can influence the effects of a chemical. Factors that may reduce the likelihood of mutagenicity or carcinogenicity in a structurally alerting compound include steric hindrance of reactive or potentially reactive substituents, metabolism, toxicity, and substituents that enhance the chemical's excretion (Ashby, 1994). Moreover, some agents that lack structural alerts may stimulate mutagenesis indirectly by mechanisms such as the generation of radicals that cause oxidative DNA damage, including strand breaks and modified bases (Clayson, et al., 1994).

The ability to identify carcinogens on the basis of structure has been tested through prospective predictions for 40 compounds tested for carcinogenicity in rodents by the NTP (Parry, 1994). Carcinogenicity or noncarcinogenicity was correctly predicted for 88 percent of the chemicals, using structural alerts, mutagenicity data from bacteria, and rodent subchronic toxicity data. The requirement for critical interpretation was clear in that several artificial intelligence systems that have been developed to predict mutagenicity and carcinogenicity fared worse than did the human appraisal, and none was correct more than 59 percent of the time (Parry, 1994).

## MUTAGENICITY ASSAYS

Mutagenicity testing has become prominent in toxicology during the last two decades. Genetic assays are used to identify germ cell mutagens, somatic cell mutagens, and potential carcinogens and encompass diverse kinds of genetic alterations that are relevant for human health. Assays for gene mutations, chromosome aberrations, and other indicators of DNA damage have been used to study the genetic effects of hundreds of chemicals. Although assays for aneuploidy are not as refined as those for gene mutations and chromosome aberrations, promising methods are being developed.

It is common for toxicologists conducting a computerized search for literature on the mutagenicity of a compound to encounter a bewildering array of assays that may include viruses, bacteria, fungi, cultured mammalian cells, plants, insects, and mammals. More than 200 assays for mutagens have been proposed, and useful information has been obtained from many of them. Data from relatively obscure assays can contribute to a judgment about the genetic activity of a compound. The great bulk of genetic toxicology testing, however, has relied on relatively few assays. This section will therefore begin with a broad overview of the assays one is apt to encounter in the genetic toxicology literature and then concentrate on those which are most extensively used in current testing.

## Survey of Assays

Table 9-1 lists assays for genotoxic effects. Any agent that causes a reproducible positive response in any of these assays or in other assays for DNA damage, gene mutations, clastogenic effects, recombinagenic effects, aneuploidy, or polyploidy may be considered genotoxic. Detailed information on assay design, testing data, necessary controls, sample sizes, and other factors in effective testing may be found in the references cited in this table. Even this extensive table does not include all assays; it is restricted to methods that have found extensive use in testing or illustrate the diversity of genetic endpoints and experimental organisms in mutagenicity assays. Methods that are used to elucidate mechanisms of mutagenesis but have not been used in mutagenicity testing are not included.

The assays in Table 9-1 range from inexpensive short-term tests that can be performed in a few days to involved assays for mutations in mammalian germ cells. To save time and money, a large proportion of mutagenicity testing is done in microorganisms and mammalian cell cultures. Even in complex multicellular organisms, however, there has been an emphasis on designing assays that detect mutations with great efficiency. Nevertheless, there remains a gradation in which an increase in relevance to human risk entails more elaborate and costly tests. Because a great deal can be learned from the simpler tests, the most expensive mammalian tests are typically reserved for agents of special importance in basic research or risk assessment.

Table 9-2 lists some of the most widely used assays. Among them, the *Salmonella*/mammalian microsome assay (i.e., the Ames test) and mammalian in vivo cytogenetic assays have come to hold a central place in genetic toxicology testing. The Ames test is the most widely used short-term genetic test and has performed reproducibly and well with hundreds of compounds in laboratories throughout the world. To supplement data from the Ames test in evaluating a chemical for mutagenicity, one often wants a system that includes mammalian in vivo metabolism and evaluates damage at the chromosomal level. Cytogenetic assays in rodents are most commonly used for this purpose. Besides these two central assays, Table 9-2 shows other assays that have found extensive use in mutagenicity testing or have special importance in the assessment of mutagenic hazards.

## Assay Design

The common genetic toxicology assays use genetic methods to detect the induction of gene mutations and small deletions on the basis of their phenotypic effects and cytological methods to observe gross chromosomal damage.

**Assays for Gene Mutations.** Two categories of gene mutation assays are those which detect forward mutations and those which detect reversion. Forward mutations alter a wild-type gene, and inactivation of the gene results in a detectable change in phenotype. In contrast, a back mutation or reversion is a mutation that restores gene function in a mutant and thus brings about a return to the wild-type phenotype.

Microbial assays have figured prominently in genetic toxicology because of their speed and low cost and the ease of detecting events that occur at low frequencies (i.e., mutations). The most common means of detecting mutations in microorganisms is to select for reversion in strains that have a specific nutritional requirement differing from that of wild-type members of the species; such strains are called *auxotrophs*. For example, in the widely used assay developed by Bruce Ames and his colleagues in *Salmonella typhimurium*, one measures the frequency of histidine-independent bacteria that arise in a histidine-requiring strain in the presence and absence of the chemical being tested. Auxotrophic bacteria are treated with the chemical of interest by one of several procedures (e.g., a plate incorporation assay or a preincubation test) and plated on medium that is deficient in histidine (Maron and Ames, 1983; Kirkland et al., 1990). The assay is conducted using several genetically different strains so that reversion by base-pair substitutions and frameshift mutations in several DNA sequence contexts can be detected and distinguished. Besides the histidine alleles that provide the target for measuring mutagenesis, the Ames tester strains contain other genes and plasmids that enhance the assay. The principal strains of the Ames test and their characteristics are summarized in Table 9-3.

Mutagenicity assays in cultured mammalian cells have some of the advantages of microbial assays and use similar methods. The most widely used assays for gene mutations in mammalian cells detect forward mutations that confer resistance to a toxic chemical (DeMarini et al., 1989). For example, mutations in the gene encoding hypoxanthine-guanine phosphoribosyltransferase (HPRT enzyme, *hprt* gene) confer resistance to the purine analogue 6-thioguanine, and thymidine kinase mutations (TK enzyme, *tk* gene) confer resistance to the pyrimidine analogue trifluorothymidine.

In principle, forward mutation assays should respond to a broad spectrum of mutagens because any mutation that interferes with gene function should confer the selected phenotype. In contrast, a reversion assay might be expected to exhibit a more restricted mutational response, because only mutations that correct or compensate for the specific mutational alteration in a particular mutant will be detected. In fact, some reversion assays respond to a broader spectrum of mutational changes than one might expect, because mutations at a site other than the original mutant site (i.e., a suppressor mutation) sometimes can confer the selected phenotype (Koch et al., 1994). Similarly, not all forward mutation assays are responsive to diverse mechanisms of mutagenesis. For example, resistance to ouabain results from a specific alteration in the target gene, and alterations that eliminate the gene function are lethal (DeMarini et al., 1989); therefore, ouabain resistance is not useful for general mutagenicity testing.

In mutagenicity testing, one must be aware of many possible sources of error. Factors to consider in the application of mutagenicity assays include the choice of suitable organisms and growth conditions, appropriate monitoring of genotypes, effective experimental design and treatment conditions, inclu-

be sure that they grow in its absence. Such pitfalls exist in all mutagenicity tests. Anyone performing mutagenicity tests must therefore have detailed familiarity with the laboratory application and literature of the assay and be observant of the responsiveness of the assay.

In vivo genetic assays involve treating intact animals and scoring specific effects in appropriate tissues. The choice of suitable doses, treatment procedures, controls, and sample sizes is critical in the conduct of in vivo tests. The design of the tests must compensate for the fact that mutation occurs at a low frequency, and even the simplest animal systems face a problem of numbers; one can easily screen millions of bacteria or cultured cells by using selection techniques, but screening large numbers of fruit flies or mice has practical limitations. Therefore, assays in animals must offer a straightforward, unequivocal identification of mutants with minimal labor.

A strength of the sex-linked recessive lethal (SLRL) test in *Drosophila* (Mason et al., 1987) is that it permits the detection of recessive lethal mutations at 600 to 800 different loci on the X chromosome by screening for the presence or absence of wild-type males in the offspring of specifically designed crosses. The spontaneous frequency of SLRLs is about 0.2 percent, and a significant increase over this frequency in lineages derived from treated males indicates mutagenesis. Although it requires screening large numbers of fruit fly vials, the SLRL test yields information about mutagenesis in germ cells that is lacking in all microbial and cell culture systems. However, means of exposure, measurement of doses, metabolism, and gametogenesis in *Drosophila* differ from those in mammalian toxicology. Mammalian assays therefore provide the best basis for assessing risks to human germ cells and hold a central place in genetic toxicology despite their expense.

The specific-locus test in mice developed by William L. Russell detects recessive mutations that produce easily scored visible phenotypes (e.g., coat color) conferred by seven defined genes (Russell and Shelby, 1985; Ehling, 1991; Russell and Russell, 1992). Mutants may be classified as having point mutations or chromosomal alterations on the basis of both phenotypic criteria and molecular analysis (Russell and Rinchik, 1993). This assay has been important in assessing the genetic risks of ionizing radiation and has been used to study various chemical mutagens. Other gene mutation assays in mouse germ cells detect recessive mutations that cause electrophoretic changes in proteins (Lewis, 1991) and dominant mutations that cause skeletal abnormalities or cataracts (Ehling, 1991).

Mammalian assays permit the measurement of mutagenesis at different germ cell stages. The late stages of spermatogenesis are often found to be sensitive to mutagenesis; however, spermatocytes, spermatids, and spermatozoa are transitory. Mutagenesis in stem cell spermatogonia and resting oocytes is of special interest in the assessment of genetic risk because of the persistence of these stages throughout reproductive life (Ehling, 1991; Russell, 1994). Chemical mutagens show considerable specificity with respect to germ cell stages. For example, ENU and chlorambucil are both potent mutagens in the mouse specific-locus test; the former induces primarily point mutations in spermatogonia, while the latter effectively induces deletions and other rearrangements in spermatids (Russell, 1994). The ratio of deletions to point mutations not only is a function of the nature of the mutagen but depends on the germ cell stage, as several mutagens induce higher proportions of gross alterations in late stages of spermatogenesis than in spermatogonia (Russell and Rinchik, 1993).

**Assays for Chromosome Aberrations.** Genetic assays are indirect in that one observes a phenotype and reaches conclusions about genes. In contrast, cytogenetic assays use microscopy for direct observation of the effect of interest. In traditional cytogenetics, metaphase analysis is used to detect chromosomal anomalies, especially chromosome and chromatid aberrations. A key factor in the design of cytogenetic assays is obtaining appropriate cell populations for treatment and analysis (Kirkland et al., 1990). Cells with a stable, well-defined karyotype, a short generation time, a low chromosome number, and large chromosomes are ideal for cytogenetic analysis. For this reason, Chinese hamster ovary (CHO) cells have been used widely in cytogenetic testing. Other cells are also suitable, and human cells, especially peripheral lymphocytes, have been used extensively. Cells should be treated during a sensitive period of the cell cycle (typically S), and aberrations should be scored in the first mitotic division after treatment so that the sensitivity of the assay is not reduced because unstable aberrations have been lost during division. Examples of chromosome aberrations are shown in Fig. 9-4.

Cytogenetic assays require careful attention to growth conditions, controls, doses, treatment conditions, and the time intervals between treatment and the sampling of cells for analysis (Kirkland et al., 1990). Data collection is a critical step in cytogenetic analysis. It is essential that enough cells be scored, because a negative result in a small sample is meaningless. The results should be recorded for specific classes of aberrations, not just as an overall index of aberrations per cell. The need for detailed data is all the more important because of nonuniformity in the classification of aberrations and disagreement on whether small achromatic (i.e., unstained) gaps in chromosomes are aberrations. Gaps should be quantified but should not be pooled with other aberrations.

In interpreting assays for the induction of chromosome aberrations in cell cultures, one must be alert to the possibility of artifacts associated with extreme culture conditions. The induction of aberrations under extreme conditions is sometimes ascribable to mechanisms that are unique to the assay conditions rather than being a reflection of general genotoxicity (Scott et al., 1991). Questionable positive results have been found at high chemical concentrations where osmolality may cause apparent genotoxic effects. Similarly, assays at highly cytotoxic doses and pH extremes warrant careful scrutiny, as do metabolic activation systems that may be genotoxic (Scott et al., 1991). While excessively high doses may lead to artifactual positive responses, failure to test to sufficiently high doses also undermines the utility of a test; therefore, testing should be extended to a dose at which some cytotoxicity is observed, such as a reduction in the mitotic index (the proportion of cells in division), or to an arbitrary limit of about 10 mM if the chemical is nontoxic (Kirkland et al., 1990).

In vivo assays for chromosome aberrations involve treating intact animals and later collecting cells for cytogenetic analysis. The main advantage of in vivo assays is that they include mammalian metabolism, DNA repair, and pharma-

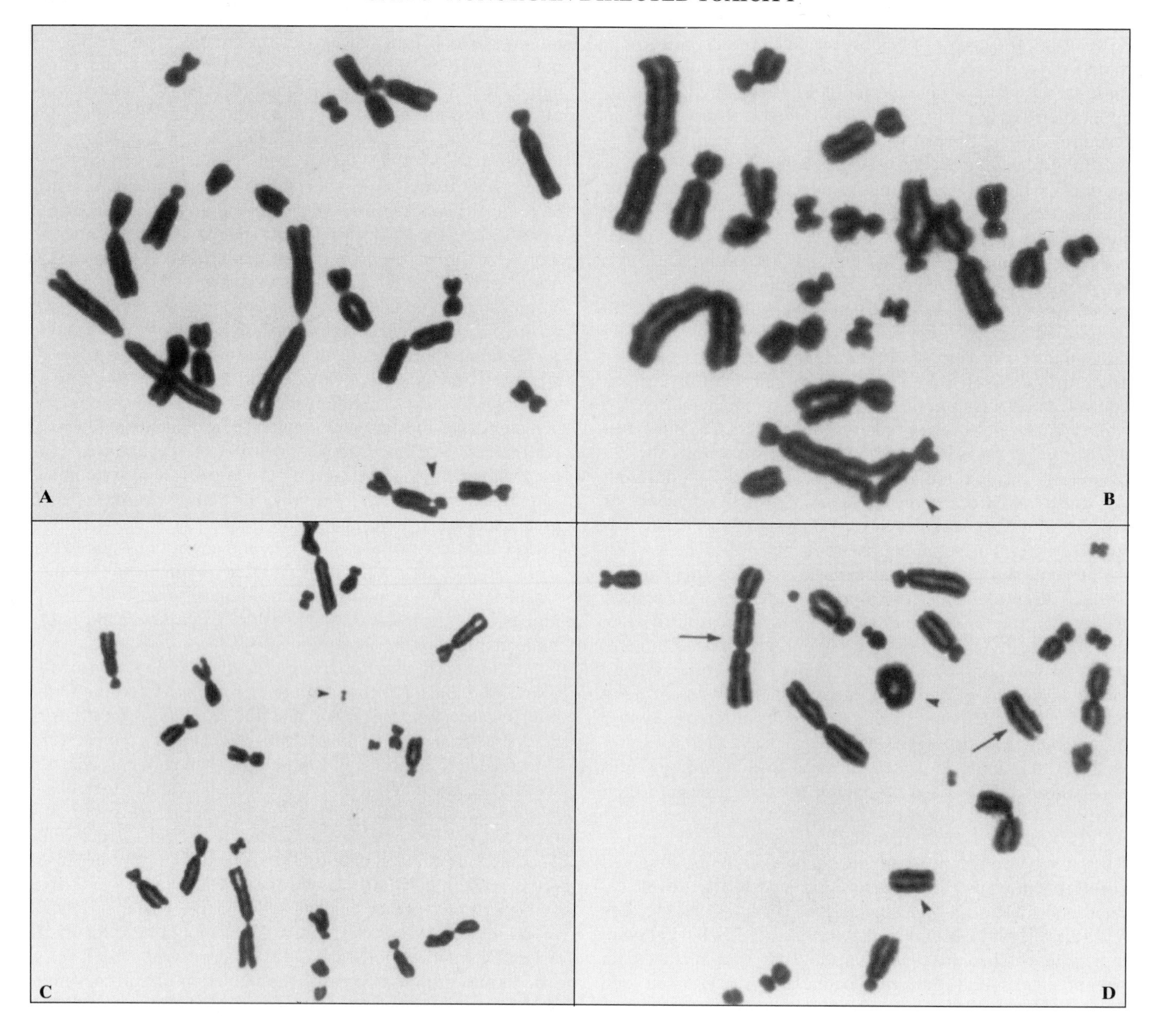


*Figure 9–4. Chromosome aberrations induced by x-rays in Chinese hamster ovary (CHO) cells.*

*A*. A chromatid deletion (➤). *B*. A chromatid exchange called a triradial (➤). *C*. A small interstitial deletion (➤) that resulted from chromosome breakage. *D*. A metaphase with more than one aberration: a centric ring plus an acentric fragment (➤) and a dicentric chromosome plus an acentric fragment (→). (Photographs courtesy of R. Julian Preston.)

codynamics. The target must be a tissue from which large numbers of dividing cells can be easily prepared for analysis, and so bone marrow from rats, mice, or Chinese hamsters is most commonly used. Effective testing requires dosages and routes of administration that ensure adequate exposure of the target cells, proper intervals between treatment and the collection of cells, and sufficient numbers of animals and cells scored (Kirkland et al., 1990).

Metaphase analysis is time-consuming and requires considerable skill; so there is interest in the prospect of developing simpler cytogenetic assays. Two promising developments are the refinement of micronucleus assays and the detection of chromosomal anomalies using fluorescence in situ hybridization (FISH).

Micronuclei are chromatin-containing bodies that represent chromosomal fragments or whole chromosomes that were not incorporated into a nucleus during mitosis. Since micronuclei usually represent fragments, they are used as simple indicators of chromosomal damage. Micronucleus assays may be conducted in vivo or in cultured cells. The in vivo assay is most often performed by counting micronuclei in immature (polychromatic) erythrocytes in the bone marrow of treated mice but also may be based on peripheral blood (Heddle et al., 1991; Hayashi et al., 1994). Micronuclei remain in the cell when the nucleus is extruded in the maturation of erythroblasts. A germ cell micronucleus assay in rodent spermatids permits the analysis of chromosomal damage induced during meiosis (Lähdetie et al., 1994).

Micronucleus assays in cultured cells have been greatly improved by the cytokinesis-block technique, in which cytoplasmic division is inhibited with cytochalasin B, resulting in binucleate and multinucleate cells (Fenech and Morley, 1989). In this assay, nondividing ($G_0$) human lymphocytes may be treated with ionizing radiation or a radiomimetic chemical and then stimulated to divide with the mitogen phytohemagglutinin. Alternatively, the lymphocytes may be exposed to the mitogen first so that the subsequent mutagenic treatment includes the S period of the cell cycle. In either case, cytochalasin B is added for the last part of the culture period, and micronuclei are counted only in binucleate cells to ensure that the cells have undergone a single nuclear division. The assay thus avoids the confusion caused by differences in cellular proliferation kinetics. Micronuclei in a binucleate human lymphocyte are shown in Fig. 9-5. Though most often used with human lymphocytes, the cytokinesis-block assay has been adapted to other mammalian cells (Lynch and Parry, 1993).

FISH entails hybridizing a nucleic acid probe to complementary sequences in chromosomal DNA. If the probe is labeled with a fluorescent dye, the chromosomal location to which it binds is rendered fluorescent and can be detected visually by fluorescence microscopy. Composite probes have been developed from sequences unique to specific human chromosomes, and so FISH provides a uniform fluorescent label over an entire chromosome. Slides prepared for standard metaphase analysis are suitable for FISH after they have undergone a simple denaturation procedure. The use of whole-chromosome probes is commonly called "chromosome painting."

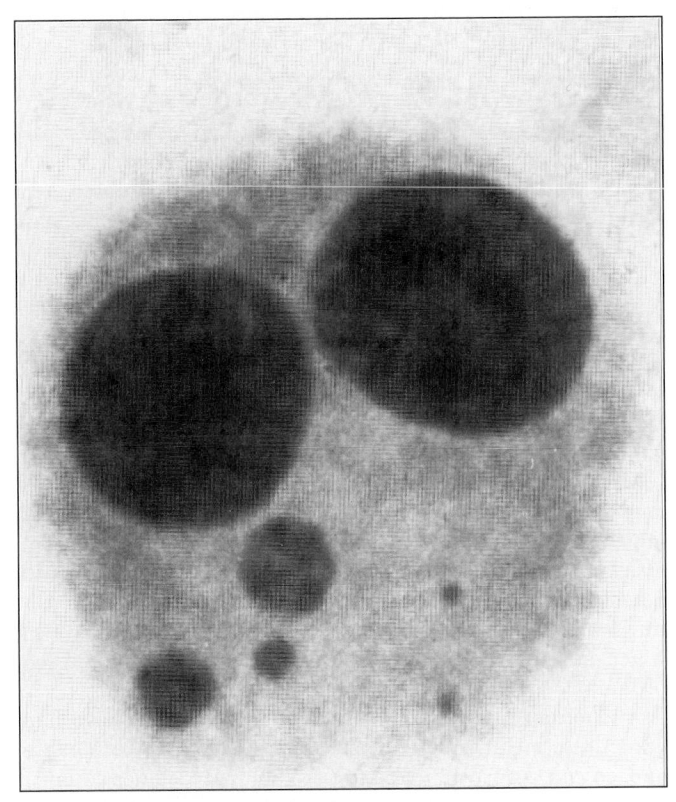

*Figure 9–5. Micronuclei in a human lymphocyte.*

In the cytokinesis-block assay, micronuclei are counted in binucleate cells to measure their frequency after a single nuclear division. This cell with five micronuclei is from a culture treated with a high concentration of the clastogenic drug bleomycin. In control cultures, fewer than 2 percent of cells contain a micronucleus, and cells with more than one micronucleus are rare.

Chromosome painting facilitates cytogenetic analysis because aberrations are easily detected by the number of fluorescent regions in a painted metaphase. For example, if chromosome 4 were painted with a probe while the other chromosomes were counterstained in a different color, one would see only the two homologues of chromosome 4 in the color of the probe in a normal cell. However, if there were a translocation or a dicentric chromosome and fragment involving chromosome 4, one would see three areas of fluorescence: one normal chromosome 4 and the two pieces involved in the chromosome rearrangement. Aberrations are detected only in the painted portion of the genome, but this disadvantage may be offset by painting a few chromosomes simultaneously with probes of different colors (Tucker et al., 1993b). FISH reduces the time and technical skill required to detect chromosome aberrations and permits the scoring of stable aberrations, such as translocations and insertions, that are not readily detected in traditional metaphase analysis of unbanded chromosomes. Moreover, frequencies of stable and unstable chromosome exchanges detected by FISH are consistent with those measured by the more laborious method of chromosome banding (Tucker et al., 1993b). FISH is a valuable research tool for studying clastogens and promises to have a substantial impact in monitoring human populations for chromosomal damage.

Knowledge of the induction of chromosome aberrations in germ cells is important in assessing risks to future generations. Although metaphase analysis of germ cells is not widely used in mutagenicity testing, it is feasible in rodent spermatogonia, spermatocytes, and oocytes (Kirkland et al., 1990; Tease, 1992). Besides cytological observation, indirect evidence of chromosome aberrations is obtained in some germ cell assays; the dominant lethal assay measures embryonic and fetal deaths in the offspring of treated mice or rats (Adler et al., 1994), and the mouse heritable translocation assay detects chromosomal rearrangements on the basis of reduced fertility in the offspring of treated males (Russell and Shelby, 1985). Cytogenetic confirmation is possible in the heritable translocation assay but not in the dominant lethal assay.

**Assays for Aneuploidy.** Assays to detect the induction of aneuploidy have been developed in fungi, plants, *Drosophila,* cultured mammalian cells, and mammals (Table 9-1). Some methods are restricted to specific targets, such as the mitotic spindle in an assay for effects on the polymerization of tubulin in vitro (Parry, 1993). Most, however, measure aneuploidy itself and should therefore encompass all relevant cellular targets. Promising assays include chromosome counting, the detection of micronuclei that contain kinetochores (Natarajan, 1993), and gross examination for abnormal spindles and spindle-chromosome associations in cells in which spindles and chromosomes have been differently stained (Warr et al., 1993).

A complication in chromosome counting is caused by the fact that a spread of metaphase chromosomes may lack chromosomes that were lost when the cell was dropped onto the microscope slide rather than having been absent from the living cell. To avoid this artifact, cytogeneticists have used extra chromosomes (i.e., hyperploidy) rather than missing chromosomes (i.e., hypoploidy) as an indicator of aneuploidy in chromosome preparations from cell cultures or mice (Galloway and Ivett, 1986; Adler, 1993). A promising means of circumventing this difficulty consists of growing and treating cells on a glass surface and then making chromosome preparations in situ rather than dropping cells onto slides from a cell suspension. By counting chromosomes in intact cells, one can collect data for both hyperploidy and hypoploidy (Natarajan et al., 1993).

Besides detecting clastogens, micronucleus assays can detect aneugens. Micronuclei that contain whole chromosomes are not readily distinguished from those containing chromosome fragments in typically stained preparations, though the former tend to be somewhat larger (Natarajan, 1993). However, the presence of the spindle attachment region of a chromosome in a micronucleus can indicate that the micronucleus contains a whole chromosome. Aneuploidy may therefore be detected by means of antikinetochore antibodies with a fluorescent label or FISH with a probe for centromere-specific DNA (Lynch and Parry, 1993; Natarajan, 1993). Micronuclei containing kinetochores or centromeric DNA may be detected both in cell culture assays (Lynch and Parry, 1993) and in vivo (Heddle et al., 1991; Adler, 1993). The frequency of micronuclei ascribable to aneuploidy and that ascribable to clastogenic effects may therefore be determined concurrently by tabulating micronuclei with and without kinetochores.

**Assays for Other Effects on the Genetic Material.** DNA damage such as adducts or strand breaks can be measured directly rather than measuring the mutational consequences of the damage. One can also determine that damage has occurred on the basis of DNA repair. For example, unscheduled DNA synthesis (UDS) is a measure of excision repair, and its occurrence indicates that DNA has been damaged. Several DNA damage and repair assays are listed in Table 9-1.

Assays for recombinagenic effects offer another indication of DNA damage. The best-characterized assays for recombinagens are those which detect mitotic crossing over and mitotic gene conversion in the yeast *Saccharomyces cerevisiae* (Zimmermann, 1992). Hundreds of chemicals have been tested for recombinagenic effects in straightforward yeast assays. In yeast strain D7, for example, mitotic crossing over involving the *ade2* locus is detected on the basis of pink and red colony color and mitotic gene conversion at the *trp5* locus is detected by selection for growth without tryptophan. Strategies also have been devised to detect recombinagenic effects in bacteria, mycelial fungi, cultured mammalian cells, plants, and mice (Hoffmann, 1994), and at least 350 chemicals have been evaluated in *Drosophila* somatic cell assays in which recombinagenic effects are detected by examining wings or eyes for regions in which recessive alleles are expressed in heterozygotes (Vogel, 1992).

Sister chromatid exchange (SCE), in which segments have been exchanged between the two chromatids of a chromosome, is visible cytologically through differential staining of chromatids. Fig. 9-6 shows SCE in human cells. Many mutagens induce SCE in cultured cells and in mammals in vivo (Tucker et al., 1993a). Despite the convenience and responsiveness of SCE assays, data on SCE are less informative than are data on chromosome aberrations. There is great uncertainty about the underlying mechanisms by which SCEs are formed and the way in which DNA damage or perturbations of DNA synthesis stimulate their formation.

## Metabolic Activation

Many compounds are not mutagenic or carcinogenic but can be converted into mutagens and carcinogens by mammalian metabolism. Such compounds are called *promutagens* and *procarcinogens*. Because microorganisms and mammalian cell cultures lack many of the metabolic capabilities of intact mammals, some provision must be made for metabolic activation to detect promutagens in many genetic assays.

A method that found much use early in the history of genetic toxicology is the host-mediated assay (Legator et al., 1982), in which test organisms, usually bacteria, are inserted in an animal (e.g., by intraperitoneal injection) before treatment of the animal. The test organisms are later recovered from the animal and assayed for mutagenicity, detecting not only the effects of the test chemical itself but also those of the mammalian metabolites that reached the test organisms in the animal. Although it has some use as a research tool, the host-mediated assay has been largely supplanted by in vitro metabolic activation systems. Heinrich Malling first combined mammalian tissue homogenates for metabolic activation with a microbial assay for mutation detection, demonstrating the activation of dimethylnitrosamine into a mutagen by mouse liver. Subsequently, many other compounds, including members of important groups such as polynuclear aromatic hydrocarbons (PAHs) and aromatic amines, have been shown to be activated into mutagens by in vitro metabolic activation systems, and metabolic activation has become a standard part of mutagenicity testing.

The most common means of providing metabolic activation in microbial and mammalian cell assays is to add a postmitochondrial supernatant from a rat liver homogenate along with appropriate buffers and cofactors (Maron and Ames, 1983; Kirkland et al., 1990). The standard liver metabolic activation system is generally called an S9 mixture to designate a supernatant formed by centrifugation at 9000 *g*. Variations based on other species or organs are sometimes used. Unlike mutagenicity assays in intact animals, most of the short-term assays in Table 9-1 require exogenous metabolic activation to detect promutagens. Exceptions are an assay for UDS in cultured hepatocytes (Madle et al., 1994) and yeast assays in which an endogenous cytochrome P-450 can activate some promutagens (Zimmermann et al., 1984).

Alternative metabolic activation systems that have had limited use include metabolism by intact hepatocytes (Langenbach and Oglesby, 1983) and a system that includes a reduction step required for the mutagenicity of some azo dyes and nitro compounds (Dellarco and Prival, 1989). An interesting development in metabolic activation is the construction of B-lymphoblastoid cell lines that express human cDNAs that encode metabolic activation enzymes (Crespi et al., 1993). Genes for at least nine human cytochrome P-450s and microsomal epoxide hydrolase have been incorporated into

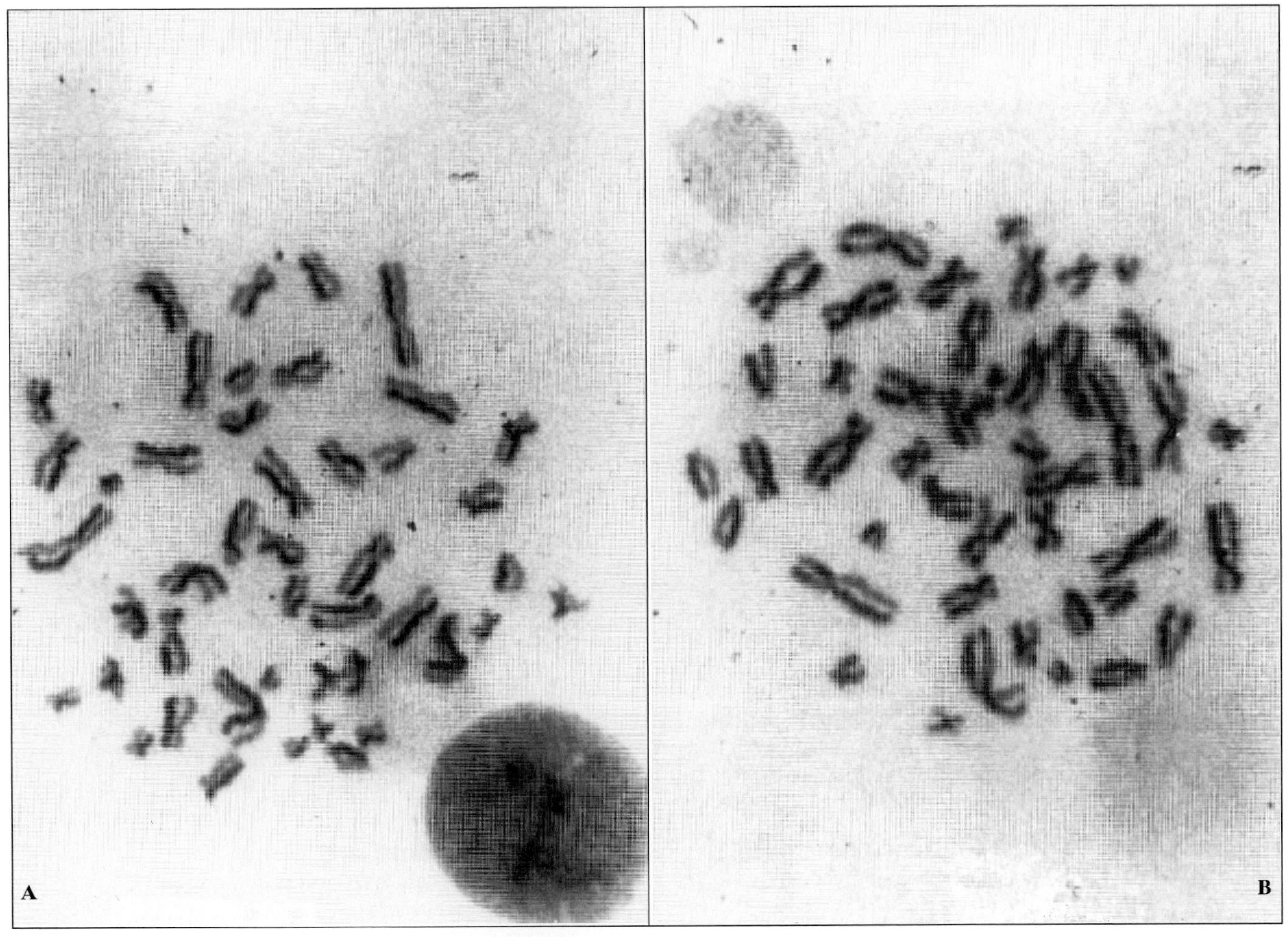


***Figure 9–6. Sister chromatid exchange in human lymphocytes.***

Differentially stained chromatids permit the counting of SCEs in untreated cells (*A*) and cells exposed to the mutagen mitomycin C (*B*).

these cells in various combinations. The cells can detect gene mutations at the *hprt* and *tk* loci and should be valuable in distinguishing the contributions of different enzymes to the metabolism of promutagens.

Despite their usefulness, metabolic activation systems do not mimic mammalian metabolism perfectly. There are differences among tissues in regard to reactions that activate or inactivate foreign compounds, and organisms of the normal flora of the gastrointestinal tract can contribute to metabolism in intact mammals. Agents that induce enzyme systems or otherwise alter the physiological state also can modify the metabolism of toxicants, and the balance between activation and detoxication reactions in vitro may differ from that in vivo.

## Transgenic Systems

Transgenic animals are products of DNA technology in which an animal contains foreign DNA sequences that have been added to the genome and are transmitted through the germ line. The foreign DNA is therefore represented in all the somatic cells of the animal. Mutagenicity assays in transgenic animals show promise for combining in vivo metabolism and pharmacodynamics with simple microbial detection systems, permitting refined analyses of mutations induced in diverse mammalian tissues (Mirsalis et al., 1994).

The transgenic animals that have figured most heavily in genetic toxicology are mice that carry *lac* genes from *E. coli*. The bacterial genes were introduced into mice by injecting a vector carrying the genes into zygotes (Mirsalis et al., 1994). The strains are commonly referred to by their commercial names: the "Big Blue Mouse" (Big Blue; Stratagene) and "MutaMouse" (Muta Mouse; Hazleton Laboratories). The former uses *lacI* as a target for mutagenesis, and the latter uses *lacZ*. The *lac* genes are easily recovered from the animal, packaged in phage $\lambda$, and transferred to *E. coli* for mutational analysis. Mutant plaques are identified on the basis of phenotype, and mutant frequencies can be calculated for different tissues of the treated animals. Figure 9-7 outlines *lacZ* and *lacI* transgenic assays.

More than 25 mutagens have been studied in transgenic mouse assays, including direct-acting alkylating agents, nitrosamines, cyclophosphamide, procarbazine, and PAHs. Mutant frequencies have been analyzed for diverse tissues, including liver, skin, spleen, kidney, bladder, small intestine, bone marrow, and testis (Morrison and Ashby, 1994). Tissue-specific mutant frequencies can be compared with the distribution of adducts among tissues and the site specificity of carcinogenesis

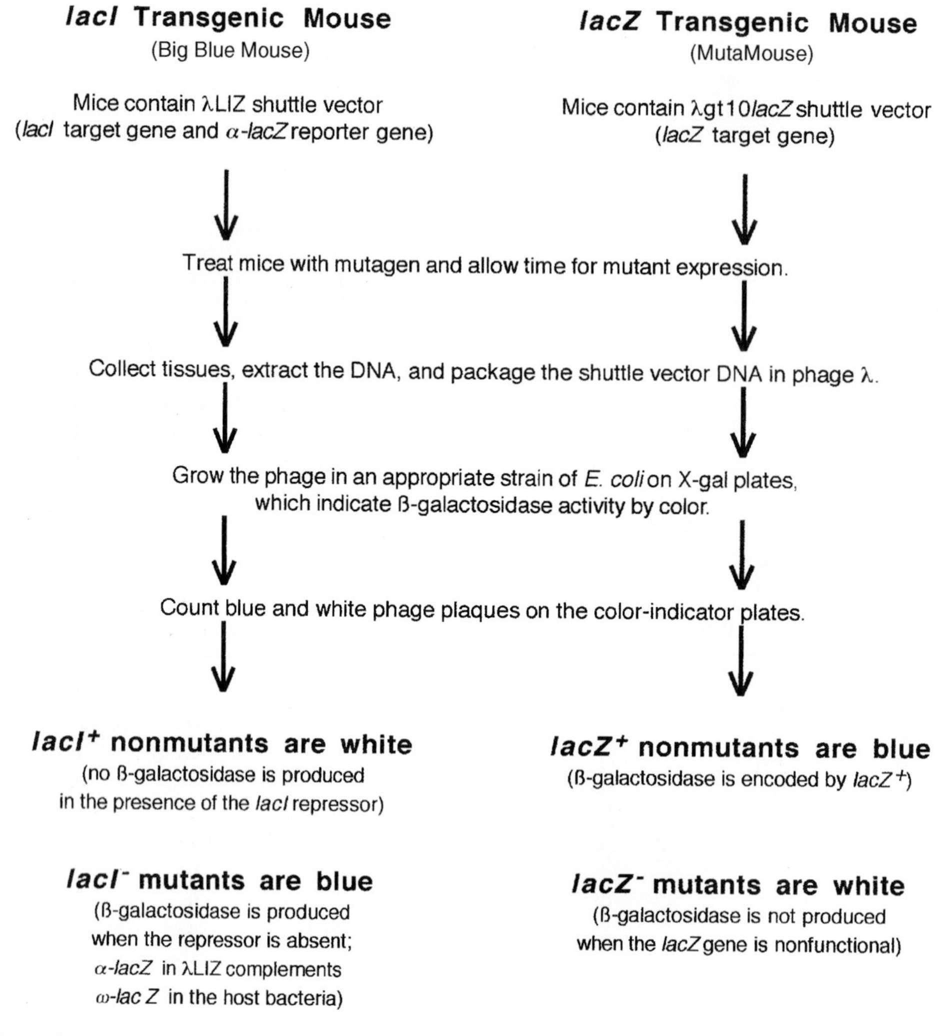


*Figure 9–7. Transgenic mouse models for the study of mutagenesis.*

(Mirsalis et al., 1994). An important issue that remains to be resolved is whether the mutational responses of transgenes are similar to those of endogenous genes. The specificity of ENU in inducing mutations in transgenes seems to differ from that in endogenous bacterial genes or in mammalian genes in vivo (Burkhart and Malling, 1993), and questions have been raised about the relevance of mutations that might be recovered from dying or dead animal tissues (Burkhart and Malling, 1994). Therefore, transgenic animals offer promising models for the study of chemical mutagenesis, but there are technical questions that need to be resolved before their place in genetic toxicology and mutation research will be clear.

## MOLECULAR ANALYSIS OF MUTATION

Molecular biology has added powerful new methods for studying mutagenesis, and modern mutation research combines genetic and molecular analysis. Some early systems for characterizing mutations at the molecular level compared mutant proteins with wild-type proteins; conclusions were reached about changes in genes on the basis of changes in the proteins they encode (Auerbach, 1976). Now, however, nucleic acids are amenable to direct analysis, and DNA technology has revolutionized mutation research.

Point mutations and deletions, which are not always distinguishable on the basis of phenotype, have traditionally been differentiated by genetic analysis. They also may be characterized directly through the use of probes for the target gene and Southern blotting (Albertini et al., 1990; Cole and Skopek, 1994). Point mutations do not alter DNA enough to be detectable on Southern blots, whereas gross structural alterations are visible. Southern analysis of restricted DNA has been used to determine the proportions of mutations ascribable to deletions and other structural alterations in several assays, including the mouse specific-locus test (Russell and Rinchik, 1993) and human *hprt* mutations (Cole and Skopek, 1994).

Point mutations can be characterized by DNA sequence analysis. Sequencing requires having many copies of a small fragment of DNA that includes the mutation. To obtain mutant DNA, one may direct the mutagenesis to a predetermined small piece of isolated DNA (Lambert et al., 1992) or induce mutations randomly and use genetic and molecular methods to localize and isolate them. Many copies of a mutation may be obtained by cloning. Cloning entails transferring the mutation to a cloning vector that serves as a carrier. When the vector is introduced into cells (usually bacteria) and allowed to replicate, the mutation is amplified along with it (Halliday and Glickman, 1991). Thus, cloning is the in vivo amplification of the sequence of interest. Mutations also may be amplified in vitro by the polymerase chain reaction (PCR).

PCR (Griffiths et al., 1993) is a powerful technique that permits the amplification of mutations directly from genomic DNA (Sierra et al., 1993; Levine et al., 1994) or from cDNA (Cole and Skopek, 1994). It is finding increasing use because it avoids some of the technical complexity and tedium of cloning. PCR is easily applied to DNA that has been genetically purified, such as that of revertants from the Ames assay that have been picked, streaked, and reisolated from single colonies on selective medium (Koch et al., 1994). When mutations are amplified by PCR from a heterogeneous population of mutants or from mutant DNA contaminated with the nonmutant sequence, they can be purified for sequence analysis by denaturing gradient gel electrophoresis (Cariello and Skopek, 1993b). Whether cloned or amplified by PCR, mutations are readily sequenced by variations on two basic methods (Griffiths et al., 1993): the Maxam-Gilbert chemical degradation method and, more commonly, the Sanger method, also called the enzymatic method or the dideoxy chain termination method.

A versatile assay for the molecular analysis of mutations in bacteria is the *lacI* system developed in *E. coli* by Jeffrey Miller and colleagues (Calos and Miller, 1981). Mutations in the *lacI* gene, which encodes the repressor of the lactose operon, are easily identified by phenotype and characterized genetically. Molecular analysis of *lacI* mutations entails transferring them from the strain in which they originated to a phage vector and cloning them for sequencing (Halliday and Glickman, 1991). Alternatively, *lacI* mutations may be amplified directly from mutant phage plaques by PCR and sequenced (Mirsalis et al., 1994). The *lacI* gene is widely used as a target for mutagenesis in *E. coli* and transgenic mice, and more than 30,000 *lacI* mutants have been sequenced (Mirsalis et al., 1994).

DNA sequencing permits the elucidation of mutation spectra. A mutation spectrum shows the distribution within a gene of base-pair substitutions, frameshifts, and small deletions, all of which are clearly defined at the molecular level. The spectrum also may include sequence changes called complex mutations that are not readily explained by single mutational events. By revealing the sequence context of mutations, mutation spectra provide information about the effects of neighboring sequences on the mutability of particular sites. For example, in the *E. coli lacI* assay, about 98 percent of the mutations induced by the acridine mustard ICR-191 are frameshifts in which a single G:C base pair has been gained or lost in a region of repetitive G:C base pairs (Calos and Miller, 1981). Thus, mutation spectra reveal highly mutable locations in a gene called hotspots. Hotspots exist for both spontaneous and induced mutations. An analysis of 729 spontaneous *lacI* mutations in *E. coli* revealed that 70 percent occurred in a region that is only 13 nucleotides long and contains the repeated sequence (5'-TGGC-3')$_3$ (Halliday and Glickman, 1991).

Molecular studies have revealed that physical alteration of the conformation of DNA can be important in mutagenesis. Both AAF and the related compound *N*-2-aminofluorene (AF) bind to the C8 position of guanine, but their adducts have different effects on DNA conformation. AAF adducts insert into the DNA, extruding a guanine and causing localized distortion of the DNA structure, whereas AF adducts remain outside the double helix or are inserted with less distortion (Heflich and Neft, 1994). In a forward mutation assay in the tetracycline-resistance gene of plasmid pBR322 in *E. coli*, AAF primarily induces frameshifts while AF mainly induces transversions. Two kinds of hotspots for AAF-induced frameshifts have been identified: −1 frameshifts in repetitive sequences (e.g., GGGGG) and −2 frameshifts in the alternating G:C base pairs of the sequence GGCGCC (Heflich and Neft, 1994). The −1 frameshifts probably arise from misalignment in the repetitive sequence when a polymerase is stalled at the site of the bulky AAF adduct (Lambert et al., 1992). The induction of −2 frameshifts also may occur through misalignment or by AAF triggering a localized conformational shift from the familiar right-handed helical structure of DNA (i.e., B-DNA) to a left-handed helix called Z-DNA that is prone to the −2 mutation (Heflich and Neft, 1994).

Further evidence for the importance of conformational changes in mutagenesis has come from the analysis of sequences involved in complex mutations, such as a frameshift and nearby base-pair substitutions that would be expected to occur at extremely low frequencies if they were independent events (Drake, 1991). Such mutations are often associated with inverted DNA repeats. The palindromic or nearly palindromic sequences can form hairpinlike loops, and some complex mutations, rather than arising from more than one independent mutation, can be explained by a single event in the metabolic processing of the hairpin. Some deletions are also associated with palindromic sequences; an example is shown in Fig. 9-8.

The importance of the Ames assay in genetic toxicology has stimulated efforts to characterize revertants in the Ames tester strains at the molecular level. The primary reversion mechanisms, which are summarized in Table 9-3, were initially determined by genetic and biochemical means (Maron and Ames, 1983; Hartman et al., 1986). Spontaneous and induced revertants have since been cloned and sequenced (Levine et al., 1994). An ingenious method called allele-specific colony hybridization has greatly facilitated the molecular analysis of revertants in the Ames assay (Koch et al., 1994). Radioactive synthetic oligonucleotide primers that correspond to major classes of revertants are hybridized to the DNA of revertant colonies that have been transferred to filters and lysed. Unbound probe is removed by washing, and autoradiography is used to detect bound probe. The hybridization is specific enough that the presence of the radioactive label indicates that the revertant has the precise sequence that is complementary to the probe. The colony hybridization technique quickly identifies the principal classes of revertants, making it unnecessary to sequence them. Revertants whose DNA sequences are not identified by colony hybridization are then subjected to PCR and sequenced (Koch et al., 1994; Levine et al., 1994). The combination of colony hybridization and PCR has proved extremely effective in determining mechanisms of reversion in the Ames assay.

Shuttle vectors have been used to study the processing of DNA damage into mutations in mammalian cells (Dixon et al., 1989). A shuttle vector consists of a target gene for detecting mutations, such as the *E. coli supF* gene, incorporated into a

```
....G-G-A-C-A-C-T-A-G-C-C-A-T-C-C-T-A-G-T-C-A-T-C....
....C-C-T-G-T-G-A-T-C-G-G-T-A-G-G-A-T-C-A-G-T-A-G....

                      ↓ ↑

                       A
                     C   T
                     C   C
                      G C
                      A T
                      T A
                      C G
                      A T
          ....G-G-A-C     C-A-T-C....
          ....C-C-T-G     G-T-A-G....
                      T A
                      G C
                      A T
                      T A
                      C G
                     G   G
                     G   A
                       T
```

*Figure 9–8. Formation of a hairpinlike secondary structure in a palindromic DNA sequence.*

Replication across the base of the hairpin can lead to deletion of the 15 base pairs in the hairpin.

plasmid or a virus-based extrachromosomal element that can replicate in mammalian cells. Mutations induced in the target gene in mammalian cells are recovered from the cells and transferred to bacteria for detection and sequencing. Inconsistencies among shuttle vector systems, such as the finding that AAF produces a different spectrum of mutations in different assays, call for further studies on the characteristics of the target genes and the processing of adducts into mutations in different cells (Heflich and Neft, 1994). Shuttle vectors also are used to analyze mutations induced in bacterial genes in transgenic mice (Mirsalis et al., 1994).

DNA sequence analysis of mutations has been extended to endogenous eukaryotic genes, including those of *Drosophila* (Sierra et al., 1993); cultured mammalian cells; and humans (Cariello and Skopek, 1993a). More than 1000 *hprt* mutations have been isolated from human cells in vitro and in vivo and analyzed. These mutations include base-pair substitutions, frameshifts, and small deletions as well as the larger deletions and other rearrangements detected by Southern blot analysis (Cole and Skopek, 1994). The *hprt* data reveal distributions of mutations among the nine coding regions of the *hprt* gene, mutation spectra for several mutagens, and hotspots for both base-pair substitutions and frameshifts (Cariello and Skopek, 1993a).

Sequence data have been obtained for many mutations in the p53 tumor suppressor gene in human cancers (Hollstein et al., 1991; Aguilar et al., 1994). More than 90 percent of these mutations are base-pair substitutions of the missense type (Harris, 1993). There are differences among cancers in that transitions predominate in lymphomas, leukemias, and tumors of the colon and brain, whereas transversions are more common in lung and liver cancers (Hollstein et al., 1991). The spectrum of p53 mutations is relevant to the etiology of the cancers in that some mutations in p53 are most readily explained as spontaneous mutations, whereas others are likely to be induced. CpG dinucleotides in p53 are hotspots for transition mutations that arise spontaneously by deamination of 5-methylcytosine (Harris, 1993). Transitions at dipyrimidine sites in skin cancers, especially a double transition of adjacent base pairs that is extremely rare except among UV-induced mutations, suggest causation by exposure to sunlight (Dumaz et al., 1994). Thus, mutation spectra can link specific cancers to mutagens. In the case of hepatocellular carcinoma, G:C $\rightarrow$ T:A transversions at codon 249 of p53 link the cancer to the carcinogen aflatoxin $B_1$ (Harris, 1993). This transversion is prevalent in regions of China and Africa where there is high exposure to aflatoxin but not in areas where there is less aflatoxin exposure; the evidence suggests a causative and early role of aflatoxin in hepatocarcinogenesis in the exposed populations (Aguilar et al., 1994).

## PREDICTIVE POWER OF MUTAGENICITY ASSAYS

Validating an assay for mutagens entails determining how well it performs with many compounds from diverse chemical classes in several laboratories. Thoroughly studied, potent mutagens offer an obvious reference point for test validation, but one must also determine whether the assay detects weak mutagens and is unresponsive to nonmutagens. An assay should be thoroughly characterized before it is applied in testing. A reproducible positive result in a well-characterized genetic assay indicates that a compound is a mutagen. In view of the clear association of mutations with genetic disease and cancer, a demonstration of mutagenicity suggests that a compound may be hazardous for humans and warrants further investigation if human exposures are known or anticipated.

### Predicting Carcinogenicity

Mutagenicity assays are often used in efforts to predict which chemicals are carcinogens. In predicting carcinogenicity, one should consider both the sensitivity and the specificity of an assay. Sensitivity refers to the proportion of carcinogens that are positive in an assay, whereas specificity refers to the proportion of noncarcinogens that are negative (Tennant et al., 1987). The word "sensitivity" also can be used to denote the ability of an assay to detect a mutagen at a low concentration or a small change in mutation frequency; so alternative usages must be recognized from the context. Sensitivity and specificity both contribute to the concordance of a short-term assay with carcinogenicity, and a useful assay must have reasonable predictive value for both carcinogens and noncarcinogens. A positive result in a short-term test is often called a false positive if the compound is noncarcinogenic, and a negative result is called a false negative if the compound is carcinogenic.

Several years ago it was commonly claimed that 90 percent of carcinogens could be detected as mutagens. Although reasonable at the time, such statements are too simplistic because carcinogenicity is not a single entity but a complex pattern of responses with diverse underlying mechanisms and because calculations of the sensitivity of genetic assays in predicting the totality of carcinogenic responses can be misleading. The prevalence of different classes of chemicals in the analysis can strongly affect the outcome (Ashby and Tennant, 1991). For example, carcinogenic metals are not effectively detected in the Ames assay (Barrett, 1993), and their inclusion among the chemicals evaluated would reduce the apparent sensitivity of the assay. In an analysis of 301 compounds, *Salmonella* detected 93 percent of aromatic amino or nitro compounds that were found to be carcinogenic in mice or rats and 100 percent of those which were carcinogenic in both species, but it detected none of the carcinogens that are nonreactive halogen compounds, including dioxins, polybrominated biphenyls, and chlordane (Ashby and Tennant, 1991).

Some chemicals exert their carcinogenic effects by mechanisms that do not involve DNA damage, and one should not expect mutagenicity tests to detect them. Such carcinogens are called nongenotoxic or epigenetic carcinogens. Carcinogens that seem to act through nongenotoxic mechanisms include estrogens (Butterworth and Slaga, 1987; Barrett, 1993), nitrilotriacetate, the peroxisome proliferator diethylhexyl phthalate, and the nonreactive halogen compounds mentioned above (Ashby and Tennant, 1991). The existence of nongenotoxic carcinogens does not negate the importance of mutagenicity in the carcinogenicity of other chemicals.

The predictive power of mutagenicity assays for identifying carcinogens is often evaluated through comparisons with carcinogenicity assays in rodents. In a study that had a substantial impact on genetic toxicology, Raymond Tennant and colleagues compared the results from four widely used short-term genetic assays with cancer bioassays of 73 chemicals in mice and rats (Tennant et al., 1987). The Ames assay, the TK assay in mouse lymphoma cells, chromosome aberrations in CHO cells, and SCE in CHO cells each showed a concordance with the carcinogenicity assays of about 60 percent, a value much lower than might have been anticipated.

The findings of Tennant and associates (1987) stimulated vigorous debate, because a possible interpretation is that short-term genetic assays are not useful in identifying carcinogens. Critics pointed out that discordance with rodent carcinogenicity may not be a failing of the mutagenicity assay, because the assumption that the carcinogenicity assay permits a correct classification of carcinogens and noncarcinogens is subject to question. In fact, many carcinogenicity results are equivocal (Prival and Dunkel, 1989), and there is often discordance among animal species in carcinogenicity tests. Concordance between mice and rats was 67 percent in the study of Tennant and associates (1987) and 71 percent in an analysis of 224 chemicals (Zeiger, 1987). In the latter study, only 46 percent of the chemicals that were carcinogenic in rats or mice were carcinogenic in both species. Besides interspecies variation, other factors can complicate the interpretation of some carcinogenesis assays, including a lack of statistical power, the high spontaneous incidence of some tumors in rodents, the absence of replicate experiments in expensive bioassays, and shortcomings in dosage regimens or other aspects of assay design (Brockman and DeMarini, 1988; Prival and Dunkel, 1989). The identification of noncarcinogens on the basis of negative results in cancer assays can be problematic (Prival and Dunkel, 1989), especially in regard to chemical classes in which structurally related compounds are carcinogenic. One must ask whether a compound is truly noncarcinogenic or whether its carcinogenicity was not detected because of factors such as the species used, the test doses, or the numbers of animals. Some putative false positives in short-term assays may actually be carcinogens that were misclassified in a carcinogenesis assay.

An analysis of data for 301 chemicals tested for carcinogenicity in mice and rats revealed that the Ames assay detected only 56 percent of the carcinogens in the entire data set but 70 percent of those that were carcinogenic in both mice and rats (Ashby and Tennant, 1991). Moreover, the *Salmonella* results showed 87 percent correspondence with structural alerts, which are substituent groups in the chemical structure that suggest DNA reactivity. When the carcinogens were partitioned into those with structural alerts and those without, it was found that *Salmonella* detected 84 percent of the former but only 4 percent of the latter. Among structurally alerting chemicals that were carcinogenic in both rats and mice, 93 percent were mutagenic in *Salmonella* (Tennant and Ashby, 1991). The analysis of a larger database that included 351 rodent carcinogens that had been tested for mutagenicity in *Salmonella* revealed that 81 percent of the chemicals that induced tumors at multiple sites in both rats and mice were *Salmonella* mutagens (Gold et al., 1993).

Taken as a whole, the data indicate that mutagenicity testing in *Salmonella*, combined with evaluation of chemical structure, allows the identification of a large proportion of genotoxic rodent carcinogens. This view is reinforced by the correct prediction of the carcinogenicity or noncarcinogenicity of 88 percent of 40 chemicals on the basis of structural alerts, *Salmonella* mutagenicity, and rodent subchronic toxicity before the carcinogenicity tests were conducted (Parry, 1994). Moreover, an analysis of 511 rodent carcinogens supports the view that genotoxicity and structural alerts are common properties of transspecies, multiple-site carcinogens, whereas putative nongenotoxic carcinogens often give responses that are more specific with respect to species, sites, and conditions (Ashby and Paton, 1993; Gold et al., 1993).

The commonly held view that deficiencies in the sensitivity or specificity of individual genetic assays can be circumvented by using complementary assays in combinations called tiers or batteries was also challenged by Tennant and associates (1987). Rather than complementing each other's strengths and weaknesses, genetic toxicology assays are often consistent with one another. This finding argues against the use of extensive tiers and batteries but suggests that these assays do detect agents that are truly mutagenic. A study based on 301 compounds (Ashby and Tennant, 1991) has confirmed that carcinogens and noncarcinogens that are incorrectly classified by the *Salmonella* assay are not readily distinguished by other short-term genetic assays. Therefore, rather than trying to assemble batteries of complementary assays, it seems prudent to emphasize mechanistic considerations in choosing assays. Such an approach would make a sensitive assay for gene mutations (e.g., the Ames assay) and an assay for clastogenic effects in mammals pivotal in the evaluation of genotoxicity.

Mutagenicity data are compared with rodent cancer bioassays because data on chemical carcinogenesis in humans are limited. The relative importance of genotoxic and nongenotoxic carcinogens for humans is difficult to ascertain, but genotoxic carcinogens are well represented among chemicals that have been identified as human carcinogens (Shelby and Zeiger, 1990). The human carcinogenicity of cyclosporin (an immunosuppressant) and some hormones, however, suggests that nongenotoxic carcinogens cannot be disregarded (Ashby and Paton, 1993). After eliminating hormones, metals, and carcinogenic fibers for being inappropriate to the assays, one finds that the combination of the Ames assay and a mouse bone marrow assay for chromosome aberrations or micronuclei detects all 21 defined human carcinogens (Shelby and Zeiger, 1990). Of the 20 organic carcinogens tested in *Salmonella*, only benzene was nonmutagenic. Mouse cytogenetic assays were positive for 17 of 18 human carcinogens, including benzene, with one compound giving inconclusive results. In addition to these defined agents, soots, tars, and oils that are human carcinogens were also mutagenic.

The linkages among mutagenicity, structural alerts, and carcinogenicity indicate that a reproducible mutagenic response must be taken seriously both as an indicator of the inherent mutagenicity of a compound and as suggestive evidence of carcinogenicity. If a chemical is found to be mutagenic in the Ames assay or in vivo cytogenetics, that response is in itself a biological effect that requires more thorough analysis. If a chemical is mutagenic in both assays, there is a high probability that it poses a genotoxic hazard for humans.

### Predicting Germ Cell Mutagenicity

Evaluating the ability of a short-term assay to predict mammalian germ cell mutagenicity is no simpler than measuring its ability to predict carcinogenicity because too few compounds have been tested for mutagenicity in mammalian germ cells. However, a positive test for mutagenicity in a well-characterized gene mutation assay in mammalian germ cells, such as a mouse specific-locus test, provides a strong suggestion that the chemical would be mutagenic in human germ cells. The induction of heritable translocations, cytogenetically detectable chromosome aberrations, or micronuclei in rodent germ cells similarly indicates that the agent is likely to be clastogenic in human germ cells. Unfortunately, negative results are more difficult to interpret because the assay conditions might not have been optimal or the scale of the study might have been insufficient to detect a small increase in mutation frequency.

## SCREENING FOR MUTAGENS

Concern about the adverse effects of mutation on human health has provided the impetus to identify environmental mutagens. Unfortunately, it is not feasible to conduct thorough tests of all the chemicals to which people are exposed. More than 50,000 distinct substances are registered with the EPA and FDA (Ehling, 1991), and new chemicals continue to be introduced. Besides commercial chemicals, many naturally occurring compounds and pollutants generated in the environment have significant toxicological effects. The inability to test all compounds necessitates setting priorities for testing. Factors such as production volumes, intended uses, the extent of human exposure, environmental distribution, and effects that may be anticipated from chemical structure or previous toxicological tests must be considered to ensure that the compounds with the greatest potential for adverse effects receive the most thorough study.

The most obvious use of genetic toxicology assays is in screening chemicals to detect mutagens. Many compounds have been tested, and the database of the Environmental Mutagen Information Center (EMIC) in Oak Ridge, Tennessee, includes more than 80,000 publications on the genetic effects of about 25,000 chemicals. Data from screening are used in setting priorities for further testing and contribute to decisions concerning the development of chemical products and regulatory processes. An important consideration in screening is that laboratory practices meet a high standard with respect to procedures, safety, and data handling (Kirkland et al., 1990). A description of specific mutagens is beyond the scope of this chapter, but general coverage of many chemical, physical (e.g., radiation), and biological (e.g., viruses and transposable genetic elements) mutagens is available elsewhere (Li and Heflich, 1991).

Besides screening pure chemicals, environmental testing has received much attention because many mutagens exist in complex mixtures (DeMarini, 1991; Lewtas, 1991). Two approaches are used: testing environmental samples for mutagenicity in the laboratory and detecting mutagenic effects in indicator organisms in the environment of interest. Most studies have relied on the former approach, using concentrated environmental samples. Even under controlled laboratory conditions, complex mixtures pose difficult problems because of their variable composition and the fact that the procedures used in the collection, extraction, concentration, fractionation, and other processing of samples can affect the outcome of the tests.

Mutagenicity tests of complex mixtures can be used in quality control and environmental monitoring (DeMarini, 1991; Lewtas, 1991). For example, products can be screened for the presence of mutagenic contaminants, and the effectiveness of pollution control technologies or containment facilities can be assessed. The Ames assay has been widely used in studies of complex mixtures because its speed and simplicity allow the testing of many samples. Complex mixtures that have been analyzed for mutagenicity include air; drinking water; other water sources; industrial emissions and effluents; automotive emissions; emissions from burning wood, coal, and oil; diverse oils and fuels; photocopy toners; foods and beverages; and tobacco smoke (DeMarini, 1991; Lewtas, 1991). Such testing is most effective when combined with analytic chemistry so that the classes of chemicals are characterized and some major mutagenic components are identified. Identifying all the components in complex mixtures is not feasible, however, as these mixtures may contain tens of thousands of compounds. Because the quantities of materials in fractionated samples are often small, modified testing procedures such as microsuspension assays in *Salmonella* have been developed to perform tests in small volumes (DeMarini, 1991; Lewtas, 1991).

An alternative to controlled laboratory exposures is in situ monitoring for mutagens (Lewtas, 1991). In in situ monitoring, one looks for evidence of mutagenic effects in organisms that are grown or occur naturally in the environment of interest. Plant assays (Table 9-1) have been the most frequently used assays for this purpose (Grant, 1994). Natural populations of organisms also can be examined for evidence of genetic damage. For example, frequencies of chlorophyll mutations in red mangroves have been correlated with concentrations of PAHs in the sediments in which the plants grow (Klekowski et al., 1994). While studies of natural populations are of obvious interest, they require the utmost precaution in characterizing the environments being compared and defining appropriate control populations.

A general toxicological principle that is especially important in the study of complex mixtures is that the effects of chemicals need not be additive. Synergistic and antagonistic effects may occur among mutagens, and nonmutagens may exhibit comutagenic and antimutagenic effects (DeMarini, 1991). Antimutagens—agents that reduce the genotoxic effects of mutagens—are being studied to elucidate the basic mechanisms underlying the interactions and explore their possible roles in protecting against mutagenesis and carcinogenesis (Ferguson, 1994).

## MONITORING HUMAN POPULATIONS

Screening people who have had known or suspected contact with mutagens can be useful in quantifying exposures and assessing risks. In some mutagen exposures, such as radiotherapy, data collected from the same individuals before exposure can serve as a baseline for comparison. Generally, however, the study population must be compared with an appropriate control population that is defined with an awareness of factors such as age, sex, smoking habits, and medical history.

### Germ Cell Mutagenesis

Monitoring for germ cell mutagenesis involves looking for genetic effects in offspring. Interpreting associations between parental exposures and effects in children is complicated by the many variables inherent in epidemiological studies, and explanations other than germ cell mutagenesis, such as transplacental exposure, can be difficult to exclude. Concentrating on paternal occupational exposures reduces the confounding influence of transplacental exposure but does not remove alternative explanations entirely from consideration, because a person may inadvertently bring toxic compounds into his home and expose his family to them. Several epidemiological studies have reported associations between occupational exposures of men and the likelihood of cancer or birth defects in their children. For example, elevated frequencies of childhood leukemias and brain cancer have been reported in the children of men occupationally exposed to paint or hydrocarbons. However, despite numerous epidemiological studies, no causal links between paternal exposure and birth defects or cancer in children have been clearly established (Savitz and Chen, 1990; Wyrobek, 1993).

No clear evidence exists for the induction of heritable alterations by radiation or chemicals in human germ cells. Even the children of obviously exposed populations such as cancer chemotherapy and radiotherapy patients, workers exposed to mustard gas, individuals accidentally exposed to ionizing radiation, and survivors of the atomic explosions in Hiroshima and Nagasaki have not provided clear evidence of germ cell mutagenesis (Neel et al., 1993; Shelby, 1994). The absence of convincing evidence stems from the technical difficulty of measuring events that occur at a low frequency in human populations; it does not indicate that the induction of mutations in human germ cells does not occur.

In principle, mutagenesis can be detected by monitoring for an increase in the frequency of sentinel phenotypes, which are characteristics that serve as indicators of new mutations. The best candidates for serving as a sentinel phenotype are severe, sporadically occurring disorders that can be ascribed to a single dominant or sex-linked mutant gene that is expressed uniformly and diagnosed easily and accurately at or near birth (Mulvihill, 1990; Neel et al., 1993). The sentinel phenotypes approach is insensitive because individual genetic diseases are rare, and large populations are required to detect an increase in the mutation rate. For example, the combined frequency of 24 sentinel phenotypes that are recognizable at birth is about $3 \times 10^{-4}$ (Neel et al., 1993). Monitoring for electrophoretic protein variants in blood samples from the offspring of a study population also could indicate mutagenic effects (Mohrenweiser, 1991; Neel et al., 1993) but would similarly require large populations. While these methods may be appropriate in a few instances of large mutagen exposures (e.g., mutagenic chemotherapy or radiotherapy), they are not suitable when the exposed population is small or the exposure is modest. A negative result in monitoring for germ cell mutagenesis is therefore likely to reflect the insensitivity of the method rather than the real absence of an effect.

While evidence of induced transmissible mutations in human germ cells is lacking, there is no real doubt that human germ cells are subject to mutagenesis. Ionizing radiation and diverse chemicals induce transmissible mutations and chromosome aberrations in laboratory animals. Moreover, there is evidence from testicular biopsy that chromosome aberrations are induced by x-rays in human spermatocytes (Shelby, 1994).

Chromosomal alterations may be observed in human germ cells by fusing human sperm with hamster oocytes. This technique allows the observation of sperm pronuclear chromosomes and suggests that about 9 to 10 percent of human sperm have structural chromosome aberrations and that about 2 percent are aneuploid (Martin, 1993b). Increased frequencies of aberrations are detected in sperm from men whose testes were irradiated in cancer radiotherapy (Martin, 1993b) or who had received cancer chemotherapy (Genescà et al., 1990). While sperm and lymphocytes both show the induction of aberrations by irradiation, they differ in the time course over which the damage appears and declines, suggesting that somatic cells may not be wholly suitable as a surrogate for germ cells in monitoring for genetic damage (Martin, 1993b). A lingering uncertainty is whether the unusual conditions of an interspecific fusion assay affect the frequency of aberrations. Aberration frequencies in sperm from control men (6 to 13 percent) are higher than those in intraspecific fertilization in rodents—1.3 percent in Chinese hamsters and 0.6 percent in mice (Genescà et al., 1990)—suggesting that the assay may cause aberrations or permit the persistence of DNA damage that might normally be repaired. Interspecific fusion is also technically difficult and time-consuming. Efforts are therefore being made to detect genetic alterations directly in human spermatozoa.

Early attempts were made to detect aneuploidy by screening quinacrine-stained human spermatozoa for fluorescent spots (Allen et al., 1986). It was proposed that spermatozoa with two spots (YFF) have two Y chromosomes. Increased frequencies of YFF sperm were reported in men who were occupationally exposed to dibromochloropropane or clinically exposed to x-rays, doxorubicin (Adriamycin), or metronidazole. The YFF method cannot be regarded as a reliable indicator of aneuploidy because it overestimates the frequency of sperm with two Y chromosomes and yields frequencies of sperm with a single fluorescent spot lower than the expected 50 percent (Robbins et al., 1993). While the YFF assay has fallen into disuse, its goal of detecting aneuploidy by counting fluorescent spots may now be realized through the application of FISH.

FISH with probes for specific chromosomes offers the prospect of detecting extra chromosomes as extra fluorescent spots in stained spermatozoa. Probes for repetitive sequences on chromosomes 1 and Y have indicated that sperm with an extra chromosome, as indicated by two fluorescent regions, occur at frequencies of about 0.05 percent for the Y chromosome and 0.14 percent for chromosome 1 (Robbins et al., 1993). Similarly, probes for chromosomes 1, 12, and X in another study have shown frequencies of aneuploidy of 0.06 percent, 0.04 percent and 0.03 percent, respectively (Martin, 1993b). All these values are compatible with those found by fusing human sperm with hamster oocytes (Martin, 1993b; Robbins et al., 1993). Thus, FISH may provide a rapid means of quantifying aneuploidy in human sperm. The interspecific fusion technique, though more laborious, offers a means of confirming the results from FISH and permits the quantification of structural chromosome aberrations.

The methods of molecular biology offer the possibility of devising novel strategies for measuring mutation rates and detecting induced mutations in human populations. Approaches that have been suggested include using denaturing gradient gel electrophoresis (Cariello and Skopek, 1993b) or single-strand conformation polymorphism analysis (Sekiya, 1993) to detect point mutations in DNA fragments that have been amplified by PCR, detecting deletions and rearrangements by Southern blotting, using high-performance liquid chromatography to detect deletions and duplications in DNA segments amplified by PCR, detecting sequence differences by means of hybridization with oligonucleotides, and analyzing for alterations in minisatellite or hypervariable DNA sequences (Neel et al., 1993; Shelby, 1994).

## Somatic Cell Mutagenesis

Methods for detecting mutagenic effects in human somatic cells are more advanced than those for detecting mutagenesis in germ cells. Cytogenetics offers a direct link between mutagenicity tests in experimental organisms and effects in humans and is the most common means of detecting human mutagen exposures (Bender et al., 1988; Sorsa et al., 1992). Chromosome aberrations, including chromatid breaks, chromatid exchanges, acentric fragments, dicentric chromosomes, ring chromosomes, and some inversions and translocations, can be scored in peripheral lymphocytes from people who have been exposed to mutagens. Elevated frequencies of aberrations have been detected after exposures to ionizing radiation (Bender et al., 1988) and diverse chemicals, including benzene, coal tars, cyclophosphamide, ethylene oxide, nickel compounds, vinyl chloride, and styrene (Sorsa et al., 1992). In the case of large radiation exposures, one can estimate doses from the frequencies of aberrations in lymphocytes (Bender et al., 1988). Micronucleus assays have found use as a surrogate for metaphase analysis in human monitoring (Sorsa et al., 1992), as they have in mutagenicity testing and research.

Like all toxicological methods, cytogenetic monitoring has limitations. Preexposure aberration frequencies are unknown in most accidental exposures and many medical exposures. It is therefore necessary to compare frequencies of aberrations with those of matched controls. Control frequencies, however, vary in different individuals and different studies (Bender et al., 1988). This variation arises both from technical factors, such as culture conditions, sampling times, preparation of slides, and slide scoring, and from differences associated with the subjects, including genetic differences and confounding variables that affect the control and study populations (Sorsa et al., 1992). The lack of baseline frequencies and variability in controls detract from the ability of cytogenetic methods to detect small increases in the frequency of aberrations.

Elevated frequencies of aberrations in lymphocytes demonstrate damage to the genetic material in human cells in vivo. At the population level, such damage identifies hazardous exposures and groups of individuals at risk for the adverse effects of mutagenesis, including cancer (Hagmar et al., 1994). Interpreting risk at the individual level is more uncertain, and it is therefore difficult to tell a subject what an elevated frequency of aberrations really means. A prospective cohort study of 1979 subjects whose lymphocytes were analyzed for chromosome aberrations between 1970 and 1988 suggests that individuals with an aberration frequency classified as high have a significantly increased risk of developing cancer (Hagmar et al., 1994). The frequency of cancer in individuals with high aberration frequencies was about 2.5-fold that in individuals with low or intermediate frequencies; the number of cancer cases (66) in the study, however, was still quite limited, and additional data are required to put the positive trend into perspective.

Chromosome painting by FISH promises to facilitate the measurement of chromosomal damage in humans because the scoring of slides is rapid and all classes of aberrations can be observed. In addition to the unstable aberrations that are quantified in traditional metaphase analysis, stable aberrations are readily detected. Stable aberrations such as translocations are more likely to persist in a cell population and may therefore be suitable indicators of damage in chronic exposures or long after exposure (Tucker et al., 1993b).

SCE is readily monitored in people (Sorsa et al., 1992; Tucker et al., 1993a). The mechanism of SCE is not well understood, but many mutagens induce SCE, and SCE assays are responsive to low doses. Moreover, the scoring of SCE is less subjective than that of aberrations. The problem of confounding variables in human populations remains, and the difficulty of explaining the results to subjects may be worse for SCE than for aberrations because of the lesser understanding of the alteration. Nevertheless, SCE can serve as an indicator of exposure even if the significance of the effect is unclear.

Gene mutations in human somatic cells in vivo may be studied through assays that detect mutant lymphocytes or erythrocytes. These assays are less advanced as monitoring techniques than are cytogenetic assays but have produced valuable information on the kinds of mutations that occur in humans.

The most refined assay for human gene mutations in vivo detects lymphocytes that are resistant to 6-thioguanine because a mutation in the *hprt* gene on the X chromosome has eliminated their HPRT activity (Albertini et al., 1990; Cole and Skopek, 1994). The mutants that arise in vivo may be cultured in vitro, and one can confirm that they originated as independent events by the heterogeneity of their T-cell receptors. Frequencies can therefore be calculated on the basis of confirmed independent mutations. The cloning of the mutants permits the molecular analysis of *hprt* mutations. About 85 percent of spontaneous *hprt* mutations in adults with no obvious mutagen exposures are point mutations, while the remainder are deletions and other structural alterations that are detectable by Southern analysis (Cole and Skopek, 1994). In contrast, newborns have a higher proportion of deletions, and the activity of V(D)J recombinase in T-lymphocyte development has been implicated in their origin. Increased frequencies of *hprt* mutations have been associated with cancer chemotherapy, radiotherapy, radioimmunoglobulin therapy, smoking, and occupational exposures to *nor*-nitrogen mustard and ethylene oxide. Compared with spontaneous *hprt* mutations, radiation-induced mutations include more deletions and other gross structural changes (Cole and Skopek, 1994). The availability of lymphocyte *hprt* assays in mice, rats, and cynomolgus monkeys offers parallel experimental systems in which experimental mutagen exposures can be made (Walker and Skopek, 1993).

Other in vivo assays in human lymphocytes are based on the genes of the major histocompatibility complex (HLA) or the CD3/T-cell receptor (TCR) complex (Cole and Skopek, 1994). The HLA assay detects mutations in the HLA-A locus on chromosome 6 by selecting against nonmutant lymphocytes with specific anti-HLA antibodies. Southern blot analysis has been used to differentiate HLA point mutations from chromosomal alterations. Since HLA-A is autosomal, this assay should permit the detection of chromosomal events, such as mitotic recombination and chromosome loss, that are not detectable at the sex-linked *hprt* locus. No results for mutagen-exposed individuals have been reported for the HLA assay (Cole and Skopek, 1994). The CD3/TCR assay uses fluorescent anti-CD3 and anti-CD4 TCR antibodies and flow cytometry to detect mutations in genes on chromosomes 7 and 14 that encode components of the CD3/TCR complex. An elevated frequency of TCR mutants was observed in patients receiving therapy with radioisotopes (Cole and Skopek, 1994).

Gene mutations that arise in vivo in the glycophorin-A gene on chromosome 4 of nucleated erythrocyte precursors can be detected in erythrocytes. Erythrocyte assays do not lend themselves to molecular analysis of mutations because the detection system is based on cells without nuclei, but the possibility of analysis at the mRNA level has been suggested (Cole and Skopek, 1994). GPA is a cell-surface glycoprotein that carries the M and N blood group antigens. Mutant erythrocytes are detected in MN heterozygotes by means of fluorescent antibodies against M and N (Grant and Bigbee, 1993). Flow cytometry is used to screen the cells, and mutants are identified by their loss of one of the fluorescent signals. Aneuploidy and mitotic recombination can be detected and seem to occur more frequently than do gene mutations in control individuals (Cole and Skopek, 1994). Elevated frequencies of GPA mutations have been detected in survivors of the atomic explosion in Hiroshima, individuals exposed to ionizing radiation in accidents in Chernobyl and Brazil, and patients who received cancer chemotherapy with Adriamycin, cyclophosphamide, and cisplatin (Grant and Bigbee, 1993). Like GPA mutations, mutations in hemoglobin genes can be detected in erythrocytes by means of fluorescent antibodies and automated detection techniques (Cole and Skopek, 1994).

Nongenetic biomarkers can provide useful indicators of mutagen exposure. Metabolites and products of DNA repair can be detected in urine, and adducts on DNA or proteins can be measured in blood and other tissues (Chang et al., 1994). DNA adducts can be detected by $^{32}$P-postlabeling, immunologic methods using antibodies against specific adducts, and fluorometric methods in the case of fluorescent compounds such as PAHs and aflatoxin. The $^{32}$P-postlabeling technique is highly sensitive and applicable to diverse mutagens and carcinogens. Adducts in DNA have been quantified by $^{32}$P-postlabeling and immunologic methods after human exposures to various chemicals, including PAHs, alkylating agents, aflatoxin, and the drugs 8-methoxypsoralen and cisplatin (Chang et al., 1994). Mutagenicity tests of concentrated urine also can indicate mutagen exposure, and urinary mutagens have been associated with cigarette smoking, occupational exposures, consumption of fried meats, and treatment with cancer chemotherapy or antiparasitic drugs (Venitt, 1988). Exposure indicators often can be correlated with biological effects in vivo. For example, adducts on hemoglobin have been used to quantify occupational exposure to ethylene oxide and are associated with increased frequencies of chromosome aberrations, micronuclei, SCE, and *hprt* mutations in lymphocytes (Ribeiro et al., 1994). PAH adducts in lymphocyte DNA from occupationally exposed foundry workers have similarly been correlated with the frequency of *hprt* mutations (Perera et al., 1993).

## ASSESSING MUTAGEN HAZARDS

The extent to which mutagens contribute to the total burden of genetic disease and cancer is unknown. A troublesome aspect of human exposure to mutagens is that there is a long time between exposure and effect, whether it is the latency period in carcinogenesis or, even more so, the separation between germ cell mutagenesis and effects in subsequent generations. Consequently, adverse effects in humans may not be observed until after further exposures have occurred, and even then the association of an effect with its cause may not be possible. Major goals in genetic toxicology are therefore the identification of mutagens in experimental organisms, assessment of the risks they pose, and prevention of unnecessary human exposures.

The fact that DNA is the hereditary material in all organisms provides a basis for extrapolating among species with respect to mutagenesis. Chemicals that are mutagens in one species usually are found to be mutagenic in others, and a positive result in any well-characterized mutagenicity assay therefore suggests that the agent may be mutagenic in humans. Such a finding calls for follow-up tests to characterize the mutagenic effect and evaluate its generality. Moreover, a reproducible finding of mutagenicity suggests that a chemical may be a carcinogen, a suggestion that requires evaluation in a carcinogenesis assay to be definitive. Despite the generality of DNA being the principal target for mutagenesis, differences among species occur, as they do in other areas of toxicology.

Microorganisms and cultured cells differ from intact mammals in terms of routes of exposure, dosimetry, distribution of toxicants, metabolism, and repair processes. The interpretation of test data with respect to human risk requires extrapolation on many levels, and mammalian tests must play a central role. Genetic toxicology therefore relies on short-term assays for screening many chemicals and mammalian assays for risk assessment and detailed study of selected mutagens.

In attempting to predict risks to future generations, the targets of interest are germ cells. Assays for mutations in germ cells therefore hold special importance in genetic toxicology. Nonmammalian assays cannot easily be extrapolated to mammalian germ cells, as even *Drosophila* germ cells do not adequately predict the sensitivity of different mammalian germ cell stages to mutagenesis (National Research Council, 1990; Bentley et al., 1994; Russell, 1994). Unfortunately, the best germ cell assays for risk assessment, such as a mouse specific-locus test, are too expensive to apply to large numbers of chemicals. Decisions on which compounds warrant analysis in costly germ cell assays therefore must be made on the basis of simpler genetic assays and other toxicological data. Indicators of DNA damage in mammalian testes such as UDS and alkaline elution assays can facilitate this process by identifying agents that reach and affect germinal tissue (Bentley et al., 1994).

Genetic risk assessment seeks to predict the increase in mutations and genetic disease in humans that would result from a particular mutagen exposure. This type of prediction is extremely complex. The induction of dominant mutations is a more immediate concern than is the induction of recessive mutations, because the latter would not be expressed for many generations (National Research Council, 1983; Sankaranarayanan, 1993). Recessive mutations on the X chromosome, however, are like dominants in that they are subject to early expression in males. Another concern about recessives is that many of them may not be recessive in the strictest sense; rather, they may be expressed to a slight degree in heterozygotes (National Research Council, 1990). For example, heterozygotes for the recessive disease ataxia-telangiectasia do not have the high cancer incidence associated with the disease but have a cancer incidence higher than that of the general population (Friedberg, 1985). Because of their effects in heterozygotes (National Research Council, 1990), recessive mutations should not be dismissed as irrelevant for genetic risk. Nevertheless, practical considerations call for an emphasis on dominant and sex-linked mutations when one is trying to quantify the impact of germ cell mutagenesis on human health.

Various strategies have been proposed for predicting risks to human germ cells on the basis of data from laboratory animals. The most rigorous efforts in risk estimation are those made over several decades for ionizing radiation (National Research Council, 1990; Ehling, 1991; Sankaranarayanan, 1993). Two principal methods have been used: the doubling dose method and the direct method. The doubling dose method uses mouse data to calculate the amount of radiation that would produce as many mutations as occur spontaneously in one generation (i.e., a doubling dose). The doubling dose of ionizing radiation is estimated to be about 1 Gy (100 rad). Calculation of the doubling dose has been based primarily on the mouse specific-locus test, but the method has been extended to other mouse assays (National Research Council, 1990). In contrast, the direct method uses rates of induction of dominant mutations that cause skeletal abnormalities or cataracts in mice to estimate risks of dominant genetic disease caused in the first generation by radiation exposure (Ehling, 1991; Sankaranarayanan, 1993).

Preferences have been expressed for the doubling dose approach (National Research Council, 1990) or the direct method (Ehling, 1991), depending on the strength of misgivings about the validity of the assumptions underlying the other method. Reservations about the doubling dose method center on its use of recessive specific-locus mutations as a basis for estimating the induction of genetic damage in the first generation and its use of spontaneous mutations as a standard (Ehling, 1991). The spectrum of mutations induced by mutagens can differ from that of spontaneous mutations, as is seen in the high proportion of deletions induced by x-rays. The direct method has been criticized for its assumption that skeletal or cataract mutations in mice are representative of all dominant mutations that cause human disease (Sankaranarayanan, 1993). Nevertheless, the risk estimates provide reasonable assurance of an adequate margin of safety (National Research Council, 1990; Sankaranarayanan, 1993), and through the debate there has emerged a growing insight into the relationships among mutation rates, mutation spectra, and genetic risk.

Extending the concept of risk analysis to chemicals introduces many complexities related to the metabolism and pharmacodynamics of the compounds and the lack of a sufficient database concerning the induction of mutations in mammalian germ cells. Efforts in radiation risk assessment provide a useful starting place for analyzing chemicals, and variations on the doubling dose and direct approaches have helped shape thinking on how to assess genetic risks from chemical mutagens. Other strategies have also emerged, including direct extrapolation from nonmammalian species under various assumptions of proportionality among mutation rates, calculation of chemical mutagenic risks in terms of radiation equivalency, and extrapolations based on molecular dosimetry (National Research Council, 1983).

Molecular dosimetry entails measuring exposure by means of a molecular lesion that can be quantified in various cells or tissues, such as DNA adducts. Data on adducts can be used to estimate mutagenic effects for which data are lacking. The general approach of estimating an unmeasured mutagenic effect on the basis of three points of data and assumptions of proportionality has been called the parallelogram approach (Anderson et al., 1994). For example, if one lacks mutation data for mammalian germ cells, one may estimate a germ cell mutagenic effect from data on adducts in mouse germ cells if one assumes that the ratio of adducts to mutations is the same as that in a simpler assay, such as a gene mutation assay in cultured cells (Anderson et al., 1994). The parallelogram approach offers the possibility of estimating effects that are not readily measured, such as human germ cell mutagenesis. Several variations on this approach have been suggested, using ratios such as mutations to adducts, somatic mutations to germ cell mutations, and mouse mutations to human mutations.

An illuminating example of the incorporation of many factors into a quantitative risk assessment can be found in an attempt to predict human germ cell risk for ethylene oxide, a mutagen used as a sterilizing agent and reactant in chemical syntheses (Rhomberg et al., 1990). The assessment, which was conducted by the EPA, was based primarily on the induction of heritable translocations in postmeiotic male germ cells of mice exposed to ethylene oxide by inhalation. Other sources of data were incorporated into the analysis, including comparisons of dosimetry among tissues and species, germ cell sensitivity, and models for high-dose to low-dose extrapolation. A range of human heritable translocation frequencies was predicted for different levels of exposure under several mathematical models whose strengths and weaknesses were evaluated. When one considers the substantial unknowns and many assumptions in the risk assessment for ethylene oxide, a compound whose effects are reasonably well understood on the basis of extensive data from laboratory organisms and human occupational exposures, one is struck by the extent to which our ability to assess human germ cell risks quantitatively remains rudimentary.

Research and testing in genetic toxicology have advanced our ability to detect mutagens and our understanding of the ways in which they affect biological systems. However, the problems posed by environmental mutagens are complex, and our ability to assess mutational risks quantitatively is still primitive. A sustained effort in genetic toxicology will be required to discern which of the many environmental mutagens that have been identified pose significant risks and which pose negligible risks. Evaluating the impact of mutagenesis on human health must encompass gene mutations, chromosome aberrations, and aneuploidy and must consider effects in both somatic cells and germ cells.

## ACKNOWLEDGMENTS

The author thanks Drs. M. D. Shelby, K. Dearfield, D. M. DeMarini, S. Galloway, H. Holden, P. Lemay, J. P. O'Neill, and X. Veaute for helpful suggestions; Dr. R. J. Preston for photographs of chromosome aberrations; and Mrs. Linda Walsh for excellent secretarial assistance.

# REFERENCES

Adler I-D: Synopsis of the in vivo results obtained with the 10 known or suspected aneugens tested in the CEC collaborative study. *Mutat Res* 287:131–137, 1993.

Adler I-D, Shelby MD, Bootman J, et al: Summary report of the working group on mammalian germ cell tests. *Mutat Res* 312:313–318, 1994.

Aguilar F, Harris CC, Sun T, et al: Geographic variation of p53 mutational profile in nonmalignant human liver. *Science* 264:1317–1319, 1994.

Albertini RJ, Nicklas JA, O'Neill JP, Robison SH: In vivo somatic mutations in humans: Measurement and analysis. *Annu Rev Genet* 24:305–326, 1990.

Allen JW, Liang JC, Carrano AV, Preston RJ: Review of literature on chemical-induced aneuploidy in mammalian germ cells. *Mutat Res* 167:123–137, 1986.

Anderson D, Sorsa M, Waters MD: The parallelogram approach in studies of genotoxic effects. *Mutat Res* 313:101–115, 1994.

Ashby J: Two million rodent carcinogens? The role of SAR and QSAR in their detection. *Mutat Res* 305:3–12, 1994.

Ashby J, Paton D: The influence of chemical structure on the extent and sites of carcinogenesis for 522 rodent carcinogens and 55 different human carcinogen exposures. *Mutat Res* 286:3–74, 1993.

Ashby J, Tennant RW: Definitive relationships among chemical structure, carcinogenicity and mutagenicity for 301 chemicals tested by the U.S. NTP. *Mutat Res* 257:229–306, 1991.

Auerbach C: *Mutation Research: Problems, Results, and Perspectives.* London: Chapman and Hall, 1976.

Barrett JC: Mechanisms of multistep carcinogenesis and carcinogen risk assessment. *Environ Health Perspect* 100:9–20, 1993.

Bender MA, Awa AA, Brooks AL, et al: Current status of cytogenetic procedures to detect and quantify previous exposures to radiation. *Mutat Res* 196:103–159, 1988.

Bentley KS, Sarrif AM, Cimino MC, Auletta AE: Assessing the risk of heritable gene mutation in mammals: *Drosophila* sex-linked recessive lethal test and tests measuring DNA damage and repair in mammalian germ cells. *Environ Mol Mutagen* 23:3–11, 1994.

Bishop JM: Molecular themes in oncogenesis. *Cell* 64:235–248, 1991.

Brockman HE, DeMarini DM: Utility of short-term tests for genetic toxicity in the aftermath of the NTP's analysis of 73 chemicals. *Environ Mol Mutagen* 11:421–435, 1988.

Brockman HE, deSerres FJ, Ong T, et al: Mutation tests in *Neurospora crassa:* A report of the U.S. Environmental Protection Agency Gene-Tox Program. *Mutat Res* 133:87–134, 1984.

Burkhart JG, Malling HV: Mutagenesis and transgenic systems: Perspective from the mutagen, N-ethyl-N-nitrosourea. *Environ Mol Mutagen* 22:1–6, 1993.

Burkhart JG, Malling HV: Mutations among the living and the undead. *Mutat Res* 304:315–320, 1994.

Butterworth BE, Slaga TJ (eds): *Nongenotoxic Mechanisms in Carcinogenesis*, Banbury Report 25. Cold Spring Harbor, NY: Cold Spring Harbor Laboratory Press, 1987.

Calos MP, Miller JH: Genetic and sequence analysis of frameshift mutations induced by ICR-191. *J Mol Biol* 153:39–66, 1981.

Cariello NF, Skopek TR: Analysis of mutations occurring at the human *hprt* locus. *J Mol Biol* 231:41–57, 1993a.

Cariello NF, Skopek TR: Mutational analysis using denaturing gradient gel electrophoresis and PCR. *Mutat Res* 288:103–112, 1993b.

Chang LW, Hsia SMT, Chan P-C, Hsieh L-L: Macromolecular adducts: Biomarkers for toxicity and carcinogenesis. *Annu Rev Pharmacol Toxicol* 34:41–67, 1994.

Clayson DB, Mehta R, Iverson F: Oxidative DNA damage—the effects of certain genotoxic and operationally non-genotoxic carcinogens. *Mutat Res* 317:25–42, 1994.

Cole J, Skopek TR: Somatic mutant frequency, mutation rates and mutational spectra in the human population in vivo. *Mutat Res* 304:33–105, 1994.

Cooper DN, Krawczak M: The mutational spectrum of single base-pair substitutions causing human genetic disease: Patterns and predictions. *Hum Genet* 85:55–74, 1990.

Crespi CL, Langenbach R, Penman BW: Human cell lines, derived from AHH-1 TK+/− human lymphoblasts, genetically engineered for expression of human cytochromes P450. *Toxicology* 82:89–104, 1993.

Dellarco VL, Prival MJ: Mutagenicity of nitro compounds in *Salmonella typhimurium* in the presence of flavin mononucleotide in a preincubation assay. *Environ Mol Mutagen* 13:116–127, 1989.

Dellarco VL, Voytek PE, Hollaender A (eds): *Aneuploidy: Etiology and Mechanisms*. New York: Plenum Press, 1985.

DeMarini DM: Environmental mutagens/complex mixtures, in Li AP,

Heflich RH (eds): *Genetic Toxicology.* Boca Raton, FL: CRC Press, 1991, pp 285–302.

DeMarini DM, Brockman HE, deSerres FJ, et al: Specific-locus mutations induced in eukaryotes (especially mammalian cells) by radiation and chemicals: A perspective. *Mutat Res* 220:11–29, 1989.

Dixon K, Roilides E, Hauser J, Levine AS: Studies on direct and indirect effects of DNA damage on mutagenesis in monkey cells using an SV40-based shuttle vector. *Mutat Res* 220:73–82, 1989.

Drake JW: Spontaneous mutation. *Annu Rev Genet* 25:125–146, 1991.

Dumaz N, Stary A, Soussi T, et al: Can we predict solar ultraviolet radiation as the causal event in human tumours by analysing the mutation spectra of the p53 gene? *Mutat Res* 307:375–386, 1994.

Ehling UH: Genetic risk assessment. *Annu Rev Genet* 25:255–280, 1991.

Elia MC, Storer R, McKelvey TW, et al: Rapid DNA degradation in primary rat hepatocytes treated with diverse cytotoxic chemicals: Analysis by pulsed field gel electrophoresis and implications for alkaline elution assays. *Environ Mol Mutagen* 24:181–191, 1994.

Evans HJ, Prosser J: Tumor-suppressor genes: Cardinal factors in inherited predisposition to human cancers. *Environ Health Perspect* 98:25–37, 1992.

Fearon ER, Vogelstein B: A genetic model for colorectal tumorigenesis. *Cell* 61:759–767, 1990.

Fenech M, Morley AA: Kinetochore detection in micronuclei: An alternative method for measuring chromosome loss. *Mutagenesis* 4:98–104, 1989.

Ferguson LR: Antimutagens as cancer chemopreventive agents in the diet. *Mutat Res* 307:395–410, 1994.

Ferguson LR, Denny WA: Frameshift mutagenesis by acridines and other reversibly-binding DNA ligands. *Mutagenesis* 5:529–540, 1990.

Ferguson LR, Denny WA: The genetic toxicology of acridines. *Mutat Res* 258:123–160, 1991.

Friedberg EC: *DNA Repair.* New York: Freeman, 1985.

Galloway SM, lvett JL: Chemically induced aneuploidy in mammalian cells in culture. *Mutat Res* 167:89–105, 1986.

Galloway SM, Aardema MJ, Ishidate M Jr, et al: Report from working group on in vitro tests for chromosomal aberrations. *Mutat Res* 312:241–261, 1994.

Gatehouse D, Haworth S, Cebula T, et al: Recommendations for the performance of bacterial mutation assays. *Mutat Res* 312:217–233, 1994.

Genescà A, Benet J, Caballín MR, et al: Significance of structural chromosome aberrations in human sperm: Analysis of induced aberrations. *Hum Genet* 85:495–499, 1990.

Gold LS, Slone TH, Stern BR, Bernstein L: Comparison of target organs of carcinogenicity for mutagenic and non-mutagenic chemicals. *Mutat Res* 286:75–l00, 1993.

Grant SG, Bigbee WL: In vivo somatic mutation and segregation at the human glycophorin A (GPA) locus: Phenotypic variation encompassing both gene-specific and chromosomal mechanisms. *Mutat Res* 288:163–172, 1993.

Grant WF: The present status of higher plant bioassays for the detection of environmental mutagens. *Mutat Res* 310:175–185, 1994.

Griffiths AJF, Miller JH, Suzuki DT, et al: *An Introduction to Genetic Analysis,* 5th ed. New York: Freeman, 1993.

Hagmar L, Brøgger A, Hansteen I, et al: Cancer risk in humans predicted by increased levels of chromosomal aberrations in lymphocytes: Nordic study group on the health risk of chromosome damage. *Cancer Res* 54:2919–2922, 1994.

Halliday JA, Glickman BW: Mechanisms of spontaneous mutation in DNA repair-proficient *Escherichia coli. Mutat Res* 250:55–71, 1991.

Hamasaki T, Sato T, Nagase H, Kito H: The genotoxicity of organotin compounds in SOS chromotest and rec-assay. *Mutat Res* 280:195–203, 1992.

Hanawalt P, Mellon I: Stranded in an active gene. *Curr Biol* 3:67–69, 1993.

Harris CC: p53: At the crossroads of molecular carcinogenesis and risk assessment. *Science* 262:1980–1981, 1993.

Hartman PE, Ames BN, Roth JR, et al: Target sequences for mutagenesis in *Salmonella* histidine-requiring mutants. *Environ Mutagen* 8:631–641, 1986.

Hayashi M, Tice RR, MacGregor JT, et al: In vivo rodent erythrocyte micronucleus assay. *Mutat Res* 312:293–304, 1994.

Heddle JA, Cimino MC, Hayashi M, et al: Micronuclei as an index of cytogenetic damage: Past, present, and future. *Environ Mol Mutagen* 18:277–291, 1991.

Heflich RH, Neft RE: Genetic toxicity of 2-acetylaminofluorene, 2-aminofluorene, and some of their metabolites and model metabolites. *Mutat Res* 318:73–174, 1994.

Hoffmann GR: Induction of genetic recombination: Consequences and model systems. *Environ Mol Mutagen* 23(Suppl 24):59–66, 1994.

Holbrook NJ, Fornace AJ Jr: Response to adversity: Molecular control of gene activation following genotoxic stress. *New Biol* 3:825–833, 1991.

Hollstein M, Sidransky D, Vogelstein B, Harris CC: p53 mutations in human cancers. *Science* 253:49–53, 1991.

Ishidate M Jr, Harnois MC, Sofuni T: A comparative analysis of data on the clastogenicity of 951 chemical substances tested in mammalian cell cultures. *Mutat Res* 195:151–213, 1988.

Jurado J, Alejandre-Durán E, Pueyo C: Mutagenicity testing in *Salmonella typhimurium* strains possessing both the His reversion and Ara forward mutation systems and different levels of classical nitroreductase or o-acetyltransferase activities. *Environ Mol Mutagen* 23:286–293, 1994.

Kier LE, Brusick DJ, Auletta AE, et al: The *Salmonella typhimurium*/mammalian microsomal assay: A report of the U.S. Environmental Protection Agency Gene-Tox Program. *Mutat Res* 168:69–240, 1986.

Kirkland DJ, Gatehouse DG, Scott D, et al (eds): *Basic Mutagenicity Tests: UKEMS Recommended Procedures.* New York: Cambridge University Press, 1990.

Klekowski EJ Jr, Corredor JE, Morell JM, Del Castillo CA: Petroleum pollution and mutation in mangroves. *Marine Pollut Bull* 28:166–169, 1994.

Koch WH, Henrikson EN, Kupchella E, Cebula TA: *Salmonella typhimurium* strain TAl00 differentiates several classes of carcinogens and mutagens by base substitution specificity. *Carcinogenesis* 15:79–88, 1994.

Lähdetie J, Keiski A, Suutari A, Toppari J: Etoposide (VP-16) is a potent inducer of micronuclei in male rat meiosis: Spermatid micronucleus test and DNA flow cytometry after etoposide treatment. *Environ Mol Mutagen* 24:192–202, 1994.

Lambert IB, Napolitano RL, Fuchs RPP: Carcinogen-induced frameshift mutagenesis in repetitive sequences. *Proc Natl Acad Sci USA* 89:1310–1314, 1992.

Langenbach R, Oglesby L: The use of intact cellular activation systems in genetic toxicology assays, in deSerres FJ (ed): *Chemical Mutagens: Principles and Methods for Their Detection.* New York: Plenum Press, 1983, vol 8, pp 55–93.

Laval J, Boiteux S, O'Connor TR: Physiological properties and repair of apurinic/apyrimidinic sites and imidazole ring-opened guanines in DNA. *Mutat Res* 233:73–79, 1990.

Legator MS, Bueding E, Batzinger R, et al: An evaluation of the host-mediated assay and body fluid analysis: A report of the U.S. Environmental Protection Agency Gene-Tox Program. *Mutat Res* 98:319–374, 1982.

Levine JG, Schaaper RM, DeMarini DM: Complex frameshift mutations mediated by plasmid pKM101: Mutational mechanisms deduced from 4-aminobiphenyl-induced mutation spectra in Salmonella. *Genetics* 136:731–746, 1994.

Lewis SE: The biochemical specific-locus test and a new multiple-endpoint mutation detection system: Considerations for genetic risk assessment. *Environ Mol Mutagen* l8:303–306, 1991.

Lewtas J: Environmental monitoring using genetic bioassays, in Li AP, Heflich RH (eds): *Genetic Toxicology.* Boca Raton, FL: CRC Press, 1991, pp 359–374.

Li AP, Heflich RH (eds): *Genetic Toxicology*. Boca Raton, FL: CRC Press, 1991.

Lindahl T: Instability and decay of the primary structure of DNA. *Nature* 362:709–715, 1993.

Littlefield LG, Hoffmann GR: Modulation of the clastogenic activity of ionizing radiation and bleomycin by the aminothiol WR-1065. *Environ Mol Mutagen* 22:225–230, 1993.

Lynch AM, Parry JM: The cytochalasin-B micronucleus/kinetochore assay in vitro: Studies with 10 suspected aneugens. *Mutat Res* 287:71–86, 1993.

Madle S, Dean SW, Andrae U, et al: Recommendations for the performance of UDS tests in vitro and in vivo. *Mutat Res* 312:263–285, 1994.

Maron DM, Ames BN: Revised methods for the *Salmonella* mutagenicity test. *Mutat Res* 113:173–215, 1983.

Marshall CJ: Tumor suppressor genes. *Cell* 64:313–326, 1991.

Martin JB: Molecular genetics of neurological diseases. *Science* 262:674–676, 1993a.

Martin RH: Detection of genetic damage in human sperm. *Reprod Toxicol* 7:47–52, 1993b.

Mason JM, Aaron CS, Lee WR, et al: A guide for performing germ cell mutagenesis assays using *Drosophila melanogaster. Mutat Res* 189:93–102, 1987.

Mirsalis JC, Monforte JA, Winegar RA: Transgenic animal models for measuring mutations *in vivo. Crit Rev Toxicol* 24:255–280, 1994.

Modrich P: Mechanisms and biological effects of mismatch repair. *Annu Rev Genet* 25:229–253, 1991.

Mohrenweiser HW: Germinal mutation and human genetic disease, in Li AP, Heflich RH (eds): *Genetic Toxicology.* Boca Raton, FL: CRC Press, 1991, pp 67–92.

Morley AA: Mitotic recombination in mammalian cells in vivo. *Mutat Res* 250:345–349, 1991.

Morrison V, Ashby J: A preliminary evaluation of the performance of the Muta™Mouse (*lacZ*) and Big Blue™ (*lacI*) transgenic mouse mutation assays. *Mutagenesis* 9:367–375, 1994.

Mulvihill JJ: Sentinel and other mutational effects in offspring of cancer survivors, in Mendelsohn ML, Albertini RJ (eds): *Mutation and the Environment, Part C.* New York: Wiley-Liss, 1990, pp 179–186.

Natarajan AT: An overview of the results of testing of known or suspected aneugens using mammalian cells in vitro. *Mutat Res* 287:113–118, 1993.

Natarajan AT, Duivenvoorden WCM, Meijers M, Zwanenburg TSB: Induction of mitotic aneuploidy using Chinese hamster primary embryonic cells: Test results of 10 chemicals. *Mutat Res* 287:47–56, 1993.

National Research Council, Committee on Chemical Environmental Mutagens: *Identifying and Estimating the Genetic Impact of Chemical Mutagens.* Washington, DC: National Academy Press, 1983.

National Research Council, Committee on the Biological Effects of Ionizing Radiations: *Health Effects of Exposure to Low Levels of Ionizing Radiation: BEIR V.* Washington, DC: National Academy Press, 1990.

Neel JV, Satoh C, Myers R: Report of a workshop on the application of molecular genetics to the study of mutation in the children of atomic bomb survivors. *Mutat Res* 291:1–20, 1993.

Parry JM: An evaluation of the use of in vitro tubulin polymerisation, fungal and wheat assays to detect the activity of potential chemical aneugens. *Mutat Res* 287:23–28, 1993.

Parry JM: Detecting and predicting the activity of rodent carcinogens. *Mutagenesis* 9:3–5, 1994.

Pastink A, Vreeken C, Vogel EW, Eeken JCJ: Mutations induced at the *white* and *vermilion* loci in *Drosophila melanogaster. Mutat Res* 231:63–71, 1990.

Perera FP, Tang DL, O'Neill JP, et al: HPRT and glycophorin A mutations in foundry workers: Relationship to PAH exposure and to PAH-DNA adducts. *Carcinogenesis* 14:969–973, 1993.

Prival MJ, Dunkel VC: Reevaluation of the mutagenicity and carcinogenicity of chemicals previously identified as "false positives" in the *Salmonella typhimurium* mutagenicity assay. *Environ Mol Mutagen* 13:1–24, 1989.

Quillardet P, Hofnung M: The SOS chromotest: A review. *Mutat Res* 297:235–279, 1993.

Rabbitts TH: Chromosomal translocations in human cancer. *Nature* 372:143–149, 1994.

Rhomberg L, Dellarco VL, Siegel-Scott C, et al: Quantitative estimation of the genetic risk associated with the induction of heritable translocations at low-dose exposure: Ethylene oxide as an example. *Environ Mol Mutagen* 16:104–125, 1990.

Ribeiro LR, Salvadori DMF, Rios ACC, et al: Biological monitoring of workers occupationally exposed to ethylene oxide. *Mutat Res* 313:81–87, 1994.

Robbins WA, Segraves R, Pinkel D, Wyrobek AJ: Detection of aneuploid human sperm by fluorescence in situ hybridization: Evidence for a donor difference in frequency of sperm disomic for chromosomes 1 and Y. *Am J Hum Genet* 52:799–807, 1993.

Russell LB: Role of mouse germ-cell mutagenesis in understanding genetic risk and in generating mutations that are prime tools for studies in modern biology. *Environ Mol Mutagen* 23(Suppl 24):23–29, 1994.

Russell LB, Rinchik EM: Structural differences between specific-locus mutations induced by different exposure regimes in mouse spermatogonial stem cells. *Mutat Res* 288:187–195, 1993.

Russell LB, Russell WL: Frequency and nature of specific-locus mutations induced in female mice by radiations and chemicals: A review. *Mutat Res* 296:107–127, 1992.

Russell LB, Shelby MD: Tests for heritable genetic damage and for evidence of gonadal exposure in mammals. *Mutat Res* 154:69–84, 1985.

Sancar A, Tang M: Nucleotide excision repair. *Photochem Photobiol* 57:905–921, 1993.

Sankaranarayanan K: Ionizing radiation, genetic risk estimation and molecular biology: Impact and inferences. *Trends Genet* 9:79–84, 1993.

Savitz DA, Chen J: Parental occupation and childhood cancer: Review of epidemiologic studies. *Environ Health Perspect* 88:325–337, 1990.

Scicchitano DA, Hanawalt PC: Intragenomic repair heterogeneity of DNA damage. *Environ Health Perspect* 98:45–51, 1992.

Scott D, Galloway SM, Marshall RR, et al: Genotoxicity under extreme culture conditions. *Mutat Res* 257:147–204, 1991.

Sekiya T: Detection of mutant sequences by single-strand conformation polymorphism analysis. *Mutat Res* 288:79–83, 1993.

Sengstag C: The role of mitotic recombination in carcinogenesis. *Crit Rev Toxicol* 24:323–353, 1994.

Shelby MD: Human germ cell mutagens. *Environ Mol Mutagen* 23(Suppl 24):30–34, 1994.

Shelby MD, Zeiger E: Activity of human carcinogens in the Salmonella and rodent bone-marrow cytogenetics tests. *Mutat Res* 234:257–261, 1990.

Shevell DE, Friedman BM, Walker GC: Resistance to alkylation damage in *Escherichia coli:* Role of the Ada protein in induction of the adaptive response. *Mutat Res* 233:53–72, 1990.

Sierra LM, Pastink A, Nivard MJM, Vogel EW: DNA base sequence changes induced by diethyl sulfate in postmeiotic male germ cells of *Drosophila melanogaster. Mol Gen Genet* 237:370–374, 1993.

Sorsa M, Wilbourn J, Vainio H: Human cytogenetic damage as a predictor of cancer risk, in Vainio H, Magee PN, McGregor DB, McMichael AJ (eds): *Mechanisms of Carcinogenesis in Risk Identification.* Lyons: International Agency for Research on Cancer, 1992, pp 543–554.

Styles JA, Penman MG: The mouse spot test: Evaluation of its performance in identifying chemical mutagens and carcinogens. *Mutat Res* 154:183–204, 1985.

Tease C: Radiation- and chemically-induced chromosome aberrations in mouse oocytes: A comparison with effects in males. *Mutat Res* 296:135–142, 1992.

Tennant RW, Ashby J: Classification according to chemical structure, mutagenicity to Salmonella and level of carcinogenicity of a further 39 chemicals tested for carcinogenicity by the U.S. National Toxicology Program. *Mutat Res* 257:209–227, 1991.

Tennant RW, Margolin BH, Shelby MD, et al: Prediction of chemical carcinogenicity in rodents from in vitro genetic toxicity assays. *Science* 236:933–941, 1987.

Tice RR, Hayashi M, MacGregor JT, et al: Report from the working group on the in vivo mammalian bone marrow chromosomal aberration test. *Mutat Res* 312:305–312, 1994.

Tucker JD, Auletta A, Cimino M, et al: Sister-chromatid exchange: Second report of the Gene-Tox program. *Mutat Res* 297:101–180, 1993a.

Tucker JD, Ramsey MJ, Lee DA, Minkler JL: Validation of chromosome painting as a biodosimeter in human peripheral lymphocytes following acute exposure to ionizing radiation *in vitro. Int J Radiat Biol* 64:27–37, 1993b.

Venitt S: The use of short-term tests for the detection of genotoxic activity in body fluids and excreta. *Mutat Res* 205:331–353, 1988.

Vogel EW: Tests for recombinagens in somatic cells of Drosophila. *Mutat Res* 284:159–175, 1992.

Walker VE, Skopek TR: A mouse model for the study of in vivo mutational spectra: Sequence specificity of ethylene oxide at the *hprt* locus. *Mutat Res* 288:151–162, 1993.

Warr TJ, Parry EM, Parry JM: A comparison of two in vitro mammalian cell cytogenetic assays for the detection of mitotic aneuploidy using 10 known or suspected aneugens. *Mutat Res* 287:29–46, 1993.

Wassom JS: Origins of genetic toxicology and the Environmental Mutagen Society. *Environ Mol Mutagen* 14(Suppl 16):1–6, 1989.

Wyrobek AJ: Methods and concepts in detecting abnormal reproductive outcomes of paternal origin. *Reprod Toxicol* 7:3–16, 1993.

Zeiger E: Carcinogenicity of mutagens: Predictive capability of the *Salmonella* mutagenesis assay for rodent carcinogenicity. *Cancer Res* 47:1287–1296, 1987.

Zimmering S, Mason JM, Osgood C: Current status of aneuploidy testing in Drosophila. *Mutat Res* 167:71–87, 1986.

Zimmermann FK: Tests for recombinagens in fungi. *Mutat Res* 284:147–158, 1992.

Zimmermann FK: A test for uniparental disomy in *Saccharomyces cerevisiae. Mutat Res* 306:187–196, 1994.

Zimmermann FK, von Borstel RC, von Halle ES, et al: Testing of chemicals for genetic activity with *Saccharomyces cerevisiae:* A report of the U.S. Environmental Protection Agency Gene-Tox Program. *Mutat Res* 133:199–244, 1984.

# CHAPTER 10

# DEVELOPMENTAL TOXICOLOGY

*John M. Rogers and Robert J. Kavlock*

## HISTORY

Developmental toxicology encompasses the study of pharmacokinetics, mechanisms, pathogenesis, and outcome after exposure to agents or conditions that lead to abnormal development. Manifestations of developmental toxicity include structural malformations, growth retardation, functional impairment, and death of the organism. The use of the term "developmental toxicity" to include all manifestations of abnormal development is relatively recent (Wilson, 1973). By this definition developmental toxicology is a relatively new science, but its roots are firmly embedded in teratology, the study of structural birth defects. As a descriptive science, teratology precedes written language. For example, a marble sculpture from southern Turkey dating back to 6500 B.C. depicts conjoined twins (Warkany, 1983), and Egyptian wall paintings of human conditions such as cleft palate and achondroplasia have been dated as early as 5000 years before the present. It is believed that mythological figures such as cyclopes and sirens originated with the birth of severely malformed infants (Thompson, 1930; Warkany, 1977). The Babylonians, Greeks, and Romans believed that abnormal infants were reflections of stellar events and as such were considered portents of the future. Indeed, the Latin word *monstrum,* from *monstrare* ("to show") or *monere* ("to warn") is derived from this perceived ability of malformed infants to foretell the future. In turn, the word "teratology" is derived from the Greek word for monster, *teras*.

Hippocrates and Aristotle thought abnormal development could originate from physical causes such as uterine trauma or pressure, but Aristotle also shared a widespread belief that maternal impressions and emotions could influence the development of the child. He advised pregnant women to gaze at beautiful statuary to increase their children's beauty. As fanciful as this theory may be, it appears in diverse cultures throughout recorded history, and we now know that maternal stress can be deleterious to the developing conceptus (Chernoff et al., 1989).

Another belief—the hybrid theory—held that interbreeding between humans and animals could be a cause of congenital malformations (Ballantyne, 1904). Again, such hybrid creatures abound in mythology, including centaurs, minotaurs, and satyrs. In 1493, Paracelsus, one of the earliest toxicologists, wrote of the basilisk, a cross between a cock and a toad. Into the seventeenth century, cohabitation of humans with demons and witches was blamed for the production of birth defects. Birth defects were also viewed as representing God's retribution on the parents of a malformed infant and on society.

In 1649, the French surgeon Ambrois Pare expanded the theory of Aristotle and Hippocrates by writing that birth defects could result from narrowness of the uterus, faulty posture of the pregnant woman, or physical trauma such as a fall. Amputations were thought to result from amniotic bands, adhesions, or twisting of the umbilical cord. This conjecture has proved to be true. With the blossoming of the biological sciences in the sixteenth and seventeenth centuries, theories about the causation of birth defects with a basis in scientific fact began to emerge. In 1651, William Harvey put forth the theory of developmental arrest, which stated that malformations result from incomplete development of an organ or structure. One example given by Harvey was harelip in humans, a condition that occurs normally at an early developmental stage. Much later, the theory of developmental arrest was solidified by the experiments of Stockard (1921), using eggs of the minnow, *Fundulus heteroclitus*. By manipulating the chemical constituents and temperature of the growth medium, he was able to produce malformations in the embryos, the nature of which depended on the stage of the insult. He concluded that developmental arrest explains all malformations except those of hereditary origin (Barrow, 1971).

With the propounding of the germ plasm theory by Weissmann in the 1880s and the rediscovery of Mendel's laws in 1900, there was acceptance of genetics as the basis for some birth defects. In 1894, Bateson published a treatise on the study of variations in animals as a tool for understanding evolution, inferring that the inheritance of such variations could be a basis for speciation. His study contains detailed descriptions and illustrations of human birth defects such as polydactyly and syndactyly, supernumerary cervical and thoracic ribs, duplicated appendages, and horseshoe (fused) kidneys. In this volume Bateson coined the term "homeosis" to denote morphological alterations in which one structure has taken on the likeness of another. The study of such alterations, especially in mutants of the fruit fly *Drosophila*, has served as the basis for much recent knowledge about the genetic control of development. *Homeobox genes* are found throughout the animal and plant kingdoms and direct embryonic pattern formation (Graham et al., 1989). Studies of inborn errors of metabolism in humans in the first decade of the twentieth century furthered the acceptance of the genetic basis of malformations.

Modern experimental teratology began in the early nineteenth century with the work of Etienne Geoffrey Saint-Hilaire and his son, Isadore Etienne. Etienne Geoffrey Saint-Hilaire produced malformed chick embryos by subjecting eggs to various environmental conditions, including physical trauma (jarring, inversion, pricking) and toxic exposures. In the latter part of the nineteenth century, Camille Dareste experimented extensively with chick embryos, producing a wide variety of malformations by administering noxious stimuli, physical trauma, or heat shock at various times after fertilization. He found that timing was more important than the nature

**Table 10–1**
**Wilson's General Principles of Teratology**

1. Susceptibility to teratogenesis depends on the genotype of the conceptus and the manner in which it interacts with adverse environmental factors.
2. Susceptibility to teratogenesis varies with the developmental stage at the time of exposure to an adverse influence.
3. Teratogenic agents act in specific ways (mechanisms) on developing cells and tissues to initiate sequences of abnormal developmental events (pathogenesis).
4. The access of adverse influences to developing tissues depends on the nature of the influence (agent).
5. The four manifestations of deviant development are death, malformation, growth retardation, and functional deficit.
6. Manifestations of deviant development increase in frequency and degree as the dose increases from no effect to the totally lethal level.

SOURCE: Wilson (1953, 1973).

of the insult in determining the type of malformation produced. Among the malformations described and illustrated by Dareste (1877, 1891) were the neural tube defects anencephaly and spina bifida, cyclopia, heart defects, situs inversus, and conjoined twins. Many of the great embryologists of the nineteenth and twentieth centuries, including Loeb, Morgan, Driesch, Wilson, Spemann, and Hertwig, performed teratological manipulations using various physical and chemical probes to deduce the principles of normal development.

Early in the twentieth century, a variety of environmental conditions (temperature, microbial toxins, drugs) were found to perturb development in avian, reptile, fish, and amphibian species. However, despite the already rich literature on nonmammalian teratological experiments, mammalian embryos were thought to be resistant to the induction of malformations and to be either killed outright or protected from adverse environmental conditions by the maternal system. The first reports of induced birth defects in mammalian species were published in the 1930s and were concerned with maternal nutritional deficiencies. Hale (1935) produced malformations including anophthalmia and cleft palate in the offspring of sows fed a diet deficient in vitamin A. Beginning in 1940, Warkany and coworkers began a series of experiments in which they demonstrated that maternal dietary deficiencies and other environmental factors can affect intrauterine development in rats (Warkany and Nelson, 1940; Warkany, 1945; Warkany and Schraffenberger, 1944; Wilson et al., 1953). These experiments were followed by many other studies in which chemical and physical agents, such as nitrogen mustard, trypan blue, hormones, antimetabolites, alkylating agents, hypoxia, and x-rays were clearly shown to cause malformations in mammalian species (Warkany, 1965).

The first human epidemic of malformations induced by an environmental agent was reported by Gregg (1941), who linked an epidemic of rubella virus infection in Austria to an elevation in the incidence of eye, heart, and ear defects as well as mental retardation. Heart and eye defects predominated with infection in the first or second month of pregnancy, whereas hearing and speech defects and mental retardation were most commonly associated with infection in the third month. Later, the risk of congenital anomalies associated with rubella infection in the first 4 weeks of pregnancy was estimated to be 61 percent; in weeks 5 to 8, 26 percent; and in weeks 9 to 12, 8 percent (Sever, 1967). It has been estimated that in the United States alone approximately 20,000 children have been impaired as a consequence of prenatal rubella infections (Cooper and Krugman, 1966).

Although the embryos of mammals, including humans, were found to be susceptible to common external influences such as nutritional deficiencies and intrauterine infections, the impact of these findings at the time was not great (Wilson, 1973). However, that changed in 1961, when the association between thalidomide ingestion by pregnant women and the birth of severely malformed infants was established (see "Scope of the Problem," below).

Principles of teratology were proposed by Jim Wilson in 1959 (Wilson et al., 1959) and in his watershed monograph, *Environment and Birth Defects* (Wilson, 1973) (Table 10-1). Wilson went on to state: "Very likely with increased understanding of teratogenic mechanisms, it will be necessary to formulate additional principles and to revise those now formulated." It is testimony both to Wilson's clarity of thought and foresight and to the difficulty of elucidating teratogenic mechanisms that over 20 years later these principles can be restated largely unchanged.

In the two decades since the publication of Wilson's monograph, a number of human developmental toxicants have been identified and animal experimentation has led to greater understanding of the mechanisms and pathogenesis of birth defects. The study of developmental functional deficits, including neurobehavioral effects, has emerged during this time. Furthermore, with the continuing elucidation of how genes direct development, we are presented with exciting opportunities to apply powerful new tools to the task of understanding the mechanisms of abnormal development. As has been true for the past two centuries, it is likely that progress in experimental embryology and teratology will continue to be intimately linked.

## SCOPE OF THE PROBLEM: THE HUMAN EXPERIENCE

The accumulated evidence suggests that successful pregnancy outcome in the general population occurs at a surprisingly low frequency. Estimates of adverse outcomes include postimplantation pregnancy loss, 31 percent; major birth defects, 4 percent at birth and increasing to 6 to 7 percent at 1 year as more manifestations are diagnosed; minor birth defects, 14 percent; low birthweight, 7 percent; infant mortality (before 1 year of age), 1.4 percent; and abnormal neurological function, 16 to 17 percent (Schardein, 1993). Thus, less than half of all human pregnancies result in the birth of a completely normal, healthy infant. The reasons for these adverse outcomes are largely unknown. Brent and Beckman (1990) attributed 15 to 25 percent of human birth defects to genetic causes, 4 percent to maternal conditions, 3 percent to maternal infections, 1 to 2 percent to deformations (e.g., mechanical problems such as umbilical cord limb amputations), less than 1 percent to chemicals and other environmental influences, and 65 percent to unknown etiologies. These estimates are not dramatically different from those suggested by Wilson (1977). Regardless of the etiology, the sum total represents a significant health burden in light of the 2 million births per year in the United States.

It has recently been estimated that more that 3300 chemicals have been tested for teratogenicity, with approximately 63 percent having been shown to be nonteratogenic, 7 percent teratogenic in more than one species, 21 percent teratogenic in most species tested, and 9 percent producing equivocal experimental results (Schardein, 1993). In contrast, only about 35 chemicals, chemical classes, or conditions (Table 10-2) have been documented to alter prenatal development in humans (Schardein and Keller, 1989; Shepard, 1992). A review of several human developmental toxicants provides both a historical view of the field of developmental toxicology and an illustration of some of key principles presented in "Principles of Developmental Toxicology," below.

## Thalidomide

In 1960, a large increase in newborns with rare limb malformations was recorded in West Germany. The affected individuals had amelia (absence of the limbs) or various degrees of phocomelia (reduction of the long bones of the limbs), usually affecting the arms more than the legs and usually involving both the left and right sides, although to differing degrees. Congenital heart disease; ocular, intestinal, and renal anomalies; and malformations of the external ears were also involved, but the limb defects were the characteristic effect. Limb reduction anomalies of this nature are exceedingly rare. At the university clinic in Hamburg, for example, no cases of phocomelia were reported between 1940 and 1959. In 1959 there was a single case; in 1960, 30 cases; and in 1961, 154 cases (Taussig, 1962). The unusual nature of the malformations was a key to unraveling the epidemic. In 1961, Lenz and McBride, working independently in Germany and Australia, identified the sedative thalidomide as the causative agent (McBride, 1961; Lenz, 1961, 1963). Thalidomide was introduced in 1956 by Chemie Grunenthal as a sedative/hypnotic and was used throughout the world as a sleep aid and to ameliorate nausea and vomiting during pregnancy. It had no apparent toxicity or addictive properties in humans or adult animals at therapeutic exposure levels. The drug was widely prescribed at an oral dose of 50 to 200 mg/day. There were a few reports of peripheral neuritis attributable to thalidomide, but only in patients with long-term use for up to 18 months (Fullerton and Kermer, 1961). After the association was established, thalidomide was withdrawn from the market at the

**Table 10–2**
**Human Developmental Toxicants**

| |
|---|
| Radiation |
| Therapeutic |
| Radioiodine |
| Atomic fallout |
| Infections |
| Rubella virus |
| Cytomegalovirus |
| Herpes virus hominis |
| Toxoplasmosis |
| Venezuelan equine encephalitis virus |
| Syphilis |
| Parvovirus B-19 |
| Maternal metabolic imbalances |
| Alcoholism |
| Cretinism |
| Diabetes |
| Folic acid deficiency |
| Hyperthermia |
| Phenylketonuria |
| Rheumatic disease |
| Virilizing tumors |
| Drugs and chemicals |
| Androgenic chemicals |
| Angiotensin-converting enzyme inhibitors |
| Captopril, enalapril |
| Antibiotics |
| Tetracyline |
| Anticancer drugs |
| Aminopterin, methylaminopterine, cyclophosphamide, busulfan |
| Anticonvulsants |
| Diphenylhydantoin, trimethadione, valproic acid |
| Antithyroid drugs |
| Methimazole |
| Chelators |
| Penicillamine |
| Chlorobiphenyls |
| Cigarette smoke |
| Cocaine |
| Coumarin anticoagulants |
| Warfarin |
| Diethylstilbesterol |
| Ethanol |
| Ethylene oxide |
| Iodides |
| Lithium |
| Metals |
| Mercury (organic) |
| Lead |
| Retinoids |
| 13-*cis*-retinoic acid |
| Etretinate |
| Thalidomide |

SOURCE: Schardein and Keller (1989) and Shepard (1992).

end of 1961 and case reports ended in mid-1962 as exposed pregnancies were completed. All told, an estimated 5850 malformed infants were born worldwide (Lenz, 1988). Quantitative estimates of malformation risks from exposure have been difficult to compile but are believed to be in the range of 1 in 2 to 1 in 10 (Newman, 1985). As a result of concerns regarding the severity of the peripheral neuritis and subsequent questions about safety in pregnancy, thalidomide did not receive U.S. marketing approval by the FDA before its removal from the world market after the epidemic.

As a result of this catastrophe, regulatory agencies in many countries began developing animal testing requirements for evaluating the effects of drugs on pregnancy outcomes that were separate from chronic toxicity studies. In the United States, the discussion ultimately led to the development of the Segment I, II, and III testing protocols (Kelsey, 1988). Details of the safety testing requirements for the assessment of pregnancy outcomes appear later in this chapter.

It is ironic that the chemical largely responsible for the advent of modern regulatory authority over potential developmental toxicants has a very complex pattern of effects in various animal species used for safety evaluations. It has been tested for prenatal toxicity in at least 19 laboratory species. Malformations and increased resorption have been observed in some studies in rats, while no effects are generally reported in studies with hamsters and in most mouse strains. Effects similar to those observed in humans have been reported for several rabbit strains and in eight of nine primate species. The potency of thalidomide ranges from approximately 1 to 100 mg/kg among sensitive species. In this ranking, the human sensitivity was estimated to be 1 mg/kg (Schardein, 1993). Research conducted to understand the species and strain differences for thalidomide has had little success. Extensive structure-activity studies involving analogues of thalidomide found strict structural requirements (e.g., an intact phthalimide or phthalimidine group) but shed little light on the potential mechanisms (Jonsson, 1972; Schumacher, 1975; Helm et al., 1981). Stephens (1988) reviewed 24 proposed mechanisms, including biochemical alterations involving vitamin B, glutamic acid, acylation, nucleic acids, and oxidative phosphorylation; cellular mechanisms, including cell death and cell-cell interactions; and tissue level mechanisms, including inhibition of nerve and blood vessel outgrowth. None was considered sufficient. The lack of success in elucidating the mechanisms of the best known human teratogen has probably had a stifling effect on the development of the scientific discipline. However, recent research on the effects of the stable thalidomide derivative EM-12 in marmosets is beginning to shed light on the issue. A reliable animal model has been produced (Merker et al., 1988) that distinguishes the activity of two enantiomers (Heger et al., 1988). Significantly, effects have been observed on the expression of cell surface markers in lymphocyte maturation that may point to a fundamental mechanism by which thalidomide alters cellular function (Neubert et al., 1993). Thalidomide also has been shown to inhibit angiogenesis in the rabbit cornea micropocket assay (D'Amato et al., 1994). The research on alterations in immune function and angiogenesis has opened the possibility of expanded use of thalidomide in several chronic disease states, including HIV infection, arthritis, diabetic retinopathy, and macular degeneration (Adler, 1994).

## Diethylstilbesterol

Diethylstilbesterol (DES) is a synthetic nonsteroidal estrogen that was widely used from the 1940s to the 1970s in the United States to prevent miscarriage by stimulating the synthesis of estrogen and progesterone in the placenta. Between 1966 and 1969, seven young women between the ages of 15 and 22 were seen at Massachusetts General Hospital with clear cell adenocarcinoma of the vagina. This tumor had never before been seen in patients younger than age 30. An epidemiological case-control study subsequently found an association with first-trimester DES exposure (reviewed in Poskranzer and Herbst, 1977). The Registry of Clear Cell Adenocarcinoma of the Genital Tract of Young Females was established in 1971 to track affected offspring. Maternal use of DES before the eighteenth week of gestation appeared to be necessary for induction of the genital tract anomalies in offspring. The incidence of genital tract tumors peaked at age 19 and declined through age 22, with the absolute risk of clear cell adenocarcinoma of the vagina and cervix estimated to be 0.14 to 1.4 per 1000 exposed pregnancies (Herbst et al., 1977). However, the overall incidence of benign alterations in the vagina and cervix was estimated to be as high as 75 percent (Poskranzer and Herbst, 1977). In male offspring of exposed pregnancies, a high incidence of epididymal cysts, hypotrophic testes, and capsular induration, along with low ejaculated semen volume and poor semen quality was observed (Bibbo et al., 1977). The recognition of the latent and devastating manifestations of the developmental toxicity of prenatal DES exposure has broadened our concept of the magnitude and scope of potential adverse outcomes of intrauterine exposures and has foreshadowed today's interest in "endocrine disruptors" (Colburn et al., 1993).

## Ethanol

Concern over the developmental toxicity of ethanol has been recurrent throughout history and can be traced to biblical times (e.g., Judges, 13:3–4). However, it is only since the description of the fetal alcohol syndrome (FAS) by Jones and Smith in the early 1970s (Jones and Smith, 1973; Jones et al., 1973) that a clear recognition and acceptance of alcohol's developmental toxicity has occurred. Since that time, there have been hundreds of clinical, epidemiological, and experimental studies of the effects of ethanol exposure during gestation.

The FAS comprises craniofacial dysmorphism, intrauterine and postnatal growth retardation, retarded psychomotor and intellectual development, and other nonspecific major and minor abnormalities (Abel, 1982). The average IQ of FAS children has been reported to be 68 (Streissguth et al., 1991a) and changes little over time (Streissguth et al., 1991b). Full-blown FAS has been observed only in children born to alcoholic mothers, and among alcoholics the incidence of FAS has been estimated at 25 per thousand (Abel, 1984). There are numerous methodological difficulties involved in attempting to estimate the level of maternal ethanol consumption associated with FAS, but estimates of a minimum of 3 to 4 oz of alcohol per day have been made (Clarren et al., 1987; Ernhart et al., 1987).

In utero ethanol exposure to lower levels of ethanol has been associated with a wide continuum of effects, including isolated components of FAS and milder forms of neurological and behavioral disorders. These more subtle expressions of the toxicity of prenatal ethanol exposure have been termed fetal alcohol effects (FAE) (Clarren, 1982). Alcohol consumption can affect birth weight in a dose-related fashion even if the mother is not alcoholic. Little (1977) studied prospectively 800 women to evaluate the effects of drinking on birth weight. After adjusting for smoking, gestational age, maternal height, age and parity, and sex of the child, it was found that for each ounce of absolute ethanol consumed per day during late pregnancy there was a 160-g decrease in birth weight. Effects of maternal alcohol consumption during pregnancy on attention, short-term memory, and performance on standardized tests have been noted in a longitudinal, prospective study of 462 children (Streissguth et al., 1944a,b). A number of alcohol intake scores were related to these effects, but the number of drinks per drinking occasion was the strongest predictor.

There have been a number of animal models employing different exposure paradigms used to study the toxicity of ethanol, including effects during pregnancy. Because ethanol has caloric value and replaces calories from other dietary sources, liquid diets are used in many of these studies (Lieber and DeCarli, 1982). One animal model of FAS in which pathogenesis of the craniofacial effects has been extensively studied involves acute intraperitoneal injection of ethanol to pregnant C57Bl/6J mice in early pregnancy when the embryos are at the gastrulation stage of development (Sulik et al., 1981; Sulik and Johnston, 1983). Following such exposures, term fetuses exhibit many of the features of FAS, including microcephaly, microphthalmia, short palpebral fissures, deficiencies of the philtral region, and a long upper lip. The specific set of craniofacial malformations produced in offspring is very sensitive to the time of exposure. The mechanisms by which ethanol exerts its teratogenic effects are not understood, but excess cell death in sensitive cell populations appears to be a common finding (Kotch and Sulik, 1992).

## Cocaine

Cocaine, a plant alkaloid derived from coca, is a local anesthetic with vasoconstrictor properties. Pharmacologically, cocaine disrupts neural transmission by blocking fast sodium channels and blocks neuronal uptake of catecholamines and 5-hydroxytryptamine. During the 1980s, cocaine abuse became an epidemic health problem as more potent forms became widely available. It has been estimated that up to 45 percent of pregnancies at an urban teaching hospital and 6 percent at a suburban hospital involved recent cocaine exposure. The effects on the fetus are complicated and controversial and demonstrate the difficulty of monitoring the human population for adverse reproductive outcomes (reviewed in Scanlon, 1991; Volfe, 1992). Accurate exposure ascertainment is difficult, as there is no simple biomarker of exposure and many confounding factors, including socioeconomic status and concurrent use of cigarettes, alcohol, and other drugs of abuse, may be involved. In addition, reported effects on the fetus and infant (neurological and behavioral changes) are difficult to identify and quantify. Nevertheless, a plethora of adverse effects appear to be reliably associated with cocaine exposure in humans, including abruptio placentae; premature labor and delivery; microcephaly; altered prosencephalic development; decreased birthweight; a neonatal neurological syndrome of abnormal sleep, tremor, poor feeding, irritability, and occasional seizures; and sudden infant death syndrome. Congenital malformations of the genitourinary tract also have been reported (Lutiger et al., 1991). Both vasoconstriction, which could inhibit placental transport and function, and the pharmacological effect have been implicated as causes of altered embryo development.

## Retinoids

The ability of excess vitamin A (retinol) to induce malformations has been known for at least 40 years (Cohlan, 1954). The effects on the developing embryo are widespread, with malformations of the face, limbs, heart, central nervous system, and skeleton predominating. Similar malformations were later shown to be induced by retinoic acid administration in the mouse (Kochhar, 1967) and the hamster (Shenefelt, 1972). Since those observations were made, an explosion of knowledge relating to the effects of retinol, retinoic acid, and structurally related chemicals that bind to and activate specific nuclear receptors which then regulate a variety of transcriptional events has occurred (Chambon, 1994; Lohnes et al., 1994; Mendelsohn et al., 1994). The teratogenic effects of vitamin A and retinoids have been reviewed (Nau et al., 1994). Beginning in 1982, one retinoid, 13-*cis*-retinoid acid (isotretinoin or Accutane), was marketed as an effective treatment for recalcitrant cystic acne. Despite clear warnings against use during pregnancy on the label of this prescription drug (FDA pregnancy Category X), an extensive physician and patient education program, and restrictive requirements for prescription to women of childbearing potential, infants with pathognomonic malformations involving the ears, heart, brain, and thymus began to be reported as early as 1983 (Rosa, 1983; Lammer et al., 1985). Among 115 exposed pregnancies that were not electively terminated, 18 percent ended in spontaneous abortion, and 28 percent of the liveborn infants had at least one major malformation (Dai et al., 1992). In another prospective study, there was nearly a doubling of the risk for premature delivery after first-trimester exposure, and about 50 percent of the exposed children had full-scale IQ scores below 85 at age 5 (Lammer, 1992). There was and remains considerable controversy over the marketing of this potent human teratogen. Teenagers constitute a large segment of the patient population, and it is recognized that this population can be sexually active without strict adherence to contraceptive measures. In light of these concerns, the Teratology Society took the unusual step of publishing a position paper that recommended further limiting of exposure among pregnant women to those who absolutely require the drug and will reliably use adequate contraception (Teratology Society, 1991).

## Valproic Acid

Valproic acid (2-propylpentanoic acid) is an anticonvulsant that was first marketed in Europe in 1967 and in the United States in 1978. In 1982, Elizabeth Robert reported that in 146 cases of spina bifida aperta detected in a birth defects surveillance system in Lyon, France, nine of the mothers had taken valproate during the first trimester. The odds ratio for this finding in a case-control study was 20.6 (95 percent confidence limits of 8.2 to 47.9). The estimated risk of a valproate-exposed woman having a child with spina bifida was estimated to be about 1.2 percent, a risk similar to that for women with a previous child with a neural tube defect (Centers for Disease Control, 1982). The report was quickly confirmed in other areas through the efforts of the International Clearinghouse of Birth Defect Registries (Centers for Disease Control, 1983). Because of the relatively low risk, the fact that epileptic women are already at an elevated risk for birth defects, and the fact that the majority of pregnant epileptics are on drug therapy (including several known teratogens), it was fortunate that several events came together that allowed the determination of valproate as a human teratogen. These events included the active birth defects registry, an interest by Robert in the genetics of spina bifida, a question about epilepsy and anticonvulsant use in Robert's survey, and the prevalence of valproate monotherapy for epilepsy in that region (Lammer et al., 1987). While these findings spurred a great deal of research on the effects of valproate in multiple species, including interesting results on the effects of enantiomers of valproate analogues, the mechanism of action, as for most developmental toxicants, has eluded investigators (Nau et al., 1991; Ehlers et al., 1992; Hauck and Nau, 1992).

### Bendectin: A Human Developmental Nontoxicant

The examples of thalidomide, DES, ethanol, cocaine, retinoids, and valproate illustrate the scientific and social aspects of identifying human developmental toxicants. Bendectin (doxylamine and pyridoxine), which was once used to alleviate morning sickness, provides an important social perspective on the difficulties of determining causality in humans. Although the vast majority of evidence supports the conclusion that Bendectin is not a human developmental toxicant, the consequences of even transiently being identified as such were far-reaching. Bendectin was taken by an estimated 25 percent of pregnant women in the United States (Holmes, 1983) and was available as an over-the-counter medication in at least 20 countries. The controversy over the safety of Bendectin began with a single case report of an infant born with a unilateral limb reduction defect after a Bendectin-exposed pregnancy. The case was litigated, and although the defendant manufacturer won, a great deal of attention was focused on the safety of the drug. Schardein (1993) reviewed 25 large epidemiology studies consisting of over 25,000 exposed pregnancies. Only five of those studies showed any association of birth defects and Bendectin exposure, and those associations were weak, inconsistent, or inconclusive. The strongest case against any risk of birth defects was made by Brent (1981, 1988) on the basis of a lack of a clear syndrome of effects, the preponderance of negative epidemiological evidence, the uncorrelated nature of increasing drug sales and the overall incidence of birth defects, the lack of supporting animal testing data showing a potential for teratogenicity, and the particular nature of the defect in the initial case report (nongenetically induced unilateral limb reduction defects are exceptionally rare). Citing the U.S. Government Accounting Office's estimate that 5 percent of all federal court filings involving product liability between 1974 and 1985 involved Bendectin, Schardein (1993) concluded: "The real tragedy of the episode was the unwarranted fear instilled in many pregnant women and the vast sums of money and time that were devoted to the matter. . . ." Reacting to the the cost of liability insurance to cover the ever-increasing numbers of lawsuits filed against it despite the overwhelming scientific evidence, Merrill-Dow ceased production of the drug in June 1983. The word "litagen" has since been used by some researchers to describe an agent regulated not on the basis of its public health concerns but rather because of the legal costs associated with liability claims.

## PRINCIPLES OF DEVELOPMENTAL TOXICOLOGY

### Critical Periods of Susceptibility and Endpoints of Toxicity

A prerequisite to an understanding of abnormal development is a firm grasp of normal development. Development is characterized by changes in size, biochemistry and physiology, and form and functionality. These changes are orchestrated by a cascade of gene transcription regulating factors, the first of which are maternally inherited and present in the egg before fertilization. In turn, these factors activate regulatory genes in the embryonic genome, and sequential gene activation continues throughout development. One family of transcription factors—the *homeobox genes*—that are widely conserved in the animal kingdom and control the basic patterning of the embryo, has received much attention in the biological literature and is illustrative of the role of selective gene activation in development (see below).

Because of the rapid changes that occur during development, the nature of the embryo/fetus as a target for toxicity is also changing. While the basic tenets of toxicology discussed elsewhere in this text apply during development, the principle of critical periods of sensitivity based on the developmental stage of the conceptus must necessarily be a primary and unique consideration. This section highlights some normal developmental stages in the context of their known and potential susceptibility to toxicants. It should be made clear, however, that development is a continuum and that these stages are used for descriptive purposes and do not necessarily represent discrete developmental events. The timing of some key developmental events in humans and experimental animal species is presented in Table 10-3.

The development of the human organism is a lifelong cycle. As a logical starting point, *gametogenesis* is the process of forming the haploid germ cells: the egg and sperm. These gametes fuse in the process of *fertilization* to form the diploid *zygote,* or one-celled embryo. Gametogenesis and fertilization are vulnerable to toxicants, but that is the topic of Chap. 19. It is now known that the maternal and paternal genomes are not functionally equivalent in their contributions to the zygotic genome. The process of *imprinting* occurs during gametogenesis, conferring to certain allelic genes a differential expressivity, depending on whether they are of maternal or paternal origin (Hall, 1990).

Exposure to toxicants during a brief period (~6 h) immediately after fertilization has been demonstrated to result in malformed fetuses for a number of chemicals, including ethylene oxide (Generoso et al., 1987), ethylmethane sulfonate, ethylnitrosourea, and triethylene melamine (Generoso et al., 1988). The mechanisms underlying these unexpected findings have not been elucidated but probably do not involve point mutations. Although it is a plausible target for toxicity, im-

**Table 10–3**
**Timing of Key Developmental Events in Some Mammalian Species**

| | RAT | RABBIT | MONKEY | HUMAN |
|---|---|---|---|---|
| Blastocyst formation | 3–5 | 2.6–6 | 4–9 | 4–6 |
| Implantation | 5–6 | 6 | 9 | 6–7 |
| Organogenesis | 6–17 | 6–18 | 20–45 | 21–56 |
| Primitive streak | 9 | 6.5 | 18–20 | 16–18 |
| Neural plate | 9.5 | — | 19–21 | 18–20 |
| First somite | 10 | — | — | 20–21 |
| First pharyngeal arch | 10 | — | — | 20 |
| Ten somites | 10–11 | 9 | 23–24 | 25–26 |
| Upper limb buds | 10.5 | 10.5 | 25–26 | 29–30 |
| Lower limb buds | 11.2 | 11 | 26–27 | 31–32 |
| Forepaw rays | 13.4 | 14.5 | 34 | 35 |
| Testes differentiation | 14.5 | 20 | — | 43 |
| Heart septation | 15.5 | — | — | 46–47 |
| Palate closure | 16–17 | 19–20 | 45–47 | 56–58 |
| Length of gestation | 22 | 32 | 165 | 267 |

Developmental ages are in days of gestation.
SOURCE: Shepard (1992).

printing is not well understood and there are no documented examples of toxicant effects on this process. Toxic effects on imprinting could conceivably play a role in paternally mediated developmental toxicity, a topic that will not be discussed here but one that has received increased attention in the recent literature (Olshan and Mattison, 1995).

After fertilization, the embryo moves down the fallopian tube and is implanted in the wall of the uterus. The *preimplantation* period involves mainly an increase in cell number through a rapid series of cell divisions with little growth in size (*cleavage* of the zygote) and cavitation of the embryo to form a fluid-filled blastocoele. This stage, termed the *blastocyst,* composed of about a thousand cells, may contain as few as three cells destined to give rise to the embryo proper (Markert and Petters, 1978), and these cells are in a region called the *inner cell mass.* The remainder of the blastocyst cells give rise to extraembryonic membranes and support structures (e.g., trophoblast and placenta). However, the fates of the cells in the early embryo are not completely determined at this stage. The relatively undifferentiated preimplantation embryo has great restorative (regulative) growth potential (Snow and Tam, 1979). As exemplified by the experiments of Moore and associates (1968), single cells from eight-celled rabbit embryos are capable of producing normal offspring.

Toxicity during preimplantation is largely thought to result in no effect or a slight effect on growth (because of regulative growth) or in death (through overwhelming damage or failure to implant). Preimplantation exposure to DDT, nicotine, or methylmethane sulfonate results in body and/or brain weight deficits and embryo lethality but not malformations (Fabro, 1973; Fabro et al., 1984). However, there are also examples of toxicant exposure during the preimplantation period leading to fetal malformations. Treatment of pregnant mice with methylnitrosourea on days 2.5, 3.5, and 4.5 of gestation resulted in neural tube defects and cleft palate (Takeuchi, 1984). Cyproterone acetate and medroxyprogesterone acetate can produce malformations when administered on day 2 of gestation (Eibs et al., 1982). Because of the rapid mitoses that occur during the preimplantation period, chemicals affecting DNA synthesis or integrity and those affecting microtubule assembly would be expected to be particularly toxic if given access to the embryo.

After implantation the embryo undergoes *gastrulation,* the process of the formation of the three primary germ layers: the *ectoderm, mesoderm,* and *endoderm.* During gastrulation, cells migrate through a structure called the *primitive streak* and through these movements set up basic morphogenetic fields in the embryo (Smith et al., 1994). A prelude to organogenesis, the period of gastrulation appears to be quite susceptible to teratogenesis. A number of toxicants administered during gastrulation produce malformations of the eye, brain, and face. These malformations are indicative of damage to the anterior neural plate, one of the regions defined by the cellular movements of gastrulation.

The formation of the neural plate in the ectoderm marks the onset of *organogenesis,* during which the rudiments of most bodily structures are established. This is a period of heightened susceptibility to malformations and extends from approximately the third week to the eighth week of gestation in humans. During this short period the embryo undergoes rapid and dramatic changes. At 3 weeks of gestation the human conceptus is in most ways indistinguishable from other vertebrate embryos, consisting of only a few cell types in a trilaminar arrangement. By 8 weeks the conceptus, which can now be termed a fetus, has a form clearly recognizable as human. The rapid changes of organogenesis require cell proliferation, cell migration, cell-cell interactions, and morphogenetic tissue remodeling. These processes are exemplified by the *neural crest* cells. These cells originate at the border of the *neural plate* and migrate to form a wide variety of structures throughout the embryo. The way in which migration patterns are controlled is not understood but may in part involve homeobox (Hox) gene expression. The Hox family of genes are involved in axial patterning of the embryo and are believed to function in a variety of structures, including the skeleton, limbs, and nervous system. The Hox genes are arranged in chromosomal clusters that are evolutionary homologues of the *Drosophila* HOM-C (ANT-C/BC-X) homeotic complex. In the mouse and human there are four clusters (A through D) that have arisen by duplication from a common ancestor (Graham et al., 1989; Duboule and Morata, 1994). Patterns of Hox gene expression and neural crest cell migration in the branchial region of the head are depicted in Fig. 10-1. Neural crest cells derived from segments of the hindbrain (*rhombomeres*) migrate to form bone and connective tissues in this region (Krumlauf, 1993). The fate of the neural crest cells is imprinted before they leave the hindbrain, and specific Hox gene expression is maintained during and after migration.

Within organogenesis, there are periods of maximum susceptibility for each forming structure. This is nicely illustrated by the work of Shenefelt (1972), who studied the developmental toxicity of carefully timed exposures to retinoic acid in the hamster. The incidence of some of the defects seen (at the fetal $LD_{50}$ for each exposure time) after retinoic acid administration at different times in development are shown in Fig. 10-2. The peak incidence of these malformations coincides with the timing of key developmental events in these structures. Thus, the specification of developmental fields for the eyes is established quite early, and microphthalmia has an early critical period. The establishment of the rudiments of the long bones of the limbs occurs later, as does susceptibility to shortened limbs. The palate has an interesting pattern, with two separate peaks of susceptibility. The first corresponds to the early establishment of the palatal folds, and the second corresponds to the later events leading to palatal closure. Note also that the total incidence of malformations at the fetal $LD_{50}$ is lower before organogenesis but increases to 100 percent by gestation day $7\frac{3}{4}$. The processes underlying the development of normal structures are poorly understood but involve a number of key events. A given toxicant may affect one or several developmental events, and so the pattern of sensitivity of a structure can change depending on the nature of the toxic insult. Cleft palate is induced in mouse fetuses after maternal exposure to methanol as early as day 5 of gestation, with a peak sensitivity around day 7 and little or no sensitivity after day 9 (Rogers et al., 1993). For most toxic agents, the peak critical period for the induction of cleft palate in the mouse lies between gestation days 11 and 13; in a large series of experiments in NMRI mice, Neubert's group found that the day of peak sensitivity to cleft palate induction was day 11 for TCDD, day 12 for 2,4,5-T, and day 13 for dexamethasone (Neubert et al., 1973). Detection of unexpected critical periods like that for induction of cleft palate by methanol may provide clues to normal developmental processes that are not understood at present.

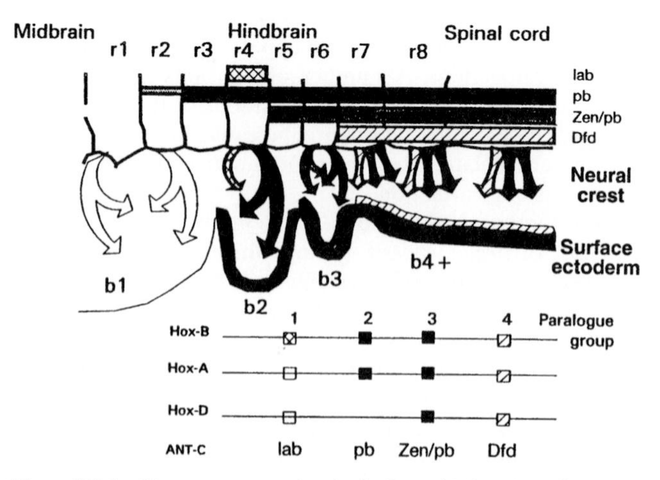


***Figure 10–1. Hox gene expression in the branchial region of a mouse embryo on gestation day 9.5.***

The Hox genes are expressed in the rhombomeres (r) of the hindbrain, migrating neural crest cell populations (arrows), and surface ectoderm after the neural crest cells have migrated into the branchial arches (b1 through b4+). Relationship of the Hox gene paralog groups to the *Drosophila* ANT-C complex is shown at the bottom. [From Krumlauf (1993), with permission.]

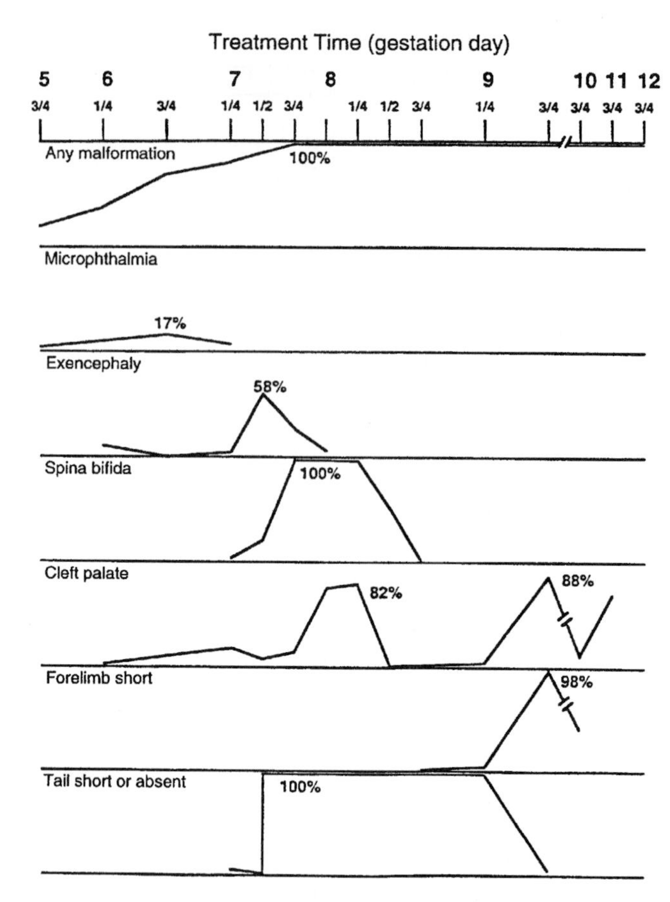


***Figure 10-2. Critical periods of sensitivity for the induction of various defects by retinoic acid in the hamster.***

Incidences of defects are estimates for the embryo/fetus $LD_{50}$ maternal dosage. Note in the top panel that fewer malformations are induced on days 5 and 6, before organogenesis, indicating that during this period embryos for the most part either die or recover. The likelihood of malformation increases rapidly during gastrulation and reaches 100 percent during organogenesis. Peak incidences for each defect are enumerated and reflect the timing of critical events in the development of each structure. [Modified after Shenefelt (1972) with permission.]

The end of organogenesis marks the beginning of the *fetal period* (from day 56 to 58 to birth in humans), which is characterized primarily by tissue differentiation, growth, and physiological maturation. This is not to say that formation of the organs is complete, but almost all the organs are present and grossly recognizable. Further development of organs proceeds during the fetal period to attain the requisite functionality before birth, including fine structural morphogenesis (e.g., neural outgrowth and synaptogenesis, branching morphogenesis of the bronchial tree and renal cortical tubules) as well as biochemical maturation (e.g., induction of tissue-specific enzymes and structural proteins).

Exposure during the fetal period is most likely to result in effects on growth and functional maturation. Functional anomalies of the central nervous system (CNS) and reproductive organs, including behavioral, mental, and motor deficits and decreases in fertility, are among the possible adverse outcomes. These manifestations are not apparent prenatally and require careful postnatal observation and testing of offspring exposed prenatally. Such postnatal functional manifestations can be sensitive indicators of in utero toxicity, and recent reviews of postnatal functional deficits of the CNS (Rodier et al., 1994), immune system (Holladay and Luster, 1994), and heart, lung, and kidneys (Lau and Kavlock, 1994) are available. Major structural alterations can occur during the fetal period, but these changes generally result from *deformations* (disruption of previously normal structures), not malformations. The extremities may be affected by amniotic bands, wrapping of the umbilical cord, or vascular disruptions, leading to the loss of distal structures.

There is a paucity of data concerning the long-term effects of toxic exposure during the fetal period. Some effects could require years to become apparent (such as those noted for DES in "Scope of the Problem," above), and others may result in the premature onset of senescence and/or organ failure later in life. The potential occurrence of such effects has not been systematically studied.

It is important to reiterate that development does not stop at birth. We have focused only on the prenatal period in this chapter because of space limitations. Special susceptibilities also exist in the neonatal, childhood, and adolescent years. For a review of toxicity concerns specific to childhood and adolescence, refer to Guzelian et al. (1992).

## Dose-Response Patterns and the Threshold Concept

The major effects of prenatal exposure observed at the time of birth in developmental toxicity studies are embryolethality, malformations, and growth retardation. Embryolethality precludes measurements of growth retardation or malformation because those two events are observed only in live fetuses. The relationship between embryolethality, malformations, and growth retardation is complex and varies with the type of agent, the timing of exposure, and the dose. For some agents these endpoints may represent a continuum of increasing toxicity, with low doses producing growth retardation and increasing doses producing malformations and then lethality. Malformations and/or death can also occur in the absence of any effect on intrauterine growth, but this is unusual. Similarly, growth retardation and embryolethality can occur without malformations. Agents that produce the latter pattern of response would be considered embryotoxic or embryolethal but not teratogenic unless it was subsequently established that death was due to a structural malformation.

Another key element of the dose-response relationship is the shape of the dose-response curve at low exposure levels. Because of the high restorative growth potential of the mammalian embryo, cellular homeostatic mechanisms, and maternal metabolic defenses, mammalian developmental toxicity has generally been considered a threshold phenomenon. The assumption of a threshold means that there is a maternal dose below which an adverse response is not elicited. Daston (1993) summarized two approaches for establishing the existence of a threshold. The first, which is exemplified by a large teratology study of 2,4,5-T (Nelson and Holson, 1978), suggests that no study is capable of evaluating the dose response at low response rates (805 litters per dose would be necessary to detect the relatively high rate of a 5 percent increase in resorptions). The other approach is to determine whether a threshold exists for the mechanism responsible for the observed effect. While relatively few mechanisms are known with any certainty for developmental toxicity, it is clear that cellular and embryonic repair mechanisms and dose-dependent kinetics could both contribute to the plausibility of a mechanistic threshold. Lack of a threshold infers that exposure to any amount of a toxic chemical, even one molecule, has the potential to cause developmental toxicity. One mechanism of abnormal development for which this might be the case is gene mutation. A point mutation in a critical gene could theoretically be induced by a single hit or a single molecule, leading to a deleterious change in a gene product and consequent abnormal development. This of course carries the assumption that the molecule could traverse the maternal system and the placenta and enter a critical progenitor cell in the embryo. An effect on a single cell might result in abnormal development at the zygote (one-cell) stage, the blastocyst stage (when only a few cells in the inner cell mass are embryo progenitors), or during organogenesis, when the organ anlagen may consist of only a few cells. However, even in the case of point mutations, the embryo has efficient repair mechanisms.

An apparent threshold for developmental toxicity that is based at least in part on cellular homeostatic mechanisms is demonstrated in studies of the biological mechanisms underlying the developmental dose response for 5-fluorouracil (Shuey et al., 1994; see also "Safety Assessment," below). This agent inhibits the enzyme thymidylate synthetase (TS), thus interfering with DNA synthesis and cell proliferation. Significant embryonal TS inhibition can be measured at maternal dosages an order of magnitude below those required to produce malformations and about five-fold below those affecting fetal growth (Fig. 10-3). The lack of developmental toxicity despite significant TS inhibition probably reflects the ability of the embryo to compensate for imbalances in cellular nucleotide pool sizes.

In the context of risk assessment for human health, it is also important to consider the distinction between individual thresholds and population thresholds. There is wide variability in the human population, and a threshold for a population is defined by the threshold of the most sensitive individual in that population (Gaylor et al., 1988). Indeed, even though the

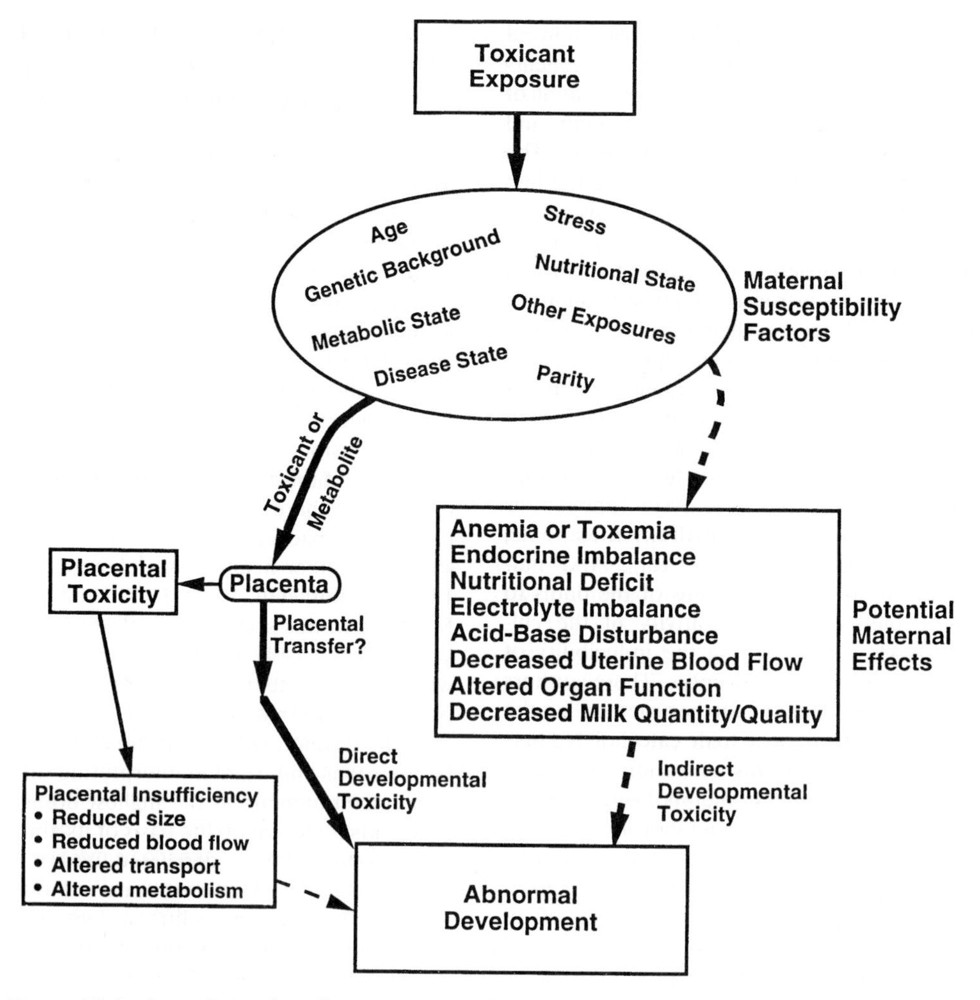


*Figure 10–8. Interrelationships between maternal susceptibility factors, metabolism, induction of maternal physiological or functional alterations, placental transfer and toxicity, and developmental toxicity.*

A developmental toxicant can cause abnormal development through any one or a combination of these pathways. Maternal susceptibility factors determine the predisposition of the mother to respond to a toxic insult, and the maternal effects listed can adversely affect the developing conceptus. Most chemicals traverse the placenta in some form, and the placenta also can be a target for toxicity. In most cases, developmental toxicity probably is mediated through a combination of these pathways.

paternal race, while the offspring of white fathers did not have a higher incidence of CL(P) than did the offspring of black fathers after correcting for maternal race.

Among experimental animals, the "A" family of inbred mice has a high spontaneous occurrence of cleft lip and palate (Kalter, 1979). Two related mouse strains, A/J and CL/Fr, produce spontaneous CL(P) at 8 to 10 percent and 18 to 26 percent frequencies, respectively. The incidence of CL(P) in offspring depends on the genotype of the mother rather than that of the embryo (Juriloff and Fraser, 1980). The response to vitamin A of murine embryos heterozygous for the curly-tail mutation depends on the genotype of the mother (Seller et al., 1983). The teratogenicity of phenytoin has been compared in several inbred strains of mice. The susceptibility of the offspring of crosses between susceptible A/J mice and resistant C57BL/6J mice was determined by the maternal genome, not the embryonic genome (Hansen and Hodes, 1983).

**Disease.** Chronic hypertension is a risk factor for the development of preeclampsia, eclampsia, and toxemia of pregnancy, and hypertension is a leading cause of pregnancy-associated maternal death. Uncontrolled maternal diabetes mellitus is a significant cause of prenatal morbidity. Certain maternal infections can adversely affect the conceptus (e.g., rubella virus, discussed earlier) through indirect disease-related maternal alterations or direct transplacental infection. Cytomegalovirus infection is associated with fetal death, microcephalus, mental retardation, blindness, and deafness (MacDonald and Tobin, 1978), and maternal infection with *Toxoplasma gondii* is known to induce hydrocephaly and chorioretinitis in infants (Alford et al., 1974).

One factor common to many disease states is hyperthermia. Hyperthermia is a potent experimental animal teratogen (Edwards, 1986), and there is a body of evidence associating maternal febrile illness during the first trimester of pregnancy with birth defects in humans, most notably malformations of the CNS (Warkany, 1986; Milunsky et al., 1992).

**Nutrition.** A wide spectrum of dietary insufficiencies ranging from protein-calorie malnutrition to deficiencies of vitamins, trace elements, and/or enzyme cofactors is known to have an adverse effect on pregnancy (Keen et al., 1993). Among the most significant findings related to human nutrition and pregnancy outcome in recent years are the results of studies in which pregnant women at risk for having infants with neural tube defects (NTDs) were supplemented with folate (Wald, 1993). The largest and most convincing study is the Medical Research Council (MRC) Vitamin Study, in which supplementation with 4 mg folic acid reduced NTD recurrence by over 70 percent (MRC, 1991). The results of these studies have prompted the U.S. Centers for Disease Control and Prevention to recommend folate supplementation for women of childbearing age.

**Stress.** Diverse forms of maternal toxicity may have in common the induction of a physiological stress response. An understanding of the potential effects of maternal stress on development may help us interpret the developmental toxicity observed in experimental animals at maternally toxic doses. Various forms of physical stress have been applied to pregnant animals in an attempt to isolate the developmental effects of stress. Subjecting pregnant rats or mice to noise stress throughout gestation can produce developmental toxicity (Geber, 1966; Geber and Anderson, 1967; Kimmel et al., 1976; Nawrot et al., 1980, 1981). Restraint stress produces increased fetal death in rats (Euker and Riegle, 1973) and cleft palate (Barlow et al., 1975), fused and supernumerary ribs, and encephaloceles in mice (Beyer and Chernoff, 1986).

Objective data on the effects of stress in humans are difficult to obtain. Nevertheless, studies investigating the relationship of maternal stress and pregnancy outcome have indicated a positive correlation between stress and adverse developmental effects, including low birthweight and congenital malformations (Stott, 1973; Gorsuch and Key, 1974).

## Placental Toxicity

The placenta is the interface between the mother and the conceptus, providing attachment, nutrition, gas exchange, and waste removal. The placenta also produces hormones critical to the maintenance of pregnancy and can metabolize and/or store xenobiotics. Placental toxicity may compromise these functions and produce or contribute to untoward effects on the conceptus. Slikker and Miller (1994) listed 46 toxicants known to be toxic to the yolk sac or chorioallantoic placenta, including metals such as cadmium (Cd), arsenic and mercury, cigarette smoke, ethanol, cocaine, endotoxin, and sodium salicylate (Daston, 1994; Slikker and Miller, 1994). Cd is among the best studied of these toxicants, and it appears that the developmental toxicity of Cd during middle to late gestation involves both placental toxicity (necrosis, reduced blood flow) and inhibition of nutrient transport across the placenta. Maternal injection of Cd during late gestation results in fetal death in rats despite the fact that little cadmium enters the fetus (Parizek, 1964; Levin and Miller, 1980). Fetal death occurs concomitantly with reduced uteroplacental blood flow within 10 h (Levin and Miller, 1980). The authors' conclusion that fetal death was caused by placental toxicity was supported by experiments in which fetuses were directly injected with Cd. Despite fetal Cd burdens almost 10-fold higher than those which followed maternal administration, only a slight increase in fetal death was observed.

Cd is a transition metal similar in its physicochemical properties to the essential metal zinc (Zn). Cadmium interferes with Zn transfer across the placenta (Samarawickrama and Webb, 1979; Sorell and Graziano, 1990), possibly via metallothionein (MT), a metal-binding protein induced in the placenta by Cd. Because of its high affinity for Zn, MT may sequester Zn in the placenta, impeding transfer to the conceptus (induction of maternal hepatic MT by Cd or other agents can also induce fetal Zn deficiency, as discussed below). Cadmium inhibits Zn uptake by human placental microvesicles (Page et al., 1992), suggesting that Cd also may compete directly with Zn for membrane transport. Cadmium also may competitively inhibit other Zn-dependent processes in the placenta. Coadministration of Zn ameliorates the developmental toxicity of administered Cd, further indicating that interference of Cd with Zn metabolism is a key to the developmental toxicity of Cd (Ferm and Carpenter, 1967; Daston, 1982).

## Maternal Toxicity

A retrospective analysis of relationships between maternal toxicity and specific types of prenatal effects found species-specific associations between maternal toxicity and specific adverse developmental effects. However, among rat, rabbit, and hamster studies, 22 percent failed to show any developmental toxicity in the presence of significant maternal toxicity (Khera, 1984, 1985). The approach of tabulating literature data suffers from possible bias in the types of studies published (e.g., negative results may not be published), incomplete reporting of maternal and developmental effects, and lack of standard criteria for the evaluation of maternal and developmental toxicity. In a study designed to test the potential of maternal toxicity to affect development, Kavlock and colleagues (1985) acutely administered 10 structurally unrelated compounds to pregnant mice at maternotoxic doses. Developmental effects were agent-specific, ranging from complete resorption to lack of effect. An exception was an increased incidence of supernumerary ribs (ribs on the first lumbar vertebra), which occurred with 7 of the 10 compounds. Chernoff and coworkers (1988) dosed pregnant rats for 10 days with a series of compounds chosen because they had exhibited little or no developmental toxicity in previous studies. When these compounds were administered at high doses, producing maternal toxicity (weight loss or lethality), a variety of developmental outcomes was noted, including increased intrauterine death (two compounds), decreased fetal weight (two compounds), supernumerary ribs (two compounds), and enlarged renal pelvises (two compounds). In addition, two of the compounds produced no developmental toxicity despite substantial maternal toxicity. These diverse developmental responses led these authors to conclude that maternal toxicity defined by weight loss or mortality is not associated with any consistent syndrome of developmental effects in the rat.

There have been a number of studies directly relating specific forms of maternal toxicity to developmental toxicity, including those in which the test chemical causes maternal effects that exacerbate the agent's developmental toxicity, and instances in which developmental toxicity is thought to be a direct result of adverse maternal effects. However, clear delineation of the relative roles of indirect maternal and direct embryo/fetal toxicity is difficult.

Acetazolamide inhibits carbonic anhydrase and is teratogenic in mice (Hirsch and Scott, 1983). Although maternal weight loss is not correlated with malformation frequency, maternal hypercapnia potentiates the teratogenicity of acetazolamide. In C57Bl/6J mice, maternal hypercapnia alone results in right forelimb ectrodactyly, the characteristic malformation induced by acetazolamide. Correction of maternal acidosis failed to reduce developmental toxicity, suggesting that the primary teratogenic factor was elevated maternal plasma $CO_2$ tension (Weaver and Scott, 1984a and b).

Diflunisal, an analgesic and anti-inflammatory drug, causes axial skeletal defects in rabbits. Developmentally toxic doses resulted in severe maternal anemia (hematocrit 20 to 24 percent versus 37 percent in controls) and depletion of erythrocyte ATP levels (Clark et al., 1984). Teratogenicity, anemia, and ATP depletion were unique to the rabbit among the species studied. A single dose of diflunisal on day 5 of gestation produced a maternal anemia that lasted through day 15. The concentration of the drug in the embryo was less than 5 percent of the peak maternal blood level, and diflunisal was cleared from maternal blood before day 9, the critical day for the induction of similar axial skeletal defects by hypoxia. Thus, the teratogenicity of diflunisal in the rabbit is probably due to hypoxia resulting from maternal anemia.

Phenytoin, an anticonvulsant, can affect maternal folate metabolism in experimental animals, and these alterations may play a role in the teratogenicity of this drug (Netzloff et al., 1979; Hansen and Billings, 1985). Further, maternal heart rates were monitored on gestation day 10 after administration to susceptible A/J mice and resistant C57Bl/6J mice (Watkinson and Millikovsky, 1983). Heart rates were depressed by phenytoin in a dose-related manner in A/J mice but not in C57Bl/6J mice. A mechanism of teratogenesis was proposed that related depressed maternal heart rate and embryonic hypoxia. Supporting studies have demonstrated that hyperoxia reduces the teratogenicity of phenytoin in mice (Millicovsky and Johnston, 1981). Reduced uterine blood flow has been proposed as a mechanism of teratogenicity caused by hydroxyurea, which produces elevated systolic blood pressure, altered heart rate, decreased cardiac output, severely decreased uterine blood flow, and increased vascular resistance in pregnant rabbits (Millicovsky et al., 1981). Embryos exhibited craniofacial and pericardial hemorrhages immediately after treatment (Millicovsky and DeSesso, 1980a), and identical embryopathies were achieved by clamping the uterine vessels of pregnant rabbits for 10 min (Millicovsky and DeSesso, 1980b).

Metallothionein (MT) synthesis can be induced by a wide variety of chemical and physical agents, including metals, alcohols, urethane, endotoxin, alkylating agents, hyper- or hypothermia, and ionizing radiation (Daston, 1994). MT synthesis is also induced by endogenous mediators such as glucocorticoids and certain cytokines (Klaassen and Lehman-McKeeman, 1989). A mechanism common to the developmental toxicity of these diverse agents may be Zn deficiency of the conceptus secondary to induction of maternal MT. Induction of MT synthesis can produce hepatic MT concentrations over an order of magnitude higher than normal, leading to substantial sequestration of circulating Zn in the maternal liver, lowered plasma Zn concentrations, and reduced Zn availability to the conceptus. Embryofetal zinc deficiency secondary to maternal hepatic MT induction has been demonstrated for diverse chemicals, including valproic acid (Keen et al., 1989), 6-mercaptopurine (Amemiya et al., 1986, 1989), urethane (Daston et al., 1991a and b), ethanol, and $\alpha$-hederin (Taubeneck et al., 1994). In a study combining data for many of these compounds, Taubeneck and coworkers (1994) found a strong positive relationship between maternal hepatic MT induction and maternal hepatic $^{65}Zn$ retention and a negative relationship between maternal MT induction and $^{65}Zn$ distribution to the litter (Fig. 10-9).

## Quantitative Comparisons of Maternal and Developmental Toxicity

Quantification of the relationship between maternal and developmental toxicity has been attempted by a number of investigators in order to identify selectively embryotoxic agents (Brent, 1964; Robson and Sullivan, 1968; Johnson 1980, 1981; Fabro et al., 1984; Platzek et al., 1982, 1983). The general approach has been to construct a ratio using as the numerator a measure of the maternal effective administered dose [(e.g., $LD_{50}$, $LD_{01}$, or maternal no observed adverse effect level (NOAEL)] and as the denominator a measure of the developmentally effective administered dose (e.g., embryonic $LD_{50}$; dose producing 5 percent, 10 percent, or 50 percent terata; or developmental NOAEL). These ratios are intended to gauge the selectivity of the agent's toxicity for the con-

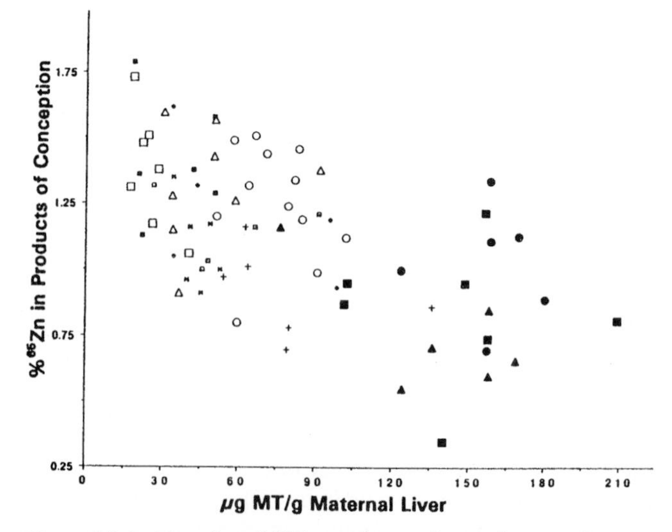


*Figure 10–9. Transfer of $^{65}Zn$ to the products of conception as a function of maternal hepatic metallothionein (MT) concentration.*

Pregnant rats were dosed on gestation day 11 with ● $\alpha$-hederin; □ dimethylsulfoxide; ■ ethanol; ▲ urethane; + melphalan; ◆ acidified alcohol; or □ styrene or were ○ food-deprived or △ food-restricted. □ = Saline control. Eight h after dosing, dams were orally gavaged with a diet slurry containing $^{65}Zn$. The amount of $^{65}Zn$ transferred to the conceptuses was inversely correlated with the degree of treatment-related maternal hepatic MT induction. [Adapted from Taubeneck et al. (1994) with permission.]

ceptus; the higher the value, the more selectively toxic the agent is to the developing organism compared with the mother. These ratios are not consistent across species (Daston et al., 1991). In addition, maternal and developmental dose-response curves are almost always nonparallel, which means that no single index can describe the relationship between the two (Rogers, 1987). Further, computer simulation studies have shown that such indexes derived from standard study designs are highly variable and are poor at predicting the relative adult and developmental responses at doses lower than those used to calculate the index (Setzer and Rogers, 1991). It is indisputable that maternal toxicity that is observed to be concomitant with developmental toxicity in testing protocols complicates the interpretation of the results for risk assessment. Thus, there is no simple way to factor in the maternal toxicity variable, and few developmental toxicologists consider such ratios useful.

## MODERN SAFETY ASSESSMENT

Experience with chemicals that have the potential to induce developmental toxicity indicates that both laboratory animal testing and surveillance of the human population (i.e., epidemiological studies) are necessary to provide adequate public health protection. Laboratory animal investigations are guided both by regulatory requirements for drug and chemical marketing and by the basic desire to understand the mechanisms of toxicity.

### In Vivo Regulatory Guidelines

Before the thalidomide tragedy, safety evaluations for reproductive effects were limited in regard to both the types of chemicals evaluated and the sophistication of the endpoints. Subsequently, the Food and Drug Administration issued more extensive testing protocols (Segments I, II, and III) for application to a broader range of agents (U.S. FDA, 1966). These testing protocols, with minor variations, were adopted by a variety of regulatory agencies around the world and remained similar for nearly 30 years. Recently, several factors, including the historical experience of testing thousands of chemicals, increased knowledge of basic reproductive processes, the ever-increasing cost of testing, the acknowledged redundancy and overlap of required protocols, a growing divergence in study design requirements in different countries, and the expanding international presence of the pharmaceutical industry, have led to the establishment of new and streamlined testing protocols that have been accepted internationally (U.S. FDA, 1994). These guidelines, which are the result of the International Conference of Harmonization of Technical Requirements for Registration of Pharmaceuticals for Human Use (ICH), specifically include considerable flexibility in implementation depending on the circumstances of the agent under evaluation. Rather than specify study and technical details, these guidelines rely on the investigator to meet the primary goal of detecting and bringing to light any indication of toxicity to reproduction. Palmer (1993) has provided a recent overview of issues relevant to implementing the new ICH guideline. Key elements of FDA Segments I, II, and III studies as well as the ICH protocols are provided in Table 10-4. In each protocol, guidance is provided on species and/or strain selection, route of administration, number and spacing of dosage levels, exposure duration, experimental sample size, observational techniques, statistical analysis, and reporting requirements. Details are available in the original publications and in several recent reviews (Manson, 1994; Francis, 1994). Variations of these protocols also exist that include extensions of exposure to early or later time points in development and extensions of observations to postnatal ages with more sophisticated endpoints. For example, the U.S. Environmental Protection Agency has promulgated a Developmental Neurotoxicity Protocol for the rat that includes exposure from gestation day 6 though lactation day 10 and observation of postnatal growth, the developmental landmarks of puberty (balanopreputial separation, vaginal opening), motor activity, auditory startle, learning and memory, and neuropathology at various ages through postnatal day 60 (U.S. EPA, 1991a and b).

The general goal of these regulatory studies is to identify the NOAEL, on the highest dosage level that does not produce a significant increase in adverse effects in the offspring. These NOAELs are then used in the risk assessment process (see below) to assess the likelihood of effects in humans under certain exposure conditions.

### Multigenerational Tests

Information pertaining to developmental toxicity also can be obtained from studies in which animals are exposed to a test substance continuously over one or more generations. For additional information on this approach, see Chap. 19.

### Alternative Testing Strategies

A variety of alternative test systems have been proposed to refine, reduce, or replace reliance on the standard regulatory guidelines for assessing prenatal toxicity (Table 10-5). They can be grouped into assays based on cell cultures, cultures of embryos in vitro (including sub-mammalian species), and short-term in vivo tests; an effort has been made to qualitatively and quantitatively compile results across both the standard and the alternative tests (Faustman, 1988; Kavlock et al., 1991). Validation of these alternative tests has constituted a major and unresolved issue (reviewed in Neubert, 1989; Welsch, 1990). Much of the validation work has used a selection of chemicals proposed by Smith et al. (1983), which has been criticized for being biased toward direct-acting cytotoxicants and for not factoring in the potential confounding of fetal effects by maternal toxicity (Johnson, 1985; Brown 1987). Without an accepted standard, assessing the significance of the sensitivity and specificity of results from these tests has been problematic. Efforts to produce a revised updated list have not proved successful, although it is now generally accepted that a validated test would have to produce information that is in some way predictive of results of full in vivo developmental toxicity protocols (Schwetz et al., 1991). While it was initially hoped that the alternative approaches would become generally applicable to all chemicals and help prioritize full-scale testing, this has not been accomplished. Indeed, given the complexity of embryogenesis and the multiple mechanisms and target sites of potential teratogens, it

**Table 10-4**
**Summary of In Vivo Regulatory Protocol Guidelines for Evaluation of Developmental Toxcity**

| STUDY | EXPOSURE | ENDPOINTS COVERED | COMMENTS |
|---|---|---|---|
| *Segment I* | | | |
| Fertility and General Reproduction Study | Males: 10 weeks before mating<br>Females: 2 weeks before mating | Gamete development, fertility, pre- and postimplantation viability, parturition lactation | Assesses reproductive capabilities of male and female after exposure over one complete spermatogenic cycle or several estrous cycles |
| *Segment II* | | | |
| Teratogenicity Test | Implantation through end of organogenesis | Viability and morphology (external, visceral, and skeletal) of conceptus just before birth | Limited exposure to prevent maternal metabolic adaptation and provide high exposure to embryo during period of heightened vulnerability associated with gastrulation and organogenesis |
| *Segment III* | | | |
| Perinatal Study | Last trimester of pregnancy through lactation | Postnatal survival, growth, and external morphology | Intended to observe effects on development of major organ functional competence during perinatal period; thus may be relatively more sensitive to adverse effects at this time |
| *ICH 4.1.1* | | | |
| Fertility Protocol | Males: 4 weeks before mating<br>Females: 2 weeks before mating | Males: reproductive organ weights and histology, sperm count and motility<br>Females: viability of conceptus at midpregnancy or later | Improved assessment of male reproductive endpoints; shorter treatment duration than Segment I |
| *ICH 4.1.2* | | | |
| Effects on Prenatal and Postnatal Development, Including Maternal Function | Implantation through end of lactation | Relative toxicity to pregnant versus nonpregnant female; postnatal viability, growth, development, and functional deficits (including behavior, maturation, and reproduction) | Similar to Segment I study |
| *ICH 4.1.3:* | | | |
| Effects on Embryo/ Fetal Development | Implantation through end of organogenesis | Viability and morphology (external, visceral, and skeletal) of fetuses just before birth | Similar to Segment II study. Usually conducted in two species (rodent and nonrodent) |

was perhaps unrealistic to have expected a single test or even a small battery to accurately prescreen the activity of chemicals in general. To date, the primary success of these tests has come from evaluating the relative potency of series of congeners when the prototype chemical has demonstrated appropriate concordance with the in vivo result (Kavlock, 1993).

The major exception to the poor acceptance of the alternative tests for prescreening for developmental toxicity is the in vivo test developed by Chernoff and Kavlock (1982). In this test, pregnant females are exposed during the period of major organogenesis to a limited number of dosage levels near those that induce maternal toxicity and offspring are evaluated over a brief neonatal period for external malformations, growth, and viability. The test has proved reliable over a large number of chemical agents and classes (Hardin et al., 1987), and a regulatory testing guideline has been developed (U.S. EPA, 1985).

## Epidemiology

Reproductive epidemiology is the study of the possible statistical associations between specific exposures of the father or the pregnant woman and her conceptus and the outcome of pregnancy. In rare situations, such as rubella, thalidomide, and isotretinoin, where a relatively high risk exists and the outcome is a relatively rare event, formal studies may not be needed to identify causes of abnormal birth outcomes. The plausibility of linking a particular exposure with a series of

**Table 10–5**
**Brief Survey of Alternative Test Methodologies**

| ASSAY | BRIEF DESCRIPTION AND ENDPOINTS EVALUATED | CONCORDANCE* | REFERENCES |
|---|---|---|---|
| Mouse ovarian tumor | Labeled mouse ovarian tumor cells added to culture dishes with concanavalin A–coated disks for 20 min. Endpoint is inhibition of attachment of cells to disks. | Sensitivity: 19/31; 19/30 Specificity: 7/13; 5/13 | Steele et al., 1988 (results from two labs) |
| Human embryonic palatal mesenchyme | Human embryonic palatal mesenchyme cell line grown in attached culture. Cell number assessed after 3 days. | Sensitivity: 21/31; 21/30 Specificity: 7/13; 5/13 | Steele et al., 1988 (results from two labs) |
| Micromass culture | Midbrain and limb bud cells dissociated from day 13 rat embryos and grown in micromass culture for 5 days. Endpoints include cell proliferation and biochemical markers of differentiation. | Sensitivity: 25/27; 20/33; 11/15 Specificity: 17/19; 18/18; 8/10 | Flint and Orton, 1984 Renault et al., 1989 Uphill et al., 1990 |
| Chick embryo neural retina cell culture | Neural retinas of day 6.5 chick embryos dissociated and grown in rotating suspension culture for 7 days. Endpoints include cellular aggregation, growth, differentiation, and biochemical markers. | Sensitivity: 36/41 Specificity: 14/17 | Daston et al. (1991) Daston et al. (1995) (concordances combined) |
| *Drosophila* | Fly larva grown in treated media from egg disposition through to hatching of adults. Adult flies examined for specific structural defects (bent bristle and notched wing). | Sensitivity: 10/13 Specificity: 4/5 | Lynch et al., 1991 |
| *Hydra* | *Hydra attenuata* cells aggregated to form an "artificial embryo" and allowed to regenerate. Dose response compared to that for adult *Hydra* toxicity. | Accuracy: >90% | Johnson and Gabel (1982) Johnson et al. (1988) |
| FETAX | Midblastula-stage *Xenopus* embryos exposed for 96 h. Embryos evaluated for viability, growth, and morphology. | Accuracy: ~ 90% | Bantle (1995) |
| Chernoff/Kavlock assay | Pregnant mice or rats exposed during organogenesis and allowed to deliver. Postnatal growth, viability, and gross morphology of litters recorded. | Sensitivity: 49/58 Specificity: 28/34 | Hardin et al., 1987 |

* Authors' interpretation. Sensitivity = correct identification of "positive" chemicals; Specificity = correct identification of "negative" compounds. Accuracy = agreement with mammalian data.

case reports increases with the rarity of the defect, the rarity of exposure in the population, a small source population, a short time span for study, and the biological plausibility of the association (Khoury et al., 1991). In other situations, such as ethanol and valproic acid, associations are sought through either a case-control approach or a cohort approach. Both approaches require accurate ascertainment of abnormal outcomes and exposure and a large enough effect and study population to detect an elevated risk. This is one of the difficulties facing epidemiologists who study abnormal reproductive outcomes. For example, it has been estimated that the monitoring of more than 1 million births would have been necessary to detect a statistically significant increase in the frequency of spina bifida after the introduction of valproic acid in the United States, where the frequency of exposure was less than 1 in 1000 pregnancies and the risk was only a doubling over the background incidence (Khoury and Holtzman, 1987). Another challenge to epidemiologists is the high percentage of human pregnancy wastage, perhaps as much as 31 percent in the periimplantation period (Wilcox et al., 1988) and an additional 15 percent that is clinically recognized. Therefore, pregnancy failures related to a particular exposure may go undetected in the general population. Furthermore, with the availability of prenatal diagnostic procedures, additional pregnancies involving malformed embryos (particularly those with neural tube defects) are electively aborted. Thus, the incidence of abnormal outcomes at birth may not reflect the true rate of abnormalities, and the term "prevalence," rather than "incidence," is preferred when the denominator is the number of live births instead of total pregnancies. Other issues particularly relevant to reproductive epidemiology include homogeneity, recording proficiency, and confounding factors. Homogeneity refers to fact that a particular outcome may be described differently by various recording units and that even with a specific outcome, there can be multiple pathogenetic origins (e.g., cleft palate could arise by a variety of mechanisms). Recording difficulties relate to inconsistencies in definitions and nomenclature and problems in ascertaining or recalling outcomes and exposures. For example, birthweights usually are determined and recalled accurately, but spontaneous abortions and certain malformations may not be. Confounding by factors such as maternal age and parity, dietary factors, diseases and drug use, and social characteristics must be accounted for to control for variables that affect both exposure and outcome (Khoury et al., 1992).

Epidemiological studies of abnormal reproductive outcomes usually are undertaken with three objectives in mind. The first objective is scientific research into the causes of abnormal birth outcomes and usually involves an analysis of case reports or clusters. The second aim is prevention and is targeted at broader surveillance of trends such as the analyses done by birth defect registries around the world. The third objective is informing the public and providing assurance. In this regard, it is informative to consider the review by Schardein (1993) of the method by which and the year in which human teratogens were detected. For 23 of 28 chemicals (including 9 cancer therapeutics, androgenic hormones, antithyroid drugs, aminoglycoside antibiotics, coumarin anticoagulants, diethylstilbestrol, dimethylmercury, hydantoins, primidone, penicillamine, lithium, vitamin A, and retinoic acid), case reports presented the first evidence in humans. For two of these chemicals (diethylstilbestrol and lithium), the case reports were soon followed by registries that provided confirmation, while for two others (dimethyl mercury and hydantoins), follow-up epidemiology studies added support. While only four chemicals—alcohol, PCBs, carbamazepine, and cocaine—did an analytic epidemiological study provide the first human evidence. Evidence for one chemical—valproic acid—was first obtained by analysis of a birth defect registry. Among the 28 chemicals in that review, human evidence of developmental toxicity preceded published animal evidence in 11 instances.

## Concordance of Data

There have been several extensive reviews of the similarity of the responses of laboratory animals and those of humans to developmental toxicants. In general, these studies support the assumption that the results from laboratory tests are predictive of potential human effects. Concordance is strongest when there are positive data from more than one test species, although even in this case the results cannot be used to extrapolate specific types of effects across species. The predictiveness of animal data for presumed negative human developmental toxicants is less than that for positive agents, a finding that probably is related to the problems associated with ascertaining a negative response in humans as well as the issue of inappropriate design or interpretation of animal studies. In a quantitative sense, the few comparisons that have been made suggest that humans tend to be more sensitive to developmental toxicants than is the most sensitive test species. While concordance among species for agents reported as positive is high, often special steps must be taken retrospectively to produce an animal model that reflects the nature of the outcome in humans (e.g., valproic acid) (Ehlers et al., 1992).

Frankos (1985) reviewed data for 38 compounds with demonstrated or suspected activity in humans; all except tobramycin, which caused otological defects, were positive in at least one species, and 76 percent were positive in more than one test species. Predictiveness was highest in the mouse (85 percent) and rat (80 percent), with lower rates for rabbits (60 percent) and hamsters (40 percent). Frankos identified 165 chemicals with no evidence of human effects; only 29 percent were negative in all species tested, while 51 percent were negative in more than one species. Schardein and Keller (1989) examined concordance by species and developmental manifestation for 51 potential human developmental toxicants that have adequate animal data (3 human developmental toxicants did not). Thalidomide received the widest testing, with data from 19 species; 53 percent had data from 3 species, and 18 percent had data from 4 or 5 species. Across all chemicals, the most common findings in humans, rabbits, and monkeys was spontaneous abortion and fetal/neonatal death followed by malformations and then growth retardation. In the rat, prenatal death, growth retardation, and then malformations constituted the typical pattern. The concordance of results is presented in Table 10-6. All species showed at least one positive response for 64 percent of the human developmental toxicants, and with only a single exception, all the potential human developmental toxicants showed a positive response in at least one species. The exception was formaldehyde, which was negative in the only two species tested: the rat and the mouse. The inclusion of formaldehyde as even a potential human developmental toxicant is questionable, as it was based on a single occupational study. Overall, the match to the human, regardless of the nature of the developmental response, was rat, 98 percent; mouse, 91 percent; hamster, 85 percent; monkey, 82 percent; and rabbit, 77 percent. Jelovsek et al. (1989) reviewed the predictiveness of animal data for 84 negative human developmental toxicants, 33 with unknown activity, 26 that were considered suspicious, and 32 that were considered positive. The variables considered included the response of each species, the number of positive and negative species, the percentage of positive and negative species, and mutagenicity and carcinogenicity. Multivariate statistics using the human effect as the classification variable were used to examine the predictiveness of the animal database. The compounds were correctly classified 63 to 91 percent of the time on the basis of animal data, depending on how the suspicious and unknown human toxicants were considered. The various models had a sensitivity of 62 to 75 percent, a positive predictive value of 75 to 100 percent, and a negative predictive value of 64 to 91 percent.

In addition to qualitative comparisons among species, several attempts at quantitative comparisons of potencies have been conducted, although they have been based on administered doses and have not attempted to factor in pharmacokinetic differences. Schardein and Keller (1989) estimated the human and animal "threshold" dosages for 21 chemicals. In only two cases—aminopterin and carbon disulfide—were developmental effects seen at doses in animal studies that were lower than those believed to cause effects in humans. For the other chemicals, ratios of the "threshold" doses in the most sensitive animals to those in humans ranged from 1.2 to 200. Newman and coworkers (1993) looked at the data for four well-characterized human developmental toxicants: valproic acid, isotreti-

**Table 10–6**
**Predictiveness of Animal Data for 51 Potential Human Developmental Toxicants**

| | | MOUSE | RAT | MONKEY | RABBIT | HAMSTER |
|---|---|---|---|---|---|---|
| Potential human developmental toxicants tested (%) | | 86 | 96 | 33 | 61 | 26 |
| Concordance by class | G* | 61 | 57 | 65 | 39 | 39 |
| | D | 75 | 71 | 53 | 52 | 54 |
| | M | 71 | 67 | 65 | 65 | 62 |
| | All | 91 | 98 | 82 | 77 | 85 |
| False positives | G | 25 | 33 | 6 | 19 | 8 |
| | D | 11 | 16 | 18 | 10 | 0 |
| | M | 14 | 12 | 6 | 7 | 15 |
| False negatives | G | 10 | 14 | 29 | 39 | 54 |
| | D | 14 | 12 | 29 | 39 | 46 |
| | M | 11 | 25 | 29 | 29 | 23 |

* G = growth retardation; D = death of conceptus; M = malformation; All = growth, death, or malformations.
SOURCE: Schardein and Keller (1989).

noin, thalidomide, and methotrexate. The monkey was the most sensitive test species for the first three chemicals, while the rabbit was the most sensitive to methotrexate. Based on the NOAEL of the most sensitive test species, human embryos were between 0.9 and approximately 10 times more sensitive.

## Elements of Risk Assessment

The extrapolation of animal test data for developmental toxicity follows two basic directions: one for drugs where exposure is voluntary and usually involves high doses and the other for environmental agents where exposure is generally involuntary and involves low levels. For drugs, a use-in-pregnancy rating is utilized (U.S. FDA, 1979). In this system the letters A, B, C, D, and X are used to classify the evidence that a chemical poses a risk to the human conceptus. For example, drugs are placed in category A if adequate, well-controlled studies in pregnant humans have not demonstrated a risk and in category X (contraindicated for pregnancy) if studies in animals or humans or investigational or postmarketing reports have shown a level of fetal risk that clearly outweighs any possible benefit to the patient. The default category is C (risks cannot be ruled out), which is given when there is a lack of human studies and animal studies are lacking or are positive for fetal risk but the benefits may justify the potential risk. Categories B and D represent areas of relatively lesser or greater concern for risk, respectively. Manson (1994) reviewed the 1992 *Physician's Desk Reference* and found that 7 percent of the 1033 drugs were in category X, 66 percent were in category C, and only 0.7 percent were in category A. The FDA categorization procedure has been criticized (Teratology Society, 1994) for being too reliant on risk-benefit comparisons, especially since the magnitude of risk is often unknown and the benefits are not an issue (e.g., after the drug in question has been taken during early pregnancy and the question is directed to the management of the exposed pregnancy).

For environmental agents, the purpose of the risk assessment process for noncancer endpoints such as developmental toxicity is generally to define the dose, route, timing, and duration of an exposure that induces effects at the lowest level in the most relevant laboratory animal model (U.S. EPA, 1991a and b). The exposure associated with this "critical effect" is then subjected to a variety of safety or uncertainty factors to derive an exposure level for humans that is presumed to be relatively safe (Chap. 4). The principal uncertainty factors include interspecies extrapolation and the possibility of uniquely susceptible subpopulations in the human population. The default value for each of these factors is 10. In the absence of firm evidence on which to base decisions about whether to extrapolate animal test data, certain default assumptions generally are made. They include the following:

1. An agent that produces an adverse developmental effect in experimental animals potentially poses a hazard to humans after sufficient exposure during development.
2. All four manifestations of developmental toxicity (death, structural abnormalities, growth alterations, and functional deficits) are of concern.
3. The types of developmental effects seen in animal studies are not necessarily the same as those which may be produced in humans.
4. The most appropriate species is used to estimate human risk when data are available (in the absence of such data, the most sensitive species is appropriate).
5. In general, a threshold is assumed for the dose-response curve for agents that produce developmental toxicity.

One of the more troubling and subjective aspects of risk assessment for developmental toxicants involves distinguishing adverse effects (defined as an unwanted effect determined to be detrimental to health) from lesser effects which, while different from those observed in control groups, are not considered significant to human health. Considerations relevant to this issue can be categorized into two areas: (1) the observation of the finding and related events in the same or associated experiments and (2) the understanding of the biology of the effect. The interpretation of reduced fetal growth in devel-

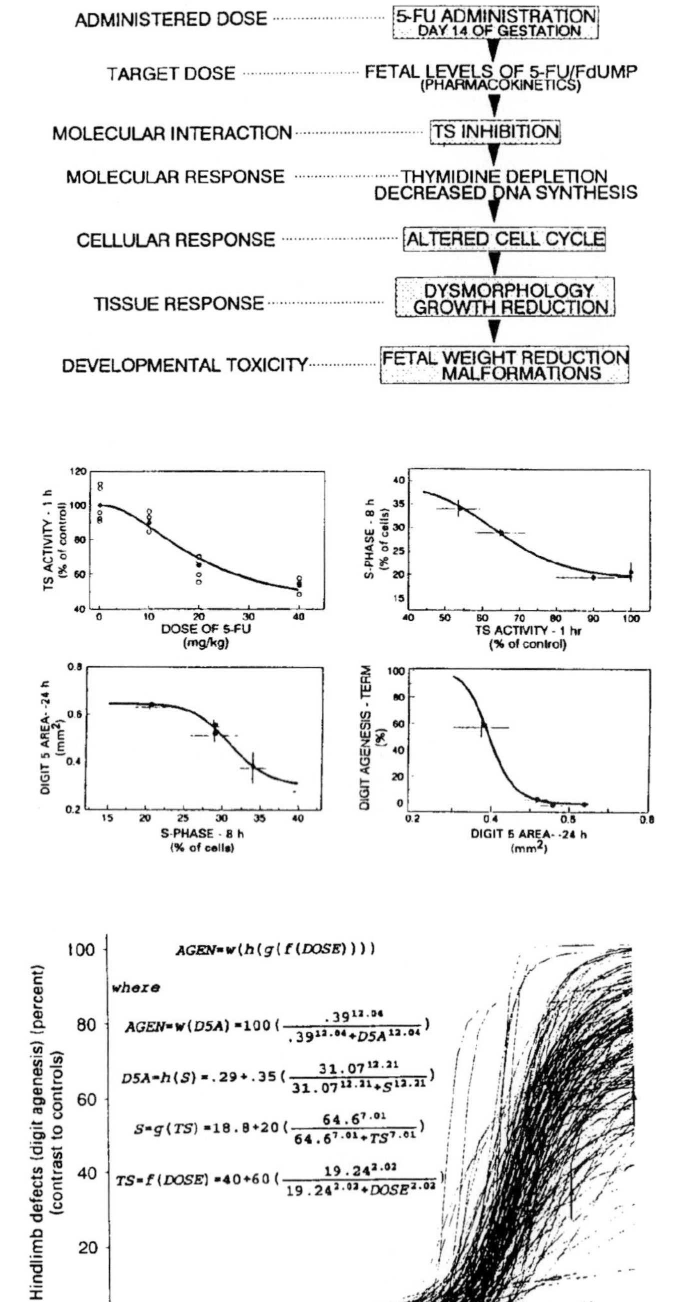


*Figure 10–10. Biologically-based dose-response modeling of the developmental toxicity of 5-fluorouracil (5-FU) after maternal administration on gestation day 14.*

*Top:* Proposed model for the developmental toxicity of 5-FU based on thymidylate synthetase (TS) inhibition, decreased DNA synthesis, cell cycle alterations, and growth deficits and hindlimb dysmorphogenesis. Shaded events were measured experimentally. *Middle:* Relationships between successive endpoints are shown in these four panels (hindlimb bud TS activity versus 5-FU dose, S-phase accumulation versus TS activity, limb digit 5 area at 24 h after dose versus proportion of cells in S phase, and digit agenesis at term versus limb digit 5 area at 24 h). Data were fitted with Hill equations. *Bottom:* Model for induction of hindlimb defects induced by 5-FU, generated by successively applying the individual Hill equations describing the relationships between model endpoints as presented in the middle panels. These individual equations are listed here, and the curves were generated by Monte Carlo simulation to estimate variability around the predicted relationship. The simulation results indicate that variability in the intermediate endpoints can account for differences between the predicted and actual dose responses. AGEN = digit agenesis at term; D5A = digit = area; S = percent of cells in S phase. [Adapted from Shuey et al. (1994).]

opmental toxicity studies illustrates most of these issues. While we have accepted definitions of very low birthweight in humans and understand how intrauterine growth retardation translates to an elevated risk of infant mortality and mental retardation, we do not have similar knowledge for fetal weight in rodents and seldom even know whether reduced fetal weight recorded in prenatal toxicity studies persists beyond birth. Further complicating matters, recent epidemiological evidence suggests that birthweight in humans is inversely associated with cardiovascular disease in adults (Osmond et al., 1993). The standardized mortality ratios (SMRs) for men were 61 for those with birthweights between 9 and 9.5 lb, 80 for those weighing 7 to 7.5 lb, and 96 for those weighing less than 5.5 lb. Importantly, the relationship was not limited to the tails of the distribution of birthweights but was almost linear across the normal range of birthweights. The authors hypothesized that fetal undernutrition is associated with changes in fetal and placental hormones and with altered hormone levels that lead to altered tissue sensitivity and, ultimately, function in the adult. Perhaps these findings will focus attention on subtle postnatal functional deficits and alter our interpretation of modest changes in fetal growth rates.

## New Approaches: The Benchmark Dose and Biologically Based Dose-Response Modeling

**The Benchmark Dose Approach.** The use of safety or uncertainty factors applied to an experimentally derived NOAEL to arrive at a presumed safe level of human exposure is predicated on the risk assessment assumption that a threshold for developmental toxicity exists (see "Principles of Developmental Toxicity," above). The threshold should not be confused with the NOAEL, as this value is dependent entirely on the power of the study and, as will be seen later, is associated with risks on the order of 5 percent over the control incidence in typical studies. Also, the value obtained by the application of uncertainty factors to NOAEL should not be confused with a threshold, as this exposure is only assumed to be without appreciable risk.

The use of NOAEL in the risk assessment process has been criticized for several reasons. For example, because NOAEL is dependent on statistical power to detect pairwise differences between a treated group and a control group, the use of larger sample sizes and more dose groups (which might better characterize the dose-response relationship) can only yield lower NOAELs; thus, better experimental designs are actually penalized by this approach. In addition, the NOAEL is limited to an experimental dose, and an experiment may have to be repeated to develop a NOAEL for risk assessment. A final point relates to the fact that because of variability in

and intrauterine development. *Am J Obstet Gynecol* 148:929–938, 1984.

Fantel AG, Greenaway JC, Juchau MR, Shepard TH: Teratogenic bioactivation of cyclophosphamide in vitro. *Life Sci* 25:67–72, 1979.

Faustman EM: Short-term tests for teratogens. *Mutat Res* 205:355–384, 1988.

Faustman EM, Allen BC, Kavlock RJ, Kimmel CA: Dose response assessment for developmental toxicity: I. Characterization of database and determination of no observed adverse effect levels. *Fundam Appl Toxicol* 23:478–486, 1994.

Ferm VH, Carpenter SJ: Teratogenic effect of cadmium and its inhibition by zinc. *Nature* 216:1123, 1967.

Fisher JW, Whitaker TA, Taylor DH, et al: Physiologically based pharmocokinetic modeling of the pregnant rat: A multiroute exposure model for trichloroethylene and its metabolite, trichloroacetic acid. *Toxicol Appl Pharmacol* 99:395–414, 1989.

Flint OP, Orton TC: An in vitro assay for teratogens with culture of rat embryo midbrain and limb bud cells. *Toxicol Appl Pharmacol* 76:383–395, 1984.

Francis BM, Rogers JM, Sulik KK, et al: Cyclophosphamide teratogenesis: Evidence for compensatory responses to induced cellular toxicity. *Teratology* 42:473–482, 1990.

Francis EZ: Testing of environmental agents for developmental and reproductive toxicity, in Kimmel CA, Buelke-Sam J (eds): *Developmental Toxicology,* 2d ed. New York: Raven Press, 1994, pp 403–428.

Frankos VH: FDA perspectives on the use of teratology data for human risk assessment. *Fundam Appl Toxicol* 5:615–622, 1985.

Fullerton PM, Kermer M: Neuropathy after intake of thalidomide. *Br Med J* 2:855–858, 1961.

Gabrielson JL, Larson KS: Proposals for improving risk assessment in reproductive toxicology. *Pharmacol Toxicol* 66:10–17, 1990.

Gabrielson JL, Paalzow LK: A physiological pharmacokinetic model for morphine disposition in the pregnant rat. *J Pharmacokinet Biopharm* 11:147–163, 1983.

Garbis-Berkvens JM, Peters PWJ: Comparative morphology and physiology of embryonic and fetal membranes, in Nau H, Scott WJ (eds): *Pharmacokinetics in Teratogenesis*, vol 1. Boca Raton, FL: CRC Press, 1987, pp 13–44.

Gaylor DW, Sheehan DM, Young JF, Mattison DR: The threshold dose question in teratogenesis. *Teratology* 38:389–391, 1988.

Geber WF: Developmental effects of chronic maternal audiovisual stress on the rat fetus. *J Embryol Exp Morphol* 16:1–16, 1966.

Geber WF, Anderson TA: Abnormal fetal growth in the fetal albino rat and rabbit induced by maternal stress. *Biol Neonat* 11:209–215, 1967.

Generoso WM, Rutledge JC, Cain KT, et al: Exposure of female mice to ethylene oxide within hours after mating leads to fetal malformations and death. *Mutat Res* 176:269–274, 1987.

Generoso WM, Rutledge JC, Cain KT, et al: Mutagen-induced fetal anomalies and death following treatment of females within hours after mating. *Mutat Res* 199:175–181, 1988.

Gorsuch RL, Key MK: Abnormalities of pregnancy as a function of anxiety and life stress. *Psychosom Med* 36:352–362, 1974.

Graham A, Papoalopulu N, Krumlauf R: The murine and Drosophila homeobox gene complexes have common features of organization and expression. *Cell* 57:367–378, 1989.

Gregg NM: Congenital cataract following German measles in the mother. *Tr Ophtalmol Soc Aust* 3:35–40.

Guenther TM, Mannering GT: Induction of hepatic monooxygenase systems of pregnant rats with phenobarbital and 3-methylcholanthrene. *Biochem Pharmacol* 26:577–584, 1977.

Guzelian PS, Henry CJ, Olin SS (eds): *Similarities and Differences between Children and Adults: Implications for Risk Assessment.* Washington, DC: ILSI Press, 1992.

Hale F: Pigs born without eyeballs. *J Hered* 27:105–106, 1935.

Hales B: Comparison of the mutagenicity of cyclophosphamide and its active metabolites, 4-hydroxycyclophosphamide, phosphoramide mustard and acrolein. *Cancer Res* 42:3018–3021, 1982.

Hales B: Relative mutagenicity and teratogenicity of cyclophosphamide and two of its structural analogs. *Biochem Pharmacol* 32:3791–3795, 1983.

Hall JG: Genetic inprinting: Review and relevance to human diseases. *Ann Hum Genet* 46:857–873, 1990.

Hansen DK, Billings RE: Phenytoin teratogenicity and effects on embryonic and maternal folate metabolism. *Teratology* 31:363–371, 1985.

Hansen DK, Hodes ME: Comparative teratogenicity of phenytoin among several inbred strains of mice. *Teratology* 28:175–179, 1983.

Hardin BD, Becker RJ, Kavlock RJ, et al: Overview and summary: Workshop on the Chernoff/Kavlock preliminary developmental toxicity test. *Teratogenesis Carcinog Mutagen* 7:119–127, 1987.

Harrison ML, Nicol CJ, Wells PJ: Tumor supressor genes and chemical teratogenesis: Benzo[a]pyrene embryopathy and cytochromes p-450 activities in p53-deficient transgenic mice. *Toxicologist* 14:246, 1994.

Hauck R-S, Nau H: The enantiomers of the valproic acid analogue 2-*n*-propylpentyoic acid (4-yn-VPA): Asymmetric synthesis and highly stereoselective teratogenicity in mice. *Pharmaceut Res* 9:850–854, 1992.

Heger W, Klug S, Schmahl H-J, et al: Embryotoxic effects of thalidomide derivatives in the non-human primate *Calithrix jacchus:* III. Teratogenic potency of the EM 12 enantiomers. *Arch Toxicol* 62:205–208, 1988.

Helene C, Toulme JJ: Specific regulation of gene expression by antisense, sense and antigene nucleic acids. *Biochim Biophys Acta* 1049:99–125, 1990.

Helm FC, Frankus E, Friderichs E, et al: Comparative teratological investigation of compounds structurally related to thalidomide. *Arnz Forsch Drug Res* 31:941–949, 1981.

Herbst AL, Cole P, Colton T, et al: Age-incidence and risk of diethylstilbestrol-related clear cell adenocarcinoma of the vagina and cervix. *Am J Obstet Gynecol* 128:43–50, 1977.

Hirsch KS, Scott WJ Jr: Searching for the mechanism of acetazolamide teratogenesis, in Kalter H (ed): *Issues and Reviews in Teratology.* New York: Plenum Press, 1983, vol 1, pp 309–347.

Holladay SD, Luster MI: Developmental immunotoxicology, in Kimmel CA, Buelke-Sam J (eds): *Developmental Toxicology,* 2d ed. New York: Raven Press, 1994, pp 93–117.

Holmes L: Teratogen update: Bendectin. *Teratology* 27:277–281, 1983.

Hytten FE: Physiologic changes in the mother related to drug handling, in Krauer B, Hytten F, del Pozo E (eds): *Drugs and Pregnancy*. New York: Academic Press, 1984, pp 7–17.

Jelovsek FR, Mattison DR, Chen JJ: Prediction of risk for human developmental toxicity: How important are animal studies for hazard identification? *Obstet Gynecol* 74:624–636, 1989.

Johnson EM: A subvertebrate system for rapid determination of potential teratogenic hazards. *J Environ Pathol Toxicol* 4:153-156, 1980.

Johnson EM: Screening for teratogenic hazards: Nature of the problems. *Annu Rev Pharmacol Toxicol* 21:417–429, 1981.

Johnson EM: A review of advances in prescreening for teratogenic hazards, in *Progress in Drug Research.* Basel: Birkhauser, 1985, vol 29, pp 121–154.

Johnson EM, Gabel BEG: Application of the hydra assay for rapid detection of developmental hazards. *J Am Coll Toxicol* 1:57–71, 1982.

Johnson EM, Newman LM, Gabel BEG, et al: An analysis of the Hydra assay's applicability and reliability as a developmental toxicity prescreen. *J Am Coll Toxicol* 7:111–126, 1988.

Jones KL, Smith DW, Ulleland CN, Streissguth AP: Pattern of malformation in offspring of chronic alcoholic mothers. *Lancet* 1:1267–1271, 1973.

Jones KL, Smith DW: Recognition of the fetal alcohol syndrome in early infancy. *Lancet* 2:999–1001, 1973.

Jonsson NA: Chemical structure and teratogenic properties. *Acta Pharm Suec* 9:521–542, 1972.

Juchau MR: Enzymatic bioactivation and inactivation of chemical teratogens and transplacental carcinogens/mutagens, in Juchau MR (ed): *The Biochemical Basis of Chemical Teratogenesis*. New York: Elsevier/North Holland, 1981, pp 63–94.

Juchau MR, Faustman-Watts EM: Pharmacokinetic considerations in the maternal-placental unit. *Clin Obstet Gynecol* 26:379–390, 1983.

Juchau MR, Lee QP, Fantel AG: Xenobiotic biotransformation/bioactivation in organogenesis-stage conceptual tissues: Implications for embryotoxicity and teratogenesis. *Drug Metab Rev* 24:195–238, 1992.

Juriloff DM, Fraser FC: Genetic maternal effects on cleft lip frequency in A/J and CL/Fr mice. *Teratology* 21:167–175, 1980.

Kalter H: The history of the A family of mice and the biology of its congenital malformations. *Teratology* 20:213–232, 1979.

Kavlock RJ: Structure-activity approaches in the screening of environmental agents for developmental toxicity: *Reprod Toxicol* 7:113–116, 1993.

Kavlock RJ, Allen BC, Faustman EM, Kimmel CA: Dose response assessment for developmental toxicity. IV. Benchmark doses for fetal weight changes. *Fundam Appl Toxicol* 26: 211–222, 1995.

Kavlock RJ, Chernoff N, Rogers EH: The effect of acute maternal toxicity on fetal development in the mouse. *Teratogenesis Carcinog Mutagen* 5:3–13, 1985.

Kavlock RJ, Greene JA, Kimmel GL, et al: Activity profiles of developmental toxicity: Design considerations and pilot implementation. *Teratology* 43:159–185, 1991.

Keen CL, Peters JM, Hurley, LS: The effect of valproic acid on $^{65}$Zn distribution in the pregnant rat. *J Nutr* 119:607–611, 1989.

Keen CL, Bendich A, Willhite CC (eds): *Maternal Nutrition and Pregnancy Outcome. Ann NY Acad Sci* 678:1–372, 1993.

Kelsey FO: Thalidomide update: Regulatory aspects. *Teratology* 38:221–226, 1988.

Kessel M, Balling R, Gruss P: Variations of cervical vertebrae after expression of a Hox-1.1 transgene in mice. *Cell* 61:301–308, 1990.

Khera KS: Maternal toxicity—a possible factor in fetal malformations in mice. *Teratology* 29:411–416, 1984.

Khera KS: Maternal toxicity: A possible etiological factor in embryo/fetal deaths and fetal malformations of rodent-rabbit species. *Teratology* 31:129–153, 1985.

Khoury MJ, Erickson JD, James LM: Maternal factors in cleft lip with or without palate: Evidence from interracial crosses in the United States. *Teratology* 27:351–357, 1983.

Khoury MJ, Holtzman NA: On the ability of birth defects monitoring systems to detect new teratogens. *Am J Epidemiol* 126:136–143, 1987.

Khoury MJ, James LM, Flanders D, Erickson JD: Interpretation of recurring weak associations obtained from epidemiologic studies of suspected human teratogens. *Teratology* 46:69–77, 1992.

Khoury MJ, James LM, Lynberg MC: Quantitative analysis of associations between birth defects and suspected human teratogens. *Am J Med Genet* 40:500–505, 1991.

Kimmel CA, Cook RO, Staples RE: Teratogenic potential of noise in rats and mice. *Toxicol Appl Pharmacol* 36:239–245, 1976.

Kimmel CA, Young JF: Correlating pharmacokinetics and teratogenic endpoints. *Fundam Appl Toxicol* 3:250–255, 1983.

Klaassen CD, Lehman-McKeeman LD: Induction of metallothionein. *J Amer Coll Toxicol* 8:1315–1321, 1989.

Kochhar DM: Teratogenic activity of retinoic acid. *Acta Pathol Microbiol Immuno Scand* 70:398–404, 1967.

Kotch LE, Sulik KK: Experimental fetal alcohol syndrome: Proposed pathogenic basis for a variety of associated facial and brain anomalies. *Am J Med Genet* 44:168–176.

Krauer B: Physiological changes and drug disposition during pregnancy, in Nau H, Scott WJ (eds): *Pharmacokinetics in Teratogenesis.* Boca Raton, FL: CRC Press, 1987, vol 1, pp 3–12.

Krumlauf R: *Hox* genes and pattern formation in the branchial region of the vertebrate head. *Trends Genet* 9:106–112, 1993.

Lammer EJ: Retinoids—interspecies comparisons and clinical results, in Sundwall A, Danielsson BR, Hagberg O, et al (eds): *Developmental Toxicology—Preclinical and Clinical Data in Retrospect,* Stockholm: Tryckgruppen, 1992, pp 105–109.

Lammer EJ, Chen DT, Hoar RM, et al: Retinoic acid induced embryopathy. *N Engl J Med* 313:837–841, 1985.

Lammer EJ, Sever LE, Oakley GP Jr: Teratogen update: Valproic acid. *Teratology* 35:465–473, 1987.

Lau C, Cameron AM, Rogers JM, et al: Development of biologically based dose-response models: Correlations between developmental toxicity of 5-fluorouracil (5-FU) and its inhibition of thymidylate synthetase (TS) activity in the rat embryo. *Teratology* 45:457, 1992.

Lau C, Kavlock RJ: Functional toxicity in the developing heart, lung and kidney, in Kimmel CA, Buelke-Sam J (eds): *Developmental Toxicology,* 2d ed. New York: Raven Press, 1994, pp 119–188.

Lavin M, Watters D (eds): *Programmed Cell Death: The Cellular and Molecular Biology of Apoptosis.* Chur, Switzerland: Harwood, 1993.

Lenz W: Kindliche Missbildungen nach Medikament-Einnahme während der gravidität? *Dtsch Med Wochenschr* 86:2555–2556, 1961.

Lenz W: Das thalidomid-syndrom. *Fortschr Med* 81:148–153, 1963.

Lenz W: A short history of thalidomide embryopathy. *Teratology* 38:203–215, 1988.

Levin AA, Miller RK: Fetal toxicity of cadmium in the rat: Maternal vs. fetal injections. *Teratology* 22:1–5, 1980.

Lieber CS, DiCarli LM: The feeding of alcohol in liquid diets: Two decades of applications and 1982 update. *Alcohol Clin Exp Res* 6:523–531, 1982.

Little RE: Moderate alcohol use during pregnancy and decreased infant birth weight. *Am J Publ Health* 67:1154–1156, 1977.

Little SA, Mirkes PE: Relationship of DNA damage and embryotoxicity induced by 4-hydroperoxydechlorocyclophosphamide in postimplantation rat embryos. *Teratology* 41: 223–231, 1990.

Little SA, Mirkes PE: Effects of 4-hydroperoxycyclophosphamide (4-OOH-CP) and 4-hydroperoxydechlorocyclophosphamide (4-OOH-deClCP) on the cell cycle of postimplantation rat embryos. *Teratology* 45:163–173, 1992.

Lohnes D, Mark M, Mendelsohn C, et al: Function of the retinoic acid receptors (RARs) during development: I. Craniofacial and skeletal abnormalities in RAR double mutants. *Development* 120:2723–2748, 1994.

Luecke RH, Wosilait WD, Pearce BA, Young JF: A physiologically based pharmacokinetics computer model for human pregnancy. *Teratology* 49:90–103, 1994.

Lutiger B, Graham K, Einarson TR, Koren G: Relationship between gestational cocaine use and pregnancy outcome: A meta-analysis. *Teratology* 44:405–414, 1991.

Lynch DW, Schuler RL, Hood RD, Davis DG: Evaluation of Drosophila for screening developmental toxicants: Test results with eighteen chemicals and presentation of new Drosophila bioassay. *Teratogenisis Carcinog Mutagen* 11:147–173, 1991.

MacAuley AM, Werb Z, Mirkes PE: Characterization of the unusually rapid cell cycles during rat gastrulation. *Development* 117:873–883, 1993.

MacDonald H, Tobin JOH: Congenital cytomegalovirus infection: A collaborative study on epidemiological, clinical and laboratory findings. *Dev Med Child Neurol* 20:271–282, 1978.

MacNeish JD, Scott WJ, Potter SS: Legless, a novel mutation found in PHT1-1 transgenic mice. *Science* 241:837–839, 1988.

Manson JM: Testing of pharmaceutical agents for reproductive toxicity, in Kimmel CA, Buelke-Sam J (eds): *Developmental Toxicology,* 2d ed. New York: Raven Press, 1994, pp 379–402.

Markert CL, Petters RM: Manufactured hexaparental mice show that

adults are derived from three embryonic cells. *Science* 202:56–58, 1978.

Marshall H, Nonchev S, Sham MH, et al: Retinoic acid alters hindbrain Hox code and induces transformation of rhombomeres 2/3 into a 4/5 identity. *Nature* 360:737–741, 1992.

Mattison DR, Blann E, Malek A: Physiological alterations during pregnancy: Impact on toxicokinetics. *Fundam Appl Toxicol* 16: 215–218, 1991.

McBride WG: Thalidomide and congenital anomalies. *Lancet* 2:1358, 1961.

Mendelsohn C, Lohnes D, Décimo, D, et al: Function of the retinoic acid receptors (RARs) during development: II. Multiple abnormalities at various stages of organogenesis in RAR double mutants. *Development* 120:2749–2771, 1994.

Merker H-J, Heger W, Sames K, et al: Embryotoxic effects of thalidomide derivatives in the non-human primate *Calithrix jacchus*: I. Effects of 3-(1,3-dihydro-1-oxo-2H-isoindol2-yl)-2,6-dioxopiperidine (EM 12) on skeletal development. *Arch Toxicol* 61:165–179, 1988.

Millicovsky G, DeSesso JM: Differential embryonic cardiovascular responses to acute maternal uterine ischemia: An in vivo microscopic study of rabbit embryos with either intact or clamped umbilical cords. *Teratology* 22:335–343, 1980a.

Millicovsky G, DeSesso JM: Cardiovascular alterations in rabbit embryos in situ after a teratogenic dose of hydroxyurea: An in vivo microscopic study. *Teratology* 22:115–124, 1980b.

Millicovsky G, DeSesso JM, Kleinman LI, Clark KE: Effects of hydroxyurea on hemodynamics of pregnant rabbits: A maternally mediated mechanism of embryotoxicity. *Am J Obstet Gynecol* 140:747–752, 1981.

Millicovsky G, Johnston MC: Maternal hyperoxia greatly reduces the incidence of phenytoin-induced cleft lip and palate in A/J mice. *Science* 212:671–672, 1981.

Milunsky A, Ulcickas M, Rothman KJ, et al: Maternal heat exposure and neural tube defects. *JAMA* 268:882–885, 1992.

Mirkes PE: Simultaneous banding of rat embryo DNA, RNA and protein in cesium trifluoroacetate gradients. *Anal Biochem* 148:376–383, 1985a.

Mirkes PE: Cyclophosphamide teratogenesis: A review. *Teratogenesis Carcinog Mutagen* 5:75–88, 1985b.

Mirkes PE: Molecular and metabolic aspects of cyclophosphamide teratogenesis, in Welsch F (ed): *Approaches to Elucidate Mechanisms in Teratogenesis.* Washington, DC: Hemisphere, 1987, pp 123–147.

Mirkes PE, Fantel AG, Greenaway JC, Shepard TH: Teratogenicity of cyclophosphamide metabolites: Phosphoramide mustard, acrolein, and 4-ketocyclophosphamide on rat embryos cultured in vitro. *Toxicol Appl Pharmacol* 58:322–330, 1981.

Mirkes PE, Greenaway JC, Hilton J, Brundrett R: Morphological and biochemical aspects of monofunctional phosphoramide mustard teratogenicity in rat embryos cultured in vitro. *Teratology* 32:241–249, 1985.

Mirkes PE, Ricks JL, Pascoe-Mason JM: Cell cycle analysis in the cardiac and neuroepithelial tissues of day 10 rat embryos and the effects of phosphoramide mustard, the major teratogenic metabolite of cyclophosphamide. *Teratology* 39:115–120, 1989.

Moore NW, Adams CE, Rowson LEA: Developmental potential of single blastomeres of the rabbit egg. *J Reprod Fertil* 17:527–531, 1968.

MRC Vitamin Study Research Group [Prepared by Wald N with assistance from Sneddon J, Densem J, Frost C, Stone R]: Prevention of neural tube defects: Results of the MRC vitamin study. *Lancet* 338:132–137, 1991.

Nau H: Species differences in pharmacokinetics and drug teratogenesis. *Environ Health Perspect* 70:113–129, 1986.

Nau H: Physicochemical and structural properties regulating placenta drug transfer, in Polin RA, Fox WW (eds): *Fetal and Neonatal Physiology.* New York: Saunders, 1992, vol 1, pp 130–149.

Nau H, Chahoud I, Dencker L, et al: Teratogenicity of vitamin A and retinoids, in Blomhoff R (ed): *Vitamin A in Health and Disease.* New York: Marcel Dekker, 1994, pp 615–664.

Nau H, Hauck R-S, Ehlers K: Valproic acid induced neural tube defects in mouse and human: Aspects of chirality, alternative drug development, pharmacokinetics and possible mechanisms. *Pharmacol Toxicol* 69:310–321, 1991.

Nau H, Scott WJ: Weak acids may act as teratogens by accumulating in the basic milieu of the early mammalian embryo. *Nature* 323: 276–278, 1986.

Nau H, Scott WJ: *Pharmacokinetics in Teratogenesis,* vols 1 and 2. Boca Raton, FL: CRC Press, 1987.

Nawrot PS, Cook RO, Hamm CW: Embryotoxicity of broadband high-frequency noise in the CD-1 mouse. *J Toxicol Environ Health* 8:151–157, 1981.

Nawrot PS, Cook RO, Staples RE: Embryotoxicity of various noise stimuli in the mouse. *Teratology* 22:279–289, 1980.

Neims AH, Warner M, Loughnan PM, Aranda JV: Developmental aspects of the hepatic cytochrome $P_{450}$ monooxygenase system. *Ann Rev Pharmacol Toxicol* 16:427–444, 1976.

Nelson CJ, Holson JF: Statistical analysis of teratologic data: Problems and recent advances. *J Environ Pathol Toxicol* 2:187–199, 1978.

Netzloff ML, Streiff RR, Frias JL, Rennert, OM: Folate antagonism following teratogenic exposure to diphenylhydantoin. *Teratology* 19:45–50, 1979.

Neubert D: In-vitro techniques for assessing teratogenic potential, in Dayan AD, Paine AJ (eds): *Advances in Applied Toxicology*. London: Taylor and Francis, 1989, pp 191–211.

Neubert D, Zens P, Rothenwallner A, Merker H-J: A survey of the embryotoxic effects of TCDD in mammalian species. *Environ Health Perspect* 5:63–79, 1973.

Neubert R, Nogueira AC, Neubert D: Thalidomide derivatives and the immune system: I. Changes in the pattern of integrin receptors and other surface markers on T lymphocyte subpopulations of marmoset blood. *Arch Toxicol* 67:1–17, 1993.

New DAT: Whole embryo culture and the study of mammalian embryos during organogenesis. *Biol Rev* 5:81–94, 1978.

Newman CGH: Teratogen update: Clinical aspects of thalidomide embryopathy—a continuing preoccupation. *Teratology* 32:133–144, 1985.

Newman LM, Johnson EM, Staples RE: Assessment of the effectiveness of animal developmental toxicity testing for human safety. *Reprod Toxicol* 7:359–390, 1993.

O'Flaherty EJ, Scott WJ, Shreiner C, Beliles RP: A physiologically based kinetic model of rat and mouse gestation: Disposition of a weak acid. *Toxicol Appl Pharmacol* 112:245–256, 1992.

Olshan A, Mattison D (eds): *Male-Mediated Developmental Toxicity.* New York: Plenum Press, 1995.

Oltvai ZN, Korsmeyer SJ: Checkpoints of dueling dimers foil death wishes. *Cell* 79:189–192, 1994.

Osmond C, Barker DJP, Winter PD, et al: Early growth and death from cardiovascular disease in women. *Br Med J* 307:1519–1524, 1993.

Page K, Abramovich D, Aggett P, et al: Uptake of zinc by human placental microvillus border membranes and characterization of the effects of cadmium on the process. *Placenta* 13:151–162, 1992.

Palmer AK: Implementing the ICH guideline for reproductive toxicity, in *Current Issues in Drug Development* II. Huntington, United Kingdom: Huntington Research Centre, 1993, pp 1–21.

Parizek J: Vascular changes at sites of estrogen biosynthesis produced by parenteral injection of cadmium salts: The destruction of the placenta by cadmium salts. *J Reprod Fertil* 7:263–265, 1964.

Platzek T, Bochert G, Scheider W, Neubert D: Embryotoxicity induced by alkylating agents: Ethylmethanesulfonate as a teratogen in mice—a model for dose-response relationships of alkylating agents. *Arch Toxicol* 51:1–25, 1982.

Platzek T, Bochert G, Rahm U: Embryotoxicity induced by alkylating agents. Teratogenicity of acetoxymethyl-methylnitrosamine: Dose-response reltaionship, application route dependency and phase specificity. *Arch Toxicol* 52:42–69, 1983.

Poskanzer D, Herbst AL: Epidemiology of vaginal adenosis and adenocarcinoma associated with exposure to stilbestrol in utero. *Cancer* 39:1892–1895 1977.

Renault J-Y, Melcion C, Cordier A: Limb bud cell culture for in vitro teratogen screening: Validation of an improved assessment method using 51 compounds. *Teratogenesis Carcinog Mutagen* 9:83–96 1989.

Robson JM, Sullivan FM: Teratology, in Boulard E, Goulding R (eds): *Modern Trends in Toxicology*. New York: Appleton, 1968, pp. 86–106.

Rodier PM, Cohen IR, Buelke-Sam J: Developmental neurotoxicology: Neuroendocrine manifestations of CNS insult, in Kimmel CA, Buelke-Sam J (eds): *Developmental Toxicology* 2d ed. New York: Raven Press, 1994, pp 65–92.

Rogers JM: Comparison of maternal and fetal toxic dose responses in mammals. *Teratogenesis Carcinog Mutagen* 7:297–306, 1987.

Rogers JM, Barbee BD, Rehnberg BF: Critical periods of sensitivity for the developmental toxicity of inhaled methanol. *Teratology* 47: 395, 1993.

Rogers JM, Mole ML, Chernoff N, et al: The developmental toxicity of inhaled methanol in the CD-1 mouse, with quantitative dose-response modeling for estimation of benchmark doses. *Teratology* 47:175–188, 1993.

Rosa FW: Teratogenicity of isotretinoin. *Lancet* 2:513, 1983.

Sadler TW, Hunter ES: Principles of abnormal development: Past, present and future, in Kimmel CA, Buelke-Sam J (eds): *Developmental Toxicology* 2d ed. New York: Raven Press, 1994, pp 53–63.

Sadler TW, Warner CW: Use of whole embryo culture for evaluating toxicity and teratogenicity. *Pharmacol Rev* 36:145S–150S, 1984.

Samarawickrama GP, Webb M: Acute effects of cadmium on the pregnant rat and embryo-fetal development. *Environ Health Perspect* 28:245–249, 1979.

Sanes JR, Rubenstein LR, Nicolas JF: Use of a recombinant retrovirus to study postimplantation cell lineage in mouse embryos. *EMBO J* 5:3133–3142, 1986.

Sanyal MK, Kitchin KT, Dixon RL: Anomalous development of rat embryos cultured in vitro with cyclophosphamide and microsomes. *Pharmacologist* 21:A231, 1979.

Sanyal MK, Naftolin F: In vitro development of the mammalian embryo. *J Exp Zool* 228:235–251, 1983.

Scanlon JW: The neuroteratology of cocaine: Background, theory, and clinical implications. *Reprod Toxicol* 5:89–98, 1991.

Schardein JL: *Chemically Induced Birth Defects*, 2d ed. New York: Marcel Dekker, 1993.

Schardein JL, Keller KA: Potential human developmental toxicants and the role of animal testing in their identification and characterization. *CRC Crit Rev Toxicol* 19:251–339, 1989.

Schumacher HJ: Chemical structure and teratogenic properties, in Shepard T, Miller R, Marois M (eds): *Methods for Detection of Environmental Agents That Produce Congenital Defects*. New York: American Elsevier, 1975, pp 65–77.

Schwetz BA, Morrissey RE, Welsch F, Kavlock RJ: In vitro teratology. *Environ Health Perspect* 94:265–268, 1991.

Seller MJ, Perkins KJ, Adinolfi M: Differential response of heterozygous curly-tail mouse embryos to vitamin A teratogenesis depending on maternal genotype. *Teratology* 28:123, 1983.

Setzer RW, Rogers JM: Assessing developmental hazard: The reliability of the A/D ratio. *Teratology* 44:653–665, 1991.

Sever JL: Rubella as a teratogen. *Adv Teratol* 2:127–138, 1967.

Shenefelt RE: Morphogenesis of malformations in hamsters caused by retinoic acid: Relation to dose and stage of treatment. *Teratology* 5:103–118, 1972.

Shepard TH: *Catalog of Teratogenic Agents,* 7th ed. Baltimore: Johns Hopkins University Press, 1992.

Shuey DL, Lau C, Logsdon TR, et al: Biologically based dose-response modeling in developmental toxicology: biochemical and cellular sequelae of 5-fluorouracil exposure in the developing rat. *Toxicol Appl Pharmacol* 126:129–144, 1994.

Slikker W, Miller RK: Placental metabolism and transfer: Role in developmental toxicology, in Kimmel CA, Buelke-Sam J (eds): *Developmental Toxicology,* 2d ed. New York: Raven Press, 1994, pp 245–283.

Smith JL, Gesteland KM, Schoenwolf GC: Prospective fate map of the mouse primitive streak at 7.5 days of gestation. *Dev Dynam* 201:279–289, 1994.

Smith MK, Kimmel GL, Kochhar DM, et al: A selection of candidate compounds for in vitro teratogenesis test validation. *Teratogenesis Carcinog Mutagen* 3:461–480, 1983.

Snow MHL, Tam PPL: Is compensatory growth a complicating factor in mouse teratology? *Nature* 279:555–557, 1979.

Sorrell TL, Graziano JH: Effect of oral cadmium exposure during pregnancy on maternal and fetal zinc metabolism in the rat. *Toxicol Appl Pharmacol* 102:537–545, 1990.

Steele VE, Morrissey RE, Elmore EL, et al: Evaluation of two in vitro assays to screen for potential developmental toxicants. *Fundam Appl Toxicol* 11:673–684, 1988.

Stephens TD: Proposed mechanisms of action in thalidomide embryopathy. *Teratology* 38:229–239, 1988.

Stockard CR: Developmental rate and structural expression: An experimental study of twins, "double monsters," and single deformities, and the interaction among embryonic organs during their origin and development. *Am J Anat* 28:115–277, 1921.

Stott DH: Follow-up study from birth of the effects of prenatal stress. *Dev Med Child Neurol* 15:770–787, 1973.

Streissguth AP, Aase JM, Clarren SK, et al: Fetal alcohol syndrome in adolescents and adults. *JAMA* 265:1961–1967, 1991a.

Streissguth AP, Barr HM, Olson HC, et al: Drinking during pregnancy decreases word attack and arithmetic scores on standardized tests: Adolescent data from a population-based prospective study. *Alcohol Clin Exp Res* 18:248–254, 1994a.

Streissguth AP, Randels SP, Smith DF: A test-retest study of intelligence in patients with fetal alcohol syndrome: implications for care. *J Am Acad Child Adolesc Psychiatry* 30:584–587, 1991b.

Streissguth AP, Sampson PD, Olson HC, et al: Maternal drinking during pregnancy: Attention and short-term memory in 14-year-old offspring—a longitudinal prospective study. *Alcohol Clin Exp Res* 18:202–218, 1994b.

Sulik KK, Cook CS, Webster WS: Teratogens and craniofacial malformations: Relationships to cell death. *Development* 103(Suppl): 213–231, 1988.

Sulik KK, Johnston MC: Sequence of developmental alterations following acute ethanol exposure in mice: Craniofacial features of the fetal alcohol syndrome. *Am J Anat* 166:257–269, 1983.

Sulik KK, Johnston MC, Webb MA: Fetal alcohol syndrome: Embryogenesis in a mouse model. *Science* 214:936–938, 1981.

Takeuchi IK: Teratogenic effects of methylnitrosourea on pregnant mice before implantation. *Experientia* 40:879–881, 1984.

Taubeneck MW, Daston GP, Rogers JM, Keen CL: Altered maternal zinc metabolism following exposure to diverse developmental toxicants. *Reprod Toxicol* 8:25–40, 1994.

Taussig HB: A study of the German outbreak of phocomelia: The thalidomide syndrome. *JAMA* 180:1106, 1962.

Teratology Society: Recommendations for isotretinoin use in women of childbearing potential. *Teratology* 44:1–6, 1991.

Teratology Society: FDA classification system of drugs for teratogenic risk. *Teratology* 49:446–447, 1994.

Thompson CJS, *Mystery and Lore of Monsters*. London: Williams and Norgate, 1930.

Uphill PF, Wilkins SR, Allen JA: In vitro micromass teratogen test: Results from a blind trial of 25 compounds. *Toxicol In Vitro* 4:623–626, 1990.

U.S. Environmental Protection Agency: Toxic Substance Control Act Testing Guidelines. Final Rules: Preliminary developmental toxicity screen. *Federal Register* 50:39428–39429, 1985.

U.S. Environmental Protection Agency: Guidelines for Developmental Toxicity Risk Assessment; Notice. *Federal Register* 56:63798–63826, 1991a.

U.S. Environmental Protection Agency: *Pesticide Assessment Guidelines, subdivision F, Hazard Evaluation: Human and domestic animals, addendum 10: Neurotoxicity*. Series 81, 82, and 83. EPA 540/09-91-123 PB 91-154617, 1991b.

U.S. Food and Drug Administration: *Guidelines for Reproduction Studies for Safety Evaluation of Drugs for Human Use*. Rockville, MD: 1966.

U.S. Food and Drug Administration: Labeling and prescription drug advertizing: Content and format for labeling for human prescription drugs. *Federal Register* 44:37434–37467, 1979.

U.S. Food and Drug Administration: International Conference on Harmonization: Guideline on Detection of Toxicity to Reproduction for Medicinal Products, Availability, Notice. *Federal Register* 59:48746–48752, 1994.

Volfe JJ: Effects of cocaine on the fetus. *N Engl J Med* 327:399–407, 1992.

Wald N: Folic acid and the prevention of neural tube defects, in Keen CL, Bendich A, Willhite CC (eds): *Maternal Nutrition and Pregnancy Outcome. Ann NY Acad Sci* 678:112–129, 1993.

Warkany J, Nelson, RC: Appearance of skeletal abnormalities in the offspring of rats reared on a deficient diet. *Science* 92:383–384, 1940.

Warkany J: Teratology: Spectrum of a science, in Kalter H (ed): *Issues and Reviews in Teratology*. New York: Plenum Press, 1983, vol 1, pp 19–31.

Warkany J: Manifestations of prenatal nutritional deficiency. *Vitam Horm* 3:73–103, 1945.

Warkany J: Development of experimental mammalian teratology, in Wilson JG, Warkany J (eds): *Teratology: Principles and Techniques*. Chicago: U. of Chicago Press, 1965, pp 1–11.

Warkany J: History of teratology, in Wilson JG (ed): *Handbook of Teratology*. New York: Plenum Press, 1977, vol 1, pp 3–45.

Warkany J: Teratogen update: Hyperthermia. *Teratology* 33:365–371, 1986.

Warkany J, Schraffenberger E: Congenital malformations induced in rats by roentgen rays. *AJR* 57:455–463, 1944.

Watkinson WP, Millicovsky G: Effects of phenytoin on maternal heart rate in A/J mice: Possible role in teratogenesis. *Teratology* 28:1–8 1983.

Weaver TE, Scott WJ Jr: Acetazolamide teratogenesis: Association of maternal respiratory acidosis and ectrodactyly in C57BL/6J mice. *Teratology* 30:187–193, 1984a.

Weaver TE, Scott WJ Jr: Acetazolamide teratogenesis: Interactions of maternal metabolic and respiratory acidosis in the induction of ectrodactyly in C57BL/6J mice. *Teratology* 30:195–202, 1984b.

Welsch F: Short term methods of assessing developmental toxicity hazard, in Kalter H (ed): *Issues and Review in Teratology*. New York: Plenum Press, 1990, vol 5, pp 115–153.

White E: Death defying acts: A meeting review on apoptosis. *Genes Dev* 7:2277–2284, 1993.

Wilcox AJ, Weinberg CR, O'Connor JF, et al: Incidence of early loss of pregnancy. *N Engl J Med* 319:189–194, 1988.

Wilson JG: Experimental studies on congenital malformations. *J Chronic Dis* 10:111–130, 1959.

Wilson JG: *Environment and Birth Defects*. New York: Academic Press, 1973.

Wilson JG: Embryotoxicity of drugs in man, in Wilson JG, Fraser FC (eds): *Handbook of Teratology*. New York: Plenum Press, 1977, pp 309–355.

Wilson JG, Roth CB, Warkany J: An analysis of the syndrome of malformations induced by maternal vitamin A deficiency: Effects of restoration of vitamin A at various times during gestation. *Am J Anat* 92:189–217, 1953.

Zakany J, Tuggle CK, Nguyen-Huu CM: The use of *lacZ* gene fusions in the studies of mammalian development: Developmental regulation of mammalian homeobox genes in the CNS. *J Physiol (Paris)* 84:21–26, 1990.

# UNIT 4

# TARGET ORGAN TOXICITY

# CHAPTER 11

# TOXIC RESPONSES OF THE BLOOD

*Roger P. Smith*

For many years hematology was considered to involve the study of only the formed elements of the blood: red cells, white cells, and platelets. An immense body of morphological information has accrued from the microscopic study of smears of peripheral blood (Bessis, 1977). The formed elements constitute a complex organ with a mass equivalent to that of the liver. Gradually, hematology expanded to include other parts of the system, such as bone marrow, spleen, lymph nodes, and reticuloendothelial tissue (phagocytic macrophages in the reticulum of various organs and in the lining of some sinuses). Obviously, the formed elements have a functional relationship with blood plasma and with the heart and lungs. Most of the biochemical and hematologically normal values used in this chapter apply to humans; Mitruka and Rawnsley (1977) have compiled an extensive anthology of biochemical and hematologic values for laboratory animals. Less elaborate compendiums are also available (Burns and de Lannoy, 1966; Calsey and King, 1980) that include data on proteins, enzymes, electrolytes, and other constituents of plasma.

## HEMATOPOIESIS

In the human fetus, several organs are sequentially involved in the production of blood cells (Fig. 11-1). For a brief period, the yolk sac produces nucleated red cells containing an embryonic hemoglobin designated as $(\alpha^{2+}\varepsilon^{2+})_2$. Subsequently, red cells are supplied by the liver, the spleen, and eventually the bone marrow. The liver is also the first organ that produces white cells and platelets. Hepatic red cells are not nucleated but contain fetal hemoglobin, $(\alpha^{2+}\gamma^{2+})_2$. The oxygen affinity of human fetal blood is higher than that of human adult blood, and this helps the fetus extract oxygen from the maternal circulation (see below).

At birth, only the marrow produces red blood cells. A slow "switchover" from the synthesis of fetal to adult hemoglobin, $(\alpha^{2+}\beta^{2+})_2$, begins at that time; it is usually complete by the fourth to sixth month of age. Up to about age 4 years, hepatic and splenic red cell production can be reactivated in response to the hypoxic demands associated with normal growth, but beyond that age, these extramedullary sites are activated only in pathophysiological states. For example, the spleen is reactivated to serve as a reserve source of red cells in rats and mice exposed to high altitude (Ou et al., 1980), but in most mammals it cannot support life after bone marrow failure. Thus, bone marrow damage is always a grave threat to survival. It is also abnormal to find nucleated red cells in the systemic circulation of adult mammals. However, birds, fish, reptiles, and amphibians always have nucleated red cells in peripheral blood (Prankerd, 1961) because the cells are formed inside blood vessels instead of in bone marrow (see below).

### The Bone Marrow

Bone marrow contains stem cells, the immature precursors of the formed elements of the blood (Figure 11-2). This multipotential stem cell pool is stimulated to differentiate into unipotential, or committed, cells that eventually mature into red cells (erythrocytes), platelets (thrombocytes), or one of several series of white cells (leukocytes). Decreased numbers of these elements in peripheral blood as determined by actual counts, usually with an electronic cell counter, are referred to, respectively, as anemia, thrombocytopenia, and leukopenia. Stimulation of the stem cell pool is carried out by bloodborne factors called *poietins* or *colony-stimulating factors*. It is likely that each circulating cell type has one or more stimulating factors.

*Erythropoiesis* refers to the process by which red cells are produced. Control over the rate of erythropoiesis is exerted primarily through the activity of a plasma hormone, *erythropoietin*. The kidney is critical in the production of erythropoietin after birth, but in the fetus, erythropoietin is produced by

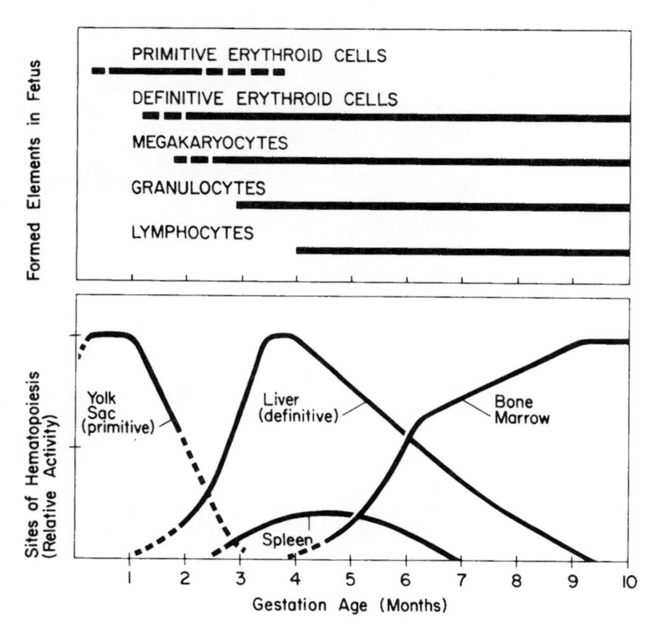


***Figure 11–1. Sites of hematopoiesis during human fetal development and the sequence of appearance of formed elements of the blood in the systemic circulation.***

Broken lines indicate doubt about the precise timing. The yolk sac produces primitive erythroid cells. The liver, spleen, and bone marrow produce definitive erythroid cells. [From Rifkind et al. (1980).]

the liver. Synthesis is stimulated by hypoxia, and it appears that the oxygen sensor is a heme protein. It has been hypothesized that when the oxygen tension in kidney decreases, the sensor is converted to its deoxyconformation, which triggers increased expression of the erythropoietin gene. As the oxygen tension rises, the sensor binds oxygen and the stimulus for erythropoietin synthesis is suppressed (Goldberg et al., 1988).

In the marrow, erythropoietin acts on the differentiation process at the stage in which a stem cell is converted to a proerythroblast (Fig. 11-2). Therefore, erythropoietin may be thought of as regulating the size of the pool of committed red cells. After several additional stages, an immature red cell is released from the marrow as a reticulocyte. This occurs in specialized marrow vessels (marrow sinuses) in which the walls consist of attenuated endothelium. Oddly, the reticulocyte passes through the cytoplasm of a single endothelial cell instead of through the space between cells. If the cell has not already actively extruded its nucleus, it is pitted out during this process (Fig. 11-3). This is the first in a long series of deformations that the cell must undergo during its life span. Thus, the endothelium forms a barrier that can exert considerable control over what enters the systemic circulation (bone marrow–blood barrier). The cell still possesses an endoplasmic reticulum (hence its name) and can synthesize small amounts of hemoglobin. Systems for aerobic metabolism are still func-

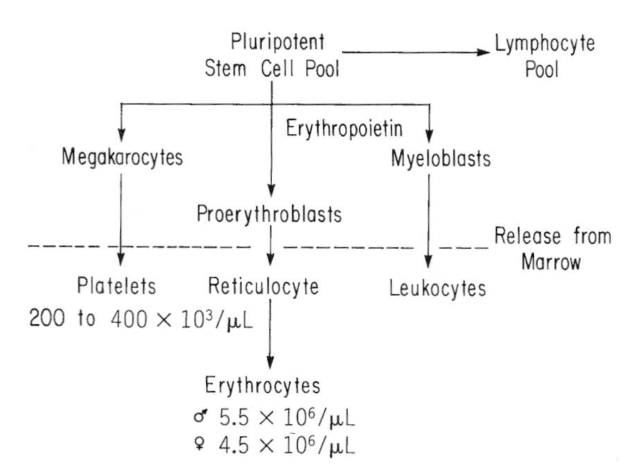


***Figure 11–2. Bone marrow differentiation into the formed elements of peripheral blood.***

See Fig. 11-4 for further differentiation and classification of lymphocytes and leukocytes.

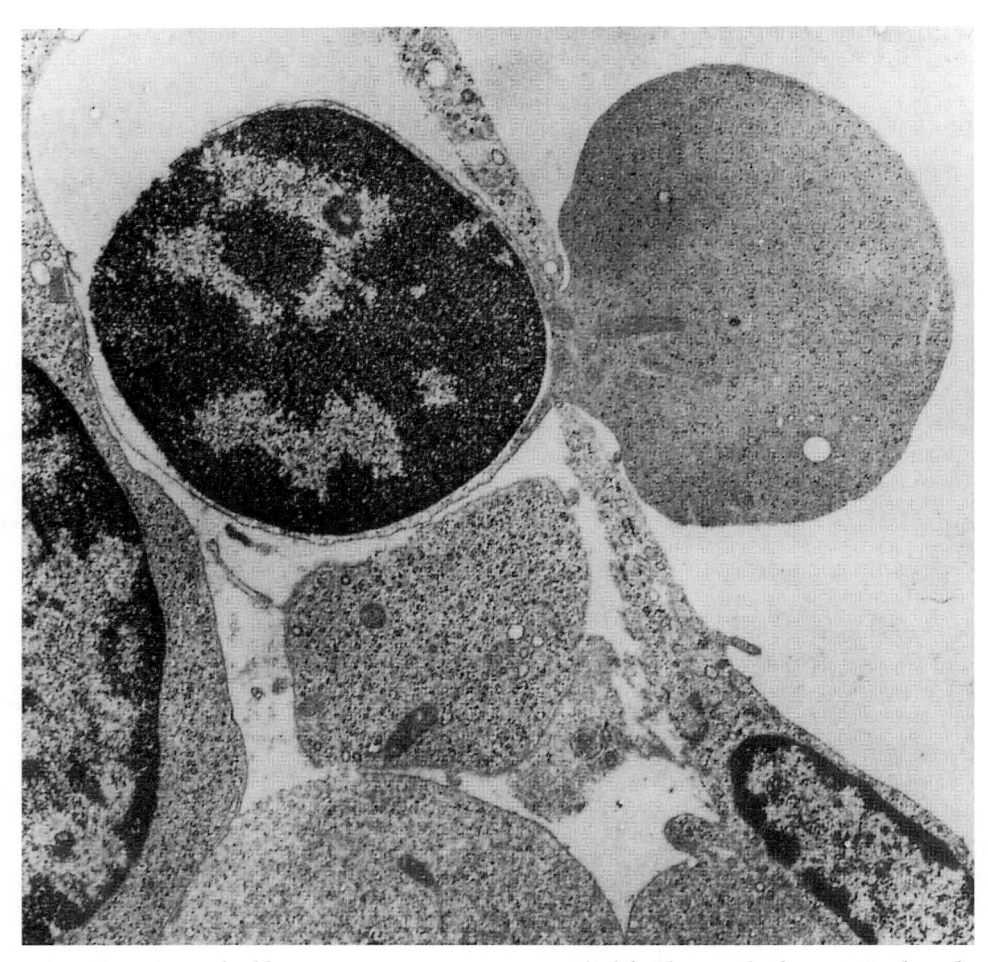

***Figure 11–3. An erythroblast in a marrow sinus is seen on the left. The vascular lumen is on the right.***

Between the two is a thin endothelial cell with an elongated nucleus *(bottom right)*. A mature but nucleated red cell is in the process of passing through the wall of the endothelial cell. The cytoplasm is completely within the lumen. The nucleus of the red cell, however, cannot pass through the aperture and must remain behind in the marrow sinus. ×8500. (From Tavassoli M, Crosby WH: Fate of the nucleus of the marrow erythroblast. *Science* 179:912–913, 1973. Copyright 1973 by AAAS.)

tional in reticulocytes but are absent in mature mammalian red cells. Maturation of reticulocytes into erythrocytes occurs over the first 24 to 36 h in the systemic circulation.

The presence of an abnormally large number of reticulocytes in the peripheral blood (>2 percent of the erythrocytes in adults or >6 percent in infants) is called *reticulocytosis,* and indicates an accelerated replacement function of the bone marrow such as might occur in chronic hemolytic disease, after exposure to hypoxia, or after an acute episode of intravascular hemolysis. Reticulocytes are easily distinguished after supravital staining of peripheral blood smears. The absolute count of reticulocytes may be reported (normal is about 60,000/$\mu$L) or it may be corrected for abnormal changes in hematocrit.

The presence of nucleated "blast" forms of immature red cells in peripheral blood may indicate an even greater demand for replacement. Megaloblastic macrocytic anemia with large oval red cells (macroovalocytes) in peripheral blood is indicative of a defect in DNA synthesis in marrow. This so-called maturation block may be a sign of a deficiency of the essential cofactors: vitamin $B_{12}$ and/or folic acid. Folic acid antagonist drugs used in cancer chemotherapy (methotrexate) or as antimalarials (pyrimethamine, chlorguanide) may induce megaloblastic anemia as a side effect because of their inhibition of DNA synthesis in marrow (Stebbins and Bertino, 1976).

In contrast, a microcytic hypochromic anemia is seen in iron deficiency as it occurs in premature infants, infants and children during rapid growth spurts, blood loss, pregnancy or lactation, or malabsorption syndromes. Oral replacement with enteric coated tablets of ferrous sulfate is effective in all these conditions except malabsorption, in which parenteral forms of iron may be required.

Bone marrow failure is characterized by inadequate production of red cells and/or other formed elements. Chemicals that are toxic to bone marrow can result in a decrease in the circulating numbers of all three major groups of formed elements, a condition called *pancytopenia.* A diagnosis of pancytopenia is based on actual cell counts in peripheral blood. Agents regularly associated with pancytopenia, if the exposure is sufficiently intense, include ionizing radiation, benzene, antimetabolites, lindane or chlordane, nitrogen mustards, arsenic, chloramphenicol, trinitrotoluene, gold salts, hydantoin derivatives, and phenylbutazone (Harris and Kellermeyer, 1970).

Damage to bone marrow may be so severe that the marrow does not proliferate normally, a condition described morphologically as *aplastic anemia.* This diagnosis is made after microscopic examination of bone marrow biopsy specimens. By contrast, in some conditions the marrow can have normal cellularity or even hypercellularity but still fail to deliver normal formed elements or normal numbers of formed elements. Ineffective erythropoiesis is a functional description of normal-appearing but unresponsive marrow.

It has been known for almost a century that benzene exposure is associated with bone marrow toxicity, and since the mid-1970s, benzene has been recognized as a human leukemogen. It is not clear whether the former is an absolute requirement for the latter. Most authorities agree that biotransformation is essential for benzene-induced bone marrow damage. The toxic metabolites are not known with certainty, although some evidence suggests that benzoquinone plays an important role. There is disagreement about whether benzene is activated in the marrow or in other tissues, such as the liver, followed by transport of the toxic metabolite or metabolites to the marrow (Snyder, 1987) (see Chap. 24). In addition to direct cytotoxic effects of chemicals such as benzene on the marrow, which usually are mediated through disturbances in DNA function, bone marrow damage may have an immunologic basis, as sometimes appears to be the case with chloramphenicol.

**Thrombocytes.** The process of differentiation into thrombocytes, the smallest formed elements in the blood, is unique. Large numbers of thrombocytes are batch produced and released from a single megakaryocyte, the largest cell type in marrow. The spent form of this giant cell is then phagocytized.

Platelets are the first line of defense against accidental blood loss. They accumulate rapidly at sites where vascular injury has exposed collagen fibers. Within seconds, the normally nonsticky circulating platelets adhere to these fibers (adhesion), undergo degranulation, and release adenosine disphosphate (ADP), which causes further adhesion but also causes platelets to stick to each other (aggregation). With the loss of individual membranes, the platelets form a viscous mass—the platelet plug—which quickly arrests bleeding, but the process is still reversible at this point. It becomes irreversible when the intrinsic and extrinsic clotting systems are activated to generate insoluble fibrin to reinforce the platelet plug. Fibroblasts then infiltrate into the area to complete the repair with scar formation.

Platelet aggregation in vivo can be studied with turbidimetric techniques in which aggregating agents are added to platelet-rich plasma; as the platelets aggregate, the optical density decreases (Born, 1962). If it is suspected that an active metabolite of a drug is involved, that drug can be given to a patient and its effects on platelet aggregation can be examined ex vivo. The primary aggregating agent in vivo is believed to be ADP, but aggregation also can be induced by epinephrine, thrombin, collagen, or other agents. Inhibition of platelet aggregation by drugs can be useful in preventing the thromboembolic complications of atherosclerosis. In 1986, the U.S. Food and Drug Administration (FDA) approved the labeling of aspirin to indicate that a single table taken daily may reduce the risk of death in patients who have already survived a myocardial infarction or have unstable angina. The effects of aspirin on prostaglandin synthesis are unique among nonsteroidal anti-inflammatory drugs because aspirin irreversibly acetylates cyclooxygenase in platelets; moreover, platelets lack the capacity to synthesize new enzyme. This irreversible effect on circulating platelets suppresses the synthesis of thromboxane $A_2$, which promotes aggregation.

Platelet aggregation is also inhibited by the so-called NO vasodilator drugs, including glyceryl trinitrate and its chemical relatives and sodium nitroprusside. Other xenobiotics in the group that are not used therapeutically as vasodilators include sodium azide, hydroxylamine hydrochloride, and sodium nitrite (Schwerin et al., 1983). These drugs owe their ability to relax vascular smooth muscle and inhibit platelet aggregation to their conversion to nitric oxide (NO). The NO is believed to activate guanylate cyclase to increase the synthesis of cGMP, which initiates a cascade of kinase or phosphorylase reactions to produce these effects.

Normal human blood contains several hundred thousand platelets per $\mu$L (Fig. 11-2). The minimal number needed for normal hemostasis is about 50,000/$\mu$L. Thrombocytopenia is defined as a count of <20,000/$\mu$L, and may be manifested by hemorrhagic disorders, the most common of which is leakage of blood from capillaries after a minor injury (purpura). Petechiae, prolonged bleeding time, and impaired clot retraction are also consequences. Thrombocytopenia accompanies a bewildering array of congenital and acquired disorders, but drugs are the most common cause. Myelosuppressive anticancer drugs may cause thrombocytopenia as part of a generalized depression of bone marrow function. Quinidine and phenacetin are recognized as causes of autoimmune thromocytopenia, resulting in increased destruction of peripheral platelets. An abnormally increased number of circulating platelets (thrombocytosis) has not been associated with chemical exposure.

**Leukocytes.** Leukocytes have the most complex organization among the formed elements. They differ from other blood cells in that they perform important functions outside the vascular compartment. Although each subtype seems to have unique functions, their primary purpose appears to be to defend the body against "foreignness." Defense against foreign organisms or extraneous materials involves two mechanisms: (1) phagocytosis and (2) antibody production as carried out by the immunocytic series (Fig. 11-4). The immunocytes are discussed at length in Chap. 12 and will not be referred to further here.

Phagocytes are subdivided into granulocytes (neutrophils, eosinophils, and basophils) and monocytes/macrophages. Subdivision of the granulocytes is accomplished on the basis of their reactivity with Wright's stain (Fig. 11-4), but these distinctions would be more valuable if their various functions were more clearly understood. Neutrophils are the most active phagocytes; eosinophils are less active. Eosinophilia occurs in some allergic diseases and infestations with large parasites. Basophils seem to be related to tissue mast cells and release histamine and other mediators in response to immunologic stimuli.

Granulocytes spend less than a day in the circulation before becoming marginated (attached to blood vessel walls); they then pass between vascular endothelial cells by means of diapedesis and are disposed of in various tissues. Mediators that increase capillary permeability are released from inflammatory lesions, and specific leukotactic factors (leukotrienes) attract granulocytes to the area of injury. Foreign particles or bacteria are phagocytized and destroyed by a "respiratory" burst that has long been thought to involve hydrogen peroxide and halide. In some cases, destruction of bacterial membranes, release of lysosomal enzymes, and formation of pyrogens may temporarily exacerbate the local inflammatory response. Pharmacological doses of glucocorticoids tend to decrease the numbers of granulocytes that diapedese and enter an inflammatory exudate because of their inhibitory effect on the synthesis of leukotrienes as well as prostaglandins. Presumably, this phenomenon accounts for the well-known increased susceptibility of patients receiving steroids to infections, since steroids do not decrease the rate of granulocyte production.

The term "granulocytopenia" is used when the total granulocyte count falls to 3000/$\mu$L (Fig. 11-4). When the count reaches 1000/$\mu$L, the patient becomes vulnerable to infection, and at 500/$\mu$L, the risk is very serious. The confusing term "agranulocytosis" refers to a condition in which both the marginated pool and the bone marrow are devoid of neutrophils (this condition is also called *neutropenia*).

Granulocytopenia is the most common manifestation of chemically induced bone marrow damage. The reaction also can be induced by ionizing radiation. Alkylating agents and antimetabolites regularly cause granulocytopenia, and phenothiazines, nonsteroidal anti-inflammatory drugs, antithyroid drugs, and certain anticonvulsants sometimes elicit the reaction (Pisciotta, 1973). Peripheral destruction of granulocytes is a much less common reaction caused by drug haptens after exposure to aminopyrine or phenylbutazone.

An excess in the number of granulocytes in peripheral blood occurs transiently after the administration of epinephrine, cortisone, and some endotoxins but is not believed to be of physiological significance. The term "granulocytosis" is used for counts above 10,000/$\mu$L. Chronic granulocytosis has not been associated with exposure to specific chemicals except when it occurs as a preliminary phase of leukemia. Leukemia is associated with counts of over 30,000/$\mu$L. In patients with advanced disease, the volume of leukocytes in blood may exceed the hematocrit, and the blood appears pale. Chronic

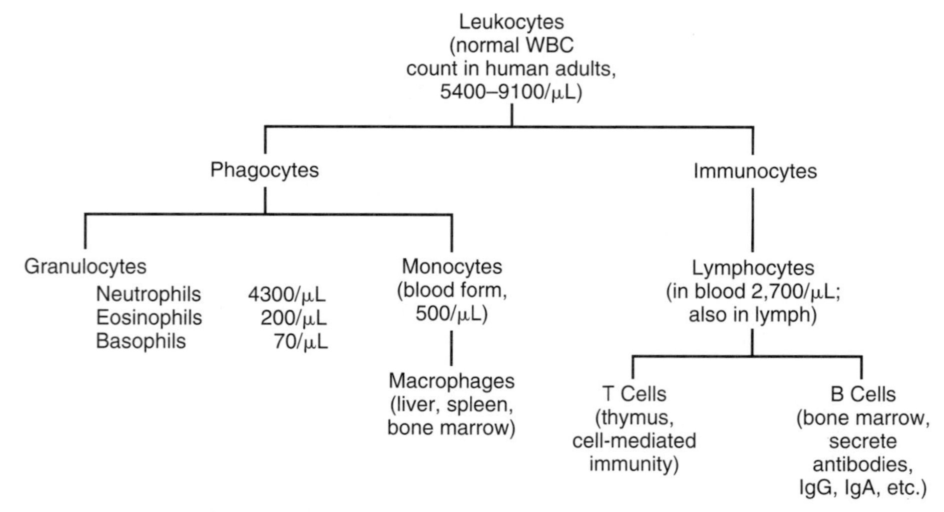


***Figure 11–4.** A classification of leukocytes and their normal values in humans.*

granulocytic leukemia has a better prognosis than does the acute form of the disease. The chronic form more commonly occurs in middle age, and although chemicals are suspected as etiologic agents, clear-cut associations have been difficult to make. The acute leukemias are rapidly fatal in the absence of effective chemotherapy. They are divided into two groups: (1) acute lymphocytic leukemia and (2) acute myelogenous leukemia, which includes all other marrow-derived leukocytes. Benzene is the only agent that definitely has been linked to acute leukemia in humans, but butadiene, ethylene oxide, and alkylating agents produce it in laboratory animals.

Monocytes circulate in the blood for 3 or 4 days. After they migrate into reticuloendothelial tissues such as the liver, spleen, and bone marrow, they are called *macrophages,* and they survive for several months in those sites. Macrophages play a role in the phagocytic response to inflammation and infection but are also responsible for the ongoing destruction of senile blood cells and the pinocytotic removal of denatured plasma proteins and lipoproteins. Macrophages also are involved in iron metabolism and have inducible heme oxidase activity for the catabolism of hemoglobin. They also contain an inducible form of NO-synthase, the enzyme that generates endogenous NO from arginine. NO-Synthase is induced by cytokines and bacterial endotoxin (lipopolysaccharide). The highly reactive NO destroys foreign particles and bacteria (Stuehr and Marletta, 1987). The condition known as septic or endotoxic shock may involve a pathological overproduction of NO (Wang et al., 1991). Neither monocytosis nor monocytopenia appears to be induced specifically by chemical injury, but either can be part of a generalized syndrome of bone marrow damage.

**Erythrocytes.** No cell type in the human body has been studied as extensively as has the red blood cell (Surgenor, 1975). This unique disk-shaped element (Fig. 11-5) has a diameter of about 8 $\mu$m, and its biconcave sides make it more than twice as thick at the periphery (about 2.4 $\mu$m) as it is in the center. The reason for its shape is not known, but the shape would tend to decrease intracellular diffusional distances. Although erythrocytes are devoid of intracellular organelles, special techniques in combination with scanning electron microscopy suggest that an internal structure may exist. As much as 30 percent of the wet weight of red cells consists of hemoglobin, which is the most extensively studied protein in the body.

Erythrocytes perform the essential function of transporting oxygen from the alveoli of the lungs to peripheral tissue, where it is used to support aerobic metabolism. On the return trip, red cells serve as a means for the transport of waste carbon dioxide for excretion via the lungs. A small amount of carbon dioxide is transported in simple solution within the cell, but the bulk (75 percent) is transported as bicarbonate through the activity of intracellular carbonic anhydrase. Another small fraction combines directly with free amino groups on hemoglobin to form carbaminohemoglobin (R—NH—COOH). An analogous reaction can occur with cyanate (see below). Hemoglobin also can accept hydrogen ions, and it accounts for about 85 percent of the buffer capacity of the blood.

Acute damage to red cells or to their content of hemoglobin can result in an impairment of oxygen transport and secondary peripheral hypoxia. The signs and symptoms in such cases are mediated through the central nervous system, the organ

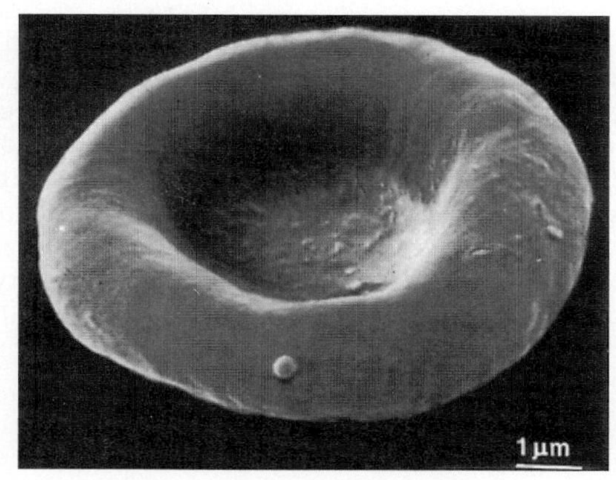


***Figure 11–5. Scanning electron micrograph of an unetched normal red blood cell. [From Stuart et al. (1969).]***

most sensitive to oxygen lack. Normally, the human erythrocyte remains in the blood for an average of 120 days before its life is ended in the spleen. Common laboratory animals (rabbits, rats, and especially guinea pigs and mice) have much shorter red cell survival times than do humans (Prankerd, 1961).

Anemia may arise if for any reason the rate of red cell destruction in the periphery exceeds the normal rate of their production in bone marrow. Some chemicals have acute and direct hemolytic effects in vivo, for example, saponin, phenylhydrazine, arsine, and naphthalene. Many other chemicals, such as primaquine, produce hemolysis only in red cells that are deficient in glucose-6-phosphate dehydrogenase (see below). In other cases, peripheral red cell destruction may involve an immunologic mechanism after sensitization by a drug such as acetanilid.

Laboratory evidence for an accelerated rate of hemolysis includes decreases in red cell life span, plasma haptoglobin levels, hematocrit, and red cell counts and increases in plasma hemoglobin (hemoglobinemia) and bilirubin (Rifkind et al., 1980). An unusual hematologic condition is characterized by hemoglobinemia in the face of polycythemia (increased hematocrit or red cell count). This reaction has been demonstrated in several species of laboratory animals exposed to chronic extreme hypoxia in the form of simulated altitude. Under these conditions, it appears that splenic, and perhaps hepatic, erythropoiesis is reactivated in an attempt to meet the demand for increased oxygen transport to peripheral tissues. At least part of this effort, however, appears to be ineffective in that the cells hemolyze shortly after or even before reaching the systemic circulation (Ou and Smith, 1978).

When hemoglobin is released into plasma, the iron of its heme groups undergoes autoxidation. The entire porphyrinic structure is labilized (see below), and it may exchange with albumin, haptoglobin, or hemopexin (Müller-Eberhard, 1970). These substances transport the heme to reticuloendothelial tissues that have inducible heme oxidase activity, which helps conserve the iron. If the rate of hemolysis is sufficient to saturate these carrier systems, free hemoglobin may be found in the urine, and hemoglobinuria is a sign of a severe hemolytic crisis that eventually may compromise renal function.

Polycythemia vera may be an acquired disease in which there is overproduction of red cells in the absence of an appropriate stimulus (altitude, cardiopulmonary disease, anemic hypoxia). It may be caused by an unusual sensitivity of the stem cell pool to erythropoietin. Cobalt ion is a known inappropriate stimulus for erythropoiesis. It was regularly seen, along with other signs, in the epidemics of beer drinker's cardiomyopathy in the 1960s. The onset of these epidemics coincided with the introduction of minute amounts of cobalt into some brands of beer to stabilize the foamy head (Gosselin et al., 1984). The tissue sensor for hypoxia (see above) also responds to cobalt ion by increasing the synthesis of erythropoietin.

## CHEMICALLY INDUCED HYPOXIA

*Hypoxia* refers to any condition in which there is a decreased supply of oxygen to peripheral tissues that is short of anoxia, but hypoxias can be subdivided into three classes with different root causes. *Arterial (anoxic) hypoxia* is characterized by lower than normal $P_{O_2}$ in arterial blood when the oxygen capacity and rate of blood flow are normal or even elevated. Among toxic insults, this type of hypoxia results from exposure to pulmonary irritants that produce airway obstruction ranging from spasm or edema of the glottis to pulmonary edema (adult respiratory distress syndrome). Opioid narcotics and other drugs that depress respiration also produce arterial hypoxia. *Anemic hypoxia* is characterized by a lowered oxygen capacity when the arterial $P_{O_2}$ and the rate of blood flow are normal or elevated. This type of hypoxia results from a decreased concentration of functional hemoglobin, a reduced number of red cells, or chemically induced alterations in hemoglobin. *Stagnant (hypokinetic) hypoxia* is characterized by a decreased rate of blood flow, as in heart failure and uncorrected vasodilatation. Sometimes a fourth condition, *histotoxic hypoxia*, is included in the classification even though in this condition the peripheral tissue oxygen tension may be normal or even elevated, and the defect lies in the ability of the cell to utilize molecular oxygen (see below).

### Oxygen Binding to Hemoglobin

Normal adult hemoglobin A is an oligomeric protein with a molecular weight of about 67,000 that contains four separate globin peptide chains: two alpha chains and two beta chains $(\alpha^{2+}\beta^{2+})_2$. Each peptide chain has a noncovalently bound porphyrinic heme group (Fig. 11-6). The globin chains have irregularly folded conformations that enclose the heme group in a hydrophobic pocket. The complete tertiary structure of hemoglobin is known (Perutz et al., 1968).

The structure of a single heme group may be represented as a square planar complex with the four nitrogens of the porphyrin ring at the angles (Fig. 11-6). The central iron atom has a hexavalent coordination shell that is analogous to the inorganic iron complexes, ferrocyanide, or nitroprusside. The two remaining coordination bonds are closely associated with imidazole (histidyl) residues from the particular globin chain to which the heme group is attached. One of these bonds is available for reversible combination with molecular oxygen, which binds between the iron and the histidyl. No ligand occupies this site in deoxyhemoglobin.

The reversible binding of oxygen by hemoglobin is called *oxygenation*; the tertiary structures of the oxygenated and deoxygenated forms of hemoglobin are known to differ. Since

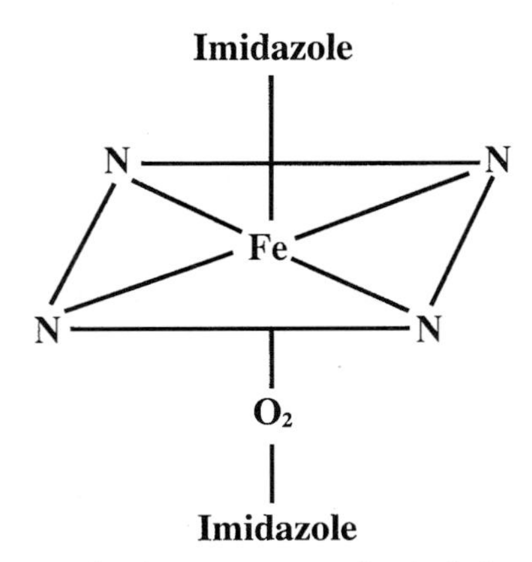


*Figure 11–6. A stylized representation of a single heme group.*

conformational changes do not occur on oxygenation of a single globin-heme unit such as myoglobin, it follows that there are interactions between the four subunits that constitute a hemoglobin molecule. These interactions are called *cooperativity*.

There are two physiological regulators of the affinity of hemoglobin for oxygen, which is usually defined in terms of $P_{50}$, or the partial pressure of oxygen necessary to half saturate the heme groups. The two regulators are hydrogen ion, which is responsible for the Bohr effect, and 2,3-diphosphoglycerate (2,3-DPG). Increasing concentrations of either substance tend to decrease the affinity of hemoglobin for oxygen, whereas increasing concentrations have the opposite effect.

Red cells can both synthesize and degrade 2,3-DPG (Fig. 11-7), and 2,3-DPG is normally present in red cells in about the same molar concentration as hemoglobin. One molecule of 2,3-DPG binds reversibly with one molecule of hemoglobin in the central cavity formed by the four subunits. This complex tends to stabilize hemoglobin in the deoxy form, so that 2,3-DPG and oxygen could be regarded as competitive ligands for hemoglobin, although they bind to different sites to exert allosteric effects. A decreased affinity of hemoglobin for oxygen shifts the oxygen dissociation curve (Fig. 11-8) in a parallel fashion to the right (increases the $P_{50}$), whereas an increased affinity produces a left-shifted dissociation curve. A number of drugs, chemicals, and manipulations are known to result in shifts in either direction (Norton and Smith, 1981).

Normal adult human hemoglobin binds 2,3-DPG more tightly than does fetal hemoglobin, accounting for the higher oxygen affinity of fetal blood that was noted above. Sickle-cell anemia is due to the inheritance of an abnormal hemoglobin with a single amino acid substitution on the $\beta$-globin chains. Hemolytic crises are triggered by hypoxia because only the deoxy form of hemoglobin S can form the polymeric structures that distort the shape of a red cell (Fig. 11-9). Irreversible carbamylation of the terminal valine residues on the globin chains by cyanate (see above) increases the oxygen affinity of hemoglobins A and S. This makes hemoglobin S less likely to exist in the deoxy form at any one time, and this decreases the incidence of hemolytic crises. Although cyanate was effective in limited clinical trials, it proved to be too neurotoxic for chronic use in human patients (Cerami and Manning, 1971). An alternative approach might be to devise some way to decrease the red cell concentration of 2,3-DPG, which would also increase the affinity of hemoglobin S for oxygen. Finally, if a safe and reliable way of reactivating the synthesis of fetal

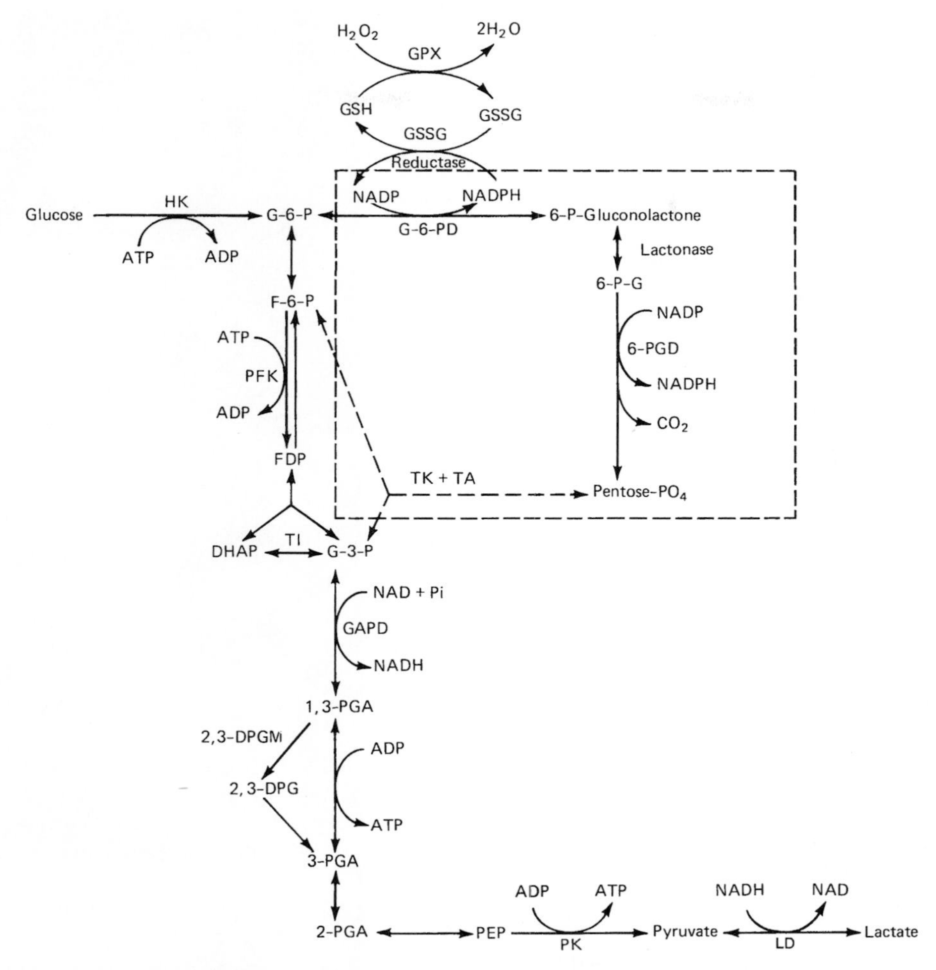


***Figure 11–7. The metabolic resources of mature mammalian red cells.***

GSH = reduced glutathione; GSSG = oxidized glutathione; G-6-P = glucose-6-phosphate; F-6-P = fructose-6-phosphate; FDP = fructose-1,6-diphosphate; DHAP = dihydroxyacetone phosphate; G-3-P = glyceraldehyde-3-phosphate; LD = lactic dehydrogenase; NADP = oxidized triphosphopyridine nucleotide; NADPH = reduced triphosphopyridine nucleotide; NAD = oxidized diphosphopyridine nucleotide; *NADH,* reduced diphosphopyridine nucleotide; 6-P-G = 6-phosphogluconate; G-6-PD = glucose-6-phosphate dehydrogenase; TK = transketolase; TA = transaldolase; Pi = inorganic phosphate; ADP = adenosine diphosphate; ATP = adenosine triphosphate; PEP = phosphoenolpyruvate; PK = pyruvic kinase; 1,3-PGA = 1,3-phosphoglyceric acid; 3-PGA = 3-phosphoglyceric acid; 2-PGA = 2-phosphoglyceric acid; 2,3-DPG = 2,3-diphosphoglyceric acid; 6-PGD = 6-phosphogluconate dehydrogenase; PFK = phosphofructokinase; HK = hexokinase; TI = trioseisomerase; GPX = glutathione peroxidase; GAPD = glyceraldehyde-3-phosphate dehydrogenase; 2,3-DPGM = 2,3-diphosphoglycerate mutase. [Modified from Harris and Kellermeyer (1970).]

hemoglobin could be devised, the higher oxygen affinity of fetal hemoglobin might benefit patients with the sickle-cell trait. In this case, the $\gamma$-globin chains would substitute for the defective $\beta$-chains on hemoglobin S (Letvin et al., 1984).

Deoxygenation of hemoglobin occurs in four separate steps, each of which has a different dissociation constant because of cooperativity changes that accompany the release of each successive oxygen molecule:

$$\begin{array}{lll} Hb(O_2)_4 \rightarrow Hb(O_2)_3 + O_2 & & K_1 \\ Hb(O_2)_3 \rightarrow Hb(O_2)_2 + O_2 & & K_2 \\ Hb(O_2)_2 \rightarrow Hb(O_2) + O_2 & & K_3 \\ Hb(O_2) \rightarrow Hb + O_2 & & K_4 \end{array}$$

The exact values for the individual dissociation constants listed above are unknown, but they represent equilibrium constants of the form

$$K_1 = \frac{[Hb(O_2)_3]\,[O_2]}{[Hb(O_2)_4]}$$

with units of mols per liter. The comparable association constant would be the reciprocal expression with units of liters per mol. The smaller the dissociation constant is, the more tightly the ligand is bound and the more stable the complex is.

When the hemoglobin molecule is fully saturated, all the oxygens may be thought of as equivalent since it is not known

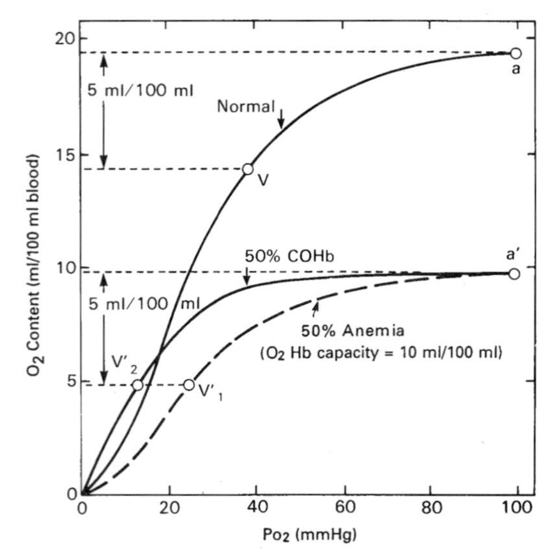


***Figure 11–8. Normal oxyhemoglobin dissociation curve and curves for the case of a 50 percent anemia and the case of a 50 percent carboxyhemoglobinemia.***

The delivery of 25 percent of the total oxygen content of fully oxygenated arterial blood (5 ml/100 ml blood) requires a drop in the $P_{O_2}$ of about 60 mmHg (from point a to point V on the normal curve). Delivery of a comparable volume of oxygen in the case of a 50 percent anemia requires a drop in the $P_{O_2}$ of more than 75 mmHg (from point a′ to point $V'_1$), but an even greater fall in the $P_{O_2}$ is required to deliver the same volume of oxygen in the case of the curve distorted by the presence of carboxyhemoglobin (from point a′ to point $V'_2$). See text for an explanation of this phenomenon. [From Bartlett (1973).]

whether the two types of globin chains play a role in sequencing deoxygenation. A fall in the ambient $P_{O_2}$ results in the release of one oxygen molecule. This release triggers a cooperativity change that greatly facilitates the release of the second oxygen molecule; thus, $K_1$ is considerably smaller than $K_2$. Similarly, the release of the second oxygen facilitates the release of the third. The release of the fourth oxygen does not occur under normal physiological conditions.

The sequence described above is responsible for the sigmoid shape of the normal oxygen dissociation curve (Fig. 11-8). Since the total oxygen content of normal blood is about 20 ml/100 ml, the release of 5 ml $O_2$/100 ml blood could be considered analogous to the release of one oxygen molecule from a single hemoglobin tetramer; in each case, it is one-fourth of the total load. That release requires a decrease in the $P_{O_2}$ of about 60 mmHg (from point a to point V). The release of an additional 5 ml $O_2$/100 ml blood (or the second molecule of $O_2$ from a tetramer) requires a further decrease in the $P_{O_2}$, but only of about 15 mmHg (from about 40 down to 25 mmHg) because of cooperativity. The release of a third increment of oxygen can then be effected by a decrease in the $P_{O_2}$ of only 10 mmHg. Thus, cooperativity facilitates the loading and unloading of large amounts of oxygen over a physiologically critical range of $P_{O_2}$.

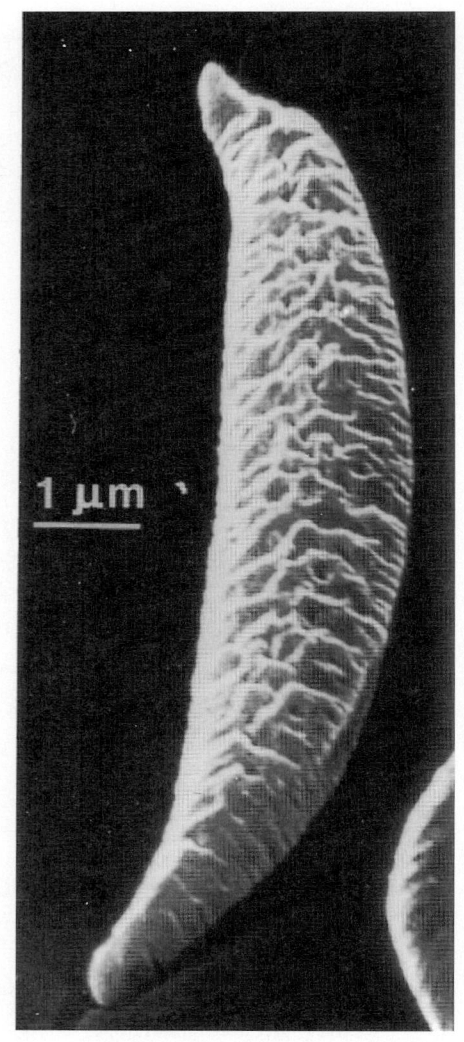


***Figure 11–9. Scanning electron micrograph of a red blood cell from a patient with sickle-cell disease after ion etching in oxygen for 5 min at 1 mtorr.***

The technique was carried out with equipment normally used for the study of metals and inorganic materials. [From Stuart et al. (1969).]

## Carbon Monoxide Binding to Hemoglobin

Carbon monoxide is the most widely studied chemical agent that can produce anemic hypoxia. The elucidation of its mechanism of action by Claude Bernard in 1865 is a classic example of the successful application of the experimental method (Bernard, 1957). Bernard's original deductions were formalized (Douglas et al., 1912) as the so-called Haldane equation, which defines quantitatively the competitive nature of oxygen and carbon monoxide for the same ferrous heme binding sites on hemoglobin:

$$\frac{[Hb(CO)_4]}{[Hb(O_2)_4]} = M\frac{[P_{CO}]}{[P_{O_2}]}$$

The constant $M$ has the value of 245 at pH 7.4 for human blood. Therefore, if the $P_{CO} = 1/245\ P_{O_2}$, the blood at equilibrium will be half saturated with oxygen and half saturated with carbon monoxide. Since air contains 21 percent oxygen by volume, exposure to a gas mixture of about 0.1 percent carbon monoxide in air would result in a 50 percent carboxyhemoglobinemia at equilibrium and at sea level. For this reason, carbon monoxide is dangerous at very low concentrations. However, the rate at which the arterial blood approaches equilibrium with the inspired gas concentration depends on factors such as the diffusion capacity of the lungs and the alveolar ventilation, both of which in turn depend on the level of exercise of the subject.

Some species variation is recognized with respect to the value of *M* in the Haldane equation, but this is not necessarily the major determinant of the sensitivity of a species to carbon monoxide. For example, the *M* value for canary blood is less than half the value for human blood. The very rapid rate of breathing needed by canaries to support a higher rate of aerobic metabolism allows them to reach equilibrium between blood and inspired carbon monoxide more rapidly than humans can. However, the canary brain appears to be less sensitive to hypoxia than is the human brain. Because of these opposing factors, canaries are more sensitive than are humans to short exposures at high concentrations of carbon monoxide, but with long exposures to low concentrations, the roles can be reversed (Spencer, 1962).

If, instead of air or oxygen, hemoglobin is exposed to pure carbon monoxide, a gradual decrease in the $P_{CO}$ allows one to derive a carboxyhemoglobin dissociation curve of the same shape as the oxyhemoglobin dissociation curve. Thus, cooperativity is a property of the hemoglobin tetramer and is not influenced by the ligands that occupy the ferrous heme binding sites; that is, the hemoglobin molecule has no intrinsic mechanism for distinguishing between oxygen and carbon monoxide.

When the ambient atmosphere contains both oxygen and carbon monoxide, another phenomenon is observed that has profound physiological significance (Fig. 11-8). If the ambient $P_{CO}$ is $\frac{1}{245}$ of the ambient $P_{O_2}$, at equilibrium, half the ferrous heme binding sites will be occupied by CO and half will be occupied by $O_2$. The distribution of the two ligands among the four heme groups on any one tetramer, however, is random. Thus, the blood will contain a distribution of hybrid species in which most tetramers contain both oxygen and carbon monoxide.

The effect of these hybrid species on the oxyhemoglobin dissociation curve in comparison with a simple 50 percent anemia is shown in Fig. 11-8. Since half the total number of ferrous heme binding sites are always going to be occupied by carbon monoxide, the total oxygen capacity is half of normal, as in simple anemia. However, the curve for a simple anemia retains a sigmoid shape because the hemoglobin is binding only oxygen. For any given value for the $P_{O_2}$ on the abscissa, the value for the oxygen content on the ordinate is half that for the normal dissociation curve. In contrast, the curve for a 50 percent carboxyhemoglobinemia is shifted to the left and loses the sigmoid shape.

The physiological significance of this phenomenon can be grasped from Fig. 11-8, where a change in the $P_{O_2}$ of 75 mmHg (from point a′ to point $V'_1$) is required to deliver 5 ml $O_2$/100 ml of blood to peripheral tissues in the case of a 50 percent anemia, whereas in the case of a 50 percent carboxyhemoglobinemia, a change in the $P_{O_2}$ of 85 mmHg (from point a′ to point $V'_2$) is required to deliver the same amount of oxygen to peripheral tissues. Obviously, a person with a 50 percent carboxyhemoglobinemia is more severely compromised than is a person with a simple 50 percent anemia. As was noted above, cooperativity remains normal in hybrid species in which both oxygen and carbon monoxide are bound to the same tetramer. Thus, the basis of the effect on the oxygen dissociation curve is simply a loss of the number of opportunities for cooperativity to facilitate the dissociation of oxygen. In the hybrid species, which contains two oxygens and two carbon monoxides, cooperativity facilitates the unloading of the second oxygen, but afterward there are no more oxygens left to unload. In contrast, in the 50 percent anemia, each tetramer has a full complement of four oxygens and cooperativity could facilitate the unloading of the third and even the fourth oxygen in times of great demand. In effect, in a 50 percent carboxyhemoglobinemia, only the top half of the normal oxyhemoglobin dissociation curve is available for use.

**Carbon Monoxide Poisoning.** The model described above illustrates the molecular mechanisms at work in terms of hemoglobin, but in intact humans and animals other factors play important roles in the pathophysiology of carbon monoxide poisoning. Changes are known to occur in cardiac output and regional blood flow. Changes in ventilation influence the rate at which equilibrium between the inspired gas concentration and the blood content is achieved. Exposure to very high ambient concentrations of carbon monoxide can result in hemoglobin saturation sufficient to produce unconsciousness or death in minutes with few, if any, premonitory signs. At low ambient concentrations, however, considerable time may be required to reach equilibrium with the blood (for example, as long as 4 h for a sedentary person exposed to 0.1 percent by volume). For these and other reasons (see below), there are sometimes surprising discrepancies between the blood carboxyhemoglobin levels and signs in poisoned patients.

Although the presence of carboxyhemoglobin can result in significant decreases in the oxygen content of blood, ambient concentrations are rarely high enough to cause a detectable decrease in the $P_{O_2}$ of arterial blood. Therefore, it is uncommon for chemoreceptor mechanisms to be triggered, and the parameters of ventilation usually remain within normal limits. Peripheral vasodilation occurs in response to a slowly developing hypoxia, necessitating an increase in cardiac output. This compensatory mechanism is limited, and fainting is more common than dyspnea in victims of carbon monoxide poisoning. Consciousness may be lost for long periods before death. Tachycardia and electrocardiographic (ECG) changes suggestive of hypoxia may be observed at 30 percent or greater carboxyhemoglobin saturation. Other symptoms include headache, weakness, nausea, dizziness, and dimness of vision. Lactic acidemia indicates a limitation on aerobic metabolism. Unconsciousness, coma, convulsions, and death are associated with 50 to 80 percent saturation.

Carbon monoxide is not a cumulative poison in the usual sense. Carboxyhemoglobin is fully dissociable, and once exposure has been terminated, the pigment reverts to oxyhemoglobin. Liberated carbon monoxide is eliminated through the lungs. Many individuals are occupationally exposed to carbon monoxide—for example, garage workers and traffic police—and may suffer acute recurring intoxications. Without an adequate history, an unwary physician may be baffled by the symptomatology. Any hypoxic insult of sufficient severity, however, including carbon monoxide poisoning, may induce permanent neurological sequelae if the victim survives.

Carboxyhemoglobin is cherry-red in color, and its presence in blood can be detected only with appropriate chemical tests. Its presence in the venous return may impart an abnormal red coloration to the skin and mucous membranes. Carbon monoxide combines in vitro with myoglobin and heme enzymes, but the significance of these reactions in acute poisonings is unknown. A considerable number of experiments have attempted to show that factors other than simple hypoxia contribute to carbon monoxide poisoning (Gosselin et al., 1984). Most of these attempts have yielded only suggestive results for cellular effects of carbon monoxide, but differential reflectance spectroscopy allows direct measurements of brain energy metabolism in intact animals. Such results have indicated that the inhibitory effects of carbon monoxide on cytochrome *c* oxidase contribute to the intoxication syndrome. More important, the impairment of energy metabolism can continue despite the elimination of carboxyhemoglobin from the blood. Recovery from inhibition was more rapid under hyperbaric than under normobaric oxygen (Brown and Piantadosi, 1992).

***Management of Carbon Monoxide Poisoning.*** The obvious and specific antagonist to carbon monoxide is oxygen. After termination of the exposure, breathing must be supported by artificial means if necessary. Advantage can be taken of the mass law to accelerate the rate of conversion of carboxy- to oxyhemoglobin in vivo by increasing the ambient $P_{O_2}$. For example, the half-recovery time in terms of blood carboxyhemoglobin in resting adults breathing air at 1 atmosphere is 320 min. When oxygen is given instead, the time is decreased to 80 min. Further reductions can be effected through the use of hyperbaric chambers to deliver pure oxygen at greater than atmospheric pressures. Current recommendations are 2.5 to 3.0 atmospheres for 90 to 120 min with one or more follow-up treatments if needed in any victim with neurological impairment regardless of the blood carboxyhemoglobin level (Piantadosi, 1990).

**Endogenous and Environmental Carbon Monoxide.** Nonsmoking human adults normally do not have more than 1 percent of their total circulating hemoglobin in the form of carboxyhemoglobin, but heavy smokers may show values as high as 5 to 10 percent saturation. Combustion of fossil fuels and automobile exhaust fumes (4 to 7 percent carbon monoxide) are other key environmental sources of exposure. However, carbon monoxide is generated endogenously in normal humans (Coburn et al., 1967). This carbon monoxide arises from the catabolism of heme proteins, principally hemoglobin, with heme enzymes contributing smaller amounts. The carbon monoxide comes from the $\alpha$-methene bridge of porphyrins and is generated in amounts that are equimolar to the bile pigment produced. The average rate of production (0.4 ml/h) is increased in hemolytic disease (National Academy of Sciences, 1977a).

## Methemoglobinemia

As opposed to oxygenation, the heme irons of hemoglobin are susceptible to chemical oxidation through the loss of an electron with a valence change from $2^+$ to $3^+$. The resulting pigment is greenish-brown to black in color, is called methemoglobin, and cannot combine reversibly with oxygen or carbon monoxide. Therefore, methemoglobinemia is another possible cause of anemic hypoxia. As in the oxidation of simple inorganic coordination complexes of iron, oxidation does not change the total number of bonds in the coordination shell (Fig. 11-6). The additional positive charge on the heme iron is satisfied in vivo by hydroxyl or chloride anion. The ferric heme iron also can combine with a variety of nonphysiological anions, and this property has been exploited for therapeutic purposes (see below).

No method has been devised to test the hypothesis that short of completely saturating concentrations, carboxyhemoglobin exists as hybrid species in which both oxygen and carbon monoxide are found on the same tetramer. In contrast, it is known with certainty that "methemoglobin" generated either in vivo or in vitro by partial oxidation of hemoglobin or partial reduction of the totally oxidized pigment consists of a mixture of two hybrid species: $(\alpha^{2+}\beta^{3+})_2$ and $(\alpha^{3+}\beta^{2+})_2$. Complete oxidation of $(\alpha^{2+}\beta^{2+})_2$ to $(\alpha^{3+}\beta^{3+})_2$ can be forced with an excess of oxidant in vitro but would certainly be fatal in vivo (Tomoda and Yoneyama, 1981). Like carboxyhemoglobinemia, methemoglobinemia both decreases the oxygen content of blood and shifts the oxygen dissociation curve to the left with a distortion of its sigmoid shape. The explanation of the effect of methemoglobinemia on oxygen dissociation is also believed to involve a decrease in the number of opportunities for cooperativity to facilitate oxygen unloading. The proof of hybrid species in the case of methemoglobin, however, lends credence to the hypothesis about carboxyhemoglobin.

Methemoglobin has an additional property that is of toxicological interest: its ability to dissociate complete heme groups as units. Free hemoglobin in plasma rapidly undergoes autoxidation to methemoglobin, which can transfer heme groups to plasma albumin to form the pigment, methemalbumin. Methemalbumin is associated with acute hemolytic crises such as transfusion reactions, severe malaria, paroxysmal nocturnal hemoglobinuria, and poisonings by chemicals such as chlorate salts. If a blood sample drawn under anaerobic conditions appears to be abnormally dark in color, inadequate oxygenation can be distinguished from oxidation simply by shaking it in air. A change in color to bright red indicates that the sample originally contained abnormally high concentrations of deoxyhemoglobin. The persistence of a dark color may indicate the presence of methemoglobin (an intraerythrocytic pigment) or methemalbumin (an extracellular pigment). Centrifugation often allows one to distinguish between the two.

**Hemoglobin Autoxidation.** A variety of chemicals greatly increase the rate of hemoglobin oxidation (see below), but oxidation also occurs spontaneously in the presence of oxygen. This autoxidation presumably accounts for the low concentrations ($<2$ percent) of methemoglobin normally found in circulating blood in humans and most other common mammals. As studied in vitro, autoxidation appears to be a first-order process with respect to the ferrous forms of hemoglobin and myoglobin. The first-order rate constants, however, depend in a complex manner on the $P_{O_2}$. The rate constant is maximal at a $P_{O_2}$ that corresponds to half saturation of the reduced pigment. Since a reaction mechanism in which a deoxygenated heme group interacts with an oxygenated one would not exhibit first-order kinetics, a multistep mechanism can be inferred. The quasi-first-order kinetics then can be explained as arising from an algebraic artifact rather than from any single intramolecular rate-determining step.

The complexity of these reactions is illustrated by studies of their stoichiometry. Both myoglobin and hemoglobin autoxidation consume many times more oxygen than can be accounted for on the basis of the reduction of an appropriate amount of oxygen to water (Smith and Olson, 1973). It has been suggested that the reduced heme may simply transfer an electron to molecular oxygen to form superoxide anion (Fridovich, 1983), but this mechanism does not account for the peculiarities noted above.

**Methemoglobin-Generating Chemicals.** Some chemicals that are capable of mediating the oxidation of hemoglobin are active both in vitro and in vivo. Others are active only in vivo, and those in a third group are much more active in lysates or solutions of hemoglobin than in intact cells in vitro (Fig. 11-10). Sodium nitrite and hydroxylamine hydrochloride are active both in vitro and in vivo; both directly relax vascular smooth muscle and are converted to NO in red cell suspensions and in mice (Kruszyna et al., 1988). Despite these similarities, they appear to oxidize hemoglobin by different mechanisms (Cranston and Smith, 1971).



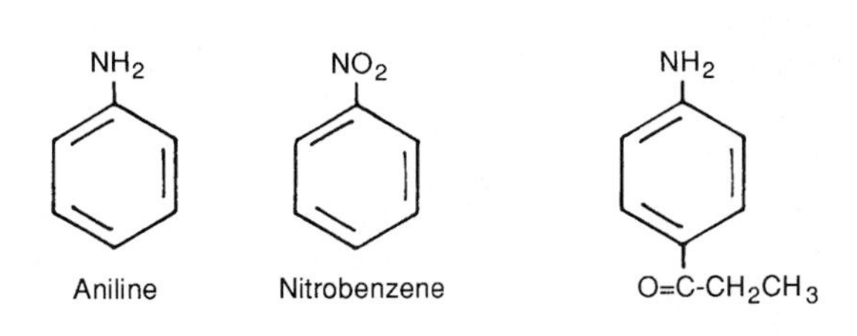


***Figure 11–10. Prototypical methemoglobin-generating chemicals.***

(1) Agents that are active in vitro and in vivo. (2) Agents that are active only in vivo. (3) Agents that are active only or primarily in lysates. [From Smith and Olson (1973).]

Under strictly anaerobic conditions, 1 mol of nitrite yields 1 mol of ferric heme and 1 mol of the ferroheme-NO complex. Under physiological conditions and in the presence of excess nitrite, complete oxidation of hemoglobin occurs, and the heme oxygen is largely consumed in the process. After a lag phase, the reaction proceeds with a pronounced autocatalytic phase that is not observed when nitrite reacts with deoxyhemoglobin. Nitrite is one of the nonphysiological anions that complex with ferric heme groups. Thus, excess nitrite can force complete oxidation, with subsequent formation of a nitrite-methemoglobin complex. The phenomenon has no toxicological significance but can produce artifacts in the in vitro spectrophotometric determination of methemoglobin (van Assendelft and Zijlstra, 1965; Smith, 1967).

Organic compounds that are active both in vivo and in vitro include some aminophenols, certain *N*-hydroxylamines, amyl nitrite and other aliphatic esters of nitrous acid, and some aliphatic esters of nitric acid, such as glyceryl trinitrate (Kiese, 1974). As tested in mice, phenylhydroxylamine and some simple homologues were all approximately equipotent in terms of the peak levels of methemoglobin generated. At the same time, they were 10 times more potent than nitrite, hydroxylamine, or simple aminophenols (Smith et al., 1967). Intraerythrocytic recycling must account for the high potency of *N*-hydroxylamines relative to the other compounds, since phenylhydroxylamine is no more potent than is nitrite in lysates. According to Kiese (1974), phenylhydroxylamine and related compounds react with hemoglobin to form methemoglobin and nitrosobenzene (Fig. 11-10). In a normal red cell, mechanisms apparently exist for the reduction of nitrosobenzene to regenerate phenylhydroxylamine. A requirement for glucose, as opposed to lactate, in this system suggests that the pentose phosphate shunt is involved; perhaps the system requires NADPH (Fig. 11-7).

Aromatic amino and nitro compounds such as aniline and nitrobenzene generate methemoglobin only in vivo. Obviously, these chemicals must be bioactivated, probably to aminophenols or to *N*-hydroxylamines, but the relative importance of these two possibilities is still not known for the two examples cited above. In contrast, the active metabolite of *p*-aminopropiophenone (PAPP), the most widely studied example of this type of agent, has been shown with certainty to be the *N*-hydroxyl metabolite in several laboratory animal species. This biotransformation is probably mediated by one of the isozymes of hepatic cytochrome P-450, but the bioactivation of nitrobenzene may be mediated by nitroreductases in the intestinal microflora of the rat (Reddy et al., 1976). Prominent species differences in potency occur with this type of chemical because of differences between the rates of activation and inactivation of the parent compound and of its metabolites.

Some aromatic amines are human carcinogens, and there is considerable interest in adducts formed between amine metabolites and the globin moiety of hemoglobin as a possible means of monitoring bioactivation or exposure to cigarette smoke and other environmental carcinogens. Significant differences between smokers and nonsmokers were found for several adducts to amines that are known to be human bladder carcinogens (Bryant et al., 1988). In rats, there seemed to be a correlation between the extent of amine adduct formation on globin and the ability of the compound to generate methemoglobin (Birner and Neumann, 1988). This approach can only serve as an index of recent exposure because of the finite life span of red cells.

Three unusual compounds are active largely or exclusively in lysates (Fig. 11-10). The first of these compounds—potassium ferricyanide—is unable to penetrate an intact red cell membrane. It is, however, the most widely used reagent for standardizing methemoglobin assays. One mol of ferricyanide mediates the oxidation of 1 mol of reduced heme whether or not oxygen is present. The ferricyanide reaction with oxyhemoglobin is unique in that ferricyanide is the only methemoglobin-generating agent known that effects a quantitative release of the heme oxygen. This phenomenon has been exploited in the laboratory determination of the oxygen content of hemoglobin. The ferrocyanide that is generated binds tenaciously to the globin chains of methemoglobin.

The second agent is molecular oxygen, which is probably equally active in intact red cells and lysates. In intact cells, however, its activity is masked because of the efficient mechanisms for reducing methemoglobin back to hemoglobin (see below and Fig. 11-11). For reasons that are not clearly understood, hemolysis virtually abolishes methemoglobin reductase activity, and the oxidized pigment accumulates until the reaction has been completed. The redox dye methylene blue is somewhat similar except that in intact cells it can activate a separate methemoglobin-reducing system that is additive to the effects of methemoglobin reductase (see below and Fig. 11-11).

Hemolysis abolishes the methemoglobin-reducing activity of methylene blue as well as the activity of methemoglobin reductase. In lysates, methylene blue actually generates methemoglobin and leucomethylene blue. The latter compound is susceptible to oxidation by molecular oxygen, so that a cyclic mechanism exists for hemoglobin oxidation in lysates in which methylene blue is as potent as phenylhydroxylamine is in intact cells, although the reaction proceeds much more slowly. It is presumed that this reaction also occurs in intact cells but is masked by the methemoglobin-reducing activity of methylene blue. Although methemoglobin never accumulates under these conditions, it is inferred that the rate of hemoglobin-methemoglobin turnover is accelerated. This may account for the weak anticyanide activity of methylene blue in vivo (see below and Smith and Thron, 1972).

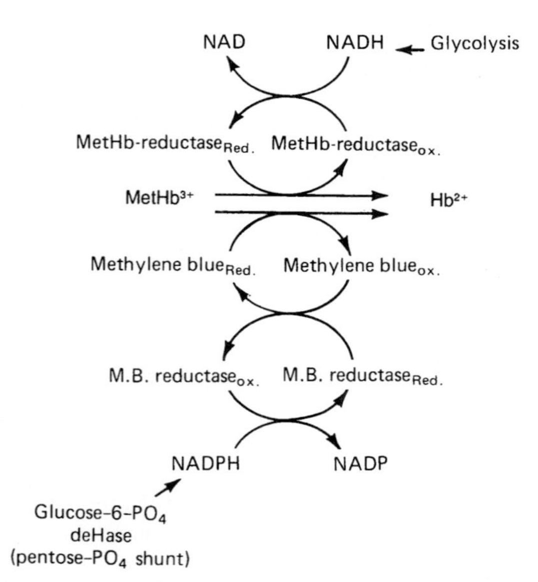


***Figure 11–11. The spontaneous (NADH) and dormant (NADPH) methemoglobin reductase systems.***

Methemoglobin (MetHb) reductase is active in intact red cells in the presence of substrates that can provide for NAD reduction. The NADPH system requires intact red cells, glucose or its metabolic equivalent, a functioning pentose phosphate shunt, and methylene blue (M.B.). M.B.-reductase reduces M.B., which in turn nonenzymatically reduces MetHb.

***Susceptibility of Mammalian Hemoglobins to Oxidation.*** Small differences are recognized among mammalian hemoglobins in regard to the rates of their oxidation by various chemicals (Bartels et al., 1963). Such differences undoubtedly reflect conformational or structural variations. Smith and Beutler (1966b) found that the conversion half-times in minutes for hemoglobin solutions exposed to the same concentration of nitrite to be about 2 for sheep, goat, and bovine hemoglobin; 3 for human hemoglobin; 4 for equine hemoglobin; and up to 7 for porcine hemoglobin. These values are low relative to the duration of a nitrite-methemoglobinemia induced in any of these species in vivo, which would be on the order of several hours.

**Pathophysiology of Methemoglobinemias.** As an experimental tool for the study of the effects of peripheral hypoxia, methemoglobinemia is much less satisfactory than simulated altitude, oxygen replacement, or even exposure to carbon monoxide. Unless the methemoglobin-generating chemical is infused continuously, it is impossible to maintain stable circulating levels of the pigment for long periods. A variety of intraerythrocytic mechanisms can reduce methemoglobin back to hemoglobin. After a single dose of the agent, methemoglobin levels rise abruptly and then decline toward normal at rates that vary widely with the species (Table 11-1) and result in wide variations in peripheral tissue oxygen tensions.

Moreover, chemicals that produce acquired methemoglobinemias have additional effects that can make important contributions to the toxic syndrome. Nitrite, hydroxylamine, aliphatic esters of nitrous and nitric acid, and nitroprusside are all vasodilators by virtue of their conversion to NO in vivo (Kruszyna et al., 1988). These compounds may produce orthostatic hypotension, reflex tachycardia, circulatory inadequacy, and cardiovascular collapse so that the anemic hypoxia is compounded by a stagnant or hypokinetic hypoxia. The aromatic amino and nitro compounds seem to have complex central and cardiac effects that may be the proximal cause of death in humans and some animal species. Intravascular hemolysis is induced by chlorate salts, arsine, large doses of hydroxylamine (Cranston and Smith, 1971), and even PAPP. The "methemoglobinemia" may be largely extracellular and may be confounded by sulfhemoglobinemia and Heinz bodies (see below). The methemoglobinemia induced by paraquat (Ng et al., 1982) is almost trivial in comparison with the devastating effects of this compound on the lungs and other organ systems.

It is doubtful that any chemical produces a "pure" methemoglobinemia that is uncomplicated by effects on other organs or tissues, but PAPP in moderate doses has few, if any,

**Table 11–1**
**Spontaneous Methemoglobin Reductase Activity of Mammalian Erythrocytes**

| | INVESTIGATORS | | | | |
|---|---|---|---|---|---|
| | (1) | (2) | (3) | (4) | (5) |
| SPECIES | *Activity in Species/Activity in Humans* | | | | |
| Pig | 0.37 | 0.37 | | 0.09 | |
| Horse | 0.75 | 0.50 | | 0.64 | |
| Cat | | 0.50 | 0.85 | 1.2 | 1.0 |
| Cow | 0.80 | 0.75 | | 1.1 | |
| Goat | 1.1 | 0.75 | | | |
| Dog | | 0.88 | 1.4 | 1.3 | 1.0 |
| Sheep | 1.4 | 1.0 | | 2.1 | |
| Rat | | 1.4 | 1.3 | 1.9 | 5.0 |
| Guinea pig | | 1.2 | 2.4 | 1.9 | 4.5 |
| Rabbit | | 3.5 | 3.3 | 3.8 | 7.5 |
| Mouse | | | | | 9.5 |

Data from various investigators using nitrited red cells with glucose as a substrate have been normalized by making a ratio of the activity of the species to the activity in human red cells. The indicated investigators are (1) Smith and Beutler, 1966b; (2) Malz, 1962; (3) Kiese and Weis, 1943; (4) Robin and Harley, 1966; (5) Stolk and Smith, 1966; Smith et al., 1967; Bolyai et al., 1972.

"side effects." Large differences exist among various agents for methemoglobin levels at death as measured in a single species (Smith and Olson, 1973). It is therefore inappropriate to suggest that there is a lethal level of methemoglobin without accounting for the particular agent and species involved.

**Metabolic Resources of the Mature Mammalian Red Cell.** The reversal of a carboxyhemoglobinemia is spontaneous and passive in accordance with the ambient partial pressure of the gas and oxygen. In contrast, energy must be expended by a red cell to reverse an acquired methemoglobinemia. Indeed, much of the total energy expenditure of red cells is directed toward that end, maintenance of the integrity of the membrane, and restoration of the shape of the cell after deformation. The metabolic resources of the red cell, however, are meager. Only two anaerobic alternatives are available for glucose metabolism: the Embden-Meyerhof glycolytic sequence and the pentose phosphate (hexosemonophosphate) shunt (Fig. 11-7).

The enzyme glucose-6-phosphate dehydrogenase (G-6-PD) occupies a key position in red cell metabolism. It introduces the pentose phosphate shunt and mediates the reduction of NADP. Another mol of NADPH is generated in the next step mediated by 6-phosphogluconate dehydrogenase. These are the only sources of NADPH for red cells. If lactate is substituted for glucose as a metabolic fuel, the cell can produce NADH through the activity of lactic dehydrogenase but not NADPH. In some mammalian red cells, stereospecificity of G-6-PD prevents the utilization of galactose by the pentose phosphate shunt, although it can be utilized by glycolysis (Smith and Beutler, 1966a).

**Methemoglobin-Reducing Systems.** ***Spontaneous Methemoglobin Reduction.*** The major system responsible for methemoglobin reduction in mammalian red cells is methemoglobin reductase, which has been identified as cytochrome $b_5$. This intracellular enzyme requires NADH as a cofactor.

Chronic congenital methemoglobinemia has been recognized in rare individuals for more than a century. This condition is due to an inherited deficiency of methemoglobin reductase (Scott and Griffith, 1959). These individuals may chronically have 10 to 50 percent of their circulating blood pigment in the form of methemoglobin. The deficit is primarily a cosmetic one, since they have a compensatory polycythemia and little in the way of pathophysiological signs or symptoms. Since the methemoglobin levels are at a steady state short of complete oxidation, alternative mechanisms for methemoglobin reduction must exist in red cells, but these individuals are particularly sensitive to methemoglobin-generating chemicals. Any additional acquired pigment persists for abnormally long periods. Newborns are also said to be unusually sensitive to methemoglobin-generating chemicals both because of a transient deficiency in methemoglobin reductase and because of a high concentration of fetal hemoglobin in their erythrocytes.

Congenital methemoglobinopathies caused by abnormal amino acid substitutions in globin chains constitute separate disease entities. The abnormal hemoglobins M and H apparently have an enhanced ability to dissociate their heme groups, making the iron more susceptible to autoxidation. These people are also more sensitive to methemoglobin-generating chemicals in that higher peak concentrations are produced, but the methemoglobin reductase system functions normally.

The duration of methemoglobinemia after an acute challenge with a chemical such as sodium nitrite depends on both the peak concentrations generated and the methemoglobin reductase activity in the red cells of the species involved. Some evidence, however, suggests that nitrite or a product of the nitrite-hemoglobin reaction may inhibit the reductase system in mice (Kruszyna et al., 1982). Mouse red cells have unusually high rates of methemoglobin reductase activity (Table 11-1), but nitrite produces a uniquely prolonged methemoglobinemia in that species in comparison with all other agents tested. In human red cells, the reductase activity is so sluggish that the methemoglobinemia was of about the same duration with all the agents tested.

As shown in Table 11-1, methemoglobin reductase activities differ by over more than an order of magnitude among the red cells of the species tested. It is presumed that these differences primarily reflect differences in methemoglobin reductase activity, but possible contributions from alternative mechanisms were not evaluated. In each case glucose was the substrate, and the data have been expressed as a ratio of the species activity to that in human red cells. To place the ratios in perspective, estimates of the reduction half-time for 80 to 100 percent levels of methemoglobin in human red cells under the same conditions range from 6 to 24 h (Bolyai et al., 1972). The data are too crude to define the elimination kinetic pattern precisely, but in general rates of reduction seemed to decrease with decreasing methemoglobin levels.

Pig and horse red blood cells have considerably slower rates of reductase activity than do human cells (Table 11-1). In vivo, both porcine and equine red cells seem to utilize plasma lactate in preference to glucose as a metabolic fuel for methemoglobin reduction (Rivkin and Simon, 1965; Robin and Harley, 1967). The rat, guinea pig, mouse, and rabbit have high rates of methemoglobin reductase activity in relation to humans, but the significance of these differences is unknown.

***The Dormant NADPH-Linked Reductase System.*** Human and most mammalian red cells have a second methemoglobin reductase system that can be activated by methylene blue and requires NADPH as a cofactor (Figure 11-11). Because of the requirement for NADPH, methylene blue does not increase the rate of methemoglobin reduction in G-6-PD-deficient cells. The physiological function of the enzyme that is capable of reducing methylene blue is unknown. In a very rare case of congenital deficiency of this enzyme, methylene blue also failed to accelerate the rate of methemoglobin reduction. However, the methemoglobin levels were normal and the propositus had no other obvious pathophysiology (Sass et al., 1967). Reduced or leucomethylene blue transfers its acquired electron in normal subjects to reduce methemoglobin nonenzymatically (Sass et al., 1969). The injection of methylene blue in patients with severe acquired methemoglobinemias can be a life-saving intervention. It also temporarily returns levels to normal in subjects with methemoglobin reductase deficiency but should not be used chronically for that purpose. Large doses of ascorbic acid on a chronic basis are sometimes effective for this cosmetic purpose.

Species differences also exist in terms of the magnitude of the response to exogenous methylene blue (Table 11-2), but all the species tested responded to 1 to 2 × $10^{-5}$ *M* dye with an increase in reductase activity over that observed with glucose alone. The data are again expressed as a ratio of the species increase to the increase observed in human cells under the same conditions. To place these data in perspective, estimates of the reduction half-time of 70 to 90 percent levels of methemoglobin in human red cells with methylene blue range from 45 to 90 min (Layne and Smith, 1969). The observations were too crude to establish the precise kinetics of the reduction, but the data were approximately linear with time.

A certain parallelism can be seen between Tables 11-1 and 11-2 in that species with high rates of spontaneous reductase activity respond more vigorously to methylene blue, with the possible exception of the rabbit. The nucleated red cells of birds, reptiles, and amphibians also have both NADH and NADPH reductase systems, but in these species the tricarboxylic acid cycle appears to be the source of the cofactors (Board et al., 1977).

**Table 11–2**
**Stimulation of Methemoglobin Reductase Activity Mammalian Erythrocytes by Methylene Blue**

| | INVESTIGATORS | | | | |
|---|---|---|---|---|---|
| | (1) | (2) | (3) | (4) | (5) |
| SPECIES | *Increased Activity, Species/ Increased Activity, Humans* | | | | |
| Pig | 0.05 | 0.03 | | 0.15 | |
| Horse | 0.10 | 0.06 | | 0.25 | |
| Goat | 0.50 | 0.03 | | | |
| Sheep | 0.38 | 0.28 | | 0.45 | |
| Cow | 0.42 | 0.34 | | 1.0 | |
| Cat | | 0.69 | 0.16 | 0.65 | 1.0 |
| Dog | | 0.41 | 0.24 | 0.85 | 1.0 |
| Rabbit | | 0.50 | 1.4 | 0.70 | 0.50 |
| Mouse | | | | | 1.1 |
| Guinea pig | | 1.3 | 0.94 | 2.4 | |
| Rat | | 2.1 | 1.0 | 2.2 | 1.9 |

Data from various sources using nitrited red cells with glucose as a substrate have been normalized by the ratio

$$\frac{(\text{activity M.B. and glucose — activity glucose})_{\text{species}}}{(\text{activity M.B. and glucose — activity glucose})_{\text{human}}}$$

See footnote to Table 11-1 for literature citation.

***Minor Pathways for Methemoglobin Reduction.*** Red cells have several minor pathways for nonenzymatic methemoglobin reduction. Reduced glutathione slowly reduces methemoglobin but can account for only 12 percent of the total reductive capacity (Scott et al., 1965). Ascorbic acid (vitamin C) is sometimes used in patients with methemoglobin reductase deficiency (above) but normally accounts for only 16 percent of the total reductive effort. Scorbutic (ascorbate-deficient) subjects and G-6-PD-deficient subjects with decreased red cell levels of reduced glutathione do not have elevated levels of methemoglobin. Primates and guinea pigs are among the rare mammals that require exogenous ascorbate. Oddly, guinea pig red cells do not respond to ascorbate as do human cells (Bolyai et al., 1972). Cysteine, ergothioneine, NADH, and NADPH also have limited capabilities for direct methemoglobin reduction.

**Management of Acquired Methemoglobinemias.** As was already noted, methemoglobin-generating chemicals usually have additional toxic effects that contribute to the intoxication syndrome. Nevertheless, a reduction in the circulating levels of methemoglobin in symptomatic patients is a desirable therapeutic goal. With agents that produce hemolysis as well, this can be accomplished only by means of exchange transfusion. If the methemoglobin is intracellular and the cells are normal, the intravenous administration of 1 to 2 mg/kg of methylene blue usually results in a dramatic response (Gosselin et al., 1984). Although methylene blue is not equally efficacious against all chemically induced methemoglobinemias as tested in vitro in human red cell suspensions, it provides unequivocal protection against death in laboratory animals with all the agents that have been tested (Smith and Layne, 1969; Smith and Olson, 1973).

A possible alternative to methylene blue that would bypass the lesion in oxygen transport might be hyperbaric oxygen. Oxygen at 4 atmospheres decreased mortality and methemoglobin levels in rats that were given nitrite. After PAPP administration to rats, however, methemoglobin levels were actually increased (Goldstein and Doull, 1971, 1973). The mechanism of the effect on nitrite poisoning is not known, but hyperbaric oxygen seems to inhibit the acetylation of PAPP, which is an important mechanism for its detoxification. The same may be true of all related aromatic amino compounds that generate methemoglobin. In mice, methylene blue and hyperbaric oxygen seem to have additive effects in preventing nitrite poisoning (Way and Sheehy, 1971).

## Oxidative Hemolysis

**Sulfhemoglobin.** The term "sulfhemoglobin" was coined more than a century ago to describe a pigment generated in vitro by passing a stream of pure hydrogen sulfide through blood. This pigment does not play a role in acute hydrogen sulfide poisoning (see below). When generated in that manner, the pigment seems to be unstable, and the solutions become so turbid that visible absorption spectra can be derived only indirectly (Drabkin and Austin, 1935–1936).

Sulfhemoglobin may have a weak absorption maximum at about 620 nm, which overlaps to some extent with the absorption maximum of methemoglobin at 630 nm. This coincidence might have contributed to confusion in the early literature. In contrast to methemoglobin, the absorption maximum of sulfhemoglobin at 620 nm is not abolished by cyanide. This difference forms the basis for methods said to be suitable for the determination of both pigments in mixtures (Evelyn and Malloy, 1938; van Kampen and Zijlstra, 1965). So-called sulfhemoglobins of high purity have been generated in vitro with hydrogen sulfide under special conditions (e.g., Nichol et al., 1968), but their relationship to the originally described pigment is unknown.

When the criterion of an absorption band at 620 nm which is stable toward cyanide was applied to large numbers of human blood samples in clinical laboratories, positive results were obtained in some patients (Evelyn and Malloy, 1938). Those patients were said to be sulfhemoglobinemic even though no source of exposure to hydrogen sulfide or even to exogenous sulfur-containing xenebiotics could be documented. All attempts to find this pigment in laboratory animals that were exposed to hydrogen sulfide failed. In retrospect, it appears likely that two unrelated phenomena have been identified by the same name for many years because of a coincidence involving the position of an absorption maximum and its stability toward cyanide (National Academy of Sciences, 1977b).

Over the years, sulfhemoglobin has come to mean an abnormal blood pigment or pigments generated either in vivo or in vitro in the absence of exogenous sulfur. Perhaps this pigment might better be called pseudosulfhemoglobin, but it is associated with three clinical conditions: (1) the ingestion of "oxidant" drugs such as phenacetin, chlorate, and naphthalene, which also may generate low levels of methemoglobin in normal subjects, (2) the presence of an abnormal hemoglobin such as M or H (Tönz, 1968), and (3) the exposure of individuals with G-6-PD deficiency to certain drugs or chemicals such as primaquine, sulfonamides, and methylene blue (see below).

It seems likely that as it is encountered in the circumstances above, sulfhemoglobin is a partially oxidized and denatured mixture of pigments arising as a result of nonspecific oxidative damage (Beutler, 1969). No mechanism exists in red cells for the reversal of sulfhemoglobinemia, but it has never been encountered in life-threatening concentrations. Either it persists until the red cell containing it is replaced by erythropoiesis, or it is part of a broader and more serious hemolytic reaction (see below).

**Heinz Body Hemolytic Anemia.** Heinz bodies are dark-staining, dense refractile granules consisting of denatured hemoglobin, possibly sulfhemoglobin (Fig. 11-12). They appear to be covalently bound to the interior surface of red cell membranes, perhaps through disulfide bridges (Jacob et al., 1968). Gross distortions in the shape of the cell may occur, resulting in premature splenic phagocytosis, or impairment of active or passive ion transport may cause changes in osmotic pressure, hyperpermeability, and intravascular hemolysis. Thus, sulfhemoglobinemia, Heinz body formation, and hemolysis represent a continuum of oxidative stress to red cells.

Some authorities believe that the triad described above is preceded by a transient methemoglobinemia (Jandl et al., 1960), but others point to a poor (or even inverse) correlation between the ability of a given chemical to generate methemoglobin and its tendency to produce Heinz bodies (Rentsch, 1968). Methemoglobinemia per se does not lead to hemolysis (Beutler, 1969), although in some cases this may simply be a matter of dose or concentration. Oxygen is necessary for Heinz body formation but not for methemoglobin generation. Hydroxylamine reacts with deoxyhemoglobin to form methemoglobin, but the reaction with oxyhemoglobin results in both sulfhemoglobin and methemoglobin formation (Cranston and Smith, 1971).

***Mechanisms of Heinz Body Formation.*** Congenital Heinz bodies are found in individuals with certain types of abnormal hemoglobins that apparently facilitate dissociation of the heme group from the globin chains. Partial or total loss of heme groups results in decreased water solubility and an increased tendency for the pigment to precipitate. The heme group can be stabilized in vitro in such pigments with the addition of cyanide (see below) or carbon monoxide (Jacob et al., 1968; Rieder, 1970). Heme dissociation, however, has not been demonstrated in acquired Heinz body anemias as in the reaction of normal red cells with phenylhydrazine or the reaction of G-6-PD-deficient cells with primaquine.

It is now thought that oxidant chemicals such as phenylhydrazine generate hydrogen peroxide in red cells either by direct reaction with molecular oxygen or by a coupled reaction with oxyhemoglobin. The peroxide can be detoxified by glutathione peroxidase (Fig. 11-7), resulting in the oxidation of reduced

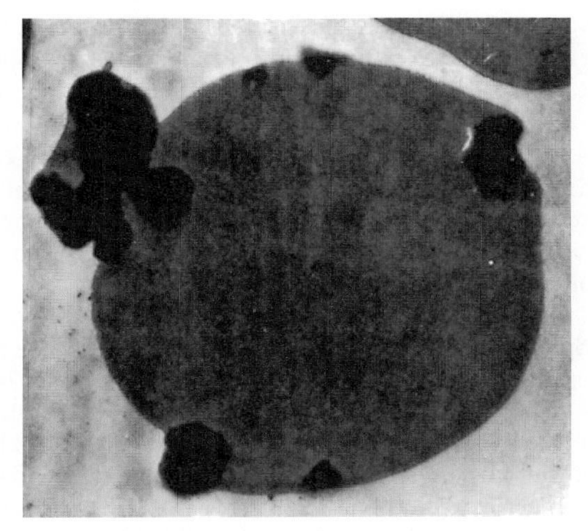

***Figure 11–12. End-stage Heinz bodies lying under and distorting the plasma membrane of a mature erythrocyte. ×26,000. [From Rifkind (1965).]***

glutathione. Oxidized glutathione is reduced by the activity of glutathione reductase, which also requires NADPH generated by G-6-PD. These three enzymes work in concert, and a deficiency in any one of them carries with it an increased sensitivity of the cell to oxidative stress. Red cells also contain catalase, but catalase-deficient red cells are not more sensitive to peroxide-induced damage. With the recent discovery that catalase also needs NADPH for maximum peroxide detoxification, it appears likely that G-6-PD deficiency compromises the activity of both glutathione peroxidase and catalase (Gaetani et al., 1989). The extent of the involvement of other active oxygen species, such as superoxide anion and superoxide dismutase, which is also present in red cells, is not clear. An early event in this reaction, whether it is induced in normal red cells or in G-6-PD-deficient ones, is a precipitous fall in the levels of glutathione. Oxidized glutathione may form mixed disulfides with free sulfhydryl groups on globin chains and thus contribute to instability and denaturation (Allen and Jandl, 1961).

***Agents Producing Heinz Bodies.*** Aniline, nitrobenzene, and related homologues produce Heinz bodies in many species. Whether the active metabolites are the same as those responsible for methemoglobin formation is not known. Prominent species differences probably relate to differences in the rates of activation and inactivation of these chemicals in vivo. Nonnitrogenous compounds also generate Heinz bodies; phenols, propylene glycol, ascorbic acid, sulfite dichromate, arsine, and stibine are examples. Hydroxylamine and chlorate salts were among the earliest agents that were recognized as eliciting this response. Ingestion of crude oil has resulted in Heinz body hemolytic anemia in marine birds (Leighton et al., 1983), and dimethyl disulfide produces this reaction in chickens (Maxwell, 1981). Perhaps Heinz body formation is a less specific oxidative process than is methemoglobin formation.

***Species Differences.*** Cat, mouse, dog, and human red cells are said to be particularly susceptible to Heinz body formation, whereas rabbit, monkey, chick, and guinea pig cells are relatively resistant. Unfortunately, these impressions are not based on systematic quantitative investigations. Indeed, there is no general agreement about how to quantify the damage in such reactions. The morphology and ultrastructure of Heinz bodies also vary between species and agents. Under certain conditions, large numbers of small bodies are seen. Perhaps these bodies eventually coalesce into larger multibodied inclusions. In the nucleated turkey red cell, phenylhydrazine-induced Heinz bodies were smaller than those produced under identical conditions in dog and horse red cells and were seen in both the nucleoplasm and the cytoplasm. Extraerythrocytic Heinz bodies were observed with suspensions of horse red cells but not dog or turkey red cells (Simpson, 1971).

**The Spleen.** Although red cells normally end their life in the spleen after 120 days in the circulation, splenectomy in humans does not result in an increase in red cell survival time. The function of senescent red cell destruction is quickly assumed by other segments of the reticuloendothelial system, such as the liver and bone marrow. The anatomic ultrastructure of the spleen, however, is particularly well suited for that task. Red cells enter the spleen via the Billroth's cord from a terminal arteriole or capillary, percolate through the fine spaces formed by reticular fibers and macrophages, and then exit by gaining access to a splenic sinusoid. This is the moment of truth, for the red cell then has to pass through fenestrations in the sinusoidal basement membrane that are smaller than its own diameter. The apertures are lined with macrophages. Cells with unusual shapes such as sickle cells, cells with Heinz bodies, and cells lacking the metabolic energy to resume their normal conformation after passage through capillaries are phagocytized, as are cells flagged with immunoglobulin or complement (Weed et al., 1969). After hemolysis, the hemoglobin is catabolized and the heme groups are degraded to bilirubin. Splenic engorgement and increased heme oxidase activity are signs of hemolytic disease because of the increased demand for these functions.

## HISTOTOXIC HYPOXIA

Semantic purists object to the term "histotoxic hypoxia" because in this condition the $P_{O_2}$ in peripheral tissues is normal or higher than normal. The lesion is characterized by an inability to utilize molecular oxygen at the cellular level. The chemicals known to have this action are the soluble salts or weak acids of sulfide and cyanide. Ballantyne and Marrs (1987) have edited an exhaustive monograph on cyanide. The key features for the case of hydrogen cyanide are illustrated in Fig. 11-13, but hydrogen sulfide is very similar. Some evidence suggests that it is the undissociated acids that actually interrupt electron transport down the chain through inhibition at the cytochrome a–cytochrome $a_3$ step (Smith et al., 1977). Since these cytochromes are isolated as a single unit, they are referred to as cytochrome $aa_3$ or cytochrome *c* oxidase. As a result of cyanide inhibition, oxidative phosphorylation and aerobic metabolism are compromised. Electron transfer from cyto-

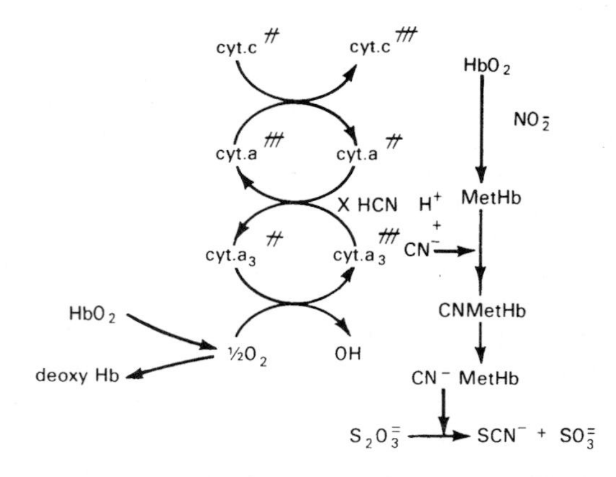


***Figure 11–13. Principles of the therapeutic management of cyanide poisoning.***

Although the exact chemical details are still unknown, the undissociated form (HCN) appears to block electron transfer in the cytochrome $aa_3$ complex. As a consequence, oxygen utilization is decreased and oxidative metabolism may slow to the point where it cannot meet metabolic demands. At the level of the brainstem nuclei, this effect may result in central respiratory arrest and death. On injection of sodium nitrite, methemoglobin is generated, which can compete effectively with cytochrome $aa_3$ for free cyanide. Note that it is the ionic form that complexes with methemoglobin. The injection of thiosulfate provides subtrate for the enzyme rhodanese, which catalyzes the biotransformation of cyanide to thiocyanate.

chrome oxidase to molecular oxygen is blocked, peripheral tissue $P_{O_2}$ begins to rise, and the unloading gradient for oxyhemoglobin is decreased. As a result, abnormally high concentrations of oxyhemoglobin are found in the venous return, imparting a flush to skin and mucous membranes that is not unlike that seen in carbon monoxide poisoning. The increased demand placed on glycolysis results in a profound lactic acidemia.

Cyanide and sulfide directly stimulate the chemoreceptors of the carotid and aortic bodies to produce a brief period of hyperpnea. Cardiac irregularities are often noted, but the heart invariably outlasts the respirations. Death is due to central respiratory arrest, which can occur within seconds or minutes of the inhalation of high concentrations of hydrogen cyanide or sulfide gas. Because of slower absorption, death may be delayed after the ingestion of cyanide salts, but the critical events still occur within the first hour.

As a strong nucleophile, cyanide probably has multiple effects. In neurons it leads to the accumulation of intracellular calcium (Johnson et al., 1986). Cyanide can initiate the release of catecholamines from the adrenals and adrenergic nerve terminals (Kanthasamy et al., 1991). It causes the release of excitatory neurotransmitters in the brain (Patel et al., 1991a and b) and inhibits enzymes that protect the brain against oxidation injury (Ardelt et al., 1989).

Other sources of cyanide have been responsible for human poisonings, such as amygdalin, a cyanogenic glycoside found in sweet almonds and apricot, peach, and other fruit pits. Amygdalin is a complex of glucose, benzaldehyde, and cyanide; the cyanide is released by the action of $\beta$-glucosidase or emulsin. Such enzymes are not found in mammalian tissues but are present in normal human intestinal microflora. For this reason, amygdalin is about 40 times more toxic by mouth than it is by intravenous injection. Thus, the quack anticancer remedy Laetrile, which consisted chiefly of amygdalin, could be given safely by parenteral routes but caused cyanide poisoning when accidentally ingested by children.

The antihypertensive drug sodium nitroprusside can cause cyanide poisoning in an overdose. Its reaction with hemoglobin results in the direct formation of cyanmethemoglobin, but in vivo most of the cyanide seems to be released by its reaction with the vascular endothelium or smooth muscle (Smith and Kruszyna, 1974; Devlin et al., 1989b). Fortunately, the therapeutic index for nitroprusside is quite high. The acute toxic effects of a series of commercially important aliphatic nitriles also appear to be due to the metabolic release of free cyanide (Willhite and Smith, 1981; Doherty et al., 1982).

## Treatment of Cyanide Poisoning

Time is of the essence in treating cyanide poisoning, and traditionally three drugs have been given. The most controversial of these drugs is amyl nitrite given by inhalation. Amyl nitrite is a poor methemoglobin former in humans, especially when given by the pulmonary route, but it seems to serve no other useful purpose (Klimmek and Krettek, 1988). This is followed by sodium nitrite given intravenously in an initial dose of 300 mg for an adult. The nitrite converts a tolerable fraction of the total circulating hemoglobin to methemoglobin (Fig. 11-13). Ferric heme groups avidly bind ionic cyanide to form the stable complex cyanmethemoglobin. As the blood concentration of free cyanide falls, it effects a dissociation of the cyanide complex with cytochrome oxidase and a resumption of oxidative metabolism. Up to this point, the same basic principles hold for sulfide as well.

Although this approach can be rapidly efficacious, there are two undesirable results to this stopgap measure. Cyanmethemoglobin is inert in terms of oxygen transport, and although the cyanide is bound very tenaciously, it is still a fully reversible complex which carries a risk of the release of free cyanide and the recurrence of the poisoning. In some species, such as rabbits and mice, cyanmethemoglobin apparently can serve as a substrate for methemoglobin reductase. Late deaths may ensue as the cyanide is released from this biologically inert store (Kruszyna et al., 1982). Permanent irreversible detoxification of cyanide is accomplished through the intravenous injection of sodium thiosulfate. Thiosulfate contains a sulfane-sulfur, one bound only to another sulfur, which can be utilized by the widely distributed enzyme rhodanese (thiosulfate-cyanide sulfurtransferase) to convert cyanide to thiocyanate. This much less toxic product is excreted in the urine. After dissociation of its cyanide for biotransformation, methemoglobin is restored to functional blood pigment by the action of methemoglobin reductase (Fig. 11-11).

It has long been believed that liver rhodanese plays the major role in cyanide detoxification, particularly when exogenous thiosulfate is provided, but rhodanese in skeletal muscle makes a significant contribution. Indeed, in the absence of thiosulfate, skeletal muscle clears more cyanide than does the liver (Devlin et al., 1989a). This observation and an inferred large redundancy of the liver enzyme may explain why surgical removal of two-thirds of the liver or severe liver damage induced by carbon tetrachloride did not increase cyanide lethality in mice whether or not thiosulfate was also given (Rutkowski et al., 1986). Prominent species differences are recognized in rhodanese activity; sheep have relatively high levels of activity, whereas dogs have relatively low levels (Aminlari and Gilanpour, 1991).

Although oxygen can do no harm, in terms of the principles summarized in Fig. 11-13, it seems to serve no useful purpose. Even hyperbaric oxygen alone had no effect on cyanide poisoning in mice (Way et al., 1972). However, oxygen further and significantly decreased mortality when it was used in combination with nitrite and thiosulfate in cyanide-poisoned mice (Way et al., 1966). Since rhodanese is not sensitive to oxygen, the mechanism for this potentiation is unknown.

## Hydrogen Sulfide Poisoning

As was noted above, hydrogen sulfide has also been established as an in vitro inhibitor of cytochrome oxidase (Smith et al., 1977). Human poisonings invariably result from exposure to the gas, but soluble salts are used experimentally by the parenteral route in laboratory animals. In either case, the signs of poisoning are similar in almost all respects to those induced by cyanide. Sulfide, however, has a greater tendency to produce local tissue reactions such as conjunctivitis (gas eye) and pulmonary edema (Lopez et al., 1989).

As was already noted, the hydrosulfide anion ($HS^-$) forms a complex with methemoglobin known as sulfmethemoglobin, which is analogous to cyanmethemoglobin. Sulfmethemoglobin is a well-characterized entity, in contrast to the confusion (see above) about the identity of sulfhemoglobin. The dissociation constant for sulfmethemoglobin is about $6 \times 10^{-6}$ mol/liter, whereas the dissociation constant for cyanmethemoglobin is on the order of $2 \times 10^{-8}$ mol/liter. Despite the lower binding affinity, a nitrite-induced methemoglobinemia provides unequivocal protection and has antidotal effects against sulfide poisoning in laboratory animals (Smith and Gosselin, 1964). The procedure has been used successfully in the resuscitation of several human victims of hydrogen sulfide poisoning (Hoidal et al., 1986; Huang and Chu, 1987; Stine et al., 1976; Peters, 1981). Neither thiosulfate nor oxygen has significant effects alone or in combination with nitrite (Smith et al., 1976), but oxygen is indicated if the victim shows signs of adult respiratory distress syndrome. Sulfide reacts rapidly to split disulfide bridges under physiological conditions; thus, oxidized glutathione and other simple disulfides have protective and possibly antidotal effects (Smith and Abbanat, 1966). Sulfide in vivo is metabolized to sulfite and sulfate.

Hydrogen sulfide can be encountered in high concentrations in natural and volcanic gases and petroleum deposits. Hydrothermal vents in certain locations on the ocean floor continuously release high concentrations, and vent tube worms in the vicinity may have blood concentrations that would be lethal to mammalian species. A primitive form of hemoglobin in their blood binds sulfide through its ability to split disulfide bonds and transports it to an organ containing symbiotic bacteria that utilize it as an energy-producing substrate (Powell and Somero, 1983).

Sewer gas, a synonym for hydrogen sulfide, refers to its presence wherever organic matter undergoes putrefaction. It is found in the emissions from industrial paper plants that use the Kraft process. The leather industry uses hydrosulfide to remove the hair from hides before tanning, and ton quantities have been employed in facilities for the production of heavy water for nuclear reactors (National Academy of Sciences, 1977b). Carbonyl sulfide, a by-product of coal hydrogenation and gasification, is metabolized in vivo to hydrogen sulfide by carbonic anhydrase (Chengelis and Neal, 1980). Rare human poisonings resemble hydrogen sulfide intoxication except for the delay in the appearance of the signs (presumably as a result of the need for metabolism) and highly labile periods of unconsciousness (Gosselin et al., 1984). One patient was successfully resuscitated, using the nitrite therapy for hydrogen sulfide descibed above (Martin et al., 1994).

# REFERENCES


Allen DW, Jandl JH: Oxidative hemolysis and precipitation of hemoglobin: II. Role of thiols in oxidant drug action. *J Clin Invest* 40:454–475. 1961.

Aminlari M, Gilanpour H: Comparative studies on the distribution of rhodanese in different tissues of domestic animals. *Comp Biochem Physiol* 99B:673–677, 1991.

Ardelt BK, Borowitz JL, Isom GE: Brain lipid peroxidation and antioxidant defense mechanisms following cyanide intoxication. *Toxicology* 56:147–154, 1989.

Ballantyne B, Marrs TC: *Clinical and Experimental Toxicology of Cyanides*. Bristol: Wright, 1987.

Bartels H, Hilpert P, Barbey K, et al: Respiratory functions of blood of the yak, llama, camel, Dybowski deer and African elephant. *Am J Physiol* 205:331–336, 1963.

Bartlett D Jr: Effects of carbon monoxide in human physiological processes. *Proceedings of the Conference on Health Effects of Air Pollutants*. Washington, DC: U.S. Government Printing Office, Serial 93–15, November 1973, pp 103–126.

Bernard C: *An Introduction to the Study of Experimental Medicine*, first 1865. Reprinted by New York: Dover, 1957.

Bessis M: *Blood Smears Reinterpreted*, transl. by G. Brecher. Berlin: Springer-Verlag, 1977.

Beutler E: Drug-induced hemolytic anemia. *Pharmacol Rev* 21:73–103, 1969.

Birner G, Neumann H-G: Biomonitoring of aromatic amines: II. Hemoglobin binding of some monocyclic amines. *Arch Toxicol* 62:110–115, 1988.

Board PG, Agar NS, Gruca M, Shine R: Methaemoglobin and its reduction in nucleated erythrocytes from reptiles and birds. *Comp Biochem Physiol* 57B:265–267, 1977.

Bolyai JZ, Smith RP, Gray CT: Ascorbic acid and chemically induced methemoglobinemias. *Toxicol Appl Pharmacol* 21:176–185, 1972.

Born GVR: Aggregation of blood platelets by adenosine diphosphate and its reversal. *Nature* 194:927–929, 1962.

Brown SD, Piantadosi CS: Recovery of energy metabolism in rat brain after carbon monoxide hypoxia. *J Clin Invest* 89:666–672, 1992.

Bryant MS, Vineis P, Skipper PL, Tannenbaum SR: Hemoglobin adducts of aromatic amines: Associations with smoking status and type of tobacco. *Proc Natl Acad Sci USA* 85:9788–9791, 1988.

Burns KF, de Lannoy CW Jr: Compendia of normal blood values of laboratory animals, with indications of variations: I. Random-sexed populations of small animals. *Toxicol Appl Pharmacol* 8:429–437, 1966.

Calsey JD, King DJ: Clinical chemical values for some common laboratory animals. *Clin Chem* 26:1877–1879, 1980.

Cerami A, Manning JM: Potassium cyanate as an inhibitor of the sickling of erythrocytes *in vitro*. *Proc Natl Acad Sci USA* 68:1180–1183, 1971.

Chengelis CP, Neal RA: Studies of carbonyl disulfide toxicity: Metabolism by carbonic anhydrase. *Toxicol Appl Pharmacol* 55:198–202, 1980.

Coburn RF, Williams WJ, White P, Kahn SB: The production of carbon monoxide from hemoglobin *in vivo*. *J Clin Invest* 46:346–356, 1967.

Cranston RD, Smith RP: Some aspects of the reactions between hydroxylamine and hemoglobin derivatives. *J Pharmacol Exp Ther* 177:440–446, 1971.

Devlin DJ, Smith RP, Thron CD: Cyanide metabolism in the isolated, perfused, bloodless hindlimbs or liver of the rat. *Toxicol Appl Pharmacol* 98:338–349, 1989a.

Devlin DJ, Smith RP, Thron CD: Cyanide release from nitroprusside in the isolated, perfused, bloodless liver and hindlimbs of the rat. *Toxicol Appl Pharmacol* 99:354–356, 1989b.

Doherty PA, Smith RP, Ferm VH: Tetramethyl substitution on succinonitrile confers pentylenetetrazole-like activity and blocks cyanide release in mice. *J Pharmacol Exp Ther* 223:635–641, 1982.

Douglas CG, Haldane JS, Haldane JBS: The laws of combination of haemoglobin with carbon monoxide and oxygen. *J Physiol (Lond)* 44:275–304, 1912.

Drabkin DL, Austin JH: Spectrophotometric studies: II. Preparations from washed blood cells; nitric oxide hemoglobin and sulfhemoglobin. *J Biol Chem* 112:51–65, 1935–1936.

Evelyn KA, Malloy HT: Microdetermination of oxyhemoglobin, methemoglobin and sulfhemoglobin in a single sample of blood. *J Biol Chem* 126:655–662, 1938.

Fridovich I: Superoxide radical, an endogenous toxicant. *Annu Rev Pharmacol Toxicol* 23:239–257, 1983.

Gaetani GF, Galiano S, Canepa L, et al: Catalase and glutathione peroxidase are equally active in detoxification of hydrogen peroxide in human erythrocytes. *Blood* 73:334–339, 1989.

Goldberg MA, Dunning SP, Bunn HF: Regulation of the erythropoietin gene: Evidence that the oxygen sensor is a heme protein. *Science* 242:1412–1415, 1988.

Goldstein GM, Doull J: Treatment of nitrite-induced methemoglobinemia with hyperbaric oxygen. *Proc Soc Exp Biol Med* 138:137–139, 1971.

Goldstein GM, Doull J: The use of hyperbaric oxygen in the treatment of *p*-aminopropiophenone-induced methemoglobinemia. *Toxicol Appl Pharmacol* 26:247–252, 1973.

Gosselin RE, Smith RP, Hodge HC: *Clinical Toxicology of Commercial Products,* 5th ed. Baltimore: Williams & Wilkins, 1984.

Harris JW, Kellermeyer RW: *The Red Cell—Production, Metabolism, Destruction: Normal and Abnormal,* rev. ed. Cambridge, MA.: Harvard University Press, 1970.

Hoidal CR, Hall AH, Robinson MD, et al: Hydrogen sulfide poisoning from toxic inhalations of roofing asphalt fumes. *Ann Emerg Med* 15:826–830, 1986.

Huang C-C, Chu N-S: A case of acute hydrogen sulfide ($H_2S$) intoxication sucessfully treated with nitrites. *J Formosan Med Assoc* 86:1018–1020, 1987.

Jacob HS, Brian MC, Dacie JV: Altered sulfhydryl reactivity of hemoglobins and red blood cell membranes in congenital Heinz body hemolytic anemia. *J Clin Invest* 47:2644–2677, 1968.

Jandl JH, Engle LK, Allen DW: Oxidative hemolysis and precipitation of hemoglobin: I. Heinz body anemias as an acceleration of red cell aging. *J Clin Invest* 39:1818–1836, 1960.

Johnson JP, Meisenheimer TL, Isom GE: Cyanide-induced neurotoxity: Role of neuronal calcium. *Toxicol Appl Pharmacol* 84:464–469, 1986.

Kanthasamy AG, Borowitz JL, Isom GE: Cyanide-induced increases in plasma catecholamines: Relationship to acute toxicity. *Neurotoxicology* 12:777–784, 1991.

Kiese M: *Methemoglobinemia: A Comprehensive Treatise*. Cleveland: CRC Press, 1974.

Kiese M, Weis B: Die Reduktion des Hämiglobins in den Erythrocyten verschiedener Tiere. *Naunyn Schmiedebergs Arch Pharmacol* 202:493–501, 1943.

Klimmek R, Krettek C: Effects of amyl nitrite on circulation, respiration and blood hemostasis in cyanide poisoning. *Arch Toxicol* 62:161–166, 1988.

Kruszyna R, Kruszyna H, Smith RP: Comparison of hydroxylamine, 4-dimethylaminophenol and nitrite protection against cyanide poisoning in mice. *Arch Toxicol* 49:191–202, 1982.

Kruszyna R, Kruszyna H, Smith RP, Wilcox DE: Generation of valency hybrids and nitrosylated species of hemoglobin in mice by nitric oxide vasodilators. *Toxicol Appl Pharmacol* 94:458–465, 1988.

Layne WR, Smith RP: Methylene blue uptake and the reversal of chemically induced methemoglobinemias in human erythrocytes. *J Pharmacol Exp Ther* 165:36–44, 1969.

Leighton FA, Peakall DB, Butler RG: Heinz body hemolytic anemia from the ingestion of crude oil, a primary toxic effect in marine birds. *Science* 220:871–873, 1983.

Letvin NL, Linch DC, Beardsley GP, et al: Augmentation of fetal hemoglobin production in anemic monkeys by hydroxyurea. *N Engl J Med* 310:869–873, 1984.

Lopez A, Prior MG, Reiffenstein RJ, Goodwin LR: Preacute toxic effects of inhaled hydrogen sulfide and injected sodium hydrosulfide on the lungs of rats. *Fundam Appl Toxicol* 12:367–373, 1989.

Malz E: Vergleichende Untersuchungen über die Methämoglobinreduktion in kernhaltigen und kernlosen Erythrozyten. *Folia Haematol (Leipz)* 78:510–515, 1962.

Martin HL, Nutt AW, Myers BL, Hightower JO: Unknown plant deconstruction hazard—toxic COS and $CS_2$ gas from torch cutting of pipe MS-94-0180. Aikers, SC: Westinghouse Savannah River Co., 1994.

Maxwell MH: Production of a Heinz body anemia in the domestic fowl after ingestion of dimethyl disulfide: A haematological and ultrastructural study. *Res Vet Sci* 30:233–238, 1981.

Mitruka BM, Rawnsley HM: *Clinical Biochemical and Hematological Reference Values in Normal Experimental Animals*. New York: Masson, 1977.

Müller-Eberhard U: Hemopexin. *N Engl J Med* 238:1090–1094, 1970.

National Academy of Sciences: *Carbon Monoxide*. Washington, D.C.: Committee on Medical and Biological Effects of Environmental Pollutants, National Research Council, 1977a.

National Academy of Sciences: *Hydrogen Sulfide*. Washington, D.C.: Committee on Medical and Biological Effects of Environmental Pollutants, National Research Council, 1977b.

Ng LL, Naik RB, Polak B: Paraquat ingestion with methaemoglobinaemia treated with methylene blue. *Br Med J* 284:1445, 1982.

Nichol AW, Hendry I, Morrell DB: Mechanism of formation of sulfhaemoglobin. *Biochim Biophys Acta* 156:97–108, 1968.

Norton JM, Smith RP: Drugs affecting the oxygen transport function of hemoglobin, in *Respiratory Pharmacology,* Section 104: *International Encyclopedia of Pharmacology and Therapeutics* (section ed., J. Widdicombe). Oxford: Pergamon Press, 1981.

Ou LC, Kim D, Layton WM Jr, Smith RP: Splenic erythropoiesis in polycythemic response of the rat to high altitude exposure. *J Appl Physiol* 48:857–861, 1980.

Ou LC, Smith RP: Hemoglobinuria in rats exposed to high altitude. *Exp Hematol* 6:473–478, 1978.

Patel MN, Yim GKW, Isom GE: Blockade of N-metyl-D-aspartate receptors prevents cyanide-induced neuronal injury in primary hippocampal cultures. *Toxicol Appl Pharmacol* 115:124–129, 1992a.

Patel MN, Yim GKW, Isom GE: Potentiation of cyanide neurotoxicity by blockade of ATP-sensitive potassium channels. *Brain Res* 593:114–116, 1992b.

Perutz MF, Muirhead H, Cox JM, Goaman LCG: Three-dimensional Fourier synthesis of horse oxyhaemoglobin at 2.8 Å resolution: The atomic model. *Nature* 219:131–139, 1968.

Peters JW: Hydrogen sulfide poisoning in a hospital setting. *JAMA* 246:1588–1589, 1981.

Piantadosi CA: Carbon monoxide poisoning, in Vincent TL (ed): *Update in Intensive Care and Emergency Medicine*. Berlin: Springer Verlag, vol 10, 1990, pp 460–471.

Pisciotta AV: Immune and toxic mechanisms in drug-induced agranulocytosis. *Semin Hematol* 10:279–310, 1973.

Powell MA, Somero GN: Blood components prevent sulfide poisoning of respiration of the hydrothermal vent tube worm *Rifitia pachytila. Science* 219:297–299, 1983.

Prankerd TAJ: *The Red Cell: An Account of Its Clinical Physiology and Pathology*. Oxford: Blackwell, 1961.

Reddy BG, Pohl LR, Krishna G: The requirement of the gut flora in nitrobenzene-induced methemoglobinemia in rats. *Biochem Pharmacol* 25:119–122, 1976.

Rentsch G: Genesis of Heinz bodies and methemoglobin formation. *Biochem Pharmacol* 17:423–427, 1968.

Rieder RF: Hemoglobin stability: Observations on the denaturation of normal and abnormal hemoglobins by oxidant dyes, heat and alkali. *J Clin Invest* 49:2369–2376, 1970.

Rifkind RA, Bank A, Marks PA, et al: *Fundamentals of Hematology,* 2d ed. Chicago: Year Book, 1980.

Rifkind RA, Danon D: Heinz body anemia—an ultrastructural study: I. Heinz body formation. *Blood* 25:885–896, 1965.

Rivkin SE, Simon ER: Comparative carbohydrate metabolism and methemoglobin reduction in pig and human erythrocytes. *J Cell Comp Physiol* 66:49–56, 1965.

Robin H, Harley JD: Factors influencing response of mammalian species to the methemoglobin reduction test. *Aust J Exp Biol Med Sci* 4:519–526, 1966.

Robin H, Harley JD: Regulation of methaemoglobinemia in horse and human erythrocytes. *Aust J Exp Biol Med Sci* 45:77–88, 1967.

Rutkowski JV, Roebuck BD, Smith RP: Liver damage does not increase the sensitivity of mice to cyanide given acutely. *Toxicology* 38:305–314, 1986.

Sass MD, Caruso CJ, Axelrod DR: Mechanism of the TPNH-linked reduction of methemoglobin by methylene blue. *Clin Chim Acta* 24:77–85, 1969.

Sass MD, Caruso CJ, Farhangi M: TPNH-methemoglobin reductase deficiency: A new red cell enzyme defect. *J Lab Clin Med* 70:760–767, 1967.

Schwerin FT, Rosenstein R, Smith RP: Cyanide prevents the inhibition of platelet aggregation by nitroprusside, hydroxylamine and azide. *Thromb Haemost* 50:780–783, 1983.

Scott EM, Duncan IW, Ekstrand V: The reduced pyridine nucleotide dehydrogenases of human erythrocytes. *J Biol Chem* 240:481–485, 1965.

Scott EM, Griffith IV: Enzymatic defect of hereditary methemoglobinemia: The diaphorase. *Biochim Biophys Acta* 34:584–586, 1959.

Simpson CF: The ultrastructure of Heinz bodies in horse, dog, and turkey erythrocytes. *Cornell Vet* 61:228–238, 1971.

Smith JE, Beutler E: Anomeric specificity of human erythrocyte glucose-6-phosphate dehydrogenase. *Proc Soc Exp Biol Med* 122:671–673, 1966a.

Smith JE, Beutler E: Methemoglobin formation and reduction in man and various animal species. *Am J Physiol* 210:347–350, 1966b.

Smith L, Kruszyna H, Smith RP: The effect of methemoglobin on the inhibition of cytochrome *c* oxidase by cyanide, sulfide and azide. *Biochem Pharmacol* 26:2247–2250, 1977.

Smith RP: The nitrite-methemoglobin complex—its significance in methemoglobin analyses and its possible role in methemoglobinemia. *Biochem Pharmacol* 16:1655–1664, 1967.

Smith RP, Abbanat RA: Protective effect of oxidized glutathione in acute sulfide poisoning. *Toxicol Appl Pharmacol* 9:209–217, 1966.

Smith RP, Alkaitis AA, Shafer PR: Chemically induced methemoglobinemias in the mouse. *Biochem Pharmacol* 16:317–328, 1967.

Smith RP, Gosselin RE: The influence of methemoglobinemia on the lethality of some toxic anions: II. Sulfide. *Toxicol Appl Pharmacol* 6:584–592, 1964.

Smith RP, Kruszyna H: Nitroprusside produces cyanide poisoning via a reaction with hemoglobin. *J Pharmacol Exp Ther* 191:557–563, 1974.

Smith RP, Kruszyna R, Kruszyna H: Management of acute sulfide poisoning: Effects of oxygen, thiosulfate, and nitrite. *Arch Environ Health,* 33:166–169, 1976.

Smith RP, Layne WR: A comparison of the lethal effects of nitrite and hydroxylamine in the mouse. *J Pharmacol Exp Ther* 165:30–35, 1969.

Smith RP, Olson MV: Drug-induced methemoglobinemia. *Semin Hematol* 10:253–268, 1973.

Smith RP, Thron CD: Hemoglobin, methylene blue and oxygen interactions in human red cells. *J Pharmacol Exp Ther* 183:549–558, 1972.

Snyder CA: Benzene, in Snyder R (ed): *Ethel Browning's Toxicity and Metabolism of Industrial Solvents,* 2d ed., vol 1: *Hydrocarbons*. Amsterdam: Elsevier, 1987.

Spencer TD: Effect of carbon monoxide on man and canaries. *Ann Occup Hyg* 5:231–240, 1962.

Stebbins R, Bertino JR: Megaloblastic anemias produced by drugs. *Clin Haematol* 5:619–630, 1976.

Stine RJ, Slosberg B, Beacham BE: Hydrogen sulfide intoxication: A case report and discussion of treatment. *Ann Intern Med* 85:756–758, 1976.

Stolk JM, Smith RP: Species differences in methemoglobin reductase activity. *Biochem Pharmacol* 15:343–351, 1966.

Stuart PR, Osborn JS, Lewis SM: The use of radio-frequency sputter ion etching and scanning electron microscopy to study the internal structure of biological material. *Proc 2nd Annual Scanning Electron Microscope Symposium*. Chicago: IIT Research Institute, April 1969.

Stuehr DJ, Marletta MA: Synthesis of nitrite and nitrate in murine macrophage cell lines. *Cancer Res* 47:5590–5594, 1987.

Surgenor DM: *The Red Blood Cell,* 2d ed. New York: Academic Press, vol I, 1974; vol II, 1975.

Tavassoli M, Crosby WH: Fate of the nucleus of the marrow erythroblast. *Science* 179:912–913, 1973.

Tomoda A, Yoneyama Y: A simple method for preparation of valency hybrid hemoglobins, $(\alpha^{3+}\beta^{2+})_2$ and $(\alpha^{2+}\beta^{3+})_2$. *Anal Biochem* 110:431–436, 1981.

Tönz O: *The Congenital Methemoglobinemias, Physiology and Pathophysiology of Hemoglobin Metabolism*. Basel: S. Karger, 1968. Published simultaneously as *Bibliotheca Haematologica,* no. 28.

Van Assendelft OW, Zijlstra WG: The formation of haemoglobin using nitrites. *Clin Chim Acta* 11:571–577, 1965.

Van Kampen EJ, Zijlstra WG: Determination of hemoglobin and its derivatives, in Sobotka H, Stewart CP (eds): *Advances in Clinical Chemistry*. New York: Academic Press, 1965, pp 142–187.

Wang Q, Jacobs J, DeLeo J, Kruszyna H, et al: Nitric oxide hemoglobin in mice and rats in endotoxic shock. *Life Sci* 49:PL55–PL60, 1991.

Way JL, End E, Sheehy M, et al: Effect of oxygen on cyanide intoxication: IV. Hyperbaric oxygen. *Toxicol Appl Pharmacol* 22:415–421, 1972.

Way JL, Gibbon SL, Sheehy M: Effect of oxygen on cyanide intoxication: I. Prophylactic protection. *J Pharmacol Exp Ther* 153:381–385, 1966.

Way JL, Sheehy M: Antagonism of sodium nitrite intoxication. *Toxicol Appl Pharmacol* 19:400–401, 1971.

Weed RI, LaCelle PL, Merritt EW: Metabolic dependence of red cell deformability. *J Clin Invest* 48:795–809, 1969.

Willhite CC, Smith RP: The role of cyanide liberation in the acute toxicity of aliphatic nitriles. *Toxicol Appl Pharmacol* 59:589–602, 1981.

# CHAPTER 12

# TOXIC RESPONSES OF THE IMMUNE SYSTEM

*Leigh Ann Burns, B. Jean Meade, and Albert E. Munson*

Immunity, by definition, is a homeostatic condition in which the body maintains protection from infectious disease. It is a series of delicately balanced, complex, multicellular, and physiological mechanisms that allow an individual to distinguish foreign material from "self" and to neutralize and/or eliminate the foreign matter. It is characterized by a virtually infinite repertoire of specificities, highly specialized effectors, complex regulatory mechanisms, and an ability to travel throughout the body. The immune system provides the means to initiate rapid and highly specific responses against a myriad of potentially pathogenic organisms. Indeed, the conditions of genetically determined immunodeficiency and of acquired immunodeficiency syndrome (AIDS) graphically highlight the importance of the immune system in the host's defense against microbial infection. In addition, evidence is rapidly building that the immune system plays a role in tumor identification and rejection (immune surveillance).

In light of the central role that the immune system plays in the maintenance of the health of the individual, the interaction of xenobiotics (pharmacological agents, environmental contaminants, and other chemicals) with the various components of the immune system has become an area of profound interest. Indeed, in some instances, the immune system has been shown to be compromised (decreased lymphoid cellularity, alterations in lymphocyte subpopulations, decreased host resistance, altered specific immune function responses) in the absence of observed toxicity in other organ systems. Decreased immunocompetence (immunosuppression) may result in repeated, more severe, or prolonged infections as well as the development of cancer. Immunoenhancement may lead to immune-mediated diseases such as hypersensitivity responses or autoimmune disease (Fig. 12-1). Because of the potentially profound effects resulting from disruption of the delicately balanced immune system, there is a need to understand the cellular, biochemical, and molecular mechanisms of xenobiotic-induced immunomodulation. With the availability of sensitive, reproducible, and predictive tests, it is now apparent that the inclusion of immunotoxicity testing may represent a sig-

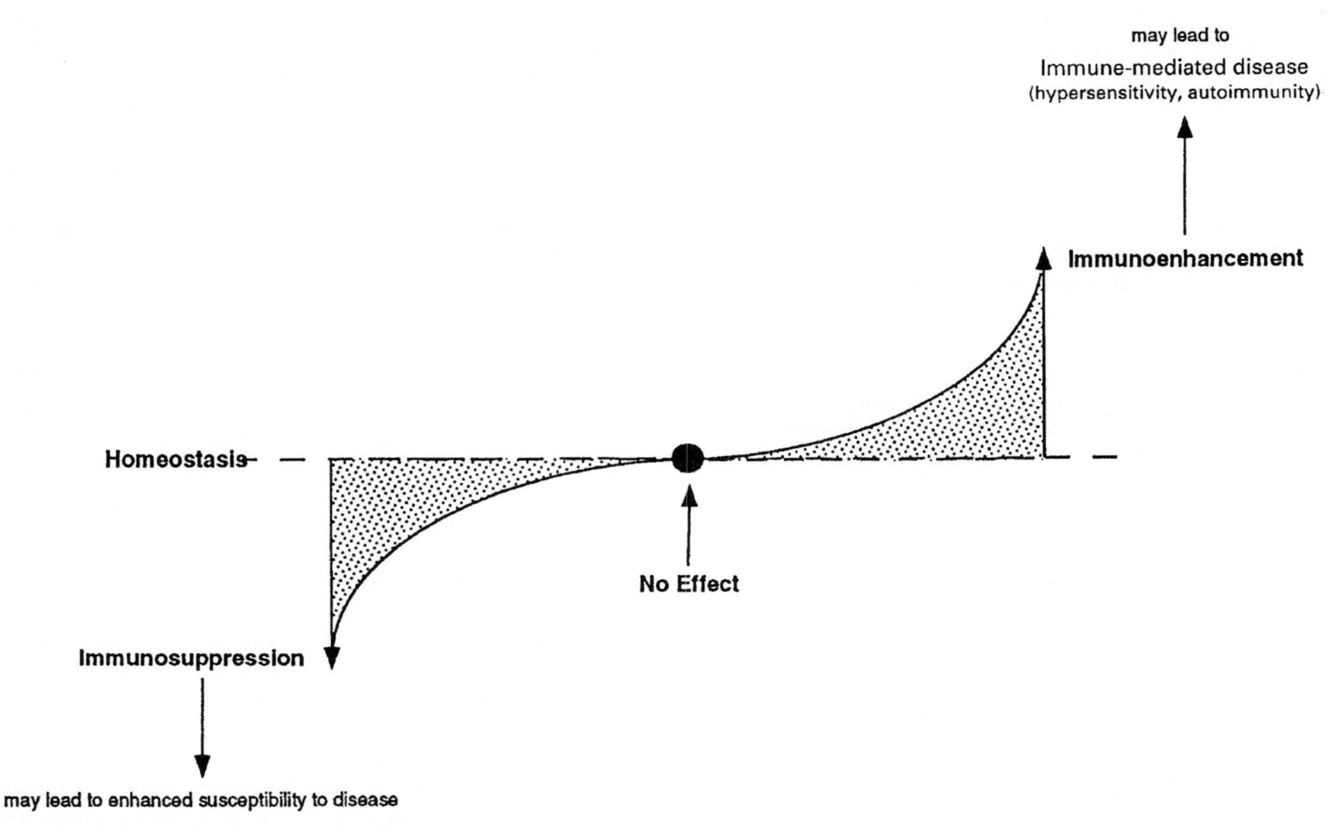


***Figure 12–1. Potential consequences of immunomodulation.***

nificant adjunct to routine safety evaluations for therapeutic agents, biological agents, and chemicals now in development.

This chapter will provide: (1) an overview of basic concepts in immunology (structure, components, and functions) which are important to the understanding of the impact xenobiotics may have on the exposed individual, (2) a summary of selected current methods utilized to assess immune function, and (3) a brief review of current information on the immunomodulation (immunosuppression, hypersensitivity, and autoimmunity) induced by a variety of xenobiotics. This chapter is not meant to be an immunology textbook nor an exhaustive review of the mechanisms of immunotoxicity of a myriad of xenobiotics. For detailed information on immunology the reader is referred to two texts, the first edited by Paul (1993), the second edited by Roitt and colleagues (1993). For a more comprehensive review of immunotoxicology the reader is referred to a text edited by Dean and colleagues (1994).

## THE IMMUNE SYSTEM

Unlike most organ systems, the immune system has the unique quality of not being confined to a single site within the body. It is comprised of numerous lymphoid organs (Table 12-1) and numerous different cellular populations with a variety of functions. The bone marrow and the thymus contain microenvironments capable of supporting the production of mature T and B lymphocytes and myeloid cells, such as macrophages and polymorphonuclear cells from nonfunctional precursors (stem cells), and are thus referred to as primary lymphoid organs. With regard to T and B cells, key events which occur in both primary and secondary organs are: (1) acquisition of the ability to recirculate and become localized in appropriate places in the periphery (homing capacity), (2) the ability to recognize antigen (rearrangement of the T-cell receptor and the B-cell antigen receptor germline genes), and (3) the ability to interact with accessory cells (through the expression of various cell-surface molecules and the development of biochemical signaling pathways) to allow differentiation into both effector and memory cell populations.

The bone marrow is the site of origination of the pluripotent stem cell, a self-renewing cell from which all other hematopoietic cells are derived (Figs. 12-2 and 12-6). During gestation, this cell is found in the embryonic yolk sack and fetal liver and subsequently migrates to the bone marrow. Within the bone marrow, the cells of the immune system developmentally "commit" to either the lymphoid or myeloid lineages. Cells of the lymphoid lineage make a further commitment to become either T cells or B cells. Because of their critical role in initiation and regulation of immune responses, T-cell precursors are programmed to leave the bone marrow and migrate to the thymus where they undergo "thymic education" for recognition of self and nonself. This will be discussed in more detail under "Cellular Components," in the sec. below titled "Acquired (Adaptive) Immunity."

**Table 12–1**
**Organization of the Immune System: Lymphoid Organs**

| CLASSIFICATION | LYMPHOID ORGANS |
|---|---|
| Primary | Bone marrow |
| | Thymus |
| Secondary | Spleen |
| | Lymph nodes |
| Tertiary | Skin-associated lymphoid tissue (SALT) |
| | Mucosal lamina propria (MALT) |
| | Gut-associated lymphoid tissue (GALT) |
| | Bronchial-associated lymphoid tissue (BALT) |
| | Cells lining the genitourinary tract |

Mature naive or virgin lymphocytes (those T and B cells which have never undergone antigenic stimulation) are first brought into contact with exogenously derived antigens within the highly organized microenvironment of the spleen and lymph nodes, otherwise known as the secondary lymphoid organs. These organs can be thought of as biological sieves. The spleen serves as a filter for the blood, removing both foreign antigens and any circulating dead cells and cellular debris. The lymph nodes are part of a network of lymphatic veins which filter antigens from the fluid surrounding the tissues of the body. Key events that occur within the secondary lymphoid organs are: (1) specific antigen recognition in the context of the major histocompatibility complex (MHC) class II, (2) clonal expansion (proliferation) of antigen-specific cells, and (3) differentiation of antigen-stimulated lymphocytes into effector and memory cells.

Lymphoid tissues associated with the skin (skin-associated lymphoid tissue; SALT) and mucosal lamina propria (mucosal-associated lymphoid tissue; MALT) can be classified as tertiary lymphoid tissues. Tertiary lymphoid tissues are primarily effector sites where memory and effector cells exert immunologic and immunoregulatory functions. Although in a broad interpretation this would include essentially all tissues of the body, tertiary lymphoid tissues are associated primarily with the surfaces lining the intestines (gut-associated lymphoid tissue; GALT), respiratory tract (bronchial-associated lymphoid tissue; BALT), and the genitourinary tract, since these tissues have access directly to the external environment.

### Innate Immunity

**General Considerations.** Mammalian immunity can be classified into two functional divisions: innate immunity and acquired (adaptive) immunity (Table 12-2). Innate immunity acts as a first line of defense against infectious agents elimating most potential pathogens before significant infection occurs. It is characterized by being *nonspecific* and includes physical and biochemical barriers both inside and outside of the body as well as immune cells designed for specific responses. Unlike acquired immunity, there is no immunologic memory associated with innate immunity. Therefore, in a normal healthy adult, the magnitude of the immune response to a foreign organism is the same for a secondary or tertiary challenge as it is for the primary exposure.

Externally, the skin provides an effective barrier, as most organisms cannot penetrate intact skin. Most infectious agents enter the body through the respiratory system, gut,

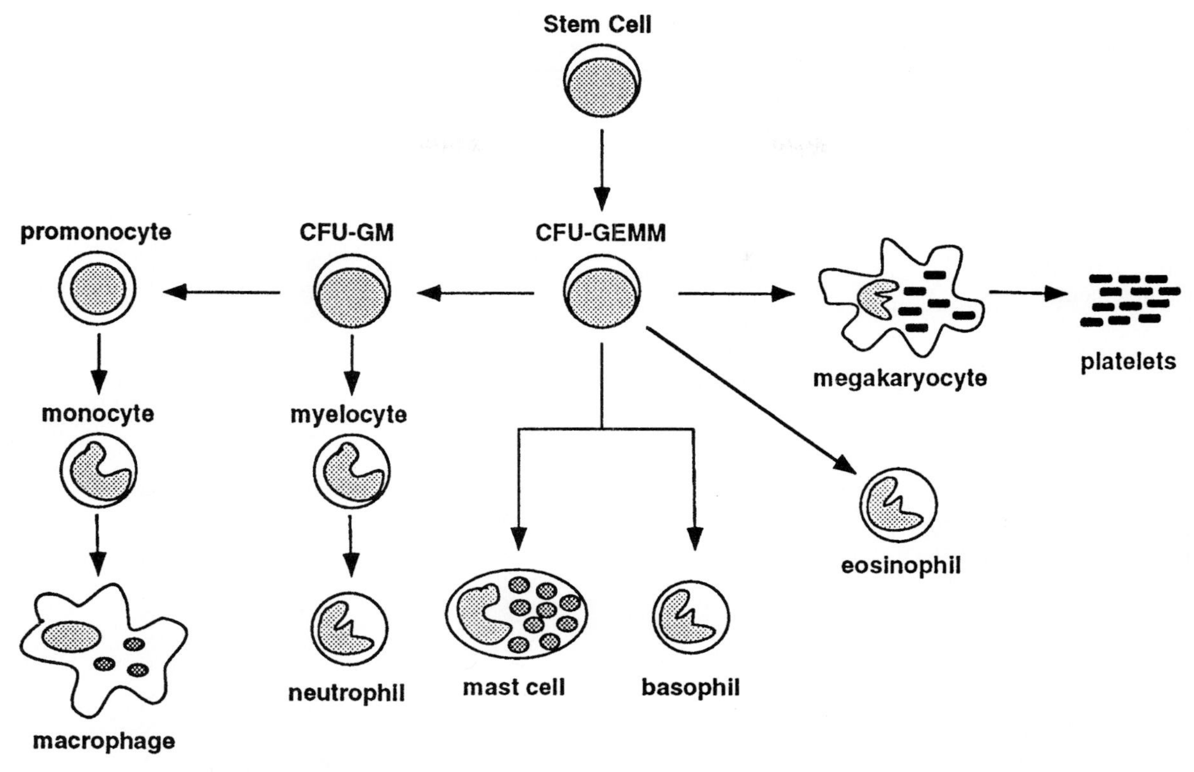


*Figure 12–2. Development of the cellular components of the immune system.*

or genitourinary tract. Innate defenses present to combat infection from pathogens entering through the respiratory system include mucus secreted along the nasopharynx, the presence of lysozyme in most secretions, and cilia lining the trachea and main bronchi. In addition, reflexes such as coughing, sneezing, and elevation in body temperature are also a part of innate immunity. Pathogens which enter the body via the digestive tract are met with severe changes in pH (acid) within the stomach and a host of microorganisms living in the intestines.

**Cellular Components: NK, PMN, MØ.** Two general types of cells are involved in nonspecific (innate) host resistance: natural killer (NK) cells and professional phagocytes (Table 12-3). Like other immune cells, NK cells are derived from the bone marrow stem cell. It is not yet clear exactly how the NK lineage progresses; however, NK cells do possess several surface markers which have been used to define T cells, suggesting that the NK cell is a derivative of a lymphoid precursor cell. The vast majority of NK cells express CD16 (Fc receptor for IgG) on their surface. Although apparently derived from a

**Table 12–2**
**Innate vs. Acquired Immunity**

| CHARACTERISTIC | INNATE IMMUNITY | ACQUIRED IMMUNITY |
|---|---|---|
| Cells involved | Polymorphonuclear cells (PMN)<br>Monocyte/macrophage<br>NK cells | T Cells<br>B Cells<br>Macrophages<br>NK Cells |
| Primary soluble mediators | Complement<br>Lysozyme<br>Acute phase proteins<br>Interferon $\alpha/\beta$<br>Cytokines | Antibody<br>Cytokines |
| Specificity of response | None | Yes<br>(very high specificity) |
| Response enhanced by repeated antigen challenge | No | Yes |

**Table 12–3**
**Characteristics of Selected Immune Cells**

| PROPERTIES | MONOCYTE/ MACROPHAGE | T CELLS | B CELLS | NK CELLS |
|---|---|---|---|---|
| Phagocytosis | Yes | No | No | No |
| Adherence | Yes | No | No | No |
| Surface receptors: | | | | |
| Antigen receptors | No | Yes | Yes | No |
| Complement | Yes | No | Yes | Yes |
| Fc Region of Ig | Yes | Some | Yes | Yes |
| Surface markers | CD64 | CD4 | Ig | CD16 |
| | CD11b | CD8 | | Asialo-GM1 (mouse) |
| | | CD3 | | CD11b |
| | | Thy-1 (mouse) | | |
| Proliferation in response to: | | | | |
| Allogeneic cells (MLR) | No | Yes | No | No |
| Lipopolysaccharide (LPS) | No | No | Yes | No |
| Phytohemagglutinin (PHA) | No | Yes | No | No |
| Concanavalin A (Con A) | No | Yes | No | No |
| Anti-Ig + IL-4 | No | No | Yes | No |
| Anti-CD3 + IL-2 | No | Yes | No | No |
| Effector functions: | | | | |
| Antibody production | No | No | Yes | No |
| Cytokine production | Yes | Yes | Yes | Yes |
| Bactericidal activity | Yes | No | No | No |
| Tumor cell cytotoxicity | Yes | Yes | No | Yes |
| Immunologic memory | No | Yes | Yes | No |

similar lineage as the T cell, NK cells do not express cell surface CD3 (T cell receptor-associated protein complex) or either chain of the T-cell receptor (TCR). NK cells are located primarily in the spleen, blood, and peritoneal exudate, although they are occasionally found in lymph node tissue as well. For their part in innate immunity, NK cells can recognize virally infected and malignant changes on the surface of cells as well as the Fc portion of IgG on an antibody-coated target cell. The latter recognition is utilized in cell-mediated immunity. Using surface receptors, the NK cell binds and undergoes cytoplasmic reorientation so that cytolytic granules (perforins and enzymatic proteins) are localized near the target cell. These granules are then expelled onto the surface of the target cell. The result of this process is the induction of apoptosis (DNA fragmentation, membrane blebbing, and cellular disintegration) of the target cell.

Phagocytic cells include polymorphonuclear cells (PMN; neutrophil) and the monocyte/macrophage (MØ). The precursors of the MØ and PMN develop from pluripotent stem cells which have become committed to the myeloid lineage (Fig. 12-2). Evidence exists that there are bipotentiating reactive precursors for PMN and MØ and that differentiation into one or the other is dependent upon the interaction with specific colony-stimulating factors (CSFs) such as macrophage-CSF (M-CSF), granulocyte-CSF (G-CSF), granulocyte-macrophage-CSF (GM-CSF), interleukin-3 (IL-3), and others (Unanue, 1993). Within the bone marrow, both cell types undergo several rounds of replication before entering the bloodstream where they circulate for about 10 h and then enter the tissues where they perform effector functions for about 1 to 2 days. PMNs are capable of passing through the cell membrane of the blood vessels and thereby represent a primary line of defense against infectious agents. They are excellent phagocytic cells and can eliminate most microorganisms. Their phagocytic activity is greatly enhanced by the presence of complement and antibody deposited on the surface of the foreign target. They are also important in the induction of an inflammatory response.

Macrophages are terminally differentiated monocytes. Upon exiting the bone marrow, monocytes circulate within the bloodstream for about 1 day. At that time, they begin to distribute to the various tissues where they can then differentiate into MØs. MØs can be found in all tissues, most notably in the liver, lung, spleen, kidney, and brain. Within different tissues, MØs have distinct properties and vary in extent of surface receptors, oxidative metabolism, and expression of MHC class II. This is likely due to the factors present within the microenvironment in which the monocyte differentiates. The liver MØs, or Kupffer cell, are primarily responsible for particulate and microbial clearance from the blood. They express high levels of MHC class II, are actively phagocytic, and release several soluble mediators. Thus, they are the primary cell responsible for the acute phase response. Alveolar MØs remove foreign particulate matter from the alveolar space. They are self-renewing and have a particularly long lifespan. These cells can be harvested by broncheoalveolar lavage and actively secrete proteases and bactericidal enzymes such as lysozyme. Splenic MØs also phagocytose particulate material and polysaccharides from the blood and tissue. However, unlike other tissue MØs, they are more diverse within the tissue and their level of expression of MHC class II and their stage of differentiation appear to be dependent upon where within the splenic architecture the MØs are located. Mononuclear phagocytes within the central nervous system (CNS) are known as microglia and are responsible for antigen presentation in immunologic diseases of the CNS. Microglia have a very slow turnover time, and thus recruitment of monocytes to areas of inflammation within the CNS is also slow.

Should PMN be unable to contain an infection, MØs are then recruited to the site of infection. Although MØs are phagocytic by nature, their bactericidal activity can be augmented by lymphokines produced by T cells which recognize a specific microbial antigen. MØs are unique cells within the immune system because they play roles in both the innate arm of immunity (as phagocytic cells) and the acquired arm (as antigen-presenting cells). They adhere well to glass or plastic, are recruited to sites of inflammation by chemotactic factors, can be activated by cytokines to become more effective killers, and can produce cytokines, such as IL (interleukin)-1, IL-6, and TNF (tumor necrosis factor), that act in a paracrine and autocrine fashion. MØs also play critical roles as scavengers in the daily turnover of senescent tissues such as red cell nuclei from maturing red cells, PMN, and plasma cells. The importance of phagocytic cells to the organism can be seen in individuals with spontaneous or induced reduction in the numbers or activity of these cells. Such individuals are associated with repeated, and sometimes fatal, bacterial and fungal infections.

**Soluble Factors: Acute Phase Proteins and Complement.** In addition to the cellular components of innate immunity, there are several soluble components as well (Table 12-2). These are the acute phase response and the complement cascade. Upon infection, MØs (Kupffer cells, in particular) become activated and secrete a variety of cytokines which are carried by the blood stream to distant sites. This global response to foreign agents is termed the *acute phase response* and consists of fever and large shifts in the types of serum proteins synthesized by hepatocytes, such as serum amyloid A, serum amyloid P, and C-reactive protein. These proteins increase rapidly to concentrations up to 100 times the normal concentration and stay elevated through the course of infection. These proteins can bind to bacteria and facilitate the binding of complement and the subsequent uptake of the bacteria by phagocytic cells. This process of protein coating to enhance phagocytosis is termed *opsonization.*

The complement system is a series of about 30 serum proteins whose primary functions are the modification of membranes of infectious agents and the promotion of an inflammatory response. The components of the complement cascade interact with each other and with other elements of both the innate and acquired arms of immunity. Complement activation occurs with each component sequentially, acting on others in a manner similar to the blood clotting cascade (Fig. 12-3). Early components of the cascade are often modified serine proteases which activate the system, but have limited substrate specificity. Several components are capable of binding to microbial membranes and serve as ligands for complement receptors associated with the membrane. The final components, which are related structurally, are also membrane-binding proteins which can insert into the membrane and disrupt membrane integrity (membrane attack complex). And finally, there are several regulatory complement proteins which are designed to protect the host from inadvertent damage.

There are two pathways that have been identified in the complement cascade. The classical pathway is involved when antibody binds to the microorganism. Because specific antibody defines the target, this is a mechanism by which complement aids effectors of the acquired side of immunity. The second, or alternative pathway, is used to assist the innate arm of immunity. For this cascade, it is not necessary for the host to have prior contact with the pathogen since several microbial proteins can alone initiate this pathway. Whatever the mechanism of activation, the results are the same. The complement-coated material is targeted for elimination by interaction with complement receptors on the surface of circulating immune cells.

## Acquired (Adaptive) Immunity

**General Considerations.** If the primary defenses against infection (innate immunity) are breached, the acquired arm of the immune system is activated and produces a specific immune response to each infectious agent, which usually eliminates the infection. This branch of immunity is also capable of remembering the pathogen and can protect the host from future infection by the same agent. Therefore, the two key features which distinguish acquired immunity are *specificity* and *memory*. This means that in a normal healthy adult, the speed and magnitude of the immune response to a foreign organism is greater for a secondary challenge than it is for the primary challenge (Table 12-2). This is the principle which is exploited in vaccination.

Acquired immunity may be further subdivided into cell-mediated immunity (CMI) and humoral immunity. CMI, in its broadest sense, includes all immunologic activity in which antibody plays a minimal role. Humoral immunity is directly dependent upon the production of antigen-specific antibody by B cells and involves the coordinated interaction of antigen-presenting cells, T cells, and B cells. A more detailed discussion of both CMI and humoral immunity appears later.

Essential to the development of specific immunity is the recognition of antigen and the generation of an antibody that can bind to it. An antigen (sometimes referred to as an immunogen or allergen) is defined functionally as a substance that can elicit the production of a specific antibody and can be specifically bound by that antibody. Antigens are usually (but not absolutely) biological molecules that can be cleaved and rearranged for presentation. They may be either proteins, carbohydrates (often bacterial), lipids, nucleic acids, or human-engineered substances, and they must be foreign (nonself) or occult (hidden, sequestered). Generally, antigens are about 10 kDa or larger in size. Smaller antigens are termed *haptens* and must be conjugated with carrier molecules (larger antigens) in order to elicit a specific response. However, once a response is made, the hapten can interact with the specific antibody in the absence of the carrier.

Antibodies are produced by B cells and are also defined functionally by the antigen with which they react (i.e., anti-sheep red blood cell IgM; anti-SRBC IgM). Because the im-

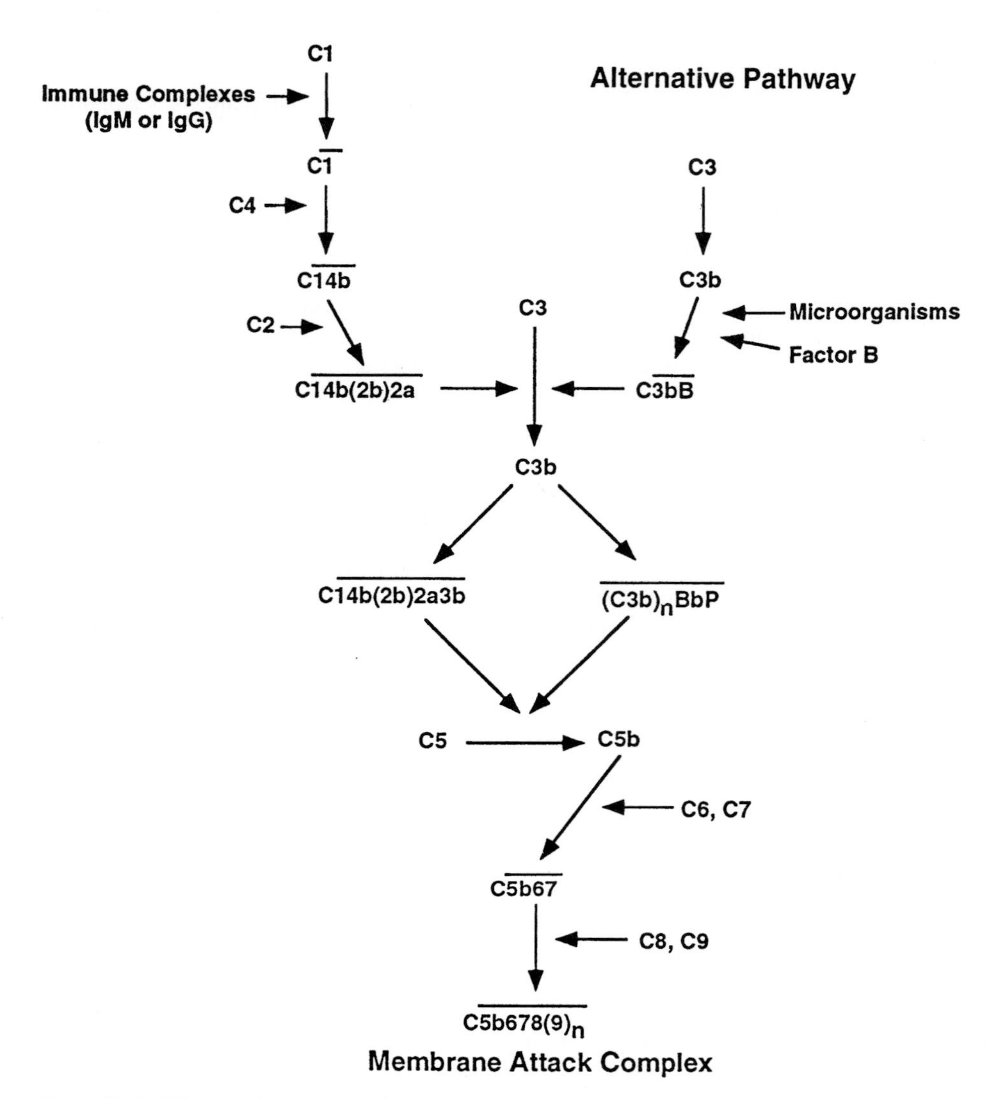


*Figure 12–3. The complement cascade.*

mune system generates antibody to thousands of antigens with which the host may, or may not, ever come into contact, general antibody of unknown specificity is referred to as *immunoglobulin* (e.g., serum immunoglobulin or serum IgM) until it can be defined by its specific antigen (e.g., anti-SRBC IgM). A simple way to view this point is that an antibody is an immunoglobulin, but immunoglobulin is not necessarily antibody. There are five types of immunoglobulin that are related structurally (Table 12-4): IgM, IgG (and subsets), IgE, IgD, and IgA. All immunoglobulins are made up of heavy and light chains, and of constant and variable regions. It is the variable regions that determine antibody specificity. In addition, the immunoglobulin molecule can be divided into the Fab [or $F(ab)'_2$] and Fc fragments (Fig. 12-4). It is the Fab region (specifically, the variable region) that interacts with antigen, while the Fc region mediates effector functions such as complement fixation (IgM and some IgG subclasses) and phagocyte binding (via Fc receptors). Antibodies subserve several functions in acquired immunity: (1) opsonization (coating of a pathogen with antibody to enhance Fc receptor-mediated endocytosis by phagocytic cells); (2) initiation of the classical pathway of complement-mediated lysis; (3) neutralization of viral infection by binding to viral particles and preventing further infection; and (4) enhancement of the specificity of effectors of CMI by binding to specific antigens on target cells which are then recognized and eliminated by effector cells such as NK or cytotoxic T lymphocytes (CTL).

During an immune response, the cells of the immune system must be able to communicate to coordinate all the activities that occur during the recognition and elimination of foreign antigens. Connecting all the cells of the immune system with each other, as well as with other nonimmune cell types within the body, is a vast network of soluble mediators: the cytokines. Nearly all immune cells secrete cytokines that may have local or systemic effects. Table 12-5 provides a brief summary of the sources and functions of cytokines of interest in the immune system. Although it would appear that many cytokines have related functions, these functions are not often

**Table 12–4**
**Properties of Immunoglobulin Classes and Subclasses**

| CLASS | MEAN SERUM CONCENTRATION, HUMAN (mg/ml) | HALF-LIFE (DAYS) | BIOLOGICAL PROPERTIES |
|---|---|---|---|
| IgG | | | Complement fixation |
| Subclasses | | | (selected subclasses) |
| $IgG_1$ | 9 | 21 | Cross-placenta |
| $IgG_2$ | 3 | 20 | heterocytotropic |
| $IgG_3$ | 1 | 7 | antibody |
| $IgG_4$ | 1 | 21 | |
| IgA | 3 | 6 | Secretory antibdy |
| IgM | 1.5 | 10 | Fix complement |
| | | | Efficient agglutination |
| IgD | 0.03 | 3 | Possible role in antigen-triggered lymphocyte differentiation |
| IgE | 0.0001 | 2 | Allergic responses (mast cell degranulation) |

identical, and a single cytokine may have multiple effects on a variety of cell types. Since cytokines work to tightly regulate immune responses, some induce synthesis of other cytokines and inflammatory mediators, while others inhibit this process. Although the actual number of cytokines (lymphokines, monokines, chemokines, etc.) may not be altogether that large, the complexity of the network is magnified severalfold by the multitude of biological actions of each cytokine and the diversity of cells secreting each mediator.

**Cellular Components: APC, T Cells, B Cells.** In order to elicit a specific immune response to a particular antigen, that anti-

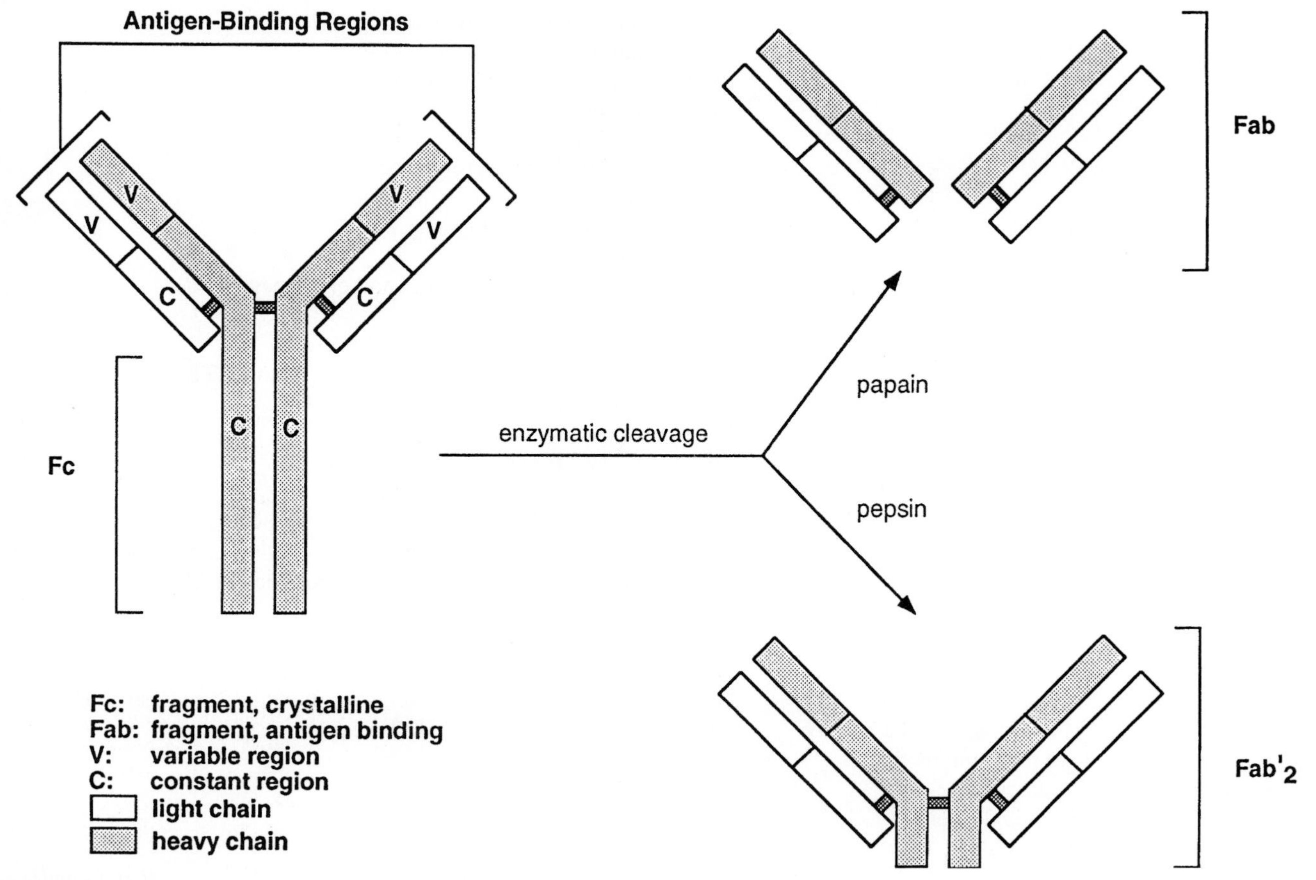


*Figure 12–4. Immunoglobulin structure and cleavage products.*

**Table 12–5**
**Cytokines: Sources and Functions in Immune Regulation**

| CYTOKINE | SOURCE | PHYSIOLOGIC ACTIONS |
|---|---|---|
| IL-1 | Macrophages<br>B Cells<br>Fibroblasts<br>Endothelial cells | Activation and proliferation of T cells<br>Pro-inflammatory<br>Induces fever and acute phase proteins<br>Induces synthesis of IL-8 and TNF$\alpha$ |
| IL-2 | T Cells | Primary T-cell growth factor<br>Growth factor for B cells and NK cells |
| IL-3 | T Cells<br>Stromal cells | Stimulates the proliferation and differentiation of progenitors of the macrophage, granulocyte, and erythroid lineages |
| IL-4 | T Cells | Proliferation of activated T and B cells<br>B-Cell differentiation and isotype switching may inhibit some macrophage functions |
| IL-5 | T Cells | Proliferation and differentiation of eosinophils and B-Cell isotype switching in B cells |
| IL-6 | Macrophages<br>Activated T cells<br>B Cells<br>Fibroblasts<br>Keratinocytes | B-Cell differentiation<br>Induction of acute phase proteins<br>Pro-inflammatory<br>Proliferation of T cells |
| IL-7 | Stromal cells | Proliferation of pre-T cells<br>Proliferation of pro- and pre-B cells |
| IL-8 | Macrophages<br>Fibroblasts<br>Platelets<br>Keratinocytes | Activation and chemotaxis of monocytes, neutrophils, and basophils<br>Pro-inflammatory |
| IL-9 | T Cells | T-Cell growth factor enhances mast cell activity<br>Stimulates growth of early erythroid progenitors |
| IL-10 | T Cells<br>Macrophages<br>B Cells | Inhibits macrophage cytolytic activity<br>General inhibitor of cytokine synthesis<br>Inhibits macrophage activation of T cells<br>Enhances proliferation of activated B cells<br>Mast cell growth<br>Enhances $CD8^+$ T cell cytolytic activity<br>Anti-inflammatory |
| IL-11 | Fibroblasts<br>Stromal cells | Megakaryocyte growth factor<br>Enhances AFC responses<br>Stimulates platelets, neutrophils, and erythrocytes<br>Induces acute-phase proteins |
| IL-12 | Macrophages<br>B Cells | Proliferation and cytolytic action of NK cells<br>Activation, proliferation, and cytolytic action of CTL<br>Stimulates production of IFN$\gamma$<br>Proliferation of activated T cells |
| IL-13 | T Cells | Stimulates class II expression on APC<br>Enhances antigen processing by APC<br>Enhances B cell differentiation and isotype switching<br>Anti-inflammatory (inhibits synthesis of pro-inflammatory cytokines)<br>Inhibits antibody-dependent cellular cytotoxicity (ADCC) |
| IL-14 | T Cells<br>Some malignant B cells | B-Cell proliferation<br>Inhibition of immunoglobulin secretion<br>Selective expansion of some B-cell subpopulations |
| IL-15 | Activated monocytes<br>Macrophages and a variety of nonimmune tissues | NK Cell activation can have effects on activated T cells, since IL-15 utilizes components of the IL-2 receptor |
| Interferon-$\alpha/\beta$ (IFN-$\alpha/\beta$) | Leukocytes<br>Epithelial cells<br>Fibroblasts | Induction of class I expression<br>Antiviral activity<br>Stimulation of NK cells |

*(Continued)*

**Table 12–5**
**Cytokines: Sources and Functions in Immune Regulation *(Continued)***

| CYTOKINE | SOURCE | PHYSIOLOGIC ACTIONS |
|---|---|---|
| Interferon γ (IFN-γ) | T Cells<br>NK Cells<br>Epithelial cells<br>Fibroblasts | Induction of class I and II<br>Activates macrophages (as APC and cytolytic cells)<br>Improves CTL recognition of virally infected cells |
| Tumor Necrosis Factor (TNF-α) and Lymphotoxin (TNF-β) | Macrophages<br>Lymphocytes<br>Mast cells | Induces inflammatory cytokines<br>Increases vascular permeability<br>Activates macrophages and neutrophils<br>Tumor necrosis (direct action)<br>Primary mediator of septic shock<br>Interferes with lipid metabolism (result is cachexia)<br>Induction of acute phase proteins |
| Transforming Growth Factor-β (TGF-β) | Macrophages<br>Megakaryocytes<br>Chondrocytes | Enhances monocyte/macrophage chemotaxis<br>Enhances wound healing: angiogenesis, fibroblast<br>Proliferation, deposition of extracellular matrix<br>Inhibits T- and B-cell proliferation<br>Inhibits macrophage cytokine synthesis<br>Inhibits antibody secretion<br>Primary inducer of isotype switch to IgA |
| GM-CSF | T Cells<br>Macrophages<br>Endothelial cells<br>Fibroblasts | Stimulates growth and differentiation of monocytes and granulocytes |
| Migration Inhibitory Factor (MIF) | T Cells | Inhibits macrophage migration |
| Erythropoietin (EPO) | Endothelial cells<br>Fibroblasts | Stimulates maturation of erythrocyte precursors |

SOURCE: Information on selected cytokines taken Paul and Seder (1994), Ruddle (1992), Quesniaux (1992), and Zurawski and de Vries (1994).

gen must be taken up and processed by accessory cells for presentation to lymphocytes. Accessory cells that perform this function are termed antigen-presenting cells (APCs) and include the macrophage (MØ), follicular dendritic cell (FDC), Langerhans-dendritic cell, and B cells. A description of the MØ is found in the section above titled "Cellular Components of Innate Immunity"; however, the MØ also plays a critical role as an APC in acquired immunity. Unique among the APCs is the FDC. Unlike hematopoietic cells, the FDC is not derived from the bone marrow stem cell. It is found in secondary lymphoid organs and binds antigen–antibody complexes, but it does not internalize and process the antigen. Instead, the primary function of the FDC is in the persistence of antigen within the secondary lymphoid tissues and the presentation of antigen to B cells. This is believed to be critical for the maintenance of memory for B cells and the induction of high-affinity B-cell clones. Although thought of more for its ability to produce immunoglobulin, the B cell can also serve as an APC, and in low antigen concentrations this cell is equally as competent as the MØ in serving this function. The Langerhans'-dendritic cell is also a bone marrow-derived cell, but its lineage is distinct from the MØ. It is found primarily in the epidermis, mucosal epithelium, and lymphoid tissues. The Langerhans'-dendritic cell can migrate into the lymphatic system where it serves as an APC in the lymph nodes. This cell plays a primary role in contact sensitization.

The interaction of APC and lymphocytes is critical for the development of an immune response. With the exception of the FDC, APCs internalize the antigen either by phagocytosis, pinocytosis, or receptor-mediated endocytosis (via antigen, Fc, or complement receptors). Following internalization, antigen is processed (intracellular denaturation and catabolism) through several cytoplasmic compartments, and a piece of the antigen (peptide fragments about 20 amino acids in length) becomes physically associated with major histocompatibility (MHC) class II (Fig. 12-5). This MHC class II-peptide complex is then transported to the surface of the cell and can interact in a specific manner with lymphocytes. For most APCs, an immunogenic determinant is expressed on the surface of the APC within an hour after internalization, although this is slightly longer for B cells (3 to 4 h). In addition to processing and presentation, pieces of processed antigen may be expelled into the extracellular space. These pieces of processed antigen can then bind in the peptide groove of empty MHC class II on the surface of other APCs for the presentation of that peptide fragment to lymphocytes.

Not only are B lymphocytes capable of serving as APCs, but they are also the effector cells of humoral immunity, producing a number of isotypes of immunoglobulin (Ig) with varying specificities and affinities. Like other immune cells, the B cell develops in the bone marrow from the pluripotent stem cell and becomes committed to the B cell lineage when the cell

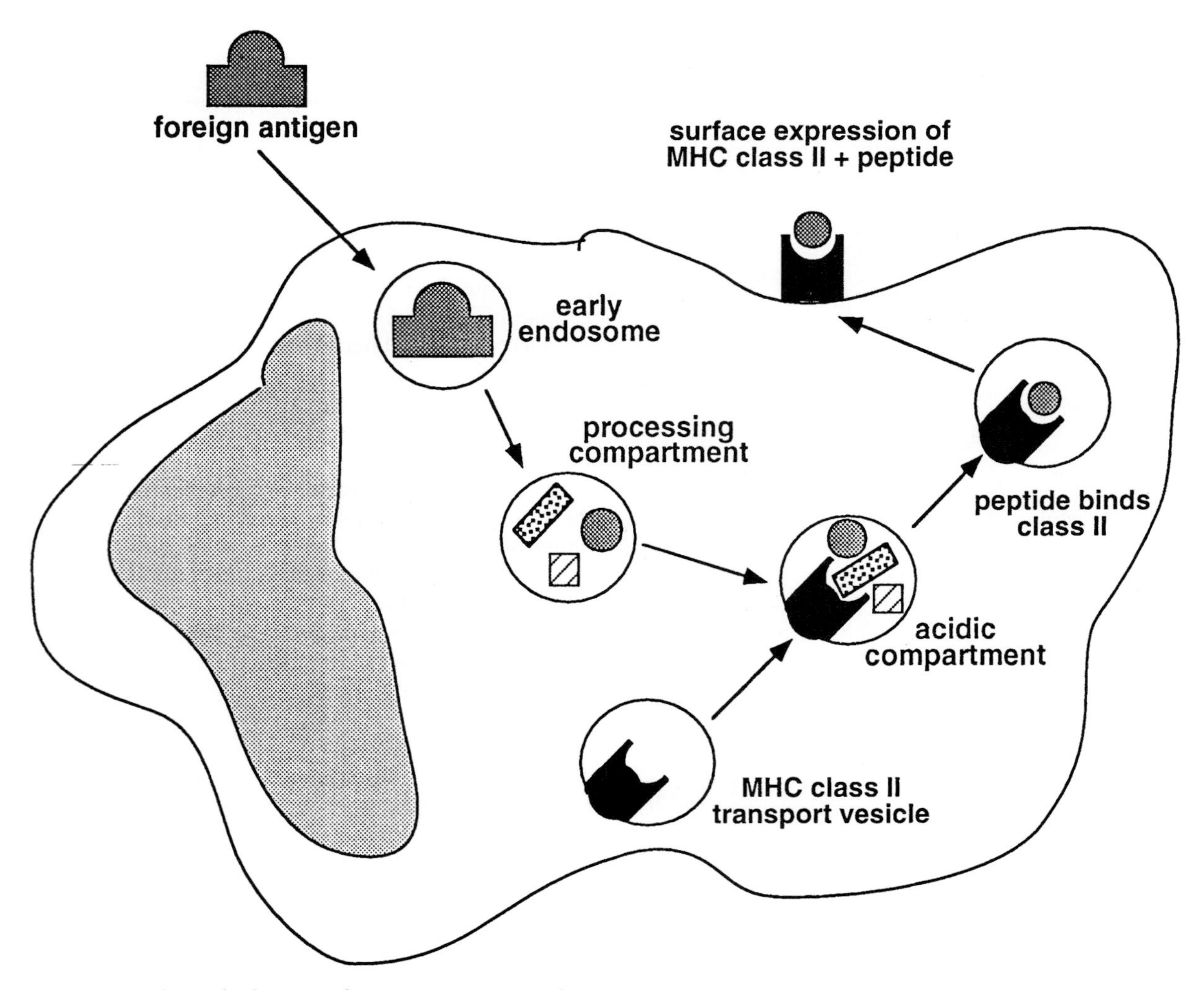


*Figure 12–5. General schematic of antigen processing and presentation.*

begins to rearrange its Ig genes (Fig. 12-6). If, after several attempts, the cell is unsuccessful at rearranging its Ig genes, it dies. Following Ig rearrangement, these cells express $\mu$ heavy chains in their cytoplasm and are termed pre-B cells. Expression of surface IgM and IgD indicates a mature B cell. Mature B cells are found in the lymph nodes, spleen, and peripheral blood. Upon antigen binding to surface Ig, the mature B cell becomes activated and, after proliferation, undergoes differentiation into either a memory B cell or an antibody-forming cell (AFC; plasma cell), actively secreting antigen-specific antibody. A broad description of several B cell characteristics can be found in Table 12-3.

At a specified time following their commitment to the T-cell lineage, pre-T cells migrate from the bone marrow to the thymus where, in a manner analogous to their B-cell cousins, they begin to rearrange their TCRs (Fig. 12-6). This receptor consists of two chains ($\alpha$ and $\beta$, or $\gamma$ and $\delta$) and is critical for the recognition of MHC + peptide on APCs. At this time, the T cells begin to express the surface marker CD8. CD8 (and CD4) are coreceptors expressed by T cells and are involved in the interaction of the T cell with the APC. T cells bearing the $\gamma/\delta$ TCR subsequently lose expression of CD8 and proceed to the periphery. T cells with the $\alpha/\beta$ TCR gain surface expression of both the TCR and CD4 and are termed *immature double-positive cells* ($CD4^+/CD8^+$). These immature cells then undergo positive selection to eliminate cells that cannot interact with MHC. Following this interaction, TCR expression increases. Any of these T cells that interact with MHC + self peptide are then eliminated (negative selection). The double-positive cells then undergo another selection process whereby they lose expression of either CD4 or CD8 and then proceed to the periphery as mature single-positive cells ($CD4^+$ or $CD8^+$) with a high level of TCR expression. This rigorous selection process produces T cells that can recognize MHC + foreign peptides and eliminates autoreactive T cells. Generally, T cells that express CD8 mediate cell killing (CTL) or suppressor activity (T suppressor cells). Lymphocytes that participate in delayed hypersensitivity (DHR) or that provide "B-cell help" in humoral responses (helper T cells; $T_H1$ and $T_H2$) express CD4 on their surface. A broad description of several T-cell characteristics can be found in Table 12-3.

**Humoral and Cell-Mediated Immunity.** The activation of antigen-specific T cells begins with the interaction of the T-cell receptor with MHC class II + peptide. This interaction is strengthened by the presence of coreceptors such as CD4, LFA-3, CD2, LFA-1, and ICAM-1 and involves the bilateral exchange of information, triggering a cascade of biochemical events that ultimately leads to the activation of not only the T

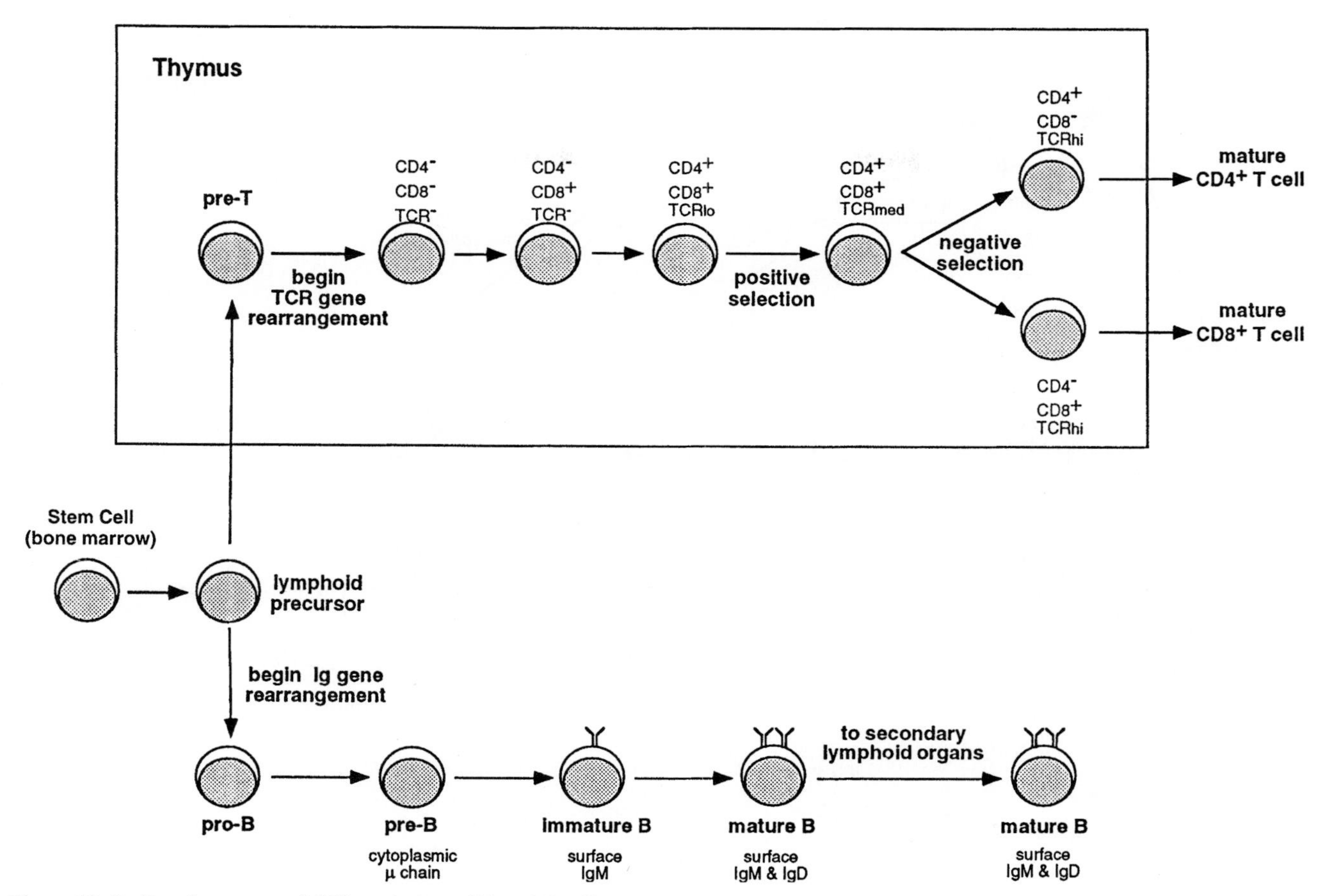


*Figure 12–6. Development and differentiation of T and B cells.*

cell but the APC as well. Although the MØ or dendritic cell is traditionally thought of as the APCs involved in humoral responses, B cells can also subserve this function. In fact, many believe that, in low antigen concentrations, the B cell serves as the primary APC because of the presence of the high-affinity Ig receptor on the surface of the B cell.

Upon activation and in the presence of IL-1 secreted by the APC, T cells begin to express high-affinity receptors for the major T-cell growth factor, IL-2. In addition, T cells begin to produce IL-2 which can act in an autocrine fashion (on IL-2 receptors on the same T cell) or paracrine fashion (IL-2 receptors on other T cells or on B cells). As T cells begin to undergo clonal expansion (proliferation), they secrete numerous lymphokines (cytokines secreted from lymphocytes; Table 12-5) which can influence (1) the strength of an immune response, (2) the down-regulation of the immune response, (3) the isotype of antibody secreted by the AFC, (4) the activation of cells involved in cell-mediated immunity, and (5) the modulation of activities of numerous immune and nonimmune cells. The next step in the generation of the humoral response is the interaction of activated T cells with B cells. This may be a direct interaction of the T cell with B cell (antigen-specific) or may simply involve the production of lymphokines (such as IL-2, IL-4, IL-6, and TNF-$\alpha$ and -$\beta$) which lead to B cell growth and differentiation into AFCs or memory B cells. A general diagram of the cellular interactions involved in the humoral immune response is given in Fig. 12-7. The production of antigen-specific IgM requires 3 to 5 days after the primary (initial) exposure to antigen (Fig. 12-8). Upon secondary antigen challenge, the B cells undergo isotype switching, producing primarily IgG antibody which is of higher affinity. In addition, there is a higher serum antibody titer associated with a secondary antibody response.

CMI, in its broadest sense, includes all immunological activity in which antibody plays a minimal role. However, for purposes of discussion here, CMI will be more specifically defined as the T-cell–mediated responses such as delayed hypersensitivity (DHR) or CTL activity, antibody-dependent cellular cytotoxicity (ADCC) mediated by NK cells, and soluble-factor–mediated macrophage cytotoxic responses. Whether or not an antigen will elicit a primarily cell-mediated or humoral response (or a combination of both) is dependent upon numerous factors. However, it should be noted that there is often an interplay between these two branches of acquired immunity. Cells are involved in the initiation of antibody responses and antibody is often an essential player in cell-mediated responses.

There are two general forms of cell-mediated immunity referred to as delayed-type hypersensitivity and cell-mediated cytotoxicity. Delayed-type hypersensitivity is presented below in this chapter in the section titled "Immune-Mediated Disease." Cell-mediated cytotoxicity responses may occur in numerous ways: (1) MHC class I-dependent recognition of specific antigens (such as viral particles) by CTL, (2) the indirect antigen-specific recognition by the binding of antibody-coated target cells to NK cells via Fc receptors on the latter, and

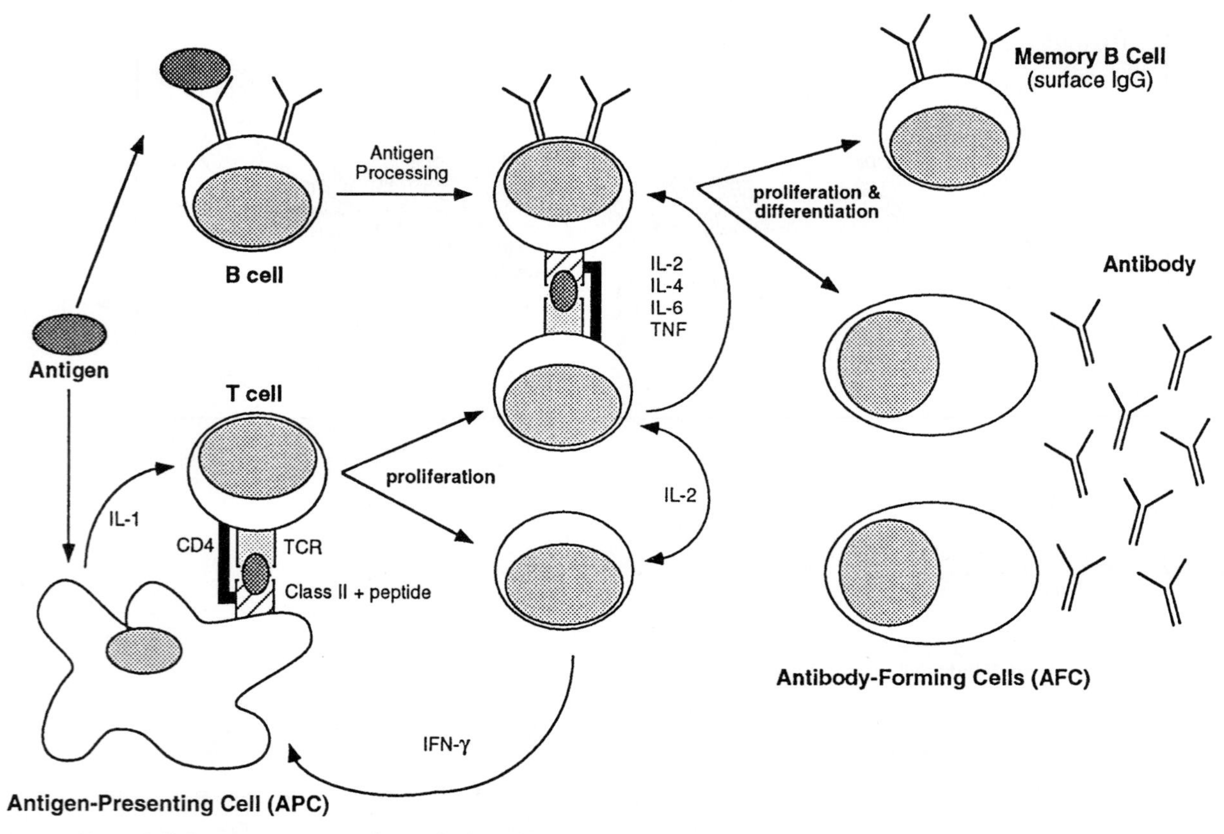


*Figure 12–7. Cellular interactions in the antibody response.*

(3) receptor-mediated recognition of complement-coated foreign targets by MØ. Let us consider the first two together, since their mechanisms of cytotoxicity are similar.

In cell-mediated cytotoxicity, the effector cell (CTL or NK) binds in a specific manner to the target cell (Fig. 12-9). The majority of CTL express CD8 and recognize either foreign MHC class I on the surface of allogeneic cells, or antigen in association with self MHC class I (e.g., viral particles). In acquired immunity, NK recognition of target cells may be considered antigen-specific because the mechanism of recognition involves

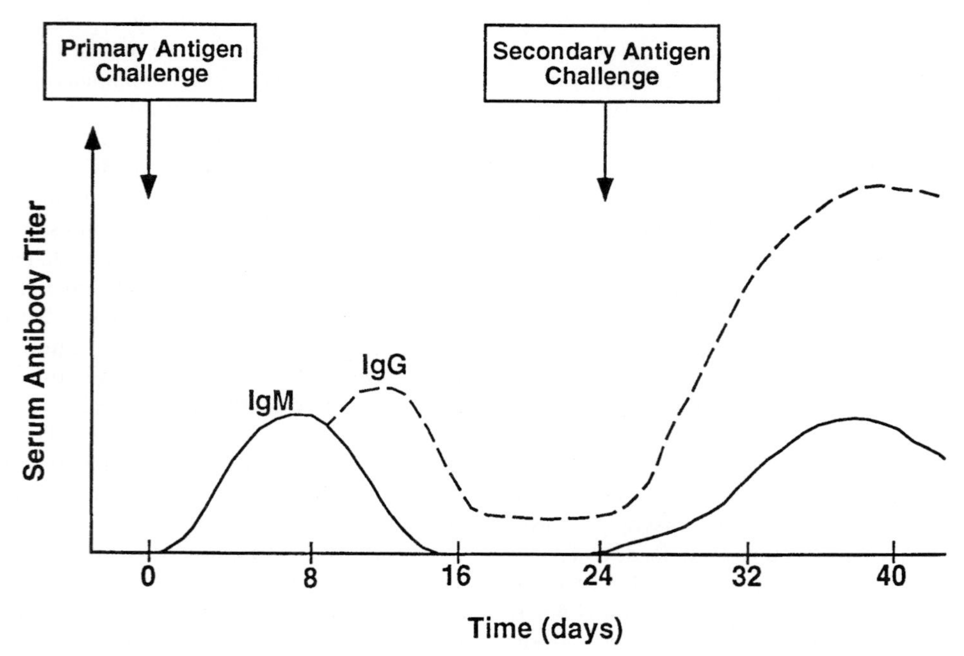


*Figure 12–8. Kinetics of the antibody response.*

1. **Identification and engagement of target by effector.**

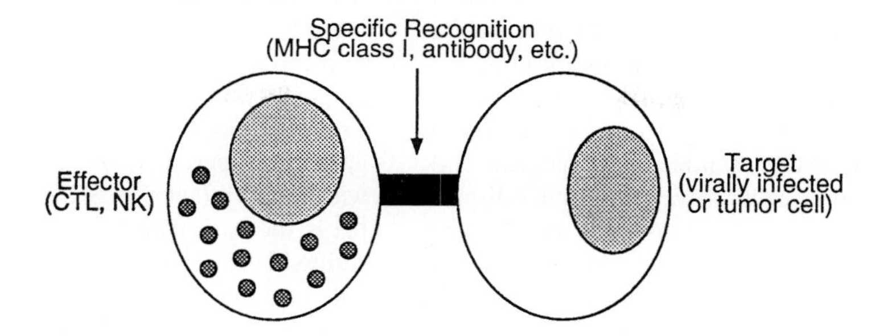


2. **Strengthening of interaction and cytoplasmic reorientation of effector.**

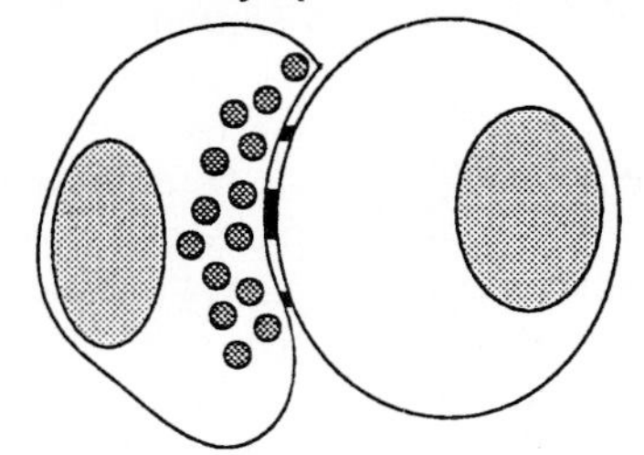

3. **Degranulation of effector onto target.**

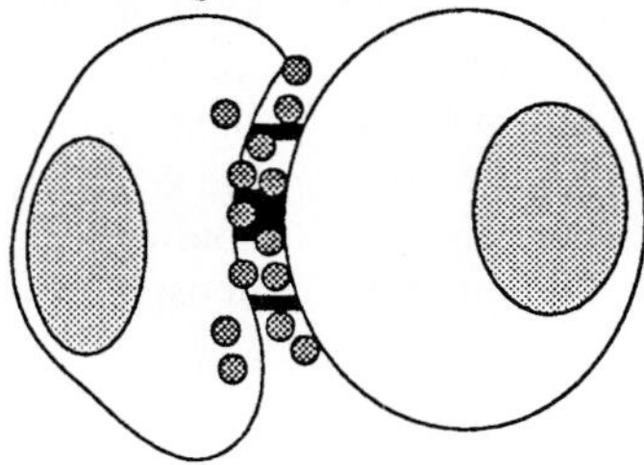

4. **Disengagement of effector and death of target.**

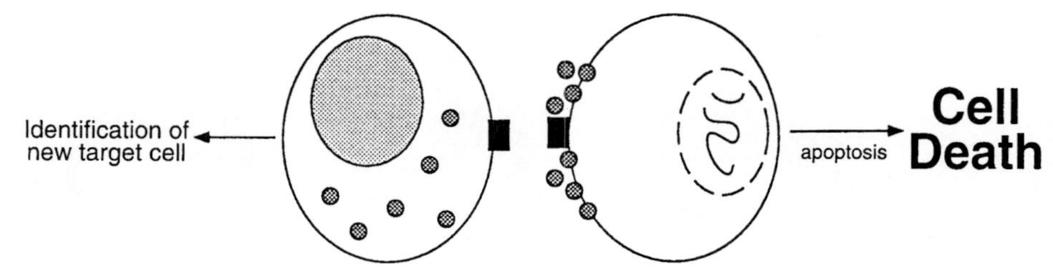


*Figure 12–9. Cell-mediated cytotoxicity.*

the binding of the Fc portion of antigen-specific antibody coating a target cell to the NK via its Fc receptors. Once the CTL or NK cell interact with the target cell, the effector cell undergoes cytoplasmic reorientation so that cytolytic granules are oriented along the side of the effector which is bound to the target. The effector cell then releases the contents of these granules onto the target cell. The target cell may be damaged by the perforins or enzymatic contents of the cytolytic granules. In addition, the target is induced to undergo programmed cell death (apoptosis). Once it has degranulated, the effector cell can release the dying target and move on to kill other target cells.

Macrophages are the most promiscuous of the immune cells in that they play roles in both innate and acquired (both humoral and cell-mediated) immunity. Their role in cell-mediated cytotoxicity involves activation by T-cell–derived lymphokines (such as interferon-gamma; IFN-$\gamma$) and subsequent recognition of complement-coated target cells via complement receptors present on the surface of the MØ. The result is enhanced phagocytic ability and the synthesis and release of hydrogen peroxide, nitric oxide, proteases, and TNF, all of which serve obvious cytolytic functions.

## ASSESSMENT OF IMMUNOLOGIC INTEGRITY

For many years, toxicologists have been aware that xenobiotics can have significant actions on the immune system. However, it has only been in recent years that the subdiscipline of immunotoxicology has come into its own with a battery of tests to evaluate immunocompetence. Among the unique features of the immune system is the ability of immune cells to be removed from the body and to function in vitro. This unique quality offers the toxicologist an opportunity to comprehensively evaluate the actions of xenobiotics on the immune system, by providing an excellent system for dissecting the cellular, biochemical, and molecular mechanisms of action of multitudes of xenobiotics. While standard toxicological endpoints such as organ weights, cellularity, and enumeration of cell subpopulations are important components in assessing immune injury, by far the most sensitive indicators of immunotoxicity are the tests that challenge the various immune cells to respond functionally to exogenous stimuli (reviewed in White, 1992). This section will focus on selected in vivo and in vitro tests currently used for evaluating immunotoxicity.

## Methods to Assess Immunocompetence

**General Assessment.** Central to any series of studies evaluating immunocompetence is the inclusion of standard toxicological studies, because any immunologic findings should be interpreted in conjunction with effects observed on other target organs. Standard toxicological studies that are usually evaluated include body and selected organ weights, general observations of overall animal health, selected serum chemistries, hematological parameters, and status of the bone marrow (ability to generate specific colony-forming units). In addition, histopathology of lymphoid organs, such as the spleen, thymus, and lymph nodes, may provide insight into potential immunotoxicants. Because of the unique nature of the immune system, there are several approaches that may be taken to assess immunotoxicity and to evaluate the mechanisms of action of xenobiotics. These are depicted in Fig. 12-10 and vary with respect to in vivo or in vitro exposure, immunologic challenge, or immunologic evaluation (immune assay). For example, immune cells may be exposed to a chemical in vivo, challenged with antigen (such as SRBCs) in vivo, and evaluated in vitro [as is the case with the plaque-forming cell (PFC) assay described below]. In contrast, splenocytes can be removed from a naive animal, exposed to xenobiotic and antigen in vitro, and evaluated in vitro. An example of this would be the in vitro-generated PFC response (Mishell-Dutton assay; Mishell and Dutton, 1967).

Using fluorescently labeled monoclonal antibodies to cell surface markers (Table 12-3) in conjunction with a flow cytometer, it is now possible to accurately enumerate lymphocyte subsets. Antibodies are available to the T-cell surface markers Thy-1 (mouse only), CD4, CD8, and CD3. Dual colored fluorochromes allow cells to be stained for two markers simultaneously. In this manner, the number of $CD4^+$ and $CD8^+$ cells can be determined simultaneously on a single sample of cells. In the thymus, this dual staining also helps determine the number of $CD4^+/CD8^+$ (double positive) and $CD4^-/CD8^-$ (double negative) cells residing in this organ. This gives the researcher insight into which specific T-cell subsets are targeted and whether the xenobiotic may affect T-cell maturation. Antibodies available to surface immunoglobulin (Ig) and to B220 (the CD45 phosphatase on B cells) help determine the numbers of B cells.

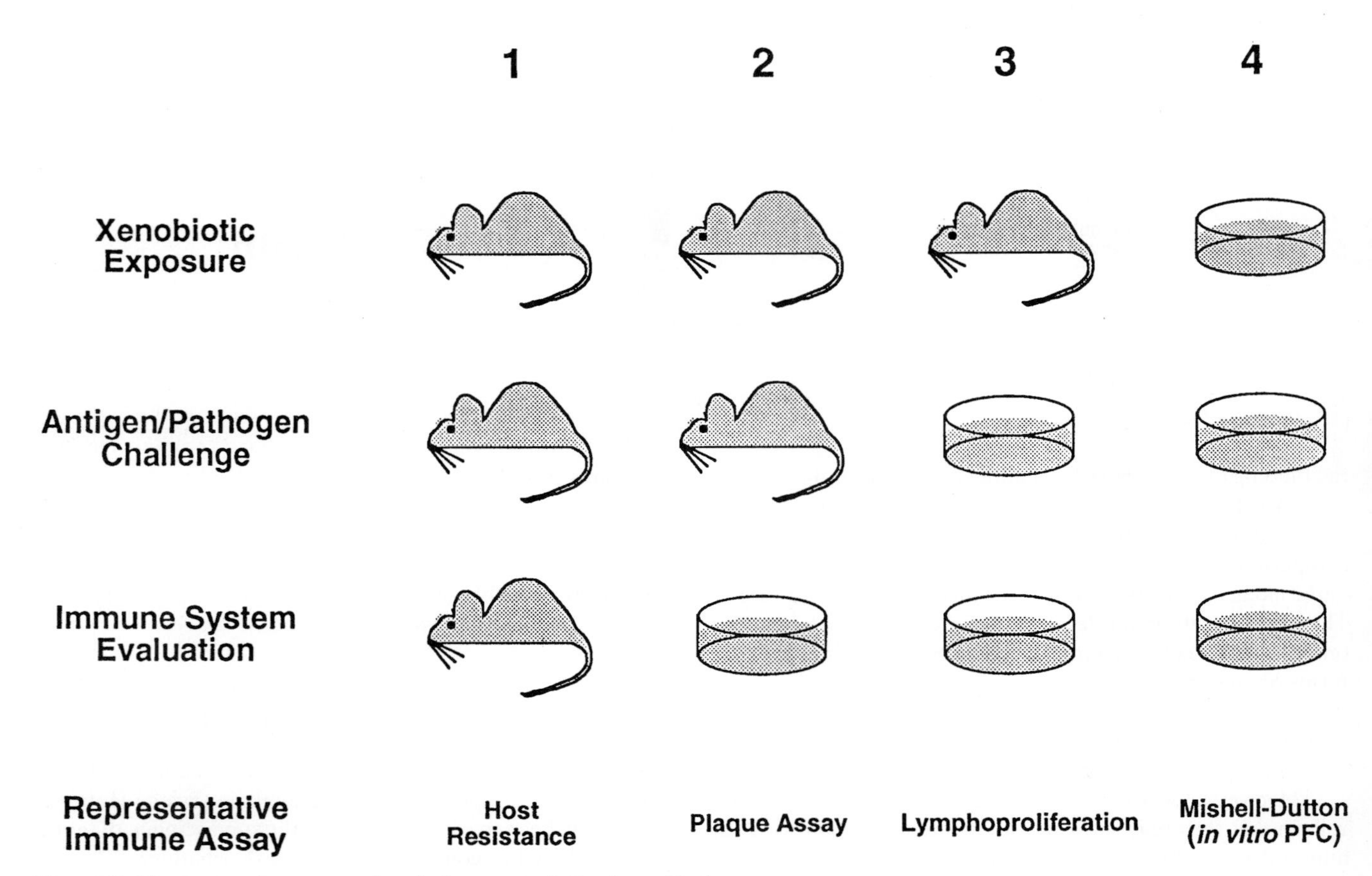


*Figure 12–10. Approaches to assessing the immunotoxicity of xenobiotics.*

Surface markers can reveal significant alterations in lymphocyte subpopulations and in many instances this is indicative of alterations in immunologic integrity. Indeed, an indicator of acquired immunodeficiency syndrome (AIDS) is the changes observed in $CD4^+$ T-cell numbers. Luster and coworkers (1992) have reported that, in conjunction with two or three functional tests, the enumeration of lymphocyte subsets can greatly enhance the detection of immunotoxic chemicals. However, it is important to keep in mind that although surface marker analysis can indicate shifts in lymphocyte populations, functional analysis of the immune system offers greater sensitivity for the detection of immunotoxicity.

**Functional Assessement.** ***Innate Immunity.*** As described earlier, innate immunity encompasses all those immunologic responses that do not require prior exposure to an antigen and that are nonspecific in nature. These responses include recognition of tumor cells by NK cells, phagocytosis of pathogens by MØs, and the lytic activity of the components of the complement cascade.

To evaluate phagocytic activity, MØs are harvested from the peritoneal cavity (peritoneal exudate, or PE, cells) and are allowed to adhere in 24-well tissue culture plates. The cells are then incubated with chromated chicken red blood cells ($^{51}$Cr-CRBCs). Following incubation, the supernatant, containing $^{51}$Cr-CRBCs that have not been bound by MØs, is removed. The CRBCs which are bound to the MØs, but which have not been phagocytized, are removed by a brief incubation with ammonium chloride. Finally, MØs are lysed with NaOH and radioactivity in the lysate is counted to determine the amount of phagocytosis that occurred. A set of control wells is needed to determine DNA content for each set of wells. Data are presented as a specific activity for adherence and phagocytosis (adhered or phagocytized cpm/DNA content) since xenobiotics altering adherence will have a significant effect on the results.

Another method to evaluate phagocytosis, but which does not require radioactivity, begins similarly to the $^{51}$Cr-CRBC assay. Peritoneal MØs are allowed to adhere to each chamber of a tissue culture slide. After adherence, MØs are washed and incubated with latex covaspheres. At the end of incubation, cells are fixed in methanol and stained in methylene chloride. Macrophages containing five covaspheres or more are counted as positive and data are expressed as a percentage of phagocytosis (the ratio of MØs with $\geq$5 covaspheres to total MØs counted).

The previous MØ assays are conducted in vitro after chemical exposure either in vivo or in vitro. If an in vivo assay of the ability of tissue MØs to phagocytose a foreign antigen is required, the functional activity of the reticuloendothelial system can be evaluated. Intravenously injected radiolabeled sheep red blood cells ($^{51}$Cr-SRBCs) are removed by the tissue MØ from the circulation and sequestered for degradation in organs such as the liver, spleen, lymph nodes, lung, and thymus. Clearance of the $^{51}$Cr-SRBCs is monitored by sampling of the peripheral blood. When steady state has been attained, animals are euthanized and organs are removed and counted in a gamma counter to assess uptake of the $^{51}$Cr-SRBCs.

Evaluation of the ability of NK cells to lyse tumor cells is achieved using the YAC-1 cell line as a tumor target for an in vitro cytotoxicity assay. YAC-1 cells are radiolabeled with $^{51}$Cr and incubated (in 96-well microtiter plates) in specific effector-to-target ratios with splenocytes from xenobiotic-exposed and nonexposed animals. During an incubation step, splenic NK cells (effectors) lyse the $^{51}$Cr-YAC-1 cells, releasing $^{51}$Cr into the supernatant. At the end of the incubation, plates are centrifuged and the supernatant is removed and counted on a gamma counter. After correcting for spontaneous release (which should be $< 10\%$), specific release of $^{51}$Cr is calculated for each effector-to-target ratio and compared to the specific release from control animals.

***Acquired Immunity: Humoral.*** The plaque- (antibody) forming cell (PFC or AFC) assay is a sensitive indicator of immunological integrity for several reasons. It is a test of the ability of the host to mount an antibody response to a specific antigen. When the particulate T-dependent antigen (an antigen that requires T cells to help B cells make antibody) sheep erythrocytes (SRBCs) is used, this response requires the coordinated interaction of several different immune cells: macrophages, T cells, and B cells. Therefore, an effect on any of these cells (e.g., antigen processing and presentation, cytokine production, proliferation, or differentiation) can have a profound impact on the ability of B cells to produce antigen-specific antibody. Other antigens, termed T cell-independent antigens, such as DNP-Ficoll or TNP-LPS (lipopolysaccharide), can be used that bypass the requirement for T cells in eliciting antibody production by B cells.

A standard PFC assay involves immunizing control and xenobiotic-exposed mice either IV or IP with the SRBC. The antigen is taken up in the spleen and an antibody response occurs. Four days after immunization, spleens are removed and splenocytes are mixed with SRBC, complement, and agar. This mixture is plated onto petri dishes and covered with a cover slip. After the agar hardens the plates are incubated for 3 h at 37°C. During this time, B cells secrete anti-SRBC IgM antibody. When the IgM and complement coat the surrounding SRBCs, areas of hemolysis (plaques) appear which can be enumerated (Fig. 12-11). At the center of each plaque is a single B cell (antibody- or plaque-forming cell; AFC or PFC). Data are usually presented as IgM AFC (or PFC) per million splenocytes. IgG AFC can also be enumerated by slight modifications of this same assay. This isotype switching (from IgM to IgG) is important in secondary responses in which memory B cells respond more quickly to an antigen.

More recently, it has become evident that the PFC assay can be evaluated in vivo using serum from peripheral blood of immunized mice and an enzyme-linked immunosorbant assay (ELISA; Fig. 12-12). Although the optimal response is delayed by 1 to 2 days (compared to the PFC assay), this assay takes into account antigen-specific antibody secreted by B cells in the spleen as well as B cells residing in the bone marrow. Like the PFC assay, mice (or other experimental animals) are immunized with SRBCs and 6 days later peripheral blood is collected. Serum from each sample is serially diluted and incubated in microtiter plates that have been coated with SRBC membranes. The membranes serve as the antigen to which SRBC-specific IgM or IgG will bind. After incubation of the test sera and a wash step, an enzyme-conjugated monoclonal antibody (the secondary antibody) against IgM (or IgG) is added. This antibody recognizes the IgM (or IgG) and binds specifically to that antibody. After incubation and a wash step,

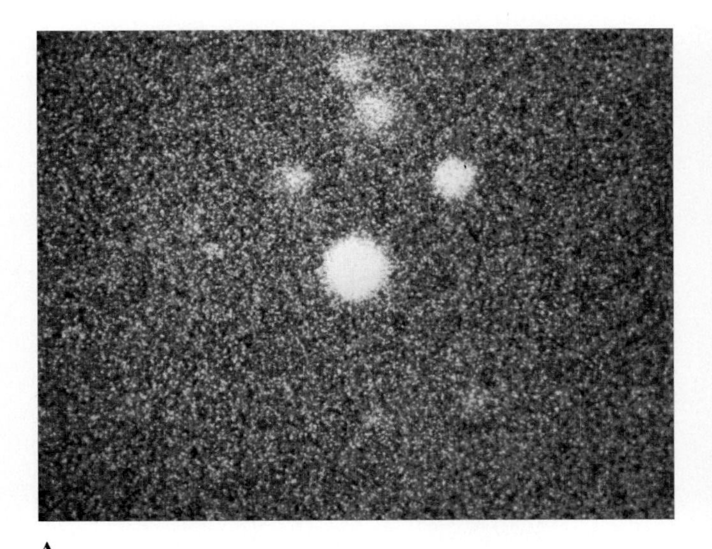

A

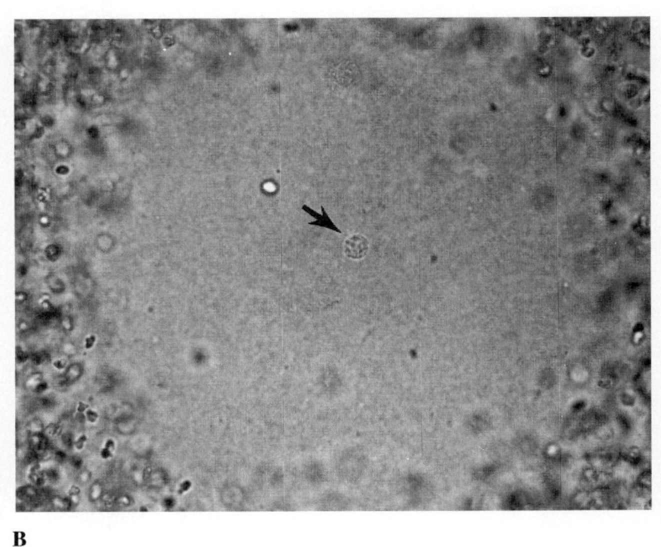

B

***Figure 12–11. The plaque-forming cell (PFC) assay.***

*A*. Demonstration of plaques (areas of hemolysis) which have formed within the lawn of sheep red blood cells ×10 magnification. *B*. ×100 magnification of a plaque from panal A showing the B cell evident in the center of the plaque. [From photos by Dr. Tracey L. Spriggs (with permission)].

the enzyme substrate (chromogen) is added. When the substrate comes into contact with the enzyme on the secondary antibody, a color change occurs which can be detected by measuring absorbance with a plate reader. Since this is a kinetic assay (color develops over time and is dependent upon concentration of anti-SRBC antibody in the test sera), it is important to establish control concentration–response curves so that data can be evaluated in the linear range of the curve. Data are usually expressed in arbitrary optical density (OD) units. Advantages of the ELISA over the PFC assay are the ability to conduct in vivo analyses and to attain a greater degree of flexibility, since serum samples can be stored frozen for analysis at a later date.

One final assay measures the ability of B cells to undergo blastogenesis and proliferation, which are critical steps in the generation of an antibody response. This is achieved in microtiter plates by stimulating splenocytes with a monoclonal antibody to surface Ig (anti-Ig) in the presence of IL-4, or with the B cell mitogen LPS. Proliferation is evaluated 2 to 3 days after stimulation by measuring uptake of $^{3}$H-thymidine into the DNA of the cultured cells. Data are usually expressed as mean cpm for each treatment group. These studies are usually done in conjunction with T-cell proliferative responses described below.

***Acquired Immunity: Cell-Mediated.*** While there are numerous assays used to assess cell-mediated immunity, three primary tests are used routinely in the National Toxicology Program (NTP) test battery: the cytotoxic T lymphocyte (CTL) assay, the delayed hypersensitivity response (DHR), and the T cell proliferative responses to antigens (anti-CD3 + IL-2), mitogens (PHA and Con A), and allogeneic cell antigens (mixed lymphocyte responses; MLR).

The CTL assay measures the in vitro ability of splenic T cells to recognize allogeneic target cells by evaluating the ability of the CTL to proliferate and then lyse the target cells. Splenocytes are incubated with P815 mastocytoma cells, which serve as target cells. These target cells are pretreated with mitomycin C so that they cannot proliferate themselves. During this sensitization phase, the CTL recognize the targets and undergo proliferation. Five days after sensitization, the CTL are harvested and incubated in microtiter plates with radiolabeled ($^{51}$Cr) P815 mastocytoma cells. During this elicitation phase, the CTL that have acquired memory recognize the foreign MHC Class I on the P815 cells and lyse the targets. At the end of the incubation, plates are centrifuged, the supernatant is removed, and radioactivity released into the supernatant is counted on a gamma counter. After correcting for spontaneous release, the percent cytotoxicity is calculated for each effector-to-target ratio and compared to that from control animals.

The DHR evaluates the ability of memory T cells to recognize foreign antigen, proliferate and migrate to the site of the antigen, and secrete cytokines which result in the influx of other inflammatory cells. Like the PFC response, this assay is conducted completely in vivo. The assay itself quantitates the influx of radiolabeled monocytes into the sensitization site. During xenobiotic exposure, mice are sensitized twice with keyhole limpet hemocyanin (KLH) subcutaneously between the shoulders. On the last day of exposure, mononuclear cells are labeled in vivo with an IV injection of $^{125}$I-5-iododeoxyuridine (IUdR). One day later, mice are challenged intradermally in one ear with KLH. Twenty-four hours after challenge, animals are euthanized, the ears are biopsied, and radiolabeled cells are counted in a gamma counter. Data are expressed as a stimulation index which represents the counts per minute (cpm) in the challenged ear divided by the cpm in the unchallenged ear.

T cells play a central role in cell-mediated immunity and the ability of T cells to undergo blastogenesis and proliferation is critical to this role. Several mechanisms exist to evaluate proliferative capacity. The mixed lymphocyte response (MLR) measures the ability of T cells to recognize foreign MHC class I on splenocytes from an MHC-incompatible mouse (allogeneic cells) and undergo proliferation. For example, splenocytes from B6C3F1 mice (responders) are incubated with

**1. Bind antigen to plate. Wash.**

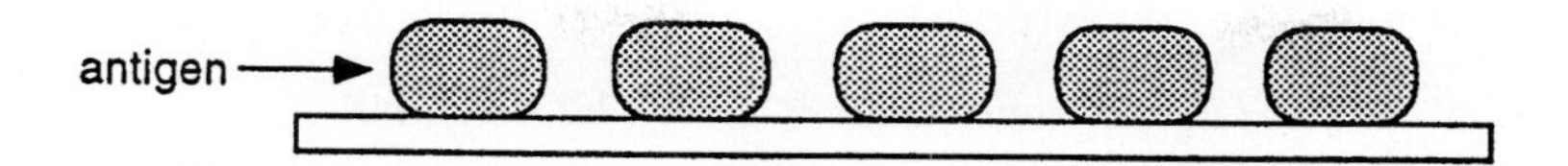


**2. Add test sera and incubate. Wash.**

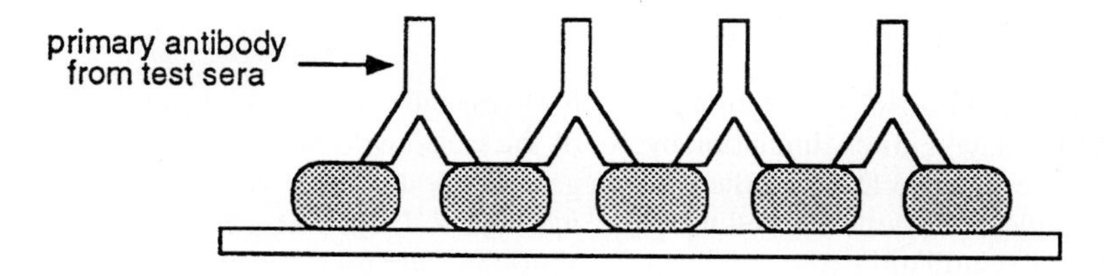


**3. Add enzyme-coupled secondary antibody. Wash.**

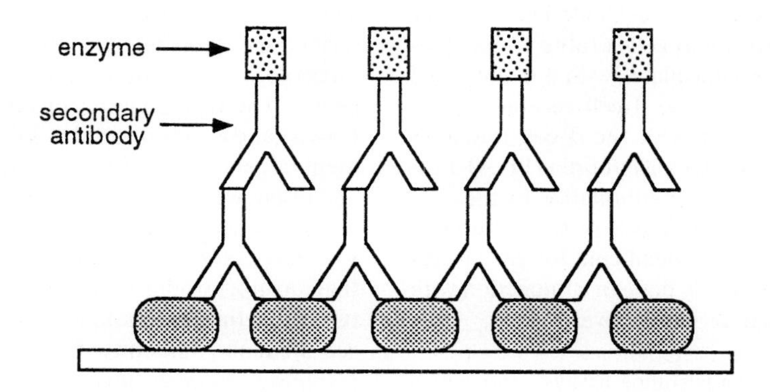


**4. Add chromogen and develop color.**

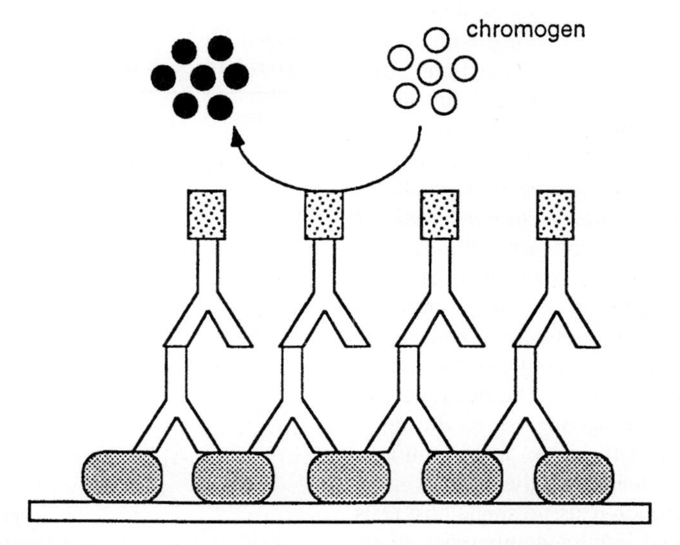


*Figure 12–12. Schematic diagram of a standard enzyme-linked immunosorbant assay (ELISA).*

**Table 12–6**
**Models of Host Resistance**

| CHALLENGE MODEL | PATHOGEN | PRIMARY FACTORS INVOLVED IN HOST RESISTANCE |
|---|---|---|
| Bacterial | *Lysteria monocytogenes* | MØ, T cell, NK |
| | *Streptococcus pneumoniae* | Complement, PMN, MØ, B cell |
| Parasite | *Plasmodium yoelii* | T Cell |
| Viral | Influenza A2 | CTL, Antibody, complement |
| Tumor | B16F10 Melanoma | NK, MØ |

SOURCE: From Bradley and Morahan (1992). See also for an extensive review of host resistance models.

splenocytes from mitomycin C-treated DBA/2 mice (stimulators). Proliferation is evaluated 4 to 5 days after stimulation by measuring uptake of $^3$H-thymidine into the DNA of the cultured responder cells. Cells are collected from each well using a cell harvester and counted in a scintillation counter. Data may be expressed as either the mean cpm for each treatment group or as a stimulation index where the index is calculated by dividing the cpm of wells containing responders + stimulators by the cpm of wells containing responders alone.

General T cell proliferation can be evaluated in a manner similar to that described above for B cells (Table 12-3). Splenocytes are stimulated in microtiter plates with a monoclonal antibody to the CD3 complex of the T-cell receptor (anti-CD3) in the presence of IL-2, or with the T-cell mitogens concanavalin A (Con A) and phytohemagglutinin (PHA). Proliferation is evaluated 2 to 3 days after stimulation by measuring uptake of $^3$H-thymidine into the DNA of the cultured T cells. Data are usually expressed as mean cpm for each treatment group. These studies are usually done in conjunction with B cell proliferative responses described above.

***Host Resistance Assays.*** Host resistance assays represent a way of assaying how xenobiotic exposure affects the ability of the host to handle infection by a variety of pathogens. Although host resistance studies provide significant insight into the mechanisms by which an immunotoxicant is acting, these assays should not be a first or only choice for evaluating immunocompetence. An example of why this is true is the actions of the semiconductor material gallium arsenide (GaAs) on the immune system. Although GaAs produces profound immunosuppression of nearly all cell types evaluated, this compound was observed to confer varying degrees of protection to challenge with *Listeria monocytogenes* and *Streptococcus pneumoniae*. It was subsequently determined that the circulating blood arsenic concentrations were sufficient to inhibit growth of both of these organisms. In host resistance studies, it is also important to consider the following: (1) strain, route of administration, and challenge size of the pathogen; (2) strain, age, and sex of the host; (3) physiological state of the host and the pathogen; and (4) time of challenge with the pathogen (prior to, during, or after xenobiotic exposure). All of these can have significant effects on the results from any individual study.

As with other immune function tests, no single host resistance model can predict overall immunocompetence of the host, primarily because each model uses different mechanisms for elimination of various pathogens. A representative list of host resistance models is shown in Table 12-6 as well as some of the cells involved in the immune response to these pathogens. Typically, three challenge levels of pathogen (approximating the $LD_{20}$, $LD_{50}$, and $LD_{80}$) for each concentration of xenobiotic are used in order to be able to detect both increases and decreases in resistance. Endpoint analyses are lethality (for bacterial and viral pathogens), changes in tumor burden, and increased or decreased parasitemia.

**The Tier Approach.** Luster and colleagues (1988) have described the selection of a battery of tests used by the National Toxicology Program to screen for potential immunotoxic agents. The result was a tier approach to assessing immunotoxicity and is summarized in Table 12-7. Tier I provides assessment of general toxicity (immunopathology, hematology, body and organ weights) as well as endline functional assays (proliferative responses, PFC assay, and NK assay). It was designed to detect potential immunotoxic compounds at concentrations that do not produce overt toxicity. Tier II was designed to further define an immunotoxic effect and includes tests for cell-mediated immunity (CTL and DHR), secondary antibody responses, enumeration of lymphocyte populations, and host resistance models. Subsequently, several testing configurations were defined that would minimize the number of immune

**Table 12–7**
**Tier Approach for Immunotoxicology Testing**

| TESTING LEVEL | PROCEDURES |
|---|---|
| Tier I | Hematology |
| | Body weight |
| | Organ weights (spleen, thymus, kidney, liver) |
| | Spleen cellularity |
| | Bone marrow cellularity and CFU |
| | Immunopathology |
| | PFC Assay |
| | Proliferative responses |
| | NK Assay |
| Tier II | Surface marker analysis |
| | Secondary (IgG) PFC assay |
| | CTL Assay |
| | DHR Assay |
| | Host resistance studies |

**Table 12–8**
**Suggested Testing Configurations: Three Tests with 100% Concordance**

| | | |
|---|---|---|
| PFC | DHR | Surface Markers |
| PFC | NK | DHR |
| PFC | NK | Thymus:body wt. |
| PFC | DHR | Thymus:body wt. |
| Surface markers | NK | DHR |
| Surface markers | DHR | T-Cell mitogens |
| Surface markers | DHR | Thymus:body wt. |
| Surface markers | DHR | LPS Response |

SOURCE: Luster et al. (1988), modified.

tests needed, yet still provide a high degree of sensitivity for detecting potential immunotoxicants. These configurations are depicted in Table 12-8.

### Selection of Animal Models

The mouse has been the animal of choice for studying the actions of xenobiotics on the immune system for several reasons: (1) because there is a vast database available on the immune system of the mouse, (2) mice are less expensive to maintain than larger animals, and (3) a wider variety of reagents (cytokines, antibodies, etc.) are available for the mouse (Vos et al., 1994). Because of the need in the industrial setting to integrate immunotoxicological assessments with routine toxicology testing, a worldwide effort has been underway to validate the rat as a model for immunotoxicology testing. With the exception of a few functional studies, the rat provides a near equal model to the mouse for assessing immunocompetence. In addition, other experimental animals including the chicken, guinea pig, and fish are being used to evaluate the immunotoxicity of xenobiotics, and many reagents that are available for studying the human immune system can also be used in Rhesus and Cynomolgous monkeys. Finally, there are promising models for assessing the mechanisms of xenobiotic-induced immunosuppression that include nude (athymic) mice and rats, transgenic mice, and SCID (severe combined immunodeficient) mice which can be engrafted with human immune cells.

### Evaluation of Mechanisms of Action

As mentioned previously, a unique quality of the immune system is the ability to remove immune cells and have them function in vitro. This is particularly important when investigating the mechanisms of action of xenobiotics. For example, it can be determined whether a compound acts either directly or indirectly on immune cells by comparing in vivo to in vitro chemical exposure. Immunotoxic compounds that act indirectly will have no effect on an in vitro-generated immune response. Compounds that require metabolism to reactive metabolites will also have no effect on in vitro-generated immune responses following in vitro exposure. However, this metabolic requirement can be mimicked in vitro by incubating the chemical with a microsomal S9 preparation prior to in vitro exposure of splenocytes. The metabolically activated compound may then be capable of suppressing in vitro-generated immune responses.

Numerous methodologies are available to evaluate cellular and molecular mechanisms of action. Xenobiotic-induced effects on specific cell types of the antibody response can be determined using antigens that require several cell types, such as MØ, T, and B cells (SRBC), macrophages, and B cells only (DNP-Ficoll), or B cells alone (LPS) for the production of antigen-specific antibody. In addition, splenocytes can be separated into the various cell populations such as adherent cells (primarily macrophages) and nonadherent cells (T and B cells), that can be individually exposed and then reconstituted in cell culture to yield an in vitro-generated immune response equal to that of unseparated cells. This separation/reconstitution analysis is an excellent way to determine specific cell targets of xenobiotic action. In addition, supernatants from in vitro-generated antibody responses can be transferred among themselves in an effort to assess xenobiotic action on soluble factors such as the cytokines, and ELISA methodology and quantitative PCR can be used to quantitate in vitro cytokine production and cytokine gene transcription, respectively, in response to various stimuli. Much of the progress in immunotoxicology research has been the result of the application of advances made in immunology and molecular biology and it is expected that this will continue as these areas of basic science progress by leaps and bounds.

## IMMUNOMODULATION BY XENOBIOTICS

### Immunosuppression

**Halogenated Aromatic Hydrocarbons.** Few classes of xenobiotics have been as extensively studied for immunotoxicity as the halogenated aromatic hydrocarbons (HAHs; reviewed by Kerkvliet and Burleson, 1994, and Holsapple, 1995). The prototypical and most biologically potent member of this family of chemicals, which includes the polychlorinated biphenyls (PCBs), the polybrominated biphenyls (PBBs), the polychlorinated dibenzofurans (PCDFs), and the polychlorinated dibenzodioxins (PCDDs), is 2,3,7,8-tetrachlorodibenzo-*p*-dioxin (TCDD; dioxin). Substantial evidence has accumulated that demonstrates the immune system to be a target for toxicity for these chemicals. Derived from a variety of animal models, primarily rodents, this evidence includes thymic atrophy, pancytopenia, cachexia, immunosuppression, and tumor promotion. There is also epidemiological evidence suggesting immunotoxicity by the HAHs can also occur in humans; however, significant immunosuppression has not been associated conclusively with specific alterations of human immune function.

Quite possibly the most important advance in recent years in the study of the HAHs has been the determination of a genetic basis for sensitivity to the toxic effects of this family of chemicals. Many of the biochemical and toxic effects of the HAHs appear to be mediated via HAH binding to an intracellular heterodimeric complex between the aryl hydrocarbon receptor (*Ah*-R) and the aromatic receptor nuclear transporter (ARNT; Hoffman et al., 1991). The *Ah*-R–ARNT complex translocates to the nucleus, binds to dioxin-responsive elements (DREs), and directs transcriptional activation (e.g.,

CYP1A1, PAI-2, *fos/jun*) and mRNA stabilization (e.g., TGF-$\alpha$, IL-1$\beta$) (Sutter et al., 1991; Sutter and Greenlee, 1992). In mice, allelic variation at the *Ah* locus has been described. These alleles code for *Ah*-Rs with differential binding affinities for TCDD. For example, the C57Bl/6 (B6) mouse represents a strain of mice ($Ah^{bb}$) which is exquisitely sensitive to TCDD (*TCDD responsive*), while the DBA/2 strain of mice ($Ah^{dd}$) is much less sensitive to the toxic effects of TCDD (*TCDD nonresponsive* or *TCDD low-responsive*). These allelic differences may ultimately explain the controversial differences in observed toxic responses between animal species and even between individual tissues within the same species.

***Polychlorinated Biphenyls.*** PCBs have seen extensive commercial use for over half a century. Their unique physical and chemical properties make PCB mixtures ideal for use as plasticizers, adhesives, and as dielectric fluids in capacitors and transformers. Mixtures of PCBs (e.g., Aroclors) have been commonly used to evaluate the immunotoxicity of PCBs and have been reported to suppress immune responses and decrease host resistance (reviewed by Kerkvliet, 1984). The first indication that PCBs produced immunotoxic effects was the observation of severe atrophy of the primary and secondary lymphoid organs in general toxicity tests and the subsequent demonstration of the reduction in numbers of circulating lymphocytes.

Studies to characterize the immunotoxic action of the PCBs have primarily focused on the antibody response. This parameter is by far the one most consistently affected by PCB exposure and effects on antibody response have been demonstrated in guinea pigs, rabbits, mice, and Rhesus monkeys. PCB-exposed monkeys exhibit chloracne, alopetia, and facial edema, all classical symptoms of HAH toxicity. In an extensive characterization of the effects of PCBs on nonhuman primates, Tryphonas and colleagues (1991a, 1991b) exposed Rhesus monkeys to Aroclor 1254 for 23 to 55 months. The only immune parameter consistently suppressed was the PFC response to SRBC (both IgM and IgG). In addition, after 55 months of exposure, lymphoproliferative responses were dose-dependently suppressed and serum complement levels were significantly elevated. The observed elevation in serum complement has also been reported in PCDD-exposed children from Seveso, Italy (Tognoni and Bonaccorsi, 1982) and in B6C3F1-exposed mice (White et al., 1986).

The effects of PCBs on CMI are far less clear and both suppression and enhancement have been reported. Exposure to Aroclor 1260 has been demonstrated to suppress delayed-type hypersensitivity (DTH) responses in guinea pigs, whereas exposure to Aroclor 1254 was reported to enhance lymphoproliferative responses in rats. In a similar study in Fischer 344 rats (Aroclor 1254), thymic weight was decreased, NK cell activity was suppressed, PHA-induced proliferative responses were enhanced, and there was no effect on the MLR proliferative response or CTL activity. Other investigators (Silkworth and Loose, 1978; 1979) have reported enhancement of graft vs. host reactivity and the MLR proliferative response. The augmentation of selected CMI assays may reflect a PCB-induced change in T-cell subsets (as described above) and thus in immunoregulation.

Studies on host resistance following exposure to PCBs indicate that the host defenses against hepatitis virus (ducks) and to herpes simplex virus, *Plasmodium berghei*, *Listeria monocytogenes*, and *Salmonella typhimurium* (mice) are suppressed (reviewed by Dean et al., 1985). PCB-induced changes in tumor defenses have not been well-defined and both augmentation and suppression have been reported. This probably reflects the variability in observed responses in CMI.

***Polybrominated Biphenyls.*** The polybrominated biphenyls (PBBs) have been used primarily as flame retardants (Firemaster BP-6 and FF-1). While it is assumed that their profile of activity is similar to that of the PCBs, few studies have actually evaluated the action of the PBBs on immunocompetence. In Michigan (in 1973) Firemaster BP-6 was inadvertently substituted for a nutrient additive in cattle feed resulting in widespread exposure of animals and humans to PBBs. Studies conducted on livestock following the incident indicated little, if any, PBB-induced alterations in immunocompetence (Kately and Bazzell, 1978; Vos and Luster, 1989). Like CMI observations involving PCBs, CMI responses in PBB-exposed individuals are not conclusive, showing both a reduction in circulating numbers of T and B cells and a suppression of selected CMI parameters or no effect on CMI at all.

***Polychlorinated Dibenzodioxins.*** By far, the majority of the investigations into the immunotoxic potential and mechanisms of action of the HAHs have focused on TCDD, primarily because this chemical is the most potent of the HAHs, binding the *Ah*-R with the highest affinity. The effects of TCDD on immune function have been demonstrated to be among the earliest and most sensitive indicators of TCDD-induced toxicity (reviewed by Holsapple et al., 1991a; 1991b). TCDD is not produced commercially, except in small amounts for research purposes. Rather, it is an environmental contaminant formed primarily as a by-product of the manufacturing process that uses chlorinated phenols or during the combustion of chlorinated materials. It is usually associated with the production of herbicides such as 2,4,5-trichlorophenoxyacetic acid (2,4,5-T), and Agent Orange [a 1:1 combination of 2,4-dichlorophenoxyacetic acid (2,4-D) and 2,4,5-T]. Other sources include pulp and paper manufacturing (chlorine bleaching), automobile exhaust (leaded gasoline), combustion of municipal and industrial waste, and the production of PCBs.

Like other HAHs, exposure to TCDD results in severe lymphoid atrophy. Because thymus-derived cells play an integral role in tumor surveillance and host resistance, the earliest studies on TCDD-induced immunotoxicity focused on changes in cell-mediated immunity. Studies on CMI have shown that this branch of acquired immunity is sensitive to the toxic effects of TCDD. CTL development and activity has been shown by numerous investigators to be significantly decreased after exposure to TCDD, an effect which appeared to be age dependent (e.g., the younger the mice when exposed, the greater the sensitivity to TCDD). In addition to suppression of CTL function, TCDD exposure also results in decreases in PHA- and Con A-induced proliferative responses, DHR, and graft vs. host responses. Enhanced proliferative responses in juvenile mice have also been observed (Lundberg et al., 1990).

Consistent with the observation that mice exposed perinatally or postnatally (developmentally younger animals) are more sensitive to the effects of TCDD, it has recently been determined that thymic involution is a result of TCDD-induced terminal differentiation of the thymic epithelium and, thus, T cells do not have a proper nutrient-filled microenvironment in which to develop (Greenlee et al., 1984; 1985). This conclusion is supported by previous observations that TCDD significantly decreased the number of immature T cells ($CD4^+/CD8^+$) in the thymus (Kerkvliet and Brauner, 1990).

Numerous investigations have demonstrated the PFC response to be exquisitely sensitive to the toxic effects of TCDD. This effect segregates with the *Ah* locus (Vecchi et al., 1983) and appears to be dependent upon duration and conditions of exposure (Holsapple et al., 1991c). Although TCDD induces profound changes in the PFC assay, no changes have been observed in splenic cellularity (numbers of $Ig^+$, $CD4^+$, or Thy-$1^+$ cells) either before or after antigen challenge. In addition, in spite of suppression of antigen-induced antibody production, TCDD has been reported to enhance total serum immunoglobulin concentrations.

Although many labs have defined $T_H$ cells as unaffected by TCDD exposure, Kerkvliet has reported suppression of T cell regulation of immune responses (Kerkvliet and Brauner, 1987; Kerkvliet et al., 1990). However, studies using separation/reconstitution or in vitro exposure techniques have elucidated the B cell as the primary immune cell target for TCDD. In addition, B-cell differentiation was identified as the stage affected. Consistent with these findings, TCDD has a selectively greater effect on immature B cells than on mature B cells. Additionally, the selective effect on B cells cannot be accounted for by induction of $T_S$.

The information presented so far implicates an effect of TCDD on lymphocyte development/maturation either in the bone marrow, thymus, or after antigenic challenge. In support of this conclusion, TCDD exposure has been shown to suppress bone marrow cellularity and stem cell proliferation in rodent neonates exposed *in utero*. TCDD also appears to alter homing patterns of lymphocytes after perinatal or postnatal exposure in Fischer 344 rats and can alter development of CFU-GM at concentrations below those which induce thymic atrophy. Using fetal thymic or bone marrow equivalent cells from birds, it has been demonstrated that TCDD severely attenuates proliferation and development of $CD4^+/CD8^+$ cells and of B cells. These data support the conclusions of Greenlee and colleagues (1984,1985) that TCDD alters the microenvironment in which lymphocytes develop.

The effects of TCDD on innate immunity are less well-studied. TCDD has been shown to inhibit some PMN functions, including cytolytic and cytostatic activities. This inhibition has been postulated to be related to PMN development in the bone marrow. Results by several investigators have shown TCDD-induced alterations in serum C3, indicating soluble mediators of innate immunity may also be targeted (White and Anderson, 1985; White et al., 1986). There have been no observed effects on macrophage-mediated cytotoxicity, NK function, or interferon production. In host resistance models, TCDD exposure has been shown to increase susceptibility to several bacterial, viral, and tumor models.

There is little doubt that TCDD and related PCDDs are immunotoxic, particularly in mice. However, extrapolation to human exposure has proven to be difficult. There are a few instances in which accidental human exposure to TCDD and related congeners has afforded the opportunity to study exposure-related human immunologic responses. In children exposed to PCDDs in Seveso, Italy (1976), nearly half of the exposed study group exhibited chloracne (a hallmark of human exposure to PCDDs) 3 years after the accident. Immune parameters measured at that time were unaffected. In a second study conducted 6 years later on different subjects, there was an increase in complement, which correlated with the incidence of chloracne, an increase in circulating T and B cells, and an increase in peripheral blood lymphocyte (PBL) mitogenic responses. A second incident occurred in 1971 in Times Beach, Missouri, when wastes containing TCDD were sprayed on roads to prevent dust formation. Both low-risk and high-risk individuals from this area were examined for DHR responses. Slight, but statistically nonsignificant alterations were observed in high-risk compared to low-risk individuals. In addition, there was a low-level increase in mitogenic responsiveness in high-risk persons. In a second study conducted 12 years later, no alterations were observed in DHR or mitogenic responses between exposed or control individuals. More recently, studies have been undertaken to evaluate the in vitro effects of TCDD on human cells. TCDD suppressed IgM secretion by human B cells in response to the superantigen toxic shock syndrome toxin-1 (TSST-1) and the proliferation and IgG secretion of human tonsillar B cells in response to LPS and cytokines.

***Polychlorinated Dibenzofurans.*** Like the PCDDs, PCDFs are not produced commercially but are true environmental contaminants associated with the production of chlorophenoxy acids, pentachlorophenol, and other PCB mixtures. Although higher concentrations are required to achieve observable effects, the immunotoxic profile of the PCDFs is similar in nature to that described for TCDD. In fact, most of what is known regarding the immunotoxicity of the PCDFs in animal models has been learned during structure–activity relationship studies comparing TCDD to congeners of the dibenzofurans. TCDF (tetrachlorodibenzofuran) exposure in most species is associated with thymic atrophy and in guinea pigs it has been shown to suppress the DHR and lymphoproliferative responses to PHA and LPS. Suppression of the PFC response to SRBC after exposure to several PCDF congeners has also been reported.

Two important case studies of human immunotoxicology involved populations accidentally exposed to HAHs. There is evidence that the PCDFs were the primary contributors to the observed toxic effects. Greater than 1850 individuals in Japan (in 1968) and in excess of 2000 people in Taiwan (in 1979) were affected when commercial rice oil was found to be contaminated with HAHs. PCDFs were observed in the tissues of the exposed populations and subsequent studies on immune status revealed a decrease in total circulating T cells, decreased DHR, and enhanced lymphoproliferative responses to PHA and pokeweed mitogen (PWM). In addition, many of the exposed individuals suffered from recurring respiratory infections, suggesting that host resistance mechanisms had been compromised.

**Polycyclic Aromatic Hydrocarbons.** The polycyclic aromatic hydrocarbons (PAHs) are a ubiquitous class of environmental contaminants. They enter the environment through many routes including the burning of fossil fuels and forest fires. In addition to being carcinogenic and mutagenic, the PAHs have been found to be potent immunosuppressants. Effects have been documented on humoral immunity, cell-mediated immunity, and on host resistance (reviewed by Ward et al., 1985, and

White et al., 1986). The most extensively studied PAHs are 7,12-dimethylbenz[a]anthracene (DMBA) and benzo[a]pyrene (BaP).

The PAHs suppress the antibody response to a variety of T-cell–dependent and T-cell–independent antigens. In addition, mice exposed to BaP exhibit suppressed lymphoproliferative responses to mitogens but not alloantigens (Dean et al., 1983). In Dean's studies, host resistance to the PYB6 tumor and to *Listeria monocytogenes* were unaffected by BaP exposure, as was the DHR response and allograft rejection, suggesting that the T cell (and CMI) was only minimally affected by BaP. Since the PFC response to T-cell–dependent and T-cell–independent antigens is markedly suppressed by BaP exposure, it would appear that BaP may target the macrophage or the B cell.

In contrast to BaP, DMBA (the more potent PAH) significantly suppresses not only PFC responses but also NK activity, CTL responses, DHR responses, and alloantigen-induced lymphoproliferative responses as well. Therefore DMBA exposure seems to result in long-lasting immunosuppression of humoral immunity (HI), CMI, and tumor resistance mechanisms in mice. Suppression of the immunologic mechanism of tumor resistance by PAHs tends to correlate with their carcinogenic properties and may contribute to their carcinogenicity.

Although it is well established that the PAHs are immunosuppressive in nature, the mechanism(s) by which they elicit this action has remained elusive until recently (reviewed by White et al., 1994). It is generally recognized that PAHs exert carcinogenic and mutagenic effects after being metabolized by P-450 enzymes to more toxic metabolites. It has recently been shown that splenocytes from unexposed mice can metabolize exogenously added DMBA via P-450 enzymes (Ladics et al., 1991). In addition, Ladics and colleagues (1992a, 1992b) demonstrated that macrophages were the primary cell capable of metabolizing PAHs, and that these cells were capable of generating 7,8-dihydroxy-9,10-epoxy-7,8,9,10-benzo[a]pyrene (BPDE), the reactive metabolite proposed to be the ultimate carcinogenic form of BaP. These data are consistent with other studies demonstrating the presence and inducibility of aryl hydrocarbon hydrolase (AHH) in cells of the macrophage lineage and with other data suggesting that the macrophage is the primary target and is functionally compromised (with respect to accessory cell help) following exposure to the PAHs.

**Metals.** Generally speaking, metals target multiple organ systems and exert their toxic effects via an interaction of the free metal with the target: enzyme systems, membranes, or cellular organelles. Although specific immunotoxic consequences of metal exposure are well-documented in the literature (see reviews by Lawrence, 1985; McCabe, 1994; Burns et al., 1994e), this section will focus on the four most well-studied immunotoxic metals: lead, arsenic, mercury, and cadmium. In considering the immunotoxicity of most metals, it is important to remember that at high concentrations, metals usually exert immunosuppressive effects; however, at lower concentrations, immunoenhancement is often observed (Koller, 1980; Vos, 1977).

***Lead.*** By far, the most consistent finding in studies evaluating the effects of metals on immune responses is increased susceptibility to pathogens. For lead (Pb), decreased resistance to the bacterial pathogens *Salmonella typhimurium*, *Escherichia coli*, and *Listeria monocytogenes* has been observed. Enhanced susceptibility to viral challenge has also been reported. Other investigators found no change in virally induced IFN production in Pb-exposed animals.

Studies on the specific effects of Pb on functional cell-mediated immunity have yielded no conclusive results, as reports range from significant suppression to no effect. Currently, these differences cannot be explained by differences in routes of exposure or dose. Suppression of humoral immunity, however, has been demonstrated. In rodents exposed to Pb, lower antibody titers have been observed. In addition, children environmentally exposed to Pb and infected naturally with *Shigella enteritis* had prolonged diarrhea, and occupationally exposed persons reported more colds and influenza and exhibited suppressed secretory IgA levels, suggesting Pb-induced suppression of humoral immunity. Pb-induced effects on myeloid cells include an increase in the number of myeloid progenitors in the bone marrow (CFU-GM) with a subsequent decrease in more mature cells. Following in vivo exposure to Pb, splenocytes displayed consistently suppressed IgM PFC responses to SRBC. Separation and reconstitution experiments indicated that this suppression is likely due to an effect on MØ function.

In recent mechanistic studies (reviewed by McCabe, 1994), an alteration in the ability of the MØ to process and present antigen to antigen-primed T cells confirmed the previous observation and suggested that Pb alters immune recognition. In contrast to other reports concerning the immunosuppressive action of Pb on PFC responses, enhancement of the in vitro-generated PFC response (in vitro exposure in Mishell–Dutton-type culture) has been reported which appeared to be the result of enhancement of B-cell differentiation. This effect may occur at the level of B-cell activation or cytokine responsiveness. And finally, in vitro addition studies indicate that Pb may have differential effects on $T_H1$ and $T_H2$ cells and can inhibit the production of IL-2. If the production or activity of other cytokines is observed to be suppressed or enhanced by metal exposure, it may be that metals can exert significant effects on immune regulation which can result in either immunoenhancement or immunosuppression.

***Arsenic.*** The literature concerning arsenic (As)-induced immunomodulation is fraught with inconsistencies due to differences in speciation of As (which plays a significant role in arsenic toxicity), the route of administration, the concentrations used, and the various species and strains of animals utilized. As with many other metals, exposure to low concentrations of As often leads to enhanced immune responses while exposure to higher concentrations results in immunosuppression (reviewed by Burns et al., 1994e). Exposure of mice to sodium arsenite ($NaAsO_2$) in the drinking water or subcutaneously was shown to decrease resistance to viral pathogens. Other investigators have shown that exposure to arsenicals offers some degree of protection against tumor incidence, although tumors that did develop grew at a much faster rate. No alterations in CMI were observed in those investigations. Interestingly, host resistance studies, conducted after exposure to the semiconductor material gallium arsenide (GaAs), revealed that GaAs afforded modest protection against infection with both *Streptococcus pneumoniae* and *Listeria monocytogenes*, although resistance to the B16F10 melanoma was reduced. It was subsequently determined that the As concentrations in the blood of these animals was high enough to offer a chemotherapeutic effect against the bacterial pathogens (arsenicals were once widely used as chemotherapeutic agents before the development of drugs with higher efficacy and lower toxicity). These studies are important because they are among the first to demonstrate the intricate interplay between the host, the pathogen, and the xenobiotic.

In addition to these holistic immune alterations, As exposure has been shown to inhibit both the PFC response in animal models and peripheral blood lymphocyte proliferation in humans. Also, substantial mechanistic information exists regarding the immunotoxicity of intratracheally instilled GaAs. Exposure results in suppression of the PFC, CTL, DHR, and MLR responses. Following instillation, both arsenic and gallium can be detected in the blood and tissues for as long as 30 days, suggesting that the lung acts as a depot for prolonged systemic exposure to dissociated gallium and arsenic. Mechanistic studies revealed that all cell types involved in the generation of an antibody response (MØ, T, and B cells) are affected by GaAs exposure. Decreased expression of Ia and ability to process and present the particulate antigen, SRBC, represent functional deficits of the MØ, while inhibition of mitogen- or receptor-driven proliferation, expression of the IL-2 receptor, and production of cytokines during the antibody response represent functional deficits of the T cell. A criticism of the studies using GaAs has been that instillation of particulate matter causes a stress response resulting in increased levels of circulating corticosteroids, known to have potent immunosuppressive activity. Studies utilizing the glucocorticoid antagonist RU-486 showed that although GaAs in the lung did increase circulating corticosterone levels, elevated corticosterone was not responsible for suppression of the AFC response. Rather, GaAs exerted direct immunosuppressive effects independent of its ability to increase serum corticosteroid levels.

***Mercury.*** Both organic and inorganic mercury (Hg) have been shown to decrease immunologic responses. Specifically, Hg exposure suppresses the PFC response and increases susceptibility to encephalomyocarditis (EMC) virus, in addition to decreasing polyclonal activation of lymphocytes by T-cell mitogens. It has also been reported that Hg can activate B cells and augment anaphylaxis by enhancing IgE production. Recently, interest in Hg has focused on the ability of this metal to induce type III hypersensitivity. Hg administration is used to induce glomerulonephritis in Brown-Norway rats (a model for induction of autoimmune disease; Sapin et al., 1981).

***Cadmium.*** Like other metals, cadmium (Cd) exposure increases susceptibility to both bacterial and viral pathogens, although enhanced resistance to tumor and EMC virus has been reported. Exposure to Cd has also been demonstrated to modulate lymphocyte proliferative responses to mitogens and allogeneic cells. Greenspan and Morrow (1984) reported decreased MØ phagocytic ability, which correlates with changes in host resistance. Humoral immunity (PFC response and serum antibody titer) and NK function have also been demonstrated to be suppressed by Cd exposure, while CTL activity appears to be enhanced.

***Other Metals.*** Organotin compounds are used primarily as heat stabilizers and catalytic agents (dialkyltin compounds) and as biocides (trisubstituted organotins). The immunotoxicity of the organotins has been extensively reviewed (Penninks et al., 1990). Since the trisubstituted organotins will be examined later (see the section titled Pesticides below, this chap.), discussion here will be limited to the dialkyltins, di-*n*-octyltin dichloride (DOTC) and di-*n*-dibutyltin dichloride (DBTC). Like tributyltin oxide (TBTO), the most outstanding action of the dibutyltins is the induction of profound, but reversible, thymic atrophy. Additionally, there is a preferential loss of $CD4^+$ cells observed in the peripheral blood. The dialkylorganotins have also been observed to decrease resistance to *Listeria monocytogenes* and to suppress the DHR and allograft rejection responses. Suppression of the PFC response to SRBC and inhibition of T-cell mitogen responses was also observed while no effect on B-cell mitogenesis or the PFC response to LPS occurred. These data suggest that the T cell may be a primary target for compounds like DOTC and DBTC. Like the trisubstituted organotins and the HAHs, the developing immune system appears to be more sensitive to the effects of these compounds than does the immune system of the adult.

Beryllium is known primarily for its ability to produce beryllium lung disease, a chronic granulomatous inflammation of the lung often observed in persons with occupational contact or environmental exposure to beryllium compounds. This metal produces a T-cell-mediated hypersensitivity and causes the in vitro transformation of PBL (from exposed, but not from nonexposed patients) into large lymphoblasts (Hanifin et al., 1970). In addition, lymphocytes from beryllium oxide-exposed individuals produce migration inhibitor factor (MIF) that inhibits the migration of MØs (Henderson et al., 1972).

Platinum compounds have been used in cancer chemotherapy and have been shown to suppress MØ chemotaxis, to inhibit humoral immunity and lymphoproliferation, and to induce hypersensitivity responses. Gold salts, used therapeutically in rheumatic disease, may cause immune complex hypersensitivity and enhance allergic reactions. While nickel has been reported to enhance anaphylaxis, it also inhibits humoral immunity, NK activity, and impairs resistance to pathogenic challenge. Chromium at low doses enhances phagocytic ability and PFC responses but appears to suppress these responses at higher concentrations. Cobalt, a constituent of vitamin $B_{12}$, has been demonstrated to suppress PMN chemotaxis and host resistance to Streptococcal infection, and to inhibit the PFC response.

**Pesticides.** Pesticides include all xenobiotics whose purpose is to specifically kill another form of life, usually insects or small rodents. These compounds can be divided into four classes: the organophosphates, organotins, carbamates, and organochlorines. While there is increasing evidence that certain pesticides can produce alterations in immune function in animal models (reviewed by Penninks et al., 1990, and Barnett and Rodgers, 1994), studies following human exposure are limited and reveal no conclusive results (Thomas et al., 1990).

***Organophosphates.*** Occupational exposure to organophosphates has been linked to decreased PMN chemotaxis and increased upper respiratory infection. Overall, there is relatively little known about the immunotoxic effects of organophosphates on the immune system. The most extensively studied are malathion, parathion, and methyl parathion. Prolonged exposure to low doses of malathion (a cumulative high dose) results in decreased humoral immunity. High doses, which have direct cholinergic effects, also suppress humoral immunity, but whether this is a direct effect of the chemical on the immune system or a stress response elicited by cholinergic effects is unclear. In contrast, acute oral exposure has been shown to enhance humoral immunity and mitogenic proliferative responses with no other immune-related effects. In vitro exposure of either human mononuclear cells or murine splenocytes to malathion results in decreased lymphoproliferative responses, suppressed CTL generation, and a decrease in the stimulus-induced respiratory burst in peritoneal cells. Moreover, after metabolism of malathion by liver S9 preparations, the metabolites of malathion were not immunosuppressive. In addition, separation and reconstitution studies revealed that the adherent population (i.e., the macrophage) is the primary cellular target for malathion. Malathion exposure also induces peritoneal mast cell degranulation and enhances macrophage phagocytosis. In light of the above findings and the fact that mast cell degranulation products can modulate leukocyte activity, it has been suggested that peritoneal mast cell degranulation following acute malathion exposure may subsequently lead to augmentation of leukocyte functions, thereby nonspecifically enhancing the generation of an immune response.

Parathion has attracted more attention than malathion, probably because it is more acutely toxic. This pesticide suppresses both humoral and cell-mediated immunity. Following exposure to methyl parathion, decreased germinal centers after antigen challenge, thymic atrophy, and suppressed DHR responses have been reported. Other experiments have shown suppression of lymphoproliferative responses as well as increased susceptibility to pathogens. In vitro exposure to parathion or paraoxon suppresses CMI in murine splenocytes, IL-2 production in rat splenocytes, and proliferative responses in human lymphocytes. Finally, exposure of human bone marrow cells to organophosphates may result in inhibition of CFU formation.

***Organochlorines.*** The organochlorines include chemicals such as chlordane, dichlorodiphenyltrichloroethane (DDT), Mirex, pentachlorophenol, aldrin, dieldrin, and hexachlorobenzene. These are among the more long-lived pesticides and they have an increased propensity for contamination of soil and ground water. The humoral immune response to both T-cell–dependent and T-cell–independent antigens is suppressed following exposure to dieldrin and macrophage functions from dieldrin-exposed animals are depressed. The apparent effect of dieldrin on MØs correlates with the increased susceptibility of dieldrin-exposed animals to murine hepatitis virus, which targets macrophages (Krzystyniak et al., 1985).

Definitive immunosuppression produced by chlordane was first reported in 1982 by Spyker-Cranmer and colleagues. *In utero* exposure resulted in decreased DHR responses in mice with no deficit in antibody production to SRBC. This correlated with an increase in resistance to influenza infection because the DHR contributes to the pathology of the infection (Menna et al., 1985). As reported for dieldrin, the primary cellular target for chlordane appears to be the macrophage. Although peritoneal exudate cells from *in utero* chlordane-exposed mice showed normal cytotoxic responses, the response is delayed by 24 to 48 h. Preliminary evidence suggests that prenatal exposure inhibits myeloid progenitor development in bone marrow, but no cause–effect relationship between this and macrophage deficits has been determined. In contrast to observations from mice exposed *in utero*, exposure of adult mice to chlordane does not result in any changes to several immune parameters, including PFC response to SRBC, MLR, DHR, or mitogenic lymphoproliferation.

DDT is one of the oldest pesticides in use today and one of the first studied for its immunotoxic potential. DDT inhibited antiovalbumin serum antibody titers in rats exposed via the drinking water (Wasserman et al., 1969). In contrast, both rats and guinea pigs fed DDT exhibited no alterations in antitoxin antibody (Gabliks et al., 1973, 1975). These animals did, however, have a suppressed anaphylactic reaction as a result of decreased numbers of mast cells. Studies by Street (1981) indicated that chickens exposed to DDT or Mirex had suppressed levels of circulating IgM and IgG, although specific antibody titers were normal. In addition, DDT exposure resulted in decreased antigen-induced germinal centers, thymic atrophy and suppressed CMI. While most studies on DDT have focused on humoral immunity, the effects of DDT on CMI, host resistance, and particularly macrophage function remain relatively unexplored.

***Organotins.*** Trisubstituted organotins such as TBTO are widely used as biocides and have recently been recognized as producing some immunotoxic effects. The action of these compounds on lymphoid tissue and immunity has been extensively reviewed (Penninks et al., 1990). The most outstanding action of TBTO is the induction of profound, but reversible, thymic atrophy. In addition, the developing immune system appears to be more sensitive to the effects of TBTO than does the immune system of the adult animal. Studies by Vos et al. (1984) demonstrated a decrease in cellularity in the spleen, bone marrow, and thymus. The decrease in splenic cellularity was associated with a concomitant loss of T lymphocytes. More specifically, oral TBTO exposure resulted in decreased serum IgG, increased serum IgM, and suppression of DHR responses to tuberculin and ovalbumin. In those studies, host resistance to *Listeria monocytogenes* was diminished. Cytotoxicity by adherent peritoneal cells was suppressed but there was no observed effect on NK cytotoxicity. In contrast, van Loveren et al. (1990) observed suppressed lung NK cytotoxicity in rats exposed orally to TBTO. In addition, the lymphoproliferative response of thymocytes to PHA, Con A, and PWM was significantly suppressed.

***Carbamates.*** Carbamate insecticides such as carbaryl (Sevin) and aldicarb have frequently been studied as immunotoxicants. Studies involving oral exposure of chickens to Sevin resulted in acute and sometimes prolonged suppression of germinal centers and antibody production. In addition, carbaryl exposure suppresses granulocyte phagocytosis, which may last for up to 9 months. However, other studies have found no indication of immunotoxicity except at near lethal concentrations. Conflicting results have also been observed in animals exposed to aldicarb or methyl isocyanate, an intermediate in carbamate pesticide production. Deo and colleagues (1987) reported alterations in T cells and lymphoproliferative responses in humans accidentally exposed to methyl isocyanate. In contrast, mice exposed to the same compound showed no significant alterations in immune status (Luster et al., 1986). More recently, Pruett and coworkers (1992a) evaluated the immunotoxicity of sodium methyldithiocarbamate, a chemical widely used for the control of weeds, fungi, and nematodes in soil. These investigators observed decreased thymus weight, depletion of the $CD4^+/CD8^+$ population of thymocytes, and profound suppression of NK activity following both oral and dermal exposure. Given the number of conflicting reports, currently there is insufficient evidence in either humans or animal models to indicate that carbamate pesticides pose a significant risk to the human population.

Naphthalene is a bicyclic aromatic hydrocarbon that is used, among other things, as an insect repellent, insecticide, and vermicide. To date, no evidence for immunotoxicity has been demonstrated despite prolonged exposure (Shopp et al., 1984). Recently it has been suggested that this lack of effect may be related to the inability of splenocytes to metabolize naphthalene and/or to relatively low concentrations of metabolites which may be generated in the liver and diffuse to the spleen (Kawabata and White, 1990).

**Inhaled Substances.** Pulmonary defenses against inhaled gases and particulates are dependent upon both physical and immunologic mechanisms. Immune mechanisms primarily involve the complex interactions between PMNs and alveolar MØs and their abilities to phagocytize foreign material and produce cytokines, which act not only as local inflammatory mediators but also serve to attract other cells into the airways.

***Urethane.*** Urethane (ethyl carbamate) was once widely used as a veterinary anesthetic until its carcinogenic potential was defined in 1948. Exposure to urethane produces severe myelotoxicity resulting in suppression of NK cell activity and antibody responses to SRBC (Luster et al., 1982; Gorelik and Heberman, 1981). In addition, urethane exposure leads to increased frequency of spontaneous lung adenomas in susceptible mouse strains and impaired resistance to B16F10 melanoma cells and metastatic tumor growth in the lungs.

***Tobacco Smoke.*** Cigarette smoke has been implicated in acute respiratory illness and chronic obstructive lung disease, but the effect of exposure to mainstream cigarette smoke has yielded ambiguous results in humans and in animal models (reviewed by Sopori et al., 1994). In humans, the number of alveolar MØs is increased threefold to fivefold in smokers compared to nonsmokers. This may be a result of increased production of IL-1 by the resident alveolar MØs, resulting in enhanced influx of other inflammatory cells (PMNs and peripheral blood mononuclear cells) into the lung. In addition to the increased numbers of MØs, the MØs present appear to be in an activated state, as evidenced by an increase in cytoplasmic inclusions, increased enzyme levels, altered surface morphology, and enhanced production of oxygen radicals. However, despite their apparent activated state, these MØs seem to have decreased phagocytic and bactericidal activity. Although the primary site of exposure of the immune system to cigarette smoke is the lung, selected immune parameters have been shown to be altered in smokers. Decreased serum immunoglobulin levels and decreased NK cell activity have been reported. Concentration-dependent leukocytosis (increased numbers of T and B cells) is well-defined in smokers when compared to nonsmokers. However, the question of whether there is a relationship between smoking and lymphocyte function is debatable.

Numerous immunological studies have been conducted in animals exposed to cigarette smoke that demonstrate suppression of antibody responses, biphasic lymphoproliferative capacity (enhanced, then suppressed with continued exposure), and enhanced susceptibility to murine sarcoma virus and influenza virus. Animal studies cannot precisely replicate human exposure conditions because of the route of exposure and the rapid chemical changes which occur to the components of tobacco smoke upon its generation.

***Asbestos.*** It is believed that alterations in both humoral and cell-mediated immunity occur in individuals exposed to asbestos and exhibiting asbestosis. Decreased DHR and fewer T cells circulating in the periphery as well as decreased T-cell proliferative responses have been reported to be associated with asbestosis (reviewed by Miller and Brown, 1985, and Warheit and Hesterberg, 1994). Autoantibodies and increased serum immunoglobulin levels have also been observed. Within the lung, alveolar MØ activity has been implicated as playing a significant role in asbestos-induced changes in immunocompetence. Fibers of asbestos that are deposited in the lung are phagocytized by MØs, resulting in MØ lysis and release of lysosomal enzymes and subsequent activation of other MØs. Recently it has been hypothesized that the development of asbestosis in animal models occurs by the following mechanism. Fibers of asbestos deposited in the alveolar space recruit MØ to the site of deposition. Some fibers may migrate to the interstitial space where the complement cascade becomes activated, releasing C5a, a potent MØ activator and chemoattractant for other inflammatory cells. Recruited interstitial and resident alveolar MØs phagocytize the fibers and release cytokines, which cause the proliferation of cells within the lung and the release of collagen. A sustained inflammatory response could then contribute to the progressive pattern of fibrosis which is associated with asbestos exposure.

***Pulmonary Irritants.*** Chemicals such as formaldehyde, silica, and ethylenediamine have been classified as pulmonary irritants and may produce hypersensitivity-like reactions. Macrophages from mice exposed to formaldehyde vapor exhibit increased synthesis of hydroperoxide (Dean et al., 1984). This may contribute to enhanced bactericidal activity and potential damage to local tissues. Although usually thought of for its potential to induce silicosis in the lung (a condition similar to asbestosis), the immunomodulatory effects of silica have also been documented (Levy and Wheelock, 1975). Silica decreased reticuloendothelial system (RES) clearance and suppressed both humoral immunity (PFC response) and the cell-mediated response (CTL) against allogeneic fibroblasts. Both local and serum factors were found to play a role in silica-induced alterations in T-cell proliferation. Silica exposure may also inhibit phagocytosis of bacterial antigens (related to RES clearance) and inhibit tumoricidal activity (Thurmond and Dean, 1988).

***Oxidant Gases.*** It is becoming increasingly clear that exposure to oxidant gases, such as ozone ($O_3$), sulfur dioxide ($SO_2$), nitrogen dioxide ($NO_2$), or phosgene, alters pulmonary immunologic responses and may increase the susceptibility of the host to bacterial infections (reviewed by Selgrade and Gilmour, 1994). Infiltration of both PMNs and MØs has been observed, resulting in the release of cellular enzyme components and free radicals which contribute to pulmonary inflammation, edema, and vascular changes. Exposure to $O_3$ has been demonstrated to impair the phagocytic function of alveolar MØs and to inhibit the clearance of bacteria from the lung. This correlated with decreased resistance to *Streptococcus zooepidemicus* and suggests that other extracellular bacteriostatic factors may be impaired following exposure to these oxidant gases. Short-term $NO_2$ exposure decreases killing of several bacterial pathogens and, like $O_3$, this decreased resistance is probably related to changes in pulmonary MØ function. A role for the products of aracadonic acid metabolism (specifically, the prostaglandins) has recently been implied. This is supported by the fact that decreased MØ functions are associated with increased $PGE_2$ production, and the fact that pretreatment with indomethacin inhibits $O_3$-induced pulmonary hyperresponsiveness and related inflammatory responses.

It is clear that exposure to oxidant gases can also augment pulmonary allergic reactions. This may be a result of increased lung permeability (leading to greater dispersion of the antigen) and to the enhanced influx of antigen-specific IgE-producing cells in the lungs. In studies involving $O_3$ exposure and challenge with *Listeria monocytogenes*, decreased resistance to the pathogen correlated not only with changes in MØ activity, but with alterations in T cell-derived cytokine production (which enhances phagocytosis) as well. In support of an effect on T cells, other cell-mediated changes were observed: changes in the T-cell to B-cell ratio in the lung, decreased DHR response, enhanced allergic responses, and changes in T-cell proliferative responses. Together, these data suggest that in addition to altering MØ functions, oxidant gases may also produce an imbalance in the $T_H1$ and $T_H2$ T-cell populations. Given the different patterns of lymphokine secretion by these T-cell subpopulations (Mosmann and Coffman, 1989) this is a very plausible explanation for some of the observed immune alterations.

**Organic Solvents and Related Chemicals.** There is limited, but substantive evidence that exposure to organic solvents and their related compounds can produce immunosuppression (reviewed by Snyder, 1994). By far the most well-characterized immunotoxic effects are those produced by benzene. In animal models, benzene induces anemia, lymphocytopenia, and hypoplastic bone marrow. In addition, it has been suggested recently that this myelotoxicity may be a result of altered differentiative capacity in bone marrow-derived lymphoid cells. Benzene exposure (oral and inhaled) alters both humoral and cell-mediated immune parameters including suppression of the anti-SRBC antibody response, decreased T- and B-cell lymphoproliferative responses (mitogens and alloantigens), and inhibition of CTL activity. Benzene exposure also appears to increase the production of both IL-1 and TNF$\alpha$ and to inhibit the production of IL-2. With these dramatic effects on immune responses, it is not surprising that animals exposed to benzene exhibit reduced resistance to a variety of pathogens. More recently, nitrobenzene (an oxidizing agent used in the synthesis of aniline and benzene compounds) has been reported to also produce immunotoxic effects (Burns et al., 1994a), with the primary targets being the peripheral blood erythrocyte and the bone marrow.

Immunomodulating activity has also been observed for toluene, although most effects occur at significantly high concentrations. When compared with benzene, toluene has little to no effect on immunocompetence. However, it should be noted that toluene exposure effectively attenuates the immunotoxic effects of benzene (probably because of competition for metabolic enzymes).

In contrast to the parent toluene, the monosubstituted nitrotoluenes (para- and meta-nitrotoluene) do significantly alter the immune system (Burns et al., 1994b, 1994c). Exposure to p-nitrotoluene has been demonstrated to suppress the antibody response to SRBC, to decrease the number of $CD4^+$ splenic T cells, and to inhibit the DHR to keyhole limpet hemocyanin (KLH). In addition, host resistance to *Listeria monocytogenes* was impaired, suggesting the T cell as a primary target. Similarly, m-nitrotoluene suppresses the antibody response to SRBC, the DHR to KLH, T-cell mitogenesis, and host resistance to *Listeria monocytogenes,* again suggesting the T cell as the cellular target. The di-substituted nitrotoluene (2,4-dinitrotoluene; DAT) is also immunosuppressive (Burns et al., 1994d), with exposure resulting in suppressed humoral immunity, NK activity, and phagocytosis by splenic MØs. Host resistance to bacterial challenge was also impaired. It would appear that DAT may perturb the differentiation and maturation of leukocytes.

Carbon tetrachloride ($CCl_4$) is widely recognized as hepatotoxic. Recent studies have revealed that $CCl_4$ is also immunotoxic. Mice exposed for 7 to 30 days to $CCl_4$ (orally or IP) exhibit a decreased T-cell dependent antibody response (SRBC), suppressed mixed lymphocyte responses (allogeneic cells), and lower lymphoproliferative capacity (T and B cells). Induction or inhibition of liver P-450 activity augmented and blocked, respectively, the immunotoxic actions of $CCl_4$, suggesting a requirement for metabolism in order for $CCl_4$ to be immunosuppressive. In contrast, Fischer 344 rats exposed orally for 10 days exhibited no immunotoxic effects, despite signs of liver toxicity. These differences may represent differences in the metabolic capabilities between these two species.

A relative paucity of information exists on other solvents and related chemicals. Exposure to dichloroethylene (in drinking water for 90 days) has been reported to suppress the anti-SRBC antibody response in male CD-1 mice and to inhibit MØ function in their female counterparts (Shopp et al., 1985). Similarly, exposure to trichloroethylene (in the drinking water for 4 to 6 months) was reported to inhibit both humoral and cell-mediated immunity and bone marrow colony-forming activity (Sanders et al., 1982). In those experiments, females were more sensitive than males. Exposure to 1,1,2-trichloroethane results in suppression of humoral immunity in both sexes. In addition, MØ function was inhibited (males only; Sanders et al., 1985). Finally, inhalation of dichloroethane, dichloromethane, tetrachloroethene, and trichloroethene has been reported to suppress pulmonary host resistance to *Klebsiella pneumoniae* (Aranyi et al., 1986; Sherwood et al., 1987), suggesting that alveolar macrophages may be affected.

**Therapeutic Agents.** Historically speaking, very few drugs used today as immunosuppressive agents were actually developed for that purpose. In fact, if one looks closely enough, nearly all therapeutic agents possess some degree of immunomodulatory activity (Descotes, 1986). The recent explosion of knowledge regarding the function and regulation of the immune system (at the cellular, biochemical, and molecular level) has provided investigators a relatively new avenue for specific drug development. The following discussion will focus on those drugs used primarily for modulating the immune system: the immunosuppressants, AIDS therapeutics, and the recombinant cytokines. Extensive reviews of these drugs can be found elsewhere (Spreafico et al., 1985; Rosenthal and Kowolenko, 1994; Talmadge and Dean, 1994).

***Immunosuppressive Drugs.*** Originally developed as an antineoplastic agent, cyclophosphamide (Cytoxan, CYP) is the prototypical member of a class of drugs known as alkylating agents. Upon entering the cell, the inactive drug is cleaved into phosphoramide mustard, a powerful DNA alkylating agent that leads to blockade of cell replication. Clinically, CYP has found use in reducing symptoms of autoimmune disease and in the pretreatment of bone marrow transplant recipients. Experimentally, this drug is often used as a positive immunosuppressive control in immunotoxicology studies because it can suppress both humoral and cell-mediated immune responses. There appears to be preferential inhibition of B-cell responses, possibly due to decreased production and surface expression of immunoglobulins. CMI activities that are suppressed include the DHR, CTL, graft vs. host (GVH) disease, and the MLR.

The immunosuppressive actions of corticosteroids has been known for years. Following binding to an intracellular receptor, these agents produce profound lymphoid cell depletion in rodent models. In nonhuman primates and humans, lymphopenia associated with decreased monocytes and eosinophils and increased PMNs is seen. Corticosteroids induce apoptosis and T cells are particularly sensitive. In addition, these agents inhibit MØ accessory cell function, the production of IL-1 from the MØs, and the subsequent synthesis of IL-2 by T-cells. In general, corticosteroids suppress the generation of CTL responses, MLR, NK activity, and lymphoproliferation. While it is clear that these drugs inhibit T-cell function, their effects on B cells are not completely clear. Corticosteroids inhibit humoral responses, but this appears to be due to effects on T cells, as antigen-specific antibody production by B cells to T-independent antigens does not appear to be affected by corticosteroid treatment.

Azathioprine (AZA), one of the antimetabolite drugs, is a purine analog that is more potent than the prototype, 6-mercaptopurine as an inhibitor of cell replication. Immunosuppression likely occurs because of the ability of the drug to inhibit purine biosynthesis. It has found widespread use in the inhibition of allograft rejection, although it is relatively ineffective in attenuating acute rejection reactions. It can also act as an anti-inflammatory drug and can reduce the number of PMNs and monocytes. Clinical use of the drug is limited by bone marrow suppression and leukopenia. AZA inhibits humoral immunity, but secondary responses (IgG) appear more sensitive than primary responses (IgM). A large range of CMI reactivities are also reduced by AZA treatment including DHR, MLR, and GVH disease. Although T-cell functions are the primary targets for this drug, inhibition of NK function and MØ activities has also been reported.

Cyclosporin A (Sandimmune, CsA) is a cyclic undecapeptide isolated from fungal organisms found in the soil. Important to its use as an immunosuppressant is the relative lack of secondary toxicity (e.g., myelotoxicity) at therapeutic concentrations (Calne et al., 1981). However, hepatotoxicity and nephrotoxicity are limiting side effects. CsA acts preferentially on T cells by inhibiting the biochemical signaling pathway emanating from the T-cell receptor (TCR). The result is inhibition of IL-2 gene transcription and subsequent inhibition of T-cell proliferation. More specifically, CsA interacts with the intracellular molecule cyclophillin, an intracellular protein with peptidyl proline isomerase activity (although this enzymatic activity probably has nothing to do with the immunosuppressive effect of CsA). The CsA–cyclophillin complex inhibits the serine/threonine phosphatase activity of a third molecule, calcineurin. Calcineurin is proposed to dephosphorylate the cytoplasmic subunit of NF-AT (nuclear factor of activated T cells) and allow the transport of NF-AT into the nucleus where it can couple with nuclear components and induce the transcription of the IL-2 gene. Inhibition of calcineurin phosphatase activity by the CsA–cyclophillin complex then prevents nuclear translocation of NF-AT and the resulting IL-2 gene transcription.

FK506 is a cyclic macrolide which is structurally distinct from CsA, but which possesses a nearly identical mechanism of action. Like CsA, FK506 binds intracellularly to proteins with peptidyl proline isomerase activity, the most abundant of which is FK506 binding protein-12 (FKBP12). The FK506–FKBP12 complex also binds to and inhibits calcineurin activity, thereby inhibiting IL-2 gene transcription. Clinically, FK506 inhibits T-cell proliferation, lacks myelotoxicity (although, like CsA, it does cause nephrotoxicity), and induces transplantation tolerance. In addition, the minimum effective dose appears to be approximately tenfold lower than that of CsA.

Rapamycin (RAP) is also a cyclic macrolide which is structurally related to FK506. However, the mechanism by which it produces inhibition of proliferation is strikingly distinct. Unlike CsA and FK506, RAP does not inhibit TCR-dependent signaling events and IL-2 gene transcription. Rather, this compound inhibits IL-2-stimulated T-cell proliferation by blocking cell-cycle progression from late $G_1$ into S phase (Morice et al., 1993; Terada et al., 1993). Like FK506, RAP binds to the intracellular protein FKBP12. But this RAP–FKBP12 complex does not bind calcinurin. Moreover, until very recently, the actual target protein(s) of this complex have remained elusive. Now it is clear that the RAP–FKBP12 complex binds to the mammalian target of rapamycin, mTOR (Sabers et al., 1995), also referred to as FRAP-1 and RAFT-1 (Brown et al., 1994; Sabatini et al., 1994). This protein, originally identified as two proteins (TOR-1 and TOR-2) in rapamycin-resistant yeast mutants (Kunz et al., 1993), have homology to the lipid kinase domain of the p110 catalytic subunit of phosphatidylinositol 3-kinase (PI3K, a biochemical signaling molecule) and VPS34 (a yeast PI3K). The function of the TOR proteins in cellular regulation (specifically cell cycle progression) remains unknown at this time. Unlike both CsA and FK506, RAP does not appear to be nephrotoxic.

Leflunomide, an isoxazole derivative, is a relatively new drug which has shown promise as an immunosuppressive agent in the treatment of rheumatic disease and transplantation (Xiao et al., 1994). Experimentally, this agent can block the generation of allo-specific antibodies, decrease the mononuclear infiltrate in grafts undergoing rejection, and reverse acute graft rejections. It has been found to be equal to or better than CsA in its ability to inhibit B cell-mediated autoimmune disease. Early mechanistic studies indicate leflunomide can directly inhibit B-cell proliferation ($IC_{50} \leq 20$ $\mu$M) and this may account for the drug's ability to inhibit both T-cell-dependent and T-cell-independent specific antibody production. Leflunomide also can inhibit T-cell proliferation ($IC_{50} = 50 - 75$ $\mu$M) induced by mitogens, antibody directed against CD3, or IL-2. IL-2 production is also attenuated, but expression of the IL-2 receptor (CD25) is not altered. Biochemical analyses indicate this drug can inhibit IL-2-dependent protein tyrosine kinase activity and suggests that the mechanism of T-cell inhibition may be at the level of T-cell responsiveness to IL-2. Although similar in broad terms, this mechanism of action is distinctly different from the mechanism of action of RAP.

***AIDS Therapeutics.*** Traditionally, antiviral therapies have not been extremely successful in their attempt to rid the host of viral infection. This may be due to the fact that these organisms target the DNA of the host. Thus, eradication of the infection means killing infected cells. Although numerous strategies have been developed to combat the AIDS virus (primarily targeting viral reverse transcriptase or viral protease, and up-regulation of other immune responses), no one drug has produced any significant advance. This is possibly because the very nature of the infection has significant immunosuppressive consequences. Without a doubt, more basic scientific knowledge about the physiology and biochemistry of the virus is required before rational drug design will yield an effective therapeutic agent.

Zidovudine (3′-azido-3′-deoxythymidine; AZT) is a pyrimidine analog that inhibits viral reverse transcriptase. It was the first drug shown to have any clinical efficacy in the treatment of HIV-1 infection. Unfortunately, its use is limited by myelotoxicity (macrocytic anemia and granulocytopenia). Animal studies have confirmed that the primary action of AZT is on innate immunity, although changes in both humoral and cell-mediated immunity have also been observed. Clinically, AZT increases the number of circulating $CD4^+$ cells and can transiently stimulate cell-mediated immune responses (lymphoproliferation, NK activity, and IFN-$\gamma$ production).

Stavudine (2′,3′-didehydro-2′,3′-dideoxythymidine; d4T) is another pyrimidine analog currently in clinical trials. Unlike its sister drug AZT, the limiting toxicity appears to be peripheral neuropathy, rather than myelotoxicity. In addition, d4T also appears to increase the number of circulating $CD4^+$ cells. Animal studies suggest that d4T does not modulate generation of CTL, NK activity, PFC responses, mitogenicity of lymphocytes, or lymphocyte subsets.

Zalcitabine (2′,3′-dideoxycytidine; ddC) is a third pyrimidine analog which has recently been approved for use. Clinically, there appears to be an increase in circulating $CD4^+$ cells and some restoration of CMI in HIV-infected persons. There also appears to be no significant myelotoxicity and, like d4T, the limiting toxic effect of ddC is peripheral neuropathy. Investigations in animals revealed no significant effect on immune status.

Videx (2′,3′-dideoxyinosine; ddI) is the first purine analog approved for use in HIV infection. In clinical trials, the dose-limiting toxicities were shown to be peripheral neuropathy and pancreatitis. There appears to also be an increase in circulating $CD4^+$ cells, some restoration of CMI, and a reversal of HIV-induced myelotoxicity. Although ddI is converted into ddA-TP, the use of ddA as an antiviral agent was ruled out due to severe nephrotoxic effects. In animal models, both ddI and ddA produce suppression of humoral immunity.

***Recombinant Cytokines.*** In recent years there has been a significant increase in the number of soluble immune mediators (i.e., cytokines and growth factors) which have been identified and cloned. Armed with the knowledge of the primary actions of these cytokines on immune function, pharmaceutical and biotechnology companies have set out to mass produce these factors (by recombinant DNA technology) and move them into clinical trials. To date, the majority have been used as immunostimulants and include IFN-$\alpha$, IFN-$\gamma$, IL-2, GM-CSF, and erythropoietin (EPO). The immunopharmacology (and toxicity) of these agents has been reviewed extensively elsewhere (Talmadge and Dean, 1994). Although some can be used alone as therapeutics, the best hope for these agents lies in their ability to be used in combination with other drugs.

**Drugs of Abuse.** Drug abuse is a social issue with far-reaching effects on the abuser as well as on friends and family. While drug paraphernalia has been directly associated with the spread of the AIDS virus, in recent years the actual abuse of some drugs has been linked to the progression, and possibly the onset, of AIDS. Although definitive scientific proof of the hypothesis is lacking, drugs which are often abused have been shown to alter immunocompetence.

***Cannabinoids.*** Much attention has been focused on the immunomodulatory effects of the cannabinoids ($\Delta^9$-tetrahydrocannabinol; THC) due to the therapeutic potential for this drug in the treatment of glaucoma and as an antiemetic used in patients undergoing cancer chemotherapy. Early studies showed exposure to THC decreases host resistance to bacterial and viral pathogens (reviewed by Kaminski, 1994). In addition, cannabinoids alter both humoral and cell-mediated immune responses. Suppression of NK and CTL activity by THC appears to be related to an effect occurring subsequent to target-cell binding. THC exposure also alters MØ morphology and some nonspecific functions, but the effects on accessory cell activities (e.g., antigen processing and presentation) are not clear. What is apparent, however, is that the suppression of humoral immunity is exquisitely dependent upon the temporal association between exposure and antigen sensitization. Oral exposure to THC during the sensitization process (in vivo antigen administration) suppresses the PFC response to SRBC. In contrast, exposure to THC *prior* to sensitization (but not during the sensitization time), resulted in no observable effects on the PFC response. This may be one of the most critical factors influencing the reported effects of THC on immune responsiveness.

Similar to the in vivo situation, for in vitro THC exposure (Mishell-Dutton cultures), the drug must be added within 2 h of the addition of antigen in order to suppress the PFC response (Schatz et al., 1992). Also, humoral responses to T-cell-dependent antigens, but not T-cell-independent antigens, are suppressed by THC exposure. Together with the fact that T-cell proliferative responses are suppressed after THC exposure in vivo, this suggests that THC affects primarily T cells and may alter early T-cell activation events (e.g., biochemical signaling). Most recently, cannabinoid receptor transcripts have been identified in human spleen, tonsils, peripheral blood lymphocytes, and MØs (Bouaboula et al., 1993; Munro et al., 1993). Additionally, murine splenocytes exhibit a high degree of saturable, specific binding of THC with a $K_d$ approximating 1 nM and a $B_{max}$ of about 1000 receptors per cell (Kaminski et al., 1992). An understanding of a potential role of this receptor in immune responses awaits identification of the endogenous ligand.

***Cocaine.*** Cocaine is a potent local anesthetic and CNS stimulant. This drug and its derivatives have been shown to alter several measures of immunocompetence, including humoral and cell-mediated immune responses and host resistance (Watson et al., 1983; Ou et al., 1989; Starec et al., 1991). Functions of PMNs including superoxide production and cell-surface receptor expression, as well as inhibition of MØ killing ability by decreasing the production of reactive oxygen intermediates, have been reported (Haines et al., 1990; Lefkowitz et al., 1993). Cocaine also induces the secretion of TGF-$\beta$, which has been linked to the observation that cocaine exposure enhances replication of the HIV-1 virus in human peripheral blood mononuclear cells (PBMC; Chao et al., 1991; Peterson et al., 1991). Holsapple et al. (1993) evaluated in vitro cocaine exposure on the generation of an antibody response against SRBCs and found effects only at concentrations that were not clinically relevant (100 $\mu$M; lethal blood concentrations are estimated to be around 6 $\mu$M). These investigators postulated that the immunosuppressive effects of cocaine in vivo were mediated by P-450-generated reactive intermediates and they subsequently demonstrated sex and strain differences in cocaine immunosuppressive activity, which correlated with well-characterized differences in metabolic capability in mice. Male B6C3F1 mice are more sensitive than females and DBA/2 females are more sensitive than B6C3F1 females.

***Opioids: Heroin and Morphine.*** Chronic morphine exposure has been associated with increased susceptibility to both bacterial and viral antigens (Arora et al., 1990; Chao et al., 1990), and it is clear that exposure to opioids can suppress immune responses. What is not clear, however, is whether this action is a direct effect of the drug on immune cells or an indirect effect resulting from drug-induced increases in circulating corticosteroids. Evaluation of the immunocompetence of heroin addicts revealed a decrease in total T cells and E-rosette capability (McDonough et al., 1980). In that study, treatment with naloxone reversed these effects, suggesting a role for an opioid receptor in mediating immune suppression. LeVier and coworkers (1994) reported that chronic morphine exposure decreased serum C3, NK activity, total leukocyte counts, the PFC response to SRBC, and RES clearance. However, because many of these effects were not dose-related (i.e., the dose–response curve was flat), these investigators concluded that these effects were not receptor-mediated, but were the result of increased circulating corticosteroids (which were significantly elevated in those animals). This conclusion is supported by the findings of other investigators as well (Pruett et al., 1992b). Morphine-induced suppression of MØ phagocytosis and cytokine production also has been reported (Eisenstein et al., 1993; Tubaro et al., 1987; LeVier et al., 1993). In the study by LeVier and colleagues (1993), the glucocorticoid antagonist RU-486 was utilized to demonstrate that while suppression of hepatic MØ function may be due in part to a receptor-mediated event, inhibition of splenic MØ activity was wholly receptor-independent.

***Ethanol.*** Until recently (reviewed by Jerrells and Pruett, 1994), data concerning the immunomodulatory effects of ethanol (EtOH) exposure have largely been based on clinical observations of alcoholic patients. A prime reason for this is that rodents (the animal model of choice for extensive immunological evaluation) do not voluntarily consume intoxicating quantities of EtOH. Thus, the criteria for the development of animal models for EtOH exposure need to be refined to assure that clinically relevant blood levels are attained and long-term exposure can be assessed. In addition, the affect of acute exposure (binge drinking) needs to be further assessed.

In humans, alcoholism is associated with increased incidence of, and mortality from, pulmonary infection. There is also an increased incidence of bacterial infection and spontaneous bacteremia in alcoholics with cirrhosis of the liver. A consistent finding in abusers of EtOH is the significant change in the mononuclear cells of the peripheral blood. In animal models, this is observed as depletion of T and B cells in the spleen and the T cells in the thymus, particularly $CD4^+/CD8^+$ cells. The latter effect may be related, in part, to increased levels of corticosteroids.

There are also numerous indications that acute EtOH exposure can also have profound immunodepressive consequences: decreased PMN chemotaxis, decreased host resistance, and inhibition of the PFC response. EtOH administration also inhibits mitogen-driven T-cell proliferation and T-cell responsiveness to IL-2. The actions of EtOH exposure on B-cell antibody production and NK cell activity are still controversial.

**Silicones.** Silicones have widespread use in consumer products such as cosmetics, toiletries, food stuffs, household products, and paints, as well as use in the medical field (e.g., lubricants in tubing and syringes and in numerous implantable devices). In recent years, significant interest has focused on the biocompatibility of silicones and the potential for these products to produce immunotoxic effects. This interest has been driven largely by the clinical literature, with reports of adverse reactions to silicone-containing medical materials, and by the claims of women possessing silicone gel-containing breast implants. Despite the fact that there has been persistent, unsubstantiated speculation that silicone breast implants may provoke connective tissue disease, no link between exposure to silicones and human disease has been unequivocally established.

Numerous studies have been conducted that both support and refute the specific actions of various silicones on the immune system. To date, only two studies have been reported that extensively evaluated immune status following exposure to silicones used in medical practice (e.g., polydimethylsiloxane, PDMS). In the first study, mice were implanted for 10 days with PDMS fluid, gel, and elastomer, as well as polyurethane as a control (Bradley et al., 1994a). There were no observable alterations in immune function (either innate or acquired immunity) in these studies. In addition, the silicones tested afforded modest protection to an approximate $LD_{50}$ challenge with *Listeria monocytogenes*. The second study evaluated the same silicone products and involved exposure (implantation) for 180 days (Bradley et al., 1994b). In those investigations, the only consistent immunologic effect observed was a modest suppression of NK cell activity. However, this did not correlate with altered susceptibility to challenge with B16F10 melanoma. These silicone products did not alter host resistance to *Listeria monocytogenes*, *Streptococcus pneumonia*, or B16F10 melanoma.

## IMMUNE-MEDIATED DISEASE

As stated earlier, the purpose of the immune system is to secure the individual from disease states, whether infectious, parasitic or cancerous, through both cellular and humoral mechanisms. In so doing, the ability to distinguish "self" from "nonself" plays a predominant role. However, situations arise in which the individual's immune system responds in a manner producing tissue damage, resulting in a self-induced disease. These disease states fall into two categories, hypersensitivity, or allergy, and autoimmunity. Figure 12-13 shows a schematic which delineates the possible cascade of effects that can occur when a chemical produces an immune-mediated disease. Hypersensitivity reactions result from the immune system responding in an exaggerated or inappropriate manner. These reactions have been subdivided by Coombs and Gell (1975) into four types, which represent four different mechanisms leading to tissue damage. In the case of autoimmunity, mechanisms of self-recognition break down and immunoglobulins and T-cell receptors react with self-antigens resulting in tissue damage and disease.

## HYPERSENSITIVITY REACTIONS

One characteristic common to all four types of hypersensitivity reactions is the necessity of prior exposure in order to elicit a reaction. In the case of types I, II and III, prior exposure to antigen leads to the production of specific antibody, IgE, IgM, or IgG, and, in the case of type IV, to the generation of memory T cells. Figure 12-14 illustrates the mechanisms of hypersensitivity reactions as classified by Coombs and Gell. Regulation of immunoglobulin production is dependant on the charactistics of the antigen, the genetics of the individual, and environmental factors. The mechanism of antibody production in hypersensitivity reactions is identical to that described earlier in the chapter (Fig. 12-7). A description of the four types of hypersensitivity reactions is presented below.

### Type I (Immediate Hypersensitivity)

Using penicillin as an example, Fig. 12-15 depicts the major events involved in a type I hypersensitivity reaction. Sensitization occurs as the result of exposure to appropriate antigens through the respiratory tract, dermally, or by exposure through the gastrointestinal tract. IgE production is highest in lymphatic tissues that drain sites of exposure (i.e., tonsils, bron-

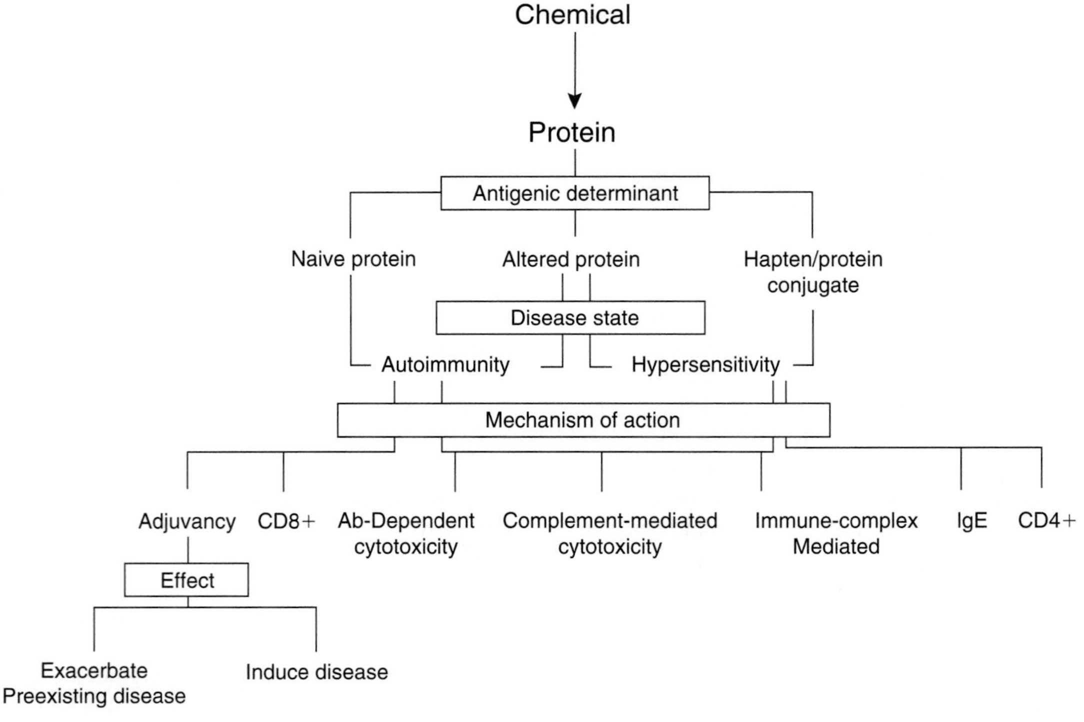


*Figure 12–13. Schematic diagram of chemical interaction leading to hypersensitivity reactions or autoimmunity.*

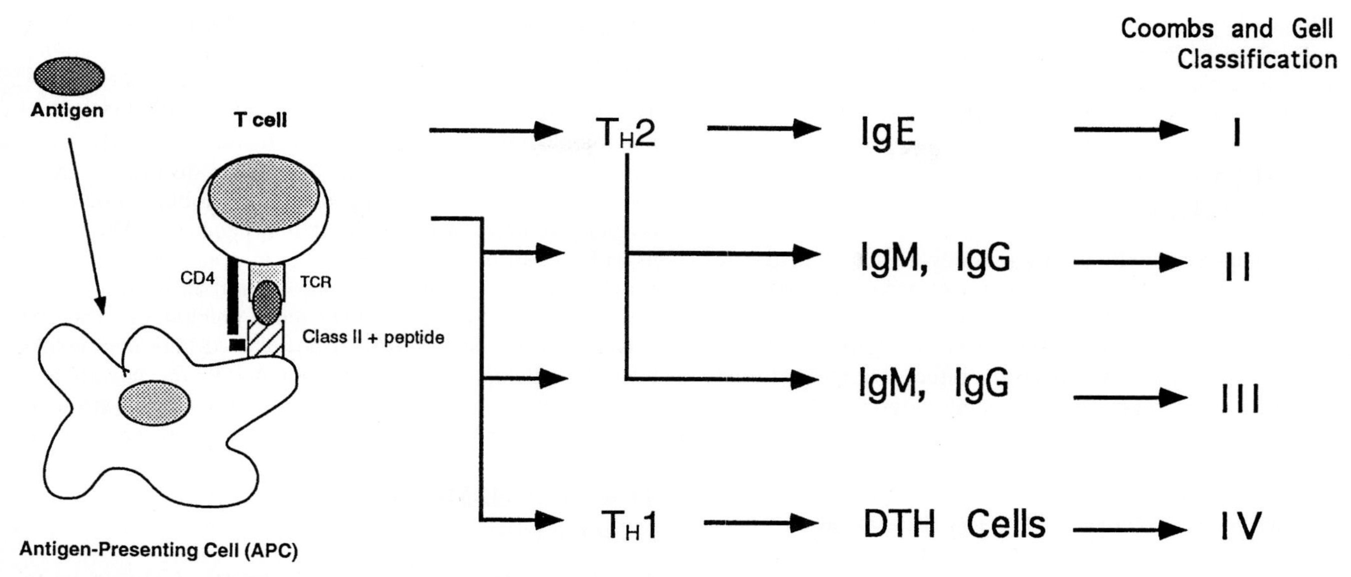


*Figure 12–14. Schematic of classification of hypersensitivity reactions.*

chial lymph nodes, and intestinal lymphatic tissues, including Peyer's Patches). It is low in the spleen. Serum concentration of IgE is low compared to other immunoglobulins, and serum half-life is short (Table 12-4). Once produced, IgE binds to local tissue mast cells before entering the circulation, where it binds to circulating mast cells, basophils, and tissue mast cells at distant sites. Once sensitized, reexposure to the antigen results in degranulation of the mast cells with the release of preformed mediators and cytokines typical of $T_H2$ cells. Synthesis of leukotrienes and thromboxanes is also induced. These mediators promote vasodilation, bronchial constriction, and inflammation. Clinical manifestations can vary from urticarial skin reactions (wheals and flares) to signs of hay fever, including rhinitis and conjuctivitis, to more serious diseases, such as

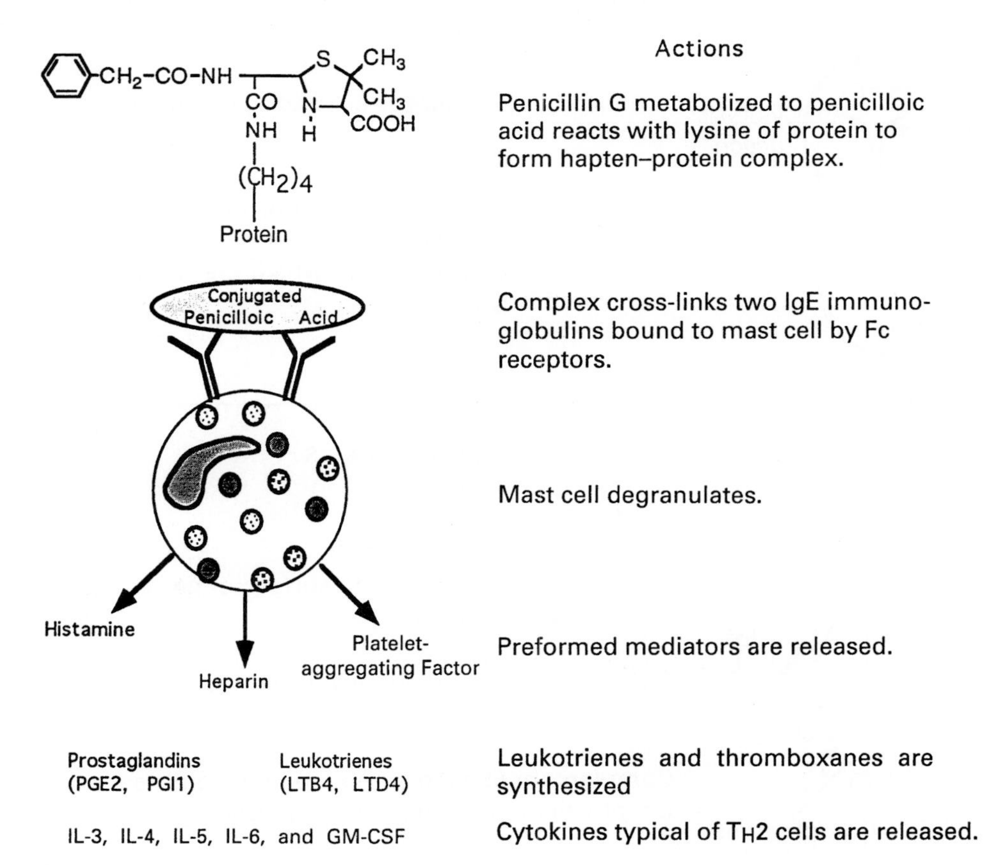


*Figure 12–15. Schematic of type I hypersensitivity reaction.*

asthma and potentially life-threatening anaphylaxis. These responses may begin within minutes of reexposure to the offending antigen and, therefore, type I hypersensitivity is often referred to as immediate hypersensitivity.

## Type II (Antibody-Dependent Cytotoxic Hypersensitivity)

Type II hypersensitivity is also antibody-mediated. Figure 12-16 shows the mechanisms of action of a complement-independent cytotoxic reaction and complement-dependent lysis. The immunoglobulin involved can be of the IgG or IgM class. Tissue damage may result from the direct action of cytotoxic cells, such as macrophages, neutrophils, or eosinophils, linked to immunoglobulin-coated target cells through the Fc receptor on the antibody or by antibody activation of the classical complement pathway. Complement activation may result in C3b or C3d binding to the target-cell surface. These act as a recognition site for effector cells. Alternatively, the C5b-9 membrane attack complex may be bound to the target cell surface resulting in cell lysis (Fig. 12-3).

## Type III (Immune-Complex-Mediated Hypersensitivity)

Type III hypersensitivity reactions may also involve IgM or IgG immunoglobulins. The distinquishing feature of type III is that, unlike type II in which immunoglobulin production is against specific tissue-associated antigen, immunoglobulin production is against soluble antigen in the serum (Fig. 12-17). This results in widely distributed tissue damage in areas where immune complexes are deposited. The most common location is the vascular endothelium in the lung, joints, and kidneys. The skin and circulatory systems also may be involved. Pathology results from the inflammatory response initiated by the activation of complement. Macrophages, neutrophils, and platelets attracted to the deposition site contribute to the tissue damage.

## Type IV (Cell-Mediated Hypersensitivity)

Type IV, or delayed hypersensitivity (DTH) responses, can be divided into two classes: contact hypersensitivity and tuber-

Complement-Independent Cytotoxic Lysis

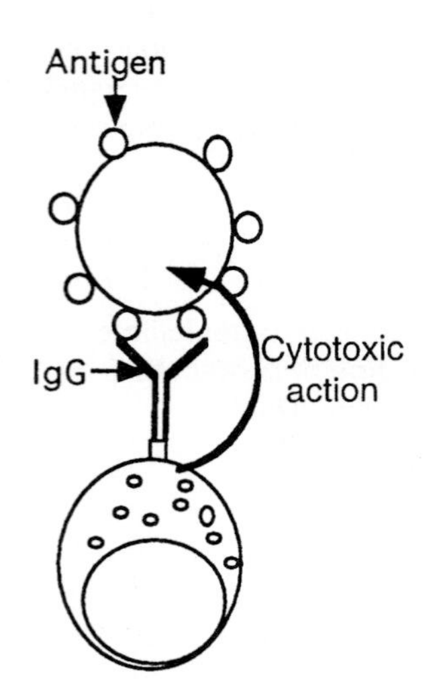


Action

Foreign antigen attaches to surface of normal cell, i.e., RBC, platelet, etc.

Antibody, IgG or IgM, is directed against foreign antigen.

Cytotoxic cell attaches to Fc portion of Ig, stimulating release of cytotoxic granules. Innocent bystander cell to which the Ag is attached is lysed.

Complement-Dependent Lysis

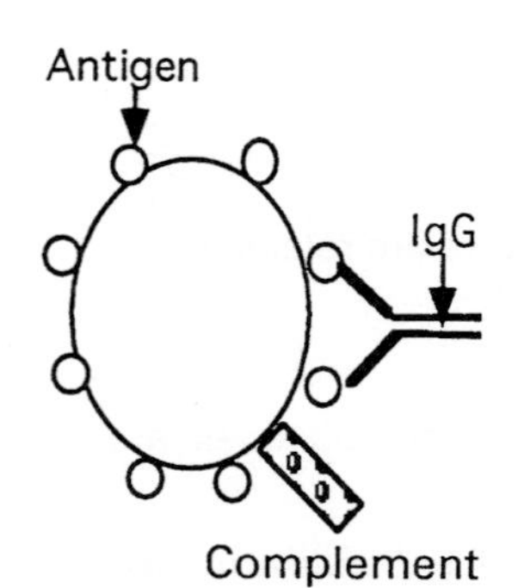


Action

Foreign antigen attaches to surface of normal cell, i.e., RBC, platelet, etc.

Antibody is directed against foreign antigen.

Complement fixes to complement receptors on target-cell membrane, inducing lysis.

*Figure 12–16. Schematic of type II hypersensitivity reactions.*

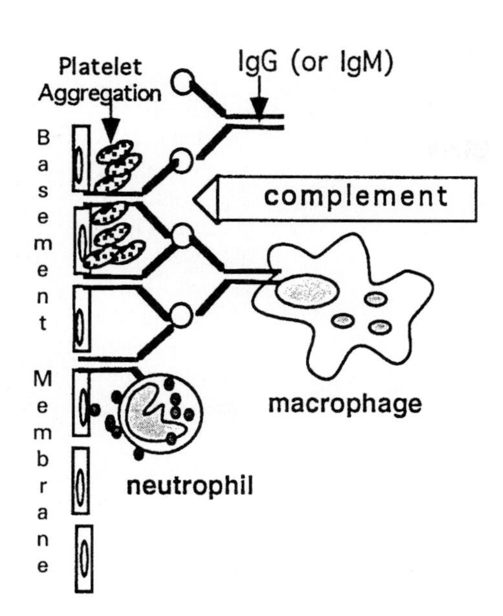


Action

IgG of IgM produced to soluble Ag, Ag–Ab complexes are deposited in tissues.

Platelets interact with immune complexes leading to aggregation and microthrombi formation.

Complement is activated leading to release of vasoactive amines and chemotactic factors.

Chemotactic factors attract inflammatory cells to site.

Local tissues damaged by lysosomal enzymes released from phagocytes.

*Figure 12–17. Schematic of type III hypersensitivity reaction.*

culin-type hypersensitivity. Contact hypersensitivity is initiated by topical exposure and the associated pathology is primarily epidermal. It is characterized clinically by an eczematous reaction at the site of allergen contact and consists of two phases: sensitization and elicitation (Figs. 12-18 and 12-19). Sensitization occurs when the hapten penetrates the epidermis and forms a complex with a protein carrier. The hapten–carrier complex is processed by Langerhans-dendritic cells which migrate out of the epidermis to the local lymph nodes. There, the APC presents the processed antigen to $CD4^+$ T cells leading to clonal expansion and the generation of memory T cells.

Upon second contact, Langerhans-dendritic cells once again migrate to the lymph nodes and present the processed hapten–carrier complex to memory T cells. These activated T cells then secrete cytokines that bring about further proliferation of T cells and induce the expression of adhesion molecules on the surface of keratinocytes and endothelial cells in the dermis. Both the expression of adhesion molecules and the secretion of proinflammatory cytokines by T cells and keratinocytes facilitate the movement of inflammatory cells into the skin resulting in erythema, papule, and vesicle formation.

Tuberculin-type hypersensitivity is primarily a dermal reaction and begins following the intradermal injection of a

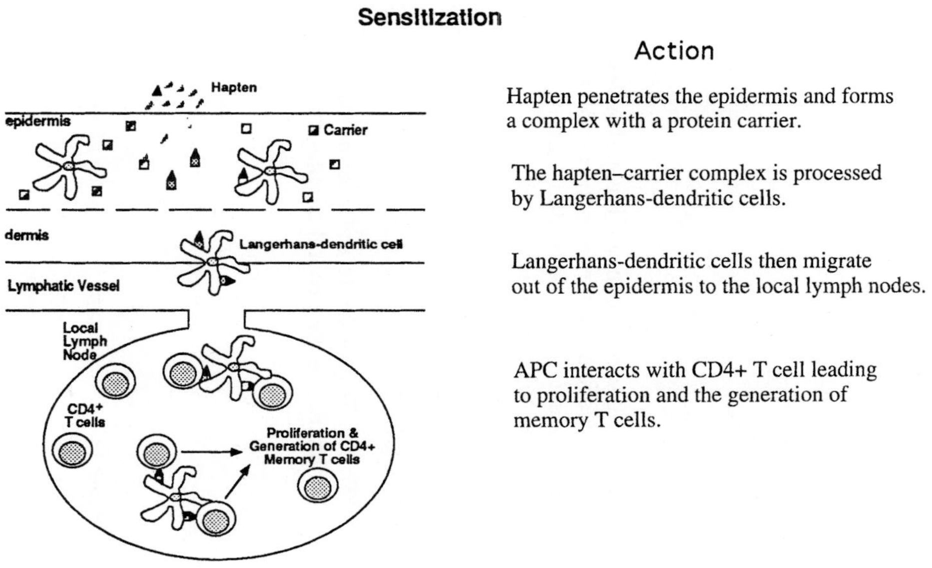

**Sensitization**

Hapten
epidermis
Carrier
dermis
Langerhans-dendritic cell
Lymphatic Vessel
Local Lymph Node
CD4+ T cells
Proliferation & Generation of CD4+ Memory T cells

Action

Hapten penetrates the epidermis and forms a complex with a protein carrier.

The hapten–carrier complex is processed by Langerhans-dendritic cells.

Langerhans-dendritic cells then migrate out of the epidermis to the local lymph nodes.

APC interacts with CD4+ T cell leading to proliferation and the generation of memory T cells.

*Figure 12–18. Schematic of sensitization phase of type IV hypersensitivity reaction.*

## Elicitation

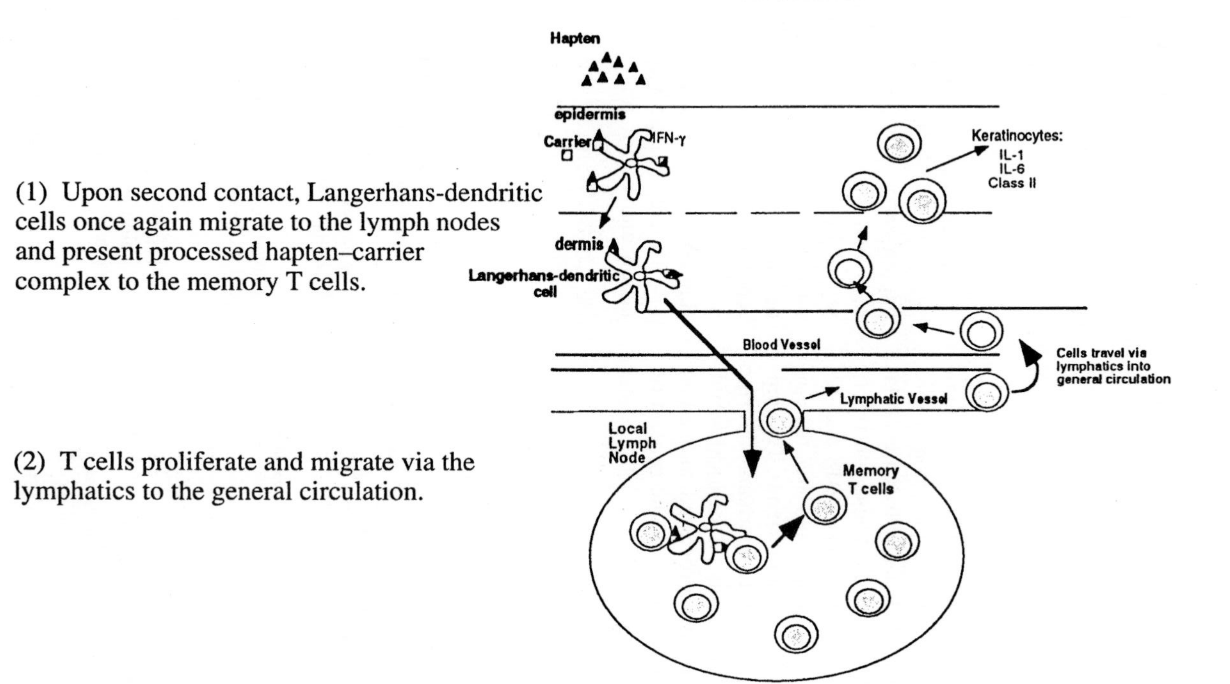


(1) Upon second contact, Langerhans-dendritic cells once again migrate to the lymph nodes and present processed hapten–carrier complex to the memory T cells.

(2) T cells proliferate and migrate via the lymphatics to the general circulation.

(3) T cells leave the general circulation and are attracted to the site of antigen exposure by the expression of adhesion molecules and chemotactic cytokines.

(4) Activated keratinocytes and T cells secrete proinflammatory cytokines attracting T cells and macrophages into the area.

*Figure 12–19. Schematic of elicitation phase of type IV hypersensitivity reaction.*

specific antigen to which the individual has been previously exposed (such as a microbial antigen). Within hours a cellular infiltrate (primarily CD4$^+$ T cells) begins to appear. This infiltration continues as MØ and Langerhans-dendritic cells begin to migrate into the area of injection. Circulation of immune cells to and from the local lymph nodes is thought to be like that in contact hypersensitivity. Also like the contact hypersensitivity response, CD4$^+$ T cells then secrete lymphokines which cause the expression of MHC Class II on the surface of MØs and keratinocytes. The result is activation of these cells, the release of proinflammatory mediators, and the generation of an area of firm, red swelling of the dermal tissue.

Separation of hypersensitivity responses into the types I–IV classification of Coombs and Gell is helpful in understanding mechanisms involved. It is important, however, to realize that this is a simplification and that often pathology is the result of a combination of these mechanisms. In addition, associated inflammation may be a nonimmune acute response and/or the result of an immune-mediated event. For example, if one looks at the pathophysiology of respiratory disease induced by the acid anhydrides, a mixture of immune and nonimmune events is found to be important. Direct toxic effects of the chemicals may lead to bronchial epithelial damage, causing cells to release cytokines that induce a nonimmune inflammatory response. Damage to epithelial cells may also expose underlying lamina propia, allowing the chemical to exert direct effects on inflammatory cells and to stimulate sensory vagal afferents, leading to reflex bronchoconstriction and hyperresponsiveness. Along with these nonimmune mechanisms, all four classes of immune-mediated hypersensitivity responses to acid anhydrides have been shown to occur (Bernstein and Bernstein, 1994).

## ASSESSMENT OF HYPERSENSITIVITY RESPONSES

One of the most important and challenging problems in the field of immunotoxicology is determining the potential for chemicals to elicit an immune reaction and, in the current context, to promote hypersensitivity reactions. Thus, it becomes essential to have validated predictive animal models and to understand the underlying mechanisms of action. The following is a review of the currently used methods of predicting types I and IV, the most frequently occurring hypersensitivity reactions to chemicals.

### Assessment of Respiratory Hypersensitivity in Experimental Animals

Methods for detecting pulmonary hypersensitivity have been reviewed by Sarlo and Karol (1994) and can be divided into two types: (1) those for detecting immunologic sensitization and (2) those for detecting pulmonary sensitization. In some cases the methodologies may overlap. Immunologic sensitization occurs, in the case of types I–III, when immunoglobulin is produced in response to exposure to an antigen or, in the case of type IV, when a population of sensitized T lymphocytes is produced. Pulmonary sensitization is determined by a change in respiratory function subsequent to the challenge of a sensitized animal or patient. In certain cases, immunological sensitization may be confirmed by detection of antigen-specific antibody; however, subsequent challenge does not produce clinical signs of respiratory distress. It is also possible to detect pulmonary sensitization in animal models where there is no detectable antigen-specific antibody production. In these cases, cell-mediated or other mechanisms may be involved or there may be a difficulty in antibody detection.

Guinea pig models are most frequently used for detection of pulmonary reactions to chemicals. In the guinea pig, as in the human, the lung is the major shock organ for anaphylactic response. Like humans, the guinea pig also demonstrates immediate- and late-onset allergic reactions, as well as bronchial hyperreactivity. The major difference in the mechanism of pulmonary responses between humans and guinea pigs is that the antibody involved in type I reactions in humans is IgE and in the guinea pig it is IgG1. Due to the lack of availability of immunologic reagents for guinea pigs, in vitro detection of antibody is difficult.

Methods utilized for respiratory exposure to chemicals are either inhalation or intratracheal administration. There are advantages and disadvantages to each. Inhalation more closely represents environmental exposure by allowing for chemical contact with the upper as well as the lower respiratory tract. However, the equipment required is expensive and difficult to maintain. In contrast, although intratracheal exposure can be performed inexpensively, only the lower respiratory tract below the bronchial bifurcation is exposed.

Generally, inhalation models consist of a period of daily exposures, usually a matter of minutes, to the test article followed by a rest period and then a daily challenge. Individual protocols may differ in the amount of antigen delivered, the amount of exposure time per day, and the number of days of exposure and the rest prior to challenge. Immunological sensitization is determined by obtaining sequential blood samples throughout the challenge period and measuring antibody titer. Guinea pig titers are generally measured by passive cutanous anaphylaxis. Pulmonary sensitization is measured by detecting the presence of pulmonary reactivity following challenge. This may be accomplished by visual inspection of the animal's respiratory pattern or more quantitatively by whole-body plethysmography. With whole-body plethysmography, the respiratory rate, tidal volume, and plethysmographic pressure can be measured. Again, expense and the time required to conduct a study are major considerations.

Intratracheal models involve the weekly administration of the test article. Animals are observed following dosing for signs of pulmonary sensitization and blood samples are collected to determine antibody titers.

Inhalation models are generally used for low-molecular-weight compounds, whereas intratracheal models are frequently used with high-molecular-weight compounds. One of the drawbacks of low-molecular-weight models is that often these compounds must conjugate with body proteins to become antigenic. Often, a challenge with the conjugated chemical is necessary to induce a pulmonary response. Adding this variable can make analyzing test results more difficult. False negative results may occur due to variability in test article conjugation. Chemical conjugates are also necessary to measure immunologic response.

## Assessment of Respiratory Hypersensitivity Responses in Humans

Listed below are methods of human type I hypersensitivity testing. These test results, in conjunction with a relevant history and physical exam, can be diagnostic of IgE-mediated pulmonary disease. Three skin tests are available for immediate hypersensitivity testing. In all three, the measured endpoint is a "wheal and flare" reaction which is the result of edema and erythema subsequent to the release of preformed mediators. The prick-and-scratch tests introduce very small amounts of antigen under the skin and are recommended as screening tests due to the reduced chance of systemic reaction. For test compounds not eliciting a reaction in the less sensitive tests, the intradermal test using dilute concentrations of antigen may be used, but there is a higher risk of anaphylaxis. For a more detailed description of testing methods, see Booth (1985) and von Krogh and Maibach (1987).

Measurement of antigen-specific IgE can be accomplished by the radioallergosorbent test (RAST). In this assay, test serum is added to a plate containing highly concentrated antigen which has been covalently bound to a cellulose disk. Serum IgE binds to the antigen and then radiolabeled anti-IgE antibody is added. Radioactivity for the test sample is compared to a standard titration curve to determine IgE antibody titer.

Bronchial provocation tests are performed by nebulizing an antigen extract into the bronchial tree and comparing its effect with that produced by nebulization of the vehicle solution. In some cases this may be the only way to demonstrate that a test article is capable of producing an asthmatic response. Care must be taken in these test situations in that it is possible to produce severe asthmatic reactions or anaphylaxis in sensitized individuals.

## Assessment of Contact Hypersensitivity in Experimental Animals

Classically, the potential for a chemical to produce contact hypersensitivity has been assessed by the use of guinea pig models. These tests vary in their method of application of the test article, in the dosing schedule, and in the utilization of adjuvants. For a description of methods employed in representative tests see Klecak (1987). The two most commonly utilized guinea pig models, the Büehler test (Büehler, 1965) and the guinea pig maximization test (Magnusson and Kligman, 1969) will be described briefly. In the Büehler test, the test article is applied to the shaven flank and covered with an occlusive bandage for 6 h. This procedure is repeated on days 7 and 14. On day 28, a challenge dose of the test article is applied to a shaven area on the opposite flank and covered with an occlusive dressing for 24 h. Twenty-four and forty-eight hours after the patch is removed, test animals are compared to vehicle-treated controls for signs of edema and erythema. The guinea pig maximization test differs in that the test article is administered by intradermal injection, an adjuvant is employed, and irritating concentrations are used. Animals are administered pairs of intradermal injections into a shaven area on the shoulders. One pair of injections contains adjuvant alone, one pair contains test article alone, and one pair contains the test article mixed with adjuvant. Seven days following injection, after reshaving the area, the test article is applied topically and an occluded patch is applied for 48 h. In cases in which the test article at the given concentration is nonirritating, the area is pretreated with 10 percent sodium lauryl sulfate 24 h before the patch is applied to produce a mild inflammatory response. Two weeks following topical application, the animals are challenged on the shaven flank with a nonirritating concentration of the test article, which remains under an occluded patch for 24 h. The test site is examined for signs of erythema and edema 24 and 48 h later. Although guinea pig models are very sensitive and reproducible, they pose some difficulties. Evaluation is subjective and it is difficult to assess irritating or colored compounds using these models.

Over the past 10 years, efforts have been made to develop and validate more quantitative and immunologically based assay methods in other species, focusing mainly on the mouse and in vitro systems. Gad and coworkers (1986) developed the mouse ear swelling test which uses a quantitative measurement of ear thickness as an endpoint. Animals are sensitized by topical application of the test article to abdominal skin which has been prepared by intradermal injection of adjuvant and tape stripping for 4 consecutive days. On day 10, the animals are challenged by topical application of the test article to one ear and of the vehicle to the contralateral ear. Measurements are made of ear thickness 24 and 48 h later. A positive response is considered anything above a 20 percent increase in thickness of the treated ear over the controlled ear. Thorne and colleagues (1991) showed that dietary supplementation with vitamin A enhanced the mouse ear swelling assay in the absence of adjuvants, injections, or occlusive patches. Kimber and colleagues have developed (Kimber et al., 1989) and validated (Kimber et al., 1991) a mouse local lymph node assay in which the sensitization phase of contact sensitization is measured by the incorporation of $^3$H-thymidine into proliferating lymphocytes in lymph nodes draining the site of test article application. Animals are dosed by topical application of the test article to the ears for 3 or 4 consecutive days. The animals are rested for 1 day and then injected intravenously with 20 $\mu$Ci of $^3$H-thymidine. Five hours later animals are sacrificed, the draining lymph nodes are dissected out, and single cell suspensions are made and radioassayed. A threefold increase in $^3$H-thymidine counts over controls is considered to be a positive response.

More recently, attempts have been made to correlate cytokine levels with contact and respiratory sensitizing potential. The differential stimulation of immune function by contact and respiratory allergens has been shown (Dearman and Kimber, 1991). Some compounds capable of producing contact sensitization also induce IgE production and subsequent respiratory hypersensitivity. As an example, using three known allergenic diisocyanates, diphenylmethane-4,4′-diisocyanate (MDI), dicyclohexylmethane-4,4′-diisocyanate (HMDI), and isophorone diisocyanate (IPDI), Dearman and coworkers (1992) showed that all three known contact sensitizers induced lymphocyte proliferation in the draining lymph node but that only MDI, a known respiratory sensitizer, induced elevated levels of serum IgE and IgG2b. As was seen in Fig. 12-14, antigens, once processed, are presented on the surface of the

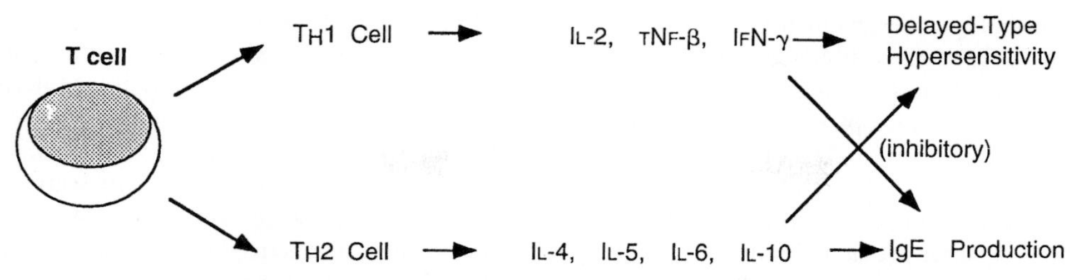


*Figure 12–20. Schematic of cytokines involved in hypersensitivity reactions.*

APC in conjuction with the MHC II antigen. Activation of either $T_H1$ or $T_H2$ cells stimulates the production of cytokines, which are instrumental in driving the system toward immunoglobulin production or the activation and proliferation of sensitized T cells (delayed-type hypersensitiviy). The specific cytokines involved are shown in Fig. 12-20. IL-2, TNF-$\beta$, and IFN-$\gamma$ are produced by $T_H1$ cells and lead to the development of delayed-type hypersensitivity, whereas, IL-4, IL-5, IL-6, and IL-10 are produced by $T_H2$ cells and lead to the production of IgE (Mosmann and Coffman, 1989; Mosmann et al., 1991). Not only does IFN-$\gamma$ promote the induction of delayed hypersensitivity, it appears to have an inhibitory effect on IgE production (Mosmann and Coffman, 1989). Likewise, IL-10, which promotes IgE production, inhibits the delayed-type hypersensitivity response (Enk et al., 1993; Schwarz et al., 1994). Measurement of cytokine levels may prove to be an important predictive tool for assessing the potential of chemicals to elicit hypersensitivity reactions.

## Assessment of Contact Hypersensitivity in Humans

Human testing for contact hypersensitivity reactions is by skin patch testing. Patch testing allows for the diagnostic production of acute lesions of contact hypersensitivity by the application of a suspected allergen to the skin. Patches containing specified concentrations of the allergen in the appropriate vehicle are applied under an occulsive patch for 48 h in most test protocols. Once the patch is removed and enough time elapses for the signs of mechanical irritation to resolve, approximately 30 min, the area is read for signs of erythema, papules, vesicles, and edema. Generally, the test is read again at 72 h and in some cases signs may not appear for up to 1 week or more. For more detailed information on patch testing, the reader is referred to Hjorth (1987).

Human repeat insult patch tests (HRIPT) are available as predictive tests in humans. Like predictive testing in animal models, many variations exist in the attempt to increase the sensitivity of these procedures. These include preparation of the induction site by either stripping, the application of an irritating concentration of sodium laury sulfate, or using high concentrations of the test article for induction of sensitization. In general, the application of multiple occlusive patches, up to 10 for 48 h each at the same site, is followed by a rest period and then challenge under an occlusive patch at a different site. Positive reactions are scored in the same manner as diagnostic patch tests.

# HYPERSENSITIVITY REACTIONS TO XENOBIOTICS

## Polyisocyanates

Polyisocyanates have a widespread use in industry and are responsible for more cases of occupationally related lung disease than any other class of low-molecular-weight (LMW) compounds. These chemicals are used in the production of adhesives, paint hardeners, elastomers, and coatings. Occupational exposure is by inhalation and skin contact. Members of the group are known to induce the full spectrum of hypersensitivity responses, types I–IV, as well as nonimmune inflammatory and neuroreflex reactions in the lung (Bernstein and Bernstein, 1994; Grammer, 1985). Sensitized individuals have shown cross reactivity between compounds in this group.

Toluene diisocyanate (TDI) is one of the most widely used and most studied members of this group. Pulmonary sensitization to this compound can occur through either topical or inhalation exposure. It is a highly reactive compound which readily conjugates with endogenous protein. A 70,000 kDa protein, laminin, has been identified as the protein that TDI conjugates in the airways. Studies with guinea pigs have confirmed the need for a threshold level of exposure to be reached in order to obtain pulmonary sensitization. This finding supports the human data in which, frequently, pulmonary sensitization is the result of exposure to a spill, whereas workers exposed to low levels of vapors for long periods of time fail to develop pulmonary sensitization. Unlike many hypersensitivity reactions, in which removal of the antigen alleviates the symptoms of disease, in many TDI-induced asthma patients symptoms may persist for up to years after cessation of exposure.

## Acid Anhydrides

The acid anhydrides comprise another group of compounds for which nonimmune and IgE, cytotoxic, immune complex, and cell-mediated reactions have been reported (Bernstein and Bernstein, 1994; Grammer, 1985). These reactive organic compounds are used in the manufacturing of paints, varnishes, coating materials, adhesives, and casting and sealing materials. Trimellitic acid anhydride (TMA) is one of the most widely used compounds in this group. Inhaled TMA fumes may conjugate with serum albumin or erythrocytes leading to subsequent exposure to a type I (TMA-asthma), type II (pulmonary disease–anemia), or type III (hypersensitivity pneumonitis) hypersensitivity reaction. Topical exposure to TMA may lead to type IV hypersensitivity reactions resulting in contact dermatitis. Also, reexposure by inhalation may lead to a cell-mediated immune response in the lung, which plays a role in the pathology seen in conjunction with types II and III pulmonary disease. Human and animal testing have supported the clinical findings in TMA-exposed workers. Levels of serum IgE can be measured in exposed workers and are predictive of the occurrence of type I pulmonary reactions. Serum titers of IgA, IgG, and IgM have been detected in patients with high levels of exposure to TMA. Similar findings have been reported in studies with Rhesus monkeys, in which exposed animals showed IgA, IgG, and IgM titers to TMA-haptenized erythrocytes. Inhalation studies with rats have produced a model corresponding to human TMA-induced pulmonary pneumonitis. Other anhydrides known to induce immune-mediated pulmonary disease include phthalic anhydride, himic anhydride, and hexahydrophthalic anhydride.

## Metals

Metals and metallic substances, including metallic salts, are responsible for producing contact and pulmonary hypersensitivity reactions. Metallic salts have been implicated in numerous immunologic and nonimmunologic pulmonary diseases. Exposure to these compounds may occur via inhalation or due to their solubility in aqueous media (they can be dissociated and transported into the lungs where damage due to sensitization or nonimmunologic events takes place). Platinum, nickel, chromium, and cobalt are the most commonly implicated salts. For details the reader is referred to the reviews by Bernstein and Bernstein (1994), Menné (1987), and Marzulli and Maibach (1987).

**Platinum.** Chloroplatinate salts are highly allergenic in comparison to other metalic salts. Exposure may occur in the mining and metallurgic industries, in chemical industries where platinum is used as a catalyst, and in the production of catalytic converters. Exposed workers are at risk of developing allergic rhinitis and asthma secondary to IgE production. Sensitized workers show positive skin tests and antigen-specific IgE by RAST testing.

**Cobalt.** Five percent of workers exposed to cobalt develop occupational asthma. These patients exhibit antigen-specific IgE and their lymphocytes proliferate in response to free cobalt or cobalt conjugated to human serum albumin.

**Nickel.** Although nickel is a common contact sensitizer, pulmonary hypersensitivity reactions to nickel salts are rare. Occupational exposure to nickel is most common in the mining, milling, smelting, and refinishing industries. Pulmonary reactions, when they occur, are most frequently due to a direct toxic effect on the CNS and lung tissues. The contact sensitizing potential of nickel has been reviewed by Marzulli and Maibach (1987) and Menné (1987). In addition to industrial contact, exposure occurs in the form of jewelry, coins, and fasteners on clothing, making nickel one of the most frequently contacted sensitizers for the general population. Studies have shown nickel sulfate to be the most frequent sensitizer when standard tray sensitizers are used, with positive results being between 6.7 and 11 percent. Nickel appears to require a long sensitization period, and studies have shown that patients may lose their hypersensitivity to nickel after long periods of avoidance.

**Chromium.** Chromium is another metal often associated with dermatoses and less frequently with respiratory disease. Occupational exposure to chromium is most frequent in industries involved in electroplating processes, leather tanning, and paint, cement, and paper pulp production. Chromium eczema (type IV hypersensitivity) is one of the most common occupationally associated skin diseases. Predictive tests on normal human subjects have shown sensitization rates to chromium sulfate as high as 48 percent. Occupational asthma from chromium exposure is less well documented and skin-prick tests have been negative. Evidence of IgE-mediated disease has been supported by immediate bronchial hyperreactivity after challenge and the identification of antigen-specific IgE antibodies. Cell-mediated (type IV) reactions have been postulated to play a role, since late asthmatic reactions following bronchial challenge have been seen.

**Beryllium.** Beryllium is a metal capable of producing both contact and tuberculin type IV hypersensitivity reactions. The role of CMI in beryllium-induced disease has been reviewed by Newman (1994). Beryllium exposure occurs most frequently in the aerospace, high-technology ceramics manufacturing, dental alloy manufacturing, electronics, nuclear weapons, and nuclear reactors industries. A major source of exposure was in the production of fluorescence light bulbs until the discontinuance of its use for this purpose. Skin contact has been found to produce lesions of contact hypersensitivity, whereas lesions produced by penetration of splinters of beryllium under the skin are granulomatous in nature. Inhalation of beryllium can result in disease ranging from acute pneumonitis, tracheobronchitis, and chronic beryllium disease, to an increase in the risk of lung cancer. Environmentally induced berylliosis was evidenced by the incidence of disease in nonfactory workers in communities around beryllium extraction plants. Exposure resulted from emissions from plants and contact with beryllium-contaminated family members' clothing.

In cases of chronic beryllium disease, there is often a latent period of up to 10 years following first exposure. Lung pathology consists of multiple granulomas with mononuclear cell infiltrates, primarily macrophages, lymphocytes, and plasma cells, and fibrosis. Although lesions are usually localized in the lungs and associated lymph nodes, granulomatous involvement of other organs has been seen. As pulmonary disease progresses, effects on pulmonary circulation may lead to right-side heart failure. Death due to berylliosis may then be due to respiratory or cardiac failure.

Unlike most hypersensitivity reactions in which removal from exposure to the offending agent usually abates the disease, removal from beryllium exposure does little to alter the course of the disease. Although the majority of beryllium is eliminated from the lung soon after inhalation, small amounts of retained beryllium are sufficient to induce and sustain the ongoing cellular immune response. Years after the last exposure, mass absorption data have shown beryllium to be present in lung granulomas.

Due to the similarities in clinical symptoms and pathology between berylliosis and other granulomatous lung diseases, immunological testing is important in definitive diagnosis. Patients with beryllium disease tested positive to patch testing with beryllium salt and often showed granulomatous lesions at the patch test site within 3 weeks. However, these test procedures proved to be unsafe. Patch tests were found to induce sensitization in some patients and often caused exacerbation of lung disease. More recently the beryllium-specific lymphocyte proliferation test (BeLT) has been utilized to detect beryllium sensitization. This test has proven to be a more sensitive indicator of early disease than patient history, physical exam, chest radiographs, or lung function test. Although this disease is not curable, the progression of the disease process can be slowed by corticosteriod therapy. BeLT allows for earlier detection of sensitization. This results in improved patient monitoring and permits earlier institution of treatment. In industry, BeLT provides a means of detecting jobs with a high risk of exposure.

## Drugs

Hypersensitivity responses to drugs represent one of the major types of unpredictable drug reactions, accounting for up to 10 percent of all adverse effects. Drugs are designed to be reactive in the body and multiple treatments are common. This type of exposure is conducive to producing an immunologic reaction. Immunologic mechanisms of hypersensitivity reactions to drugs include types I–IV. For a detailed review of drug allergy see DeSwarte (1985). Penicillin is the most common agent involved in drug allergy and will be discussed here as an example. Exposure to penicillin is responsible for 75 percent of the deaths due to anaphylaxis in the United States. The route of administration, dosage, and length of treatment all appear to play a role in the type and severity of hypersensitivity reaction elicited. Severe reactions are less likely following oral administration as compared to parenteral, and prolonged treatment with high doses increases the risk of acute interstitial nephritis and immune hemolytic anemia. The high incidence of allergic reaction to penicillin is in part due to widespread exposure to the compound. Not only has there been indiscriminant use of the drug, but exposure occurs through food products including milk from treated animals and the use of penicillin as an antimicrobial in the production of vaccines. Efforts have been made to reduce unnecessary exposure.

Reactions to penicillin are varied and may include any of the four types of hypersensitivity reactions. The most commonly seen clinical manifestation of type I reactions is urticaria; however, anaphylactic reactions occur in about 10 to 40 of every 100,000 patients receiving injections. Clinical signs of rhinitis and asthma are much less frequently observed. Blood dyscrasias can occur due to the production of IgG against penicillin metabolites bound to the surface of red blood cells (type II reaction). Penicillin has also been implicated in type III reactions leading to serum-sickness-like symptoms. Due to the high frequency of type IV reactions when penicillin is applied topically, especially to inflamed or abraded skin, products are no longer available for topical application. Type IV reactions generally result in an eczematous skin reaction, but, infrequently, a life-threatening form of dermal necrosis may result. In these cases there is severe erythema and a separation of the epidermis at the basal layer. This reaction, which gives the clinical appearance of severe scalding, is thought to be a severe delayed reaction.

## Pesticides

Pesticides have been implicated as causal agents in both contact and immediate hypersensitivity reactions. Definitive diagnosis is often difficult or lacking in reported cases and animal and human predictive data often do not correlate well. Pesticide hypersensitivity responses have been reviewed by Thomas and coworkers (1990) and will be described briefly below.

One of the difficulties in obtaining good epidemiological data to document reactions to pesticides is the nature of exposure. Agricultural workers are among those most commonly exposed and the fact that workers are exposed to multiple chemicals as well as harsh environmental factors makes diagnosis difficult. Furthermore, diagnositic follow-up among this group is infrequent.

In the case of barban, a carbamate insecticide, the reported incidence of contact sensitivity due to exposure is rare; however, predictive testing with the guinea pig maximization test (GPMT) and the diagnostic human patch test indicates this pesticide to be a potent sensitizer. Likewise, malathion, captan, benomyl, maneb, and naled have been identified as strong-to-extreme sensitizers using the GPMT. Human predictive data, diagnostic patch testing, and the reported incidence in the literature of toxicity with the use of these compounds often are not in agreement with the animal data.

Pesticides have been implicated in cases of immediate hypersensitivity, including rhinitis, conjunctivitis, asthma, and anaphylaxis. However, there has been no definitive proof of the association. It is possible that observed reactions are of an irritant nature rather than an immunologic response. It has been shown that the asthmatic response to organophosphate insecticides is not due to the acetylcholinesterase activity, since the administration of atropine, a cholinergic antagonist, failed to block the response. Animal studies show some evidence to support the role of immediate hypersensitivity responses to pesticides. Mice injected intraperitoneally with malathion or 2,4-dichlorophenoxyacetic acid conjugates developed IgE antibody. However, antibody was not detected to these chemicals when they were applied topically. More epidemiological and mechanistic studies are needed in the area of pesticide hypersensitivity to further define these relationships.

## Others

**Cosmetics and Personal Hygiene Products.** Contact dermatitis and dermatoconjuctivitis may result from exposure to many cosmetic and personal hygiene products, including makeup, deodorants, hair sprays, hair dyes and permanent solutions, nail polish, soaps, face cream, and shampoos (Liberman et al.,1985). These agents contain coloring agents, lanolin, paraffin, petrolatum, vehicles, perfumes, and antimicrobials such as paraben esters, sorbic acid, phenolics, organic mercurials, quaternary ammonium compounds, EDTA, and formaldehyde. Applicators used to apply these products may also induce an allergic reaction. Diagnosis may be accomplished by patch testing; however, it is often necessary to use products used by the patient in patch testing in addition to those on a standard test tray. In cases of dermatoconjunctivitis, false-negative testing may occur. The skin of the eyelids may be more sensitive to agents than that of the forearm or back, making patch testing unreliable. Elimination-provocation procedures may be helpful in the diagnosis of difficult cases. All suspect offending agents must be removed from the patient's environment, and once clinical signs have resolved, agents may be reintroduced one at a time while observing for the recurrence of signs.

**Enzymes.** Enzymes are another group capable of eliciting type I hypersensitivity responses (Gutman, 1985). Subtilin, a proteolytic enzyme derived from Bacillus subtilis, is used in laundry detergents to enhance cleaning ability. Both individuals working in the environment where the product is made and individuals using the product may become sensitized. Subsequent exposure may produce signs of rhinitis, conjunctivitis, and asthma. An alveolar hypersensitivity reaction associated with precipitation antibodies and an Arthus-type reaction from skin testing has also been seen. Papain is another enzyme known to induce IgE-mediated disease. It is a high-molecular-weight sulfhydryl protease obtained from the fruit of the papaya tree. It is most commonly used as a meat tenderizer and as a clearing agent in the production of beer, but is also used in the production of tooth powders, laxatives and contact lens cleansers.

**Formaldehyde.** Formaldehyde was discussed above as one of the components of cosmetics capable of causing a contact hypersensitivity reaction. Formaldehyde exposure also occurs in the textile industry where it is used to improve wrinkle resistance, and in the furniture, auto upholstery, and resins industries. The general public may be exposed to low levels of formaldehyde in products as ubiquitous as newspaper dyes and photographic films and paper. This low-molecular-weight compound is extremely soluble in water and it haptenates human proteins easily (Maibach, 1983). Human predictive testing with 1 to 10 percent formalin (formalin is 37 percent formaldehyde) for induction and 1 percent formalin for challenge showed sensitization rates of 4.5 to 7.8 percent (Marzulli and Maibach, 1974). Occupational exposure to formaldehyde has been associated with the occurrence of asthma, although it has been difficult to demonstrate antibodies to formaldehyde in these individuals (Hendrick et al., 1982).

For further information and a listing of chemicals known to cause hypersensitivity reactions affecting the respiratory system and skin, see Chaps. 15 and 18.

## AUTOIMMUNE REACTIONS

In the section on "Hypersensitivity Reactions" presented above, we discussed two mechanisms, types II and III, by which host tissues are damaged by their own immune system, creating autoimmune-like disease. In these situtations unaltered self antigens are not the target of the immune mechanisms but damage occurs to cells bearing hapten on membranes or to innocent bystander cells in close proximity to antigen–antibody complexes. For example, damage produced in autoimmune Goodpasture's disease is similar to that seen in type III hypersensitivity reactions in the lung due to TMA. Although the resulting pathology may be the same for autoimmune reactions and hypersensitivity, mechanisms of true autoimmune disease are distinquished from hypersensitivity. In cases of autoimmunity, self antigens are the target, and in the case of chemical-induced autoimmunity, it is a modification of host tissues or immune cells by the chemical and not the chemical acting as an antigen/hapten that induces the disease state.

## MECHANISMS OF AUTOIMMUNITY

The immunopathogenesis of autoimmune disease has been reviewed by Rose (1994) and will be described briefly below as background information for understanding how chemicals may induce autoimmunity. Three types of molecules are involved in the process of self-recognition, immunoglobulins (Igs), T-cell receptors (TCRs) and the products of major histocompatibility complex (MHC). Igs and TCRs are expressed clonally on B and T cells, respectively, whereas MHC molecules are present on all nucleated cells. The ability of lymphocytes to distinquish one molecule from another stems from the antigen binding a specific lymphocyte receptor. In B cell lines, through rearrangement of heavy and light Ig chains, tremendous diversity, $10^6$ to $10^7$ specificities, occurs among Ig recognition structures. Likewise, a similar number of specific TCRs are produced as the result of gene rearrangement in T cells induced by peptide hormones produced by thymic epithelial cells. Two major types of B and T cells are produced. B cells expressing CD5 predominate in embryonic life and are later found mostly in the intestinal mucosa. These cells produce high levels of IgM and much of it is autoantibody. Although most B cells do not express CD5 prior to class switching, they do express high levels of IgM. Influenced by cytokines produced by interacting T cells following antigen stimulation, these cells produce primarily IgG, IgA, or IgE. Similarly, T cells develop from one of two lineages, those with $\alpha\beta$TCRs and those with $\gamma\delta$TCRs. Although most mature T cells express $\alpha\beta$TCRs, $\gamma\delta$TCRs are predominant on mucosal surfaces. As described earlier in the chapter, $\alpha\beta$TCRs continue differentiation into $CD4^+$ or $CD8^+$ T cells. $CD4^+$ cells have primarily helper and inducer functions and recognize antigens in the context of MHC class II molecules. $CD8^+$ T lymphocytes are mainly cytotoxic cells and recognize antigenic determinants in conjunction with MHC class I molecules.

The process of negative selection against autoreactive T cells in the thymus is important in the prevention of autoimmune disease. T cells expressing $\alpha\beta$TCRs that fit self MHC molecules with high affinity undergo apoptosis (programmed cell death) at an accelerated rate, whereas those with a low affinity for self antigen and a high affinity for foreign antigen undergo positive selection and proliferate in the thymus, eventually migrating to the peripheral lymphatics. Although negative selection greatly reduces the numbers of self-reactive T cells, some of these cells do leave the thymus and remain in circulation in a state of anergy. These cells are able to bind their designated antigen but do not undergo proliferation due to a lack of necessary second signal. This second signal is generally provided by an antigen-presenting cell in the form of a cytokine, IL-2, or a cell-surface receptor which interacts with the T cell.

Reactive $CD4^+$ T cells only recognize processed antigen presented by antigen-presenting cells, generally macrophages,

B cells, or dendritic cells, in conjunction with MHC class II molecules. These antigen-presenting cells take up exogenous antigens, cleave them with proteolytic enzymes, and express them on their cell surface. In contrast, intracellular antigens are processed and presented on cell surfaces in conjunction with MHC class I molecules. These antigens may be the products of malignant or normal cells or may result from infection with bacterial, viral, or other intracellular pathogens. The processed antigen–MHC class I complex is recognized by a specific TCR on a $CD8^+$ lymphocyte.

Several mechanisms are available that may break down self-tolerance leading to autoimmunity: (1) Exposure to antigens not available in the thymus during embryonic development. Therefore, the antigen-specific T-cell reactive lymphocytes not subjected to negative selection could induce an autoimmune reaction. Examples include myelin and organ-specific antigens such as thyroglobulin. Breakdown of self-tolerance to these antigens may be induced by exposure to adjuvants or by exposure to another antigenically related protein. (2) Overcoming T-cell anergy by chronic lymphocyte stimulation. (3) Finally, interference with normal immunoregulation by $CD8^+$ T-cell suppressor cells may create an environment conducive to the development of autoimmune disease.

Effector mechanisms involved in autoimmune disease can be the same as those described earlier for types II and III hypersensitivity or, in the case of pathology associated with solid tissues including organs, may involve $CD8^+$ cytotoxic T cells. Tissue damage associated with $CD8^+$ cells may be the result of direct cell-membrane damage and lysis induced by binding or the results of cytokines produced and released by the T cell. TNF-$\beta$ has the ability to kill susceptible cells and IFN-$\gamma$ may increase the expression of MHC class I on cell surfaces, making them more susceptible to $CD8^+$ cells. Cytokines also may be chemotactic for macrophages which can cause tissue damage directly or indirectly through the release of proinflammatory cytokines. As is the case with hypersensitivity reactions, autoimmune disease is often the result of more than one mechanism working simultaneously. Therefore, pathology may be the result of antibody-dependent cytotoxicity, complement-dependent antibody-mediated lysis, or direct or indirect effects of cytotoxic T cells.

Genetic and environmental factors appear to affect the susceptibility of individuals to autoimmune disease. Familial predisposition to autoimmune disease has been found, as well as a similarity in MHC genetic traits among individuals involved. Certain chemicals and drugs are known to induce autoimmune disease in genetically predisposed individuals and examples of these will be discussed below. The role of environmental pollutants is uncertain and more study is needed in this area. One point of interest is that in all known cases of drug-induced autoimmunity, the disease has abated once the offending chemical was removed.

## ASSESSMENT OF AUTOIMMUNE RESPONSES

There are few models available for accessing the potential of a chemical to induce autoimmune disease and those have major limitations. The most commonly used models include graft-vs.-host disease (GVHD), the popliteal lymph node (PLN) model in mice, and human lymphocyte transformation assays. Although these models may have some predictive value, at this point, immunohistopathology is the only definitive diagnostic tool.

There are numerous reports of chemicals that have been associated with autoimmunity. These relationships may be causative through direct mechanisms or they may be indirect, acting as an adjuvant. They may also serve to exacerbate a preexisting autoimmune state (reviewed by Kilburn and Warshaw, 1994; Coleman and Sim, 1994). In the area of autoimmunity, exact mechanisms of action are not always known. Table 12-9 lists chemicals known to be associated with autoimmunity, showing the proposed self antigenic determinant or stating adjuvancy as the mechanism of action. A brief discussion of selected drug and nondrug chemicals is provided.

**Table 12–9**
**Chemical Agents Known to Be Associated with Autoimmunity**

| CHEMICAL | CLINICAL MANIFESTATIONS | PROPOSED ANTIGENIC DETERMINANT | REFERENCE |
|---|---|---|---|
| Drugs | | | |
| Methyl dopa | Hemolytic anemia | Rhesus antigens | Murphy and Kelton (1991) |
| Hydralazine | SLE-like syndrome | Myeloperoxidase | Cambridge et al. (1994) |
| Isoniazid | SLE-like syndrome | Myeloperoxidase | Jiang et al. (1994) |
| Procainamide | SLE-like syndrome | DNA | Totoritis et al. (1988) |
| Halothane | Autoimmune hepatitis | Liver microsomal proteins | Kenna et al. (1987) |
| Non-drug chemicals | | | |
| Vinyl Chloride | Scleroderma-like syndrome | Abnormal protein synthesized in liver | Ward et al. (1976) |
| Mercury | Glomerular neuropathy | Glomerular basement membrane protein | Pelletier et al. (1994) |
| Silica | Scleroderma | Most likely acts as an adjuvant | Pernis and Paronetto (1962) |

## AUTOIMMUNE REACTIONS TO XENOBIOTICS

### Methyldopa

Methyldopa is a centrally acting sympatholytic drug that has been widely used for the treatment of essential hypertension. With the advent of newer antihypertensive drugs the use of methyldopa has declined. Platelets and erythrocytes are targeted by the immune system in individuals treated with this drug. In the case of thrombocytopenia, antibodies are detected against platelets, which is indicative of immune recognition of a self or altered self antigen. Hemolytic anemia occurs in at least 1 percent of individuals treated with Methyldopa and up to 30 percent of these individuals develop antibodies to erythrocytes as manifested in a positive Coombs test. The antibodies are not directed against the chemical or a chemical membrane conjugate.

### Hydralazine, Isoniazid, and Procainamide

Hydralazine, isoniazid, and procainamide produce autoimmunity, which is manifested as a sytemic lupus erythematosus (SLE)-like syndrome. Antibodies to DNA have been detected in individuals showing this syndrome. Hydralazine is a direct-acting vasodilator drug used in the treatment of hypertension. Isoniazid is an antimicrobial drug used in the treatment of tuberculosis. Procainamide is a drug that selectively blocks NA+ channels in myocardial membranes, making it useful in the treatment of cardiac arrhythmias. Studies with hydralazine and isoniazid indicate that the antigenic determinant is myeloperoxidase. Immunoglobulins are produced against myeloperoxidase in individuals treated with these drugs. DNA is the apparent antigenic determinant for procainamide. For these three drugs, there is no evidence indicating that the immune system is recognizing the chemical or a chemical conjugate. In addition, these drugs have also been shown to produce hypersensitivity responses not associated with the SLE syndrome.

### Halothane

Halothane, one of the most widely studied of the drugs inducing autoimmunity, is an inhalation anesthetic that can induce autoimmune hepatitis. The incidence of this iatrogenic disease in humans is about 1 in 20,000. The pathogenesis of the hepatitis results from the chemical altering self (a specific liver protein) to such a degree that the immune system recognizes the altered self and antibodies are produced. Studies using rat microsomes show that Halothane has to be oxidized by cytochrome P-450 enzymes to trifluoroacetylhalide before it binds to the protein. Investigations indicate that in affected individuals antibodies to specific microsomal proteins are produced.

### Vinyl Chloride

Vinyl chloride, which is used in the plastics industry as a refrigerant and in synthesis of organic chemicals, is a known carcinogen and is also associated with a schlerodermalike syndrome. The disease affects multisystemic collagenous tissues, manifesting itself as pulmonary fibrosis, skin sclerosis, and/or fibrosis of the liver and spleen. Ward and coworkers (1976) reported on 320 exposed workers, showing that 58 (18 percent) had a schlerodermalike syndrome. The individuals that showed the disease were in a group genetically similar (i.e. HLA-DR5) to classic idiopathic schleroderma patients. Although the exact mechanism whereby this chemical produces autoimmunity is unclear, it is presumed that vinyl chloride acts as an amino acid and is incorporated into protein. Since this would produce a structurally abnormal protein which would be antigenic, an immune response would be directed against tissues with the modified protein present.

### Mercury

This widely used metal is now known to have several target systems, including CNS and renal system. Mercury also has two different actions with respect to the immune system. The first action is direct injury, which was described previously. Mercury also produces an autoimmune disease demonstrated as glomerular nephropathy. Antibodies produced to laminin are believed to be responsible for damage to the basement membrane of the kidney. Mice and rats exposed to mercury also show antinuclear antibodies. The role of these antibodies in the autoimmune disease is not clear. However, they represent a known biomarker of autoimmunity. Studies in the Brown Norway rat point to a mercury-induced autoreactive $CD4^+$ cell as being responsible for the polyclonal antibody response. Mercury chloride induces an increase in the expression of MHC class II molecules on B lymphocytes as well as shifting the T helper cell population along the $T_H2$ line. It is the $T_H2$ cell that promotes antibody production. The imbalance between $T_H1$ and $T_H2$ cells is believed to be caused by the depletion of cysteine and the reduced form of gluthathione in $T_H1$ cells. These chemical groups are known to be important in synthesis and responsiveness to IL-2 in T cells. Thus, $T_H1$ cells that synthesize and respond to IL-2 would be at a greater risk than $T_H2$ cells.

Mercury-induced autoimmunity has a strong genetic component. This has been extensively studied in the rat. Some strains of rats are completely resistant, such as the Lewis rat while others, such as the Brown Norway, are exquisitely sensitive. Susceptibility appears to be linked to three or four genes, one of which is the major histocompatibility complex. An excellent review of mercury and autoimmunity is provided by Pelletier and coworkers. (1994).

### Silica

Crystalline silica (silicon dioxide) is a primary source of elemental silicon and is used commercially in large quantities as a constituent of building materials, ceramics, concretes, and glasses. Experimental animals as well as humans exposed to silica may have perturbations in the immune system. Depending on the length of exposure, dose, and route of administration of silica, it may kill macrophages or may act as an immunostimulant. Silica has been shown to be associated with an increase in scleroderma in silica-exposed workers (reviewed by Kilburn and Warshaw, 1994). This effect is believed to be mediated via an adjuvant mechanism. Adjuvancy as a mechanism of causing autoimmunity has been implicated with a number of other chemicals including paraffin and silicones. Inherent in adjuvancy as a mechanism of producing autoim-

**Table 12–10**
**Chemicals Implicated in Autoimmunity**

| MANIFESTATION | IMPLICATED CHEMICAL | REFERENCE |
|---|---|---|
| Scleroderma | Solvents (toluene, xylene) | Walder (1983) |
| | Tryptophan | Silver et al. (1990) |
| | Silicones | Fock et al. (1984) |
| Systemic lupus erythromatosus | Phenothiazines | Canoso et al. 1990 |
| | Penicillamine | Harpey et al. (1971) |
| | Propylthiouracil | DeSwarte (1985) |
| | Quinidine | Jiang et al. 1994 |
| | L-Dopa | DeSwarte (1985) |
| | Lithium carbonate | Ananth et al. (1989) |
| | Trichloroethylene | Kilburn and Washaw (1992) |
| | Silicones | Fock et al. (1984) |

munity is that the population affected by these chemicals must already be at risk for the autoimmune disease. This is supported by the data indicating a genetic component to many autoimmune diseases.

Table 12-10 shows chemicals that have been implicated in autoimmune reactions, but in these cases the mechanism of autoimmunity has not been as clearly defined or confirmed. The list includes both drug and nondrug chemicals. The heterogeneity of these structures and biological activities illustrate the breadth of potential for the induction of chemically mediated autoimmune disease.

### Multiple Chemical Sensitivity Syndrome

Multiple chemical sensitivity syndrome (MCS) has been associated with hypersensitivity responses to chemicals. The disease associated with MCS is characterized by multiple subjective symptoms related to more than one system. The more common symptoms are nasal congestion, headaches, lack of concentration, fatigue, and memory loss. Many mechanisms have been put forth to explain how chemicals cause these symptoms; however, there remains considerable controversy as to a cause–effect relationship. Clinical ecologists, the major proponents of MCS, have focused on immunologic mechanisms to explain the etiology. They hypothesize that MCS occurs when chemical exposure sensitizes certain individuals, and, upon subsequent exposure to exceedingly small amounts of these or unrelated chemicals, the individual exhibits an adverse response. Controlled studies on the immunologic status of individuals with MCS have shown no alterations in their immune system or any indication that MCS results from impairment of the immunity including inappropriate immune response to chemicals. The search for a theoretical basis for MCS is now being focused on the nervous system. Two untested hypotheses have emerged. The first involves a nonspecific inflammatory response to low-level irritants known as "neurogenic inflammation." The second involves induction of lasting changes in limbic and neuronal activity (via kindling) that alter a broad spectrum of behavioral and physiological functions. The reader is referred to a review by Sikorski and colleagues (1995) for details and references concerning MCS.

## CONCLUDING COMMENT AND FUTURE DIRECTIONS

Our understanding of the immune system as a target for toxicity, whether it be via xenobiotic-induced immune injury or immune-mediated disease, continues to progress in concert with our knowledge of the biochemistry and physiology of the immune system. The balance between immune recognition and destruction of foreign invaders and the proliferation of these microbes and/or cancer cells can be a precarious one. Xenobiotics that alter the immune system can upset this balance giving the edge to the invader. Furthermore, new xenobiotics continuously being introduced represent the potential for increased hypersensitivity and/or autoimmune responses. Validated methods are in place to detect xenobiotics that produce adverse effects related to the immune system. Once identified, fundamental principles of toxicology can be applied leading to risk assessment and determination of no effect levels. These methods must continually be improved using the latest knowledge and technologies in order to provide a safe environment.

# REFERENCES

Ananth J, Johnson R, Kataria P, et al: Immune dysfunctions in psychiatric patients. *Psychiatr J* 14(4):542–546, 1989.

Aranyi C, O'Shea W, Graham J, Miller F: The effects of inhalation of organic chemical air contaminants on murine lung host defenses. *Fundam Appl Toxicol* 6:713–720, 1986.

Arora PK, Fride E, Petitto J, et al: Morphine-induced immune alterations in vivo. *Cell Immunol* 126:343–353, 1990.

Barnett JB, Rodgers KE: Pesticides, in Dean JH, Luster MI, Munson AE, Kimber I (eds): *Immunotoxicology and Immunopharmacology*, 2d ed. New York: Raven Press, 1994, pp 191–212.

Bernstein JA, Bernstein IL: Clinical aspects of respiratory hypersensitivity to chemicals, in Dean JH, Luster MI, Munson AE, Kimber I (eds): *Immunotoxicology and Immunopharmacology*, 2d ed. New York: Raven Press, 1994, pp 617–642.

Buehler EV: Delayed contact hypersensitivity in the guinea pig. *Arch Dermatol* 91:171–177, 1965.

Booth BH: Diagnosis of immediate hypersensitivity, in Patterson R (ed): *Allergic Diseases, Diagnosis and Management*, 3d ed. Philadelphia: Lippincott, 1985, pp 102–122.

Bouaboula M, Rinaldi M, Carayon P, et al: Cannabinoid receptor expression in human leukocytes. *Eur J Biochem* 214:173–180, 1993.

Bradley SG, Munson AE, McCay JA et al: Subchronic 10 day immunotoxicity of polydimethylsiloxane (silicone) fluid, gel and elastomer and polyurethane disks in female B6C3F1 mice. *Drug and Chemical Toxicol* 17(3):175–220, 1994a

Bradley SG, White KL Jr, McCay JA et al: Immunotoxicity of 180 day exposure to polydimethylsiloxane (silicone) fluid, gel and elastomer and polyurethane disks in female B6C3F1 mice. *Drug and Chemical Toxicol* 17(3):221–269, 1994b.

Brown EJ, Albers MW, Shin TB, et al: A mammalian protein targeted by $G_1$-arresting rapamycin receptor complex. *Nature* 369:756–758, 1994.

Burns LA, Bradley SG, White KL, et al: Immunotoxicology of nitrobenzene in female B6C3F1 mice. *Drug and Chemical Toxicol* 17(3):271–315, 1994a.

Burns LA, Bradley SG, White KL, et al: Immunotoxicology of nitrotoluenes in female B6C3F1 mice. I. Para-nitrotoluene. *Drug and Chemical Toxicol* 17(3):359–399, 1994b.

Burns LA, Bradley SG, White KL, et al: Immunotoxicology of nitrotoluenes in female B6C3F1 mice. II. Meta-nitrotoluene. *Drug and Chemical Toxicol* 17(3):401–436, 1994c.

Burns LA, Bradley SG, White KL, et al: Immunotoxicology of 2,4-diaminotoluene in female B6C3F1 mice. *Drug and Chemical Toxicol* 17(3):317–358, 1994d.

Burns LA, LeVier DG, Munson AE: Immunotoxicology of Arsenic, in Dean JH, Luster MI, Munson AE, Kimber I (eds): *Immunotoxicology and Immunopharmacology*, 2d ed. New York: Raven Press, 1994e, pp 213–225.

Calne RY, Rolles K, White DJ, et al: Cyclosporin A in clinical organ grafting. *Transplant Proc* 13:349–358, 1981.

Cambridge G, Wallace H, Bernstein RM, Leaker B: Autoantibodies to myeloperoxidase in idiopathic and drug-induced systemic lupus erythematosus and vasculitis. *Br J Rheumatol* 33(2):109–114, 1994.

Canoso RT, de Oliveira RM, Nixon RA: Neuroleptic-associated autoantibodies. A prevalence study. *Biol Psychiatry* 27(8):863–870, 1990.

Chao CC, Molitor TW, Gekker G, et al: Cocaine-mediated suppression of superoxide production by human peripheral blood mononuclear cells. *J Pharmacol Exp Ther* 256:255–258, 1991.

Chao CC, Sharp BM, Pomeroy C, et al: Lethality of morphine in mice infected with Toxoplasma gondii. *J Pharmacol Exp Ther* 252:605–609, 1990.

Coleman JW, Sim E: Autoallergic responses to drugs: Mechanistic aspects, in Dean JH, Luster MI, Munson AE, Kimber I (eds): *Immunotoxicology and Immunopharmacology*, 2d ed., New York: Raven Press, 1994, pp 553–572.

Coombs RRA, Gell PGH: Classification of allergic reactions responsible for clinical hypersensitivity and disease, in Gell PGH, Coombs RRA, Lachmann PJ (eds): *Clinical Aspects of Immunology*, Oxford: Oxford University Press, 1975, p 761.

Dean JH, Luster MI, Boorman GA: Immunotoxicology, in Sirois P, Rola-Pleszcynski M (eds): *Immunopharmacology*. Amsterdam: Elsevier, 1982, pp 349–397.

Dean JH, Luster MI, Boorman GA, et al: Selective immunosuppression resulting from exposure to the carcinogenic congener of benzopyrene in B6C3F1 mice. *Clin Exp Immunol* 52:199–206, 1983.

Dean JH, Luster MI, Munson AE, Amos H (eds): *Immunotoxicology and Immunopharmacology*. New York: Raven Press, 1985.

Dean JH, Luster MI, Munson AE, Kimber I (eds): *Immunotoxicology and Immunopharmacology*, 2d ed. New York: Raven Press, 1994.

Dearman RJ, Kimber I: Differential stimulation of immune function by respiratory and contact chemical allergens. *Immunology* 72:563–570, 1991.

Dearman RJ, Spence LM, Kimber I: Characterization of murine immune responses to allergenic diisocyanates. *Toxicol Appl Pharmacol* 112:190–197, 1992.

Deo MG, Gangal S, Bhisey AN, et al: Immunological, mutagenic, and genotoxic investigations in gas-exposed population of Bhopal. *Indian J Med Res* 86:63–76, 1987.

Descotes J (Ed): *Immunotoxicology and Drugs and Chemicals*. Amsterdam: Elsevier, 1986.

DeSwarte RD: Drug allergy, in Patterson R (ed): *Allergic Diseases, Diagnosis and Management,* 3d ed. Philadelphia: Lippincott, 1985, pp 505–661.

Eisenstein TK, Bussiere JL, Rogers TJ, Adler MW: Immunosuppressive effects of morphine on immune responses in mice. *Adv Exp Med Biol* 335:41–52, 1993.

Enk AH, Angeloni VL, Udey MC, Katz SI: Inhibition of Langerhans cell antigen-presenting function by IL-10. *J Immunol* 151:2390–2398, 1993.

Fock KM, Feng PH, Tey BH: Autoimmune disease developing after augmentation mammoplasty: Report of 3 cases. *J Rheumatol* 11:98–100, 1984.

Gabliks J, Al-zubaidy T, Askari E: DDT and immunological responses. 3. Reduced anaphylaxis and mast cell population in rats fed DDT. *Arch Environ Health* 30:81–84, 1975.

Gabliks J, Askari EM, Yolen N: DDT and immunological responses. I. Serum antibodies and anaphylactic shock in guinea pig. *Arch Environ Health* 26:305–309, 1973.

Gad SC, Dunn BJ, Dobbs DW, et al: Development and validation of an alternative dermal sensitization test: The mouse ear swelling test (MEST). *Toxicol Appl Pharmacol* 84:93–114, 1986.

Gorelik E, Heberman R: Susceptibility of various strains of mice to urethane-induced lung tumors and depressed natural killer activity. *J Natl Cancer Inst* 67:1317–1322, 1981.

Grammer LC: Occupational immunologic lung disease, in Patterson R (ed): *Allergic Diseases, Diagnosis and Management*, 3d ed. Philadelphia: Lippincott, 1985, pp 691–708.

Greenlee WF, Dold KM, Irons RD, Osborne R: Evidence for a direct action of 2,3,7,8-tetrachlorodibenzo-p-dioxin (TCDD) on thymic epithelium. *Toxicol Appl Pharmacol* 79:112–120, 1985.

Greenlee WF, Dold KM, Osborne R: A proposed model for the actions of TCDD on epidermal and thymic epithelial target cells, in Poland A, Kimbrough RD (eds): *Banbury Report 18: Biological Mechanisms of Dioxin Action*. Cold Spring Harbor Laboratory, 1984, pp 435ff.

Greenspan BJ, Morrow PE: The effects of in vitro and aerosol exposures to cadmium on phagocytosis by rat pulmonary macrophages. *Fundam Appl Toxicol* 4:48–57, 1984.

Gutman AA: Allergens and other factors important in atopic disease, in Patterson R (ed): *Allergic Diseases, Diagnosis and Management*, 3d ed. Philadelphia: Lippincott, 1985, pp 123–175.

Haines KA, Reibman J, Callegari PE, et al: Cocaine and its derivatives blunt neutrophil functions without influencing phosphorylation of a 47-kilodalton component of the reduced nicotinamide-adenine dinucleotide phosphate oxidase. *J Immunol* 144:4757–4764, 1990.

Hanifin JM, Epstein WL, Cline MJ: In vitro studies of granulomatous hypersensitivity to beryllium. *J Invest Dermatol* 55:284–288, 1970.

Harpey JP, Caille B, Moulias R, Goust JM: Lupus-linked syndrome induced by D-penicillamine in Wilson's Disease. *Lancet* 1:292, 1971.

Henderson WR, Fukuyama K, Epstein WL, Spitler LE: In vitro demonstration of delayed hypersensitivity in patients with beryliosis. *J Invest Dermatol* 58:5–8, 1972.

Hendrick DJ, Rando RJ, Lane DJ, Morris MJ: Formaldhyde asthma: Challenge exposure levels and fate after five years. *J Occup Med* 24:893–897, 1982.

Hjorth N: Diagnostic patch testing, in Marzulli FN, Maibach HI (eds): *Dermatotoxicology*, 3d ed. Washington, DC: Hemisphere Publishing, 1987, pp 307–317.

Hoffman EC, Reyes H, Chu F-F, et al: Cloning of a factor required for activity of the Ah (dioxin) receptor. *Science* 252:954, 1991.

Holsapple MP: Immunotoxicity of halogenated aromatic hydrocarbons, in Smialowicz R, Holsapple MP (eds): *Experimental Immunotoxicology*. Boca Raton, FL: CRC Press, 1995, pp 257–297.

Holsapple MP, Matulka RA, Stanulis ED, Jordan SD: Cocaine and immunocompetence: Possible role of reactive metabolites. *Adv Exp Med Biol* 335:121–126, 1993.

Holsapple MP, Morris DL, Wood SC, Snyder NK: 2,3,7,8-tetrachlorodibenzo-*p*-dioxin-induced changes in immunocompetence: Possible mechanisms. *Ann Rev Pharmacol Toxicol* 31:73–100, 1991a.

Holsapple MP, Snyder NK, Wood SC, Morris DL: A review of 2,3,7,8-tetrachlorodibenzo-*p*-dioxin-induced changes in immunocompetence. *Toxicology* 69:219–255, 1991b.

Holsapple MP, Snyder NK, Gokani V, et al: Role of Ah receptor in suppression of in vivo antibody response by 2,3,7,8-tetrachlorodibenzo-*p*-dioxin (TCDD) is dependent on exposure conditions. *Fed Am Soc Exp Biol J* 5(4):A508, 1991c.

Jerrells TR, Pruett SB: Immunotoxic effects of ethanol, in Dean JH, Luster MI, Munson AE, Kimber I (eds): *Immunotoxicology and Immunopharmacology*, 2d ed. New York: Raven Press, 1994, pp 323–347.

Jiang X, Khursigara G, Rubin RL: Transformation of lupus-inducing drugs to cytotoxic products by activated neutrophils. *Science* 266(5186):810–813, 1994.

Kaminski NE: Mechanisms of immune modulation by cannabinoids, in Dean JH, Luster MI, Munson AE, Kimber I (eds): *Immunotoxicology and Immunopharmacology*, 2d ed. New York: Raven Press, 1994, pp 349–362.

Kaminski NE, Abood ME, Kessler FK, et al: Identification of a functionally relevant cannabinoid receptor on mouse spleen cells involved in cannabinoid-mediated immune modulation. *Mol Pharmacol* 42:736–742, 1992.

Kately JR, Bazzell SJ: Immunological studies in cattle exposed to polybrominated biphenyl. *Environ Health Perspect* 23:750, 1978.

Kawabata TT, White KL Jr: Effects of naphthlene metabolites on the in vitro humoral immune response. *J Toxicol Environ Health* 30:53–67, 1990.

Kenna JG, Neuberger J, Williams R: Identification by immunoblotting of three halothane-induced microsomal polypeptide antigens recognized by antibodies in sera from patients with halothane-associated hepatitis. *J Pharmacol Exp Ther* 242:733–740, 1987.

Kerkvliet NI, Brauner JA: Flow cytometric analysis of lymphocyte subpopulations in the spleen and thymus of mice exposed to an acute immunosuppressive dose of 2,3,7,8-tetrachlorodibenzo-*p*-dioxin (TCDD). *Environ Res* 52:146–164, 1990.

Kerkvliet NI, Brauner JA: Mechanisms of 1,2,3,4,6,7,8-Heptachlorodibenzo-*p*-dioxin (HpCDD)-induced humoral immune suppression: Evidence of primary defect in T cell regulation. *Toxicol Appl Pharmacol* 87:18–31, 1987.

Kerkvliet NI, Burleson GR: Immunotoxicity of TCDD and related halogenated aromatic hydrocarbons, in Dean JH, Luster MI, Munson AE, Kimber I (eds): *Immunotoxicology and Immunopharmacology*, 2d ed. New York: Raven Press, 1994, pp 97–121.

Kerkvliet NI: Halogenated aromatic hydrocarbons (HAH) as immunotoxicants, in Kende M, Gainer J, Chirigos M (eds): *Chemical Regulation of Immunity in Veterinary Medicine*. New York: Alan R. Liss, 1984, pp 369–387.

Kerkvliet NI, Steppan LB, Brauner JA, et al: Influence of the Ah locus on the humoral immunotoxicity of 2,3,7,8-tetrachlorodibenzo-*p*-dioxin: Evidence for Ah receptor-dependent and Ah receptor-independent mechanisms of immunosuppression. *Toxicol Appl Pharmacol* 105:26–36, 1990.

Kilburn KH, Warshaw RH: Prevalence of symptoms of systemic lupus erythematosus (SLE) and of fluorescent antinuclear antibodies associated with chronic exposure to trichlorethylene and other chemicals in well water. *Environ Res* 57:1–9, 1992.

Kilburn KH, Warshaw RH: Chemical-induced autoimmunity, in Dean JH, Luster MI, Munson AE, Kimber I (eds): *Immunotoxicology and Immunopharmacology*, 2d ed. New York: Raven Press, 1994, pp 523–538.

Kimber IA, Hilton J, Weisenberger C: The murine local lymph node assay for identification of contact allergens: A preliminary evaluation of in situ measurement of lymphocyte proliferation. *Contact Dermatitis* 21:215–220, 1989.

Kimber IA, Hilton J, Botham PA, et al: The murine local lymph node assay: Results of an inter-laboratory trial. *Toxicol Lett* 55:203–213, 1991.

Klecak G: Identification of contact allergens: Predicitive tests in animals, in Marzulli FN, Maibach HI (eds): *Dermatotoxicology*, 3d ed. Washington, DC: Hemisphere Publishing, 1987, pp 227–290.

Koller LD: Immunotoxicology of heavy metals. *Int J Immunopharmacol* 2:269–279, 1980.

Krzystyniak K, Hugo P, Flipo D, Fournier M: Increased susceptibility to mouse hepatitis virus 3 of peritoneal macrophages exposed to dieldrin. *Toxicol Appl Pharmacol* 80:397–408, 1985.

Kunz J, Henriquez R, Schneider U, et al: Target of rapamycin in yeast, TOR2, is an essential phosphatidylinositol kinase homolog required for G1 progression. *Cell* 73:585–596, 1993.

Ladics GS, Kawabata TT, White KL Jr: Suppression of the in vitro humoral immune response of mouse splenocytes by 7,12-dimethylbenz[a]anthracene metabolites and inhibition of suppression by a-naphthoflavone. *Toxicol Appl Pharmacol* 110:31–44, 1991.

Ladics GS, Kawabata TT, Munson AE, White KL Jr: Metabolism of benzo[a]pyrene by murine splenic cell types. *Toxicol Appl Pharmacol* 116:248–257, 1992a.

Ladics GS, Kawabata TT, Munson AE, White KL Jr: Generation of 7,8-dihydroxy-9,10-epoxy-7,8,9,10-tetrahydrobenzo[a]pyrene by murine splenic macrophages. *Toxicol Appl Pharmacol* 115:72–79, 1992b.

Lawrence DA: Immunotoxicity of heavy metals, in Dean JH, Luster MI, Munson AE, Amos H (eds): *Immunotoxicology and Immunopharmacology*. New York: Raven Press, 1985, pp 341–353.

Lefkowitz SS, Vaz A, Lefkowitz DL: Cocaine reduces macrophage killing by inhibiting reactive oxygen intermediates. *Int J Immunopharmacol* 15:717–721, 1993.

LeVier DG, Brown RD, McCay JA, et al: Hepatic and splenic phagocytosis in female B6C3F1 mice implanted with morphine sulfate pellets. *J Phamacol Exp Ther* 367:357–363, 1993.

LeVier DG, McCay JA, Stern ML, et al: Immunotoxicological profile of morphine sulfate in B6C3F1 mice. *Fundam Appl Toxicol* 22:525–542, 1994.

Levy MH, Wheelock EF: Effects of intravenous silica on immune and non-immune functions of the murine host. *J Immunol* 115:41–48, 1975.

Liberman P, Crawford L, Drewry RD Jr, Tuberville A: Allergic diseases of the eye and ear, in Patterson R (ed): *Allergic Diseases, Diagnosis and Management*, 3d ed. Philadelphia: Lippincott, 1985, pp 374–407.

Lundberg K, Grovnick K, Goldschmidt TJ, et al: 2,3,7,8-tetrachlorodibenzo-*p*-dioxin (TCDD) alters intrathymic T cell development in mice. *Chem-Biol Interact* 74:179, 1990.

Luster MI, Dean JH, Boorman GA, et al: Host resistance and immune functions in methyl and ethyl carbamate treated mice. *Clin Exp Immunol* 50:223–230, 1982.

Luster MI, Munson AE, Thomas PT, et al: Development of a testing battery to assess chemical-induced immunotoxicity: National Toxicology Program's guidelines for immunotoxicity evaluation in mice. *Fundam Appl Toxicol* 10:2–9, 1988.

Luster MI, Portier C, Pait DG, et al: Risk assessment in immunotoxicology. I. Sensitivity and predictability of immune tests. *Fundam Appl Toxicol* 18:200–210, 1992.

Luster MI, Tucker JA, Germolec DR, et al: Immunotoxicity studies in mice exposed to methyl isocyanate. *Toxicol Appl Pharmacol* 86:140–144, 1986.

Magnusson B, Kligman AM: The identification of contact allergens by animal assay. The quinea pig maximization test. *J Invest Dermatol* 52:268–276, 1969.

Maibach H: Formaldehyde: Effects on animal and human skin, in Gibson J (ed): *Formaldehyde Toxicity*. New York: Hemisphere Publishing, 1983, pp 166–174.

Marzulli FN, Maibach HI: The use of graded concentrations in studying skin sensitizers: Experimental contact sensitization in man. *Food Cosmet Toxicol* 12:219–227, 1974.

Marzulli FN, Maibach HI: Contact allergy: Predictive testing in humans, in Marzulli FN, Maibach HI (eds): *Dermatotoxicology,* 3d ed. Washington, DC: Hemisphere Publishing, 1987, pp 319–340.

McCabe MJ Jr: Mechanisms and consequences of immunomodulation by lead, in Dean JH, Luster MI, Munson AE, Kimber I (eds): *Immunotoxicology and Immunopharmacology*, 2d ed. New York: Raven Press, 1994, pp 143–162.

McDonough RJ, Madden JJ, Falck A, et al: Alteration of T and null lymphocyte frequencies in the peripheral blood of human opiate addicts: In vivo evidence for opiate receptor sites on T lymphocytes. *J Immunol* 125:2539–2543, 1980.

Menna JH, Barnett JB, Soderberg LSF: Influenze type A infection of mice exposed *in utero* to chlordane: Survival and antibody studies. *Toxicol Lett* 24:45–52, 1985.

Menné T: Reactions to systemic exposure to contact allergens, in Marzulli FN, Maibach HI (eds): *Dermatotoxicology*, 3d ed. Washington, DC: Hemisphere Publishing, 1987, pp 535–552.

Miller K, Brown RC: The immune system and asbestos-associated disease, in Dean JH, Luster MI, Munson AE, Amos H (eds): *Immunotoxicology and Immunopharmacology*. New York: Raven Press, 1985, pp 429–440.

Mishell RI, Dutton RW: Immunization of dissociated mouse spleen cell culture from normal mice. *J Exp Med* 126:423–442, 1967.

Morice WG, Brunn GJ, Wiederrecht G, et al: Rapamycin-induced inhibition of $p34^{cdc2}$ kinase activation is aoociated with $G_1/S$ phase growth arrest in T lymphocytes. *J Biol Chem* 268:3734–3738, 1993.

Mosmann TR, Coffman RL: Heterogeneity of cytokine secretion patterns and function of helper T cells. *Adv Immunol* 46:111–147, 1989.

Mosmann TR, Schumacher JH, Street NF, et al: Diversity of cytokine synthesis and function of mouse $CD4^+$ T cells. *Immunol Rev* 123:209–229, 1991.

Munro S, Thomas KL, Abu-Shaar M: Molecular characterization of peripheral receptor for cannabinoids. *Nature* 365:61–65, 1993.

Murphy WG, Kelton JG: Immune haemolytic anaemia and thrombocytopaenia with drugs and antibodies. *Biochem Soc Trans* 19:183–186, 1991.

Newman LS: Beryllium lung disease: The role of cell-mediated immunity in pathogenesis, in Dean JH, Luster MI, Munson AE, Kimber I (eds): *Immunotoxicology and Immunopharmacology*, 2d ed. New York: Raven Press, 1994, pp 377–394.

Ou D, Shen ML, Luo YD: Effects of cocaine on the immune system of BALB/c mice. *Clin Immun Immunopath* 52:305–312, 1989.

Paul WE (ed): *Fundamental Immunology*, 3d ed. New York: Raven Press, 1993.

Paul WE, Seder RA: Lymphocyte responses and cytokines. *Cell* 76:241–251, 1994.

Pelletier L, Castedo M, Bellon B, Druet P: Mercury and autoimmunity, in Dean JH, Luster MI, Munson AE, Kimber I (eds): *Immunotoxicology and Immunopharmacology*, 2d ed. New York: Raven Press, 1994, pp 539–552.

Penninks AH, Snoeij NJ, Pieters RHH, Seinen W: Effect of organotin compounds on lymphoid organs and lymphoid functions: An overview, in Dayan AD, Hentel RF, Heseltine E, Kazantzis G, Smith EM, Vander Venne MT (eds): *Immunotoxicity of Metals and Immunotoxicology*. New York: Plenum Press, 1990, pp 191–207.

Pernis B, Paronetto F: Adjuvant effect of silica (tridymite) on antibody production. *Proc Soc Exp Biol Med* 110:390–392, 1962.

Peterson PK, Gekker G, Chao CC, et al: Cocaine potentiates HIV-1 replication in human peripheral blood mononuclear cell cultures. Involvement of transforming growth factor-b. *J Immunol* 146:81–84, 1991.

Pruett SB, Barnes DB, Han YC, Munson AE: Immunotoxicological characteristics of sodium methyldithiocarbamate. *Fund Appl Toxicol* 18:40–47, 1992a.

Pruett SB, Han Y, Fuchs BA: Morphine suppresses primary humoral immune responses by a predominantly indirect mechanism. *J Pharmacol Exp Ther* 262:923–928, 1992b.

Quesniaux VFJ: Interleukins 9, 10, 11, and 12, and kit ligand: A brief overview. *Res Immunol* 143:385–400, 1992.

Roitt I, Brostoff J, Male D (eds): *Immunology*, 3d ed. London: Mosby, 1993.

Rosenthal GJ, Kowolenko M: Immunotoxicologic manifestations of AIDS therapeutics, in Dean JH, Luster MI, Munson AE, Kimber I (eds): *Immunotoxicology and Immunopharmacology*, 2d ed. New York: Raven Press, 1994, pp 227–247.

Rose RN: Immunopathogenesis of autoimmune diseases, in Dean JH, Luster MI, Munson AE, Kimber I (eds): *Immunotoxicology and Immunopharmacology*, 2d ed. New York: Raven Press, 1994, pp 513–522.

Ruddle NH: Tumor necrosis factor (TNF$\alpha$) and lymphotoxin (TFN$\beta$). *Curr Opin Immunol* 4:327–332, 1994.

Sabatini DM, Erdjument-Bromage H, Lui M, et al: A mammalian protein that binds to FKBP12 in a rapamycin-dependent fashion and is homologous to yeast TORs. *Cell* 78:35–43, 1994.

Sabers CJ, Martin MM, Brunn GJ, et al: Isolation of a protein target of the FKBP12–rapamycin complex in mammalian cells. *J Biol Chem* 270(2):815–822, 1995.

Sanders VM, Tucker AN, White KL Jr, et al: Humoral and cell-mediated immune status in mice exposed to trichloroethylene in the drinking water. *Toxicol Appl Pharmacol* 62:358–368, 1982.

Sanders VM, White KL Jr, Shopp GM, Munson AE: Humoral and cell-mediated immune status of mice exposed to 1,1,2-trichloroethane. *Drug Chem Toxicol* 8(5):357–372, 1985.

Sapin C, Mandet C, Druet E, et al: Immune complex type disease induced by $HgCl_2$: Genetic control of susceptibility. *Transplant Proc* 13:1404–1406, 1981.

Sarlo K, Karol MH: Guinea pig predictive tests for respiratory allergy, in Dean JH, Luster MI, Munson AE, Kimber I (eds): *Immunotoxicology and Immunopharmacology*, 2d ed. New York: Raven Press, 1994, pp 703–720.

Schatz AR, Kessler FK, Kaminski NE: Inhibition of adenylate cyclase by $\Delta$9-tetrahydrocannabinol in mouse spleen cells: A potential mechanism for cannabinoid-mediated immunosuppression. *Life Sci* 51:25–30, 1992.

Schwarz A, Grabbe S, Reimann H, et al: In vivo effects of interleukin-10 on contact hypersensitivity and delayed-type hypersensitivity reactions. *J Invest Dematol* 103:211–216, 1994.

Selgrade MJK, Gilmour MI: Effects of gaseous air pollutants on immune responses and susceptibility to infectious and allergic diseases, in Dean JH, Luster MI, Munson AE, Kimber I (eds): *Immunotoxicology and Immunopharmacology*, 2d ed. New York: Raven Press, 1994, pp 395–411.

Sherwood R, O'Shea W, Thomas P, et al: Effects of inhalation of ethylene dichloride on pulmonary defenses of mice and rats. *Toxicol Appl Pharmacol* 91:491–496, 1987.

Shopp GM, Sanders VM, Munson AE: Humoral and cell-mediated immune status of mice exposed to trans-1,2-dichloroethylene. *Drug Chem Toxicol* 8(5):393–407, 1985.

Shopp GM, White KL Jr, Holsapple MP, et al: Naphthlene toxicity in CD-1 mice: General toxicology and immunotoxicology. *Fundam Appl Toxicol* 4:406–419, 1984.

Sikorski EE, Kipen HM, Selner JC, et al: Roundtable Summary: The Question of Multiple Chemical Sensitivity. *Fundam Appl Toxicol* 24:22–28, 1995.

Silkworth JB, Loose LD: Cell-mediated immunity in mice fed either Aroclor 1016 or hexachlorobenzene. *Toxicol Appl Pharmacol* 45:326–327, 1978.

Silkworth JB, Loose LD: PCB and HCB induced alteration of lymphocyte blastogenesis. *Toxicol Appl Pharmacol* 49:86, 1979.

Silver RM, Heyes MP, Maize JC, et al: Scleroderma, fasciitis and eosinophilia associated with the ingestion of tryptophan *N Engl J Med* 322:874–881, 1990.

Snyder CA: Organic solvents, in Dean JH, Luster MI, Munson AE, Kimber I (eds): *Immunotoxicology and Immunopharmacology*, 2d ed. New York: Raven Press, 1994, pp 183–190.

Sopori ML, Goud NS, Kaplan AM: Effects of tobacco smoke on the immune system, in Dean JH, Luster MI, Munson AE, Kimber I (eds): *Immunotoxicology and Immunopharmacology*, 2d ed. New York: Raven Press, 1994, pp 413–434.

Spreafico F, Allegrucci M, Merendino A, Luini W: Chemical immunodepressive drugs: Their action on the cells of the immun system and immune mediators, in Dean JH, Luster MI, Munson AE, Amos H (eds): *Immunotoxicology and Immunopharmacology*. New York: Raven Press, 1985, pp 179–192.

Spyker-Cranmer JM, Barnett JB, Avery DL, Cranmer MF: Immunoteratology of chlordane: Cell-mediated and humoral immune responses in adult mice exposed *in utero*. *Toxicol Appl Pharmacol* 62:402–408, 1982.

Starec M, Rouveix B, Sinet M, et al: Immune status and survival of opiate- and cocaine-treated mice infected with Friend virus. *J Pharmacol Exp Ther* 259:745–750, 1991.

Street JC: Pesticides and the immune system, in Sharma RP (ed): *Immunologic Considerations in Toxicology*. Boca Raton, FL: CRC Press, 1981, pp 46–66.

Sutter TR, Greenlee WF: Classification of members of the Ah gene battery. *Chemosphere*. 25:223, 1992.

Sutter TR, Guzman K, Dold KM, Greenlee WF: Targets for dioxin: Genes for plasminogen activator inhibitor-2 and interleukin-1b. *Science* 254:415, 1991.

Talmadge JE, Dean JH: Immunopharmacology of recombinant cytokines, in Dean JH, Luster MI, Munson AE, Kimber I (eds): *Immunotoxicology and Immunopharmacology*, 2d ed. New York: Raven Press, 1994, pp 227–247.

Terada N, Lucas JJ, Szepesi A, et al: Rapamycin blocks cell cycle progression of activated T cells prior to events characteristic of the middle to late $G_1$ phase of the cycle. *J Cell Physiol* 154:7–15, 1993.

Thomas PT, Busse WW, Kerkvliet NI, et al: Immunologic effects of pesticides, in Baker SR, Wilkinson CF (eds): *The Effects of Pesticides on Human Health*. New York: Princeton Scientific Publishers, 1990, Vol 18, pp 261–295.

Thorne PS, Hawk C, Kaliszewski SD, Guiney PD: The noninvasive mouse ear swelling assay. I. Refinements for detecting weak contact sensitizers. *Fundam Appl Toxicol* 17:790–806, 1991.

Thurmond LM, Dean JH: Immunological responses following inhalation exposure to chemical hazards, in Gardner EE, Crapo JD, Massaro EJ (eds): *Toxicology of the Lung*. Raven Press, New York, 1988, pp 375–406.

Tognoni G, Boniccorsi A: Epidemiological problems with TCDD. A critical review. *Drug Metab Rev* 13:447–469, 1982.

Totoritis MC, Tan EM, McNally EM, Rubin RL: Association of antibody to histone complex H2A-H2B with symptomatic procainamide-induced lupus. *N Engl J Med* 318(22):1431–1436, 1988.

Tryphonas H, Luster MI, Schiffman G, et al: Effect of chronic exposure of PCB (Aroclor 1254) on specific and nonspecific immune paramemters in the Rhesus (*Macaca mulatta*) monkey. *Fund Appl Toxicol* 16:773–786, 1991a.

Tryphonas H, Luster MI, White KL Jr, et al: Effect of chronic exposure of PCB (Aroclor 1254) on specific and nonspecific immune paramemters in the Rhesus (*Macaca mulatta*) monkey. *Int J Immunopharmacol* 13:639–648, 1991b.

Tubaro E, Santiangeli C, Belogi L, et al: Methadone vs. morphine: Comparison of their effect on phagocytic functions. *Int J Immunopharmacol* 9:79–88, 1987.

Unanue E: Macrophages, antigen-presenting cells, and the phenomena of antigen handling and presentation, in Paul WE (ed): *Fundamental Immunology*, 3d ed. New York: Raven Press, 1993, pp 111–144.

van Loveren H, Krajnc E, Rombout PJA, et al: Effects of ozone, hexachlorobenzene and bis(tri-*n*-butyltin)oxide on natural killer activity in the rat lung. *Toxicol Appl Pharmacol* 102:21–33, 1990.

Vecchi A, Sironi M, Canegrati MA, et al: Immunosuppressive effects of 2,3,7,8-tetrachlorodibenzo-*p*-dioxin in strains of mice with different susceptibility to induction of aryl hydrocarbon hydroxylase. *Toxicol Appl Pharmacol* 68:434–441, 1983.

von Krogh G, Maibach HI: The contact urticaria syndrome, in Marzulli FN, Maibach HI (eds): *Dermatotoxicology*, 3d ed. Washington, DC: Hemisphere Publishing, 1987, pp 341–362.

Vos JG, Luster MI: Immune alterations, in Kimbrough RD, Jensen AA (eds): *Halogenated Biphenyls, Terphenyls, Napthalenes, Dibenzodioxins, and Related Products*. Amsterdam: Elsevier, 1989, pp. 295–322.

Vos JG: Immune suppression as related to toxicology. *CRC Crit Rev Toxicol* 5:67–101, 1977.

Vos JG, de Klerk A, Krajnc FI, et al: Toxicity of bis(tri-*n*-butyltin)oxide in the rat. II. Suppression of thymus-dependent immune responses and of paramemters of non-specific resistance after short-term exposure. *Toxicol Appl Pharmacol* 75:387–408, 1984.

Vos JG, Smialowicz RJ, Van Loveren H: Animal models for assessment, in Dean JH, Luster MI, Munson AE, Kimber I (eds): *Immunotoxicology and Immunopharmacology*, 2d ed. New York: Raven Press, 1994, pp 19–30.

Walder BK: Do solvents cause scleroderma? *Int J Dermatol 22*:157–158, 1983.

Ward AM, Udnoon S, Watkins J, et al: Immunological mechanisms in the pathogenesis of vinyl chloride disease. *Br Med J* 1:936–938, 1976.

Ward EC, Murray MJ, Dean JH: Immunotoxicity of non-halogenated polycyclic aromatic hydrocarbons, in Dean JH, Luster MI, Munson AE, Amos H (eds): *Immunotoxicology and Immunopharmacology*. New York: Raven Press, 1985, pp 291–303.

Warheit DB, Hesterberg TW: Asbestos and other fibers in the lung, in Dean JH, Luster MI, Munson AE, Kimber I (eds): *Immunotoxicology and Immunopharmacology*, 2d ed. New York: Raven Press, 1994, pp 363–376.

Wasserman M, Wasserman D, Gershon Z, Zellermayer L: Effects of organochlorine insecticides on body defense systems. *Ann NY Acad Sci* 160:393–401, 1969.

Watson ES, Murphy JC, ElSohly HN, et al: Effect of the administration of coca alkaloids on the primary immune responses of mice: Interaction with $\Delta^9$-tetrahydrocannabinol and ethanol. *Toxicol Appl Pharmacol* 71:1–13, 1983.

White KL Jr, Anderson AC: Suppression of mouse complement activity by contaminants of technical grade pentachlorophenol. *Agents Actions* 16(5):385, 1985.

White KL Jr: Specific immune function assays, in Miller K, Turk JL, Nicklin S (eds): *Principles and Practice of Immunotoxicology*. Boston: Blackwell, 1992, pp 304–323.

White KL Jr, Kawabata TT, Ladics GS: Mechanisms of polycyclic aromatic hydrocarbon immunotoxicity, in Dean JH, Luster MI, Munson AE, Kimber I (eds): *Immunotoxicology and Immunopharmacology*, 2d ed. New York: Raven Press, 1994, pp 123–142.

White KL Jr, Lysy HH, McCay JA, Anderson AC: Modulation of serum complement levels following exposure to polychlorinated dibenzo-p-dioxins. *Toxicol Appl Pharmacol* 84:209–219, 1986.

Xiao F, Chong AS-F, Bartlett RR, Williams JW: Leflunomide: A promising immunosuppressant in transplantation, in Thomas AW, Starzyl TE (eds): *Immunosuppressive Drugs: Developments in Anti-Rejection Therapy*. Boston: Edward Arnold, 1994, pp 203–212.

Zurawski G, de Vries JE: Interleukin 13, an interleukin 4-like cytokine that acts on monocytes and B cells, but not T cells. *Immunol Today* 15(1):19–26, 1994.

# CHAPTER 13

# TOXIC RESPONSES OF THE LIVER

*Mary Treinen Moslen*

Hepatotoxicity is a field with long-standing recognition that is characterized by intense investigation. Many industrial compounds and therapeutic agents are well established as injurious to the liver. Consequently, the use of such chemicals has been eliminated or restricted. For example, carbon tetrachloride was once commonly used in unventilated garages to degrease automobile engines. Plastic industry workers without any protective equipment once crawled into giant vats coated with a residue containing vinyl chloride (Kramer, 1974). Now exposures to these potent hepatotoxins are tightly regulated. However, each year new chemicals are found to damage the liver, such as the promising drug fialuridine, whose clinical trial as a form of therapy for chronic hepatitis was terminated suddenly in 1993 when patients started to die from liver failure (Macilwain, 1993). Humans and animals continue to ingest environmental hepatotoxins in foods, teas, and contaminated waters. The serious problem of chemically induced liver damage has inspired several excellent books (Zimmerman, 1978; Meeks et al., 1991; Farrell, 1994).

Our understanding of hepatic functions and cell injury has been advanced by observations on hepatotoxicants. New techniques in molecular biology, immunochemical probes, and imaging have enhanced the value of hepatotoxins as tools to probe basic physiological and pathological processes. Scientists have identified mechanisms by which chemicals injure specific populations of liver cells. Factors are known that determine why the liver, as opposed to other organs, is the dominant target site of specific toxins. However, questions remain. Although excessive consumption of ethanol is an established cause of hepatic cirrhosis, not all the factors responsible for the greater vulnerability of females versus males to ethanol are known (Lieber, 1994). Immune-mediated responses to adducts between chemicals and hepatic proteins are a frequently postulated, but poorly documented cause of the liver damage observed after repeated exposure to drugs that cause liver damage only sporadically (Farrell, 1994).

Toxicologists regard the phrase "produces liver injury" as vague, since liver cells respond in many different ways to acute and chronic insults by chemicals. A basic understanding of chemical hepatotoxicity requires an appreciation of the physiology and anatomy of the liver. Key aspects for appreciation are (1) the major functions of the liver, (2) the structural organization of the liver, and (3) the processes involved in the excretory function of the liver, namely, bile formation. These aspects contribute to the vulnerability of hepatic cells to chemical insults.

## PHYSIOLOGY AND PATHOPHYSIOLOGY

### Hepatic Functions

Residing between the intestinal tract and the rest of the body, the liver is strategically positioned to perform its task of maintaining the body's metabolic homeostasis (Table 13-1). Venous blood from the stomach and intestines flows into the portal vein and then through the liver before entering the systemic circulation. Thus, the liver is the first organ to encounter ingested nutrients, vitamins, metals, drugs, and environmental toxicants as well as the waste products of bacteria that enter the portal blood. Efficient scavenging or uptake processes extract these absorbed materials from the blood for catabolism, storage, and/or excretion into bile.

All the major functions of the liver can be detrimentally altered by liver injury resulting from acute or chronic exposure to toxicants (Table 13-1). Alcohol abuse is the major cause of liver diseases in most western countries (Crawford, 1994); thus, ethanol provides a highly relevant example of a toxin with multiple functional consequences (Lieber, 1994). The early stages of ethanol abuse are characterized by lipid accumulation (fatty liver) caused by the diminished use of lipids as fuels and an impaired ability to synthesize the lipoproteins that transport lipids out of the liver. As alcohol-induced liver disease progresses, the functioning mass of the liver is replaced by scar tissue and the hepatic capacity for the biotransformation of certain drugs progressively declines (Sotaniemi et al., 1977). People with hepatic cirrhosis resulting from chronic alcohol abuse frequently become deficient at detoxifying both the ammonia formed by the catabolism of amino acids and the bilirubin derived from the breakdown of hemoglobin. Uncontrollable hemorrhage caused by inadequate synthesis of clotting factors is a common fatal complication of alcoholic cirrhosis. A consequence of liver injury that merits emphasis is the fact that the loss of liver functions can lead to aberrations in other organ systems and to death.

### Structural Organization

Two concepts exist for the organization of the liver into operational units: the lobule and the acinus. Classically, the liver was divided into hexagonal lobules oriented around terminal hepatic venules (also known as central veins). At the corners of the lobule are the portal triads (or portal tracts), which contain a branch of the portal vein, a hepatic arteriole, and a bile duct

**Table 13–1**
**Major Functions of Liver and Consequences of Impaired Hepatic Functions**

| TYPE OF FUNCTION | EXAMPLES | CONSEQUENCES OF IMPAIRED FUNCTION |
|---|---|---|
| Nutrient homeostasis | Glucose storage and synthesis | Hypoglycemia, confusion |
| | Cholesterol uptake | Hypercholesterolemia |
| Filtration of particulates | Products of intestinal bacteria, e.g., endotoxin | Endotoxemia |
| Protein synthesis | Clotting factors | Excess bleeding |
| | Albumin | Hypoalbuminemia, ascites |
| | Transport proteins (e.g., very low density lipoprotein) | Fatty liver |
| Biotransformation and detoxification | Bilirubin and ammonia | Jaundice, hyperammonemia-related coma |
| | Steroid hormones | Loss of secondary male characteristics |
| | Xenobiotics | Diminished drug metabolism |
| Formation of bile and biliary excretion | Bile acid-dependent uptake of dietary lipids and vitamins | Fatty diarrhea, malnutrition, vitamin E deficiency |
| | Bilirubin and cholesterol | Jaundice, hypercholesterolemia |
| | Metals, e.g., Cu and Mn | Mn-induced neurotoxicity |
| | Xenobiotics | Delayed drug clearance |

(Fig. 13-1). Blood entering the portal tract through the portal vein and hepatic artery is mixed in the penetrating vessels, enters the sinusoids and percolates along the cords of parenchymal cells (hepatocytes), eventually flows into terminal hepatic venules, and exits the liver through the hepatic vein. The lobule is divided into three regions: the centrolobular, midzonal, and periportal regions. The acinus is preferred as a concept of a functional hepatic unit. The base of the acinus is formed by the terminal branches of the portal vein and hepatic artery that extend out from the portal tracts. The acinus has three zones: zone 1 is closest to the entry of blood, zone 3 abuts the terminal hepatic vein, and zone 2 is interme-

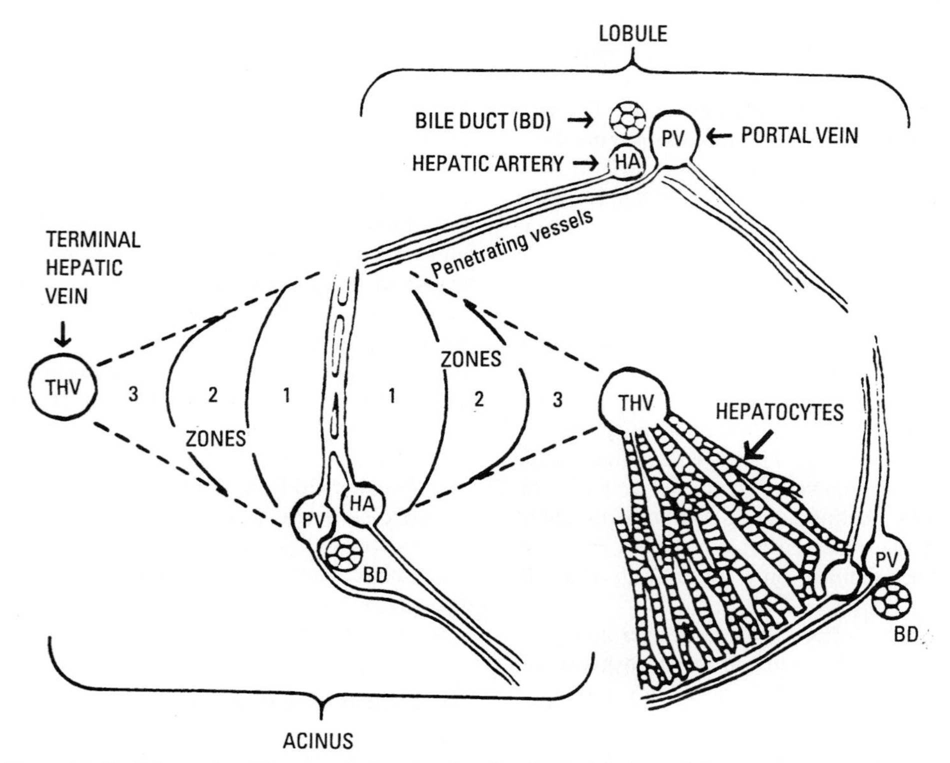


*Figure 13–1. Schematic of liver operational units: the classic lobule and the acinus.*

The lobule is centered on the terminal hepatic vein (central vein), where the blood drains out of the lobule. The acinus has as its base the penetrating vessels where blood supplied by the portal vein and hepatic artery flows down the acinus past the cords of hepatocytes. Zones 1, 2, and 3 of the acinus represent metabolic regions that are increasingly distant from the blood supply.

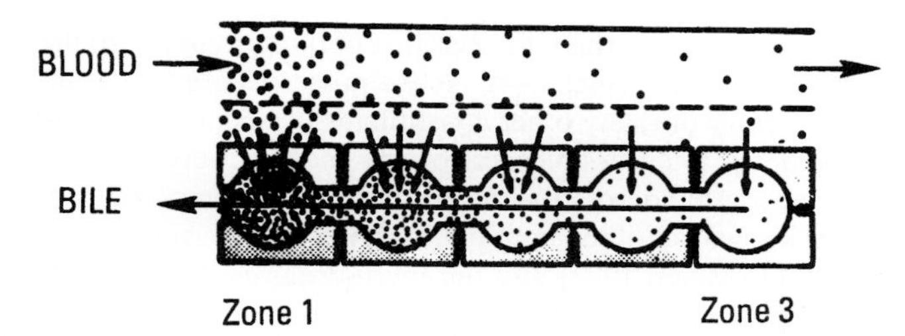


*Figure 13–2. Schematic of the acinar gradient of bile acids.*

Efficient uptake of bile acids by zone 1 hepatocytes results in very low levels of bile acids in the blood that flows past zone 3 hepatocytes. A less steep gradient exists for the uptake of bilirubin and other organic anions.

diate. Despite the utility of the acinar concept, lobular terminology is still used to describe regions of pathological lesions of hepatic parenchyma. Fortunately, the three zones of the acinus roughly coincide with the three regions of the lobule (Fig. 13-1).

Acinar zonation is of considerable functional consequence in regard to the gradients of components both in blood and in hepatocytes (Traber et al., 1988; Jungermann and Katz, 1989). Blood entering the acinus consists of oxygen-depleted blood from the portal vein (60 to 70 percent of hepatic blood flow) and oxygenated blood from the hepatic artery (30 to 40 percent). En route to the terminal hepatic venule, oxygen rapidly leaves the blood to meet the high metabolic demands of the parenchymal cells. Approximate oxygen concentrations in zone 1 are 9 to 13 percent $O_2$ compared with only 4 to 5 percent $O_2$ in zone 3. Therefore, hepatocytes in zone 3 are exposed to substantially lower concentrations of oxygen than are hepatocytes in zone 1. In comparison to other tissues, zone 3 is hypoxic. Another well-documented acinar gradient is that of bile acids (Groothuis et al., 1982). Physiological concentrations of bile acids are extracted efficiently by zone 1 hepatocytes, with little bile acid left in the blood that flows past zone 3 hepatocytes (Fig. 13-2).

Heterogeneities in the protein levels of hepatocytes along the acinus generate gradients of metabolic functions. Hepatocytes in the mitochondria-rich zone 1 are predominant in fatty acid oxidation, gluconeogenesis, and ammonia detoxification to urea. Gradients of enzymes involved in the bioactivation and detoxification of xenobiotics have been observed along the acinus by immunohistochemical techniques (Jungermann and Katz, 1989). Notable gradients for hepatotoxins are the higher levels of glutathione in zone 1 and the greater amounts of cytochrome P-450 proteins in zone 3, particularly the CYP-2E1 isozyme, which is inducible by ethanol (Tsutsumi et al., 1989).

Hepatic sinusoids are the channels between cords of hepatocytes where blood percolates on its way to the terminal hepatic vein. Sinusoids are larger and more irregular than normal capillaries. The three major types of cells in the sinusoids are endothelial cells, Kupffer cells, and Ito cells (Fig. 13-3). Sinusoids are lined by thin, discontinuous endothelial cells with small and large fenestrae (pores). Very little, if any, basement membrane separates the endothelial cells from the hepatocytes. The numerous fenestrae and the lack of a basement membrane facilitate exchanges of fluids and molecules such as albumin between the sinusoids and hepatocytes but hinder the movement of particles larger than chylomicron remnants. Endothelial cells are important in the scavenging of lipoproteins and denatured proteins. Hepatic endothelial cells also secrete cytokines.

Kupffer cells are the resident macrophages of the liver and constitute approximately 80 percent of the fixed macrophages in the body. Kupffer cells are situated within the lumen of the sinusoid. The primary function of these cells is to ingest and degrade particulate matter. These cells also are a source of cytokines and can act as antigen-presenting cells (Laskin, 1990). Ito cells, which also are known by the more descriptive terms "fat-storing cells" and "stellate cells," are located in the

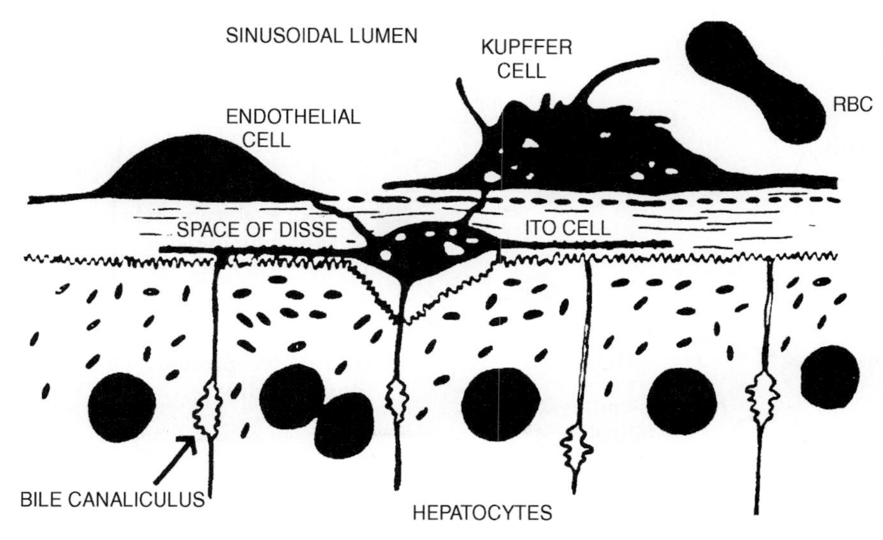


*Figure 13–3. Schematic of liver sinusoidal cells.*

Note that the Kupffer cell resides in the sinusoidal lumen. The Ito cell is located in the space of Disse between the thin, fenestrated endothelial cells and the cord of hepatocytes. [Modified from Ramadori G, Rieder H, Knittell T: Biology and pathobiology of sinusoidal liver cells, in Travoloni N, Berk PD (eds): *Hepatic Transport and Bile Secretion: Physiology and Pathophysiology*. New York: Raven Press, 1993, pp 83–102.]

space of Disse between endothelial cells and hepatocytes. Ito cells synthesize collagen and are the major site for vitamin A storage in the body.

## Bile Formation

Bile is a yellow fluid that contains bile acids, glutathione, phospholipids, cholesterol, bilirubin and other organic anions, proteins, metals, ions, and xenobiotics (Klaassen and Watkins, 1984). The formation of this fluid is a specialized function of the liver. Adequate bile formation is essential for the uptake of lipid nutrients from the small intestine and the excretion of endogenous and xenobiotic compounds (Table 13-1). Hepatocytes begin the process by transporting bile acids, glutathione, and other solutes into the canalicular lumen, which is a space formed by specialized regions of the plasma membrane between adjacent hepatocytes (Fig. 13-3). Tight junctions seal the canalicular lumen from materials in the sinusoid. The structure of the biliary tract is analogous to the roots and trunk of a tree, where the tips of the roots are equivalent to the canalicular lumens. Canaliculi form channels between hepatocytes that connect to a series of larger and larger channels or ducts in the liver. The large extrahepatic bile ducts merge into the common bile duct. Bile can be stored and concentrated in the gallbladder before its release into the duodenum. However, the gallbladder is not essential to life and is absent in several species, including the horse, whale, and rat.

Our understanding of bile formation is rapidly evolving from a descriptive orientation toward the identification of specific cellular and subcellular processes (Meier, 1993). Transporters on the sinusoidal and canalicular membranes of hepatocytes are responsible for the uptake of bile acids and bilirubin from blood and then the secretion of those solutes into the canalicular lumen (Fig. 13-4). Active processes are important for the entry of many other constituents of bile. Leukotriene metabolites, phospholipids, estrogens, and a variety of drugs are transported across the canalicular by membrane by proteins known as the multiple organic anion transporter (MOAT) (Meier, 1993) and the multi-drug-resistant (MDR) P-glycoproteins (Smit et al., 1993; Gosland et al., 1993). Fluids and ions enter bile by paracellular diffusion and endocytic transcytosis. Metals are excreted into bile by a series of partially understood processes that include uptake across the sinusoidal membrane by facilitated diffusion or receptor-mediated endocytosis, storage in binding proteins or lysosomes, and into the canaliculus secretion via lysosomes, a glutathione-coupled event, or a specific canalicular membrane transporter (Ballatori, 1991). Biliary excretion is important in the homeostasis of Cu, Mn, Fe, Zn, Au, Al, and Hg. Species and age differences are known for the biliary excretion of several toxic metals; for example, rats excrete arsenic into bile much faster than dogs do (Klaassen, 1976).

Canalicular lumen bile is pushed forward into larger channels by dynamic ATP-dependent contractions of the pericanalicular cytoskeleton (Watanabe et al., 1991). Bile ducts are no longer regarded as passive conduits, since bile can be modified by active processes of absorption or secretion while traveling through the bile ducts (Lira et al., 1992). Biliary excretion usually is a prelude to excretion in feces or urine. However, a few toxins are known to be absorbed from the biliary tract. Extensive absorption of methylmercury from the gallbladder is thought to contribute to the long biological half-life and toxicity of methylmercury (Dutczak et al., 1991).

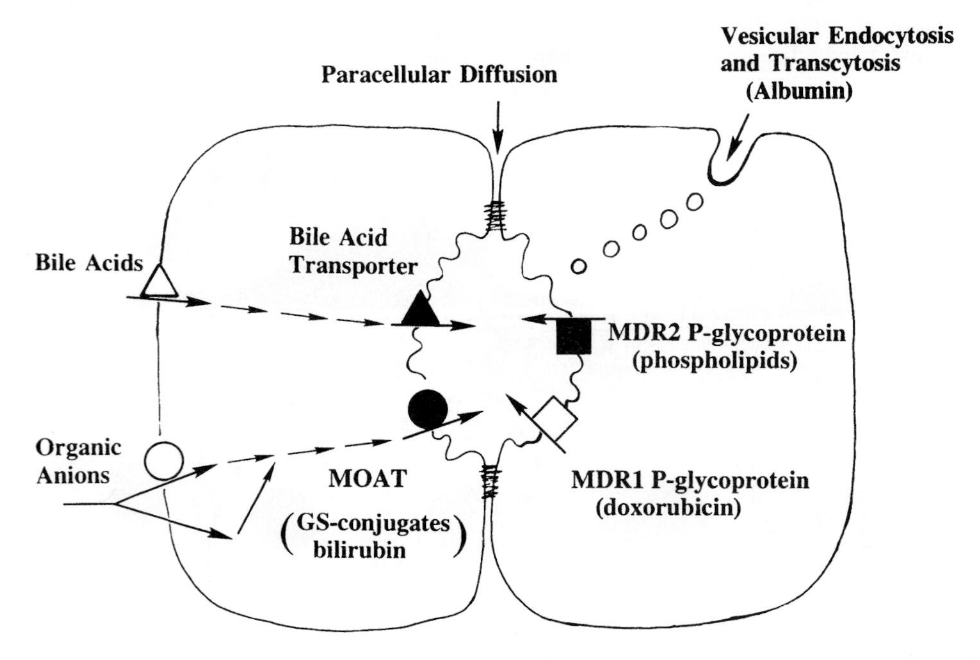


***Figure 13–4. Processes involved in hepatocyte uptake and secretion of bile acids, organic anions, endogenous compounds (bilirubin, proteins, and phospholipids), and exogenous compounds (drugs and conjugates of glutathione with xenobiotics).***

Of particular relevance to the canalicular secretion of toxic chemicals are the canalicular MOAT (multiple organic anion transporter) system and the family of MDR (multi-drug-resistant) P-glycoproteins.

## TYPES OF INJURY AND TOXIC CHEMICALS

Hepatic responses to insults by chemicals depend on the intensity of the insult, the population of cells affected, and whether the exposure is acute or chronic. Acute poisoning with carbon tetrachloride causes lipid accumulation rapidly before necrosis is evident. Some chemicals produce a very specific type of damage; other chemicals, notably ethanol, produce sequential types of damage or combinations of damage (Table 13-2). Note that the representative hepatotoxins listed in Table 13-2 include drugs (valproic acid, cyclosporin A, dacarbazine), a vitamin (vitamin A), metals (Fe, Cu, Mn), hormones (estrogens and androgens), industrial chemicals (dimethylformamide, methylene dianiline), compounds found in teas (germander) or foods (phallodin), and toxins produced by fungi (sporidesmin) and algae (microcystin). See Fig. 13-5 for the structures of representative hepatotoxic chemicals.

### Fatty Liver

Fatty liver, also known as steatosis, is defined biochemically as an increase in the hepatic lipid content to greater than 5 percent by weight. Histologically, in standard paraffin-embedded and solvent-extracted sections, hepatocytes containing excess fat appear to have multiple round, empty vacuoles which displace the nucleus to the periphery of the cell. Frozen sections and special stains readily document the contents of the vesicles as fat. Fatty liver can stem from one or more of the following events: oversupply of free fatty acids to the liver, interference with the triglyceride cycle, increases in the synthesis or esterification of fatty acids, decreased fatty acid oxidation, decreased apoprotein synthesis, and decreased synthesis or secretion of very low density lipoproteins.

Steatosis is a common response to acute exposure to many but not all hepatotoxins (Farrell, 1994). An exception is provided by acetaminophen. A compound that produces steatosis associated with lethality is the drug valproic acid (Hall, 1994). However, toxin-induced steatosis often is reversible and does not necessarily lead to the death of hepatocytes. The metabolic inhibitors ethionine, puromycin, and cycloheximide cause fat accumulation without causing the death of cells. Many other conditions besides toxin exposure, such as obesity, are associated with marked fat accumulation in the liver. Therefore, assumptions about cause-and-effect relationships in regard to toxins and steatosis should be made judiciously.

### Hepatocyte Death

Hepatocytes can die by two different modes: necrosis and apoptosis. *Necrosis* is associated with cell swelling, leakage, nuclear disintegration, and an influx of inflammatory cells. *Apoptosis* is associated with cell shrinkage, nuclear fragmentation, the formation of apoptotic bodies, and a lack of inflammation. Apoptosis is more difficult to detect histologically because of the rapid removal of affected cells (Corcoran et al., 1994). Lysed debris of necrotic cells can persist for days when large numbers of cells die.

When necrosis occurs in hepatocytes, the associated plasma membrane leakage can be detected biochemically by assaying plasma (or serum) for liver cytosol-derived enzymes, including lactate dehydrogenase and the transaminases [alanine aminotransferase (ALT) and aspartate aminotransferase (AST)]. Biochemical assays provide a relatively simple method for screening populations for potential liver necrosis caused by occupational or environmental toxins. A careful occupational health study by Redlich and associates (1988, 1990) in a New Haven, Connecticut, plant with primitive systems for worker protection found that exposure to dimethylformamide was associated with liver damage. Transaminase levels were appreciably elevated in most of the exposed workers; however, liver biopsies indicated that a substantial cause of the liver damage in one of the workers was an infectious agent. Thus, a limitation of biochemical indexes of liver necrosis is their inability to distinquish between chemically induced effects and other causes, such as the hepatitis virus.

Hepatocyte death can occur in a focal, zonal, or panacinar (panlobular) pattern. Focal cell death is characterized by the randomly distributed death of single hepatocytes or small clusters of hepatocytes. Zonal necrosis refers death to hepatocytes predominantly in zone 1 (periportal) or zone 3 (centrolobular). Many toxins cause zone 3 necrosis, while fewer agents are known to specifically damage cells in zone 1 or zone 2. Information about the zonal location of injury by a given chemical helps identify a sensitive biochemical index of liver injury. For example, in vivo cytochrome P-450–dependent metabolism of the drug aminopyrine is lowered after zone 3 damage but not after zone 1 damage (Farag and Volicer, 1985).

**Table 13–2**
**Types of Hepatic Injury**

| INJURY TYPE | REPRESENTATIVE TOXINS |
|---|---|
| Fatty liver | $CCl_4$, ethanol, valproic acid |
| Hepatocyte death | Acetaminophen, Cu, dimethylformamide, ethanol, Fe, germander, microcystin |
| Canalicular cholestasis | Chlorpromazine, cyclosporin A, 1,1-dichloroethylene, estrogens, ethanol, Mn, phalloidin |
| Bile duct damage | ANIT, methylene dianiline, sporidesmin |
| Cirrhosis | Arsenic, ethanol, pyrrolizidine alkaloids, vitamin A |
| Vascular disorders | Arsenic, dacarbazine, pyrrolizidine alkaloids, microcystin |
| Tumors | Aflatoxins, androgens, thorium dioxide, vinyl chloride |

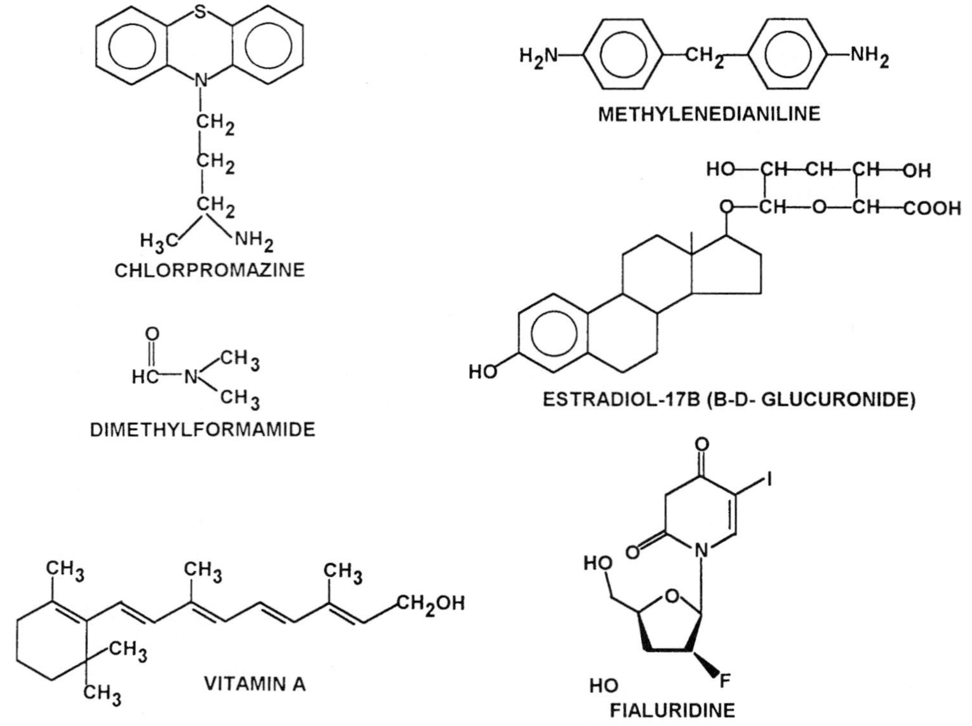

*Figure 13–5. Structures of representative hepatotoxic chemicals.*

Some reasons for the zonal specificity of chemical toxins will be discussed in the subsequent section on "Factors in Liver Injury." Zone 3 necrosis can affect only a narrow rim of cells around the central vein or can extend into zone 2. Panacinar necrosis refers to massive death of hepatocytes with only a few if any remaining survivors. An intermediate form of substantial necrosis is called bridging necrosis because the extensive zones of cell lysis become confluent with each other. The mechanisms of acute toxin-induced necrosis include lipid peroxidation, binding to cell macromolecules, mitochondrial damage, disruption of the cytoskeleton, and massive calcium influx. A mechanism for hepatoycte death after repeated chemical exposure is antibody-mediated immune attack.

## Canalicular Cholestasis

Canalicular cholestasis is defined physiologically as a decrease in the volume of bile formed or an impaired secretion of specific solutes into bile. Cholestasis is characterized biochemically by elevated serum levels of compounds that normally are concentrated in bile, particularly bile acids and bilirubin. When biliary excretion of the yellowish bilirubin pigment is impaired, this pigment accumulates in the skin and eyes, producing jaundice, and spills into urine, coloring the urine bright yellow or dark brown. Dyes that are excreted in bile, such as bromsulphalein (BSP), have been used to assess biliary function. The histological features of cholestasis can be very subtle and difficult to detect without ultrastructural studies. Structural changes include dilation of bile canaliculis and the presence of bile plugs in bile ducts and canaliculi. Chemical-induced cholestasis can be transient or chronic; when substantial, it is associated with cell necrosis. Many different types of chemicals, including metals, hormones, and drugs, cause cholestasis (Table 13-2); some provide valuable experimental models (Table 13-3).

## Bile Duct Damage

Another name for damage to the intrahepatic bile ducts is cholangiodestructive cholestasis (Cullen and Ruebner, 1991). A useful biochemical index of bile duct damage is leakage of enzymes localized to bile ducts, particularly alkaline phosphatase. In addition, serum levels of bile acids and cholesterol are elevated, as is observed with canalicular cholestasis. The initial lesions after a single dose of cholangiodestructive agents include swollen biliary epithelium, debris of damaged cells in ductal lumens, and inflammatory cell infiltration of portal tracts. Chronic administration of toxins that cause bile duct destruction can lead to biliary duct proliferation and fibrosis resembling biliary cirrhosis. Another response to hepatotoxic drugs is the loss of bile ducts; this is known as the vanishing bile duct syndrome. A noteworthy cause of bile duct damage is methylene dianiline, a compound used to make epoxy resins. Epidemiological studies have established this chemical as the causal agent of "Epping jaundice," which was an outbreak of jaundice and severe hepatobiliary disease in more than 80 residents of the English village of Epping; the affected villagers had eaten bread made from flour contaminated with methylene dianiline (Kopelman et al., 1966). Small doses of methylene dianiline produce selective bile duct injury and thus

**Table 13–3**
**Experimental Hepatotoxicants**

| | |
|---|---|
| Acetaminophen | Diethylnitrosamine |
| Allyl alcohol | Estrogens |
| ANIT | Methylene dianiline |
| Vitamin A ± $CCl_4$ | Microcystin |
| 1,1-Dichloroethylene | Mn plus bilirubin |

provide an experimental model for studying the mechanisms of chemically induced bile duct damage (Kanz et al., 1992).

### Cirrhosis

Cirrhoses is the end stage of chronic liver injury in which extensive amounts of fibrous tissue, specifically collagen fibers, are deposited in response to direct injury or inflammation. Fibrosis can develop around central veins or portal tracts or may be deposited in the space of Disse, which limits the diffusion of material from the sinusoid. With repeated chemical insults, destroyed hepatic cells are replaced by fibrotic scars. With continuing fibrosis, the architecture of the liver is disrupted by interconnecting fibrous scars. When the liver becomes subdivided by scar tissue surrounding nodules of regenerating hepatocytes, this is termed cirrhosis. Cirrhosis is not reversible and has a poor prognosis for survival. Cirrhosis is usually a result of repeated exposure to chemical toxins.

### Vascular Disorders

Vascular disorders can occur in sinusoids or in large vessels. When sinusoids are affected, the fenestrae enlarge to such an extent that red blood cells are trapped in the fenestrae or pass through the fenestrae to become trapped in the space of Disse. Such changes have been illustrated by scanning electron microscopy after large doses of the drug acetaminophen (Walker et al., 1983). A consequence is that the liver becomes engorged with blood cells while the rest of the body goes into shock; microcystin produces this effect within hours in rodents (Hooser et al., 1989). Microcystin dramatically deforms hepatocytes by altering cytoskeleton actin filaments but does not affect sinusoidal cells (Hooser et al., 1991). Thus, the deformities that microcystin produces on the cytoskeleton of hepatocytes probably produce a secondary change in the structural integrity of the sinusoid as a result of the close proximity of hepatocytes to sinusoidal endothelial cells (Fig. 13-3).

Another form of vascular injury is veno-occlusive disease, which results from nonthrombotic obstruction of the terminal hepatic venules and the smaller intrahepatic veins. A potential aspect of the pathogenesis is destruction of the endothelium of hepatic venules (Farrell, 1994). Dacarbazine, an alkylating chemotherapeutic drug, is an established cause of veno-occlusive disease; in vitro studies indicate that the selective toxicity of dacarbazine to sinusoidal endothelial cells is related to a greater imbalance between bioactivation and detoxification in this cell type than in hepatocytes (DeLeve, 1994).

### Tumors

Chemical-induced neoplasia can involve hepatocellular tumors that are derived from hepatocytes or the rare, highly malignant angiosarcomas that are derived from sinusoidal lining cells. Androgens and alflatoxins are linked to hepatocellular tumors. Angiosarcomas have been closely associated with occupational exposure to vinyl chloride, arsenic, and thorium dioxide (Farrell, 1994). The history of thorium dioxide is a tale of a useful agent with a very detrimental effect because of its site of accumulation. Between 1920 and 1950 at least 50,000 people were given suspensions of thorium dioxide, known as thorotrast, as a radioactive contrast medium. This compound accumulates in Kupffer cells, the resident macrophages of the sinusoids, and emits radioactivity throughout its very extended half-life. Thus, it is not surprising that liver tumors found in patients who were given thorium dioxide are derived from sinusoidal cells.

## FACTORS IN LIVER INJURY

Why is the liver the target site for so many chemicals with diverse structures? Our understanding of this fundamental question is incomplete, yet several key factors are known. Location is a determining factor for hepatotoxicity. A high biotransformation capacity is a critical factor for many xenobiotics, especially since hepatic biotransformation processes are readily modified by exposure to other chemicals. In the last decade, a new appreciation has emerged for factors that concern the interrelationships between hepatocytes and sinusoidal cells and the critical influence of inflammatory cells.

### Uptake, Accumulation, and Excretion

The location of the liver downstream of portal blood flow from the gastrointestinal tract positions it for "first-pass" uptake of ingested toxic chemicals. Lipophilic compounds, particularly drugs and environmental pollutants, readily diffuse into hepatocytes because the fenestrated epithelium of the sinusoid facilitates close contact between circulating molecules and the hepatocyte membrane. Thus, the membrane-rich liver concentrates lipophilic compounds. Other toxins are rapidly extracted from portal blood because they are substrates for sinusoidal transport processes that are specific for the liver.

Phalloidin and microcystin are illustrative examples of hepatotoxins which target the liver as a consequence of extensive uptake into hepatocytes by the sinusoidal bile acid transporters (Frimmer, 1992; Eriksson et al., 1990). Ingestion of the mushroom *Amanita phalloides* is a common cause of severe, acute hepatotoxicity in continental Europe and North America; outbreaks of hepatotoxicity have occurred in sheep and cattle after they drank water containing the blue-green algae *Microcystis aeruginosa* (Farrell, 1994). An early clue to preferential uptake as a factor in the target organ specificity of phalloidin was the observation that bile duct ligation, which elevates systemic bile acid levels, protects rats against phalloidin-induced hepatotoxicity in association with an 85 percent decrease in hepatic uptake of phalloidin (Walli et al., 1981). Subsequent in vitro studies found that coexposure to other substrates for the bile acid transport system (e.g., cyclosporin A, rifampicin) prevented the hepatotoxicity of phalloidin and microcystin (Ziegler and Frimmer, 1984; Ericksson et al., 1990).

Accumulation in liver cells by processes that facilitate uptake and storage is a determining factor in the hepatotoxicity of vitamin A and several metals. Ito cells actively extract and store vitamin A. When large doses of this vitamin are taken, Ito cells become engorged and hyperplastic and protrude into the sinusoid. Prolonged ingestion of vitamin A at doses therapeutic for dermatologic problems produces severe liver damage, including fatal cirrhosis (Geubel et al., 1991).

Hepatocytes regulate the homeostasis of Fe and Cu by extracting those metals from the sinusoid by receptor-medi-

**Table 13–4**
**Mechanisms of Zonal Injury**

| TOXICANT | MECHANISM OF CELL INJURY | POTENTIAL EXPLANATION FOR ZONAL INJURY |
|---|---|---|
| *Zone 1* | | |
| Fe overload | Stimulation of lipid peroxidation | Zone 1 stores more Fe than does zone 3. |
| Allyl alcohol | Oxidation to acrolein | Zone 1 has more $O_2$. |
| *Zone 3* | | |
| $CCl_4$ | P-450 activation to $\cdot CCl_3$ free radical | Zone 3 has more P-450 and less $O_2$. |
| Acetaminophen | Imbalance between cytochrome P-450 activation and glutathione detoxification | Zone 3 has more P-450 and less glutathione |

ated processes. The metals are stored in specific proteins (ferritin or metallothionein), with excess amounts stored in lysosomes (Bacon and Britton, 1989; Gollan, 1990). Acute Fe toxicity is most commonly observed in young children who accidentally ingest iron tablets, while acute Cu toxicity is due to accidental or suicidal ingestion (Farrell, 1994). The cytotoxicity of free Fe and free Cu is attributed to their function as electron donors for the formation of reactive oxygen species that initiate destructive lipid peroxidation reactions. The accumulation of excess Fe or Cu is initially evident in zone 1 hepatocytes, which have first contact with blood entering the acinus. Thus, the zone 1 pattern of hepatocyte damage after acute iron poisoning is attributable to both location for preferential Fe uptake and higher oxygen concentrations that facilitate the subsequent injurious process of lipid peroxidation (Table 13-4).

Less is known about excretion processes as factors in hepatoxicity than is known about the impact of uptake or accumulation. Excretion has been proposed as the phase III reaction to xenobiotics after phase I activation and phase II conjugation reactions (Ishikawa, 1992). Defects in the excretion of Fe and Cu lead to progressive accumulation of toxic levels in hepatocytes in the genetic disorders hemochromatosis and Wilson's disease, respectively. The molecular defect in Wilson's disease consists of an inability to transport Cu across the bile canalicular membrane (Gollan, 1990; Bull et al., 1993).

## Bioactivation and Detoxification

Hepatocytes have very high constituitive activities of many phase I enzymes that convert xenobiotics to reactive electrophiles, including cytochrome P-450 isozymes, alcohol dehydrogenases, and quinone reductases. Also, hepatocytes have a rich collection of phase II enzymes that add a polar group to a molecule and thus enhance its removal from the body. Phase II reactions usually yield stable, nonreactive metabolites. In general, the balance between phase I and phase II reactions governs whether a compound initiates liver cell injury or is safely detoxified. The balance can be shifted toward liver injury by preexposure to conditions that enhance bioactivation processes or impair detoxification processes. Potent enhancing conditions include drug- or pollutant-related induction of activating enzymes and depletion of antioxidants.

Cytochrome P-450–dependent conversion of $CCl_4$ to $\cdot CCl_3$ and then to $CCl_3OO\cdot$ is the classic example of xenobiotic biotransformation to a free radical that initiates lipid peroxidation by abstracting a hydrogen atom from the polyunsaturated fatty acid of a phospholipid (Recknagel, 1967). Many treatments and conditions modulate the extent of liver damage produced by $CCl_4$. Protective situations include: baby animals with little cytochrome P-450, treatments with compounds that inhibit cytochrome P-450, pretreatment with a small dose of the same toxin that diminishes cytochrome P-450 levels, and hyperoxia, since $O_2$ competes with $CCl_4$ for electrons from cytochrome P-450 (Reynolds and Moslen, 1980; Burk et al., 1986). Augmenting situations include pretreatment with other chemicals, notably ethanol and acetone, that induce CYP 2E1, the isozyme most effective in the activation of $CCl_4$; hypoxia; diabetes; pretreatment with aliphatic alcohols; and diets low in vitamin E, since this antioxidant scavenges lipid peroxide radicals (Hewitt et al., 1980; Lindros et al., 1990). $CCl_4$-induced injury is of interest as a readily reproducible model for lipid peroxidation and subsequent events, including alterations in the intracellular Ca pool and injury to the endoplasmic reticulum. Investigations of this classic toxin helped clarify factors critical to the injury produced by other agents which also cause lipid peroxidation.

Cytochrome P-450–dependent bioactivation of acetaminophen to a reactive electrophile (Fig. 13-6) is a serious clinical problem and a well-characterized model of cell damage linked to the formation of stable adducts between a chemical and macromolecules, which often is called covalent binding (Farrell, 1994). Typical therapeutic doses of acetaminophen are not hepatotoxic, since the dominant pathway of biotransformation is conjugation with glucuronide or sulfate (Fig. 13-6). Ethanol induction of the cytochrome P-450 isozyme CYP 2E1 shifts the balance toward the bioactivation reaction and is consistent with the marked enhancement of acetaminophen toxicity in alcoholics (Lieber, 1994). Injury after large doses of acetaminophen is enhanced by fasting and other conditions that de-

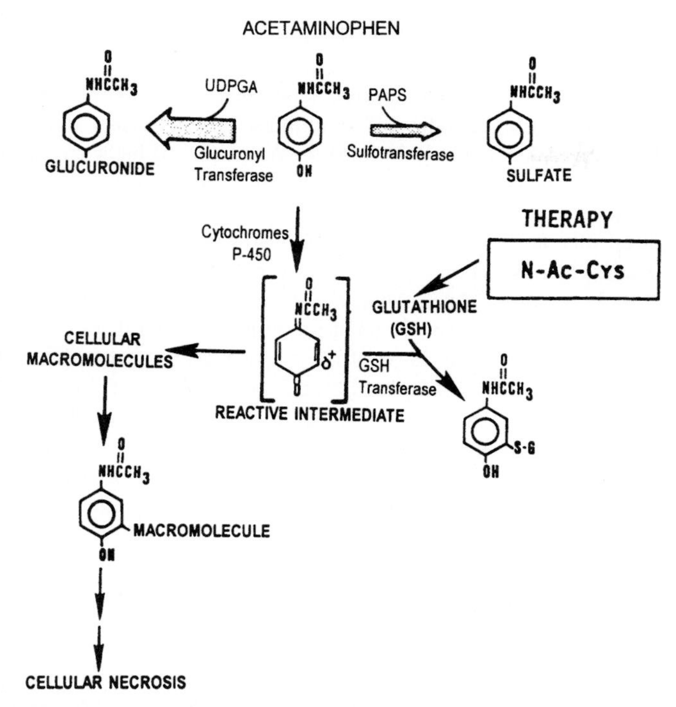


*Figure 13–6. Biotransformation of acetaminophen.*

As indicated by the larger arrows, the dominant pathways lead to glucuronide and sulfate conjugates, while the pathway leading to adducts with macromolecules is a minor pathway. Therapy with the glutathione precursor *N*-acetyl-cysteine (N-Ac-Cys) facilitates detoxification of the reactive intermediate. (Modified from To EAC, Wells PG: Biochemical changes associated with potentiation of acetaminophen hepatotoxicity by brief anesthesia with diethyl ether. *Biochem Pharmacol* 35:4139–4152, 1986.)

plete glutathione and is minimized by treatments that enhance hepatocyte synthesis of glutathione, particularly cysteine, the rate-limiting amino acid in glutathione synthesis. The introduction of interventive therapy with *N*-acetylcysteine, a well-tolerated source of intracellular cysteine, has saved the lives of many people who took overdoses of acetaminophen, usually in suicide attempts (Smilkstein et al., 1988).

Close parallels between the glutathione status, the extent of adduct formation, and the magnitude of liver injury provide strong evidence that adduct formation is associated with the toxicity of acetaminophen (Mitchell et al., 1973). The introduction of antibodies that recognize adducts of acetaminophen to macromolecules demonstrated that limited numbers of hepatic proteins are targets of acetaminophen binding, and that adduct formation precedes cell leakiness (Fig. 13-7) and occurs predominantly in zone 3, where histological injury occurs (Bartolone et al., 1989; Roberts et al., 1991). A difficulty researchers have encountered in establishing cause-and-effect relationships between adducts and liver damage lies in finding an appropriate time to measure adduct formation, since adduct formation usually preceeds detectable injury and damaged cells leak adducted proteins as well as enzymes indicative of tissue-specific injury (e.g., ALT) (Fig. 13-7). A persisting question is whether adduct formation is the critical event in acetaminophen toxicity.

The hepatotoxicity of the anesthetic halothane involves bioactivation either to a free radical that initiates lipid peroxidation or to a reactive electrophile (an acid chloride) that forms adducts with liver proteins. The use of halothane as an anesthetic for adult humans has decreased as a result of its replacement by other compounds that are less prone to bioactivation, but halothane is still used for some human pediatric

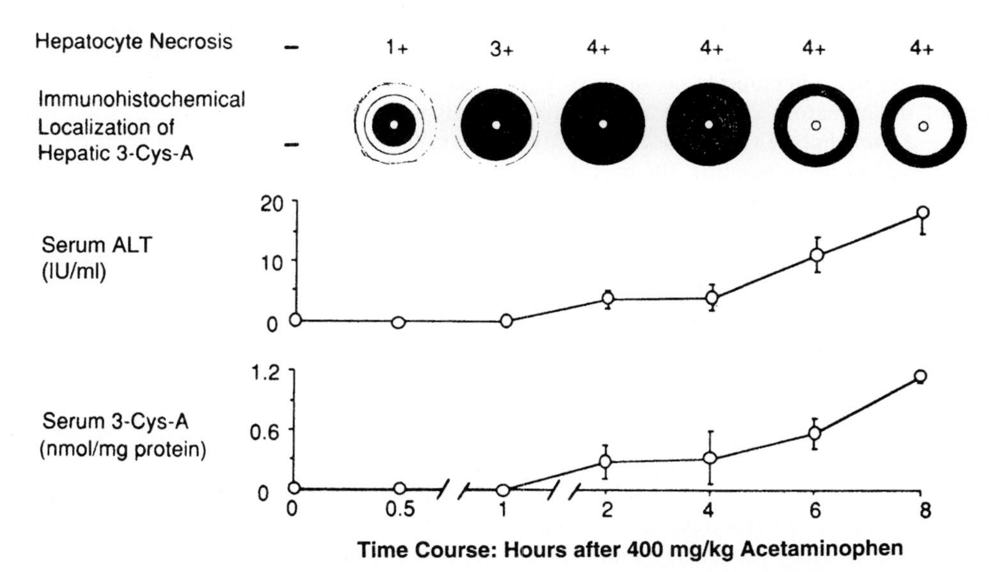


*Figure 13–7. Time course for acetaminophen hepatotoxicity and immunochemical detection of adducts between acetaminophen and proteins (3-Cys-A) in mice given 400 mg/kg acetaminophen.*

The scale for the extent of hepatocyte necrosis above the control of (−) (no pathology) is 1+ (minimal necrotic area) to 4+ (very extensive necrosis). The progressive changes in the intensity and relative density of immunohistochemically detectable acetaminophen-protein adducts are represented by circular symbols of varying diameter and density around terminal hepatic venules. The time course for leakage of the transaminase ALT into the serum parallels the rise in the serum content of the acetaminophen-protein adducts. Note that the adducts were first observed in a narrow inner ring of zone 3 cells but later became less prominent around the terminal hepatic vein as the hepatocytes became leaky. [From Roberts et al. (1991).]

and veterinary procedures. The hepatotoxicity of halothane is dependent on cytochrome P-450 bioactivation. Conditions associated with enhancement of halothane hepatotoxicity include hypoxia, hyperthyroidism, cytochrome P-450 induction, and obesity (Reynolds and Moslen, 1980; Farrell, 1994). Localization of hepatocyte injury to zone 3 after $CCl_4$ or halothane is consistent with the predominant expression of cytochrome P-450 isozmes in zone 3 (Table 13-4).

The importance of cytochrome P-450 to the bioactivation of liver toxins must be emphasized, since new instances regularly appear. The hepatotoxicity of the plant germander (*Teucrium chamaedrys* L) was recently found to be dependent on metabolism by certain cytochrome P-450 isozymes to reactive species that are detoxified by conjugation with glutathione (Loeper et al., 1994). Germander was considered a safe component of herbal teas until the consumption of capsules containing large amounts of germander for weight control was linked to multiple cases of hepatic damage in France (Larrey et al., 1992; Loeper et al., 1994). Other enzymes also convert chemicals to hepatotoxic metabolites. Alcohol dehydrogenase converts allyl alcohol to the reactive metabolite acrolein in an oxygen-dependent manner (Badr et al., 1986) that is consistent with the in vivo pattern of zone 1 injury (Table 13-3). The hepatotoxicity of allyl alcohol varies with age and sex according to the balance between acrolein formation and subsequent detoxification by aldehyde dehydrogenases (Rikans and Moore, 1987).

## INFLAMMATORY AND IMMUNE RESPONSES

The migration of neutrophils, lymphocytes, and other inflammatory cells into regions of damaged liver is a well-recognized feature of the hepatotoxicity produced by many chemicals. In fact, the potentially confusing term "hepatitis" refers to hepatocyte damage by any cause when hepatocyte death is associated with an influx of inflammatory cells. The progressive phase of alcohol-induced liver disease (between simple fatty liver and cirrhosis) is called alcoholic hepatitis. The liver damage occasionally observed after multiple exposures to the anesthetic halothane is known as halothane hepatitis.

A relevant question in regard to chemically induced acute damage to the liver is: Does the influx of inflammatory cells facilitate beneficial removal of debris from damaged liver cells, or does it contribute in a detrimental way to the extent of liver damage after chemical injury? Detrimental effects are plausible, since activated neutrophils release cytotoxic proteases and reactive oxygen species. Depletion of neutrophils was found to diminish the hepatotoxic and cholestatic effects of $\alpha$-napthylisothiocyanate (ANIT), an extensively studied compound that causes histological damage to hepatocytes and bile ducts (Dahm et al., 1991). Pretreatments with prostaglandins and other compounds with anti-inflammatory activity have been reported to reduce the acute hepatotoxicity of ANIT, $CCl_4$, and other compounds (Ruwart et al., 1984; Divald et al., 1985; Farrell, 1994). These observations merit further investigation.

Immune responses are considered to be factors in the hepatotoxicity that is observed occasionally after repeated exposure to chemicals, usually drugs. The most compelling evidence concerns the liver damage observed after multiple exposures to halothane (Pohl, 1990). The assumed scenario is as follows: During an initial exposure to halothane, biotransformation leads to adducts between halothane and liver proteins. These adducts leak out of injured hepatocytes, serve as antigens, and lead to the formation of antibodies. On reexposure to halothane, adducts are again formed. When the adducts are located on the plasma membrane of hepatocytes, such cells are vulnerable to antibody-mediated immune lysis. Immune-mediated mechanisms of liver damage also may occur for other drugs which occasionally produce liver damage upon reexposure. For example, diclofenac, a nonsteroidal anti-inflamatory drug which is extensively used for musculoskeletal diseases, occasionally produces hepatotoxicity after weeks to months of use (Sallie et al., 1991). Hepatic biotransformation of diclofenac leads to the formation of adducts on hepatocyte membrane proteins which are recognized by antibodies (Hargus et al., 1994). Shifts in the balance between activation and detoxification processes probably are also a critical factor in immune-mediated chemical hepatotoxicity.

## MECHANISMS OF LIVER INJURY

### Cholestasis

Chemicals impair bile formation by a variety of different mechanisms (Vore, 1991; Reichen, 1993) at different sites (Fig. 13-8). An increase in the leakiness of the junctions that form the structural barrier between the blood and the canalicular lumen allows solutes to leak out of the canalicular lumen. These paracellular junctions provide a size and charge barrier to the diffusion of solutes between the blood and the canalicular lumen, while water and small ions diffuse across these junctions. One hepatotoxin that causes tight junction leakage is ANIT (Krell et al., 1987).

Chemicals that disrupt the structural or functional integrity of the cytoskeleton affect bile formation by diminishing the rate and force of canalicular contractions or the rate of transcytosis across hepatocytes (Fig. 13-8). Phalloidin, a mushroom toxin that binds to cytoskeletal actin microfilaments, was observed to cause a dose-dependent slowing of canalicular contraction by elegant time-lapse photomicrographic studies of couplets of hepatocytes (Watanabe and Phillips, 1986). Colchicine, which inhibits the polymerization of tubulin into microtubules, inhibits protein secretion into bile by diminishing the microtubule-dependent transcytosis of vesicles (Vore, 1991).

Inhibition of the transporters involved in bile formation is a documented mechanism for the cholestatic effects of the immunosuppressive drug cyclosporin (Farrell, 1994). Increases in serum bile acid and bilirubin levels and a reduction in bile flow are frequent side effects of systemic cyclosporin therapy in humans and experimental animals. Recent careful studies of hepatocyte membrane fractions demonstrated that cyclosporin preferentially inhibits the ATP-dependent bile acid transporter on the canalicular membrane (Bohme et al., 1994).

Compounds that produce cholestasis do not necessarily act by a single mechanism at one site. Chlorpromazine impairs canalicular contractility and bile acid uptake (Farrell, 1994). Multiple alterations have been documented for estrogens, a well-known cause of reversible canalicular cholestasis (Vore, 1991; Bossard et al., 1993). Problems occur with both synthetic estrogens and metabolites of endogenous estrogens, particularly *D*-ring glucuronides. Estrogens decrease bile acid uptake

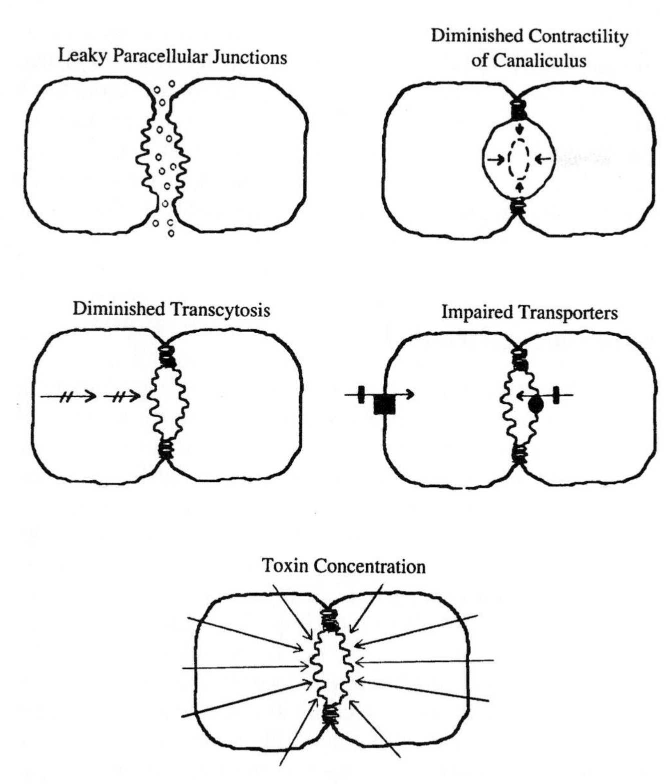


***Figure 13–8. Schematic of five potential mechanisms for cholestasis: leakiness of the junctions that seal off the canlicular lumen from the blood, diminished contractility of the canaliculus, diminished transcytosis, impairments of transporter-mediated processes on the sinusoidal and canalicular membranes, and concentration of toxic chemicals or their metabolites in the pericanalicular area.***

through their effects at the sinusoidal membrane, including a decrease in the Na/K-ATPase necessary for Na-dependent transport of bile acids across the plasma membrane and changes in the lipid components of this membrane. At the canalicular membrane, estrogens diminish the transport of glutathione conjugates and reduce the number of bile acid transporters.

An additional mechanism for canalicular cholestasis is concentration of the reactive forms of chemicals in the pericanalicular area. Most chemicals that cause canalicular cholestasis are excreted in bile; thus, the proteins and lipids in the canalicular region must encounter a high concentration of these chemicals. Observations consistent with this concentration mechanism have been reported for Mn and diclofenac. Manganese is a known cholestatic agent in humans and experimental animals (Lustig et al., 1982). Treatments that modify the extent of Mn-induced cholestasis produce consonant changes in the amount of Mn recovered in the canalicular membrane fraction (Ayotte and Plaa, 1985). Localization of drug-protein adducts to canalicular proteins is a prominent response of the liver to the drug diclofenac, whose hepatotoxicity is frequently associated with cholestasis (Hargus et al., 1994). A postulated mechanism for the bile canaliculus as the target site of 1,1-dichloroethylene is congregation of its reactive thioether glutathione conjugates (Liebler et al., 1988) in the pericanalicular region (Moslen and Kanz, 1993).

Concentration within a confined region is also a plausible factor in the target site selectivity of chemicals that damage bile ducts, since all recognized bile duct toxins are excreted in bile. Sporidesmin, a fungus-derived bile duct toxin, is concentrated in bile up to 100-fold (Farrell, 1994). The formation of a semistable conjugate of ANIT with glutathione has been postulated to promote biliary secretion of this bile duct toxicant (Carpenter-Deyo et al., 1991). Bile ducts are not passive conduits. Bile duct cells have cytochrome P-450 for bioactivation but relatively low (compared with hepatocytes) levels of glutathione and glutathione transferases (Parola et al., 1990). Thus, the balance between bioactivation and detoxification is a factor in the vulnerability of bile duct cells to chemical injury.

## Activation of Sinusoidal Cells

Acute responses to a number of chemical toxins are modifed by prior exposures to other chemicals that affect sinusoidal Kuppfer cells. A series of studies by Laskin and colleagues demonstrated that the hepatotoxicity of acetaminophen could readily be enhanced or diminished by agents that, respectively, activated or inactivated Kuppfer cells (Laskin, 1990). Similarly, Kupffer cell activation by vitamin A profoundly enhances the acute liver necrosis produced by a small dose of carbon tetrachloride (ElSisi et al., 1993). A plausible way for activated Kuppfer cells to augment hepatic injury is through the release of reactive oxygen species (Fig. 13-9). The administration of antioxidant enzymes was found to abrogate the vitamin A–enhanced hepatotoxicity of carbon tetrachloride (ElSisi et al., 1993).

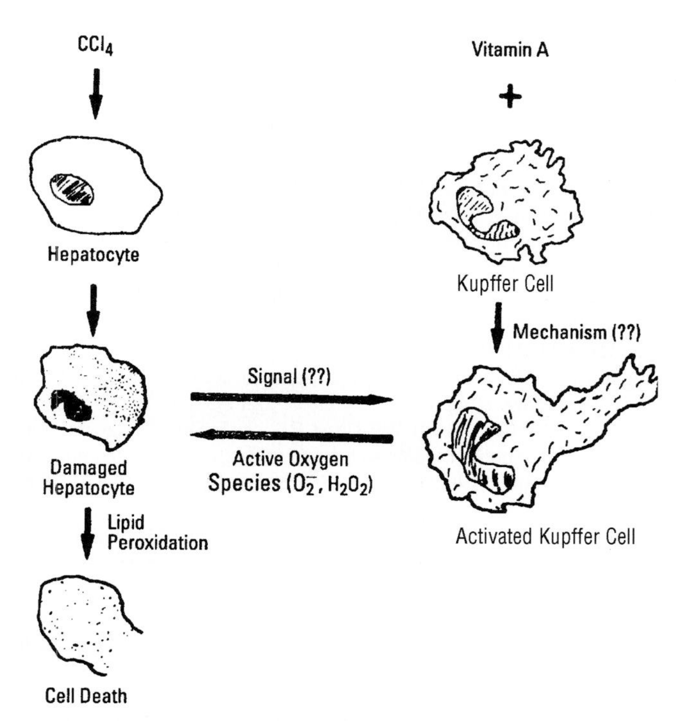


***Figure 13–9. Proposed mechanism by which pretreatment with vitamin A potentiates the hepatotoxicity of a low dose of $CCl_4$.***

Vitamin A activates Kupffer cells, and $CCl_4$ injures hepatocytes. The activated Kupffer cells respond to a signal from the injured hepatocytes by releasing active oxygen species that promote a destructive process of lipid peroxidation in the hepatocytes. [From ElSisi et al., (1993).]

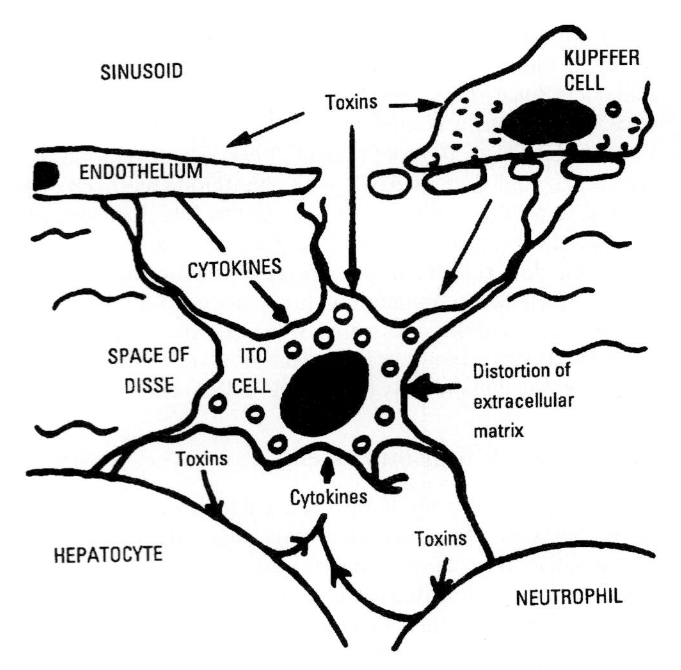


***Figure 13–10. Proposed mechanism by which toxins and other factors stimulate collagen production by Ito cells in cirrhosis.***

Toxins could directly stimulate Ito cells or could exert their effects indirectly by provoking the release of cytokines from endothelial cells, Kupffer cells, or hepatocytes. [Modified from Crawford (1994).]

Activation of sinusoidal lining cells is also a known factor in the fibrotic and cirrhotic responses of the liver to chronic exposures to chemical toxins. Toxic chemicals are thought to stimulate collagen synthesis by Ito cells either directly or indirectly via cytokines released from other liver cells or lymphoctyes (Fig. 13-10). This stimulation is important since Ito cells become the major source of the excess collagen fiber (scar tissue) that is a central feature of cirrhosis.

## Experimental Models

Our understanding of the mechanisms and critical factors in chemically mediated hepatotoxicity will improve because of model systems that allow the observation of events at the level of the cell, organnelle, and molecule. Advances in the area of cholestasis are possible using highly purifed canalicular membranes and hepatocyte couplets that secrete bile. The consequences of damage to specific parts of the liver will be clarified through experiments with chemicals that have defined target sites (Table 13-4). Important interrelationships between sinusoidal cells and other types of liver cells can be identified by using coculture systems or treatments that modify the functions of sinusoidal cells. Transgenic mice and other applications of molecular biology will provide insight into the roles of biotransformation and excretion processes in hepatotoxicity.

# REFERENCES


Ayotte P, Plaa GL: Hepatic subcellular distribution of manganese in manganese and manganese-bilirubin induced cholestasis. *Biochem Pharmacol* 34:3857–3865, 1985.

Bacon BR, Britton RS: The pathology of hepatic iron overload: A free radical-mediated process? *Hepatology* 11:127–137, 1990.

Badr MZ, Belinsky SA, Kauffman FC, Thurman RG: Mechanism of hepatotoxicity to periportal regions of the liver lobule due to allyl alcohol: Role of oxygen and lipid peroxidation. *J Pharmacol Exp Ther* 238:1138–1142, 1986.

Ballatori N: Mechanisms of metal transport across liver cell plasma membranes. *Drug Metab Rev* 23:83–132, 1991.

Bartolone JB, Beirschmitt WP, Birge RB, et al.: Selective acetaminophen metabolite binding to hepatic and extrahepatic proteins: An in vivo and in vitro analysis. *Tox Appl Pharmacol* 99:240–249, 1989.

Bohme M, Muller M, Leier I, et al.: Cholestasis caused by inhibition of the adenosine triphosphate-dependent bile salt transporter in rat liver. *Gastroenterology* 107:255–265, 1994.

Bossard R, Stieger B, O'Neill B, et al.: Ethinylestradiol treatment induces multiple canalicular membrane transport alterations in rat liver. *J Clin Invest* 91:2714–2720, 1993.

Bull PC, Thomas GR, Rommens JM, et al.: The Wilson disease gene is a putative copper transporting P-type ATPase similar to the Menkes gene. *Nature Genet* 5:327–337, 1993.

Burk RF, Reiter R, Lane JM: Hyperbaric oxygen protection against carbon tetrachloride hepatotoxicity in the rat: Association with altered metabolism. *Gastroenterology* 90:812–818, 1986.

Carpenter-Deyo L, Marchand DH, Jean PA, et al.: Involvement of glutathione in α-napthylisothiocyanate (ANIT) metabolism and toxicity to isolated hepatocytes. *Biochem Pharmacol* 42:2171–2180, 1991.

Corcoran GB, Fix L, Jones DP, et al.: Apoptosis: Molecular control point in toxicity. *Toxicol Appl Pharmacol* 128:169–191,1994.

Crawford JM: The liver and the biliary tract, in Cotran RS, Kumar V, Robbins SL (eds): *Robbins: Pathological Basis of Disease,* 5th ed. Philadelphia: Saunders, 1994, pp 831–896.

Cullen JM, Ruebner BH: A histopathologic classification of chemical-induced injury of the liver, in Meeks RG, Harrison SD, Bull RJ (eds): *Hepatotoxicology.* Boca Raton, FL: CRC Press, 1991, pp 67–92.

Dahm LJ, Schultze AE, Roth RA: An antibody to neutrophils attenuates α-napthylisothiocyanate-induced liver injury. *J Pharmacol Exp Ther* 256:412–420, 1991.

DeLeve LD: Dacarbazine toxicity in murine liver cells: A model of hepatic endothelial injury and glutathione defense. *J Pharmacol Exp Ther* 268:1261–1270, 1994.

Divald A, Ujhelyi E, Jeney A, et al.: Hepatoprotective effects of prostacyclins on $CCl_4$-induced liver injury in rats. *Exp Mol Pathol* 42:163–166, 1985.

Dutczak WJ, Clarkson TW, Ballatori N: Biliary-hepatic recycling of a xenobiotic: Galbladder absorption of methyl mercury. *Am J Physiol* 260:G873–G880, 1991.

ElSisi AED, Earnest DL, Sipes IG: Vitamin A potentiation of carbon-tetrachloride hepatotoxicity: Role of liver macrophages and active oxygen species. *Toxicol Appl Pharmacol* 119:295–301, 1993.

Eriksson JE, Gronberg L, Nygard S, et al.: Hepatocellular uptake of $^3$H-dihydromicrocystin-LR, a cyclic peptide toxin. *Biochim Biophys Acta* 1025:60–66, 1990.

Farag MM, Volicer L: Aminopyrine breath test and zonal hepatic damage in rats. *Pharmacology* 31:309–317, 1985.

Farrell GC: *Drug-Induced Liver Disease*. Edinburgh: Churchill Livingstone, 1994.

Frimmer M: Organotropism by carrier-mediated transport. *Trends Pharmacol Sci* 3:395–397, 1982.

Geubel AP, De Galocsy C, Alves N, et al.: Liver damage caused by therapeutic vitamin A administration: Estimate of dose-related toxicity in 41 cases. *Gastroenterology* 100:1701–1709, 1991.

Gollan JL: Copper metabolism, Wilson's disease, and hepatic copper toxicosis, in Zakim D, Boyer TD (eds): *Hepatology: A Textbook of Liver Disease. Philadelphia: Saunders, 1990, pp 1249–1272.*

Gosland M, Tsuboi C, Hoffman T, et al: 17 $\beta$-Estradiol glucuronide: An inducer of cholestasis and a physiological substrate for the multidrug resistance transporter. *Cancer Res* 53:5382–5385, 1993.

Groothuis GMM, Hardonk MJ, Keulemans KPT, et al.: Autoradiographic and kinetic demonstration of acinar heterogeneity of taurocholate transport. *Am J Physiol* 243:G455–G462, 1982

Hall P: Histopathology of drug-induced liver disease, in Farrell GC (ed): *Drug-Induced Liver Disease*. Edinburgh: Churchill Livingstone, 1994, pp 115–151.

Hargus SJ, Amouzedeh HR, Pumford NR, et al.: Metabolic activation and immunochemical localization of liver protein adducts of the nonsteroidal anti-inflammatory drug diclofenac. *Chem Res Toxicol* 7:575–582, 1994.

Hewitt WR, Miyajima H, Cote MG, Plaa GL: Modification of haloalkane-induced hepatotoxicity by exogenous ketones and metabolic ketosis. *Fed Proc* 39:3118–3123, 1980

Hooser SB, Beasley VR, Lovell RA, et al.: Toxicity of microcystin LR, a cyclic heptapeptide hepatotoxin from *Microcystis aeruginosa*, to rats and mice. *Vet Pathol* 26:246–252, 1989.

Hooser SB, Beasley VR, Waite LL, et al.: Actin filament alterations in rat hepatocytes induced in vivo and in vitro by microcystin-LR, a hepatotoxin from the blue green alga, *Microcystis aeruginosa*. *Vet Pathol* 28:259–266, 1991.

Ishikawa T: The ATP-dependent glutathione S-conjugate export pump. *Trends Biol Sci* 17:462–468, 1992.

Jungermann K, Katz N: Functional specialization of different hepatocyte populations. *Pharmacol Rev* 69:708–764, 1989

Kanz MF, Kaphalia L, Kaphalia BS, et al.: Methylene dianiline: Acute toxicity and effects on biliary function. *Toxicol Appl Pharmacol* 117:88–97, 1992.

Klaassen CD: Biliary excretion of metals. *Drug Metab Rev* 5:165–193,1976.

Klaassen CD, Watkins JB: Mechanisms of bile formation, hepatic uptake, and biliary excretion. *Pharmacol Rev* 36:1–67, 1984.

Kopelman H, Scheuer PJ, Williams R: The liver lesion of the Epping jaundice. *Q J Med* 35:553–564, 1966.

Kramer B: Vinyl-chloride risks were known by many before first deaths. *Wall Street Journal*, October 2, 1974.

Krell H, Metz J, Jaeschke H, et al.: Drug-induced intrahepatic cholestasis: Characterization of different pathomechanisms. *Arch Toxicol* 60:124–130, 1987.

Larrey D, Vial T, Pauwels A, et al.: Hepatitis after germander (*Teucrium chamaedris*) ingestion: Another instance of herbal medicine hepatotoxicity. *Ann Intern Med* 117:129–132, 1992

Laskin DL: Nonparenchymal cells and hepatoxicity. *Semin Liver Dis* 10:293–304, 1990.

Lieber CS: Alcohol and the liver: 1994 update. *Gastroenterology* 106:1085–1105, 1994.

Liebler DC, Latwesen DG, Reeder TC: S-(2-chloroacetyl) glutathione, a reactive glutathione thiol ester and a putative metabolite of 1,1-dichloroethylene. *Biochemistry* 27:3652–3657, 1988.

Lindros KO, Cai Y, Penttila KE: Role of ethanol-inducible cytochrome P-450 IIE1 in carbon tetrachloride-induced damage to centrilobular hepatocytes from ethanol-treated rabbits. *Hepatology* 5:1092–1097, 1990.

Lira M, Schteingart CD, Steinbach JH, et al.: Sugar absorption by the biliary ductular epithelium of the rat: Evidence for two transport systems. *Gastroenterology* 102:563–571, 1992.

Loeper J, Descatoire V, Letteron P, et al: Hepatotoxicity of germander in mice. *Gastroenterology* 106:464–472, 1994.

Lustig S, Pitlik SD, Rosenfeld JB: Liver damage in acute self-induced hypermanganemia. *Arch Intern Med* 142:405–406, 1982

Macilwain C: NIH, FDA seeks lessons from hepatitis B drug trial deaths. *Nature* 364:275, 1993

Meeks RG, Harrison SD, Bull RJ: *Hepatoxicology*. Boca Raton, FL: CRC Press, 1991.

Meier PJ: Canalicular membrane transport processes, in Tavoloni N, Berk PD (eds): *Hepatic Transport and Bile Secretion: Physiology and Pathophysiology*. New York: Raven Press, 1993, pp 587–596.

Mitchell JR, Jollow DJ, Potter WZ, et al.: Acetaminophen-induced hepatic necrosis: IV. Protective role of glutathione. *J Pharmacol Exp Ther* 187:211–217, 1973.

Moslen MT, Kanz MF: Biliary excretion of marker solutes by rats with 1,1-dichloroethylene-induced bile canalicular injury. *Toxicol Appl Pharmacol* 122:117–130, 1993.

Parola M, Cheeseman KH, Biocca ME, et al.: Menadione and cumene hydroperoxide induced cytotoxicity in biliary epithelial cells isolated from rat liver. *Biochem Pharmacol* 39:1727–1734, 1990.

Pohl LR: Drug induced allergic hepatitis. *Semin Liver Dis* 10:305–315, 1990.

Recknagel RO: Carbon tetrachloride hepatotoxicity. *Pharmacol Rev* 19:145–208, 1967.

Redlich CA, Beckett WS, Sparer J, et al.: Liver disease associated with occupational exposure to the solvent dimethylformamide. *Ann Intern Med* 108:680–686, 1988.

Redlich CA, West AB, Fleming L, et al.: Clinical and pathological characteristics of hepatotoxicity associated with occupational exposure to dimethylformamide. *Gastroenterology* 99:748–757, 1990.

Reichen J: Mechanisms of cholestasis, in Travoloni N, Berk PD (eds): *Hepatic Transport and Bile Secretion: Physiology and Pathophysiology.* New York: Raven Press, 1993, pp 665–672.

Reynolds ES, Moslen MT: Environmental liver injury: Halogenated hydrocarbons, in Farber E, Fisher MM (eds): *Toxic Injury of the Liver*. New York: Marcel Dekker, 1980, pp 541–596.

Rikans LE, Moore DR: Effect of age and sex on allyl alcohol hepatoxicity in rats: Role of liver alcohol and aldehyde dehydrogenase activities. *J Pharmacol Exp Ther* 243:20–26, 1987.

Roberts DW, Bucci TJ, Benson RW, et al.: Immunohistochemical localization and quantification of the 3-(cystein-S-yl)-acetaminophen protein adduct in acetaminophen hepatotoxicity. *Am J Pathol* 138:359–371, 1991.

Ruwart MJ, Rush BD, Friedle NM, et al.: 16,16-Dimethyl-$PGE_2$ protection against $\alpha$-napthylisothiocyanate-induced experimental cholangitis in the rat. *Hepatology* 4:658–660, 1984.

Sallie RW, McKenzie T, Reed WD, et al.: Diclofenac hepatitis. *Aust N Z J Med* 21:251–255, 1991.

Smilkstein MJ, Knapp GL, Kulig KW, Rumack BH: Efficacy of oral *N*-acetylcysteine in the treatment of acetaminophen overdose: Analysis of the National Multicenter Study (1976–1985). *N Engl J Med* 319:1557–1562, 1988.

Smit JJM, Schlinkel AH, Oude Elferink RPJ, et al.: Homozygous disruption of the murine mdr2 P-glycoprotein gene leads to a complete absence of phospholipid from bile and to liver disease. *Cell* 75:451–462, 1993.

Sotaniemi EA, Ahlqvist RO, Pelkonen RO, et al.: Histologic changes in the liver and indices of drug metabolism in alcoholics. *Eur J Clin Pharmacol* 11:295–303, 1977.

Traber PG, Chianale J, Gumucio JJ. Physiologic significance and regulation of hepatocellular heterogeneity. *Gastroenterology* 95: 1130–1143, 1988.

Tsutsumi M, Lasker JM, Shimizu M, et al.: The intralobular distribution of ethanol-inducible P450IIE1 in rat and human liver. *Hepatology* 10:437–446, 1989.

Vore M: Mechanisms of cholestasis, in Meeks RG, Harrison SD, Bull RJ (eds) *Hepatotoxicology*. Boca Raton, FL: CRC Press, 1991 pp 525–568.

Walker RM, Racz WJ, McElligott TF: Scanning electron microscopic examination of acetaminophen-induced hepatoxicity and congestion in mice. *Am J Pathol* 113:321–330, 1983.

Walli AK, Wieland E, Wieland TH: Phalloidin uptake by the liver of cholestatic rats in vivo, in isolated perfused liver and isolated hepatocytes. *Naunyn-Schmiedebergs Arch Pharmacol* 316:257-261, 1981.

Watanabe N, Phillips MJ: Acute phalloidin toxicity in liver hepatocytes: Evidence for a possible disturbance in membrane flow and for multiple functions for actin in the liver cell. *Am J Pathol* 122:101–111, 1986.

Watanabe N, Tsukada N, Smith CR, et al.: Permeabilized hepatocyte couplets: Adenosine triphosphate-dependent bile canalicular contractions and a circumferential pericanalicular microfilament belt demonstrated. *Lab Invest* 65:203–213, 1992.

Ziegler K, Frimmer M: Cyclosporin A protects liver cells against phalloidin: Potent inhibition of the inward transport of cholate and phallotoxins. *Biochim Biophys Acta* 805:174–180, 1984.

Zimmerman HJ: *Hepatotoxicity.* New York: Appleton-Century-Crofts, 1978.

# CHAPTER 14

# TOXIC RESPONSES OF THE KIDNEY

*Robin S. Goldstein and Rick G. Schnellmann*

The functional integrity of the mammalian kidney is vital to total body homeostasis, as the kidney plays a principal role in the excretion of metabolic wastes and in the regulation of extracellular fluid volume, electrolyte composition, and acid–base balance. In addition, the kidney synthesizes and releases hormones, such as renin and erythropoietin, and metabolizes vitamin $D_3$ to the active 1,25-dihydroxy vitamin $D_3$ form. A toxic insult to the kidney therefore could disrupt any or all of these functions and could have profound effects on total body metabolism. Fortunately, the kidneys are equipped with a variety of detoxification mechanisms and have considerable functional reserve and regenerative capacities. Nonetheless, the nature and severity of the toxic insult may be such that these detoxification and compensatory mechanisms are overwhelmed, and renal failure ensues. The outcome of renal failure can be profound; permanent renal damage may result, requiring chronic dialysis treatment or kidney transplantation.

## FUNCTIONAL ANATOMY

Gross examination of a sagittal section of the kidney reveals three clearly demarcated anatomical areas: the cortex, medulla, and papilla. The cortex constitutes the major portion of the kidney and receives a disproportionately higher percentage (90 percent) of blood flow compared to the medulla (~6–10 percent) or papilla (1–2 percent). Thus, when a blood-borne toxicant is delivered to the kidney, a high percentage of the material will be delivered to the cortex and will have a greater opportunity to influence cortical, rather than medullary or papillary functions. Nonetheless, medullary and papillary tissues are exposed to higher lumenal concentrations of toxicants for prolonged periods of time, a consequence of the more concentrated tubular fluid and the more sluggish flow of blood and filtrate in these regions.

The functional unit of the kidney, the nephron, may be considered in three portions: the vascular element, the glomerulus, and the tubular element.

### Renal Vasculature and Glomerulus

The renal artery branches successively into interlobar, arcuate, and interlobular arteries. The latter gives rise to the afferent arterioles which supply the glomerulus; blood then leaves the glomerular capillaries via the efferent arteriole. Both the afferent and efferent arterioles, arranged in a series before and after the glomerular capillary tuft, respectively, are ideally situated to control glomerular capillary pressure and glomerular plasma flow rate. Indeed, these arterioles are innervated by the sympathetic nervous system, and contract in response to nerve stimulation, angiotensin II, vasopressin, endothelin, prostanoids, and cytokines, affecting glomerular pressures and blood flow. The efferent arterioles draining the cortical glomeruli branch into a peritubular capillary network, whereas those draining the juxtamedullary glomeruli form a capillary loop, the vasa recta, supplying the medullary structures (Fig. 14-1). These postglomerular capillary loops provide an efficient arrangement for delivery of nutrients to the postglomerular tubular structures, delivery of wastes to the tubule for excretion, and return of reabsorbed electrolytes, nutrients, and water to the systemic circulation.

The glomerulus is a complex specialized capillary bed composed primarily of endothelial cells that are characterized by an attenuated and fenestrated cytoplasm, visceral epithelial cells characterized by a cell body (podocyte) from which many trabeculae and pedicles (foot processes) extend, and a glomerular basement membrane (GBM) which is a trilamellar structure sandwiched between the endothelial and epithelial cells (Fig. 14-2). A portion of the blood entering the glomerular capillary network is fractionated into a virtually protein-free and cell-free ultrafiltrate which passes through Bowman's space and into the tubular portion of the nephron. The formation of such an ultrafiltrate is the net result of the Starling forces that determine fluid movement across capillary beds; that is, the balance between transcapillary hydrostatic pressure and colloid oncotic pressure (Maddox and Brenner, 1991). Filtration is therefore favored when transcapillary hydrostatic pressure exceeds plasma oncotic pressure. An additional determinant of ultrafiltration is the effective hydraulic permeability of the glomerular capillary wall; in other words, the ultrafiltration coefficient ($K_f$) which is determined by the total surface area available for filtration and the hydraulic permeability of the capillary wall. Consequently, chemically induced decreases in glomerular filtration rate (GFR) may be related to (1) decreases in transcapillary hydrostatic pressure and glomerular plasma flow due to increased afferent arteriolar resistance or to (2) decreases in the surface area available for filtration, resulting from decreases in the size and/or number of endothelial fenestrae or detachment or effacement of foot processes.

Although the glomerular capillary wall permits a high rate of fluid filtration (approximately 20 to 40 percent of blood entering the glomerulus is filtered), it provides a significant barrier to the transglomerular passage of macromolecules. Experiments using a variety of charged and neutral tracers have established that this barrier function is based on the ability of the glomerulus to act as a size-selective and charge-selective filter (Brenner et al., 1977). In general, the filtration of macromolecules is inversely proportional to the molecular weight of a substance; thus, small molecules such as inulin (MW=5000) are freely filtered while large molecules such as albumin (MW=60,000–70,000) are restricted. Filtration of anionic

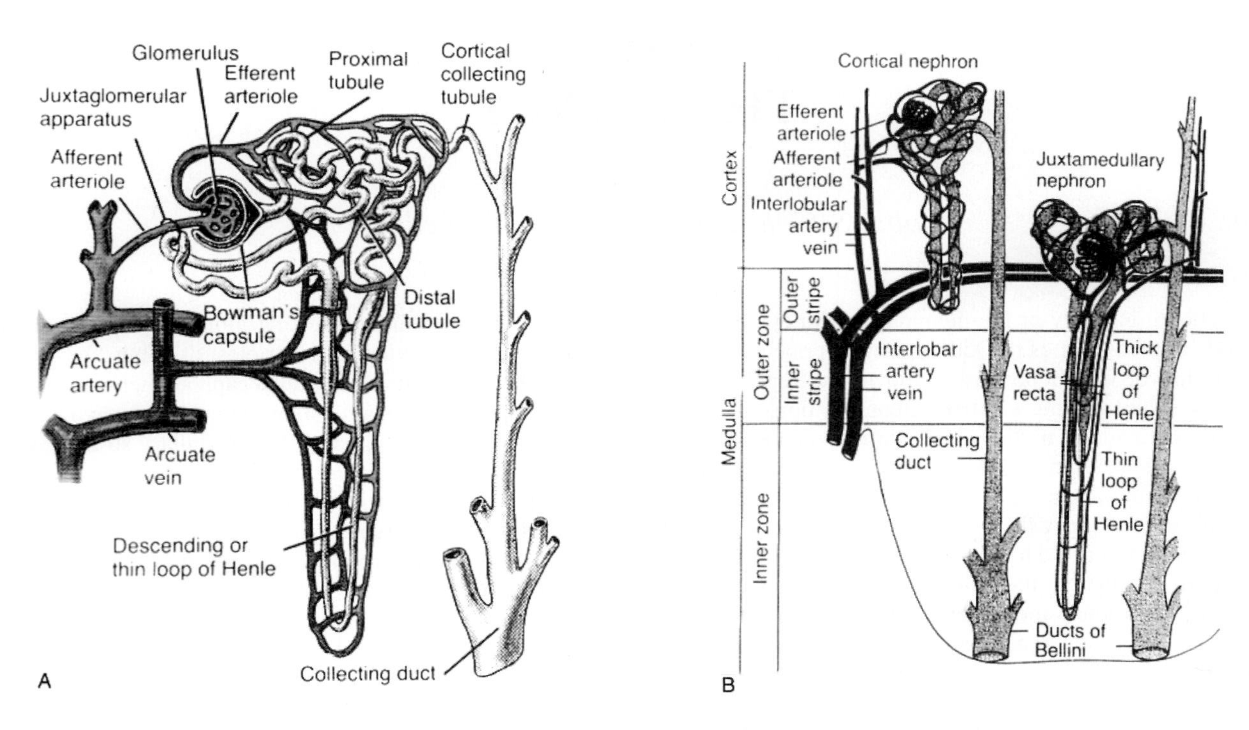


*Figure 14–1. A. The anatomy of the nephron, illustrating the vascular, glomerular, and tubular components. B. The tubular and vascular arrangement in cortical and juxtamedullary nephrons. [From Guyton, AC(ed): Textbook of Medical Physiology. Philadelphia, Saunders, 1991, p 287.]*

molecules tend to be restricted compared to neutral or cationic molecules of the same size. These permselective properties of the glomerulus appear to be directly related to the physicochemical properties of the different cell types within the glomerulus (Kanwar et al., 1991). In particular, charge-selective properties of the glomerulus appear to be related to the anionic groups of the GBM coupled with the anionic coating of the epithelial and endothelial cells. These highly anionic components produce electrostatic repulsion and hinder the circulation of polyanionic macromolecules, thereby markedly retarding passage of these molecules across the filtration barrier. Toxicants that neutralize or reduce the number of fixed anionic charges on glomerular structural elements therefore will impair the charge- and/or size-selective properties of the glomerulus, resulting in urinary excretion of polyanionic and/or large-molecular-weight proteins.

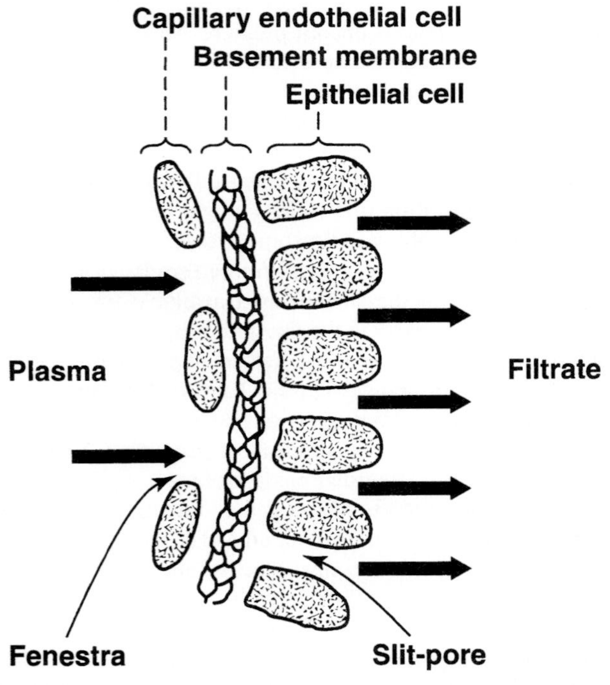

*Figure 14–2. The structure of the glomerulus. [From Guyton (1991), p 290.]*

## Proximal Tubule

The proximal tubule consists of three discrete segments: the $S_1$ (pars convoluta), $S_2$ (transition between pars convoluta and pars recta), and $S_3$ (the pars recta) segments (Tisher and Madsen, 1991) (Fig. 14-3). The $S_1$ segment is the initial portion of the proximal convoluted tubule and is characterized by a tall brush border and a well-developed vacuolar lysosomal system. The basolateral membrane is extensively interdigitated and many long mitochondria fill the basal portion of the cell, characteristic of $Na^+$-transporting epithelia. The $S_2$ segment comprises the end of the convoluted segment and the initial portion of the straight segments. These cells possess a shorter brush border, fewer apical vacuoles and mitochondria, and less basolateral interdigitation compared to the $S_1$ cells. The $S_3$ segment comprises the distal portion of proximal segments and extends to the junction of the outer and inner stripe of the outer medulla. The $S_3$ cells have a well-developed brush border, but fewer and smaller lysosomes and mitochondria than $S_1$ and $S_2$ cells.

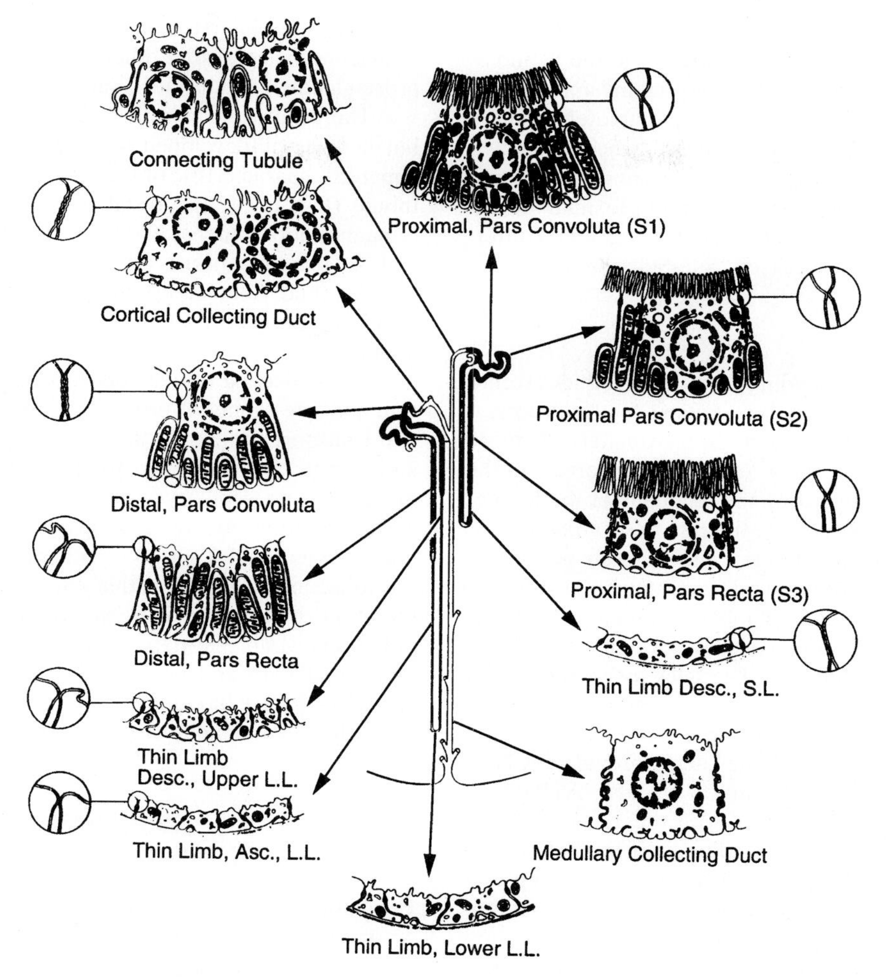


***Figure 14–3. The morphologic characteristics of the different regions of the renal tubule.***

Note that the $S_1$ segment is characterized by a tall, well-developed brush border and abundant mitochondria: the $S_2$ segment has a shorter microvillus brush border and fewer mitochondria, and the $S_3$ segment is characterized by an intermediate-sized brush border but fewer and more spherical mitochondria. All other cell types lack a brush border. [From Bulger RE, Hebert SC: Structural–functional relationships in the kidney, in Schrier RW, Gottschalk CW (eds): *Diseases of the Kidney*. Boston: Little, Brown, 1988, vol 1, pp 3–65.]

The formation of urine is a highly complex and integrated process in which the volume and composition of the glomerular filtrate is progressively altered as fluid passes through each of the different tubular segments. The proximal tubule is the workhorse of the nephron as it reabsorbs approximately 60 to 80 percent of solute and water filtered at the glomerulus. Toxicant-induced injury to the proximal tubule therefore will have major consequences to water and solute balance. Water reabsorption is an isoosmotic passive process driven primarily by $Na^+$ reabsorption, mediated by $Na^+$ $K^+$-ATPase localized in the basolateral plasma membrane. In addition to active $Na^+$ reabsorption, the proximal tubule reabsorbs other electrolytes such as $K^+$, $HCO_3^-$, $Cl^-$, $PO_4^{3-}$, $Ca^{2+}$ and $Mg^{2+}$. The proximal tubule contains numerous transport systems capable of driving concentrative transport of many metabolic substrates, including amino acids, glucose, and citric acid cycle intermediates. The proximal tubule also reabsorbs virtually all of the filtered low-molecular-weight proteins (LMWP) by specific endocytotic protein reabsorption processes. In addition, small linear peptides may be hydrolyzed by peptidases associated with the proximal tubular brush border. An important excretory function of the proximal tubule is secretion of weak organic anions and cations by specialized transporters that drive concentrative movement of these ions from postglomerular blood into proximal tubular cells, followed by secretion into tubular fluid. Toxicant-induced interruptions in the production of energy for any of these active transport mechanisms or the function of critical membrane-bound enzymes or transporters can profoundly affect proximal tubular and whole kidney function.

The different segments of the proximal tubule exhibit marked biochemical and physiological heterogeneity (Goldstein, 1993). For example, filtered $HCO_3^-$, LMWP, amino acids, and glucose are primarily reabsorbed by the $S_1$ segment. Transport capacities for these substances in the $S_2$ and $S_3$ segments are appreciably less; for example, glucose reabsorption in the $S_2$ and $S_3$ segments is about 50 percent and 10 percent of that in the $S_1$ segment, respectively. In contrast, the principle site of organic anion and cation secretion is in the $S_2$ and $S_1/S_2$ segments, respectively. Oxygen consumption, $Na^+$, $K^+$-ATPase activity, and gluconeogenic capacity are greater in the $S_1$ and $S_2$ segments than in the $S_3$ segment. Catabolism and apical transport of glutathione (GSH) occurs to a much greater extent in the $S_3$ segment, where the brush broder enzyme, γ-glutamyltranspeptidase (GGT), is present in greater amounts. Chemically induced selective injury to the different proximal tubular segments therefore may be related in part to segmental differences in biochemical properties (see "Site-Selective Injury").

## Loop of Henle

The thin descending and ascending limbs and the thick ascending limb of the loop of Henle are critical to the processes involved in urinary concentration. Approximately 20 to 30 percent of the filtered $Na^+$ and $K^+$ and 15 to 20 percent of the filtered water are reabsorbed by the segments of the loop of Henle. The tubular fluid entering the thin descending limb is isoosmotic to the renal interstitium; water is freely permeable and solutes, such as electrolytes and urea, may enter from the interstitium. The thin ascending limb, in contrast, is relatively impermeable to water. Sodium chloride but not urea, is reabsorbed here by passive diffusion. The thick ascending limb is impermeable to water. This segment of the loop is involved in the active transport of $Na^+$ and $Cl^-$ mediated by a $Na^+$-$K^+$-$Cl^-$ cotransport mechanism with the energy provided by $Na^+$, $K^+$-ATPase. The relatively high rates of $Na^+$, $K^+$-ATPase activity and oxygen demand, coupled with the meager oxygen supply in the medullary thick ascending limb, are believed to contribute to the vulnerability of this segment of the nephron to hypoxic injury. The close interdependence between metabolic workload and tubular vulnerability has been demonstrated in studies by Brezis and Epstein (1993), indicating that selective damage to the thick ascending limb in the isolated perfused kidney can be blunted by reducing tubular work and oxygen consumption (via inhibition of $Na^+$, $K^+$-ATPase with ouabain) or by increasing oxygen supply (via provision of an oxygen carrier, hemoglobin). Conversely, increasing the tubular workload (via an ionophore, amphotericin B) exacerbates hypoxic injury to this segment (Brezis et al., 1984).

## Distal Tubule and Collecting Duct

Specialized cells of the distal tubule, commonly referred to as the macula densa, are located between the end of the thick ascending limb and the early distal tubule, in close proximity to the afferent arteriole. This anatomic arrangement is ideally suited for a feedback system whereby a stimulus received at the macula densa is transmitted to the arterioles of the same nephron. Under normal physiological conditions, increased solute delivery or concentration at the macula densa triggers a signal, resulting in afferent arteriolar constriction leading to decreases in GFR (and hence decreased solute delivery). Thus, increases in fluid/solute out of the proximal tubule, due to impaired tubular reabsorption, will activate this feedback system, referred to as tubuloglomerular feedback (TGF), resulting in decreases in the filtration rate of the same nephron. This regulatory mechanism is viewed as a powerful volume-conserving mechanism, designed to decrease GFR in order to prevent massive losses of fluid/electrolytes due to impaired tubular reabsorption. Humoral mediation of TGF by the renin-angiotensin system has been proposed and several lines of evidence suggest that other substances, such as adenosine, prostaglandins, and intracellular calcium, may be involved.

The distal tubular cells contain numerous mitochondria but lack a well-developed brush border and an endocytotic apparatus characteristic of the pars convoluta of the proximal tubule (Fig. 14-3). The distal tubule reabsorbs most of the remaining intralumenal $Na^+$ in exchange for $K^+$ and $H^+$; $H^+$ and $K^+$ secretory processes are driven by $Na^+$ reabsorption. Tubular fluid volume is reduced an additional 20 to 30 percent during transit through the distal tubular segments of the nephron.

The collecting tubule and duct perform the final regulation and fine-tuning of urinary volume and composition. Active transport systems in the collecting tubule reabsorb $Na^+$ and secrete $K^+$ and $H^+$. Additionally, the combination of medullary and papillary hypertonicity generated by countercurrent multiplication and the action of antidiuretic hormone (vasopressin, ADH) serves to enhance water permeability of the collecting duct. Agents that interfere with ADH synthesis, secretion, or action therefore may impair concentrating ability. Additionally, since urinary concentrating ability is dependent upon medullary and papillary hypertonicity, agents that increase medullary blood flow may impair concentrating ability by dissipating the medullary osmotic gradient.

# ASSESSMENT OF NEPHROTOXICITY

Evaluation of the effects of a chemical on the kidney can be accomplished using a variety of both in vivo and in vitro methods (Davis and Berndt, 1994; Foulkes, 1993). Initially, nephrotoxicity can be assessed by evaluating serum chemistry and urinalyses following treatment with the chemical in question. The standard battery of noninvasive tests includes measurement of urine volume and osmolality, pH, and urinary composition (e.g., electrolytes, glucose, protein). Although specificity is often lacking in such an assessment, urinalysis provides a relatively easy and noninvasive assessment of overall renal functional integrity and can provide some insight into the nature of the nephrotoxic insult. For example, chemically induced increases in urine volume, accompanied by decreases in osmolality, may suggest an impaired concentrating ability, possibly via a defect in ADH synthesis, release, and/or action. To determine whether the impaired concentrating ability is due to an altered tubular response to ADH, concentrating ability can be determined before and after an exogenous ADH challenge. Glucosuria may reflect chemically induced defects in proximal tubular reabsorption of sugars; however, because glucosuria also may be secondary to hyperglycemia, measurement of serum glucose concentrations also must be evaluated. Urinary excretion of high-molecular-weight proteins, such as albumin, is suggestive of glomerular damage, whereas excretion of LMWP, such as $\beta_2$-microglobulin, suggests proximal tubular injury (Christensen and Nielsen, 1991) (Fig. 14-4). Urinary excretion of enzymes localized in the brush border (e.g., alkaline phosphatase, GGT) may reflect brush border damage, whereas urinary excretion of other enzymes (e.g., lactate dehydrogenase) may reflect more generalized cell damage. Enzymuria is often a transient phenomenon, as chemically induced damage may re-

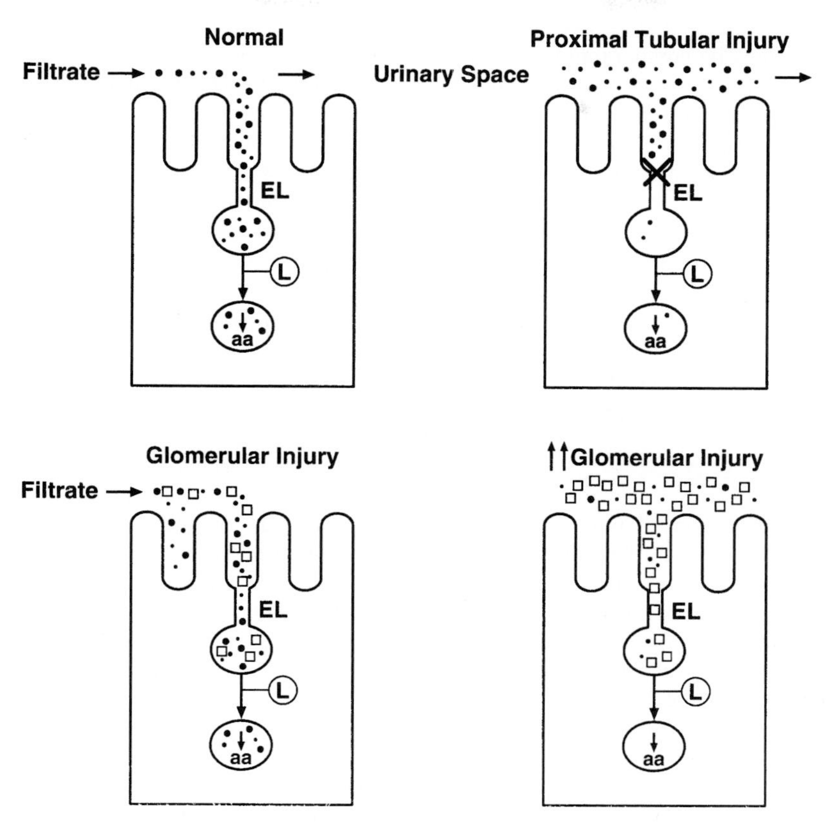


*Figure 14–4. Mechanisms of glomerular and tubular proteinuria.*

In the normal, healthy kidney, LMWP are filtered by the glomerulus and reabsorbed by an endocytotic mechanism to form an endosome (EL), which in turn fuses with lysosomes (L) where proteins are catabolized to their constituent amino acids (aa) (*upper left*). Following proximal tubular injury, formation and internalization of endocytotic vesicles may be impaired, resulting in decreased reabsorption and increased urinary excretion of LMWP (*upper right*). In mild glomerular injury, large-molecular-weight proteins, such as albumin, which traverse the glomerular barrier, may be taken up by the proximal tubule (*bottom left*); however with severe glomerular injury, proximal tubular transport of albumin is saturated, resulting in albuminuria (*bottom right*).

sult in an early loss of most (if not all) of the enzyme available. Thus, the absence of enzymuria does not necessarily reflect an absence of damage.

Serial blood samples may be obtained and blood urea nitrogen (BUN) and serum creatinine concentrations determined to assess the potential effects of a chemical on GFR. These substances are normally filtered by the glomerulus; therefore, increased serum concentrations suggest decreases in GFR. However, both serum creatinine and BUN are rather insensitive indices of GFR; a 50 to 70 percent decrease in GFR must occur before increases in serum creatinine and BUN develop. Chemically induced increases in BUN and/or serum creatinine may not necessarily reflect renal damage but rather may be secondary to dehydration, hypovolemia, and/or protein catabolism. These extrarenal events should be taken into consideration when evaluating BUN/serum creatinine as potential endpoints of renal toxicity and/or when correlating these endpoints with renal histopathology. Histopathologic evaluation of the kidney following treatment is crucial in identifying the site, nature, and severity of the nephrotoxic lesion. Assessment of chemically induced nephrotoxicity therefore should include urinalysis, serum clinical chemistry, and histopathology to provide a reasonable profile of the functional and morphological effects of a chemical on the kidney.

Once a chemical has been identified as a nephrotoxicant in vivo, a variety of in vitro techniques may be used to elucidate underlying mechanisms. Tissue obtained from naive animals may be used in the preparation of isolated perfused kidneys, kidney slices, suspensions of renal tubules, cells or subcellular organelles, or primary cultures. The reader is referred to several excellent reviews for further details on the utility and limitations of these preparations (Davis and Berndt, 1994; Tarloff and Goldstein, 1994; Ford and Williams, 1992). Such approaches may be used to distinguish between an effect on the kidney due to a direct chemical insult and one caused by extrarenal effects such as extrarenally generated metabolites, hemodynamic effects, immunological effects, and so forth. Care must be taken to ensure that the cell type affected in the in vitro model is the same as that affected in vivo. In addition, concentrations of the nephrotoxicant to be used in in vitro preparations must be comparable to that observed in vivo, as different mechanisms of toxicity may be operative at concentrations that saturate metabolic pathways or overwhelm detoxification mechanisms. Once a mechanism has been identified in vitro, the postulated mechanism needs to be tested in vivo. Thus, appropriately designed in vivo and in vitro studies should provide a complete characterization of the biochemical, functional, and morphological effects of a chemical on the kidney and an understanding of the underlying mechanisms in the target cell population(s).

## PATHOPHYSIOLOGICAL RESPONSES OF THE KIDNEY

### Acute Renal Failure

One of the most common manifestations of nephrotoxic damage is acute renal failure (ARF), characterized by an abrupt decline in GFR with resulting azotemia (Table 14-1). The course of ARF can be divided into three distinct phases: the initiation phase involving exposure of the kidney to the offending agent with marked changes in renal function, the maintenance phase characterized by the sustained loss of renal function, and, if damage is not too severe, the recovery phase marked by cell proliferation and restoration of structure and function. Importantly, there may be different pathogenic mechanisms underlying hypofiltration during these different phases.

The pathogenesis of ARF is complex (Badr and Ichikawa, 1988; Lieberthal and Levinksy, 1990; Brezis and Epstein, 1993) and may involve prerenal factors (i.e., hypovolemia, insufficient cardiac output, obstruction of renal arteries) or postrenal factors (i.e., ureteral or bladder obstruction) (Fig. 14-5). Intrarenal mechanisms mediating nephrotoxic ARF may be associated with chemically induced glomerular damage. For example, decreases in $K_f$, occurring secondary to decreases in the size and number of endothelial fenestrae or in the detachment and/or effacement of epithelial cell foot processes, will lead to decreases in GFR (Fig. 14-5). Importantly, mechanisms underlying nephrotoxicant-induced decreases in GFR are not limited to effects on the glomerulus. In fact, in most instances, ARF is associated with increased renal vascular resistance and/or tubular damage (Table 14-1). Renal vasoconstriction appears to play a contributory role in hypofiltration associated with cyclosporine (Kopp and Klotman, 1990; Racusen and Solez, 1993), amphotericin B (Sawaya et al., 1991; Tolins and Raij, 1988; Sabra and Branch, 1991), cisplatin (Borch, 1993), and radiocontrast agents (Bakris, 1993; Barrett, 1994). The exact mechanisms by which these agents induce vasoconstriction are not known but may relate in part to an imbalance in the release of vasoconstrictor and vasodilator substances. Increased release of vasoconstrictors such as endothelin and/or thromboxanes has been implicated in both cyclosporine and amphotericin B nephrotoxicity (Perico et al., 1986; Smeesters et al., 1988; Kon et al., 1990; Nambi et al., 1990; Kivlighn et al., 1994). Direct vascular damage, by causing endothelial cell swelling and by stimulating endothelin release, also may reduce blood flow. Alternatively, activation of TGF, triggered by impaired tubular reabsorption of electrolytes/fluid, may result in profound afferent arteriolar constriction, leading to a marked decline in GFR. Although renal blood flow (RBF) is recognized as a contributing factor in the pathogenesis of ARF, a number

**Table 14–1**
**Classification of Nephrotoxic Injury**

| | PATHOGENESIS | PRIMARY MECHANISM | SELECT NEPHROTOXICANTS |
|---|---|---|---|
| Acute renal failure | Hypoperfusion/ Hypofiltration | Renal vasoconstriction Glomerular injury | Amphotericin B, aminoglycosides, cyclosporine, NSAIDs, radiocontrast agents |
| | Acute tubular necrosis | Direct tubular injury | Aminoglycosides, amphotericin B, acetaminophen, $\beta$-lactams, cisplatin, halogenated hydrocarbons, heavy metals, mycotoxins, polymyxin, radiocontrast agents, vancomycin |
| | Obstruction | Intratubular obstruction | Radiocontrast agents |
| | Tubulointerstitial nephritis | Immunologic, inflammatory | $\beta$-Lactams, NSAIDs, sulfonamides, tetracycline |
| Chronic renal failure | Chronic tubulointerstitial nephritis | Immunologic, inflammatory | Analgesics, cisplatin, cyclosporine, lithium, cadmium, lead |
| | Papillary necrosis | Ischemia, cell injury | Analgesics, NSAIDs |

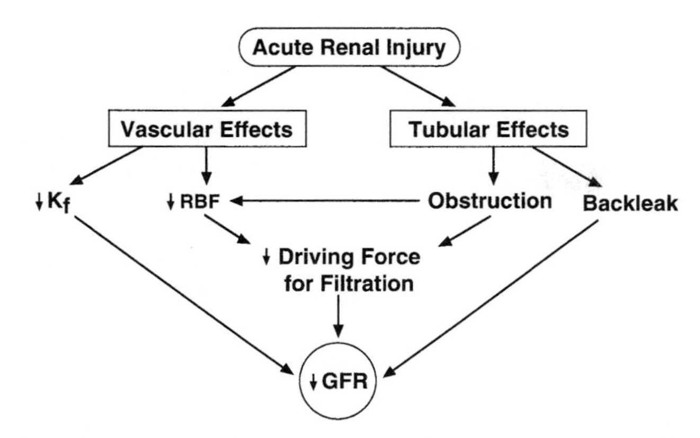


***Figure 14–5. The mechanisms contributing to decreased glomerular filtration rate (GFR) in acute renal failure.***

$K_f$, ultrafiltration coefficient; RBF, renal blood flow. [From Brezis M, et al (1993), pp 129–152.]

of observations suggest that reductions in RBF alone are unlikely to be the sole causative factor as in many cases, the decrease in GFR, particularly during the maintenance phase, is disproportionately greater than that of RBF.

Nephrotoxicant-induced decreases in GFR also may be secondary to tubular damage (Fig. 14-5). Chemically induced tubular necrosis may increase tubular permeability, resulting in diffusion and backleak of the fitrate across the tubular basement membrane back into the interstitium and circulation, leading to an apparent decrease in GFR. Under these circumstances, backleak of filtrate results in decreased excretion and increased retention of nitrogenous wastes. Tubular backleak is a contributing factor in mercuric chloride and cisplatin nephrotoxicity. Another mechanism by which tubular injury may result in hypofiltration is related to sloughing of necrotic tubular epithelium into the lumen, resulting in tubular obstruction and increased intratubular pressure, effects which will oppose the forces governing filtration.

The maintenance of tubule integrity is dependent on cell-to-cell and cell-to-matrix adhesion; these interactions are mediated in part by the integrins and cell adhesion molecules. The observation that some renal tubular cells in urine of patients with ARF are viable and not necessarily necrotic has led Goligorsky and colleagues to postulate that cell-to-matrix detachment and cell-to-cell adhesion play significant roles in ARF (Goligorsky et al., 1993). Specifically, it has been hypothesized that shortly after a nephrotoxic insult, adhesion of nonlethally damaged cells to the basement membrane is compromised, leading to their detachment from the basement membrane and appearance in the urine. Morphologically, such an event would lead to gaps in the epithelial cell lining, potentially resulting in backleak of filtrate and diminished GFR. These detached cells may aggregate in the tubular lumen (cell-to-cell adhesion) and/or adhere or re-attach to adherent epithelial cells downstream, potentially resulting in tubular obstruction. Further, it has been proposed that the loss of expression of integrins on the basolateral membrane is responsible for the exfoliation of proximal tubular cells and that redistribution of integrin receptors from the basolateral to the apical membrane facilitates adhesion of detached cells to the in situ epithelium (Goligorsky et al., 1993).

Other studies have indicated that leukocyte adhesion molecules play a critical role in ARF, possibly because of the ability of activated leukocytes to release cytokines and reactive oxygen species, resulting in capillary damage/leakage which may lead to the vascular congestion often observed in ARF. Bonventre and colleagues have demonstrated that treatment of rats with either monoclonal antibodies against the integrins, CD11a and CD11b, or with a monoclonal antibody against ICAM-1 (a ligand for CD11a) conferred significant protection against renal ischemic injury (Kelly et al., 1994; Rabb et al., 1994), suggesting a critical role for leukocyte–endothelial adhesion in the pathophysiology of ischemic ARF.

While nephrotoxicant-induced ARF can be initiated by proximal tubular cell injury, nephrotoxicants also may inhibit cellular proliferation and migration, thereby protracting the maintenance phase of ARF and delaying renal functional recovery. For example, Leonard et al. (1994) demonstrated that cisplatin impaired tubular regeneration resulting in prolonged renal dysfunction, effects that were in contrast to the regenerative response and renal functional recovery following tobramycin-induced nephrotoxicity. More recently, Counts et al. (1995) reported that following mechanically induced injury to a proximal tubule monolayer, proliferation and migration were inhibited by mercuric chloride ($HgCl_2$), the mycotoxin fumonisin $B_1$, and dichlorovinyl-L-cysteine (DCVC), suggesting that these nephrotoxicants may inhibit/delay the regenerative process.

## Adaptation Following Toxic Insult

Fortunately, the kidney has a remarkable ability to compensate for a loss in renal functional mass. Micropuncture studies have revealed that following unilateral nephrectomy, GFR of the remnant kidney increases by approximately 40 to 60 percent, an effect associated with early compensatory increases in glomerular plasma flow rate and glomerular hydraulic pressure. Compensatory increases in single-nephron GFR are accompanied by proportionate increases in proximal tubular water and solute reabsorption; glomerulotubular balance therefore is maintained and overall renal function appears normal by standard clinical tests. Consequently, chemically induced changes in renal function may not be detected until these compensatory mechanisms are overwhelmed by significant nephron loss and/or damage.

In addition to compensatory hypertrophy, there are a number of cellular and molecular responses to a nephrotoxic insult which ameliorate or prevent cell damage or death (Fig. 14-6). Two of the most notable responses are metallothionein induction (see "Cadmium" below) and the heat shock response. Heat shock proteins (Hsp) have been classified into different families based on molecular mass, are highly conserved in eukaroytes, and are induced in response to a number of pathophysiological states (Jaattela and Wissing, 1992; Hightower, 1991) such as heat shock, anoxia, oxidative stress, toxicants, heavy metal exposure, and tissue trauma. These proteins are believed to play an important housekeeping role in the maintenance of normal protein structure and/or the degradation of damaged proteins and thereby provide a defense mechanism against toxicity and/or facilitate recovery and repair. Hsp induction in renal tissue has been demonstrated following renal ischemia (Van Why et al., 1992; Enami et al. 1991), and treatment with nephrotoxicants such as gentamicin

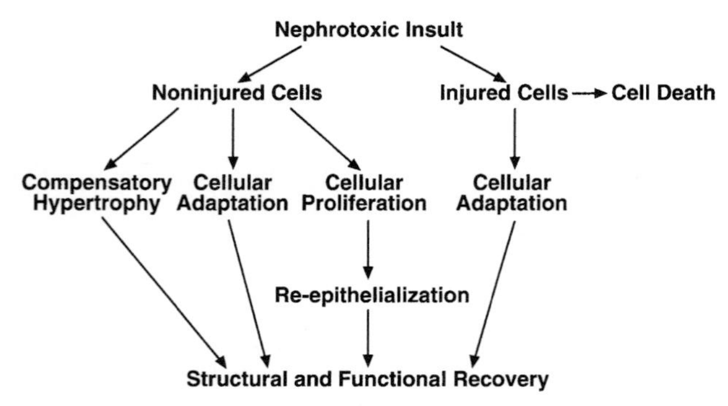


*Figure 14–6. Physiological and biochemical responses to a nephrotoxic insult.*

(Komatsuda et al., 1993), puromycin aminonucleoside (Komatsuda et al., 1992), cysteine conjugates (Chen et al., 1992), and $HgCl_2$(Goering et al., 1992). Interestingly, proximal tubular Hsps have been identified as molecular targets of the reactive metabolites of the halogenated cysteine conjugate, tetrafluoroethyl-L-cysteine (TFEC) (Bruschi et al., 1993), an effect that could alter the normal housekeeping functions of the proximal tubule and thereby potentially contribute to and exacerbate TFEC nephrotoxicity.

Recovery from a nephrotoxic injury requires tissue repair and regeneration in which viable cells adjacent to the site of injury undergo dedifferentiation, proliferation, migration, and differentiation (Fig. 14-6). Typically, there is an early and transient increase in renal DNA synthesis following injury. Growth factors delivered to renal epithelial cells from local and systemic sources help orchestrate the proliferative repair of the nephron after cellular necrosis. Several growth factors such as epidermal growth factor (EGF), insulin-like growth factor-1 (IGF-1), hepatocyte growth factor (HGF), fibroblast growth factors, and transforming growth factors $\alpha$ and $\beta$ have been implicated in proximal tubular regeneration (Hammerman and Miller, 1994). Interestingly, exogenous administration of EGF, HGF, or IGF-1 accelerates renal repair following ischemic-, gentamicin-, bromohydroquinone-, and/or $HgCl_2$-induced ARF. However, it is not clear which endogenous growth factors are required for tubular regeneration.

## Chronic Renal Failure

Progressive deterioration of renal function associated with chronic tubulointerstitial nephropathy may occur with long-term analgesic, lithium, or cyclosporine treatment (Table 14-1). It is generally believed that progression to end-stage renal failure is not simply a function of the primary renal insult *per se* but rather is related to secondary pathophysiological processes triggered by the initial injury. The progression of chronic renal disease, for example, has been postulated by Brenner and his colleagues (1982) to be a consequence of the glomerular hemodynamic response to renal injury. That is, following nephron loss, there are adaptive increases in glomerular pressures and flows which increase the single-nephron GFR of remnant viable nephrons. Although these compensatory mechanisms serve to maintain whole-kidney GFR, evidence has accumulated to suggest that, with time, these alterations are maladaptive and foster the progression of renal failure. Glomerular sclerosis eventually develops in these glomeruli and may lead to obliteration of the capillary loops. Consequently, glomerulosclerosis in these nephrons will perpetuate the cycle of triggering further compensatory increases in the hemodynamics of less damaged nephrons, contributing in turn to their eventual destruction. Although the underlying mechanisms are not precisely known, Brenner and his colleagues have suggested that sustained, compensatory increases in glomerular pressures and flows of the remnant glomeruli may result in (a) mechanical damage to the capillaries due to increased shear stress on the endothelium, (b) damage to the glomerular capillary wall, leading to altered permeabilities, and (c) mesangial thickening due to increased transcapillary flux and local deposition of macromolecules (Dunn et al., 1986). More recent evidence, however, suggests that altered glomerular hemodynamics are unlikely to be the sole factor in the pathogenesis of chronic renal failure. Glomerular hypertrophy (Ichikawa et al., 1988), tubulointerstitial injury (Bertani et al., 1986) and hyperlipidemia also have been suggested to play a pathogenic role in the progression of renal failure.

# THE SUSCEPTIBILITY OF THE KIDNEY TO TOXIC INJURY

## The Incidence and Severity of Toxic Nephropathy

A wide variety of drugs, environmental chemicals, and metals can cause nephrotoxicity (Tables 14-2, 14-3). In the early 1970s, the incidence of nephrotoxic ARF due to drugs was approximately 5 to 9 percent and it has risen to an estimated 20

**Table 14–2**
**Examples of Nephrotoxic Therapeutic Agents***

| | |
|---|---|
| Antiinfectives | Diuretics |
| Aminoglycosides | Organic mercurials |
| $\beta$-Lactams | |
| Vancomycin | |
| Sulfonamides | |
| Demeclocycline | |
| Amphotericin B | |
| Polymyxin B, E | |
| Antineoplastics | Immunosuppressants |
| Adriamycin | d-Penicillamine |
| Cisplatin | Cyclosporine A |
| Nitrosureas | FK-506 |
| Mitomycin C | |
| Methotrexate | |
| Analgesics/anti-inflammatory | Radiocontrast Agents |
| Acetaminophen | Diatrizoates |
| NSAIDs† | Iodohippurates |
| | Iodothalamates |
| CNS/Anesthetics | |
| Enflurane | |
| Methoxyflurane | |
| Lithium | |

* Examples represent some but not all commonly cited nephrotoxicants.
† NSAIDs, Nonsteroidal anti-inflammatory drugs.

**Table 14–3**
**Examples Of Environmental Nephrotoxicants***

| | |
|---|---|
| Mycotoxins/botanicals | Metals |
| Aflatoxin B | Cadmium |
| Citrinin | Gold |
| Monocrotaline | Bismuth |
| Pyrrolizidine alkaloids | Gallium |
| Rubratoxin B | Indium |
| Fumonisin $B_1$ | Lead |
| | Mercury |
| | Nickel |
| | Chromium |
| Halogenated Aliphatic Hydrocarbons | Herbicides |
| Bromobenzene | Paraquat |
| Bromodichloromethane | Diquat |
| Carbon tetrachloride | Succinimides |
| Chloroform | 2,4,5-Trichlorophenoxyacetate |
| Dibromochloropropane | |
| 1,2 Dibromoethane | |
| 1,2 Dichloroethane | |
| Hexachlorobutadiene | Organic Solvents |
| Pentachloroethane | Ethylene glycol |
| Trichloroethylene | Diethylene glycol |
| Tetrachloroethylene | Toluene |
| Tetrafluoroethylene | |
| Tris (2,3-dibromopropyl)-phosphate | |
| Chemicals causing $\alpha_{2u}$-globulin nephropathy | Miscellaneous |
| Decalin | p-Aminophenol |
| Unleaded gasoline | Benzidine |
| d-Limonene | d-Serine |
| 2,2,4-Trimethylpentane | d-Lysine |
| 1,4-Dichlorobenzene | Maleic acid |
| Lindane | Bromoethanamine |
| JP Jet fuels | Phenylanthranillic acid |
| Tetrachloroethylene | Puromycin aminonucleoside |

* Examples represent some but not all commonly cited nephrotoxicants.

percent (Société de Nephrologie, 1985). Nephrotoxicity is a recognized clinical liability of certain classes of drugs; in particular, antibiotics represent the major class of nephrotoxic drugs, followed by glafenin, nonsteroidal anti-inflammatory drugs (NSAIDs), and radiocontrast media. Nephrotoxicity has been reported to occur in as many as 10 to 26 percent of patients receiving aminoglycosides, in 16 percent of those receiving NSAIDs, in 25 percent of patients receiving cisplatin in early clinical trials, and in approximetly 80 percent of patients receiving amphotericin B (Kovach et al., 1973; Kleinknecht and Fillastre, 1986; Butler et al., 1964). A myriad of risk factors appear to contribute to the incidence/severity of ARF, including volume depletion, septic shock, dehydration, hypotension, age, diabetes, and preexisting renal disease (Bennett and Porter, 1993; Porter, 1989). The consequences of ARF can be profound, as permanent renal damage may result, and dialysis or renal transplantation may be required.

Chronic renal failure leading to end-stage renal failure has been associated with long-term abuse of analgesics. The incidence of analgesic nephropathy has been reported to be as high as 20 to 25 percent in certain countries (e.g., Switzerland). Other agents such as lithium, cyclosporine, NSAIDs, lead, and cadmium may produce chronic tubulointerstitial nephropathy with progressive loss of renal function.

## Reasons for the Susceptiblity of the Kidney to Toxicity

The unusual susceptibility of the mammalian kidney to the toxic effects of noxious chemicals can be attributed in part to the unique physiological and anatomic features of this organ. Although the kidneys constitute only 0.5 percent of total body mass, the kidneys receive about 20 to 25 percent of the resting cardiac output. Consequently, any drug or chemical in the systemic circulation will be delivered to this organ in relatively high amounts. The processes involved in forming a concentrated urine also serve to concentrate potential toxicants in the tubular fluid. As water and electrolytes are reabsorbed from the glomerular filtrate, chemicals in the tubular fluid also may be concentrated, thereby driving passive diffusion of toxicants into tubular cells. Therefore, a nontoxic concentration of a chemical in the plasma may reach toxic concentrations in the kidney. Progressive concentration of toxicants along the nephron may result in intralumenal precipitation of relatively insoluble compounds, causing ARF secondary to tubular obstruction. Finally, renal transport, accumulation, and metabolism of xenobiotics contribute significantly to the susceptibility of the kidney (and specific nephron segments) to toxic injury (see "Site-Selective Injury" below).

In addition to intrarenal factors, the incidence and/or severity of chemically induced nephrotoxicity may be related to the sensitivity of the kidney to circulating vasoactive substances. For example, nephrotoxicity due to NSAIDs is known to result in ARF if patients are suffering from hypotension, hypovolemia, and/or cardiac insufficiency (Brezis et al., 1991). Under these conditions, vasoconstrictors such as angiotensin II or vasopressin are increased. Normally, the actions of high circulating levels of vasoconstrictor hormones are counterbalanced by the actions of increased vasodilatory prostaglandins; thus, RBF and GFR are maintained. However, when prostanglandin synthesis is suppressed by NSAIDS, RBF declines markedly and ARF ensues, due to the unopposed actions of vasoconstrictors. Another example of predisposing risk factors relates to the clinical use of the angiotensin-converting enzyme (ACE) inhibitor, captopril. Captopril has been reported to produce ARF primarily in patients with severe hypertension, due to either bilateral renal artery stenosis or renal artery stenosis in a solitary kidney. Under these conditions, glomerular filtration pressure is dependent on angiotensin II-induced efferent arteriolar constriction. ACE inhibitors will block this vasoconstriction, resulting in a precipitous decline in filtration pressure and causing ARF.

## Site-Selective Injury

Many nephrotoxicants have their primary effects on discrete segments or regions of the nephron. For example, the proximal tubule is the primary target for most nephrotoxic antibiotics, antineoplastics, halogenated hydrocarbons, mycotoxins, and heavy metals, whereas the glomerulus is the primary site for immune complexes, the loop of Henle/collecting ducts for fluoride ions, and the medulla/papilla for chronically consumed analgesic mixtures. The reasons underlying this site-selective injury are complex but can be attributed in part to site-specific differences in: blood flow, transport and accumulation of chemicals, physicochemical properties of the epithelium, reactivity of cellular/molecular targets, balance of bioactivation/detoxification reactions, cellular energetics, and/or regenerative/repair mechanisms.

## Glomerular Injury

Although the glomerulus is an initial site of chemical exposure within the nephron, only a few nephrotoxicants produce structural injury to this segment. In certain instances, the susceptibility of the glomerulus may be attributed to chemical interactions with the fixed anionic charges on the glomerular elements. For example, gentamicin-induced decreases in GFR are believed to be due in part to electrostatic interactions between the polycationic aminoglycoside and the anionic sites of the endothelium, resulting in a reduction in the size and number of endothelial fenestrae and thereby decreasing $K_f$ (Maita et al., 1984). Similarly, albuminuria following administration of the polycationic molecule hexadimethrine (HDM) has been attributed to defects in the charge- and size-selective properties of the glomerulus, resulting from neutralization of glomerular polyanions by HDM (Hunsicker et al., 1981; Bertolatus et al., 1984).

Other agents that damage glomerular structure and/or function include the antineoplastic *mitomycin* and the immunosuppressant *cyclosporine*, both of which are injurious to the endothelial cell and the glomerular capillary tuft, and *puromycin aminonucleoside* (PAN) and *adriamcyin*, which produce epithelial cell injury. Although the mechanisms of PAN- and adriamycin-induced glomerular injury are poorly understood, intraglomerular generation of reactive oxygen species (ROS) has been suggested to play a role (Shah, 1991). It is now well-recognized that glomerular epithelial cells release oxidants and GBM-degrading proteinases which may be involved in producing epithelial cell injury (Johnson et al., 1994).

Chemically induced glomerular injury also may be mediated by extrarenal factors. Circulating immune complexes may be trapped within the glomeruli and binding of complement, attraction of neutrophils, and phagocytosis may result. Neutrophils and macrophages are commonly observed within glomeruli in glomerulonephritis and the local release of cytokines and ROS may contribute to glomerular injury. Chemicals may function as a hapten attached to some native protein (e.g., tubular antigens released secondary to toxicity) or as a complete antigen, particularly if sequestered within the glomerulus via electrostatic interactions, and elicit an antibody response. Antibody reactions with cell-surface antigens (e.g., GBM) lead to immune deposit formation within the glomeruli, mediator activation, and subsequent injury to glomerular tissue. A variety of mediators of immunologic glomerular injury have been identified and they include both cellular and soluble elements (Schreiber and Groggel, 1994).

## Proximal Tubular Injury

The proximal tubule is the most common site of toxicant-induced renal injury. The reasons for this relate in part to the selective accumulation of xenobiotics into this segment of the nephron. For example, in contrast to the distal tubule, which is characterized by a relatively tight epithelium with high electrical resistance, the proximal tubule is a leaky epithelium, favoring the flux of compounds into proximal tubular cells. Furthermore, and perhaps more importantly, tubular transport of organic anions and cations, LMWP and peptides, GSH conjugates, and heavy metals is localized primarily (if not exclusively) to the proximal tubule. Thus, transport of these molecules will be greater in the proximal tubule than in other segments, resulting in proximal tubular accumulation and toxicity of these xenobiotics. Indeed, segmental differences in transport and accumulation appear to play a significant role in the onset and development of proximal tubular toxicity associated with certain drugs such as aminoglycosides, $\beta$-lactam antibiotics and cisplatin, environmental chemicals such as ochratoxin, haloalkene S-conjugates, d-limonene, and 2,4,4-trimethylpentane, and metals such as cadmium and mercury. Although correlations between proximal tubular transport, accumulation, and toxicity suggest that the site of transport is a crucial determinant of the site of toxicity, transport is unlikely to be the sole criterion. For example, the $S_2$ segment is the primary site of transport and toxicity of cephaloridine and several lines of evidence suggest a strong correlation between transport, accumulation, and nephrotoxicity of this antibiotic. However, when a variety of cephalosporins are considered, the rank order of accumulation does not follow the rank order of nephrotoxicity; for example, renal cortical concentrations of the potent nephrotoxicant, cephaloglycin, are comparable to that of the relatively nontoxic cephalexin. These data suggest that site-specific transport and accumulation is a necessary but not sufficient factor in the proximal tubular toxicity of cephalosporins. Once taken up and sequestered by the proximal tubular cell, the nephrotoxic potential of these drugs ultimately may be dependent upon the intrinsic reactivity of the drug with subcellular or molecular targets.

In addition to segmental differences in transport, segmental differences in cytochrome P-450 and cysteine conjugate $\beta$-lyase activity also are contributing factors to the enhanced susceptibility of the proximal tubule. Both enzyme systems are localized almost exclusively in the proximal tubule with negligible (if any) activity in the glomerulus, distal tubules, or collecting ducts. Thus, nephrotoxicity requiring P-450 and $\beta$-lyase-mediated bioactivation will most certainly be localized in the proximal tubule. Indeed, the site of proximal tubular bioactivation contributes at least in part to the proximal tubular lesions produced by chloroform (via cytochrome P-450) and by haloalkene S-conjugates (via cysteine $\beta$-lyase).

Finally, proximal tubular cells appear to be more susceptible to ischemic injury when compared to distal tubular cells. Therefore, the proximal tubule likely will be the primary site of toxicity for chemicals that interfere with renal blood flow, cellular energetics and/or mitochondrial function.

### Loop of Henle/Distal Tubule/Collecting Duct Injury

Compared to the proximal tubule, chemically induced injury to the more distal tubular structures is an infrequent occurrence. Functional abnormalities at these sites manifest primarily as impaired concentrating ability and as an acidification defect. Drugs that have been associated with acute injury to the more distal tubular structures include amphotericin B, cisplatin and methyoxyflurane. Each of these drugs induces an ADH-resistant polyuria, suggesting that the concentrating defect occurs at the level of the medullary thick ascending limb and/or the collecting duct. However, the mechanisms mediating these drug-induced concentrating defects appear to be different. Amphotericin B is highly lipophilic and interacts with lipid sterols such as cholesterol, resulting in the formation of transmembrane channels or pores and disrupting membrane permeability (Sabra and Branch, 1990). Thus, amphotericin effectively transforms the tight distal tubular epithelium into one that is leaky to water and ions and impairs reabsorption at these sites. The mechanisms mediating cisplatin-induced polyuria are not completely understood but may be related to dissipation of the corticopapillary solute gradient (Safirstein et al., 1981), impaired NaCl reabsorption at the level of the proximal tubule and medullary thick ascending limb (secondary to inhibition of $Na^+$, $K^+$-ATPase activity) (Seguro et al., 1989), and/or direct cytotoxicity to the inner medullary collecting duct (Brady et al., 1993). Methoxyflurane nephrotoxicity is known to be mediated by the inhibitory effects of the metabolite, fluoride, on solute and water reabsorption. Fluoride inhibits NaCl reabsorption by the thick ascending limb and, in addition, inhibits ADH-mediated reabsorption of water and urea, effects possibly due to disruption in cAMP metabolism.

### Papillary Injury

The renal papilla is susceptible to the chronic injurious effects of abusive consumption of analgesics. Although the exact mechanisms underlying selective damage to the papilla by analgesics are not known, the intrarenal gradient for prostaglandin H synthase activity is likely to be a contributing factor. Prostaglandin H synthase activity is greatest in the medulla and least in the cortex. The prostaglandin hydroperoxidase component metabolizes acetaminophen and phenacetin to reactive intermediates capable of covalent binding to cellular macromolecules. Other factors may contribute to this site-selective injury, including high papillary concentrations of potential toxicants and inhibition of vasodilatory prostaglandins, compromising renal blood flow to the renal medulla/papilla and resulting in tissue ischemia (Bach and Gregg, 1985).

## BIOCHEMICAL MECHANISMS/MEDIATORS OF RENAL CELL INJURY

### Cell Death

In many cases, renal cell injury may culminate in cell death. In general, cell death is thought to occur through either necrosis or apoptosis (Wyllie, 1993; Corcoran and Ray, 1992). The morphological and biochemical characteristics of necrosis and apoptosis are very different. Apoptosis is a tightly controlled organized process that usually affects scattered individual cells. The organelles retain integrity while cell volume decreases. Ultimately, the cell breaks into small fragments that are phagocytized by adjacent cells or macrophages without producing an inflammatory response. In some cases DNA fragmentation occurs through an endonuclease-mediated cleavage of the DNA at internucleosomal linker regions which can be visualized as a ladderlike pattern, following agarose gel electrophoresis. In contrast, necrosis often affects many contiguous cells, and the organelles swell, cell volume increases, and the cell ruptures with the release of cellular contents followed by inflammation. In general, most nephrotoxicants are thought to produce cell death through necrosis. However, very little information is available concerning apoptosis in the kidney.

### Mediators of Toxicity

A chemical can initiate cell injury by a variety of mechanisms. In some cases the chemical may initiate toxicity due to its intrinsic reactivity with cellular macromolecules. For example, amphotericin B reacts with the plasma membrane, increasing membrane permeability; fumonisin $B_1$ inhibits sphinganine (sphingosine) N-acyltransferase; and mercury binds to sulfhydryl groups on cellular proteins. In contrast, some chemicals are not toxic until they are biotransformed to a reactive intermediate. Biologically reactive intermediates, also known as alkylating agents, are electron-deficient compounds (electrophiles) that bind to cellular nucleophiles (electron-rich compounds) such as proteins and lipids. For example, acetaminophen and chloroform are metabolized in the mouse kidney by cytochrome P-450 to the reactive intermediates, N-acetyl-p-benzoquinonimine and phosgene, respectively (see "Chloroform" and "Acetaminophen" below). The covalent binding of the reactive intermediate to critical cellular macromolecules is thought to interfere with the normal biological activity of the macromolecule and thereby initiate cellular injury. In other instances, extrarenal biotransformation may be required prior to the delivery of the penultimate nephrotoxic species to the proximal tubule where it is metabolized further to a reactive intermediate.

Finally, chemicals may initiate injury indirectly by inducing oxidative stress via increased production of ROS, such as superoxide anion, hydrogen peroxide, and hydroxyl radicals. ROS can react with a variety of cellular constituents to induce toxicity. For example, ROS are capable of: (1) inducing lipid peroxidation which may result in altered membrane fluidity, enzyme activity, and membrane permeability and transport characteristics; (2) inactivating cellular enzymes by directly oxidizing critical protein sulfhydryl or amino groups; (3) depolymerizing polysaccharides; and (4) inducing DNA strand breaks and chromosome breakage. Each of these events could lead to cell injury and/or death. Oxidative stress has been proposed to contribute, at least in part, to the nephrotoxicity associated with $HgCl_2$ (Fukino et al., 1984; Lund et al., 1993), cisplatin (Sugihara et al., 1987; Hanneman and Baumann, 1988), cyclosporine (Wang and Salahudeen, 1994), cephaloridine (Tune, 1993), and haloalkene cysteine conjugates (Chen et al., 1990; Groves et al., 1991).

## Cellular/Subcellular and Molecular Targets

A number of cellular targets have been identified to play a role in necrotic cell death (Weinberg, 1993). It is generally thought that an intracellular interaction (e.g., an alkylating agent or ROS with a macromolecule) initiates a sequence of events that leads to cell death. Somewhere along this sequence a "point of no return" is reached in which the cell will die irrespective of any intervention. The idea of a single sequence of events is probably simplistic for most toxicants, given the extensive number of targets available for alkylating species and ROS. Rather, multiple pathways, each with a distinct sequence of events, may lead to cell death.

## Cell Volume and Ion Homeostasis

Cell volume and ion homeostasis are tightly regulated and are critical for the reabsorptive properties of the tubular epithelial cells. Toxicants generally disrupt cell volume and ion homeostasis by interacting with the plasma membrane and increasing ion permeability or by inhibiting energy production. The loss of ATP, for example, results in the inhibition of membrane transporters which maintain the internal ion balance and drive transmembrane ion movement. Following ATP depletion, $Na^+$,$K^+$-ATPase activity decreases, resulting in $K^+$ efflux, $Na^+$ and $Cl^-$ influx, cell swelling, and ultimately cell lysis. Miller and Schnellmann (1993, 1995) have proposed that ATP depletion in rabbit renal proximal tubule segments initially results in $K^+$ efflux and $Na^+$ influx followed by a lag period before $Cl^-$ influx occurs. $Cl^-$ influx occurs during the late stages of cell injury produced by a diverse group of toxicants and does not appear to be due to currently characterized renal chloride transporters. $Cl^-$ influx may be a trigger for cell swelling, because decreasing $Cl^-$ influx decreased cell swelling and cell death, and inhibition of cell swelling decreased cell lysis but not $Cl^-$ influx.

## Cytoskeleton and Cell Polarity

Toxicants may cause early changes in membrane integrity such as loss of the brush border, blebbing of the plasma membrane, or alterations in membrane polarity. These changes can result from toxicant-induced alterations in cytoskeleton components and cytoskeletal–membrane interactions, or they may be associated with perturbations in energy metabolism or calcium and phospholipid homeostasis. Recent work by Molitoris and colleagues (1993) have demonstrated marked changes in the polarity of tubular epithelium following an ischemic insult. Under normal conditions the tubular epithelial cell is polarized with respect to certain transporters and enzymes. Molitoris (1993) has demonstrated that during in vivo ischemia and in vitro ATP depletion there is a dissociation of $Na^+$, $K^+$-ATPase from the actin cytoskeleton and redistribution from the basolateral membrane to the apical domain in renal proximal tubule cells. The redistribution of this enzyme has been postulated to explain decreased $Na^+$ and water reabsorption during ischemic injury.

## Mitochondria

Many cellular processes depend on mitochondrial ATP and, thus, become compromised simultaneously with inhibition of respiration. Conversely, mitochondrial dysfunction may be a consequence of some other cellular process altered by the toxicant. Therefore, it is often difficult to develop cause-and-effect relationships to determine whether mitochondrial dysfunction plays a direct role in the cell injury produced by a compound. Numerous nephrotoxicants cause mitochondrial dysfunction (Schnellman and Griner, 1994). For example, following in vivo exposure, $HgCl_2$ altered isolated renal cortical mitochondrial function and mitochondrial morphology prior to proximal tubule necrosis (Weinberg et al., 1982a). Furthermore, $HgCl_2$ produced similar changes in various respiratory parameters when added to isolated rat renal cortical mitochondria (Weinberg et al., 1982b). Different toxicants also may produce different types of mitochondrial dysfunction. For example, pentachlorobutadienyl-L-cysteine initially uncouples oxidative phosphorylation in renal proximal tubular cells by dissipating the proton gradient, while TFEC does not uncouple oxidative phosphorylation but rather inhibits state 3 respiration by inhibiting sites I and II of the electron transport chain (Schnellmann et al., 1987, 1989; Wallin et al., 1987; Hayden and Stevens, 1990).

## Lysosomes

Lysosomes are key subcellular targets of aminoglycosides, unleaded gasoline, and d-limonene and are believed to induce cellular injury via rupture and release of lysosomal enzymes and toxicants into the cytoplasm following excessive accumulation of reabsorbed toxicant(s) and lysosomal overload. $\alpha_{2u}$-Globulin is normally reabsorbed in the proximal tubule and degraded in the lysosomes. $\alpha_{2u}$-Nephropathy occurs in male rats when compounds such as d-limonene and constituents of unleaded gasoline bind to $\alpha_{2u}$-globulin, inhibiting normal lysosomal degradation and resulting in the accumulation of $\alpha_{2u}$-globulin in the proximal tubule. The size and number of lysosomes increase and a characteristic protein-droplet morphology is observed. Ultimately, this leads to single-cell necrosis and regenerative hyperplasia.

The aminoglycosides also induce lysosomal dysfunction following tubular reabsorption of aminoglycosides and accumulation in lysosomes. The size and number of lysosomes increase and electron-dense lamellar structures called myeloid bodies appear. The myeloid bodies contain undegraded phospholipids and are thought to occur through the inhibition of lysosomal hydrolases and phospholipases by the aminoglycosides.

## Calcium Homeostasis

$Ca^{+2}$ is a second messenger and plays a critical role in a variety of cellular functions. The distribution of $Ca^{+2}$ within renal cells is complex and involves binding to anionic sites on macromolecules and compartmentation within subcellular organelles. The critically important cellular calcium pool for regulation is the free $Ca^{+2}$ present in the cytosol. The concentration of this pool is approximately 100 nM and is maintained at this level against a large extracellular/intracellular gradient (10,000 : 1) by a series of pumps and channels located on the plasma membrane and endoplasmic reticulum. In addition, the proximal tubular cells reabsorb approximately 50 to 60 percent of the filtered load of calcium and thus must maintain low cytosolic $Ca^{+2}$ concentrations during a large calcium flux.

Sustained elevations or abnormally large increases in cytosolic free $Ca^{+2}$ can exert a number of detrimental effects on the cell. For example, an increase in intracellular free $Ca^{+2}$ can activate a number of degradative $Ca^{+2}$-dependent enzymes, such as phospholipases and proteinases, and can produce aberrations in the structure and function of cytoskeletal and contractile elements. The precise role of calcium in toxicant-induced injury remains unclear and controversial. Mitochondria are known to accumulate $Ca^{+2}$ in lethally injured cells through a low-affinity, high-capacity $Ca^{+2}$ transport system. While this system plays little if any role in normal cellular $Ca^{+2}$ regulation, under injurious conditions the uptake of calcium may predispose mitochondria to ROS damage (Malis and Bonventre, 1986).

## Phospholipases

Phospholipase $A_2$ ($PLA_2$) consists of a family of enzymes that hydrolyze the acyl bond at the sn-2 position of phospholipids resulting in the release of arachidonic acid and lysophospholipid. The enzymes within this family have different biochemical characteristics, substrate preferences, and calcium dependencies. $PLA_2$ activation has been suggested to play a role in various forms of cell injury through a variety of mechanisms. A supraphysiological increase in $PLA_2$ activity could result in the loss of membrane phospholipids and consequently impair membrane function. The increase in $PLA_2$ activity may be secondary to an increase in cytosolic $Ca^{+2}$, since many $PLA_2$ enzymes are $Ca^{+2}$-dependent. Cell membranes are rich with polyunsaturated fatty acids and as such are susceptible to lipid peroxidation. Peroxidized lipids are predisposed to degradation by $PLA_2$, resulting in increased $PLA_2$ activity and the formation of arachidonic acid metabolites and lysophospholipids. Lysophospholipids are toxic to cells and can alter membrane permeability characteristics and uncouple mitochondrial respiration. Furthermore, the eicosanoid products of arachidonic metabolism are chemotactic for neutrophils which also may contribute to tissue injury.

The actual role of $PLA_2$ in renal cell injury has been controversial, as it is unclear whether changes in $PLA_2$ are a cause or consequence of cell injury or death. Further difficulties arise because inhibitors of $PLA_2$ are not very selective. Portilla and colleagues (1992) reported an increase in $PLA_2$ activity in rabbit renal proximal tubule cells subjected to anoxia, and Bunnachak and coworkers (1994) showed that the phospholipase inhibitors mepacrine and dibucaine decreased hypoxia-induced rat renal proximal tubule cell death. In contrast, Schnellmann and colleagues (1994) did not observe a release in arachidonic acid from rabbit renal proximal tubules exposed to the mitochondrial inhibitor antimycin A or cytoprotection by mepacrine and dibucaine. When tubules were exposed to the oxidant *t*-butylhydroperoxide, arachidonic acid was released prior to the onset of cell death, and mepacrine and dibucaine decreased arachidonic acid release and cell death. These results suggest that $PLA_2$ may play a role in hypoxic and/or oxidant-induced renal proximal tubule injury.

## Endonucleases

The activation of endonucleases has been suggested to play a role in cell death. DNA laddering, a marker of endonuclease activation, has been observed following in vivo renal ischemia (Schumer et al., 1992) and in vitro exposure of LLC-PK1 cells to hydrogen peroxide (Ueda and Shah, 1992) but not following in vitro exposure of proximal tubules to mitochondrial inhibitors, the oxidant *t*-butylhydroperoxide, or the calcium ionophore ionomycin (Schnellmann et al., 1993). A recent study by Iwata and colleagues (1994) demonstrated minimal DNA laddering that was associated with necrosis, not apoptosis, in postischemic rat kidneys and posthypoxic isolated rat proximal tubule segments. These results, in addition to a recent study describing the artifactual appearance of DNA laddering during renal DNA isolation (Enright et al., 1994), suggest that endonuclease activation does not uniformly occur following renal cell injury.

## Proteinases

Supraphysiological activation of proteinases could disrupt normal membrane and cytoskeleton function and lead to cell death. One source of proteinases is the lysosomes where proteins are normally degraded by acid hydrolases. Under conditions of cell injury, the lysosomal membrane could rupture, releasing hydrolases into the cytosol to degrade susceptible proteins. However, several studies suggest that proximal tubular cell death does not necessarily involve lysosomal rupture (Weinberg, 1993). Wilson and Hartz (1991) observed that E64, a cysteine proteinase inhibitor, protected primary cultures of individually microdissected human and rabbit renal proximal tubules from cyclosporine A-induced cell death. There was no evidence of lysosomal rupture prior to cell death nor beneficial effects of lysosomal enzyme depletion. Likewise Yang and Schnellmann (1995) showed that a variety of cysteine and serine proteinase inhibitors were ineffective in protecting rabbit renal proximal tubule segments from antimycin A, TFEC, bromohydroquinone and t-butylhydroperoxide. Only E64 demonstrated any cytoprotective properties following exposure to antimycin A and TFEC, and the cytoprotection was not associated with the inhibition of lysosomal cysteine proteinases. These results suggest that nonlysosomal cysteine proteinases play an important role in cell death.

The calcium-activated neutral proteinases are likely candidates for a role in cell death because they are cysteine proteinases, they are activated by calcium, and they have cytoskeletal proteins, membrane proteins, and enzymes as substrates (see Saido et al., 1994 for a review). In a preliminary report, Schnellmann and coworkers (1994) showed that the calpain inhibitors I or II decreased the cell death produced by a variety of toxicants, suggesting that calpains may play an important role in the cell death produced by a diverse range of toxicants. The mechanisms and targets of calpains in cell injury remain to be determined.

## SPECIFIC NEPHROTOXICANTS

### Heavy Metals

Many metals, including cadmium, chromium, lead, mercury, platinum, and uranium, are nephrotoxic. It is important to recognize that the nature and severity of metal nephrotoxicity varies with respect to its form. For example, salts of inorganic mercury produce a greater degree of renal injury and a lesser degree of neurotoxicity compared to organic mercury compounds, an effect that has been associated with the greater degree of lipophilicity of organic mercury compounds (Conner and Fowler, 1993; Zalups and Lash, 1994). In addition, different metals have different primary targets within the kidney. For example, potassium dichromate primarily affects the $S_1$ and $S_2$ segments of the proximal tubule, while mercuric chloride affects the $S_2$ and $S_3$ segments (Zalups and Lash, 1994).

Metals may cause toxicity through their ability to bind to sulfhydryl groups. For example, the affinity of mercury for sulfhydryl groups is very high and is about ten orders of magnitude higher than the affinity of mercury for carbonyl or amino groups (Ballatori, 1991). Thus, metals may cause renal cellular injury through their ability to bind to sulfhydryl groups of critical proteins within the cells and thereby inhibit their normal function.

### Mercury

Humans and animals are exposed to elemental mercury vapor, inorganic mercurous and mercuric salts, and organic mercuric compounds through the environment. Administered elemental mercury is rapidly oxidized in erythrocytes or tissues to inorganic mercury, and thus the tissue distribution of elemental and inorganic mercury is similar. Due to its high affinity for sulfhydryl groups, virtually all of the inorganic mercury found in blood is bound to cells, albumin, other sulfhydryl containing proteins, glutathione, and cysteine.

The kidneys are the primary target organ for accumulation of inorganic mercury, and the $S_3$ segment of the proximal tubule is the initial site of toxicity. As the dose or duration of treatment increases, the $S_1$ and $S_2$ segments may be affected. Renal uptake of mercury is very rapid with as much as 50 percent of a nontoxic dose of inorganic mercury found in the kidneys within a few hours of exposure. Considering the fact that virtually all of the inorganic mercury found in blood is bound to an endogenous ligand, it is likely that the luminal and/or basolateral transport of mercury into the proximal tubular epithelial cell is through cotransport of mercury with an endogenous ligand such as glutathione, cysteine, or albumin, or through some plasma membrane mercury-ligand complex. Current evidence indicates that at least two mechanisms are involved in the proximal tubular uptake of mercury (Fig. 14-7). One mechanism appears to involve the apical activity of $\gamma$-glutamyltranspeptidase (GGT), and the other mechanism appears to be linked to the basolateral organic anion transport system (Zalups, 1995).

The acute nephrotoxicity induced by inorganic mercury is characterized by proximal tubule necrosis and ARF within 24 to 48 h after administration. Early markers of $HgCl_2$-induced renal dysfunction include an increase in the urinary excretion of brush border enzymes such as alkaline phosphatase and GGT, suggesting that the brush border may be an initial target of $HgCl_2$. Subsequently, when tubular injury becomes severe, intracellular enzymes such as lactate dehydrogenase and aspartate aminotransferase increase in the urine. As injury progresses, tubular reabsorption of solutes and water decreases and there is an increase in the urinary excretion of glucose, amino acids, albumin, and other proteins. Associated with the increase in injured proximal tubules is a decrease and progressive decline in the GFR. For example, GFR was reduced 35 percent in rats within 6 h of $HgCl_2$ administration and continued to decline to 32 percent and 16 percent of controls at 12 and 24 h, respectively (Eknoyan et al., 1982). The reduction in GFR results from the glomerular injury, tubular injury, and/or vasoconstriction. Interestingly, there is an early decrease in RBF, secondary to the vasoconstriction. RBF may return to normal within 24 to 48 h while GFR continues to decline. If the decline in renal function is not too severe, the remaining proximal tubular cells undergo a proliferative response and renal function returns over time.

As stated above, mercury has a very high affinity for protein sulfhydryl groups and this interaction is thought to play an important role in the toxicity of mercury at the cellular level. Changes in mitochondrial morphology and function are very early events following $HgCl_2$ administration, supporting the hypothesis that mitochondrial dysfunction is an early and important contributor to inorganic mercury-induced cell death along the proximal tubule. Other studies have suggested that oxidative stress plays an important role in $HgCl_2$-induced renal injury. For example, Fukino and colleagues (1984) observed increased thiobarbituric acid reactive substances, a marker of lipid peroxidation, in renal cortical homogenates following $HgCl_2$ administration, suggesting that oxidative stress did occur. Recent studies by Lund and coworkers (1993) showed that mitochondria isolated from rats treated with $HgCl_2$ exhibited elevated hydrogen peroxide formation and thus was a possible source of ROS. Finally, $HgCl_2$ increases intracellular free cal-

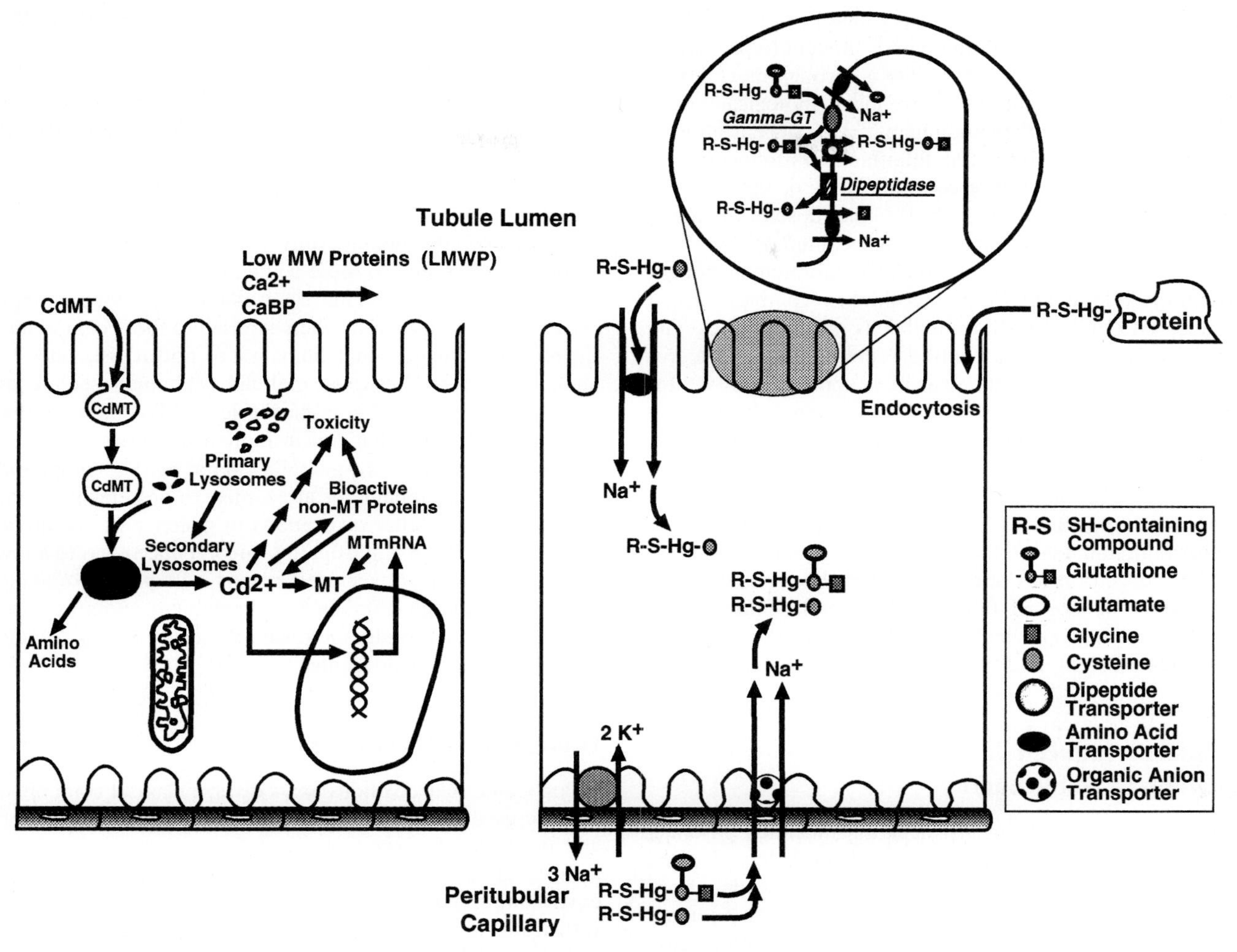


*Figure 14–7.* **Left:** ***Proximal tubular uptake of cadmium-metallothionein (CdMT).***

Reabsorbed CdMT is degraded by the renal lysosome, resulting in release of Cd and subsequent MT induction (left). Once the MT pool is saturated, Cd is available to interact with other molecular targets to produce toxicity. [From Conner and Fowler (1993), modified.]

**Right:** ***Proximal tubular uptake of mercury.***

Mercury transport may involve: (1) a dipeptide or amino acid transporter on the luminal membrane, (2) $Na^+$-dependent, probenecid and p-aminohippurate (PAH)-sensitive organic anion transport on the basolateral membrane, and (3) endocytosis of inorganic mercury bound to the sulfhydryl group of filtered proteins. (Courtesy of Dr. R.K. Zalups.)

cium in primary cultures of rabbit renal tubular cells (Smith et al., 1987) and may activate a variety of degradative pathways that contribute to proximal tubular injury.

Several animal studies have shown that chronic exposure to inorganic mercury results in an immunologically mediated membranous glomerular nephritis, secondary to the production of antibodies against the glomerular basement membrane and the deposition of immune complexes (Bigazzi et al., 1988).

## Cadmium

Chronic exposure of nonsmoking humans and animals to cadmium is primarily through food and results in nephrotoxicity. In the workplace, inhalation of cadmium-containing dust and fumes is the major route of exposure. Cadmium has a half-life of greater than 10 years in humans and thus accumulates in the body over time. Approximately 50 percent of the body burden of cadmium can be found in the kidney. Cadmium produces proximal tubule dysfunction ($S_1$ and $S_2$ segments) and injury characterized by increases in urinary excretion of glucose, amino acids, calcium, and cellular enzymes. This injury may progress to a chronic interstitial nephritis.

Numerous studies have tried to identify markers to predict the nephrotoxic effects of cadmium in humans. These include but are not limited to urinary cadmium, calcium, amino acids, albumin, $\beta_2$-microglobulin, N-acetyl-$\beta$-D-glucosaminidase, and retinol-binding protein concentrations. Lauwerys and coworkers (1994) have recently suggested that cadmium concentrations in the urine greater than 5 and 2 nmol/mmol creatinine for adult male workers and the general population, respectively, are associated with tubular dysfunction.

A very interesting aspect of cadmium nephrotoxicity is the role of metallothionein. Metallothionein is a low-molecular-weight, cysteine-rich, metal binding protein that has a high affinity for cadmium and other heavy metals. In general, the mechanism by which metallothionein is thought to play a role in cadmium and heavy metal toxicity is through its ability to bind to a heavy metal and thereby render it biologically inactive. This assumes that the unbound or "free" concentration of the metal is the toxic species. Metallothionein production can be induced by low, nontoxic concentrations of metals. Subsequently, animals challenged with a higher dose of the metal will not exhibit toxicity compared to naive animals.

Following an oral exposure to $CdCl_2$, cadmium is thought to reach the kidneys as a Cd-metallothionein complex formed and released either from intestinal cells or hepatocytes. The Cd-metallothionein complex is freely filtered by the glomerulus and is reabsorbed by the proximal tubule (Fig. 14-7). Inside the tubular cells it is thought that lysosomal degradation of the cadmium-metallothionein results in the release of "free" cadmium, which in turn induces renal metallothionein production. Once the renal metallothionein pool is saturated, "free" cadmium initiates injury. The mechanism by which cadmium produces injury at the cellular level is not clear; however, low concentrations of cadmium have been shown to interfere with the normal function of several cellular signal transduction pathways, including inositol triphosphate, cytosolic free calcium, and protein kinase C (Beyersmann et al., 1994; Smith et al., 1989).

## Chemically Induced $\alpha_{2u}$-Globulin Nephropathy

A diverse group of chemicals including unleaded gasoline, d-limonene, 1,4-dichlorobenzene, tetrachloroethylene, decalin, and lindane causes $\alpha_{2u}$-globulin nephropathy or hyaline droplet nephropathy (Borghoff et al., 1990; Lehman-McKeeman, 1993; Swenberg, 1993; Melnick, 1992). This nephropathy occurs in male but not in female rats, is characterized by the accumulation of protein droplets in the $S_2$ segment of the proximal tubule, and results in single-cell necrosis, the formation of granular casts at the junction of the proximal tubule and the thin loop of Henle, and cellular regeneration. Chronic exposure to these compounds results in progression of these lesions and, ultimately, chronic nephropathy. With compounds such as unleaded gasoline, chronic exposure results in an increased incidence of renal adenomas/carcinomas by nongenotoxic mechanisms.

As the name implies, the expression of this nephropathy requires the presence of the $\alpha_{2u}$-globulin protein. $\alpha_{2u}$-Globulin is synthesized in the liver of male rats and is under androgen control. Due to its low molecular weight (18.7), $\alpha_{2u}$-globulin is freely filtered by the glomerulus with approximately half being reabsorbed via endocytosis in the $S_2$ segment of the proximal tubule (Fig. 14-8). Many of the compounds that cause $\alpha_{2u}$-globulin nephropathy bind to $\alpha_{2u}$-globulin in a reversible manner and decrease the ability of lysosomal proteases in the proximal tubule to breakdown $\alpha_{2u}$-globulin. This results in the accumulation of $\alpha_{2u}$-globulin in the proximal tubule with an increase in the size and number of lysosomes and the characteristic protein-droplet morphology. A proposed mechanism of $\alpha_{2u}$-globulin nephropathy is that cellular necrosis secondary to lysosomal overload leads to a sustained increase in cell proliferation, which in turn results in the promotion of spontaneously or chemically initiated cells to form preneoplastic and neoplastic foci (Lehman-McKeeman, 1993, Swenberg, 1993).

$\alpha_{2u}$-Globulin nephropathy appears to be sex- and species-specific. That is, it occurs in male rats but not female rats and in male or female mice, rabbits, or guinea pigs because they do not produce $\alpha_{2u}$-globulin. Furthermore, it does not occur in male Black Reiter rats which lack $\alpha_{2u}$-globulin (Dietrich and Swenberg, 1991). Considering the diversity of compounds that cause $\alpha_{2u}$-globulin nephropathy and renal tumors and that humans are exposed to these compounds regularly, the question arises whether humans are at risk for $\alpha_{2u}$-globulin nephropathy and renal tumors when exposed to these compounds. Current data suggest that humans are not at risk since (1) humans do not synthesize $\alpha_{2u}$-globulin, (2) humans secrete less proteins in general and in particular less LMWP in urine than the rat; (3) LMWP that are in human urine are either not related structurally to $\alpha_{2u}$-globulin, do not bind to compounds that bind to $\alpha_{2u}$-globulin, or are similar to proteins in female rats, male Black Reiter rats, rabbits, or guinea pigs that do not exhibit $\alpha_{2u}$-globulin nephropathy; and (4) mice excrete a low-molecular-weight urinary protein that is 90 percent homologous to $\alpha_{2u}$-globulin, but they do not exhibit $\alpha_{2u}$-globulin-nephropathy and renal tumors following exposure to $\alpha_{2u}$-globulin-nephropathy-inducing agents.

## Halogenated Hydrocarbons

Halogenated hydrocarbons are a diverse class of compounds and are used extensively as chemical intermediates, solvents, and pesticides. Consequently, humans are exposed to these compounds not only in the workplace but also through the environment. Numerous toxic effects have been associated with acute and chronic exposure to halogenated hydrocarbons, including nephrotoxicity (Elfarra, 1993).

**Chloroform.** Chloroform produces nephrotoxicity in a variety of species, with some species being more sensitive than others. The primary cellular target is the proximal tubule with no primary damage to the glomerulus or the distal tubule. Proteinuria, glucosuria, and increased blood urea nitrogen levels are all characteristic of chloroform-induced nephrotoxicity. The nephrotoxicity produced by chloroform is linked to its metabolism by renal cytochrome P-450 and the formation of a reactive intermediate that binds covalently to nucleophilic groups on cellular macromolecules. Cytochrome P-450 biotransforms chloroform to trichloromethanol, which is unstable and releases HCl to form phosgene. Phosgene can react with: (1) water to produce 2 HCl + $CO_2$; (2) two molecules of glutathione to produce diglutathionyl dithiocarbonate; (3) cysteine to produce 2-oxothizolidine-4-carboxylic acid; or (4) cellular macromolecules to initiate toxicity. The sex differences observed in chloroform nephrotoxicity appear to be related to differences in renal cytochrome P-450 isozyme contents. For example, castration of male mice decreased renal cytochrome P-450 and chloroform-induced nephrotoxicity (Smith et al., 1984). Likewise, testosterone pretreatment of female mice increased cytochrome P-450 content and rendered female mice susceptible to the nephrotoxic effects of chloroform. Cytochrome P-450 isozymes 2B1 and 2E1 are present in male mice and are expressed in female mice treated with testosterone

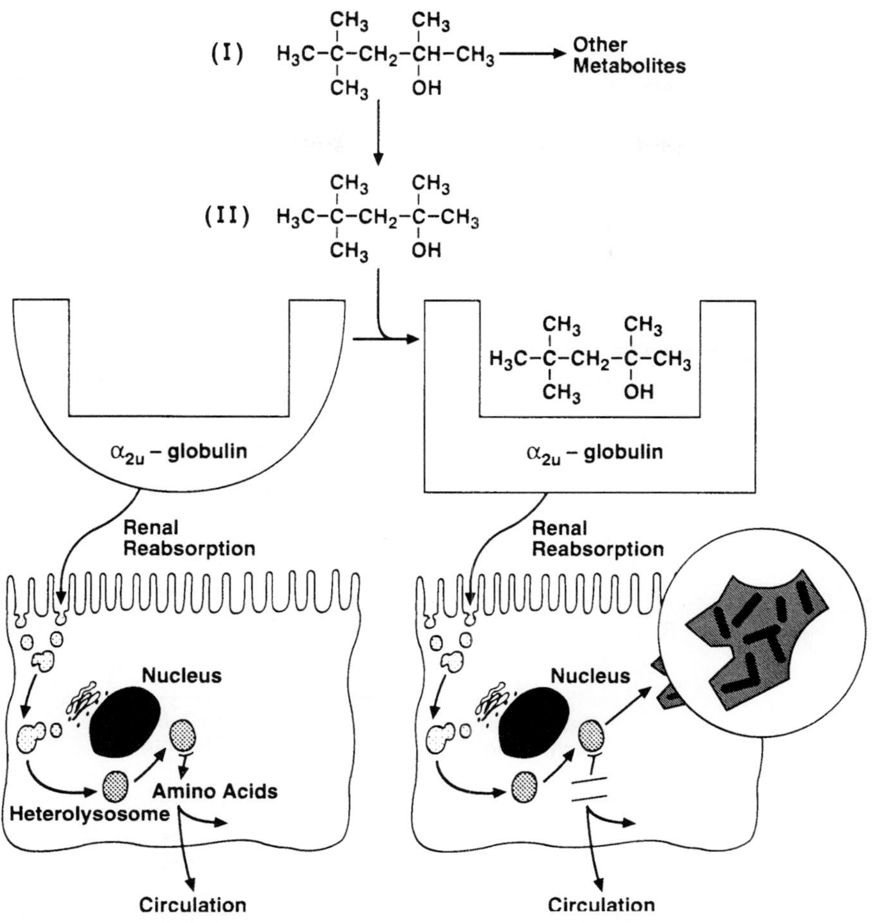


*Figure 14–8. Proposed mechanisms for $\alpha_{2u}$ nephropathy in male rats.*

In the normal healthy kidney, $\alpha_{2u}$ is taken up into the proximal tubular cells via an endocytotic mechanism and ultimately catabolized by lysosomal enzymes. The nephrotoxic chemical reversibly binds to $\alpha_{2u}$, altering the structure of the protein and decreasing its lysosomal catabolism in proximal tubular cells. This results in $\alpha_{2u}$ accumulation, lysosomal overload, and cytotoxicity. Sustained increases in regenerative cell proliferation with chronic exposure result in promotion of initiated cells to renal tumors. (From Swenberg JA, Short B, Borghoff S, et al. The comparative pathobiology of $\alpha_{2u}$-globulin nephropathy. *Toxicol Appl Pharm* 97:35-46, 1989.)

(Lock, 1994). Thus, these isozymes may play a role in chloroform-induced nephrotoxicity.

**Tetrafluoroethylene.** Tetrafluoroethylene is metabolized in the liver by GSH-S-transferases to S-(1,1,2,2-tetrafluoroethyl)-glutathione. The GSH conjugate is secreted into the bile and small intestine where it is degraded to the cysteine S-conjugate (TFEC), reabsorbed, and transported to the kidney. The mercapturic acid also may be formed in the small intestine and reabsorbed. Alternatively, the glutathione conjugate can be transported to the kidney and biotransformed to the cysteine conjugate by GGT and a dipeptidase located on the brush border (Fig. 14-9). The mercapturic acid is transported into the proximal tubule cell by the organic anion transporter while cysteine conjugates are transported by the organic anion transporter and the sodium-independent L and T transport systems. The cysteine S-conjugate of these compounds is thought to be the penultimate nephrotoxic species. Following transport into the proximal tubule, which is the primary cellular target for haloalkenes and haloalkanes, the cysteine S-conjugate is a substrate for the cytosolic and mitochondrial forms of the enzyme cysteine conjugate $\beta$-lyase. In the case of the N-acetyl-cysteine S-conjugate, the N-acetyl group must be removed by a deacetylase for it to be a substrate for cysteine conjugate $\beta$-lyase. The products of the reaction are ammonia, pyruvate, and a reactive thiol that is capable of binding covalently to cellular macromolecules. There is a correlation between the covalent binding of the reactive thiol of the cysteine conjugate with renal protein and nephrotoxicity. Hayden and colleagues (1991) and Bruschi and coworkers (1993) have shown that biotransformation of TFEC results in difluorothioamidyl-L-lysine–protein adducts in mitochondria and that two of the targeted proteins may belong to the heat shock family of proteins. Hayden and colleagues (1992) also have shown that halogenated thioamide adducts of phosphatidylethanolamine are formed in mitochondria following cysteine conjugate $\beta$-lyase biotransformation of TFEC.

The nephrotoxicity produced by haloalkenes is charac-

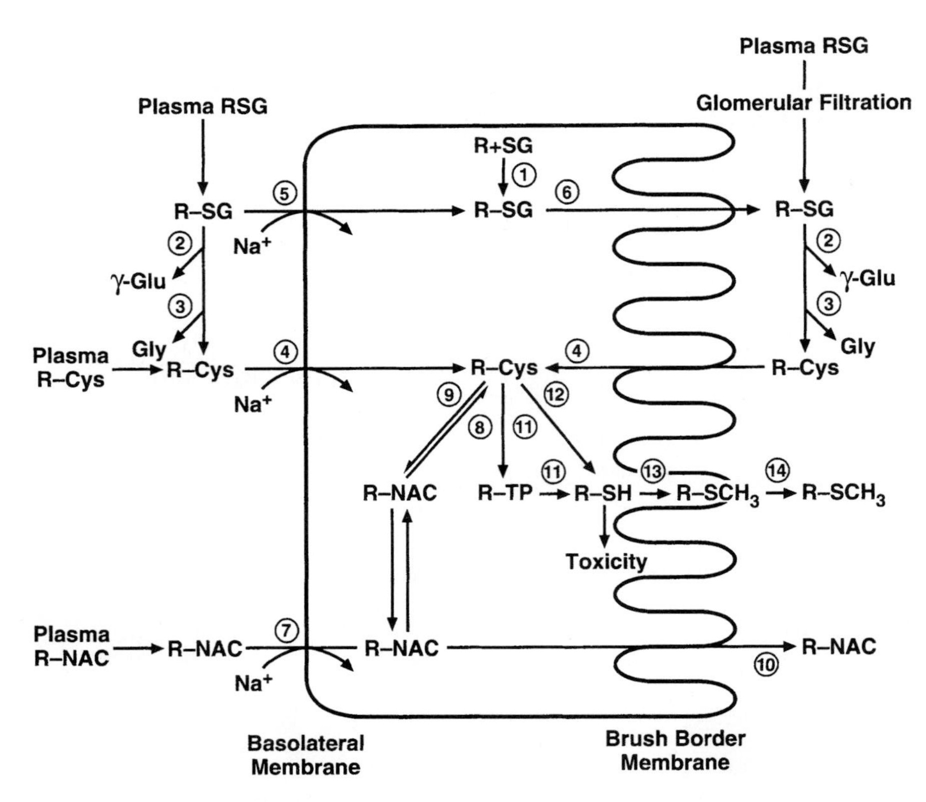


***Figure 14–9. Renal tubular uptake and metabolism of GSH conjugates.***

(1) Intracellular formation of GSH conjugates (R-SG) catalyzed by renal GSH S-transferase(s); (2) $\gamma$-GT-mediated catabolism of R-SG and formation of the corresponding S-cysteinylglycine conjugate; (3) formation of the corresponding cysteine conjugate (R-Cys); (4) $Na^+$-coupled transport of R-Cys into the renal proximal tubular cell; (5) $Na^+$-coupled transport of RSG across the basolateral membrane; (6) translocation of RSG and excretion across the brush border membrane into the tubular lumen; (7) $Na^+$-coupled and probenecid-sensitive transport of the mercapturate (R-NAC) across the basolateral membrane; (8) deacetylation of R-NAC to R-Cys and (9) acetylation of R-Cys to R-NAC; (10) excretion of the mercapturate into the tubular lumen; (11) thiol formation (R-TP) via the intermediate formation of the thiopyruvic acid conjugate (R-TP) or (12) via $\beta$-lyase; (13) methylation of the reactive thiol and (14) excretion of the methyl thiol into the urine. [From Monks TJ, Lau SS: Commentary: Renal transport processes and glutathione conjugate-mediated nephrotoxicity. *Drug Metab Dispos* 15:437–441, 1987, (Modified.)]

terized morphologically by proximal tubule necrosis, primarily affecting the $S_3$ segment, and functionally by increases in urinary glucose, protein, cellular enzymes, and BUN. Following in vivo and in vitro exposures to TFEC, the mitochondrion appears to be a primary target. In rabbit renal proximal tubules and isolated mitochondria there is a marked decrease in state 3 respiration (respiration associated with maximal ATP formation), following TFEC exposure (Groves et al., 1993). Furthermore, the decrease in mitochondrial function occurs prior to the onset of cell death. Oxidative stress also may play a contributing role in TFEC-induced cell death since lipid peroxidation products were formed prior to the onset of cell death, and antioxidants and iron chelators ameliorated cytotoxicity (Chen et al., 1990; Groves et al., 1991).

**Bromobenzene.** In addition to their hepatotoxic effects, bromobenzene and other halogenated benzenes also produce nephrotoxicity. Like the haloalkenes, the biotransformation of these compounds is critical for the expression of the nephrotoxicity. In a series of studies, Lau and Monks demonstrated that bromobenzene must be oxidized by hepatic cytochrome P-450 to bromophenol and then further oxidized to bromohydroquinone (BHQ) (Lau and Monks, 1993). BHQ is conjugated to glutathione, forming 2-bromodiglutathion-*S*-ethylhydroquinone and three positional isomers of 2-bromo-monoglutathion-S-ethylhydroquinone. The diglutathione conjugate is approximately a thousandfold more potent than bromobenzene in producing nephrotoxicity, while it produces the same morphological changes in the $S_3$ segment and increases the amount of protein, glucose, and cellular enzymes in the urine. The glutathione conjugates of BHQ are substrates for renal GGT activity and may ultimately be converted to cysteine and *N*-acetyl-cysteine conjugates of BHQ. Monks and coworkers (1994) have proposed a sequence of pathways for the renal disposition of 2-bromocysteine-*S*-ethylhydroquinones and identified possible toxic reactive intermediates. The cysteine conjugate may undergo N-acetylation, $\beta$-elimination via cysteine conjugate $\beta$-lyase or oxidation. The oxidation pathway is probably the primary one and results in the formation of an arylating species and the generation of ROS. The exact mechanism by which these compounds produce proximal tubular cell death remains to be determined.

## Mycotoxins

The nephrotoxicity of two mycotoxins, ochratoxin A and citrinin, have been studied extensively and recently reviewed by Berndt (1993). Citrinin and ochratoxin A are found on a variety of cereal grains. Citrinin administration to rats may result in either anuric renal failure and death or nonoliguric renal failure with complete recovery within 8 days. In contrast, ochratoxin A only produces renal dysfunction after repeated injections of small doses and is characterized by glucosuria, ketonuria, proteinuria, and polyuria. One or both of these mycotoxins have been implicated in Balkan nephropathy in humans, although the data to support this are less than clear.

Fumonisins (mycotoxins produced by the fungus *Fusarium moniliforme* and other Fusarium species) are commonly found on corn and corn products and recently have been shown to produce nephrotoxicity in rats (Riley et al., 1994). Histological examination of the kidney revealed disruption of the basolateral membrane and mitochondrial swelling, increased numbers of clear and electron-dense vacuoles, and cells with opaque cytoplasm. The fumonisins are structurally similar to sphingoid bases and are thought to produce their toxicity through the inhibition of sphinganine (sphingosine) N-acyltransferase. Inhibition of this enzyme results in an increase in the ratio of free sphinganine to free sphingosine and a decrease in complex sphingolipids. However, the mechanism by which these sphingolipid alterations results in cell death is unknown.

## Therapeutic Agents

**Acetaminophen.** Large doses of the antipyretic and analgesic acetaminophen (APAP) are commonly associated with hepatoxicity. However, large doses of APAP also can cause nephrotoxicity in humans and animals. APAP nephrotoxicity is characterized by proximal tubule necrosis with increases in BUN and plasma creatinine, decreases in GFR and para-aminohippurate clearance, increases in the fractional excretion of water, sodium, and potassium, and increases in urinary glucose, protein, and brush border enzymes. There appears to be a marked species difference in the nature and mechanism of APAP nephrotoxicity (Emeigh Hart et al., 1994). Morphologically, the primary targets in the mouse kidney are the $S_1$ and $S_2$ segments of the proximal tubule, while in the rat kidney the $S_3$ segment is the target. In the mouse, renal cytochrome P-450 activates APAP to a reactive intermediate, N-acetyl-p-amino-benzoquinoneimine, that arylates proteins in the proximal tubule and initiates cell death. Renal CYP2E1 has been associated with renal APAP bioactivation and covalent binding of *N*-acetyl-benzoquinoneimine to two renal proteins of 58 kDa and 44 kDa have sequence homology similar to a selenium-binding protein, whose function is unknown, and to glutamine synthetase, respectively (Emeigh Hart at al., 1994; Bartolone et al., 1992; Pumford et al., 1992; Khairallah et al., 1993). The mechanism, however, by which protein adducts initiate proximal tubule cell death and ultimately nephrotoxicity remains to be determined. While renal cytochrome P-450 plays a role in APAP activation and nephrotoxicity, glutathione conjugates of APAP also may contribute to APAP nephrotoxicity. Evidence for this pathway was provided by experiments in which GGT or organic anion transport was inhibited and APAP-induced nephrotoxicity decreased (Emeigh Hart et al., 1990)

In contrast to its effects in the mouse, a critical and early step in APAP nephrotoxicity in the rat is the conversion of APAP to para-aminophenol (PAP) (Newton et al., 1985). PAP is also a metabolite of phenacetin and aniline and is a known toxicant to the $S_3$ segment of the proximal tubule in the rat. The steps following PAP formation and the expression of nephrotoxicity are less clear. PAP or a metabolite must be further oxidized to a benzoquinoneimine or other oxidized reactive intermediate for nephrotoxicity to occur, and there is an association between covalent binding of a PAP equivalent to renal protein and nephrotoxicity (Crowe et al., 1979; Fowler et al., 1993). The mitochondrion may be an intracellular target of PAP because renal mitochondrial dysfunction has been observed following in vivo and in vitro exposures to PAP (Crowe et al., 1977; Lock et al., 1993). Although GSH conjugates of PAP have been isolated from rats treated with PAP (Klos et al., 1992) and have been shown to be nephrotoxic when administered (Fowler et al., 1991), the exact role they play in PAP nephrotoxicity is not clear. For example, inhibition of GGT or organic anion transport did not ameliorate PAP-induced nephrotoxicity (Anthony et al., 1993; Fowler et al., 1993), while bile duct cannulation and GSH depletion partially attenuated PAP-induced nephrotoxicity (Gartland et al., 1990).

## Nonsteroidal Anti-Inflammatory Drugs (NSAIDS)

NSAIDS such as aspirin, ibuprofen, naproxen, and indomethacin are extensively used as analgesics and anti-inflammatory agents and produce their therapeutic effects through the inhibition of prostaglandin synthesis. At least three different types of nephrotoxicity have been associated with NSAID administration (Murray and Brater, 1993). Acute renal failure (ARF) may occur within hours of a large dose of a NSAID, is usually reversible upon withdrawal of the drug, and is characterized by decreased RBF and GFR and by oliguria. When the normal production of vasodilatory prostaglandins is inhibited by NSAIDs, vasoconstriction induced by circulating catecholamines and angiotensin II are unopposed, resulting in decreased RBF and ischemia.

In contrast, chronic consumption of NSAIDs and/or APAP ($>$3 yrs) results in an often irreversible form of nephrotoxicity known as analgesic nephropathy. The incidence of analgesic nephropathy varies widely in the western world, ranging from less than 1 to 36 percent of patients who present with end-stage renal disease requiring dialysis (Murray and Brater, 1993). The primary lesion in this nephropathy is papillary necrosis with chronic interstitial nephritis. Initial changes include necrosis of the medullary loops of Henle and medullary capillaries followed by necrosis throughout the papillae. The mechanism by which NSAIDs produce analgesic nephropathy is not known but may result from chronic medullary/papillary ischemia secondary to renal vasoconstriction. Other studies have suggested that a reactive intermediate is formed in the cells that in turn initiates an oxidative stress or binds covalently to critical cellular macromolecules. APAP is metabolized to an arylating metabolite in vitro by an arachidonic acid-dependent pathway (Moldeus and Rahimtula, 1980; Mohandas et al., 1981; Boyd and Eling, 1981). In vitro arachidonic acid-dependent covalent binding of APAP was greatest in the papilla and least in the cortex, which is consistent with the known distribution of prostaglandin H synthase in the kidney. Furthermore, inhibitors of prostaglandin synthesis and antioxidants decreased the covalent binding.

The third, albeit rare type of nephrotoxicity associated with NSAIDs is an interstitial nephritis (Murray and Brater, 1993) which is characterized by a diffuse interstitial edema with infiltration of inflammatory cells. Patients normally present with elevated serum creatinine and proteinuria. If NSAIDs are discontinued, renal function improves in 1 to 3 months.

## Aminoglycosides

The aminoglycoside antibiotics are so named because they consist of two or more amino sugars joined in a glycosidic linkage to a central hexose nucleus. While they are drugs of choice for many gram-negative infections, their use is primarily limited by their nephrotoxicity. The incidence of renal dysfunction following aminoglycoside administration ranges from 5 to 26 percent but seldom leads to a fatal outome (Laurent et al., 1990; Fillastre and Godin, 1994; Kacew and Bergeron, 1990).

Renal dysfunction by aminoglycosides is characterized by a nonoliguric renal failure with reduced GFR and an increase in serum creatinine and BUN. Polyuria is an early event following aminoglycoside administration and may be due to inhibition of chloride transport in the thick ascending limb (Kidwell et al., 1994). Within 24 h increases in urinary brush border enzymes, glucosuria, aminoaciduria, and proteinuria are observed. Histologically, lysosomal alterations are noted initially, followed by damage to the brush border, endoplasmic reticulum, mitochondria, and cytoplasm, ultimately leading to tubular cell necrosis. Interestingly, proliferation of renal proximal tubule cells can be observed early after the onset of nephrotoxicity.

Aminoglycosides are highly polar cations and they are almost exclusively filtered by the glomerulus and excreted unchanged. Filtered aminoglycosides undergo proximal tubular reabsorption by binding to anionic phospholipids in the brush border, followed by endocytosis and sequestration in lysosomes of the $S_1$ and $S_2$ segments of the proximal tubules (Fig. 14-10). Basolateral membrane binding and uptake also may occur, but is a minor contribution to the total proximal tubular uptake of aminoglycosides. The earliest lesion observed following clinically relevant doses of aminoglycosides is an increase in the size and number of lysosomes. These lysosomes contain *myeloid bodies*, which are electron-dense lamellar structures containing undegraded phospholipids. The renal phospholipidosis produced by the aminoglycosides is thought to occur through their inibition of lysosomal hydrolases, such as sphingomyelinase and phospholipases.

While phospholipidosis plays an important role in aminoglycoside nephrotoxicity, the steps between the phos-

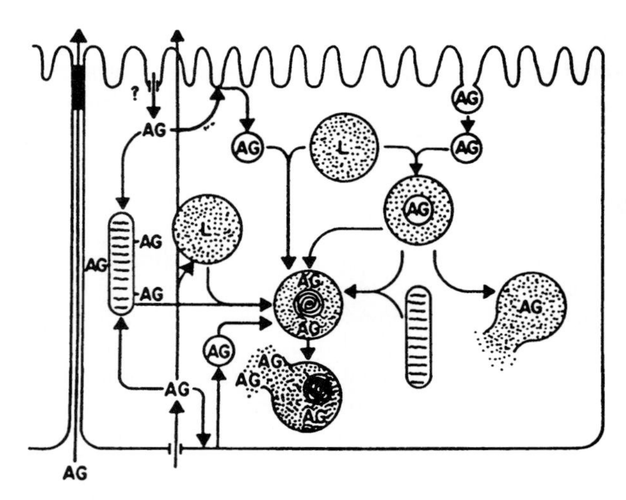


***Figure 14–10. Proposed pathways by which aminoglycoside (AG) antibiotics are transported across the basolateral membrane, accumulated within the lysosomes (L), and subsequently released within proximal tubular cells.***

The accumulation of AG within lysosomes may impair phospholipase degradation of phospholipid, resulting in formation of myeloid bodies, lysosomal overload, and release of lysosomal enzymes and AG into the cytoplasm. The released AG and lysosomal enzymes may interact with other molecular targets to produce toxicity. (From Kaloyanides GJ: *Aminoglycoside nephrotoxicity, in Schrier RW, Gottschalk CW (eds): Diseases of the Kidney, 5th ed. Boston: Little, Brown, 1993, vol 2, p 1138.)*

pholipid accumulation in the lysosomes and tubule cell death are less clear. One hypothesis proposed by Kaloyanides (1992) suggests that the lysosomes become progressively distended until they rupture, releasing lysosomal enzymes and high concentrations of aminoglycosides into the cytoplasm (Fig. 14-10). There the released lysosomal contents can interact with various membranes and organelles and trigger cell death. Other postulated mechanisms of aminoglycoside nephrotoxicity include inhibition of $Na^+$, $K^+$-ATPase, oxidative stress, and perturbations in signal transduction pathways (e.g., the phosphoinositide pathway), mitochondrial function, and/or calcium homeostasis.

## Amphotericin B

Amphotericin B is a very effective antifungal agent whose clinical utility is limited by its nephrotoxicity (Carlson and Condon, 1994). Renal dysfunction associated with amphotericin B treatment is dependent on cumulative dose and is due to both hemodynamic and tubular effects. Amphotericin B nephrotoxicity is characterized by ADH-resistant polyuria, renal tubular acidosis, hypokalemia, and either acute or chronic renal failure. Amphotericin B nephrotoxicity is unusual in that it impairs the functional integrity of the glomerulus and of the proximal and distal portions of the nephron.

Amphotericin B administration is associated with decreases in RBF and GFR secondary to renal arteriolar vasoconstriction or activation of TGF. In animals the calcium channel blocker verapamil blocks the acute amphotericin B-induced renal vasoconstriction, suggesting that the vasoconstriction may be mediated through increased calcium levels in vascular smooth muscle cells (Tolins and Raij, 1988a). However, verapamil did not completely block the acute decrease in GFR, suggesting that the decrease in GFR is not exclusively due to vasoconstriction. Cotreatment with diltiazem ameliorated amphotericin B-induced decreases in RBF and GFR observed during chronic treatment (Tolins and Raij, 1991). Thus, renal vasoconstriction is an important component in amphotericin B-induced chronic renal failure.

Some of the renal tubular cell effects of amphotericin B are due to the ability of this polyene to bind to cholesterol in the plasma membrane and form aqueous pores (Steinmetz and Husted, 1982). In the presence of amphotericin B, cells of the turtle and rat distal tubule do not produce a normal net outward flux of protons due to an increase in proton permeability (Steinmetz and Husted, 1982; Gil and Malnic, 1989). This results in impaired proton excretion and renal tubular acidosis. The hypokalemia observed with amphotericin B may be due to an increase in lumenal potassium ion permeability in the late distal tubule and the cortical collecting duct and the loss of potassium ions in the urine. While the increased ion permeability produced by amphotericin B may account for the hypokalemia and renal tubular acidosis, Sokol-Anderson and colleagues (1986) have proposed that amphotericin B produces cellular toxicity through oxidative stress.

## Cyclosporin A

Cyclosporin A (CsA) is an important immunosuppressive agent and is widely used to prevent graft rejection in organ transplantation. CsA is a fungal cyclic polypeptide and acts by selectively inhibiting T-cell activation. Nephrotoxicity is a critical side effect of CsA, with nearly all patients who receive the drug exhibiting some form of nephrotoxicity. Clinically, CsA-induced nephrotoxicity may be manifested as: (1) acute reversible renal dysfunction, (2) acute vasculopathy, and (3) chronic nephropathy with interstitial fibrosis (Racusen and Solez, 1993).

Acute renal dysfunction is characterized by dose-related decreases in RBF and GFR and increases in BUN and serum creatinine. These effects are lessened by reducing the dosage or by cessation of therapy. The decrease in RBF and GFR is related to marked vasoconstriction induced by CsA, and it is probably produced by a number of factors, including an imbalance in vasoconstrictor and vasodilatory prostaglandin production. In particular, increased production of the vasoconstrictor thromboxane appears to play a role in CsA-induced ARF (Remuzzi and Bertani, 1989). Endothelin may contribute to the afferent arteriole constriction since endothelin receptor antagonists inhibit CsA-induced vasoconstriction (Lanese and Conger, 1993). While a number of studies have explored possible direct effects of CsA on tubular cells, it is still not clear whether a direct effect of CsA on tubular cells plays a role in the nephrotoxicity.

Acute vasculopathy or thrombotic microangiopathy is a rather unusual nephrotoxic lesion which affects arterioles and glomerular capillaries, without an inflammatory component, following CsA treatment. Hyaline and/or fibroid changes, often with fibrinogen deposition, is observed in arterioles, while thrombosis with endothelial cell desquamation affects the glomerular capillaries (Racusen and Solez, 1993). The pathogenesis of this lesion is poorly understood. While the characteristics of this lesion differ from the vascular changes of acute rejection, under the clinical transplant setting a variety of factors may contribute to this lesion.

Long-term treatment with CsA can result in chronic nephropathy with interstitial fibrosis. Modest elevations in serum creatinine and decreases in GFR occur along with hypertension, proteinuria, and tubular dysfunction. Histological changes are profound; they are characterized by arteriolopathy, global and segmental glomerular sclerosis, striped interstitial fibrosis, and tubular atrophy. These lesions may not be reversible if CsA therapy is discontinued and may result in end-stage renal disease. While the mechanism of chronic CsA nephropathy is not known, vasoconstriction probably plays a contributing role. A recent study by Wang and Salahudeen (1994) indicated that rats treated with CsA and an antioxidant lazaroid for 30 days exhibited increased GFR and RBF and less tubulointerstitial fibrosis and lipid peroxidation than rats treated with CsA alone, suggesting that oxidative stress plays a role in CsA nephrotoxity in rats. The marked interstitial cell proliferation and increased procollagen secretion that occurs following CsA administration may contribute to the interstitial fibrosis (Racusen and Solez, 1993). Recently, the use of another immunosuppressive agent, FK 506, has been associated with nephrotoxicity.

## Cisplatin

Cisplatin is a valuable drug in the treatment of solid tumors with nephrotoxicity limiting its clinical use. The kidney is not only responsible for the majority of cisplatin excretion but is also the primary site of accumulation (Borch, 1993). The effects of cisplatin on the kidney are severalfold and include acute and chronic renal failure, renal magnesium wasting, and polyuria.

ARF, characterized by decreases in RBF and GFR, enzymuria, $\beta_2$-microglobulinuria, and inappropriate urinary losses of magnesium, was identified in early clinical trials of cisplatin. Although the primary cellular target associated with ARF is the proximal tubule $S_3$ segment in the rat, in humans the $S_1$ and $S_2$ segments, distal tubule, and collecting ducts also can be affected. The chronic renal failure observed with cisplatin is due to prolonged exposure and is characterized by focal necrosis in numerous segments of the nephron, without a significant effect on the glomerulus. Considerable effort has been expended in the development of measures to prevent cisplatin nephrotoxicity. These efforts include the use of extensive hydration and mannitol diuresis, the development of less nephrotoxic platinum compounds such as tetraplatin, and the identification of compounds that may bind or chelate platinum.

The mechanism by which cisplatin produces cellular injury is not known but may involve metabolites of cisplatin. Interestingly, the trans isomer of cisplatin is not nephrotoxic even though similar concentrations of platinum are observed in the kidney after dosing. Thus, it is not the platinum atom per se that is responsible for the toxicity but rather the geometry of the complex or the metabolite. The antineoplastic and perhaps the nephrotoxic effects of cisplatin may be due to its intracellular hydrolysis to the reactive mono-chloro-mono-aquo-diammine-platinum or diaquo-diammine-platinum species and the ability of these metabolites to alkylate purine and pyrimidine bases. In vitro studies using primary cultures of rabbit renal proximal tubule cells showed that while DNA synthesis, protein synthesis, glucose transport, $Na^+$-$K^+$-ATPase activity, and cell viability were all inhibited, DNA synthesis was the most sensitive to the effects of cisplatin (Courjault et al., 1993). These results suggest that cisplatin may produce nephrotoxicity through its ability to inhibit DNA and protein synthesis as well as transport functions. Furthermore, the lack of complete return of renal function following cisplatin treatment in vivo may result from the interference of cisplatin with the normal proliferative response that occurs after injury.

Like other heavy metals, platinum can bind to sulfhydryl groups of proteins such as renal ATPase and GGT, inhibiting their activity and resulting in toxicity. Mitochondrial injury in proximal tubules is an early event following in vitro and in vivo exposures to cisplatin and may result in adenine nucleotide depletion and cell death (Gordon and Gattone, 1986; Brady et al., 1993). The mitochondrial injury is associated with the loss of mitochondrial protein sulfhydryl groups subsequent to decreases in mitochondrial glutathione concentrations (Zhang and Lindup, 1993). Oxidative stress also has been implicated as a mechanism of cisplatin-induced nephrotoxicity (Sugihara et al., 1987; Hanneman and Baumann, 1988; Brady et al., 1993; Zhang and Lindup, 1993). Lipid peroxidation products have been identified in vivo and in vitro following cisplatin treatment, and pretreatment with antioxidants decreased cisplatin-induced lipid peroxidation and injury. Interestingly, antioxidants do not reverse the mitochondrial glutathione and protein sulfhydryl group depletion, suggesting that lipid peroxidation and mitochondrial injury are mediated through distinct mechanisms.

### Radiocontrast Agents

Iodinated contrast media are used for the imaging of tissues with two major classes of compounds currently in use. The ionic compounds, diatrizoate derivatives, are (1) ionized at physiological pH, (2) not significantly bound to protein, (3) restricted to the extracellular space, (4) almost entirely eliminated by the kidney, and (5) freely filtered by the glomerulus and neither secreted nor reabsorbed. These agents have a very high osmolality (>1200 mOsm/L) and are potentially nephrotoxic, particularly in patients with existing renal impairment, diabetes, heart failure, or who are receiving other nephrotoxic drugs. The newer class of contrast agents (e.g., iotrol, iopamidol) is nonionic, due to the addition of an organic side chain, low osmolality, and is less nephrotoxic.

The nephrotoxicity of these agents is due to both hemodynamic alterations and tubular injury (Bakris, 1993; Barrett, 1994). Numerous studies have demonstrated that contrast media injection leads to a brief phase of increased RBF followed by a longer period of reduced RBF secondary to vasoconstriction. However, given the degree of reduced RBF, it is unlikely that this pathway alone plays a significant role in the renal dysfunction. Radiocontrast agents also produce proximal tubular necrosis and desquamation leading to tubular obstruction and ARF.

## REFERENCES


Anthony ML, Beddell CR, Lindon JC, Nicholson JK: Studies on the effects of L(*aS,5S*)-*a*-amino-3-chloro-4,5-diphydro-5-isoxazoleacetic acid (AT-125) on 4-aminophenol-induced nephrotoxicity in the Fischer 344 rat. *Arch Toxicol* 67:696–705, 1993.

Bach PH, Gregg NJ: Experimentally induced renal papillary necrosis and upper urothelial carcinoma. *Int Rev Exp Pathol* 301–350, 1985.

Badr KF, Ichikawa I: Prerenal failure: A deleterious shift from renal compensation to decompensation. *N Engl J Med* 319:623–629, 1988.

Bakris GL: Pathogenesis and therapeutic aspects of radiocontrast-induced renal dysfunction, in Hook BH, Goldstein RS (eds): *Toxicology of the Kidney*, 2d ed. New York: Raven Press, 1993, pp 361–386.

Ballatori N: Mechanisms of metal transport across liver cell plasma membrane. *Drug Metab Rev* 23:83–132, 1991.

Barrett BJ: Contrast nephrotoxicity. *J Am Soc Nephrology* 5:125–137, 1994.

Bartolone JB, Birge RB, Bulera SJ, et al: Purification, antibody production, and partial amino acid sequence of the 58-kDa acetaminophen-binding liver proteins. *Toxicol Appl Pharmacol* 113:19–29, 1992.

Bennett WM, Porter GA: Overview of clinical nephrotoxicity, in Hook JB, Goldstein RS (eds): *Toxicology of the Kidney,* 2d ed., New York: Raven Press, 1993, pp 61–97.

Berndt WO: Effects of selected fungal toxins on renal function, in Hook JB, Goldstein RS (eds): *Toxicology of the Kidney*, 2d ed. New York: Raven Press, 1993, pp 459–475.

Bertani T, Cutillo F, Zoja C, et al: Tubulointerstitial lesions mediate renal damage in adriamycin glomerulopathy. *Kidney Int* 30:488–496, 1986.

Bertolatus HA, Foster SJ, Hunsicker LG: Stainable glomerular basement membrane polyanions and renal hemodynamics during hexadimethrine-induced proteinuria. *J Lab Clin Med* 103:632–642, 1984.

Beyersmann D, Block C, Malviya N: Effect of cadmium on nuclear protein kinase C. *EHP Suppl* 3:177–180, 1994.

Bigazzi PE: Autoimmunity induced by chemicals. *Clin Toxicol* 26:125–156, 1988.

Borch RF: The nephrotoxicity of antineoplastic drugs, in Hook JB, Goldstein RS (eds): *Toxicology of the Kidney*, 2d ed. New York: Raven Press, 1993, pp 283–301.

Borghoff SJ, Short BG, Swenberg JA: Biochemical mechanisms and pathobiology of $a_{2\mu}$-globulin nephropathy. *Annu Rev Pharmacol Toxicol* 30:349–367, 1990.

Boyd JA, Eling TE: Prostaglandin endoperoxide synthetase-dependent cooxidation of acetaminophen to intermediates which covalently bind in vitro to rabbit renal medullary microsomes. *J Pharmacol Exp Ther* 219:659–664, 1981.

Brady HR, Zeidel ML, Kone BC, et al: Differential actions of cisplatin on renal proximal tubule and inner medullary collecting duct cells. *J Pharmacol Exp Ther* 265:1421–1428, 1993.

Brenner BM, Bohrer MP, Baylis C, Deen WM: Determinants of glomerular permselectivity: insights derived from observations in vivo. *Kidney Int* 12:229–237, 1977.

Brenner BM, Meyer TH, Hotstetter TH: Dietary protein intake and the progressive nature of kidney disease: The role of hemodynamically mediated glomerular injury in the pathogenesis of glomerular sclerosis in agina, renal ablation and intrinsic renal disease. *N Engl J Med* 307: 652–659, 1982.

Brezis M, Epstein FH: Pathophysiology of acute renal failure, in Hook JB, Goldstein RS (eds): *Toxicology of the Kidney*, 2d ed. New York: Raven Press, 1993, pp 129–152.

Brezis M, Rosen S, Epstein FH: Acute renal failure, in Brenner BM, Rector FJ (eds): *The Kidney*, 4th ed. Philadelphia, Saunders, 1991, pp 993–1061.

Brezis M, Rosen S, Silva P: Transport activity modifies thick ascending limb damage in isolated perfused kidney. *Kidney Int* 25:65–72, 1984.

Bruschi SA, West K, Crabb JW, et al: Mitochondrial HSP60 (P1 protein) and a HSP-70 like protein (mortalin) are major targets for modification during S-(1,1,2,2-tetrafluorethyl)-L-cysteine induced nephrotoxicity. *J Biol Chem* 268:23157–23161, 1993.

Bunnachak D, Almeida AR, Wetzels JF, et al: $Ca^{2+}$ uptake, fatty acid, and LDH release during proximal tubule hypoxia: Effects of mepacrine and dibucaine. *Am J Physiol* 266:196–201, 1994.

Butler WT, Bennett JE, Alling DW, et al: Nephrotoxicity of amphotericin B: Early and late effects in 81 patients. *Ann Intern Med* 61:175–187, 1964.

Carlson MA, Condon RE: Nephrotoxicity of amphotericin B. *J Am Coll Surg* 179:361–381, 1994.

Chen Q, Jones TW, Brown PC, Stevens JL: The mechanism of cysteine conjugate cytotoxicity in renal epithelial cells. *J Biol Chem* 265:21603–21611, 1990.

Chen Q, Yu K, Stevens JL: Regulation of the cellular stress response by reactive electrophiles: The role of covalent binding and cellular thiols in transcriptional activaiton of the 70Kd heat shock protein gene by nephrotoxic cysteine conjugates. J Biol Chem 267: 24322–24327, 1992.

Christensen EI, Nielsen S: Structural and functional features of protein handling in the kidney proximal tubule. *Sem Nephrol* 11: 414–439, 1991.

Clarkson TW: Molecular and ionic mimicry of toxic metals. *Annu Rev Pharmacol Toxicol* 32:545–571, 1993.

Conner EA, Fowler BA: Mechanisms of metal-induced nephrotoxicity, in Hook JB, Goldstein RS (eds): *Toxicology of the Kidney,* 2d ed. New York: Raven, pp 437–457, 1993.

Corcoran GB, Ray SD: The role of the nucleus and other compartments in toxic cell death produced by alkylating hepatotoxicants. *Toxicol Appl Pharmacol* 113:167–183, 1992.

Counts RS, Nowak G, Wyatt RD, Schnellmann RG: Nephrotoxicants inhibition of renal proximal tubule cell regeneration. *Am J Physiol* 269:F274–F281, 1995.

Courjault F, Leroy D, Coquery I, Toutain H: Platinum complex-induced dysfunction of cultured renal proximal tubule cells. *Arch Toxicol* 67:338–346, 1993.

Crowe CA, Calder IC, Madsen NP, et al: An experimental model of analgesic-induced renal damage—some effects of p-aminophenol on rat kidney mitochondria. *Xenobiotica* 27:345–356, 1977.

Crowe CA, Yong AC, Calder IC, et al: The nephrotoxicity of *p*-aminophenol. I. The effect on microsomal cytochromes, glutathione and covalent binding in kidney and liver. *Chem Biol Interact* 27:235–243, 1979.

Davis ME, Berndt WO: Renal methods for toxicology, in Hayes AW (ed): *Principles and Methods of Toxicology*, 3d ed. New York: Raven, pp 871–894, 1994.

Dietrich DR, Swenberg JA: The presence of $\alpha_{2u}$-globulin is necessary for d-limonene promotion of male rat kidney tumors. *Cancer Res* 51:3512–3521, 1991.

Dunn RB, Anderson S, Brenner B: The hemodynamic basis of progressive renal disease. *Sem Nephrol* 6:122–138, 1986.

Eknoyan G, Bulger RE, Dobyan DC: Mercuric chloride-induced acute renal failure in the rat. I. Correlation of functional and morphologic changes and their modification by clonidine. *Lab Invest* 46:613–620, 1982.

Elfarra AA: Aliphatic halogenated hydrocarbons, in Hook JB, Goldstein RS (eds): *Toxicology of the Kidney*, 2d ed. New York: Raven Press 1993, pp 387–413.

Emeigh Hart SGE, Beierschmitt WP, Wyand DS, et al: Acetaminophen nephrotoxicity in CD-1 Mice. I. Evidence of a role for in situ activation in selective covalent binding and toxicity. *Toxicol Appl Pharmacol* 126:267–275, 1994.

Emeigh Hart SG, Wyand DS, Khairallah EA, Cohen SD: A role for the glutathione conjugate and renal cytochrome P450 in acetaminophen (APAP) induced nephrotoxicity in the CD-1 mouse. *Toxicologist* 11:57, 1990.

Enami A, Schwartz JH, Borkan SC: Transient ischemia or heat stress induces a cytoprotectant protein in rat kidney. *Am J Physiol* 260: F479–F485, 1991.

Enright H, Hebbel RP, Nath KA: Internucleosomal cleavage of DNA as the sole criterion for apoptosis may be artifactual. *J Lab Clin Med* 124:63–68 1994

Fillastre JP, Godin M: An overview of drug-induced nephropathies, in Goldstein RS, (ed): *Mechanisms of Injury in Renal Disease and Toxicity*. Boca Raton, FL: CRC, 1991, pp 123–147.

Ford SM, Williams PD: Primary proximal tubule culture for screening nephrotoxicants, in Watson RR (ed): *In Vitro Methods of Toxicology. Boca Raton, FL: CRC, 1992, pp 123–141.*

Foulkes EC: Functional assessment of the kidney, in Hook JB, Goldstein RS (eds): *Toxicology of the Kidney*, 2d ed. New York: Raven, 1993, pp 37–60.

Fowler LM, Foster JR, Lock EA: Nephrotoxicity of 4-aminophenol glutathione conjugate. *Hum Exp Toxicol* 10:451–459, 1991.

Fowler LM, Foster JR, Lock EA: Effect of ascorbic acid, acivicin and probenecid on the nephrotoxicity of 4-aminolphenol in the Fischer 344 rat. *Arch Toxicol* 67:613–621, 1993.

Fukino H, Hirai M, Hsueh YM, Yamane Y: Effect of zinc pretreatment on mercuric chloride-induced lipid peroxidation in the rat kidney. *Toxicol Appl Pharmacol* 73:395–401, 1984.

Gartland KPR, Eason CT, Bonner FW, Nicholson JK: Effects of biliary cannulation and buthionine sulphoximine pretreatment on the nephrotoxicity of para- aminophenol in the Fischer 344 rat. *Arch Toxicol* 64:14–25, 1990.

Gil FZ, Malnic G: Effect of amphotericin B on renal tubular acidification in the rat. *Pflugers Arch* 413:280–286, 1989.

Goering PL, Fisher BR, Chaudhary PP, Dick CA: Relationship between stress protein induction in rat kidney by mercuric chloride and nephrotoxicity. *Toxicol Appl Pharmacol* 113:184–191, 1992.

Goldstein RS: Biochemical heterogeneity and site-specific tubular injury, in Hook JB, Goldstein RS (eds): *Toxicology of the Kidney*, 2d ed. New York: Raven Press, 1993, pp 201–248.

Goligorsky MS, Lieberthal W, Racusen L, Simon EE: Integrin receptors in renal tubular epithelium: New insights into pathophysiology of acute renal failure. *Am J Physiol* 264:F1–F8, 1993.

Gordon JA, Gattone VH: Mitochondrial alterations in cisplatin induced acute renal failure. *Am J Physiol* 250:F991–F998, 1986.

Groves CE, Hayden PJ, Lock EA, Schnellmann RG: Differential cellular effects in the toxicity of haloalkene and haloalkane cysteine conjugates to rabbit renal proximal tubules. *J Biochem Toxicol* 8:49–56, 1993.

Groves CE, Lock EA, Schnellmann RG: The role of lipid peroxidation in renal proximal tubule cell death induced by haloalkene cysteine conjugates. *J Toxicol Appl Pharmacol* 107:54–62, 1991

Hammerman MR, Miller SB: Therapeutic use of growth factors in renal failure. *J Am Soc Nephrol* 5:1–11, 1994.

Hannemann J, Baumann K: Cisplatin-induced lipid peroxidation and decrease of gluconeogenesis in rat kidney cortex: Different effects of antioxidants and radical scavengers. *Toxicology* 51:119–132, 1988.

Hayden PJ, Stevens JL: Cysteine conjugate toxicity, metabolism and binding to macro-molecules in isolated rat kidney mitochondria. *Mol Pharmacol* 37:468–476, 1990.

Hayden PJ, Welsh CJ, Yang Y, et al: Formation of mitochondrial phospholipid adducts by nephrotoxic cysteine conjugate metabolites. *Chem Res Toxicol* 5:231–237, 1992.

Hayden PJ, Yang Y, Ward AJ, et al: Formation of diflourothionoacetyl-protein adducts by S-(1,1,2,2-tetrafluoroethyl)-L-cysteine metabolites: Nucleophilic catalysis of stable lysyl adduct formation by histidine and tyrosine. *Biochemistry* 30:5935–5943, 1991.

Hightower LE: Heat shock, stress proteins, chaperones and proteotoxicity. *Cell* 66:191–197, 1991.

Hunsicker LG, Shearer TP, Shaffer SJ: Acute reversible proteinuria induced by infusion of the polycation hexadimethrine. *Kidney Int* 20:7–17, 1981.

Ichikawa I, Yoshida Y, Fogo A: Glomerular hyperfiltration, hyperperfusion or hypertension does not mediate the hypertrophy of glomeruli which predisposes to sclerosis. *Kidney Int* 33:377, 1988.

Iwata M, Myerson D, Torok-Storb B, Zager RA: An evaluation of renal tubular DNA laddering in response to oxygen deprivation and oxidant injury. *J Am Soc Nephrol* 5:1307–1313, 1994.

Jaattela M, Wissing D: Emerging role of heat shock proteins in biology and medicine. *Ann Med* 24:249–258, 1992.

Johnson RJ, Lovett D, Lehrer RI, et al: Role of oxidants and proteases in glomerular injury. *Kidney Int* 45:352–359, 1994.

Kacew S, Bergeron S: Pathogenic factors in aminoglycoside-induced nephrotoxicity. *Toxicol Lett* 51:241–259, 1990.

Kaloyanides GJ: Drug-phospholipid interactions: Role in aminoglycoside nephrotoxicity. *Renal Fail* 14:351–357, 1992.

Kanwar YS, Liu ZZ, Kashihara N, Wallner EI: Current status of the structural and functional basis of glomerular filtration and proteinuria. *Sem Nephrol* 11:390–413, 1991.

Kelly KJ, Williams WW, Colvin RB, Bonventre JV: Antibody to intercellular adhesion molecule 1 protects the kidney against ischemic injury. *Proc Natl Acad Sci USA* 91:812–816, 1994.

Khairallah EA, Bulera SJ, Cohen SD: Identification of the 44-kDa acetaminophen binding protein as a subunit of glutamine synthetase. *Toxicologist* 13:361, 1993.

Kidwell DT, KcKeown JW, Grider JS, et al: Acute effects of gentamicin on thick ascending limb function in the rat. *Eur J Pharmacol, Environ Toxicol Pharmacol Section* 270:97–103, 1994.

Kivlighn SD, Gabel RA, Siegl PKS: Effects of BQ-123 on renal function and acute cyclosporine-induced renal dysfunction. *Kidney Int* 45:131–136, 1994.

Kleinknecht D, Fillastre JP: Clinical aspects of drug-induced tubular necrosis in man, in Bertani T, Remuzzi G, Garrattini S (eds): *Drugs and Kidney*. New York: Raven Press, 1986, pp 123-136.

Klos C, Koob M, Kramer C, Dekant W: *p*–Amininophenol nephrotoxicity. Biosynthesis of toxic glutathione conjugates. *Toxicol Appl Pharmacol* 115:98–106, 1992.

Komatsuda A, Wakui H, Ima H, et al: Renal localization of the constitutive 73-kDa heat shock protein in normal and PAN rats. *Kidney Int* 41:1204–1212, 1992.

Komatsuda A, Wakui H, Satoh K, et al: Altered localization of 73-kilodalton heat shock protein in rat kidneys with gentamicin-induced acute tubular injury. *Lab Invest* 68:687–695, 1993.

Kon V, Sugiura M, Inagami T, et al: Role of endothelin in cyclosporine-induced glomerular dysfunction. *Kidney Int* 37:1487–1491, 1990.

Kopp JB, Klotman PE: Cellular and molecular mechanisms of cyclosporin nephrotoxicity. *J Am Soc Nephrol* 1:162–179, 1990.

Kovach JS, Moertel CG, Shutt AJ: Phase II study of cis-diamminedichloroplatinum (NSC-119875) in advanced carcinoma of the large bowel. *Cancer Chemother Rep* 57:337–359, 1973.

Lanese DM, Conger JD: Effects of endothelin receptor antagonist on cyclosporine-induced vasoconstriction in isolated rat renal arterioles. *J Clin Invest* 91:2144–2149, 1993.

Lau SS, Monks TJ: Nephrotoxicity of bromobenzene: The role of quinine-thioethers, in Hook JB, Goldstein RS (eds): *Toxicology of the Kidney,* 2d ed. New York: Raven Press, 1993, pp 415–436.

Laurent G, Kishore BK, Tulkens PM: Aminoglycoside-induced renal phospholipidosis and nephrotoxicity. *Biochem Pharmacol* 40:2383–2392, 1990.

Lauwerys RR, Bernard AM, Roels HA, Buchet J-P: Cadmium: Exposure markers as predictors of nephrotoxic effects. *Clin Chem* 40:1391–1394, 1994.

Lehman-McKeeman LD: Male rat-specific light hydrocarbon nephropathy, in Hook JB, Goldstein RS (eds): *Toxicology of the Kidney*, 2d ed. New York: Raven Press, 1993, pp 477–494.

Leonard I, Zanen J, Nonclercq D, et al: Modification of immunoreactive EGF and EGF receptor after acute tublular necrosis induced by tobramycin or cisplatin. *J Renal Fail* 16:583–608, 1994.

Lieberthal W, Levinksy NG: Treatment of acute tubular necrosis. *Sem Nephrol* 10:571–583, 1990.

Lock EA: Renal drug metabolizing enzymes in experimental animals and humans, in Goldstein RS (ed): *Mechanisms of Injury in Renal Disease and Toxicity.* Boca Raton, FL: CRC, 1994, pp 173–206.

Lock EA, Cross TJ, Schnellmann RG: Studies on the mechanism of 4-aminophenol-induced toxicity to renal proximal tubules. *Hum Exp Toxicol* 12:383–388, 1993.

Lund BO, Miller DM, Woods JS: Studies in Hg(II)-induced $H_2O_2$ formation and oxidative stress in vivo and in vitro in rat kidney mitochondria. *Biochem Pharmacol* 45:2017–2024, 1993.

Maddox DA, Brenner BM: Glomerular ultrafiltration, in Brenner BM, Rector FC (eds): *The Kidney*, 4th ed. Philadelphia: Saunders, 1991, pp 205–244.

Maita K, Cojocel C, Dociu N, et al: Effects of aminoglycosides on glomerular ultrastructure. *Pharmacology* 29:292–300, 1984.

Malis CD, Bonventre JV: Mechanism of calcium potentiation of oxygen free radical injury to renal mitochondria. A model for post ischemic and toxic mitochondrial damage. *J Biol Chem* 261:14201–14208, 1986.

Melnick R: An alternative hypothesis on the role of chemically induced protein droplet ($\alpha 2\mu$-Globulin) nephropathy in renal carcinogenesis. *Reg Toxicol Pharmacol* 16:111–125, 1992.

Miller GW, Schnellmann RG: Cytoprotection by inhibition of chloride channels: The mechanism of action of glycine and strychnine. *Life Sci* 53:1211–1215, 1993.

Miller GW, Schnellmann RG: Inhibitors of renal chloride transport do not block toxicant-induced choloride influx in the proximal tubule. *Toxicol Lett* 76:179–184, 1995.

Mohandas J, Duggin GG, Horvath JS, Tiller DJ: Metabolic oxidation of acetaminophen (paracetamol) mediated by cytochrome P-450 mixed function oxidase and prostaglandin endoperoxidase synthetase in rabbit kidney. *Toxical Appl Pharmacol* 61:252–259, 1981.

Moldeus P, Rahimtula A: Metabolism of paracetamol to a glutathione conjugate catalyzed by prostaglandin synthetase. *Biochem Biophys Res Commun* 96:469–475, 1980.

Molitoris BA: $Na^+$-$K^+$-ATPase that redistributes to apical membrane during ATP depletion remains functional. *Am J Physiol* 34:693–697, 1993.

Monks TJ, Lo HH, Lau SS: Oxidation and acetylation as determinants of 2-bromocystein-S-ylhydroquinone-mediated nephrotoxicity. *Chem Res Toxicol* 7:495–502, 1994.

Murray MD, Brater DC: Renal toxicity of the nonsteroidal anti-inflammatory drugs. *Annu Rev Pharmacol Toxicol* 32:435-465, 1993.

Nambi PM, Pullen LC, Contino LC, Brooks DP: Upregulation of renal endothelin receptors in rats with cyclosporine A-induced nephrotoxicity. *Eur J Pharmacol* 187:113–116, 1990.

Newton JF, Kuo CH, DeShone DM, et al: The role of *p*-aminophenol in acetaminophen-induced nephrotoxicity: Effect of bis(*p*-nitrophenol)phosphate on acetaminophen and *p*-aminophenol nephrotoxicity and metabolism in Fischer 344 rats. *Toxicol Appl Pharmacol* 81:416–430, 1985.

Perico N, Zoja C, Benigni A, et al: Effect of short-term cyclosporine administration in rats on renin-angiotensin and thromboxane $A_2$:

Possible relevance to the reduction in glomerular filtration rate. *J Pharmacol Exp Ther* 239:229–235, 1986.

Porter GA: Risk factors for toxic nephropathies. *Toxicol Lett* 46:269–279, 1989.

Portilla D, Mandel LJ, Bar-Sagi D, Millington DS: Anoxia induces phospholipase $A_2$ in rabbit renal proximal tubules. *Am J Physiol* 262:F354, 1992.

Pumford NR, Martin BM, Hinson JA: A metabolite of acetaminophen covalently binds to the 56 kDa selenium binding protein. *Biochem Biophys Res Comm* 182:1348–1355, 1992.

Rabb H, Mendiola CC, Dietz J, et al: Role of CD11a and CDllb in ischemic acute renal failure in rats. *Am J Physiol* 267:F1052–F1058, 1994.

Racusen LC, Solez K: Nephrotoxicity of cyclosporine and other immunotherapeutic agents, in Hook JB, Goldstein RS (eds): *Toxicology of the Kidney*, 2d ed. New York: Raven Press, 1993, pp 319–360.

Remuzzi G, Bertani T: Renal vascular and thrombotic effects of cyclosporine. *Am J Kidney* Dis 13:261–272, 1989.

Riley RT, Hinton DM, Chamberlain WJ, et al: Dietary fumonisin $B_1$ induces disruption of sphindolipid metabolism in Sprague-Dawley rats: A new mechanism of nephrotoxicity. *J Nutr* 124:594–603, 1994.

Sabatini S: Anagesic-induced papillary necrosis. *Sem Nephrol* 8:41–54, 1988.

Sabra R, Branch RA: Amphotericin B nephrotoxicity. *Drug Saf* 5:94–108, 1990.

Sabra R, Branch RA: Mechanisms of amphotericin B-induced decrease in glomerular filtration rate in rats. *Antimicrob Agents Chemother* 35:2509–2514, 1991.

Safirstein R, Miller P, Dikman S, et al: Cisplatin nephrotoxicity in rats. Defect in papillary hypertonicity. *Am J Physiol* 241:F175–F185, 1981.

Saido TC, Sorimachi H, Suzuki K: Calpain: New perspectives in molecular diversity and physiological-pathological involvement. *FASEB J* 8:814–822, 1994.

Sawaya BP, Weihprecht H, Campbell WR, et al: Direct vasoconstriction as a possible cause for amphotericin B-induced nephrotoxicity in rats. *J Clin Invest* 87:2097–2107, 1991.

Schnellmann RG, Cross TJ, Lock EA: Pentachlorabutadienyl-L-cysteine uncouples oxidative phosphorylation by dissipating the proton gradient. *Toxicol Appl Pharmacol* 100:498–505, 1989.

Schnellmann RG, Griner RD: Mitochondrial mechanisms of tubular injury, in Goldstein RS (ed): *Mechanisms of Injury in Renal Disease and Toxicity*. Boca Raton, FL: CRC, 1994, pp 247–265.

Schnellmann RG, Swagler AR, Compton MM: Absence of endonuclease activation acute cell death in renal proximal tubules. *Am J Physiol* 265:C485–C490, 1993.

Schnellmann RG, Yang X, Carrick JB: Arachidonic acid release in renal proximal tubule cell injuries and death. *J Biochem Toxicol* 9:211–217, 1994.

Schnellmann RG, Yang X, Cross TJ: Calpains play a critical role in renal proximal tubule (RPT) cell death. *Can J Physiol Pharm* 72:602, 1994.

Schreiber BD, Groggel GC: Immunologic mechanisms in renal disease, in Goldstein, R.S. (ed): *Mechanisms of Injury in Renal Disease and Toxicity*. Boca Raton, FL: CRC, 1994, pp 103–122.

Schumer M, Columbel MC, Sawczuk IS: Morphologic, biochemical, and molecular evidence of apoptosis during the reperfusion phase after brief periods of renal ischemia. *Am J Pathol* 140:831–838, 1992.

Seguro AC, Shimizu MHM, Kudo LH, Rocha A: Renal concentrating defect induced by cisplatin. *Am J Nephrol* 9:59–65, 1989.

Shah SV: Oxidant mechanisms in glomerulonephritis. *Sem Nephrol* 11:320–326, 1991.

Smeesters C, Chaland P, Giroux L, et al: Prevention of acute cyclosporine A nephrotoxicity by a thromboxane synthetase inhibitor. *Transpl Proc* 20:658–664, 1988.

Smith JB, Dwyer SD, Smith L: Cadmium evokes inositol polyphosphate formation and calcium mobilization. *J Biol Chem* 256:7115–7118, 1989.

Smith JH, Maita K, Sleight SD, Hook JB: Effect of sex hormone status on chloroform nephrotoxicity and renal mixed function oxidases in mice. *Toxicology* 30:305–316, 1984.

Smith MW, Ambudkar IS, Phelps PC, et al: $HgCl_2$-induced changes in cytosolic $Ca^{2+}$ of cultured rabbit renal tubular cells. *Biochem Biophys Acta* 931:130–142, 1987.

Société de Nephrologie. Kleinknecht D, Laudais P, Goldfarb B: Drug-associated acute renal failure. A prospective multicentre report. *Proc EDTA-ERA* 22:1002–1007, 1985.

Sokol-Anderson ML, Brajtburg J, Medoff G: Amphotericin B-induced oxidative damage and killing of Candida Albicans. *J Infect Dis* 154:76–83, 1986.

Steinmetz PR, Husted RF: Amphotericin B toxicity for epithelial cells, in Porter GA (ed): *Nephrotoxic Mechanisms of Drugs and Environmental Toxins.* New York, London: 1982, pp 95-98.

Sugihara K, Nakano S, Gemba M: Stimulatory effect of cisplatin on production of lipid peroxidation in renal tissues. *Jpn J Pharmacol* 43:247–252, 1987.

Swenberg JA: $a_{2u}$-Globulin nephropathy: Review of the cellular and molecular mechanisms involved and their implications for human risk assessment. *Environ Health Perspect Suppl* 6:39–44, 1993.

Tarloff JB, Goldstein RS: In vitro assessment of nephrotoxicity, in Gad SC (ed): *In Vitro Toxicology*, New York: Raven Press, 1994, pp 149–193.

Tisher CC, Madsen KM: Anatomy of the kidney, in Brenner BM, Rector FC (eds): *The Kidney*, 4th ed. Philadelphia: Saunders, 1991, pp 3–75.

Tolins JP, Raij L: Adverse effect of amphotericin B administration on renal hemodynamics in the rat. Neurohumoral mechanisms and influence of calcium channel blockade. *J Pharmacol Exp Ther* 245:594–599, 1988.

Tolins JP, Raij L: Chronic amphotericin B nephrotoxicity in the rat: Protective effect of prophylactic salt loading. *Am J Kidney Dis* 11:313–317, 1988.

Tolins JP, Raij L: Chronic amphotericin B nephrotoxicity in the rat: protective effect of calcium channel blockade. *J Am Soc Nephrol* 2:98–102, 1991.

Tune BM: The nephrotoxicity of $\beta$-Lactam Antibiotics, in Hook JB, Goldstein RS (eds): *Toxicology of the Kidney*, 2d ed. New York: Raven Press, 1993, pp 257–281.

Ueda N, Shah SV: Endonuclease-induced DNA damage and cell death in oxident injury to renal tubular epithelial cells. *J Clin Invest* 90:2593–2597, 1992.

Van Why SK, Friedhelm H, Ardito T, et al: Induction and intracellular localization of HSP-72 after renal ischemia. *Am J Physiol* 263:F769–F775, 1992.

Wallin A, Jones TW, Vercesi AE, et al: Toxicity of S-pentachorobutadienyl-L-cysteine studied with isolated rat renal cortical mitochondria. *Arch Biochem Biophys* 258:365–372, 1987.

Wang C, Salahudeen AK: Cyclosporine nephrotoxicity: Attenuation by an antioxidant-inhibitor of lipid peroxidation in vitro and in vivo. *Transplantation* 58:940–946, 1994.

Weinberg JM: The cellular basis of nephrotoxicity, in Schrier RW, Gottschalk CW (eds): *Diseases of the Kidney*, 5th ed. Boston, Toronto, London: Little, Brown, vol 2, pp 1031–97, 1993.

Weinberg JM, Harding PG, Humes HD: Mitochondrial bioenergetics during the initiation of mercuric chloride-induced renal injury. II. Functional alterations of renal cortical mitochondria isolated after mercuric chloride treatment. *J Biol Chem* 257:68–74, 1982a.

Weinberg JM, Harding PG, Humes HD: Mitochondrial bioenergetics during the intitiation of mercuric chloride-induced renal injury. I. Direct effects of in vitro mercuric chloride on renal cortical mitochondrial function. *J Biol Chem* 257:60–67, 1982b.

Wilson PD, Hartz PA: Mechanisms of cyclosporine A toxicity in defined cultures of renal tubule epithelia: a role for cysteine proteases. *Cell Biol Int Rep* 15:1243–1258, 1991.

Wyllie AH: Apoptosis. *Br J Cancer* 67:205-208, 1993.

Yang X, Schnellmann RG: Proteinases in renal cell death. *J Toxicol Env Hlth* (in press).

Zalups RK: Organic anion transport and action of $\gamma$-glutamyl-transpeptidase in kidney linked mechanistically to renal tubule uptake of inorganic mercury. *Toxicol Appl Pharmacol* 132:289–289, 1995.

Zalups RK, Lash LH: Advances in understanding the renal transport and toxicity of mercury. *J Toxicol Environ Health* 42:1-44, 1994.

Zhang J-G, Lindup WE: Role of mitochondria in cisplatin-induced oxidative damage exhibited by rat renal cortical slices. *Biochem Pharmacol* 45:2215–2222,1993.

# CHAPTER 15

# TOXIC RESPONSES OF THE RESPIRATORY SYSTEM

*Hanspeter R. Witschi and Jerold A. Last*

Initially, lung injury caused by chemicals was primarily associated with certain professions and occupations. In his classical treatise of 1713, the Italian physician Bernardino Ramazzini provided detailed and harrowing accounts of the sufferings of miners, whose ailments had been known and described since antiquity. Two of Ramazzini's quotations are noteworthy. With regard to miners of metals, he stated that "the lungs and brains of that class of workers are badly affected, the lungs especially, since they take in with the air mineral spirits and are the first to be keenly aware of injury." Ramazzini also was aware of the important concept of exposure: "They (workers who shovel, melt, and cast and refine mined material) are liable of the same diseases, though in less acute form, because they perform their tasks in open air." Thus, exposure to chemicals by inhalation can have two effects: on the lung tissues and on distant organs that are reached after chemicals enter the body by means of inhalation. Indeed, "inhalation toxicology" refers to the route of exposure, whereas "respiratory tract toxicology" refers to target organ toxicity, in this case abnormal changes in the respiratory tract produced by airborne (and on occasion bloodborne) agents. We now know of numerous lung diseases prompted by occupational exposures, many crippling and some fatal. Examples include black lung in coal miners, silicosis and silicotuberculosis in sandblasters and tunnel miners, and asbestosis in shipyard workers and asbestos miners. Occupational exposures to asbestos or metals such as nickel, beryllium, and cadmium also can cause lung cancer. In the twentieth century, it has become obvious that disease caused by airborne agents may not be limited to certain trades. The ubiquitous presence of airborne chemicals is a matter of concern, since "air pollution" adversely affects human health and may be an important contributor to mortality (Schenker, 1993).

To better understand environmental lung disease, we need more precise knowledge about the doses of toxic inhalants delivered to specific sites in the respiratory tract and an understanding of the extent to which repeated and often intermittent low-level exposures eventually may initiate and propagate chronic lung disease. Lung tissue can be injured directly or secondarily by metabolic products from organic compounds. However, the most important effect of many toxic inhalants is to place an undue oxidative burden on the lungs. Observations made in humans and animals provide strong evidence that the sequelae of oxidative stress may be instrumental in initiating and propagating ailments such as chronic bronchitis, emphysema, interstitial disorders (fibrosis) and cancer (Crapo et al., 1992).

Respiratory tract toxicology is a field in which collaboration involving epidemiologists, physiologists studying human lung function, and toxicologists has become close and fruitful. Epidemiologists now use a variety of pulmonary function tests to assess decrements in lung function in workers and populations exposed to air pollutants. These pulmonary function tests have been adapted for animal studies and are used by many investigators to examine the mechanisms responsible for the pulmonary effects of air pollutants. When similar data can be obtained in both experimental animals and human subjects (for example, studies of mucociliary clearance of particles or responsiveness to bronchoconstrictive agents), these direct comparisons assist in extrapolating from animals to humans. Progress has been made in understanding some of the mechanisms that underlie the response of the lungs to toxic agents. In response to toxic insult, pulmonary cells are known to release a variety of potent chemical mediators that may critically affect lung function. Biochemical data from the study of cells taken from exposed animals and in vitro exposure of cells in culture are also useful in assessing the toxic potential of many agents. Bronchoalveolar lavage is now widely used in experimental animals and human subjects to examine respiratory airways' contents (cellular and acellular) after exposure. This chapter will discuss how pulmonary toxicologists use these methods to study the biochemical, structural, and functional changes produced by the inhalation of pollutant gases and particles.

## LUNG STRUCTURE AND FUNCTION

### Nasal Passages

Air enters the respiratory tract through the nasal and oral regions. Many species, particularly small laboratory rodents, are obligatory nose breathers in which air passes almost exclusively through the nasal passages. Other species, including humans, monkeys, and dogs, can inhale air both through the nose and through the mouth (oronasal breathers). Air is warmed and humidified while passing through the nose. The nasal passages function as a filter for particles, which may be collected by diffusion or impaction on the nasal mucosa. Highly water soluble gases are absorbed efficiently in the nasal passages, which reach from the nostril to the pharynx.

The nasal passages are lined by distinctive epithelia: stratified-squamous epithelium in the vestibule, nonciliated cuboidal/columnar epithelium in the anterior chamber, ciliated pseudostratified respiratory epithelium, and olfactory epithelium. The greater part of the internal nasal passages is covered by respiratory epithelium containing goblet cells, ciliated cells, nonciliated columnar cells, cuboidal cells, brush cells, and basal cells. Located in the superior part is the olfactory epithelium, which contains sensory cells. Nerve endings in the nasal passages are associated mostly with the fifth cranial (trigeminal) nerve.

Nasal epithelia are competent to metabolize foreign compounds (Dahl and Lewis, 1993). Hydrogen cyanide is readily produced from organonitriles; the presence of rhodanase mitigates the potential toxic effects caused by cyanide. Nasal tissue has been found to activate nitrosamines to mutagenic compounds. P-450 isozymes 1A1, 2B1, and 4B1 have been localized in the nose of several species by immunohistochemical procedures. The nasal cavity is thus a ready target site for metabolite-induced lesions. The olfactory epithelium appears to be particularly vulnerable. Metabolism by the olfactory epithelium may play a role in providing or preventing access of inhalants directly to the brain; for example, inhaled xylene may be converted to metabolites that move to the brain by axonal transport.

## Conducting Airways

The proximal airways—the trachea and bronchi—have a pseudostratified epithelium containing ciliated cells and two types of nonciliated cells: mucous and serous cells. Mucous cells (and glandular structures) produce respiratory tract mucus, a family of high-molecular-weight glycoproteins with a sugar content of 80 percent or more that coat the epithelium with a viscoelastic sticky protective layer that traps pollutants and cell debris. Serous cells produce a fluid in which mucus may be dissolved. The action of the respiratory tract cilia, which beat in synchrony under the control of the central nervous system (CNS), continuously drives the mucus layer toward the pharynx, where it is removed from the respiratory system by swallowing or expectoration. The mucus layer is also thought to have antioxidant, acid-neutralizing, and free radical–scavenging functions that protect the epithelial cells.

Conducting airways have a characteristic branched bifurcating structure, with successive airway generations containing approximately twice the number of bronchi with a successively decreasing internal diameter. Thus, the conducting airways contain a continuously increasing total surface area from the trachea to the distal airways. Bifurcations have flow dividers at branch points that serve as sites of impaction for particles, and successively narrower diameters also favor the collection of gases and particles on airway walls. Eventually a transition zone is reached where cartilaginous airways (bronchi) give way to noncartilaginous airways (bronchioles), which in turn give way to gas exchange regions, respiratory bronchioles, and alveoli. Mucus-producing cells and glands give way to Clara cells in the bronchiolar epithelium. There are important structural and cellular differences between the conductive airways of humans and these of many commonly studied laboratory animals, as will be discussed later in this chapter.

## Gas Exchange Region

Human lungs are divided into five lobes: the superior and inferior left lobes and the superior, middle, and inferior right lobes. In small laboratory animals such as rats, mice, and hamsters, the left lung consists of a single lobe, whereas the right lung is divided into four lobes: cranial, middle, caudal, and ancillary. In the guinea pig and rabbit, the left lung is divided into two lobes. Dogs have two left and four right lobes. The lung can be further subdivided at the periphery of the bronchial tree into distinct anatomic bronchopulmonary segments, then into lobules, and finally into acini. An acinus includes a terminal bronchiole and all its respiratory bronchioles, alveolar ducts, and alveolar sacs. An acinus may be made up of two to eight ventilatory units. A ventilatory unit is defined as an anatomical region that includes all alveolar ducts and alveoli distal to each bronchiolar-alveolar duct junction (Mercer and Crapo, 1991). The ventilatory unit is important because it represents the smallest common denominator when the distribution of inhaled gases to the gas-exchanging surface of the lung is modeled (Fig. 15-1). While the human lung contains respiratory bronchioles—small conducting airways with occasional outpockets of alveoli—normal rat lungs have an abrupt transition from nonrespiratory bronchioles to alveolar ducts (Phalen and Oldham, 1983).

Gas exchange occurs in the alveoli, which represent approximately 80 percent to 90 percent of the total parenchymal lung volume; adult human lungs contain an estimated 300 million alveoli. The ratio of total capillary surface to total alveolar surface is slightly less than 1. Within the alveolar septum, capillaries are organized in a single sheet. Capillaries, blood plasma,

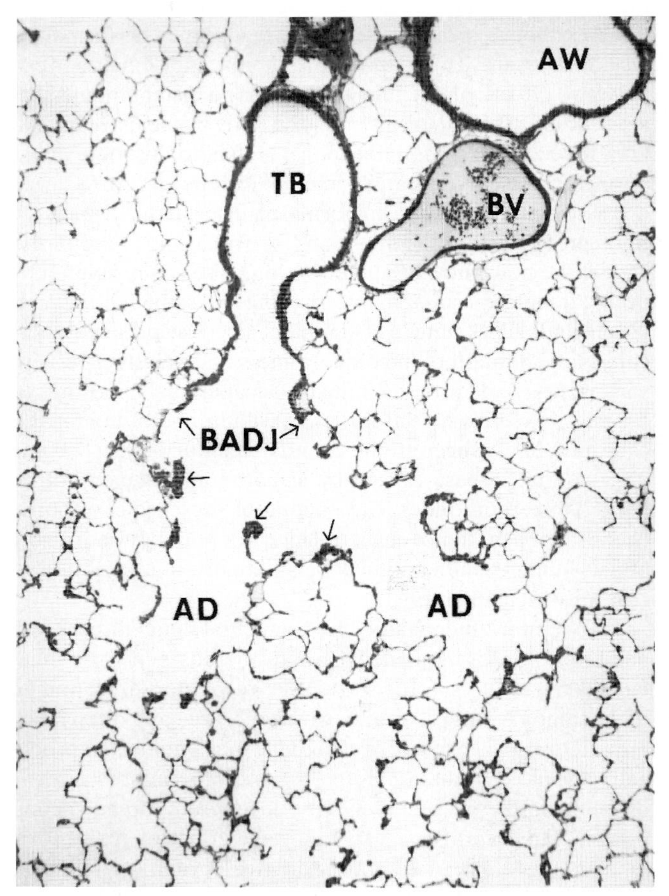


***Figure 15–1. Centriacinar region (ventilatory unit) of the lung.***

An airway and an arteriole [blood vessel (BV)] are in close proximity to the terminal bronchiole (TB) opening into alveolar ducts (AD) at the bronchiole–alveolar duct junction (BADJ). A number of the alveolar septal tips (arrows) close to the BADJ are thickened after a brief (4 h) exposure to asbestos fibers, indicating localization of fiber deposition. Other inhalants, such as ozone, produce lesions in the same locations. (Photograph courtesy of Dr. Kent E. Pinkerton, University of California, Davis.)

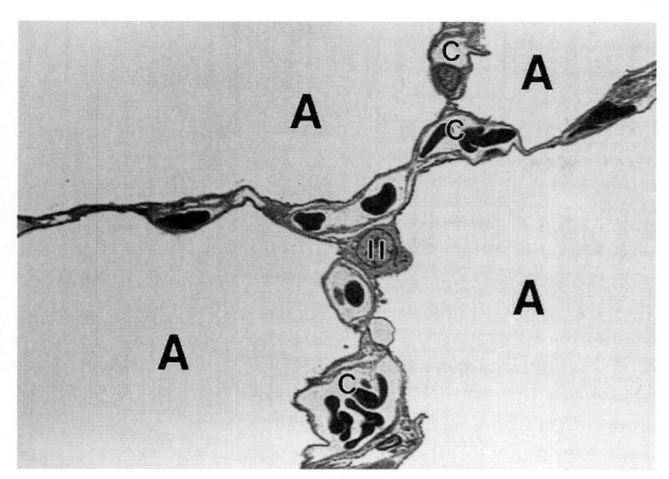


*Figure 15–2. Micrograph of four alveoli (A) separated by the alveolar septum.*

The thin air-to-blood tissue barrier of the alveolar septal wall is composed of squamous alveolar type I cells and occasional alveolar type II cells (II), a small interstitial space, and the attenuated cytoplasm of the endothelial cells that form the wall of the capillaries (C). (Photograph courtesy of Dr. Kent E. Pinkerton, University of California, Davis.)

and formed blood elements are separated from the air space by a thin layer of tissue formed by epithelial, interstitial, and endothelial components (Pinkerton et al., 1991).

Type I and type II alveolar cells represent approximately 25 percent of all the cells in the alveolar septum (Fig. 15-2). Type III epithelial cells, also called brush cells, are relatively rare. Type I cells cover a large surface area (approximately 90 percent of the alveolar surface). They have an attenuated cytoplasm and appear to be poor in organelles but probably are as metabolically competent as are the more compact type II cells. Preferential damage to type I cells by various agents may be explained by the fact that they constitute a large target. Type II cells are cuboidal and show abundant perinuclear cytoplasm. They produce surfactant and, in case of damage to the type I epithelium, may undergo mitotic division and replace damaged cells. The shape of type I and type II cells is independent of alveolar size and is remarkably similar in different species. A typical rat alveolus (14,000 $\mu m^2$ surface) contains an average of two type I cells and three type II cells, whereas a human alveolus with a surface of 200,000 to 300,000 $\mu m^2$ contains 32 type I cells and 51 type II cells (Pinkerton et al., 1991).

The mesenchymal interstitial cell population consists of fibroblasts that produce collagen and elastin, pericytes, monocytes, and lymphocytes. Macrophages reside in the interstitium before they enter the alveoli. Endothelial cells have a thin cytoplasm and cover about one-fourth of the area covered by type I cells. Clara cells are located in the terminal bronchioles and have a high content of xenobiotic metabolizing enzymes.

## Gas Exchange

The principal function of the lung is gas exchange, which consists of ventilation, perfusion, and diffusion. The lung is superbly equipped to handle its main task: bringing essential oxygen to the organs and tissues of the body and eliminating its most abundant waste product, $CO_2$ (Weibel, 1983).

**Ventilation.** During inhalation, fresh air is moved into the lung through the upper respiratory tract and conducting airways and into the terminal respiratory units when the thoracic cage enlarges and the diaphragm moves downward; the lung passively follows this expansion. After diffusion of oxygen into the blood and that of $CO_2$ from the blood into the alveolar spaces, the air (now enriched in $CO_2$) is expelled by exhalation. Relaxation of the chest wall and diaphragm diminishes the internal volume of the thoracic cage, the elastic fibers of the lung parenchyma contract, and air is expelled from the alveolar zone through the airways. Any interference with the elastic properties of the lung, for example, the decrease in elastic fibers that occurs in emphysema, adversely affects ventilation, as do decreases in the diameters of or blockage of the conducting airways, as in asthma.

The total volume of air in an inflated human lung, approximately 5700 $cm^3$, represents the total lung capacity (TLC). After a maximum expiration, the lung retains approximately 1200 $cm^3$ of air, the residual volume (RV). The air volume moved into and out of the lung with a maximum inspiratory and expiratory movement, which is called the vital capacity (VC), is thus approximately 4500 $cm^3$. Under resting conditions, only a fraction of the vital capacity, the tidal volume (TV), is moved into and out of the lung. In resting humans, the TV measures approximately 500 $cm^3$ with each breath (Fig. 15-3). The respiratory frequency, or the number of breaths per minute, is approximately 12 to 20. If an augmented metabolic demand of the body requires the delivery of increased amounts of oxygen, for example, during heavy and prolonged exercise, both the TV and the respiratory rate can be greatly increased. The amount of air moved into and out of the human lung may increase to up to 60 liters per minute. Increased ventilation in a polluted atmosphere increases the deposition of inhaled toxic material. For this reason, it is often stated that people, particularly children, should not exercise during episodes of heavy air pollution.

The TLC, as well as the ratio of RV to VC, changes when the lung is diseased. In emphysema, the alveoli overextend and

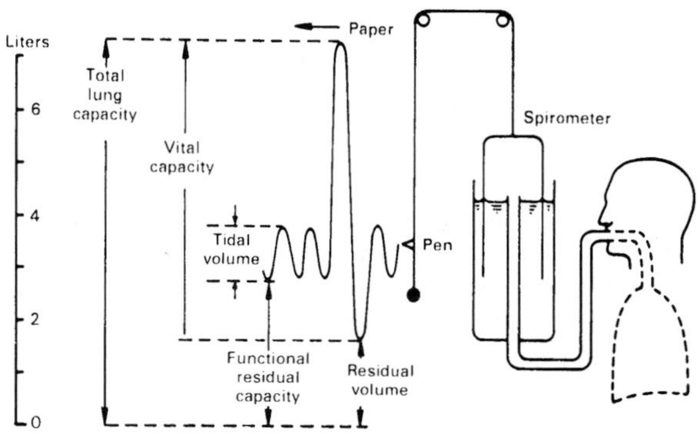

Liters
6
4
2
0
Paper
Total lung capacity
Vital capacity
Tidal volume
Functional residual capacity
Residual volume
Pen
Spirometer

*Figure 15–3. Lung volumes.*

Note that the functional residual capacity and residual volume cannot be measured with spirometer. (From West JB: *Respiratory Physiology—The Essentials.* ©1994 The Williams & Wilkins Co., Baltimore.)

more air is trapped. While the TLC may stay the same or even increase, the volume of air that is actually moved during breathing is diminished. This results in decreased VC with a concomitant increase in RV. If part of the lung collapses or becomes filled with edema fluid, TLC and VC are reduced. Pulmonary function tests give quantitative information on such changes.

**Perfusion.** The lung receives the entire output from the right ventricle, approximately 70 to 80 $cm^3$ of blood per heartbeat, and thus may be exposed to substantial amounts of toxic agents carried in the blood. An agent placed onto or deposited under the skin (subcutaneous injection) or introduced directly into a peripheral vein (intravenous injection) travels through the venous system to the right ventricle and then comes into contact with the pulmonary capillary bed before distribution to other organs or tissues in the body.

**Diffusion.** Gas exchange takes place across the entire alveolar surface. Contact to airborne toxic agent thus occurs over a surface (approximately 140 $m^2$) (Pinkerton et al., 1991) that is second only to the small intestine (approximately 250 $m^2$) (Guyton, 1991) and considerably larger than the skin (approximately 1.75 $m^2$) (Ritschel, 1986), two other organs that are in direct contact with the outside world. A variety of abnormal processes may thicken the alveolar septum and adversely affect the diffusion of oxygen to the erythrocytes. Such processes may include accumulation of liquid in the alveolar space and an abnormal thickening of the pulmonary epithelium. It is often seen as a result of chronic toxicity because of an abnormal accumulation of tissue constituents in the interstitial space through proliferation of interstitial cells. Increased formation and deposition of extracellular substances such as collagen or because of the interstitial accumulation of edema fluid has similar consequences.

## GENERAL PRINCIPLES IN THE PATHOGENESIS OF LUNG DAMAGE CAUSED BY CHEMICALS

### Oxidative Burden

An important type of injury to the lung is thought to be caused by an undue oxidative burden that often is mediated by free radicals, such as those generated by ozone, $NO_2$, tobacco smoke, and lung defense cells. Evidence for the role of free radicals in lung damage includes a wide variety of observations. Numerous studies have reported increases in the activity of free radical–scavenging enzymes in the lungs of animals exposed to $O_3$, $NO_2$, and other toxicants, indirectly supporting this hypothesis. Treatment with various hydroxyl radical scavengers can protect rats from pulmonary edema induced by high doses of thiourea and otherwise lethal levels of gamma irradiation. Other studies have shown protection against hyperoxia by superoxide dismutase or catalase stabilized by encapsulation in liposomes (Turrans et al., 1984).

Theories of lung oxidant toxicity relate to the formation of reactive and unstable free radicals, with subsequent chain reactions leading to uncontrolled destructive oxidation. Recent work has emphasized the pivotal roles of superoxide, nitric oxide, peroxynitrate, hydroxyl radicals, and perhaps singlet oxygen in mediating tissue damage. Reduction of $O_2$ to active $O_2$ metabolites normally occurs as a by-product of cellular metabolism during both microsomal and mitochondrial electron transfer reactions; considerable amounts of superoxide anion are generated by NADPH–cytochrome P-450 reductase reactions. Because these oxidant species are potentially cytotoxic, they may mediate or promote the actions of various pneumotoxicants. Such mechanisms have been proposed for paraquat- and nitrofurantoin-induced lung injury. When cellular injury of any type occurs, the release of otherwise contained cellular constituents such as microsomes and flavoproteins into the extracellular space may lead to extracellular generation of deleterious reactive $O_2$ species.

Among mammalian cells, neutrophils, monocytes, and macrophages seem particularly adept at converting molecular $O_2$ to reactive $O_2$ metabolites; this probably is related to their phagocytosis and antimicrobial activities. As a by-product of this capability, toxic $O_2$ species are released (possibly by the plasmalemma itself) into surrounding tissues. As most forms of toxic pulmonary edema are accompanied by phagocyte accumulation in the lung microcirculation (pulmonary leukostasis) and parenchyma, oxidative damage may represent a significant component of all types of pneumotoxic lung injury accompanied by a phagocyte-mediated inflammatory component.

Chemotactic and phagocytic "activation" processes result in a substantial increase in the release of potent oxidants by stimulated phagocytes; these radicals cause oxidative damage to the surrounding tissues. A key role of hydrogen peroxide as the mediator of the extracellular cytotoxic mechanism of "activated" phagocytes has been well documented. Phenomena occurring at the phagocyte surface, such as those which may occur in endogenous lung phagocytes after exposure to dusts and toxic gases, or in circulating phagocytes before their accumulation in the lung or after to their attachment to normal or damaged lung endothelium seem to be important in determining their degree of enhanced oxidative activity, which is otherwise at a much lower basal level in the unstimulated cell. It also has been long appreciated that phagocytes may cause lysosomal enzyme release and tissue damage. The significance of these events in initiating or amplifying lung injury and edema, however, has not been completely characterized.

Although steroids appear to inhibit the generation of toxic oxygen metabolites by "activated" phagocytes, there is little convincing evidence that steroids limit pneumotoxin-induced pulmonary edema. The fact that oxidative processes are complex is suggested by the finding that phagocytic production of active oxygen species causes inactivation of proteinase inhibitors and degranulation of mast cells. The production of oxygen radicals by phagocytes is enhanced not only by interactions of cell surface membranes with various appropriate stimuli but also by hyperoxia. Platelets (and platelet microthrombi) also have the ability to generate activated $O_2$ species.

The lung can respond with specific defense mechanisms that may be acquired over time and may be stimulated by constant exposure to numerous species of airborne microorganisms as well as by a variety of low- and high-molecular-weight antigenic materials. The immune system can mount either cellular or humorally mediated responses to these inhaled antigens that can add to the nonspecific mechanisms of lung defense. Direct immunologic effects occur when inhaled foreign material sensitizes the respiratory system to further exposure to the same material. The mammalian lung has a well-developed immune system. Lymphocytes reside in the hilar or mediastinal lymph nodes, lymphoid aggregates, and lymphoepithelial nodules as well as in aggregates or as single cells throughout the airways. Bronchoconstriction and chronic pulmonary disease can result from the inhalation of materials that appear to act wholly or partly through an allergic response. In some instances, these reactions are caused by spores of molds or bacterial contaminants. Frequently, chemical components of the sensitizing dusts or gases are responsible for the allergic response. Low-molecular-weight compounds can act as haptens that combine with native proteins to form a complex that is recognized as an antigen by the immune system. Further exposure to the sensitizing compound can result in an allergic reaction that is characterized by the release of various inflammatory mediators that produce an early and/or a late bronchoconstrictor response. Such a response is observed in sensitized workers exposed to toluene diisocyanate (TDI), a chemical widely used in the manufacture of polyurethane plastics (Karol et al., 1994).

Indirect immune effects occur when exposure to air pollutants either suppresses or enhances the immune response to other materials. Both sulfur dioxide ($SO_2$) and ozone can boost the response of the respiratory system to inhaled foreign material, at least in experimental animals (guinea pigs). It is not known whether these effects occur in humans, but they form the bases for concerns about increased susceptibility of asthmatic individuals to air pollutants such as ozone and sulfur dioxide.

## Toxic Inhalants, Gases, and Dosimetry

The sites of deposition of gases in the respiratory tract define the pattern of toxicity of those gases. Water solubility is the critical factor in determining how deeply a given gas penetrates into the lung. Highly soluble gases such as $SO_2$ do not penetrate farther than the nose and are therefore relatively nontoxic to animals, especially obligatory nose breathers such as the rat. When $SO_2$ is inhaled with particles or aerosols that can adsorb the gas, it can bypass the nasopharynx, penetrate to the deep lung, and elicit toxic responses (Amdur, 1974). Relatively insoluble gases such as ozone and $NO_2$ penetrate deeply into the lung and reach the smallest airways and the alveoli (centriacinar region), where they can elicit toxic responses. Mathematical models of gas entry and deposition in the lung that are based solely on the aqueous solubility of a gas predict sites of lung lesions fairly accurately. These models may be useful for extrapolating findings made in laboratory animals to humans (Overton et al., 1987; Kimbell et al., 1993). Very insoluble gases such as CO and $H_2S$ efficiently pass through the respiratory tract and are taken up by the pulmonary blood supply to be distributed throughout the body.

## Particle Deposition and Clearance

The site of deposition of solid particles or droplets in the respiratory tract, along with their chemical makeup, is important. Particle size is usually the critical factor that determines the region of the respiratory tract in which a particle or an aerosol will be deposited. Deposition of particles on the surface of the lung and airways is brought about by a combination of lung anatomy and the patterns of airflow in the respiratory system (Fig. 15-4).

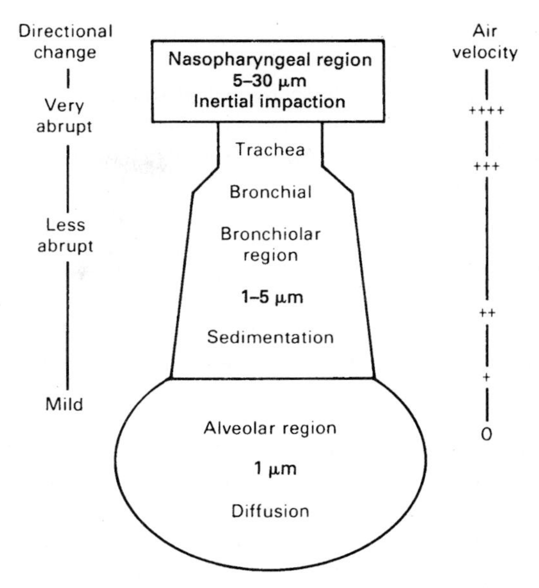


***Figure 15-4. Parameters influencing particle deposition.** [From Casarett, LJ: The vital sacs: Alveolar clearance mechanisms in inhalation toxicology, in Blood FR (ed): Essays in Toxicology. New York: Academic Press, 1972, vol 3.]*

**Particle Size.** Inhaled aerosols are most frequently polydisperse in regard to size. The size distribution of many aerosols approximates a log-normal distribution that may be described by the *median* or *geometric mean* and the *geometric standard deviation*. A plot of the frequency of occurrence of a given size against the log of the size produces a bell-shaped probability curve. Particle data frequently are handled by plotting the cumulative percentage of particles smaller than a stated size on log-probability paper. This results in a straight line that may be fitted by eye or mathematically. In actual practice, it is not unusual to have some deviation from a straight line at the largest or smallest particle sizes measured. The geometric mean is the 50 percent size as the mean bisects the curve. The geometric standard deviation ($\sigma g$) is calculated as

$$\sigma g = \frac{84.1\%\text{size}}{50\%\ \text{size}}$$

The $\sigma g$ of the particle size distribution is a measure of the polydispersity of the aerosol. In the laboratory, values for $\sigma g$ of 1.8 to 3.0 are encountered frequently. In the field, values for $\sigma g$ may range up to 4.5. An aerosol with a $\sigma g$ below 1.2 may be considered monodisperse.

The median diameter that is determined may reflect the number of particles, as in the count median diameter (CMD), or reflect mass, as in the mass median aerodynamic diameter (MMAD). The larger the number and mass of particles capable of penetrating the lung, the greater the probability of a toxic effect. The size distribution in relation to other factors, such as particle shape and surface area, also may be of interest. Surface area is of special importance when toxic materials are adsorbed on the surfaces of particles and thus are carried to the lung.

Particles that are nonspherical in shape are frequently characterized in terms of equivalent spheres on the basis of equal mass, volume, or aerodynamic drag. The *aerodynamic diameter* takes into account both the density of the particle and aerodynamic drag. It represents the diameter of a unit density sphere with the same terminal settling velocity as the particle, regardless of its size, shape, and density. Aerodynamic diameter is the proper measurement for particles that are deposited by impaction and sedimentation. For very small particles, which are deposited primarily by diffusion, the critical factor is particle size, not density. It must be kept in mind that the size of a particle may change before its deposition in the respiratory tract. Materials that are hygroscopic, such as sodium chloride, sulfuric acid, and glycerol, take on water and grow in size in the warm, saturated atmosphere of the lower respiratory tract.

**Deposition Mechanisms.** Deposition of particles occurs primarily by interception, impaction, sedimentation, and diffusion (brownian movement). Interception occurs only when the trajectory of a particle brings it near enough to a surface so that an edge of the particle contacts the airway surface. Interception is important for the deposition of fibers. Whereas fiber diameter determines the probability of deposition by impaction and sedimentation, interception is dependent on fiber length. Thus, a fiber with a diameter of 1 μm and a length of 200 μm will be deposited in the bronchial tree primarily by interception rather than impaction.

As a result of inertia, particles suspended in air tend to continue to travel along their original path. In a bending airstream, such as at an airway bifurcation, a particle may be impacted on the surface. At relatively symmetrical bifurcations, which typically occur in the human lung, the deposition rate is likely to be high for particles that move in the center of the airway. Generalizations regarding the site of deposition of particles of a given size are problematic. However, in the average adult, most particles larger than 10 μm in aerodynamic diameter are deposited in the nose or oral pharynx and cannot penetrate to tissues distal to the larynx. Recent data have shown that very fine particles (0.01 μm and smaller) are also trapped relatively efficiently in the upper airways by diffusion. Particles that penetrate beyond the upper airways are available to be deposited in the bronchial region and the deeper-lying airways. Therefore, the alveolar region has significant deposition efficiencies for particles smaller than 5 μm and larger than 0.003 μm.

Sedimentation brings about deposition in the smaller bronchi, the bronchioles, and the alveolar spaces, where the airways are small and the velocity of airflow is low. As a particle moves downward through air, buoyancy and the resistance of air act on the particle in an upward direction while gravitational force acts on the particle in a downward direction. Eventually, the gravitational force equilibrates with the sum of the buoyancy and the air resistance, and the particle continues to settle with a constant velocity known as the terminal settling velocity. Sedimentation is not a significant route of particle deposition when the aerodynamic diameter is below 0.5 μm.

Diffusion is an important factor in the deposition of submicrometer particles. A random motion is imparted to these particles by the impact of gas molecules. This brownian motion increases with decreasing particle size, and so diffusion is an important deposition mechanism in the nose and in other airways and alveoli for particles smaller than about 0.5 μm.

An important factor in particle deposition is the pattern of breathing. During quiet breathing, in which the TV is only two to three times the volume of the anatomic dead space (i.e, the volume of the conducting airways where gas exchange does not occur), a large proportion of the inhaled particles may be exhaled. During exercise, when larger volumes are inhaled at higher velocities, impaction in the large airways and sedimentation and diffusion in the smaller airways and alveoli increase. Breath holding also increases deposition from sedimentation and diffusion. Factors that modify the diameter of the conducting airways can alter particle deposition. In patients with chronic bronchitis, the mucous layer is greatly thickened and extended peripherally and may partially block the airways in some areas. Jets formed by air flowing through such partially occluded airways have the potential to increase the deposition of particles by impaction and diffusion in the small airways. Irritant materials that produce bronchoconstriction tend to increase the tracheobronchial deposition of particles. Cigarette smoking has been shown experimentally to produce such an effect.

**Particle Clearance.** The clearance of deposited particles is an important aspect of lung defense. Rapid removal lessens the time available to cause damage to the pulmonary tissues or permit local absorption. The specific mechanisms available for the removal of particles from the respiratory tract vary with the site of the deposition. It is important to emphasize that clearance of particles from the respiratory tract is not synonymous with clearance from the body. Depending on the specific clearance mechanism used, particles are cleared to (1) the stomach and gastrointestinal (GI) tract, (2) the lymphatics and lymph nodes, where they may be dissolved and enter the venous circulation, or (3) the pulmonary vasculature. The only mechanisms by which the respiratory system can truly remove deposited particles from the body are coughing and blowing the nose.

***Nasal Clearance.*** Particles deposited in the nose are cleared by various mechanisms, depending on their site of deposition and solubility in mucus. The anterior portion of the nose is lined with relatively dry squamous epithelium, and so particles deposited there are removed by extrinsic actions such as wiping and blowing. The other regions of the nose are largely covered by a mucociliary epithelium that propels mucus toward the glottis, where it is swallowed. Insoluble particles generally are cleared from this region in healthy adults and swallowed within an hour of deposition. Particles that are soluble in mucus may dissolve and enter the epithelium and/or blood before they can be mechanically removed. Uncertainties still remain about the clearance of particles that are deposited on olfactory regions or areas that are damaged by acute infection, chronic illnesses, or toxic injury.

***Tracheobronchial Clearance.*** The mucus layer covering the tracheobronchial tree is moved upward by the beating of the underlying cilia. This mucociliary escalator transports deposited particles and particle-laden macrophages upward to the oropharynx, where they are swallowed and pass through the GI tract. Mucociliary clearance is relatively rapid in healthy individuals and is completed within 24 to 48 h for particles deposited in the lower airways. Infection and other injuries can greatly impair clearance.

***Pulmonary Clearance.*** There are several primary ways by which particulate material is removed from the lower respiratory tract once it has been deposited:

1. Particles may be directly trapped on the fluid layer of the conducting airways by impaction and cleared upward, in the tracheobronchial tree via the mucociliary escalator.
2. Particles may be phagocytized by macrophages and cleared via the mucociliary escalator.
3. Particles may be phagocytized by alveolar macrophages and removed via the lymphatic drainage.
4. Material may dissolve from the surfaces of particles and be removed via the bloodstream or lymphatics.
5. Small particles may directly penetrate epithelial membranes.

Minutes after particles are inhaled, they may be found in alveolar macrophages. Many alveolar macrophages are ultimately transported to the mucociliary escalator. It is possible that macrophages are carried to the bronchioles with the alveolar fluid that contributes to the fluid layer in the airways. Other particles may be sequestered in the lung for very long periods, often in macrophages located in the interstitium.

**Airway Reactivity.** Large airways are surrounded by bronchial smooth muscles, which help maintain airway tone and diameter during expansion and contraction of the lung. Bronchial smooth muscle tone is normally regulated by the autonomic nervous system. Reflex contraction occurs when receptors in the trachea and large bronchi are stimulated by irritants such as cigarette smoke and air pollutants. Bronchoconstriction can be provoked by cholinergic drugs such as acetylcholine, a phenomenon that serves as the basis for a sensitive measure (bronchoprovocation testing) of whether a toxicant can cause bronchoconstriction in animals or humans primed by a prior dose of an acetylcholinelike agent. These agents bind to cell surface receptors (cholinergic receptors) and trigger an increase in the intracellular concentration of cyclic guanosine monophosphate (cGMP), which in turn facilitates smooth muscle contraction. The actions of cGMP can be antagonized by cyclicadenosine monophospate (cAMP), which has bronchodilatory activity, and can be increased by agents that bind to beta-adrenergic receptors on the cell surface. Other important mediators of airway smooth muscle tone include histamine, various prostaglandins and leukotrienes, substance P, and nitric oxide. The bronchial smooth muscles of individuals with asthma contract with much less provocation than do those of normal subjects. Bronchoconstriction causes a decrease in airway diameter and a corresponding increase in resistance to airflow. Characteristic associated symptoms include wheezing, coughing, a sensation of chest tightness, and dyspnea. Exercise potentiates these problems. A major cause of concern about ambient air pollution is whether asthmatic individuals represent a population that is particularly susceptible to the adverse health effects of sulfur dioxide, ozone, nitrogen dioxide, other respiratory irritant gases, and respirable particles. Since the major component of airway resistance usually is contributed by large bronchi, inhaled agents that cause reflex bronchoconstriction are generally irritant gases with moderate solubility. Demonstrations of the bronchoconstrictive effects of gases in laboratory animals often are performed in guinea pigs, which seem to represent a natural animal model of asthmatic humans with respect to innate airway reactivity.

**Pulmonary Edema.** Toxic pulmonary edema represents an acute, exudative phase of lung injury that generally produces an increase in the alveolar-capillary barrier. Edema fluid, when present, alters ventilation-perfusion relationships and limits diffusive transfer of $O_2$ and $CO_2$ even in otherwise structurally normal alveoli. Edema is often a sign of acute lung injury.

The biological consequences of toxic pulmonary edema not only induce acute compromise of lung structure and function but also may include abnormalities that remain after resolution of the edematous process. After exposure to some toxic agents in which the alveolar-capillary surface is denuded (such as alloxan), recovery is unlikely, whereas in situations of more modest injury (such as histamine administration), full recovery is readily achievable. Between these two extremes there are forms of severe lung injury accompanied by amplified inflammatory damage and/or exaggerated restorative-reparative processes (e.g., after paraquat ingestion). In these severe forms, the extensive interstitial and intraalveolar inflammatory exudate resolves via fibrogenesis, an outcome that may be beneficial or damaging to the lung. Accumulation and turnover of inflammatory cells and related immune responses in an edematous lung probably play a role in eliciting both mitogenic activity and fibrogenic responses.

Pulmonary edema is customarily quantified in experimental animals by some form of gravimetric measurement of lung water content. Very commonly, the wet (undesiccated) weight of the whole lung or that of a single lung lobe is determined. This value is often normalized to the weight of the animal from which the lung was taken. Alternatively, some investigators determine lung water content by weighing whole lungs or lung slices before and after complete drying in an oven or desiccator. Commonly used methods for expressing such data include (1) percentage water content [$100 \times$ (wet weight $-$ dry weight)/(wet weight)], (2) percentage dry weight [$100 \times$ (dry weight)/(wet weight)], and (3) water content $\approx$[(ml of water)/(dry weight)].

**Respiratory Tract Injury.** Airborne agents can contact cells lining the respiratory tract from the nostrils to the gas-exchanging region. The sites of interaction of toxicants in the respiratory tract have important implications for evaluation of the risk to humans posed by inhalants. For example, rats have much more nasal surface on a per body weight basis than do humans. Measurement of DNA-protein cross-links formed in nasal tissue by the highly reactive gas formaldehyde has demonstrated that rats, which readily develop nasal tumors, have many more DNA cross-links per unit of exposure (concentration of formaldehyde $\times$ duration of exposure) than do monkeys. Because the breathing pattern of humans resembles that of monkeys more than that of rats, it was concluded that extrapolation of tumor data from rats to humans on the basis of formaldehyde concentration may overestimate doses of formaldehyde to humans. Instead, measurement of DNA cross-links was deemed an appropriate biomarker of the delivered dose (U.S. EPA, 1991). Patterns of animal activity can affect dose to the lung; nocturnally active animals such as rats receive a greater dose per unit of exposure at night than during the day, whereas humans show the opposite diurnal relationships of exposure concentration to dose.

Certain gases and vapors stimulate nerve endings in the nose, particularly those of the trigeminal nerve (Nielsen and Alarie, 1991). The result is holding of the breath or changes in breathing patterns, to avoid or reduce further exposure. If continued exposure cannot be avoided, many acidic or alkaline irritants produce cell necrosis and increased permeability of the alveolar walls. Other inhaled agents can be more insidious; inhalation of HCl, $NO_2$, $NH_3$, or phosgene may at first produce very little apparent damage in the respiratory tract. The epithelial barrier in the alveolar zone, after a latency period of several hours, begins to leak, flooding the alveoli and producing a delayed pulmonary edema that is often fatal.

A different pathogenetic mechanism is typical of highly reactive molecules such as ozone. It is unlikely that ozone as such can penetrate beyond the layer of fluid covering the cells of the lung. Instead, ozone lesions are propagated by a cascade of secondary reaction products, such as aldehydes and hydroxyperoxides produced by ozonolysis of fatty acids and other substrates in the lung's lining fluid, and by reactive oxygen species arising from free radical reactions. Reactive oxygen species also have been implicated in pulmonary bleomycin toxicity, pulmonary oxygen toxicity, paraquat toxicity, and the development of chronic lesions such as the fibrogenic and carcinogenic effects of asbestos fibers.

Metabolism of foreign compounds can be involved in the pathogenesis of lung injury. The balance of activation and detoxification plays a key role in determining whether a given chemical ultimately will cause damage. The lung contains most of the enzymes involved in xenobiotic metabolism that have been identified in other tissues, such as the liver. While the overall levels of these enzymes tend to be lower in lung than in liver, they often are highly concentrated in specific cell populations of the respiratory tract. Moreover, their specific content of particular cytochrome P-450 isozymes may be much higher in lung. Thus, the turnover of a substrate for a lung P-450 may be far more rapid than occurs in liver. Many isozymes of the cytochrome P-450 complex have been identified in and isolated from the lungs of rabbits, rats, hamsters and humans. Cytochrome P-450 1A1 is present in low amounts in normal rat and rabbit lungs but is highly inducible by polycyclic aromatic hydrocarbons, flavones, and mixtures of polyhalogenated biphenyls. This isozyme also is present in human lungs and is thought to be involved in the metabolic activation of the polycyclic aromatic hydrocarbons that are present in cigarette smoke. By inference, this P-450 isozyme may play a role in the pathogenesis of lung cancer. Attempts have been made to use the expression of cytochrome P-450 1A1 as a biomarker of exposure and sensitivity to cigarette smoke in humans, although the precise relationships remain unclear. Cytochrome P-450 2B1, which is readily inducible in rat liver by phenobarbital, is not inducible in lung tissue. Other isozymes identified in human lung are cytochrome P-450 2F1, 4B1, and 3A4. Further microsomal enzymes found in the lung include NADPH–cytochrome P-450 reductase, epoxide hydrolase, and flavin-containing monoxygenases. Finally, two important cytosolic enzymes involved in lung xenobiotic metabolism are glutathione-*S*-transferase and glutathione peroxidase (Guengerich, 1993). Adult human lungs appear to contain several forms of glutathione-*S*-transferase.

## Mediators of Lung Toxicity

Advances in cell culture techniques have allowed investigators to examine the role of specific signal molecules in toxicant-induced lung damage; this is a very active area of research. Such studies are often guided by results obtained by analysis of cytokines and other mediators in lung lavage fluid from animals or human volunteers exposed to inhaled toxic agents (Devlin et al., 1991).

For example, platelet-derived growth factor (PDGF), transforming growth factor (TGF-beta), and tumor necrosis factor (TNF-alpha) have all been implicated in the cascade of reactions that is thought to be responsible for the pathogenesis of pulmonary fibrosis (Piguet et al., 1989; Broekelmann et al., 1991). Similarly, several of the 13 described members of the interleukin family, especially IL-1, IL-2, and IL-6, are thought to be essential components of the lung's response to epithelial cell injury. Various specific prostaglandins, especially $PGE_2$, and leukotrienes have been implicated in intracellular signaling pathways in the lung. The roles of cell surface adhesion molecules and their interaction with cell matrix components and with control of inflammatory cell migration (particularly neutrophil influx to the lung) have been studied intensively.

Analysis of normal lung homogenates suggests that the lung contains large amounts of endogenous cytokines and inflammatory mediators, far more than enough for these potent compounds to elicit effects. Thus, these agents must be compartmentalized in a healthy lung to control their potent bioactivity. How these processes are regulated normally, what exactly goes wrong with homeostasis in a damaged lung, the temporal and geographic relationship of different cytokines in the amplification of an initial injurious event, and detailed mechanisms of resolution of lung injury are not well understood and represent the current focus of much research on mechanisms of lung injury by toxic agents. The reader is referred to reviews of these topics (Kelley, 1990; Elias et al., 1990; Pilewski and Albelda, 1993) for more details on specific mediators and toxic agents in this rapidly changing research area.

**Cell Proliferation.** The effects of toxicants on the lung may be reversible or irreversible. Postexposure progression of lung fibrosis has been demonstrated in rats exposed to ozone, mice exposed to cyclophosphamide, and hamsters exposed to bleomycin or bleomycin plus oxygen. The mechanisms for exacerbating lung damage or repairing such damage during a postexposure period in which filtered air alone is inhaled are not obvious. Examination of the time course and cellular components of reepithelialization of the alveolar ducts and walls during the postexposure period would be especially important in this regard. To avoid misinterpretation of data as a result of altered growth rates in exposed and control animals, the use of appropriate (pair-fed) controls in experiments with growing animals exposed to high levels of toxicants is required. Research on the postexposure effects of inhaled toxicants is an important area for further study.

The lung parenchyma repairs itself remarkably efficiently. In mice exposed to 90 percent oxygen for 6 days, large portions of the alveolar epithelium become severely damaged. If the animals are allowed to recover in air, type II alveolar epithelial cells divide and eventually transform into type I epithelial cells, which recover the denuded alveolar basement membrane. Other cells in the alveolar zone, such as capillary endothelial cells, interstitial cells, and alveolar macrophages, also proliferate. A similar sequence of events occurs in lungs damaged by inhaled $CdCl_2$ or bloodborne butylated hydroxytoluene or methylcyclopentadienyl manganese tricarbonyl. Epithelial recovery may be delayed in acute lung damage produced by cytostatic drugs (Witschi, 1991). Damage to the epithelium is repaired by division of Clara cells and other nonciliated cells in the conducting airways (Shami and Evans, 1991)

Originally it was thought that the epithelial labeling index in the pulmonary parenchyma is directly proportional to the extent of injury suffered by the type I cell population. However, the migration of mobile blood cells such as leukocytes across the pulmonary capillaries into the alveolar lumen can be sufficient to trigger a mitotic response. This observation is important, since it may explain the increased cell proliferation seen in the lung without concomitant parenchymal damage. In the nose, labeled cells provide indexes of exposure in the absence of other histopathologic signs.

## CHRONIC RESPONSES OF THE LUNG TO INJURY

### Fibrosis

Defined clinically, lung fibrosis refers to the type of interstitial fibrosis that is seen in the later stages of idiopathic pulmonary fibrosis (also called cryptogenic fibrosing alveolitis in the United Kingdom). In this disease, the hallmark of pulmonary fibrosis seen by the pathologist is increased focal staining of collagen fibers in the alveolar interstitium. Fibrotic lungs from humans with acute or chronic pulmonary fibrosis contain increased amounts of collagen as evaluated biochemically, in agreement with the histological findings.

In lungs damaged by toxicants, the response resembles adult or infant respiratory distress syndrome more closely than it resembles chronic interstitial fibrosis. Excess lung collagen is usually observed not only in the alveolar interstitium but also throughout the centriacinar region, including the alveolar ducts and respiratory bronchioles. The relationship between increased collagen deposition around small airways and lung mechanics is not understood either theoretically or empirically.

At least 13 genetically distinct collagen types are known to occur in all mammals, of which at least 7 have been found in normal lungs or synthesized by isolated lung cells. Two types predominate in the lung, representing about 90 percent or more of the total lung collagen. Type I and type III collagen are major interstitial components and are found in the normal lungs of all mammals in an approximate ratio of 2:1. Type I collagen is the material that stains histologically as "collagen," whereas type III collagen is appreciated histologically as reticulin. Some types of toxicant-induced pulmonary fibrosis, including that induced by $O_3$, involve abnormalities in the type of collagen made. For example, there is an increase in type I collagen relative to type III collagen in patients with idiopathic pulmonary fibrosis. Similar shifts have been demonstrated in the lungs of adults and infants dying of acute respiratory distress syndrome. It is not known whether shifts in collagen types, compared with absolute increases in collagen content, account for the increased stiffness of fibrotic lungs. Type III collagen is much more compliant than is type I; thus, an increasing proportion of type I relative to type III collagen may result in a stiffer lung, as is observed in pulmonary fibrosis. Changes in collagen cross-linking in fibrotic lungs also may contribute to the increased stiffness. It is unclear whether the observed increase in stainable collagen is due solely to the increase in the collagen content of the lungs observed biochemically or whether altered collagen types or cross-linking might also contribute to the histological changes.

Increased collagen type I:type III ratios also have been observed in newly synthesized collagen in several animal models of acute pulmonary fibrosis. Although the mechanism for this shift in collagen types is unknown, there are many possible explanations. Clones of fibroblasts responsive to recruitment and/or proliferation factors may preferentially synthesize type I collagen compared with the action of the fibroblasts normally present. Alterations in the extracellular matrix resulting from inflammatory mediators secreted by various effector cells also may cause the fibroblasts to switch the collagen phenotype that is synthesized.

Collagen associated with fibrosis also may be abnormal with respect to cross-linking. Alterations in cross-links in experimental silicosis and bleomycin-induced fibrosis have been described. As in the case of alterations in collagen type ratios, it is unclear whether the mechanisms can be ascribed to changes in the clones of fibroblasts that actively synthesize collagen or to changes in the milieu that secondarily affect the nature of the collagen made by a given population of lung fibroblasts.

### Emphysema

In many ways emphysema can be viewed as the opposite of fibrosis in terms of the response of the lungs to an insult: The lungs become larger and too compliant rather than becoming smaller and stiffer. Destruction of the gas-exchanging surface area results in a distended, hyperinflated lung that no longer effectively exchanges oxygen and carbon dioxide as a result of both loss of tissue and air trapping. The currently accepted pathological definition of emphysema is "a condition of the lung characterized by abnormal enlargement of the airspaces distal to the terminal bronchiole, accompanied by destruction of the walls, without obvious fibrosis" (Snider et al., 1985). The major cause of human emphysema is, by far, cigarette smoke inhalation, although other toxicants also can elicit this response. A feature of toxicant-induced emphysema is severe or recurrent inflammation, especially alveolitis with release of proteolytic enzymes by participating leukocytes.

A unifying hypothesis that explains the pathogenesis of emphysema has emerged from studies by several investigators. Early clinical research on screening blood protein phenotypes identified a rare mutation giving rise to a hereditary deficiency of the serum globulin alpha$_1$-antitrypsin (Laurell and Eriksson, 1963). Homozygotes for this mutation had no circulating levels of this protein, which can prevent the proteolytic activity of serine proteases such as trypsin. Thus, alpha$_1$-antitrypsin (now called alpha$_1$-antiprotease) is one of the body's main defenses against uncontrolled proteolytic digestion by this class of enzymes, which includes elastase. There is a clinical association between the genetic lack of this important inhibitor of elastase and the development of emphysema at an extraordinarily young age. Further studies in smokers led to the hypothesis that neutrophil (and perhaps alveolar macrophage) elastases can break down lung elastin and thus cause emphysema; these elastases usually are kept in check by alpha$_1$-antiprotease that diffuses into the lung from the blood. As the individual ages, an accumulation of random elastolytic events can cause the emphysematous changes in the lungs that are normally associated with aging. Toxicants that cause inflammatory cell influx and thus increase the burden of neutrophil elastase can accelerate this process. In accordance with this hypothesis are a large number of experimental studies in animals instilled intratracheally with pancreatic or neutrophil elastase or with other proteolytic enzymes that can digest elastin in which a pathological condition develops that has some of the characteristics of emphysema, including destruction of alveolar walls and airspace enlargement in the lung parenchyma.

An additional clue to the pathogenesis of emphysema is provided by the observation that transgenic mice that overexpress the gene for human collagenase develop emphysema of extremely early onset (D'Armiento et al., 1992). This new animal model suggests that enzymes other than elastase may play an important role in the pathogenesis of emphysema and that in its simplest form the elastase-antiprotease model alone cannot fully explain the detailed biochemical mechanisms that underlie the etiology of emphysema.

## Lung Cancer

Lung cancer, an extremely rare disease around the turn of the century, is now the leading cause of death from cancer among men and women. Because lung cancer was initially such an unusual illness, a rise in its incidence during the 1930s was noticed by clinicians and pathologists. Cigarette smoking, which had become popular during World War I, was suspected as a possible cause. Retrospective and, more conclusively, prospective epidemiological studies confirmed a causal association between tobacco smoking and lung cancer. Smoking of cigarettes is the most important single risk factor for the development of lung cancer. It has been estimated that approximately 80 percent to 90 percent of lung cancers (and several other cancers, such as cancer of the bladder, esophagus, oral cavity, and pancreas) are caused by this habit. Average smokers have a 10-fold, and heavy smokers a 20-fold, increased risk of developing lung cancer compared with nonsmokers.

Inhalation of asbestos fibers and metallic dusts or fumes, such as arsenic, beryllium, cadmium, chromium, and nickel, encountered in smelting and manufacturing operations has been associated with cancer of the respiratory tract. Workers who manufacture chloromethyl ether or mustard gas also have an increased risk of developing lung cancers, as do men exposed to effluent gases from coke ovens. Radon gas is a known human lung carcinogen. Formaldehyde is a probable human respiratory carcinogen. Silica, human-made fibers, and welding fumes are suspected carcinogens (International Agency for Research on Cancer, 1987, 1993). Smokers who inhale radon or asbestos fibers increase their risk of developing lung cancer severalfold, suggesting a synergistic interaction between the carcinogens. Whether common air pollutants such as ozone, nitrogen dioxide, sulfur dioxide, and fumes emanating from power plants and oil refineries contribute to the development of lung cancer in the general population is not known; epidemiological studies on rural-urban differences in lung cancer incidence remain equivocal, as do animal studies (Samet, 1994). Indoor air pollution, including environmental tobacco smoke, increases the risk of developing lung cancer in nonsmokers (U.S. EPA, 1992).

Human lung cancers may have a latency period of 20 to 40 years, making the relationship to specific exposures difficult to establish. Most lung cancers in humans appear to originate from the cells lining the airways (lung cancer originating from such sites is often referred to as bronchogenic carcinoma); peripheral lung tumors (bronchoalveolar carcinomas) occur less frequently. Compared with cancer in the lung, cancer in the upper respiratory tract is less common. Malignant lesions of the nasal passages, which are seen frequently in experimental animals, are comparatively rare in humans. They are associated with certain occupations, including chromate workers, nickel refiners, mustard gas makers, isopropyl alcohol workers, makers of wooden furniture, and boot and shoe workers. Possible carcinogens include hexavalent chromium compounds, metallic nickel and nickel subsulfide, nickel oxide, and certain wood and leather dusts.

The potential mechanisms of lung carcinogenesis have been studied extensively by means of analysis of tumor material and in studies of human bronchial cells maintained in culture. Damage to DNA is thought to be a key mechanism. An activated carcinogen or its metabolic product, such as alkyldiazonium ions derived from *N*-nitrosamines, may interact with DNA. Persistence of $O^6$-alkyldeoxyguanosine in DNA appears to correlate with carcinogenicity. However, tumors do not always develop when adducts are present, and adduct formation may be a necessary but not sufficient condition for carcinogenesis. DNA damage caused by active oxygen species is another potentially important mechanism. Ionizing radiation leads to the formation of superoxide, which is converted through the action of superoxide dismutase to hydrogen peroxide. In the presence of Fe and other transition metals, hydroxyl radicals may be formed which then cause DNA strand breaks. Cigarette smoke contains high quantities of active oxygen species and other free radicals. Additional oxidative stress may be placed on the lung tissue of smokers by the release of superoxide anions and hydrogen peroxide by activated macrophages, metabolism of carcinogens, and lipid peroxidation caused by reactive aldehydes (Church and Pryor, 1991).

In laboratory animals, spontaneously occurring malignant lung tumors are uncommon unless the animals reach a very advanced age. Exposure to carcinogens by the inhalation route or by intratracheal instillation or systemic administration readily produces lung tumors in many laboratory species, such as mice, rats, hamsters, and dogs. There are several differences between lung tumors in animals and bronchogenic cancer in humans. In animals, particularly rodents, most tumors are in the periphery rather than arising from the bronchi. The incidence of benign lung tumors such as adenomas is often very high, and carcinomas seem to require more time to develop. Lung tumors in animals do not metastasize as aggressively, if they do so at all, as do human lung cancers (Hahn, 1989). Cancer of the nasal passages is readily induced in experimental animals in inhalation studies.

Because lung tumors in mice and rats are often seen in carcinogenesis bioassays, they deserve special mention. Murine lung tumors are mostly benign-appearing adenomas originating from alveolar type II cells or bronchiolar Clara cells. Some eventually assume malignant features, although it is not clear whether adenocarcinomas arise from adenomas or represent a new tumor generation. Certain mouse strains, such as strain A and the Swiss-Webster mouse, have a high incidence of spontaneously occurring lung tumors. These animals respond with increased numbers of tumors to the inhalation or injection of many carcinogens. Other strains are much more resistant. Lung tumors in strain A mice have become valuable tools for studing the genetic factors that determine susceptibility (Malkinson, 1992). They contain frequent mutations in the *K-ras* gene. Methylating nitrosamines (NNK and DMN) produce mutations consistent with the formation of $O^6$-methylguanine and ethylating nitrosamines (ENU and DEN) and mutations consistent with the formation of $O^4$-ethylthymidine. Other agents, such as urethane, create unexpected mutations. In strains less susceptible than the A/J mouse, chemicals such as tetranitromethane, 1,3-butadiene, DMN, and NNK generate tumors with mutations consistent with the result of DNA adduct formation, whereas other chemicals (acetylaminofluorene, methylene chloride) did not produce tumors with carcinogen-specific mutations.

Lung tumors in rats exposed to airborne carcinogens consist mostly of peripheral adenocarcinomas and squamous cell carcinomas. In addition, rat lungs on occasion contain lesions that are characterized by an epithelium surrounding a space filled with keratin. The mass may compress the surrounding lung parenchyma and occasionally invades it. These lesions are classified by some pathologists as bona fide tumors, whereas other pathologists characterize this type of lesion as a cyst filled with keratin. Classification of such a lesion as a tumor is important because these lesions often are found in long-term tests in animals that have been exposed to agents that are not considered carcinogens, such as carbon black, titanium dioxide, and certain human-made fibers (Carlton, 1994).

## AGENTS KNOWN TO PRODUCE LUNG INJURY IN HUMANS

The prevention and treatment of acute and chronic lung disease will eventually be based on a knowledge of the cellular and molecular events that determine lung injury and repair. During the past 20 years, a large body of evidence has accumulated. Table 15-1 lists common toxicants that are known to produce acute and chronic lung injury in humans. In the following sections, a few examples of our current understanding of lung injury at the mechanistic level are discussed, with emphasis on agents directly responsible for human lung disease.

### Airborne Agents That Produce Lung Injury in Humans

**Asbestos.** The term "asbestos" describes silicate minerals in fiber form. The most commonly mined and commercially used asbestos fibers include the serpentine chrysotile asbestos and the amphiboles crocidolite, anthophyllite, amosite, actinolite, and tremolite. Exposure to asbestos fibers occurs in mining operations and in the construction and shipbuilding industries, where asbestos was at one time widely used for its highly desirable insulating and fireproofing properties. During the last few years, concern about asbestos in older buildings has led to the removal of asbestos-based insulating material; abatement workers may now represent an additional population at risk.

Asbestos causes three forms of lung disease in humans: asbestosis, lung cancer, and malignant mesothelioma. Asbestosis is characterized by a diffuse increase of collagen in the alveolar walls (fibrosis) and the presence of asbestos fibers, either free or coated with a proteinaceous material (asbestos bodies). Malignant mesothelioma (a tumor of the cells covering the surface of the visceral and parietal pleura), a tumor that otherwise occurs only extremely rarely in the general population, is unequivocally associated with asbestos exposure. There is some discrepancy between human observations and animal data. In animal experiments, chrysotile produces mesothelioma much more readily than do the amphibole fibers. In humans, amphibole fibers are implicated more often even when the predominant exposure is to chrysotile asbestos. Chrysotile breaks down much more readily than do the amphiboles. It is possible that in small laboratory animals chrysotile fibers, even if broken down, are retained longer relative to the life span of the animal than they are in humans, thus explaining the higher rate of mesothelioma development.

The hazards associated with asbestos exposure depend on fiber length. Fibers 2 $\mu$m in length may produce asbestosis; mesothelioma is associated with fibers 5 $\mu$m long, and lung cancer with fibers larger than 10 $\mu$m. Fiber diameter is another critical feature. Fibers with diameters larger than approximately 3 $\mu$m do not readily penetrate into the peripheral lung. For the development of mesothelioma, fiber diameter must be less than 0.5 $\mu$m, since thinner fibers may be translocated from their site of deposition via the lymphatics to other organs, including the pleural surface.

Once asbestos fibers have been deposited in the lung, they may become phagocytized by alveolar macrophages. Short fibers are completely ingested and subsequently removed via the mucociliary escalator. Longer fibers are incompletely ingested, and the macrophages become unable to leave the alveoli. Activated by the fibers, macrophages release mediators such as lymphokines and growth factors, which in turn attract immunocompetent cells or stimulate collagen production. Asbestos-related lung disease thus may be mediated through the triggering of an inflammatory sequence of events or the production of changes that eventually lead to the initiation (DNA damage caused by reactive molecular species) or promotion (increased rate of cell turnover in the lung) of the carcinogenic process.

The surface properties of asbestos fibers appear to be an important mechanistic element in toxicity. The protection afforded by superoxide dismutase or free radical scavengers in asbestos-related cell injury in vitro suggests that the generation of active oxygen species and concomitant lipid peroxidation are important mechanisms in asbestos toxicity. The interaction of iron on the surface of asbestos fibers with oxygen may lead to the production of hydrogen peroxide and the

**Table 15–1**
**Industrial Toxicants That Produce Lung Disease**

| TOXICANT | COMMON NAME OF DISEASE | OCCUPATIONAL SOURCE | ACUTE EFFECT | CHRONIC EFFECT |
|---|---|---|---|---|
| Asbestos | Asbestosis | Mining, construction, shipbuilding, manufacture of asbestos-containing material | | Fibrosis, pleural calcification, lung, cancer, pleural mesothelioma |
| Aluminum dust | Aluminosis | Manufacture of aluminum products, fireworks, ceramics, paints, electrical goods, abrasives | Cough, shortness of breath | Interstitial fibrosis |
| Aluminum abrasives | Shaver's disease, corundum smelter's lung, bauxite lung | Manufacture of abrasives, smelting | Alveolar edema | Interstitial fibrosis, emphysema |
| Ammonia | | Ammonia production, manufacture of fertilizers, chemical production, explosives | Upper and lower respiratory tract irritation, edema | Chronic bronchitis |
| Arsenic | | Manufacture of pesticides, pigments, glass, alloys | Bronchitis | Lung cancer, bronchitis, laryngitis |
| Beryllium | Berylliosis | Ore extraction, manufacture of alloys, ceramics | Severe pulmonary edema, pneumonia | Fibrosis, progressive dyspnea, interstitial granulomatosis, lung cancer, cor pulmonale |
| Cadmium oxide | | Welding, manufacture of electrical equipment, alloys, pigments, smelting | Cough, pneumonia | Emphysema, cor pulmonale |
| Carbides of tungsten, titanium, tantalum | Hard metal disease | Manufacture of cutting edges on tools | Hyperplasia and metaplasia of bronchial epithelium | Peribronchial and perivascular fibrosis |
| Chlorine | | Manufacture of pulp and paper, plastics, chlorinated chemicals | Cough, hemoptysis, dyspnea, tracheobronchitis, bronchopneumonia | |
| Chromium (VI) | | Production of Cr compounds, paint pigments, reduction of chromite ore | Nasal irritation, bronchitis | Lung cancer, fibrosis |
| Coal dust | Pneumoconiosis | Coal mining | | Fibrosis |
| Cotton dust | Byssinosis | Manufacture of textiles | Chest tightness, wheezing, dyspnea | Reduced pulmonary function, chronic bronchitis |
| Hydrogen fluoride | | Manufacture of chemicals, photographic film, solvents, plastics | Respiratory irritation, hemorrhagic pulmonary edema | |
| Iron oxides | Siderotic lung disease; silver finisher's lung, hematite miner's lung, arc welder's lung | Welding, foundry work, steel manufacture, hematite mining, jewelry making | Cough | Silver finisher's lung: sub pleural and perivascular aggregations of macrophages; hematite miner's lung: diffuse fibrosislike pneumonconiosis; arc welder's lung: bronchitis |
| Isocyanates | | Manufacture of plastics, chemical industry | Airway irritation, cough, dyspnea | Asthma, reduced pulmonary function |

**Table 15–1**
**Industrial Toxicants That Produce Lung Disease *(Continued)***

| TOXICANT | COMMON NAME OF DISEASE | OCCUPATIONAL SOURCE | ACUTE EFFECT | CHRONIC EFFECT |
|---|---|---|---|---|
| Kaolin | Kaolinosis | Pottery making | | Fibrosis |
| Manganese | Manganese pneumonia | Chemical and metal industries | Acute pneumonia, often fatal | Recurrent pneumonia |
| Nickel | | Nickel ore extraction, smelting, electronic electroplating, fossil fuels | Pulmonary edema, delayed by 2 days (NiCO) | Squamous cell carcinoma of nasal cavity and lung |
| Oxides of nitrogen | | Welding, silo filling, explosive manufacture | Pulmonary congestion and edema | Bronchiolitis obliterans |
| Ozone | | Welding, bleaching flour, deodorizing | Pulmonary edema | Fibrosis |
| Phosgene | | Production of plastics, pesticides, chemicals | Edema | Bronchitis, fibrosis |
| Perchloro-ethylene | | Dry cleaning, metal degreasing, grain fumigating | Edema | Cancer, liver and lung |
| Silica | Silicosis, pneumoconiosis | Mining, stone cutting, construction, farming, quarrying, sand blasting | Acute silicosis | Fibrosis, silicotuberculosis |
| Sulfur dioxide | | Manufacture of chemicals, refrigeration, bleaching, fumigation | Bronchoconstriction, cough, chest tightness | Chronic bronchitis |
| Talc | Talcosis | Rubber industry, cosmetics | | Fibrosis |
| Tin | Stanosis | Mining, processing of tin | | Widespread mottling of x-ray without clinical signs |
| Vanadium | | Steel manufacture | Airway irritation and mucus production | Chronic bronchitis |

highly reactive hydroxyl radical, events that have been associated with asbestos toxicity (Lippmann, 1993).

**Silica.** Silicosis in humans may be acute or chronic; this distinction is important conceptually because the pathological consequences are manifested quite differently. Acute silicosis occurs only in subjects exposed to a very high level of aerosol containing particles small enough to be respirable (usually less than 5 $\mu$m) over a relatively short period, generally a few months to a few years. These patients have worsening dyspnea, fever, cough, and weight loss. There is rapid progression of respiratory failure, usually ending in death within a year or two. No known treatment modality influences the relentless course of acute silicosis.

Chronic silicosis has a long latency period, usually more than 10 years. Uncomplicated silicosis is almost entirely asymptomatic; little alteration is shown on routine pulmonary function tests even after the disease is radiographically demonstrable. The x-ray picture presents fibrotic nodules, generally in the apical portion of lung. The hilar lymph nodes have peripheral calcifications known as eggshell calcifications. Simple silicosis may progress into complicated silicosis, which is defined as the presence of conglomerate nodules larger than 1 cm in diameter. These nodules usually occur in the upper and midlung zones. At an advanced stage they may be surrounded by emphysematous bullae. Chronic silicosis is associated with an increased incidence of tuberculosis.

Crystalline silica is a major component of the earth's crust; after oxygen, silicon is the most common element. As a pure mineral, silicon exists primarily in the form of its dioxide, silica ($SiO_2$), which has a crystalline form in which a central silicon atom forms a tetrahedron with four shared oxygen atoms. The three principal crystalline isomeric forms are quartz, tridymite, and cristobalite. The tetrahedral structure is linked to fibrogenic potential. Stishovite, a rare crystalline variant without the tetrahedral conformation, is biologically inert. Amorphous forms of silica such as kieselguhr and vitreous silica have very low fibrogenic potential. The ubiquitous presence of silica has made it an occupational hazard ever since humans began shaping tools from stone, and silicosis remains a significant industrial hazard throughout the world in occupations such as mining and quarrying, sandblasting, and foundry work. The main factors that affect the pathogenicity of silica both in vivo and in vitro, in addition to its structure, are particle size and concentration. Many studies have examined the relationship of silica particle size to fibrogenicity. In studies with humans, the most fibrogenic particle size appears to be about 1 $\mu$m (range 0.5 to 3$\mu$m). In animal experiments (rats, hamsters), the comparable values appear to be 1 to 2 μm (range 0.5 to 5 μm). In animal models, there appears to be a direct relationship between the concentration of silica dust to which an animal is exposed and the intensity and rapidity of the histological reaction in the lung.

The pathophysiological basis of pulmonary fibrosis in chronic silicosis is probably better understood than is the etiology of any other form of lung fibrosis. The role of pulmonary alveolar macrophages in the ingestion of silica as an initiating event has been established. Apparently, as part of the cytotoxic response of a macrophage to silica ingestion, the macrophage may release cytokines and other substances that cause fibroblasts to replicate and/or increase their rate of collagen biosynthesis. The role of inflammatory cells other than alveolar macrophages in this process is unknown. Also not understood is the role of the host's immune response and the roles of lymphocyte factors in stimulating fibroblast proliferation and/or collagen synthesis by fibroblasts in lung fibrogenesis.

**Lung Overload Caused by Particles.** Investigators studying the kinetics of the pulmonary clearance of particles have observed a slowing of the rate of alveolar clearance when deposited lung burdens are high. At about the same time, investigators evaluating inhaled particles in carcinogenesis bioassays observed excess tumors in animals that inhaled very high concentrations of apparently inert so-called nuisance dusts, which were included in such experiments as negative controls. From these observations came a unifying hypothesis (Morrow, 1992) that clearance mechanisms in the deep lung depending predominantly if not completely on phagocytosis and migration of pulmonary alveolar macrophages can be overwhelmed by quantities of respirable dusts far in excess of physiological loads. As a consequence, lung burdens of these dusts persist for months or years, and completely unphysiological mechanisms of disease pathogenesis may come into play. Especially noteworthy in this regard are controversies with respect to the putative carcinogenesis of diesel soot. Diesel exhaust particles produce lung tumors in rats on chronic exposure to concentrations 100-fold to 1000-fold in excess of realistic ambient concentrations. Carbon black particles have produced lung tumors in rats. The issue of whether particle overloading defines a threshold in such experiments remains unresolved.

**Naphthalene.** Naphthalene occurs in tars and petroleum and is a widely used precursor chemical for synthetic tanning agents, phthalic acid anhydride, carbaryl, and 2-naphthol. It is present in ambient air. Smokers inhale substantial amounts of naphthalene in cigarette smoke. In experimental animals, inhaled or parenterally administered naphthalene has shown remarkable species and tissue specificity: it produces extensive and selective necrosis in the bronchiolar epithelium of the mouse but much less necrosis in rats and hamsters.

Animals treated with small doses of naphthalene or inhibitors of microsomal oxidases show little or no tissue damage, implicating metabolism in the toxicity of this chemical. Metabolism to the oxide is mediated through cytochrome P-450 1A1 and 2F2. Naphthalene epoxides may subsequently be conjugated with glutathione and form adducts that presumably are not toxic. It is also possible that the epoxides undergo rearrangement to 1-naphthol with subsequent metabolism to quinones, which are potentially toxic compounds. In rats and other species, probably including humans, conversion of naphthalene is less stereospecific and rates of formation of the epoxide are much slower than in mice. This may explain the species differences that were noted previously (Franklin et al., 1993).

**Oxygen.** In infants who are given oxygen therapy after birth, a syndrome known as bronchopulmonary dysplasia may develop. Lung pathology is characterized by necrotizing bronchiolitis, fibroblast proliferation, squamous metaplasia of the bronchial lining, and destruction of alveolar ducts. In animals exposed to 95 percent to 100 percent oxygen, diffuse pulmonary damage develops and is usually fatal after 3 to 4 days. There is extensive damage to the cells of the alveolar-capillary septum. Type I epithelial cells and capillary endothelial cells develop necrotic changes. Capillary damage leads to leakage of proteinaceous fluid and formed blood elements into the alveolar space. Hyaline membranes formed by cellular debris and proteinaceous exudate are a characteristic sign of pulmonary oxygen toxicity. In animals returned to air after the development of acute oxygen toxicity, there is active cell proliferation (Fisher, 1988).

Oxygen toxicity is mediated though increased production of partially reduced oxygen products such as superoxide anion, perhydroperoxy and hydroxyl radicals, and possibly singlet molecular oxygen. A fascinating recent development is the finding that pulmonary oxygen toxicity can be mitigated greatly in transgenic mice that express human Mn-type superoxide dismutase in their pulmonary epithelial cells (Wispe et al., 1993).

## Bloodborne Agents That Cause Pulmonary Toxicity in Humans

**Paraquat.** The bipyridylium compound paraquat, a widely used herbicide, produces extensive lung injury when ingested by humans. In patients who survive the first few days of acute paraquat poisoning, progressive and eventually fatal lung lesions can develop. Paraquat lung disease is characterized by diffuse interstitial and intraalveolar fibrosis. The initial damage consists of widespread necrosis of both type I and type II epithelial cells of the alveolar region. Extensive proliferation of fibroblasts in the alveolar interstitium and the largely collapsed alveoli follows. Paraquat accumulates in the cells of the lung through the polyamine uptake system. Once inside the cells, paraquat continuously cycles from its oxidized form to the reduced form, with the concomitant formation of active oxygen species (Chap. 3). In vitro, paraquat produces extensive lipid peroxidation. An alternative but not mutually exclusive hypothesis to explain the mechanism of action of paraquat involves oxidation of cellular NADPH and eventual depletion of the NADPH content of pulmonary cells (Smith, 1987).

**Monocrotaline.** Monocrotaline is a pyrrolizidine alkaloid, one of many structurally related naturally occurring products of plants that have been used in herbal teas. These compounds produce liver toxicity (hepatocellular necrosis and veno-occlusive disease). Although metabolism is usually completed 24 h after the administration of a single dose, pyrrolizidine alkaloids are known to cause delayed lung injury. The lesion is characterized by a remodeling of the vascular bed with hyperplasia of capillary endothelial cells, thickening of the arterial media, formation of microthrombi, and eventually capillary occlusion with resulting hypertension of the pulmonary arterial system and hypertrophy of the right side of the heart. The alkaloids propagate changes in the contractile response of arterial smooth muscle, changes in smooth muscle Na/K-ATPase activity, release of platelet factors, and decreased serotonin transport by vascular endothelial cells.

Monocrotaline is metabolized in the liver to a highly reactive pyrrole or possibly to pyrrole conjugates with glutathione or cysteine. The pyrrole is released from the liver and travels to other organs, such as the kidney and the lung, where it initiates endothelial injury. Why the reactive molecule survives in the bloodstream is not entirely clear. It is possible that it is somehow transported in a relatively inert form in the red blood cells and, upon arrival in the capillaries of the lung, is activated to a reactive aldehyde (Wilson et al., 1992).

**Bleomycin.** Bleomycin, a mixture of several structurally similar compounds, is a widely used cancer chemotherapeutic agent. Pulmonary fibrosis, often fatal, represents the most serious form of toxicity. The sequence of damage includes necrosis of capillary endothelial and type I alveolar cells, edema formation and hemorrhage, delayed (after 1 to 2 weeks) proliferation of type II epithelial cells, and eventually thickening of the alveolar walls by fibrotic changes.

In many tissues, the cytosolic enzyme bleomycin hydrolase inactivates bleomycin. In lung and skin, two target organs for bleomycin toxicity, the activity of this enzyme is low compared with that in other organs. Bleomycin stimulates the production of collagen in the lung. Before increased collagen biosynthesis, steady-state levels of mRNA coding for fibronectin and procollagens are increased, presumably subsequent to a bleomycin-mediated release of cytokines such as TGF beta and TNF. Bleomycin also combines with Fe (II) and molecular oxygen; when it combines with DNA, single- and double-strand breaks are produced by a free radical reaction (Lazo et al., 1993).

**Cyclophosphamide and 4-Ipomeanol.** Cyclophosphamide is widely used as an anticancer and immunosuppressive agent. The undesirable side effects include hemorrhagic cystitis and pulmonary fibrosis. Cyclophosphamide is metabolized by the cytochrome P-450 system to two highly reactive metabolites: acrolein and phosphoramide mustard. In the lung, cooxidation with the prostaglandin H synthase system, which has high activity in the lung, is a possibility. Although the exact mechanism of action for causing lung damage has not been established, studies with isolated lung microsomes have shown that cyclophosphamide and its metabolite acrolein initiate lipid peroxidation (Patel, 1993). 4-Ipomeanol, a toxicant found in moldy sweet potatoes, is another agent that is converted to a toxic metabolite by cytochrome P-450. It produces extensive Clara cell damage and is being investigated as a potential anticancer drug (Gram, 1993).

**1,3 Bis (2-Chloroethyl)-1-Nitrosourea.** Carmustine (BCNU) is an effective chemotherapeutic agent that exerts its antitumor properties by reacting with cellular macromolecules and forms inter- and intrastrand cross-links with DNA. In humans, a dose-related pulmonary toxicity is often noticed first by a decrease in diffusion capacity. Pulmonary fibrosis caused by this drug can be fatal. The mechanism of action is not entirely clear. It is possible that BCNU inhibits pulmonary glutathione disulfide reductase, an event that may lead to a disturbed GSH/GSSG state in pulmonary cells. Eventually, this state leaves the cell unable to cope with oxidant stress. High concentrations of oxygen in the inspired air may enhance the pulmonary toxicity of BCNU and also that of the other anticancer drugs known to affect lung tissue: cyclophosphamide and bleomycin (Smith, 1993).

**Cationic Amphophilic Drugs.** Several drugs with similar structural characteristics that are called cationic amphophilic drugs (CADs) produce pulmonary lipidosis. The antiarrhythmic amiodarone and the anorexic chlorphentermine elicit such changes in humans. Pulmonary lipidosis is characterized by the intracellular presence, particularly in macrophages, of large concentric membranous structures now known to be secondary lysosomes. CADs inhibit phospholipases A and B, presumably because these drugs combine with phospholipids and form indigestible complexes. Degradation of pulmonary surfactant is impaired, and the material accumulates in phagocytic cells. In humans, amiodarone may cause dyspnea and cough. In animals and humans, the condition is fully reversible on drug withdrawal (Reasor, 1989).

## METHODS FOR STUDYING LUNG INJURY

### Inhalation Exposure Systems

The generation of a gas available in high purity as a compressed "tank gas," for example, $SO_2$, $O_2$, or $NO_2$, is relatively straightforward, and metering and dilution produce appropriate concentrations for exposure. Monitoring and quantifying gaseous pollutants require either expensive detectors that need frequent calibration (and usually a computer to process the tremendous amount of data generated) or very labor intensive wet chemical analysis procedures after sampled gases from the chambers are bubbled through traps. Particle generation is difficult, and specialized references must be consulted (Phalen, 1984: McClellan and Henderson, 1989).

Exposure chambers must allow for the rapid attainment of the desired concentrations of toxicants, maintenance of desired levels homogeneously throughout the chamber, adequate capacity for experimental animals, and minimal accumulation of undesired products associated with animal occupancy (usually ammonia, dander, heat, and carbon dioxide). Modern chambers tend to be fabricated from inert materials (usually glass, stainless steel, and Teflon) and have flow patterns that are designed to promote mixing and homogeneity of the chamber atmosphere and prevent a buildup of undesirable contaminants. A major concern with regard to exposure to acid aerosols has been the putative buildup of ammonia in chambers because of microbial action on animal excreta. Thus, maximal loading factors and sanitation also must be considered in chamber usage. As a general rule, the total body volume of the animals should not exceed 5 percent of the chamber volume. Nose-only exposure chambers avoid some of these problems. Finally, concern for the environment and the safety of facility personnel suggest prudence in how chambers are exhausted (Phalen et al., 1984).

In inhalation studies, selection of animals with a respiratory system similar to that of humans is particularly desirable. The respiratory system of monkeys most closely resembles that of humans. However, the availability and cost of animals and the necessity for special facilities for housing monkeys and performing long-term exposures, along with ethical considerations, including the confinement of primates in small exposure chambers for prolonged periods, severely limit the use of primates. Rats are widely used, although fundamental differences in respiratory anatomy (for example, lack of respiratory bronchioles) and function (rats are obligate nose breathers) can complicate the extrapolation of effects to humans. Guinea pigs and rabbits have accurately predicted the response of humans to sulfuric acid (Amdur, 1989).

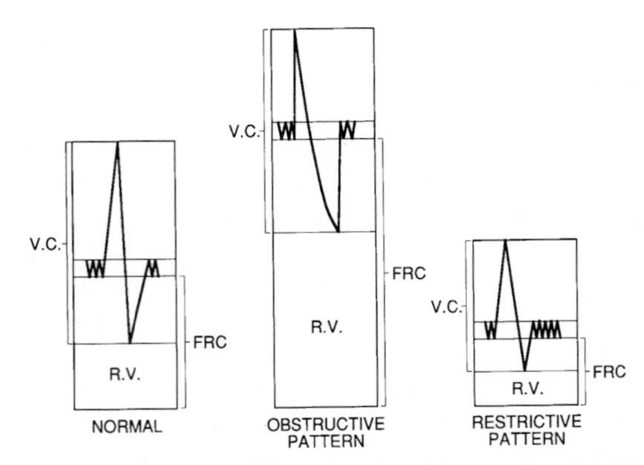


***Figure 15–5. Typical lung volume measurements from individuals with normal lung function, obstructive airways disease, or restrictive lung disease.***

Note that there is (1) a slowing of forced expiration in addition to gas trapping (an increase in residual volume) in obstructive disease and (2) a general decrease in lung volumes in restrictive disease. Note that the measurements read from left to right.

## Pulmonary Function Studies

Numerous tests are available with which to study pulmonary function and gas exchange in humans and experimental animals. Commonly used tests include measurement of VC, TLC, functional residual volume, TV, airway resistance, and maximum flow (Fig. 15-5). Additional tests evaluate the distribution of ventilation, lung and chest wall compliance, diffusion capacity, and the oxygen and carbon dioxide content of the arterial and venous blood (Costa et al., 1991).

Many pulmonary function tests require active collaboration by the subject examined, for example, the so-called $FEV_1$ (forced expiratory volume) during the first second of an active exhalation. This is an easy test to administer to humans, does not require sophisticated equipment or a hospital setting, and is completely noninvasive. The subject is asked first to inhale deeply and then to exhale the air as quickly as possible. The test is often used in epidemiological studies or controlled clinical studies designed to assess the potential adverse effects of air pollutants. A reduction in $FEV_1$ is usually indicative of impaired ventilation such as that found in restrictive (increased lung stiffness) or obstructive (obstructed airflow) lung disease. Experimental animals, by contrast, cannot be made to maximally inhale or exhale at the investigator's will. In experimental animals, $FEV_1$ can be obtained, but the test is done under anesthesia. Expiration is forced by applying external pressure to the thorax or negative pressure to the airways (Mauderly, 1991).

Analysis of breathing patterns has been widely used to assess the effects of irritants. This technique allows one to differentiate between sensory or upper airway irritants and "pulmonary" irritants. Highly water soluble irritants such as ammonia, chlorine, and formaldehyde produce upper respiratory tract irritation, whereas less soluble gases such as nitrogen dioxide and ozone generate pulmonary irritation. The sensory irritant pattern has been described as slowing down respiratory frequency while increasing TV. Pulmonary irritants usually increase respiratory frequency and decrease minute volume. The result is rapid, shallow breathing.

Analysis of volume-pressure curves of the lung provides some indication of lung compliance. Compliance (volume/pressure) is measured as the slope of the volume-pressure curve; it gives some indication of the intrinsic elastic properties of the lung parenchyma and, when measured in vivo, the thoracic cage. This is a comparatively easy test to perform in animals, requiring little specialized apparatus. Cannulation of the excised lungs and attachment to a syringe and manometer to measure volume and pressure are all that is needed. Volume-pressure curves can be obtained from lungs filled with air or physiological saline. The latter test is much more sensitive to structural changes in lung parenchyma, as the effects of surfactant are eliminated in a saline-filled lung.

To accomplish proper oxygenation of venous blood and elimination of $CO_2$, the gases have to diffuse across the air-blood barrier. Gas exchange may be hindered by the accumulation of fluids or cellular elements in the alveoli (edema, pneumonic infiltrates), thickening of the alveolar wall (fibrosis), insufficient ventilation of the alveolar region (emphysema), or insufficient presence of oxygen transport elements (reduced alveolar blood volume or reduced amount of hemoglobin in the blood). Gas exchange can be evaluated by measuring the arterial partial pressure of both oxygen and $CO_2$. In experimental animals, the collection of arterial blood may require the presence of indwelling catheters.

In general, blood gas analysis is a comparatively insensitive assay for disturbed ventilation because of the organism's buffering and reserve capacities. While it is a useful tool in clinical medicine, in animals, only the most severe obstructive or restrictive pulmonary alterations cause signs of impaired gas exchange. Measurement of diffusion capacity with CO, a gas that binds with 250 times higher affinity to hemoglobin than does oxygen, is more sensitive. The test is comparatively easy to perform in both humans and laboratory animals and is widely used in toxicology studies.

## Morphological Techniques

The pathology of acute and chronic injury may be described after examination of the respiratory tract by gross inspection and under the microscope. Morphological evaluation should not be limited to the peripheral lung; nasal passages, the larynx, and major airways must be examined as carefully as is the lung parenchyma. For example, formaldehyde produces nasal tumors but not deep lung tumors in the rat. In hamsters ex-

been associated with a potentially irreversible limbic-cerebellar syndrome in humans and similar behavioral changes in primates (Besser et al., 1987, Reuhl et al., 1985). Trimethyltin gains access to the NS where, by an undefined mechanism, it leads to diffuse neuronal injury. Many neurons of the NS begin to accumulate cytoplasmic bodies composed of Golgi-like structures, followed by cellular swelling and necrosis (Bouldin et al., 1981). The hippocampus is particularly vulnerable to this process; following acute intoxication the cells of the *fascia dentata* degenerate, and with chronic intoxication, the cells of the *corpus ammonis* are lost. Several hypotheses seek the mechanism of trimethyltin neurotoxicity, including energy deprivation and excitotoxic damage. The role of stannin, a protein present in trimethyltin-sensitive neurons (Toggas et al., 1992), remains to be established.

## Hydroxydopamine and Catecholamine Toxicity

The progressive loss of catecholaminergic neurons that occurs with age has been postulated to derive from the toxicity of the oxidation products of catecholamines as well as from the products of the partial reduction of oxygen. The oxidation of catecholamines by monoamine oxidase (MAO) yields $H_2O_2$, a known cytotoxic metabolite. The metal ion-catalyzed autoxidation of catecholamines, especially dopamine, results in the production of catecholamine-derived quinones as well as superoxide anion ($O_2^{\cdot-}$), $H_2O_2$ from $O_2^{\cdot-}$ dismutation, and OH· from the Fenton reaction (Fig. 16-3) (Cohen and Heikkila, 1977). Cellular glutathione affords protection from the flux of quinones, glutathione peroxidase from $H_2O_2$, and superoxide dismutase from $O_2^{\cdot-}$. Among the naturally occurring catecholamines, dopamine is the most cytotoxic, because of both its greater ease of autoxidation and the greater reactivity of its orthoquinone oxidation product (Graham et al., 1978).

The analog of dopamine, 6-hydroxydopamine, is extremely potent in leading to a chemical sympathectomy. This compound fails to cross the blood–brain barrier, so its site of action is limited to the periphery. In addition, it does not cross into peripheral nerves and gains access to nerves only at their terminals. 6-Hydroxydopamine is actively transported into nerve terminals with an uptake mechanism for the structurally similar catecholamines in sympathetic terminals. The uptake of 6-hydroxydopamine results in an injury to sympathetic neurons due to an oxidative process of this catecholamine analog similar to that of dopamine (Fig. 16-3). The result is selective

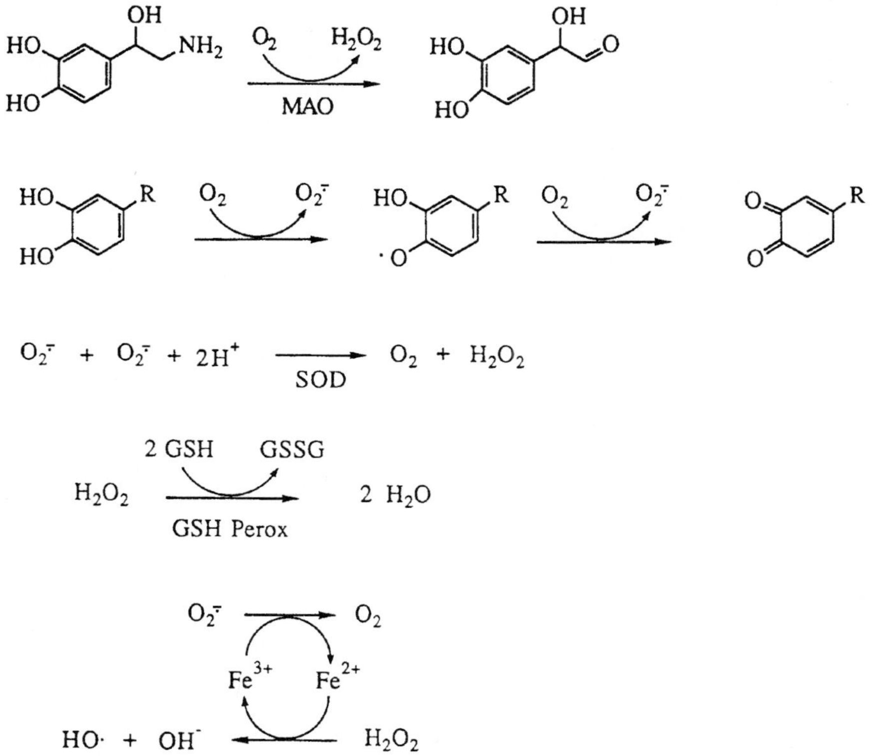

$$O_2^{\cdot-} + O_2^{\cdot-} + 2H^+ \xrightarrow[\text{SOD}]{} O_2 + H_2O_2$$

$$H_2O_2 \xrightarrow[\text{GSH Perox}]{2\ \text{GSH} \rightarrow \text{GSSG}} 2\ H_2O$$

$$O_2^{\cdot-} \rightarrow O_2 \quad (Fe^{3+} \rightarrow Fe^{2+});\quad H_2O_2 \rightarrow HO\cdot + OH^- \quad (Fe^{2+} \rightarrow Fe^{3+})$$

***Figure 16–3. Catecholamine oxidation and activated oxygen species.***

Both the enzyme-catalyzed oxidation of catecholamines, here illustrating the action of monoamine oxidase (MAO) on norepinephrine, and the nonenzymatic oxidation of catecholamines generate activated oxygen species, hydrogen peroxide, and superoxide. There are intracellular enzymes that handle the flux of superoxide (superoxide dismutase, SOD) and hydrogen peroxide (glutathione peroxidase, GSH Perox). The hydroxyl radical (HO·) is a highly reactive molecule that may react with lipids, proteins, and nucleic acids. Although originally thought to arise through the direct reaction of peroxide and superoxide, it appears that the only likely source of hydroxyl radical is through the metal-catalyzed Fenton reaction. In addition, the autoxidation of catecholamines generates the semiquinone and the catecholamine-derived quinone, which is a strong electrophile and reacts with available sulfhydryls.

destruction of sympathetic innervation (Malmfors, 1971). The sympathetic fibers degenerate, resulting in an uncompensated parasympathetic tone, a slowing of the heart rate, and hypermotility of the gastrointestinal system. It is noteworthy that neurobiologists employ 6-hydroxydopamine to destroy specific groups of catecholaminergic neurons. For example, stereotaxic injection of 6-hydroxydopamine into the caudate nucleus, which is rich in dopaminergic synapses, leads to neurite degeneration; if injected into the *substantia nigra*, then the cell bodies of the dopamine neurons are destroyed (Marshall et al., 1983).

## MPTP

Because of a chemist's error, people who injected themselves with a meperidine derivative, or "synthetic heroin," also received a contaminant, 1-methyl-4-phenyl-1,2,3,6-tetrahydropyridine (MPTP). Over hours to days, dozens of these patients developed the signs and symptoms of irreversible Parkinson's disease (Langston and Irwin, 1986), some becoming almost immobile with rigidity.

It is not only surprising that a compound like MPTP is neurotoxic, it is also surprising that MPTP is a substrate for the B isozyme of monoamine oxidase (MAO-B). It appears that MPTP, an uncharged species at physiological pH, easily crosses the blood–brain barrier and diffuses into cells, including astrocytes. The MAO-B of astrocytes catalyzes the two electron oxidation to yield the corresponding dihydropyridinium ion, $MPDP^+$ (Trevor et al., 1987). A further two-electron oxidation yields the pyridinium ion, $MPP^+$ (Fig. 16-4). $MPP^+$ enters dopaminergic neurons of the *substantia nigra* via the dopamine uptake system, resulting in injury or death of the neuron. Noradrenergic neurons of the *locus ceruleus* are also vulnerable to repeated exposures of MPTP (Langston and Irwin, 1986), although they are less affected by single exposures than the dopaminergic neurons. Once inside neurons,

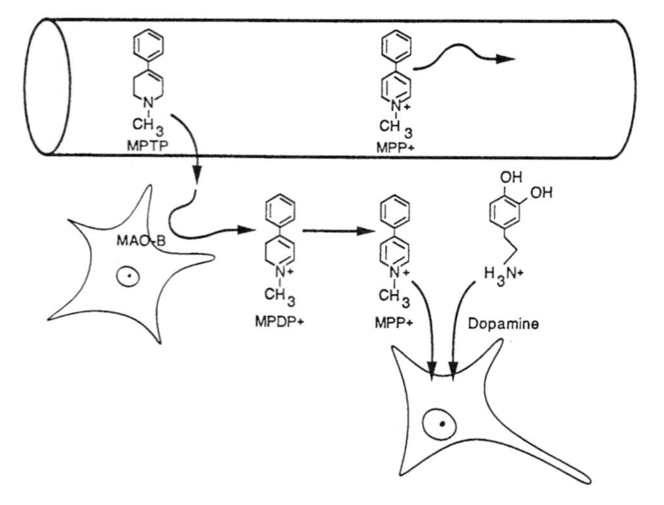


***Figure 16–4. Diagram of MPTP toxicity.***

$MPP^+$, either formed elsewhere in the body following exposure to MPTP or injected directly into the blood, is unable to cross the blood–brain barrier. In contrast, MPTP gains access and is oxidized in situ to $MPDP^+$ and $MPP^+$. The same transport system that carries dopamine into the dopaminergic neurons also transports the cytotoxic $MPP^+$.

$MPP^+$ acts as a general mitochondrial toxin, blocking respiration at complex I (Kopin, 1992). In fact, the general toxicity of $MPP^+$ itself is great when administered to animals, although systemic exposure to $MPP^+$ does not result in neurotoxicity because it does not cross the blood–brain barrier.

Although not identical, MPTP neurotoxicity and Parkinson's disease are strikingly similar. The symptomatology of each reflects a disruption of the nigrostriatal pathway: masked facies, difficulties in initiating and terminating movements, resting "pill-rolling" tremors, rigidity, and bradykinesias are all features of both conditions. Pathologically, there is an unusually selective degeneration of neurons in the substantia nigra and depletion of striatal dopamine in both diseases (Kopin, 1988). These parallels have spurred research into the molecular mechanisms of Parkinson's disease and efforts to identify other, more widespread environmental toxicants that may operate through a similar mechanism (Kopin, 1992).

It has been observed that individuals exposed to insufficient MPTP to result in immediate parkinsonism have developed early signs of the disease years later (Calne et al., 1985). This observation presents a frightening specter that the onset of a neurotoxicologic disease may follow toxic exposure by many years. It does not seem likely that an early sublethal injury to dopaminergic neurons later becomes lethal. Rather, smaller exposures to MPTP may cause a decrement in the population of neurons within the substantia nigra. Such a loss would most likely be silent because the symptoms of Parkinson's disease do not develop until approximately 80 percent of the substantia nigra neurons are lost. Then, in these predisposed individuals, the neurological picture of Parkinson's disease develops at an earlier age than in unexposed individuals, as a further loss of catecholaminergic neurons occurs during the process of aging.

## AXONOPATHIES

The neurotoxic disorders termed "axonopathies" are those in which the primary site of toxicity is the axon itself. The axon degenerates, and with it the myelin surrounding that axon; however, the neuron cell body remains intact (Fig. 16-2). John Cavanagh coined the term "dying-back neuropathy" as a synonym for axonopathy (Cavanagh, 1964). The concept of "dying-back" postulated that the focus of toxicity was the neuronal cell body itself and that the distal axon degenerated progressively from the synapse, back toward the cell body with increasing injury. It now appears that, in the best-studied axonopathies, a different pathogenetic sequence occurs; the toxicant results in a "chemical transection" of the axon at some point along its length, and the axon distal to the transection, biologically separated from its cell body, degenerates.

Because longer axons have more targets for toxic damage than shorter axons, one would predict that longer axons would be more affected in toxic axonopathies. Indeed, such is the case. The involvement of long axons of the CNS, such as ascending sensory axons in the posterior columns or descending motor axons, along with long sensory and motor axons of the PNS, prompted Spencer and Schaumburg (1976) to suggest that the toxic axonopathies in which the distal axon was most vulnerable be called "central peripheral distal axonopathies," which, though cumbersome, accurately depicts the pathologic sequence.

A critical difference exists in the significance of axonal degeneration in the CNS compared to that in the PNS: peripheral axons can regenerate, whereas central axons cannot. Thus partial recovery, or in mild cases complete recovery, can occur after axonal degeneration in the PNS, whereas the same event is irreversible in the CNS.

Axonopathies, then, can be considered to result from a chemical transection of the axon. The number of axonal toxicants is staggering (Table 16-2); however, they may be viewed as a group, all of which result in the pathologic loss of axons with the survival of the cell body. Because the axonopathies pathologically resemble the actual physical transection of the axon, axonal transport appears to be a likely target in many of the toxic axonopathies. Furthermore, as these axons degenerate, the result is most often the clinical condition of peripheral neuropathy, in which sensations and motor strength are first impaired in the most distal extent of the axonal processes, the feet and hands. With time and continued injury, the deficit progresses to involve more proximal areas of the body and the long axons of the spinal cord. The potential for regeneration is great when the insult is limited to peripheral nerves and may be complete in axonopathies in which the initiating event can be determined and removed.

## γ-Diketones

Since the late 1960s and early 1970s, it has been appreciated that humans develop a progressive sensorimotor distal axonopathy when exposed to high concentrations of a simple alkane, *n*-hexane, day after day in work settings (Yamamura, 1969), or after repeated intentional inhalation of hexane-containing glues. This axonopathy can be reproduced in its entirety in rats and larger species after weeks to months of exposure to *n*-hexane or its oxidative metabolites (Krasavage et al., 1980).

The observation in a fabric printing plant in Ohio (Allen et al., 1980) that methyl *n*-butyl ketone (2-hexanone) resulted in a neuropathy identical to that caused by *n*-hexane prompted elucidation of the metabolism of these two 6-carbon compounds. The ω-1 oxidation of the carbon chain (Fig. 16-5) results ultimately in the γ-diketone, 2,5-hexanedione (HD). That HD is the ultimate toxic metabolite of both *n*-hexane and methyl *n*-butyl ketone is shown by the fact that other γ-diketones or γ-diketone precursors are similarly neurotoxic, while α- and β-diketones are not (Krasavage et al., 1980).

The elucidation of the pathogenetic mechanism of γ-diketone neuropathy has come from an understanding of the biology of the axon and the chemistry of γ-diketone reactivity. The γ-diketones react with amino groups in all tissues to form pyrroles (DeCaprio et al., 1982; Graham et al., 1982; Amarnath et al., 1991a). That pyrrole formation is an actual step in the pathogenesis of this axonopathy has been established by two observations. First, 3,3-dimethyl-2,5-hexanedione, which cannot form a pyrrole, is not neurotoxic (Sayre et al., 1986). Second, the *d,l*-diastereomer of 3,4-dimethyl-2,5-hexanedione (DMHD) both forms pyrroles faster than *meso*-DMHD and is more neurotoxic than *meso*-DMHD (Genter et al., 1987).

While all proteins are derivatized by γ-diketones, the cytoskeleton of the axon, and especially the neurofilament, are very stable proteins, making it the toxicologically significant target in γ-diketone intoxication. The cellular changes are identical in rats and humans: the development of neurofilament aggregates in the distal, subterminal axon, which, as they grow larger, form massive swellings of the axon, often just proximal to nodes of Ranvier. The neurofilament-filled axonal swellings result in marked distortions of nodal anatomy, including the retraction of paranodal myelin. Following labeling of neurofilament proteins with radioactive amino precursors, the neurofilament transport is impaired in the γ-diketone model (Griffin et al., 1984; Pyle et al., 1994). With continued intoxication swellings are seen more proximally and there is degeneration of the distal axon along with its myelin. Long axons in the CNS also develop neurofilament-filled swellings distally, but axonal degeneration is seen much less often. The attribute of the neurofilament that seemingly determines it as the toxicologically relevant target is its slow rate of transport down the axon (Baitinger et al., 1982; Nixon and Sihag, 1991), predisposing it to progressive derivatization and cross-linking.

Hexane neuropathy is one of the best understood of the toxic neuropathies, and much of this understanding has stemmed from controversy over whether pyrrole formation alone is the injury (an arylation reaction) or whether subsequent oxidation of pyrroles leading to covalent protein cross-linking is a necessary step (Graham et al., 1982; DeCaprio et al., 1983; Sayre et al., 1985; Amarnath et al., 1994). The question was apparently resolved in experiments with a novel γ-diketone, 3-acetyl-2,5-hexanedione (AcHD) (St. Clair et al., 1988). AcHD results in very rapid pyrrole formation both in vitro and in vivo. However, the electron-withdrawing acetyl group renders the resulting pyrrole essentially inert, so that it does not undergo oxidation. Despite massive pyrrole derivatization, AcHD results in neither clinical nor morphologic evidence of neurotoxicity. Thus pyrrole derivatization is not sufficient to produce the neurofilamentous swellings; pyrrole oxidation, followed by nucleophilic attack and neurofilament cross-linking seem to be necessary for neurotoxicity.

The pathologic processes of neurofilament accumulation and degeneration of the axon are followed by the emergence of a clinical peripheral neuropathy. Experimental animals become progressively weak, beginning in the hindlimbs. With continued exposure, the axonopathy may progress, leading to successive weakness in more proximal muscle groups. This is precisely the sequence of events in humans as well, and the initial stocking-and-glove distribution of sensory loss progresses to involve more proximal sensory and motor axons.

## Carbon Disulfide

The most significant exposures of humans to $CS_2$ have occurred in the vulcan rubber and viscose rayon industries. Manic psychoses were observed in the former setting and were correlated with very high levels of exposure (Seppäläinen and Haltia, 1980). In recent decades, interest in the human health effects has been focused on the NS and the cardiovascular system, where injury has been documented in workers exposed to much higher levels than those that are allowed today.

What is clearly established is the capacity of $CS_2$ to cause a distal axonopathy that is identical pathologically to that caused by hexane. There is growing evidence that covalent cross-linking of neurofilaments also underlies $CS_2$ neuropathy through a series of reactions that parallel the sequence of events in hexane neuropathy. While hexane requires metabo-

**Table 16–2**
**Compounds Associated with Axonal Injury (Axonopathies)**

| NEUROTOXICANT | NEUROLOGICAL FINDINGS | CELLULAR BASIS OF NEUROTOXICITY | |
|---|---|---|---|
| Acrylamide | Peripheral neuropathy (often sensory) | Axonal degeneration, axon terminal affected in earliest stages | 2,3 |
| *p*-Bromophenylacetyl urea | Peripheral neuropathy | Axonal degeneration in PNS and CNS | 3 |
| Carbon disulfide | Psychosis (acute), peripheral neuropathy (chronic) | Axonal degeneration, early stages include neurofilamentous swelling | 2,3 |
| Chlordecone (Kepone) | Tremors, incoordination | Insufficient data (humans); axonal swelling and degeneration (exper. animals) | 3<br>3 |
| Chloroquine | Peripheral neuropathy | Axonal degeneration, inclusions in dorsal root ganglion cells | 2 |
| Clioquinol | Encephalopathy, subacute myelo-optic neuropathy | Axonal degeneration, spinal cord, PNS, optic tracts | 2,3 |
| Colchicine | Peripheral neuropathy | Axonal degeneration, neuronal perikaryal filamentous aggregates | 2,3 |
| Dapsone | Peripheral neuropathy, predominantly motor | Axonal degeneration | 2 |
| Dichlorophenoxy-acetate | Peripheral neuropathy (delayed) | Insufficient data | 3 |
| Dimethylaminopropio-nitrile | Peripheral neuropathy, urinary retention | Axonal degeneration (both myelinated and unmyelinated axons) | 3 |
| Disulfiram | Peripheral neuropathy, predominantly sensory | Axonal degeneration, swellings in distal axons | 2 |
| Ethylene oxide | Peripheral neuropathy | Axonal degeneration | 2 |
| Glutethimide | Peripheral neuropathy (predominantly sensory) | Insufficient data | 3 |
| Gold | Peripheral neuropathy (may have psychiatric problems) | Axonal degeneration, some segmental demyelination | 2,3 |
| Hexane | Peripheral neuropathy, severe cases have spasticity | Axonal degeneration, early neurofilamentous swelling, PNS and spinal cord (severe) | 2,3 |
| Hydralazine | Peripheral neuropathy | Insufficient data | 3 |
| 3,3′-Iminodipropio-nitrile | No data in humans; excitatory movement disorder (rats) | Axonal swellings, degeneration of olfactory epithelial cells, vestibular hair cells | 2 |

| | | | |
|---|---|---|---|
| Isoniazid | Peripheral neuropathy, ataxia (high doses) | Axonal degeneration, myelinated and unmyelinated fibers | 2,3 |
| Lithium | Lethargy, tremor, ataxia (reversible) | Insufficient data | 3 |
| Methyl *n*-butyl ketone | Peripheral neuropathy | Axonal degeneration, early neurofilamentous swelling, PNS and spinal cord | 2,3 |
| Metronidazole | Sensory peripheral neuropathy, ataxia, seizures | Axonal degeneration, mostly affecting myelinated fibers; lesions of cerebellar nuclei | 2 |
| Misonidazole | Peripheral neuropathy | Axonal degeneration | 2,3 |
| Nitrofurantoin | Peripheral neuropathy | Axonal degeneration | 3 |
| Organophosphorus compounds | Headache, abdominal pain (acute anticholinesterase) | No anatomic changes (related to neurotransmitter effect) | 1,2 |
| | Delayed peripheral neuropathy (motor), spasticity | Axonal degeneration (delayed after single exposure), PNS and spinal cord | 1,2,3,4 |
| Platinum | Ototoxicity with tinnitus, peripheral neuropathy | Axonal degeneration, axonal loss in posterior columns of spinal cord | 2 |
| Polybrominated biphenyls | Blurred vision, fatigue | Insufficient data | 3 |
| Pyridinethione | No reported human toxicity; weakness (exper. animals) | Axonal degeneration, early stages with membranous arrays in axon terminals | 2,3 |
| Pyrethroids | Movement disorders (tremor, choreoathetosis) | Axonal degeneration (variable) | 1 |
| Taxol | Peripheral neuropathy | Axonal degeneration; microtubule accumulation in early stages | 2 |
| Trichloroethylene | Cranial (most often trigeminal) neuropathy | Insufficient data | 3 |
| Vincristine | Peripheral neuropathy, variable autonomic symptoms | Axonal degeneration (PNS), neurofibrillary changes (spinal cord, intrathecal route) | 2,3 |

1. *Handbook of Neurotoxicology,* Chang LW and Dyer RS, eds. New York, Marcel Dekker, Inc., 1995.
2. *Greenfield's Neuropathology, 5th Edition,* Adams JH, Duchen LW, eds. New York, Oxford University Press, 1992.
3. *Experimental and Clinical Neurotoxicology,* Spencer PS and Schaumburg HH, eds. Baltimore, Williams and Wilkins, 1980.
4. *Neurotoxicology,* Abou-Donia MB, ed. Boca Raton, CRC Press, 1993.
5. *Neurotoxicity: Identifying and Controlling Poisons of the Nervous System,* U.S. Congress, Office of Technology Assessment (OTA-BA-436). Washington DC, U. S. Government Printing Office, 1990.

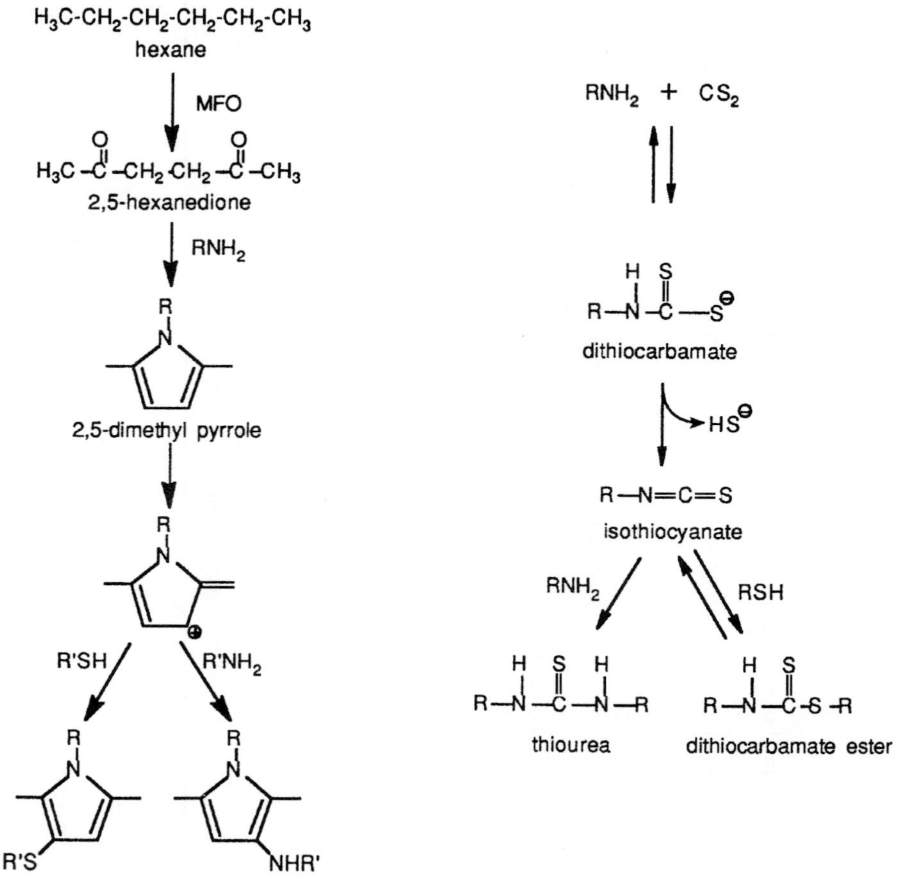

***Figure 16–5. Molecular mechanisms of protein crosslinking in the neurofilamentous neuropathies.***

Both 2,5-hexanedione, produced from hexane via $\omega$-1 oxidation function of mixed function oxidase (MFO), and $CS_2$, are capable of crosslinking proteins. Pyrrole formation from 2,5-hexanedione is followed by oxidation and reaction with adjacent protein nucleophiles. Dithiocarbamate formation from $CS_2$ is followed by formation of the protein-bound isothiocyanate, and subsequent reaction with adjacent protein nucleophiles.

lism to 2,5-hexanedione, $CS_2$ is itself the ultimate toxicant, reacting with protein amino groups to form dithiocarbamate adducts (Lam and DiStefano, 1986). The dithiocarbamate adducts of lysyl amino groups undergo decomposition to isothiocyanate adducts, electrophiles that then react with protein nucleophiles to yield covalent cross-linking (Fig. 16-5). The reaction of the isothiocyanate adducts with cysteinyl sulfhydryls to form *N,S*-dialkyldithiocarbamate ester cross-links is reversible, while the reaction with protein amino functions forms thiourea cross-links irreversibly. Over time, the thiourea cross-links predominate and are most likely the most biologically significant (Amarnath et al., 1991b; Valentine et al., 1992, 1995; DeCaprio et al., 1992; Graham et al., 1995).

As with hexane neuropathy, it has been postulated that the stability and long transport distance of the neurofilament determine that this protein is the toxicologically relevant target in chronic $CS_2$ intoxication. Nonetheless, proteins throughout the organism are derivatized and cross-linked as well. The cross-linking of erythrocyte spectrin appears to have excellent potential as a biomarker of absorbed dose, suggesting that quantification of spectrin dimers in workers exposed chronically to $CS_2$ could allow identification of those in danger of developing neurotoxicity. Similarly, the neuropathy derived from $CS_2$ released from dithiocarbamate pesticides or from dithiocarbamates employed in metal chelation, cancer chemotherapy, or alcohol aversion therapy may be prevented through careful monitoring of levels of dimerization of erythrocyte spectrin (Valentine et al., 1993; Graham et al., 1995).

The clinical effects of exposure to $CS_2$ in the chronic setting are very similar to those of hexane exposure, with the development of sensory and motor symptoms occurring initially in a stocking-and-glove distribution. In addition to this chronic axonopathy, $CS_2$ can also lead to aberrations in mood and signs of diffuse encephalopathic disease. Some of these are transient at first and subsequently become more long lasting, a feature that is common in vascular insufficiency in the NS. This fact, in combination with the knowledge that $CS_2$ may accelerate the process of atherosclerosis, suggests that some of the effects of $CS_2$ on the CNS are vascular in origin.

## IDPN

$\beta,\beta'$-Iminodipropionitrile (IDPN) is a bifunctional nitrile that causes a bizarre "waltzing syndrome" which appears to result from degeneration of the vestibular sensory hair cells (Llorens et al., 1993). In addition, administration of IDPN is followed by massive neurofilament-filled swellings (Griffin and Price, 1980) of the proximal, instead of the distal, axon (Fig. 16-6). The possibility that the nitrile groups undergo bioactivation to generate a bifunctional cross-linking reagent is suggested by the effects of deuterium substitution on the potency and metabolism of IDPN (Denlinger et al., 1992, 1994). The similarity of the neurofilament-filled swellings to those seen with the $\gamma$-diketones and carbon disulfide is a striking feature of this model neurotoxicant, underscoring this possibility. Axonal swellings do not occur in neurofilament-deficient quails, supporting the notion that the disorder is caused by a selective effect of IDPN on neurofilaments (Mitsuishi et al., 1993)

Understanding of the similarities between the $\gamma$-diketones and IDPN was extended when the potency of the $\gamma$-diketones was increased through molecular modeling. DMHD (3,4-dimethyl-2,5-hexanedione) is an analog of 2,5-hexanedione that accelerates the rates of both pyrrole formation and oxidation of the pyrrole. DMHD is 20 to 30 times more potent as a neurotoxicant and, in addition, the neurofilament-filled swellings occur in the proximal axon (Anthony et al., 1983a), as in IDPN intoxication. In these models of proximal neurofilamentous axonopathies, there is a block of neurofilament transport down the axon; thus in this situation the accumulation of neurofilaments results from blockage of the slow component A of axonal transport (Griffin et al., 1978, 1984). Decreasing the rate of intoxication with DMHD changes the location of the swellings to more distal locations, suggesting that the neurofilamentous axonopathies have a common mechanism and that the position of the neurofilamentous swellings along the axon reflects the rate at which this process occurs (Anthony et al., 1983b).

An important difference is seen between the two proximal neurofilamentous axonopathies caused by IDPN and DMHD, however. After DMHD intoxication, animals become progressively paralyzed in all four limbs, corresponding with marked degeneration of the axon distal to the swellings. By contrast, the axon distal to IDPN-induced swellings undergoes atrophy, not degeneration, and the animal does not experience

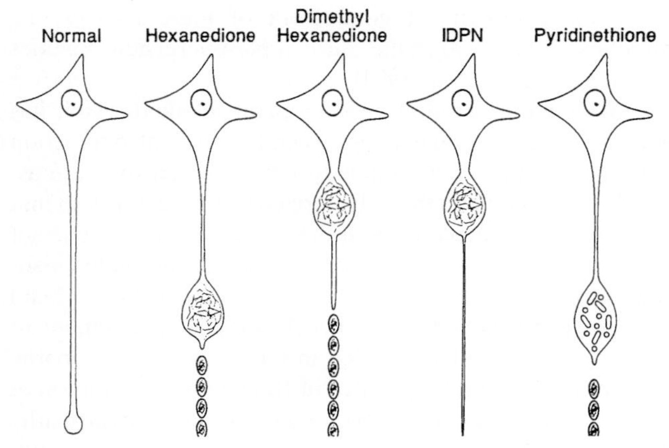


***Figure 16–6. Diagram of axonopathies.***

While 2,5-hexanedione results in the accumulation of neurofilaments in the distal regions of the axon, 3,4-dimethyl-2,5-hexanedione results in identical accumulation within the proximal segments. These proximal neurofilamentous swellings are quite similar to those that occur in the toxicity of $\beta,\beta'$-iminodipropionitrile (IDPN), although the distal axon does not degenerate in IDPN axonopathy, but becomes atrophic. Pyridinethione results in axonal swellings that are distended with tubulovesicular material, followed by distal axonal degeneration.

the same muscle weakness or paralysis. This observation suggests not only that axonal degeneration is required before muscle weakness develops but also that the presence of neurofilamentous aggregates in the proximal axon is not incompatible with the survival of the distal axon.

## Acrylamide

Acrylamide is a vinyl monomer used in the manufacture of paper products, as a flocculant in water treatment, as a soil-stabilizing and waterproofing agent, and for making polyacrylamide gels in the research laboratory. While cautious handling of acrylamide in the laboratory should be encouraged, human poisonings have been largely limited to factory and construction workers exposed to high doses (Kesson et al., 1977; Myers and Macun, 1991; Collins et al., 1989). The neuropathy induced by acrylamide is a toxic distal axonopathy, beginning with degeneration of the nerve terminal. Continued intoxication results in degeneration of the more proximal axon, a sequence of events that recapitulates what one would expect in a "dying-back" process. The neuropathy appears identical whether acrylamide is administered in a single dose (Miller and Spencer, 1984) or in multiple smaller doses. The earliest changes are seen in the Pascinian corpuscles, then in muscle spindles and motor nerve terminals (Schaumburg et al., 1974). Within nerve terminals early events include decreased densities of synaptic vesicles and mitochondria (Tsujihata et al., 1974) and accumulations of neurofilaments and tubulovesicular profiles (DeGrandechamp et al., 1990), along with evidence for terminal sprouting (DeGrandechamp and Lowndes, 1990). Multifocal accumulations of membranous bodies, mitochondria and neurofilaments are observed in the distal axon (Brismar et al., 1987), suggesting abnormal axonal transport. Indeed, retrograde fast transport has been shown to be impaired by acrylamide exposure (Miller and Spencer, 1984; Padilla et al., 1993) before any morphological changes are evident in axons or their terminals. Abnormalities in fast axonal transport have been observed and may be limited to transport of glycoproteins and/or the glycosylation of proteins carried in fast anterograde transport (Harry et al., 1992).

Recent studies employing chick or rat embryo neuron cultures have demonstrated that both anterograde and retrograde fast axonal transport are inhibited by acrylamide (Harris et al., 1994). These effects are clearly not the result of ATP depletion, nor do they appear to reflect direct inhibition of kinesin or dynein (Martenson et al., 1995b). In addition, specific alterations of growth cone structure, including loss of filopodial elements, follow exposure to acrylamide, and these are separable from the effects of ATP depletion and sulfhydryl alkylation (Martenson et al., 1995a). Because the growth cone of growing neurites in culture has many similarities to the axon terminal in vivo, it has been suggested that the growth cone alterations are a good model for the initial reactions of acrylamide with its axon terminal target(s).

## Organophosphorus Esters

Many toxicologists and most physicians who practice in rural areas are aware of the acute cholinergic poisoning induced by certain organophosphorus esters. These compounds, which are used as pesticides and as additives in plastics and petroleum products, inhibit acetylcholinesterase and create a cholinergic excess. However, as tens of thousands of humans could attest, tri-*ortho*-cresyl phosphate (TOCP) may also cause a severe central peripheral distal axonopathy without inducing cholinergic poisoning. An epidemic of massive proportion occurred during Prohibition in the United States, when a popular drink (Ginger Jake) was contaminated with TOCP (Kidd and Langworthy, 1933). Another outbreak occurred in Morocco when olive oil was adulterated with TOCP. Human cases of paralysis have also occurred after exposure to the herbicides and cotton defoliants EPN (*O*-ethyl *O*-4-nitrophenyl phenylphosphonothioate) and leptophos [*O*-(4-bromo-2,5-dichlorophenyl) *O*-methyl phenylphosphonothioate] (Abou-Donia and Lapadula, 1990).

The hydrophobic organophosphorus compounds readily enter the NS, where they alkylate or phosphorylate macromolecules and lead to delayed-onset neurotoxicity. There are probably multiple targets for attack by organophosphorus esters, but which targets are critically related to axonal degeneration is not clear. Not all of the organophosphorus esters that inhibit acetylcholinesterase lead to a delayed neurotoxicity. While these "nontoxic" organophosphorus esters inhibit most of the esterase activity of the NS, there is another esterase activity, or "neuropathy target esterase" (NTE), that is inhibited by the neurotoxic organophosphorus esters. Furthermore, there is a good correlation between the potency of a given organophosphorus ester as an axonal toxicant and its potency as an inhibitor of NTE, both in vivo and in culture systems (Funk et al., 1994). Neither the normal function for this enzyme activity nor its relation to axonal degeneration is understood (Davis and Richardson, 1980; Johnson, 1982; Lotti et al., 1993).

The degeneration of axons does not commence immediately after acute organophosphorus ester exposure but is delayed for 7 to 10 days between the acute high-dose exposure and the clinical signs of axonopathy. The axonal lesion in the PNS appears to be readily repaired, and the peripheral nerve becomes refractory to degeneration after repeated doses (Abou-Donia and Graham, 1978). By contrast, axonal degeneration in the long tracks of the spinal cord is progressive, resulting in a clinical picture that may resemble multiple sclerosis.

## Pyridinethione

Zinc pyridinethione has antibacterial and antifungal properties and is a component of shampoos that are effective in the treatment of seborrhea and dandruff. Because the compound is directly applied to the human scalp, it caused some concern when it was discovered that zinc pyridinethione is neurotoxic in rodents. Rats, rabbits, and guinea pigs all develop a distal axonopathy when zinc pyridinethione is a contaminant of their food (Sahenk and Mendell, 1979). Fortunately, however, zinc pyridinethione does not penetrate skin well, and it has not resulted in human injury to date.

Although the zinc ion is an important element of the therapeutic action of the compound, only the pyridinethione moiety is absorbed following ingestion, with the majority of zinc eliminated in the feces. In addition, sodium pyridinethione is also neurotoxic, establishing that it is the pyridinethione that is responsible for the neurotoxicity (Collum and Winek, 1967). Pyridinethione chelates metal ions and, once oxidized to the disulfide, may lead to the formation of mixed disulfides with proteins. However, which of these properties, if either, is the molecular mechanism of its neurotoxicity remains unknown.

Although these molecular issues remain to be resolved, pyridinethione appears to interfere with the fast axonal transport systems. While the fast anterograde system is less affected, pyridinethione impairs the turnaround of rapidly transported vesicles and slows the retrograde transport of vesicles (Sahenk and Mendell, 1980). This aberration of the fast axonal transport systems is the most likely physiologic basis of the accumulation of tubular and vesicular structures in the distal axon (Fig. 16-6). As these materials accumulate in one region of the axon, they distend the axonal diameter, resulting in axonal swellings filled with tubulovesicular profiles. As in many other distal axonopathies, the axon degenerates in its more distal regions beyond the accumulated structures. The earliest signs are diminished grip strength and electrophysiologic changes of the axon terminal, with normal conduction along the proximal axon in the early stages of exposure (Ross and Lawhorn, 1990). Ultimately, the functional consequence of the axonal degeneration in this exposure is similar to that of other axonopathies—a peripheral neuropathy.

## Microtubule-Associated Neurotoxicity

The role of microtubules in axonal transport and in the maintenance of axonal viability is still being elucidated; however, the biochemistry and toxicity of several alkaloids isolated from plants have greatly aided the understanding of these processes. The first of these historically are the vinca alkaloids and colchicine which bind to tubulin and inhibit the association of this protein subunit to form microtubules. Vincristine, one of the vinca alkaloids, has found clinical use in the treatment of leukemia due to the antimitotic activity of its microtubule-directed action. Colchicine, in contrast, is used primarily in the treatment of gout. Both of these microtubule inhibitors also have been the cause of peripheral neuropathies in patients (Casey et al., 1973).

Much more recently another plant alkaloid, taxol, has been described that has a significantly different interaction with microtubules. Taxol binds to tubules when they are assembled and stabilizes the polymerized form of tubules so that they remain assembled even in the cold or in the presence of calcium, conditions under which microtubules normally dissociate into tubulin subunits (Schiff and Horwitz, 1981). Taxol has also found its way into clinical usage as a treatment of certain cancers and has resulted in sensorimotor axonopathy in patients receiving large doses of this compound (Lipton et al., 1989; Sahenk et al., 1994), or in autonomic neuropathy (Jerian et al., 1993).

It is fascinating that both the depolymerization of tubules by colchicine and the vinca alkaloids and the stabilization of tubules by taxol lead to an axonopathy. It has been known for some time that microtubules are in a state of dynamic equilibrium in vitro, with tubules existing in equilibrium with dissociated subunits. This process almost certainly occurs in vivo as well, even as tubulin migrates down the axon. Thus, the tubules are constantly associating and dissociating. It is within this dynamic equilibrium that taxol and the vinca alkaloids exert their toxic effects, preventing the interchange of the two pools of tubulin (Fig. 16-7).

The morphology of the axon is of course different in the two situations. In the case of colchicine, the axon appears to undergo atrophy and there are fewer microtubules within the axons. In contrast, following exposure to taxol, microtubules are present in great numbers and are aggregated to create arrays of microtubules (Roytta et al., 1984; Roytta and Raine, 1986). Both situations probably interfere with the process of fast axonal transport, although this has not yet been demonstrated definitively with taxol. In both situations, the resultant clinical condition is a peripheral neuropathy.

## MYELINOPATHIES

Myelin provides the electrical insulation of neuronal processes, and its absence leads to a slowing of conduction and aberrant conduction of impulses between adjacent processes, so-called ephaptic transmission (Rasminsky, 1980; Delio et al., 1987). Toxicants exist that result in the separation of the myelin lamellae, termed intramyelinic edema, and in the selective loss of myelin, termed demyelination (Fig. 16-2). Intramyelinic edema may be caused by alterations in the transcript levels of myelin basic protein-mRNA (Veronesi et al., 1991) and early in its evolution is reversible. However, the initial stages may progress to segmental demyelination, with loss of myelin from the axon. Segmental demyelination may also result from direct toxicity to the myelinating cell. After segmental demyelination, remyelination of naked internodes by Schwann cells is often seen in the PNS, whereas remyelination in the CNS occurs to only a limited extent. Interestingly, remyelination after segmental demyelination in peripheral nerve involves multiple Schwann cells and results, therefore, in internodal lengths (the distances between adjacent nodes of Ranvier) that are much shorter than normal and a permanent record of the demyelinating event.

The compounds in Table 16-3 each lead to a myelinopathy. Some of these compounds have created problems in humans, and many have been used as tools to explore the process of myelination of the NS and the process of remyelination following toxic disruption of myelin. In general terms, the functional consequences of demyelination depend on the extent of the demyelination and whether it is localized within the CNS, the PNS, or is more diffuse in its effects. Those toxic myelinopathies in which the disruption of myelin is diffuse generate a global neurologic deficit, whereas those that are limited to the PNS produce the symptoms of peripheral neuropathy.

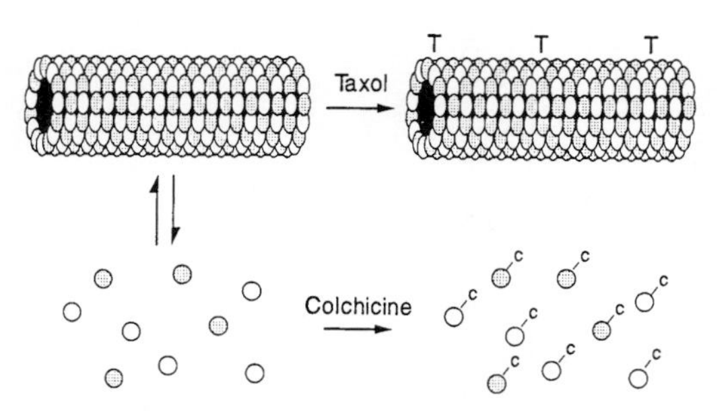


***Figure 16–7. Neurotoxicants directed toward microtubules.***

Colchicine leads to the depolymerization of microtubules by binding to the tubulin monomers and preventing their association into tubules. Taxol stabilizes the microtubules, preventing their dissociation into subunits under conditions in which they would normally dissociate. Both compounds interfere with the normal dynamic equilibrium that exists between tubulin and microtubules, and both are neurotoxic.

### Hexachlorophene

Hexachlorophene, or methylene 2,2′-methylenebis(3,4,6-trichlorophenol), resulted in human neurotoxicity when newborn infants, particularly premature infants, were bathed with the compound to avoid staphylococcal infections (Mullick, 1973). Following skin absorption of this hydrophobic compound, hexachlorophene enters the NS and results in intramyelinic edema, splitting the intraperiod line of myelin in both the CNS and the PNS. Experimental studies with erythrocyte membranes show that hexachlorophene binds tightly to cell membranes, resulting in the loss of ion gradients across the membrane (Flores and Buhler, 1974). It may be that hexachlorophene results in loss of the ability to exclude ions from between the layers of myelin and that, with ion entry, water also separates the myelin layers as "edema." Another, perhaps related effect is the uncoupling of mitochondrial oxidative phosphorylation by hexachlorophene (Cammer and Moore, 1974) because this process is dependent on a proton gradient. Intramyelinic edema is reversible in the early stages, but with increasing exposure hexachlorophene causes segmental demyelination, and the addition of water and ions to myelin adds to the volume of the brain. Swelling of the brain causes increased intracranial pressure which may be fatal in and of itself. With high-dose exposure, axonal degeneration is seen, along with degeneration of photoreceptors in the retina. It has been postulated that the pressure from severe intramyelinic edema may also injure the axon, leading to axonal degeneration, and endoneurial pressure measurements support this idea (Myers et al., 1982). The toxicity of hexachlorophene expresses itself functionally in diffuse terms that reflect the diffuse process of myelin injury. Humans exposed acutely to hexachlorophene may have generalized weakness, confusion, and seizures. Progression may occur to include coma and death.

### Tellurium

Although human cases have not been reported, neurotoxicity of tellurium has been demonstrated in animals. Young rats exposed to tellurium in their diet develop a severe peripheral neuropathy. Within the first 2 days of beginning a diet containing tellurium, the synthesis of myelin lipids in Schwann cells displays some striking changes (Harry et al., 1989). There is a decreased synthesis of cholesterol and cerebrosides, lipids richly represented in myelin, whereas the synthesis of phosphatidylcholine, a more ubiquitous membrane lipid, is unaffected. Myelin protein mRNA steady state levels are down-regulated (Morell et al., 1994). The synthesis of free fatty acids and cholesterol esters increases to some degree, and there is a marked elevation of squalene, a precursor of cholesterol. These biochemical findings demonstrate that there are a variety of lipid abnormalities, and the simultaneous increase in squalene and decrease in cholesterol suggest that tellurium or

**Table 16–3**
**Compounds Associated with Injury of Myelin (Myelinopathies)**

| NEUROTOXICANT | NEUROLOGICAL FINDINGS | CELLULAR BASIS OF NEUROTOXICITY | |
|---|---|---|---|
| Acetylethyltetramethyl tetralin (AETT) | Not reported in humans; hyperexcitability, tremors (rats) | Intramyelinic edema; pigment accumulation in neurons | 2,3 |
| Amiodarone | Peripheral neuropathy | Axonal degeneration and demyelination; lipid-laden lysosomes in Schwann cells | 2 |
| Cuprizone | Not reported in humans; encephalopathy (exper. animals) | Status spongiosis of white matter, intramyelinic edema | 2,3 |
| Cyanate | Peripheral neuropathy | Segmental demyelination, axonal degeneration | 3 |
| Ethidium bromide | Insufficient data (humans) | Intramyelinic edema, status spongiosis of white matter | 3 |
| Hexachlorophene | Irritability, confusion, seizures | Brain swelling, intramyelinic edema in CNS and PNS | 2,3 |
| Lysolecithin | Effects only on direct injection into PNS or CNS | Selective demyelination | 2 |
| Perhexilene | Peripheral neuropathy | Demyelinating neuropathy, membrane-bound inclusions in Schwann cells | 2,3 |
| Tellurium | Hindlimb paralysis (exper. animals) | Demyelinating neuropathy, lipofuscinosis (data for exper. animals only) | 2 |
| Triethyltin | Headache, photophobia, vomiting, paraplegia (irreversible) | Brain swelling (acute) with intramyelinic edema | 1,2,3 |

1. *Handbook of Neurotoxicology,* Chang LW and Dyer RS, eds. New York, Marcel Dekker, Inc., 1995.
2. *Greenfield's Neuropathology, 5th Edition,* Adams JH, Duchen LW, eds. New York, Oxford University Press, 1992.
3. *Experimental and Clinical Neurotoxicology,* Spencer PS and Schaumburg HH, eds. Baltimore, Williams and Wilkins, 1980.
4. *Neurotoxicology,* Abou-Donia MB, ed. Boca Raton, CRC Press, 1993.
5. *Neurotoxicity: Identifying and Controlling Poisons of the Nervous System,* U.S. Congress, Office of Technology Assessment (OTA-BA-436). Washington DC, U. S. Government Printing Office, 1990.

one of its derivatives may interfere with the normal conversion of squalene to cholesterol.

At the same time as these biochemical changes are occurring, lipids are accumulating in Schwann cells within intracytoplasmic vacuoles, and shortly afterwards, these Schwann cells lose their ability to maintain myelin. Axons and the myelin of the CNS are impervious to the effects of tellurium. However, individual Schwann cells in the PNS disassemble their concentric layers of myelin membranes, depriving the adjacent intact axon of its electrically insulated status. Not all Schwann cells are equally affected by the process, but rather those Schwann cells that encompass the greatest distances appear to be the most affected. These cells are associated with the largest diameter axons, encompass the longest intervals of myelination, and provide the thickest layers of myelin. Thus, it appears that these vulnerable cells are those with the largest volume of myelin to support (Bouldin et al., 1988).

As the process of remyelination begins, several cells cooperate to reproduce the myelin layers that were previously formed by a single Schwann cell. Perhaps this diminished demand placed upon an individual cell is the reason that remyelination occurs even in the presence of continued exposure to tellurium (Bouldin et al., 1988). The expression of the neurologic impairment is also short in duration, reflecting the transient cellular and biochemical events. The animals initially develop severe weakness in the hindlimbs but then recover their strength after 2 weeks on the tellurium-laden diet.

### Lead

Lead exposure in animals results in a peripheral neuropathy with prominent segmental demyelination, a process that bears a strong resemblance to tellurium toxicity (Dyck et al., 1977). However, the neurotoxicity of lead is much more variable in humans than in rats, and there are also a variety of manifestations of lead toxicity in other organ systems.

The neurotoxicity of lead has been appreciated for centuries. In current times, adults are exposed to lead in occupational settings through lead smelting processes and soldering and in domestic settings through lead pipes or through the consumption of "moonshine" contaminated with lead. In addition, even in the absence of definable exposures, some areas contain higher levels of environmental lead resulting in higher blood levels in the inhabitants. Children, especially those younger than 5 years, have higher blood levels of lead than adults in the same environment due to mouthing objects and the consumption of substances other than food. The most common acute exposure in children, however, is through the consumption of paint chips containing lead pigments (Perlstein and Attala, 1966).

In young children, acute massive exposures result in severe cerebral edema, perhaps from damage to endothelial cells. Children seem to be more susceptible to this lead encephalopathy than adults; however, adults may also develop an acute encephalopathy in the setting of massive lead exposure.

Chronic lead intoxication in adults results in peripheral neuropathy that is often accompanied by manifestations outside the NS, such as gastritis, colicky abdominal pain, anemia, and the prominent deposition of lead in particular anatomic sites, creating lead lines in the gums and in the epiphyses of long bones in children. The effects of lead in the peripheral nerve of humans is not entirely understood. Electrophysiological studies have demonstrated a slowing of nerve conduction (Buchthal and Behse, 1979). While this observation is consistent with the segmental demyelination that develops in experimental animals, pathologic studies in humans with lead neuropathy typically have demonstrated an axonopathy (Buchthal and Behse, 1979). Another curious finding in humans is the predominant involvement of motor axons, creating one of the few clinical situations in which patients present with a predominantly motor neuropathy.

Although the manifestations of acute and chronic exposures to lead have been long established, it is only in recent years that the concept has emerged that extremely low levels of exposure to lead in "asymptomatic" children may have an effect on their intelligence. Initial reports noted a relationship between mild elevations of blood lead in children and school performance; more recently correlations between elevated lead levels in decidual teeth and performance on tests of verbal abilities, attention, and behavior (nonadaptive) have been demonstrated (Needleman and Gatsonis, 1990; Needleman, 1994). Although there is a clear association between lead level and intellectual performance, there has been some controversy as to whether lead is causal. Children with higher blood levels tend to share certain other environmental factors, such as socioeconomic status and parental educational level. However, in spite of these complex human situations, it appears that lead exposure has an adverse effect on the intellectual abilities of children (Needleman, 1994), an association between lead exposure and brain dysfunction which has received experimental support in animal models (Gilbert and Rice, 1987).

## NEUROTRANSMISSION-ASSOCIATED TOXICITY

Many neurotoxicants destroy cellular structures within the NS, providing anatomic footprints of their toxicity. In some instances, however, dysfunction of the NS may occur without evidence of altered cellular structures; rather, the neurotoxicity expresses itself in terms of altered behavior or impaired performance on neurologic tests. In fact, many of the neurotoxic agents that lead to anatomic evidence of cellular injury were first demonstrated to be neurotoxic through the detection of neurologic dysfunction.

Molecular mechanisms are not understood for some of these agents; however, there is a group of such compounds in which the chemical basis of their action is clear. These are the toxicants that impair the process of neurotransmission. A wide variety of naturally occurring toxins, as well as synthetic drugs, interact with specific mechanisms of intercellular communication. At times, interruption of neurotransmission is beneficial to an individual, and the process may be viewed as neuropharmacology. However, excessive or inappropriate exposure to compounds that alter neurotransmission may be viewed as one of the patterns of neurotoxicology.

This group of compounds may interrupt the transmission of impulses, block or accentuate transsynaptic communication, or interfere with second-messenger systems. In general, the acute effects of these compounds are directly related to the immediate concentration of the compound at the active site, which bears a direct relationship to the level of the drug in the blood. The structural similarity of many compounds with similar actions has led to the recognition of specific categories of drugs and toxins. For example, some mimic the process of neurotransmission of the sympathetic nervous system and are termed the *sympathomimetic compounds*. As the targets of these drugs are located throughout the body, the responses are not localized; however, the responses are stereotyped in that each member of a class tends to have similar biologic effects. In terms of toxicity, most of the side effects of these drugs may be viewed as short-term interactions that are easily reversible with time or that may be counteracted by the use of appropriate antagonists. However, some of the toxicity associated with long-term use is irreversible. For example, phenothiazines, which have been used to treat chronic schizophrenia for long periods of time, may lead to the condition of tardive dyskinesia in which the patient is left with a permanent disability of prominent facial grimaces (DeVeaugh-Geiss, 1982). Both reversible acute high-dose toxicity and sustained effects following chronic exposure are common features of the agents that interact with the process of neurotransmission.

## Nicotine

Widely available in tobacco products and in certain pesticides, nicotine has diverse pharmacologic actions and may be the source of considerable toxicity. These toxic effects range from acute poisoning to more chronic effects. Nicotine exerts its effects by binding to a subset of cholinergic receptors, the nicotinic receptors. These receptors are located in ganglia, at the neuromuscular junction, and also within the CNS where the psychoactive and addictive properties most likely reside. Smoking and "pharmacologic" doses of nicotine accelerate heart rate, elevate blood pressure, and constrict blood vessels within the skin. Because the majority of these effects may be prevented by the administration of $\alpha$- and $\beta$-adrenergic blockade, these consequences may be viewed as the result of stimulation of the ganglionic sympathetic nervous system (Benowitz, 1986). At the same time, nicotine leads to a sensation of "relaxation" and is associated with alterations of electroencephalographic (EEG) recordings in humans. These effects are probably related to the binding of nicotine with nicotinic receptors within the CNS, and the EEG changes may be blocked with an antagonist, mecamylamine.

Acute overdose of nicotine has occurred in children who accidentally ingest tobacco products, in tobacco workers exposed to wet tobacco leaves (Gehlbach et al., 1974), or workers exposed to nicotine-containing pesticides. In each of these settings, the rapid rise in circulating levels of nicotine leads to excessive stimulation of nicotinic receptors, a process that is followed rapidly by ganglionic paralysis. Initial nausea, rapid heart rate, and perspiration are followed shortly by marked slowing of heart rate with a fall in blood pressure. Somnolence and confusion may occur, followed by coma; if death results, it is often the result of paralysis of the muscles of respiration.

Such acute poisoning with nicotine fortunately is uncommon. Exposure to lower levels for longer duration, in contrast, is very common and the health effects of this exposure are of considerable epidemiologic concern. In humans, however, it has been impossible so far to separate the effects of nicotine from those of other components of cigarette smoke. The complications of smoking include cardiovascular disease, cancers (especially malignancies of the lung), chronic pulmonary disease, and attention deficit disorders in children of women who smoke during pregnancy. Nicotine may be a factor in some of these problems. For example, an increased propensity for platelets to aggregate is seen in smokers and this platelet abnormality correlates with the level of nicotine. Nicotine also places an increased burden on the heart through its acceleration of heart rate and blood pressure, suggesting that nicotine may play a role in the onset of myocardial ischemia (Benowitz, 1986). In addition, nicotine also inhibits apoptosis and may play a direct role in tumor promotion and tobacco-related cancers (Wright et al., 1993)

It seems more clear that chronic exposure to nicotine has effects on the developing fetus. Along with decreased birth weights, attention deficit disorders are more common in children whose mothers smoke cigarettes during pregnancy, and nicotine has been shown to lead to analogous neurobehavioral abnormalities in animals exposed prenatally to nicotine (Lichensteiger et al., 1988). Nicotinic receptors are expressed early in the development of the NS, beginning in the developing brain stem and later expressed in the diencephalon. The role of these nicotinic receptors during development is unclear; however, it appears that prenatal exposure to nicotine alters the development of nicotinic receptors in the CNS (van de Kamp and Collins, 1994), changes that may be related to subsequent attention and cognitive disorders in animals and children.

## Cocaine

Cocaine differs from nicotine in the eyes of the law, a feature of the compound that affects the willingness of users to discuss their patterns of use. Nonetheless, it has been possible to obtain estimates of the number of users. In 1972, approximately 9 million college-age adults were using the drug; in 1982, approximately 33 million (Fishburne et al., 1983). In urban settings, from 10 to 45 percent of pregnant women take cocaine (Volpe, 1992), and cocaine metabolites can be detected in as many as 6 percent of babies born at suburban hospitals (Schutzman et al., 1991).

Cocaine blocks the reuptake of catecholamines at nerve terminals, and its entry into the CNS across the blood–brain barrier allows a central effect that accounts for the euphoric sensation and the addictive properties. Acute toxicity due to excessive intake, or overdose, may result in unanticipated deaths. While the tragic accounts of celebrities' overdoses may attract media attention, it is the chronic "recreational" consumption of cocaine that is of greatest epidemiologic concern. Perhaps the most alarming of these trends, considering the youth of the population who uses cocaine, is the potential for cocaine-induced effects on the fetus.

Although cocaine increases maternal blood pressure during acute exposure, in pregnant animals, the blood flow to the uterus actually diminishes. Depending on the level of the drug in the mother, the fetus may develop marked hypoxia as a result of the diminished uterine blood flow (Woods et al., 1987). In a study of women who used cocaine during pregnancy, there were more miscarriages and placental hemorrhages (abruptions) than in drug-free women (Chasnoff et al., 1985). Impaired placental function may be the cause for the increase in infarctions and hemorrhages in the newborn infant who has been exposed to cocaine (Volpe, 1992). In addition, the newborn infants of cocaine users were less interactive than normal newborns and exhibited a poor response to stimuli in the environment (Chasnoff et al., 1985).

## Excitatory Amino Acids

Glutamate and certain other acidic amino acids are excitatory neurotransmitters within the CNS. The discovery that these excitatory amino acids are neurotoxic at concentrations that are low relative to their concentrations in the brain has generated a great amount of interest in these "excitotoxins." In vitro systems have established that the toxicity of glutamate can be blocked by certain glutamate antagonists (Rothman and Olney, 1986), and the concept is rapidly emerging that the toxicity of excitatory amino acids may be related to such divergent conditions as hypoxia, epilepsy, and neurodegenerative diseases (Meldrum, 1987; Choi, 1988; Lipton and Rosenberg, 1994).

Glutamate is the main excitatory neurotransmitter of the brain and its effects are mediated by several subtypes of receptors (Schoepfer et al., 1994; Hollmann and Heinemann, 1994; Lipton and Rosenberg, 1994). The two major subtypes of glutamate receptors are those that are ligand-gated directly to ion channels (ionotropic) and those that are coupled with G proteins (metabotropic). Ionotropic receptors may be further subdivided by their specificity for binding kainate, quisqualate and *a*-amino-3-hydroxy-5-methylisoxazole-4-propionic acid (AMPA), and *N*-methyl-*D*-aspartate (NMDA). The entry of glutamate into the CNS is regulated at the blood–brain barrier and, following an injection of a large dose of glutamate in infant rodents, glutamate exerts its effects in the area of the brain in which the blood–brain barrier is least developed, the circumventricular organ. Within this site of limited access, glutamate injures neurons, apparently by opening glutamate-dependent ion channels, ultimately leading to neuronal swelling and neuronal cell death (Olney, 1978; Coyle, 1987). The toxicity affects the dendrites and neuronal cell bodies but seems to spare axons. The only known related human condition is the "Chinese restaurant syndrome," in which consumption of large amounts of monosodium glutamate as a seasoning may lead to a burning sensation in the face, neck, and chest.

The cyclic glutamate analog, kainate, was initially isolated from a seaweed in Japan as the active component of an herbal treatment for ascariasis. Kainate is extremely potent as an excitotoxin, being a hundred-fold more toxic than glutamate, and is selective at a molecular level for the kainate receptor (Coyle, 1987). Like glutamate, kainate selectively injures dendrites and neurons and shows no substantial effect on glia or axons. As a result, this compound has found great use in neurobiology as a tool (McGeer et al., 1978). Injected into a region of the brain, kainate can destroy the neurons of that area without disrupting all of the fibers that pass through the same region (Coyle, 1987). Neurobiologists, as a result of this neurotoxic tool, are able to study the role of neurons in a particular area independent of the axonal injuries that occur when similar lesioning experiments are performed by mechanical cutting.

Recently there has been renewed interest in the possibility that another excitotoxin, *a*-amino-methylaminopropionic acid (or *β*-*N*-methylamino-L-alanine, BMAA), present in the seeds of *Cycas circinalis* (Kisby et al., 1992), is responsible for the neuronal degenerative disease amyotrophic lateral sclerosis-parkinsonism-dementia (ALS/PD) complex, which developed in the 1940s and 1950s in the Chamorro population of Guam. Kurland proposed that Guamanian ALS/PD was due to a component of the diet, and evaluations of the diet at that time suggested the disorder may be related to the cycad (Kurland, 1963). However, acute exposures of rats to the cycad failed to reveal a neurodegenerative disorder, and the topic was not studied further until recently.

With the intervening years, however, several epidemiologic facts provide support for the idea that ALS/PD of Guam may be due to an environmental agent. First, the incidence of ALS/PD has decreased substantially, a finding compatible with an environmental factor. Second, ALS/PD of Guam has occurred in immigrants to Guam who adopted the lifestyle of the Chamorros (Garruto et al., 1981). Initial attempts to identify an environmental agent focused on heavy metals, and attention was drawn to concentrations of aluminum in Guam and in the brains of patients dying of ALS/PD (Rodgers-Johnson et al., 1986). However, if aluminum plays a role in this disease, it is not likely to be the only factor because the manifestations and pathologic features are very different from "dialysis dementia," which appears to have a clear relationship to excessive exposure to aluminum in dialysis fluid (Elliott et al., 1978).

While evidence for aluminum as the putative toxicant in Guamanian ALS/PD appears thin, a toxicity associated with the cycad, or specifically with BMAA as an excitatory amino acid peculiar to the cycad, is attractive in explaining the regional and temporal distributions of ALS/PD on Guam. During World War II, the cycad was used as a source of food by the Chamorros, and it has long been suspected that this disease may be the delayed onset of cycad-related toxicity. BMAA has been isolated from the cycad and is excitotoxic, producing seizures in animals. The toxicity of BMAA is similar to that of glutamate in vitro and can be blocked by certain glutamate antagonists (Nunn et al., 1987). Studies in vivo, however, have not yet demonstrated a clear etiologic relationship between BMAA and ALS/PD. To date, the only evidence in whole animals that BMAA may be related to the disorder is the finding of motor symptoms in macaques exposed to BMAA in their diet (Spencer et al., 1987; Hugon et al., 1988) and the neuronal degeneration in rats that is specific for GABAergic cells (Seawright et al., 1990). It therefore remains to be resolved what role BMAA and cycad consumption play in developing Guamanian ALS/PD; however, it seems likely that the disorder is due to an environmental agent and may be considered a form of neurotoxicity (Duncan, 1992).

The growing field of the excitotoxic amino acids embodies many of the same attributes that characterize the more general discipline of neurotoxicology. Neurotoxicology is generally viewed as the study of compounds that are deleterious to the NS, and the effects of glutamate and kainate may be viewed as this type of deleterious toxicity. Exposure to these excitotoxic amino acids leads to neuronal injury and when of sufficient degree may kill neurons. However, the implications of these findings, as with the entire field of neurotoxicology, extend beyond the direct toxicity of the compounds in exposed populations. With kainate, as with many other neurotoxic compounds, has come a tool for neurobiologists who seek to explore the anatomy and function of the NS. Kainate, through its selective action on neuronal cell bodies, has provided a greater understanding of the functions of cells within a specific region of the brain while previous lesioning techniques addressed only regional functions. Finally, the questions surrounding BMAA, the cycad, aluminum, and Guamanian ALS/PD serve to remind the student of neurotoxicology that the causes of many neurologic diseases remain unknown. This void in understanding and the epidemiologic evidence that some neurodegenerative diseases may have environmental etiologies provide a heightened desire to appreciate more fully the effects of elements of our environment on the NS.

# REFERENCES


Abel EL, Jacobson S, Sherwin BT: *In utero* alcohol exposure: Functional and structural brain damage. *Neurobehav Toxicol Teratol* 5:363–366, 1983.

Abou-Donia MB, Graham DG: Delayed neurotoxicity of *O*-ethyl *O*-4-nitrophenyl phenylphosphonothioate: subchronic (90 days) oral administration in hens. *Toxicol Appl Pharmacol* 45:685–700, 1978.

Abou-Donia MB, Lapadula DM: Mechanisms of organophosphorus ester-induced delayed neurotoxicity: Type I and Type II. *Annu Rev Pharmacol Toxicol* 30:405–440, 1990.

Allen N, Mendell JR, Billmaier DJ, et al: Toxic polyneuropathy due to methyl *n*-butyl ketone: an industrial outbreak. *Arch Neurol* 32:209–218, 1975.

Amarnath V, Anthony DC, Amarnath K, et al; Intermediates in the Paal-Knorr synthesis of pyrroles. *J Org Chem* 56:6924–6931, 1991a.

Amarnath V, Anthony DC, Valentine WM, Graham DG: The molecular mechanism of the carbon disulfide mediated crosslinking of proteins. *Chem Res Toxicol* 4:148–150, 1991b.

Amarnath V, Valentine WM, Amarnath K, et al: The mechanism of nucleophilic substitution of alkylpyrroles in the presence of oxygen. *Chem Res Toxicol* 7:56–61, 1994.

Anthony DC, Boekelheide K, Anderson CW, Graham DG: The effect of 3,4-dimethyl substitution on the neurotoxicity of 2,5-hexanedione. II. Dimethyl substitution accelerates pyrrole formation and protein crosslinking. *Toxicol Appl Pharmacol* 71:372–382, 1983a.

Anthony DC, Boekelheide K, Graham DG: The effect of 3,4-dimethyl substitution on the neurotoxicity of 2,5-hexanedione. I. Accelerated clinical neuropathy is accompanied by more proximal axonal swellings. *Toxicol Appl Pharmacol* 71:362–371, 1983b.

Atchison WD, Hare MF: Mechanisms of methylmercury-induced neurotoxicity. *FASEB J* 8:622–629, 1994.

Baitinger C, Levine J, Lorenz T, et al: Characteristics of axonally transported proteins, in Weiss DG (ed): *Axoplasmic Transport.* Berlin: Springer-Verlag, 1982, pp 110–120.

Bakir F, Damluji SF, Amin-Zaki L, et al: Methylmercury poisoning in Iraq. *Science* 181:230–241, 1973.

Becking GC, Boyes WK, Damstra T, MacPhail RC: Assessing the neurotoxic potential of chemicals—a multidisciplinary approach. *Environ Res* 61:164–175, 1993.

Benowitz NL: Clinical pharmacology of nicotine. *Annu Rev Med* 37:21–32, 1986.

Besser R, Kramer G, Thumler R, et al: Acute trimethyltin limbic-cerebellar syndrome. *Neurology* 37:945–950, 1987.

Bouldin TW, Gaines ND, Bagnell CR, Krigman MR: Pathogenesis of trimethyltin neuronal toxicity. *Am J Pathol* 104:237–249, 1981.

Bouldin TW, Samsa G, Earnhardt TS, Krigman MR: Schwann cell vulnerability to demyelination is associated with intermodal length in tellurium neuropathy. *J Neuropathol Exp Neurol* 47:41–47, 1988.

Brady ST, Lasek RJ: The slow components of axonal transport: movements, compositions and organization, in Weiss DG (ed): *Axoplasmic Transport.* Berlin: Springer-Verlag, 1982, pp 206–217.

Braun PE: Molecular architecture of myelin, in Morrell P (ed): *Myelin.* New York: Plenum Press, 1977, pp 91–115.

Braun PE, Pereyra PM, Greenfield S: Myelin organization and development: a biochemical perspective, in Hashim GA (ed): *Myelin: Chemistry and Biology*. New York: Alan R. Liss, 1980, pp 1–17.

Brierley JB, Brown AW, Caverley J: Cyanide intoxication in the rat—physiological and neuropathological aspects. *J Neurol Neurosurg Psychiatry* 39:129–140, 1976.

Brierley JB, Graham DI: Hypoxia and vascular disorders of the central nervous system, in Adams JH, Corsellis JAN, Duchen LW (eds): *Greenfield's Neuropathology*, 4th ed. New York: John Wiley & Sons, 1984, pp 125–156.

Brightman MW: The anatomic basis of the blood–brain barrier, in Neuwelt EA (ed): *Implications of the Blood–Brain Barrier and Its Manipulation*. New York: Plenum Press, 1989, vol 1, pp 53–83.

Brismar T, Hildebrand C, Tegner R: Nodes of Ranvier in acrylamide neuropathy: voltage clamp and electron microscopic analysis of rat sciatic nerve fibres at proximal levels. *Brain Res* 423:135–143, 1987.

Brouillet E, Jenkins BG, Hyman BT, et al: Age-dependent vulnerability of the striatum to the mitochondrial toxin 3-nitropropionic acid. *J Neurochem* 60:356–359, 1993.

Buchthal F, Behse F: Electrophysiology and nerve biopsy in men exposed to lead. *Br J Ind Med* 36:135–147, 1979.

Burbacher TM, Sackett GP, Mottet NK: Methylmercury effects on the social behavior of *Macaca fascicularis. Neurotoxicol Teratol* 12:65–71, 1990.

Calne DB, Langston JW, Martin WR, et al: Positron emission tomography after MPTP: observations relating to the cause of Parkinson's disease. *Nature* 317:246–248, 1985.

Cammer W, Moore CL: The effect of hexachlorophene on the respiration of brain and liver mitochondria. *Biochem Biophys Res Commun* 46:1887–1894, 1972.

Carpenter MB, Sutin J: *Human Neuroanatomy*, 8th ed. Baltimore: Williams & Wilkins, 1983, pp 85–133.

Casey EB, Jeliffe AM, LeQuesne PM, Millett YL: Vincristine neuropathy: clinical and electrophysiological observations. *Brain* 96:69–86, 1973.

Cavanagh JB: The significance of the "dying-back" process in experimental and human neurological disease. *Int Nat Rev Exp Pathol* 7:219–267, 1964.

Cavanagh JB: Towards the molecular basis of toxic neuropathies, in Galli CL, Manzo L, Spencer PS (eds): *Recent Advances in Nervous System Toxicology.* New York: Plenum Press, pp 23–42, 1984.

Chasnoff IJ, Burns WJ, Schnoll SH, Burns KA: Cocaine use in pregnancy. *N Engl J Med* 313:666–669, 1985.

Cheung MK, Verity MA: Experimental methyl mercury neurotoxicity: Locus of mercurial inhibition of brain protein synthesis in vivo and in vitro. *J Neurochem* 44:1799–1808, 1985.

Cho ES: Toxic effects of Adriamycin on the ganglia of the peripheral nervous system: A neuropathological study. *J Neuropathol Exp Neurol.* 36:907–915, 1977.

Cho ES, Spencer PS, Jortner BS, Schaumburg HH: A single intravenous injection of doxorubicin (Adriamycin) induces sensory neuropathy in rats. *Neurotoxicology* 1:583–590, 1980.

Choi DW: Glutamate neurotoxicity and diseases of the nervous system. *Neuron* 1:623–634, 1988.

Cohen G, Heikkila RE: In vivo scavenging of superoxide radicals by catecholamines, in Michelson AM, McCord JM, Fridovich I (eds): *Superoxide and Superoxide Dismutases.* London: Academic Press, 1977, pp 351–365.

Collins JJ, Swaen GMH, Marsh GM, et al: Mortality patterns among workers exposed to acrylamide. *J Occup Med* 31: 614–617, 1989.

Collum WD, Winek CL: Percutaneous toxicity of pyridinethiones in a dimethylsulfoxide vehicle. *J Pharm Sci* 56:1673–1675, 1967.

Coyle JT: Kainic acid: insights into excitatory mechanisms causing selective neuronal degeneration, in Bock G, O'Connor M (eds): *Selective Neuronal Death.* New York: John Wiley, 1987, pp 186–203.

Davis CS, Richardson RJ: Organophosphorus compounds, in Spencer PS, Schaumburg HH (eds): *Experimental and Clinical Neurotoxicology.* Baltimore: Williams & Wilkins, 1980, pp 527–544.

Davson H: History of the blood–brain barrier concept, in Neuwelt EA (ed): *Implications of the Blood–Brain Barrier and Its Manipulation.* New York: Plenum Press, 1989, vol 1 , pp 27–52.

DeCaprio AP, Olajas EJ, Weber P: Covalent binding of a neurotoxic *n*-hexane metabolite: Conversion of primary amines to substituted pyrrole adducts by 2,5-hexanedione. *Toxicol Appl Pharmacol* 65:440–450, 1982.

DeCaprio AP, Spink DC, Chen X, et al: Characterization of isothiocyanates, thioureas, and other lysine adduction products in carbon disulfide-treated peptides and protein. *Chem Res Toxicol* 5:496–504, 1992.

DeGrandchamp RL, Lowndes HE: Early degeneration and sprouting at the rat neuromuscular junction following acrylamide administration. *Neuropathol Appl Neurobiol* 16:239–254, 1990.

DeGrandchamp RL, Reuhl KR, Lowndes HE: Synaptic terminal degeneration and remodeling at the rat neuromuscular junction resulting from a single exposure to acrylamide. *Toxicol Appl Pharmacol* 105:422–433, 1990.

Delio DA, Gold BG, Lowndes HE: Crosstalk between intraspinal elements during progression of IDPN neuropathy. *Toxicol Appl Pharmacol* 90:253–260, 1987.

Denlinger RH, Anthony DC, Amarnath K, et al: Metabolism of 3,3′-iminodipropionitrile and deuterium-substituted analogs: Potential mechanisms of detoxification and activation. *Toxicol Appl Pharmacol* 124:59–66, 1994.

Denlinger RH, Anthony DC, Amarnath V, Graham, DG: Comparison of location, severity, and dose response of proximal axonal lesions induced by 3,3′-iminodipropionitrile and deuterium substituted analogs. *J Neuropathol Exp Neurol* 51:569–576, 1992.

DeVeaugh-Geiss J: Tardive dyskinesia: phenomenology, pathophysiology, and pharmacology, in *Tardive Dyskinesia and Related Involuntary Movement Disorders.* Boston: John Wright PSG, 1982, pp 1–18.

Duncan ID, Hammang JP, Trapp BD: Abnormal compact myelin in the myelin deficient rat: Absence of proteolipid protein correlates with a defect in the intraperiod line. *Proc Natl Acad Sci USA* 84:6287–6291, 1987.

Duncan MW: $\beta$-Methylamino-L-alanine (BMAA) and amyotrophic lateral sclerosis-parkinsonism dementia of the western Pacific. *Ann NY Acad Sci* 648:161–168, 1992.

Dyck PJ, O'Brien PC, Ohnishi A: Lead neuropathy. 2. Random distribution of segmental demyelination among "old internodes" of myelinated fibers. *J Neuropathol Exp Neurol* 36:570–575, 1977.

Ehrlich P: *Das Sauerstoff-Bedurfnis des Organismus. Eine Farbenanalytische Studie,* Berlin: Hershwald, 1885, pp 69–72.

Elliott HL, Dryburgh F, Fell GS, et al: Aluminum toxicity during regular haemodialysis. *Br Med J* 1:1101–1103, 1978.

Ernsting J: Some effects of brief profound anoxia upon the central nervous system, in Schadé JP, McMenemey WM (eds): *Selective Vulnerability of the Brain in Hypoxemia.* Oxford: Blackwell Scientific, 1963, pp 41–45.

Farrell CL, Risau W: Normal and abnormal development of the blood–brain barrier. *Microsc Res Tech* 27:495–506, 1994.

Federal Register: *Principles of Neurotoxicity Risk Assessment.* Environmental Protection Agency Final Report. US Government Printing Office, Washington, DC: pp. 42360–42404, 1994, vol 59, no 158.

Fishburne PM, Abelson HI, Cisin I: *National Household Survey on Drug Abuse: National Institute of Drug and Alcohol Abuse Capsules, 1982.* Dept of Health and Human Services, 1983.

Flores G, Buhler DR: Hemolytic properties of hexachlorophene and related chlorinated biphenols. *Biochem Pharmacol* 23:1835–1843, 1974.

Fowler BA, Woods JS: The transplacental toxicity of methylmercury to fetal rat liver mitochondria. *Lab Invest* 36:122–130, 1977.

Frenkel GD, Harrington L: Inhibition of mitochondrial nucleic acid synthesis by methylmercury. *Biochem Pharmacol* 28:651–655, 1979.

Funk KA, Liu CH, Higgins RJ, Wilson BW: Avian embryonic brain reaggregate culture system. II. NTE activity discriminates between effects of a single neuropathic or nonneuropathic organophosphorus compound exposure. *Toxicol Appl Pharmacol* 124:159–163, 1994.

Garruto RM, Gajdusek DC, Chen KM: Amyotrophic lateral sclerosis and parkinsonism-dementia among Filipino migrants to Guam. *Ann Neurol* 10:341–350, 1981.

Gehlbach SH, Williams WA, Perry LD, Woodall JS: Green-tobacco sickness: An illness of tobacco harvesters. *JAMA* 229:1880–1883, 1974.

Genter MB, Szákal-Quin G, Anderson CW, et al: Evidence that pyrrole formation is a pathogenetic step in $\gamma$-diketone neuropathy *Toxicol Appl Pharmacol* 87:351–362, 1987.

Gilbert SG, Rice DC: Low-level lifetime lead exposure produces behavioral toxicity (spatial discrimination reversal) in adult monkeys. *Toxicol Appl Pharmacol* 91:484–490, 1987.

Goldberger ME, Murray M: Recovery of function and anatomical plasticity after damage to the adult and neonatal spinal cord, in Cotman CW (ed): *Synaptic Plasticity*. New York: Guilford Press, 1985, pp 77–110.

Grafstein B, Forman D: Intracellular transport in neurons. *Physiol Rev* 60:1167–1218, 1980.

Graham DG, Amarnath V, Valentine WM, et al: Pathogenetic studies of hexane and carbon disulfide neurotoxicity. *CRC Critical Reviews in Toxicology*, 25:91–112, 1995.

Graham DG, Anthony DC, Boekelheide K, et al: Studies of the molecular pathogenesis of hexane neuropathy. II. Evidence that pyrrole derivatization of lysyl residues leads to protein crosslinking *Toxicol Appl Pharmacol* 64:415–422, 1982.

Graham DG, Tiffany SM, Bell WR Jr, Gutknecht WF: Autoxidation versus covalent binding of quinones as the mechanism of toxicity of dopamine, 6-hydroxydopamine and related compounds for C1300 neuroblastoma cells in vitro. *Mol Pharmacol* 14:644–653, 1978.

Griffin JW, Anthony DC, Fahnestock KE, et al: 3,4-Dimethyl-2,5-hexanedione impairs the axonal transport of neurofilament proteins. *J Neurosci* 4:1516–1526, 1984.

Griffin JW, Hoffman PN, Clark AW, et al: Slow axonal transport of neurofilament proteins: impairment by $\beta,\beta'$-iminodipropionitrile administration. *Science* 202:633–635, 1978.

Griffin JW, Price DL: Proximal axonopathies induced by toxic chemicals, in Spencer PS, Schaumburg HH (eds): *Experimental and Clinical Neurotoxicology.* Baltimore: Williams & Wilkins, 1980, pp 161–178.

Harris CH, Gulati AK, Friedman MA, Sickles DW: Toxic neurofilamentous axonopathies and fast axonal transport. V. Reduced bidirectional vesicle transport in cultured neurons by acrylamide and glycidamide. *J Toxicol Environ Health* 42:343–356, 1994.

Harry GJ, Goodrum JF, Bouldin TW, et al: Tellurium-induced neuropathy: metabolic alterations associated with demyelination and remyelination in rat sciatic nerve. *J Neurochem* 52:938–945, 1989.

Harry GJ, Morell P, Bouldin TW: Acrylamide exposure preferentially impairs axonal transport of glycoproteins in myelinated axons. *J Neurosci Res* 31:554–560, 1992.

Hoffman PN, Lasek RJ: The slow component of axonal transport: identification of major structural polypeptides of the axon and their generality among mammalian neurons. *J Cell Biol* 66:351–366, 1975.

Hollmann M, Heinemann S: Cloned glutamate receptors. *Ann Rev Neurosci* 17:31–108, 1994.

Hugon J, Ludolph A, Roy DN, et al: Studies on the etiology and pathogenesis of motor neuron diseases. II. Clinical and electrophysiologic features of pyramidal dysfunction in macaques fed *Lathyrus sativus* and IDPN. *Neurology* 38:435–442, 1988.

Jerian SM, Sarosy GA, Link CJ Jr, et al: Incapacitating autonomic neuropathy precipitated by taxol. *Gynecol Oncol* 51:277–280, 1993.

Johnson KA: Pathway of the microtubule-dynein ATPase and the structure of dynein: A comparison with actomyosin. *Annu Rev Biophys Biophys Chem* 14:161–188, 1985.

Johnson MK: The target for initiation of delayed neurotoxicity by organophosphorus esters: Biochemical studies and toxicological applications, in Hodgson E, Bend JR, Philpot RM (eds): *Reviews in Biochemical Toxicology*. New York: Elsevier, vol 4, 1982, pp 141–212.

Kesson CM, Baird AW, Lawson DH: Acrylamide poisoning. *Postgrad Med J* 53:16–17, 1977.

Kidd JG, Langworthy OR: Paralysis following the ingestion of Jamaica ginger extract adulterated with tri-*ortho*-cresyl phosphate. *Johns Hopkins Med J* 52:39–60, 1933.

Kinney HC, Brody BA, Kloman AS, Gilles FH: Sequence of central nervous system myelination in human infancy. II. Patterns of myelination in autopsied infants. *J Neuropathol Exp Neurol* 47:217–234, 1988.

Kisby GE, Ellison M, Spencer PS: Content of the neurotoxins cycasin (methylazoxymethanol beta-D-glucoside) and BMAA (beta-N-methylamino-L-alanine) in cycad flour prepared by Guam Chamorros. *Neurology* 42:1336–1340, 1992.

Klaassen CD: Absorption, distribution and excretion of zinc pyridinethione in rabbits. *Toxicol Appl Pharmocol* 35:581–587, 1976.

Kondo A, Inoue T, Nagara H, et al: Neurotoxicity of Adriamycin passed through the transiently disrupted blood–brain barrier by mannitol in the rat brain. *Brain Res* 412:73–83, 1987.

Kopin IJ: MPTP effects on dopamine neurons. *Ann NY Acad Sci* 537:451–461, 1988.

Kopin IJ: Mechanisms of 1-methyl-4-phenyl-1,2,3,6-tetrahydropyridine induced destruction of dopaminergic neurons, in Herken H, Hucho F (eds): *Handbook of Experimental Pharmacology, Selective Neurotoxicity.* New York, 1992, vol 102.

Krasavage WJ, O'Donoghue JL, DiVincenzo GD, Terhaar CJ: The relative neurotoxicity of MnBk, *n*-hexane, and their metabolites. *Toxicol Appl Pharmacol* 52:433–441, 1980.

Kurland LT: Epidemiological investigations of neurological disorders in the Mariana islands, in Pemberton J (ed): *Epidemiology Reports on Research and Teaching*. Oxford and New York: Oxford University Press, 1963, pp 219–223.

Kurland LT, Faro SN, Siedler J: Minamata disease. *World Neurol* 1:370–395, 1960.

Lam G-W, DiStefano V: Characterization of carbon disulfide binding in blood and to other biological substances. *Toxicol Appl Pharmacol* 86:235–242, 1986.

Langston JW, Irwin I: MPTP: Current concepts and controversies. *Clin Neuropharmacol* 9:485–507, 1986.

Lichensteiger W, Ribary U, Schlumpf M, et al: Prenatal adverse effects of nicotine on the developing brain, in Boer GJ, Feenstra MGP, Mirmiran M, Swaab DF, Van Haaren F (eds): *Progress in Brain Research.* Amsterdam: Elsevier, 1988, vol 73, pp 137–157.

Lipton RB, Apfel SC, Dutcher JP, et al: Taxol produces a predominantly sensory neuropathy. *Neurology* 39:368–373, 1989.

Lipton SA, Rosenberg PA: Excitatory amino acids as a final common pathway for neurologic disorders. *N Engl J Med* 330:613–622, 1994.

Llorens J, Dememes D, Sans A: The behavioral syndrome caused by 3,3′-iminodipropionitrile and related nitriles in the rat is associated with degeneration of the vestibular sensory hair cells. *Toxicol Appl Pharmacol* 123:199–210, 1993.

Lorenz T, Willard M: Subcellular fractionation of intra-axonally transported polypeptides in the rabbit visual system. *Proc Natl Acad Sci USA* 75:505–509, 1978.

Lotti M, Moretto A, Capodicasa E, et al: Interactions between neuropathy target esterase and its inhibitors and the development of polyneuropathy. *Toxicol Appl Pharmacol* 122:165–171, 1993.

Lucey JF, Hibbard E, Behrman RE, et al: Kernicterus in asphyxiated newborn Rhesus monkeys. *Exp Neurol* 9:43–58, 1964.

Ludolf AC, He F, Spencer PS, et al: 3-Nitropropionic acid—exogenous animal neurotoxin and possible human striatal toxin. *Can J Neurol Sci* 18:492–498, 1991.

Ludolf AC, Seelig M, Ludolf A, et al: 3-Nitropropionic acid decreases cellular energy levels and causes neuronal degeneration in cortical explants. *Neurodegeneration* 1:155–161, 1992.

Malmfors T: The effects of 6-hydroxydopamine on the adrenergic nerves as revealed by fluorescence histochemical method, in Malmfors T, Thoenen H (eds): *6-Hydroxydopamine and Catecholaminergic Neurons.* Amsterdam: North-Holland, 1971, pp 47–58.

Marshall JF, Drew MC, Neve KA: Recovery of function after mesotelencephalic dopaminergic injury in senescence. *Brain Res* 259:249–260, 1983.

Martenson CH, Odom A, Sheetz MP, Graham DG: Effect of acrylamide and other sufhydryl alkylators on the ability of dynein and kinesin to translocate microtubules in vitro. *Toxicol Appl Pharmacol*, in press, 1995b.

Martenson CH, Sheetz MP, Graham DG: In vitro acrylamide exposure alters growth cone morphology. *Toxicol Appl Pharmacol*, 131:119–129, 1995a.

McGeer EG, Olney JW, McGeer PL (eds): *Kainic Acid as a Tool in Neurobiology*. New York: Raven Press, 1978.

Meldrum B: Excitatory amino acid antagonists as potential therapeutic agents, in Jenner P (ed): *Neurotoxins and Their Pharmacological Implications.* New York: Raven Press, 1987, pp 33–53.

Miller MS, Spencer PS: Single doses of acrylamide reduce retrograde transport velocity. *J Neurochem* 43:1401–1408, 1984.

Mitsuishi K, Takahashi A, Mizutani M, et al: beta,beta′-Iminodipropionitrile toxicity in normal and congenitally neurofilament-deficient Japanese quails. *Acta Neuropathol* 86:578–581, 1993.

Morell P, Toews AD, Wagner M, Goodrum JF: Gene expression during tellurium-induced primary demyelination. *Neurotoxicology* 15:171–180, 1994.

Moser VC, Anthony DC, Sette WF, MacPhail RC: Comparison of subchronic neurotoxicity of 2-hydroxyethyl acrylate and acrylamide in rats. *Fundament Appl Toxicol* 18:343–352, 1992.

Moser VC, MacPhail RC: Comparative sensitivity of neurobehavioral tests for chemical screening. *Neurotoxicology*, 11:335–344, 1990.

Mullick FG: Hexachlorophene toxicity: Human experience at the AFIP. *Pediatrics* 51:395–399, 1973.

Myers JE, Macun I: Acrylamide neuropathy in a South African factory: An epidemiologic investigation. *Amer J Indust Med* 19:487–493, 1991.

Myers RR, Mizisin AP, Powell HC, Lampert PW: Reduced nerve blood flow in hexachlorophene neuropathy: relationship to elevated endoneurial pressure. *J Neuropathol Exp Neurol* 41:391–399, 1982.

Needleman HL: Childhood lead poisoning. *Curr Opin Neurol* 7:187–190, 1994.

Needleman HL, Gatsonis CA: Low-level lead exposure and the IQ of children. A meta-analysis of modern studies. *JAMA* 263:673–678, 1990.

Nixon RA, Sihag RK: Neurofilament phosphorylation: A new look at regulation and function. *TINS* 14:501–506, 1991.

Nunn PB, Seelig M, Zagoren JC, Spencer PS: Stereospecific acute neurotoxicity of "uncommon" plant amino acids linked to human motor system diseases. *Brain Res* 410:375–379, 1987.

Olney JW: Neurotoxicity of excitatory amino acids, in McGeer EG, Olney JW, McGeer PL (eds): *Kainic Acid as a Tool in Neurobiology.* New York: Raven Press, 1978, pp 95–122.

O'Shea KS, Kaufman MH: The teratogenic effect of acetaldehyde: implications for the study of fetal alcohol syndrome. *J Anat* 128:65–76, 1979.

Padilla S, Atkinson MB, Breuer AC: Direct measurement of fast axonal organelle transport in the sciatic nerve of rats treated with acrylamide. *J Toxicol Environ Health* 39:429–445, 1993.

Paterson RA, Usher DR: Acute toxicity of methylmercury on glycolytic intermediates and adenine nucleotides in rat brain. *Life Sci* 10:121–128, 1971.

Penny DG: Acute carbon monoxide poisoning: animal models: a review. *Toxicology* 62:123–160, 1990.

Perlstein MA, Attala R: Neurologic sequelae of plumbism in children. *Clin Pediatr* 5:292–298, 1966.

Pham-Dinh D, Popot JL, Boespflug-Tanguy O, et al: Pelizaeus-Merzbacher disease: a valine to phenylalanine point mutation in a putative extracellular loop of myelin proteolipid. *Proc Natl Acad Sci USA* 88:7562–7566, 1991.

Plum F, Posner JB: Neurobiologic essentials, in Smith LH Jr, Thier SO (eds): *Pathophysiology: The Biological Principles of Disease.* Philadelphia: W.B. Saunders, 1985, pp 1009–1036.

Pyle SJ, Graham DG, Anthony DC: Dimethylhexanedione impairs the movement of neurofilament protein subunits, NFM and NFL, in the optic system. *Neurotoxicology* 15:279–286, 1994.

Rasminsky M: Ephaptic transmission between single nerve fibers in the spinal nerve roots of dystrophic mice. *J Physiol (Lond)* 305:151–169, 1980.

Readhead C, Schneider A, Griffiths I, Nave KA: Premature arrest of myelin formation in transgenic mice with increased proteolipid protein gene dosage. *Neuron* 12:583–595, 1994.

Reese TS, Karnovsky MJ: Fine structural localization of a blood–brain barrier to exogenous peroxidase. *J Cell Biol* 34:207–217, 1967.

Reuhl KR, Chang LW: Effects of methylmercury on the development of the nervous system: A review. *Neurotoxicology* 1:21–55, 1979.

Reuhl KR, Gilbert SG, Mackenzie BA, et al: Acute trimethyltin intoxication in the monkey (*Macaca fascicularis*). *Toxicol Appl Pharmacol* 79:436–452, 1985.

Rodgers-Johnson P, Garruto RM, Yanagihara R, et al: Amytrophic lateral sclerosis and parkinsonism-dementia on Guam: A 30-year evaluation of clinical and neuropathological trends. *Neurology* 36:7–13, 1986.

Ross JF, Lawhorn GT: ZPT-related distal axonopathy: Behavioral and electrophysiologic correlates in rats. *Neurotoxicol Teratol* 12:153–159, 1990.

Rothman SM, Olney JM: Glutamate and the pathophysiology of hypoxic-ischemic brain damage. *Ann Neurol* 19:105–111, 1986.

Roytta M, Horwitz SB, Raine CS: Taxol-induced neuropathy: short-term effects of local injection. *J Neurocytol* 13:685–701, 1984.

Roytta M, Raine CS: Taxol-induced neuropathy: chronic effects of local injection. *J Neurocytol* 15:483–496, 1986.

Sahenk Z, Barohn R, New P, Mendell JR: Taxol neuropathy: Electrodiagnostic and sural nerve biopsy findings. *Arch Neurol* 51:726–729, 1994.

Sahenk Z, Mendell JR: Ultrastructural study of zinc pyridinethione-induced peripheral neuropathy. *J Neuropathol Exp Neurol* 38:532–550, 1979.

Sahenk Z, Mendell JR: Axoplasmic transport in zinc pyridinethione neuropathy: evidence for an abnormality in distal turn-around. *Brain Res* 186: 343–353, 1980.

Sayre LM, Autilio-Gambetti L, Gambetti P: Pathogenesis of experimental giant neurofilamentous axonopathies: a unified hypothesis based on chemical modification of neurofilaments. *Brain Res Rev* 10:69–83, 1985.

Sayre LM, Shearson CM, Wongmongkolrit T, et al: Structural basis of $\gamma$-diketone neurotoxicity: non-neurotoxicity of 3,3-dimethyl-2, 5-hexanedione, a $\gamma$-diketone incapable of pyrrole formation. *Toxicol Appl Pharmacol* 84:36–44, 1986.

Schaumburg HH, Wisniewski HM, Spencer PS: Ultrastructural studies of the dying-back process. 1. Peripheral nerve terminal and axon degeneration in systemic acrylamide intoxication. *J Neuropathol Exp Neurol* 33:260–284, 1974.

Schiff PB, Horwitz SB: Taxol assembles tubulin in the absence of exogenous guanosine 5′-triphosphate or microtubule-associated proteins. *Biochemistry* 20:3242–3252, 1981.

Schnapp BJ, Reese TS: Dynein is the motor for retrograde axonal transport of organelles. *Proc Natl Acad Sci USA* 86:1548–1552, 1989.

Schnapp BJ, Vale RD, Sheetz MP, Reese TS: Single microtubules from squid axoplasm support bidirectional movement of organelles. *Cell* 40:455–462, 1985.

Schoepfer R, Monyer H, Sommer B, et al: Molecular biology of glutamate receptors. *Prog Neurobiol* 42:353–357, 1994.

Schutzman DL, Frankenfield-Chernicoff M, Clatterbaugh HE, Singer J: Incidence of intrauterine cocaine exposure in a suburban setting. *Pediatrics* 88: 825–827, 1991.

Seawright AA, Brown AW, Nolan CC, Cavanagh JB: Selective degeneration of cerebellar cortical neurons caused by cycad neurotoxin, L-beta-methylaminoalanine (L-BMAA), in rats. *Neuropathol Appl Neurobiol* 16:153–169, 1990.

Seppäläinen AM, Haltia M: Carbon disulfide, in Spencer PS, Schaumburg HH (eds): *Experimental and Clinical Neurotoxicology.* Baltimore: Williams & Wilkins, 1980, pp 356–373.

Shiraki, H: Neuropathological aspects of organic mercury intoxication, including Minimata disease, in Vinken PJ, Bruyn GW (eds): *Handbook of Clinical Neurology*. Amsterdam: North-Holland, 1979, vol 36, pp 83–145.

Spencer PS, Nunn PB, Hugon J, et al: Guam amyotrophic lateral sclerosis-parkinsonism-dementia linked to a plant excitant neurotoxin. *Science* 237:517–522, 1987.

Spencer PS, Schaumburg HH: Central-peripheral distal axonopathy: the pathology of dying-back polyneuropathies, in Zimmerman H (ed): *Progress in Neuropathology*. New York: Grune & Stratton, 1976, vol 3, pp 253–295.

St. Clair MBG, Amarnath V, Moody MA, et al: Pyrrole oxidation and protein crosslinking are necessary steps in the development of $\gamma$-diketone neuropathy *Chem Res Toxicol* 1:179–185, 1988.

Stoltenburg-Didinger G, Spohr HL: Fetal alcohol syndrome and mental retardation: spine distribution of pyramidal cells in prenatal alcohol exposed rat cerebral cortex. *Brain Res* 11:119–123, 1983.

Takeuchi T, Morikawa H, Matsumoto H, Shiraishi Y: A pathological study of Minamata disease in Japan. *Acta Neuropathol* 2:40–57, 1962.

Tilson HA: Neurobehavioral methods used in neurotoxicological research. *Toxicol Lett* 68:231–240, 1993.

Toews AD, Lee SY, Popko B, Morell P: Tellurium-induced neuropathy: a model for reversible reductions in myelin protein gene expression. *J Neurosci Res* 26:501–507, 1990.

Toggas SM, Krady JK, Billingsley ML: Molecular neurotoxicology of trimethyltin: Identification of stannin, a novel protein expressed in trimethyltin-sensitive cells. *Mol Pharmacol* 42:44–56, 1992.

Trevor AJ, Singer TP, Ramsay RR, Castagnoli NE Jr: Processing of MPTP by monoamine oxidases: Implications for molecular toxicology. *J Neural Transm (Suppl)* 23:73–89, 1987.

Tsujihata M, Engel AG, Lambert EH: Motor end-plate fine structure in acrylamide dying-back neuropathy: A sequential morphometric study. *Neurology* 24:849–856, 1974.

Vale RD, Reese TS, Sheetz MP: Identification of a novel force-generating protein, kinesin, involved in microtuble-based motility. *Cell* 42:39–50, 1985.

Valentine WM, Amarnath V, Amarnath K, et al : Carbon disulfide-mediated protein cross-linking by *N,N*-diethyldithiocarbamate. *Chem Res Toxicol,* 8:96–102, 1995.

Valentine WM, Amarnath V, Graham DG, Anthony DC: Covalent cross-linking of proteins by carbon disulfide. *Chem Res Toxicol* 5:254–262, 1992.

Valentine WM, Graham DG, Anthony DC: Covalent cross-linking of erythrocyte spectrin in vivo. *Toxicol Appl Pharmacol* 121:71–77, 1993.

van de Kamp JL, Collins AC: Prenatal nicotine alters nicotinic receptor development in the mouse brain. *Pharmacol Biochem Behav* 47:889–900, 1994.

Veronesi B, Jones K, Gupta S, et al: Myelin basic protein-messenger RNA (MBP-mRNA) expression during triethyltin-induced myelin edema. *Neurotoxicol*ogy 12:265–276, 1991.

Volpe JJ: Effect of cocaine use on the fetus. *N Engl J Med* 327:399–407, 1992.

Williamson AM: The development of a neurobehavioral test battery for use in hazard evaluations in occupational settings. *Neurotoxicol Teratol* 12:509–514, 1990.

Winneke G: Cross species extrapolation in neurotoxicology: Neurophysiological and neurobehavioral aspects. *Neurotoxicology* 13:15–25, 1992.

Woods JR, Plessinger MA, Clark KE: Effect of cocaine on uterine blood flow and fetal oxygenation. *JAMA* 257:957–961, 1987.

Wright SC, Zhong J, Zheng H, Larrick JW: Nicotine inhibition of apoptosis suggests a role in tumor production. *FASEB J* 7:1045–1051, 1993.

Yamamura Y: *n*-Hexane polyneuropathy. *Folia Psychiatr Neurol* 23:45–57, 1969.

# CHAPTER 17

# TOXIC RESPONSES OF THE HEART AND VASCULAR SYSTEMS

*Kenneth S. Ramos, Enrique Chacon, and Daniel Acosta, Jr.*

The cardiovascular system has two major components: the myocardium and a diverse network of vascular vessels consisting of arteries, capillaries, and veins. Both units of the cardiovascular system have important functions in supplying the tissues and cells of the body with appropriate nutrients, respiratory gases, hormones, and metabolites and removing the waste products of tissue and cellular metabolism as well as foreign matter such as invading microorganisms. In addition, the cardiovascular system, through its circulation of blood and fluids to every tissue in the body, is responsible for maintaining the optimal internal homeostasis of the body as well as for critical regulation of body temperature and maintenance of tissue and cellular pH. Thus, the cardiovascular system plays a critical role in the well-being and survival of the other major organs of the body, especially highly vascularized organs that are dependent on nutrients and oxygen carried by the blood. If the cardiovascular system is injured by disease or toxic chemicals, this damage has a far-reaching impact on the survival of the organism.

The discipline of cardiovascular toxicology is concerned with the adverse effects of drugs, chemicals, and xenobiotics on the heart and circulatory system of a living organism. The introduction of drugs or xenobiotics into the body eventually leads to their absorption into the bloodstream and transport to the heart; toxic interactions with the cardiovascular system usually are determined by the concentration of a xenobiotic in contact with the myocardium or vasculature and by the duration of exposure. A wide spectrum of xenobiotics, including drugs, natural products, industrial chemicals, and environmentally introduced agents, may interact directly with the cardiovascular system to cause structural and/or functional changes. There also may be indirect actions secondary to changes in other organ systems, especially the central and autonomic nervous systems and selective actions of the endocrine system. Functional alterations that affect the rhythmicity and contractility of the heart, if severe enough, may lead to lethal arrhythmias without major evidence of structural damage to the myocardium. Drugs that may produce arrhythmic effects in the myocardium include phenothiazines, tricyclic antidepressants, and emetine. Structural alterations such as degenerative necrosis and inflammatory reactions are often caused by direct effects of chemicals on the myocardium. Large doses of catecholaminelike agents may induce myocardial necrosis in ways similar to the pathological processes associated with myocardial ischemic injury secondary to atherosclerotic occlusion of the coronary arteries. Thus, toxicologists have been instrumental in developing a chemical model of myocardial ischemic injury with catecholamines and gaining a better understanding of the cell injury process in ischemic myocardium. Figure 17-1 illustrates the direct and indirect dynamic interactions of a toxicant on the cardiovascular system.

This chapter reviews chemical agents that have major toxic effects on the myocardium and vascular system to provide a better understanding of the mechanisms by which these chemicals are toxic to the cardiovascular system. The classification of cardiovascular toxicants is not a simple matter because a wide variety of chemical and drug classes have pharmacological as well as toxicological actions on the heart and circulatory system. We have arbitrarily classified the cardiovascular toxicants into three major categories: (1) pharmaceuticals, including antineoplastics, anesthetics, psychotropics, and antibiotics, (2) industrial chemicals such as heavy metals, solvents, and alcohols, and (3) natural products such as peptides and hormones. To better understand how these chemical

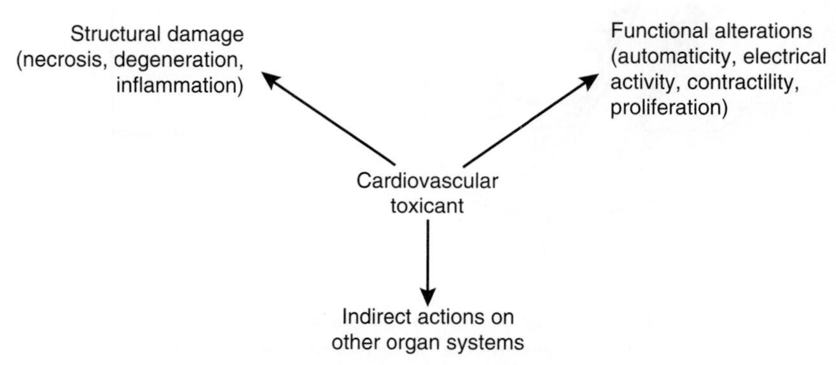


***Figure 17–1. Direct and indirect actions of a cardiovascular toxicant.***

agents injure the cardiovascular system, several biochemical mechanisms of the toxicity are discussed. These biological mechanisms have generated much interest and research activity, especially when they help explain general processes of cell injury associated with pathological conditions and diseases (e.g., myocardial ischemic injury).

## OVERVIEW OF CARDIAC PHYSIOLOGY

An understanding of the normal anatomy and physiology of the heart provides the basis for understanding the effects of xenobiotics on cardiac function. Figure 17-2 illustrates the basic anatomy of the heart. The main purpose of the heart is to pump blood to the lungs and the systemic arteries to provide oxygen and nutrients to all the tissues of the body. The heart consists of four pumping chambers: the right and left atria and the right and left ventricles. Venous blood from the systemic circulation enters the right atrium and right ventricle, where it is then pumped into the lungs to become oxygenated. The left atrium and ventricle then receive the oxygenated blood via the pulmonary veins and pump it to the systemic arteries via the aorta. Each contraction cycle consists of an orchestrated series of events that result in the blood-pumping action of the heart.

### Basic Electrophysiology

The cardiac cycle begins in pacemaker cells that spontaneously depolarize in an autorhythmic fashion and pass a depolarizing electrical current to neighboring cells. Pacemaker cells do not contract but are responsible for initiating and conducting action potentials to the muscle cells in the heart. Autorhythmic cell excitation is different from nerve and muscle excitation in that pacemaker cells do not remain at a constant resting potential. Instead, a pacemaker cell's membrane potential slowly depolarizes or drifts toward threshold as a result of a decreased $K^+$ efflux that is superimposed on a slow inward leak of $Na^+$. Overall, there is a gradual buildup of positive ions inside the cells, causing the inside of the cells to become less negative relative to the extracellular space. This gradual depolarization or drift toward threshold eventually gives rise to an action potential. Once a threshold is reached, $Ca^{2+}$ channels open, leading to a rapid influx of $Ca^{2+}$ and production of the characteristic action potential (Fig. 17-2).

This specialized autorhythmic property can be found in various regions throughout the heart (Fig. 17-2): the sinoatrial node (SA node), the atrioventricular node (AV node), the bundle of His (atrioventricular bundle), and Purkinje fibers. SA node cells exhibit the fastest rate of action potential discharge (70 to 80 action potentials per minute) and thus set the pace of the heart (hence the term "pacemaker"). If the SA node is damaged or inhibited, the next fastest depolarizing cells (AV node) assume the pacemaking activity. The AV node cells depolarize at a rate of approximately 40 to 60 action potentials per minute. The bundle of His and Purkinje fibers fire at a rate of approximately 20 to 40 action potentials per minute. The non-SA nodal autorhythmic cells are referred to as latent pacemakers and can take over to set the cardiac pace if the normal pacemaker cells fail. However, because of decreased rates of firing in the latent pace-

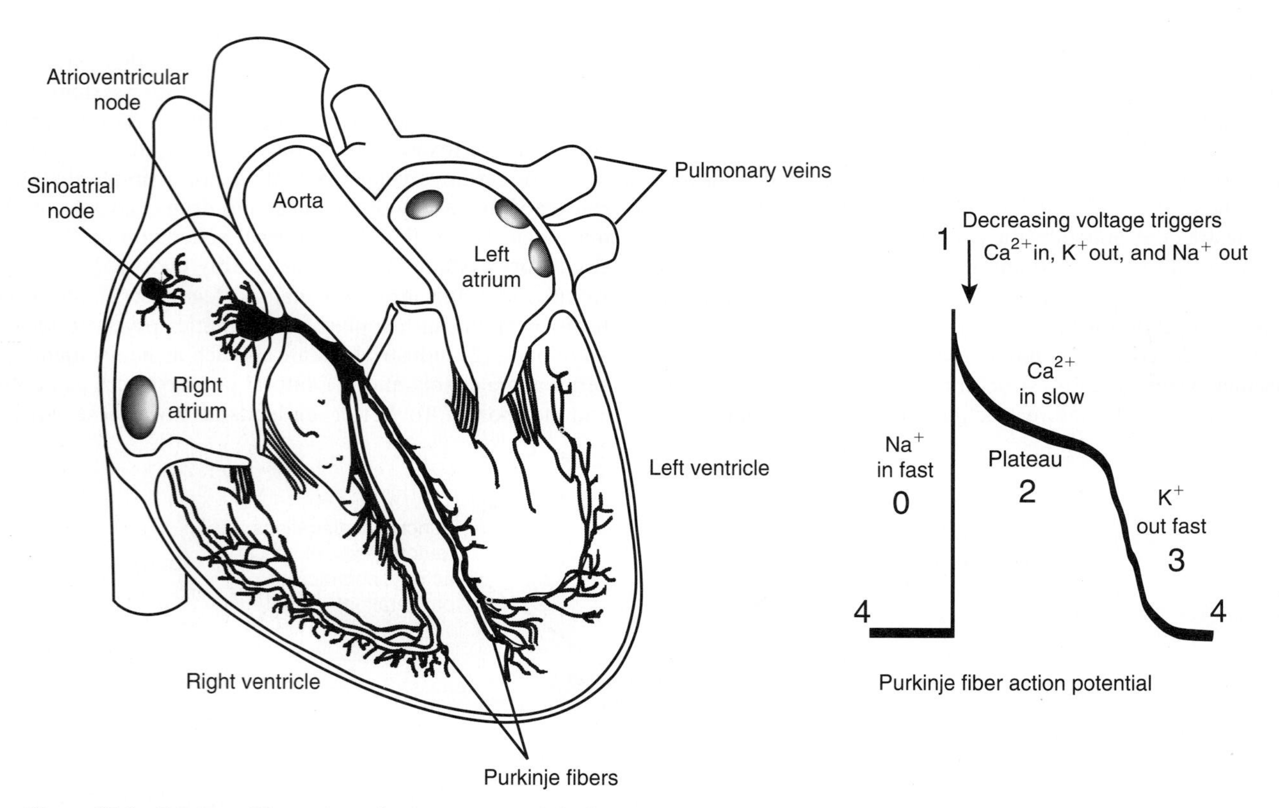


*Figure 17–2. Diagram illustrating a basic anatomy of the heart and a characteristic action potential recording of Purkinje cells. A Purkinje cell action potential is characterized by a sequence of events (phases) that correspond with ion movements across the sarcolemma.*

maker cells, normal cardiac function is compromised as a result of slower firing rates.

Normally, the initiation of the cardiac cycle begins with the autorhythmic depolarization of cells in the SA node as a result of their rapid firing rate. The electrical impulse propagates through the atrial muscle cells to the AV node. The dense fibrous tissue of the AV node causes the electrical impulse to slow down. This delayed transfer of current between the atria and the ventricles allows the atria to complete contraction before depolarization of the ventricles. The AV node impulse is then sent down the bundle of His, the bundle branches, and the Purkinje network, causing depolarization and contraction of muscle cells in the ventricles.

Electrical cardiac activity is regulated by the peripheral autonomic nervous system (ANS). The ANS enhances or restrains pacemaker cellular activity. The efferent, or motor, side of the ANS influences heart rate and contractility in accordance with the body's demand. The efferent ANS consists of postganglionic adrenergic fibers (sympathetic fibers) and postganglionic cholinergic fibers (parasympathetic fibers). The chemical transmitter of the sympathetic system is norepinephrine (noradrenaline). The chemical transmitter of the parasympathetic system is acetylcholine (ACh). Sympathetic fibers are found in the SA and AV nodes as well as in the atrial and ventricular walls. Parasympathetic fibers (vagal fibers) are found in the SA and AV nodes as well as in atrial muscle. Thus, norepinephrine and similar sympathomimetics stimulate the rate of depolarization and the rate of impulse transmission, resulting in an increase in the cardiac rate and the contractility of the myocardium. The major effect of parasympathomimetics is to enhance the vagal tone of the SA and AV nodes and the atrial muscle and thus decrease the rate of depolarization with only a slight decrease in ventricular contractility.

**Basic Review of Action Potential.** The ionic basis of membrane activity is represented by the transmembrane potential. At any given time, the potential across the sarcolemma is a reflection of the ion concentration gradients across the membrane: calcium ($Ca^{2+}$), sodium ($Na^{+}$), and potassium ($K^{+}$). The characteristic appearance of the Purkinje fiber action potential demonstrates how ion currents result in changes in the membrane potential (Fig. 17-2). In a resting cell, the density of the electrical charge on both sides of the sarcolemma is referred to as phase 4 or the diastolic potential. When an action potential is initiated (phase 0), there is a rapid influx of sodium that depolarizes the cell from approximately −70 mV (nonpacemaker cardiac cells) to slightly greater than 0 mV. Calcium begins an inward flux at approximately −35 mV (phase 1: early fast repolarization). As the sodium current dissipates, calcium continues to enter the cell, giving rise to the characteristic plateau appearance of phase 2. Repolarization of the cell (phase 3) gives rise to the resting potential.

## Basic Cardiac Structure

Contraction in cardiac muscle cells is similar to contraction in skeletal muscle cells. A brief review showing the structural organization of muscle tissue can be summarized as follows (Fig. 17-3):

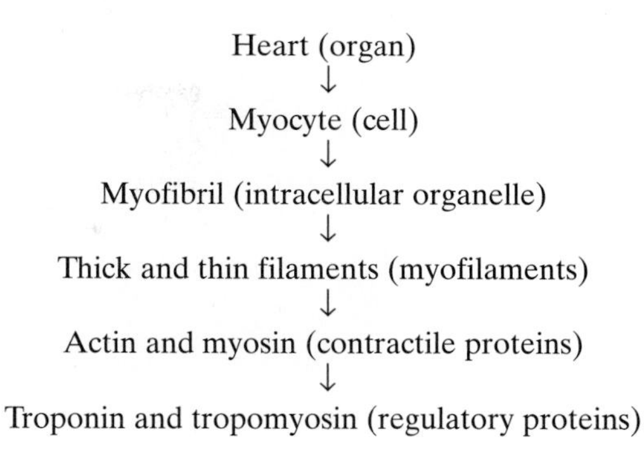


Each myofibril consists of a number of smaller filaments (the thick and thin myofilaments). The thick filaments are special assemblies of the protein myosin, whereas the thin filaments are made up primarily of the protein actin. These essential structural components of myocardial contraction display alternating dark bands (A bands) and light bands (I bands). Visible in the middle of the I band is a dense vertical Z line. The area between two Z lines is called a sarcomere, the fundamental unit of muscle contraction. About 50 percent of each cardiac cell is composed of myofibrils. The remaining intracellular space contains mitochondria (33 percent), one or more nuclei (5 percent), the sarcoplasmic reticulum (2 percent), lysosomes (very low), glycogen granules, a Golgi network, and cytosol (12 percent) (Opie, 1986a).

**Contraction.** Contraction occurs when an action potential causes the release of calcium from the sarcoplasmic reticulum (SR). Released calcium then binds with the inhibitory proteins troponin and tropomysin, which allow actin to slide on myosin. Energy for contraction is obtained from the splitting of adenosine triphosphate (ATP) by hydrolysis via an ATPase site on myosin. Each mole of ATP hydrolyzed liberates about 30 kJ (kilojoules) of energy. The heart contains about 3 mg ATP per gram wet weight (5 $\mu$mol/g) and approximately a pool of creatine phosphate that is three times larger; this accounts for a minimal reserve sufficient to last only about 50 to 75 beats (Opie, 1986b). Since the majority of ATP for contraction is provided by the mitochondria, it is not surprising that mitochondria occupy a large portion of each heart cell and maintain integrity to support myocardial function.

## Cardiac Function

Cardiac function is measured in stroke volume, cardiac output, and blood pressure. During each cardiac cycle, muscle fibers shorten in length. The force and length of myofibril contraction are converted into changes in blood pressure and volume. The amount of blood pumped out of each ventricle with each contraction is known as the stroke volume (SV). Cardiac output (CO) is the volume of blood pumped by each ventricle per minute. Thus, cardiac output is a function of heart rate and stroke volume, as described by the formula

$$\text{Cardiac output} = \text{heart rate} \times \text{stroke volume}$$

where average cardiac output is approximately 5 liters/min, average heart rate is approximately 70 beats per minute, and the average stroke volume is about 70 ml per beat (Sherwood, 1993)

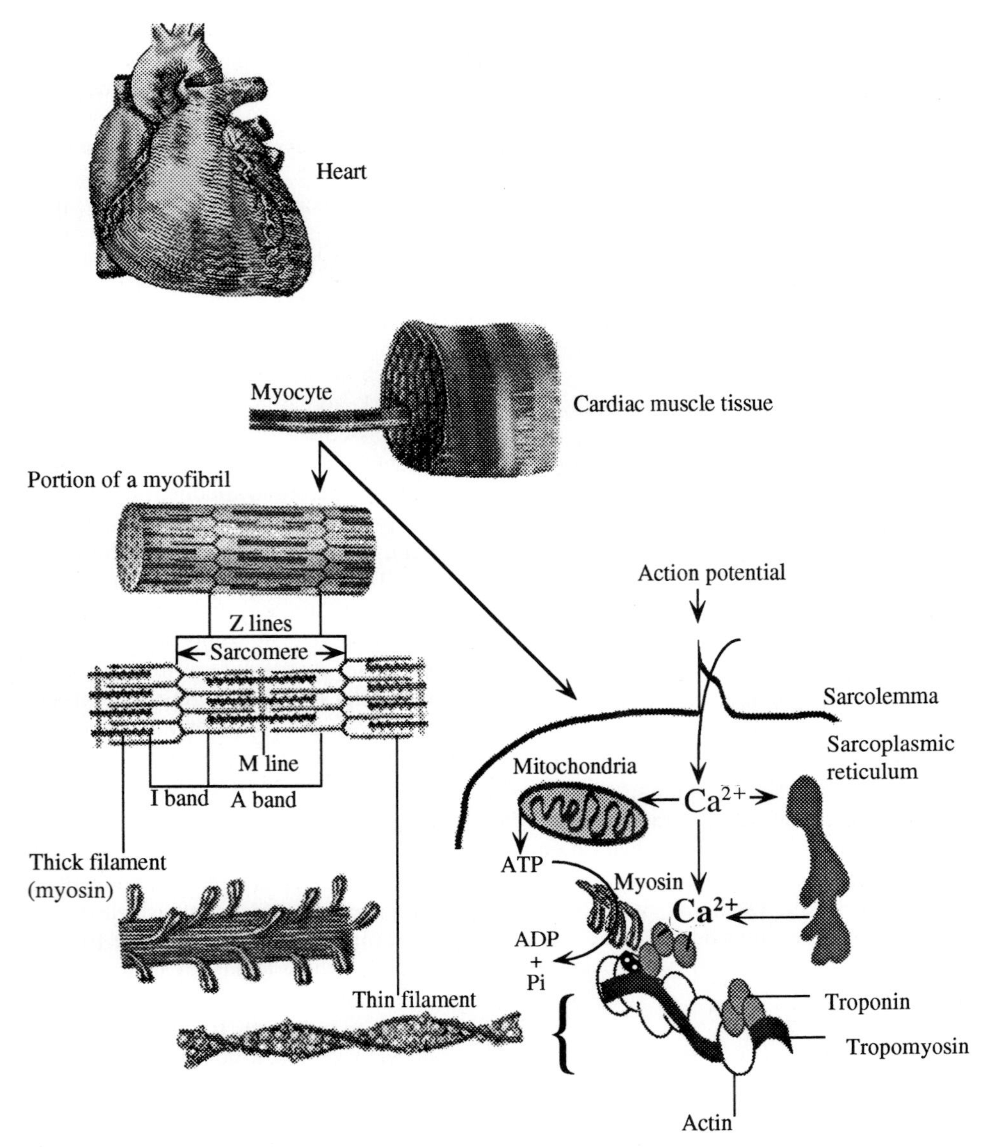


***Figure 17–3. Structural organization of cardiac muscle tissue and basic review of action potential–induced contraction.***

## DISTURBANCES IN CARDIAC FUNCTION

Xenobiotics affect cardiac function in accordance with their inherent mechanisms of action. Typical chemical-induced cardiac disorders consist of effects on heart rate (chronotropic), contractility (inotropic), conductivity (dromotropic), and excitability (bathmotropic).

In the myocardium, electrical activity is converted to mechanical activity. Thus, abnormal electrical activity results in abnormal contractile activity of the heart. Electrical currents generated during depolarization and repolarization spread throughout the heart, body fluids, and body surface, where they can be detected by recording electrodes to produce the characteristic electrocardiogram (ECG). Examination of ECG patterns is useful for diagnosing abnormal heart rates, arrhythmias, and damage of heart muscle (Fig. 17-4).

### Abnormalities in Rate

A rapid heart rate above 100 beats per minute is known as tachycardia (Greek *tachys*, "rapid"), whereas a slow heart rate below 60 beats per minute is known as bradycardia (Greek *bradys*, "slow").

### Abnormalities in Rhythm

Any variation from normal rhythm is termed an arrhythmia. Arrhythmias are classified on the basis of their origin (supraventricular or ventricular). Supraventricular arrhythmias (atrial in origin) are further divided into two categories: (1) supraventricular tachycardia based on defects in AV nodal reentry circuits or anatomic bypass tracts and (2) atrial fibrillation, where there is some form of atrial damage. Ventricular

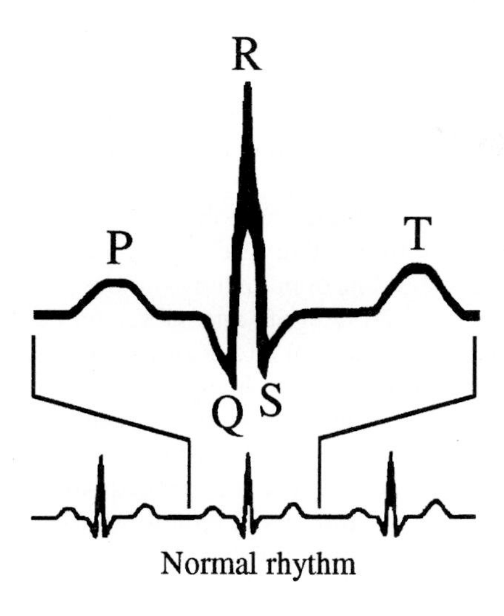


Abnormal Rate

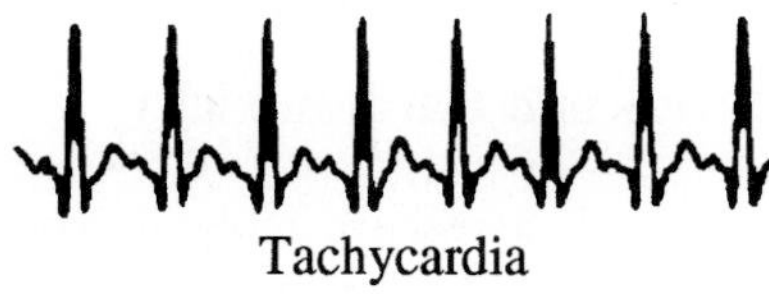


Abnormal Rhythms

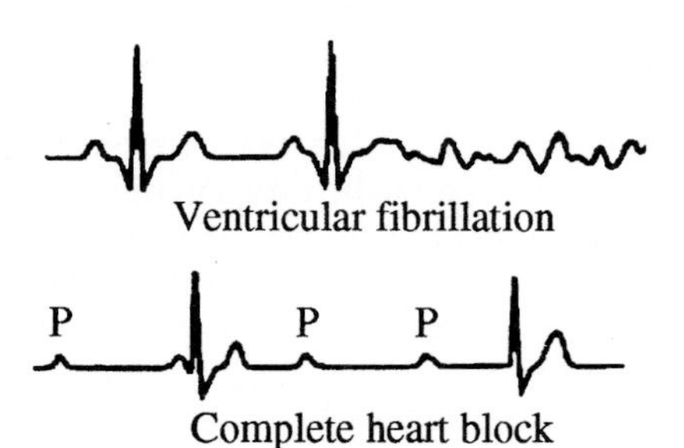


Cardiac Myopathies

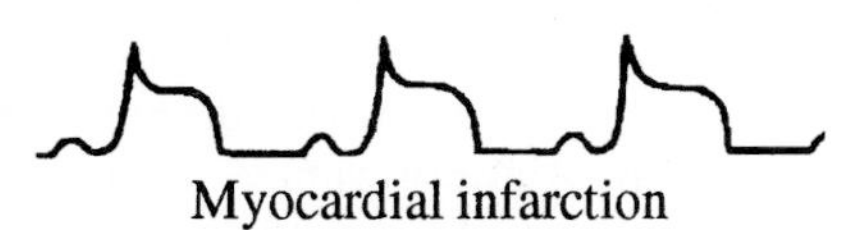


***Figure 17–4. Characteristic ECG patterns that are useful for diagnosing abnormal heart rates, arrhythmias, and damage of heart muscle.***

arrhythmias are often based on defects resulting from an infarcted or ischemic region.

Arrhythmias occur as a result of alterations in impulse rate, depolarizations that originate in abnormal sites, or velocity of impulse conduction. The most common arrhythmia is the ectopic beat that is characteristic of a skipped heartbeat in response to excitement. Ectopic beats are usually harmless but have the potential to initiate supraventricular tachycardias. Other abnormalities in rhythm are atrial flutter, atrial fibrillation, ventricular fibrillation, and heart block.

**Atrial Flutter.** Atrial flutter is characterized by a rapid and regular beat of atrial depolarizations between 200 and 380 beats per minute. However, because of the longer refractory period of the AV node and ventricles, the ventricles typically are unable to synchronize their depolarization with the rapidly firing atria. In fact, during atrial flutter, only one of every two to three atrial depolarizations passes through the AV node to depolarize the ventricles.

**Atrial Fibrillation.** Atrial fibrillation is characterized by rapid, randomized, and uncoordinated depolarizations of the atria. This erratic depolarization results in regularly shaped QRS complexes without a definite P wave (atrial repolarization). Atrial contractions are unsychnchronized, and AV conduction is also irregular. The AV irregularity causes irregular ventricular rhythm and subsequent inefficiency in ventricular filling. Less ventricular filling time results in diminished blood pumping to the extent that the pulse rate may be depressed. Under normal circumstances, pulse rate coincides with heart rate.

**Ventricular Fibrillation.** Ventricular fibrillation is a life-threatening abnormal rhythm characterized by repetitive, rapid, and randomized excitation of the ventricles, usually as a result of ectopic foci in the ventricles. Impulses travel chaotically around the ventricles. Hence, the ventricles become inefficient as pumps and death is inevitable unless normal rhythm is reestablished through the use of electrical defibrillation or cardiac compression.

**Heart Block.** Heart block is due to impairments in the cardiac conducting system. Typically, the atria maintain regular beating rates, but the ventricles occasionally fail to depolarize. For example, only every second or third atrial impulse may pass to depolarize the ventricles. Heart blocks are classified on the basis of their degree of depression of the conduction system. Complete heart block is characterized by complete block of conduction between the atria and ventricles. Under complete heart block, the atria beat regularly but the ventricles begin their own pacemaker activity at a much slower rate. Thus, the P wave (atrial depolarization) exhibits normal rhythm, while the QRS and T waves exhibit a slower rhythm that is independent of the P wave rhythm.

## Cardiac Myopathies

Cardiac myopathy is characterized by any type of damage to heart muscle. The mechanism of a myocardial defect can be attributed to a number of factors, such as ischemia-induced necrosis, metabolic toxicities, endocrine disturbances, and a variety of idiopathic diseases. Abnormal ECG patterns also can be used to assess the extent of cardiac damage. For example, prominent abnormalities in the QRS complex are seen when necrotic regions of the heart exist (Fig. 17-4). Typically, xenobiotic-induced cardiomyopathies require chronic exposure. The most frequent causes of xenobiotic-induced cardiac myopathies are described below.

**Alcoholic Cardiomyopathy.** Chronic ethanol consumption and its implications in cardiac disease were first reported in the early 1960s. After years of investigation, it was proposed that the metabolite acetaldehyde is responsible for some of the cardiac damage associated with ethanol consumption. The metabolic enzyme responsible for the conversion of ethanol to acetaldehyde is alcohol dehydrogenase, which is absent in cardiac myocytes. However, studies have indicated that the impaired liver function of alcoholics may be sufficient to generate quantities of acetaldehyde that can reach the heart. The direct effects of acetaldehyde on the myocardium include inhibition of protein synthesis, inhibition of calcium sequestration by the sarcoplasmic reticulum, alterations in mitochondrial respiration, and disturbances in the association of actin and myosin. The exact mechanism of alcoholic cardiomyopathy is unresolved. It has been suggested that a combination of multiple factors is involved and that certain conditions may predispose an individual to cardiac damage from ethyl alcohol. Factors such as chronic ethanol consumption, malnutrition, cigarette smoking, systemic hypertension, and beverage additives have all been implicated as potential contributors that can result in alcoholic cardiomyopathy (Ahmed and Regan, 1992). Further discussion on the mechanism of cardiotoxicity of alcohol is found in "Biochemical Mechanisms of Cardiotoxicity," below.

**Catecholamine Cardiomyopathy.** The most widely studied cardiotoxic catecholamines are epinephrine (adrenaline), norepinephrine, and isoproterenol. Isoproterenol is a synthetic derivative of the naturally occurring sympathomimetic amines epinephrine and norepinephrine. The cardiotoxicity of these compounds represents an exaggeration of cardiac beta-agonist activity. Of the three compounds, isoproterenol is the only agent that has been shown to produce myocardial necrosis that closely resembles infarction. Hence, myocardial injury from isoproterenol is used as a model for myocardial infarction. Typically, catecholamine cardiomyopathy is considered an experimentally induced phenomenon. However, clinical relevance may exist for individuals on chronic high-dose beta-agonist therapy for asthma and patients who have a pheochromocytoma. Numerous hypotheses have been suggested to account for the mechanism of cardiac damage by isoproterenol. Several subcellular organelles have been implicated as targeted sites. The major site appears to involve the sarcolemma, which is essential for maintaining cell integrity. In particular, increased plasma membrane permeability to $Ca^{2+}$ and other ions results in ionic imbalances followed by subsequent rupture of the sarcolemma that is coincident with cell death. The mechanism by which the sarcolemma becomes more permeable has not been defined. Further discussion on isoproterenol's mechanism of cardiotoxicity can be found in other sections below.

**Anthracycline Cardiomyopathies.** Anthracycline antibiotics such as doxorubicin and daunorubicin are very effective antitumor agents. However, their clinical utility is limited by their cardiotoxicity (Havlin, 1992). Both acute and chronic cardiotoxic effects have been described. The acute effects mimic anaphylactic-type responses such as tachycardia and various arrhythmias; these effects are clinically manageable and most likely are due to the potent release of histamine from mast cells that is sometimes observed in acute dosing. Acutely, large doses can also cause left ventricular failure that responds to digitalis, isoproterenol, and high perfusions of $Ca^{2+}$, suggesting an acute mechanism of toxicity that involves low levels of cytosolic calcium. A greater limiting factor of the anthracyclines lies in their long-term exposure, which usually results in the development of cardiomyopathies; in severe stages, this results in congestive heart failure (Havlin, 1992). Morphologically, there is vacuolization of the sarcoplasmic reticulum, myofibrillar loss, and swelling of the mitochondria.

Four major hypotheses have been suggested to account for the onset of anthracycline cardiomyopathies: (1) oxidative stress from redox cycling or mitochondrial $Ca^{2+}$ cycling, (2) defects in mitochondrial integrity and subsequent deterioration of myocardial energetics, (3) alterations in both SR $Ca^{2+}$ currents and mitochondrial $Ca^{2+}$ homeostasis, and (4) selective inhibition of cardiac gene expression. The cause-and-effect relationships of the proposed mechanisms of cardiotoxicity have not been determined. No single theory adequately explains the exact mechanism for anthracycline-induced cardiomyopathy. Further discussion on the anthracyclines is found below.

## GENERAL BIOCHEMICAL MECHANISMS OF CARDIOTOXICITY

### Oxidative Stress and Cardiotoxicity

**Myocardial Injury.** If a reactive molecule contains one or more unpaired electrons, the molecule is termed a free radical. In recent years, much interest has been focused on the biochemistry of oxygen activation and the biological significance of reactive oxygen species. Highly reactive oxygen species are intermediates formed as a normal consequence of a variety of essential biochemical reactions. For example, the univalent stepwise reduction of molecular oxygen to water results in the formation of several potentially toxic intermediates, including superoxide radical anion, hydrogen peroxide, and hydroxyl radical (i.e., prooxidants). Oxidases and electron transport systems are prime and continuous sources of intracellular reactive oxygen species.

Oxidative stress denotes a shift in the prooxidant/antioxidant balance in favor of the prooxidants, and thus oxidative damage inflicted by reactive oxygen species has been called oxidative stress (Sies, 1991). The extent of tissue damage depends on the balance between the free oxygen radicals generated and the antioxidant protective defenses of the tissue. Antioxidant enzymes such as superoxide dismutase, catalase, and glutathione peroxidase are preventive antioxidants because they inactivate or remove the oxygen species involved in lipid peroxidative damage of membranes, inactivation of sulfhydryl-containing enzymes, and cross-linking of integral proteins. Small-molecule antioxidants such as glutathione, ascorbate, and the tocopherols interact directly with free oxygen radicals to detoxify them. Under normal conditions, reactive oxygen species are broken down rapidly by these tissue defensive mechanisms to protect cells against their deleterious effects. The toxic effects of reactive oxygen species are observed only when their rates of formation exceed their rates of inactivation. Figure 17-5 depicts the formation of these reactive oxygen species and their inactivation by specific enzyme systems.

A number of studies have indicated that reactive oxygen species are generated during myocardial ischemia and at the time of reperfusion (Simpson and Lucchesi, 1987; Bolli, 1988). In cardiovascular diseases such as atherosclerosis, oxidative

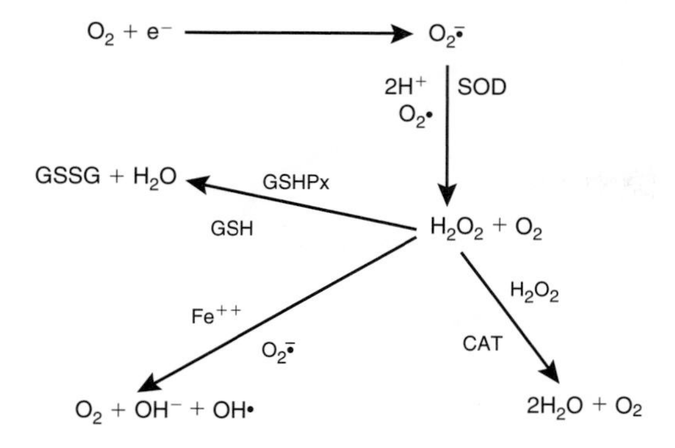


*Figure 17–5. Formation and inactivation of reactive oxygen species.*

Single-electron reduction of oxygen results in the formation of superoxide anion radical ($O_2^{\bar{\cdot}}$), which is maintained at low intracellular concentrations by spontaneous dismutation and/or catalytic breakdown by the enzyme superoxide dismutase (SOD) to form hydrogen peroxide ($H_2O_2$). Three possible events may occur with $H_2O_2$: (1) In the presence of $O_2^{\bar{\cdot}}$ or transition metals such as iron and copper, it is reduced to the hydroxyl radical (OH·), (2) it may be catalyzed by catalase (CAT) to form water and oxygen, and (3) it may be detoxified by glutathione peroxidase (GSHPx) in the presence of glutathione (GSH) to form water and oxidized glutathione (GSSG).

alteration of low-density lipoprotein is thought to be involved in the formation of atherosclerotic plaques. As was mentioned above, a primary mechanism that has been proposed to explain cell injury induced by reactive oxygen species involves the formation of lipid peroxides in the sarcolemma and organellar membranes. Among the major reactive oxygen species, the hydroxyl radical is thought to be the most toxic, reacting with a wide variety of membranes and leading to increased membrane fluidity and permeability and loss of membrane integrity. Upon reperfusion of ischemic myocardium, the production of oxygen free radicals has been associated with arrhythmias, myocardial stunning, and myocardial necrosis. However, it is controversial whether oxygen free radicals contribute significantly to myocyte necrosis in the clinical setting (Kloner and Przyklenk, 1992). At the subcellular and biochemical levels, reactive oxygen species have been shown to alter the activities of enzymes such as $Na^+$-$K^+$-ATPase, phospholipase D, glucose-6-phosphatase, and cytochrome oxidase. Calcium homeostasis is also altered by reactive oxygen species, as reflected by modifications in $Na^+$-$Ca^{2+}$ exchange, sarcoplasmic reticular $Ca^{2+}$ transport, and mitochondrial $Ca^{2+}$ uptake. Figure 17-6 summarizes the adverse effects of reactive oxygen radicals generated during myocardial ischemia and reperfusion.

**Reactive Oxygen Species and Drug-Induced Cardiotoxicity.** Two drugs—doxorubicin and ethanol—have been shown to have prominent cardiotoxic effects which have been associated with the production of reactive oxygen species. Doxorubicin, an anthracycline antibiotic, is an efficient antineoplastic agent that is used against human carcinomas, although congestive heart failure resulting from degenerative cardiomyopathy limits its clinical therapeutic effectiveness (Doroshow, 1991). Although several hypotheses have been proposed to explain the mechanism of the cardiotoxicity of doxorubicin, the free radical hypothesis has received the most attention. The formation of reactive oxygen species by doxorubicin (schematically shown in Fig. 17-7) has been attributed to a redox cycling of the drug (Powis, 1989). The quinonelike structure of doxorubicin permits this molecule to accept an electron and form a semiquinone radical. Oxidation of the semiquinone back to the parent quinone by molecular oxygen results in superoxide

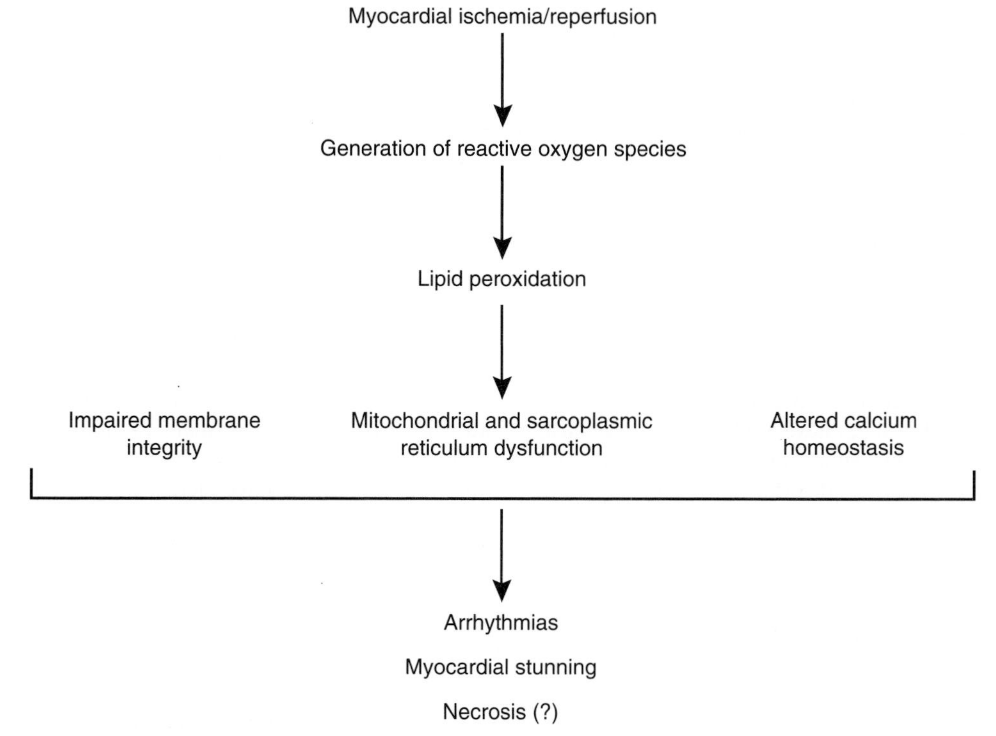


*Figure 17–6. Deleterious effects of reactive oxygen species in myocardial ischemia and reperfusion.*

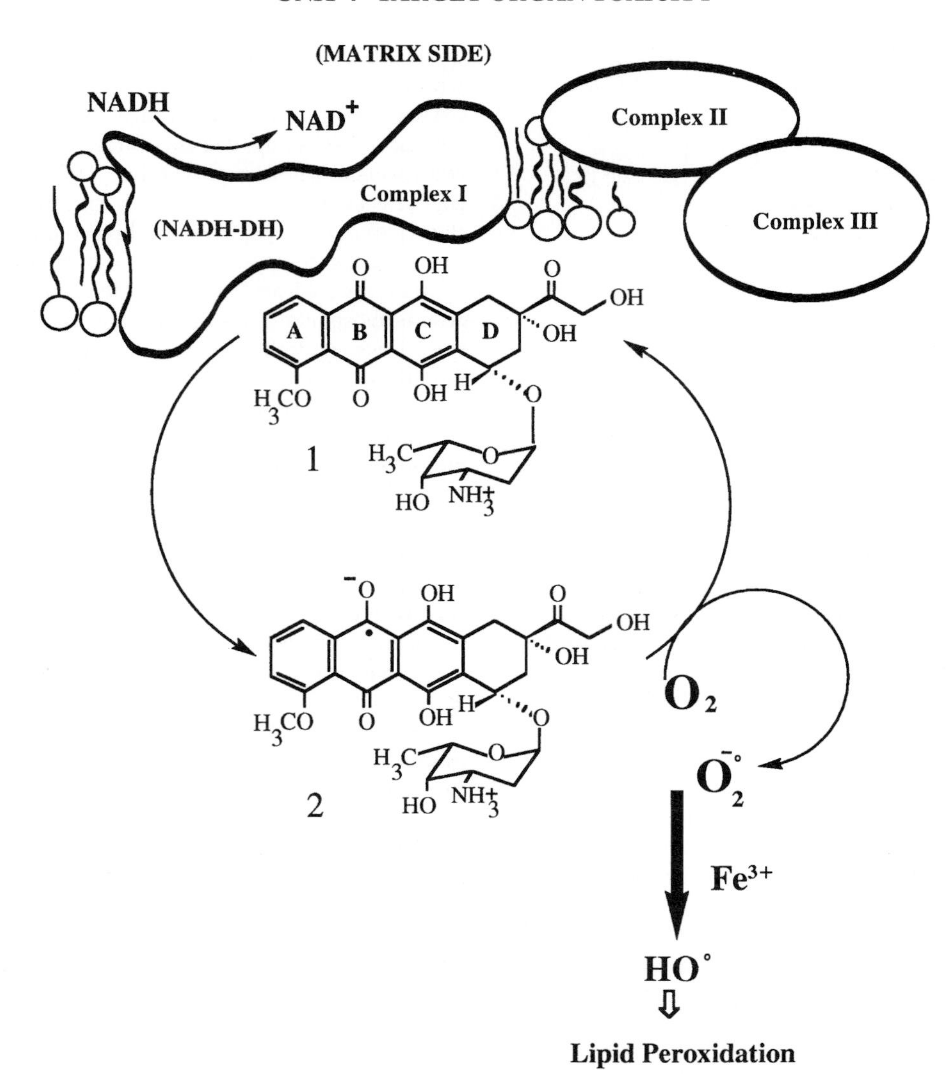


***Figure 17–7. Production of superoxide radical anions by oxidation-reduction cycling of doxorubicin at the level of the mitochondria.***

NADH dehydrogenase (NAD-DH), which is located within complex I, has been proposed as the enzyme that catalyzes the one-electron reduction of doxorubicin (1) to a semiquinone radical (2). The semiquinone then may be reoxidized back to the parent compound by means of the reduction of molecular oxygen to superoxide.

radical ions that are believed to initiate oxidative stress. The enzymatic reduction that is believed to be responsible for the generation of superoxide by doxorubicin (at the level of the mitochondria) has been proposed to occur between complexes I and III of the mitochondrial respiratory chain. Doxorubicin has high affinity for cardiolipin, a phospholipid found on the inner mitochondrial membrane, where NADH dehydrogenase converts the drug to a semiquinone radical (Marcillat et al., 1989). In the presence of oxygen, this radical is responsible for the generation of reactive oxygen species, which then may peroxidize unsaturated membrane lipids and initiate myocardial cell injury. Nonetheless, several observations appear to be inconsistent with the free radical–induced cardiotoxicity of doxorubicin (Olson and Mushlin, 1990). Other hypotheses for explaining the cardiotoxicity of doxorubicin are discussed in the section on cardiotoxicants, below.

The chronic consumption of ethanol by humans has been associated with myocardial abnormalities and dysfunction, a condition or syndrome known as alcoholic cardiomyopathy, and is closely related to congestive cardiomyopathy. However, for a long time the role of alcohol in the pathogenesis of the syndrome was not widely understood, mainly because heart dysfunction was attributed to thiamine deficiency secondary to alcoholism (beriberi heart disease) and other types of malnutrition or to specific additives found in alcoholic beverages, such as cobalt (beer drinker's cardiomyopathy). However, more recent studies have clearly suggested that cardiac dysfunction in alcoholics can be dissociated from nutritional deficiencies and beriberi heart disease. In addition, the withdrawal of alcohol from patients with myocardial dysfunction may reverse many of the clinical symptoms, providing more evidence that alcohol is involved in the pathogenesis of the cardiomyopathy.

There is suggestive evidence that the generation of reactive oxidative metabolites from the metabolism of ethanol may lead to lipid peroxidation of myocardial cells or oxidation of cytosolic and membraneous protein thiols (Ribiere et al., 1992). Additional evidence that reactive oxidative metabolites derived from ethanol may be involved in the pathogenesis of alcoholic cardiomyopathy is provided by the report by Redetzki et al. (1983), who showed that pretreatment of rodents with alpha-tocopherol before an acute dose of ethanol prevented increases in lactate dehydrogenase isoenzymes in the plasma and reduced ultrastructural evidence of myocardial damage. Because alpha-tocopherol can serve as an antioxidant and a free radical scavenger, this study suggests that alcohol-induced heart injury may be mediated by the generation of free radicals from ethanol metabolism. Other investigations have shown that ethanol administration may increase the conversion of xanthine dehydrogenase to xanthine oxidase, an enzyme involved in the generation of superoxide anions, and may enhance the activity of peroxisomal acyl-CoA oxidase and catalase in rat myocardium. These two enzymes may increase the production of hydrogen peroxidase and acetaldehyde, which may contribute to myocardial lipid peroxidation by ethanol treatment. Although oxidative stress and lipid peroxidation are attractive hypotheses for explaining alcohol-induced cardiotoxicity, other hypotheses have been proposed (for further discussion, see "Cardiotoxicants," below).

## Ischemic Reperfusion Injury

Intracellular acidosis, inhibition of oxidative phosphorylation, and ATP depletion are consequences of myocardial ischemia. Reperfusion of ischemic tissue results in cell death. Several mechanisms have been proposed to account for the reperfusion injury, including the generation of toxic oxygen radicals ($O_2$ paradox, as described above), $Ca^{2+}$ overload ($Ca^{2+}$ paradox), uncoupling of mitochondrial oxidative phosphorylation, and physical damage to the sarcolemma. However, none of these mechanisms adequately explains the cell injury associated with reperfusion injury.

A more recent hypothesis to explain the mechanism of cell death associated with reperfusion injury is the pH paradox (Lemasters et al., 1995). After reperfusion, reoxygenation, $Ca^{2+}$ loading, and a return to physiological pH occur and correspond with cell death. Inhibition of $Na^+/H^+$ exchange across the sarcolemma during reperfusion maintains intracellular acidosis and prevents cell killing despite reoxygenation or $Ca^{2+}$ overload. The pH paradox suggests that the acidosis of ischemia is generally protective and that a return to physiological pH precipitates cell injury. Thus, rescue of ischemic myocardium may be possible to a much greater extent than is generally assumed, provided that the tissue is reperfused at acidotic pH, followed by a gradual return of pH to normal levels.

## Sarcolemmal Injury, Calcium Overload, and Cardiotoxicity

The role of calcium in the regulation and control of various cellular functions has been an area of productive research during the last several years (Carafoli, 1987). The calcium messenger system may be considered an integral function of several systems and is highly influenced by homeostatic mechanisms. All cells contain elaborate systems for the regulation of calcium ions in the cell. Therefore, it is not surprising that a great deal of interest has been directed at studying alterations in calcium homeostasis and the way in which such effects may contribute to cell injury.

Understanding the mechanisms of chemically induced cell injury has been a principal quest of toxicologists. Alterations of calcium by toxicants may perturb the regulation of cellular functions beyond the normal range of physiological control. Intracellular calcium overload has been proposed to result in a breakdown of high-energy phosphates. Other cytotoxic effects induced by calcium include blebbing of the plasma membrane, activation of calcium-dependent phospholipases, stimulation of calcium-dependent neutral proteases, and calcium-activated DNA fragmentation. Because calcium may act as an intracellular messenger, alterations in calcium-mediated processes may be a critical cellular event which may prove deleterious to the cell.

**Sarcolemmal Injury and Calcium Alterations by Catecholamines.** A prominent hypothesis to explain the cardiotoxicity of catecholamines such as isoproterenol is derangement of electrolyte homeostasis of myocardial cells at the level of the sarcolemma and other subcellular membrane sites. Electrolyte shifts in magnesium and potassium have been suggested as possible factors in the myocardial dysfunction and necrosis associated with isoproterenol administration. For example, magnesium may serve as a cofactor in the regulation of phosphate transfers and may cause a decrease in the uptake of calcium by isolated respiring mitochondria.

However, the use of the concept of calcium overload to explain isoproterenol-induced cardiac necrosis has generated much interest (Fleckenstein et al., 1974). These investigators showed that there was a six- to sevenfold increase in the rate of calcium uptake and a doubling of the net myocardial calcium content. It was suggested that this excessive calcium overload may initiate a loss of high-energy phosphates through increased activation of calcium-dependent intracellular ATPase and impaired mitochondrial oxidative phosphorylation. Accumulation of large amounts of calcium in myocardial cells may alter the integrity and function of several membrane systems. In addition to affecting mitochondrial energy production, calcium may activate neutral proteases and phospholipases. Activation of these degradative enzymes may inhibit membrane-bound enzymes such as $Na^+/K^+$-ATPase. As a result, there is an increase in $Na^+$ levels and a loss of cytoplasmic $K^+$. The increased $Na^+$ content would further enhance calcium accumulation through the $Na^+$-$Ca^{2+}$ exchange system. The summation of these alterations leads to cellular dysfunction and cardiotoxicity.

Recently, it has been suggested that oxidative degeneration of membrane lipids may result in increased sarcolemmal calcium permeability. Because isoproterenol may form oxidative by-products, these metabolites could interact with the lipid bilayer, cause sarcolemmal injury, and alter calcium regulatory mechanisms. A discussion of these other actions of isoproterenol and catecholamines is found in "Cardiotoxicants," below.

## Mitochondrial Dysfunction and Cardiotoxicity

Cells are continuously engaged in various biochemical reactions. In particular, the synthesis of the major cell components requires energy. The energy to do work is derived from food by oxidizing the nutrients and channeling them into the formation of high-energy phosphate compounds such as adenosine triphosphate (ATP). ATP is the immediate energy source for doing work in most biological systems and is obtained mainly through the oxidative phosphorylation of adenine diphosphate (ADP). Oxidative phosphorylation (ATP formation) occurs as a function of cellular respiration (Chap. 3). Mitochondria possess an inner membrane and an outer membrane and are subcellular organelles in aerobic eukaryotic cells that are sites of cellular respiration. In essence, mitochondria are the energy producers within a cell. In a highly energy demanding tissue such as the heart, mitochondria occupy a large proportion of the cell.

Cellular respiration which gives rise to the formation of ATP is dependent on electron transfer reactions and is measured as oxygen consumption (Scarpa, 1979). Various oxidative pathways in a cell utilize coenzymes such as nicotinamide adenine dinucleotide ($NAD^+$) and flavin adenine dinucleotide ($FAD^+$) as electron acceptors, giving rise to their reduced states (NADH and $FADH_2$, respectively). The availability of oxidized coenzymes ($NAD^+$ and FAD) for use as electron acceptors depends on reoxidation of the reduced coenzymes. Molecular oxygen functions as the terminal electron acceptor for coenzyme oxidation. However, the free-energy change for the direct oxidation of NADH or $FADH_2$ by oxygen is larger than that which is usually encountered in biological reactions, and so the electrons are not passed directly to oxygen. The electrons are transferred in a stepwise fashion by means of a series of reversible oxidizable electron acceptor proteins in the inner mitochondrial membrane. These proteins make up the mitochondrial respiratory chain (electron transport chain). Hence, the total free energy available between reduced coenzymes and oxygen is distributed along the respiratory chain. More specifically, the energy of electron transport is used to build up and maintain an electrochemical potential across the inner membrane, establishing the mitochondrial membrane potential.

The process of electron transfer coupled with oxidative phosphorylation is a phenomenon described as coupling (Scarpa, 1979). Electron flow and consequently the rate of oxygen consumption in the presence of substrate and ADP are maximally stimulated (state 3 respiration). After the ADP has been consumed, electron flow and rates of oxygen consumption are low (state 4 respiration). The respiratory control ratio (RCR), which is calculated as the ratio of state 3 to state 4 respiration, can be used to determine the extent of coupling, which provides an index of mitochondrial function and integrity. Mitochondria which show no difference between state 3 and state 4 respiration are termed uncoupled. The synthesis of ATP occurs at the expense of the free energy available at three distinct sites (Fig. 17-8) designated as site I (between NADH and coenzyme Q), site II (between cytochrome b and cytochrome c), and site III (between cytochrome oxidase and oxygen). Because oxygen consumption and ATP synthesis pro-

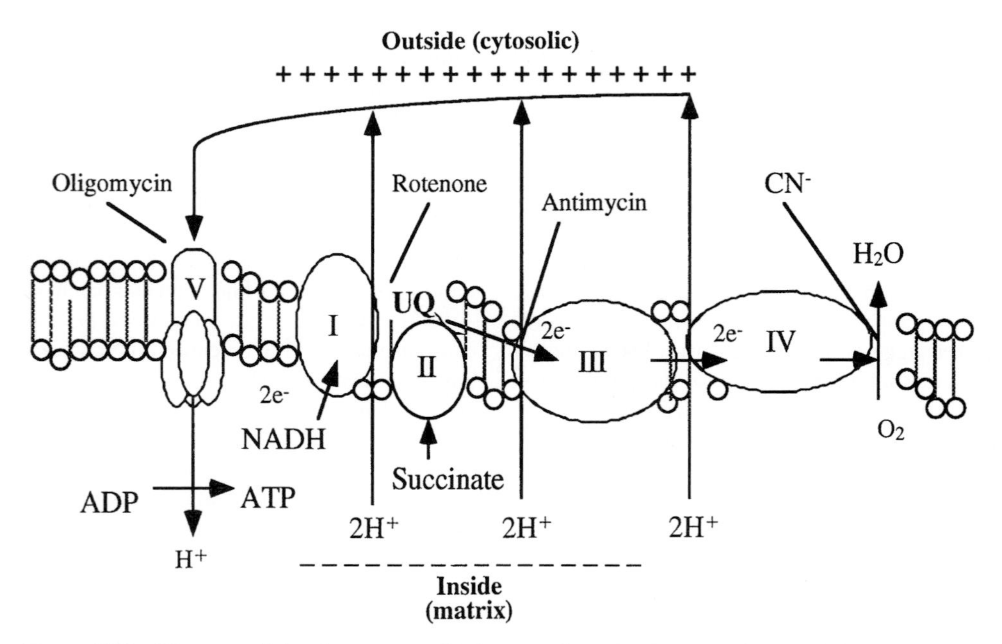


*Figure 17–8. Diagram of the electron-transferring complexes I, II, III, and IV and the ATPase (V) present in the inner mitochondrial membrane.*

The respective complexes are I, NADH: ubiquinone oxidoreductase; II, succinate: ubiquinone oxidoreductase; III, ubiquinol: ferrocytochrome c oxidoreductase; IV, ferrocytochrome c: oxygen oxidoreductase; V, ATP synthesase. UQ = ubiquinone or coenzyme Q. The mitochondrial electron transport chain is coupled at three points so that the electron transfer between carriers is sufficiently exergonic to drive the transport of protons and to establish an electrochemical proton gradient on which ATP formation depends. Various inhibitors and their sites are also noted.

ceed in parallel, substrates entering the respiratory chain at site I give rise to the formation of three molecules of ATP (P/O ratio of 3). Hence, substrates entering the respiratory chain at complex II produce only two molecules of ATP (P/O ratio of 2). The P/O ratio can be calculated by the amount of ATP synthesized (nmoles of ADP added) divided by the nano atoms of oxygen in state 3 respiration.

Oxidative phosphorylation can be affected by several chemical agents (Scarpa, 1979). Respiration can be inhibited at various sites along the respiratory chain by using different chemical inhibitors (Fig. 17-8). Rotenone is an inhibitor which blocks electron transfer between NADH and coenzyme Q (site I). Antimycin A blocks electron transport between coenzyme Q and cytochrome c (site II). Cyanide and carbon monoxide block the final step of electron transfer from cytochrome oxidase to oxygen (site III). Conversely, uncouplers stimulate electron flow and respiration but prevent the formation of ATP by short-circuiting the proton current. Uncouplers such as 2,4-dinitrophenol are lipophilic weak acids that may migrate through the lipid membrane and shuttle protons across the membrane, bypassing the normal flow of protons through the ATP synthetase.

In the evaluation of the various cardiac toxicants discussed below (see "Cardiotoxicants," below), mitochondrial injury or dysfunction may be an important element in explaining the mechanism of cardiotoxicity. Often, no single biochemical event can explain the process by which a chemical agent is cardiotoxic. Thus, several of the biochemical mechanisms discussed in this section may be interrelated and may help explain the cardiotoxicity of selected chemical agents.

## MAJOR CATEGORIES OF CARDIOTOXICANTS

Because there is no obvious system for classifying chemicals or drugs in regard to their cardiotoxic actions, we have arbitrarily categorized the cardiovascular toxicants into three major groups: (1) pharmaceutical agents, (2) industrial chemicals, and (3) natural products and other miscellaneous agents. Wherever possible, we will emphasize the major biochemical mechanisms of cardiotoxicity proposed for the agents under discussion.

### Pharmaceutical Agents

The cardiotoxicity of a pharmacologically active cardiovascular drug often represents an overexpression of its principal pharmacological effect on the heart. For example, digitalis, quinidine, and procainamide may induce cardiac arrhythmias as an exaggerated pharmacological action of the drugs. In contrast, other cardiovascular drugs may produce cardiotoxicity by actions that are not necessarily related to their pharmacological effects. For instance, in addition to their pharmacological actions on the myocardium and because of their pronounced sympathomimetic actions, the catecholamines may exert other cardiotoxic effects through their biochemical effects on certain cellular and subcellular processes (e.g., oxidative stress and calcium overload). Furthermore, other pharmaceutical agents, such as antibacterial antibiotics, anthracyclines, and other antineoplastic agents, may produce myocardial necrosis and other cardiotoxic effects which are not related to their therapeutic and pharmacological uses. The pharmaceutical agents selected for discussion purposes will emphasize, if appropriate, cardiotoxic effects not necessarily related to their principal pharmacological actions on the heart and vascular system.

**Antibacterial Antibiotics.** Although the clinical use of antibiotics usually presents limited cardiovascular problems in routine therapy for uncomplicated infections in normal patients, one should be aware that the use of certain antibiotics may result in adverse cardiac effects, especially in instances of overdosage and in patients with preexisting cardiovascular dysfunction. Keller and associates (1992) have presented an excellent review of key antibiotics which may have adverse cardiovascular effects. The aminoglycoside class of antibiotics, which includes agents such as streptomycin, gentamicin, kanamycin, and amikacin, is associated with direct cardiodepressant actions in a number of species. Gentamicin, a representative aminoglycoside, has been thoroughly investigated for its calcium-related myocardial depressant actions. The preliminary findings showed that gentamicin's negative inotropic actions can be antagonized by excess calcium and that gentamicin has an inhibitory action on slow inward calcium channels in heart muscle. It has been proposed that aminoglycosides inhibit the uptake or binding of calcium at sarcolemmal sites, thus reducing the concentration of membrane-bound calcium available for movement into the myoplasm during depolarization of the sarcolemma. Other investigators have confirmed these observations and have reported other data that suggest that gentamicin's principal mechanism of cardiodepression is the dislocation of calcium from slow channel binding sites on the external surface of the sarcolemma, which results in a blockade of the channels (Hino et al., 1982).

Other antibiotics have been shown to produce cardiac dysfunction, but their mechanisms have not been investigated as extensively as those of the aminoglycosides (Keller et al., 1992). Erythromycin use is associated with cardiac dysrhythmias characterized by an unusual tachyarrhythmia known as torsades de pointes. Tetracycline and chloramphenicol have been reported to depress myocardial contractility by direct myocardial cell interaction or an indirect effect that lowers calcium concentrations in the plasma or extracellular spaces, respectively. Some of the polyene group of antifungal agents (e.g., amphotericin B) may depress myocardial contractility by blocking activation of slow calcium channels and inhibiting the influx of sodium.

**Anthracyclines and Other Antineoplastic Agents.** Cardiotoxicity is now recognized as a serious side effect of chemotherapy for malignant cancers, especially with well-known antitumor agents such as 5-fluorouracil, cyclophosphamide, doxorubicin, and daunorubicin. Havlin (1992) has published an excellent review of some of these important antitumor agents and their cardiotoxic effects. Clinical evidence of fluorouracil cardiotoxicity ranges from mild precordial pain and ECG abnormalities (ST segment elevation, high peaked T waves, T-wave inversions, and sinus tachycardia) to severe hypotension, atrial fibrillation, and abnormalities of ventricular wall motion. A principal mechanism proposed for the cardiotoxicity of fluorouracil is myocardial ischemia precipitated by coronary spasm, but this finding has been disputed because of the short half-life of fluorouracil. More recent studies suggest that the cardiotoxicity of fluorouracil can be attributed to impurities present in commercial products of the drug, one of which is metabolized to fluoroacetate, a highly cardiotoxic agent.

High doses of cyclophosphamide (CP) given to cancer or transplant patients may lead to severe hemorrhagic cardiac necrosis. The mechanism of the cardiotoxicity of this agent is not clear, but there is suggestive evidence that the toxic metabolite of CP, 4-hydroperoxycyclophosphamide (4-HC), may alter the ionic homeostasis of cardiomyocytes, resulting in increased sodium and calcium content and reduced potassium levels (Levine et al., 1993). Furthermore, the same investigators showed that the cytotoxicity of 4-HC is markedly altered by the cellular glutathione concentration.

The anthracyclines—doxorubicin and daunorubicin—are widely used antineoplastics for the treatment of leukemias and a variety of solid tumors. Unfortunately, these agents can cause acute cardiotoxicity manifested by electrocardiographic changes, resulting in a dose-dependent cardiomyopathy (Havlin, 1992). As alluded to in "General Biochemical Mechanisms of Cardiotoxicity," above, doxorubicin can undergo a futile redox cycling that results in the production of oxygen free radicals; these reactive oxygen species may then oxidize proteins, lipids, and nucleic acids and potentially cause DNA strand scission. Other possible mechanisms to explain the cardiotoxicity include calcium overload that overwhelms intracellular homeostatic processes, increased production of prostaglandins and platelet-activating factor, increased release of histamine, and the formation of a toxic metabolite of doxorubicin (Olson and Mushlin, 1990).

An alternate hypothesis to explain the cardiotoxicity of doxorubicin implicates a disruption of mitochondrial calcium homeostasis without necessarily involving pronounced calcium overload (Chacon and Acosta, 1991; Chacon et al., 1992; Solem et al., 1994). This hypothesis suggests that doxorubicin induces a cycling of mitochondrial calcium that is associated with the production of reactive oxygen species and a dissipation in the mitochondrial membrane potential, which in turn may result in a depletion of cellular ATP. Because ruthenium red, an inhibitor of the mitochondrial calcium uniport, decreased the production of reactive oxygen species induced by doxorubicin in mitochondria and isolated myocardial cells and protected the cardiomyocytes from doxorubicin-induced cell killing, disruption of mitochondrial calcium homeostasis may be an important mechanism for understanding the cardiotoxicity of doxorubicin. Furthermore, cyclosporin A, a selective inhibitor of the calcium-dependent calcium release channel in mitochondria, inhibited the calcium-induced depolarization of mitochondrial membrane potential of mitochondria isolated from rats chronically treated with doxorubicin. These results suggest that doxorubicin may induce a futile cycling of calcium across the mitochondrial membrane and that this may be responsible for the formation of reactive oxygen species rather than or in addition to a redox cycling of the quinone moiety.

**Centrally Acting Drugs.** There are numerous examples of central nervous system (CNS)-acting drugs that have considerable effects on the cardiovascular system. Some of the more cardiotoxic agents that have a major pharmacological action on the brain and nervous system include tricyclic antidepressants, general anesthetics, some of the opioids, and antipsychotic drugs. Other drugs, such as cocaine and ethanol, are discussed in separate sections (see below). Standard tricyclic antidepressants (amitriptyline, imipramine, desipramine, doxepin, and protriptyline) have significant cardiotoxic actions in cases of overdose, including ST segment elevation, Q-T prolongation, and ventricular and supraventricular arrhythmias. In addition, as a result of peripheral alpha-adrenergic blockade, they may cause postural hypotension. Although many of these adverse effects are related to the quinidinelike actions, anticholinergic effects, and adrenergic actions of these agents, the tricyclics also may have direct cardiotoxic actions on cardiomyocytes, including depression of calcium influx and loss of ATP content.

The general anesthetics, as exemplified by halothane, methoxyflurane, enflurane, and isoflurane, may have adverse cardiac effects, including reducing cardiac output by 20 to 50 percent, depression of contractility, and production of arrhythmias (generally benign in healthy myocardium but more serious in cardiac disease). These anesthetics may sensitize the heart to the arrhythmogenic effects of endogenous epinephrine or to beta-receptor agonists. Investigations suggest that halothane, as a prototype, may block the L-type calcium channel by interfering with its dihydropyridine binding sites, may disrupt calcium homeostasis associated with the sarcoplasmic reticulum, and may modify the responsiveness of the contractile proteins to activation by calcium (Bosnjak, 1991).

Antipsychotic agents (e.g., the phenothiazines) may cause negative inotropism and quinidinelike antiarrhythmic effects on the heart. Some ECG changes include prolongation of the Q-T and P-R intervals, blunting of T waves, and depression of the ST segment.

**Local Anesthetics.** Because of their ability to block conduction in nerve axons, local anesthetics interfere with the conduction or transmission of impulses in other excitable organs, including the heart and circulatory system. In general, local anesthetics such as lidocaine and mepivacaine have few undesirable cardiovascular effects. However, when high systemic concentrations of cocaine and procainamide are attained, these agents may have prominent adverse effects on the heart. Because cocaine is abused by a significant number of individuals, its adverse effects on the myocardium will be described in more detail. Some of the more severe cardiotoxic effects of cocaine include cardiac arrhythmias, myocardial ischemia or infarction, systemic hypertension, and congestive heart failure.

The cardiotoxicity of cocaine is usually explained by its general pharmacological actions on excitable tissues, which include its ability to act as a local anesthetic and block conduction in nerve fibers by reversibly inhibiting sodium channels and stopping the transient rise in sodium conductance. In the heart, cocaine decreases the rate of depolarization and the amplitude of the action potential, slows conduction speed, and increases the effective refractory period. The other major pharmacological action of cocaine is its ability to inhibit the reuptake of norepinephrine and dopamine into sympathetic nerve terminals (sympathomimetic effect). Cocaine will, indirectly through its actions on catecholamine reuptake, stimulate beta- and alpha-adrenergic receptors, leading to increased cyclic AMP and inositol triphosphate levels. These second messengers will in turn provoke a rise in cytosolic calcium, which causes sustained action potential generation and extrasystoles. The local anesthetic action, as described above, impairs conduction and creates a condition for reentrant circuits. The net effect of these two pharmacological actions is to elicit and maintain ventricular fibrillation.

Whereas the sympathomimetic and local anesthetic actions of cocaine are plausible mechanisms to explain the cardiac arrhythmias experienced by some cocaine abusers, it is still not clear how myocyte necrosis (myocardial infarction) may develop with cocaine use. The usual explanation is that the increased levels of catecholamines caused by cocaine's inhibition of their reuptake leads to myocardial ischemia resulting from coronary artery vasoconstriction by the catecholamines. However, while the adverse actions of cocaine have been documented in humans with advanced coronary artery disease, the majority of cocaine users are young and have normal coronary arteries. Whether coronary constriction by cocaine and the catecholamines is sufficient to lead to myocardial ischemia and/or myocardial infarction in a normal human population is not known.

A third explanation for the cardiotoxicity of cocaine is that it may be directly toxic to the myocardium. Peng and coworkers (1989) ultrastructurally examined endomyocardial biopsy specimens from seven patients with a history of cocaine abuse and found that more than 70 percent of the patients showed multifocal myocyte necrosis. There was extensive loss of myofibrils, and marked sarcoplasmic vacuolization was observed. Peng and coworkers suggested that these toxic manifestations were not secondary to myocardial ischemic events because the amount of myocardial necrosis was small and focal and usually involved individual cells that were occasionally surrounded by inflammatory cell infiltrates, changes that are not associated with myocardial ischemia. In addition, these cardiotoxic manifestations produced by cocaine are similar to those seen in doxorubicin cardiotoxicity, an agent known for its direct toxicity to myocardial cells.

The mechanism by which cocaine directly injures myocardial cells is not clear. However, this drug may significantly inhibit mitochondrial electron transport, especially in the NADH dehydrogenase region (Fantel et al., 1990). Alterations in calcium homeostasis by excess catecholamine release induced by cocaine or by the direct effects of cocaine on sarcolemmal integrity also may be involved in myocyte necrosis. Thus, a combination of actions involving mitochondrial dysfunction and calcium disturbances may contribute to direct injury of the myocardium by cocaine.

**Catecholamines and Related Drugs.** Catecholamines represent a chemical class of neurotransmitters synthesized in the adrenal medulla (epinephrine and norepinephrine) and in the sympathetic nervous system (norepinephrine). Because of their ability to activate alpha- and beta-receptors, especially in the cardiovascular system, a number of synthetic catecholamines have been developed for the treatment of cardiovascular disorders and conditions such as asthma and nasal congestion. However, high circulating concentrations of epinephrine and norepinephrine and high doses of synthetic catecholamines such as isoproterenol may induce toxic effects on the heart, including myocardial necrosis. The pathogenesis of catecholamine-induced cardiotoxicity is, however, unclear. Dhalla and colleagues (1992) have written a comprehensive review of the cardiotoxicity of catecholamines and related agents. Some of the more important hypotheses that explain the cardiotoxicity of catecholamines are discussed below.

A prominent early hypothesis about catecholamine cardiotoxicity was the pronounced pharmacological actions of these compounds at high concentrations on the cardiovascular system, including an increased heart rate, enhanced myocardial oxygen demand, and an overall increase in systolic arterial blood pressure. In the case of isoproterenol, there is a fall in blood pressure. These actions may cause myocardial hypoxia and, if severe enough, lead to the production of necrotic lesions in the heart. Because isoproterenol has greater cardiotoxicity than does epinephrine or norepinephrine, it was suggested that the hypotension produced by isoproterenol is a major factor in lesions produced in the myocardium. However, subsequent investigations revealed that hypotension is nonessential for the production of cardiac necrosis by isoproterenol.

Other possible mechanisms for the cardiotoxicity of high concentrations of catecholamines include coronary insufficiency resulting from spasm, decreased levels of high-energy phosphate stores caused by mitochondrial dysfunction, increased sarcolemmal permeability leading to electrolyte alterations, altered lipid metabolism resulting in the accumulation of fatty acids, and intracellular $Ca^{2+}$ overload. Although these mechanisms have received support through the years, there are conflicting studies which argue against one or more of these proposed mechanisms (Dhalla et al., 1992).

However, as was indicated in "General Biochemical Mechanisms of Cardiotoxicity," above, oxidative stress as a factor in myocardial cell injury induced by selected xenobiotics has been recognized by several investigators (Dhalla et al., 1992). Because the oxidation of catecholamines may result in the formation of aminochromes and oxygen free radicals, oxidative stress may play a significant role in catecholamine-induced cardiotoxicity. Antioxidants such as vitamin E and ascorbic acid have been shown to provide protection against the cardiotoxicity of isoproterenol and other catecholamines. Figure 17-9 illustrates the role of oxidative stress in the development of catecholamine-induced myocardial damage and dysfunction.

**Miscellaneous Drugs.** A significant number of other pharmaceutical agents have been reported to have cardiotoxic effects. For instance, many of the cardiac drugs used for the treatment of cardiovascular diseases may have toxic effects when an overdose occurs. Several of the antiarrhythmic drugs, as discussed in "Local Anesthetics," above, may have cardiotoxic actions as a result of their pharmacological effects on sodium channel blockade (e.g., lidocaine, procainamide, quinidine, and phenytoin). Other antiarrhythmic agents, such as amiodarone, prolong the action potential duration and the effective refractory period of Purkinje fibers and ventricular muscle cells as their principal antiarrhythmic mechanism. However, amiodarone may have cardiotoxic effects by stimulating excessive calcium uptake, especially in the presence of procaine (Gotzsche and Pederson, 1994).

Recently, there has been an association of cardiotoxicity with the use of the second-generation $H_1$ receptor antagonists or antihistamines (Simons, 1994). For example, terfenadine and astemizole have been shown to have a number of adverse effects on the electrophysiology of the heart, including altered repolarization, notched inverted T waves, prominent TU waves, increased $QT_c$ interval, first- and second-degree AV

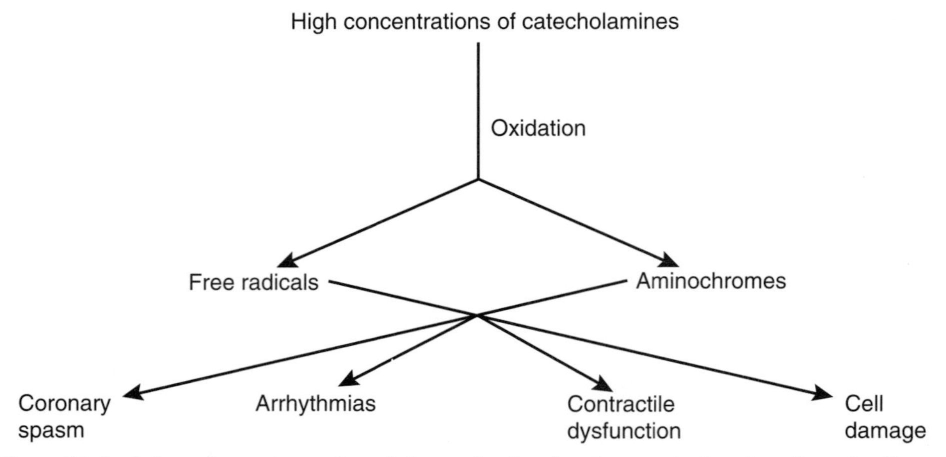


***Figure 17–9.*** ***Schematic representation of the mechanism for the genesis the of cardiotoxic effects of high concentrations of catecholamines. [Reprinted with permission from Dhalla et al. (1992).]***

block, ventricular tachycardia or fibrillation, and pause-dependent torsades de pointes. It has been postulated that these $H_1$ blockers produce cardiac arrhythmias by blocking the delayed rectifier potassium channel in cardiomyocytes.

Sperelakis (1992) has provided an excellent review of how some cardiotoxic agents affect the heart by acting on ion channels, electrical properties of the sarcolemma, and the excitation-contraction coupling sequence. Pharmaceutical agents discussed in that review include salicylates, cardiac glycosides, methylxanthines, calcium channel blockers, and the compounds discussed above.

Table 17-1 provides a summary of key pharmaceutical agents with their prominent cardiotoxic effects and proposed mechanisms of cardiotoxicity.

## Industrial Agents

**Industrial Solvents.** Cardiotoxicity from industrial solvents can involve multiple mechanisms. Their inherent liophilicity allows them to act on the CNS, which in turn is responsible for regulating cardiac electrical activity. In addition, because of their their high lipid solubility, solvents may disperse into cell membranes and affect membrane fluidity that is crucial for cellular functions, such as second messenger membrane signaling and oxidative phosphorylation. Hence, solvents may affect physiological functions such as contraction and energy production; sympathetic and parasympatheic control of the heart may be disrupted by solvents either directly or indirectly. Their influence on cardiac function also may involve the release of circulating hormones such as catecholamines, vasopressin, and serotonin. From a more general prespective, industrial solvents typically produce a depressant effect on the CNS and an attenuation of myocardial contractility. Moreover, chronic exposure to solvents in sublethal doses may result in subtle toxicities that may be apparent only after prolonged exposure. For a more comprehensive review of industrial agents and their cardiotoxic potential, the reader is referred to Zakhari (1992).

***Alcohols and Aldehydes.*** On a molar basis, there is a relationship between increased carbon chain length of the alcohol and cardiotoxicity. Metabolic oxidation of alcohols yields aldehydes. Aldehydes have sympathomimetic activity as a result of their effect on releasing catecholamines. Unlike alcohols, the sympathomimetic activity of aldehydes decreases with increased chain length. The acute cardiodepressant effects of alcohols and aldehydes are related to a putative inhibition of intracellular calcium transport.

Ethanol cardiotoxicity can be divided into two categories: acute and chronic (alcoholism). From an industrial point of view, the acute toxicity of ethanol is presented. For a more detailed review of the chronic effects of ethanol, the reader is referred to the section on alcoholic cardiomyopathy and the references cited there. Ethanol has been shown to produce a negative dromotropic effect and a decreased threshold for ventricular fibrillation. Oxidation of ethanol to acetaldehyde proceeds at a rate that is independent of blood concentration. Arrhythmias are prominent only after long-term exposure.

Methanol (methyl alcohol or wood alcohol) is a common industrial solvent whose effects on the heart are similar to those of ethanol. Methanol is metabolized by alcohol dehydrogenase and aldehyde dehydrogenase to formaldehyde and formic acid. As with ethanol, oxidation of methanol proceeds at a rate that is independent of blood concentration. However, the rate of oxidation is about one-seventh that of ethanol, and complete elimination requires several days. Clinically, blood pressure is usually unaffected but pulse may be slow.

Isopropyl alcohol is a common industrial and household solvent whose effects on the heart are similar to those of ethanol. Isopropyl alcohol–induced toxicity typically occurs from ingestion or inhalation. Isopropanol is a potent CNS depressant that causes cardiovascular depression in large doses. Isopropanol is metabolized to acetone, which is also believed to potentiate and lengthen the duration of CNS depression. Acetone is metabolized to formic acid and acetic acid, which have the potential to induce mild acidosis. Tachycardia is the most prominent clinical finding.

Acetaldehyde, a hepatic metabolite of ethanol, has negative inotropic effects at concentrations that can be obtained with moderate alcohol consumption. At higher blood levels, acetaldehyde has sympathomimetic effects.

***Halogenated Alkanes.*** Halogenated alkanes encompass a wide range of industrial and pharmaceutical agents. Their highly lipophilic nature allows them to cross the blood-brain

**Table 17–1**
**Cardiotoxicity of Key Pharmaceutical Agents**

| AGENT OR CHEMICAL CLASS | CARDIOTOXIC MANIFESTATIONS | PROPOSED MECHANISMS OF CARDIOTOXICITY |
|---|---|---|
| *Antibacterial agents* | | |
| Aminoglycosides (e.g., gentamicin) | Cardiodepressant action: negative inotropy | Inhibition of calcium uptake or binding at sarcolemma |
| Erythromycin | Cardiac dysrhythmias (e.g., torsades de pointes) | Blockade of fast $Na^+$ channel (see $H_1$ receptor antagonists, below) |
| Lincomycin | Arrhythmias; hypotension | Decreased excitability and conduction velocity |
| Chloramphenicol | Cardiodepressant action: negative inotropy and chronotropy | Direct myocardial cell interaction (?) |
| Tetracycline | Cardiodepressant action | Decreased calcium concentration in plasma |
| Amphotericin B | Cardiodepressant action | Decreased activation of slow calcium channels; inhibition of sodium influx |
| *Antineoplastic agents* | | |
| Anthracyclines (e.g., doxorubicin) | ECG alterations; cardiomyopathy | Lipid peroxidation; calcium overload; formation of toxic metabolite; altered mitochondrial calcium homeostasis |
| 5-Fluorouracil | ECG abnormalities; hypotension; arrhythmias | Coronary spasm leading to myocardial ischemia (?); product impurities: fluoroacetate formation |
| Cyclophosphamide | Hemorrhagic cardiac necrosis | Formation of toxic metabolite; increased sodium and calcium levels and decreased potassium |
| *Centrally acting drugs* | | |
| Tricyclic antidepressants (e.g., amitriptyline) | Ventricular and supraventricular arrhythmias; postural hypotension | Depression of calcium influx and decreased ATP levels |
| General anesthetics (halothane, methoxyflurane, enflurane, isoflurane) | Reduced cardiac output; depression of contractility; sensitize heart to arrhythmogenic effects of catecholamines | Blockade of L-type calcium channel; disruption of SR calcium homeostasis |
| Phenothiazines | Orthostatic hypotension; ECG disturbances; negative inotropy; arrhythmias | Slowed recovery of fast sodium channels |
| *Local anesthetics* | | |
| Cocaine | Arrhythmias; myocardial infarction; systemic hypertension; congestive heart failure | Coronary vasoconstriction; inhibition of mitochondrial electron transport; altered calcium homeostasis |

**Table 17–1**
**Cardiotoxicity of Key Pharmaceutical Agents *(Continued)***

| AGENT OR CHEMICAL CLASS | CARDIOTOXIC MANIFESTATIONS | PROPOSED MECHANISMS OF CARDIOTOXICITY |
|---|---|---|
| *Catecholamines and related drugs* | Myocardial necrosis | Exaggerated beta-receptor actions in toxic doses; coronary spasm; mitochondrial dysfunction; altered lipid metabolism; calcium overload; oxidative stress |
| *Miscellaneous drugs* | | |
| Amiodarone | Arrhythmias | Stimulation of excessive calcium uptake |
| $H_1$ receptor antagonists (terfenadine and astemizole) | ECG disturbances; ventricular fibrillation; torsades de pointes | Blockade of the delayed rectifier potassium channel; exacerbated by inhibition of liver cytochrome P-450 enzymes (3A4) with compounds such as erythromycin and ketoconazole |

barrier readily. This action, coupled with their CNS depressant activity, makes these compounds ideally suited for anesthetics (halothane, methoxyfluorane, and enflurane). Halogenated hydrocarbons depress heart rate, contractility, and conduction. The number of halogen atoms and unsaturated bonds influences the relative potency of these agents. In addition, some of these agents sensitize the heart to the arrhythmogenic effects of beta-agonists such as endogenous epinepherine. Fluorocarbons (freons) have been reported to have this sensitizing effect on the myocardium. Trichlorofluoromethane is one of the most toxic fluorocarbons. Table 17-2 summarizes some halogenated hydrocarbons that have been reported to have arrhythmogenic properties. Chronic exposure to halogenated hydrocarbons has been postulated to have degenerative cardiac effects.

**Heavy Metals.** The most common heavy metals that have been associated with cardiotoxicity are cadmium, lead, and cobalt. These metals exhibit negative inotropic and dromotropic effects and also can produce structural changes in the heart. Chronic exposure to cadmium has been reported to cause cardiac hypertrophy. Lead has an arrhythmogenic sensitizing effect on the myocardium. In addition, lead has been reported to cause degenerative changes in the heart. Cobalt has been reported to cause cardiomyopathy. The cardiotoxic effects of heavy metals are attributed to their ability to form complexes with intracellular macromolecules and their ability to antagonize intracellular $Ca^{2+}$.

Other metals that have been reported to affect cardiac function are manganese, nickel, and lanthanum. Their mechanism of action appears to be the blocking of $Ca^{2+}$ channels. The concentrations reported to block $Ca^{2+}$ channels are approximately 1 m*M*. Barium is another metal that can affect cardiac function. Barium chloride given intravenously to rabbits at 5 mg/kg has been reported to induce arrhythmias. This arrhythmogenic effect of barium chloride has been utilized to screen antirrhythmic agents.

Table 17-3 provides a summary of selected industrial agents with their prominent cardiotoxic effects and proposed mechanisms of cardiotoxicity.

## Natural Products

The compounds discussed in this section are chemical agents that are synthesized by humans, animals, or plants and that have significant cardiotoxic effects. These natural products include steroid hormones and some synthetic hormonelike compounds (oral contraceptives and anabolic steroids), cytokines, animal toxins, and plant toxins. Because of the diverse nature of these natural compounds, representative examples will be used to illustrate key toxicological actions on the cardiovascular system. Limited discussion will be provided on plant and animal toxins; the reader is directed to Chaps. 26 and 27 for more detailed information on the cardiovascular toxicity of these natural products.

**Steroid Hormones.** The principal steroid hormones produced by humans are the estrogens, progestins, androgens, and adrenocortical steroids. In general, the estrogens and progestins have limited physiological actions on the cardiovascular system under normal conditions. However, the use of synthetic estrogens and progestins as oral contraceptives has been associated with several cardiovascular disorders. See the section on vasculotoxic agents for more information.

**Table 17–2**
**Halogenated Hydrocarbons Reported to Have Arrhythmogenic Properties**

| | |
|---|---|
| Carbon tetrachloride | |
| Chloroform | Methyl bromide |
| Chloropentafluoroethane | Methyl chloride |
| 1,2-Dibromotetrafluoromethane | Methylene chloride |
| Dichlorodifluoromethane | Monochlorodifluoroethane |
| *cis*-Dichloroethylene | Monochlorodifluoromethane |
| *trans*-Dichloroethylene | Octafluorocyclobutane |
| 1,2-Dichloropropane | Propyl chloride |
| Dichlorotetrafluroethane | 1,1,1-Trichloroethane |
| Difluoroethane | Trichloroethane |
| Ethyl bromide | Trichloroethylene |
| Ethyl chloride | Trichlorofluoromethane |
| Fluorocarbon 502 | Trichloromonofluoroethylene |
| 1,2-Hexafluoroethane | Trichlorotrifluoroethane |
| Isopropyl chloride | Trifluorobromethane |

SOURCE: Reprinted with permission from Zakhari S: Cardiovascular toxicology of halogenated hydrocarbons and other solvents, in Acosta D (ed): *Cardiovascular Toxicology*, 2d ed. New York: Raven Press, 1992.

The principal androgens are testosterone, which is synthesized in the testis, the ovary, and the adrenal cortex, and its active metabolite, dihydrotestosterone, which serves as an intracellular mediator of most androgen actions. Synthetic androgens used as anabolic steroids include nandrolone, danazol, and stanozol. In general, androgens are relatively nontoxic to the cardiovascular system. However, the use of anabolic steroids has been suggested to be a factor in the increased incidence of cardiovascular risks, primarily morbid circulatory events such as thrombosis (Rockhold, 1993). However, there are limited human data, and so it is difficult to make positive correlations and critically evaluate incidence rates.

Long-term therapy with corticosteroids, especially aldosterone and cortisol, has a prominent effect on sodium retention and the production of hypertension. The genesis of hypertension has not been totally clarified or explained.

**Cytokines.** Cytokines represent a diverse and heterogeneous group of proteins with important functions in cellular and humoral immune responses. Some of these cytokines—inter-

**Table 17–3**
**Cardiotoxicity of Selected Industrial Agents**

| AGENT OR CHEMICAL CLASS | CARDIOTOXIC MANIFESTATIONS | PROPOSED MECHANISMS OF CARDIOTOXICITY |
|---|---|---|
| *Solvents* | | |
| Toluene (paint products) | Arrhythmogenic | Decreased parasympathetic CNS activity with enhanced sensitivity to epinephrine |
| Halogenated hydrocarbons (aerosols, refrigerants) | Arrhythmogenic<br>Decreased myocardial contractility | Decreased parasympathetic CNS activity with enhanced sensitivity to epinephrine |
| Ketones (acetone, methyl ethyl ketone, etc.) | Arrhythmogenic | Decreased parasympathetic CNS activity with enhanced sensitivity to epinephrine |
| Glycol ethers and esters (diethylene glycol monoethyl ether) | Potentially teratogenic | Mechanisms unresolved; glycols with shorter alkyl chain ethers are more prone to cause embryotoxicity than are those with longer chains |
| *Heavy metals* | | |
| Arsenic | Arteriosclerosis<br>Vascular lesions | Mechanisms unresolved |
| Mercury | Aortic lesions | Inhibition of amino acid uptake; calcium overload |

feron and interleukins—have been reported to produce adverse cardiovascular effects. For instance, interleukin-2 may decrease the mechanical performance and metabolic efficiency of the heart; these myocardial effects may be related to changes in nitric oxide synthesis and $Na^+/H^+$ exchange. Interferon administration may result in cardiac arrhythmias, dilated cardiomyopathy, and signs of myocardial ischemia. However, human data are limited for both cytokines, and the risks of cardiac toxicity are not clearly defined.

**Animal and Plant Toxins.** Animal toxins in the venom of snakes, spiders, scorpions, and marine organisms have profound effects on the cardiovascular system. There are also a number of plants, such as foxglove, oleander, and monkshood, that contain toxic constituents and have adverse effects on the cardiovascular system. A description of these toxic cardiovascular effects is found in Chaps. 26 and 27.

## OVERVIEW OF VASCULAR PHYSIOLOGY

The vascular system consists of a complex network of vessels of varying size and complexity that serve as the circuitry for the delivery of oxygen and nutrients to tissues throughout the body and for the removal of the waste products of cellular metabolism. Oxygenated blood returning from the lungs to the heart is emptied into the aorta, a large conduit vessel, which gradually branches off, giving rise to smaller vessels that reach individual organs (Fig. 17-10). Although the distribution of the cardiac output among different organs depends on their relative resistance to blood flow, in most instances the blood flow to critical regions such as the brain and the kidney remains constant despite changes in arterial pressure or cardiac output. The movement of blood through the vascular network is governed by the general laws of hydrodynamics, although the properties of the blood and those of the vessels impose some modifications. Blood returns to the heart for reoxygenation through the venous system before the reinitiation of subsequent cycles.

Large and medium-size blood vessels in mammals are organized into three morphologically distinct layers (Fig. 17-11). The innermost layer is referred to as the tunica intima and consists of a single layer of endothelial cells resting on a thin basal lamina and a subendothelial layer. Luminal endothelial cells are flat and elongated, with the long axis parallel to blood flow. These cells act as a semipermeable barrier between the blood and underlying components of the vessel wall. The subendothelial layer is formed by connective tissue bundles and elastic fibrils in which a few cells of smooth muscle origin may be oriented parallel to the long axis of the vessel. The subendothelial layer is seen only in large elastic arteries such as the

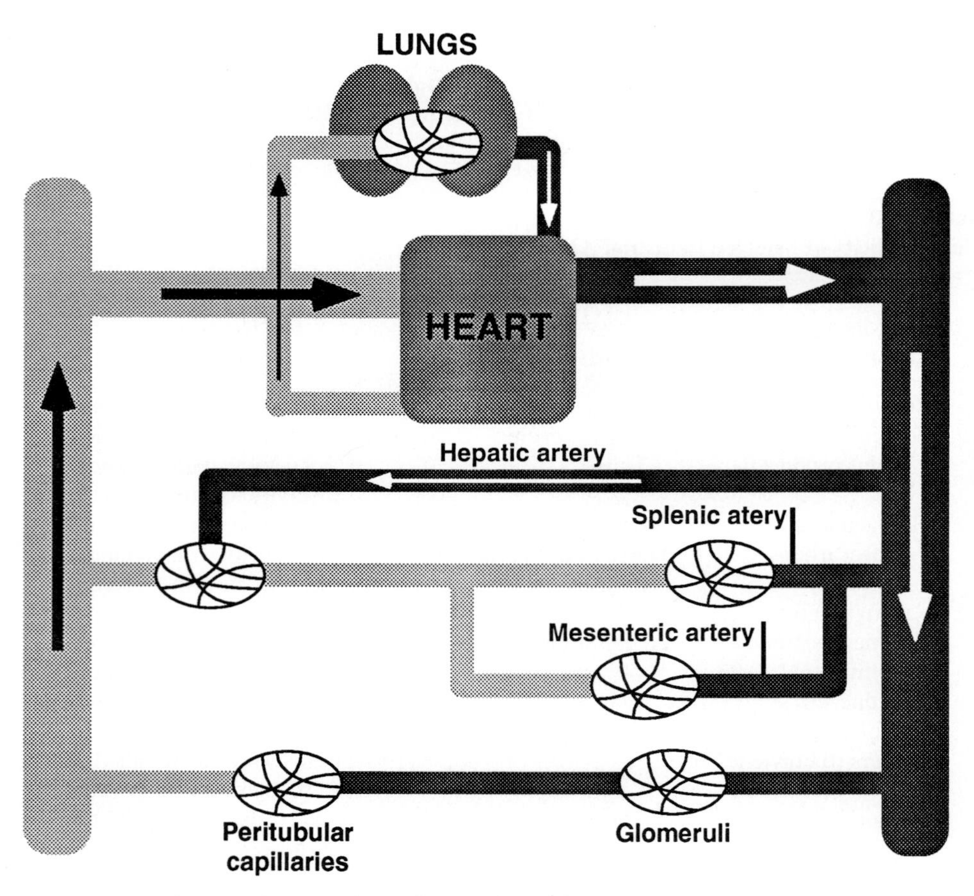


*Figure 17–10. Schematic diagram of vascular supply to selected organs.*

The capillary beds are represented by thin lines connnecting the arteries (*right*) with the veins (*left*), and the distribution of the vasculature in several organs (liver, kidney, lung) indicates the importance of the vascular system in toxicology.

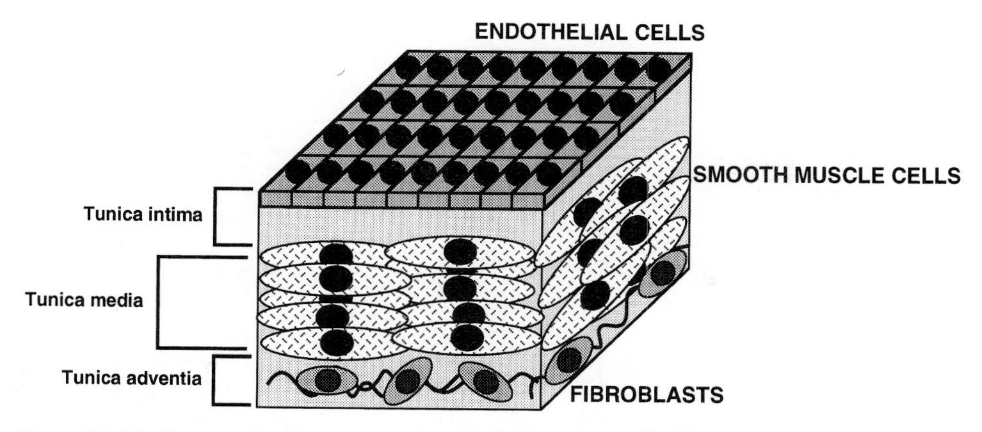


*Figure 17–11. Cross-sectional representation of the vascular wall of large and medium-size blood vessels.*

The tunica intima is composed of endothelial cells facing the vessel lumen that rest on a thin basal lamina. The tunica media consists mainly of vascular smooth muscle cells interwoven with collagen and elastin. The tunica adventia is a layer of fibroblasts, collagen, elastin, and glycosaminoglycans.

human aorta and is not clearly defined in smaller species. The medial layer, or tunica media, is composed of elastin and collagen interwoven between multiple layers of smooth muscle cells. In the majority of vascular beds smooth muscle cells dominate the media, but these cells also may be present in the intima of some arteries and veins, and in the adventitia of veins. The media is separated from the outermost layer, the tunica adventitia, by a poorly defined external lamina. The adventitial layer consists of a loose layer of fibroblasts, collagen, elastin, and glycosaminoglycans. With the exception of capillaries, the walls of smaller vessels also have three distinct layers. However, in smaller vessels the tunica media is less elastic and consists of fewer layers of smooth muscle cells. As described for the muscular arteries, venules are structurally similar to their arteriolar counterparts. Because muscular venules are larger than arterioles, a large fraction of blood is contained in these so-called capacitance vessels. Capillaries are endothelial tubes measuring 4 to 8 mm in diameter that rest on a thin basal lamina to which pericytes often are attached. When one capillary converges with another, the vessel formed is referred to as a postcapillary venule. The capillary and the pericytic venule are the principal sites of exchange between the blood and tissues.

Vascular endothelial cells play an integral role in the regulation of hemostasis, vascular tone, and angiogenesis. Angiogenesis involves the formation of blood vessels secondary to the migration, proliferation, and differentiation of vascular cells. Endothelial cells also are involved in the regulation of macromolecular transport across the vessel wall, attachment and recruitment of inflammatory cells, synthesis of connective tissue proteins, and generation of reactive oxygen species. Medial smooth muscle cells are responsible for the regulation of vascular tone. The contractile response of blood vessels is mediated by receptors located primarily on the plasma membrane of smooth muscle cells. Activation of these receptors brings about changes in calcium conductance that lead to activation of the contractile apparatus. Calcium homeostasis is controlled by the interplay of multiple regulatory mechanisms (Fig. 17-12). In contrast to cardiac myocytes, where relatively large stores of calcium are found, vascular smooth muscle depends primarily on extracellular calcium sources for con-

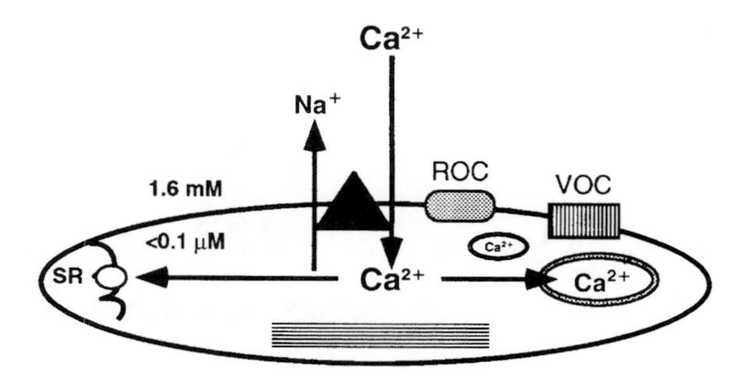


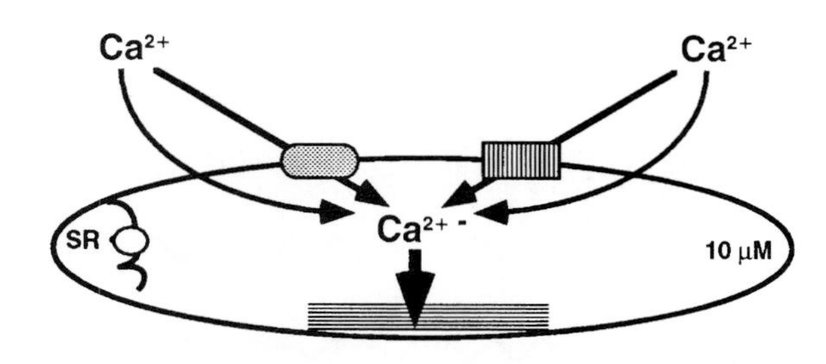


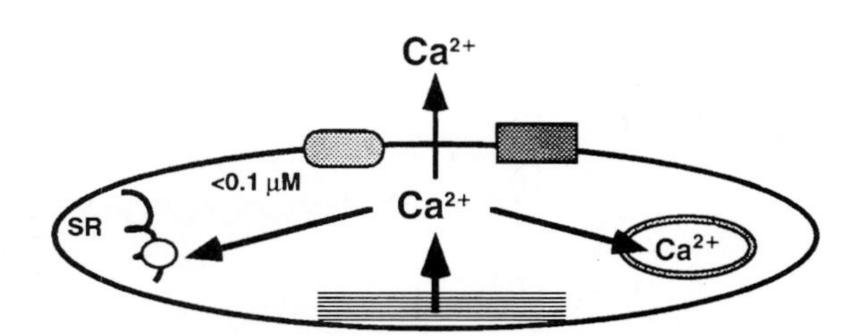


*Figure 17–12. Calcium regulation and homeostasis in vascular smooth muscle cells.*

Intracellular calcium is sequestered primarily in the sarcoplasmic reticulum (SR), but contraction of smooth muscle cells is initiated by an influx of extracellular calcium through receptor-operated channels (ROC) or voltage-operated channels (VOC).

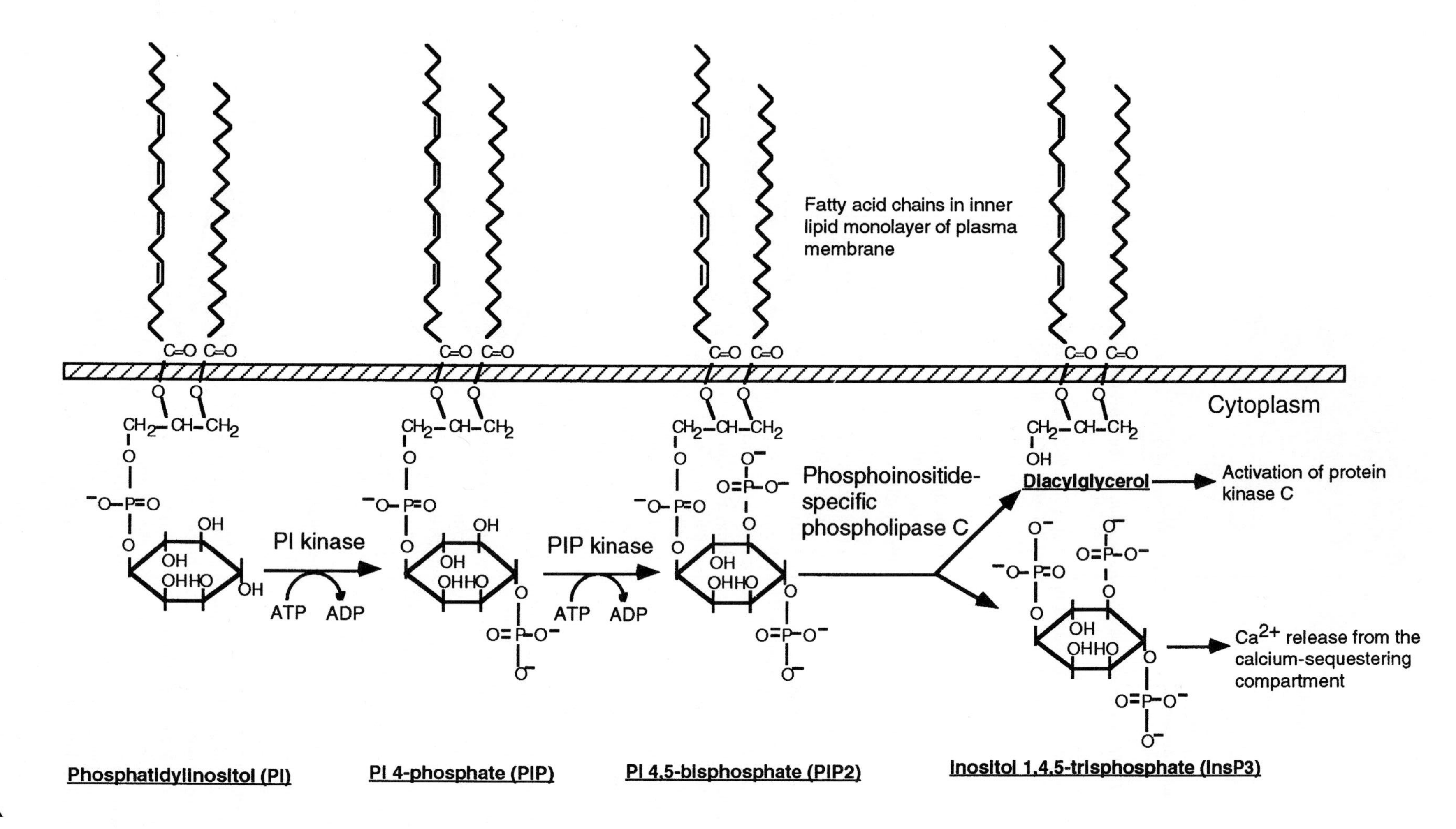

Fatty acid chains in inner lipid monolayer of plasma membrane
Cytoplasm
PI kinase
ATP
ADP
PIP kinase
ATP
ADP
Phosphoinositide-specific phospholipase C
Diacylglycerol
Activation of protein kinase C
Ca2+ release from the calcium-sequestering compartment
Phosphatidylinositol (PI)
PI 4-phosphate (PIP)
PI 4,5-bisphosphate (PIP2)
Inositol 1,4,5-trisphosphate (InsP3)


A

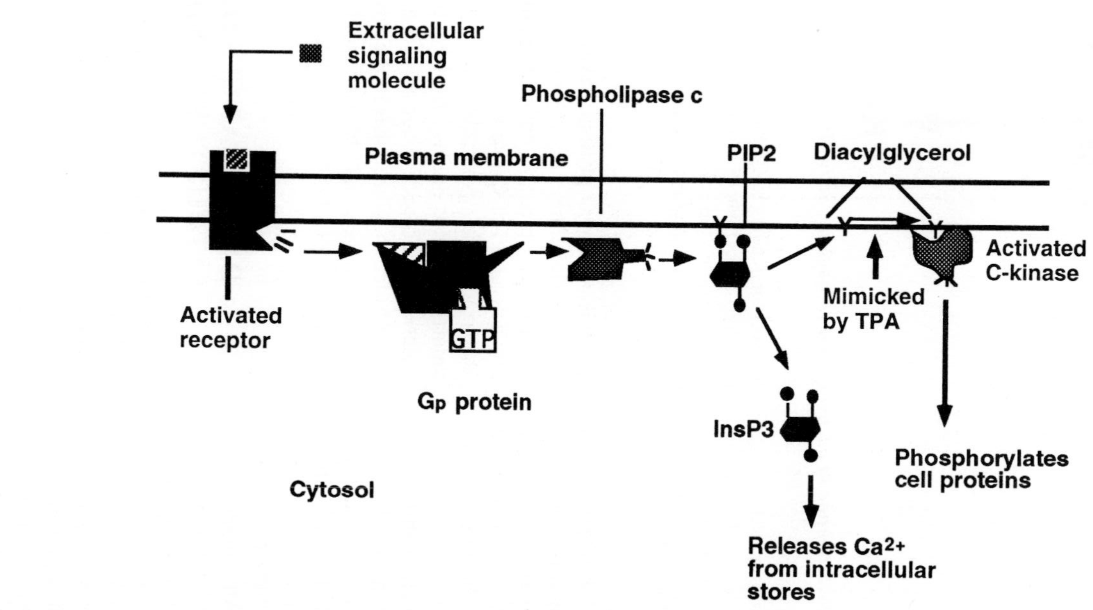


B

***Figure 17–13. Phosphatidylinositol metabolism and subsequent production of intracellular second messengers in vascular smooth muscle cells.***

Inositol 1,4,5-trisphosphate (InsP3), which elicits intracellular $Ca^{2+}$ release, is generated from phosphatidylinositol (PI) by the sequential actions of PI kinase, PIP kinase, and phospholipase C (*A*). PI 4,5-bisphosphate (PIP2) can also be cleaved by phospholipase C to form diacylglycerol, which activates protein kinase C (*B*).

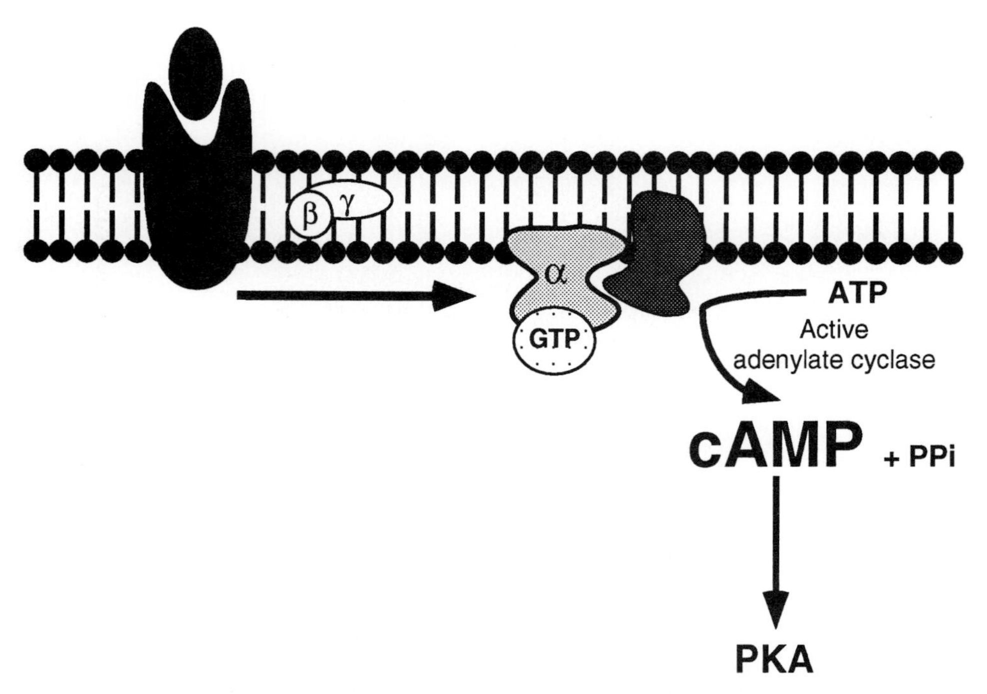


***Figure 17–14. Depiction of the activation of adenyl cyclase through the activation of a beta$_2$-adrenergic receptor.***

Ligand binding results in a conformational change in the receptor, leading to GTP displacement of GDP on the *a* subunit of the receptor-linked G protein. The binding of GTP elicits the release of the *β* and *γ* subunits and the binding of the *a* subunit to adenyl cyclase, activating the enzyme. Cyclic AMP (cAMP) is produced, and this can lead to various events, including the activation of protein kinse A.

traction. Increases in cytoplasmic calcium often involve the influx of calcium through either receptor- or voltage-operated channels. Cytoplasmic $Ca^{2+}$ activates a calmodulin-dependent protein kinase that in turn phosphorylates myosin to allow the interaction of myosin and actin and the shortening of the sarcomere.

Catecholamines influence vascular function through the activation of surface receptors, among which the alpha$_1$ and beta$_2$ receptors have been the most extensively characterized. Activation of alpha$_1$ receptors in smooth muscle cells increases contractility, while activation of beta$_2$ receptors decreases it. Two alpha$_1$-adrenergic receptor subtypes—alpha$_{1A}$ and the alpha$_{1B}$—have been identified. Alpha$_{1B}$-adrenergic stimulation elicits smooth muscle contraction by activating phospholipase-mediated hydrolysis of phosphatidylinositol-4,5-bisphosphate to yield diacylglycerol and inositol-1,4,5-trisphosphate (Fig. 17-13). Diacylglycerol binds to and activates protein kinase C, while inositol-1,4,5-trisphosphate binds to an intracellular receptor on the sarcoplasmic reticulum to initiate the release of calcium stores. The alpha$_{1A}$-adrenergic receptor mediates extracellular calcium entry through voltage-sensitive L-type calcium channels. Activation of beta$_2$ receptors leads to G protein–mediated activation of adenylyl cyclase and the production of cyclic AMP (Fig. 17-14). Beta$_2$ agonists induce a conformational change in the receptor, resulting in dissociation of the *a* subunits from the *βγ* subunits of the G protein. The *a* subunit in turn achieves a biologically active conformation that modulates adenylyl cyclase activity after displacement of GDP by GTP. Inactivation occurs through hydrolysis of GTP by the intrinsic GTPase activity of the G protein. Several other neurohormones, such as acetylcholine, angiotensin II, arginine-vasopressin, histamine, thrombin, and endothelin, modulate contractile events by activation of G protein-coupled receptors. Smooth muscle cells also are responsible for the synthesis of extracellular matrix proteins during arterial repair, the metabolism and/or secretion of bioactive substances, and the regulation of monocyte function. Fibroblasts in the adventitial layer secrete some of the collagen and glycosaminoglycans needed to give structural support to the vessel wall.

## DISTURBANCES OF VASCULAR STRUCTURE AND FUNCTION

Human epidemiological studies have established a positive correlation between injury to a blood vessel wall and the occurrence of vascular diseases such as atherosclerosis and hypertension (Rosenman, 1990). Atherosclerosis is a major structural change in the vessel wall that leads to deleterious consequences to the vessel as well as the other organs involved. This disease is a degenerative process involving focal intimal thickenings formed after migration of smooth muscle cells to the intima and uncontrolled proliferation. Extracellular matrix components such as collagen and elastin, intra- and extracellular lipids, complex carbohydrates, blood products, and calcium accumulate to varying degrees as the lesion advances. The plaque also contains inflammatory cells, such as infiltrated monocytes and leukocytes, which participate in the progression of the pathological response. Figure 17-15 shows two pathways that can mediate

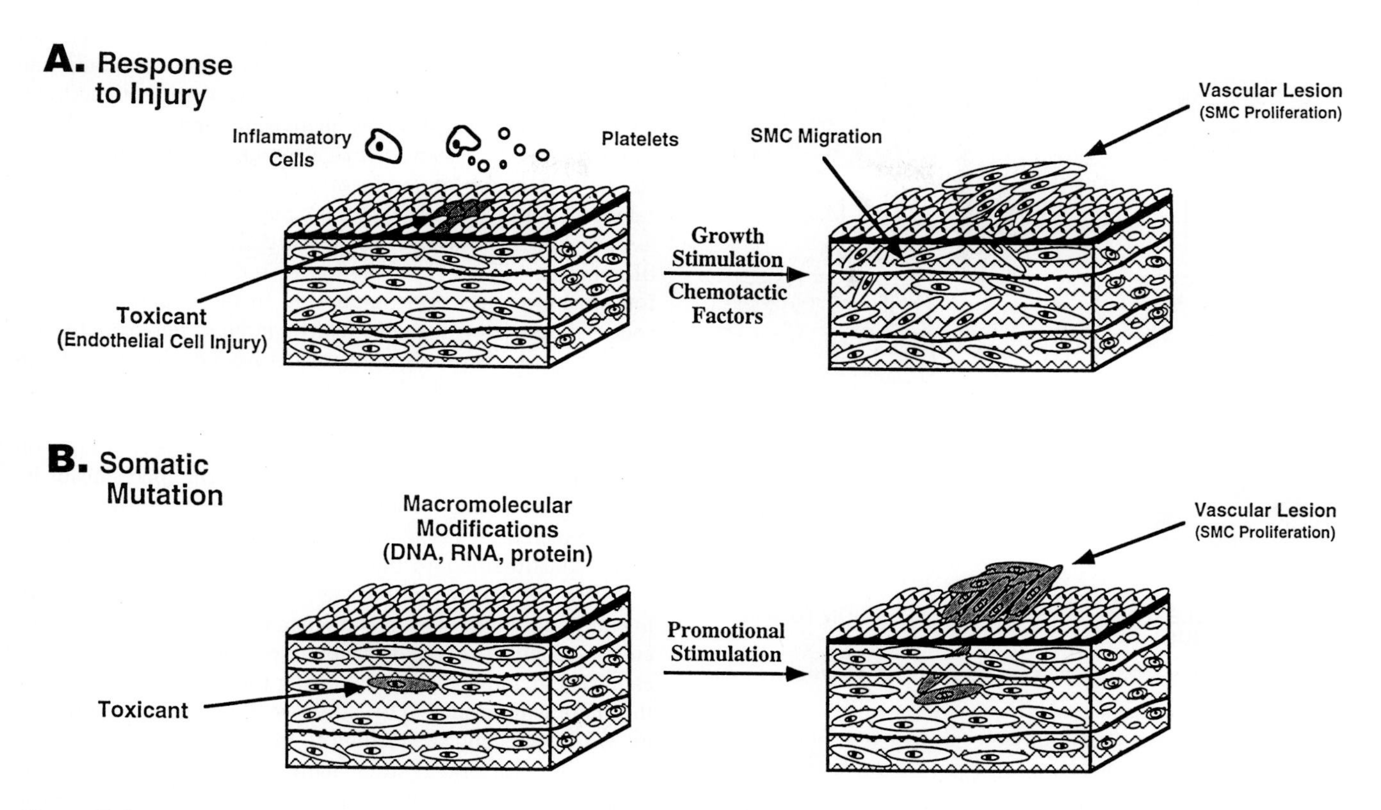


***Figure 17–15. Representation of the two major hypotheses for the molecular and cellular events that lead to atherosclerosis.***

The response to injury hypothesis initially proposed by Ross and subsequently modified (1993) states that injury of endothelial cells triggers a response involving recruitment of platelets and inflammatory cells that stimulate smooth muscle cell migration and proliferation. In contrast, Benditt and Benditt (1973) proposed that atherosclerotic lesions are a result of the monoclonal expansion of a mutated smooth muscle cell. [Reprinted with permission from Ramos et al. (1994). Copyright Taylor and Francis, 1994.]

the initiation and/or promotion of the atherosclerotic process by toxic chemicals. Lesions generally occur in large and medium-sized blood vessels such as the aorta and the coronary, carotid, and femoral arteries. In young human subjects, atherosclerotic lesions are distributed in the region of the aortic valve ring. The aortic arch and the thoracic and abdominal aorta become more severely affected as a function of age. The principal consequence of atheroma formation is progressive narrowing of the arterial lumen that leads to a restricted blood supply to distal sites. Such changes can result in renal hypertension, stroke, and myocardial ischemia and infarction.

Toxic chemicals can induce or enhance atheroma formation by several mechanisms involving injury to luminal endothelial cells and/or medial smooth muscle cells (Ramos et al., 1994). Such lesions often result from chronic cycles of vascular injury and repair and typically require long latency periods. Mechanical or toxic injury to the endothelium has been associated with initiation of the atherogenic response. Agents such as acrolein, butadiene, cyclophosphamide, heavy metals, and homocysteine have been identified as endothelial toxins. In a wide variety of animal species (including rabbits and rats), vascular endothelial cell injury potentiates the atherogenic process and in some instances precedes the development of atherosclerotic plaques. In humans and animals, a hypercholesterolemic diet causes an increase in plasma lipoproteins, damages the endothelium, and results in proliferation of smooth muscle cells. As part of the repair process, smooth muscle cell mitogens and chemotatic agents are released from one or more cell types. Atherosclerotic lesions also can develop as a result of injury to medial smooth muscle cells. Agents such as allylamine, benzo*(a)*pyrene, dinitrotoluenes, and hydrazines have been identified as smooth muscle cell toxins. Proliferation may be secondary to regenerative repair or to genetic changes in a small population of medial cells. After studying the monotypism of glucose-6-phosphate dehydrogenase, Benditt and Benditt (1973) proposed over 20 years ago that smooth muscle cells in the atherosclerotic plaque are the progeny of a single smooth muscle cell. Thus, the atherosclerotic process would resemble benign neoplastic growth of smooth muscle tumors (leiomyomas) (Fig. 17-16). Upon exposure to a toxic agent, smooth muscle cells may exist in a genetically altered state that gives rise to lesions after exposure to chemotatic/growth-promoting factors. Alternatively, mutations could induce the constitutive production of growth factors in smooth muscle cells, resulting in autocrine stimulation of growth. DNA isolated from human atherosclerotic plaques is capable of transforming NIH3T3 cells and producing tumors in nude mice, a finding that suggests that atherosclerotic cells possess intrinsic transforming potential.

Changes in blood pressure are often seen during acute poisonings. Hypotension—a sustained reduction of systemic arterial pressure—is common in poisonings with CNS depressants or antihypertensive agents as well as during anaphylactic reactions. Postural hypotension, particularly in elderly people,

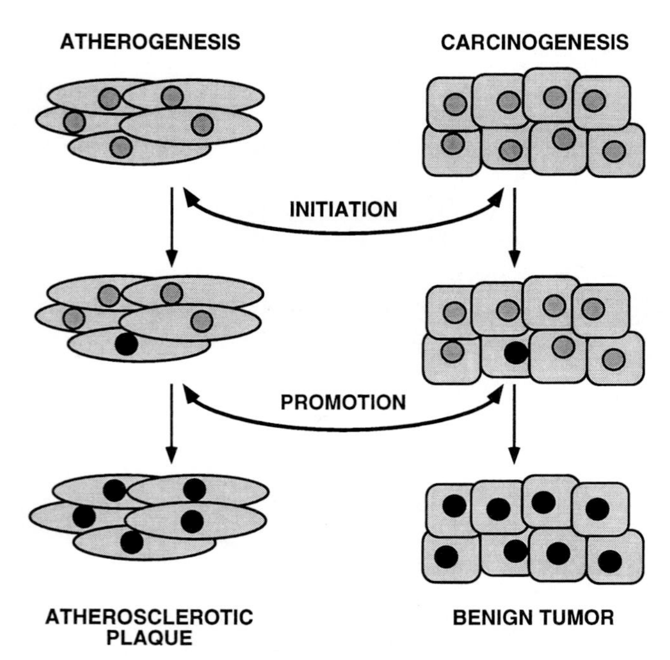


***Figure 17–16. Representation of the links between atherogenesis and carcinogenesis.***

Both disease processes may involve the initiation of a target cell and subsequent promotional events to result in a full response.

can be induced by therapeutic agents such as drugs that lower cardiac output or decrease blood volume. These agents include depressants of the vasomotor center such as morphinelike compounds, antihypertensive agents, sedatives, neuroleptics, and antiparkinsonian agents. In addition, agents that inhibit noradrenaline production and reuptake, such as methyldopa or antidepressants, respectively, also induce postural hypotension. Circulatory insufficiency can be delayed or even prevented by increased sympathoadrenal activity. However, poisonings associated with extreme loss of body fluids caused by persistent vomiting or diarrhea and conditions resulting in marked reductions in plasma, such as hemorrhage, lead to a state of circulatory insufficiency (shock). Other causes of shock include inadequate myocardial contraction resulting from severe arrhythmia and inadequate peripheral circulation brought about by altered vasomotor tone resulting from the effects of chemical mediators, such as histamine, leukotriene, and kinins. Vasodilation, which is mediated by activation of H1 and H2 receptors located throughout the resistance vessels, is the most prominent action of histamine in humans. Histamine tends to constrict the larger blood vessels.

Hypertension may result from an increased concentration of circulating vasoconstrictors such as angiotensin II and catecholamines or from disturbances of local regulation mediated by metabolic, myogenic, or angiogenic mechanisms. Increased vascular resistance has been associated with an overall increase in wall thickness caused at least in part by hypertrophy and proliferation of smooth muscle cells. A sustained elevation in blood pressure also has been associated with destruction of capillaries at the tissue level and compensatory angiogenesis. Arterial hypertension may occur in the course of an overdose of sympathomimetic and anticholinergic drugs. Sudden drug-induced hypertension can cause cerebrovascular accidents when diseased blood vessels cannot adapt to high perfusion pressures. Mineralocorticoids can cause excessive sodium retention and lead to sustained elevation of blood pressure by increasing circulatory volume. Licorice, which contains glycyrrhizin, an aldosteronelike substance that exerts mineralocorticoid activity, can cause sustained hypertension. Agents that cause hyperreninemia, such as cadmium, can raise blood pressure through the generation of angiotensinogen II. Depletion of renomedullary vasodilator substances has been implicated in the hypertensive episodes associated with analgesic drug-induced nephropathy. Increased synthesis of angiotensinogen has been considered an important factor in the hypertension produced by high doses of estrogen-containing oral contraceptives. Sustained hypertension is the most important risk factor predisposing a person to coronary and cerebral atherosclerosis. The mechanisms by which hypertension produces vascular degenerative lesions involve increased vascular permeability that leads to entry of blood constituents into the vessel wall.

The vascular toxicity of some therapeutic agents, including antimicrobial drugs and anticoagulants, often involves vasculitis secondary to hypersensitivity reactions. Some chemicals can cause hemorrhage by damaging the large vessels, such as the aneurysms produced by lathyrogens. Damage to capillaries by cytotoxic chemicals leading to petechial hemorrhages are seen in several organs after acute poisonings. A chemically induced defect in the blood-clotting mechanism increases the probability that a hemorrhage will occur. Thrombosis—the formation of a semisolid mass from blood constituents in the circulation—can occur in both arteries and veins as a result of toxicant exposure. Predisposition to thrombosis occurs by means of induction of platelet aggregation, an increase in their adhesiveness, or creation of a state of hypercoagulability through an increase in or activation of clotting factors, as seen with large doses of epinephrine. Other chemicals may lead to thrombosis by interfering with antithrombin III (oral contraceptive steroids) or inhibiting fibrinolysis (corticosteroids, mercurials). Sudden changes in blood flow brought about by excessive vasoconstriction or decreased peripheral resistance can trigger arterial thrombosis. Venous stasis contributes to the development of venous thrombosis. Table 17-4 provides a partial list of thrombogenic agents and their putative mechanisms of action. Injury to the vessel wall by intravenous infusion of an irritating drug produces generalized endothelial damage and leads to thromboses at the sites of lesions. Portions of a thrombus may be released and travel in the vascular system until arrested as an embolus in a vessel with a caliber even smaller than that of its origin. The consequence depends on the site of arrest, but a thrombus can result in death. The most important drugs known to produce thromboembolisms are the contraceptive steroids.

## GENERAL BIOCHEMICAL MECHANISMS OF VASCULAR TOXICITY

Epidemiological and experimental evidence has established a correlation between exposure to toxic chemicals and the incidence of cardiovascular morbidity and mortality. Such a correlation is best exemplified by the role of tobacco smoke as a

**Table 17–4**
**Compounds Producing Thrombosis**

| AGENT | MECHANISM OF ACTION AND SPECIFIC EFFECTS |
|---|---|
| *Endothelial Damage* | |
| Homocysteine | Deendothelialization |
| Endotoxin | Deendothelialization |
| Sodium acetriozate | Disseminated thrombosis in capillaries and veins |
| *Pathophysiological Circulatory Dynamics* | |
| Ergotamine | Profound vasoconstriction in peripheral arteries |
| Pitressin | Profound vasoconstriction in coronary and mesenteric arteries |
| Oral contraceptives | Venous stasis in lower extremities |
| Acetylcholine and autonomic blockers | Hypovolemic hypotension and stasis |
| Sympathomimetic agents | Elevated blood pressure; distension of vessels to produce endothelial damage |
| *Effects on Platelets* | |
| Serotonin | Increase in platelet count (above $10^6$/mm$^3$) |
| Progesterone | |
| Testosterone | |
| Somatotropic hormone | |
| Vinblastine | |
| Vincristine | |
| Congo Red | |
| Ristocetin | |
| Thrombin | |
| Epinephrine | |
| Adenosine diphosphate | Increase in platelet adhesiveness |
| Thrombin | |
| Evan's Blue | |
| *Effects on Clotting Factors* | |
| Epinephrine | Increase in factors VIII and IX |
| Guanethidine | Secondary effects caused by release of epinephrine |
| Debrisoquin | |
| Tyramine | |
| Lactic acid (IV infusion) | Activation of Hageman factor |
| Long-chain fatty acids (iv infusion) | Activation of contact factors |
| Catecholamines | Elevation in circulating levels of fatty acids |
| ACTH | |
| Thymoleptics | |
| Nicotine | |
| Oral contraceptives | Decrease in antithrombin III levels |
| Mercuric chloride | Inhibition of fibrinolysis |
| Corticosteroids | |
| ε-Aminocaproic acid | Plasminogen antiactivator |
| Aprotinine | Proteinase inhibitors |

major contributor to myocardial infarction, sudden cardiac death, arteriosclerotic peripheral vascular disease, and atherosclerotic aneurysm of the aorta. Angiotoxic chemicals are found in the ambient environment as a result of anthropogenic activity or occur as natural variations in the environment, such as fungal toxins in food supplies. Chemicals absorbed through the respiratory, cutaneous, gastrointestinal, and intravenous routes by necessity come in contact with vascular cells before reaching other sites in the body. This property alone puts the vascular system at increased risk of toxic insult. Although this relationship has long been ignored, the recognition that many target organ toxicities involve a significant microvascular component has become more prevalent recently.

Chemicals can produce degenerative or inflammatory changes in blood vessels as a consequence of an excessive pharmacological effect. For example, ergotamine, a naturally occurring alkaloid, causes sustained arterial vasoconstriction that leads to peripheral arterial lesions involving intimal proliferation and medial degenerative changes. Degenerative or inflammatory changes can also occur secondary to the interaction of chemicals or their reactive metabolites with a structural and/or functional component of the vessel wall. For example, endothelial cell death and atherosclerosis can be induced by homocysteine, a sulfur-containing amino acid produced in the biosynthesis of cysteine from methionine. The reactivity of the sulfhydryl group of homocysteine has been implicated in the atherogenic response. Injury to the endothelium leads to recruitment of white blood cells into the affected sites as part of the inflammatory response. The inflammatory response is directed by a variety of signaling molecules that are produced locally by mast cells, nerve endings, platelets, and white blood cells as well as by the activation of complement. In the case of medial smooth muscle cells, injury is associated with degenerative changes in the media of blood vessels. For example, allylamine toxicity is associated primarily with medial changes, but changes in endothelial cells also have been noted. Repeated cycles of vascular injury by this amine result in smooth muscle hyperplasia and coronary artery and aortic lesions that mimic those found in atherosclerotic vessels. Changes in the collagen of large arteries leading to localized dilation (aneurysms) occur in lathyrism and can be reproduced experimentally by administration of $\beta$-aminopropionitrile.

Angiotoxicity may be expressed at the mechanical, metabolic, or genetic level and in general involves interactions of multiple cellular elements (Table 17-5). Endothelial cells represent the first cellular barrier to the movement of bloodborne toxins from the lumen of the vessel to deeper layers of the wall. This location makes these regions particularly susceptible to toxic insult. Endothelial injury also occurs as a result of the production of oxygen free radicals during reperfusion injury in transplanted organs. Toxic chemicals reaching the subendothelial space may cause injury to medial smooth muscle cells

**Table 17–5**
**Cell Types Implicated in the Vasculotoxic Response**

| CELL TYPE | FUNCTION |
|---|---|
| Endothelial cells | First barrier to bloodborne toxins; synthesis and release of endothelium-derived relaxing factor; synthesis of pro- and antiaggregatory factors; attachment and recruitment of inflammatory cells; synthesis of connective tissue proteins; generation of oxygen-derived free radicals and other radical moieties |
| Smooth muscle cells | Maintenance of vasomotor tone; synthesis of extracellular matrix proteins, including collagen and elastin; synthesis of prostaglandins and other biologically active lipids; regulation of monocyte function; formation of free radicals |
| Fibroblasts | Synthesis of extracellular matrix proteins, including collagens; structural support to the vessel wall |
| Monocytes/macrophages | Scavenger potential; synthesis of macrophage-derived growth factor; generation of reactive oxygen species; lymphocyte activation; progenitor of foam cells |
| Platelets | Synthesis of proaggregatory substances and smooth muscle mitogens such as platelet-derived growth factor |
| Lymphocytes | Release of activated oxygen species; cellular immunity; production of immunoglobulins |

SOURCE: Reprinted with permission from Ramos KS, in Acosta D (ed): *Cardiovascular Toxicology*, 2d ed. New York: Raven Press, 1992.

and/or adventitial fibroblasts. Adventitial and medial cells in large elastic arteries such as the human aorta also may be reached via the vasa vasorum, the intrinsic blood supply to the vessel wall. The vasculotoxic response is also dependent on the influence of (1) extracellular matrix proteins that influence cell behavior, (2) coagulation factors that dictate the extent of hemostatic involvement, (3) hormones and growth factors that regulate vascular function, and (4) plasma lipoproteins, some of which modulate cellular metabolism and facilitate the transport and delivery of hydrophobic substances (Ferrario et al., 1985).

Common mechanisms of vascular toxicity include (1) selective alterations of vascular reactivity, (2) vessel-specific bioactivation of protoxicants, (3) erratic detoxification of the parent chemical or its metabolites, and (4) preferential accumulation of the active toxin in vascular cells (Fig. 17-17). Multiple mechanisms often operate simultaneously in the course of the toxic response. Interestingly, although vascular injury by toxic chemicals often involves different mechanisms, the modulation of growth and differentiation in vascular cells is a common toxicologic endpoint.

Vascular reactivity is regulated by the transfer of signals from the surface to the interior of the cell and/or direct modulation of the structure and function of contractile protein. Usually, disorders of vascular reactivity involve generalized disturbances of ionic regulation. Nontoxic chemicals can be converted by vascular enzymes to reactive species that cause injury to both intra- and extracellular targets. Enzyme systems that are present in vascular cells and are involved in the bioactivation of vascular toxins include amine oxidases, cytochrome P-450 monooxygenases, and prostaglandin synthetase. Amine oxidases are copper-containing enzymes that catalyze the oxidative removal of biogenic amines from blood plasma, the cross-linking of collagen and elastin in connective tissue, and the regulation of intracellular spermine and spermidine levels.

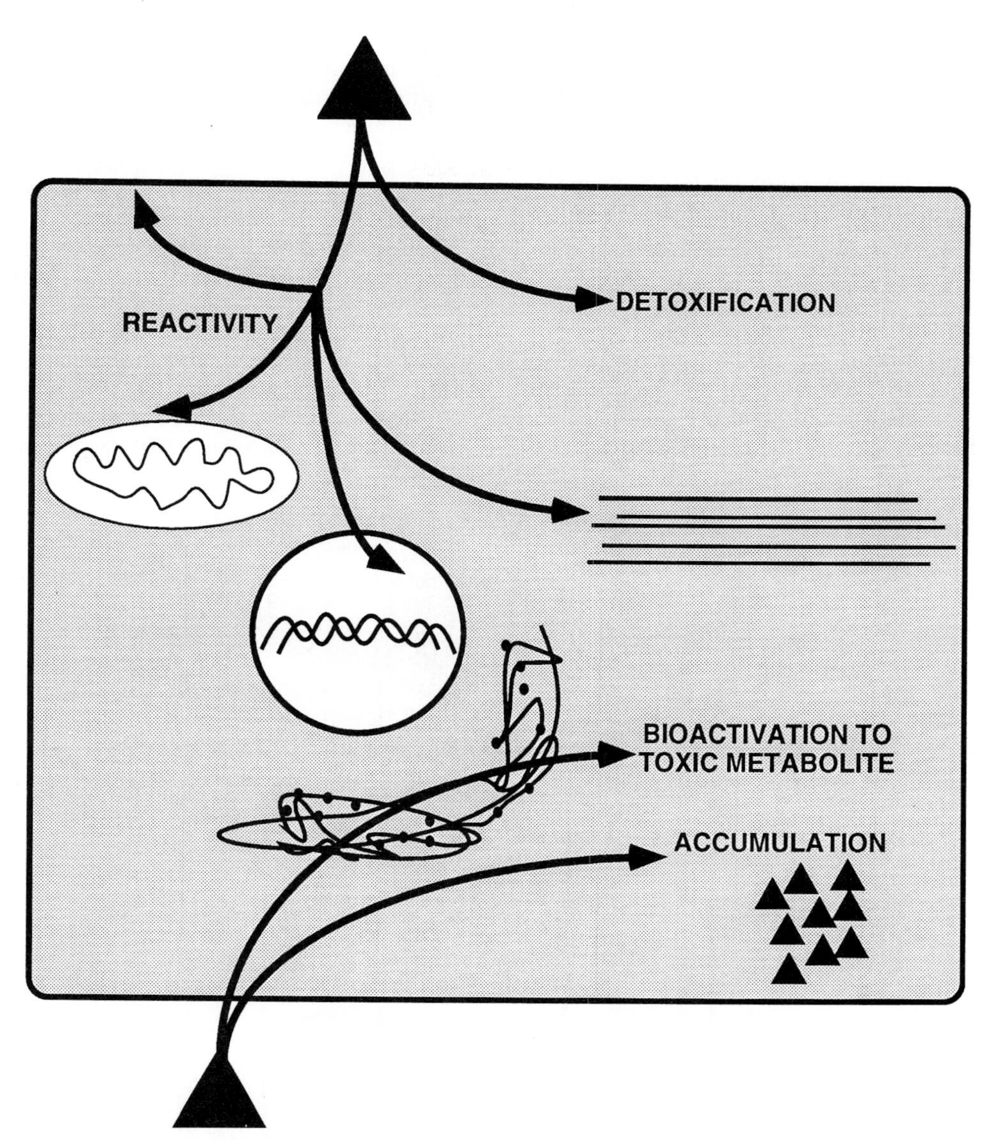


***Figure 17-17. Toxic injury to vascular cells may involve four common mechanisms.***

Alterations in vascular reactivity may include disruption of cellular membranes or the contractile apparatus of smooth muscle cells by a toxicant. Additionally, vascular cells may bioactivate protoxicants in a vessel-specific manner or aberrant detoxification may lead to cell injury. Vascular cells also may preferentially accumulate potential toxins.

These microsomal enzyme systems are involved in the bioactivation of allylamine to acrolein and hydrogen peroxide. The occurrence of several cytochrome P-450 metabolites of arachidonic acid involved in the regulation of vascular tone and sodium pump activity has also been noted. For instance, cytochrome P-450 1A1 in endothelial and smooth muscle cells metabolizes benzo*(a)*pyrene and other polycyclic aromatic hydrocarbons to toxic and genotoxic intermediates. A complex of microsomal enzymes collectively referred to as prostaglandin synthetase catalyzes the formation of biologically active lipids, including prostacyclin and thromboxane $A_2$. Prostacyclin, the major arachidonic acid metabolite in blood vessels, is a strong vasodilator and an endogenous inhibitor of platelet aggregation, while thromboxane $A_2$, the major arachidonic acid metabolite in platelets, is a potent vasoconstrictor and a promoter of platelet aggregation. The bioactivation of vascular toxins need not be confined to vascular tissue. Evidence that angiotoxic chemicals can be bioactivated by the liver and lung, with the activated metabolites leaving the metabolizing sites and reaching vascular targets through the systemic circulation, has been presented. Vascular toxicity also may be due to deficiencies in the capacity of target cells to detoxify the active toxin or handle prooxidant states. Key components of the endogenous antioxidant defense system, including the glutathione/glutathione reductase/glutathione peroxidase system, superoxide dismutase, and catalase, are operative in vascular cells.

Oxidative metabolism is critical to the preservation of vascular function, as is best exemplified by the role of oxidation in the metabolism and cytotoxicity of plasma lipoproteins. Low-density lipoproteins are oxidized by oxygen free radicals released by arterial cells, and this reaction is considered to be critical in the initiation and progression of the atherosclerotic process (Fig. 17-18). Modified low-density lipoproteins attract macrophages and prevent their migration from the tissues (Ross, 1993). Oxidation of low-density lipoproteins generates activated oxygen species, which can directly injure endothelial cells and increase adherence and the migration of monocytes and T lymphocytes into the subendothelial space. Subsequent release of growth modulators from endothelial cells and/or macrophages can promote smooth muscle cell proliferation and the secretion of extracellular matrix proteins. In the vasculature, free radicals in vivo can be generated secondary to anoxic/reoxygenation injury, metabolism of xenobiotics, neutrophil/monocyte-mediated inflammation, and oxidative modification of low-density lipoproteins. Superoxide anions inactivate endothelium-derived relaxing factor, while hydrogen peroxide and hydroxyl radicals cause direct vasodilation and stimulate the synthesis and release of relaxation factors. Oxygen radicals are considered important mediators of vascular damage in acute arterial hypertension and experimental brain injury (Wei et al., 1985). Acute exposure of rats to angiotensin II results in a hypertensive episode that results from irregular constriction patterns and in vascular hyperpermeability in small arteries and arterioles (Wilson, 1990). The treatment of hypertensive rats with free radical scavengers inhibits the vascular hyperpermeability and cellular damage associated with angiotensin II–induced hypertension. The release of superoxide from endothelial cells may modulate endothelial functions as well as the functions of other constituents of the vascular wall. In this context, activated endothelial cells have been reported to produce and secrete proteases in association with vessel penetration into surrounding connective tissue in response to angiogenic stimuli (Gross et al., 1983).

Vascular toxicity may be due to selective accumulation of chemicals in the vascular wall. Although the mechanisms re-

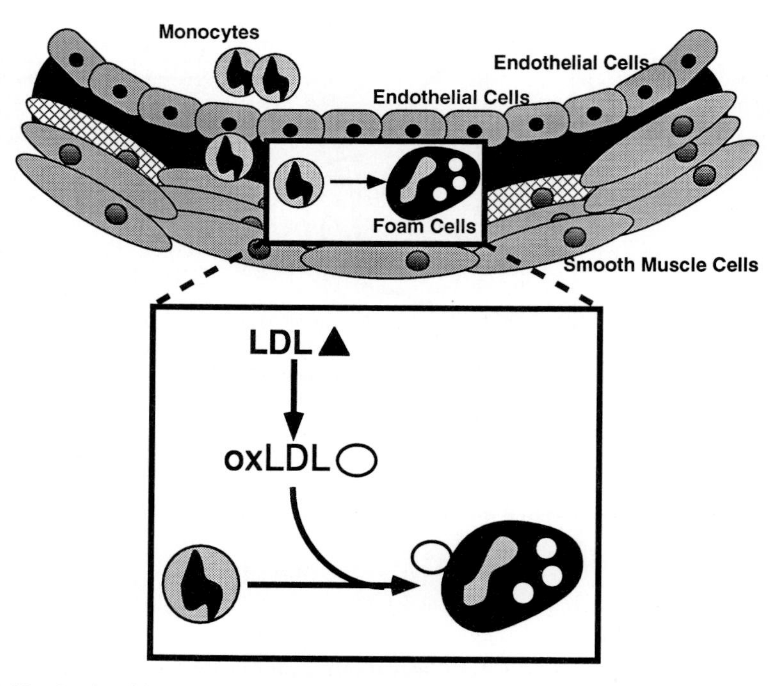


***Figure 17–18. Oxidized lipoproteins participate in the progression of atherosclerosis.***

Low-density lipoproteins (LDL) are oxidized within the vasculature. The uptake of oxLDL by macrophage scavenger receptors results in the formation of foam cells, an important cell type found in atherosclerotic plaques.

sponsible for preferential accumulation of toxins in the vessel wall are not known, receptor-mediated internalization of low-density lipoproteins may be critical in this process. This process appears to be critical in the deposition of aromatic hydrocarbons and other ubiquitous environmental contaminants, including organic acids, aldehydes, alcohols, and esters, in the vessel wall (Ferrario et al., 1985). Agents such as nonenal, naphthalene, propylfuranacetaldehyde, DDT, and hexachlorobenzene have been identified in atherosclerotic plaques. The deposition of these toxicants could be accounted for by chemical partitioning into the lipid phase of the atherosclerotic plaques. The consequences of vasculotoxic insult are dictated by the interplay between vascular and nonvascular cells and by noncellular factors such as extracellular matrix proteins, coagulation factors, hormones, immune complexes, and plasma lipoproteins. Furthermore, the toxic response can be modulated by mechanical and hemodynamic factors such as arterial pressure, shear stress, and blood viscosity. An additional consideration is the fact that kinetic and pharmacodynamic differences among different animal species also may alter the toxicological profile of a toxicant.

## CLASSIFICATION OF VASCULOTOXIC AGENTS

### Industrial Agents

**Alkylamines.** Aliphatic amines such as allylamine (3-aminopropene) are utilized in the synthesis of pharmaceutical and commercial products. Several allylamine analogues are being developed as antifungal agents for human and veterinary use. Allylamine is more toxic than are other unsaturated primary amines of higher molecular weight. Exposure to allylamine by a variety of routes in various animal species is associated with selective cardiovascular toxicity (Boor et al., 1979; Ramos and Thurlow, 1993). Hines and associates (1960) reported that acute intragastric administration of allylamine causes congestion of blood vessels in rats. The multiple organ toxicities observed after chronic inhalation of allylamine are characterized by a prominent vascular component (Lalich, 1969) involving mesenteric, pancreatic, testicular, and pulmonary artery hypertrophy and occasional alveolar hemorrhage and pulmonary edema. The specificity of the vasculotoxic response may be related to the accumulation of allylamine in elastic and muscular arteries upon administration in vivo. Gross lesions are evident in the myocardium, aorta, and coronary arteries of animals exposed to allylamine. Chronic administration is associated with the development of atheroscleroticlike lesions characterized by proliferation of smooth muscle cells and fibrosis.

Boor and associates (1990) first proposed that allylamine toxicity results from bioactivation of the parent compound to a toxic aldehyde. The oxidative deamination of allylamine results in the formation of acrolein and hydrogen peroxide, metabolites that mediate the acute and long-term toxic effects of allylamine (Fig. 17-19). Vascular-specific bioactivation of allylamine is a prerequisite for toxicity (Ramos et al., 1988). Benzylamine oxidase, which is also known as semicarbazide-sensitive amine oxidase, is believed to catalyze the oxidative deamination of allylamine. This enzyme is found in cardiovascular tissue in higher concentrations than is any other tissue. Allylamine preferentially injures smooth muscle cells relative to other cell types in the vascular wall. Mitochondria have been identified as early targets of allylamine toxicity, an observation that is consistent with the enrichment of amine oxidase activity in this subcellular compartment. Because the cytotoxic response also involves alterations in cellular glutathione status that compromise the integrity of membrane compartments (Ramos and Thurlow, 1993), modulation of glutathione status by acrolein and/or hydrogen peroxide also may disrupt mitochondrial function.

Acrolein is a highly reactive aldehyde that disrupts the thiol balance of target cells, including vascular cells (Ramos and Cox, 1987); denatures proteins; and interferes with nucleic acid synthesis. Although many molecules react with acrolein under physiological conditions, the main reaction products result from nucleophilic addition at the terminal ethylenic carbon. Acrolein toxicity also may involve conversion by NADPH-dependent microsomal enzymes to glycidaldehyde, a known mutagen and carcinogen. Acrolein is a ubiquitous toxic chemical that is found in engine exhaust and cigarette smoke. Using Dahl hypertension-resistant and hypertension-sensitive rat strains, Kutzman and colleagues (1984) demonstrated that exposure to acrolein for 62 days is more toxic to hypertension-sensitive animals than to their hypertension-resistant counterparts. The indirect sympathomimetic activity of aldehydes, including acrolein, acetaldehyde, and formaldehyde, may contribute to the enhanced sensitivity of hypertension-prone animals.

Repeated cycles of vascular injury upon in vivo exposure of rats to allylamine modulate medial aortic smooth muscle cells from a quiescent to a proliferative state (Cox and Ramos, 1990). Because cells from allylamine-treated rats maintain this altered phenotype after serial propagation in vitro, phenotypic modulation probably involves genotypic alterations secondary to chemical insult. The enhanced capacity for proliferation in allylamine cells is associated with modulation of phospholipid metabolism, enhanced protein kinase C activity, increased *c-Ha-ras* proto-oncogene expression, and differential secretion and deposition of extracellular matrix components (Ramos et al., 1993). Enhanced secretion of a 45-kD protein corresponding in size to osteopontin characterizes the proliferative phenotype induced by allylamine (Parrish and Ramos, 1995). Osteopontin is a secreted phosphoprotein that has effects on gene expression, $Ca^{2+}$ regulation, and nitric oxide production, presumably mediated through the $\alpha_v\beta_3$ integrin. Osteopontin has been associated with arterial smooth muscle cell proliferation and migration and is present in atherosclerotic lesions. Although a major contributory role in adhesion and migration has been established with a fair degree of certainty, additional studies are needed to determine whether this protein participates in the deregulation of smooth muscle cell proliferation by allylamine.

**Heavy Metals.** The vascular toxicity of food- and water-borne elements (selenium, chromium, copper, zinc, cadmium, lead, and mercury) as well as airborne elements (vanadium and lead) is thought to be mediated by reactions of metals with sulfhydryl, carboxyl, or phosphate groups. Metals such as cobalt, magnesium, manganese, nickel, cadmium, and lead also interact with and block calcium channels. Evidence suggesting that intracellular calcium-binding proteins such as calmodulin

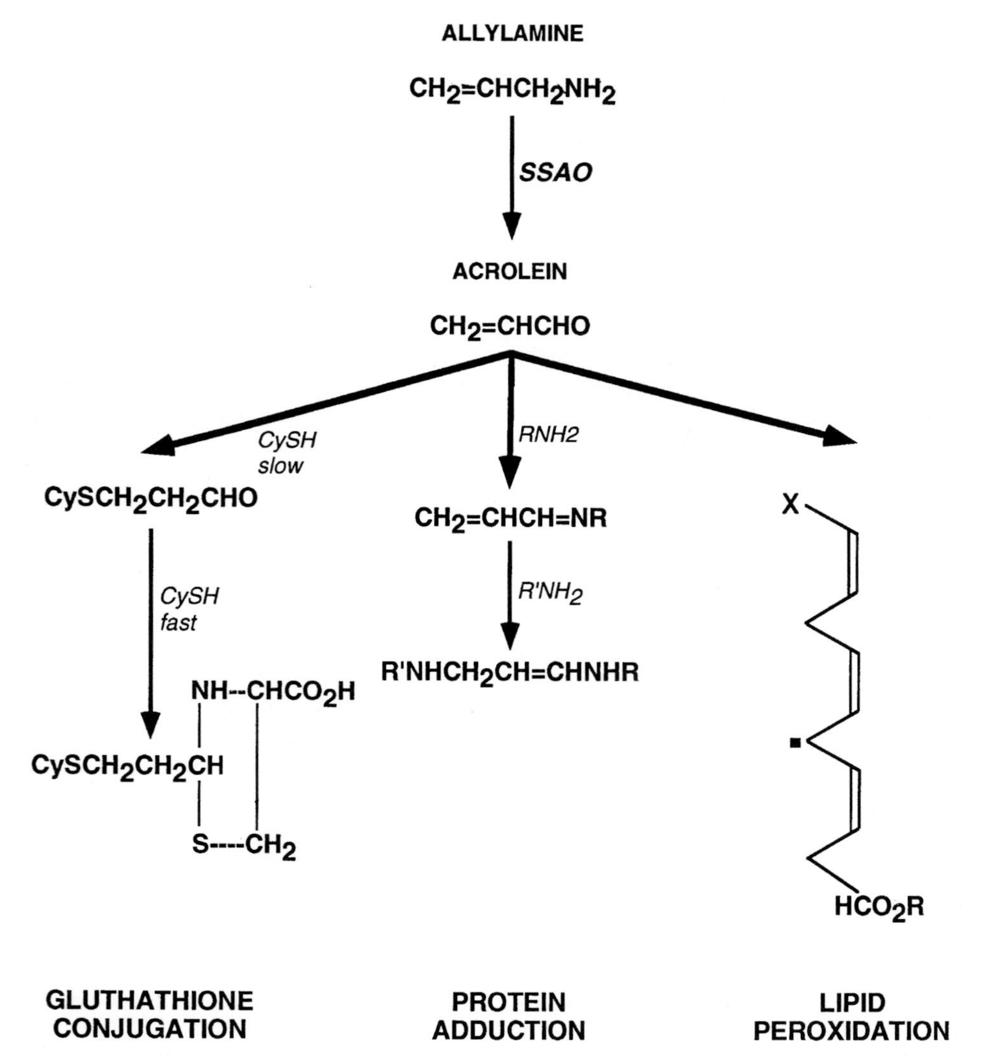


***Figure 17–19. Metabolism of allylamine to acrolein by semicarbazide-sensitive amine oxidase in vascular smooth muscle cells.***

Acrolein may be conjugated to gluthathione by the action of glutathione-S-transferase or may interact with intracellular proteins to form protein adducts. In addition, acrolein may initiate intracellular lipid peroxidation, which may lead to genotoxic or cell damage.

are biologically relevant targets of heavy metals, including mercury and lead, has been presented. The contribution of this mechanism to the toxic effects of metals has been questioned because of the inability of beryllium, barium, cobalt, zinc, and cadmium to bind readily to calmodulin in vitro.

To date, the vascular effects of cadmium have been studied in the greatest detail. Although cadmium is not preferentially localized in blood vessels relative to other tissues, when present, cadmium is thought to be localized in the elastic lamina of large arteries, with particularly high concentrations at arterial branching points (Perry et al., 1989). A large portion of the cadmium that accumulates in the body is tightly bound to hepatic and renal metallothionein, a known detoxification mechanism. The low metallothionein levels in vascular tissue may actually predispose a person to the toxic effects of cadmium (Perry et al., 1989). Long-term exposure of laboratory animals to low levels of cadmium has been associated with the development of atherosclerosis and hypertension in the absence of other toxic effects. Selenium and zinc inhibit, while lead potentiates, the hypertensive effects of cadmium. Concentrations of cadmium that increase blood pressure do not raise blood pressure in the presence of calcium. In contrast, the protective effects of zinc and selenium may be related to their ability to increase the synthesis of cadmium-binding proteins and thus enhance detoxification. Cadmium increases sodium retention, induces vasoconstriction, increases cardiac output, and produces hyperreninemia. Any one of these mechanisms could account for the putative hypertensive effects of cadmium. In rats, chronic administration of cadmium caused renal arteriolar thickening as well as diffuse fibrosis of capillaries. In fact, a recent study has suggested that low-level cadmium intake is associated with a higher frequency of atherosclerosis in humans (Houtman, 1993). Similar vascular changes are also responsible for the development of testicular damage and atrophy. The hypertensive effects of cadmium remain questionable, since population studies in humans have not confirmed the associations made in studies of laboratory animals.

Much less work has been conducted to evaluate the vasculotoxic effects of other heavy metals. Because hypertension is not commonly observed during clinical lead intoxication, many investigators consider the existing evidence to be conflicting and inconclusive. Epidemiological studies have shown that a large percentage of patients with essential hypertension have increased body stores of lead (Batuman et al., 1983). Elevated blood pressure also has been observed during childhood lead poisoning. Although in these children the level of lead burden was not severe, a significant increase in blood pressure was seen on the tenth day of poisoning and persisted for the remainder of the study. The direct vasoconstrictor effect of lead may be related to the putative hypertensive response. This effect can be complemented by the ability of lead to activate the renin-angiotensin-aldosterone system.

Inorganic mercury produces vasoconstriction of preglomerular vessels. In addition, the integrity of the blood-brain barrier may be disrupted by mercury. The opening of the blood-brain barrier results in extravasation of plasma protein across vascular walls into adjoining brain tissues. Mercury added to platelet-rich plasma causes a marked increase in platelet thromboxane $B_2$ production and platelet responsiveness to arachidonic acid. Although it is unlikely that mercury and lead compete with calcium for intracellular binding sites, their accessibility to the intracellular compartment appears to be calcium-dependent (Tomera and Harakal, 1986). Acute lead-induced neuropathy may be due to cerebral capillary dysfunction. Inorganic lead alters arterial elasticity and causes sclerosis of renal vessels. Lead intoxication has been linked to hypertension in humans, but its exact role is questionable.

Acute arsenic poisoning causes vasodilation and capillary dilation. These actions have been associated with extravasation, transudation of plasma, and decreased intravascular volume. It has been proposed that high levels of arsenic in the soil and water of Taiwan are responsible for blackfoot disease, a severe form of arteriosclerosis. Blackfoot disease is an endemic peripheral vascular occlusive disease that exhibits arteriosclerosis obliterans and thromboangiitis. The ability of arsenic to induce these changes has been attributed to its effects on vascular endothelial cells. Arsenic has been reported to cause noncirrhotic portal hypertension in humans. Chromium appears to play an important role in the maintenance of vascular integrity. A deficiency of this metal in animals results in elevated serum cholesterol levels and increased atherosclerotic aortic plaques. Autopsies of humans have revealed virtually no chromium in the aortas of individuals who died of atherosclerotic heart disease compared with individuals dying of other causes.

**Nitroaromatics.** Dinitrotoluene is used as a precursor in the synthesis of polyurethane foams, coatings, elastomers, and explosives. The manufacture of dinitrotoluene generates a technical-grade mixture that consists of 75.8 percent 2,4-dinitrotoluene, 19.5 percent 2,6-dinitrotoluene, and 4.7 percent other isomers. Several chronic toxicity studies in laboratory animals have shown that 2,4- and/or 2,6-dinitrotoluene can cause cancers of the liver, gallbladder, and kidney as well as benign tumors of the connective tissues. In humans, however, retrospective mortality studies in workers exposed daily to dinitrotoluene have shown that dinitrotoluenes cause circulatory disorders of atherosclerotic etiology. As with other chronic occupational illnesses, increased mortality from cardiovascular disorders upon exposure to dinitrotoluenes has been related to the duration and intensity of exposure.

The atherogenic effects of dinitrotoluenes have been examined experimentally. Repeated in vivo exposure of rats to 2,4- or 2,6-dinitrotoluene is associated with dysplasia and rearrangement of aortic smooth muscle cells (Ramos et al., 1990). Dinitrotoluenes are metabolized in the liver to dinitrobenzylalcohol, which is then conjugated to form a glucuronide conjugate that is excreted in bile or urine. This conjugate is thought to be hydrolyzed by intestinal microflora and subsequently reduced to a toxic metabolite or the precursor of a toxic metabolite. Dent and colleagues (1981) have shown that rat cecal microflora convert dinitrotoluene to nitrosonitrotoluenes, aminonitrotoluenes, and diaminotoluenes. In vitro exposure of rat aortic smooth muscle cells to 2,4- or 2,6-diaminotoluene inhibited DNA synthesis, a response comparable to that seen in medial smooth muscle cells isolated from dinitrotoluene-treated animals.

**Aromatic Hydrocarbons.** Aromatic hydrocarbons, including polycyclic aromatic hydrocarbons and polychlorinated dibenzo-*p*-dioxins, are persistent toxic environmental contaminants. Several aromatic hydrocarbons have been identified as vascular toxins that can initiate and/or promote the atherogenic process in experimental animals (Ou and Ramos, 1992a and b). Much of the work involved in investigating the vascular toxicity of aromatic hydrocarbons has focused on the polycyclic aromatic hydrocarbons, of which benzo*(a)*pyrene has been examined in the greatest detail. Exposure of avian species to benzo*(a)*pyrene and 7,12-dimethylbenz[*a*]anthracene causes atherosclerosis without altering serum cholesterol levels. The atherogenic effects of these carcinogens have been associated with cytochrome P-450–mediated conversion of the parent compound to toxic metabolic intermediates. The majority of the activity responsible for the biotransformation of these chemicals is associated with the smooth muscle layers of the aorta, although cytochrome P-450–dependent monoxygenase activity that can bioactivate carcinogens also has been localized in the aortic endothelium. Interestingly, the activity of aortic aryl hydrocarbon hydroxylase has been correlated with the degree of susceptibility to atherosclerosis in avian species, and Ah-responsive mice are more susceptible to atherosclerosis than are Ah-resistant mice.

3-Methylcholantrene increases both the number and the size of lipid-staining lesions in the aorta of animals that are fed an atherogenic diet for 8 weeks, suggesting that aromatic hydrocarbons can also initiate the atherogenic process. Furthermore, focal proliferation of intimal smooth muscle cells can be produced by an initiation-promotion sequence using 7,12-dimethylbenz*[a]*anthracene and the alpha-$_1$ selective adrenergic agonist methoxamine. In contrast, Albert and coworkers (1977) and Penn and Snyder (1988) have reported that treatment with several polycylic hydrocarbons increases the size but not the frequency of atherosclerotic lesions. These observations suggest that polycyclic aromatic hydrocarbons act as promoters of the atherosclerotic process. Although additional studies are required to define the "initiating" versus "promotional" actions of polycyclic aromatic hydrocarbons, their ability to readily associate with plasma lipoproteins may play a critical role in vascular toxicity. In fact, the localization of these and other lipophilic chemicals in blood vessels may depend on lipoprotein-mediated transport.

The enhanced proliferative and migratory potential of smooth muscle cells induced by benzo*(a)*pyrene may involve a mutagenic process, as predicted by the monoclonal theory of atherogenesis (Benditt and Benditt, 1973). Thus, "initiation" of the atherogenic process by benzo*(a)*pyrene and related chemicals would involve mutation of target genes, while promotion would involve modulation of mitogenic signaling, including growth-related gene expression and protein phosphorylation. Because a promotional mechanism of atherogenesis implies the existence of an "initiated" resident cell population in the vessel wall, information about the cellular heterogeneity of vascular smooth muscle cells in the vessel wall is needed.

Benzo*(a)*pyrene modulates protein kinase C signal transduction in aortic smooth muscle cells of atherosclerosis-susceptible (quail) and atherosclerosis-resistant (rat) species (Ou et al., 1995). Other aromatic hydrocarbons, such as 2,3,7,8-tetrachlorodibenzo-*p*-dioxin, share with benzo*(a)*pyrene the ability to inhibit protein kinase C in aortic smooth muscle cells, but the mechanisms appear to be different. As atherogenesis ultimately involves enhanced smooth muscle cell proliferation, the role of protein kinase C inhibition and the associated suppression of cell growth appears to involve phosphorylation-dependent changes in DNA repair efficiency. Genotoxic actions of metabolites formed in situ probably contribute to the growth inhibitory response of benzo*(a)*pyrene because sister chromatid exchanges, mutations, and unscheduled DNA synthesis in cultured rat and rabbit aortic smooth muscle cells have been noted (Zwijsen et al., 1990).

In summary, benzo*(a)*pyrene elicits alterations of smooth muscle cell proliferation through several mechanisms, including enhanced transcription of growth-related genes through aryl hydrocarbon receptor-mediated pathways, interaction and inactivation of protein kinase C, and conversion of the parent molecule to metabolites that can form covalent DNA adducts (Fig. 17-20).

## Gases

**Carbon Monoxide.** Carbon monoxide induces focal intimal damage and edema in laboratory animals at 180 ppm, a concentration to which humans may be exposed from environmental sources such as automobile exhaust, tobacco smoke, and fossil fuels. Because most sources of carbon monoxide are complex mixtures of chemicals, attempts to distinguish the direct effects of carbon monoxide from those of chemicals such as sulfur oxides, nitrogen oxides, aldehydes, and hydrocarbons have not yielded clear results. This is exemplified by the prominent vasculotoxic effects observed upon exposure of laboratory animals to other complex gas mixtures. For instance, automobile exhaust causes structural changes in the myocardium and aorta of guinea pigs and hemorrhage and infarct in the hemispheres and basal ganglia of spontaneously hypertensive rats. In addition, composition and deposition of lipids in the wall of the aorta of rats can be affected. However, it is not clear which of the many chemicals present in these mixtures mediate the atherogenic effect. Degenerative changes of myocardial arterioles have been produced experimentally in dogs that are forced to smoke. Similar changes have also been detected in humans who were heavy smokers and died of noncardiac causes (Wald and Howard, 1975; Auerbach and Carter, 1980). Tobacco smoke not only exerts a direct atherogenic effect (endothelial injury, changes in lipid profiles, and proliferation of smooth muscle cells) but also facilitates thrombosis by modulation of platelet function and vascular spasm.

Short-term exposure to carbon monoxide has been associated with direct damage to vascular endothelial and smooth muscle cells. Injury to endothelial cells increases intimal permeability and allows the interaction of blood constituents with underlying components of the vascular wall. This response may account in part for the ability of carbon monoxide to induce atherosclerotic lesions in several animal species. Although carbon monoxide enhances total arterial deposition of cholesterol in animals fed a lipid-rich diet, its vascular effects appear to be independent of serum cholesterol levels. The toxic effects of carbon monoxide have been attributed to its reversible interaction with hemoglobin. The formation of carboxyhemoglobin in vivo is favored because binding of carbon monoxide to hemoglobin is more cooperative than the binding

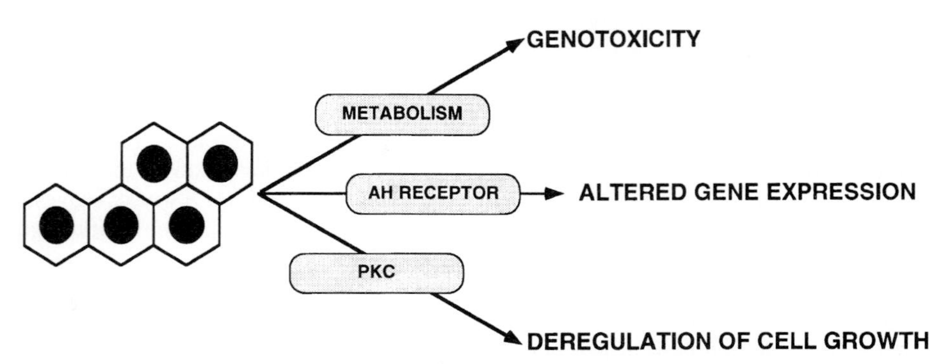


***Figure 17–20. Cellular and molecular targets of benzo(a)pyrene in vascular smooth muscle cells.***

Benzo*(a)*pyrene may be metabolized to reactive intermediates that bind covalently to DNA. Additionally, benzo*(a)*pyrene may bind to cytosolic receptors that act as ligand-activated transcription factors to regulate gene expression. Benzo*(a)*pyrene and/or its metabolites also may interact with protein kinase C to deregulate cell growth.

of oxygen. As a result of this interaction, carboxyhemoglobin decreases the oxygen-carrying capacity of blood and shifts the oxyhemoglobin saturation curve to the left. These actions make it more difficult to unload oxygen and eventually cause functional anemia resulting from reduced oxygen availability. More recently, evidence has been presented that carbon monoxide interacts with cellular proteins such as myoglobin and cytochrome *c* oxidase and that carbon monoxide elicits a direct vasodilatory response of the coronary circulation.

**Oxygen.** The administration of oxygen to a premature newborn can cause irreversible vasoconstriction and obliteration of retinal vasculature, resulting in permanent blindness. In squirrel monkeys, exposure to 100 percent oxygen for 50 to 117 h increases vascular permeability with leakage and edema of the retina, but these effects are largely reversible. In the pulmonary capillary bed, the volume and thickness of capillary endothelium decrease and perivascular edema is present. Exposure to high oxygen pressures for relatively short periods (less than 8 h) damages pulmonary endothelial cells in several species. Ozone affects the pulmonary vasculature, and the injuries usually take the form of pulmonary arterial lesions that lead to thickening of the artery walls.

**Carbon Disulfide.** Carbon disulfide (dithiocarbonic anhydride) occurs in coal tar and crude petroleum and is commonly utilized in the manufacture of rayon and soil disinfectants. This chemical has been identified as an atherogenic agent in laboratory animals. In humans, a two- to threefold increase in coronary heart disease has been reported. Although the mechanism of toxicity is not known, alterations of glucose and/or lipid metabolism and blood coagulation have been suggested. The mechanism for $CS_2$-atheroma production also may involve direct injury to the endothelium coupled with hypothyroidism, because thiocarbamate (thiourea), a potent antithyroid substance, is a principal urinary metabolite of $CS_2$.

**1,3-Butadiene.** Studies have shown that 1,3-butadiene, a chemical used in the production of styrene-butadiene, increases the incidence of cardiac hemangiosarcomas, which are tumors of endothelial origin (Miller and Boorman, 1990). Although hemangiosarcomas have also been observed in the liver, lung, and kidney, cardiac tumors are a major cause of death in animals exposed to this chemical. The toxic effects of 1,3-butadiene are dependent on its metabolic activation by cytochrome P-450 to toxic epoxide metabolites. The ultimate outcomes of exposure probably are influenced by the rates of glutathione-mediated detoxification of oxidative metabolites. Although 1,3-butadiene is a carcinogen in rats and mice, mice are considerably more sensitive than are rats to this carcinogenicity. This difference in susceptibility has been attributed to differences in the formation of the toxic mono- and diepoxide metabolites.

## Pharmaceutical Agents

### Autonomic Agents

***Sympathomimetic Amines.*** The sympathomimetic amines, including epinephrine, norepinephrine, dopamine, and isoproterenol, can damage the arterial vasculature by a variety of mechanisms. Amphetamine, a noncatecholamine sympathomimetic, damages cerebral arteries in experimental animal models. Large doses of norepinephrine produce toxic effects on the endothelium of the thoracic aorta of rabbits. Degenerative changes in the aortic arch have taken the form of increased numbers of microvilli and many focal areas of unusual endothelial cytoarchitecture. Repeated exposure to catecholamines induces atherosclerotic lesions in several animal species. The atherosclerotic effect of catecholamines probably is related to their ability to induce endothelial cell injury and/or modulate the proliferation of vascular cells. Evidence is available suggesting that the proliferative disturbances induced by catecholamines are mediated via alpha-receptors because prasozin, an alpha-receptor antagonist, effectively prevents the toxic response (Nakaki et al., 1989). However, potentiation of the atherosclerotic process by sympathetic activation is inhibited by beta-adrenergic receptor blockade. Smooth muscle cells exposed to atherosclerotic risk factors such as diabetes, hypertension, and balloon injury are more susceptible to the effects of catecholamines. Thus, the formation of arteriosclerotic lesions in certain forms of hypertension may be initiated and/or supported by high levels of circulating catecholamines.

***Nicotine.*** Nicotine, an alkaloid found in various plants, mimics the actions of acetylcholine at nicotinic receptors throughout the body. At pharmacological concentrations, nicotine increases heart rate and blood pressure as a result of stimulation of sympathetic ganglia and the adrenal medulla. Epidemiological and experimental studies have suggested that nicotine is a causative or aggravating factor in myocardial and cerebral infarction, gangrene, and aneurysm. Bull and associates (1985) have shown that repeated subcutaneous infusion of nicotine for 7 days is associated with reduced prostacyclin production in aortic segments. Reduced prostacyclin production has been observed in isolated rabbit hearts, rabbit aortas, human veins, rat aortas, and rat umbilical arteries when incubated with nicotine in vitro. It has been suggested that the effects of nicotine are due to competitive inhibition of cyclooxygenase, which precludes the formation of prostaglandin endoperoxides in vivo.

***Cocaine.*** Cardiovascular disorders are among the most common complications associated with cocaine abuse. The central actions of cocaine trigger an increase in the circulating levels of catecholamines and a generalized state of vasoconstriction. Hypertension and cerebral strokes are common vascular complications. In pregnant women, cocaine-induced vascular changes have been associated with abortions and abruptio placentae.

**Psychotropic Agents.** Several agents in the psychotropic class of drugs have been identified as potential atherogens. For instance, trifluoperazine and chlorpromazine have been shown to cause intracellular cholesterol accumulation in cultured cells of the aortic intima (Iakushkin et al., 1992). Enalapril has been shown to cause angioedema in humans. Aside from the atherogenic effects, postural hypotension has been identified as the most common cardiovascular side effect of tricyclic antidepressants.

**Antineoplastic Agents.** The vasculotoxic responses elicited by antineoplastic agents range from asymptomatic arterial lesions to thrombotic microangiopathy. Pulmonary veno-occlusive disease has been reported after the administration of various agents, including 5-fluorouracil, doxorubicin, and mitomycin. Long latencies characterize the occurrence of this disorder. Cyclophosphamide causes cerebrovascular and viscerovascular lesions, resulting in hemorrhages. In studies with 5-fluoro-2-deoxyuridine in dogs, chronic infusions into the hepatic artery resulted in gastrointestinal hemorrhage and portal vein thrombosis.

**Analgesics and Nonsteroidal Anti-Inflammatory Agents.** Aspirin can produce endothelial damage as part of a pattern of gastric erosion. Studies in rats have shown early changes in the basement membrane of endothelial cells of the capillaries and postcapillary venules, leading to obliteration of small vessels and ischemic infarcts in the large intestine. Regular use of analgesics containing phenacetin has been associated with an increased risk of hypertension and cardiovascular morbidity. Nonsteroidal anti-inflammatory drugs may induce hypertension as a result of interference with prostaglandin-mediated regulation of vascular tone.

**Oral Contraceptives.** Oral contraceptive steroids can produce thromboembolic disorders. An increased incidence of deep vein phlebitis and pulmonary embolism has been reported in young women who use oral contraceptives. Intracranial venous thrombosis and secondary increases in the risk of stroke have also been noted. A combination of cholesterol and estradiol given to experimental animals produced severe degenerative atherosclerotic effects on coronary arteries as well as lipid deposition along the ascending aorta. In an epidemiological review, Stolley and colleagues (1989) summarized the risks of vascular disease associated with the use of oral contraceptives. Oral contraceptive users have an increased risk of myocardial infarction relative to nonusers, a correlation that is markedly exacerbated by smoking. Oral contraceptive users experience an increased risk of cerebral thrombosis, hemorrhage, venous thrombosis, and pulmonary embolism. Although this has not been established with certainty, several groups have proposed that an immunologic mechanism mediates the vasculotoxic actions of oral contraceptives. However, the mechanism by which oral contraceptives increase the risk of vascular disease is unclear.

**Radio Contrast Dyes.** The iodinated radio contrast dyes used for visualization of blood vessels in angiography can cause thrombophlebitis. The cyanoacrylate adhesives used in repairing blood vessels and other tissues have produced degenerative changes in the arteries of dogs. Certain rapidly polymerizing polyurethane preparations used for transcatheter embolization techniques in surgery have produced dissolution of arterial walls. Dermal microvascular lesions have been reported after plastic film wound dressings were applied in various animal species.

**Phosphodiesterase Inhibitors.** The class of compounds that includes phosphodiesterase inhibitors is associated with toxicity in medium-size arteries of the mesentery, testis, and myocardium. Other reports showing that theophylline, an inhibitor of phosphodiesterase, causes cardiovascular lesions in mesenteric arterioles and that isomazole and indolidan cause periarteritis of the media and adventitia of small and medium-size arteries have been presented (Sandusky et al., 1991).

## Natural Products

**Bacterial Endotoxins.** Bacterial endotoxins produce a variety of toxic effects in many vascular beds. In the liver, they cause swelling of endothelial cells and adhesion of platelets to sinusoid walls. In the lung, endotoxins produce increased vascular permeability and pulmonary hypertension. Infusion of endotoxin into experimental animals produces thickening of endothelial cells and the formation of fibrin thrombi in small veins. In piglets, severe coronary artery damage has been demonstrated. These changes include disappearance of endothelial cells (exfoliation) followed by necrosis of medial smooth muscle cells. The terminal phase of the effects of endotoxin on the systemic vasculature results in marked hypotension. The ability of vitamin E to prevent disseminated intravascular coagulation induced by bacterial endotoxins in the rat suggests that this disorder is related to free radical–mediated mechanisms.

**Hydrazinobenzoic Acid.** Hydrazinobenzoic acid is a nitrogen-nitrogen bonded chemical that is present in the cultivated mushroom *Agaricus bisporus*. McManus and associates (1987) reported that this hydrazine derivative causes smooth muscle cell tumors in the aorta and large arteries of mice when administered over the life span of the animals. These tumors had the characteristic appearance and immunocytochemical features of vascular leiomyomas and leiomyosarcomas. Smooth muscle cell lysis with vascular perforation apparently precedes malignant transformation. The ability of hydrazinobenzoic acid to cause vascular smooth muscle cell tumors is shared by other synthetic and naturally occurring hydrazines. Although angiomyomas (or vascular leiomyomas) derived histogenetically from the media of blood and lymph vessels occur most commonly in the oral cavity and skin, primary leiomyosarcomas occur in the abdominal aorta.

**T-2 Toxin.** Trichothece mycotoxins, commonly classified as tetracyclic sesquiterpenes, are naturally occurring cytotoxic metabolites of *Fusarium* species. These mycotoxins, including T-2 toxin (4$\beta$,15diacetoxy-8$\alpha$-(3-methylbutyryloxy)-3$\alpha$-hydroxy 12,13-epoxytrichothec-9-ene), are major contaminants of foods and animal feeds and may cause illness in animals and humans. Acute parenteral administration of T-2 toxin to laboratory animals induces shock, hypothermia, and death from cardiovascular and respiratory failure. Wilson and coworkers (1982) reported that intravenous infusion of T-2 toxin in rats causes an initial decrease in heart rate and blood pressure, followed by tachycardia and hypertension and finally by bradycardia and hypotension. These actions may be related to a central effect on blood pressure and catecholamine release. Acute T-2 toxin exposure causes extensive destruction of myocardial capillaries, while repeated dosing promotes thickening of large coronary arteries.

**Vitamin D.** Vitamin D hypervitaminosis causes medial degeneration, calcification of the coronary arteries, and smooth muscle cell proliferation in laboratory animals. The toxic effects of vitamin D may be related to its structural similarity to 25-hydroxycholesterol, a potent vascular toxin.

A summary of selected agents and their vascular effects can be found in Tables 17-6 through 17-9.

**Table 17–6**
**Vasculotoxic Agents: Heavy Metals**

| AGENT | PROMINENT VASCULAR EFFECTS | ASSOCIATED DISEASES |
|---|---|---|
| Arsenic | Arteriosclerosis | Peripheral vascular disease; noncirrhotic portal hypertension; pulmonary edema |
| Beryllium | Decreased hepatic flow; hemorrhage | |
| Cadmium | Aortic endothelial damage; lesions to uterine endothelial cleft; effects on microcirculation | |
| Chromium (deficiency) | Atherosclerotic aortic plaques | Elevated serum cholesterol |
| Copper | | |
| (Chronic) | Acceleration of atherosclerosis | |
| (Acute) | Hypotension | |
| Copper (deficiency) | Aortic aneurysms | |
| Germanium | Hemorrhage; edema in lungs and gastrointestinal tract | |
| Indium | Hemorrhage and thrombosis in the kidney and liver | |
| Lead | Damage to endothelial cells with changes in blood-brain barrier permeability; changes in arterial elasticity; effects on ground substance; sclerosis of vessels in the kidney | Encephalopathy; hypertension |
| Mercury | Preglomerular vasoconstriction; glomerular immune complex deposits; lesions of the aorta; opening of blood-brain barrier | Glomerulonephritis |
| Selenium | Atherosclerotic plaques | |
| Thallium | Perivascular cellular infiltration in the brain | |

## VASCULOTOXIC RESPONSES IN VITAL ORGANS

The toxic responses of multiple organs can involve a significant microvascular component. In fact, the metabolic deficiency associated with disease states such as diabetes mellitus leads to disturbances in skin, kidney, lymphatic, and large vessel microcirculation.

### Brain

The microvasculature of the brain is the most important anatomic and physiological component of the blood-brain barrier. Brain capillary endothelial cells are responsible for the formation of the blood-brain barrier and thus are accessible to potentially harmful circulating compounds. Alterations in microvascular integrity can be precipitated by cerebral injuries, brain hypoxia, chronic alcohol exposure, and aging. The integrity of the blood-brain barrier relies on the structural and functional integrity of the endothelial cells and the tightness of the junctions between them. Anoxia and ischemia of the brain cause swelling of endothelial cells and opening of the junctions. Agents such as divalent cations, high concentrations of norepinephrine and serotonin, and chemically induced convulsions (e.g., metrazole) increase cerebrovascular permeability. A variety of cytolytic agents such as lipid solvents, cobra venom, surfactants, and high concentrations of sulfhydryl inhibitors can break down the blood-brain barrier by disrupting cell membranes and capillaries.

Alcohol administration for 30 min has been associated with dose-dependent vasoconstriction of rat cortical arterioles. Doses above 300 mg/dl cause reversible arteriolar spasms that often result in vessel rupture. Chronic alcohol consumption may activate the cytochrome P-450 ethanol oxidizing system and thus increase oxygen consumption. The production of free radicals arising from these oxidative processes could induce brain cell damage and compensatory vascularization.

Lead produces encephalopathy with brain edema by exerting its toxic effects on endothelial cells. These changes may actually precede those involving neurons and glia. Acute lead

**Table 17–7**
**Vasculotoxic Agents: Industrial and Environmental Agents**

| AGENT | PROMINENT VASCULAR EFFECTS | ASSOCIATED DISEASES |
|---|---|---|
| Allylamine | Bioactivation of parent compound by amine oxidase to acrolein and hydrogen peroxide, resulting in smooth muscle cell injury; intimal smooth muscle cell proliferation in larger arteries | Atherosclerosis |
| β-Aminopropionitrile | Damage to vascular connective tissue; aortic lesions; atheroma formation | Aneurysm |
| Boron | Hemorrhage; edema; increase in microvascular permeability of the lung | Pulmonary edema |
| Butadiene | Hemangiosarcomas in several organs | Cancer |
| Carbamylhydrazine | Tumors of pulmonary blood vessels | Cancer |
| Carbon disulfide | Microvascular effect on ocular fundus and retina; direct injury to endothelial cells; atheroma formation | Coronary vascular disease<br>Atherosclerosis |
| Chlorophenoxy herbicides | | Hypertension |
| Dimethylnitrosamine | Decreased hepatic flow; hemorrhage; necrosis | Occlusion of veins |
| Dinitrotoluenes | Deregulation of vascular smooth muscle cell proliferation | Atherosclerosis |
| 4-Fluoro-10-methyl-12-benzyanthracene | Pulmonary artery lesions; coronary vessel lesion | |
| Glycerol | Strong renal vasoconstriction | Acute renal failure |
| Hydrogen fluoride | Hemorrhage; edema in the lungs | Pulmonary edema |
| Hydrazinobenzoic acid | | Vascular tumors |
| Paraquat | Vascular damage in lungs and brain | Cerebral purpura |
| Polycyclic aromatic hydrocarbons | Deregulation of vascular smooth muscle cell proliferation; endothelial injury | Atherosclerosis; cancer |
| Pyrrolizidine alkaloids | Pulmonary vasculitis; damage to vascular smooth muscle cells; proliferation of endothelium and vasular connective tissue in liver | Pulmonary hypertension; hepatic veno-occlusive disease |
| Organophosphate pesticides | | Cerebral arteriosclerosis |
| T-2 toxin | Smooth muscle cell injury | Atherosclerosis |

**Table 17–8**
**Vasculotoxic Agents: Gases**

| AGENT | PROMINENT VASCULAR EFFECTS | ASSOCIATED DISEASES |
|---|---|---|
| Auto exhaust | Hemorrhage and infarct in cerebral hemispheres; atheroma formation in aorta | Atherosclerosis |
| Carbon monoxide | Damage to intimal layer; edema; atheroma formation | Atherosclerosis |
| Nitric oxide | Vacuolation of arteriolar endothelial cells; edema; thickening of alveolar-capillary membranes | Pulmonary edema |
| Oxygen | Vasoconstriction retinal damage; increased retinal vascular permeability edema; increased pulmonary vascular permeability edema | Blindness in neonate; shrinking of visual field in adults; edema |
| Ozone | Arterial lesion in the lung | Pulmonary edema |

**Table 17–9**
**Vasculotoxic Agents: Therapeutic Agents and Related Compounds**

| AGENT | PROMINENT VASCULAR EFFECTS | ASSOCIATED DISEASES |
|---|---|---|
| | *Antibiotic-Antimitotics* | |
| Cyclophosphamide | Lesions of pulmonary endothelial cells | |
| 5-Fluorodeoxyuridine | Gastrointestinal tract hemorrhage; portal vein thrombosis | |
| Gentamicin | Long-lasting vasoconstriction | Renal failure |
| | *Vasoactive Agents* | |
| Amphetamine | Cerebrovascular lesions secondary to drug abuse | Disseminated arterial lesions similar to periarteritis nodosa |
| Dihydroergotamine | Spasm of retinal vessels | |
| Ergonovine | Coronary artery spasm | Angina |
| Ergotamine | Vasospastic phenomena with and without thrombosis; medial atrophy | Gangrene of the peripheral tissues |
| Epinephrine | Peripheral arterial thrombi in hyperlipidemic rats | Participates in thrombogenesis |
| Histamine | Coronary spasm; damage to endothelial cells in hepatic portal vein | |
| Methysergide | Intimal proliferation; vascular occlusion of coronary arteries | Coronary artery disease |
| Nicotine | Alteration of cytoarchitecture of aortic endothelium; increase in microvilli | |
| Nitrites and nitrates | "Aging" of coronary arteries | Repeated vasodilation |
| Norepinephrine | Spasm of coronary artery; endothelial damage | |
| | *Metabolic Affectors* | |
| Alloxan | Microvascular retinopathy | Diabetes; blindness |
| Chloroquine | Retinopathy | |
| Fructose | Microvascular lesions in retina | Diabeteslike condition |
| Iodacetates | Vascular changes in retina | |
| | *Anticoagulants* | |
| Sodium warfarin, warfarin | Spinal hematoma; subdural hematoma; vasculitis | Uncontolled bleeding; hemorrhage |
| | *Radio Contrast Dyes* | |
| Metrizamide; metrizoate | Coagulation; necrosis in celiac and renal vasculature | |
| | *Cyanoacrylate Adhesives* | |
| 2-Cyano-acrylate-*n*-butyl | Granulation of arteries with fibrous masses | |
| Ethyl-2-cyanoacrylate | Degeneration of vascular wall with thrombosis | |
| Methyl-2-cyanoacrylate | Vascular necrosis | |
| | *Miscellaneous* | |
| Aminorex fumarate | Intimal and medial thickening of pulmonary arteries | Pulmonary hypertension |
| Aspirin | Endothelial damage; gastric erosion of small vessels; ischemic infarcts | |
| Cholesterol; oxygenated derivatives of cholesterol; noncholesterol steroids | Atheroma formation; arterial damage | Atherosclerosis |

**Table 17–9**
**Vasculotoxic Agents: Therapeutic Agents and Related Compounds *(Continued)***

| AGENT | PROMINENT VASCULAR EFFECTS | ASSOCIATED DISEASES |
|---|---|---|
| Homocysteine | Increase of vascular fragility; loss of endothelium; proliferation of smooth muscle cells; promotion of atheroma formation | Atherosclerosis |
| Oral contraceptives | Thrombosis in cerebral and peripheral vasculature | Thromboembolic disorders |
| Penicillamine | Vascular lesion in connective tissue matrix of arterial wall; glomerular immune complex deposits; inhibition of synthesis of vascular connective tissue | Glomerulonephritis |
| Talc and other silicates | Pulmonary arteriolar thrombosis; emboli | |
| Tetradecylsulfate sodium, | Sclerosis of veins | |
| Thromboxane $A_2$ | Extreme cerebral vasoconstriction | Cerebrovascular ischemia |

exposure may cause brain tissue swelling, edema, hemorrhage, necrosis, and altered capillary permeability. Autoradiographic studies in developing rats have suggested that brain capillary endothelial cells are a major site of lead accumulation.

## Heart

A high number of endogenous substances (e.g., epinephrine, angiotensin, histamine, thromboxane, and leukotrienes) cause constriction of the coronary arteries, which can result in myocardial hypoxia and death in patients with preexisting heart disease. Nitroglycerin has profound effects on the systemic as well as the cardiac microcirculation; its actions are mediated by stimulation of soluble guanylate cyclase in vascular smooth muscle cells. Long-term exposure of industrial workers to nitrates has been associated with withdrawal symptoms and sudden death from cardiovascular accidents.

Ethanol affects myocardial capillary density (Mall et al., 1982). Mall and associates have investigated ethanol-induced capillary proliferation as assessed by capillary density, capillary diameter, and endothelial cell nuclei in rats. After 3 weeks of ethanol administration, capillary density and diameter remained constant but capillary endothelial cell nuclei increased. After 5 months of ethanol exposure, there was increased density of myocardial capillaries with a decrease in capillary diameter.

## Kidney

Proper renal function requires intact glomerular function. Blood travels through renal arterioles into the glomerular capillary loops, resulting in high hydrostatic pressures in the glomerulus. Acute glomerulonephritis is characterized by proteinuria, edema, hematuria, renal failure, and hypertension. One or more of these phenomena may involve free radical formation. The mechanisms by which high cholesterol levels are thought to induce glomerular injury include enhanced mesangial deposition of lipoproteins, hyperlipidemia-induced proliferation of mesangial cells, enhanced glomerular macrophage activity, and alterations in the glomerular basement membrane. High serum cholesterol levels have been associated with increased renal vascular resistance in isolated kidneys (Kasiske et al., 1988).

Several nephrotoxins affect renal blood vessels and can induce constriction of renal arteries. Peroxidative damage induced by oxygen free radicals in rabbits is associated with capillary enlargement, subendothelial swelling, detachment of the endothelium from the basement membrane, mesangiolysis, and microaneurysms (Stratta et al., 1989). Mesanagiolysis is defined as dissolution of the mesangial matrix and degeneration of mesangial cells. A tubuloglomerular feedback control mediated by the vasoconstrictor effect of adenosine shuts down glomerular vessels after necrosis of the tubular epithelium. Nephropathies induced by cadmium, lead, and certain analgesics may produce systemic arterial hypertension by affecting one or more components of the renal blood pressure regulatory system. Structural changes in the renal vessels consisting of diffuse fibrosis of the capillaries have been reported after chronic exposure to cadmium in experimental animals. Immune complex deposits on the basement membranes of glomerular capillaries are characteristic of hypersensitivity reactions induced by many chemicals, including gold salts and *d*-penicillamine in humans and $HgCl_2$ in experimental animals.

## Liver

Anatomically, the liver is a conglomeration of several cell types, including hepatocytes and Kupffer's cells, along with an extensive vascular network composed of endothelial and smooth muscle cells. Acute exposure of humans to ethanol results in depressed reticuloendothelial function as well as alterations in the immune response. Elevated levels of circulating endotoxin have been observed in humans intoxicated with ethanol and during alcohol-related liver disease (Bode et al., 1987). The increase in circulating endotoxin in alcoholics has been attributed to a spillover of intestine-derived endotoxin that is no longer cleared by depressed Kupffer's cells. Studies have investigated the acute effects of ethanol on the hepatic microvasculature in mice (McCuskey et al., 1988). Ethanol given at a dose of 4 g/kg elicited hepatocellular damage, as evidenced by the formation of vacuoles and/or swollen organelles, vascular endothelial cellular swelling, and transient plugging of sinusoidal blood flow by leukocytes. These events parallel the intravascular events seen in sepsis and/or those seen upon the administration of tumor necrosis factor.

Hepatotoxins that produce hemorrhagic necrosis (e.g., dimethylnitrosamine) ultimately produce occlusion of veins. Pyrrolizidine alkaloids produce identical effects, resulting in hepatic veno-occlusive disease. The initial lesion consists of a proliferation of the endothelium in the small efferent veins followed by a proliferation of the vascular connective tissue, leading to occlusion of these veins. Oral contraceptives have produced thrombosis in the portal circulation that involve proliferation and thickening of the intima. A rare condition—peliosis—is induced by estrogenic and androgenic steroids. This lesion consists of islands of dilated portal sinusoids, and fatal bleeding may occur from their rupture. Endotoxins produce swelling of Kupffer's cells and endothelial cells as well as adhesion of platelets to sinusoid walls, all of which affect the microcirculation. Chronic hepatitis induced by oxyphenacetin or nitrofurantoin and cirrhosis induced by ethanol, arsenicals, or methotrexate lead to the development of portal hypertension. Tumors of the hepatic vasculature have been induced by thorium dioxide and vinyl chloride; hemangioendotheliomas and hemangiosarcomas, respectively, have been reported.

## Lungs

Pulmonary endothelial cells show ultrastructural evidence of damage after paraquat administration. Giri and associates (1981) found that intraperitoneal administration of paraquat to mice increases pulmonary vascular permeability and causes pulmonary edema. Monocrotaline is a carcinogenic alkaloid derived from the seeds of *Crotalaria spectabilis*. This alkaloid causes cellular hypertrophy and proliferation primarily of the pulmonary arterioles, although changes in the right ventricle of the heart and the larger vessels have also been noted. Monocrotaline causes medial thickening of pulmonary arteries and arterioles and pulmonary hypertension (Roth and Reindel, 1991). In [$^3$H]-thymidine labeling studies, monocrotaline-induced thickening of medial and advential layers was associated with enhanced labeling of rat pulmonary arterial smooth muscle, fibroblasts, and endothelial cells (Meyrick and Reid, 1982). Enhanced thymidine uptake is also observed in endothelial cells from alveolar capillaries.

Alveolar capillary fragility and permeability changes result in pulmonary edema, often after inhalation of irritant gases. Excessive intravenous infusion of fluid is the most frequent cause of iatrogenic pulmonary edema, especially after the replacement of blood loss by electrolyte solutions. Opiates (heroin, methadone) can produce delayed pulmonary edema after intravenous administration; neurogenic alterations of capillary permeability are implicated. Drug addicts who self-administer dissolved tablets intravenously develop pulmonary embolism and thrombosis because of the talc vehicle. Pulmonary thromboembolism has been associated with the use of high doses of oral contraceptive estrogens in women who are predisposed to thrombosis.

# REFERENCES


Ahmed SS, Regan TJ: Cardiotoxicity of acute and chronic ingestion of various alcohols, in Acosta D (ed.): *Cardiovascular Toxicology*, 2d ed. New York: Raven Press, 1992, pp 345–407.

Albert RE, Vanderlaan M, Burns FJ, Nishiizumi M: Effects of carcinogens on chicken atherosclerosis. *Cancer Res* 37:2232–2235, 1977.

Auerbach O, Carter HW: Smoking and the heart, in Bristow MR (ed): *Drug-Induced Heart Disease*. Amsterdam: Elsevier, North-Holland, 1980, pp 359–376.

Batuman V, Landy E, Maesaka JK, Wedeen RP: Contribution of lead to hypertension with renal impairment. *N Engl J Med* 309:17–21, 1983.

Benditt EP, Benditt JM: Evidence for a monoclonal origin of human atherosclerotic plaques. *Proc Natl Acad Sci USA* 70:1753–1756, 1973.

Bode C, Kugler V, Bode JC: Endotoxemia in patients with alcoholic and non-alcoholic cirrhosis and in subjects with no evidence of chronic liver disease following acute alcohol excess. *J Hepatol* 4:8–14, 1987.

Bolli R: Oxygen-derived free radicals and postischemic myocardial dysfunction ("stunned myocardium"). *J Am Coll Cardiol* 12:239–249, 1988.

Boor PJ, Hysmith RM, Sanduja R: A role for a new vascular enzyme in the metabolism of xenobiotic amines. *Circ Res* 66(1):249–252, 1990.

Boor PJ, Moslen MJ, Reynolds ES: Allylamine cardiotoxicity: I. Sequence of pathologic events. *Toxicol Appl Pharmacol* 50:581–592, 1979.

Bosnjak ZJ: Cardiac effects of anesthetics, in Blanck TJJ, Wheeler DM (eds): *Mechanisms of Anesthetic Action in Skeletal, Cardiac, and Smooth Muscle*. New York: Plenum Press, 1991, pp 91–96.

Bull HA, Pittilo RM, Blow DJ, et al: The effects of nicotine on $PGI_2$ production by rat aortic endothelium. *Thromb Haemost* 54(2):472–474, 1985.

Carafoli E: Intracellular calcium homeostasis. *Annu Rev Biochem* 56: 395–433, 1987.

Chacon E, Acosta D: Mitochodrial regulation of superoxide by $Ca^{2+}$: An alternate mechanism for the cardiotoxicity of doxorubicin. *Toxicol Appl Pharmacol* 107:117–128, 1991.

Chacon E, Ulrich R, Acosta D: A digitized-fluorescence-imaging study of mitochondrial $Ca^{2++}$ increase by doxorubicin in cardiac myocytes. *Biochem J* 281: 871–878, 1992.

Cox LR, Ramos K: Allylamine-induced phenotypic modulation of aortic smooth muscle cells. *J Exp Path* 71:11–18, 1990.

Dent JG, Schnell SR, Guest D: Metabolism of 2,4-dinitrotoluene in rat hepatic microsomes and cecal flora, in Snyder R, Park DV, Kocsis JJ, et al (eds): *Proceedings of the Second International Symposium on Biologically Reactive Intermediates: Chemical Mechanisms and Biologic Effects*. New York: Plenum Press, 1981, pp 431–436.

Dhalla NS, Yates JC, Naimark B, et al: Cardiotoxicity of catecholamines and related agents, in Acosta D (ed): *Cardiovascular Toxicology*, 2d ed. New York: Raven Press, 1992, pp 239–282.

Doroshow JH: Doxorubicin-induced cardiac toxicity. *New Eng J Med* 324:843–845, 1991.

Fantel AG, Person RE, Burroughs-Gleim CJ, Mackler B: Direct embryotoxicity of cocaine in rats: Effects on mitochondrial activity, cardiac function, and growth and development in vitro. *Teratology* 42:35–43, 1990.

Ferrario JB, DeLeon IR, Tracy RE: Evidence for toxic anthropogenic chemicals in human thrombogenic coronary plaques. *Arch Environ Contam Toxicol* 14:529–534, 1985.

Fleckenstein A, Janke J, Doring HJ, Pachinger O: Calcium overload as the determinant factor in the production of catecholamine-induced myocardial lesions, in Bajusz E, Rona G (eds): *Recent Advances in Studies on Cardiac Structure and Metabolism*. Baltimore: University Park Press, 1973, pp 455–460.

Giri SN, Hollinger MA, Schiedt MJ: The effects of paraquat and superoxide dismutase on pulmonary vascular permeability and edema in mice. *Arch Environ Health* 36:149–154, 1981.

Gotzsche LS, Pederson EM: Dose-dependent cardiotoxic effect of amiodarone in cardioplegic solutions correlates with loss of dihydropyridine binding sites: In vitro evidence for a potentially lethal interaction with procaine. *J Cardiovasc Pharmacol* 23:13–23, 1994.

Gross JL, Moscatelli D, Rifkin DB: Increased capillary endothelial cell protease activity in response to angiogenic stimuli in vitro. *Proc Natl Acad Sci USA* 80:2623–2627, 1983.

Havlin KA: Cardiotoxicity of anthracyclines and other antineoplastic agents, in Acosta D (ed): *Cardiovascular Toxicology*, 2d ed. New York: Raven Press, 1992, pp 143–164.

Hines CH, Kodama JK, Guzman RJ, Loquvam GS: The toxicity of allylamines. *Arch Environ Health* 1:343–352, 1960.

Hino N, Ochi R, Yanagisawa T: Inhibition of the slow inward current and the time-dependent outward current of mammalian ventricular muscle by gentamicin. *Pflugers Arch* 394:243–249, 1982.

Houtman JP: Prolonged low-level cadmium intake and atherosclerosis. *Sci Total Environ* 138:31–36, 1993.

Iakushkin VV, Baldenov GN, Tertov VV, Orekhov AN: Atherogenic properties of phenothiazine drugs manifesting in cultured cells of the human aortic intima. *Kardiologiia* 32:66–68, 1992.

Kasiske BL, O'Donnell MP, Cleary MP, Keane WF: Treatment of hyperlipidemia reduces glomerular injury in obese Zucker rats. *Kidney Int* 33:667–672, 1988.

Keller RS, Parker JL, Adams HR: Cardiovascular toxicity of antibacterial antibiotics, in Acosta D (ed): *Cardiovascular Toxicology*, 2d ed. New York: Raven Press, 1992, pp 165–195.

Kloner RA, Przyklenk K: Reperfusion injury to the heart. Is it a real phenomenon? in Acosta D (ed): *Cardiovascular Toxicology*, 2d ed. New York: Raven Press, 1992, pp 131–140.

Kutzman RS, Wehner RW, Haber SB: Selected responses of hypertension-sensitive and resistant rats to inhaled acrolein. *Toxicology* 31:53–65, 1984.

Lalich JJ: Coronary artery hyalinosis in rats fed allylamine. *Exp Mol Pathol* 10:14–26, 1969.

Lemasters JJ, Bond JM, Harper IS, et al: The pH paradox in reperfusion injury to heart cells, in Lemasters JJ, Oliver C (eds): *Cell Biology of Trauma*. Boca Raton, FL: CRC Press, 1995, pp 149–162.

Levine ES, Friedman HS, Griffith OW, et al: Cardiac cell toxicity by 4-hydroperoxycyclophosphamide is modulated by glutathione. *Cardiovasc Res* 27:1248–1253, 1993.

Mall G, Mattfeldt T, Rieger P, Volk B, et al: Morphometric analysis of the rabbit myocardium after chronic ethanol feeding-early capillary changes. *Basic Cardiol* 77:57–67, 1982.

Marcillat O, Zhang Y, Davies KJA: Oxidative and non-oxidative mechanisms in the inactivation of cardiac mitochondrial electron transport chain components by doxorubicin. *Biochem J* 259:181–189, 1989.

McCuskey RS, Urbaschek R, McCuskey PA, Urbaschek B: Microvascular responses to tumor necrosis factor. *FASEB J*, 2:A1873, 1988.

McManus BM, Toth B, Patil KD: Aortic rupture and aortic smooth muscle tumors in mice: Induction by p-hydrazinobenzoic acid hydrochloride of the cultivated mushroom Agaricus bisporus. *Lab Invest* 57(1):78–85, 1987.

Meyrick BO, Reid LM: Crotalaria-induced pulmonary hypertension. *Am J Pathol* 106:84–94, 1982.

Miller RA, Boorman GA: Morphology of neoplastic lesions induced by 1,3-butadiene in B6C3$F_1$ mice. *Environ Health Perspect* 86:37–48, 1990.

Nakaki T, Nakayama M, Yamamoto S, Kato R: $\alpha_1$-Adrenergic stimulation and $\beta_2$-adrenergic inhibition of DNA synthesis in vascular smooth muscle cells. *Mol Pharmacol* 37:30–36, 1989.

Olson RD, Mushlin PS: Doxorubicin cardiotoxicity: Analysis of prevailing hypothesis. *FASEB J* 4:3076–3086, 1990.

Opie L: Heart cells and organelles, in Opie L (ed): *The Heart*. New York: Harcourt Brace Jovanovich, 1986a, pp 15–29.

Opie L: The mechanism of myocardial contraction, in Opie L (ed): *The Heart*. New York: Harcourt Brace Jovanovich, 1986b, pp 98–107.

Ou X, Ramos KS: Proliferative responses of quail aortic smooth muscle cells to benzo[a]pyrene: Implications in PAH-induced atherogenesis. *Toxicology* 74:243–258, 1992a.

Ou X, Ramos KS: Modulation of aortic protein phosphorylation by benzo[a]pyrene: Implications in PAH-induced atherogenesis. *J Biochem Toxicol* 7:147–154, 1992b.

Ou X, Weber TJ, Chapkin RS, Ramos KS: Interference with protein kinase C-related signal transduction in vascular smooth muscle cells by benzo(a)pyrene. *Arch Biochem Biophys* 760:354–356, 1995.

Parrish AR, Ramos KS: Osteopontin mRNA expression in a chemically-induced model of atherogenesis. *Proc NY Acad Sci* 760:354–356, 1995.

Peng SK, French WJ, Pelikan PCD: Direct cocaine cardiotoxicity demonstrated by endomyocardial biopsy. *Arch Pathol Lab Med* 113: 842–845, 1989.

Penn A, Snyder C: Arteriosclerotic plaque development is "promoted" by polynuclear aromatic hydrocarbons. *Carcinogenesis* 9(12): 2185–2189, 1988.

Perry MH, Erlanger MW, Gustafsson TO, Perry EF: Reversal of cadmium-induced hypertension by D-myo-inositol-1,2,6-triphosphate. *J Toxicol Environ Health* 28:151–159, 1989.

Powis G: Free radical formation by antitumor quinones. *Free Radic Biol Med* 6:63–101, 1989.

Ramos KS, Bowes RC III, Ou X, Weber TJ: Responses of vascular smooth muscle cells to toxic insult: Cellular and molecular perspectives for environmental toxicants. *J Toxicol Environ Health* 43:419–440, 1994.

Ramos K, Cox LR: Primary cultures of rat aortic endothelial and smooth muscle cells: I. An in vitro model to study xenobiotic-induced vascular cytotoxicity. *In Vitro Cell Dev Biol* 21:495–504, 1987.

Ramos K, Grossman SL, Cox LR: Allylamine-induced vascular toxicity in vitro: Prevention by semicarbizide-sensitive amine oxidase inhibitors. *Toxicol Appl Pharmacol* 96:61–71, 1988.

Ramos K, McMahon KK, Alipui C, Demick D: Modulation of smooth muscle cell proliferation by dinitrotoluene, in Witmer CM, Snyder RR, Jollow DJ, et al (eds): *Biologic Reductive Intermediates.* New York: Plenum Press,vol V, 1990, pp 805–807.

Ramos KS, Thurlow CH: Comparative cytotoxic responses of cultured avian and rodent aortic smooth muscle cells to allylamine. *J Toxicol Environ Health* 40:61–76, 1993.

Ramos KS, Weber TJ, Liau G: Altered protein secretion and extracellular matrix deposition is associated with the proliferative phenotype induced by allylamine in aortic smooth muscle cells. *Biochem J* 289:57–63, 1993.

Redetzki JE, Guiswold KE, Nopajaroonsei C, Redetzki HM: Amelioration of cardiotoxic effects of alcohol by vitamin E. *J Toxicol Clin Toxicol* 20:319–331, 1983.

Ribiere C, Hininger I, Rouach H, Nordmann R: Effects of chronic ethanol administration on free radical defence in rat myocardium. *Biochem Pharmacol* 44: 1495–1500, 1992.

Rockhold RW: Cardiovascular toxicity of anabolic steroids. *Annu Rev Pharmacol Toxicol* 33: 497–520, 1993.

Rosenman KD: Environmentally related disorders of the cardiovascular system. *Med Clin North Am* 74:361–375, 1990.

Ross R: The pathogenesis of atherosclerosis, a perspective for the 1990s. *Nature* 362:801–809, 1993.

Roth RA, Reindel JF: Lung vascular injury from monocrotaline pyrrole, a putative hepatic metabolite. *Adv Exp Med Biol* 283:477, 1991.

Sandusky G E, Vodicnik MJ, Tamura RN: Cardiovascular and adrenal proliferative lesions in Fischer 344 rats induced by long-term treatment with type III phosphodiesterase inhibitors (positive inotropic agents), isomazole and indolidan. *Fundam Appl Toxicol* 16:198–209, 1991.

Scarpa A: Transport across mitochondrial membranes, in Giebisch G, Tosteson DC, Ussing HH (eds): *Membrane Transport in Biology.* New York: Springer, 1979, pp 263–355.

Sherwood L: Cardiac physiology, in Sherwood L (ed): *Human Physiology*. Minneapolis/St. Paul: West Publishing, 1993, pp 258–298.

Sies H: Oxidative stress: From basic research to clinical application. *Am J Med* 91:315–385, 1991.

Simons FER: The therapeutic index of newer $H_1$-receptor antagonists. *Clin Exp Allergy* 24:707–723, 1994.

Simpson PJ, Lucchesi BR: Free radicals and myocardial ischemia and reperfusion injury. *J Clin Lab Med* 110:13–30, 1987.

Solem LE, Henry TR, Wallace KB: Disruption of mitochondrial calcium homeostasis following chronic doxorubicin administration. *Toxicol Appl Pharmacol* 129:214–222, 1994.

Sperelakis N: Chemical agent actions on ion channels and electrophysiology of the heart, in Acosta D (ed): *Cardiovascular Toxicology*, 2d ed. New York: Raven Press, 1992, pp 283–338.

Stolley PD, Strom BL, Sartwell PE: Oral contraceptives and vascular disease. *Epidem Rev* 11:241–243, 1989.

Stratta P, Canavese C, Mazzucco G, et al: Mesangiolysis and endothelial lesions due to peroxidative damage in rabbits. *Nephron* 51:250–256, 1989.

Tomera JF, Harakal C: Mercury and lead-induced contraction of aortic smooth muscle in vitro. *Arch Int Pharmacody Ther* 283:295–302, 1986.

Wald N, Howard S: Smoking, carbon monoxide and disease. *Ann Occup Hyg* 18:1–14, 1975.

Wei EP, Christman CW, Kontos HA, Povlishock JT: Effects of oxygen radicals on cerebral arterioles. *Am J Physiol* 248:H157–H162, 1985.

Wilson CA, Everard DM, Schoental R: Blood pressure changes and cardiovascular lesions found in rats given T-2 toxin, a trichothecene secondary metabolite of certain Fusarium microfungi. *Toxicol Lett* 10:35–40, 1982.

Wilson SK: Role of oxygen-derived free radicals in acute angiotensin II-induced hypertensive vascular disease in the rat. *Circ Res* 66:722, 1990.

Zakhari S: Cardiovascular toxicology of halogenated hydrocarbons and other solvents, in Acosta D (ed): *Cardiovascular Toxicology*. New York: Raven Press, 1992, pp 409–454.

Zwijsen RML, van Kleef EM, Alink GM: A comparative study on the metabolic activation of 3,4-benzo(a)pyrene to mutagens by aortic smooth muscle cells of rat and rabbit. *Mutat Res* 230:111–117, 1990.

CHAPTER 18

# TOXIC RESPONSES OF THE SKIN

*Robert H. Rice and David E. Cohen*

As the body's first line of defense against external insult, the skin's enormous surface area (1.5–2 $m^2$) is exposed routinely to chemical agents and may inadvertently serve as a portal of entry for topical contactants. Recognizing the potential hazards of skin exposure, the National Institute of Occupational Safety and Health (NIOSH) characterized skin disease as one of the most pervasive occupational health problems in the United States. In 1982 NIOSH placed skin disease in the top ten leading work-related diseases based on frequency, severity, and the potential for prevention. Data from the Bureau of Labor Statistics indicate that skin disease attributed to workplace exposures accounts for more than 30 percent of all reported occupational disease. Incidence data from 1990 indicate a rate of 7.9 cases per 10,000 or about 61,000 new cases per year. Exposures in the agricultural and manufacturing industries were responsible for the greatest volume of disease, with incidence rates of 86 and 41/10,000, respectively. Skin conditions resulting from exposures to consumer products or occupational illnesses not resulting in lost work time are poorly recorded and tracked. Hence the incidence of such skin diseases is grossly underestimated.

## SKIN AS A BARRIER

A large and highly accessible human organ, the skin protects the body against external insults to maintain internal homeostasis. Its biological sophistication allows it to perform a myriad of functions above and beyond that of a suit of armor. Physiologically, the skin participates directly in thermal, electrolyte, hormonal, metabolic, and immune regulation, without which a human would perish. Rather than merely repelling noxious physical agents, the skin may react to them with a variety of defensive mechanisms that serve to prevent internal or widespread cutaneous damage. If an insult is severe or sufficiently intense to overwhelm the protective function of the skin, acute or chronic injury becomes readily manifest in a variety of ways (Lever and Schaumburg-Lever, 1990). The specific presentation depends on a variety of intrinsic and extrinsic factors including body site, duration of exposure, and other environmental conditions (Table 18-1).

### Skin Histology

The skin consists of two major components—the outer epidermis and the underlying dermis which are separated by a basement membrane (Fig. 18-1). The junction ordinarily is not flat but has an undulating appearance (rete ridges). In addition, epidermal appendages (hair follicles, sebaceous glands, and eccrine glands) span the epidermis and are embedded in the dermis. In thickness, the dermis comprises approximately 90 percent of the skin and has largely a supportive function. It has a high content of collagen and elastin secreted by scattered fibroblasts, thus providing the skin with elastic properties. Separating the dermis from underlying tissues is a layer of adipocytes, whose accumulation of fat has a cushioning action. The blood supply to the epidermis originates in the capillaries located in the rete ridges at the dermal–epidermal junction. Capillaries also supply the bulbs of the hair follicles and the secretory cells of the eccrine (sweat) glands. The ducts from these glands carry a dilute salt solution to the surface of the skin, where its evaporation provides cooling.

The interfollicular epidermis is a stratified squamous epithelium consisting primarily of keratinocytes. These cells are tightly attached to each other by desmosomes and to the basement membrane by hemidesmosomes. Melanocytes are interspersed among the basal cells and distributed sparsely in the dermis with occasional concentrations beneath the basal lamina and in the papilla of hair follicles. In the epidermis, these cells are stimulated by ultraviolet light to produce melanin granules. The granules are extruded and taken up by the surrounding epidermal cells, which thereby become pigmented. Migrating through the epidermis are Langerhans' cells, which are important participants in the skin's immune response to foreign agents.

Keratinocytes of the basal layer comprise the germinative compartment. When a basal cell divides, one of the progeny detaches from the basal lamina and migrates outward. As cells move toward the skin surface, they undergo a remarkable program of terminal differentiation. They gradually express new protein markers and accumulate keratin proteins, from which the name of this cell type is derived. The keratins form insoluble intermediate filaments accounting for nearly 40 percent of the total cell protein in the spinous layer. At the granular layer, the cells undergo a striking morphological transformation, becoming flattened and increasing in volume nearly 40-fold. Lipid granules fuse with the plasma membrane, replacing the aqueous environment in the intercellular space with their contents. Meanwhile, the plasma membranes of these cells become permeable, resulting in the loss of their reducing environment and consequently in extensive disulfide bonding among keratin proteins. Cell organelles are degraded, while a protein envelope is synthesized immediately beneath the plasma membrane. The membrane is altered characteristically by the loss of phospholipid and the addition of sphingolipid.

This program of terminal differentiation, beginning as keratinocytes leave the basal layer, produces the outermost layer of the skin, the stratum corneum. No longer viable, the mature cells (called *corneocytes*) are approximately 80-percent keratin in content. They are gradually shed from the surface and replaced from beneath. The process typically

**Table 18–1**
**Factors Influencing Cutaneous Responses***

| VARIABLE | COMMENT |
|---|---|
| Body site | |
| Palms/Soles | Thick stratum corneum—good physical barrier |
| | Common site of contact with chemicals |
| | Occlusion with protective clothing |
| Intertriginous areas (axillae, groin, neck, finger webs, umbilicus, genitalia) | Moist, occluded areas |
| | Chemical trapping |
| | Enhanced percutaneous absorption |
| Face | Exposed frequently |
| | Surface lipid interacts with hydrophobic substances† |
| | Chemicals frequently transferred from hands |
| Eyelids | Poor barrier function—thin epidermis |
| | Sensitive to irritants |
| Postauricular region | Chemical trapping |
| | Occlusion |
| Scalp | Chemical trapping |
| | Hair follicles susceptible to metabolic damage‡ |
| Predisposing cutaneous illnesses | |
| Atopic dermatitis | Increased sensitivity to irritants |
| | Impaired barrier function |
| Psoriasis | Impaired barrier function |
| Genetic factors | Predisposition to cutaneous skin disorders |
| | Variation in sensitivity to irritants |
| | Susceptibility to contact sensitization |
| Temperature | Vasodilation—improved percutaneous absorption |
| | Increased sweating—trapping |
| Humidity | Increased sweating—trapping |
| Season | Variation in relative humidity |
| | Chapping and wind-related skin changes |

* Adapted from Fitzpatrick TB et al. (1993).
† Downing DT et al.(1993).
‡ Lavker RM et al. (1993).

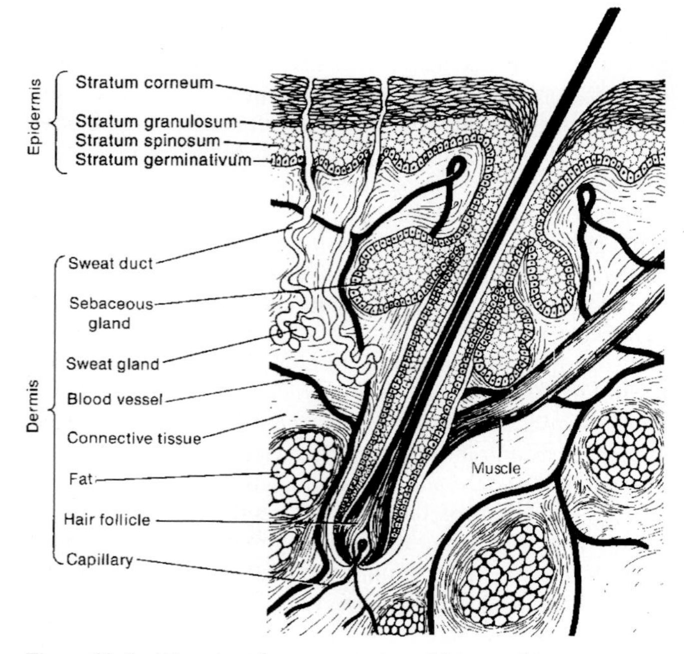


*Figure 18–1. Diagram of a cross-section of human skin.*

takes 2 weeks for basal cells to reach the stratum corneum and another 2 weeks to be shed from the surface. In the skin disease psoriasis, the migration of cells to the surface is nearly tenfold faster than normal, resulting in a stratum corneum populated by cells that are not completely mature. In instances in which the outer layer is deficient due to disease or physical or chemical trauma, the barrier to the environment that the skin provides is inferior to that provided by normal, healthy skin.

## Percutaneous Absorption

Until the turn of the century, the skin was believed to provide an impervious barrier to exogenous substances. Gradually, the ability of substances to penetrate the skin, though this process generally is very slow, became appreciated. During the past 50 years, the stratum corneum has been recognized as the primary barrier (Scheuplein and Blank, 1971). Diseases (e.g., psoriasis) or other conditions (e.g., abrasion, wounding) in which this barrier is compromised can permit greatly increased uptake of poorly permeable substances as does removal of the stratum corneum by tape stripping (Shaw et al., 1991). The viable layer of epidermis provides a much less effective barrier, because hydrophilic agents readily diffuse into the intercellular water, while hydrophobic agents can partition into cell membranes, and each can diffuse readily to the blood supply in the rete ridges of the dermis.

Probably the best-known biological membrane for this purpose, the stratum corneum prevents water loss to underlying tissues by dehydration. Its hydrophobic character reflects the lipid content of the intercellular space, approximately 15 percent of the total volume (Elias, 1992). The lipids, a major component being sphingolipids, have a high content of long-chain ceramides, removal of which seriously compromises barrier function as measured by transepidermal water loss (Grubauer et al., 1989). The stratum corneum ordinarily is hydrated (typically 20 percent water), the moisture residing in corneocyte protein, but it can take up a great deal more water upon prolonged immersion, thereby reducing the effectiveness of the barrier to agents with a hydrophilic character. Indeed, occlusion of the skin with plastic wrap, permitting the retention of perspiration underneath, is a commonly employed technique to enhance uptake of agents applied to the skin surface.

Finding the rate at which the uptake of agents through the skin occurs is important for estimating the consequences of exposure to many agents we encounter in the environment. Indeed, a regulatory strategy permitting bathing in water considered barely unfit for drinking was revised when it was realized that exposure from dermal/inhalation uptake during bathing could be comparable to that from drinking 2 liters of the water (Brown et al., 1984). Uptake through the skin is now incorporated in pharmacokinetic modeling to estimate potential risks from exposures (McKone, 1993). The degree of uptake depends upon the details of exposure conditions, being proportional to solute concentration (assuming it is dilute), time, and the amount of skin surface exposed. In addition, two intrinsic factors contribute to the absorption rate of a given compound: its hydrophobicity, which affects its ability to partition into epidermal lipid, and its rate of diffusion through this barrier. A measure of the first property is the commonly used octanol/water partitioning ratio ($K_{ow}$). An alternative has been to measure the uptake from aqueous solution into powdered human stratum corneum (Wester et al., 1987). This is particularly relevant for exposure to contaminated water, such as occurs when bathing or swimming. However, partitioning of an agent into the skin is greatly affected by its solubility in or adhesion to the medium in which it is applied (including soil). The second property is an inverse function of molecular weight (MW) or, more accurately, of molecular volume (Potts et al., 1992). Thus, hydrophobic agents of low molecular weight permeate the skin better than those of high molecular weight or those that are hydrophilic.

Although only small amounts of agents may penetrate the stratum corneum, those of high potency may still be very dangerous. For example, the hydrophobic organophosphorus pesticide parathion can be lethal by skin contact. Considerable empirical information has been collected on some compounds of especial interest (including pharmaceuticals, pesticides, and pollutants) for use in quantifying these relationships. From such information, relations can be obtained for skin penetration ($P_{cw}$) using empirically derived constants ($C_1$, $C_2$, $C_3$) that have the form shown below (Potts and Guy, 1992).

$$\log P_{cw} = C_1 - C_2(MW) + C_3 \log K_{ow}$$

Such relations describe steady-state conditions, in which an agent leaves the stratum corneum at the same rate it enters. Because rates of diffusion are slow, saturation of the stratum corneum provides a depot, leading to continued penetration into the body for relatively long time periods after external exposure to an agent stops.

Diffusion through the epidermis is considerably faster at some anatomical sites than others. A list in order of decreasing permability gives the following hierarchy: foot sole > scrotum > palm > forehead > abdomen (Scheuplein and Blank, 1971). Under ordinary conditions, absorption through the epidermal appendages is generally neglected, despite the ability of agents to bypass the stratum corneum by this route, because the combined appendageal surface area is such a small fraction of the total available for uptake. However, because loading of the stratum corneum is slow (Cleek and Bunge, 1993), penetration through the appendages can constitute an appreciable fraction of the total for short exposures. In some cases, the effects of appendages can even be dominant. For instance, benzo(a)pyrene penetrates the skin of haired mice severalfold faster than that of hairless strains (Kao et al., 1988).

**Transdermal Drug Delivery.** The ability of the stratum corneum to serve as a reservoir for exogenously applied agents is well illustrated by the recent development of methods to exploit this property for the delivery of pharmaceuticals. Application of drugs to the skin can produce systemic effects, a phenomenon observed fortuitously before the ability of the skin to serve as a delivery system was appreciated. For example, many years ago estrogen creams applied to the scalp proved ineffective in alleviating male pattern baldness, but they did induce lipid accumulation in estrogen-responsive tissues elsewhere in the body. Specially designed patches are currently in use to deliver estradiol, nitroglycerin, scopolamine, clonidine, fentanyl, and nicotine for therapeutic purposes, and others are under development. The advantages of this approach include providing a steady dosage for extended periods (typically 1–7 days), avoiding large peak plasma concentrations from loading doses, and preventing first-pass removal by the liver, if that occurs with oral dosing. The contrast in plasma concentration kinetics between different methods of delivery is particularly evident for agents that are rapidly metabolized, such as nitroglycerin, which has a half-life of minutes (Ledger et al., 1992).

**Measurements of Penetration.** For many purposes, including risk assessment and pharmaceutical design, the most useful subject for experimentation is human skin. Volunteers are dosed, plasma concentrations are measured at suitable intervals, and amounts excreted from the body are estimated. For most compounds, however, this option is not available. Excised split-thickness skin can be employed in special diffusion chambers, though care is needed to preserve the viability of the living layer of epidermis. The agent is removed from the underside by a fluid into which it partitions, thereby permitting continued penetration instead of reverse diffusion. The phamacokinetic approach with intact subjects is most commonly employed with experimental animals. Without verification using human skin, such measurements are subject to large uncertainties due to species differences in density of epidermal appendages, stratum corneum properties (e.g., thickness, lipid composition), and biotransformation rates. To simplify determination of penetration kinetics, skin flaps may be employed and the capillary blood flow monitored to measure penetration. For this purpose, pig skin has particular utility (Riviere, 1993). A promising variation minimizing species differences is to use skin grafts on experimental animals for these measurements. Human skin persists well on athymic mice and retains its normal barrier properties (Kreuger and Pershing, 1993).

## Biotransformation

The ability of the skin to metabolize agents that diffuse through it contributes to its barrier function. This influences the potential biological activity of xenobiotics and topically applied drugs, leading to their degradation or their activation as skin sensitizers or carcinogens. To this end, the epidermis and pilosebaceous units are the most relevant and, indeed, are the major sources of such activity in the skin. On a body-weight basis, phase I metabolism in this organ usually is only a small fraction (≈2 percent) of that in the liver, but its importance should not be underestimated. For example, when the epidermis of the neonatal rat is treated with benzo(a)pyrene or Aroclor 1254, the arylhydrocarbon hydroxylase (P450) activity in the skin can exceed 20 percent of that in the whole body (Mukhtar and Bickers, 1981). As illustrated in this example, cytochrome P4501A1 is inducible in the epidermis by agents that are inducers in other tissues—TCDD (tetrachlorodibenzo-*p*-dioxin), polycyclic aromatic hydrocarbons, PCBs (polychlorinated biphenyls), and crude coal tar, which is used in dermatological therapy (Chap. 6). Thus, exposure to such inducers could influence skin biotransformation and even sensitize epidermal cells to other agents that are not good inducers themselves, a phenomenon observable in cell culture (Walsh et al., 1992).

Biotransformation of a variety of compounds in the skin has been detected, including arachidonic acid derivatives, steroids, retinoids, and 2-amino-anthracene, suggesting that multiple P450 activities are expressed. Evidence has been presented for P4502A1 and 2B1 in rat skin, for example, using specific substrates, immunoblotting of the protein, and polymerase chain reaction techniques (Pham et al., 1989; Mukhtar, 1992). These and other P450s are expressed in murine skin, and at least some of them are stimulated by glucocorticoids, commonly used therapeutic agents on human skin (Jugert et al., 1994). The TCDD-inducible isozyme P4501B1 has been reported in human keratinocytes and is expressed in a variety of other tissues as well (Sutter et al., 1994). Species differences are apparent in the amounts of P450 activities detectable. For example, measured ethoxycoumarin-O-deethylase activity is 20-fold higher in mouse than human (or rat) skin. Differences of such magnitude help rationalize the observation that the rate of penetration of ethoxycoumarin is sufficient to saturate its metabolism in some species (e.g., the human) but not in others (e.g., the mouse or guinea pig) (Storm et al., 1990).

Enzymes participating in phase II metabolism are expressed in skin. For example, multiple forms of epoxide hydrolase and UDG glucuronosyl transferase have been detected in human and rodent skin (Pham et al., 1989; Pham et al., 1990). In general, this activity occurs at a much lower rate than observed in the liver, but exceptions are evident, as in the case of quinone reductase (Khan et al., 1987). Human and rodent skin exhibit qualitatively similar phase II reactions, but rodent skin often has a higher level of activity. An additional consideration is that different species express different relative amounts of the various isozymes, which could alter their target specificities or degree of responsiveness. Glutathione transferase, for instance, catalyzes the reaction of glutathione with exogenous nucleophiles or provides intracellular transport of bound compounds in the absence of a reaction. It also facilitates the reaction of glutathione with endogenous products of arachidonate lipoxygenation (leukotrienes) to yield mediators of anaphylaxis and chemotaxis, which are elements of the inflammatory response in the skin. Of the three major transferase forms characterized in the liver, the major form in the skin of humans and rodents is the $\pi$ isozyme (Chap. 6). Human skin also expresses the $\alpha$ isozyme, while rat and mouse skin express the $\mu$ isozyme and, in much smaller amounts, the $\alpha$ isozyme (Raza et al., 1992).

A variety of other metabolic enzyme activites have also been detected in human epidermal cells, including sulfatases, $\beta$-glucuronidase, and reductases (Pham et al., 1990). The intercellular region of the stratum corneum has catabolic activities (e.g., proteases, lipases, glycosidases, phosphatase) supplied by the lamellar bodies along with their characteristic lipid (Elias, 1992). The influence of hydroxysteroid dehydrogenases and microsomal reductase activities during percutaneous absorption is evident in studies on mouse skin in organ culture. In one study (Kao and Hall, 1987), 8 hours after topical application of testosterone, 59 percent of the permeated steroid was collected unchanged and the rest was transformed into metabolites. In parallel, estrone was converted substantially to estradiol (67 percent), while only 23 percent was collected as the parent compound. By contrast, estradiol was metabolized to a much lower extent (21 percent).

# CONTACT DERMATITIS

Of all occupational skin disease, contact dermatitis accounts for over 90 percent of reported causes (American Academy of Dermatology, 1994). As the single most prevalent occupational skin disease, it is one of the most important occupational illnesses affecting American workers. It comprises two distinct inflammatory processes caused by adverse exposure of the skin, *irritant dermatitis* and *allergic contact dermatitis.* These syndromes usually have indistinguishable clinical characteristics. Classically, erythema (redness), induration (thickening and firmness), scaling (flaking), and vesiculation (blistering) are present on areas directly contacting the chemical agent. Paraffin-embedded biopsies from affected sites reveal a mixed-cell inflammatory infiltrate of lymphocytes and eosinophils and the hallmark finding of spongiosis (intercellular edema). Unfortunately, these histopathologic features are not sufficient to differentiate allergic from irritant contact dermatitis, atopic dermatitis, or certain other common syndromes. Because their etiology is different, as supported by subtle but clear differences in the inflammatory responses (Mihm et al., 1976), the two syndromes are presented separately.

## Irritant Dermatitis

Irritant dermatitis is a nonimmune related response caused by the direct action of an agent on the skin. Extrinsic variables such as concentration, pH, temperature, duration, repetitiveness of contact, and occlusion impact significantly on the appearance of the eruption. Suffice it to say, chemicals such as strong acids, bases, solvents, and unstable or reactive chemicals rank high among the many possible human irritants.

Strongly noxious substances, such as those with extreme pH, can produce an immediate irreversible and potentially scarring dermatitis following a single exposure. This acute irritant phenomenon is akin to a chemical burn and has been described as an "etching" reaction (Bjornberg, 1987). More commonly, single exposures to potentially irritating chemicals will not produce significant reactions, and repeated exposures are necessary to elicit clinically noticeable changes. Such repeated exposures eventually result in either an eczematous dermatitis with clinical and histopathologic changes characteristic of allergic contact dermatitis, or a fissured, thickened eruption without a substantial inflammatory component. Chemicals inducing the latter two reactions are termed *marginal irritants.*

Because the thresholds for irritant reactions vary greatly from person to person, a genetic component to the response has been considered. Monozygotic twins have shown greater concordance than dizygotic twins in their reactions to irritant chemicals like sodium lauryl sulfate and benzalkonium chloride (Holst and Moller, 1975). While young individuals with fair complexion appear more sensitive to irritant chemicals than their respective counterparts, sex does not appear to be a significant factor (Bjornberg, 1975). Attempts to predict the relative irritancy of substances based upon their chemical relatedness to other irritants have been unsuccessful.

Divergent etiologies make it difficult to assign a specific mechanism for the pathophysiology of irritant dermatitis. Direct corrosives, protein solvents, oxidizing and reducing agents, and dehydrating agents act as irritants by disrupting the keratin ultrastructure or directly injuring critical cellular macromolecules or organelles. Marginal irritants require multifactorial variables to create disease and may not be capable of producing reactions under all circumstances. The varying time courses necessary to produce dermatitis by different known irritants result not merely from differing rates of percutaneous absorption but also depend on the specific agent selected. Thus, as Patrick and coworkers have observed (1987), "Chemicals do not produce skin irritation by a common inflammatory pathway." Supporting this view, tetradecanoylphorbol acetate (the major active ingredient of croton oil, a potent irritant) induced a tenfold increase in prostaglandin $E_2$ ($PGE_2$) in cultured human keratinocytes, whereas another irritant, ethylphenyl propriolate, induced no change in $PGE_2$ (Bloom et al., 1987). Kanauchi and coworkers demonstrated that numbers of Langerhans' cells (LCs), antigen-presenting cells in the skin critical for directing an immune response against a specific antigen, are not increased in guinea pig epidermis following provocation with croton oil. This finding contrasts with findings about other inflammatory skin lesions, like those present in human systemic lupus erythematosus and in skin lesions of MRL/1pr mice, in which LCs are increased (Kanauchi et al., 1989). Also, the intercellular adhesion molecule-1 (ICAM-1), which is important for the interaction of keratinocytes with leukocytes recruited to the site of an inflammatory response in the skin, was not up-regulated in experimentally induced irritant contact dermatitis, in contrast to experimentally induced allergic contact dermatitis in which ICAM-1 was up-regulated (Vejlsgaard et al., 1989). Although evidence suggests that irritant contact dermatitis does not occur as a result of classic immunologic mechanisms involving the recognition of antigen-presenting cells by activated T lymphocytes, other mechanisms, including secretion of inflammatory mediators such as interleukin-6 (IL-6) and tumor necrosis factor alpha (TNF-$\alpha$) by epidermal cells (Oxholm, 1992), appear to play an important role in recruiting lymphocytes to participate in the ensuing inflammatory response.

No single testing method has been successful in determining the irritancy potential of specific chemicals. Several tests exploit various contributory factors necessary to elicit irritant contact dermatitis. These tests involve either a single or repeated application of the same material to the skin. As discussed below, the single application patch test has been in use for almost 100 years in the United States and is utilized for the determination of allergic-type reactions. The use of animals in testing of potentially irritant chemicals is based on a variety of epicutaneous (epidermal surface) methods and has been utilized for decades. Generally, both intact and abraded skin of albino rabbits is tested for a reaction to various materials under occluded patches. The patches are removed in 24 h and the tested areas of the skin are evaluated at this time and again in 1–3 days.

In the Repeat Insult Patch Test, used primarily in humans for the evaluation of potential allergic sensitization, chemicals are placed on the skin under occlusion for 3 to 4 weeks. The test materials are replaced every 2 to 3 days to maintain an adequate reservoir in the patch site (Shelanski and Shelanski, 1953). The test is functionally similar to the Cumulative Irritancy Test, in which daily patches are applied under occlusion for 2 weeks in parallel with control substances (Patrick and Maibach, 1991). The Chamber Scarification Test modifies the aforementioned tests by abrading the skin to expose the upper dermis (Frosch and Kligman, 1976). All of these provocative tests rely on overt clinical changes such as erythema and induration at the site of challenge with a potential irritant. Transepidermal water loss, which is not visually observable, can increase as an early response to irritation and can be directly measured with an evaporometer. Hence, subtle changes can be documented even if overt clinical changes cannot be induced (Lammintausta et al., 1988).

## Chemical Burns

Extremely corrosive and reactive chemicals may produce immediate coagulative necrosis that results in substantial tissue damage with ulceration and sloughing. This is distinct from irritant dermatitis because the lesion is the direct result of the chemical insult and does not rely heavily on secondary inflammation to manifest the cutaneous signs of injury. In addition to the direct effects of the chemical, necrotic tissue can act as a chemical reservoir resulting in either continued cutaneous damage or percutaneous absorption and systemic injury after exposure. Table 18-2 lists selected corrosive chemicals that are important clinically.

## Allergic Contact Dermatitis

Allergic contact dermatitis represents a delayed (type IV) hypersensitivity reaction (Landsteiner and Jacobs, 1935). Because such a reaction represents a true allergy, only minute quantities of material are necessary to elicit overt reactions. This is distinct from irritant contact dermatitis where the in-

**Table 18–2**
**Selected Chemicals Causing Skin Burns***

| CHEMICAL | COMMENT |
|---|---|
| Ammonia | Potent skin corrosive<br>Contact with compressed gas can cause frostbite |
| Calcium oxide (CaO) | Severe chemical burns<br>Extremely exothermic reaction—dissolving in water can cause heat burns |
| Chlorine | Liquid and concentrated vapors cause cell death and ulceration |
| Ethylene oxide | Solutions and vapors may burn<br>Compressed gas can cause frostbite |
| Hydrogen chloride (HCl) | Severe burning with scar formation |
| Hydrogen fluoride (HF) | Severe, painful, slowly healing burns in high concentration<br>Lower concentration causes delayed cutaneous injury<br>Systemic absorption can lead to electrolyte abnormalities and death<br>Calcium containing topical medications and quaternary ammonium compounds are used to limit damage |
| Hydrogen peroxide | High concentration causes severe burns and blistering |
| Methyl bromide | Liquid exposure produces blistering, deep burns |
| Nitrogen oxides | Moist skin facilitates the formation of nitric acid causing severe yellow-colored burns |
| Phosphorous | White phosphorous continues to burn on skin in the presence of air |
| Phenol | Extremely corrosive even in low concentrations<br>Systemic absorption through burn sites may result in cardiac arrhythmias, renal disease, and death |
| Sodium hydroxide | High concentration causes deep burns, readily denatures keratin |
| Toluene diisocyanate | Severe burns with contact<br>Skin contact rarely may result in respiratory sensitization |

* Adapted from *Managing Hazardous Materials Incidents, Medical Management Guidelines for Acute Chemical Exposures*. U.S. Department of Health and Human Services, Agency for Toxic Substances and Disease Registry, 1991, vol III.

tensity of the reaction is proportional to the dose applied. An estimated 20 percent of all contact dermatitis is allergic in nature. Currently ≈2,800 chemicals have been described as potential allergens (American Academy of Dermatology, 1994). For allergic contact dermatitis to occur, one must first be sensitized to the potential allergen. Subsequent contact elicits the classical clinical and pathologic findings. Evidence dating back to the 1940s indicates that the ability to be sensitized to specific agents has a genetic component (Chase, 1941). Recent work has linked the presence of specific human leucocyte antigen (HLA) alleles to an allergy to nickel, chromium, and cobalt (Emtestam et al., 1993). Thus, to mount an immune reaction to a sensitizer, one must be genetically able to become sensitized, have a sufficient contact with a sensitizing chemical, and then have repeated contact later.

In general, low-molecular-weight chemicals (haptens) are responsible for causing allergic contact dermatitis. Most are less than 1,000 daltons and are electrophilic or hydrophilic. Some of these molecules are not inherently allergenic and must undergo metabolic transformation before participating in an allergic response (Andersen and Maibach, 1989). Because the skin has substantial metabolic capabilities, including many phase I and phase II enzymes, such biotransformation may occur in the skin at the site of contact with the chemical. Haptens, which are not intrinsically allergenic, must penetrate the stratum corneum and form a link with epidermal carrier proteins to form a complete allergen (Baer, 1986). The linkage between haptens and epidermal proteins is usually covalent, although metallic haptens may form stable noncovalent linkages with carrier proteins (Belsito, 1989). Current evidence suggests that these binding proteins are probably cell-surface molecules on the LC, most likely class II antigens encoded by genes of the HLA-DR (HLA "D-related") locus (Reinherz et al., 1983).

For sensitization to occur, the hapten/carrier protein complex is incorporated into the cytoplasm of an LC by pinocytosis for intracellular processing (Hanau et al., 1985). The LC subsequently migrates to a regional lymph node to present the processed antigen to helper T cells (CD4 cells). An LC bearing HLA-DR antigen and the hapten on its surface may present this package to a helper T cell which also must bear an antigen-specific receptor (CD3-Ti) and the cell surface molecule CD4. Concurrent with the antigen presentation, the LC produces interleukin-1 (IL-1) which directly stimulates the T cell to produce interleukin-2 (IL-2) and interferon-$\gamma$. IL-2 activates and causes proliferation of T cells specifically sensitized to that antigen. The production of other cytokines, including interferons, activates T-cell subsets that lead to the epidermal changes characteristic of contact dermatitis at the site of chemical exposure (Belsito, 1989). This scheme admittedly simplifies a complex loop of events. Keratinocytes themselves play an active role in the pathogenesis of allergic contact dermatitis. They are capable of not only producing a legion of cytokines, including IL-1 and IL-2, but also expressing HLA-DR antigen under certain circumstances. Hence, the keratinocyte is vital in the amplification process during the sensitization and elicitation phases of allergic contact dermatitis (Baer, 1990). Once induction of sensitization occurs, subsequent contact with the identical antigen initiates the same cascade of events as the aforementioned sensitization process. Now, however, sensitized T cells are present in the skin so that the immune response occurs with alacrity.

Contact dermatitis may occur upon exposure to any number of the thousands of allergens that people are potentially exposed to in the course of a day. Table 18-3 lists frequent allergens based on common exposure patterns, and Fig. 18-2 illustrates some potent sensitizers. Typical nonoccupational sources of exposure include the use of topical medications, personal hygiene products, rubber materials, textiles, cosmetics, glues, pesticides, nickel, and plastics. Contact with esoteric allergens frequently occurs in the workplace (cf, Adams, 1983). Table 18-4 lists the index of sensitivity for many common allergens in a group of 3974 individuals who were recently patch tested by the North American Contact Dermatitis Group. Such individuals generally are evaluated because they are already affected by contact dermatitis. Thus, the epidemiologic data generated, because it is not based on blinded cross-sectional evaluations, may not be representative of the general population. Nevertheless, such data permit recognition of allergens with high sensitizing potential and aid in devising strategies for their replacement by substances with low sensitizing potential.

Inspection of the chemicals listed in Tables 18-3 and 18-4 indicates that common causes of allergic contact dermatitis are ubiquitous in the materials that touch human skin regularly. There are, however, several allergens like nickel, chromium, cobalt, and some food flavorings that are also ingested with great frequency. In cases where an individual has a contact sensitivity to an agent that is systemically administered (orally), a generalized skin eruption with associated symptoms such as headache, malaise and arthralgia may occur. Less dramatic

**Table 18–3**
**Common Contact Allergens**

| SOURCE | COMMON ALLERGENS | |
|---|---|---|
| Topical medications/ Hygiene products | **Antibiotics** | **Therapeutics** |
| | Bacitracin | Benzocaine |
| | Neomycin | Fluorouracil |
| | Polymyxin | Idoxuridine |
| | Aminoglycosides | *α*-Tocopherol (Vit E) |
| | Sulfonamides | Corticosteroids |
| | **Preservatives** | **Others** |
| | Benzalkonium chloride | Cinnamic aldehyde |
| | Formaldehyde | Ethylenediamine |
| | Formaldehyde releasers | Lanolin |
| | Quaternium 15 | *p*-Phenylenediamine |
| | Imidazolidinyl urea | Propylene glycol |
| | Diazolidinyl urea | Benzophenones |
| | DMDM Hydantoin | Fragrances |
| | Methylchloroisothiazolone | Thioglycolates |
| Plants and trees | Abietic acid | Pentadecylcatechols |
| | Balsam of Peru | Sesquiterpene lactone |
| | Rosin (colophony) | Tuliposide A |
| Antiseptics | Chloramine | Glutaraldehyde |
| | Chlorhexidine | Hexachlorophene |
| | Chloroxylenol | Thimerosal (Merthiolate) |
| | Dichlorophene | Mercurials |
| | Dodecylaminoethyl glycine HCl | Triphenylmethane dyes |
| Rubber products | Diphenylguanidine | Resorcinol monobenzoate |
| | Hydroquinone | Benzothiazolesulfenamides |
| | Mercaptobenzothiazole | Dithiocarbamates |
| | p-Phenylenediamine | Thiurams |
| Leather | Formaldehyde | Potassium dichromate |
| | Glutaraldehyde | |
| Paper products | Abietic acid | Rosin (Colophony) |
| | Formaldehyde | Triphenyl phosphate |
| | Nigrosine | Dyes |
| Glues and bonding agents | Bisphenol A | Epoxy resins |
| | Epichlorohydrin | *p*-(*t*-butyl)formaldehyde resin |
| | Formaldehyde | Toluene sulfonamide resins |
| | Acrylic monomers | Urea formaldehyde resins |
| | Cyanoacrylates | |
| Metals | Chromium | Mercury |
| | Cobalt | Nickel |

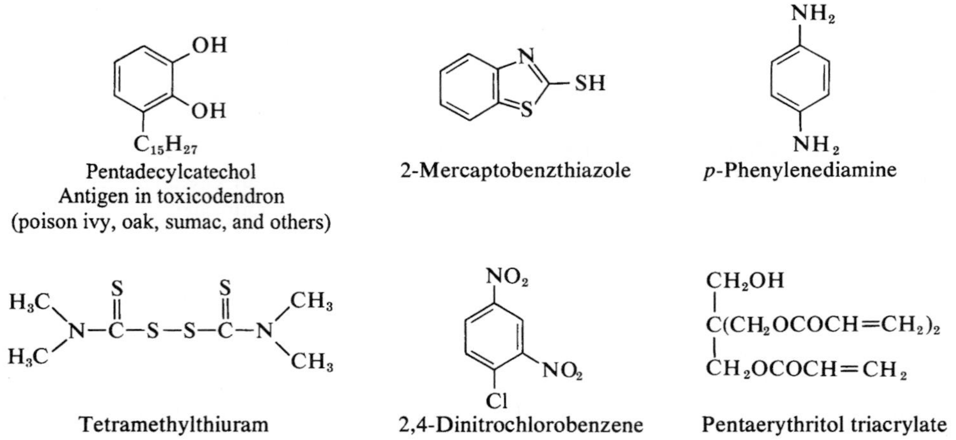

Pentadecylcatechol
Antigen in toxicodendron
(poison ivy, oak, sumac, and others)

2-Mercaptobenzthiazole

*p*-Phenylenediamine

Tetramethylthiuram

2,4-Dinitrochlorobenzene

Pentaerythritol triacrylate

*Figure 18–2. Structural formulas of some potent contact sensitizers.*

**Table 18–4**
**Index of Sensitivity to Selected Allergens***

| CHEMICAL | RESPONSE RATE (% POSITIVE) |
|---|---|
| Nickel sulfate | 10.5 |
| Thimerosal | 8.7 |
| Neomycin sulfate | 7.2 |
| Formaldehyde | 6.8 |
| *p*-Phenylenediamine | 6.4 |
| Quaternium-15 | 6.2 |
| Thiuram mix | 5.5 |
| Balsam of Peru | 5.1 |
| Cinnamic alcohol | 4.8 |
| Ethylenediamine dihydrochloride | 3.8 |
| Cinnamic aldehyde | 3.1 |
| Carba mix† | 3.1 |
| Mercapto mix‡ | 2.5 |
| Potassium dichromate | 2.4 |
| Diazolidinyl urea | 2.4 |
| Diaminophenylmethane | 2.3 |
| Benzoyl peroxide | 2.3 |
| Rosin | 2.2 |
| Mercaptobenzothiazole | 2.1 |
| Imidazolidinyl urea | 2.1 |
| Epoxy resin | 2.1 |
| Black rubber mix§ | 2.1 |
| Benzocaine | 2.1 |
| *p*-(*t*-Butyl)phenol formaldehyde resin | 1.6 |
| Wood alcohol | 1.5 |

* Adapted from Nethercott JR, Holness DL, Adams RM, et al: Multivariate analysis of the effect of selected factors on the elicitation of patch test response to 28 common environmental contactants in North America. *Am J Contact Dermatitis* 5:13–18, 1994.

† Diphenylguanidine, zinc diethyldithiocarbamate, zinc dibutyldithiocarbamate.

‡ Cyclohexyl-2-benzothiazolesulfenamide, 2,2′-benzothazyl disulfide, 4-morpholinyl-2-benzothiazyl disulfide.

§ p-Phenylenediamine congeners.

eruptions may include flaring of a previous contact dermatitis to the same substance, vesicular hand eruptions, and an eczematous eruption in flexural areas. One unusual clinical presentation has been termed the baboon syndrome, in which a pink-to-dark-violet eruption occurs around the buttocks and genitalia. Systemic contact dermatitis may produce a delayed-type hypersensitivity reaction and/or deposition of immunoglobulins and complement components in the skin. Such deposits are potent inducers of a secondary inflammatory response and are responsible for the initial pathophysiology of many blistering and connective tissue diseases of the skin (Menne et al., 1994).

Cross-reactions between chemicals may occur if they share similar functional groups critical to the formation of complete allergens (hapten plus carrier protein). These reactions may cause difficulties in controlling contact dermatitis because avoidance of known allergens and potentially cross-reacting substances is necessary for improvement. Table 18-5 lists common cross-reacting substances, and Fig. 18-3 illustrates three cross-reactors. Proper diagnosis can be hampered by concomitant sensitization to two different chemicals in the same product or simultaneous sensitization to two chemicals in different products.

## Testing Methods

**Predictive.** As with irritant dermatitis, animals have been used to determine the allergenicity of chemicals with the hope of correlating the data to humans. The Draize Test is an intradermal test in which induction of sensitization is accomplished by ten intracutaneous injections of a specific test material. Consequent challenges are performed by the same method and local reactions are graded by their clinical appearance. The Guinea Pig Maximization Test attempts to induce allergy by serial intradermal injections of an agent with the addition of Freund's complete adjuvant, an immune enhancer consisting of mycobacterial proteins. Subsequent challenge with the agent alone under an occluded chamber is graded clinically. Variations on this form of provocative testing have been done, as well as performing many of these variations on human volunteers. It should be noted that Freund's adjuvant is not

**Table 18–5**
**Common Cross-Reacting Chemicals**

| CHEMICAL | CROSS-REACTOR |
|---|---|
| Abietic acid | Pine resin (colophony) |
| Balsam of Peru | Pine resin, cinnamates, benzoates |
| Bisphenol A | Diethylstilbestrol, hydroquinone monobenzyl ether |
| Canaga oil | Benzyl salicylate |
| Chlorocresol | Chloroxylenol |
| Diazolidinyl urea | Imidazolidinyl urea, formaldehyde |
| Ethylenediamine di-HCl | Aminophylline, piperazine |
| Formaldehyde | Arylsulfonamide resin, chloroallyl-hexaminium chloride |
| Hydroquinone | Resorcinol |
| Methyl hydroxybenzoate | Parabens, hydroquinone monobenzyl ether |
| *p*-Aminobenzoic acid | *p*-Aminosalicylic acid, sulfonamide |
| Phenylenediamine | Parabens, *p*-aminobenzoic acid |
| Propyl hydroxybenzoate | Hydroquinone monobenzyl ether |
| Phenol | Resorcinol, cresols, hydroquinone |
| Tetramethylthiuram disulfide | Tetraethylthiuram mono- and disulfide |

approved for use in humans; however, other techniques, such as use of higher induction concentrations can be used to boost sensitization. For chemicals with higher allergenicity, epicutaneous skin testing can be performed, thus obviating the need for percutaneous (through the epidermis) sensitization. A variety of animal models have been described, utilizing intact and abraded skin to induce sensitization and subsequent elicitation upon rechallenges. The Buehler Test, Guinea Pig Maximization Test, and Epicutaneous Maximization Test utilize this form of testing and may occasionally add Freund's complete adjuvant to enhance sensitization (Guillot and Connet, 1985). The aforementioned tests have been used successfully to predict the allergenicity of strongly sensitizing substances in human beings. However, weaker allergens are often not discovered until they reach a large human population.

**Diagnostic.** Determining the cause of a contact dermatitis requires a careful evaluation of possible chemical exposures, history of the illness, and distribution of lesions. This alone will only hone in on groups or classes of allergens but will be insufficient to identify the specific offending chemical. Such evaluation is imperative because without strict avoidance, the dermatitis will continue. Diagnostic patch testing has been utilized in the United States for almost one hundred years. Since its introduction, little has changed in the procedure and its usefulness (Sulzberger, 1940). Standardized concentrations of material dissolved or suspended in petrolatum or water are placed on stainless steel chambers adhering to acrylic tape. Most testing material is commercially available, and the concentrations have been tested in a sufficiently large population to establish a nonirritancy threshold. Chambers are left in place for 48 h, and an initial reading is performed at the time the patches are removed. A subsequent reading 24–96 h later is also made because delayed reactions commonly occur. Reactions are graded as positive if erythema (redness) and induration (skin thickening) occur at the test site. Strict adherence to established protocols is necessary to draw conclusions about the clinical relevance of the reactions (Cronin, 1980). Mere redness without infiltration of the site or the presence of an irritant morphology are not considered significant reactions. Assigning relevance to a positive reaction is difficult in some situations but it is vital that the reaction be interpreted because many "positive" reactions correlate falsely with the presence of the irritant for which a subject is being tested. Relevance is determined through the patient's history of chemical contactants, from the distribution of the eruption on the body, and through provocative use tests. Use tests or open epicutaneous tests simulate everyday exposures better than other skin tests. With the use test a product containing a suspect allergen is applied to the same area of the skin for several days. Erythema with induration of the area denotes a positive test and contributes to the determination of relevance. Avoidance of the allergen and the substitution of the offending agent with a functional equivalent will lead to improvement in the majority of cases in a few weeks.

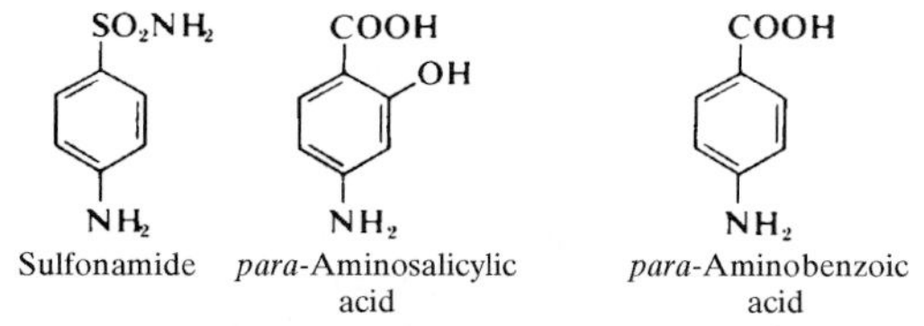

The adequate predictive and diagnostic abilities of all of the aforementioned tests rest on the use of a human or animal subject with an intact immune system. In vitro models, such as the macrophage migration inhibition assay and the lymphocyte transformation/blastogenesis assay, have been of some value for a few strong allergens such as dinitrochlorobenzene (Kashima et al., 1993), but their use in predicting chemical allergenicity or their role as a diagnostic tool is quite limited at this time.

$SO_2NH_2$ / $NH_2$ — Sulfonamide; $COOH$, $OH$ / $NH_2$ — *para*-Aminosalicylic acid; $COOH$ / $NH_2$ — *para*-Aminobenzoic acid

***Figure 18–3. Structural formulas of selected para-amino compounds that show cross-reactions in allergic contact sensitization.***

## PHOTOTOXICOLOGY

In the course of life the skin is exposed to radiation that spans the electromagnetic spectrum, including ultraviolet (UV), visible, and infrared radiation from the sun, artificial light sources, and heat sources. In general the solar radiation reaching the earth that is most capable of inducing skin changes extends from 290 nm to 700 nm, the UV and visible spectra. Wavelengths on the extremes of this range are either significantly filtered by the earth's atmosphere or are insufficiently energetic to cause cutaneous pathology. Adequate doses of artificially produced radiation such as UVC (<290 nm) or x-ray can produce profound physical and toxicological skin changes. For any form of electromagnetic radiation to produce a biological change, it must first be absorbed. The absorption of light in deeper, more vital structures of the skin is dependent on a variety of optical parameters (e.g., chromophores, epidermal thickness, and water content) that differ from region to region on the body. Melanin is a significant chromophore in the skin because it is capable of absorbing a broad range of radiation from UVB (290–320 nm) through the visible spectrum. Other chromophores in the skin include amino acids and their breakdown products, such as tryptophan and urocanic acid, which are able to absorb light in the UVB band. Biologically, the most significant chromophore is DNA because the resultant damage from radiation may have lasting effects on the structure and function of the tissue (Kochever, 1993).

## Adverse Responses to Electromagnetic Radiation

After exposure, the skin manifests injury in a variety of ways, including both acute and chronic responses (Lim and Soter, 1993). The most evident acute feature of UV radiation exposure is erythema (redness or sunburn). The minimal erythema dose (MED), the smallest dose of UV light needed to induce an erythematous response, varies greatly from person to person. The vasodilation responsible for the color change is accompanied by significant alterations in inflammatory mediators such as prostaglandins $D_2$, $E_2$, and $F_{2a}$, leukotriene $B_4$, and prostacyclin $I_2$ (Soter, 1993). Also, IL-1 activity is elevated within hours of exposure to UVB and may be responsible for several of the systemic symptoms associated with sunburn such as fever, chills, and malaise. This cytokine may be released from local inflammatory cells as well as directly from injured keratinocytes. UVB (290–320 nm) is the solar band most effective in causing erythema in human skin. Environmental conditions that affect UV-induced injury include duration of exposure, season, altitude, body site, skin pigmentation, and previous exposure (Harber and Bickers, 1989). A substantially greater dosage of UVA (320–400) reaches the earth compared to UVB (up to 100-fold); however, its efficiency in generating erythema in humans is about 1,000-fold less than that of UVB (Morrison, 1991). Overt pigment darkening is another typical response to ultraviolet exposure. This may be accomplished by enhanced melanin production by melanocytes or by photo-oxidation of melanin. Tanning or increased pigmentation usually occurs within 3 days of UV light exposure, while photo-oxidation is evident immediately. The tanning response is most readily produced by exposure in the UVB band, although longer wavelengths of light are also capable of eliciting this response to a lesser degree. Immediate pigment darkening is characteristic of UVA and visible light exposure. The tanning response serves to augment the protective effects of melanin in the skin; however, the immediate photo-oxidation darkening response does not confer improved photoprotection.

Commensurate with melanogenesis, UV radiation will provoke skin thickening primarily in the stratum corneum. For light-skinned individuals in whom melanin is not a major photoprotectant or in conditions in which melanin is completely absent (i.e., albinism or vitiligo), this response lends a significant defense against subsequent UV insult (Everett, 1961).

Chronic exposure to radiation may induce a variety of characteristic skin changes. For UV light, these changes depend greatly on the baseline skin pigmentation of the individual as well as the duration and location of the exposure. Lighter skinned people tend to suffer from chronic skin changes with greater frequency than darker individuals, and locations such as the head, neck, hands, and upper chest are more readily involved due to their routine exposures. Pigmentary changes such as freckling and hypomelanotic areas, wrinkling, telangiectasias (fine superficial blood vessels), actinic keratoses (precancerous lesions), and malignant skin lesions, such as basal and squamous cell carcinomas and malignant melanomas, are all consequences of chronic exposure to UV light. One significant pathophysiologic response of chronic exposure to UV light is the pronounced decrease of epidermal LCs. Chronically sun-exposed skin may have up to 50 percent fewer LCs compared to photoprotected areas. This decrease may result in lessened immune surveillance of neoantigens on malignant cells and thus allow such transformation to proceed unabated (Gilchrest and Rogers, 1993). Exposures to ionizing radiation may produce a different spectrum of disease depending upon the dose delivered. Large acute exposures will result in local redness, blistering, swelling, ulceration, and pain. After a latent period or following subacute chronic exposures, characteristic changes such as epidermal thinning, freckling, telangiectasias, and nonhealing ulcerations may occur. Also, a variety of skin malignancies have been described years after skin exposure to radiation (Arnold et al., 1990).

Aside from the toxic nature of electromagnetic radiation, natural and environmental exposures to certain bands of light are vital for survival. UV radiation is critical for the conversion of 7-dehydrocholesterol to previtamin $D_3$, without which normal endogenous production of vitamin D would not take place. Blue light in the 420-490 nm range can be lifesaving due to its capacity to photoisomerize bilirubin (a red blood cell breakdown product) in the skin. Infants with elevated serum bilirubin have difficulty clearing this byproduct because of its low water solubility. Its presence in high serum concentrations can be neurotoxic. The photoisomerization by blue light renders bilirubin more water soluble; hence, excretion in the urine is markedly augmented. In addition, the toxic effects of UV light have been exploited for decades through artificial light sources for the treatment of hyperproliferative skin disorders such as psoriasis.

## Photosensitivity

Described as an abnormal sensitivity to UV and visible light, photosensitivity may result from endogenous or exogenous factors. Illustrating the former, a variety of genetic diseases impair the cell's ability to repair UV light-induced damage. The autoimmune disease lupus erythematosus also features abnormal sensitivity to UV light. In hereditary or chemically-induced porphyrias, enzyme abnormalities disrupt the biosynthetic pathways producing heme (the prosthetic group of hemoglobin), leading to accumulation of porphyrin precursors or derivatives throughout the body, including the skin. These compounds in general fluoresce when exposed to UV light of 400–410 nm (Soret band), and in this excited state they interact with cellular macromolecules or with molecular oxygen to generate toxic free radicals (Lim and Sassa, 1993). Chlorinated aromatic hydrocarbons such as hexachlorobenzene and TCDD are known to induce this syndrome (Goldstein et al., 1977).

**Phototoxicity.** Phototoxic reactions from exogenous chemicals may be produced by systemic or topical administration or exposure. In acute reactions, the skin may appear red and blister within minutes to hours after UV light exposure and resemble a bad sunburn. Chronic phototoxic responses may result in hyperpigmention and thickening of the affected areas. UVA (320–400 nm) is most commonly responsible; however, UVB may occasionally be involved (Johnson and Ferguson, 1990).

Agents most often associated with phototoxic reactions are listed in Table 18-6. These chemicals readily absorb UV light and assume a higher-energy excited state, as described for porphyrins. The oxygen-dependent photodynamic reaction is the most common as these excited molecules return to the ground state. In this scenario, excited triplet-state molecules transfer their energy to oxygen, forming singlet oxygen, or become reduced and form other highly reactive free radicals. These reactive products are capable of damaging cellular components and macromolecules and causing cell death. The resulting damage elaborates a variety of immune mediators from keratinocytes and local white blood cells that recruit more inflammatory cells to the skin, yielding the clinical signs of phototoxicity.

Nonphotodynamic mechanisms have been described in the pathogenesis of phototoxicity, psoralens being the prime examples. Upon entering the cell, psoralens intercalate with DNA in a nonphotodependent interaction. Subsequent excitation with UVA provokes a photochemical reaction that ultimately results in a covalently linked cycloadduct between the psoralen and pyrimidine bases. This substantially inhibits DNA synthesis and repair, resulting in clinical phototoxic reactions (Laskin, 1994). Psoralens may be found in sufficiently high concentrations in plants (e.g., limes and celery), such that contact with their fruit and leaves in the presence of sunlight can cause a significant blistering eruption called phytophotodermatitis.

**Table 18–6**
**Selected Phototoxic Chemicals**

| |
|---|
| Furocoumarins |
|   8-Methoxypsoralen |
|   5-Methoxypsoralen |
|   trimethoxypsoralen |
| Polycyclic aromatic hydrocarbons |
|   Anthracene |
|   Fluoranthene |
|   Acridine |
|   Phenanthrene |
| Tetracyclines |
|   Demethylchlortetracycline |
| Sulfonamides |
| Chlorpromazine |
| Nalidixic acid |
| Nonsteroidal antiinflammatory drugs |
|   Benoxaprofen |
| Amyl *o*-dimethylaminobenzoic acid |
| Dyes |
|   Eosin |
|   Acridine orange |
| Porphyrin derivatives |
|   Hematoporphyrin |

**Photoallergy.** In contrast to phototoxicity, photoallergy represents a true type IV delayed hypersensitivity reaction. Hence, while phototoxic reactions can occur with the first exposure to the offending chemical, photoallergy requires prior sensitization. Induction and subsequent elicitation of reactions may result from topical or systemic exposure to the agent. If topical, the reactions are termed *photocontact dermatitis*, while systemic exposures are termed *systemic photoallergy*. In most situations, systemic photoallergy is the result of the administration of medications. Photocontact dermatitis was described over 50 years ago following the use of topical antibacterial agents. Thousands of cases were reported in the 1960s after halogenated salicylanilides were used in soaps as antibacterial additives. Tetrachlorosalicylanilide and tribromosalicylamide were quickly withdrawn from the market after numerous reports of photoallergy surfaced (Cronin, 1980). Generally, the mechanisms of photocontact dermatitis and that of systemic photoallergy are the same as those described above for allergic contact dermatitis. In the context of photocontact dermatitis, however, UV light is necessary to convert a potential photosensitizing chemical into a hapten that elicits an allergic response (Deleo, 1992).

Testing for photoallergy is similar to patch testing for allergic contact dermatitis. Duplicate allergens are placed on the back under occlusion with stainless steel chambers. Approximately 24 h later, one set of patches is removed and irradiated with UVA. All patches are removed and clinical assessments of patch test sites are made 48 h and then 1 week following placement. A reaction to an allergen solely on the irradiated side is deemed photocontact dermatitis. Reactions occurring simultaneously on the irradiated and unirradiated sides are consistent with an allergic contact dermatitis. There is disagreement about the likelihood of coexisting allergic contact and photocontact dermatitis to the same agent, since a photopatch test may occasionally exhibit greater reactivity on the irradiated side compared to the unirradiated side. Table 18-7 lists potential photoallergens used in photopatch testing at New York University Medical Center.

## ACNE

As Plewig and Kligman state (1993), "Acne is the pleomorphic disease par excellence. Its expressions are multifarious and eloquent." Despite the multifactorial etiology of acne, the influence of sebum, hormones, bacteria, genetics, and environmental factors are well known. In many situations, one of these factors has an overwhelmingly greater influence in the genesis of lesions than the others. Among the literally dozens of different kinds of acne that have been described

**Table 18–7**
**Photo-Allergen Series for Photo-Patch Testing***

| |
|---|
| p-Aminobenzoic acid |
| Bithionol (thiobis-dichlorophenol) |
| Butyl methoxydibenzoylmethane |
| Chlorhexidine diacetate |
| Chlorpromazine hydrochloride |
| Cinoxate |
| Dichlorophen |
| 4,5-Dibromosalicylanide |
| Diphenhydramine hydrochloride |
| Eusolex 8020 (1-(4-Isopropylphenyl)-3-phenyl-1,3-propandione) |
| Eusolex 6300 (3-(4-Methylbenzyliden)-camphor) |
| Fenticlor (thiobis-chlorophenol) |
| Hexachlorophene |
| Homosalate |
| Menthyl anthranilate |
| 6-Methylcoumarin |
| Musk ambrette |
| Octyl dimethyl p-aminobenzoic acid |
| Octyl methoxycinnamate |
| Octyl salicylate |
| Oxybenzone |
| Petrolatum control |
| Promethazine |
| Sandalwood oil |
| Sulfanilamide |
| Sulisobenzone |
| Tetrachlorocarbanilide |
| Thiourea |
| Tribromosalicylanilide |
| Trichlorocarbanilide |
| Triclosan |

* Used at New York University Medical Center (January 1995).

over the decades, this section concentrates on acne venenata (L. *venenum* poison).

Chemicals able to induce lesions of acne are termed comedogenic. The clinical hallmark of acne is the comedone, which may be open or closed (a blackhead or whitehead, respectively, in the vernacular). Additionally papules, pustules, cysts, and scars may complicate the process. Hair follicles and associated sebaceous glands become clogged with compacted keratinocytes that are bathed in sebum. The pigmentary change most evident in open comedones is from melanin (Plewig and Kligman, 1993). Most commonly, lesions are present on the face, back, and chest, but for acne venenata, the location of the lesions may be characteristic, based on the route of topical or systemic exposure.

Oil acne is caused by a variety of petroleum, coal tar, and cutting oil products. In animal models the application of comedogenic oil will result in biochemical and physiologic alteration in the hair follicle and cell structure leading to the development of comedones (Zimmermann, 1990). In practical situations, the skin is contaminated with oil that is permitted to remain long enough for adequate penetration into the hair follicle, resulting in acneiform alterations.

**Table 18–8**
**Causes of Chloracne**

| |
|---|
| Polyhalogenated dibenzofurans |
| Polychlorodibenzofurans (PCDFs), especially tri-, tetra- (TCDFs), penta- (PCDFs), and hexachlorodibenzofuran |
| Polybromodibenzofurans (PBDFs), especially tetrabomodibenzofuran (TBDF) |
| Polychlorinated dibenzodioxins (PCDDs) |
| 2,3,7,8-Tetrachlorodibenzo-*p*-dioxin (TCDD) |
| Hexachlorodibenzo-*p*-dioxin |
| Polychloronaphthalenes (PCNs) |
| Polyhalogenated biphenyls |
| Polychlorobiphenyls (PCBs) |
| Polybromobiphenyls (PBBs) |
| 3,4,3′,4′-Tetrachloroazoxybenzene (TCAOB) |
| 3,3′,4,4′-Tetrachloroazobenzene (TCAB) |

## Chloracne

Chloracne, one of the most disfiguring forms of acne in humans, is caused by exposure to halogenated aromatic hydrocarbons. Table 18-8 lists several chloracnegens, and Fig. 18-4 illustrates some structures. Chloracne is a relatively rare disease; however, its recalcitrant nature and preventability make it an important occupational and environmental illness. Typically, comedones and straw-colored cysts are present behind the ears, around the eyes, shoulders, back, and genitalia. In addition to acne, hypertrichosis (increased hair in atypical locations), hyperpigmentation, brown discoloration of the nail, conjunctivitis and eye discharge may be present. Because chloracnegens commonly affect many organ systems, concurrent illness in the liver and nervous system may accompany the integumentary findings (U.S. Department of Health and Human Services, 1993). Histologically, chloracne is distinct from other forms of acne with progressive degeneration of sebaceous units, transition of sebaceous gland cells to keratinizing cells, and prominent hyperkeratosis in the follicular canal (Moses and Prioleau, 1985).

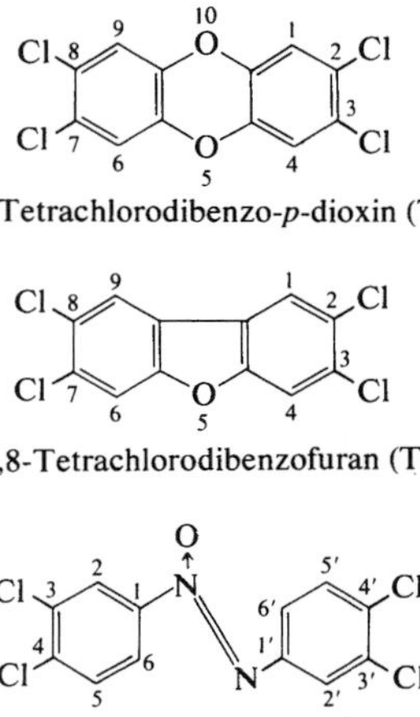

2,3,7,8-Tetrachlorodibenzo-*p*-dioxin (TCDD)

2,3,7,8-Tetrachlorodibenzofuran (TCDF)

3,3′4,4′-Tetrachloroazoxybenzene (TCAB)

*Figure 18–4. Structural formulas of certain potent chloracnegens.*

The effects of chloracnegens on humans have become well-recognized over the past 4 decades through a series of industrial disasters. In 1953 a chemical plant in Ludwigshafen exploded, discharging 2,4,5-trichlorophenol; in 1976 in Sevesco, Italy, a reactor explosion liberated TCDD; in 1968 and 1979 in Japan and Taiwan, respectively, rice cooking oil was contaminated with PCBs, polychlorinated dibenzofurans (PCDFs), and polychlorinated quaterphenols; and in 1973 in Michigan, cattle were inadvertently fed a hexabrominated biphenyl flame retardant. These incidents represent only a few of the dozens relating to human poisonings (Wolff et al., 1982). Chloracne was noted soon after exposure in these instances and has remained manifest even decades after exposure ceased (Urabe and Asahi, 1985). While reports from such events have indicated that these halogenated hydrocarbons may affect a variety of organs, such as the gastrointestinal, central nervous, reproductive, immune, and cardiovascular systems, epidemiologic studies have failed to demonstrate reproducibly organ-specific illness. Similarly, evidence pointing to human carcinogenicity from the multitude of PCB and TCDD species is also inconclusive. In contrast, chloracne has been an extremely reliable indicator of PCB and TCDD exposure in the large populations that have been studied (Caputo et al., 1988; James et al., 1993). Several incidents of accidental exposure to PCBs probably included other polyhalogenated species because PCDFs and dioxins may be formed from the combustion of PCBs during fires and explosions (Hutzinger et al., 1985).

Chlorinated dioxins and PCBs have significant and reproducible effects on cellular function. TCDD is one of the most potent known inducers of certain cytochrome P450 isozymes by virtue of its high affinity for the Ah receptor controlling their expression (Silbergeld and Gasiewicz, 1989). Some studies have suggested a more frequent association of chloracne with the more highly chlorinated congeners of PCBs than with those with lower chlorine content (Fischbein et al., 1982). Most levels of chlorination, however, have been associated with this skin problem to some degree. Given the high lipid solubility of these chemicals and their recalcitrance to metabolic clearance, their half-life in humans is long. Highly chlorinated PCBs can have a serum half-life of 15 years, and less chlorinated PCBs of 5–9 years (Wolff et al., 1992). Serum concentrations of PCBs in patients with chloracne are elevated, but the degree of elevation cannot be correlated directly with disease activity.

## PIGMENTARY DISTURBANCES

Several factors influence the appearance of pigmentation on the skin. Melanin is produced through a series of enzymatic pathways beginning with tyrosine. Errors in this pathway due to genetically deranged enzymes (i.e., albinism) or through tyrosine analogs result in abnormal pigmentation ( Fig. 18-5). Other factors such as the thickness of the epidermis and regional blood flow impact greatly on the appearance of skin color. Hyperpigmentation results from increased melanin production or deposition of endogenous or exogenous pigment in the upper dermis. Endogenous materials are usually melanin and hemosiderin (a breakdown product of hemoglobin), while exogenous hyperpigmentation can arise from deposition of metals and drugs in dermal tissue. Conversely, hypopigmentation is a loss of pigmentation either from melanin loss, melanocyte damage, or vascular abnormalities. Leukoderma and depigmentation denote complete loss of melanin from the skin, imparting a porcelain-white appearance. Many drugs and chemicals are capable of interfering with the normal formation and clearance of pigments as well as being directly toxic to melanocytes. The phenols and catechols are particularly potent melanocidal chemicals and can produce disfiguring depigmented regions. Table 18-9 lists common chemicals capable of causing alterations in pigmentation.

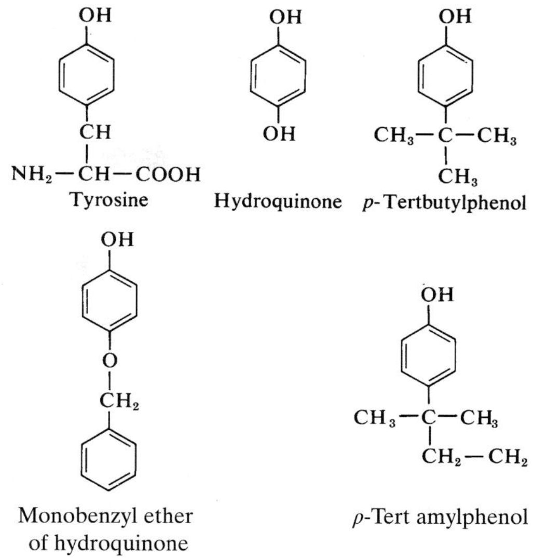

Tyrosine — Hydroquinone — p-Tertbutylphenol

Monobenzyl ether of hydroquinone — p-Tert amylphenol

***Figure 18–5. Chemical structure of tyrosine and of selected hypopigmenting and depigmenting agents.***

## GRANULOMATOUS DISEASE

A variety of dermatologic illnesses have the histopathologic findings of granulomatous inflammation. In general, a granuloma is an immune mechanism to "wall off" an adverse injury. It is seen in the skin in infectious diseases (e.g., leprosy, tuberculosis), foreign body reactions, and idiopathic illnesses. Foreign body reactions may be secondary to a primary irritant phenomenon such as traumatic introduction of talc, silica, or wood into the dermis. More rarely, sensitization may drive a granulomatous reaction as is the case for beryllium, zirconium, cobalt, mercury, and chromium, sometimes occurring in response to tatoo dyes. The pathophysiology of these granulomatous reactions is not dissimilar to those occurring in other organ systems, such as berylliosis in the lung (Lever and Schaumburg-Lever, 1990).

## URTICARIA

Urticaria (hives) represents an immediate type I hypersensitivity reaction primarily driven by histamine and vasoactive peptide release from mast cells. The mechanism of release may be immune-mediated through IgE allergen binding or by nonimmune mechanisms. Potential nonimmune releasers of histamine from mast cells include curare, aspirin, azo dyes, benzoates, and toxins from plants and animals. The majority of urticarial responses occur either from systemically ingested substances to which the person has a specific allergy or from

**Table 18–9**
**Selected Causes of Cutaneous Pigmentary Disturbances**

- I. Hyperpigmentation
  - Ultraviolet light exposure
  - Post-inflammatory changes (melanin and/or hemosiderin deposition)
  - Hypoadrenalism
  - Internal malignancy
  - Chemical exposures
    - Coal tar volatiles
    - Anthracene
    - Picric acid
    - Mercury
    - Lead
    - Bismuth
    - Furocoumarins (psoralens)
    - Hydroquinone (paradoxical)
  - Drugs
    - Chloroquine
    - Clofazimine
    - Amiodarone
    - Bleomycin
    - Zidovudine (AZT)
    - Minocycline
- II. Hypopigmentation/Depigmentation/Leukoderma
  - Post-inflammatory pigmentary loss
    - Vitiligo
    - Chemical leukoderma/hypopigmentation
      - Hydroquinone
      - Monobenzyl, monoethyl, and monomethyl ethers of hydroquinone
      - *p*-(*t*-Butyl)phenol
      - Mercaptoamines
      - Phenolic germicides
      - *p*-(*t*-Butyl)catechols
      - Butylated hydroxytoluene

completely idiopathic mechanisms. Occasionally, epicutaneous contact with a substance can elicit urticaria and is termed *contact urticaria*. Benzoic acid, cobalt chloride, butylhydroxyanisol (BHA), butylhydroxytoluene (BHT), diphenyl guanidine, and menthol are reported causes of this form. Recently, contact urticaria and deaths from systemic allergy have been reported from exposure to latex rubber (Gold et al., 1991). Natural latex rubber contains an incompletely characterized water soluble protein capable of inducing type I allergic responses. Mere contact with rubber products, such as gloves, can cause widespread hiving, asthma, anaphylaxis, and death. Many hospitals have established protocols for diagnosing latex allergy and implementing a latex avoidance program for affected individuals.

## TOXIC EPIDERMAL NECROLYSIS

Toxic epidermal necrolysis (TEN) represents one of the most immediately life-threatening dermatologic diseases and is most often caused by drugs and chemicals. It is characterized by full-thickness necrosis of the epidermis accompanied by widespread detachment of this necrotic material. After the epidermis has sloughed only dermis remains, thus severely compromising heat, fluid, and electrolyte homeostasis. Though controversy exists as to their relationship, TEN and severe erythema multiforme (Stevens Johnson syndrome), another serious reaction to drugs and infections, are often considered part of the same spectrum of disease (Roujeau and Revuz, 1994). Its etiology has remained elusive with immunologic and metabolic mechanisms popularly entertained. A recent study evaluating TEN induced by carbamazepine (an anticonvulsive drug) revealed reduced lymphocyte capacity to metabolize cytotoxic carbamazepine intermediates. Lymphocyte toxicity was not demonstrated with native carbamazepine but was found with carbamazepine metabolized by liver microsomes. Abnormalities in epoxide hydrolase and glutathione transferase may be responsible for the metabolism of the purported toxin, which may be an arene oxide. The inflammatory reaction of CD8 lymphocytes in TEN has suggested that a cytotoxic immune-mediated reaction is induced by the abnormal presence of this drug intermediate (Friedmann et al., 1994).

## CARCINOGENESIS

### Radiation

Skin cancer is the most common neoplasm in humans, accounting for nearly one third of all cancers diagnosed each year. At present the major cause of skin cancers (half a million new cases per year in the United States) is sunlight, which damages epidermal cell DNA. UV rays (290–320 nm) induce pyrimidine dimers, thereby eliciting mutations in the p53 tumor suppressor gene that select for initiated cells (Ziegler et al., 1994). They also produce immunosuppressive effects that may help skin tumors survive by inhibiting both antigen-presenting cell activation and expansion of helper T cells (Elmets, 1992). Susceptibility to the immunosuppressive effects appears to have a genetic basis (Streilein et al., 1994). The resulting cancer incidence is highest in the tropics and is highest in pale-complexioned whites, particularly at sites on the head and neck that receive the most intense exposure. Individuals who are deficient in certain DNA repair pathways (e.g., the xeroderma pigmentosum syndrome) must scrupulously avoid sun exposure to prevent the occurrence of premalignant lesions that progress with continued exposure. Even when it does not cause cancer in normal individuals, sun exposure leads to premature aging of the skin. For this reason, sunbathing is discouraged and the use of sunblock lotions is encouraged, especially those that remove wavelengths up to 400 nm.

In the recent past, ionizing radiation was an important source of skin cancer. With the discovery of radioactive elements at the turn of the century came the observation that x-rays can cause severe burns and squamous cell carcinomas of the skin. By the 1920s, basal cell carcinomas were also noted. For several decades thereafter, ionizing radiation was used to treat a variety of skin ailments (acne, atopic dermatitis, psoriasis, and ringworm) and for hair removal. The levels of exposure led to an increased risk of skin cancer and sometimes produced atrophy of the dermis (radiodermatitis) from the death or premature aging of fibroblasts which secrete elastic supporting fibrous proteins.

## Polycyclic Aromatic Hydrocarbons

A landmark epidemiological investigation by Percival Pott in 1775 connected soot with the scrotal cancer prevalent among chimney sweeps in England. Since that time, substances rich in polycyclic aromatic hydrocarbons (coal tar, creosote, pitch, and soot) have become recognized as skin carcinogens in humans and animals. The polycyclic aromatic compounds alone are relatively inert chemically, but they would tend to accumulate in membranes and thus perturb cell function if they were not removed. They are hydroxylated by a number of cytochrome P450 isozymes, primarily 1A1 in epidermal cells, and conjugated for disposal from the body. Oxidative biotransformation, however, produces electrophilic epoxides that can form DNA adducts. Phenols, produced by rearrangement of the epoxides, can be oxidized further to quinones, yielding active oxygen species, and they are also toxic electrophiles. Occupations at risk of skin cancer from exposure to these compounds (e.g., roofing) often involve considerable sun exposure, an additional risk factor.

## Arsenic

An abundant element in the earth's crust, arsenic is encountered routinely in small doses in the air, water, and food. High exposures from smelting operations and from well water derived from rock strata with a high arsenic content are associated with arsenical keratoses (premalignant lesions), blackfoot disease (a circulatory disorder reflecting endothelial cell damage), and squamous cell carcinoma of the skin and several internal epithelia (Wu et al., 1989). In earlier times, high exposures occurred from the medication Fowler's solution (potassium arsenite) and from certain pesticides. Arsenite (+3 oxidation state) avidly binds vicinal thiols, thereby inhibiting DNA ligase activity (Li and Rossman, 1989), while arsenate (+5 oxidation state) can replace phosphate in macromolecules such as DNA, but the resulting esters are unstable (Westheimer, 1987). By such means, both forms give chromosomal breaks and gene amplification (Lee et al., 1988), a plausible basis for their ability to cause transformation of cultured cells and to assist tumor development.

Considerable uncertainty exists regarding the shape of the dose–response curve for skin cancer from arsenic, an important issue in view of the estimated 100,000 Americans whose water supplies contain arsenic near the 50 ppb standard for drinking water. This value, set in 1942 and currently under review, may entail substantial risk of skin cancer (Brown et al., 1989; Smith et al., 1992). Further information is needed on the actions of arsenate and arsenite and their interconversion. Reduction of the former to the latter by glutathione is demonstrable in vitro (Scott et al., 1993) and is important in the subsequent methylation pathway (Thompson, 1993). The liver appears to be the major site of arsenic biotransformation. Partial reduction of arsenite to arsenate is observed in fibroblast-like cells (Bertolero et al., 1987) but may not occur effectively in other cell types, including erythrocytes (Delnomdedieu et al., 1994) and keratinocytes (Kachinskas et al., 1994). The slope of the dose–response relation may be much higher at high doses, where the body's ability to detoxify arsenite by methylating it to cacodylate is overtaxed. Low doses, then, may be less dangerous than estimated by simple linear extrapolations (Petito and Beck, 1991). In the absence of a suitable animal model, pharmacokinetic and mechanistic studies are directed to reducing the uncertainty of such predictions.

## Mouse Skin Tumor Promotion

Through the work of numerous investigators over the past 50 years, mouse skin has been developed as an important target for carcinogenicity testing. The observed incidence of squamous cell carcinomas has been helpful in providing a biological basis for conclusions from epidemiological studies. For instance, mouse skin carcinogenicity of tobacco smoke condensate and constituents (Wynder and Hoffman, 1967) strongly supported the conclusion that tobacco smoke is carcinogenic in humans (Report of the Surgeon General, 1979). Inferences about the sensitivity of human skin to a given agent are difficult to make from such test results, but carcinogenicity in mouse skin is taken as evidence of a more general carcinogenic risk for humans. Much has been learned about the pathogenesis of squamous cell carcinomas in this system that does have general applicability to human squamous cell carcinomas of the skin and other anatomic sites (Yuspa and Dlugosz, 1991). The further development of models for basal cell carcinoma and especially for melanoma as seen in human skin would be desirable.

A complete carcinogen induces tumors by itself at high doses but not at sufficiently low doses. The response is often nonlinear, and one explanation for this is that a large dose does more than initiate carcinogenesis by damaging the DNA in cells. It is also toxic, killing some cells and thereby stimulating a regenerative response in the surviving basal cells. Tumor promoters are agents that do not cause cancer themselves but induce tumor development in skin that has been initiated by a low dose of a carcinogen. Their promoting power generally is parallel to their ability to give sustained hyperplasia of the epidermis with continued treatment. Selective stimulation of tumor growth is envisioned to occur due to differential stimulation of initiated cells or due to the insensitivity of initiated cells to toxicity or to terminal differentiation induced by the promoter (DiGiovanni, 1992).

An advantage of the experimental model of mouse skin carcinogenesis is the ability to separate the neoplastic process into stages of initiation, promotion, and progression. With this model, the skin is treated once with a low dose of an initiator, a polycyclic aromatic hydrocarbon, for example. The skin does not develop tumors unless it is subsequently treated with a promoter, which must be applied numerous times at frequent intervals (e.g., twice per week for 3 months). Application of the promoter need not start immediately after initiation, but if it is not continued long enough, or if it is applied before or without the initiator, tumors do not develop. A consequence of promotion then is a tendency to linearize the dose–response curve for the initiator. Although an important aspect of promotion is its epigenetic nature (Yuspa and Dlugosz, 1991), papillomas are characteristically aneuploid (DiGiovanni, 1992). Mutations in the *c-H-ras* gene are commonly found in papillomas, particularly those initiated by polycyclic aromatic hydrocarbons. Eventually some of the resulting papillomas become autonomous, continuing to grow without the further addition of the promoter. Genetic damage accumulates in the small fraction of tumors that progress to malignancy.

A number of natural products are tumor promoters, many of which alter phosphorylation pathways. The best-studied example, and one of the most potent, is the active ingredient of croton oil, 12-O-tetradecanoylphorbol-13-acetate. This is a member of a diverse group of compounds that give transitory stimulation followed by chronic depletion of protein kinase C in mouse epidermis (Fournier and Murray, 1987). Another group of agents, an example of which is okadaic acid, consists of phosphatase inhibitors. Compounds acting by other routes are known, including thapsigargin (calcium channel modulator) and benzoyl peroxide (free radical generator). Sensitivity to tumor promotion is an important factor in the relative sensitivity to skin carcinogenesis among different mouse strains and even among other laboratory animal species (DiGiovanni, 1992). To cite an intriguing example, TCDD is 100-fold more potent than tetradecanoylphorbol acetate in certain hairless mouse strains but virtually inactive in nonhairless strains (Poland et al., 1982). By elucidating the genetic basis for this difference, we may improve our understanding of TCDD's activity as a promoter.

# REFERENCES


Adams RM: *Occupational Skin Disease.* New York: Grune and Stratton, 1983, pp 1–26.

American Academy of Dermatology: *Proceedings of the National Conference on Environmental Hazards to the Skin*. Schaumburg, IL: American Academy of Dermatology, 1994, pp 61–79.

Andersen KE, Maibach HI: Utilization of Guinea pig sensitization data in office practice. *Immunol Allergy Clinics N America* 9:563–577, 1989.

Arnold HL, Odom RB, James WD: *Andrew's Diseases of the Skin*. Philadelphia: W.B. Saunders, 1990, pp 22–50.

Baer RL: The mechanism of allergic contact hypersensitivity, in Fisher AA (ed): *Contact Dermatitis,* 3d ed. Philadelphia: Lea and Febiger, 1986, pp 1–8.

Baer RL: Allergic contact dermatitis: A historical view of its mechanism. *Am J Contact Dermatitis* 1:7–12, 1990.

Belsito DV: Mechanisms of allergic contact dermatitis. *Immunol Allergy Clinics N America* 9:579–595, 1989.

Bertolero F, Pozzi G, Sabbioni E, Saffioti U: Cellular uptake and metabolic reduction of pentavalent to trivalent arsenic as determinants of cytotoxicity and morphological transformation. *Carcinogenesis* 8:803–808, 1987.

Bjornberg A: Skin reactions to primary irritants in men and women. *Acta Dermato-Venereol* 55:191–194, 1975.

Bjornberg A: Irritant dermatitis, in Maibach HI (ed): *Occupational and Industrial Dermatology,* 2d ed. Chicago: Year Book Medical Publishers, 1987, pp 15–21.

Bloom E, Goldyne M, Maibach HI, et al: In vitro effects of irritants using human skin cell and organ culture models. *J Invest Dermatol* 88:478, 1987.

Brown HS, Bishop DR, Rowan CA: The role of skin absorption as a route of exposure for volatile organic compounds (VOCs) in drinking water. *Am J Public Health* 74:479–484, 1984.

Brown KG, Boyle KE, Chen CW, Gibb HJ: A dose–response analysis of skin cancer from inorganic arsenic in drinking water. *Risk Anal* 9:519–528, 1989.

Caputo R, Monti MD, Ermacora E, et al: Cutaneous manifestations of tetrachlorodibenzo-*p*-dioxin in children and adolescents. *J Am Acad Dermatol* 19:812–819, 1988.

Chase MW: Inheritance in guinea pigs of the susceptibility to skin sensitization with simple chemical compounds. *J Experimental Med* 73:711–726, 1941.

Cleek RL, Bunge AL: A new method for estimating dermal absorption from chemical exposure. 1. General approach. *Pharm Res* 10:497–506, 1993.

Cronin E: *Contact Dermatitis*. New York: Churchill-Livingstone, 1980.

Deleo VA (ed): *Photosensitivity.* New York: Igaku-Shoin, 1992, pp 1–19.

Delnomdedieu M, Basti MM, Styblo M, et al: Complexation of arsenic species in rabbit erythrocytes. *Chem Res Toixicol* 7:621–627, 1994.

DiGiovanni J: Multistage carcinogenesis in mouse skin. *Pharmacol Therap* 54:63–128, 1992.

Downing DT, Stewart ME, Wertz PW, Strauss JS: Lipids of the epidermis and the sebaceous glands, in Fitzpatrick TB, Eisen AZ, Wolff K, et al (eds): *Dermatology in General Medicine*, 4th ed. New York: McGraw-Hill, 1993, pp 216–217.

Elias PM: Role of lipids in barrier function of the skin, in Mukhtar H (ed): *Pharmacology of the Skin.* Boca Raton, FL: CRC Press, 1992, pp 29–38.

Elmets CA: Cutaneous photocarcinogenesis, in Mukhtar H (ed): *Pharmacology of the Skin*. Boca Raton, FL: CRC Press, 1992, pp 389–416.

Emtestam L, Zetterquist H, Olerup O: HLA-DR, -DQ, and -DP alleles in nickel, chromium, and/or cobalt-sensitive individuals: Genomic analysis based on restriction fragment length polymorphisms. *J Invest Dermatol* 100:271–274, 1993.

Everett MA: Protection from sunlight in vitiligo. *Arch Dermatol* 84:997–998, 1961.

Fischbein A, Thornton J, Wolff MS, et al: Dermatological findings in capacitor manufacturing workers exposed to dielectric fluid containing polychlorinated biphenyls. *Arch Environ Health* 37:69–74, 1982.

Fitzpatrick TB, Eisen AZ, Wolff K, et al (eds): *Dermatology in General Medicine*, 4th ed. New York: McGraw-Hill, 1993.

Fournier A, Murray AW: Application of phorbol ester to mouse skin causes a rapid and sustained loss of protein kinase C. *Nature* 330:767–769, 1987.

Friedmann PS, Strickland I, Pirmohamed M, Park BK: Investigation of the mechanisms in toxic epidermal necrolysis induced by carbamazepine. *Arch Dermatol* 130:598–604, 1994.

Frosch PJ, Kligman AM: The chamber scarification test for irritancy. *Contact Dermatitis* 2:314–324, 1976.

Gilchrest BA, Rogers GS: Photoaging, in Lim HW, Soter NA (eds): *Clinical Photomedicine*. New York: Marcel Dekker, 1993, pp 95–111.

Gold M, Swartz JS, Braude BM, et al: Intraoperative anaphylaxis: An association with latex sensitivity. *J Allergy Clin Immunol* 87:662–666, 1991.

Goldstein JA, Friesen M, Linder RE, et al: Effects of pentachlorophenol on hepatic drug-metabolizing enzymes and porphyria related to contamination with chlorinated dibenzo-*p*-dioxins and dibenzofurans. *Biochem Pharmacol* 26:1549–1557, 1977.

Grubauer G, Feingold KR, Harris RM, Elias PM: Lipid content and lipid type as determinants of the epidermal permeability barrier. *J Lipid Res* 30:89–96, 1989.

Guillot JP, Gonnet JF: The epicutaneous maximization test. *Curr Prob Dermatol* 14:220–247, 1985.

Hanau D, Fabre M, Lepoittevin JP, et al: Adsorptive pinocytosis, disappearance of membranous ATPase activity and appearance of

Langerhans granules are observable in Langerhans cells during the first 24 hours following epicutaneous application of DNCB in guinea pigs. *J Invest Dermatol* 84:434, 1985.

Harber LC, Bickers DR: *Photosensitivity Diseases. Principles of Diagnosis and Treatment*, 2d ed. Toronto: BC Decker, 1989, pp 115–117.

Holst R, Moller H: One hundred twin pairs patch tested with primary irritants. *Br J Dermatol* 93:145–149, 1975.

Hutzinger O, Choudhry GG, Chittim BG, Johnston LE: Formation of polychlorinated dibenzofurans and dioxins during combustion, electrical equipment fires and PCB incineration. *Environ Health Perspect* 60:3–9, 1985.

James RC, Busch H, Tamburro CH, et al: Polychlorinated biphenyl exposure and human disease. *J Occupational Med* 35:136–148, 1993.

Johnson BE, Ferguson J: Drug and chemical photosensitivity. *Sem Dermatol* 9:39–46, 1990.

Jugert FK, Agarwal R, Kuhn A, et al: Multiple cytochrome P450 isozymes in murine skin: Induction of P450 1A, 2B, 2E, and 3A by dexamethasone. *J Invest Dermatol* 102:970–975, 1994.

Kachinskas DJ, Phillips MA, Qin Q, et al: Arsenate perturbation of human keratinocyte differentiation. *Cell Growth Differ* 5:1235–1241, 1994.

Kanauchi H, Furakawa F, Imamura S: Evaluation of ATPase-positive Langerhans' cells in skin lesions of lupus erythematosus and experimentally induced inflammations. *Arch Dermatol Res* 281:327–332, 1989.

Kao J, Hall J: Skin absorption and cutaneous first pass metabolism of topical steroids: In vitro studies with mouse skin in organ culture. *J Pharmacol ExpTherap* 241:482–487, 1987.

Kao J, Hall J, Helman G: In vitro percutaneous absorption in mouse skin: Influence of skin appendages. *Toxicol Appl Pharmacol* 94:93–103, 1988.

Kashima R, Okada J, Ikeda Y, Yoshizuka N: Challenge assay in vitro using lymphocyte blastogenesis for the contact hypersensitivity assay. *Food Chem Toxicol* 31:759–766, 1993.

Khan WA, Das M, Stick S, et al: Induction of epidermal NAD(P)H:quinone reductase by chemical carcinogens: A possible mechanism for the detoxification. *Biochem Biophys Res Commun* 146:126–133, 1987.

Kochever IE: Basic principles in photomedicine and photochemistry, in Lim HW, Soter NA (eds): *Clinical Photomedicine.* New York: Marcel Dekker, 1993, pp 1–19.

Kreuger GG, Pershing LK: Human skin xenografts to athymic rodents as a system to study toxins delivered to or through skin, in Wang RGM, Knaak JB, Maibach HI (eds): *Health Risk Assessment. Dermal and Inhalation Exposure and Absorption of Toxicants.* Boca Raton, FL: CRC Press, 1993, pp 413–452.

Lammintausta K, Maibach HI, Wilson D: Susceptibility to cumulative and acute irritant dermatitis: An experimental approach in human volunteers. *Contact Dermatitis* 19:84–90, 1988.

Landsteiner K, Jacobs J: Studies on the sensitization of animals with simple chemical compounds: II. *J Exp Med* 61:625–639, 1935.

Laskin JD: Cellular and molecular mechanisms in photochemical sensitization: Studies on the mechanism of action of psoralens. *Food Chem Toxicol* 32:119–27, 1994.

Lavker RM, Miller S, Wilson C, et al: Hair follicle stem cells: Their location, role in hair cycle, and involvement in skin tumor formation. *J Invest Dermatol* 101:16S–26S, 1993.

Ledger PW, Gale R, Yum SI: Transdermal drug delivery systems, in Mukhtar H (ed): *Pharmacology of the Skin.* Boca Raton, FL: CRC Press, 1992, pp 73–85.

Lee TC, Tanaka N, Lamb PW, et al: Induction of gene amplification by arsenic. *Science* 241:79–81, 1988.

Lever WF, Schaumburg-Lever G: *Histopathology of the Skin.* New York: Lippincott, 1990, pp 243–248.

Li J-H, Rossman TG: Inhibition of DNA ligase activity by arsenite: A possible mechanism of its comutagenesis. *Molec Toxicol* 2:1–9, 1989.

Lim HW, Soter NA (eds): *Clinical Photomedicine.* New York: Marcel Dekker, 1993, pp 1–269.

Lim HW, Sassa S: The porphyrias, in Lim HW, Soter NA (eds): *Clinical Photomedicine.* New York: Marcel Dekker, 1993, pp 241–268.

McKone TE: Linking a PBPK model for chloroform with measured breath concentrations in showers: Implications for dermal exposure models. *J Exp Analysis Environ Epidemiol* 3:339–365, 1993.

Menne T, Veien N, Sjolin KE, Maibach HI: Systemic contact dermatitis. *Am J Contact Dermatitis* 5:1–12, 1994.

Mihm MC, Soter NA, Dvorak HF, Austen KF: The structure of normal skin and the morphology of atopic eczema. *J Invest Dermatol* 67:305–312, 1976.

Morrison WL: *Phototherapy and Photochemotherapy of Skin Disease,* 2d ed. New York: Raven Press, 1991.

Moses M, Prioleau PG: Cutaneous histologic findings in chemical workers with and without chloracne with past exposure to 2,3,7,8-tetrachlorodibenzo-*p*-dioxin. *J Am Acad Dermatol* 12:497–506, 1985.

Mukhtar H: Cutaneous cytochrome P-450, in Mukhtar H (ed): *Pharmacology of the Skin.* Boca Raton, FL: CRC Press, 1992, pp 139–147.

Mukhtar H, Bickers DR: Comparative activity of the mixed function oxidases, epoxide hydratase, and glutathione-S-transferase in liver and skin of the neonatal rat. *Drug Metab Dispos* 9:311–314, 1981.

Oxholm A: Epidermal expression of interleukin-6 and tumour necrosis factor-alpha in normal and immunoinflammatory skin state in humans. *APMIS Suppl* 24:1–32, 1992.

Patrick E, Burkhalter A, Maibach HI: Recent investigations of mechanisms of chemically induced skin irritation in laboratory mice. *J Invest Dermatol* 88:124S–131S, 1987.

Patrick E, Maibach HI: Predictive skin irritation tests in animals and humans in dermatotoxicology, in Marzulli FN, Maibach HI (eds): *Dermatotoxicology,* 4th ed. New York: Hemisphere, 1991, pp 211–212.

Petito CT, Beck BD: Evaluation of evidence of nonlinearities in the dose–response curve for arsenic carcinogenesis, in Hemphill DE, Cothern ER (eds): *Trace Substances in Environmental Health.* Northwood; Science Reviews Ltd, 1991, pp 143–176.

Pham M-A, Magdalou J, Siest G, et al: A novel model for the study of drug metabolism in human epidermis. *J Invest Dermatol* 94:749–752, 1990.

Pham M-A, Magdalou J, Totis M, et al: Characterization of distinct forms of cytochrome P-450, epoxide metabolizing enzymes and UDP-glucuronosyltransferases in rat skin. *Biochem Pharmacol* 38:2187–2194, 1989.

Plewig G, Kligman AM: *Acne and Rosacea.* New York: Springer-Verlag, 1993, pp 3–121.

Poland A, Palen D, Glover E: Tumor promotion by TCDD in skin of HRS/J hairless mice. *Nature* 300:271–273, 1982.

Potts RO, Bommannan DB, Guy RH: Percutaneous absorption, in Mukhtar H (ed): *Pharmacology of the Skin.* Boca Raton, FL: CRC Press, 1992, pp 13–27.

Potts RO, Guy RH: Predicting skin permeability. *Pharmacol Res* 9:663–669, 1992.

Raza H, Agarwal R, Mukhtar H: Cutaneous glutathione S-transferases, in Mukhtar H (ed): *Pharmacology of the Skin.* Boca Raton, FL: CRC Press, 1992, pp 131–137.

Reinherz EL, Meuer SC, Schlossman SF: The delineation of antigen receptors on human T lymphocytes. *Immunol Today* 4:5–9, 1983.

Report of the Surgeon General: *Smoking and Health.* Washington, US DHEW, 1979.

Riviere JE: The isolated perfused porcine skin flap, in Wang RGM, Knaak JB, Maibach HI (eds): *Health Risk Assessment. Dermal and Inhalation Exposure and Absorption of Toxicants.* Boca Raton, FL: CRC Press, 1993, pp 439–452.

Roujeau JC, Revuz J: Toxic epidermal necrolysis: An expanding field of knowledge. *J Amer Acad Dermatol* 31:301–302, 1994.

Scheuplein RJ, Blank IH: Permeability of the skin. *Physiol Rev* 51: 702–747, 1971.

Scott N, Hatlelid KM, MacKenzie NE, Carter DE: Reactions of arsenic (III) and arsenic (V) species with glutathione. *Chem Res Toxicol* 6:102–106, 1993.

Shaw JE, Prevo M, Gale R, Yum SI: Percutaneous absorption, in Goldsmith LA (ed): *Physiology, Biochemistry, and Molecular Biology of the Skin*, 2d ed. New York: Oxford University Press, 1991, pp 1447–1479.

Shelanski HV, Shelanski MV: A new technique of human patch tests. *Proc Scient Sect Toilet Goods Assn* 19:46, 1953.

Silbergeld EK, Gasiewicz TA: Dioxins and the Ah receptor. *Am J Indust Med* 16:455–474, 1989.

Smith AH, Hopenhayn-Rich C, Bates MN, et al: Cancer risks from arsenic in drinking water. *Environ Health Perspect* 97:259–267, 1992.

Soter NA: Acute effects of ultraviolet radiation on the skin, in Lim HW, Soter NA (eds): *Clinical Photomedicine.* New York: Marcel Dekker, 1993, pp 73–94.

Storm JE, Collier SW, Stewart RF, Bronaugh RL: Metabolism of xenobiotics during percutaneous penetration: Role of absorption rate and cutaneous enzyme activity. *Fund Appl Toxicol* 15:132–141, 1990.

Streilein JW, Taylor JR, Vincek V, et al: Relationship between ultraviolet radiation-induced immunosuppression and carcinogenesis. *J Invest Dermatol* 103:107S–111S, 1994.

Sulzberger MB: *Dermatologic Allergy.* Baltimore: Charles C. Thomas, 1940, pp 87–128.

Sutter TR, Tang YM, Hayes CL, et al: Complete cDNA sequence of a human dioxin-inducible mRNA identifies a new gene subfamily of cytochrome P450 that maps to chromosome 2. *J Biol Chem* 269:13092–13099, 1994.

Thompson DJ: A chemical hypothesis for arsenic methylation in mammals. *Chem Biol Interact* 88:89–114, 1993.

Urabe H, Asahi M: Past and current dermatological status of Yusho patients. *Environ Health Perspect* 59:11–15, 1985.

U.S. Department of Health and Human Services. Skin lesions and environmental exposures, in *Case Studies in Environmental Medicine.* Atlanta, GA: Agency for Toxic Substances and Disease Registry. May, 1993, vol 28.

Vejlsgaard GL, Ralfkiaer E, Avnstorp C, et al: Kinetics and characterization of intercellular adhesion molecule-1 (ICAM-1) expression on keratinocytes in various inflammatory skin lesions and malignant cutaneous lymphomas. *J Am Acad Dermatol* 20:782–90, 1989.

Walsh AA, Hsieh DPH, Rice RH: Aflatoxin toxicity in cultured human epidermal cells: Stimulation by 2,3,7,8-tetrachlorodibenzo-p-dioxin. *Carcinogenesis* 13:2029–2033, 1992.

Wester RC, Maboyen M, Maibach HI: In vivo and in vitro absorption and binding to powdered human stratum corneum as methods to evaluate skin absorption of environmental chemical contaminants from ground and surface water. *J Toxicol Environ Health* 21:367–374, 1987.

Westheimer FH: Why nature chose phosphate. *Science* 235: 1173–1178, 1987.

Wolff MS, Fischbein A, Selikoff IJ: Changes in PCB serum concentrations among capacitor manufacturing workers. *Environ Res* 59:202–216, 1992.

Wolff MS, Anderson HA, Selikoff IJ: Human tissue burdens of halogenated aromatic chemical in Michigan. *JAMA* 247:2112–2116, 1982.

Wu MM, Kuo TL, Hwang Y, Chen CJ: Dose–response relation between arsenic concentration in well water and mortality from cancers and vascular diseases. *Am J Epidemiol* 130:1123–1132, 1989.

Wynder EL, Hoffman D: *Tobacco and Tobacco Smoke: Studies in Experimental Carcinogenesis*. New York: Academic Press: 1967, pp 138–143.

Yuspa SH, Dlugosz AA: Cutaneous carcinogenesis: Natural and experimental, in Goldsmith LA (ed): *Physiology, Biochemistry, and Molecular Biology of the Skin*, 2d ed. New York: Oxford University Press, 1991, pp 1365–1402.

Ziegler A, Jonason AS, Leffell DJ, et al: Sunburn and p53 in the onset of skin cancer. *Nature* 372:773–776, 1994.

Zimmermann R: The rabbit ear model as comedogenic test. 3. *Dermatologische Monatasschrift* 176:55–61, 1990.

# CHAPTER 19

# TOXIC RESPONSES OF THE REPRODUCTIVE SYSTEM

*John A. Thomas*

The endocrine function of the gonads is primarily concerned with perpetuation of the species. The survival of any species depends on the integrity of its reproductive system. Sexual reproduction involves a very complex process for the gonads. Genes located in the chromosomes of the germ cells transmit genetic information and modulate cell differentiation and organogenesis. Germ cells ensure the maintenance of structure and function in the organism in its own lifetime and from generation to generation.

The twentieth century has undergone an industrial renaissance, and through scientific and technical advances there has been a significant extension in life expectancy and generally an enhanced quality of life. Concomitant with this industrial renaissance has come an estimated 50,000 to 60,000 chemicals into common use. Approximately 600 or more new chemicals enter commerce each year. The production of synthetic organic chemicals has risen from less than one billion pounds in 1920 to over 20 billion pounds in 1945, from 75 billion pounds in 1960 to over 200 billion pounds in the late 1980s (Lave and Ennever, 1990). There are several endocrine disorders associated with industrial chemicals (cf. Barsano and Thomas, 1992). Overall, occupational diseases in the U.S. may be responsible for about 60,000 deaths per year (Baker and Landrigan, 1990). The impact of new chemicals (or drugs) on the reproductive system was tragically accentuated by the thalidomide incident in the 1960s (Fabrio, 1985). This episode led to an increased awareness of the potential hazards of chemical and drug toxicity in the reproductive system and brought forth laws and guidelines world wide, pertaining to reproductive system safety and testing protocols. This new awareness of reproductive hazards in the workplace has led to corporate policies and legal considerations (Bond, 1986; McElveen, 1986). In 1985, the American Medical Association (AMA) Council on Scientific Affairs charged an advisory panel on Reproductive Hazards in the Work Place to consider over 100 chemicals with the intent to estimate their imminent hazards (AMA Council on Scientific Affairs, 1985).

Large numbers and large quantities of endocrine-disrupting chemicals (e.g., o,p,-DDT—dichlorodiphenyltrichloroethane) have been released into the environment since World War II (Colborn et al., 1993). Exposure to endocrine-disrupting chemicals has been linked with abnormal thyroid function in birds and fish, diminished fertility in birds, fish, shellfish, and mammals, and demasculinization and defeminization in fish, gastropods, and birds. The significance of endocrine-disrupting chemicals, also known as environmental estrogens or xenoestrogens, is unknown at this time (Safe, 1994). It is noteworthy that there are considerable quantities of phytoestrogens consumed in the diet and that there are many environmental anti-estrogens (e.g., TCDD—2,3,7,8-tetrachlorodibenzo-*p*dioxin) that can potentially affect the reproductive system in mammals and nonmammals.

Concern for reproductive hazards is not a new concern but dates back to the Roman empire (Gilfillan, 1965). Lead, found in high concentration in pottery and water vessels, probably played a role in the increased incidence of stillbirths. Lead is now known to be an abortifacient as well as being capable of producing teratospermias. In the United States, male factory workers occupationally exposed to 1,2-dibromo-3-chloropropane (DBCP) became sterile, as evidenced by oligospermia, azoospermia, and germinal aplasia. Factory workers in battery plants in Bulgaria, lead mine workers in the state of Missouri, and workers in Sweden who handle organic solvents (toluene, benzene, and xylene) suffer from low sperm counts, abnormal sperm, and varying degrees of infertility. Diethylstilbestrol (DES), lead, chlordecone, methylmercury, and many cancer chemotherapeutic agents have been shown to be toxic to the male and female reproductive system and possibly capable of inflicting genetic damage to germ cells (Barlow and Sullivan, 1982; Office of Technology Assessment Report, 1985).

The etiology of many adverse reproductive outcomes among humans is poorly understood. Generally, epidemiologic and reproductive outcomes have focused upon maternal factors (Olshan and Faustman, 1993). Relatively speaking, only recently have studies begun to examine the role of chemical perturbation of paternal exposures. Male-mediated developmental toxicity has received some recent attention. It has become increasingly clear that reproductive toxicity involves both the male and female (Mattison et al., 1990). Also noteworthy is the fact that nonreproductive endocrine organs can be adversely affected by drugs and chemicals (Thomas, 1994).

The potential hazard chemicals pose to reproduction and the risks to humans from chemical exposure are difficult to assess because of the complexity of the reproductive process, the unreliability of laboratory tests, and the quality of human data. In the human, it is estimated that one in five couples are involuntarily sterile; over one-third of early embryos die, and about 15 percent of recognized pregnancies abort spontaneously. Among the surviving fetuses, at birth approximately 3 percent have developmental defects (not always anatomic) and, with increasing age, over twice that many defects become detectable. It should be obvious from this description that even under normal physiological conditions the reproductive system does not function in a optimal state. Not surprisingly, the imposition of chemicals (or drugs) on this system can further interfere with a number of biological processes or events.

## GENERAL REPRODUCTIVE BIOLOGY

The developing gonad is very sensitive to chemical insult, with some cellular populations being more vulnerable than others to an agent's toxic actions. Further, the developing embryo is uniquely sensitive to changes in its environment, whether such changes are caused by exposure to foreign chemicals or to certain viruses. The toxicologist must be mindful of the teratogenic potential of a chemical as well as being aware of its potential deleterious actions on maternal biochemical processes. The development of normal reproductive capacity may offer particularly susceptible targets for toxins. Environmental factors might alter the genetic determinants of gonadal sex, the hormonal determinants of phenotypic sex, fetal gametogenesis, and reproductive tract differentiation, as well as postnatal integration of endocrine functions and other processes essential for the propagation of the species. The effects of environmental agents on sexual differentiation and the development of reproductive capacity are largely unknown. Of the chemicals that have been studied, it is noteworthy that they possess a wide diversity in molecular structure and that they may affect specific cell populations within the reproductive system.

## SEXUAL DIFFERENTIATION

An understanding of reproductive physiology requires consideration of the process of sexual differentiation or that pattern of development of the gonads, genital ducts, and external genitalia (cf. Simpson, 1980; De La Chapelle, 1987; Goldberg, 1988).

### Gonadal Sex

A testes-determining gene on the Y chromosome is responsible for determining gonadal sex (cf., De La Chapelle, 1987). It converts an undifferentiated gonad into a testes. The organization of the gonadal anlage into the seminiferous or spermatogenic tubules of the male may be mediated by testes-determining genes. The H-Y antigen is a surface glycoprotein present in all male cells (Goldberg, 1988). The testes produces two separate hormones: the müllerian inhibiting factor (MIF) and testosterone. Testosterone-induced masculine differentiation is modulated by androgen receptors regulated by genes on the X chromosome. Alterations of the sex chromosomes may be transmitted by either one of the parents (gonadal dysgenesis) or may occur in the embryo itself. Failure of the sex chromosomes of either of the parents to separate during gametogenesis is called *nondisjunction* and can result in gonadal agenesis. Klinefelter's syndrome is characterized by testicular dysgenesis with male morphology and an XXY karyotype; Turner's syndrome includes ovarian agenesis with female morphology, an XO karyotype, and a single X chromosome.

Hermaphroditism (true and pseudo) may occur secondary to nondisjunction of sex chromosomes during the initial cleavage mitosis of the egg. Such a condition results in sex mosaics of XY/XX or XY/XO. Pseudohermaphrodites are characterized by secondary sex characteristics that differ from those predicted by genotype.

Chemically induced nondisjunction is a common genetic abnormality. Nondisjunction of Y chromosomes may be detected by the presence or absence of fluorescent bodies on the chromatin of sperm (YFF spermatozoa). The number of YFF sperm is elevated in patients treated with certain antineoplastic agents as well as with x-rays.

### Genotypic Sex

The normal female chromosome complement is 44 autosomes and 2 sex chromosomes, XX. The 2 X chromosomes contained in the germ cells are necessary for the development of a normal ovary. Apparently, autosomes also are involved in ovarian development, differentiation of the genital ducts, and external genitalia characteristic of a normal female. This requires that only a single X chromosome be involved in genetic events within the cell. Generally speaking, the second X chromosome of a normal XX female is genetically inactive in nongonadal cells, although it has been shown that the tip of the short arm of the chromosome is genetically active.

The Y chromosome is consistent with the male determinant. The normal male has a chromosome complement of 44 autosomes and 2 sex chromosomes, X and Y. An additional X chromosome does not change the fundamental maleness caused by the Y chromosome, but the gonads are often dysfunctional (e.g., Klinefelter's syndrome). Genetic coding on the X chromosome may be involved in transforming the gonad into a testis.

The presence of chromatin material on the short (p) arm of the ($Y_p$) chromosome directs the development of the testes. Chromatin material ($Y_q$) on the long (q) arm directs the development of spermatogenesis.

### Phenotypic (Genital) Sex

During the early stages of fetal development, sexual differentiation does not require any known hormonal products. The differentiation of the genital ducts and the external genitalia, however, requires hormones. The onset of testosterone synthesis by the male gonad is necessary for the initiation of male differentiation. Although the testes are required in male differentiation, the embryonic ovaries are not needed to attain the female phenotype. Female characteristics develop in the absence of androgen secretion.

Two principal types of hormones are secreted by the fetal testes, an androgenic steroid responsible for male reproductive tract development and a nonsteroid factor that causes regression of the müllerian ducts. Sertoli cells are the likely source of MIF or antimüllerian hormone (AMH). Leydig cell differentiation and regression correspond well with the onset and subsequent decline in testosterone synthesis by the fetal testis. Thus the embryonic testis suppresses the development of the müllerian ducts, allows the development of the wolffian duct and its derivatives, and thereby imposes the male phenotype on the embryo.

There are three periods for testosterone production important to sexual differentiation. The first period occurs during days 14 to 17 of gestation in the rat and during weeks 4 to 6 in the human. The second period occurs from about day 17 of gestation to about 2 weeks postnatal age in the rat and, in the human, from month 4 of pregnancy to 1 to 3 months of postnatal age. The third period follows a long period of testicular inactivity in both species when testosterone production is reinitiated between 40 and 60 days of age in the rat and between 12 to 14 years of age in the human.

The dynamics of testosterone and dihydrotestosterone production and cellular interactions are an important prerequisite to knowing which chemicals might affect sexual differentiation. Factors that reduce the ability of testosterone to be synthesized, activated, enter the cell, and/or affect the cell nucleus' ability to regulate the synthesis of androgen-dependent proteins would have a potential to alter sexual differentiation. Some of these factors are summarized in Table 19-1. Chemicals are capable of exerting a testosterone-depriving action on the developing systems. These include effects on the feedback regulation of gonadotropin secretion, gonadotropin effectiveness, testosterone and dihydrotestosterone synthesis, plasma binding, as well as cytoplasmic receptor and nuclear chromatin binding.

Insufficient amounts of androgens can feminize the male fetus with otherwise normal testes and an XY karyotype. Slight deficiencies affect only the later stages of differentiation of the external genital organs and result in microphallus, hypospadia (i.e., the urethra opens on the undersurface of the penis), and valviform appearance of the scrotum with masculine general morphology. However, a severe androgen deficiency (or resistance) allows the müllerian system to persist and results in external genital organs of a female type (vagina and uterus) that coexist with ectopic testes and normal male efferent ducts. A lack of androgen receptors can also lead to a testicular feminization-type syndrome, even when normal levels of testosterone are present. Finally, sexual behavior also appears to be "imprinted" in the central nervous system by androgens from the testis and could be affected by endogenous and exogenous chemicals.

Estrogens exert an important developmental effect. Nearly 20 years have elapsed since the association between maternal diethylstilbestrol administration and vaginal adenocarcinoma in female offspring was reported. Diethylstilbestrol, or DES, a synthetic estrogen, has been used extensively both in human medicine and formerly in the feed of livestock. Other nonsteroidal estrogens, namely, the insecticides chlordecone and DDT (and its metabolites) exhibit uterotropic actions in experimental animals (Thomas, 1975). The estrogenicity of chlordecone was first described in workers at a pesticide-producing plant (Cohn et al., 1978). Several so-called xenoestrogens, including herbicides, fungicides, insecticides, and nematocides have been identified (cf. Colborn et al., 1993). Similarly, polychlorinated biphenyls (PCBs) are uterotropic. Zearalenones, which are plant mycotoxins, also exhibit female sex hormone properties. Environmental hormone disrupters (viz., xenoestrogens) are not restricted to only females. Indeed, vinclozolin, a dicarboximide fungicide, has metabolites that can act as androgen antagonists (Kelce et al., 1994).

**Table 19–1**
**Factors Affecting Androgen Effectiveness**

| TARGET | EFFECT | EXAMPLE |
|---|---|---|
| Hypothalamic-pituitary interaction | Feedback control of LHRH-mediated gonadotropin secretion | Estrogens, progestins |
| Gonadotropin action | Disrupt reproductive control processes involving gonadotropins | LH-FSH antibodies |
| Androgen synthesis | Inhibit key enzymes, e.g., cholesterol desmolase, 17 $\alpha$-hydroxylase, 3 $\beta$-hydroxysteroid oxidoreductase, 5 $\alpha$-reductase | Steroid analogues, diphenylmethylanes (amphenone B,DDD), pyridine derivatives (SU series), disubstituted glutartic acid imides (glutethimides), triazines, hydrazines, thiosemicarbazones |
| DHT synthesis | Inhibit 5 $\alpha$-reductase in target tissue | Androstene-17-carbosylic acid, progesterone |
| Plasma binding | Alter ratio of bound and free androgen in systemic circulation | Estrogens |
| Cytoplasmic receptors | Alter effect on target tissue by affecting binding to cytoplasmic receptors | Cyproterone acetate, 17 $\alpha$-methyl-$\beta$-testosterone, flutamide |
| DHT cellular binding | Block DHT effect on target tissue | Cyproterone acetate, spironolactone, dihydroprogesterone, RU-22930 |

SOURCE: Dixon, 1982.

## GONADAL FUNCTION

Regardless of sex, the gonads possess a dual function: an endocrine function (i.e., the secretion of sex hormones) and a nonendocrine function (i.e., the production of germ cells, or gametogenesis). The testes secrete male sex steroids, including testosterone and dihydrotestosterone. The testes also secrete small amounts of estrogens. The ovaries, depending on the phase of the menstrual cycle, secrete various amounts of estrogens and progesterone. Estradiol is the principal steroid estrogen secreted by the ovary in most mammalian species. The ovary is the chief source of progesterone secretion. The corpus luteum and the placenta are also primary sites of secretion of progesterone.

Gametogenic and secretory functions of either the ovary or testes are dependent on the secretion of adenohypophyseal gonadotropins, follicle-stimulating hormone (FSH), and luteinizing hormone (LH). In the male, LH is also referred to as ICSH (interstitial cell stimulating hormone). In the female, FSH stimulates follicular development and maturation in the ovary. In the male, FSH stimulates the process of spermatogenesis. Sertoli cells are the target cells for the action of FSH in the testes of mammals. FSH receptors are present on the Sertoli cells, and the gene for the FSH receptor is probably expressed only in these cells (cf. Heckert and Griswold, 1993). The secretion of pituitary FSH and LH are modulated by gonadal hormones. Sex steroids secreted by the testes or ovaries regulate the secretion of pituitary gonadotropins. The Sertoli cell of the testes secretes small amounts of estrogen and a proteinaceous hormone called inhibin. Inhibin aids in the modulation of spermatogenesis. ICSH(LH) provokes the process of steroidogenesis in the testes (Herbert et al., 1995).

The onset of puberty results in the cyclic secretion of pituitary gonadotropins in the female. The cyclic secretion establishes the normal menstrual cycle. In males, puberty is evidenced by the continuous and noncyclic secretion of gonadotropins.

## TESTICULAR FUNCTION

There are several subpopulations of cells in the mammalian testes, and all are subject to some degree of local regulation (Maddocks et al., 1990; Spiteri-Grech and Nieschlag, 1993). These local regulatory factors include peptide growth factors, pre-opiomelanocortin derivatives, neuropeptides and steroids (Table 19-2). There are many complex cell-to-cell communications, any one of which could serve as a site for chemical or heavy metal perturbation. Many agents that can affect either spermatogenesis or steroidogenesis can also affect leukocytes and other testes-regulating factors produced by cells of the immune system (Murdoch, 1994). The paracrine or local regulation of testicular function is an interesting concept, yet the nature of the testicular architecture and the multiple interactions that can occur at various cellular levels renders this biological system not only complex but very difficult to study from both a physiologic or a toxicologic standpoint. Nevertheless, these local testicular factors are very important in modulating the paracrine control of the male gonad.

**Table 19–2**
**Growth Factors Isolated From the Testis**

| GROWTH FACTOR* | TESTICULAR ORGAN | PROPOSED MITOGENIC TARGET IN THE TESTIS |
|---|---|---|
| IGF-I | Sertoli cells | NI |
| IGF-II | Germ cells | NI |
| TGF-$\beta$ | Sertoli cells<br>Peritubular cells | NI |
| Inhibin | Sertoli cells | NI |
| SGF | Sertoli cells | Sertoli cells? |
| $b$FGF | NI | NI |
| TGF-$\alpha$ | Sertoli cells<br>Peritubular cells | |
| SCSGF (=TGF-$\alpha$?) EGF | Sertoli cells | Germ cells? |
| RTFGF | Rete testis fluid | NI |
| IL-1 | Sertoli cells | Germ cells |
| NGF-$\beta$ | Germ cells | NI |

* Abbreviations: IGF I and II, insulinlike growth factor I and II; TGF-$\alpha$ and -$\beta$, transforming growth factor; SCSGF, Sertoli cell secreted growth factor; EGF, epidermal growth factor; RTFGF, rete testis fluid derived growth factor; tIL-1, testicular interleukin-1-like factor; NGF-$\beta$, nerve growth factor-$\beta$. NI, no information available.

SOURCE: Maddocks et al., 1990; Spiteri-Grech and Nieschlag, 1993; Shioda et al., 1994.

### Spermatogenesis

*Spermatogenesis* is a unique process in which the timing and stages of differentiation are known with a considerable degree of certainty. The dynamics of the process of spermatogenesis as well as its kinetics have been studied extensively and have recently been reviewed by Foote and Berndtson (1992). In producing spermatozoa by the process of spermatogenesis, the germinal epithelium has a dual function: It must produce millions of spermatozoa each day and also continuously replace the population of cells that give rise to the process, the spermatogonia (Amann, 1989).

Sperm are among the smallest human cells. The length of a sperm is about 50 $\mu$m or only about one-half the diameter of the ovum, the largest cell of the human female. The relative volume of a sperm is about 1/100,000 that of the egg. The sperm has a head, middle piece, and tail, which correspond, respectively, to the following functions: activation and genetics, metabolism, and motility.

Whereas only a few hundred human ova are released as cells ready for fertilization in a lifetime, millions of motile sperm are formed in the spermatogenic tubules each day. Several physiological factors affect the regulation of sperm motility (e.g., spermine, spermidine, "quiescence" factor, cAMP, motility stimulating factor, etc.) (Lindemann and Kanous, 1989). Oogenesis and spermatogenesis are compared in Fig. 19-1.

Spermatogenesis starts at puberty and continues almost throughout life. The primitive male germ cells are spermatogonia, which are situated next to the basement membrane of the seminiferous tubules. Following birth, spermatogonia are dormant until puberty, when proliferative activity begins again. The onset of spermatogenesis accompanies functional matura-

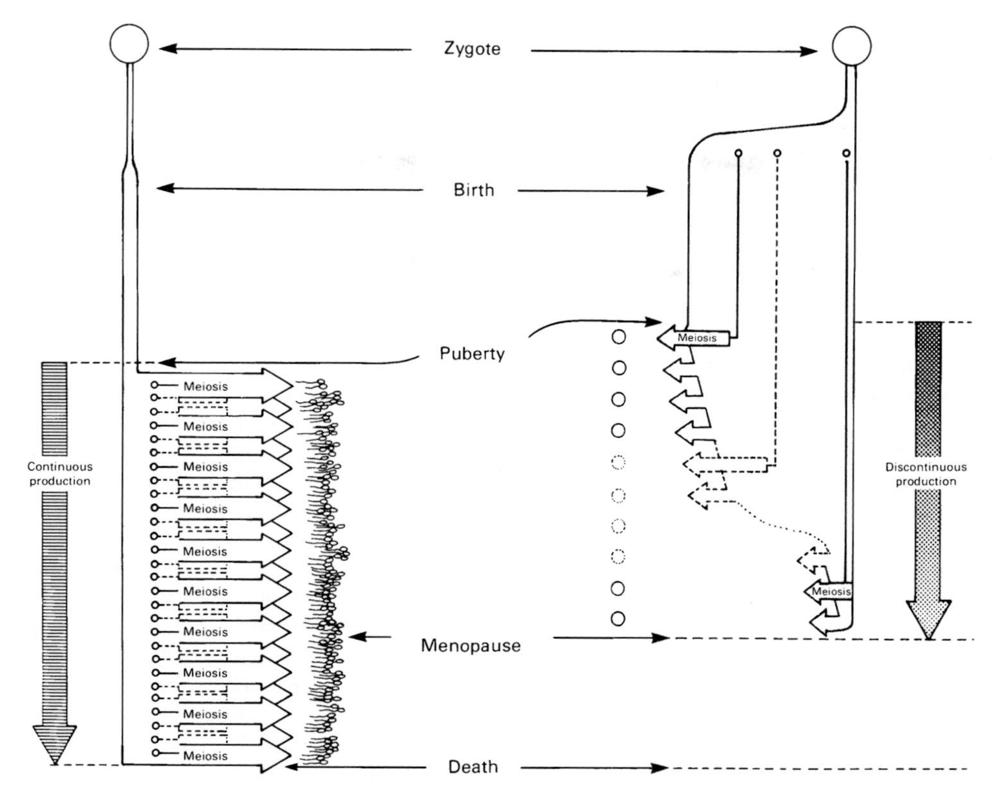


*Figure 19–1. Chronology of gametogenesis. (Modified after Tuchmann-Duplessis et al., 1972.)*

tion of the testes. Two major types of spermatogonia are present—type A, which generates other spermatogonia, and type B, which becomes a mature sperm. The latter type develops into primary spermatocytes, which undergo meiotic divisions to become secondary spermatocytes. The process of meiosis results in the reduction of the normal complement of chromosomes (diploid) to half this number (haploid) (Fig. 19-2). Meiosis ensures the biologic necessity of evolution through the introduction of controlled variability. Each gamete must receive one of each pair of chromosomes. Whether it receives the maternal or paternal chromosome is a matter of chance. In the male, meiosis is completed within several days. In the female, meiotic division begins during fetal life but then is suspended until puberty. Meiosis may be the most susceptible stage for chemical insult (Herbert et al., 1995).

Secondary spermatocytes give rise to spermatids. Spermatids complete their development into sperm by undergoing a period of transformation (spermiogenesis) that involves extensive nuclear and cytoplasmic reorganization. The nucleus condenses and becomes the sperm head; the two centrioles

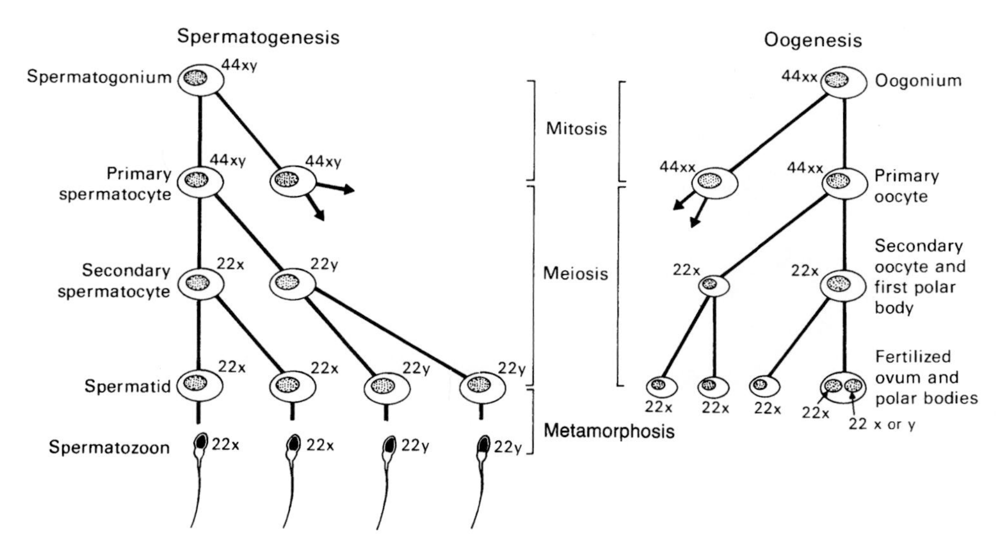


*Figure 19–2. Cellular replication (mitosis) and cellular reductive divisions (meiosis) involved in spermatogenesis, oogenesis, and fertilization.*

give rise to the flagellum or axial filament. Part of the Golgi apparatus becomes the acrosome, and the mitochondria concentrate into a sheath located between two centrioles.

Seminiferous tubules contain germ cells at different stages of differentiation and Sertoli cells. In a cyclical fashion, spermatogonia A of certain areas of a tubule become committed to divide synchronously, and the cohorts of the resulting cells differentiate in unison. Thus, a synchronous population of developing germ cells occupies a defined area within a seminiferous tubule. Cells within each cohort are connected by intercellular bridges.

The anatomical relationships of the mammalian testes reveal that the process of spermatogenesis occurs within the seminiferous tubules (Fig. 19-3). The germ cells, along with the Sertoli cells, are contained within the membranous boundaries of the seminiferous tubules. Conversely, the Leydig cells are situated in the interstitium or outside the seminiferous tubules. It may be seen that in several different species the seminiferous tubules contain a single cellular association. In humans, however, such cellular associations differ from one another but are intermingled in a mosaiclike pattern. Though this pattern varies among species, several aspects of cellular associations may be detected. Each cellular association contains four or five types of germ cells organized in a specific, layered pattern. Each layer represents one cellular generation. Fourteen cellular associations are observed in the seminiferous epithelium of the rat (LeBlond and Clermont, 1952; Heller and Clermont, 1964).

Presuming a fixed point within the seminiferous tubule could be viewed in the developing germ cell, there would be a sequential appearance of each of these cellular associations that would be characteristic of the particular specie. This progression through the series of cellular associations would continue to repeat itself in a predictable fashion. The interval required for one complete series of cellular associations to appear at one point within a tubule is termed *the duration of the cycle of the seminiferous epithelium*. The duration of one cycle of the seminiferous epithelium depends on, and is thus equal to, the cell turnover rate of spermatogonia. Thus, the duration of the cycle of seminiferous epithelium varies among mammals, being a low of about 9 days in the mouse to a high of about 16 days in humans (Table 19-3) (Galbraith et al., 1982). Spermatids, emanating from spermatogonia committed to differentiate approximately 4.5 cycles earlier, are continuously released from the germinal epithelium.

Maturation changes occur in the sperm as they traverse the tubules of the testes and the epididymides. During this passage, sperm acquire the capacity for fertility and become more motile. There is a progressive dehydration of the cytoplasm, decreased resistance to cold shock, and there are changes in metabolism and variations in membrane permeability. Each ejaculate contains a spectrum of normal sperm as well as those that are either abnormal or immature.

Normalcy of spermatogenesis can be evaluated from two standpoints: the number of spermatozoa produced per day and the quality of spermatozoa produced. The number of spermatozoa produced per day is defined as daily sperm production (Amann, 1981). The efficiency of sperm production is the number of sperm produced per day per gram of testicular parenchyma. The efficiency of sperm production in humans is only about 20 to 40 percent of that in other mammals (Amann, 1986). Sperm production in a young man is about 7 million sperm per day per gram, and by the fifth to ninth decade of life it drops to approximately one-half that amount, or about 3.5 million per day per gram (Johnson, 1986).

Blazak et al. (1985) have provided an assessment of the effects of chemicals on the male reproductive system using several parameters including sperm production, sperm number, sperm transit time, and sperm motility. These authors

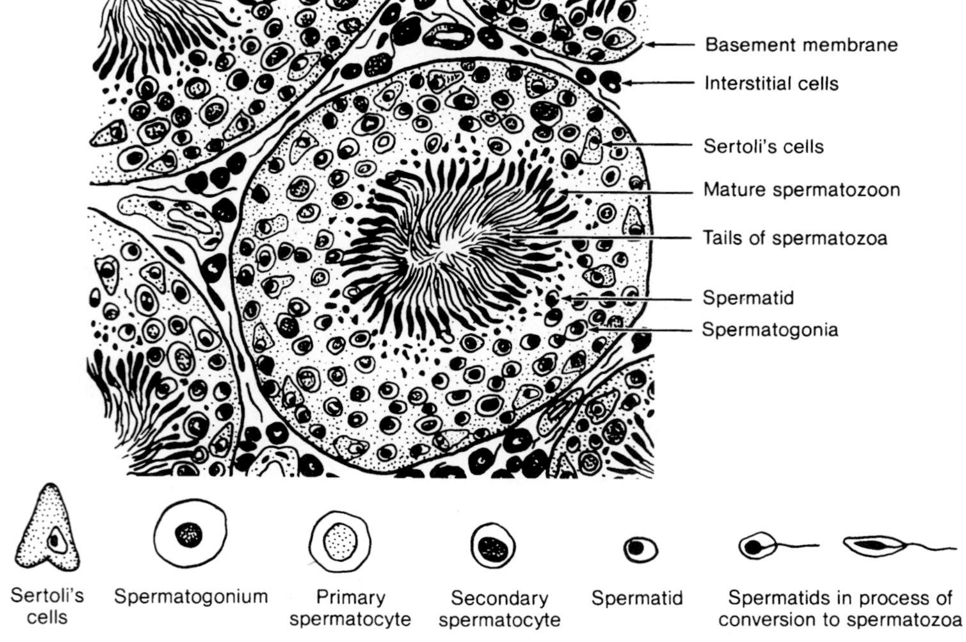


***Figure 19–3. Schematic cross-section of seminiferous tubules of testes. Morphology of the Sertoli cell along with the cellular events involved in spermatogenesis (spermatogonium through spermatid).***

**Table 19–3**
**Criteria for Spermatogenesis in Laboratory Animals and Man**

| | MOUSE | RAT | RABBIT (NEW ZEALAND WHITE) | DOG (BEAGLE) | MONKEY (RHESUS) | MAN |
|---|---|---|---|---|---|---|
| Duration of cycle of seminiferous epithelium (days) | 8.6 | 12.9 | 10.7 | 13.6 | 9.5 | 16.0 |
| Life span of: | | | | | | |
| B-type spermatogonia (days) | 1.5 | 2.0 | 1.3 | 4.0 | 2.9 | 6.3 |
| L + Z* spermatocytes (days) | 4.7 | 7.8 | 7.3 | 5.2 | 6.0 | 9.2 |
| P + D* spermatocytes (days) | 8.3 | 12.2 | 10.7 | 13.5 | 9.5 | 15.6 |
| Golgi spermatids (days) | 1.7 | 2.9 | 2.1 | 6.9 | 1.8 | 7.9 |
| Cap spermatids (days) | 3.5 | 5.0 | 5.2 | 3.0 | 3.7 | 1.6 |
| Fraction of a life span as: | | | | | | |
| B-type spermatogonia | 0.11 | 0.10 | 0.08 | 0.19 | 0.19 | 0.25 |
| Primary spermatocyte | 1.00 | 1.00 | 1.00 | 1.00 | 1.00 | 1.00 |
| Round spermatid | 0.41 | 0.40 | 0.43 | 0.48 | 0.35 | 0.38 |
| Testes wt (g) | 0.2 | 3.7 | 6.4 | 12.0 | 49 | 34 |
| Daily sperm production: | | | | | | |
| Per gram testis ($10^6$/g) | 28 | 24 | 25 | 20 | 23 | 4.4 |
| Per male ($10^6$) | 5 | 86 | 160 | 300 | 1100 | 125 |
| Sperm reserves in caudia (at sexual rest: $10^6$) | 49 | 440 | 1600 | ?† | 5700 | 420 |
| Transit time (days) through (at sexual rest): | | | | | | |
| Caput + corpus epididymides | 3.1 | 3.0 | 3.0 | ? | 4.9 | 1.8 |
| Cauda epididymides | 5.6 | 5.1 | 9.7 | ? | 5.6 | 3.7 |

* L = leptotene, Z = zygotene, P = pachytene, D = diplotene.
† A question mark indicates unclear or inadequate data.
SOURCE: Galbraith et al., 1982.

concluded that testes weights and epididymal sperm numbers were unreliable indicators of sperm production rates.

## Sertoli Cells

The Sertoli cell is now recognized as playing an important role in the process of spermatogenesis (Foster, 1992). In early fetal life, the Sertoli cells secrete AMH. The exact physiological role is not understood, but after puberty they begin to secrete the hormone inhibin, which may aid in modulating pituitary FSH.

The Sertoli cell junctions form the blood–testis barrier that partitions the seminiferous epithelium into a basal compartment, containing spermatogonia and early spermatocytes, and an adluminal compartment, containing more fully developed spermatogenic cells. An ionic gradient is maintained between the two tubular compartments. Nutrients, hormones, and other chemicals must pass either between or through Sertoli cells in order to diffuse from one compartment to another. Germinal cells are found either between adjacent pairs of Sertoli cells or inside their luminal margin.

Sertoli cells secrete a number of hormones and/or proteins. These secretory products can be used to measure Sertoli function in the presence of chemical insult. The Sertoli cells secrete tissue plasminogen activator, androgen-binding protein (ABP), inhibin, AMH, transferrin, and other proteases. ABP is a protein similar to plasma sex steroid-binding globulin (SSBG). In rodents, ABP acts as a carrier for testosterone and dihydrotestosterone. Sertoli cells probably synthesize estradiol and estrone in response to FSH stimulation.

Normal spermatogenesis requires Sertoli cells. Many chemicals affecting spermatogenesis act indirectly through their effect on the Sertoli cell (e.g., DBCP, monoethylhexyl phthalate [MEHP]) rather than directly on the germ cells (Chapin et al., 1988). Tetrahydrocannabinol (THC) acts at several sites in the reproductive system, including the Sertoli cell where it acts by inhibiting FSH-stimulated cAMP (adenosine monophosphate) accumulation (Heindel and Keith, 1989).

## Interstitium

The Leydig cells or interstitial cells are the primary site of testosterone synthesis (Fig. 19-3) (Ewing, 1992). These cells are closely associated with the testicular blood vessels and the lymphatic space. The spermatic arteries to the testes are tortuous, and their blood flows parallel to, but in the opposite direction of, blood in the pampiniform plexus of the spermatic veins (Fig. 19-8). This anatomic arrangement seems to facilitate a countercurrent exchange of heat, androgens, and other chemicals.

LH stimulates testicular steroidogenesis. Androgens are essential to spermatogenesis, epididymal sperm maturation, the growth and secretory activity of accessory sex organs, somatic masculinization, male behavior, and various metabolic processes. Surprisingly, there are a large number of diverse chemicals/drugs that can cause Leydig cell hyperplasia/neoplasia. This chemically induced proliferation of Leydig cells is particularly evident in the rodent (Table 19-4) (Thomas, 1995b).

## POSTTESTICULAR PROCESSES

The end product of testicular gametogenesis is immature sperm. Posttesticular processes involve ducts that move maturing sperm from the testis to storage sites where they await ejaculation. A number of secretory processes exist that control fluid production and ion composition; secretory organs contribute to the chemical composition (including specific proteins) of the semen.

### Efferent Ducts

The fluid produced in the seminiferous tubules moves into a system of spaces called the rete testis. The chemical composition of the rete testis fluid is unique and has a total protein concentration much lower than that of the blood plasma. The efferent ducts open into the caput epididymis.

Although the rete testis fluid normally contains inhibin, ABP, transferrin, myoinositol, steroid hormones, amino acids, and various enzymes, only ABP and inhibin appear to be specific products and useful indicators of the functional integrity of the seminiferous epithelium or Sertoli cells (Mann and Lutwak-Mann, 1981). However, relative concentrations of other constituents may indicate alterations in membrane barriers or active transport processes. The concentration of chemicals in the rete testis fluid relative to unbound plasma concentration has been used to estimate the permeability of the blood–testis barrier for selected chemicals (Okumura et al., 1975).

### Epididymides

The epididymis is a single, highly coiled duct measuring approximately 5 meters in humans. It is arranged anatomically into three parts called the caput, the corpus, and the cauda epididymides (Amann, 1987).

From the rete testis, testicular fluid first enters efferent ducts and then the epididymides. Here the sperm are subjected to a changing chemical environment as they move through the organ.

The first two sections together (the caput plus the corpus) are regarded as making up that part of the epididymis involved with sperm maturation, whereas the terminal (the cauda) segment is regarded as the site of sperm storage. There are, however, differences in the position and extent of the segments in various species of mammals.

From 1.8 to 4.9 days are required for sperm to move through the caput to the corpus epididymis where maturation takes place. In contrast, the transit time for sperm through the cauda epididymis in sexually rested males differs greatly among species and ranges from 3.7 to 9.7 days. Average sperm

**Table 19–4**
**Chemicals/Drugs Causing Leydig Cell Hyperplasia/Neoplasia in Rodents**

| AGENT/CHEMICAL/DRUG | AGENT CLASS OR BIOLOGIC ACTIVITY |
|---|---|
| Cadmium | Heavy metal |
| Estrogen | Hormone |
| Linuron | Herbicide |
| S0Z-200-110, Isradine | Calcium channel blocker |
| Flutamide | Anti-androgen |
| Gemfibrozil | Hypolidemic agent |
| Finasteride | 5 $\alpha$-Reductase inhibitor |
| Cimetidine | Histamine ($H_2$) receptor blocker |
| Hydralizine | Anti-hypertensive agent |
| Carbamazepine | Anticonvulsant/analgesic |
| Vidarabine | Anti-viral agent |
| Mesulegine | Dopamine ($D_2$) agonist-antagonistic |
| Clomiphene | Treatment of infertility |
| Perfluoroctanoate | Industrial ingredient (plasticizers, lubricant-wetting agent(s) |
| Dimethylformide | Industrial use (tannery and leathergoods, metal dyes) |
| Diethylstibesterol | Synthetic hormone |
| Nitrosamine | Industrial uses |
| Methoxychlor | Pesticide with estrogenic properties |
| Oxolinic acid | Antimicrobial agent |
| Reserpine | Antihypertensive |
| Metronidazole | Antiprotozoal |
| Cyclophosphamide | Antineoplastic |
| Methylcholanthrene | Experimental carcinogen |

SOURCES: Ewing, 1992; Bosland, 1994; Prentice et al., 1992; Thomas, 1995b.

transit time for a 21- to 30-year-old man is 6 days. The number of sperm in the caput and corpus epididymis is similar in sexually rested males and in males ejaculating daily. The number of sperm in the cauda epididymis is more variable, being lower in sexually active males.

Active transport processes affect the amount of fluid flowing through the epididymis. Because much of the fluid produced by the testis is apparently absorbed in the epididymis, the relative concentration of sperm is increased.

Hence, important functions of the epididymis are reabsorption of rete testis fluid, metabolism, epithelial cell secretions, sperm maturation, and sperm storage. The chemical composition of the epididymal plasma plays an important role in both sperm maturation and sperm storage. Environmental chemicals perturb these processes and can produce adverse effects.

## Accessory Sex Organs

The anatomical relationship of accessory sex organs in the male rodent is depicted in Fig. 19-4. Most mammals possess seminal vesicles (with the exception of cats and dogs) and most have prostate glands. However, the physiological and anatomical characteristics of the prostate gland may vary considerably among mammals (Wilson, 1995).

The seminal plasma functions as a vehicle for conveying the ejaculated sperm from the male to the female reproductive tract. The seminal plasma is produced by the secretory organs of the male reproductive system, which, along with the epididymides, include the prostate, seminal vesicles, bulbourethral (Cowper's) glands, and urethral (Littre's) glands. Any abnormal function of these organs can be reflected in altered seminal plasma characteristics. Seminal plasma is normally an isotonic, neutral medium, which, in many species, contains

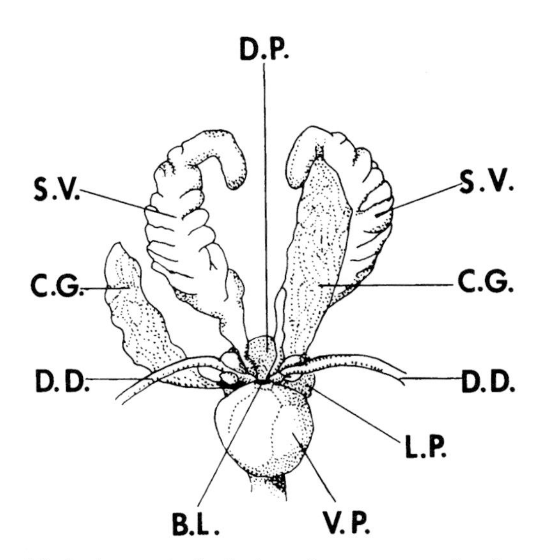


*Figure 19–4. Anatomical relation of components of rodent sex accessory glands. D.D., ductus deferens; B.L., bladder; V.P., ventral prostate; L.P., lateral prostate; C.G., coagulating gland (also called anterior prostate); S.V., seminal vesicle; D.P., dorsal prostate. (From Thomas JA et al.: Hormone assays and endocrine function, in Hayes AW: Principles and Methods of Toxicology. New York: Raven Press, 1982.)*

sources of energy such as fructose and sorbitol that are directly available to sperm. Functions of the other constituents such as citric acid and inositol are not known. In general, the secretions from the prostate and seminal vesicles contribute little to fertility (Mann and Lutwak-Mann, 1981).

The accessory sex organs are androgen dependent. They serve as indicators of the Leydig cell function and/or androgen action. The weights of the accessory sex glands are an indirect measure of circulating testosterone levels. The ventral prostate of rats has been used to study the actions of testosterone and to investigate the molecular basis of androgen-regulated gene function.

Human semen emission initially involves the urethral and Cowper's glands, with the prostatic secretion and sperm coming next and the seminal vesicle secretion delivered last. There is a considerable overlap between the presperm, sperm-rich, and postsperm fractions. Therefore, even if an ejaculate is collected in as many as six split-ejaculate fractions, it is rarely possible to obtain a sperm-free fraction consisting exclusively of prostatic or vesicular secretions.

Acid phosphatase and citric acid are markers for prostatic secretion; fructose is an indicator for seminal vesicle secretion. It is estimated that about one-third of the entire human ejaculate is contributed by the prostate and about two-thirds by the seminal vesicles. Both the vas deferens and the seminal vesicles apparently synthesize prostaglandins. Semen varies both in volume and composition between species. Human, bovine, and canine species have a relatively small semen volume (1 to 10 ml); semen of stallions and boars is ejaculated in much larger quantities. Sperm move from the distal portion of the epididymis through the vas deferens (ductus deferens) to the urethra. Vasectomy is the surgical removal of the vas deferens or a portion of it. The semen of some animals, including rodents and man, tends to coagulate on ejaculation. The clotting mechanism (e.g., "copulatory plug") involves enzymes and substrates from different accessory organs.

Although all mammals have a prostate, the organ differs anatomically, physiologically, and chemically among species, and lobe differences in the same species may be pronounced. The rat prostate is noted for its complex structure and its prompt response to castration and androgen stimulation. The human prostate is a tubuloalveolar gland made up of two prominent lateral lobes that contribute about one-third of the ejaculate.

Prostate secretion in men and many other mammal species contains acid phosphatase, zinc, and citric acid. The prostatic secretion is the main source of acid phosphatase in human semen; its concentration provides a convenient method for assessing the functional state of the prostate. The human prostate also produces spermine. Certain proteins and enzymes (acid phosphatase, $\gamma$-glutamyl transpeptidase, glutamicoxaloacetic transaminase), cholesterol, inositol, zinc, and magnesium have also been proposed as indicators of prostatic secretory function. Radioactive zinc ($^{65}Zn$) uptake by rodent prostate glands has been used as an index for androgenic potency (Gunn and Gould, 1956). An ionic antagonism exists between zinc and cadmium. Cadmium can induce metallothionein in the prostate glands of experimental animals (Waalkes et al., 1982; Waalkes et. al., 1992).

The anatomical structure of the seminal vesicle varies among animals. The seminal vesicle is a compact glandular tissue arranged in the form of multiple lobes that surround secretory ducts. Like the prostate, the seminal vesicle is responsive to androgens and is a useful indicator of Leydig cell function. The vesicular glands can be used as a gravimetric indicator for androgens.

In the human male, the seminal vesicle contributes about 60 percent of the seminal fluid. The seminal vesicles also produce more than half of the seminal plasma in laboratory and domestic animals such as the rat, guinea pig, and bull. In human males and in bulls, rams, and boars (but not in rats), most of the seminal fructose is secreted by the seminal vesicles, and, consequently, in these species the chemical assay of fructose in semen is a useful indicator of the relative contribution of the seminal vesicles toward whole semen. Seminal vesicle secretion is also characterized by the presence of proteins and enzymes, phosphorylcholine, and prostaglandins.

### Erection and Ejaculation

These physiologic processes are controlled by the central nervous system (CNS) but are modulated by the autonomic nervous system. Parasympathetic nerve stimulation results in dilatation of the arterioles of the penis, which initiates an erection. Erectile tissue of the penis engorges with blood, veins are compressed to block outflow, and the turgor of the organ increases. In the human male, afferent impulses from the genitalia and descending tracts, which mediate erections in response to erotic psychic stimuli, reach the integrating centers in the lumbar segments of the spinal cord. The efferent fibers are located in the pelvic splanchnic nerves.

Ejaculation is a two-stage spinal reflex involving emission and ejaculation. Emission is the movement of the semen into the urethra; ejaculation is the propulsion of the semen out of the urethra at the time of orgasm. Afferent pathways involve fibers from receptors in the glans penis that reach the spinal cord through the internal pudendal nerves. Emission is a sympathetic response effected by contraction of the smooth muscle of the vas deferens and seminal vesicles. Semen is ejaculated out of the urethra by contraction of the bulbocavernosus muscle. The spinal reflex centers for this portion of the reflex are in the upper sacral and lowest lumbar segments of the spinal cord; the motor pathways traverse the first to third sacral roots of the internal pudendal nerves.

Little is known concerning the effects of chemicals on erection or ejaculation (Woods, 1984). Pesticides, particularly the organophosphates, are known to affect neuroendocrine processes involved in erection and ejaculation. Many drugs act on the autonomic nervous system and affect potency (Table 19-5) (Papadopoulas, 1980; Buchanan and Davis, 1984; Stevenson and Umstead, 1984). Impotence, the failure to obtain or sustain an erection, is rarely of endocrine origin; more often the cause is psychological. The occurrence of nocturnal or early-morning erections implies that the neurologic and circulatory pathways involved in attaining an erection are intact and suggests the possibility of a psychological cause.

## OVARIAN FUNCTION

### Oogenesis

Ovarian germ cells with their follicles have a dual origin: The theca or stromal cells arise from fetal connective tissues of the ovarian medulla and the granulosa cells from the cortical mesenchyme (Fig. 19-5).

About 400,000 follicles are present at birth in each human ovary. After birth, many undergo atresia, and those that survive are continuously reduced in number. Any agent that damages the oocytes will accelerate the depletion of the pool and can lead to reduced fertility in females. About one-half of the number of oocytes present at birth remain at puberty; the number is reduced to about 25,000 by 30 years of age. About 400 primary follicles will yield mature ova during a woman's reproductive life span (Fig. 19-1). During the approximately three decades of fecundity, follicles in various stages of growth can always be found. After menopause, follicles are no longer present in the ovary.

Follicles remain in a primary follicle stage following birth until puberty, when a number of follicles start to grow during each ovarian cycle. However, most fail to achieve maturity. For the follicles that continue to grow, the first event is an increase in size of the primary oocytes. During this stage, fluid-filled spaces appear among the cells of the follicle, which unite to form a cavity or antrum, otherwise known as the Graafian follicle.

**Table 19–5**
**Drug-Induced Impotence**

| | AGENT | CN | ANS | ENDO. |
|---|---|---|---|---|
| Narcotics | Morphine | + | + | ? |
| | Ethanol | + | | |
| Psychotropic | Chlorpromazine | | + | |
| | Diazepam | + | | |
| | Tricyclic antidepressants | | + | ? |
| | MAO inhibitors | | + | |
| Hypotensives | Methyldopa | + | + | + |
| | Clonidine | + | + | |
| | Reserpine | + | + | |
| | Guanethidine | | ++ | |
| Hormones/antagonists | Estrogens | | | + |
| | Cyproterone | | | + |

SOURCE: Millar, 1979. Also Buchanan and Davis, 1984.

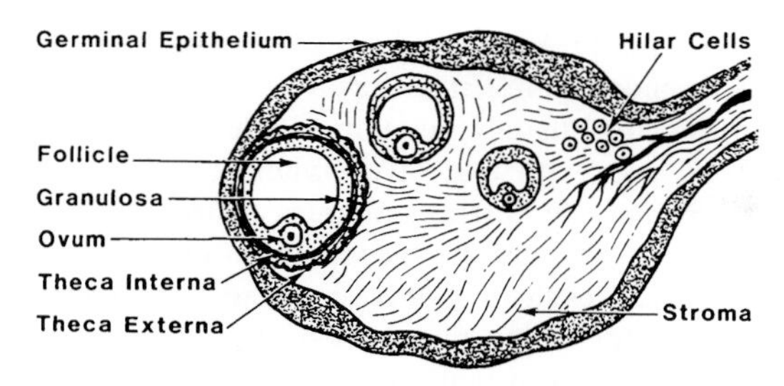


*Figure 19–5. Schematic representation of ovarian morphology. (From Thomas and Keenan, 1986.)*

Primary oocytes undergo two specialized nuclear divisions, which result in the formation of four cells containing one-half the number of chromosomes (Fig. 19-2). The first meiotic division occurs within the ovary just before ovulation, and the second occurs just after the sperm fuses with the egg. In the first stage of meiosis, the primary oocyte is actively synthesizing DNA and protein in preparation for entering prophase. The DNA content doubles as the prophase chromosomes each produce their mirror image. Each doubled chromosome is attracted to its homologous mate to form tetrads. The members of the tetrads synapse or come to lie side by side. Before separation, the homologous pairs of chromosomes exchange genetic material by a process known as "crossing over." Thus, qualitative differences occur between the resulting gametes. Subsequent meiotic stages distribute the members of the tetrads to the daughter cells in such a way that each cell receives the haploid number of chromosomes. At telophase, one secondary oocyte and a polar body have been formed, which are no longer genetically identical.

The secondary oocyte enters the next cycle of division very rapidly; each chromosome splits longitudinally; the ovum and the three polar bodies now contain the haploid number of chromosomes and half the amount of genetic material. Although the nuclei of all four eggs are equivalent, the cytoplasm is divided unequally. The end products are one large ovum and three rudimentary ova known as polar bodies, which subsequently degenerate. The ovum is released from the ovary at the secondary oocyte stage; the second stage of meiotic division is triggered in the oviduct by the entry of the sperm.

### The Ovarian Cycle

The cyclic release of pituitary gonadotropins involving the secretion of ovarian progesterone and estrogen is depicted in Fig. 19-6. These female sex steroids determine ovulation and prepare the female accessory sex organs to receive the male sperm. Sperm ejaculated into the vagina must make their way through the cervix into the uterus where they are capacitated. Sperm then migrate into the oviducts where fertilization takes place. The conceptus subsequently returns from the oviducts to the uterus and implants into the endometrium.

## POSTOVARIAN PROCESSES

Female accessory sex organs function to bring together the ovulated ovum and the ejaculated sperm. Chemical composition and viscosity of reproductive tract fluids, as well as the

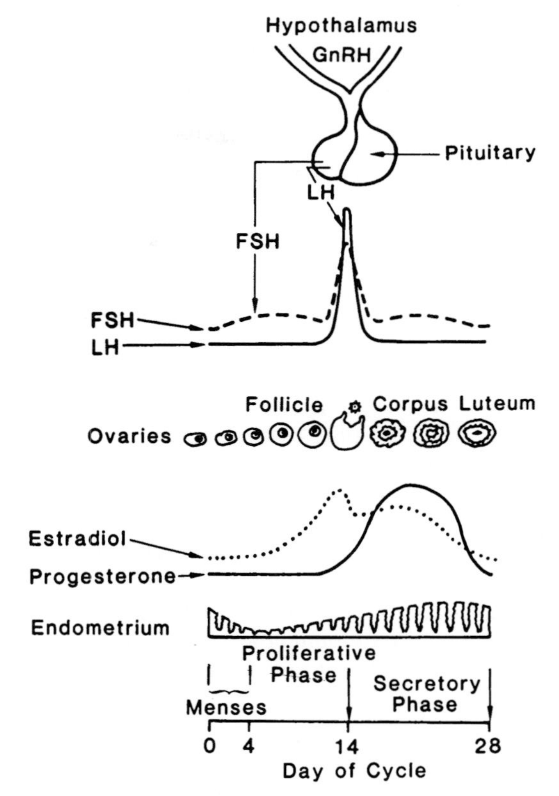


*Figure 19–6. Hormonal regulation of menstrual function. FSH, follicle stimulating hormone; GnRH, gonadotropin releasing hormone; LH, luteinizing hormone. (From Thomas and Keenan, 1986.)*

epithelial morphology of these organs, are controlled by ovarian (and trophoblastic) hormones.

### The Oviducts

The oviducts provide the taxis of the fimbria, which is under muscular control. The involvement of the autonomic nervous system in this process, as well as in oviductal transport of both the male and female gametes, raises the possibility that pharmacologic agents known to affect the autonomic nervous system may alter function and, therefore, fertility.

### The Uterus

The uterine endometrium reflects the cyclicity of the ovary as it is prepared to receive the conceptus. The myometrium's major role is contractile. In primates, at the end of menstruation, all but the deep layers of the endometrium are sloughed. Under the influence of estrogens from the developing follicle, the thickness of the endometrium increases rapidly. The uterine glands increase in length but do not secrete to any degree. These endometrial changes are called proliferative. After ovulation, the endometrium becomes slightly edematous, and the actively secreting glands become tightly coiled and folded under the influence of estrogen and progesterone from the corpus luteum. These are secretory (progestational) changes (Fig. 19-6).

When fertilization fails to occur, the endometrium is shed and a new cycle begins. Only primates menstruate. Other mammals have a sexual or estrus cycle. Female animals come into "heat" (estrus) at the time of ovulation. This is generally the only time during which the female is receptive to the male. In spontaneously ovulating species (e.g., rodents), the endocrine events are comparable with those in the menstrual cycle. In the rabbit, ovulation is a reflex produced by copulation.

### The Cervix

The mucosa of the uterine cervix does not undergo cyclic desquamation, but there are regular changes in the cervical mucus. Estrogen, which makes the mucus thinner and more alkaline, promotes the survival and transport of sperm. Progesterone makes the mucus thick, tenacious, and cellular. The mucus is thinnest at the time of ovulation and dries in an arborizing, fernlike pattern on a slide. After ovulation and during pregnancy, it becomes thick and fails to form the fern pattern. Disruptions of the cervix may be expressed as disorders of differentiation (including neoplasia), disturbed secretion, and incompetence. Exfoliative cytologic (e.g., Papanicolaou's stain) and histologic techniques are currently used to assess disorders of differentiation. Various synthetic steroids (*e.g.*, oral contraceptives) can affect the extent and pattern of cervical mucus.

### The Vagina

Estrogen produces a growth and proliferation of vaginal epithelium. The layers of cells become cornified and can be readily identified in vaginal smears. Vaginal cornification has been used as an index for estrogens. Progesterone stimulation produces a thick mucus; the epithelium proliferates, becoming infiltrated with leukocytes. The cyclic changes in the vaginal smear in rats are easily recognized. The changes in humans and other species are similar but less apparent. Analysis of vaginal fluid or cytologic studies of desquamated vaginal cells (quantitative cytochemistry) reflects ovarian function. Vaginal sampling of cells and fluid might offer a reliable and easily available external monitor of internal function and dysfunction. Alteration in vaginal flora can be a toxicologic condition associated with the use of vaginal tampons [viz., toxic shock syndrome (TSS)].

## FERTILIZATION

During fertilization, the ovum contributes the maternal complement of genes to the nucleus of the fertilized egg and provides food reserves for the early embryo. The innermost portion of the egg is the vitelline membrane. Outside the ovum proper lies a thick, tough, and highly refractile capsule termed the zona pellucida, which increases the total diameter of the human ovum to about 0.15 mm. Beyond the zona pellucida is the corona radiata derived from the follicle; it surrounds the ovum during its passage into the oviduct.

Formation, maturation, and union of a male and female germ cell are all preliminary events leading to a combined cell or zygote. Penetration of ovum by sperm and the coming together and pooling of their respective nuclei constitute the process of fertilization.

Only minutes are required for the sperm to penetrate the zona pellucida after passing through the cumulus oophorus in vitro and probably sooner in vivo. The sperm traverse a curved oblique path. Entering the perivitelline space, the sperm head immediately lies flat on the vitellus; its plasma membrane fuses with that of the vitellus and then embeds into the ovum. The cortical granules of the egg disappear, the vitellus shrinks, and the second maturation division is reinitiated, which results in extrusion of the second polar body. A specific factor in the ovum appears to trigger the development of the male pronucleus; the chromatin of the ovum forms a female pronucleus.

As syngamy approaches, the two pronuclei become intimately opposed but do not fuse. The nuclear envelopes of the pronuclei break up; nucleoli disappear and chromosomes condense and promptly aggregate. The chromosomes mingle to form the prometaphase of the first spindle, and the egg divides into two blastomeres. From sperm penetration to first cleavage usually requires about 12 h in laboratory animals.

From a single fertilized cell (the zygote), cells proliferate and differentiate until more than a trillion cells of about 100 different types are present in the adult organism.

## IMPLANTATION

The developing embryo migrates through the oviduct into the uterus. Upon contact with the endometrium, the blastocyst becomes surrounded by an outer layer or syncytiotrophoblast, a multinucleated mass of cells with no discernible boundaries, and an inner layer of individual cells, the cytotrophoblast. The syncytiotrophoblast erodes the endometrium, and the blastocyst implants. Placental circulation is then established and trophoblastic function continues. The blastocysts of most mammalian species implant about day 6 or 7 following fertilization. At this stage, the differentiation of the embryonic and extraembryonic (trophoblastic) tissues is apparent.

Trophoblastic tissue differentiates into cytotrophoblast and syncytiotrophoblast cells. The syncytiotrophoblast cells produce chorionic gonadotropin, chorionic growth hormones, placental lactogen, estrogen, and progesterone, which are needed to achieve independence from the ovary in maintaining the pregnancy. Rapid proliferation of the cytotrophoblast serves to anchor the growing placenta to the maternal tissue.

The developing placenta consists of proliferating trophoblasts, which expand rapidly and infiltrate the maternal vascular channels. Shortly after implantation, the syncytiotrophoblast is bathed by maternal venous blood, which supplies nutrients and permits an exchange of gases. Histotrophic nutrition involves yolk sac circulation; hemotrophic nutrition involves the placenta. Placental circulation is established relatively early in women and primates and, in relative terms much later in rodents and rabbits. Interestingly, placental dysfunction due to vascular compromise caused by cocaine leads to increased fetal risk, causing growth retardation and prematurity. Fetal loss due to abruptio placentae may occur (Doering et al., 1989).

Morphologically, the placenta may be defined as the fusion or opposition of fetal membranes to the uterine mucous membrane (Slikker and Miller, 1994). In humans, the placenta varies considerably throughout gestation. The integral unit of the placenta is the villous tree. The core of the villous tree contains the fetal capillaries and associated endothelium.

Placentation varies considerably among various domestic animals, experimental animals, and primates (Slikker and Miller, 1994). Man and monkey possess a hemochorial placenta. Pigs, horses, and donkeys have an epitheliochorial type of placenta, whereas sheep, goats, and cows have a syndesmochorial type of placenta. In laboratory animals (e.g., rat, rabbit, and guinea pig), the placenta is termed a *hemoendothelial* type. Among the various species, the number of maternal and fetal cell layers ranges from six layers (e.g., pig, horse) to a single layer (e.g., rat, rabbit). Primates, including man, have three layers of cells in the placenta that a substance must pass across. Thus, the placentas of some species are "thicker" than others.

Generally, the placenta is impermeable to chemicals/drugs with molecular weights of 1000 daltons or more. Most medications have molecular weights of 500 daltons or less. Hence, molecular size is rarely a factor in denying a drug's entrance across the placenta and into the embryo/fetus. Placental permeability to a chemical is affected by placental characteristics including thickness, surface area, carrier systems, and lipid-protein concentration of the membranes. The inherent characteristics of the chemical itself, such as its degree of ionization, lipid solubility, protein binding ability, and molecular size also affect its transport across the placenta.

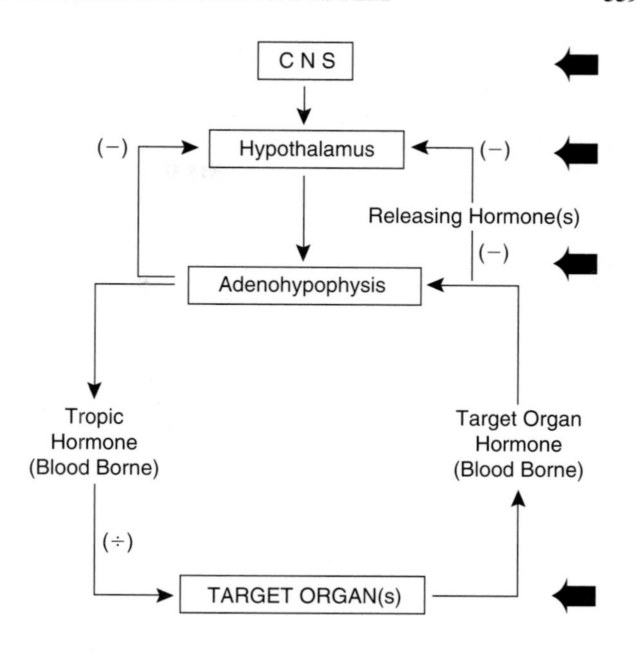


***Figure 19–7. Relation between adenohypophyseal-hypothalamic axis and hormone target organs.** (From Thomas JA et al.: Hormone assays and endocrine function, in Hayes, AW: Principles and Methods of Toxicology. New York, Raven Press, 1982.)*

# INTEGRATIVE PROCESSES

## Hypothalamo-Pituitary-Gonadal Axis

FSH and LH are glycoproteins synthesized and released from a subpopulation of the basophilic gonadotropic cells of the pituitary gland. Hypothalamic neuroendocrine neurons secrete specific releasing or release-inhibiting factors into the hypophyseal portal system, which carries them to the adenohypophysis where they act to stimulate or inhibit the release of anterior pituitary hormones. Luteinizing hormone-releasing hormone (LHRH) acts on gonadotropic cells, thereby stimulating the release of FSH and LH. LHRH and follicle stimulating hormone-releasing hormone (FSHRH) appear to be the same substance. Native and synthetic forms of LHRH stimulate the release of both gonadotrophic hormones; thus it has been proposed to call this compound gonadotropin-releasing hormone (GnRH).

The neuroendocrine neurons have nerve terminals containing monoamines (norepinephrine, dopamine, serotonin) that impinge on them. Reserpine, chlorpromazine, and monoamine oxidase (MAO) inhibitors modify the content or actions of brain monoamines that affect gonadotropins.

FSH probably acts primarily on the Sertoli cells, but it also appears to stimulate the mitotic activity of spermatogonia. LH stimulates steroidogenesis. A defect in the function of the testis (in the production of spermatozoa or testosterone) will tend to be reflected in increased levels of FSH and LH in serum because of the lack of the "negative feedback" effect of testicular hormones (Fig. 19-7).

The hypothalamo-pituitary-gonadal feedback system is a very delicate modulated hormonal process. Several sites in the endocrine process can be perturbed by drugs (e.g., oral contraceptives) and by different chemicals (Fig. 19-7). Gonadotoxic agents may act on neuroendocrine processes in the brain or they may act directly on the target organ (e.g., the gonad). Toxicants that adversely or otherwise alter the hepatic and/or renal biotransformation of the endogenous sex steroid might be expected to interfere with the pituitary feedback system.

## Puberty

From the early newborn period to the onset of puberty, the testes remain hormonally dormant. After birth, the androgen-secreting Leydig cells in the mammalian fetal testes become quiescent, and a period follows in which the gonads of both sexes await final maturation of the reproductive system.

The onset of puberty begins with the secretion of increasing levels of gonadotropins. The physiological trigger for puberty is poorly understood, but somehow a hypothalamic gonadostat changes the rate of secretion of LHRH, resulting in increases in LH. As puberty approaches, a pulsatile pattern of LH and FSH secretion is observed. The gonad itself is not required for activating FSH or LH at the onset of puberty. It is a CNS phenomenon. Female puberty is affected by a wide range of influences including climate, race, heredity, athletic activity, and degree of adiposity.

# SEXUAL BEHAVIOR AND LIBIDO

Physiologic processes that account for sexual behavior are poorly understood. The external environment greatly affects sexual behavior, and the libido's contribution to reproductive activity depends on a close interplay between neural and endocrine events. For example, a correlation of behavior and receptivity for insemination is attained by complex neuroendocrine mechanisms involving the brain, the pituitary, and sex steroid hormones. This complexity varies even among higher vertebrates. Thus, in reproductive studies involving rodents, the investigator must determine whether the animals actually mate. In the rat, this can be determined by inspecting females each day for vaginal plugs. The number of mountings, thrusts, and ejaculations each can be quantified as indicators of reproductive behavior. It is also important to determine whether the male animal mounts females or other males. If the male copulates and is sterile, indicators of male fertility such as testicular function should be considered. Failure to copulate suggests either a neuromuscular and/or behavioral defect in the experimental animal.

## GENERAL TOXICOLOGIC/PHARMACOLOGIC PRINCIPLES

Many of the principles that govern absorption, distribution, metabolism, and excretion of a chemical or drug also apply to the reproductive system. There are, however, some rather unique barriers that affect a chemical's action on the mammalian reproductive system. The maternal–fetal interface occurring at the placenta represents a barrier to chemicals coming in contact with the developing embryo. Unfortunately the placenta is not so restrictive as to prevent most chemicals from crossing the placenta. Most chemicals are not denied entry into a number of compartments or secretions of the reproductive tract. Indeed, xenobiotic substances and certain drugs can be readily detected in uterine secretions, in the milk of the lactating mother, and in seminal fluid (Mann and Lutwak-Mann, 1981). No specialized barriers appear to prevent chemicals or drugs from acting on the ovary. Several drugs are known to interfere with ovarian function (Table 19-6) (Gorospe and Reinhard, 1995). Unlike the female gonad, a somewhat specialized barrier is present in the male gonad. This specialized biological barrier is referred to as the blood–testis barrier.

## THE BLOOD–TESTIS BARRIER

There are a number of specialized anatomic barriers in the body. Tissue permeability barriers include the blood–brain barrier, and the blood–thymus barrier. Important barriers within the endocrine system are the placental barrier and the blood–testis barrier. The blood–testis barrier is situated somewhere between the lumen of an interstitial capillary and the lumen of a seminiferous tubule (Neaves, 1977). Several anatomically related structures intervene between the two luminal spaces, including the capillary endothelium, the capillary basal lamina, the lymphatic endothelium, the myoid cells, the basal lamina of the seminiferous tubule, and the Sertoli cells. The barrier that impedes or denies the free exchange of chemicals/drugs between the blood and the fluid inside the seminiferous tubules is located in one or more of these structures. The apparent positioning of space (distance) relative to transepithelial permeability can affect the passage (or blockage) of a substance through the blood–testis barrier. These epithelial cell anatomic relationships can affect the tightness of fit between cells and the extent to which a chemical's passsage can occur. Such junctions or cell unions are often leaky and may allow for a substance's passage. These so-called gap junctions may even be less developed in the immature or young mammalian testes, hence affording greater opportunities for foreign chemicals to permeate the seminiferous tubule. Steinberger and Klinefelter (1993) have developed a two-compartment model for culturing testicular cells that simulates a blood–testis barrier. This culture model has been proposed for studying Sertoli and Leydig cell dysfunction in vitro.

Setchell and coworkers (1969) first demonstrated that immunoglobulins and iodinated albumin, inulin, and a number of small molecules were excluded from the seminiferous tubules by the blood–testis barrier. Dym and Fawcett (1970) suggested that the primary permeability barrier for the seminiferous tubules was composed of the surrounding layers of myoid cells, while specialized Sertoli cell-to-Sertoli cell junctions within the seminiferous epithelium constituted a secondary cellular barrier. Certain classes of adhesive molecules (e.g., E- and N-cadherin, $\alpha$- and $\beta$-catenin, plakoglobin, etc.) may act to promote Sertoli cell-to-Sertoli cell adhesion and tight junction formation (Byers et al., 1994).

Okumura and coworkers (1975) quantified permeability rates for nonelectrolytes and for certain chemicals/drugs. Small-molecular weight molecules (e.g., water, urea) can readily cross the blood–testis barrier; larger-sized substances (e.g., inulin) are impeded from crossing. The degree of lipid solubility and ionization are important determinants as to whether a substance can permeate the blood–testis barrier. A number of factors are known to affect the permeability of the blood–testis barrier, including ligation of the efferent ductules, autoimmune orchiditis, and vasectomy (Sundaram and Witorsch, 1995).

## BIOTRANSFORMATION OF EXOGENOUS CHEMICALS

The mammalian gonad is capable of metabolizing a host of foreign chemicals that have traversed the blood–testis barrier. While mixed-function oxidases and epoxide-degrading enzymes may not be as active as hepatic systems, they are nevertheless present. Cytochromes P-450 (arylhydrocarbon hydroxylases) are present in the testes. Cytochrome P-450, in general, is fairly sensitive to the effects of a number of chemicals. Gonadal cytochrome P-450 is no exception. Arylhydrocarbon hydroxylase (AHH) is present in testicular microsomes (Lee et al., 1981). Consequently, the pathways for steroidogenesis contain a number of enzymes that are affected by chemicals or drugs (Table 19-7). Like the process of steroidogenesis in the gonads, the adrenal cortex is also vulnerable to chemical insult

**Table 19–6**
**Chemotherapeutic Agents and Ovarian Dysfunction**

| | |
|---|---|
| Prednisone | Busulfan |
| Vincristine | Methotrexate |
| Vinblastine | Cytosine arabinoside |
| 6-Mercaptopurine | L-Asparginase |
| Nitrogen mustard | 5-Fluorouracil |
| Cyclophosphamide | Adriamycin |
| Chlorambucil | |

SOURCE: Haney, 1985.

**Table 19–7**
**Inhibitors of Steroidogenic Enzymes**

| ENZYME | INHIBITOR |
|---|---|
| Cholesterol side chain cleavage | Aminoglutethimide, 3-methoxybenzidine, cyanoketone, estrogens, azastene, danazol |
| Aromatase | 4-Acetoxy-androstene-3,17-dione, 4-hydroxy-androstene-3,17-dione, 1,4,6-androstatriene-3,17-dione, 6-bromoandrostene-3,17-dione, 7α(4′amino)phenylthioandrostenedione, δ′-testolactone, fenarimol*, MEHP† |
| 11-Hydroxylase | Danazol, metyrapone |
| 21-Hydroxylase | Danazol, spironolactone |
| 17-Hydroxylase | Danazol, spironolactone |
| 17,20-Desmolase | Danazol, spironolactone |
| 17-Hydroxysteroid dehydrogenase | Danazol |
| 3-Hydroxysteroid dehydrogenase | Danazol |
| c-17-L-20-lyase | Ketoconozole‡ |

* Hirsch *et al.*, 1987.
† Davis et al., 1989.
‡ Effendy and Krause, 1989.
SOURCE: Haney, 1985 (modified).

(Colby, 1988). Both the parent compound and its metabolite(s) can adversely affect the gonad (Table 19-8). Whether biotransformation occurs gonadally or extragonadally, the end result can be interference with spermatogenesis and/or steroidogenesis. Their mechanism(s) of toxicity varies considerably. The microsomal oxidation of *n*-hexane yields 2,5-hexanedione (2,5-HD). *n*-Hexane, an environmental toxicant, causes peripheral polyneuropathy and testicular atrophy (Boekelheide, 1987, 1988). 2,5-HD produces gonadal toxicity by altering testicular tubulin. In this work, Boekelheide suggested that damage to the microtubules of the Sertoli cell results in germ cell loss in 2,5-HD-treated rats. More recently, it has been reported that 2,5-HD disrupts Sertoli cell seminiferous tubule secretion as well as interfering with this cell's microtubular system (Richburg et al., 1994). Ethylene glycol monoethyl ether, along with its metabolites, is a gonadal toxin (Nagano et al., 1979). 2-Methoxyacetaldehyde (MALD) produces specific cellular toxicity to pachytene spermatocytes (Foster et al., 1986). Vinclozolin, a fungicide, when it undergoes biotransformation produces at least two major metabolites that can effectively act as antagonists of the androgen receptor (Kelce et al., 1994). Diethylhexyl phthalate (DEHP) and its metabolite(s) MEHP are both gonadal toxicants whose mechanism(s), in part, is due to depletion of testicular zinc. DEHP and other plasticizers can adversely affect spermatogenesis (Thomas and Thomas, 1984). Gray and Beamand (1984) have proposed that the mechanism of DEHP-induced testicular atrophy involves a membrane alteration leading to separation of the germ cells (spermatocytes and spermatids) from the underlying Sertoli cells. The action of MEHP has been attributed to the ability of this phthalate to reduce FSH binding to Sertoli cell membranes (Grasso et al., 1993). The separation of spermatocytes and spermatids would interfere with the transfer of nutrients from the Sertoli cells, leading to death and disintegration of the germ cells. MEHP, and not DEHP, is most likely the principal testicular toxicant (Albro et al., 1989). DEHP exposure in rats significantly suppresses preovulatory follicle granulosa cell estradiol production (Davis et al., 1994a, 1994b). While dietary zinc deficiency in humans causes an inhibition of spermatogenesis, there are no reports of phthalate-induced zinc deficiency causing infertility in human males. Epichlorohydrin, a highly reactive electrophile used in the manufacture of glycerol and epoxy resins, produces spermatozoal metabolic lesions (Toth et al., 1989). Tri-*o*-cresyl phosphate (TOCP), an industrial chemical used as a plasticizer in lacquers and varnishes, decreases epididymal sperm motility and density. TOCP interferes with spermatogenic processes and sperm motility directly and not via an androgenic mechanism or decreased vitamin E (Somkuti et al., 1987).

The male reproductive system can be adversely affected by TCDD (Bjerke and Peterson, 1994). TCDD can alter germ cells at all developmental stages in the testes (Chahoud et al., 1992). Dioxin can reduce Leydig cell volume at doses that do not appear to affect spermatogenesis (Johnson et al., 1992). In rodents, TCDD is both embryotoxic and teratogenic (Dickson and Buzik, 1993). TCDD has an avidity for the estrogen receptor (Hruska and Olson, 1989) and other receptors (e.g., the Ah receptor). Recently, the safety assessment of PCBs, with particular reference to reproductive toxicity, has been reviewed (Battershill, 1994).

2-Methoxylethanol (2-ME), an industrial solvent, is toxic to both the male and female reproductive system (Mebus et al., 1989). 2-ME must be metabolized to 2-methoxyacetic acid (2-MAA) by alcohol and aldehyde dehydrogenases in order to attain its testicular toxicity. All stages of spermatocyte development and some stages of spermatid development are affected by 2-ME, but it seems to be more selective in destroying early-and late-stage pachytene primary spermatocytes. 2-ME is also embryotoxic and teratogenic in several species (Hanly

**Table 19–8**
**Representative Drugs, Chemicals, and Their Metabolites and Their Ability to Exert Toxic Actions Upon the Male Gonad**

| PARENT COMPOUND | METABOLITE | REFERENCE |
|---|---|---|
| Amiodarone (antiarrhythmic drug) | Desethylamiodarone | Holt et al., 1984 |
| Cephalosporin analogues (antimicrobial drug) | *N*-Methyltetrazolethiol* | Comereski et al., 1987 |
| Valproic acid (antiepileptic drug) | Isomers of 2-ethyl hexanol (?)† | Ritter et al., 1987 |
| Diethylhexyl phthalate (DEHP; plasticizer) | Mono-ethylhexyl phthalate and 2-ethyl hexanol (?)† | Thomas et al., 1982 |
| Dibromochloropropane‡ (DBCP; fungicide) | Dichloropropene(s) derivatives (?)† | Torkelson et al., 1961 |
| Ethylene glycol monoethyl ether (industrial solvent) | 2-Methoxyacetaldehyde | Foster et al., 1986 |
| *n*-Hexane (environmental toxicant) | 2,5-Hexanedione | Boekelheide, 1987 |
| Acrylamide (industrial use) | *N*-Methylacrylamide, *N*-isopropylacrylamide | Sakamoto and Hashimoto, 1986 |
| Vinclozolin (fungicide) | Butenoic acid derivative and an enanilide metabolite | Kelce et al., 1994 |

* Only substituent is a testicular toxin, not cephalosporin.
† Questionable testicular toxin but probably teratogenic.
‡ Radiometabolities of ($^3$H)-DBCP are not preferentially labeled in the testes (Shemi et al., 1987).
SOURCE: Thomas and Ballantyne (1990) (modified).

et al., 1984). 2-ME (also known as methyl cellosolve) when applied dermally can produce a decline in epididymal sperm and testicular spermatid counts in rats (Feuston et al., 1989). Ethanol also causes delayed testicular development and may affect the Sertoli cell and/or the Leydig cell (Anderson et al., 1989). Trifluoroethanol and trifluoroacetaldehyde produce specific damage to pachytene and dividing spermatocytes and round spermatids in rats (Lloyd et al., 1988). Ethane dimethane sulfonate (EDS) effectively eradicates Leydig cells and endogenous testosterone (cf. Bremner et al., 1994).

Metabolites of cephalosporin reportedly cause testicular toxicity in rats (Comereski et al., 1987). Testicular degeneration from analogues of cephalosporin is most likely to occur with cefbuperazone, cefamandole, and cefoperazone. Cyclosporin can also inhibit testosterone biosynthesis in rat testes (Rajfer et al., 1987). Amiodarone and its desethyl metabolite can be detected in high concentrations in the testes and semen, but their action(s) on spermatogenesis or sperm motility is (are) not known (Holt et al., 1984).

Like the testes, the ovaries possess the metabolic capability to biotransform certain exogenous substrates. Furthermore the process of ovarian steroidogenesis, like the testes and the adrenal cortex (Colby, 1988), is susceptible to different agents that interfere with the biosynthesis of estrogens (Table 19-6). Less is known about how chemicals or drugs interfere with ovarian metabolism. The ovaries have not been studied as extensively as the testes because of their more difficult and complex hormonal relationships. Nevertheless, several chemotherapeutic agents can inhibit ovarian function (Table 19-5). Recently, Faustman et al. (1989) have studied the toxicity of direct-acting alkylating agents on rodent embryos. Their findings failed to reveal any specific structural activity patterns among various alkylating agents. As in the testes, mixed-function oxidases and various cytochrome systems are found in the ovaries. Certain chemicals or drugs (Haney, 1985) may exert a toxic effect on the primordial oocytes, as well as on other sites of action.

## DNA REPAIR

Depending on the species, there are variations in the capacity for spermatogenic cells to repair DNA damage due to environmental toxicants (Lee, 1983). It is well known that UV and x-rays can damage DNA molecules; lethal mutation (i.e., cell death) and mutation resulting from transformed cells can also occur. Spermatogenic cells can be used to study unscheduled DNA synthesis (Dixon and Lee, 1980). Unscheduled DNA repair in spermatogenic cells is dose and time dependent. Spermiogenic cells are less able to repair DNA damage resulting from alkylating agents. This DNA repair system provides a protective mechanism from certain toxicants; it is also a sensitive index of chromosome damage.

Drug-induced unscheduled DNA synthesis in mammalian oocytes reveals that female gametes possess an excision repair capacity (Pedersen and Brandriff, 1980; Lee, 1983). Unlike mature sperm, the mature oocyte maintains a DNA repair ability. However, this ability decreases at the time of meiotic maturation.

Different occupational risks have been seen to result in characteristic types and degrees of chromosomal aberrations

**Table 19–9**
**Occupational Exposure to Lead and its Relationship to Chromosomal Aberrations**

| EXPOSED SUBJECTS | TYPE OF ABERRATION |
|---|---|
| *Positive findings* | |
| Lead oxide factory workers | Chromatid and chromosome breaks |
| Chemical factory workers | Chromatid gaps, breaks |
| Zinc plant workers | Gaps, fragments, rings, exchanges, dicentrics |
| Blast-furnace workers, metal grinders, scrap metal workers | Gaps, breaks, hyperploidy, structural abnormalities |
| Battery plant workers and lead foundry workers | Gaps, breaks, fragments |
| Lead oxide factory workers | Chromatid and chromosome aberrations |
| Battery melters, tin workers | Dicentrics, rings, fragments |
| Ceramic, lead, and battery workers | Breaks, fragments |
| Smelter workers | Gaps, chromatid and chromosome aberrations |
| Battery plant workers | Chromatid and chromosome aberrations |
| *Negative findings* | |
| Policemen | |
| Lead workers | |
| Shipyard workers | |
| Smelter workers | |
| Volunteers (ingested lead) | |
| Children (near a smelter) | |

SOURCE: Thomas and Brogan, 1983.

(Table 19-9). In particular, lead toxicity can induce a variety of chromatid and chromosome breaks. Lead was one of the earliest substances to be associated with deleterious effects on the reproductive system (Thomas and Brogan, 1983). Lead poisoning has been associated with reduced fertility, miscarriages, and stillbirths since antiquity (Gilfillan, 1965, Lancranjan et al., 1975). Lead salts are among the oldest known spermicidal agents; lead has long been known to be an abortifacient (Hildebrand et al., 1973). Lead exposure results in a general suppression of the hypothalamic-pituitary-testicular axis in rats (Klein et al., 1994) and possibly in men occupationally exposed to this heavy metal (Rodamilans et al., 1988).

## TARGETS FOR CHEMICAL TOXICITY

There are several sites of chemicals' interference with the mammalian reproductive system (Fig. 19-7). Drugs and chemicals can act directly on the CNS, particularly the hypothalamus and the adenohypophysis. A number of drugs (e.g., tranquilizers, sedatives, etc.) can modify the CNS, leading to alterations in the secretion of hypothalamic-releasing hormones and/or gonadotropins (Table 19-4). Synthetic steroids (viz., 19-nortestosterones) are very effective in suppressing gonadotropin secretion and hence block ovulation.

The gonads are also targets for a host of drugs and chemicals (Table 19-10) (Chapman, 1983; Thomas and Keenan, 1986). The majority of these agents are representatives from major chemical classes of cancer chemotherapeutic agents, particularly the alkylating agents. A number of endocrine agents are of value in the treatment of certain cancers. Anti-estrogens (e.g., Tamoxifen), aromatase inhibitors (e.g., aminoglutethimide), GNRH agonists and antagonists, and anti-androgens (e.g., Flutamide) have the capability of interfering with the endocrine system (Lonning and Lien, 1993). Procarbazine, an antineoplastic drug, causes severe damage to the acrosomal plasma membrane and the nucleus of the sperm head in hamsters (Singh et al., 1989). Alkylating agents are effective against rapidly dividing cells. Not surprisingly, cellular division of germ cells is also affected, leading to the arrest of spermatogenesis.

Different cell populations of the mammalian testis exhibit somewhat different thresholds of sensitivity to different toxi-

**Table 19–10**
**Drugs That Are Gonadotoxic in Humans**

| MALES | FEMALES |
|---|---|
| Busulfan | Busulfan |
| Chlorambucil | Chlorambucil |
| Cyclophosphamide | Cyclophosphamide |
| Nitrogen mustard | Nitrogen mustard |
| Adriamycin | |
| Corticosteroids | |
| Cytosine-arabinoside | |
| Methotrexate | |
| Procarbazine | |
| Vincristine | |
| Vinblastine | Vinblastine |

SOURCE: Chapman, 1983.

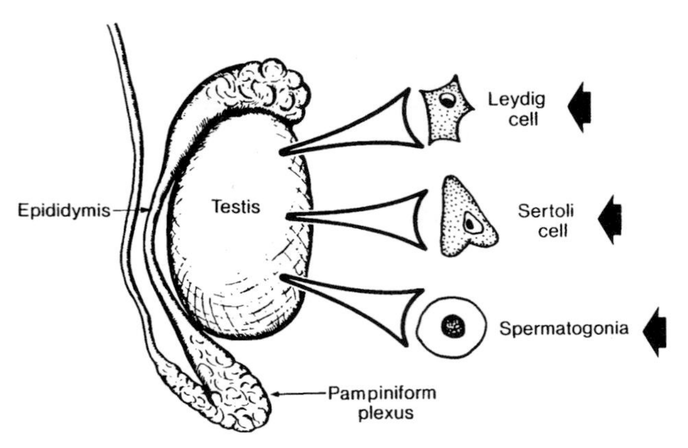


*Figure 19–8. Some possible sites of action of selected gonadotoxins. (From Thomas et al., 1982.)*

cants (Fig. 19-8). Thus, the germ cells are most sensitive to chemical insult (i.e., spermatogenesis). The Sertoli cells possess an intermediate sensitivity to chemical inhibition; Leydig cells are more resistant to environmental toxicants. Cell-specific testicular toxicants have been employed to evaluate the distribution of creatinine in the rete testis (Moore et al., 1992). Creatinine is associated with cells of the seminiferous epithelium—elevated urinary excretion of creatinine may provide a noninvasive marker for testicular toxicity in vivo.

DBCP, a fumigent, causes infertility in a number of species, including man. DBCP causes sterility but it may do so by acting on the Sertoli cell. DBCP may also inhibit sperm carbohydrate metabolism at the NADH dehydrogenase step in the mitochondrial electron transport chain (Greenwell et al., 1987). Despite DBCP's propensity to cause degeneration of the seminiferous tubules, toxicokinetic studies fail to reveal any preferential uptake of DBCP by the testes (Shemi et al., 1987). DBCP gonadotoxicity appears to be sex specific since only testicular injury has been reported; it does not cause comparable adverse effects in the female rat (Shaked et al., 1988). Analogues of DBCP cause testicular necrosis as well as DNA damage in the rat (Soderlund et al., 1988).

The production of lactate and pyruvate are indicators of Sertoli cell function (Williams and Foster, 1988). Either dinitrobenzene (DNB) or mono-(2-ethylhexyl) phthalate (MEHP) can affect lactate (and pyruvate) production by rat Sertoli cell cultures. The Sertoli cell appears to be a prime target for the toxic actions of DNB (Blackburn et al., 1988). Chapin and coworkers (1988) have also indicated that MEHP adversely affects the mitochondria of the Sertoli cell in vitro. Likewise, for dinitrotoluene (DNT) the locus of toxic action is the Sertoli cell (Bloch et al., 1988). Dinitrobenzene initially damages Sertoli cells with a subsequent degeneration and exfoliation of germ cells.

Anti-LH peptides can affect Leydig cell steroidogenesis. LHRH analogues (e.g., buserelin) can reduce testicular and uterine weights in rats (Donaubauer et al., 1987).

In some species, the pampiniform plexus, which functions as an effective heat exchange system to ensure that the blood supplying the testes is at a temperature compatible with spermatogenesis, is destroyed by cadmium, leading to necrosis of the blood vessels supplying the testes. Another anatomical structure of the testes, namely the epididymis, is less vulnerable to chemical insult, although halogenated hexoses and substituted glycerol moieties can alter electrolyte passage and sugar transport.

The liver and the kidney contain enzyme systems that affect the biological half-life of steroids and other hormones. Hence, xenobiotics that interfere with excretory processes might be expected to alter the endocrine system. For example, a number of hepatic steroid hydroxylases can be induced by either organophosphates or organochlorine pesticides. Such hydroxylation reactions can be expected to render the endogenous steroid more polar and hence more readily excreted by the kidney.

## EVALUATING REPRODUCTIVE FUNCTION

A number of hormone assays are available to assess endocrine function (Thomas and Thomas, 1994). The endocrine system of the female is more complex and dynamic than that of the male. Hence, evaluating reproductive function in the female is more difficult. Immediate distinctions must also be made between the pregnant and the nonpregnant female. Regardless of sex, both behavioral and physiologic factors must be considered in evaluating reproductive toxicity. The physiologic events involved in reproduction have inherent time factors that are species specific. Oftentimes evaluating a chemical's or drug's potential to affect the reproductive system is costly and time-consuming. Furthermore, many of the endpoints used to evaluate the reproductive system are not always reliable and have limitations (Table 19-11).

The fact that such a wide variety of chemicals or drugs can perturb the reproductive system adds another dimension of difficulty in the attempt to evaluate reproductive toxicity. Not only is there considerable diversity in the chemical configuration of the toxicants, but sites of action and mechanisms of action can be very different (Fig. 19-7).

Several classes of therapeutic agents can affect the male reproductive system (Table 19-12) as well as the female reproductive system (Table 19-13). Some of these agents act on the neutral component of the endocrine system, whereas others act directly on the gonad.

**Table 19–11**
**Advantages and Limitations of Standard Reproductive Procedures**

| ENDPOINT | LIMITATIONS | VALUE |
|---|---|---|
| Fertility | Insensitive | Integrates all reproductive functions |
| Testicular histology | Subjective; not quantitative | Information on target cell |
| Testis weights | Less sensitive than sperm counts; affected by edema | Rapid; quantitative |

SOURCE: Meistrich, 1989.

**Table 19–12**
**Agents Reported to Affect Male Reproductive Capacity**

*Steroids*
Natural and synthetic androgens (antiandrogens), estrogens (antiestrogens), and progestins

*Antineoplastic, Agents*
Alkaloids—vinca alkaloids (vinblastine, vincristine)
Alkylating agents—esters of methanesulfonic acid (MMS, EMS, busulfan); ethylenimines (TEM, TEPA); hydrazines (procarbazine): nitrogen mustards (chlorambucil, cyclophosphamide); nitrosoureas (CCNU, BCNU, MNU)
Antimetabolites—azauridine, 5-bromodeoxyuridine, cytosine arabinoside, 5-fluorouracil, 6-mercaptopurine
Antitumor antibiotics—actinomycin D, adriamycin, bleomycin, daunomvcin, mitomycin C

*Drugs That Modify the Nervous System*
Alcohols
Anesthetic gases and vapors—enflurane, halothane, methoxyflurane, nitrous oxide
Antiparkinsonism drugs—levodopa
Appetite suppressants
Narcotic and nonnarcotic analgesics—opioids
Neuroleptics—phenothiazines, imipramine, and amitriptyline
Tranquilizers—phenothiazines, reserpine, monoamine oxidase inhibitors
Antiadrenergic drugs—clonidine, methyldopa, guanethidine, bretylium, reserpine

*Other Therapeutic Agents*
Alcoholism—tetraethylthiuram disulfide (antabuse)
Analgesics and antipyretics—phenacetin
Anticonvulsants—diphenylhydantoin (phenytoin)
Antiinfective agents—amphotericin B, hexachlorophene, hycanthode, nitrofurans
Antischistosomal agents—niridazole, hycanthone
Antiparasitic drugs—quinine, quinacrine, chloroquine
Diuretics—aldactone, thiazides
Gout suppressants—colchicine
Histamines and histamine antagonists—chlorcyclizine, cimetidine
Oral hypoglycemic agents—chlorpropamide
Xanthines—caffeine, theobromine

*Metals and Trace Elements*
Al, boranes, boron, Cd, Co, Pb, Hg, methylmercury, Mo, Ni, Ag, U

*Insecticides*
Benzene hexachlorides—lindane
Carbamates—carbaryl
Chlorobenzene derivatives—chlorophenothane (DDT), methoxychlor
Indane derivatives—aldrin, chlordane, dieldrin
Phosphate esters (cholinesterase inhibitors)—dichlorvos (DDVP), hexamethylphosphoramide
Miscellaneous—chlordecone (kepone)

*Herbicides*
Chlorinated phenoxyacetic acids—(2,4-D), (2,4,5-T)
Quaternary ammonium compounds—diquat, paraquat

*Rodenticides*
Metabolic inhibitors—fluoroacetate (fluoroacetamide)

*Fungicides, Fumigants, and Sterilants*
Apholate, captan, carbon disulfide, dibromochloropropane (DBCP), ethylene dibromide, ethylene oxide, thiocarbamates (cinch, maneb), triphenyltin, carbendazim

*Food Additives and Contaminants*
Aflatoxins, cyclamate, diethylstilbestrol (DES), dimethylnitrosamine, gossypol, metanil yellow, monosodium glutamate, nitrofuran derivatives

*Industrial Chemicals*
Chlorinated hydrocarbons—hexafluoroacetone, PBBS, PCBS, dioxin (TCDD)
Hydrazines—dithiocarbamoylhydrazine
Monomers—vinyl chloride, chloroprene
Polycyclic aromatic hydrocarbons (PAHs)—dimethylbenzanthracene (DMBA), benzo[a]pyrene
Solvents—benzene, carbon disulfide, glycol ethers, hexane, thiophene, toluene, xylene

*(Continued)*

**Table 19–12**
**Agents Reported to Affect Male Reproductive Capacity *(Continued)***

*Miscellaneous*
Personal habits—alcohol consumption, tobacco smoking
Agents of abuse—marijuana, heroin, cocaine, anabolic steroids, etc.
Physical factors—heat, light, hypoxia
Radiation—$\alpha$, $\beta$ and $\gamma$ radiation: x-rays
Stable isotopes—deuterium oxide

**Table 19–13**
**Agents Reported to Affect Female Reproductive Capacity**

*Steroids*
Natural and synthetic androgens (antiandrogens), estrogen (antiestrogens), and progestins

*Antineoplastic Agents*
Alkylating agents—cyclophosphamide, busulfan
Antimetabolites—folic acid antagonists (methotrexate)

*Other Therapeutic Agents*
Anesthetic gases and vapors—enflurane, halothane, methoxyflurane
Antiparkinsonism drugs—levodopa
Antiparasitic drugs—quinacrine
Appetite suppressants
Narcotic and nonnarcotic analgesics—opioids
Neuroleptics—phenothiazines, imipramine, and amitriptyline
Serotonin
Sympathomimetic amines—epinephrine, norepinephrine, amphetamines
Tranquilizers—phenothiazines, reserpine, monoamine oxidase inhibitors

*Metals and Trace Elements*
Arsenic, lead, lithium, mercury and methylmercury, molybdenum, nickel, selenium, thallium

*Insecticides*
Benzene hexachlorides—lindane
Carbamates—carbaryl
Chlorobenzene derivatives—chlorophenothane (DDT), methoxychlor
Indane derivatives—aldrin, chlordane, dieldrin
Phosphate esters (cholinesterase inhibitors)—parathion
Miscellaneous—chlordecone (kepone), mirex, hexachlorobenzene, ethylene oxide

*Herbicides*
Chlorinated phenoxyacetic acids—(2,4-D), (2,4,5-T)

*Food Additives and Contaminants*
Cyclohexylamine, diethylstilbestrol (DES), dimethylnitrosamines, monosodium glutamate, nitrofuran ($AF_2$), nitrosamines, sodium nitrite

*Industrial Chemicals*
Building materials—formaldehyde
Chlorinated hydrocarbons—chlorinated biphenyls (PCBs), chloroform, trichloroethylene
Paints and dyes—aniline
Plastic monomers—caprolactam, styrene, vinyl chloride
Polycyclic aromatic hydrocarbons (PAHs)—benzo[a]pyrene
Rubber manufacturing—chloroprene
Solvents—benzene, carbon disulfide, chloroform, ethanol, glycol ethers, hexane, toluene, trichloroethylene, xylene
Miscellaneous—cyanoketone, hydrazines

*Consumer Products*
Flame retardants—TRIS, polybrominated biphenyls (PBBs)
Plasticizers—phthalic acid ester (DEHP)

*Miscellaneous*
Ethanol, nicotine, marijuana, cocaine, heroin

## TESTING MALE REPRODUCTIVE CAPACITY

A host of tests have been used or proposed for evaluating the male reproductive system (Table 19-14). Several cellular sites or processes are vulnerable to chemical and/or drug insult. A single exposure to a toxicant(s) seldom perturbs many of the endocrine or biochemical events associated with the male reproductive system. Rather, multiple exposures over an extended period of time are most likely required to detect male reproductive toxicity. Most of the tests are not generally acceptable for use in humans as they are invasive, hence our knowledge relies on animal models. Indeed in humans the noninvasive approaches to assesing male fertility/sterility involve sperm counts, measuring blood gonadotrophin levels, and previous success in impregnating a partner. Testicular biopsy can be used in selected circumstances to evaluate spermatogenesis (i.e., infertility/sterility), but this procedure is obviously invasive. Azoospermia can be caused by a chemical or pharmaceutical agent, by a genetic disorder (e.g., Klinefelter's syndrome), by an infection (e.g., mumps), by exposure to radiation, and by hormonal defects. Dietary deficiencies are well known to cause spermatogenic arrest (Table 19-15). Similarly, lead exposure can produce infertility, sterility, and varying abnormalities in sperm function and morphology (Table 19-16). Pogach et al. (1989) have reported that *cis*-platinum causes Sertoli cell dysfunction in rodents. These changes in Sertoli cell function appear to be responsible for *cis*-platinum-induced impairment in spermatogenesis. Other heavy metals such as cobalt, iron, cadmium, mercury, molybdenum, and silver can adversely affect spermatogenesis and accessory sex organ function. Dietary zinc deficiency can produce sterility (Prasad et al., 1967). Likewise, chemically induced zinc depletion (e.g., phthalates) can produce testicular damage as evidenced by sterile seminiferous tu-

**Table 19–14**
**Potentially Useful Test of Male Reproductive Toxicity for Laboratory Animals and/or Man**

- Testis
  - Size in situ
  - Weight
  - Spermatid reserves
  - Gross and histologic evaluation
  - Nonfunctional tubules (%)
  - Tubules with lumen sperm (%)
  - Tubule diameter
  - Counts of leptotene spernatocytes
- Epididymis
  - Weight and histology
  - Number of sperm in distal half
  - Motility of sperm, distal end (%)
  - Gross sperm morphology, distal end (%)
  - Detailed sperm morphology, distal end (%)
- Biochemical assays
- Accessory Sex Glands
  - Histology
  - Gravimetric
- Semen
  - Total volume
  - Gel-free volume
  - Sperm concentration
  - Total sperm/ejaculate
  - Total sperm/day of abstinence
  - Sperm motility, visual (%)
  - Sperm motility, videotape (% and velocity)
  - Gross sperm morphology
  - Detailed sperm morphology
- Endocrine
  - Luteinizing hormone
  - Follicle stimulating hormone
  - Testosterone
  - Gonadotropin-releasing hormone
- Fertility
- Ratio exposed: pregnant females
- Number embryos or young per pregnant female
- Ratio viable embryos: corpora lutea
- Number 2-8 cell eggs
- Sperm per ovum
- In Vitro
  - Incubation of sperm in agent
  - Hamster egg penetration test
- Other Tests Considered
  - Tonometric measurement of testicular consistency
  - Qualitative testicular histology
  - Stage of cycle at which spermiation occurs
  - Quantitative testicular histology
- Sperm Motility
  - Time-exposure photography
  - Multiple-exposure photography
  - Cinemicrography
  - Videomicrography
  - Sperm membrane characteristics
  - Evaluation of sperm metabolism
  - Fluorescent Y bodies in spermatozoa
  - Flow cytometry of spermatozoa
  - Karyotyping human sperm pronuclei
  - Cervical mucus penetration test

See Galbraith et al. (1982) for complete table and discussion of the relative usefulness of these tests.

**Table 19–15**
**Dietary Deficiency(s) and Spermatogenic Arrest**

| DEFICIENCY(S) | SPECIES |
|---|---|
| Manganese | Rats and rabbits |
| Vitamin A | Mice, rats, and guinea pigs |
| Vitamin B (pyridoxine) | Rats |
| Vitamin E | Rats, hamsters, and guinea pigs |
| Zinc | Mice, rats, dogs, and sheep |

SOURCE: Mann and Lutwak-Mann, 1981.

**Table 19–16**
**Some Actions of Lead on the Male Reproductive System**

| SPECIES | EFFECT |
|---|---|
| Rat | Infertility |
| Rat | Germinal epithelial damage |
| Rat | Oligospermia and testicular degeneration |
| Rat | Decreased sperm motility and prostate hyperplasia |
| Mouse | Infertility |
| Mouse | Abnormal sperm |
| Human | Teratospermia, hypospermia, and asthenospermia |

SOURCE: Bell and Thomas, 1980.

bules (Thomas et al., 1982). In experimental animals, zinc prevents cadmium carcinogenicity in the rat testes (Koizumi and Waalkes, 1989). The major preventive effect of zinc against cadmium-induced testicular tumors may be due to its ability to reduce the cytotoxicity of cadmium in interstitial cells. Different heavy metals seem to exert their toxicity upon different subpopulations of testicular cells (Table 19-17). Mechanisms of heavy metal toxicity vary and not only include different cell sensitivities, but also direct vs. indirect actions. Furthermore, it appears that primary damage to one cell type may secondarily affect other cell types in the testes.

Sensitivity of the various parameters used to evaluate the male reproductive system varies considerably. There are advantages as well as limitations to a number of standard reproductive procedures. Testicular weights are a rapid quantitative index, but this measurement is less sensitive than sperm counts and is affected by water imbibition (edema). In normal males, the number of sperm produced per day per testis is largely determined by testicular size. In many mammals, the size of the testis correlates positively with daily sperm production. Fertility as an index is fairly insensitive, although it does incorporate all reproductive functions. Fertility profiles using serial mating studies to assess the biologic status of sperm cells have constituted a useful test for both dominant lethal mutations (Epstein et al., 1972) and male reproductive capacity (Lee and Dixon, 1972). Testicular histology provides information on target cell morphology, although it too is subjective and not particularly quantitative. Histologic evaluation of the seminiferous tubules can establish the cellular integrity and provide information about the process of spermatogenesis (Fig. 19-9). It is more difficult to detect morphologic changes in Leydig cells and to some extent Sertoli cells. Leydig cell function is better determined by evaluating androgen levels (or gonadotropins) or, in the case of Sertoli cells, the measurement of androgen-binding protein (ABP).

Flow cystometric analyses of the testes can be used to evaluate specific cell populations (Selden et al., 1989). This technique has the advantage of being able to assess simultaneously multiple characteristics on a cell-to-cell basis with the results being rapidly correlated for each cell type or property. Cell size, cell shape, cytoplasmic granularity and pigmentation, along with measurements of surface antigens, lectin binding, DNA/RNA, and chromatin structure, are among some of the intrinsic and extrinsic parameters that can be evaluated. The

**Table 19–17**
**Summary of Cellular Sites(s) of Action of Excess Heavy Metals on the Male Reproductive System**

| METAL | EVIDENCE FOR HYPOTHALAMIC ADENOHYPOPHYSIAL EFFECTS | EVIDENCE FOR TESTICULAR TOXICITY (PRIMARY OR SECONDARY) | | | MECHANISM/COMMENT |
|---|---|---|---|---|---|
| | | GC | LC | SC | |
| Cadmium | None | ◐ | ◐ | ◐ | Hypoxia/Ischemia (Endothelial Cells) |
| Zinc | None | ○ | ◐ | ○ | Toxicity due to Deficiency |
| Lead | Possible suppression of FSH and LH | ● | ● | ◐ ? | Endocrine and Paracrine Toxicity |
| Chromium | None | ● | | | Unknown? |
| Cobalt | None | ◐ | | ◐ | Toxicity due to General Hypoxia |
| Platinum | None | ● | ● | ● | Inhibits DNA Synthesis |
| Vanadium | None | ●? | | | |

●, Evidence for direct cellular action.
◐, Evidence for some direct action, but possibly secondarily mediated.
○, Deficiency of metal causes cellular toxicity.
SOURCE: Thomas, 1995a.

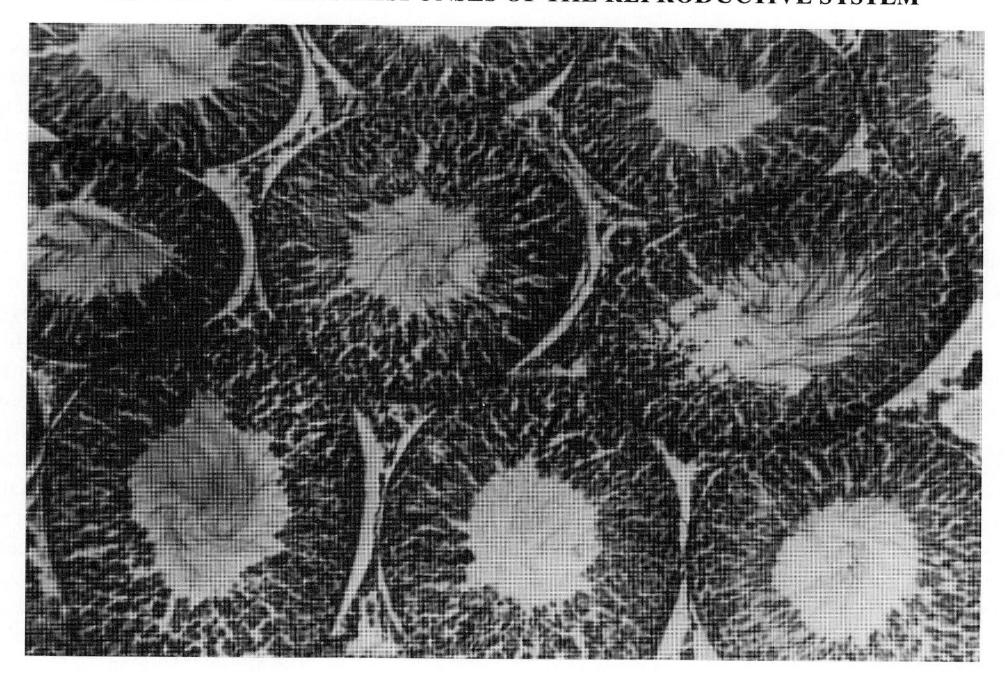

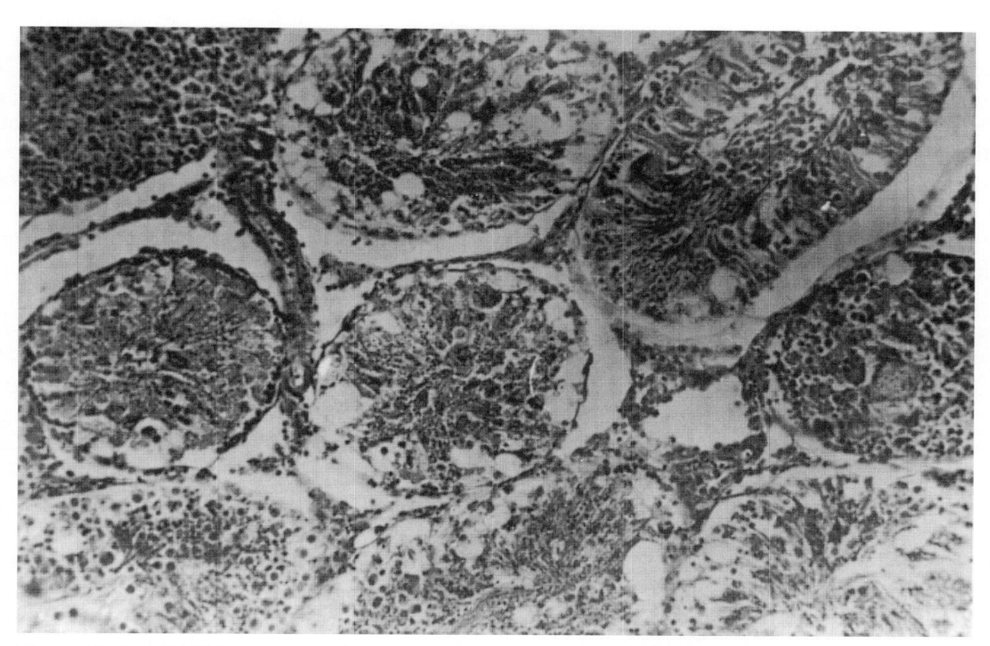

***Figure 19–9. Histology section of rat testes.*** **Above:** ***Normal H&E section revealing morphologic integrity of seminiferous tubules.*** **Below:** ***Chemical-induced testicular damage resulting in vacuolation of seminiferous tubules. Note partially sterile tubules. (From Thomas et al., 1982.)***

toxicity of thiotepa on mouse spermatogenesis has been determined using dual-parameter flow cytometry. The dual parameters of DNA stainability versus RNA content provide excellent resolution of testicular cell types (Evenson et al., 1986). Flow cytometry has also been used to study the effects of methyl-benzimidazol-2-yl-carbamate (MBC) on mouse germ cells. MBC exposure results in an altered ratio of testicular cell types, abnormal sperm head morphology, and altered sperm chromatin structure (Evenson et al., 1987).

Oxidative damage to spermatogenic cells has also been associated with reproductive dysfunction in laboratory animals, and this too can provide an index for assessing risk. Angioli et al. (1987) have proposed an in vitro spermatogenic cell model for assessing reproductive toxicity that involves the ability of bleomycin to reduce oxidative changes in male germ cell populations.

Penetration of zona-free hamster eggs by human sperm has also been suggested as a useful chemical test to assess male fertility. Recently, this assay has also been recommended as a prognostic indicator in in vitro fertilization programs (Nahhas and Blumenfeld, 1989).

The epididymis and the accessory sex organs can also be used to evaluate the status of male reproductive processes. While the epididymis has an important physiologic role in the male reproductive tract, it is less useful as a parameter for assessing gonadotoxins. Its histologic integrity may be examined, but the most meaningful determinations are the number of sperm stored within the cauda epididymis and a measure of sperm motility and morphology. Epididymal sperm may be extruded onto a glass slide and viewed under the microscope for motility and abnormalities. They may also be extruded, diluted with saline in a hemocytometer, and counted. Sperm morphology may be evaluated using either wet preparations or properly prepared, stained smears but this requires an appropriate classification scheme (Wyrobek, 1983; Wyrobek et al., 1983). Chromosomal analysis is used in the laboratory and clinic to diagnose genetic diseases. Accessory sex organs, usually the prostate (e.g., ventral lobes in the rodent) and the seminal vesicles (empty), are a rapid and quantitative measure of the male reproductive processes that are androgen dependent. Chemical indicators such as fructose and citric acid in accessory sex glands have also been used to evaluate male sex hormone function (Mann and Lutwak-Mann, 1981).

Semen analysis can be used as an index of testicular and posttesticular organ function. Semen can be collected from a number of experimental and domestic animals using an artificial vagina. Electroejaculatory techniques and chemically induced ejaculations have also been employed to produce semen samples, particularly in animal husbandry. In the human male, several trace elements, including Ca, Cd, Co, Cr, Cu, Fe, Mg, Mn, Mo, Ni, Pb, Rb, Se, Vd, and Zn can be detected in seminal plasma (Abou-Shakra et al., 1989).

Both quantitative and qualitative characteristics of more than one ejaculate must be evaluated to ensure that conclusions concerning testicular function are valid. Since semen represents contributions from accessory sex glands as well as the testes and epididymides, only the total number of sperm in an ejaculate is a reliable estimate of sperm production. The number of sperm introduced into the pelvic urethra during emission and the volume of fluid from the accessory sex glands are independent. The potential sources of error in measuring ejaculate volume, concentration, and the seminal characteristics necessary to calculate total sperm per ejaculate must be considered (Amann, 1981).

Several factors affect the number of sperm in an ejaculate including age, testicular size, frequency, degree of sexual arousal, and season (particularly in domestic animals). Although ejaculation frequency or the interval since the last ejaculation alters the total number of sperm present in each ejaculate, ejaculation frequency does not influence daily sperm production. However, because of epididymal storage, frequent ejaculation is necessary if the number of sperm counted in ejaculated semen is to reflect sperm production accurately. If only one or two ejaculates are collected weekly, a 50 percent reduction in sperm production probably would remain undetected. Ejaculates should be collected daily (or every other day) over a period of time. The analysis of isolated ejaculate of or even several ejaculates collected at irregular intervals cannot estimate daily sperm production or output. The first several ejaculates in each series contain more sperm than subsequent ejaculates because the number of sperm available for ejaculation is being reduced.

There have been recent advances in the automation of semen analysis (Boyers et al., 1989). Semiautomated measures of sperm motility may be categorized as indirect or direct methods. Indirect methods of sperm analysis estimate mean swimming speed of cells by measuring properties of the whole sperm suspension. Spectrometry or turbidimetric methods record changes in optical density. Direct methods involve visual assessment of individual sperm cells and stem from early efforts to quantitate sperm swimming speed. Such direct measurements may include photographic methods like time-exposure photography, multiple-exposure photography, and cinematography. Computer-aided sperm motion analysis (CASMA) may be applied to morphology, physiology, motility, or flagellar analysis. CASMA allows visualization of both digitized static and dynamic sperm images. Semen analysis and fertility assessment should recognize statistical power and experimental design for toxicologic studies (Williams et al., 1990).

Androgen receptors for testosterone and dihydrotestosterone (DHT) have also been used to evaluate the effects of various gonadotoxins. A number of divalent metal ions (Zn, Hg, Cu, Cd, etc.) can inhibit Androgen-receptor binding in rodent prostate glands (Donovan et al., 1980).

Efforts have been made to identify so-called testicular marker enzymes as indicators of normal or abnormal cellular differentiation in the gonad (Hodgen, 1977; Shen and Lee, 1977; Chapin et al., 1982). At least eight enzymes—namely, hyaluronidase (H); lactate dehydrogenase isoenzyme-X (LDH-X); and the dehydrogenases of sorbitol (SDH), $\alpha$-glycerophosphate (GPDH), glucose-6-phosphate (G6PDH), malate (MDH), glyceraldehyde-3-phosphate (G3PDH), and isocitrate (ICDH)-have been studied with regard to their usefulness as predictors of gonadal toxicity. Several genes are expressed exclusively in male germ cells (Heckert and Griswold, 1993).

A number of secretory products of the Sertoli cell hold some potential for evaluating male reproductive function. Of the several secretory products of the Sertoli cell (e.g., transferrin, ceruloplasmin, tissue plasminogen activator, sulfated glycoproteins), androgen-binding protein (ABP) has perhaps received the most attention as a potential indicator for detecting gonadal injury. Sertoli cell ABP and testicular transferrin may be affected by similar regulatory agents (e.g., FSH, insulin) (Skinner et al., 1989). Leydig cell cultures can also be considered as a potential indicator to evaluate endocrine function of the gonad (Brun et al, 1991). Pig Leydig cell culture can be used to distinguish between specific and nonspecific inhibitors of steroidogenesis. Leydig cells, like Sertoli cells, secrete a number of proteins, peptides, and other substances (e.g., $\beta$-endorphin, corticotropin-releasing factor [CRF]) (Eskeland et al., 1989). The testis contain various neuropeptides and growth factors. These include LHRH, TRH, POMC, oxytocin, vasopressin and still other peptide precursors (Shioda et al., 1994; Spiteri-Grech and Nieschlag, 1993). Many of these factors are involved in the autocrine or paracrine regulation of the testes (Table 19-18). Other than observing the inhibitory actions of DBCP on Sertoli cell ABP secretions, neither this cell and its secretions nor the Leydig cell has been used in reproductive toxicological evaluation.

## TESTING FEMALE REPRODUCTIVE CAPACITY

Evaluating female mammalian reproductive processes is far more complex than in the male. Female reproductive processes involve oogenesis, ovulation, the development of sexual

**Table 19–18**
**Local Factors Modulating the Function of Testicular Cells**

| *Modulating Factors* | *Cell of Origin* | *Action** | *Secretory Factors* | *Cell of Origin* | *Action** |
|---|---|---|---|---|---|
| GERM CELL (GC) | | | | | |
| IGF-1 | (SC)** | — | NGF | (SC) | — |
| IL-1 | (SC) | — | | | |
| Inhibin | (SC) | — | | | |
| SCF | (SC) | Inhibits | | | |
| Activin | (LC) | Stimulates | | | |
| LEYDIG CELL (LC)† | | | | | |
| IGF-1 | (SC) | Stimulates | $\beta$-Endorpin | (SC) | Inhibits |
| IL-1 | (SC) | Stimulates/Inhibits? | ACTH | (SC) | Stimulates |
| Inhibin | (SC) | Stimulates | CRF | (SC) | — |
| SCF | (SC) | Stimulates | Testosterone | (SC) | Stimulates |
| $TGF_{\alpha}$ | (SC) | Inhibits | Activin | (SC) | ? |
| IGF-1 | (PT) | Stimulates | Testosterone | (PT) | Stimulates |
| $TGF_{\alpha}$ | (PT) | Inhibits | Oxytocin | (PT) | Stimulates |
| $TGF_{\beta}$ | (PT) | Inhibits | Activin | (PT) | Stimulates |
| PERITUBULAR CELL (PT) | | | | | |
| $TGF_{\alpha}$ | (SC) | Stimulates | P-MOD-S | (SC) | Stimulates |
| Testosterone | (LC) | Stimulates | | | |
| Oxytocin | (LC) | Stimulates | | | |
| IGF-1 | (Serum) | — | | | |
| SERTOLI CELL (SC)‡ | | | | | |
| NGF | (GC) | Stimulates | $TGF_{\alpha}$ | (PT) | Stimulates |
| P-MOD-S | (PT) | Stimulates | $TGF_{\beta}$ | (PT) | Inhibits |
| ACTH | (LC) | Stimulates | NGAG | (PT) | Inhibits |
| MSN | (LC) | Stimulates | IGF-1 | (GC) | — |
| CRH | (LC) | — | $IL\text{-}1_{\alpha}$ | (GC) | — |
| Testosterone | (LC) | Stimulates | SGF | (GC) | Stimulates |
| $\beta$-Endorpin | (LC) | Inhibits | LHRH | (LC) | Stimulates |
| | | | SCF | (LC) | Stimulates |
| | | | $TGF_{\beta}$ | (LC) | Inhibits |
| | | | IL-1 $TGF_{\alpha}$ | (LC) | Stimulates |
| | | | IGF-1 | (LC) | Stimulates |
| | | | Inhibin | (LG) | Stimulates |
| | | | $\beta$-FGF | (LC) | Stimulates |
| | | | Estrogen | (LC) | Inhibits |

* Stimulates, denotes known stimulatory action; inhibits, denotes known inhibitory action on respective cell(s).
** Letters in parentheses denote cell of origin of the various factors (e.g., SC, Sertoli Cell; GC, Germ Cell, etc.)
† Leydig Cells (LC) are also influenced by serum-derived factors (e.g., glucocorticoids, ANF, etc), ICSH, and autoregulatory factors (e.g., estrogen, angiotensis II, $\beta$-endorphin, CRF, etc.)
‡ Sertoli Cells (SC) are also influenced by serum-derived factors (e.g., retinol, EGF, insulin, etc.), FSH, and autoregulatory factor (e.g., IGF-1, $\beta$-FGF, etc.)
SOURCE: Thomas, 1995a.

receptivity, coitus, gamete and zygote transport, fertilization, and implantation of the concepters. All these processes or events are potential sites of chemical or drug interference.

Evaluation of the female reproductive tract for toxicologic perturbations not surprisingly may overlap with testing methods for assessing teratogenicity and mutagenicity. Indeed, reproductive endpoints that indicate dysfunction in the female (Table 19-19), including perinatal parameters, often overlap with developmental toxicity end points (Table 19-20). The neonate is particularly sensitive to a variety of drugs and chemicals (Thomas, 1989).

Gross pathology (e.g., gravimetric responses of the ovary, uterus, etc.) and histopathology are important to reproductivity and should be evaluated (Ettlin and Dixon, 1985). Both light microscopy and electron (transmission and scanning) may be useful in assessing ovarian and pituitary ultrastructure. As in the male (Table 19-14), there are a number of useful tests to evaluate the female reproductive system (Table 19-21).

**Table 19–19**
**Reproductive Endpoints to Indicate Reproductive Dysfunction**

- Decreased libido; impotence
- Sperm abnormalities: decreased number/motility; morphology
- Subfecundity: abnormal gonads/ducts of external genitalia; abnormal pubertal development; infertility of male/female; amenorrhea; anovulatory cycles; delay in conception
- Illness during pregnancy/parturition: toxemia; hemorrhage
- Early fetal loss (to 28 weeks)
- Late fetal loss (after 28 weeks)/stillbirth
- Intrapartum death
- Death in first week
- Decreased birth weight
- Gestational age at delivery: prematurity; postmaturity
- Altered sex ratio; chromosome abnormalities
- Multiple births; birth defects
- Infant death
- Childhood morbidity; childhood malignancies

**Table 19–20**
**Developmental Toxicity Endpoints**

*Type I Changes*
(Outcomes Permanent, Life-Threatening, and Frequently Associated with Gross Malformations)
- Reduction of number of live births (litter size)
- Increased number of stillbirths
- Reduced number of live fetuses (litter size)
- Increased number of resorptions
- Increased number of fetuses with malformations

*Type II Changes*
(Outcomes Nonpermanent, Non-Life-Threatening, and Not Associated with Malformations)
- Reduced birth weights
- Reduced postnatal survival
- Decreased postnatal growth, reproductive capacity
- Increased number of fetuses with retarded development

SOURCE: Frankos, 1985.

**Table 19–21**
**Potentially Useful Test of Female Reproductive Toxicity**

Body Weight

Ovary
- Organ weight
- Histology
- Number of oocytes
- Rate of follicular atresia
- Follicular steroidogenesis
- Follicular maturation
- Oocyte maturation
- Ovulation
- Luteal function

Hypothalamus
- Histology
- Altered synthesis and release of neurotransmitters, neuromodulators, and neurohormones

Pituitary
- Histology
- Altered synthesis and release of trophic hormones

Endocrine
- Gonadotropin
- Chorionic gonadotropin levels
- Estrogen and progesterone

Oviduct
- Histology
- Gamete transport
- Fertilization
- Transport of early embryo

Uterus
- Cytology and histology
- Luminal fluid analysis (xenobiotics, proteins)
- Decidual response
- Dysfunctional bleeding

Cervix/Vulva/Vagina
- Cytology
- Histology
- Mucus production
- Mucus quality (sperm penetration test)

Fertiliy
- Ratio exposed: pregnant females
- Number of embryos or young per pregnant female
- Ratio viable embryos: corpora lutea
- Ratio implantation: corpora lutea
- Number 2–8 cell eggs

In Vitro
- In vitro fertilization of superovulated eggs, either exposed to chemical in culture or from treated females

These tests can be performed with a wide variety of endpoints, at different anatomical sites, and can include both biochemical, hormonal, or morphologic parameters.

Methods to assess directly the effects of test compounds on oogenesis and/or folliculogenesis include histologic determination of oocytes and/or follicle number (Dobson et al., 1978). Chemical effects on oogenesis can be measured indirectly by determining fertility of the offspring (McLachlan et al., 1981; Kimmel et al., 1995). Other indirect measures of ovarian toxicity in animals include assessment of age at vaginal opening, onset of reproductive senescence, and total reproductive capacity (Gellert, 1978; Khan-Dawood and Satyaswaroop, 1995).

Morphologic tests can quantify and assess primordial germ cell number, stem cell migration, oogonial proliferation, and urogenital ridge development. In vitro techniques can be used to evaluate primordial germ cell proliferation, migration, ovarian differentiation, and folliculogenesis (Ways et al., 1980; Thompson, 1981).

Serial oocyte counts can monitor oocyte and/or follicle destruction in experimental animals (Pedersen and Peters, 1968). This approach is a reliable means of quantifying the effects of chemicals on oocytes and follicles.

Follicular growth may be assayed in experimental animals using ($^{3}$H)-thymidine uptake, ovarian response to gonadotropins, and follicular kinetics (Hillier et al., 1980). These approaches identify both direct and indirect effects on follicular growth and identify drugs and other environmental chemicals that are ovotoxic (Mattison and Nightingale, 1980).

Serum levels of estrogen or estrogenic effects on target tissues are indicators of normal follicular function. Tissue and organ responses include time of vaginal opening in immature rats, uterine weight, endometrial morphology, and/or serum levels of FSH and LH. Granulosa cell culture techniques provide direct screens of the ability of chemicals to inhibit cell proliferation and/or estrogen production (Zeleznik et al., 1979). The biosynthesis of estradiol and its metabolism to estrone and estriol by the ovary constitutes another indicator of the reproductive process. The peripheral catabolism of these steroids is principally a function of the liver.

Nuclear and cytoplasmic estrogen/progesterone may provide important toxicologic applications. Estradiol and progesterone receptors are especially important since chemicals (e.g., DDT and other organochlorine pesticides) compete for these receptors and perhaps alter their molecular conformation (Thomas, 1975; Eckols et al., 1989).

Ovulation differs among various mammalian species. Some animals ovulate spontaneously upon copulation (e.g., the rabbit), whereas other species (e.g., humans and subhuman primates) have a hormonally dependent cycle. Several steroidal and nonsteroidal agents can interfere with this neuroendocrine process of ovulation. In the estrus cycle of rodents, ovulation occurs at intervals from 4 to 5 days. Ovulation occurs during estrus and can be readily detected by cornification of the vaginal epithelium. The rat's estrus cycle can be divided into four stages and can be recognized by changes in vaginal cytology: proestrus, estrus, metestrus, and diestrus.

The processes of fertilization and implantation can be affected by both chemicals and drugs. The formation, maturation, and union of germ cells compose a complex physiologic event that is sensitive to foreign substances. Fertilization can also be achieved in vitro with sperm and ova extradited from a variety of different mammalian species, including humans.

Reproductive performance is best assessed by pregnancy, and this represents a successful index for evaluating endocrine toxicity (or lack thereof). Mating studies using rats is a fundamental procedure that determines total reproductive capacity.

## REPRODUCTIVE TESTS AND REGULATORY REQUIREMENTS

Some regulatory agencies have adopted standard toxicologic testing programs for drugs, food additives, and pesticides (Table 19-22) (Lamb, 1985; Lamb et al., 1986). Both the U.S. Food and Drug Administration (FDA) and the U.S. Environmental Protection Agency (EPA) have established study designs to assess the reproductive risks of chemicals and drugs. The FDA imposes guidelines for drugs that include three different protocols on development, fertility, and general reproductive performance. Segment I includes fertility and reproductive function in males and in females. Segment II involves studies pertaining to developmental toxicology and teratology, whereas Segment III encompasses perinatal and postnatal studies. Segment I studies are initial studies usually requiring additional protocols leading to conventional teratology experiments that emphasize detection of any morphological defects in the offspring of laboratory animals. By using pregnant animals (Segment III) treated with the substance under review for the last third of their period of gestation, including lactation and weaning, an assessment of the effects of chemi-

**Table 19–22**
**Summary of Reproductive Toxicity Testing Used by U.S. Regulatory Agencies and by the National Toxicology Program**

| AGENCY | TEST(S) |
|---|---|
| FDA | Segment I: fertility and reproductive function in male and female |
| FDA | Segment II: development toxicology and teratology |
| FDA | Segment III: perinatal and postnatal toxicity |
| FDA | Multigenerational (three-generation) (e.g., drugs) |
| EPA | Two-generation (e.g., pesticides) |
| NTP | Fertility Assessment by Continuous Breeding (FACB) |

SOURCE: Lamb, 1985 (modified).

cals/drug exposure on late fetal development, particularly lactation and offspring survival, can be made.

The FDA uses multigenerational studies of food additives to evaluate chemical effects on fertility, gestation, parturition, lactation, and the developmental and reproductive processes of offspring. Such assessments of reproductive toxicity provide important information about chemical safety, but they require at least a year to complete. Such tests can therefore be very expensive.

The EPA has adopted a set of test guidelines for assessing reproductive toxicity, particularly as they apply to pesticides. In general, EPA tests are less costly and of shorter duration than those required by the FDA, in particular, the FDA's requirement for multigenerational testing. The EPA test guidelines necessitate that the highest dose level reveals some toxicologic manifestations but not mortality. Such a procedure gives a degree of assurance that a chemical is not a reproductive toxicant, when toxicity is detected, but the reproductive system is unaffected. It is important that guidelines for reproductive toxicology be harmonized (Christian, 1992).

The US National Toxicology Program (NTP) adopted the Fertility Assessment by Continuous Breeding (FACB) protocol in the early 1980s. The FACB protocol was introduced by McLachlan et al. (1981) and was designed to reduce the time for reproductive toxicity testing yet still provide data comparable with other testing systems. FACB tests take no longer than the improved and shortened EPA test designs. The FACB protocol uses more animals per group and, in general, increases the statistical power of the assay. In the late 1980s, Morrissey et al. (1988) evaluated the effectiveness of continuous breeding reproduction studies. Their subtle modification of the FACB design is important, since fertility is an especially important indicator of reproductive toxicity, and it is one of the least sensitive indicators in the assessment of the reproductive system (Schwetz et al., 1980). Experimental design for toxicological studies, particularly in studies involving semen analysis and fertility assessment, must recognize statistical power (Williams et al., 1990).

Reproductive toxicity studies extending over multiple generations are scientifically and logistically difficult to manage, interpret, and finance (Johnson, 1986). While the FDA's tests (Segments I-III) are collectively very meaningful in assessing reproductive toxicity (or safety), no single one of these batteries can replace another, even though the multigenerational evaluation has considerable scientific merit, an argument justifying its expense. However, current multigenerational protocols could be revised in order to improve on the toxicological information collected. FDA reproductive testing guidelines requiring preclinical animal testing for each new drug vary according to how women might be exposed to each drug. The FDA identifies five different drug categories, depending on potential risk (e.g., category A—no evidence of human developmental toxicity—to category D, with *x* number of demonstrated birth defects) (Frankos, 1985). Present FDA Bureau of Foods testing guidelines recommend a two-generation reproductive study, including a teratology phase, to be undertaken for food additives and color additives.

The classic three-generation reproductive system study requires continuous exposure of the parent generation ($F_0$) and the offspring of each succeeding generation to the test chemical (Collins, 1978). Mating indices can be calculated:

Mating index

$$= \frac{\text{Number of copulations}}{\text{Number of estrus cycles required}} \times 100$$

Fecundity index

$$= \frac{\text{Number of pregnancies}}{\text{Number of copulations}} \times 100$$

Male fertility index

$$= \frac{\text{Number of males impregnating females}}{\text{Number of males exposed to fertile nonpregnant females}} \times 100$$

Female fertility index

$$= \frac{\text{Number of females conceiving}}{\text{Number of females exposed to fertile males}} \times 100$$

Incidence of parturition

$$= \frac{\text{Number of parturitions}}{\text{Number of pregnancies}} \times 100$$

Pups are examined for physical abnormalities at birth. The numbers of viable, stillborn, and cannibalized members of each litter are recorded. Observations for clinical signs are made daily. The number of survivors on days 1, 4, 12, and 21 postparturition is recorded. The following survival indices can be calculated:

Live birth index

$$= \frac{\text{Number of viable pups born}}{\text{Total number of pups born}} \times 100$$

24-hour survival index

$$= \frac{\text{Number of pups viable at lactation day 1}}{\text{Number of viable pups born}} \times 100$$

4-day survival index

$$= \frac{\text{Number of pups viable at lactation day 4}}{\text{Number of viable pups born}} \times 100$$

12-day survival index

$$= \frac{\text{Number of pups viable at lactation day 12}}{\text{Number of pups viable at lactation day 4}} \times 100$$

21-day survival index

$$= \frac{\text{Number of pups viable at lactation day 21}}{\text{Number of pups retained at lactation day 4}} \times 100$$

Recently, the International Life Sciences Institute–Nutrition Foundation convened to discuss criteria for listing substances that might be developmental toxicants under the provisions of California's Safe Drinking Water and Toxic Enforcement Act of 1986 ("Proposition 65"). Such criteria are very difficult to establish, but they should emphasize relevancy to humans and biological plausibility (Mattison et al., 1989). Likewise, the European community has classified chemicals according to their reproductive toxicity (Sullivan, 1992).

It is evident that a number of test systems are available to assess the degree of changes to the reproductive system induced by pharmaceuticals, chemicals, and food additives. Some such tests utilize many animals and follow their reproductive histories for more than one generation, whereas others employ a cell systems approach that may be taken as modeling of the molecular level in determining the mechanism(s) of toxicological action(s).

## HUMAN RISK FACTORS AFFECTING FERTILITY

Most humans are exposed to a vast number of chemicals that may be hazardous to their reproductive capacity (Faber and Hughes, 1995). Many chemicals have been identified as reproductive hazards in laboratory studies (Clegg et al., 1986; Zenick and Clegg, 1986; Working, 1988). Although the extrapolation of data from laboratory animals to humans is inexact, a number of these chemicals also have been shown to exert detrimental effects on human reproductive performance. The list includes drugs, especially steroid hormones and chemotherapeutic agents; metals and trace elements; pesticides; food additives and contaminants; industrial chemicals; and consumer products.

Fertility in humans, like that in experimental animals, is susceptible to environmental and/or industrial chemicals. Infertility is a problem of increasing concern among industrialized countries. Levine (1983) has suggested methods for detecting occupational causes of male infertility. The purported decrease in sperm quality occurring over the past 50 years (Carlsen et al., 1992) has been refuted, attributed instead to lowering of reference standards (cf. Bromwich et al., 1994). Furthermore, a comparison of the production of spermatozoa from the testes of different species reveals that the output of human sperm is approximately four times lower than in other mammals, in terms of the number of sperm produced per gram of tissue (Amann and Howard, 1980).

It has also been suggested that the human male is more vulnerable to environmental and occupational toxins than other mammals (Overstreet, 1984; Overstreet et al., 1988). Reproductive hazards and reproductive risks have led to the formulation of policies for reproductive protection in certain occupations (Perrolle, 1993; Sattler, 1992; Thomas and Barsano, 1994). The fragile nature of the male reproductive system in relation to occupational exposure to the fungicide DBCP was reinforced when Whorton et al. (1977) described its injurious actions upon the testes. Fortunately, recovery from severe oligospermia after DBCP exposure has been reported by Lantz et al., (1981). However, Levine et al. (1983) have indicated that reproductive histories are superior to sperm counts in assessing male infertility caused by DBCP.

It has been extremely difficult to correlate directly human exposure to occupational chemicals with alterations in the reproductive system. A particularly complicating factor(s) in this puzzling difficulty is that even normal reproductive processes seldom operate at a physiologic optimum. For example, as many as 15 percent of all married couples in the United States are defined as being clinically infertile (MacLeod, 1971), whereas another 25 percent of women exhibit impaired fecundity (Mosher, 1981). At least 30 percent of early human conceptions and up to 15 percent of recognized pregnancies are terminated by spontaneous abortions (Haney, 1985). Of the 15 percent recognized pregnancies terminating as spontaneous abortions, about 25 percent have abnormalities of genetic etiology and another 7 percent are caused by so-called environmental agents. The greatest number, by far, of spontaneous abortions in recognized pregnancies are due to unknown factors, and this constitutes about 70 percent of all cases of spontaneous abortion.

Many other factors can affect the normalcy of the female reproductive system, as evidenced by variations in the menstrual process. Physiological, sociological, and psychological factors have been linked with menstrual disorders. Factors that are known to affect menstruation yet are for the most part unrelated to occupational settings include age, body weight extremes, liver disease, thyroid dysfunction, intrauterine devices (IUDs), stress, exercise, and marital status. It is therefore obvious that a number of factors can affect menstruation, that before one even considers the affects of therapeutic drugs (Selevan et al., 1985), so-called recreational drugs, or potentially toxic substances present in occupational environments. Even the choice of control populations in studies involving adverse effects on the reproductive system can affect the risk estimates. Environmental chemical exposures can produce reproductive dysfunction in males and in females (Table 19-23).

### Extrapolation of Animal Data to Humans

The exclusive use of animal experimental results to predict outcomes in humans still represents an uncertainty. This uncertainty can be somewhat relieved if findings from multiple species are known, particularly subhuman primates, and there are epidemiologic studies that help substantiate laboratory experiments. While there are many general similarities among mammals with respect to their response to drugs and/or chemicals, there are nevertheless some notable differences. Many of these species differences can be attributed to toxicokinetics, especially biotransformation. Greater predictability can be seen in results from well-validated animal models. A model for estimating human reproductive risk from animal data that is shown in Fig. 19-10. Zenick and Clegg (1989), Buiatti et al. (1984), and Paul (1988) have reviewed several factors that are important in assessing risk to the male reproductive system. It is considerably easier to extrapolate controlled drug studies in animals to exact therapeutic regimens in humans than it is to simulate a chemical's exposure in an animal to a presumed environmental exposure in humans. Occupational exposures are inexact, and environmental levels are even more difficult to document (Lemasters and Selevan, 1984). Exposures usually involve mixtures of chemicals, and individuals may not be aware of all the chemicals with which they come into contact. Thus the effect of individual chemicals is difficult to assess, and cause-and-effect relationships are nearly impossible to establish.

**Table 19–23**
**Environmental Chemical Exposure Associated with Reproductive Function**

| MALES | FEMALES |
|---|---|
| Carbon disulfide | Anesthetic gases (operating room personnel) |
| Chlordecone (Kepone) | Aniline |
| Chloroprene | Benzene |
| Dibromochloropropane (DBCP) | Carbon disulfide |
| Ethylene dibromide | Chloroprene |
| Ethylene oxide | Ethanol consumption |
| Ethanol consumption | Ethylene oxide |
| Glycol ethers | Glycol ethers |
| Hexane | Formaldehyde |
| Inorganic lead (smelter emissions) | Inorganic lead (smelter emissions) |
| Organic lead | Organic lead |
| Pesticides (occupational exposure) | Methyl mercury |
| Vinyl chloride | Pesticides (occupational exposure) |
| | Phthalic acid esters (PAEs) |
| | Polychlorinated biphenyls (PCBs) |
| | Styrene |
| | Tobacco smoking |
| | Toluene |
| | Vinyl chloride |

SOURCES: Barlow and Sullivan, 1982; Thomas, 1981; 1994).

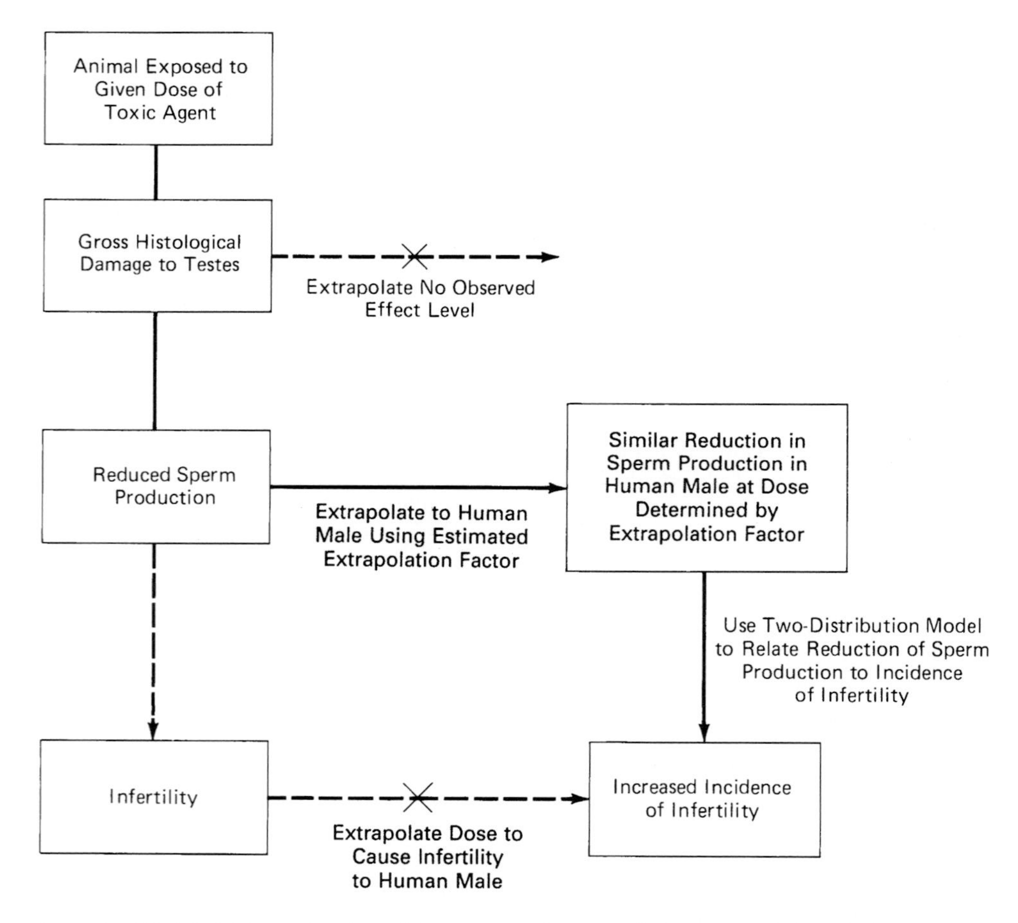


***Figure 19-10. Model for estimation of human reproductive risk from animal data. Solid lines with arrows indicate useful approaches. Dashed lines indicate approaches that are not useful, and a cross on the line indicates that extrapolation in this manner is not useful. (From Meistrich, 1989.)***

### Epidemiologic Studies

Epidemiology is increasingly important in establishing cause-and-effect relationships (Scialli and Lemasters, 1995). Epidemiology and risk assessment are inextricably related. Reproductive surveillance programs are important underpinnings for monitoring endocrine processes. By closely monitoring worker exposures to industrial/environmental toxicants, safer conditions will be established.

If exposure to a chemical has occurred in a human population or if concern surrounds the use of a certain chemical epidemiologic studies may be used to identify possible effects on reproduction. Sheikh (1987) has pointed out factors that are important in selecting control populations for studying adverse reproductive effects in occupational environments. The design of epidemiologic studies may involve either retrospective or prospective gathering of data. Statistical aspects to be considered in epidemiologic studies include power, sample size, significance level, and the magnitude of the effect.

# REFERENCES


Abou-Shakra FR, Ward NI, Everard DM: The role of trace elements in male infertility. *Fertil Steril*, 52(2):307–310, 1989.

Albro PW, Chapin RE, Corbett JT, et al: Mono-2-ethylhexyl phthalate, a metabolite of di-(2-ethylhexyl) phthalate, causally linked to testicular atrophy in rats. *Toxicol Appl Pharmacol* 100:193–200, 1989.

AMA Council on Scientific Affairs: Effects of toxic chemicals on the reproductive system. *JAMA* 253:3431–3437, 1985.

Amann RP: A critical review of methods for evaluation of spermatogenesis from seminal characteristics. *J Androl* 2:37–58, 1981.

Amann RP: Detection of alterations in testicular and epididymal function in laboratory animals. *Environ Hlth Perspect* 70:149–158, 1986.

Amann RP: Function of the epididymis in bulls and rams. *J Reprod Fertil* (Suppl):115–131, 1987.

Amann RP: Structure and function of the normal testis and epididymis. *J Am Coll Toxicol* 8:457–471, 1989.

Amann RP, Howard SS: Daily spermatozoal production and epididymal spermatozoal reserves of the human male. *J Urol* 124:211–219, 1980.

Anderson RA Jr, Berryman SH, Phillips JF, et al: Biochemical and structural evidence for ethanol-induced impairment of testicular development: apparent lack of Leydig cell involvement. *Toxicol Appl Pharmacol* 100:62-85, 1989.

Angioli MP, Ramos K, Rosenblum IY: Interactions of bleomycin with reduced and oxidized ion in rat spermatogenic cells. *In Vitro Toxicol* 1:45–54, 1987.

Baker DB, Landrigan PJ: Occupationally related disorders. *Med Clin of No Amer* 74(2):441–460, 1990.

Barlow SM, Sullivan FM: *Reproductive Hazards of Industrial Chemicals.* London: Academic Press, 1982.

Barsano CP, Thomas JA: Endocrine disorders of occupational and environmental origin. *Occupat Med: State of the Art Reviews* 7(3):479–502, 1992.

Battershill JM: Review of the safety assessment of polychlorinated biphenlyls (PCBs) with particular reference to reproductive toxicity. *Human and Exper Toxicol* 13(58):581–587, 1994.

Bell JU, Thomas JA: Effects of lead on the reproductive system, in Singhal RL, Thomas JA (eds.): *Basic and Clinical Toxicity of Lead.* Baltimore: Urban and Schwarzenberg Medical Publishers, 1980, pp 169–189.

Bjerke DJ, Peterson RE: Reproductive toxicity of 2,3,7,8-Tetrachlorodibenzo-*p*-dioxin in male rats: Different effects of in utero versus lactational exposure. *Toxicol and Appl Pharmacol* 127:241–249, 1994.

Blackburn DM, Gray AJ, Lloyd SC, et al: A comparison of the effects of the three isomers of dinitrobenzene on the testis in the rat. *Toxicol Appl Pharmacol* 92:54–64, 1988.

Blazak WF, Ernest TL, Stewart BE: Potential indicators of reproductive toxicity: testicular sperm production and epididymal sperm number, transit time, and motility in Fischer 344 rats. *Fund Appl Toxicol* 5:1097–1103, 1985.

Bloch E, Gondos B, Gatz M, et al: Reproductive toxicity of 2,4-dinitrobenzene in the rat. *Toxicol Appl Pharmacol* 94:466–472, 1988.

Boekelheide K: 2,5-Hexanedione alters microtubule assembly. I. Testicular atrophy, not nervous system toxicity, correlates with enhanced tubulin polymerization. *Toxicol Appl Pharmacol* 88:370–382, 1987.

Boekelheide K: Rat testis during 2,5-hexanedione intoxication and recovery. II. Dynamic of pyrrole reactivity, tubulin content, and microtubule assembly. *Toxicol Appl Pharmacol* 92:28–33, 1988.

Bond MB: Role of corporate policy on reproductive hazards of the workplace. *J Occup Med* 28:193–199, 1986.

Bosland MC: Male reproductive system. *Carcinogenesis* 339–402, 1994.

Boyers JN, Davis LU, Katz DF: Automated semen analysis. *Curr Probl Obstet Gynecol Fertil* Sept/Oct:169–195, 1989.

Bremner WJ, Millar MR, Sharpe RM, Saunders PTK: Immunohistochemical localization of androgen receptors in the rat testis: Evidence for stage-dependent expression and regulation by androgens. *Endocrinology* 135(3):1227-1353, 1994.

Bromwich P, Cohen J, Stewart J, Walker A: Decline in sperm counts: An artifact of changed reference range of "normal"? *Brit Med J* 309:10–20, 1994.

Brun HP, Leonard JF, Moronvalle V, et al: Pig Leydig cell culture: A useful in vitro test for evaluating the testicular toxicity of compounds. *Toxicol Appl Pharmacol* 108:307–320, 1991.

Buchanan JF, Davis LJ: Drug-induced infertility. *Drug Intellig Clin Pharm* 18:122–132, 1984.

Buiatti E, Barchielli A, Geddes M, et al: Risk factors in male infertility: a case-control study. *Arch Environ Health* 39:266–270, 1984.

Byers SW, Sujarit S, Jegou B, et al: Caherins and Cadherin-associated molecules in the developing and maturing rat testis. *Endocrinology* 134(2):630–639.

Carlsen E, Giwercman A, Keiding N, Skakkebaek NE: Evidence for decreasing quality of semen during past 50 years. *Brit Med J* 305:609–612, 1992.

Chahoud I, Hartmann J, Rune GM, Neubert D: Reproductive toxicity and toxicokinetics of 2,3,7,8-tetrachlorodibenzo-*p*-dioxin. *Arch Toxicol* 66:567–572, 1992.

Chapin RE, Gray TJB, Phelps JL, Dutton SL: The effects of mono-(2-ethylhexyl)-phthalate on rat Sertoli cell-enriched primary cultures. *Toxicol Appl Pharmacol* 92:467–479, 1988.

Chapin RE, Norton RM, Popp JA, Bus JS: The effects of 2,5-hexanedione on reproductive hormones and testicular enzyme activities in the F-344 rat. *Toxicol Appl Pharmacol* 62:262–272, 1982.

Chapman RM: Gonadal injury resulting from chemotherapy. *Am J Ind Med* 4:149–161, 1983.

Christian MS: Harmonization of reproductive guidelines: Perspective from the International Federation of Teratology Societies. *J Amer Coll of Toxicol* 11(3):299–302, 1992.

Clegg ED, Sakai CS, Voytek PE: Assessment of reproductive risks. *Biol Reprod* 34:5–16, 1986.

Colborn T, vom Saal FS, Soto AM: Developmental effects of endocrine-disrupting chemicals in wildlife and humans. *Environ Hlth Persp* 101(5):378–384, 1993.

Colby H: Adrenal gland toxicity: chemically-induced dysfunction. *J Am Coll Toxicol* 7:45–69, 1988.

Collins TFX: Reproduction and teratology guidelines: review of deliberations by the National Toxicology Advisory Committee's reproduction panel. *J Environ Pathol Toxicol* 2:141–147, 1978.

Comereski CR, Bergman CL, Buroker RA: Testicular toxicity of N-methyltetrazolethiol cephalosporin analogues in the juvenile rat. *Fund Appl Toxicol* 8:280–289, 1987.

Davis BJ, Maronpot RR, Heindel JJ: Di-(2-ethylhexyl) Phthalate suppresses estradiol and ovulation in cycling rats. *Toxicol Appl Pharmacol* 128:216–223, 1994a.

Davis BJ, Weaver R, Gaines LJ, Aeindel JT: Mono-(2-ethylhexyl) Phthalate suppresses estradiol production independent of FSH-cAMP Stimulation in rat granulosa cells. *Toxicol Appl Pharmacol* 128:224-228, 1994b.

De La Chapelle A: The Y-chromosomal and autosomal testis-determining genes, in Goodfellow PN, Craig IW, Smith JC, Wolfe J (eds): *The Sex-Determining Factor. Development 101* (Suppl). 1987, pp 33–38.

Dickson LC, Buzik SC: Health risks of "dioxins": A review of environmental and toxicological considerations. *Vet Hum Toxicol* 35(1):68–77, 1993.

Dixon RL: Potential of environmental factors to affect development of reproductive system. *Fund Appl Toxicol* 2:5–12, 1982.

Dixon RL, Lee IP: Pharmacokinetic and adaptation factors in testicular toxicity. *Fed Proc* 39:66–72, 1980.

Dobson RL, Koehler CG, Felton JS, et al: Vulnerability of female germ cells in developing mice and monkeys to tritium, gamma rays, and polycyclic aromatic hydrocarbons, in Mahlum DD, Sikor MR, Hackett PL, Andrew FD (eds): *Developmental Toxicology of Energy-Related Pollutants.* Conference 771017. Washington, DC: U.S. Department of Energy Technical Information Center, 1978.

Doering PL, Davidson CL, LaFauce L, Williams CA: Effects of cocaine on the human fetus: a review of clinical studies. *Drug Intellig Clin Pharm* 23:639–645, 1989.

Donaubauer AH, Kramer M, Krein K, et al: Investigations of the carcinogenicity of the LH-RH analog buserelin (HOE 766) in rats using the subcutaneous route of administration. *Fund Appl Toxicol* 9:738–752, 1987.

Donovan MP, Schein LG, Thomas JA: Inhibition of androgen–receptor interaction in mouse prostate gland cytosol by divalent metal ions. *Molec Pharmacol* 17:156–162, 1980.

Dym M, Fawcett DW: The blood–testis barrier in the rat and the physiological compartmentation of the seminiferous ephithelium. *Biol Reprod* 3:300–326, 1970.

Eckols K, Williams J, Uphouse L: Effects of chlordecone on progesterone receptors in immature and adult rats. *Toxicol Appl Pharmacol* 100:506–516, 1989.

Effendy I, Krause W: In vivo effects of terbinafine and ketoconazole on testosterone plasma levels in healthy males. *Dermatologica* 178:103–106, 1989.

Epstein SS, Arnold E, Andrea J, et al: Detection of chemical mutagens by the dominant lethal assay in mice. *Toxicol Appl Pharmacol* 23:288–325, 1972.

Eskeland NL, Lugo DI, Pintar JE, Schachter BS: Stimulation of beta-endorphin secretion by corticotropin-releasing factor in primary rat Leydig cell cultures. *Endocrinology* 124:2914–2919, 1989.

Evenson DP, Baer RK, Jost LK, Gesch RW: Toxicity of thiotepa on mouse spermatogenesis as determined by dual-parameter flow cytometry. *Toxicol Appl Pharmacol* 82:151–163, 1986.

Evenson DP, Janca FC, Jost LK: Effects of the fungicide methylbenzimidazol-2-yl carbamate (MBC) on mouse germ cells as determined by flow cytometry. *J Toxicol Environ Hlth* 20:387–399, 1987.

Ewing LL: The Leydig Cell, in Scialli AR, Clegg ED (eds): *Reversibility in Testicular Toxicity Assessment.* Boca Raton, FL: CRC Press, 1992, pp 89–126.

Faber KA, Hughes CL Jr: Clinical aspects of reproductive toxicology, in Witorsch RJ (ed): *Reproductive Toxicology*, 2d ed. New York: Raven Press, 1995, pp 217–240.

Fabrio S: On predicting environmentally-induced human reproductive hazards: an overview and historical perspective. *Fund Appl Toxicol* 5:609–614, 1985.

Faustman EM, Kirby Z, Gage D, Varnum M: In vitro developmental toxicity of five direct acting alkylating agents in rodent embryos: structure-activity patterns. *Teratology* 40:199–210, 1989.

Feuston MH, Bodnar KR, Kerstetter SL, et al: Reproductive toxicity of 2-methoxyethanol applied dermally to occluded and nonoccluded sites in male rats. *Toxicol Appl Pharmacol* 100:145–161, 1989.

Foote RH, Berndtson WE: The germinal cells, in Scialli AR, Clegg ED (eds): *Reversibility in Testicular Toxicity Assessment.* Boca Raton FL: CRC Press, 1992.

Foster PMD: The Sertoli cell, in Scialli AR, Clegg ED (eds): *Reversibility in Testicular Toxicity Assessment.* Ann Arbor, Boca Raton, London, Tokyo: CRC Press, 1992.

Foster PMD, Blackburn DM, Moore RB, Lloyd SC: Testicular toxicity of 2-methoxyacetaldehyde, a possible metabolite of ethylene glycol monomethyl ether in the rat. *Toxicol Lett* 32:73–80, 1986.

Frankos VH: FDA perspectives on the use of teratology data for human risk. *Fund Appl Toxicol* 5:615–625, 1985.

Galbraith WM, Voytek P, Ryon MG: *Assessment of Risks to Human Reproduction and to Development of the Human Conceptus from Exposure to Environmental Substances*. Springfield, Va: Oak Ridge National Laboratory, U.S. Environmental Protection Agency, National Technical Information Service, 1982.

Gellert RJ: Uterotrophic activity of polychlorinated biphenyls (PCB) and induction of precocious reproductive aging in neonatally treated female rats. *Environ Res* 16:123–130, 1978.

Gilfillan SC: Lead poisoning and the fall of Rome. *J Occup Med* 7:53–60, 1965.

Goldberg EH: H-Y antigen and sex determination. *Philos Trans R Soc Lond [Biol.]* 322:73–81, 1988.

Gorospe WC, Reinhard M: Toxic effects on the ovary of the nonpregnant female, in Witorsch RJ (ed): *Reproductive Toxicology,* 2d ed. New York: Raven Press, 1995, pp 141–157.

Grasso P, Heindel JJ, Powell CJ, Reichert LE Jr: Effects on mono(2-ethylhexyl) phthalate, a testicular toxicant, on follicle-stimulating hormone binding to membranes from cultured rat sertoli cells. *Biol of Reprod* 48:454–459, 1993.

Gray TJB, Beamand JA: Effect of some phthalate esters and other testicular toxins on primary cultures of testicular cells. *Food Cosmet Toxicol* 22:123–131, 1984.

Greenwell A, Tomaszewski KE, Melnick RL: A biochemical basis for 1,2-dibromo-3-chloropropane-induced male infertility: inhibition of sperm mitochondrial electron transport activity. *Toxicol Appl Pharmacol* 91:274–280, 1987.

Gunn SA, Gould TC: Difference between dorsal and lateral components of dorsolateral prostate in $Zn^{65}$ uptake. *Proc Soc Exp Biol Med* 92:17–20, 1956.

Haney AF: Effects of toxic agents on ovarian function, in Thomas JA, Korach KS, McLachlan JA (eds): *Endocrine Toxicology*. New York: Raven Press, 1985.

Hanly JR Jr, Yano BL, Nitschke KD, John JA: Comparison of the teratogenic potential of inhaled ethylene glycol monomethyl ether in rats, mice and rabbits. *Toxicol Appl Pharmacol* 75:409–422, 1984.

Heckert L, Griswold MD: Expression of the FSH receptor in the testis. *Rec Prog in Horm Res* 48:61–82, 1993.

Heindel JJ, Keith WB: Specific inhibition of FSH-stimulated cAMP accumulation by delta-9 tetrahydro-cannabinol in cultures of rat Sertoli cells. *Toxicol Appl Pharmacol* 101:124–134, 1989.

Heller CG, Clermont Y: Kinetics of the germinal epithelium in man. *Recent Prog Horm Res* 20:545–575, 1964.

Herbert DC, Supakar PC, Roy AR: Male reproduction, in Witorsch RJ (ed): *Reproductive Toxicology,* 2d ed. New York: Raven Press, 1995, pp 3–21.

Hildebrand DC, Der R, Griffin WT, Fahim MS: Effect of lead acetate on reproduction. *Am J Obstet Gynecol* 115:1058–1065, 1973.

Hillier SG, Zeleznik AJ, Knazek RA, Ross GT: Hormonal regulation of preovulatory follicle maturation in the rat. *J Reprod Fertil* 60:219–229, 1980.

Hirsch KS, Weaver DE, Black LJ, et al: Inhibition of central nervous system aromatase activity: a mechanism for Fenarinol-induced infertility in the male rat. *Toxicol Appl Pharmacol* 91:235–245, 1987.

Hodgen GD: Enzyme markers of testicular function, in Johnson AD, Gomes WR (eds): *The Testis: Advances in Physiology, Biochemistry, and Function.* New York: Academic Press, 1977, vol 4.

Holt DW, Adams PC, Campbell RWJ, et al: Amiodarone and its desethyl metabolite: tissue distribution and ultrastructural changes in amiodarone-treated patients. *Br J Clin Pharmacol* 17:195–196, 1984.

Hruska RE, Olson JR: Species differences in estrogen receptors and in response to 2,3,7,8-tetrachlorodibenzo-*p*-dioxin exposure. *Toxicol Lett* 48:289–299, 1989.

Johnson L, Dickerson R, Safe SH, et al: Reduced Leydig cell volume and function in adult rats exposed to 2,3,7,8-tetrachlorodibenzo-*p*-dioxin without a significant effect on spermatogenesis. *Toxicology* 76:103–118, 1992.

Johnson EM: The scientific basis for multigeneration safety evaluations. *J Am Coll Toxicol* 5:197–201, 1986.

Kelce WR, Monosson E, Gamcsik MP, et al: Environmental hormone disruptors: Evidence that vinclozolin developmental toxicity is mediated by antiandrogenic metabolites. *Toxicol Appl Pharmacol* 126:276–285, 1994.

Khan-Dawood FS, Satyaswaroop PG: Toxic effects of chemicals and drugs on the sex accessory organs in the nonpregnant female, in Witorsch RJ (ed): *Reproductive Toxicology*, 2d ed. New York: Raven Press, 1995, pp 59–173.

Kimmel GL, Clegg ED, Crisp TM: Reproductive toxicity testing: a risk assessment perspective, in Witorsch RJ (ed): *Reproductive Toxicology*, (2d ed). New York: Raven Press, 1995, pp 75–98.

Klein D, Wan YY, Kamyab S, et al: Effects of toxic levels of lead on gene regulation in the male axis: Increase in messenger ribonucleic acids and intracellular stores on gonadotrophs within the central nervous system. *Biol of Reprod* 50:802–811, 1994.

Koizumi T, Waalkes MP: Effects of zinc on the distribution and toxicity of cadmium in isolated interstitial cells of the rat testis. *Toxicology* 56:137–146, 1989.

Lamb JC: Reproductive toxicity testing: evaluating and developing new testing systems. *J Am Coll Toxicol* 4:163–178, 1985.

Lamb JC, Ross MD, Chapin RE: Experimental methods for studying male reproductive function in standard toxicology studies. *J Am Coll Toxicol* 5:225–234, 1986.

Lancranjan I, Papescu HI, Gavanescu O, et al: Reproductive ability of workmen occupationally exposed to lead. *Arch Environ Health* 30:396–401, 1975.

Lantz GD, Cunningham GR, Huckins C, Lipshultz LI: Recovery from severe oligospermia after exposure to dibromochloropropane. *Fertil Steril* 35:46–53, 1981.

Lave LB, Ennever FK: Toxic substances control in the 1990s: Are we poisoning ourselves with low-level exposures? *Ann Rev of Pub Hlth* 11:69–87, 1990.

LeBlond CP, Clermont Y: Definition of the stages of the cycle of the seminiferous epithelium of the rat. *Ann NY Acad Sci* 55:548–571, 1952.

Lee IP, Dixon RL: Effects of procarbazine on spermatogenesis studied by velocity sedimentation cell separation and serial mating. *J Pharmacol Exp Ther* 181:219–226, 1972.

Lee IP, Suzuki K, Nagayama J: Metabolism of benzo(a)pyrene in rat prostate glands following 2,3,7,8-tetrachlorodibenzo-p-dioxin exposure. *Carcinogenesis* 2:823–831, 1981.

Lee JP: Adaptive biochemical repair response toward germ cell DNA damage. *Am J Ind Med* 4:135–147, 1983.

Lemasters GK, Selevan SG: Use of exposure data in occupational reproductive studies. *Scand J Work Environ Hlth* 10:1–6, 1984.

Levine RJ: Methods for detecting occupational causes of male infertility. *Scand J Work Environ Hlth* 9:371–376, 1983.

Levine RJ, Blunden PB, DalCorso RD, et al: Superiority of reproductive histories to sperm counts in detecting infertility at a DBCP manufacturing plant. *J Occup Med* 25:591–597, 1983.

Lindemann CB, Kanous KS: Regulation of mammalian sperm motility. *Arch Androl* 23:1–22, 1989.

Lloyd SC, Blackburn DM, Foster PMD: Trifluoroethanol and its oxidative metabolites: comparison of in vivo and in vitro effects in rat testis. *Toxicol Appl Pharmacol* 92:390–401, 1988.

Lonning PE, Lien EA: Pharmacokinetics of anti-endocrine agents. *Cancer Surveys* 17:343–370, 1993.

MacLeod J: Human male infertility. *Obstet Gynecol Surv* 26:335–351, 1971.

Maddocks S, Parvinen M, Soder O, et al: Regulation of the testis. *J Reprod Immunol* 18:33–50, 1990.

Mann T, Lutwak-Mann C: *Male Reproductive Function and Semen.* New York: Springer-Verlag, 1981.

Mattison DR, Hanson JW, Kochhar DM, Rao KS: Criteria for identifying and listing substances known to cause developmental toxicity under California's Proposition 65. *Reprod Toxicol* 3:3–12, 1989.

Mattison DR, Nightingale MS: The biochemical and genetic characteristics of murine ovarian aryl hydrocarbon (benzo[a]pyrene)hydroxylase activity and its relationship to primordial oocyte destruction by polycyclic aromatic hydrocarbons. *Toxicol Appl Pharmacol* 56:399–408, 1980.

Mattison DR, Plowchalk DR, Meadows MJ, et al: Reproductive toxicity: Male and female reproductive systems as targets for chemical injury. *Med Clin of N Amer* 74(2):391–411, 1990.

McElveen JC Jr: Reproduction hazards in the workplace: some legal considerations. *J Occup Med* 28:103–110, 1986.

McLachlan JA, Newbold RR, Korach KS, et al: Transplacental toxicology: prenatal factors influencing postnatal fertility, in Kimmel CA, Buelke-Sam J (eds): *Developmental Toxicology*. New York: Raven Press, 1981.

Mebus CA, Welsch F, Working PK: Attenuation of 2-methoxyethanol-induced testicular toxicity in the rat by simple physiological compounds. *Toxicol Appl Pharmacol* 99:110–121, 1989.

Meistrich ML: Evaluation of reproductive toxicity by testicular sperm head counts. *J Am Coll Toxicol* 8:551–567, 1989.

Millar JGB: Drug-induced impotence. *Practitioner* 223:634–639, 1979.

Moore NP, Creasy DM, Gray TJB, Timbrell JA: Urinary creatine profiles after administration of cell-specific testicular toxicants to the rat. *Arch Toxicol* 66:435–442, 1992.

Morrissey RE, Lamb JC IV, Schwetz BA, et al: Association of sperm, vaginal cytology, and reproductive organ weight data with results of continuous breeding reproduction studies in Swiss (CD-1) mice. *Fund Appl Toxicol* 11:359–371, 1988.

Mosher WD: Contraceptive utilization: United States. *Vital Hlth Stat* 23:1–58, 1981.

Murdoch WJ: Immunoregulation of mammalian fertility. *Life Sciences* 55:1871–1886, 1994.

Nagano K, Nakayama E, Koyano M, et al: Testicular atrophy of mice induced by ethylene glycol monoakyl ethers. *Jpn J Ind Health* 21:29–35, 1979.

Nahhas F, Blumenfeld F: Zona-free hamster egg penetration assay and prognostic indicator in an IVF program. *Arch Androl* 23:33–37, 1989.

Neaves WB: The blood–testis barrier, in Johnson AD, Gomes WR (eds): *The Testis.* New York: Academic Press, 1977, vol 6, pp 125–153.

Office of Technology Assessment Report. *Reproductive Health Hazards in the Workplace.* Washington, DC: U.S. Government Printing Office, 1985.

Okumura K, Lee IP, Dixon RL: Permeability of selected drugs and chemicals across the blood-testis barrier of the rat. *J Pharmacol Exp Ther* 194:89–95, 1975.

Olshan AF, Faustman EM: Male-mediated developmental toxicity. *Annu Rev Publ Hlth* 14:159–181.

Overstreet JW: Reproductive risk assessment. *Terat Carcin Mut* 4:67–75, 1984.

Overstreet JW, Samuels SJ, Day P, et al: Early indicators of male reproductive toxicity. *Risk Analysis* 8:21–26, 1988.

Papadopoulas C: Cardiovascular drugs and sexuality. *Arch Intern Med* 140:1341–1345, 1980.

Paul ME: Reproductive fitness and risk. *Occup Med State Art Rev* 3:323–340, 1988.

Pedersen I, Peters H: Proposal for a classification of oocytes and follicles in the mouse ovary. *J Reprod Fertil* 17:555–557, 1968.

Pedersen RA, Brandriff B: Radiation- and drug-induced DNA repair in mammalian oocytes and embryos, in Generoso WM, Shelby MD, DeSerres FJ (eds): *DNA Repair and Mutagenesis in Eukaryotes.* New York: Plenum Press, 1980.

Perrolle JA: Reproductive hazards: A model protection policy for the chemical industry. *Occupat Med: State of the Art Reviews* 8(4):755–786, 1993.

Pogach LM, Lee Y, Gould S, et al: Characterization of cis-platinum-induced Sertoli cell dysfunction in rodents. *Toxicol Appl Pharmacol* 98:350–361, 1989.

Prasad AS, Obeleas D, Wolf P, Horowitz JP: Studies on zinc deficiency: changes in trace element and enzyme activities in tissues of zinc-deficient rats. *J Clin Invest* 46:549–557, 1967.

Prentice DE, Siegel RA, Donatsch P, et al: Mesulergine induced Leydig cell tumors, a syndrome involving the pituitary-testicular axis of the rat. *Arch Toxicol* 15:197–204, 1992.

Rajfer J, Sikka SC, Lemmi C, Koyle MA: Cyclosporine inhibits testosterone biosynthesis in the rat testis. *Endocrinology* 121:586–589, 1987.

Richburg JH, Redenbach DM, Boekelheide K: Seminferous tubule fluid secretion is a Sertoli cell microtubule-dependent process inhibited by 2,5-Hexanedione exposure. *Toxicol Appl Pharmacol* 128:302–309, 1994.

Ritter EJ, Scott WJ Jr, Randall JL, Ritter JM: Teratogenicity of di(ethylhexyl) phthalate, 2-ethylhexanol, 2-ethylhexanoic acid, and valproic acid, and potentiation by caffeine. *Teratology* 35:41–46, 1987.

Rodamilans M, Osaba MJM, To-Figueras J, et al: Lead toxicity on endocrine testicular function in an occupationally exposed population. *Human Toxicol* 7:125–128, 1988.

Safe SH: Dietary and environmental estrogens and antiestrogens and their possible role in human disease. *Environ Sci Pollut Res* 1(1):29–33, 1994.

Sakamoto J, Hashimoto K: Reproductive toxicity of acrylamide and related compounds in mice—effects on fertility and sperm morphology. *Arch Toxicol* 59:201–205, 1986.

Sattler B: Rights and realities: A critical review of the accessibility of information on hazardous chemicals. *Occupat Med: State of the Art Reviews* 7(2):189–196, 1992.

Schrag SD, Dixon RL: Occupational exposure associated with male reproductive dysfunction. *Annu Rev Pharmacol Toxicol* 25:567–592, 1985.

Schwetz BA, Roa KS, Park CN: Insensitivity of tests for reproductive problems. *J Environ Pathol Toxicol* 3:81–98, 1980.

Scialli AR, Lemasters GK: Epidemiologic aspects of reproductive toxicology, in Witorsch RJ (ed): *Reproductive Toxicology,* 2d ed. New York: Raven Press, 1995, pp 241-263.

Selden JR, Robertson RT, Miller JE, et al: The rapid and sensitive detection of perturbations in spermatogenesis: assessment by quantitative dual parameter (DNA/RNA) flow cytometry. *J Am Coll Toxicol* 8:507–523, 1989.

Selevan SG, Lindhohm ML, Hornung RW, Hemminki K: A study of occupational exposure to antineoplastic drugs and fetal loss in nurses. *New Engl J Med* 313:1173–1178, 1985.

Setchell BP, Vogimayr JK, Waites GMH: A blood–testis barrier restricting passage from blood lymph into rete testis fluid but not into lymph. *J Physiol* 200:73–85, 1969.

Shaked I, Sod-Moriah UA, Kaplanski J, Potashnik G: Reproductive performance of dibromochloropropane-treated female rats. *Int J Fertil* 33:129–133, 1988.

Sheikh K: Choice of control population in studies of adverse reproductive effects of occupational exposures and its effect on risk estimates. *Br J Indust Med* 44:244–249, 1987.

Shemi D, Sod-Moriah UA, Kaplanski J, et al: Gonadotoxicity and kinetics of dibromochloropropane in male rats. *Toxicol Lett* 36:209–212, 1987.

Shen RS, Lee IP: Developmental patterns of enzymes in mouse testis. *J Reprod Fertil* 48:301–305, 1977.

Shioda S, Legradi G, Leung W, et al: Localization of pituitary adenylate cyclase-activating polypeptide and its messenger ribonucleic acid in the rat testis by light and electron microscopic immunocytochemistry and in situ hybridization. *Endocrinology* 135(3):818–825, 1994.

Simpson JL: Genes, chromosomes, and reproductive failure. *Fertil Steril* 33:107–116, 1980.

Singh H, Kozel T, Jackson S: Effect of procarbazine on sperm morphology in Syrian hamsters. *J Toxicol Environ Health* 27:107–121, 1989.

Skinner MK, Schlitz SM, Anthony CA: Regulation of Sertoli cell differentiated function: testicular transferrin and androgen-binding protein expression. *Endocrinology* 124:3015–3024, 1989.

Slikker W Jr, Miller RK: Placental metabolism and transfer role in developmental toxicology, in Kimmel CA, Buelke JS (eds): *Developmental Toxicology,* 2d ed. New York: Raven Press, 1994, pp 245–283.

Soderlund EJ, Brunborg G, Omichinski JG, et al: Testicular necrosis and DNA damage caused by deuterated and methylated analogues of 1,2-dibromo-3-chloropropane in the rat. *Toxicol Appl Pharmacol* 94:437–447, 1988.

Somkuti SG, Lapadula DM, Chapin RE, et al: Reproductive tract lesions resulting from subchronic administration (63 days) of tri-o-cresyl phosphate in male rats. *Toxicol Appl Pharmacol* 89:49–63, 1987.

Spiteri-Grech J, Nieschlag E: Paracrine factors relevant to the regulation of spermatogenesis. *J of Reprod Fert* 98:1–4, 1993.

Steinberger A, Klinefelter G, Sensitivity of Sertoli and Leydig cells to xenobiotics in *in vitro* models. *Reprod Toxicol* 7:23–37, 1993.

Stevenson JG, Umstead GS: Sexual dysfunction due to antihypertensive agents. *Drug Intellig Clin Pharm* 18:113–121, 1984.

Sullivan FM: The European Community classification of chemicals for reproductive toxicity. *Toxicol Lett* 64/65:183–189, 1992.

Sundaram K, Witorsch RJ: Toxic effects on the testes, in Witorsch RJ (ed): *Reproductive Toxicology,* 2d ed. New York: Raven Press, 1995, pp 99–121.

Thomas JA: Effects of pesticides on reproduction, in Thomas JA, Singhal RL (eds): *Molecular Mechanisms of Gonadal Hormone Action.* Baltimore: University Park Press, 1975, pp 205-223.

Thomas JA: Reproductive hazards and environmental chemicals: a review. *Toxic Substances J* 2:318–348, 1981.

Thomas JA: Survey of reproductive hazards. *J Am Coll Toxicol* 5:203–207, 1986.

Thomas JA: Pharmacologic and toxicologic responses in the neonate. *J Am Coll Toxicol* 5:957–962, 1989.

Thomas JA: Actions of drugs/chemicals on nonreproductive endocrine organs. *Toxic Substances J* 13:187–200, 1994.

Thomas JA: Testes-specific metal toxicology, in Goyer RA, Waalkes MP, Klassen CD (eds): *Organ Specific Metal Toxicology.* Orlando, FL: Academic Press, 1995a (in press).

Thomas JA: Actions of chemicals and other factors on Leydig cell growth and proliferation, in *Endocrine Toxicology.* New York: Raven Press, 1995b (in press).

Thomas JA, Ballantyne B: Occupational reproductive risks: Sources, surveillance and testing. *J Occup Med* 32:547–554, 1990.

Thomas JA, Barsano CP: Occupational reproductive risks, in Cheremisnoff PN (ed): *Encyclopedia of Environmental Control Technology*. Houston: Gulf, 1994, pp 195–215.

Thomas JA, Brogan WC: Some actions of lead on the sperm and on the male reproductive system. *Am J Indust Med* 4:127–134, 1983.

Thomas JA, Curto KA, Thomas MJ: MEHP/DEHP gonadal toxicity and effects on rodent accessory sex organs. *Environ Hlth Perspect* 45:85–92, 1982.

Thomas JA, Keenan EJ: *Principles of Endocrine Pharmacology.* New York: Plenum Press, 1986, pp 1–290.

Thomas JA, Thomas MJ: Biological effects of di-(2-ethylhexyl) phthalate and other phthalic acid esters. *Crit Rev Toxicol* 13:283–317, 1984.

Thomas MJ, Thomas JA: Hormone assays and endocrine function, in Wallace HA (ed): *Principles and Methods of Toxicology,* 3d ed. New York: Raven Press, 1994, pp 1039–1063.

Thompson EA Jr: The effects of estradiol upon the thymus of the sexually immature female mouse. *J Steroid Biochem* 14:167–174, 1981.

Torkelson RR, Sadek SE, Rowe VK: Toxicologic investigations of 1,2-dibromo-3-chlorpropane. *Toxicol Appl Pharmacol* 3:545–557, 1961.

Toth GP, Zenick H, Smith MK: Effects of epichlorohydrin on male and female reproduction in Long-Evan rats. *Fund Appl Pharmacol* 13:16–25, 1989.

Tuchmann-Duplessis H, David G, Haegel P: *Illustrated Human Embryology.* New York: Springer-Verlag, 1972.

Waalkes MP, Coogan TP, Barter RA: Toxicological principles of metal carcinogenesis with special emphasis on cadmium. *Crit Rev Toxicol* 22:175–201, 1992.

Waalkes MP, Donovan MP, Thomas JA: Cadmium-induced prostate metallothionein in the rabbit. *Prostate* 3:23–25, 1982.

Ways SC, Blair PB, Bern HA, Staskawicz MD: Immune responsiveness of adult mice exposed neonatally to diethylstilbestrol, steroid hormones, or vitamin A. *J Environ Pathol* 3:207–227, 1980.

Whorton DM, Kraus RM, Marshall S, Milby TH: Infertility in male pesticide workers. *Lancet* 2:1259–1267, 1977.

Williams J, Foster PMD: The production of lactate and pyruvate as sensitive indices of altered rat Sertoli cell function in vitro following the addition of various testicular toxicants. *Toxicol Appl Pharmacol* 94:160–170, 1988.

Williams J, Gladen BC, Schrader SM, et al: Semen analysis and fertility assessment in rabbits: Statistical power and design considerations for toxicology studies. *Fund Appl Toxicol* 15:651–665, 1990.

Wilson MJ: Toxicology of the male accessory sex organs and related glands, in Witorsch RJ (ed): *Reproductive Toxicology,* 2d ed. New York: Raven Press, 1995, pp 123–139.

Woods JS: Drug effects on human sexual behavior, in Woods NF (ed): *Human Sexuality in Health and Illness,* 3d ed. St. Louis: C. V. Mosby, 1984.

Working PK: Male reproductive toxicology: comparison of the human to animal models. *Environ Hlth Perspect* 77:37–44, 1988.

Wyrobek AJ: Methods for evaluating the effects of environmental chemicals on human sperm production. *Environ Hlth Perspect* 48:53–59, 1983.

Wyrobek AJ, Gordon LA, Burkhart JG, et al: An evaluation of the mouse sperm morphology test and other sperm tests in nonhuman mammals: A report of the U.S. Environmental Protection Agency Gene-Tox Program. *Mutat Res* 115:1–72, 1983.

Zeleznik AJ, Hillier SG, Knazek RA, et al: Production of long-term steroid producing granulosa cell cultures by cell hybridization. *Endocrinology* 105:156–162, 1979.

Zenick H, Clegg ED: Tissues in risk assessment in male reproduction toxicology. *J Am Coll Toxicol* 5:249–261, 1986.

Zenick H: Assessment of male reproductive toxicity: a risk assessment approach, in Hayes AW (ed): *Principles and Methods of Toxicology,* 2d ed. New York: Raven Press, 1989, pp 275–309.

# CHAPTER 20

# TOXIC RESPONSES OF THE EYE

*Albert M. Potts*

Our objective in this, as in earlier editions, is to present pertinent material at the graduate textbook level. An exhaustive treatment of the subject would require one or more sizable volumes. Such references include Galezowski (1878), Uhthoff (1911), Lewin and Guillery (1913), Duke-Elder and MacFaul (1972), Grant (1986), and Fraunfelder (1989).

The boundaries of ophthalmic toxicology are narrowly defined by the anatomic and physiological facts pertaining to the eye and by the conditions under which harmful substances may exert their effects.

The eye, despite its small mass, contains derivatives of surface ectoderm (corneal epithelium and conjunctiva) and of mesoderm (choroid, iris, and ciliary body stroma). It contains true neural tissue (the inner retinal layer and optic nerve) and a highly specific light-sensitive modification of neural tissue (the photoreceptors). It contains two relatively large avascular areas (the lens and cornea), which are bounded by unique active transport systems responsible for maintaining a steady state of hydration and hence transparency. It contains a small private cerebrospinal fluid system (the aqueous system) where ciliary body processes are analogous to the choroid plexus, where the barrier to circulating blood is as specific as that of the brain, and where the outflow system is so critical that loss of sight is the price of dysfunction. Unique chemical substances in significant concentrations are the organ-specific lens proteins; the (at least) four photosensitive pigments; and the avid electron acceptor, melanin, present in ocular tissues at higher levels than anywhere else in the human body. These unique features in a small physical compass make for a multiplicity of types of reactions to injury and a potentially high sensitivity to toxic substances.

The activities of the worldwide chemical industries turn out new categories of chemical substances at a dizzy pace. It is inevitable that some of these will exert toxic effects on the eye. New substances will be discussed here under the name of the anatomic subdivision upon which they act. In addition, the discussion in this chapter takes into account (1) poisonings that have claimed epidemic numbers of victims with eye effects and (2) phenomena that have produced very large numbers of publications.

## Epidemics

**Two Pseudotoxic Epidemics: Tobacco-Alcohol Amblyopia.** A 1992 report from China (Wang et al., 1992) described eight subjects with tobacco-toxic optic neuropathy (TTON) and loss of central vision. The authors described a background of "long term heavy smoking, drinking, emaciation and malnutrition bodies, with low serum zinc levels." To complement this are two reports from Cuba—one by Tucker and Hedges (1993) and a second by Sadun and coworkers (1994). The 1993 paper described cases of optic neuropathy appearing in a western province of Cuba from late 1991 to mid-1993 and extending throughout the island until an estimated 50,000 cases were reported. All of the usual suspects were accused of causing the problem. Tucker and Hedges discussed compromised nutritional status and connected it with the loss of the Eastern Bloc as trading partners. Sadun and coworkers named the condition "Cuban epidemic optic neuropathy."

Despite a review published 20 years ago that demonstrated that such epidemics are due to dietary deficiency and are not toxic in origin (Potts, 1973), cases such as those cited are still labeled "tobacco-toxic" and "tobacco-alcohol amblyopia."

**Bhopal Revisited.** The Bhopal accident, said to have been the world's worst industrial disaster, involved the liberation of 40 metric tons of methyl isocyanate on the night of December 2, 1984. There were 3000 deaths from pulmonary edema. The review by Varma and Guest (1993) describes residual toxic findings in survivors, reported over the ensuing 10 years. Among the effects on multiple organ systems, residual eye burns were prominent.

**Mustard Gas in Kurdish Iraq.** It is reliably reported that 5000 people with no protection died of mustard gas toxicity in the city of Halabja. The eye burns of survivors are described by Mohammed-Ali (1992).

**Hydrogen Fluoride in Texas City, Texas.** There is an epidemiological follow-up report on the oil refinery accident that released 40,000 lb of hydrogen fluoride (HF). Two years after the accident a door-to-door survey found breathing and eye symptoms in the exposed population (Dayal et al., 1992).

## CORNEA, CONJUNCTIVA, AND NEIGHBORING TISSUES

### Special Considerations

The cornea (Fig. 20-1) and its neighboring partial analogue, the conjunctiva, are the portions of the eye directly exposed to external insults. The cornea must maintain its transparency to remain functional. A scar, the normal body reparative process, with or without vascularization, is tolerated by other body structures with no adverse effects. In the case of the cornea, a scar or vascularization can destroy function completely. Hence, a very small amount of corrosive substance—an amount of no consequence elsewhere on the body—can be the

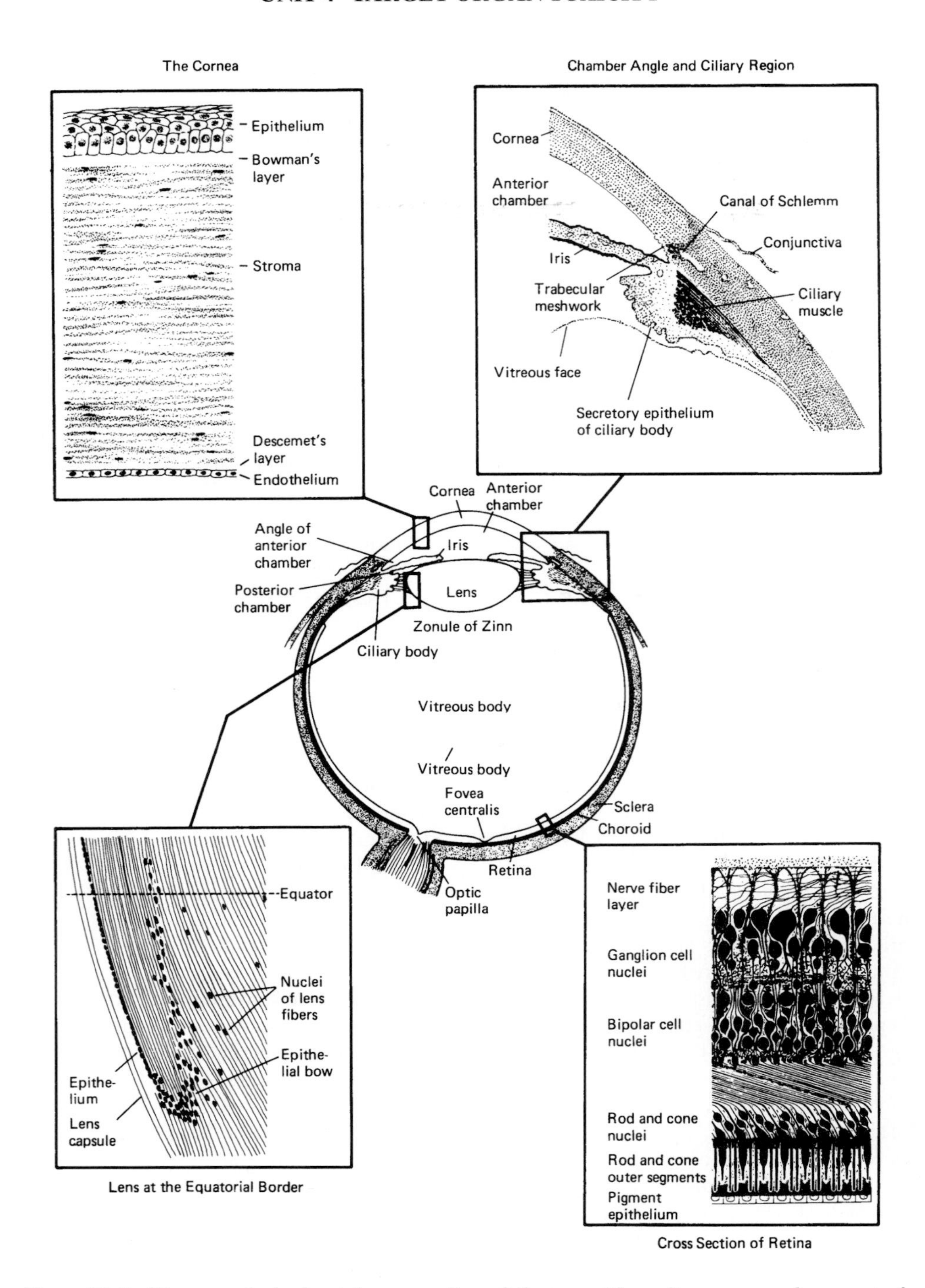


***Figure 20–1.*** ***Digrammatic horizontal cross section of the eye, with medium-power enlargement of details in cornea, chamber angle, lens, and retina. [The enlarged retina diagram (lower right) is taken from Polyak (1941). With permission of Mrs. Stephen Polyak.]***

cause of blindness if it reaches the cornea. There is convincing evidence that corneal transparency is maintained by the boundary layers of epithelium and endothelium, which have a small mass and relatively high metabolic activity (Maurice, 1969). Thus, death of these boundary layers—20 to 25 mg of tissue in the adult eye—is responsible for imbibition of water and loss of transparency. The stoichiometric implications of these minute quantities are impressive.

## External Contact Agents

**Acids.** A splash of acid in the eye is a medical emergency and offers a poor setting for gathering scientific data. We must rely on adequately controlled experimental studies for much of our knowledge of corneal burns. An excellent set of studies was performed during World War II under the auspices of the Office of Scientific Research and Development and was reported by Friedenwald and coworkers (1944, 1946). These authors established standard techniques for applying acids (and bases) to the eye and set standards by which damage could be evaluated. Their results bore out the clinical impression that damage by acid is a dual function of pH and of the capacity of the anion in question to combine with protein. Acid burns vary in severity from those that heal completely to those that cause complete opacity or even perforation of the globe.

It was assumed in the past that the degree of damage seen shortly after an acid burn is an accurate indicator of the eventual result to be expected. In view of some of the new developments in the treatment of alkali burns (see below), it may be that we will be able to abort the late sequelae of acid burns more effectively than in the past.

Special aspects of some acids complicate the picture. The dehydrating effect of concentrated sulfuric acid, as well as the high heat of hydration, adds to its acid properties in determining the severity of the burn. The affinity of the anion for the corneal tissue also plays a role in the severity of damage. Friedenwald and coworkers (1946) showed that buffered solutions of picric, tungstic, and tannic acids produced lesions of significant severity in the rabbit eye and with no great differences in severity from pH 1.5 to 9.

This effect was in sharp contrast to that of hydrochloric acid, which caused severe damage at pH 1, with virtually no effect at pH 3 and above. As the pH of buffered solutions applied to the human eye is decreased from 7.4, the onset of discomfort begins at about pH 4.5. Between pH 4.5. and 3.5, one creates punctate breaks in the corneal epithelium that are stainable with fluorescein but heal in a few hours' time.

It is universally agreed that the one best treatment for acid burns is rapid irrigation with large volumes of water. The reduction of concentration, including hydrogen ion concentration, by dilution is most important. Mechanical removal from the site of injury by the stream of water is accomplished simultaneously. Attempts to obtain some special buffered solution or mildly alkaline wash only delay the start of treatment. Washing should begin as close in time and place to the site of the accident as possible. All industrial safety personnel should know this fact and be prepared to begin treatment by washing. Even in the case of concentrated sulfuric acid burns, where it is expected that the addition of water will generate heat, the water wash is best, using a large enough volume and a fast enough rate to dissipate heat as well as wash out acid.

**Strong Alkalies: Ammonia, Collagenase.** In addition to considerations of pH, there are several factors specific to alkali burns. First, alkalies in concentrations that can cause serious eye burns exist in many homes. Household ammonia and sodium hydroxide-containing drain cleaners are the chief offenders. The second problem specific to alkalies is the serious late effects of alkali burns. Even burns that at the time of injury appear to be mild can go on to opacification, vascularization, ulceration, or perforation (Hughes, 1946a,b). The photographs presented in Hughes's experimental paper (Hughes, 1946b) are eloquent on this subject. It should be noted that in experimental animals Hughes produced burns of all degrees of severity by exposure of the cornea to isotonic *N*/20 sodium hydroxide. Exposure for 30 s followed by washing caused signs that lasted for several weeks only and usually cleared with no residues. Exposure to the same agent for 3 min followed by washing caused severe early opacification, marked vascularization at 3 months, and residues of opacity, pigment, and vessels after 10 months. Irrigation with *N*/20 NaOH for more than 3 min could cause catastrophic changes in the cornea and surrounding tissues, leading to complete opacification and purulent infiltration within a week or 10 days with ulceration and perforation.

One of the exceptions to the uniform behavior of alkali cations is that of ammonia. Of all the alkali cations measured, ammonium ion as ammonium hydroxide penetrates epithelium, stroma, and anterior chamber more rapidly than any other. Grant speculates on whether this is due to the fat solubility of nonionized $NH_3$, to rapid diffusion, or to the ability of $NH_4OH$ to injure corneal epithelium (Grant, 1986). However, this last explanation may be the case, as it has been shown that ammonia is detectable in the anterior chamber 15 s after exposure of the cornea to concentrated $NH_4OH$ (Siegrist, 1920). Uveitis may be an early manifestation in ammonia burns.

**The Special Case of Lime Burns.** The second exception to the generalizations about cations is the case of calcium oxide, known popularly as unslaked lime. This substance, a component of Portland cement and of most commercial wall plasters, absorbs water to form calcium hydroxide with the liberation of heat. Calcium hydroxide is sparingly soluble in water, but in solution (saturated solution, 0.15% pH $\neq$ 12.4) it causes the usual alkali burn. In addition to the generation of heat, the special problem in lime burns is that lime, plaster, or cement, on reaching the eye, tends to react with the moisture and protein found there and form clumps of moist compound, very difficult to remove by the usual irrigation. Such clumps tend to lodge deep in the cul-de-sacs inferiorly and superiorly and act as reservoirs for the liberation of $Ca(OH)_2$ over long periods of time. This is why physicians were especially concerned about lime burns in the past and why special care must be taken in treatment of this condition. As Grant (1986) has reported, this treatment consists of (1) rapid irrigation, to remove as much material as can be quickly washed away; (2) debridement, to remove physically whatever gross particles of lime can be seen on the cornea and in the cul-de-sacs; and (3) use of a complexing agent, preferably ethylenediaminetetraacetic acid disodium salt (EDTA), to remove the remainder of the $Ca(OH)_2$-generating material that cannot be handled grossly. With observation of these extra requirements, lime burns can be made to follow the pattern of other alkali burns.

***The Late Effects.*** The fact that early appearance of an alkali burn is not an adequate guide to prognosis and the possible appearance of infiltration, ulceration, and perforation about a week after the injury have caused much speculation about the mechanism of these late serious sequelae.

Relatively recent recent reviews dealing with alkali burns are those of Pfister and Koski (1982) and Reim and Schmidt-Martens (1982). Earlier reviewers emphasized (1) delayed epithelial repair after severe stromal burns; (2) rapid and prolonged rise of intraocular pressure secondary to prostaglandin release (Pfister and Burstein, 1976); (3) the release of lytic enzymes, particularly collagenase, from polymorphonuclear leukocytes presumably attracted to the site by the prostaglandins. This chain of events clarifies the finding by Slansky and coworkers (1968), confirmed by Brown and colleagues

(1969), that significant amounts of collagenase are present in alkali-burned cornea. The amount is greater than that present in normal corneal epithelium and was correctly attributed by the Brown group to exogenous neutrophils (1970). The use of locally applied collagenase inhibitors improved the treatment of alkali burns measurably (Brown et al., 1972). (4) The observation that ascorbic acid in the aqueous humor falls to 30% of its normal value (normal = 15 to 20 times plasma) in alkali burns (Levinson et al., 1976) has led the Pfister group to postulate that the lower ascorbate causes localized scurvy of the cornea with inhibition of formation of repair collagen (Pfister and Paterson, 1977; Pfister et al., 1978). These two reports found significant reduction of corneal ulceration and perforation in alkali-burned rabbits when ascorbate was given subcutaneously or topically.

Another report from the Pfister group on alkali burns in the rabbit suggests that for established corneal ulcers 10% citrate is demonstrably therapeutic; ascorbate is not (Pfister et al., 1988).

Aspects of the Reim and Schmidt-Martens (1982) review are (1) an extended discussion of the appropriateness of anti-inflammatory steroids as therapy in alkali burns and the conclusion—based on Reim's work, and contrary to generally held opinion in the United States—that the use of steroids is indicated; (2) consideration not only of collagenase inhibitors but also of inhibitors of prostaglandin synthesis as therapeutic agents. This introduces the whole category of nonsteroidal anti-inflammatory agents, but of these only topical indomethacin is mentioned as having a clinical trial. Anderson and coworkers (1982) advocate such a trial for 2-(2-fluoro-4-biphenylyl) propionic acid, flurbiprofen, on the basis of animal experiments.

An item of additional interest is the report of Nirankari et al. (1981) suggesting that the mechanism of action of ascorbate is as a superoxide radical scavenger and that both superoxide dismutase and ascorbate are effective in preventing ulceration after standard alkali burns.

Adding to the catalog of enzyme activities liberated from neutrophils in the alkali-burned cornea is the report of Chayakul and Reim (1982) on beta-*N*-acetylglucosaminidase. In addition to this enzyme, Reim and colleagues (1993) identify cathepsin D as another leucocyte lysosomal marker enzyme representing what may be a panoply of lytic enzymes that are responsible for the late destructiveness of alkali burns.

Thus, renewed interest in the subject has revealed new mechanisms of injury, which, in turn, point to new therapeutic approaches.

**Organic Solvents.** Neutral organic solvents such as ethanol, acetone, ethyl ether, ethyl acetate, hexane, benzol, and toluene may contact the eye in industrial or laboratory accidents. These substances have in common their ability to dissolve fats. As a result, they cause pain on contacting the eye, and examination after a generous splash of solvent shows dulling of the cornea. The epithelium will show punctate staining with fluorescein. The damage appears to be scattered loss of epithelial cells due to solution of some of the fats that occur in these cells. The sensation is due to trauma of some of the populous and sensitive corneal nerve endings. Damage is never extensive or long-lasting if the splash is at room temperature. Hot solvents of low volatility add the problem of thermal burn to that of solvent action, and the end result is potentially more serious and less predictable.

One must note an industrial hazard introduced by the needs of high technology. Trichlorosilane ($SiHCl^3$) is used to clean the surface of silicon wafers in the manufacture of microcircuit chips. The solvent has a low flash point; the mixture of its vapors with air is highly explosive; it decomposes violently in contact with water, giving off voluminous HCl-containing vapors with eye burn capability. The report of Hübner and coworkers (1979) deals with a thermal burn plus chemical burn but serves to underline the existence of the hazard.

**Detergents.** An increasing number of substances are used in technology as detergents, emulsifying agents, wetting agents, antifoaming agents, and solubilizers. They have the common property of lowering the surface tension of aqueous solutions, and they possess discrete nonpolar and polar portions in the same molecule. The nonpolar portion is frequently a long aliphatic chain. The polar portion can be cationic, anionic, or nonionic.

Curiously, there appears to be no relation between surface tension-lowering ability and the amount of damage caused by any given detergent, and the mechanism of damage is not at all clear.

In general, cationic detergents are more damaging than anionic agents, and both of these more than nonionics. For a rabbit eye test that has become the U.S. Food and Drug Administration (FDA) standard and for a table of the maximum tolerated concentrations of 23 surface-active agents, see Draize and Kelley (1952). It is remarkable that such tolerated concentrations vary from 0.5% for the cationic lauryl dimethylbenzyl ammonium chloride through 20% for sodium laurylsulfate to 100% for the nonionic sorbitan monolaurate or monooleate. Note that one-third of the animals in the rabbit test have no washing of the eye after instillation of 0.1 ml of test substance, one-third have the eye washed after 2 s, and one-third have the eye washed after 4 s. A "tolerated concentration" is one in which there is no residual irritation after 7 days.

## Surrogate Test Objects

The wrath of animal rights activists directed against the Draize test was duly noted in the previous edition of this text. It was anticipated that the virtual impossibility of obtaining valid substitute toxicity tests using less than whole animals would dawn on protesters and researchers alike. On the contrary, research funds have become available for searches for surrogates, and the literature has put on weight as a result.

One significant benefit from this activity is reexamination of the specifics of the Draize test. It was typical of a bureaucratic government department that the test should be engraved in stone and that the full number of animals should be required equally for face lotion and oven cleaner. Several suggestions have been made for most efficient use of fewer animals by Gupta and coworkers (1993) and Osgood and colleagues (1990), for example.

The animal rights activists, as a group, have no notion or concern about how many in vitro tests would be needed, how they would be validated, or how great the cost. In addition, it would be a considerable inducement to the soap and cosmetics manufacturers if they could be freed from the strictures and costs of the Draize test. In 1989 the Soap and Detergent Association reviewed nine in vitro test systems (Booman, 1989). They are (1) the corneal plasminogen activator assay (cultured rabbit corneal epithelium); (2) the chorioallantoic membrane assay (chick; size of lesion; 3 days); (3) the chorioallantoic membrane vascular assay (30 min exposure); (4) the "SIRC" cytotoxicity assay (cloning efficiency of rabbit corneal epithelium); (5) the uridine uptake inhibition assay (Balb/c 3T3 cells); (6) the cell protein accumulation assay (cell protein via biorad dye [NHEK cells]); (7) the neutral red uptake assay (measure of membrane damage); (8) the tetrahymena motility test (inhibition of motility of the protozoan *Tetrahymena thermophila*); (9) the chromium release test (release of $Cr^{51}$ from P815 mouse mastocytoma cells). A review that appeared 6 years later lists six different chorioallantoic membrane tests, 70 cytotoxicity tests, and five evaluations based on physicochemical structure-activity relationships (Herzinger et al., 1995). An interesting new substrate for cytotoxicity testing consists of several layers of human foreskin-derived, metabolically active fibroblasts, grown on nylon mesh. The preparation is sold commercially as Skin 2 by a La Jolla, California, firm.

There appears to be no valid scientific exit from the dilemma as stated.

## Antipersonnel Agents

Because of their military significance, new information on vesicants and other substances that affect the eyes is not being published. No attempt will be made to review the scant literature that is available. The older literature was discussed in earlier editions of this text. A single authoritative review that deserves special attention is that of G. Koelle (1994), which deals with the organophosphates.

Current political unrest makes crowd control agents of continuing interest, but the author finds no striking new substances in the spotlight.

Typical lacrimators are as follows (see Jacobs, 1942).

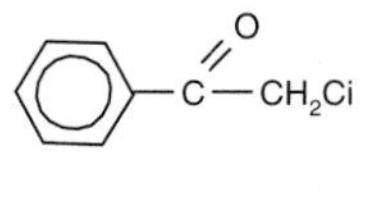

$C_6H_5$—C(=O)—$CH_2$Ci

α-Chloroacetophenone

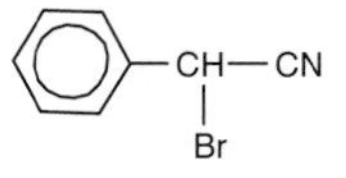

$C_6H_5$—CH(Br)—CN

α-Brombenzyl cyanide

$C_2H_5$—OC(=O)—$CH_2$I

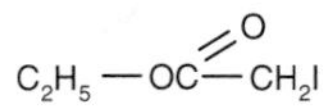

Ethyl iodoacetate

Lacrimator eye damage is complicated by the method of delivery. The two most common forms of delivery are the pencil-like tear-gas gun, purchasable by individuals in many states, and the aerosol can, used by law enforcement agencies under the trade name Mace. The pencil gun has a charge of powdered α-chloroacetophenone propelled by the equivalent of a 22-caliber blank cartridge. When the gun is discharged near the eye, the force of the propellant can drive the powdered lacrimator deep into the cornea. The cartridge wadding can also strike the eye with force, causing mechanical injury (Levine and Stahl, 1968). The chemical alone causes mechanical damage, and its concentration in the eye exceeds the lacrimatory threshold by many, many times. This type of injury may lead to permanent corneal opacity. A similar but less severe injury can result if an aerosol can containing dissolved chloroacetophenone is discharged close to the eye instead of at a distance of several feet or more as recommended by the manufacturer (Thatcher et al., 1971). In recent years the lacrimator of choice appears to be *o*-chlorobenzylidine nitrile (Athanaselis et al., 1990). The exquisite sensitivity of corneal nerve endings to lacrimators suggests that a specific agent–receptor reaction is involved. So far such a reaction has not been identified.

The urgent stimulus for reinvestigation of the subject of lacrimators is the present ubiquity of photochemical smog. Not to be confused with industrial smog, this entity results from the interaction of automobile exhaust emissions and ultraviolet radiation from sunlight. It was first noticed in the Los Angeles area in the 1940s about the time when the last definitive work on chemical warfare lacrimators reached print.

It is now a major blight in every metropolitan area of the United States. We appear to be dealing with substances formed by ultraviolet-activated oxygen, with oxides of nitrogen, and the olefins, aromatics, and perhaps aliphatic hydrocarbons of automobile exhaust. Of the products, the major identified component is the class of peroxyacyl nitrates, which have distinct lacrimator action. This is not the whole story, however, for artificially generated smog used in laboratory studies is several times more active a lacrimator than is peroxyacetyl nitrate. For a competent review of this subject, see Jaffe (1967).

Despite tightened emission control standards for new cars, and despite the avoidance of urban respiratory disasters with their help, the harder problems of chronic respiratory disease and chronic eye irritation have not been tackled. Still more remote, the esthetic problem of visibly clean air stands little chance of near-term solution when the short-term costs to large commercial interests are significant. Thus, half measures and extended studies are likely to be the order of the day. The promised very low emission automobiles have not yet materialized. At this writing, national standards for permissible emissions of oxides of nitrogen do not exist. The solar vehicle and the electric-powered vehicle are not purchasable today. As a result, our knowledge of the eye effects of photochemical smog will continue to be of pressing interest, and it may be that we will be required to restudy the general problem of lacrimators with new urgency.

**Miscellaneous Substances.** ***Metallic Salts.*** Heavy metal ions combine with protein functional groups. In high enough concentration, metal salts cause tissue destruction. Thus, workers with such materials live with the hazard of corneal opacity and ulceration, should a splash hit the eye. Adequate protection is indicated.

The more subtle deposition of metal components in the tissues of cornea, conjunctiva, and lids secondary to chronic overuse of antibacterial solutions for therapeutic purposes is a phenomenon of the recent preantibiotic past when heavy-metal salts were the only available antibacterial agents. The tissue discoloration is a striking cosmetic defect. The chief offenders in the United States have been mild silver proteinate and yellow oxide of mercury (Wheeler, 1947; Wilkes, 1953). Outside of the United States there have been reports of argyrosis secondary to a silver-containing eyelash dye (Velhagen, 1953).

***Hydroquinone.*** In many industries, a fine dust of particles can be generated, and in the absence of adequate exhaust velocity, these particles can reach the eye. This set of events can occur in the manufacture of any noxious solid substance. A particularly striking report was that of Anderson (1947) on workers engaged in the manufacture of hydroquinone for many years. The colorless hydroquinone dust, on reaching the eye (with a distribution corresponding to the palpebral fissure), oxidizes to brown benzoquinone. This material is stored in large granules in or near the basal layer of the corneal epithelium and in smaller granules in the more superficial epithelium. It is visible as a brown-band keratopathy.

***Dichloroethane.*** A remarkable note on species specificity is provided by the reaction of the dog cornea to the systemic administration of 1,2-dichloroethane. Milky-white opacity results after exposure to 1000 ppm for 7 h. This appears not to be related to direct contact of the eye with the agent but is due to secondary action of the drug or a metabolic product on the corneal endothelium. Of many species of vertebrates tested, only the dog and the fox show the effect. For a report on a number of experiments, see the review by Heppel and coworkers (1944).

## Corneal Involvement by Internally Administered Substances

Uncommonly, a systemic drug may affect the cornea selectively.

**Quinacrine.** The antimalarial quinacrine (Atabrine) is such a substance, and the effect is corneal edema. A typical report is that of Chamberlain and Boles (1946). This edema was a relatively rare occurrence in the Pacific theater during World War II, where some 25 cases were recognized among many thousands of men taking the usual daily 100-mg prophylactic dose. The precise mechanism of action is unclear, though it is tempting to postulate a specific effect on the corneal endothelium.

**Chloroquine.** A second antimalarial substance affecting the cornea after oral administration is chloroquine. However, just as with the retinal lesions (see below), chloroquine keratopathy is seen chiefly in patients receiving 250 to 500 mg/day for rheumatoid arthritis or systemic lupus. The subjective symptoms are intolerance to glare and halos around lights. At ordinary levels of illumination, vision is not impaired. Slit lamp examination shows grayish turbidity in the deep layers of the epithelium. Biopsy has shown that these particles fluoresce; so they are presumably chloroquine or a metabolic product. The involvement disappears on cessation of drug administration. For a good early report, see Calkins (1958). For retinal effects of chloroquine, see below.

**Chlorpromazine.** The eye effects of chlorpromazine are minimal, but in patients who have received daily doses of 500 mg or more for at least 3 years, granular deposits have been noted on the corneal endothelium and the lens capsule. These findings were first reported by Greiner and Berry (1964) in 12 of 70 patients. DeLong and coworkers (1965) described an additional series of 49 involved patients in a series of 131. In this latter series, only patients who received a cumulative dose of 1000 g or more of the drug showed corneal changes.

It is reasonable to assume that these chlorpromazine effects are due to the compound coming out of solution in the aqueous humor and depositing on surfaces bathed in the aqueous. A second type of deposition exists where the compound appears to come out of tear solution and deposit on corneal epithelium. This appears to be the case with tamoxifen and amiodarone (see the end of the retina section this chap.).

## Lids and the Lacrimal Apparatus

Another function that may be disturbed by lid damage is the drainage of tears through the lacrimal puncta at the inner nasal margins of the upper and lower lids. The normal tear flow enters the lacrimal canaliculi in the lid margins via the puncta and continues on through common canaliculus, lacrimal sac, and nasolacrimal duct into the nasopharynx. Action of any of the corrosives discussed above can cause scarring shut of the puncta or canaliculi or both, with obstruction of tear flow and annoying epiphora (tears running down the cheek). Indeed, the scar need not even obstruct the drainage system. If it distorts lid position enough so that the lacrimal punctum is everted and no longer in contact with the tear film, this is enough to cause epiphora. Because the drainage system of the upper lid is often inefficient, sometimes involvement of the lower lid alone is enough to cause epiphora. Other effects of scarring can be turning in of the lids (entropion) with abrasion of the cornea by eyelashes. Turning out of the lids (ectropion) can cause desiccation of the cornea if it is exposed. The surgical correction of these scarring effects is difficult and not uniformly successful.

The toxicology of the sclera is peculiar in that for practical purposes it does not exist. Externally applied corrosives reach the cornea before the sclera. Since loss of transparency of the cornea is accomplished by relatively low concentrations of corrosives and since cornea and sclera are equally susceptible to extreme burns that might cause perforation, selective scleral damage by corrosives just does not happen. Similarly, when collagen synthesis is inhibited as in lathyrism, the greater exposure of the cornea makes it more susceptible to perforation, other things being equal.

The very real threat of cicatricial lid disease posed by the beta-adrenergic blocker practolol has turned out to be a property of that drug and not of the group as a whole. In the United

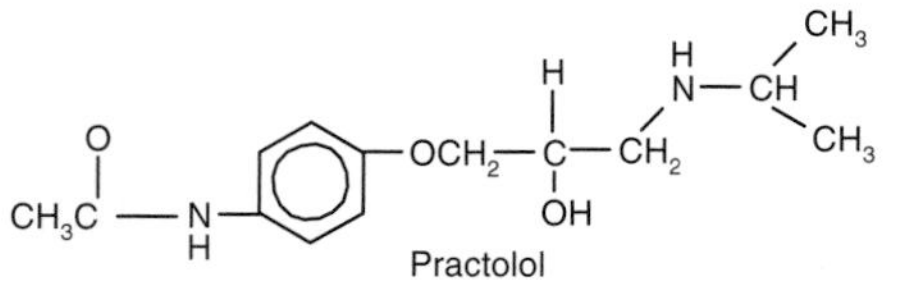

Practolol

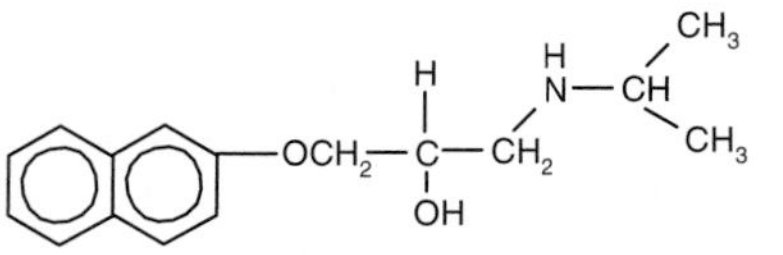

Propranolol

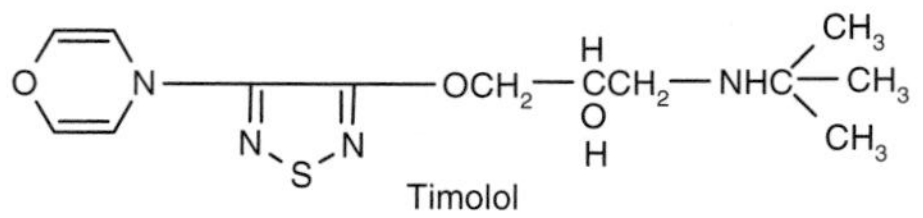

Timolol

States, propranolol has been used without reliably reported adverse ocular effects. Timolol (Timoptic), a topically applied beta blocker, has proved an effective antiglaucoma medication with minimal ocular side effects.

In a limited number of patients, practolol causes an "oculocutaneous syndrome" with atrophy of the lacrimal gland, corneal ulceration, and even corneal perforation. Because of its appearance and immunologic behavior, the syndrome has been called ocular cicatricial pemphigoid (Van Joost et al., 1976).

Elevated antinuclear antibodies caused by practolol have been demonstrated by Garner and Rahi (1976) and by Jachuck and coworkers (1977). Considering the structure of practolol versus that of innocuous propranolol, it would appear that the $\beta$-blocking property is conferred by *N*-isopropyl propanolamine side chains, ether-linked to an aromatic nucleus. This suggests that the disease-producing property of practolol resides in the dissimilar portion of the molecule. The *p*-acetamidophenol of practolol suggests similarity to the sulfonamide moiety, which can cause the oculocutaneous Stevens-Johnson syndrome.

Apparently unrelated to hypersensitivity is the cicatricial ectropion reported to occur secondary to prolonged systemic 5-fluorouracil therapy (Straus et al., 1977). The condition is reversible if the patient ceases taking the drug.

## THE IRIS: AN INDICATOR OF AUTONOMIC ACTIVITY

### Peripheral Effects

The special aspect of the iris (Fig. 20-1) for pharmacology is its double innervation (sympathetic for dilator and parasympathetic for sphincter) and its being behind a transparent window, the cornea. Thus, as one would expect, sympathomimetic and parasympatholytic substances dilate the pupil, and parasympathomimetic and sympatholytic substances constrict the pupil—events easily observed in the intact subject. Allowing for the poor ocular penetration of very polar substances and for the coexistence of centrally initiated impulses, the pupil is an excellent indicator of autonomic activity of topically or systemically administered drugs and poisons.

The eye effects of extracts of mandragora and hyoscyamus were known to Galen in the second century A.D. These effects in sixteenth century Venice gave rise to the plant name belladonna (Matthiolus, 1598). The early experiments of Thomas Fraser on physostigma (Fraser, 1863) and those of T. R. Elliott on epinephrine (Elliott, 1905) drew on observations of the iris in intact animals.

The greatest potential, happily unrealized, for observation of these types of effects in human toxicology is from the effects of so-called nerve gases in combat. (See the review of Koelle, 1994.)

A somewhat odd iris effect has been labeled "cornpicker's pupil." It is mydriasis caused by operating farm machinery in a cornfield containing jimson weed, *Datura stramonium*. Enough hyoscyamine and related parasympatholytic substances from the plant reach the eye to dilate the pupil over a period of days (Goldey et al., 1966).

It is understood that accidental poisoning by any of the agents in the autonomic group will, if severe enough, cause pupillary signs that may be helpful in establishing a diagnosis.

### Central Effects

Not all pupillary changes due to toxic substances are demonstrably direct effects on the iris. The markedly constricted pupil characteristic of morphine poisoning appears to be due to central reinforcement of the physiological light reflex. Constriction of the pupil caused by morphine is abolished by section of the optic nerve. The consensual reflex caused in the optic nerve-sectioned eye by light stimulation of the intact eye is enhanced by systemic administration of morphine. There is a small residual pupillary constriction caused by morphine in the absence of light. This may be a direct action on the pupillary constrictor center or on the muscle itself, but this effect is small in comparison to light reflex enhancement (McCrea et al., 1942).

Similarly, any drug effects observed in the alert animal are algebraically additive with centrally originating reflexes, such as sympathetic dilation in the startle reflex or pupillary constriction that accompanies concentration on a near object. These tend to be transient and are able to be sorted out from toxic drug effects. Similarly, the effects of general anesthetics in first constricting, then dilating the pupil are superimposed on other pharmacological and toxicological effects.

### Inflammatory Iris Reactions

The highly vascular iris is quite sensitive to physical and chemical trauma. Its response to all types of insults is nonspecific and consists primarily of increase in vascular permeability. The result of this is, first, liberation of protein into the normally low-protein aqueous humor. Both serum proteins and fibrin can enter the anterior chamber, and fibrin coagulum can eventually cause blockage of outflow of the aqueous humor (see "The Aqueous Outflow System," below). The second reaction to insult is entry of leukocytes from inflamed iris vessels into the aqueous humor. Subsequent fibroblast metaplasia is again a threat to the aqueous outflow system.

Any of the corrosive substances discussed earlier can cause iritis if they reach the cornea in sufficient concentrations to penetrate the anterior chamber or if they rapidly destroy the corneal epithelial barrier and then penetrate. In a special category are the relatively fat-soluble bases like ammonia and pyridine and acids or acid anhydrides such as sulfur dioxide, acetic acid, and acetic anhydride. These penetrate intact corneal epithelium rapidly and reach the iris in concentrations high enough to cause iritis.

The ciliary body (see "The Ciliary Body," below) is a pigmented vascular structure, protected by the iris from initial assault by harmful substances penetrating the cornea but susceptible to leakage of protein and leukocytes if sufficient concentrations of a noxious agent reach it. The vessels of the iris plus the ciliary body constitute the *blood-aqueous barrier*. Evidence is adequate to implicate prostaglandins in the disruption of this barrier by corrosive substances or, more gently, by rapid lowering of the intraocular pressure. The latter experimental situation was used by van Haeringen and coworkers (1982) to test the effectiveness of nonsteroidal anti-inflammatory agents, presumably in their role as inhibitors of prostaglandin synthesis.

In recent years the evidence has been accumulating that *endogenous uveitis* (inflammation of the iris and ciliary body with potentially serious consequences), whose etiology had not been identified previously, is an autoimmune disease. The use of immunosupressive agents, such as cyclosporin, is accompanied by potential toxicity with systemic use (for a review see Nussenblatt, 1992).

Some insults to the iris are severe enough to cause loss of cellular integrity. This is most easily observable as the liberation of melanin granules from the highly pigmented posterior iris epithelium into the aqueous humor. These granules may contribute to blockage of the aqueous outflow channels with consequent secondary glaucoma. The deposits on corneal endothelium and anterior lens capsule caused by high doses of phenothiazines resemble very tiny pigment granules. It seemed, on personal observation, that the white granules reported by others were diffraction halos around the tiny pigment particles as seen in the slit lamp. The remarkable storage of phenothiazines in the pigmented structures of the eye has already been reported (Potts, 1962b). It seems highly probable, in view of this storage and in view of the fact that the chlorpromazine opacities are confined to surfaces bathed by the aqueous humor, that (1) the drug is responsible for very chronic and very low-grade loss of posterior pigment epithelial cells of the iris, and (2) the pigment granules liberated from these cells accumulate on corneal endothelium and lens capsule and even may be eventually incorporated into these structures, giving rise to the clinical effects of chlorpromazine on the anterior segment.

## THE AQUEOUS OUTFLOW SYSTEM

### General Considerations

As was mentioned at the beginning of this chapter, the eye, a small segregated portion of the central nervous system, has its own equivalent of the cerebrospinal fluid system. Disturbances of this system are disastrous to the eye, just as disturbances of the cerebrospinal fluid system are to the brain. The ocular equivalent of cerebrospinal fluid is the aqueous humor, which is actively secreted into the posterior chamber by the double epithelial layer covering the ciliary processes (Fig. 20-1). The aqueous humor flows between the posterior surface of the iris and the anterior lens surface, enters the anterior chamber through the pupillary aperture, and leaves the eye at the anterior chamber angle via the trabecular meshwork, the canal of Schlemm, and the aqueous veins (Fig. 20-1). Although pathways have not yet been worked out completely, there appears to be a homeostatic mechanism that maintains normal intraocular pressure within the physiological limits of approximately 10 to 22 mmHg. However, the mechanism does not have the capacity for 100 percent modulation, for when the aqueous outflow system becomes severely incompetent due to disease, aqueous secretion is not shut off and intraocular pressure rises. When this pressure exceeds 28 to 30 mmHg, ischemic damage occurs to the optic nerve fibers just before they pierce the lamina cribrosa to exit from the eye. This damage due to increased intraocular pressure is glaucoma and may lead to complete blindness unless treated.

There are two major mechanisms by which glaucoma may originate. The first involves gradual diminution of the ability of the trabecular meshwork—canal of Schlemm—system to pass fluid, as with the inflammatory changes discussed above (see "Inflammatory Iris Reactions"). This type of disease is characterized by an insidious rise in pressure into the 30 to 40-mmHg range, an absence of pain, and a slow loss of peripheral visual field, usually unnoticed by the patient. This type of disease is known as *chronic simple glaucoma* or *chronic open-angle glaucoma*. When it follows an identifiable inflammatory episode such as a chemical burn, it may be called *secondary*, but it is still in the open-angle glaucoma category. The second mechanism is operative only in certain susceptible individuals who because of an inherited narrow chamber angle or an angle narrowed by a swelling cataractous lens can experience sudden and complete occlusion of the chamber angle filtration system by the most peripheral portion of the iris on iris dilation (cf. Fig. 20-1). This type of disease is characterized by a rapid rise in intraocular pressure to 60, 70, or even 100 mmHg, severe pain, conjunctival and deep scleral injection, and rapid loss of vision. It is known as *acute congestive* or *angle-closure* glaucoma.

### Open-Angle Glaucoma

Glaucoma of the first type, open-angle glaucoma, can occur secondary to any toxic inflammation. Burns by acid, alkali, and vesicant gases have been documented as initiators of open-angle disease (Duke-Elder, 1969). A more unusual cause of open-angle glaucoma is *epidemic dropsy*, reported from India. Individuals show edema of the extremities, gastrointestinal disturbances, and cardiac hypertrophy as well as glaucoma (Maynard, 1909). The occurrence has been attributed to contamination of cooking oil by oil from the seeds of *Argemone mexicana*, and the offending agent has been said to be the alkaloid sanguinarine from the argemone oil (S. L. Sarkar, 1926; S. N. Sarkar, 1948). Claims have been made in the past that the disease could be reproduced in experimental animals by argemone oil and by sanguinarine administration (Hakim, 1954). A recent reevaluation of the problem suggests that administration of sanguinarine orally, intravenously, or by cardiac puncture to rabbits, cats, and chickens does not reproduce the effects of epidemic dropsy; however, administration of argemone oil to chickens does cause edema of wattles (Dobbie and Langham, 1961).

There seems little question that the disease is attributable to contaminated cooking oil. One of the problems is that since the first reports of epidemic dropsy the term *sanguinarine* has changed its meaning from an impure mixture of substances obtained from *Sanguinaria canadensis*, the Canadian bloodroot (Dana, 1828), to a pure chemical substance—a naphthaphenanthridine alkaloid (Manske, 1954). It is by no means impossible that in this process the actual toxic agent of argemone oil has been lost and that we have been defeated by a change in semantics. Thus, although sanguinarine is probably not the toxic agent, some component of argemone oil is. This does not make the problem less real or less deserving of reinvestigation.

Another type of open-angle glaucoma that has been recognized is that caused by long-term topical administration of anti-inflammatory corticosteroids for eye disease (François, 1961; Goldmann, 1962; Armaly, 1963). Armaly showed further that eyes already glaucomatous had greater rises in intraocular tension after corticoids than did normal eyes. Not only can steroid glaucoma be caused by topical application to the eye, but it may be caused by systemic administration as well (see Bernstein et al., 1963a, for early literature references). The additional hazard with systemic administration is that therapy for allergic, rheumatic, and other disease will not be conducted by an ophthalmologist, and the idea of checking intraocular pressure or visual field may not occur to the physician until severe damage has occurred.

### Surgical Treatment of Open-Angle Glaucoma

Ordinarily, open-angle glaucoma can be treated successfully with topical medication. However, a small number of cases do not respond adequately to pressure-lowering medication, and these cases must be treated surgically. A limbus-based conjunctival flap is reflected, a small piece of limbal sclera is excised creating an opening into the anterior chamber, and the flap is sutured back in place. After successful surgery the aqueous humor uses both the inadequate normal channels plus the new subconjunctival route to leave the eye, and pressure is normalized. On occasion the healing of the new operative outflow channel is so complete that outflow through it slows to a halt, and intraocular pressure rises to an unacceptable level. A prophylactic measure introduced recently consists of applying cytotoxic agents to the filtering area to slow fibroblast formation. The agents of choice are 5-fluorouracil and mitomycin-C. A review by Costa and coworkers (1993) presents 222 references. The report of Lamping and Belkin (1995) suggests that these two agents are equally effective in modulating the glaucoma filtering procedure required in the presence of aphakia with a posterior chamber pseudophakos.

### Angle-Closure Glaucoma

The second type of glaucoma, angle-closure glaucoma, can be induced in an individual who is susceptible because of a genetically narrow anterior chamber angle or who has an angle narrowed by intraocular changes. This disease is frequently iatrogenic, and the precipitating event is often mydriasis for eye examination or for the treatment of iritis. The most commonly offending drug is atropine because of the effectiveness of its action and its difficult reversibility. However, any mydriatic can be the precipitating cause, and all have been implicated at one time or another. (For a partial list, see Duke-Elder, 1969.)

## THE CILIARY BODY

The ciliary body, which lies just posterior to the root of the iris (Fig. 20-1), is a structure with a dual function. By means of the collagenous zonular fibers that stretch from lens to ciliary processes, the ciliary body acts as the structure physically supporting the lens. An increase in tension of the radially directed and parasympathetically innervated ciliary muscle transmits tension to the lens capsule. This, paradoxically, seems to make the lens more spherical and to change the focus of the retinal image from distant to near objects (Schachar et al., 1993). This is the mechanism of accommodation that is stimulated by parasympathomimetic agents and paralyzed by parasympatholytic agents. Thus, in poisoning by cholinesterase inhibitors, the small pupil through the action of acetylcholine on the iris sphincter, is accompanied by spasm of accommodation due to action on the ciliary muscle. This causes blurring of distant objects that were previously in focus. The converse is true in atropine poisoning. The pupil is wide and accommodation is paralyzed, making it difficult to see near objects. When atropine or other parasympatholytics are used as medication in gastrointestinal disease, it is rare that the dose is high enough to cause measurable pupillary effects. However, it is not uncommon, particularly in a patient whose accommodation is already limited by presbyopia, that the medication will cause discomfort in near vision.

There are numerous medications said to cause blurring of vision, in which the mechanism of action is less understandable. One such instance is the blurring experienced from large doses of phenothiazines. It appears to be possible, at least, that the blurring described is due to ciliary muscle weakness secondary to very high concentrations of the drug in the ciliary body, due to storage of the polycyclic phenothiazine on melanin pigment in the ciliary body.

The second function of the ciliary body depends on its vascularity and on the two specialized layers of epithelium that cover it. The epithelium secretes aqueous humor at the rate of approximately 1 μL/min. Although it is problematic whether any substance can increase aqueous secretion, there is evidence that both epinephrine and carbonic anhydrase inhibitors, such as acetazolamide, can decrease aqueous humor formation. Diuretics based on the property of carbonic anhydrase inhibition can lower intraocular pressure as a side effect, but there is no record of any of them causing serious difficulty, such as permanent hypotony.

## THE LENS

### Description

**Normal Function and Composition.** The lens (Fig. 20-1) is an avascular, transparent tissue surrounded by an elastic, acellular, collagenous capsule. It has the property of acting with the transparent cornea as an essential element in the image-forming system of the eye.

Water and protein are the primary chemical constituents of the lens (Paterson, 1972). The fibers are mostly composed of the soluble proteins $\alpha$-, $\beta$-, and $\gamma$-crystallin and the insoluble protein albuminoid. These proteins are unique in being organ-specific, not species-specific, immunologically. With such a great proportion of protein, it is not surprising that the lens actively synthesizes proteins; in fact, lenticular growth and development depend on a continuous and abundant supply of biosynthetic proteins (Waley, 1969). Protein synthesis may also be the prime consumer of energy generated in the lens, which is necessary in the synthetic mechanics itself and in actively transporting amino acids against a concentration gradient from the aqueous humor into the epithelium (Kuck, 1970b).

Maintenance of an ionic equilibrium with a high intracellular $Na^+/K^+$ ratio through active transport of $K^+$ across the epithelium into the lens, and $Na^+$ out of the lens, expends a large quantity of energy. The flow of these ions through the lens has been attributed to the existence of a *pump-leak* mechanism (van Heyningen, 1969; Kuck, 1970b; Paterson, 1972). The high level of $K^+$ in the lenticular epithelium as a result of active transport from the aqueous humor favors diffusion of $K^+$ along a concentration gradient across the posterior capsule and into the vitreous. In contrast, the high vitreal content of $Na^+$ favors diffusion of $Na^+$ in the opposite direction, proceeding toward the epithelial cell layer, where it is actively transported out of the lens and into the aqueous humor. The enzyme presumed to be associated with active transport, $Na^+K^+$-activated adenosine triphosphatase, is almost exclusively located in the epithelium. The energy necessary to drive active transport and other endergonic reactions is derived from the metabolism of glucose and primarily from anerobic glycolysis (van Heyningen, 1969; Kuck, 1970b). However, glucose degradation via the Krebs cycle with subsequent synthesis of adenosine triphosphate (ATP) by the mitochondrial respiratory chain located solely in the anterior epithelium and superficial cortical fibers may possibly contribute as much as 30 percent to the total lenticular energy output (van Heyningen, 1969; Trayhurn and van Heyningen, 1971a; Trayhurn, 1971b).

Other biochemical reactions important to lenticular metabolism include nucleic acid synthesis in areas undergoing mitosis, the pentose shunt pathway supplying reduced nicotinamide adenine dinucleotide phosphate, the sorbitol pathway, and the $\alpha$-glycerophosphate cycle. Other cellular constituents include small amounts of lipids and glycoproteins, ophthalmic acid, and a relatively large quantity of reduced glutathione, whose role in lenticular metabolism has not been fully evaluated. Small amounts of $Ca^{2+}$ are also necessary to maintain membrane integrity.

## Cataract

Normal lenses are transparent, permitting light to pass through and allowing it to be focused on the retina. Transparency is dependent not only on the highly ordered cellular arrangement but also on fiber size, uniformity of dimension and shape, molecular structure, and regularity of packing (Kuck, 1970a,c). In fact, the primary function of lenticular metabolism appears to be directed toward maintaining this organized structure and resulting transparency. Interference with normal lens metabolism, interference with active transport across the cell boundaries, breakage of the lens capsule, and many other types of insult cause alteration in optical properties.

Cataracts can be caused by a variety of unrelated circumstances (van Heyningen, 1969), for example, senile cataract due to age, congenital cataracts possibly related to immunologic reactions or pathological infections, inborn errors of metabolism such as in galactosemia, endocrine cataracts as in diabetes, and drug-induced cataracts. It is this latter category that will be described here, although similarities in the mechanism of cataract formation may exist in all of the above classes.

**2,4-Dinitrophenol.** In addition to a variety of toxic effects, systemic administration of 2,4-dinitrophenol (DNP) causes cataracts in some individuals. The classic instances of human dinitrophenol poisoning occurred during 1935 to 1937 when the substance was introduced as an antiobesity agent and was sold without prescription. Several hundred human cataracts resulted. For a review of these events, see Horner (1942). Lenticular opacity first develops in the anterior capsule and eventually spreads to include the cortex and the nucleus. Although cataracts may develop only after months of treatment or after drug withdrawal, the subcapsular and the posterior poles of the lens are the more severely affected. Vision is not immediately hindered but rapidly deteriorates as the cataract develops.

Experimental animals are insensitive to the cataractogenic activity of DNP, with the exception of young fowl and rabbits. A reversible cataract can be induced in chicks within 1 h after systemic treatment. Analysis of aqueous humor, vitreous humor, and the lens after a dose of DNP indicated a higher DNP concentration present in the young animal than in the adult, suggesting a possible explanation for both species and age sensitivity for DNP cataractogenic activity (Gehring and Buerge, 1969b). Within 4 to 6 h after feeding a diet containing 0.25 percent DNP, vacuolization of the anterior lens can be induced in ducklings and chicks. In vitro incubation of lens with DNP forms cataracts (Gehring and Buerge, 1969a), with an increase in sodium influx and potassium efflux and swelling prior to cortical opacification (Ikemoto, 1971).

The cataractogenic activity of DNP may be related to its ability to uncouple oxidative phosphorylation, that is, to inhibit ATP synthesis without influencing electron transfer along the mitochondrial respiratory chain. Although experimental studies with other species indicate that lens metabolism is essentially anerobic, because ATP synthesis depends on glycolysis and is therefore insensitive to DNP, mitochondrial oxidative phosphorylation in the epithelial cells may play a greater role in ATP synthesis in fowl and human lenses (Kuck, 1970b). As with any cell, removal of sodium ions from the lenticular cells may be the major energy-utilizing reaction, in order to maintain proper ionic balances (Trayhurn and van Heyningen, 1971a). Other inhibitors of mitochondrial respiration, such as cyanide and amytal, also lead to increases in lenticular sodium content, which would be followed by decreases in ATP concentration, swelling, and opacification of the fibers.

**Steroids.** The first controlled study on the cataractogenic activity of corticosteroids was reported in 1960 (Black et al., 1960). Thirty-nine percent of patients receiving prolonged therapy with cortisone, prednisone, or dexamethasone for rheumatoid arthritis developed posterior subcapsular cataracts. A good correlation existed between cataract formation and dose and duration of therapy. No cataracts were observed in patients receiving low doses for a year or longer and medium or high doses for less than a year. In this study, there was no serious impairment of vision. Further investigation revealed that corticosteroid-induced cataracts could be distinguished by clinical morphology from cataracts caused by diabetes, 2,4-dinitrophenol, and trauma but could not be distinguished from cataracts caused by intraocular disease and ionizing radiation (Oglesby et al., 1961a). Later reports confirmed the etiology and morphology, and a correlation was clearly established between the incidence of posterior subcapsular opacities and having received 15 mg of prednisone per day or equivalent for a year or longer (Oglesby et al., 1961a; Crews, 1963; Williamson et al., 1969; Williamson, 1970). In contrast, four children developed posterior subcapsular cataracts after receiving 1 to 3 mg of prednisolone or an equivalent dose of paramethazone for only 3 to 10 months, suggesting either a genetic or an age-dependent sensitivity (Loredo et al., 1972). The clinical progression of the posterior subcapsular opacity has been graded I to IV by Williamson and coworkers (1969). Once vacuoles have formed, they are not reversible even if the drug is withdrawn during the early phases of opacification, although further progression to advanced stages will not occur (Lieberman, 1968). Grade III has been established as the point at which visual difficulties become evident and vacuole extension into the cortex will progress in spite of drug withdrawal (Williamson, 1970). Similar findings have been reported after topical administration of corticosteroids (Becker, 1964). A useful review is that of Lubkin (1977).

Steroidal cataracts were first observed experimentally in two out of four rabbits receiving 2 mg of betamethasone subconjunctivally for 41 weeks (Tarkkanen et al., 1966). Long-term topical administration of several steroids also caused lenticular changes that were confined to the anterior subcapsular and cortical areas (Wood et al., 1967) and therefore different from human cataracts. In contrast, short- or long-term systemic administration of prednisone or prednisolone did not result in cataracts when administered alone, although it did potentiate the cataractogenic activity of 2,4-dinitrophenol (Bettman et al., 1964) and galactose (Bettman et al., 1968) but not xylose, triparanol, or radiation. Betamethasone, applied topically, did enhance the formation of galactose cataracts (Cotlier and Becker, 1965).

The mechanism of steroid-induced cataracts has not been sufficiently investigated. In vitro studies (Ono et al., 1971, 1972b) indicated that the lens not only can accumulate cortisol but also can biotransform it to its sulfate and glucuronide conjugates. Cortisol also binds to the soluble proteins $\beta$-crystallin and $\alpha$-crystallin (Ono et al., 1972b). Alterations in $Na^+$ and $K^+$ ion transport have been reported resulting in increased hydration of the lens (Harris and Gruber, 1962). Inhibition of the synthesis of lenticular proteins has been suggested as a possible mechanism of steroidal cataracts (Ono et al., 1972a). It has been known since the work of Axelsson and Holmberg (1966) that long-acting cholinesterase inhibitors cause anterior and posterior subcapsular cataracts. This has been amply confirmed in humans and in monkeys (Shaffer and Hetherington, 1966; Kaufman et al., 1977a). The mechanism of cataractogenesis is unknown. A curious finding is that topical application of atropine prevents the experimental cataract in monkeys (Kaufman et al., 1977b).

**Chlorpromazine.** It was noted in the cornea section above that pigment granules appear on the anterior lens surface as well as the corneal endothelium in individuals who have received large doses of chlorpromazine over long periods of time. Although these granules are almost certainly exogenous to the lens in origin, they become incorporated into lens substance and cause loss of transparency. By these criteria, this phenomenon produces a cataract and should be mentioned here.

**Thallium.** The soluble salts of thallium acetate and thallium sulfate have been used as insecticides, as rodenticides, and at one time as a systemic or topical depilatory agent. Thallous ion ($Tl^+$) is readily absorbed through the skin or gastrointestinal epithelium. Ingestion or application causes a variety of toxic symptoms, such as disturbances of the gastrointestinal tract, hair loss, polyneuritis of feet and legs, weakness or paralysis of the legs, psychic disturbances, neuritis of the optic nerve (described in "The Ganglion Cell Layer and Optic Nerve," below), and in rare instances, cataracts (Duke-Elder, 1969; Grant, 1986). Thallium acetate induces cataracts in rats within 6 weeks after initiating a daily dose of 0.1 mg, appearing first as radial striations in the anterior cortex between the sutures and the equator. While the early phases will remain stationary if thallium administration ceases, development of subcapsular opacities will occur if administration continues. Microscopic examination reveals areas of proliferation or deletion of the subcapsular epithelium and accumulation of a homogeneous or granular material axially to the fibers (Duke-Elder, 1969). The nuclear region is spared.

Thallous ion rapidly accumulates in the lens both in vivo (Potts and Au, 1971) and in vitro (Kinsey et al., 1971), possibly by an active transport mechanism dependent on the action of $Na^+$-$K^+$-ATPase. Thallium especially accumulates in those tissues with high $K^+$ levels, suggesting a competition for the same cellular transport mechanisms. In fact, thallium substitutes for potassium in many enzymes requiring $K^+$ for activity but is effective at a concentration ten times lower than is needed for $K^+$. Examples of some enzymes studied are the following: (1) brain $K^+$-activated phosphatases (Inturrisi, 1969a), (2) brain microsomal $Na^+$-$K^+$-ATPase (Inturrisi, 1969b), (3) muscle pyruvate kinase (Kayne, 1971), and (4) skin $Na^+$-$K^+$-ATPase (Maslova et al., 1971). Whether any of the above reactions are affected in the lens has not been reported, but substitution for $K^+$ in the frog skin $Na^+$-$K^+$-ATPase results in inhibition of the $Na^+$ pump. Electron microscopic examination of the kidney, liver, and intestine from rats chronically receiving subacute doses (10 to 15 mg $Tl^+$ per kg) as thallium acetate reveals a possible primary lesion of the mitochondria, exhibiting swelling, loss of cristae, deposition of granular material, and aggregation of mitochondrial granules (Herman and Bensch, 1967). Additional morphological changes include disruption of the endoplasmic reticulum and formation of autophagic vacuoles.

**Busulfan.** Busulfan (Myleran) is a 1,4-bis(methanesulphonyloxy)-butane alkylating agent used in treating chronic myeloid leukemia. Posterior subcapsular opacities or irregularities may result following chronic busulfan therapy (Podos and Canellos, 1969; Ravindranathan et al., 1972; Grant, 1986; Hamming et al., 1976), although the incidence or conditions surrounding these cataracts have not been fully investigated.

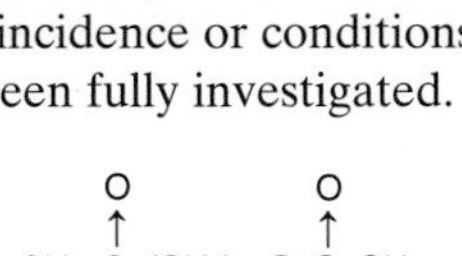

$$CH_3 \cdot \overset{O}{\overset{\uparrow}{\underset{\downarrow}{\underset{O}{S}}}} \cdot (CH_2)_4 \cdot O \cdot \overset{O}{\overset{\uparrow}{\underset{\downarrow}{\underset{O}{S}}}} \cdot CH_3$$

Busulfan (Myleran)

Experimentally induced cataracts can be produced by feeding rats a diet containing 7.5 to 20.0 mg/kg of busulfan. An irreversible cataract is completely developed in 5 to 7 weeks (Solomon et al., 1955; von Sallmann, 1957). The earliest observation includes an increased mitotic activity of the epithelium primarily in the equatorial region, which eventually returns to and drops below normal levels. White dots or small vacuoles appear in the posterior and anterior lens, rapidly followed by opacification progressing from the equator to the posterior and anterior subcapsular zones. Similarities have been drawn between busulfan and ionizing radiation cataracts, suggesting that those species with the slowest lens mitotic activity will develop cataracts more slowly (von Sallmann, 1957). The underlying mechanism may involve altered epithelial cell division. Injection of a single 12.5 mg/kg dose intraperitoneally reveals that busulfan acts during the relatively long G phase (Grimes et al., 1964) of the cell cycle (Harding et al., 1971), permitting normal synthesis of DNA but preventing subsequent mitosis. Consequently, the affected epithelial cells accumulate in preprophase, containing bizarre clumps of nuclear chromatin and twice the normal DNA content. Some of these cells undergo nuclear fragmentation and disintegration, while the remainder return to interphase with a tetraploid level of DNA. A similar mechanism occurs after chronic administration of busulfan (Grimes and von Sallmann, 1966). Following each cycle of DNA synthesis, mitosis is inhibited; and since the cells in the equatorial zone have the shortest intermitotic time (19 days), they are affected first. The cells in the equatorial zone normally migrate through the meridional rows and differentiate into lens fibers. However, death of these cells occurs after 3 days of busulfan treatment, leading to a decrease in cell density and disorganization of the meridional rows, and finally, opacification. Continuous administration of this drug results in a depletion in the number of epithelial cells and complete disruption of the equatorial zone.

**Triparanol.** Triparanol (MER-29) was developed in the late 1950s as a blood cholesterol-lowering agent. Subsequent experiments in rats revealed decreased serum and tissue cholesterol levels and concomitant elevation in desmosterol levels. Triparanol inhibits cholesterol synthesis by inhibiting the $C^{24,25}$ double-bond reduction in desmosterol (Avigan et al., 1960; Steinberg and Avigan, 1960). Two reports published prior to the removal of triparanol from the market due to other toxicities confirmed the development of posterior and anterior subcapsular opacities following a dose of at least 250 mg per day for 15 to 18 months (Kirby et al., 1962; Laughlin and Carey, 1962).

Triparanol can induce cataracts in rats fed a diet containing 0.1 percent of the drug (von Sallmann et al., 1963). Small sudanophilic vesicles form on the fibers and eventually aggregate into large clusters. Prior to central and peripheral opacification, triparanol causes a tenfold increase in lens sodium content, causing hydration and swelling (Harris 1969, 1972). Upon returning to a normal diet, the cataracts are reversed as new fibers are laid down in the periphery, excess $Na^+$ and water are pumped out, and $K^+$ levels return to normal. Morphologic alterations have been observed under the electron microscope with other tissues sensitive to triparanol toxicity. Abnormalities consist of crystalloid and membranous intracytoplasmic inclusion bodies in neurons (Schutta and Neville, 1968), mitochondrial swelling, and rupture and fragmentation of the endoplasmic reticulum in the liver (Otto, 1971). Because cholesterol is an essential component of cellular membranes, inhibition of its synthesis could result in an overall inhibition of membrane synthesis (Rawlins and Uzmana, 1970), involving all subcellular membranous structures, including mitochondria. Changes in mitochondrial oxidative metabolism (Otto, 1971) could conceivably result in deficiencies of the $Na^+$-pump mechanism in extruding intracellular $Na^+$ from the lens and consequently lead to $Na^+$ accumulation in the lens. Further experimental evidence concerning the mechanism by which triparanol cataracts are formed is lacking.

**Naphthalene.** The biochemical basis for naphthalene cataract has been investigated (van Heyningen and Pirie, 1967) and shown to be related to the liver metabolite of naphthalene, 1,2-dihydro-1,2-dihydroxynaphthalene. Lenticular catechol reductase biotransforms 1,2-dihydro-1,2-dihydroxynaphthalene to 1,2-dihydroxynaphthalene, which in turn is autooxidized in air at neutral pH to 1,2-naphthoquinone and hydrogen peroxide. Ascorbic acid reverses the latter reaction and forms dehydroascorbic acid, which can be reduced by glutathione. Because ascorbic acid diffuses out of the lens very slowly, it accumulates in the lens of the naphthalene-fed rabbit and in the lens incubated in vitro with 1,2-dihydro-1,2-dihydroxynaphthalene (van Heyningen, 1970a). The sequence of reactions involves reduction of ascorbic acid by 1,2-naphthoquinone in the aqueous humor to dehydroascorbic acid, which rapidly penetrates the lens and is reduced by glutathione. Oxidized glutathione and 1,2-naphthoquinone may compete for the enzyme glutathione reductase, which normally maintains high lenticular levels of reduced glutathione. A reduction in the concentration of these coupled with the removal of oxygen from the aqueous humor due to the autooxidation of 1,2-dihydroxynaphthalene may make the lens sensitive to naphthoquinone toxicity. Other diols that do not form quinones in similar in vitro experiments do not result in lenticular opacities or increased ascorbic acid levels (van Heyningen, 1970b).

**Galactose.** The mechanism of galactose- and other sugar-related cataracts has been explained by excessive hydration of the lens observed as early as 12 h after initiating a galactose-enriched diet. Galactose and other sugars are transported across the capsule and epithelial cell membrane by facilitated transport and diffusion (Elbrink and Bihler, 1972), and on entering the lens, galactose is either slowly phosphorylated to galactose-6-phosphate or reduced by the NADPH-dependent aldose reductase to dulcitol. While other sugar alcohols formed by aldose reductase are converted by polyol-NADP oxidoreductase to readily diffusible products, dulcitol is not further biotransformed. Since it diffuses out of the lens only very slowly, dulcitol accumulates to high levels and consequently exerts a strong osmotic force, drawing water into the lens in order to maintain osmotic equilibrium. Therefore, increases in dulcitol levels are accompanied by a parallel increase in water content (Kinoshita, 1965; van Heyningen, 1971). If dulcitol synthesis is depressed by inhibiting aldose reductase with 3,3-tetramethyleneglutaric acid, water uptake and fiber vacuolization are prevented (van Heyningen, 1971). Furthermore, feeding young Carworth Farms Webster (CFW) mice a galactose-enriched diet does not produce cataracts, because lenses of this strain fail to biotransform galactose to dulcitol (Kuck, 1970c). Therefore, lenticular hydration resulting from the osmotic force due to dulcitol accumulation and retention explains fiber vacuolization and the initial structural alterations in galactose cataracts. Further investigations verified the lack of or very low activity of other lenticular enzymes that could biotransform dulcitol, such as galactokinase or 1-gulonate NADP oxidoreductase (van Heyningen, 1971).

Experimentally induced galactose cataract has its counterpart in human physiology. Galactosemia is an autosomal recessive genetic deficiency in galactose metabolism. Affected infants on a milk diet show high blood and urine galactose levels, hepatomegaly, splenomegaly, eventual mental retardation, and cataracts. The genetic defect is a deficiency in the enzymes galactose-1-phosphate-uridyl transferase or galactokinase (Kinoshita, 1965; Monteleone et al., 1971; Nordmann, 1971; Levy et al., 1972). These enzymes are necessary in transforming unusable galactose into usable glucose-1-phosphate. Galactose or galactose-1-phosphate reaches excessive levels in the blood and aqueous humor, triggering dulcitol synthesis in the lens and subsequent fibril vacuolization (van Heyningen, 1969). Removal of galactose from the diet can reverse the symptoms.

The multiple causes of cataracts suggest multiple mechanisms rather than a final common pathway. This, in turn, suggests that we are not close to the multiple solutions required, even though the sugar cataract problem appears to be solved brilliantly.

## THE VITREOUS CAVITY

In recent years we have been learning the ground rules governing how we may invade the vitreous cavity with impunity. The *pars plana vitrectomy* seems to be executable without inevitable disaster. A natural consequence of the procedure (accomplished by simultaneous aspiration of the vitreous contents and replacement with fluid) is the investigation of how the composition of the replacement fluid will affect the structures that line the vitreous cavity, particularly the retina.

In the past, expandable gases have been used with partial success to ensure the juxtaposition of the detached retina to underlying layers. More recently silicone oil has been used (Blumenkrantz, 1988). There has been little attention paid to the nature of the monomer or the presence of contaminants. There has been a high incidence of complications, but it is difficult to evaluate what success rate is expected in such a desperate situation. Later reports incriminate low-molecular-weight components of silicone oil (Nakamura et al., 1991) and emulsification of the silicone oil (Ohira et al., 1991) as contributors to toxicity. The report of Peyman and coworkers (1992) suggests that silicone gel polymerized from the monomer in the vitreous cavity might be tolerated well. One questions whether the toxicity of the polymerizing agent will not become manifest eventually. More recently we have seen accounts of the use of the high-specific-gravity, relatively nonreactive, perhalogenated molecules for tamponade of the retina. The list includes perfluorooctyl bromide, perfluoro-tri-*N*-propylamine, perfluorooctane, perfluoropolyether, perfluorotributylamine, perfluorodecalin, and perfluorohydrophenanthrene. The ultimate is a report from Louisiana State University in which perfluorohydrophenanthrene (Vitreon) was used in 40 eyes (Tanji et al., 1993). In four of these eyes Vitreon was used for the inferior tamponade, and simultaneously silicone oil was used for the superior tamponade. In every case in which tamponade fluids were used they had to be removed in a matter of months to prevent damage from the fluid. Thus, we are making laudable progress in a class of vitreoretinal disease that was considered hopeless in the recent past. However, if there is a magic combination of techniques, we have not yet found it.

A second reason for exploring tolerance to medications within the vitreous cavity is the search for an effective inhibitor of proliferative retinopathy, the mechanism of destruction in diabetic retinopathy. Antineoplastic fluorouracil was examined for toxicity when placed in the vitreous space. Stern and coworkers (1983) found that 0.5 mg fluorouracil in the vitreous cavity of rabbits was tolerated every 24 h for 7 days with no signs of damage. On the same schedule, 1.25 mg caused marked damage. According to Burrada and colleagues (1984), fluorouracil was tolerated by primate eyes in a single dose of 750 $\mu$g. Figures were also presented by these authors on fluorouracil combined with etopside and also with vincristine. Apparently, 0.5 $\mu$g/mL of vincristine in the vitreous perfusion fluid of primates was well tolerated. The later report of Orr and coworkers (1986) dealt with recovery of $^{14}C$-labeled fluorouracil from the rabbit eye. Recovery was greatest if both vitrectomy and lensectomy had been done. The presence of silicone oil reduced the extent of recovery.

Thinking along similar lines, Kirmani and colleagues (1983) devised a test object for proliferative vitreoretinopathy by injecting cultured rabbit dermal fibroblasts into the rabbit vitreous. Six cytotoxic drugs were tested using this test object. Daunomycin at 10 nanomoles per eye stopped cellular proliferation and prevented subsequent traction detachment. Equivalent doses of actinomycin C, colchicine, cytosine arabinoside, 5-fluorodeoxyuridine, and vinblastine sulfate showed no such effect. Therapeutic use was recommended against by these authors, just as the use of doxorubicin was recommended against by Sunalp and coworkers (1985). However, the availability of dimethyl adriamycin, which lacks the mutagenicity and carcinogenicity of its parent, adriamycin (doxorubicin), has allowed Steinhorst and coworkers (1993a) to overcome completely the proliferative retinopathy in a rabbit model. A second paper from the Steinhorst group (Steinhorst et al., 1993b) avoids histologically detectable retinal toxicity from daunomycin by using divided doses in the rabbit model. However, there is a significant decline in the b-wave of the electroretinogram (ERG) in the eyes that were experimented upon.

A third reason for invading intraocular space is the possibility of treating intraocular inflammatory disease which would be otherwise inaccessible to medication. Establishing toxicity levels for this application modality is imperative.

Several specific cautions have been recorded. Zemel and coworkers (1993) have pointed out that Depo-Medrol, a favored long-acting anti-inflammatory preparation, may not be used for intraocular injection because of the toxicity of its preservative, myristyl gamma-picolinium chloride. On the basis of experiments with rabbit eyes, Oum and colleagues (1992) point out that for drug regimens involving aphakic and vitrectomized eyes, toxicity figures obtained with single injections are invalid for multiple injections. Doses must be revised downward.

Moxalactam, a third-generation, semisynthetic, cephalosporinlike antibiotic, enters the eye when given parenterally, but vitreous concentrations are disappointing (Fett et al., 1984). The rabbit retina tolerates 1.25 mg injected into the vitreous, but higher doses damage the retina. A related compound, cefoperazone, is harmless when a single dose of 8 mg is injected into the vitreous of Dutch Belted rabbits. Doses of 16 mg and higher cause retinal damage (O'Hara et al., 1986). In the same series ceftriaxone was tolerated in a maximum intravitreal dose of 20 mg (Shockley et al., 1984). Still in the same series, ceftazidine showed transient decrease of the b-wave of the ERG. The injection of 2 mg ceftazidine into the vitreous of a phakic rabbit gave what are judged to be bactericidal levels for at least 72 h (Jay et al., 1987).

The aminoglycoside antibiotics were tested for toxicity on intravitreal injection by D'Amico and coworkers (1985). Their injections began at the level of 100 $\mu$g per eye. They found gentamycin the most toxic, followed by netlimycin and tobramycin (about equal), followed by amikacin and kanamycin (also about equal).

A morphological study on the toxic manifestations of gentamycin in pig eyes showed that the changes were not pH-related; that neurons and glia of the inner retina are the site of abnormality; and that interference with retinal perfusion may play a role (Hines et al., 1993).

By light microscopy and ERG in rabbit eyes vancomycin was tolerated in vitrectomy infusion solution at 8, 16, and 32 $\mu$g/mL. At 100 $\mu$g/mL both histological and ERG abnormalities were noted (Borhani et al., 1993). A single dose of 1 mg of vancomycin into the vitreous of rabbits caused no ERG abnormality; 10 mg made the ERG nonrecordable (Mochizuki et al., 1991).

The semisynthetic beta lactam antibiotic imipinem was found by Derick and colleagues (1987) to be tolerated in vitrectomy infusion fluid at concentrations of up to 16 $\mu$g/mL in rabbits.

Pflugfelder and coworkers (1987) found that otherwise resistant strains of gram-positive organisms isolated from endophthalmitis eyes were sensitive to vancomycin. Vitrectomized rabbit eyes appeared to tolerate up to 2 mg of the drug without damage. Furthermore, the effect of vancomycin plus gentamycin appeared to be additive.

Several studies have been made on intravitreous introduction of ciprofloxacin. Marchese and coworkers (1993) performed midvitreous injections of ciprofloxacin in rabbit eyes. A single dose of 250 $\mu$g produced no ophthalmoscopic or ERG abnormalities; 500 $\mu$g of the drug produced focal areas of retinitis, and 1000 $\mu$g caused reduction of b-wave amplitudes as well. A second study on 39 rabbit eyes showed no ophthalmoscopic damage even with a 3200-$\mu$g dose, but optical microscopy showed vacuolization at 800 $\mu$g and above (Rootman et al., 1992). Both groups are in the same order of magnitude with regard to the maximum tolerated dose.

Note should be taken of the use by Alghadyan and colleagues (1988) of liposome-bound cyclosporine with a view toward reducing toxicity; 500 $\mu$g injected into the vitreous cavity was tolerated with no damage to rabbit retina.

## ANTIVIRAL AGENTS FOR IMMUNOCOMPROMISED AND IMMUNOCOMPETENT SUBJECTS

The rapid spread of the human immunodeficiency virus (HIV) problem has presented ophthalmologists with a significant number of immunocompromised patients who have acquired retinal cytomegalovirus infections. In the light of our present inability to treat acquired immunodeficiency syndrome (AIDS) effectively, these patients have no hope of a successful outcome. However, the ability to subdue cytomegalovirus (CMV) infection promises to provide a better quality of life and functional vision. At least one of the opportunistic invaders can be restrained.

A number of publications have dealt with intravitreal tolerance to antiviral agents. Pulido and coworkers (1984) recommended using up to 30 $\mu$g vidarbine intraocularly or 8 to 16 $\mu$g/mL in infusion fluid. For acyclovir, the recommendation was 80 $\mu$g intraocularly or 40 $\mu$g/mL in infusion fluid. Acyclovir has weak anti-CMV activity.

Hydroxyacyclovir was evaluated in the same laboratory a year later (Pulido et al., 1985). These workers found no changes from intravitreal doses as high as 400 $\mu$g. The effectiveness of this drug against CMV was pointed out as a special application.

In recent years two drugs have emerged as agents of choice against CMV. The first of these is gancyclovir (available as Cytovene, Syntex; Buhles et al., 1988). Gancyclovir is 9-(1,3 dihydroxy-2-propoxymethyl) guanine. The drug is supplied as a lyophylized powder to be dissolved and diluted. The side effects are granulocytopenia and thrombocytopenia, and they are not rare. For eye disease in the absence of systemic involvement, the physician has an enormous advantage if he or she is able to administer a therapeutic dose directly into the vitreous. The second drug of choice is foscarnet (available as Foscavir, Astra). The molecule is phosphonoformic acid trisodium salt, an organic analog of pyrophosphate. It inhibits replication of all known herpes viruses in vitro. It acts by selective inhibition at the pyrophosphate binding sites of virus-specific DNA polymerases and reverse transcriptases at concentrations that do not affect cellular DNA polymerases. CMV strains resistant to gancyclovir may be sensitive to foscarnet. The chief side effect of foscarnet is renal impairment, and roughly a third of patients on systemic therapy show significant elevation of serum creatinine. Once more, if we are dealing with ocular disease alone, there is enormous advantage in being able to apply medication to the eye alone and avoid the serious systemic complications.

During the years 1991–1994 more than a dozen publications appeared on the optimization of intravenous dosages of gancyclovir or foscarnet or both. A typical report was that of Jacobson and colleagues (1994). Dosage levels were successfully adjusted so that CMV was successfully supressed; dose-limiting toxicity attributable to foscarnet appeared in only 7 percent of 29 patients, and there was no dose-limiting nephrotoxicity. This held for the evaluation time of 12 weeks. Recurrences were characteristic of longer studies.

### Intravitreal Injection

During the same period a number of expedients, including direct injection, were being explored for introduction of anti-CMV medications directly into the vitreous. Turrini and colleagues (1994) used injection of 3.6 mg of foscarnet as many as six times in the rabbit vitreous with no ill effects. Berthe and coworkers (1994) used intravitreal injection in rabbits and came to similar conclusions. Human subjects were treated by intravitreal injections by Diaz-Llopis and coworkers (1994). In the hands of these workers 2400 μg of foscarnet was injected into the vitreous of 15 eyes. Over a mean period of 16 weeks, 304 injections were given. Complete resolution was seen in two-thirds of the cases; the remainder showed partial resolution. However, one-third showed relapse on maintenance therapy, and 2 out of 15 eyes went on to loss of vision.

Pang and coworkers (1992) measured the tolerance of the rabbit eye for trifluorothymidine injected into the vitreous. Their dose of 200 μg was well tolerated, and the $ID_{50}$ was maintained for 30 h (dose to inhibit 50 percent of cytopathic activity as against control CMV cultures). The question arises whether this statistic is significant for those of us for whom clinical success means complete eradication of the virus (cf. Pang et al., 1986).

## Efforts to Slow Diffusion

As reflected in the discussions above, intravitreal injection was greatly superior to systemic treatment for disease restricted to the eye, but there were difficulties with the physical trauma of the many injections required when a drug diffuses rapidly from the eye. It goes without saying that drug toxicity limits the size of the initial dose. Others have sought a solution for slowing down a rapidly diffusing drug in various ways. Moritera and coworkers (1992) delivered adriamycin to inhibit proliferative retinopathy in biodegradable polymer microspheres injected into the vitreous. Rubsamen and colleagues (1994) administered fluorouracil for experimental proliferative retinopathy in a 6 × 0.9 mm cylindrical biodegradable implant. A sustained-release *intraocular device* for insertion into the vitreous of CMV patients to liberate gancyclovir was described by Anand and coworkers (1993). The device was inserted through an inferotemporal full-thickness circumferential sclerotomy and anchored to the incision. Seven eyes obtained 16 to 82 days after death were sectioned and examined by light and electron microscopy. All seven eyes were stabilized clinically, and none showed gancyclovir toxicity. Still another approach, tried in rabbits only, was transscleral iontophoresis of foscarnet. The conditions specified (1) a probe tip of 2 $mm^2$, (2) a current of 1 mA, (3) a duration of 10 min, (4) a starting solution of 24 mg/mL provided a peak intraocular concentration of 200 micromolar. Therapeutic levels were maintained for up to 60 h. No toxicity was reported for this set of conditions. One wonders why this approach was not carried forward to human eyes; it appears to be the least traumatic method tried to date. Perhaps it is less applicable to gancyclovir (Sarraf et al., 1993).

## Additional Anti-CMV Drugs

To increase the tilt in favor of the patient still more, some new compounds have been introduced. The diethanolammonium salt of 2′-nor-cyclic GMP is a cyclic phosphate derivative of gancyclovir. On intravitreal injection of 10 μg in rabbits, no toxic effects are observed. Toxicity is apparent at 50 μg and higher. Inclusion of the drug in liposomes gives an in vitro drug release halftime of 1000 h (Shakiba et al., 1993).

Yet another drug with anti-CMV potential is (*S*)-1-(3-hydroxy-2-phosphonylmethoxypropyl) cytosine (HPMPC) (Dolnak et al., 1992). Tests of toxicity were done by direct injection into rabbit vitreous. No retinal damage was detected at the 100 μg level; half-life of the drug was 24.4 h. These results are impressive, but no mention was made of auxillary techniques to stretch out the duration of action.

## Additional Vitreous Toxicity Studies

Yoshizumi and coworkers (1986) applied vidarbine intravitreally dissolved in DMSO. The tolerated dose was 100 μg/mL in the infusion fluid. The drug has in vitro effectiveness against herpes simplex virus. The innocuousness of two separate foreign substances must be proved.

In anticipation of being able to treat vitreoretinal non-Hodgkin's lymphoma with cytarabine [1(beta-D-arabinofuranosyl)cytosine], toxicity of the drug was tested in rabbit eyes (Diets-Ouwehand et al., 1992). The eyes tolerated two daily doses of 300 μg without detectable damage. Higher doses were toxic.

Similarly, ara-M (6-methoxypurine arabinoside) was hoped to be a selective and potent inhibitor against varicella-zoster virus and was tested in rabbit eyes (Karacorlu et al., 1992). Doses up to 400 μg injected into the vitreous caused no detectable retinal toxicity.

In the same order of magnitude of toxicity is trifluorothymidine. It is tolerated at a single dose of 200 μg and at a level of 60 μg/mL on perfusion (Pang et al., 1986). The same laboratory reports that gancyclovir, active against CMV, is tolerated in infusion fluid at levels of 30 μg/mL or less (Kao et al., 1987). Further, it appears that in combinations of antiviral drugs, toxicity is not additive. Useful combinations must be defined (Small et al., 1987).

Publications on antifungal agents have been fewer in number. However, the upper therapeutic level of 5-fluorocytosine has been found to be 100 μg on intravitreal injection (Yoshizumi and Silverman, 1985). A comparable single dose of fluconazole (anticandida) is tolerated in similar conditions (Schulman et al., 1987).

The unique immunosuppressive cyclosporin is tolerated at 100 μg intravitreally; 200 μg causes histological damage (Grisolano and Peyman, 1986).

# THE RETINA AND CHOROID

The retina is the very compact and highly complex neural structure responsible for transducing the ocular light image and doing considerable preprocessing of the neural impulses before sending them toward the brain (Fig. 20-1). The layer of rods and cones—modified neural structures containing photosensitive pigments—is the receptor of the light image. The receptor cells synapse with bipolar cells, which in turn synapse with ganglion cells. In addition, lateral synapses occur with horizontal cells and feedback synapses occur with amacrine cells. The Müller cells, the glial equivalent in the retina, have nuclei near the center of the retinal thickness and long processes that extend through the whole retinal thickness. Finally, the single layer of retinal pigmented epithelium underlies the receptors and sends processes that envelop the receptor outer segments. It should be evident from these relationships—all of which exist in the 100- to 500-$\mu$m retinal thickness—that studies on the overall biochemistry and physiology of such a structure are likely to be confusing and misleading.

To dispel any lingering hope that the retinal layers are uniform metabolically if not morphologically, one need only read below, in this section, about how specific toxic substances affect specific retinal layers. After one has recognized with Warburg (1926) that the retina as a whole is the most actively metabolizing structure in the normal body, one must view metabolic studies on whole retina with healthy skepticism. The extremely compact structure of the retina creates a real dilemma when one wishes to study a single cell type. One solution is that worked out by Lowry and coworkers (1956, 1961), who microdissected freeze-dried retina and picked out nuclei of each cell type for metabolic studies. Other approaches utilize microelectrodes on micrometer carriers, but the respiration of mammals destroys any precision, and the experimenter must use curare, an open chest, and artificial respiration. It is somewhat frustrating to see the study of toxic mechanisms in the retina lagging because of the admittedly difficult territory that the retina presents.

The choroid is a vascular layer whose chief constituents in addition to the blood vessels are collagenous connective tissue and cells containing large numbers of melanin granules. The latter are important because of the affinity of melanin for polycyclic aromatic compounds. In primates, which have a well-established retinal blood supply, the choroid is responsible for nutrition of the receptor cell layer only. In lower vertebrates the choroidal vasculature supplies all of the retina. In any case the retinal pigment epithelium prevents easy ophthalmoscopic access to the choroid. Access using albino animals or infrared photography has its own difficulties.

Because of the physical proximity of these two structures, many diseases primary in the choroid cause retinal damage and some diseases primary in the retina cause choroidal damage. Thus, *chorioretinitis* is a commonly encountered term. It is based on clinical observation and does not imply which structure is primary for the disease process.

## Chloroquine

The 4-aminoquinoline chloroquine is effective as (1) an antimalarial, requiring doses of 500 mg per week for 3 to 4 weeks, with the maintenance dose at 250 mg per week, and (2) an anti-inflammatory agent, requiring doses of at least 250 mg per day to be effective. The low-dose therapy used for malaria is essentially free from any toxic side effects; however, the chronic, high-dose therapy used for rheumatoid arthritis and discoid and systemic lupus erythematosus frequently causes a number of side effects, the most serious of which involves an irreversible loss of retinal function. In 1959, the first cases of chloroquine-induced retinopathy were reported (Hobbs et al., 1959), but since then numerous reports have confirmed the etiology of similar sets of symptoms as resulting from chloroquine therapy (see reviews by Nylander, 1967; Duke-Elder and MacFaul, 1972). Hydroxychloroquine also has been reported to cause a similar retinopathy (Crews, 1967; Shearer and Dubois, 1967), although the incidence of toxicity may be less (Shearer and Dubois, 1967; Sassaman et al., 1970).

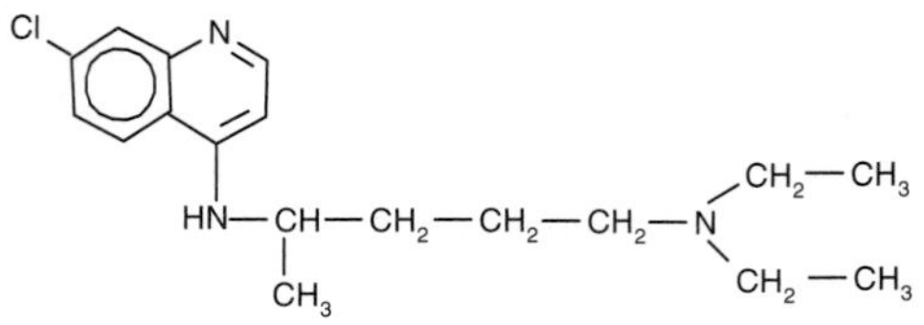

Chloroquine

The clinical findings accompanying chloroquine retinopathy generally may be thought of in terms of early and late phenomena. Among the early findings are (1) a "bull's-eye retina," visualized as a dark, central pigmented area involving the macula, surrounded by a pale ring of depigmentation, which in turn is surrounded by another ring of pigmentation; (2) diminished electrooculogram; (3) possible granular pigmentation of the peripheral retina; and (4) subjective visual disturbances, observed as blurred vision and difficulty in reading, with words or letters missing in long sentences or long words. Late findings are (1) progressive scotoma, (2) constriction of the peripheral fields commencing in the upper temporal quadrant, (3) narrowing of the retinal artery, (4) color and night blindness, (5) absence of a typical pigment pattern, and (6) abnormal electrooculograms and electroretinograms; these symptoms are irreversible. Indeed, there have been reports of irreversible chloroquine retinopathy in which the entire development of the disease has occurred after cessation of the drug (Burns, 1966).

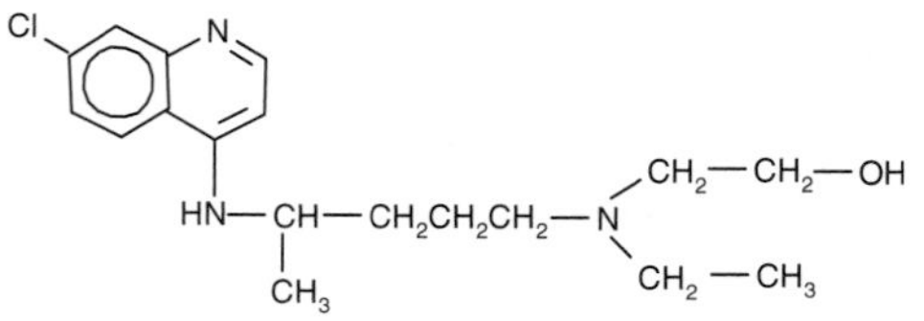

Hydroxychloroquine

It is generally recognized that the incidence of these chloroquine-induced toxic effects increases as the daily dose, total dose, and duration of therapy increase. Absence of permanent damage has been reported in patients receiving not more than 250 mg of chloroquine or 200 mg of hydroxychloroquine per day (Scherbel et al., 1965). Nevertheless, utilization of sensitive testing methods such as "macular dazzling" and retinal threshold tests has indicated some degree of retinal malfunction in all patients receiving even small doses of these drugs (Carr, 1968). Thus, there is a qualitative difference between the depression of visual function observed in all patients and the specific damage seen in relatively few individuals. Approximately 20 to 30 percent of the patients receiving higher doses of chloroquine will exhibit some type of retinal abnormality, while 5 to 10 percent show severe changes in retinal function (Butler, 1965; Crews, 1967; Nylander, 1967). One interesting paradox is worth noting. Despite severe retinopathy and "extinguished" ERG, normal or nearly normal dark adaptation performance is characteristic of chloroquine toxicity. This is in marked contrast to phenothiazine retinopathy (see "Phenothiazines," below) (Krill et al., 1971).

Experimentally induced chloroquine retinopathy was first produced in the cat after long-term, oral administration of subtoxic doses, 1.5 to 6.0 mg daily (Meier-Ruge, 1965b). A light pigmentation appeared in the cat's fundus 4 to 7 weeks after the daily dosage schedule, and the retinopathy was fully developed after 8 weeks. Histological and histochemical analysis revealed a thickening of the pigment epithelial cell layer, increases in the mucopolysaccharide and sulfhydryl group content, decreases in enzymatic activity of the pigment epithelium, migration of pigment into the outer nuclear layer, and finally total atrophy of the photoreceptors (Meier-Ruge, 1968). Similar findings were observed in rabbits (Dale et al., 1965; Meier-Ruge, 1965a; François and Maudgal, 1967) and humans (Bernstein and Ginsberg, 1964; Wetterholm and Winter, 1964).

A report on miniature pigs fed chloroquine at 1000 times the human therapeutic level describes massive storage of gangliosides in the central nervous system (CNS) and in retinal ganglion cells (Klinghardt et al., 1981). Early in the 200-day feeding program, epileptic and myoclonic fits were observed. Later, "visual impairment" was observed. One wonders whether this finding is more related to the "myeloid bodies" seen in the retinal ganglion cells of experimental animals within a week of beginning chloroquine (e.g., Kolb et al., 1972) than it is to the retinotoxicity of humans.

Because of its high affinity for melanin, the mechanism of chloroquine-induced retinopathy has been related to the extremely high concentrations that are attained in the pigmented eye and that remain at these high levels (Bernstein et al., 1963b; Potts, 1964a,b) long after other tissue levels have been depleted. Both hydroxychloroquine and desethylchloroquine, the major metabolite of chloroquine, behave similarly (McChesney et al., 1965, 1967). Accumulation of chloroquine in the pigmented structures of the human choroid and pigmented epithelium has been reported, and the amount depends on dosage and duration of drug therapy (Lawwill et al., 1968). In addition, small amounts of chloroquine and its metabolites are excreted in the urine years after cessation of drug treatment (Bernstein, 1967). The prolonged exposure of the retinal cell layers to chloroquine probably explains the irreversible nature of human retinopathy, which may not only progress (Okun et al., 1963) but also develop after chloroquine has been withdrawn (Burns, 1966).

Investigations concerning the primary retinotoxic lesion caused by chloroquine have led to two schools of thought. Based on the histological and histochemical findings and the melanin-binding property of chloroquine described above, one theory indicates a primary biochemical lesion in the pigmented epithelium cell layer of the retina. It is clear that storage in pigment in itself is not a sufficient cause for toxicity. It is simply that a toxic substance such as chloroquine, like any other poison, increases its effect as the concentration in tissue multiplied by time of exposure ($C \times T$) increases. Storage on melanin causes enormous increases in this $C \times T$ factor for the melanin-containing tissue—in this case, the retinal pigment epithelium.

Many biochemical reactions can be inhibited by chloroquine (reviewed by Bernstein, 1967; Mackenzie, 1970). Inhibition of protein metabolism of the pigment epithelium has been proposed as the primary cause for the retinotoxic effects of chloroquine (Meier-Ruge, 1968). In vitro experiments utilizing only whole-pigment epithelial cells have indicated that chloroquine and hydroxychloroquine markedly inhibit amino acid incorporation in protein (Gonsaun and Potts, 1972).

A late observation by Doly and coworkers (1993) suggests that platelet-activating factor (PAF) antagonists may block the toxic effect of chloroquine on neural retina. They pretreated normal rats with the PAF antagonist BN 50730 at a dose of 30 mg/kg per day given IP for 5 days. Retinas were removed from treated and untreated rats and were perfused with a chloroquine solution ($10^{-6}$ M). The untreated retinas showed a rapid and marked decrease in b-wave amplitude. The retinas from treated animals showed no such decrease. It will require more refined experiments to determine whether the locus of ocular chloroquine poisoning is in the neural retina or the retinal pigment epithelium or both.

## Phenothiazines

The potency of phenothiazines as tranquilizers is related to the chemical constituent attached to the N-atom of the three-ring base: Group I compounds possessing an aminopropyl side chain are least potent; group II compounds with a piperidine group in the side chain are more potent; and group III drugs composed of a piperazine group in the side chain are the most potent antipsychotic drugs (Boet, 1970). Successful remission of psychotic states requires persistent drug therapy at relatively high doses. Therefore, it is not surprising that many side effects are associated with long-term high-dose phenothiazine therapy. Ocular complications may involve the cornea and the lens, described above in "The Cornea, Conjunctiva, and Neighboring Tissues" and "The Lens," and the retina, described in this section ("The Retina and Choroid"). The availability of newer antipsychotic medications with no ocular side effects at therapeutic levels decreases the clinical importance of antipsychotic phenothiazines but as long as such drugs are available, their misuse remains a hazard. Furthermore, each toxic mechanism offers a wedge in the understanding of the complexities of retinal function.

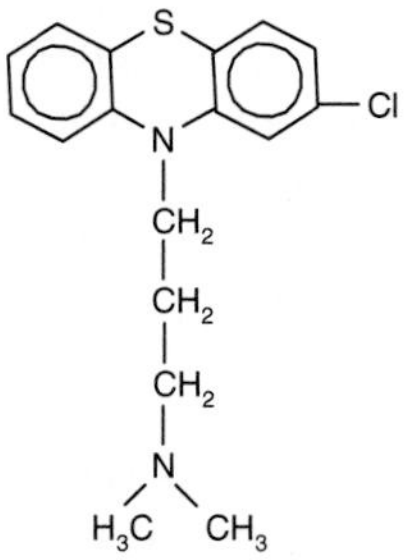

Chlorpromazine
(aminopropyl side chain)

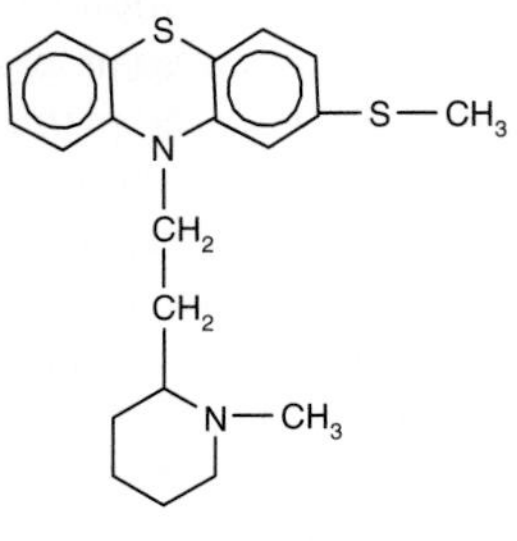

Thioridazine
(piperidyl group in the side chain)

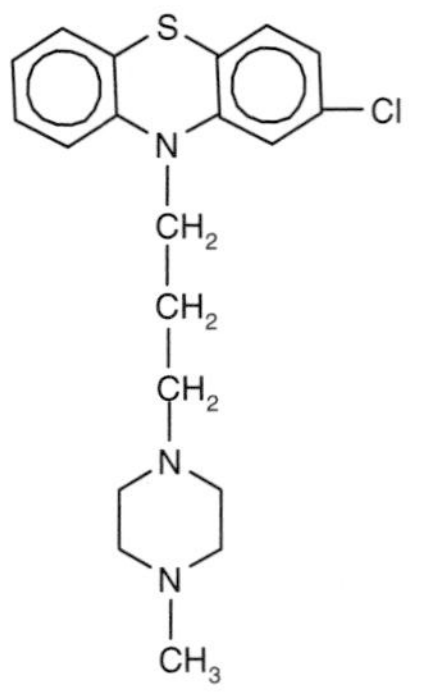

Prochlorperazine
(piperazinyl group in the side chain)

The first phenothiazine derivative reported to alter retinal function belonged to group II: piperidylchlorophenothiazine (Sandoz NP-207). During clinical trials, the initial symptoms of visual disturbances were observed as an impaired adaptation to dim light. Further disturbances involved reduced visual acuity, constricted visual fields, and abnormal pigmentation of the retina appearing in the periphery or macula as fine salt-and-pepper clumps of pigment (Kinross-Wright, 1956). Abnormalities in dark adaptation, color vision, and the ERG, coupled with severe pigment clumping during the advanced stages, indicated toxic effects in both rod and cone receptors. Disturbances of retinal function usually developed within 2 to 3 months after receiving 400 to 800 mg of the drug per day and a total of 20 to 30 g. Higher dosages required only 30 days to develop toxic symptoms. On withdrawal of the drug, some symptoms may be reversed, although pigment clumping remains visible in the fundus. However, total reversal is not possible, and in some cases, severe visual loss and blindness result. The strong evidence that NP-207 was the causative agent in these visual disturbances resulted in its removal from clinical study (Boet, 1970). One must ask whether pigment changes like those above are not a sign of retinal pigment epithelium damage whenever they are encountered.

Replacement of the 2-chlorine of NP-207 with a methylmercapto group yields thioridazine, a phenothiazine derivative effective in treating schizophrenia and nonpsychotic severe anxiety without possessing some of the side effects common to the aminopropyl phenothiazines. Thioridazine also causes pigmentary and visual disturbances similar to those caused by NP-207, but dosages of over 1200 mg per day for 30 days are required to affect retinal function (Weekley et al., 1960). Initially, a loss of visual acuity is observed, followed by night blindness, difficulty in adapting to average light conditions after being exposed to bright sunlight, and, finally, retinal pigmentary changes. In severe toxicity, excessive pigment deposition and an extinguished ERG are found. Usually, cessation of the medication is accompanied by complete or partial restoration of retinal function, although the pigmentary disturbances remain (Potts, 1968). Additional reports of thioridazine-induced retinopathy have been summarized by Siddall (1966), Boet (1970), and Cameron and colleagues (1972). Normal dosages do not cause disturbances in retinal function even after years of treatment.

The group I phenothiazine chlorpromazine is generally free from retinotoxic effects. Rare cases have been reported (Siddall, 1965, 1966, 1968) of a reversible, fine granular pigmentation in the retinal background after 2.4 g of chlorpromazine per day for 2 years following 1 to 2 g per day for 6 to 28 months. Only one patient recorded heavy pigmentation.

The piperazine derivatives (group III) have not been reported to affect retinal function (Duke-Elder and MacFaul, 1972). Because these drugs are the most potent phenothiazine derivatives, less drug is needed to control the psychotic individual, strongly suggesting that therapeutic effect and toxic effects invoke different mechanisms.

Experimentally induced phenothiazine retinopathy was accomplished by orally administering NP-207 to cats; the initial dose of 10 mg/kg per day was slowly increased to 120 mg/kg per day (Meier-Ruge and Cerletti, 1966; Cerletti and Meier-Ruge, 1967). The first retinal changes appeared as fine grayish-blackish spots on the fundus after 4 to 5 weeks of treatment. A partial explanation for the retinal changes was made by the finding that phenothiazine derivatives accumulate in very high concentrations in the uveal tract (Potts, 1962a,b). Experiments utilizing labeled chlorpromazine, prochlorperazine, and NP-207 have indicated binding of these drugs to the melanin-containing tissues of the eye, allowing high concentrations to accumulate and remain in the eye for extended periods of time (Potts, 1962a,b; Green and Ellison, 1966; Cerletti and Meier-Ruge, 1967). In vitro studies employing isolated choroidal melanin granules or synthetic melanin (Potts, 1964a,b) have indicated that several phenothiazine derivatives bind to melanin, therefore verifying the result obtained in vivo that tissue melanin content is the essential component responsible for concentrating these *N*-substituted phenothiazines. As stated above for chloroquine, concentration on pigmented structures merely gets the phenothiazine to the tissue in high concentrations. Both toxic and nontoxic phenothiazines participate in this effect. After storage the specific toxic activity (possibly one of the effects detailed in this section) is probably the cause of tissue damage.

Histological examination of retinas from NP-207-treated cats has shown initial posterior vacuolization of outer segments 1 to 2 weeks after retinal pigmentation, followed by disorganization of the entire lamellar structure of the receptor outer segments and, finally, atrophy and disintegration of the rods and cones. Other cellular layers appear normal with the exception of a proliferative pigment epithelium (Cerletti and Meier-Ruge, 1967). Despite the plethora of metabolic actions attributable to phenothiazines (e.g., Guth and Spirtes, 1964), no specific activity has been identified that is not shared by both retinotoxic substances and the innocuous ones. Thus, a pathophysiological mechanism for the toxic effect is not readily apparent.

## Indomethacin

Administration of the anti-inflammatory drug indomethacin in dosages of 50 to 200 mg per day for 1 to 2 years may result in decrease of visual acuity, visual field changes, and abnormalities in dark adaptation, ERG, and the electrooculogram (EOG) (C. A. Burns, 1966, 1968; Henkes and van Lith, 1972; Henkes et al., 1972). In one study of 34 patients (C. A. Burns, 1968), all exhibited a decreased retinal sensitivity, manifested as a lowered ERG or an altered threshold for dark adaptation. Ten of these patients had macular area disturbances, evidenced by paramacular depigmentation varying from mottled depigmentation to areas of pigment atrophy. Greater decreases in the scotopic component of the ERG than in the phototopic component have been reported (Palimeris et al., 1972). However, visual function improves upon cessation of drug treatment, accompanied by a return to normal amplitudes in the a- and b-waves of the ERG.

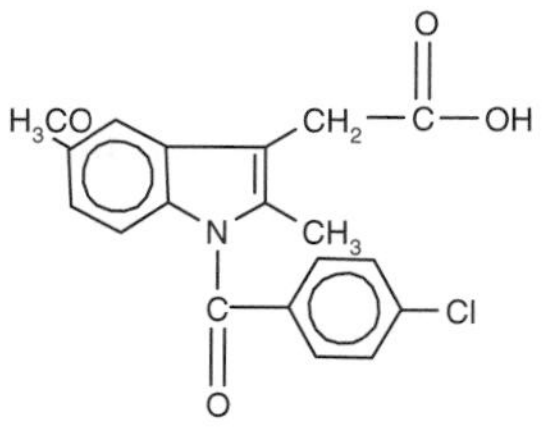

Indomethacin

Like the other nonsteroidal anti-inflammatory agents, indomethacin inhibits the prostaglandin-forming cyclooxygenase; it prevents the release of lysosomal enzymes and stabilizes liver lysosomes when exposed to labilizing conditions (Ignarro, 1972). Inhibition of $Ca_{21}$ accumulation in injured tissue (Northover, 1972) and $Ca_{21}$ influx into stimulated smooth muscle by indomethacin (Northover, 1971) have been reported. However, it is unclear whether one of these properties or some as yet unidentified property is responsible for retinal toxicity.

## Oxygen

The therapeutic use of oxygen in concentrations greater than in ambient air has increased year by year. Therapy with hyperbaric oxygen, despite its complexity, is practiced at centers with little expertise to recommend them save that they possess the equipment. Healthy adults can usually tolerate breathing pure oxygen for up to 3 h without exhibiting any uncomfortable symptoms; however, further inhalation at atmospheric pressure or short-term inhalation of high concentrations of oxygen at 2 to 3 atmospheres results in bilateral progressive constriction of the peripheral fields, impaired central vision, mydriasis, and constriction of the retinal vasculature (Grant, 1986; Nichols and Lambertsen, 1969; Mailer, 1970). All the symptoms are reversible upon inhalation of air. Severe irreversible retinal damage in adults is rare.

Although adults are not seriously affected by breathing high concentrations of oxygen, this is not true for premature infants. Frequently, premature infants are placed in incubators and breathe oxygen in concentrations greater than in air. On removal from hyperoxia, they develop an irreversible bilateral ocular disease known as retrolental fibroplasia. Critical in the development of this oxygen-induced disease is the embryological nature of the human retinal vasculature. Beginning with the fourth month of gestation, the retinal vascular system develops from the hyaloid vascular stalk in the optic nerve, and by the eighth month, the retina is vascularized only in its nasal periphery. Development into the peripheral retina is not complete until after birth of a full-term infant (Patz, 1969–70). Only the incompletely developed retinal circulation is susceptible to toxic levels of oxygen, whereas a mature retinal vascular system and other incompletely formed circulations are not sensitive to oxygen toxicity. Within 6 h after an infant is placed in a high-oxygen-containing atmosphere, vasoconstriction of the immature vessels occurs. This is reversible if the child is immediately returned to air but is irreversible if hyperoxia therapy is continued (Beehler, 1964). Obliteration of the capillary lumen takes place as the vessel walls adhere to each other. This is followed by degeneration of the capillary endothelial cells and depression of the normal anterior forward growth of the retinal vessels. Immediately after returning to a normal oxygen atmosphere, vessels adjacent to the damaged area rapidly proliferate, invade the retina, penetrate the internal limiting membrane, and enter the vitreous. During the advanced stages, retinal fibrosis may cause retinal detachment. The opaque retrolental mass causes leukocoria (Beehler, 1964; Patz, 1969–70).

Experimental investigations with kittens have indicated a similar and selective degeneration and proliferation of the developing retinal capillary endothelium. The vasoconstriction and lumen obliteration are directly related to the degree of immaturity of the retinal vascular system and to the concentration and duration of exposure to oxygen (Ashton and Pedler, 1962; Ashton, 1966, 1970; Patz, 1969–1970; Flower and Patz, 1971). While hyperoxia is selectively toxic to the immature retinal vascular system, no toxic effects are evident on the retina itself. Glycolytic and respiratory rates are unchanged (Graymore, 1970). These results contrast with the oxygen-induced photoreceptor atrophy observed in adult animals. This disparity is puzzling, but it may simply indicate that early damage was not detectable by gross anatomical or biochemical measurement.

High concentrations of oxygen inhibit a number of enzymatic paths (Davies and Davies, 1965). Inhibition of respiration, electron transport, ATP synthesis, glycolysis, and a number of enzyme and coenzyme functions requiring free sulfhydryl groups for activity have been reported (reviewed by Haugaard, 1965, 1968; Menzel, 1970). The toxicity induced during maturation of the retinal vascular system, causing retrolental fibroplasia, may be explained by any of the above deficiencies, although no specific mechanism has been proposed. However, the toxicity on the mature photoreceptor cells may be explained by inhibition of glycolysis, which is essential for retinal function.

Even with recognition of the need to reduce oxygen concentrations gradually for low-birth-weight babies, retinopathy of prematurity (i.e., retrolental fibroplasia) presents an insoluble dilemma as a toxic iatrogenic disease.

## Epinephrine

In eyes that are aphakic, postcataract extraction cystoid macular edema has been described after the use of epinephrine (Kolker and Becker, 1968; Obstbaum et al., 1976). Recovery is expected, but not invariably, on cessation of the drug.

## Iodate

In the preantibiotic era of the 1920s, attempts were made to combat systemic septic disease, such as septicemia, by intravenous injection of inorganic antiseptics. It was found after the use of one of these—concentrated Pregl solution, known under the trade name of Septojod—that a number of individuals became blind (Riehm, 1927). It was demonstrated by Riehm (1929) that the primary retinal involvement was of the pigment epithelium and that this disease could be induced experimentally by injecting Septojod into pigmented rabbits. Vito

(1935) was able to demonstrate that the actual toxic agent involved was sodium iodate. However, the exact way in which iodate causes degeneration and the reason for the particular susceptibility of the pigment epithelium have not been adequately worked out. Although iodate is known to be a relatively stable oxidizing agent, and though the probability of this mechanism of action is reinforced by the fact that the iodate effect can be completely neutralized by the reducing agent, cysteine (Sorsby and Harding, 1960), the effect has not been reproduced by other oxidizing agents, such as manganese dioxide, perborate, and persulfate (Sorsby, 1941). It is true, however, that none of these agents has the relative stability of iodate, and a dose comparable with that of iodate could not be given intravenously without killing the experimental animals.

Various experiments verified a primary effect of iodate on the pigment epithelium cell layer, followed by a secondary lesion and degeneration of the rod outer segments. Within hours after the administration of iodate, the thickness of the pigment epithelium layer is reduced, accompanied by loss of cellular limits, loss of definition, and formation of a granular cytoplasm (Graymore, 1970). Because the pigment epithelium cell layer lies between the choroidal vasculature and photoreceptors, it is responsible for the exchange of nutrients and metabolites from the blood to the visual cells. Iodate-induced interruption in this flow of nutrients by possibly affecting the energy supply of the pigment epithelium or the rhodopsin cycle in the pigment epithelium would subsequently lead to photoreceptor degeneration.

## Sparsomycin

The antibiotic sparsomycin, prepared from *Streptomyces sparsogenes*, has been used as an anticancer drug. One report (McFarlane et al., 1966) described two patients who received sparsomycin intravenously and developed pigmentary disturbances corresponding to bilateral ring scotomas. Perhaps because of this toxicity it has not been employed extensively. It may still serve as a tool in elucidating ocular toxicity.

## Retinoids

Derivatives of the naturally occurring retinol, retinal, retinoic acid family appear to be useful in dermatological disease but not without some ocular side effects. Isoretinoin, which is 13-*cis* retinoic acid, is effective against cystic acne, but a small percentage of patients develop poor night vision and glare sensitivity (Weleber et al., 1986). Although various tests of retinal function show abnormalities, there is no correlation between the medication and a single test. Etretinate is an aromatic retinoid, effective against acne. However, a few patients show decreased rod sensitivity, reduced amplitudes of the scotopic ERG, and a deutan color vision abnormality (Weber et al., 1988). The hypothesis that the drug substitutes for the retinoids of the normal photoreceptors has yet to be substantiated.

## Tamoxifen

This drug, which is a triphenylethylene derivative, has marked antiestrogen properties and appears to be effective in certain circumstances against carcinoma of the breast. Kaiser-Kupfer and Lippman (1978) reported perimacular deposits and macular edema in four patients who had received high doses of tamoxifen for more than a year. Vinding and Nielsen (1983) reported similar lesions in 2 of 17 patients who received tamoxifen at a total dose some 10 percent of that reported previously. The nature of these lesions in uncertain.

It appears that tamoxifen is effective and is likely to be used increasingly. This is the more likely since the current method of preparation—extraction from the bark of the Pacific yew—is to be replaced by a laboratory synthetic.

In addition, both sets of authors describe subepithelial corneal deposits of granules in a whorl configuration. This corneal phenomenon is most reminiscent of the findings in patients receiving the antiarrythmic drug amiodarone (Wilson et al., 1980; Hirst et al., 1982; Kaplan and Cappaert, 1982). The author of this chapter has observed several such cases and is convinced that the whorls originate because the drug is relatively insoluble in tears and that the whorls are created by the successive positions of the lid margins as the tear film evaporates.

Opinion differs on the significance of ocular toxicity. Pavlidis and coworkers (1992) described retinopathy and/or keratopathy in 4 of 63 cancer patients who received 20 mg per day over the course of 25 months. Heier and colleagues (1994) note the early reports of ocular involvement with high doses, but in 135 patients of their series on a dosage schedule similar to that of Pavlidis and coworkers (1992), only two patients showed refractile crystals in the retina, and there was no visual impairment at all. They conclude that special screening for ocular toxicity when currently accepted dosage levels are used is not indicated.

## Experimental Retinopathy

**Iodoacetate.** An important technique used in examining metabolic interrelationships between the different cell layers in the retina and also in determining which cells contribute to the components of the ERG is to destroy selectively individual cell layers in experimental animals. A most potent tool for such studies is iodoacetate, which in carefully controlled doses rapidly and thoroughly obliterates receptor cells in rabbits (Schubert and Bornschein, 1951; Noell, 1952).

Graymore and Tansley (1959) were able to reproduce the effect in rats with the help of sodium maleate in addition to the iodoacetate. Examination of the fundus of rabbits, cats, or monkeys indicates the development of a grayish retinal opacity after the first day of treatment, which persists for about a week. Retinal pigmentation, superficially similar to human retinitis pigmentosa, appears about a week following the initial dose. Electron microscopic examination of rabbit retinas indicates lesions in the rod and cone outer segments within 3 h after treatment with iodoacetate in albino rabbits and within 12 h after iodoacetate treatment in pigmented rabbits, with marked disintegration of outer segments in albinos observed after 12 h (Lasansky and de Robertis, 1959). Disorganization of the outer segment through vesiculation and lysis of the membrane structure is accompanied by swelling and vacuolization of the endoplasmic reticulum and Golgi apparatus in the inner segment, by disintegration of mitochondria in the ellipsoid, by pyknosis of the nuclei, and by lysis of the synaptic vesicles. Widespread capillary closure rapidly follows destruction of the photoreceptor cell layer (Dantzker and Gerstein,

1969). Iodoacetate causes an irreversible decrease in the amplitudes of the a-, b-, and c-waves of the ERG (Noell, 1959; François et al., 1969a). All the evidence points to a selective retinotoxic effect of iodoacetate on the photoreceptor cells, because even 1 week after a small dose both the pigment epithelium and inner nuclear cell layers are intact (Dantzker and Gerstein, 1969).

The mechanism of iodoacetate-induced retinopathy may be twofold. Iodoacetate inhibits glyceraldehyde-3-phosphate dehydrogenase and therefore prevents the conversion of 1,3-diphosphoglyceraldehyde into 1,3-glyceric acid, a necessary reaction in pyruvate and lactate production during the glycolytic catabolism of glucose (Noell, 1959). Glycolysis provides the major source of energy to the photoreceptor cells, and inhibition of this reaction would necessarily lead to cell destruction. Moreover, anerobic glycolysis was inhibited 75 percent after 10 min of treatment with iodoacetate in a dose that yielded visual cell damage (Graymore, 1970). However, this theory is inconsistent with other experimental observations. The ERG is diminished within minutes after infusion of iodoacetate (Noell, 1959), and decreases in enzyme activity do not always appear prior to morphological and structural changes of these cells. Alteration in the free sulfhydryl group content of the visual cells has been reported (Reading and Sorsby, 1966), suggesting that damage to the membrane structure of the photoreceptor cells and outer segments may be the primary retinotoxic effect of iodoacetate. An additional effect on glycolysis may contribute to the irreversible nature of iodoacetate toxicity.

**Dithizone.** Administration of the diabetogenic (Kadota, 1950; Okamoto, 1955) chemical dithizone intravenously to rabbits in doses between 17.5 and 40 mg/kg causes retinal lesions (Grignolo et al., 1952; Weitzel et al., 1954; Sorsby and Harding, 1960). Ophthalmoscopic and histological examination reveal severe retinal edema developing within 24 to 48 h, followed by the appearance of red islets indicating recovery from edema and pigmentary disturbances in the fundus. When the edema finally disappears, usually in 6 to 8 days, the irregular pigmentation has spread throughout the retina (Sorsby and Harding, 1962). While the rabbit receptors appear to be the cell layer most sensitive to dithizone toxicity, there is swelling of the nerve fiber layer. The diffuseness of the lesion is reflected in the decreased amplitudes of the ERG and the EOG (Babel and Ziv, 1957, 1959; François et al., 1969a), initially observed as a suppression of the a-wave (Wirth et al., 1957) and b-wave amplitudes (Babel and Ziv, 1957). Eventually, the entire ERG is completely obliterated. Finally, as the retina becomes disorganized, optic atrophy (François et al., 1969b) and proliferation of the pigment epithelium (Karli, 1963) are observed. Pretreatment of rabbits with cysteine does not protect against the retinotoxic action of dithizone as it does against iodate and iodoacetate poisoning (Sorsby and Harding, 1960). This suggests a difference in mechanisms between the three retinotoxic agents.

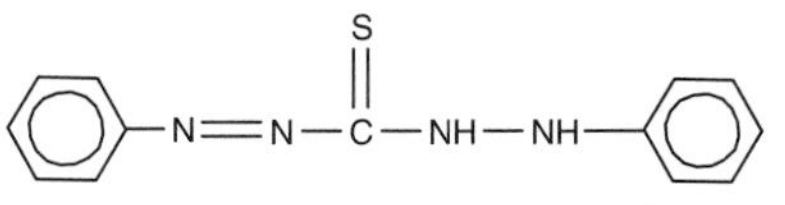

Dithizone (diphenylthiocarbazone)

**Diaminodiphenoxyalkanes.** A set of toxic substances that appear to be specific for pigment epithelium is the family of the diaminodiphenoxyalkanes. The series, in which $n = 5, 6,$ and 7 are the most active, was originally synthesized for schistosomacidal properties. No human use was ever reported, but in susceptible animals—monkey, dog, and cat—a single oral or intravenous dose causes eventual pigmented retinopathy (Edge et al., 1956; Sorsby and Nakajima, 1958) and complete loss of the ERG within a few days (Nakajima, 1958). There is selective action on the pigmented epithelium, but when these cells are destroyed, the overlying receptor cells also degenerate (Ashton, 1957). This is similar to the situation with iodate discussed above ("Iodate," this chap.).

# THE GANGLION CELL LAYER AND OPTIC NERVE

## General Considerations

The attribute that separates the ganglion cell (Fig. 20-1) from the remainder of the retina is that it is the cell body of a neuron that extends into the depth of the central nervous system. The axons from the ganglion cell layer form the nerve fiber layer of the retina and exit from the eye at the optic papilla. Most of the fibers, carrying visual information, travel some 120 mm from the globe via optic nerve, optic chiasm, and optic tract to the point where they synapse in the lateral geniculate body of the midbrain. Like any other central nervous system neuron, the optic nerve fiber degenerates in both directions from a cut. Thus, the ganglion cell of the retina may be damaged by direct action upon it, the cell body, or it may degenerate secondary to toxic destruction of the optic nerve. Instances of both types of damage will be cited below.

A second unique property of the ganglion cell–optic nerve is its behavior as a physiologically dual structure. The central 5 percent of the field of vision is the sole portion that possesses high visual acuity. This corresponds to an area of retinal receptors of 1.5-mm diameter centered on the fovea centralis. Although there is considerable preprocessing of visual information in the retina, there is still correspondence between receptor location and ganglion cell type or ganglion cell location or both. The result of this correspondence is that the information from that central, most acute 5 percent of the visual field runs in an identifiable bundle of fibers—the so-called papillomacular bundle—whose position can be identified by myelin degeneration stains at each position in the optic nerve and optic tract after damage to the central retina (Brouwer and Zeeman, 1926). Moreover, this fiber bundle acts as a separate entity in its behavior toward a number of toxic substances as well as toward some diseases.

It is not clear why this should be the case. We do know that papillomacular fibers are predominantly small fibers (Potts et al., 1972). It is possible that these fibers with the greatest ratio of surface area to volume have the highest metabolic demand of all optic nerve fibers. However, in the case of some toxic substances the papillomacular bundle is spared and the peripheral fibers are hit. Thus, it appears that specific chemical affinities may play a role. The opposite effect, the loss of the peripheral visual field to the action of a toxic substance, may not represent a case of selective affinity at all. If the substance has its primary action on the ganglion cell and if there is a uniform loss of an absolute number of cells across the entire retinal area, the peripheral retina will be wiped out. The macular area will survive with, at most, a decrease in acuity, because there are so many more cells in the macular area. Whatever mechanism is responsible for the independence of the papillomacular bundle, some toxic substances affect the ganglion cell body; others affect the fibers of the papillomacular bundle; others affect peripheral fibers only. In each case, death of a portion of the neuron means death of the entire neuron and loss of that specific information transmission channel. To take cognizance of this attribute, whereby damage to a retinal cell body can cause loss of function through an entire tract, we will designate this section as dealing with the ganglion cell neuron (GCN).

One other special consideration deals with a clinical entity, which is pallor of the disk. When any considerable number of optic nerve fibers die, their lack of demand for nutrition is somehow conveyed to the surrounding capillaries. These disappear over a period of months. In the one place where optic nerve capillaries may be inspected with ease, the optic papilla, the nerve head becomes abnormally pale on ophthalmoscopic inspection, owing to the loss of capillary supply. There is a very good correlation between the pallor observed after the loss of a large number of fibers and optic atrophy. The association is recognized as the point where many clinicians report "optic atrophy" on ophthalmoscopic examination when they mean "pale disk." Such an examination in marginal cases or one performed by a poor observer could lead to erroneous results. It is important for the reader of a report on toxicology to know whether the description of optic atrophy is a clinical or a histological one.

## Specific Substances

**Methanol.** A well-publicized and uniquely American poison affecting the GCN is methanol. The first practical distillation process that created a preparation potable by the unwary, and the clinical report of the first 275 cases of methanol poisoning, appeared in the United States (Wood and Buller, 1904). Thus, in sufficiently high doses methanol has profound systemic effects. Lest anyone think that human methanol poisoning is no longer with us, one should consult the *Arizona Star* for December 16, 1994, and February 4, 1995. In Temixco, Mexico, 31 deaths were reported with another five deaths in Tlayacapan nearby. Studies in the 1950s showed that methanol poisoning was a primate disease (Gilger and Potts, 1955) and that it was a palimpsest of three different diseases (Potts et al., 1955). Those diseases are (1) organic solvent poisoning (the only one of the three shown in subprimates), (2) systemic acidosis, and (3) central nervous system effects, including changes in the eye and the basal ganglia. It was shown that the $LD_{90}$ for primates gave only transient solvent toxicity signs and that a lucid interval set in, followed by systemic acidosis. Acidosis was enough to kill the animal unless it was combatted with base. If the acidosis was treated, the animal died later of the CNS disease. In many monkeys at the peak of the CNS signs, retinal edema was a common finding. In its most severe form, it covered the entire retina and produced the rhesus equivalent of the cherry-red spot.

Because methanol poisoning in humans is a medical emergency and it is usually impossible to determine the dose ingested, this kind of unified picture is difficult to come by. However, all the phases seen in the rhesus disease are seen in human disease, even to the basal ganglion lesion (Orthner, 1950).

The specific eye effects are definite as far as they go. Everyone agrees that nerve-head pallor is a constant finding in human cases who recover from methanol poisoning with permanent visual impairment. In monkeys, marked demyelination of the temporal retina has been demonstrated, along with a marginal loss of ganglion cells (Potts et al., 1955). Thus, optic atrophy is a definite finding in methanol poisoning, but there is some question of whether the disease is primary in the ganglion cell layer. The proximal toxic agent has been thought to be the methanol oxidation product formaldehyde (Potts, 1952; Cooper and Kini, 1962). It has now been established after some controversy that the mechanism of oxidation of methanol differs in primates and subprimates. In primates the principal metabolic pathway is via alcohol dehydrogenase (Kini and Cooper, 1961). In subprimates the favored pathway is via the catalase system (Tephly et al., 1963).

The report of Martin-Amat and coworkers (1978) that optic disk edema may be produced by infusions of formate in the monkey reopens the question of the proximal toxic agent in methanol poisoning. Since their experimental conditions require constant infusions of formate, it is difficult to design an experiment of long enough duration to determine whether the other criteria observed in human methanol poisoning can be met—that is, death with destruction of the basal ganglia. It is commendable to work out the enzymic details of methanol oxidation, as Neimeyer and Tephly (1994) have. It is not commendable to try to force the biological findings into a mold predicted by the chemical findings. Clearly, more work on the one-carbon metabolism of the primate is called for.

The treatment of methanol poisoning involves both combatting acidosis and preventing methanol oxidation. With the general availability of hemodialysis in the United States, prompt hemodialysis appears to be the method of choice in preventing methanol oxidation by removing it from the body. For a review of the literature on human cases treated by hemodialysis, see the report by Gonda and coworkers (1978). Comparison of small groups of patients by Keyvan-Larijarni and Tannenberg (1974) appears to demonstrate that peritoneal dialysis is measurably less effective than hemodialysis.

Where dialysis is not available or is delayed, prevention of methanol oxidation may be achieved by administration of ethanol, which competes successfully for alcohol dehydrogenase. This allows time for methanol to be excreted unoxidized in urine and breath. The value of ethanol administration during dialysis is marginal because it is removed from blood at about the same rate as methanol. However, because dialysis requires a finite period of time for completion, there may be some benefit in attempting to maintain a blood ethanol level.

It was suggested by Gilger and coworkers (1956) that treatment for a 70-kg man should be 4.5 oz of 50 percent ethanol initially, followed by 3.0 oz every 4 h for 48 h or until blood methanol reaches negligible levels. In a number of sporadic cases, this has appeared to be effective therapy.

A curious addendum to the methanol literature in the 1980s was caused by the rediscovery of the typical lesions of the basal ganglia. These had been described by Orthner in humans (Orthner, 1950) and in monkeys by this author (Potts et al., 1955) some 30 years earlier. The new factor was the availability of computerized tomography (CT) scan. With it there was no prerequirement for a fatal outcome plus autopsy. Neurologists examining survivors of severe methanol poisoning became aware for the first time of diminished density in the region of the putamen. They correlated this finding with the observation of extrapyramidal symptoms and with typical hemorrhagic necrosis in the basal ganglia of those patients who died and came to be autopsied (Bourrat et al., 1986; Henze et al., 1986; Wagner, 1986; Friedman et al., 1987; Guillaume et al., 1987; Rosenberg, 1987; Betta and Forno, 1988; Koopmans et al., 1988; Phang et al., 1988).

It may be that at long last the information conveyed by rhesus experiments will be appreciated. Methanol poisoning can only be understood as the composite of three separate diseases.

**Ethambutol.** This substance was found by in vivo screening to be most effective against tuberculosis in mice (Thomas et al., 1961). The drug, because of its relatively good tolerance by humans and its efficacy against isoniazid-resistant tuberculosis, has become an established member of the antituberculosis armamentarium. In some 10 percent of patients receiving 25 to 50 mg/kg per day, loss of vision appears 1 to 7 months after the start of this dosage (Carr and Henkind, 1962; Place and Thomas, 1963). (For a thorough review of human and animal toxicity, see Leibold, 1966; Place et al., 1966; Schmidt, 1966.)

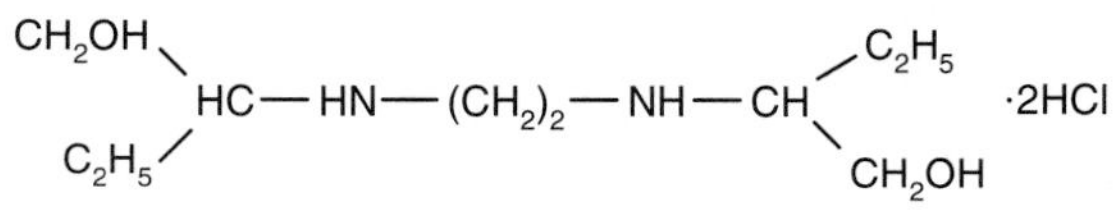

$$\begin{matrix} CH_2OH \\ C_2H_5 \end{matrix} > HC{-}HN{-}(CH_2)_2{-}NH{-}CH < \begin{matrix} C_2H_5 \\ CH_2OH \end{matrix} \cdot 2HCl$$

*d*-2-2′-(Ethylenediimino)-di-1-butanol dihydrochloride

The typical toxic phenomenon is *retrobulbar neuritis* in the sense that there is visual field involvement without obvious swelling of the nerve head. However, in addition to central scotoma, which is thought of as the typical finding in retrobulbar neuritis, a smaller proportion of patients show loss of peripheral field with preservation of central vision (Leibold, 1966). All visual symptoms are dose-related. Figures collected from various sources in the literature by Citron (1969) suggest:

| DOSAGE (mg/kg/day) | CASES | INCIDENCE OF COMPLICATIONS |
|---|---|---|
| 50 | 60 | 15% |
| >35 | 59 | 18% |
| <30 | 59 | 5% |
| 25 | 130 | 3% |
| 15 | — | Negligible |

Visual disturbances appear to regress completely on cessation of drug administration.

The mechanism of therapeutic action and the mechanism of toxicity are far from clear. Ethambutol is a chelating agent that will remove zinc from the tapetum lucidum of dogs. However, it does not cause the pigmentary retinopathy that a chelating agent such as dithizone causes (Figueroa et al., 1971). When *Mycobacterium smegmatis* is used as a model for *M. tuberculosis*, ethambutol-inhibited cells become deficient in RNA. As a consequence, protein synthesis is inhibited (Forbes et al., 1965). A recent recommendation in favor of substituting biweekly high-dose therapy for daily intermediate-dose therapy is said to eliminate visual system toxicity (Trumbull et al., 1977).

**Carbon Disulfide.** This inflammable and volatile liquid (BP = 46.3°C) was important in the past as a solvent for sulfur in the rubber industry and as a solvent for alkali-treated cellulose in the viscose process for rayon and cellophane. Improved ventilation and the substitution of other solvents have made classical carbon disulfide poisoning a thing of the past. The impressive complex of central scotoma, a drop in visual acuity, widespread peripheral neuritis, personality changes, vascular encephalopathy, and generalized arteriosclerosis with cardiovascular and renal sequelae is not seen. However, there are recent disquieting reports from Japan and from Finland of subtle eye effects, seen at solvent levels that do not produce the classic symptoms and that until now were thought to be safe (Raitta and Tolonen, 1980; Sugimoto and Goto, 1980).

Curiously, the retinopathy seen in Japan, which consists of microaneurysms and small hemorrhages, was not observed in Finnish workers to exceed the incidence in controls. In Finland the positive findings were delayed peripapillary filling on fluorescein angiography, widening of retinal arterioles, and lower peak to the ocular pulse wave. Clearly, carbon disulfide in industry needs another look.

A curious aspect of $CS_2$ poisoning is the lack of correspondence between anatomic and physiological findings (Birch-Hirschfeld, 1900; Ide, 1958). One possible reason for this is restriction of the experimental situation to rodents, which do not appear to have a dual optic nerve. Much experimentation will be required to exploit the little we now know of carbon disulfide poisoning.

**Thallium.** Considerable clinical experience in thallium poisoning has arisen from the use of thallous acetate in the 1920s as an epilating agent by dermatologists and its use as a rat poison (Celio Paste) with consequent accidental and intentional poisonings. For a short time in the early 1930s, a cosmetic depilatory cream (Koremlu) caused additional chronic cases. (For reviews of this material, see Heyroth, 1947; Prick et al., 1955). Systemic symptoms in thallium poisoning include gastroenteritis, polyneuritis, and allopecia. Ocular involvement is seen in cataracts, especially in rats, and in optic neuritis in humans.

The unifying concept that made the behavior of lens and optic nerve understandable was developed in the 1960s, when it became apparent that the thallous ion is in many ways a stand-in for the potassium ion. For a review of this discovery, see Gehring and Hammond (1967). The University of Chicago laboratory was able to show that the lens and optic nerve, two high-potassium tissues, were also able to store $Tl^+$ (Potts and Au, 1971). The ionic similarities are great enough that $Tl^+$ can activate ($Na^+$-$K^+$)-activated ATPase (Britten and Blank, 1968). Kinsey and coworkers (1971) demonstrated that thallous ion accumulation in the lens was by active transport and by the alkali metal-transporting system. An additional and unexpected finding was high storage of $Tl^+$ in melanin-containing eye structures (Potts and Au, 1971). Although $Tl^+$ can act for $K^+$ in many systems, it is clear that it cannot do so in every case. It seems logical that accumulation of thallium where potassium should normally be, without its being able to substitute for potassium in every enzyme system, is the basis for thallium toxicity. It is not clear which parts of the GCN are most affected.

Needless to say, prophylaxis is the only practical therapy in thallium poisoning.

**Pentavalent Arsenic.** Pentavalent arsenicals have been found in the past to be effective against trypanosomiasis (Thomas, 1905).

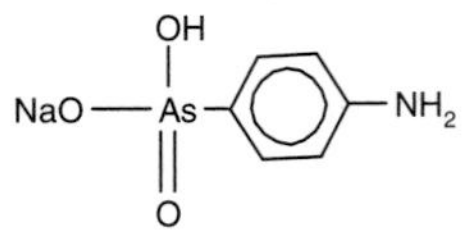

Sodium arsanilate (Atoxyl®)

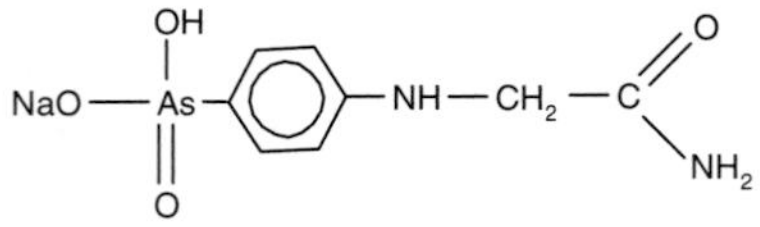

Sodium *N*-(carbamoylmethyl)-arsanilite (Tryparsamide®)

The same ability to pass the blood-brain barrier that allowed effectiveness against trypanosomes also made possible the treatment of neurosyphilis. Numerous derivatives of sodium arsanilate were synthesized by Ehrlich in his early investigations of trypanocidal and spirochetocidal activity. Tryparsamide, a substance of relatively low toxicity, was synthesized at the Rockefeller Institute (Jacobs and Heidelberger, 1919) and introduced into tropical medicine shortly thereafter (Pearce, 1921). Tryparsamide was then found effective against neurosyphilis (Henrichsen, 1939).

Eye effects were a constant accompaniment to the use of pentavalent arsenicals and were a prime reason for their eventual abandonment. The clinical figures of Neujean and coworkers (1948) suggest that 3 to 4 percent of trypanosomiasis cases treated with Tryparsamide show visual effects, and a third of these—for example, 1 percent of all cases—show peripheral contraction of visual fields. There are anatomic findings to accompany the clinical symptoms, and here the peripheral area of the ganglion cell layer is most severely involved (Birch-Hirschfeld and Köster, 1910). There is considerable evidence that at the cellular level all the arsenicals reach the same oxidation state, whatever their form at introduction (Ehrlich, 1909).

Interest has been maintained in organic arsenicals in recent years with the finding that when they are included in the feed of poultry and swine the animals thrive and gain weight. Errors on the farm can expose the animals and the growers to a toxic hazard. Studies like the thesis of Ledet (1979) should be extended.

**Quinine.** Although the massive use of quinine decreased abruptly with the advent of new synthetic antimalarials in the 1940s, plasmodia resistant to these new compounds appeared rapidly. Quinine is the drug of choice in these situations (Nieuwveld et al., 1982). Thus quinine has an established place in today's pharmacopoeia. An additional therapeutic effect is said to be the relief of nocturnal recumbency leg cramps. The availability of the drug allows its ingestion in excessive doses for intended abortion and intended suicide, as in the past. Hence quinine poisoning is still with us, as are the poorly understood eye effects.

It is now clear that there are two dosage levels at which quinine (and its congeners) may be toxic. The first is a very low level caused by a single dose of as little as 12 mg (Belkin, 1967). The symptoms are those of thrombocytopenic purpura. The cause is an immune reaction in which the drug acts as a haptene. This phenomenon was treated exhaustively by Shulman (1958), reporting on cases in which the offender was quinidine. The visual system is affected as much or as little as it would be in purpura caused by any other haptene. Its blood vessels are subject to hemorrhage secondary to thrombocytopenia as any set of vessels would be, but there is no specific selectivity for the eye.

The usual therapeutic regime for malaria is 1.3 g per day in four divided doses for seven days. Experiments on human volunteers have shown that eye effects of blurring, a decrease of visual acuity, and loss of the peripheral field occur with single doses of 2.5 to 4.0 g (Duke-Elder and MacFaul, 1972). A single dose of 8.0 g can be fatal. It is doses of 2.5 g and above that have specific eye effects. The eye effects have been attributed by some to arteriolar constriction, by others to direct action on the ganglion cell body, and by still others to effects on the whole retina. See the reports of François and coworkers (1967), Cibis and colleagues (1973), Brinton and colleagues (1980), and Gangitano and Keltner (1980) for the various arguments adduced and additional literature reviews. In cats given a sublethal dose of quinine sulfate, early electroretinographic changes that show whole-retina involvement are transient. Early peripapillary and retinal edema, which suggests ganglion cell involvement, is also transient. The earliest anatomic changes that become permanent are pyknosis and then generalized loss of retinal ganglion cells. This is almost certainly the locus of high-dose-specific eye effects.

Hemodialysis has been recommended as the treatment of choice, but some reservations are expressed by Dickinson and coworkers (1981).

**Glutamate.** An experimental entity involving the ganglion cell neuron is glutamate poisoning. Lucas and Newhouse (1957) reported that administration of high doses of sodium 1-glutamate to suckling mice caused degeneration of the retinal ganglion cell layer and the failure of formation of the inner nuclear layer. Freedman and Potts (1962) were able to reproduce this phenomenon in newborn albino rats. They showed that glutaminase I was repressed in the retinas of these animals and postulated this as the mechanism of glutamate toxicity.

Later work has revealed an extensive series of compounds related to glutamate that have neuroexcitatory or neurotoxic properties or both. The term "excitotoxin," which implies that there is a relation between the two properties, has been coined. At any event, the entire subject area is in flux; some feel for this situation may be obtained from the review by Olney (1982).

Perhaps most important is the fact that whereas glutamate affects the developing retina only, some of the newer compounds cause selective cell loss when injected intravitreally in mature animals. This represents no human hazard but promises to be a powerful experimental tool. DL-2-Aminoadipic acid, the next higher homologue of glutamic acid, destroys Müller cells and in high doses causes swelling of astrocytes and oligodendrocytes (Pedersen and Karlsen, 1979; Ishikawa and Mine, 1983). Kainic acid, a sterically hindered analogue of glutamic acid, destroys the "displaced amacrine cells" of the chicken retina (Ehrlich and Morgan, 1980).

**MNC.** In research performed during World War II on the vesicant methylnitrosocarbamate, it was found that there was selective chromatolysis and destruction of the retinal ganglion cell layer. The experiments were done in cats that were allowed to inhale the vapor at a concentration of 50 $\mu$g/L for 10 min (Gates and Renshaw, 1946). The compound is an alkylating agent like the nitrogen mustards, and it alkylates functional groups of proteins and nucleic acids in a more or less random manner. Unlike the amino acid series described above, this compound represents a hazard to its user during synthesis and during exposure of the test animal.

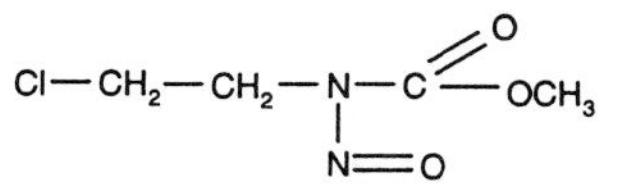

$$Cl-CH_2-CH_2-N(N{=}O)-C({=}O)-OCH_3$$

Methyl *N*-*b*-chlorethyl-*N*-nitrosocarbamate

**SMON.** Special mention should be made of the optic nerve damage (accompanying widespread demyelination in the CNS) caused by 7-iodo-5-chloro-8-hydroxyquinoline, iodochlorhydroxyquin known as Clioquinol, Entero-Vioform, and Vioform.

The drug is an effective amebicide and is useful in the treatment of amebiasis when given at the level of 500 to 750 mg three times a day for 10 days. An 8-day interval must be observed before a second 10-day course is given.

However, this drug has been available over the counter outside the United States principally to combat "traveler's diarrhea" in cases in which a specific diagnosis has not been made and in which physician control of the dosage is lacking. Particularly in Japan, an entity has been recognized and labeled "subacute myeloopticoneuropathy" (SMON) attributable to the use of this substance. It is said that from 1955 to 1970, 10,000 cases of SMON were diagnosed in Japan. A national commission was formed by the Japanese government, and in 1970 the sale of the drug was prohibited. (For a bibliography of the Japanese literature, see Shigematsu, 1975.)

The entity is characterized clinically by paresthesias and numbness of the extremities, ataxia, and weakness in the legs. Twenty-seven percent of SMON patients have visual disturbances attributed to demyelination of the optic nerve (Sobue and Ando, 1971).

The extremely high incidence of SMON in Japan has not been explained satisfactorily. High dosage levels, the additive effects of environmental pollutants, and as-yet-unidentified factors have all been invoked. A representative of the manufacturer claims that since 1935 only 50 cases of SMON with a history of iodochlorhydroxyquin consumption have been identified in the rest of the world (Burley, 1977).

The disease can be reproduced in experimental animals by feeding them the drug, and optic nerve demyelination is demonstrable in dogs and cats (Tateishi and Otsuki, 1975).

## ORGANOMERCURIALS

Metallic mercury has been recognized to present a relatively low-level hazard to the individual and the eye. The eye does not appear to be involved in poisoning by inorganic salts of mercury. This is treated well by Grant (1986). The marked toxicity of organic compounds of mercury and their effects on vision have been known since the report of Edwards (1866), but this remained a laboratory caution until the multiple epidemics of the last decades. The presently accepted site of damage to the visual system, the visual cortex, puts the subject beyond the avowed scope of this chapter, but its importance requires that it be treated here.

Epidemics of organomercurial poisoning have originated in two major and diverse manners. The earliest cases of both series were found in 1956. The subtler, hence the more difficult, of the two to identify occurred in Japan, and in retrospect cases seen in 1951 were part of the epidemic. To summarize years of active research sponsored by the Japanese government, the hazard originated when metallic mercury, used as a catalyst in the acetaldehyde plant near Minamata Bay, was discharged into the bay as waste sludge. The aquatic plant life in the bay was able to convert elemental mercury to organomercurials, especially to methylmercury. The fish and shellfish of the bay acquired methylmercury from the plants and the contaminated water. The local inhabitants, many of whom were fishermen, were poisoned by the contaminated seafood and began to ask for treatment for neurological complaints at the local hospitals. In February 1963, the disease was identified as organomercurial poisoning. From 1965 to 1974, a series of 520 patients was seen in Nigata prefecture who were identified as having organomercurial poisoning. The source of the epidemic was a similar factory. The excellent account of the findings edited by Tsubaki and Irukayama (1977), entitled *Minamata Disease*, is a model of reporting.

The second type of epidemic arose in multiple sites and always with the same causation. Seed grain treated with an organomercurial antifungal agent was used by peasant farmers to make bread. Iraq had epidemics in 1956, 1960, and 1971–72 (Bakir et al., 1973). The last caused 6530 people being admitted to hospitals, of whom 459 died. Similar but lesser outbreaks are recorded for Guatemala in 1963 to 1965, for Pakistan in 1961 and 1969, and for Ghana in 1967.

The textbook description of organomercurial poisoning is that of Hunter, Bomford, and Russell (1940); the disease complex is often designated "Hunter-Russell syndrome." The components are (1) ataxia, (2) impairment of speech, and (3) constriction of the visual field. The Minamata cases also showed a high incidence of hearing loss and somatosensory change.

Histopathology was done on monkeys by Hunter and coworkers (1940) and by Shaw and colleagues (1975) and by Takeuchi and Ito (1977) (in Tsubaki and Irukayama, 1977) on the Minamata deaths. All of them agree that eye findings are negligible and that the major and consistent finding is necrosis of neurons in the cerebral cortex, particularly in the depth of the sulci, and most particularly in the calcarine fissure of the visual cortex.

Clinically there is some description of disk hyperemia and later disk pallor in Iraqi patients (Sebelaish and Hilmi, 1976). A curious and disturbing finding is the remarkable bilateral symmetry of the reported visual field defects, presumably caused by two parallel but separate pathological events in the right and left calcarine cortex. One might expect some asymmetry and some difference in projection of the two hemifields to the right and left eye. This has not been reported.

## The Special Case of Protein Moieties

Today's technology allows the isolation and characterization of protein (and nucleic acid) fragments. Recombinant techniques make possible the preparation of significant quantities of these substances. Where there are potential or realized therapeutic applications, toxicity studies are obligatory.

Tissue plasminogen activator (tPA) has been employed by several groups to lyse intraocular fibrin membranes. Moon and coworkers (1992) treated postcataract fibrin membranes with success and with no eye damage. Maeno and colleagues (1991) treated postvitrectomy pupillary membranes. They attributed postoperative inflammation to decomposed fibrin products and recommended fluid-gas exchange. Boldt and coworkers (1992) reported a similar application in which 3 $\mu$g of tPA was effective. Animal toxicity studies at 25 $\mu$g showed retinal damage.

Recombinant human basic fibroblast growth factor caused an increased corneal epithelial healing rate and was nontoxic on local application (Mazue et al., 1991).

Platelet-activating factor antagonist (BN50730) prevented the loss of a b-wave in isolated rat retina perfused with a chloroquine solution (Meyniel et al., 1992).

Recombinant rabbit interferon injected into the vitreous in doses of $10^4$ units decreased detachments caused by intravitreal injection of dermal fibroblasts in rabbit eyes. Doses of $10^6$ units caused panuveitis (Hjelmeland et al., 1992).

These reports herald the appearance of a class of new therapies with far-reaching potential. By the same token, the implications for potential toxicity are equally great, and each substance requires careful study.

# REFERENCES


Alghadyan AA, Peyman GA, Khoobehi B, Lin KR: Liposome-bound cyclosporine: Retinal toxicity after intravitreal injection. *Int Ophthalmol* 12:105–107, 1988.

Anand R, Font RL, Fish RH, Nightingale SD: Pathology of cytomegalovirus retinitis treated with sustained release intravitreal gancyclovir. *Ophthalmology* 100(7):1032–1039, 1993.

Anderson B: Corneal and conjunctival pigmentation among workers engaged in the manufacture of hydroquinone. *Arch Ophthalmol* 38:812–826, 1947.

Anderson JA, Chen CC, Vita JB, Shackleton M: Disposition of topical flurbiprofen in normal and aphakic rabbit eyes. *Arch Ophthalmol* 100:642–645, 1982.

Armaly M: Effect of corticosteroids on intraocular pressure and fluid dynamics. *Arch Ophthalmol* 70:482–491, 492–499, 1963.

Ashton N: Degeneration of the retina due to 1:5-di(-aminophenoxy) pentane dihydrochloride. *J Pathol Bacteriol* 74:103–112, 1957.

Ashton N: Oxygen and the growth and development of retinal vessels: *Vivo and vitro studies. Am J Ophthalmol* 62:412–435, 1966.

Ashton N: Some aspects of the comparative pathology of oxygen toxicity in the retina. *Ophthalmologica* 160:54–71, 1970.

Ashton N, Pedler C: Studies on developing retinal vessels: IX. Reaction of endothelial cells to oxygen. *Br J Ophthalmol* 46:257–276, 1962.

Athanaselis S, Poulos L, Mourtzinis D, Koutselinis A: Lacrimatory agents: Self-defense devices or dangerous weapons? *J Toxicol—Cutan Ocular Toxicol* 9:3–8, 1990.

Avigan J, Steinberg D, Vroman HE, et al: Studies on cholesterol biosynthesis: I. The identification of desmosterol in serum and tissues of animals and man treated with MER-29. *J Biol Chem* 235:3123–3126, 1960.

Axelsson U, Holmberg A: The frequency of cataract after miotic therapy. *Acta Ophthalmol* 44:421–429, 1966.

Babel J, Ziv B: L'action du dithizone sur la rétine du lapin étude electrophysiolôgique. *Experientia* 13:122–123, 1957.

Babel J: L'action du métabolisme des hydrates de carbone sur l'électrorétinogramme du lapin. *Ophthalmologica* 137:270–281, 1959.

Bakir F, Damluji SF, Amin-Zaki L, et al: Methylmercury poisoning in Iraq. *Science* 181:230–241, 1973.

Becker B: Cataracts and topical corticosteroids. *Am J Ophthalmol* 58:872–873, 1964.

Beehler CC: Oxygen and the eye. *Surv Ophthalmol* 9:549–560, 1964.

Belkin GA: Cocktail purpura: An unusual case of quinine sensitivity. *Ann Intern Med* 66:583–585, 1967.

Bernstein HN: Chloroquine ocular toxicity. *Surv Ophthalmol* 12:415–477, 1967.

Bernstein HN, Ginsberg J: The pathology of chloroquine retinopathy. *Arch Ophthalmol* 71:238–245, 1964.

Bernstein HN, Mills DW, Becker B: Steroid-induced elevation of intraocular pressure. *Arch Ophthalmol* 70:15–18, 1963a.

Bernstein HN, Zvaifler N, Rubin M, Mansour Sister AM: The ocular deposition of chloroquine. *Invest Ophthalmol* 2:384–392, 1963b.

Berthe P, Badouin C, Garaffo R, et al: Toxicologic and pharmacokinetic analysis of intravitreal injections of foscarnet, either alone or in combination with gancyclovir. *Invest Ophthalmol Vis Sci* 35(3):1038–1045, 1994.

Betta PG, Forno G: Necrosi emorragica del putamen da intossicatione acuta da alcool metilico. *Patologica* 80:215–218, 1988.

Bettman JW, Fung WE, Webster RG, et al: Cataractogenic effect of corticosteroids on animals. *Am J Ophthalmol* 65:581–586, 1968.

Bettman JW, Noyes P, DeBoskey R: The potentiating action of steroids in cataractogenesis. *Invest Ophthalmol* 3:459, 1964.

Birch-Hirschfeld A: Beitrag zur Kenntnis der Netzhautganglienzellen unter physiologischen und pathologischen Verhältnissen. *Graefes Arch Ophthalmol* 50:166–246, 1900.

Birch-Hirschfeld A, Köster G: Die Schädigung des Auges durch Atoxyl. *Graefes Arch Ophthalmol* 76:403–463, 1910.

Black RL, Oglesby RB, von Sallmann L, Bunim JL: Posterior subcapsular cataracts induced by corticosteroids in patients with rheumatoid arthritis. *JAMA* 174:166–171, 1960.

Blumenkrantz MS: Management of complicated retinal detachment, in Tso MOM (ed): *Retinal Diseases*. Philadelphia: Lippincott, 1988.

Boet DJ: Toxic effects of phenothiazines on the eye. *Doc Ophthalmol* 28:1–69, 1970.

Boldt HC, Abrams GW, Murray TG, et al: The lowest effective dose of tissue plasminogen activator for fibrinolysis of postvitrectomy fibrin. *Retina* 12(Suppl 3):S75–79, 1992.

Booman KA: The SDA alternatives program: Comparison of *in vitro* data with Draize Test data. *J Toxicol—Cutan Ocular Toxicol* 8(1):35–49, 1989.

Borhani H, Peyman GA, Wafapoor H: Use of vancomycin in vitrectomy infusion solution and evaluation of retinal toxicity. *Int Ophthalmol* 17(2):85–88, 1993.

Bourrat C, Ribouliard L, Flocard F, et al: Intoxication volontaire par le methanol. *Rev Neurol (Paris)* 142:530–534, 1986.

Brinton GS, Norton EWD, Zahn JR, Knighton RW: Ocular quinine toxicity. *Am J Ophthalmol* 90:403–410, 1980.

Britten JS, Blank W: Thallium activation of the ($Na^+$-$K^+$) activated ATPase of rabbit kidney. *Biochim Biophys Acta* 159:160–166, 1968.

Brouwer B, Zeeman WPC: The protection of the retina in the primary optic neuron in monkeys. *Brain* 49:1–35, 1926.

Brown SI, Tragakis MP, Pearce DB: Treatment of the alkali-burned cornea. *Am J Ophthalmol* 74:316–320, 1972.

Brown SI, Weller CA, Akiya S: Pathogenesis of ulcers of the alkali-burned cornea. *Arch Ophthalmol* 83:205–208, 1970.

Brown SI, Weller CA, Wassermann HE: Collagenolytic activity of alkali-burned corneas. *Arch Ophthalmol* 81:370–373, 1969.

Buhles WC, et al: Treatment of life- or sight-threatening cytomegalovirus infection: Experience in 314 immunocompromised patients. *Rev Infect Dis* 10:495–506, 1988.

Burley D: Clioquinol: Time to act. *Lancet* 1:1256, 1977.

Burns CA: Ocular effects of indomethacin. Slit lamp and electroretinographic (ERG) study. *Invest Ophthalmol* 5:325, 1966.

Burns CA: Indomethacin, reduced retinal sensitivity and corneal deposits. *Am J Ophthalmol* 66:825–835, 1968.

Burns RP: Delayed onset of chloroquine retinopathy. *N Engl J Med* 275:693–696, 1966.

Burrada A, Peyman GA, Case J, et al: Evaluation of intravitreal 5-fluorouracil, vincristine, VP-16, doxorubicin and thiotepa in primate eyes. *Ophthalmic Surg* 15:767–769, 1984.

Butler I: Retinopathy following the use of chloroquine and allied substances. *Ophthalmologica* 149:204–208, 1965.

Calkins LL: Corneal epithelial changes occurring during chloroquine (Aralen) therapy. *Arch Ophthalmol* 60:981–988, 1958.

Cameron ME, Lawrence JM, Obrich JG: Thioridazine (Mellaril) retinopathy. *Br J Ophthalmol* 56:131–134, 1972.

Car RE: Chloroquine and organic changes in the eye. *Dis Nerv Syst* 29 (Suppl):36–39, 1968.

Carr RE, Henkind P: Ocular manifestations of ethambutol. Toxic amblyopia after administration of an antituberculous drug. *Arch Ophthalmol* 67:566–571, 1962.

Cerletti A, Meier-Ruge W: Toxicological studies on phenothiazine induced retinopathy. In *Toxicity and Side Effects of Psychotropic Drugs. Proc Eur Soc Drug Toxic* 9:170–188, 1967.

Chamberlain WP Jr, Boles DJ: Edema of cornea precipitated by quinacrine (Atebrine). *Arch Ophthalmol* 35:120–134, 1946.

Chayakul V, Reim M: Enzymatic activity of beta-*N*-acetylglucosaminidase in the alkali-burned rabbit cornea. *Graefes Arch Klin Exp Ophthalmol* 218:149–152, 1982.

Cibis GW, Burian HM, Blodi FC: Electroretinogram changes in acute quinine poisoning. *Arch Ophthalmol* 90:307–309, 1973.

Citron KM: Ethambutol: A review with special reference to ocular toxicity. *Tubercle* 50(Suppl):32–36, 1969.

Cooper JR, Kini MM: Biochemical aspects of methanol poisoning. *Biochem Pharmacol* 11:405–416, 1962.

Costa VP, Spaeth GL, Eiferman RA, Orengo-Nania S: Wound healing modulation in glaucoma filtration surgery. [Review.] *Ophthalmic Surg* 24(3):152–170, 1993.

Cotlier E, Becker R: Topical steroids and galactose cataracts. *Invest Ophthalmol* 4:806–814, 1965.

Crews SJ: Posterior subcapsular lens opacities in patients on long-term corticosteroid therapy. *Br Med J* 1:1644–1646, 1963.

Crews SJ: The prevention of drug induced retinopathies. *Trans Ophthalmol Soc UK* 86:63–76, 1967.

Dale AJ, Parkhill EM, Layton DD: Studies on chloroquine retinopathy in rabbits. *JAMA* 193:241–243, 1965.

D'Amico DJ, Caspers-Velu L, Libert J, et al: Comparative toxicity of intravitreal aminoglycoside antibiotics. *Am J Ophthalmol* 100:264–275, 1985.

Dana: Sanguinarin, ein neues organisches Alkali in Sanguinaria. *Mag Pharm* 23:124, 1828.

Dantzker DR, Gerstein DD: Retinal vascular changes following toxic effects on visual cells and pigment epithelium. *Arch Ophthalmol* 81:106–114, 1969.

Davies HC, Davies RE: Biochemical aspects of oxygen poisoning. In Fenn WD, Rahn H (eds): *Handbook of Physiology* Washington, DC: American Physiological Society, 1965, vol 2, sect 3.

Dayal HH, Brodwick M, Morris R, et al: A community-based epidemiologic study of health sequellae of exposure to hydrofluoric acid. *Ann Epidemiol* 2(3):213–230, 1992.

DeLong SL, Poley BJ, McFarlane JR Jr: Ocular changes associated with long-term chloropromazine therapy. *Arch Ophthalmol* 73:611–617, 1965.

Derick RJ, Paylor R, Peyman GA: Toxicity of imipenen in vitreous replacement fluid. *Ann Ophthalmol* 19:338–339, 1987.

Diaz-Llopis M, Espana E, Munoz G, et al: High dose intravitreal foscarnet in the treatment of cytomegalovirus retinitis in AIDS. *Br J Ophthalmol* 78(2):120–124, 1994.

Dickinson P, Sabto J, West RH: Management of quinine toxicity. *Trans Ophthalmol Soc NZ* 3356–3358, 1981.

Diets-Ouwehand JJ, de Keizer RJ, Vrensen GF, Groen-Jansen S, van Best JA: Toxicity of 1-(beta-D-arabinofuranosyl)cytosine after intravitreal injection in the rabbit eye. *Graefes Arch Clin Exp Ophthalmol* 230(5):488–495, 1992.

Dixon M: Reactions of lachrymators with enzymes and proteins. *Biochem Soc Symp* 2:39–49, 1948.

Dobbie GC, Langham ME: Reaction of animal eyes to sanguinarine argemone oil. *Br J Ophthalmol* 45:81–95, 1961.

Dolnak DR, Munguia D, Wiley CA, et al: Lack of retinal toxicity of the anticytomegalovirus drug (S)-1-(3-hydroxy-2-phosphonylmethoxypropyl) cytosine. *Invest Ophthalmol Vis Sci* 33(5):1557–1563, 1992.

Doly M, Cluzel J, Millerin M, et al: Prevention of chloroquine-induced electroretinographic damage by a new platelet-activating factor antagonist, BN 50730. *Ophthalmic Res* 25(5):314–318, 1993.

Draize JH, Kelley EA: Toxicity to eye mucosa of certain cosmetic preparations containing surface active agents. *Proc Sci Sect Toilet Goods Assoc* 17:1–4, 1952.

Duke-Elder Sir S: Cataract, in Duke-Elder Sir S (ed): *System of Ophthalmology. Diseases of the Lens and Vitreous: Glaucoma and Hypotony*. London: Henry Kimpton, London, 1969, vol 11.

Duke-Elder Sir S, MacFaul PA: Injuries, in Duke-Elder Sir S (ed): *System of Ophthalmology*. St. Louis: C. V. Mosby, 1972, vol 14, pt 2, pp 1011–1356.

Edge ND, Mason DFJ, Wein R, Ashton N: Pharmacological effects of certain diaminodiphenoxy alkanes. *Nature (Lond)* 178:806–807, 1956.

Edwards GN: *St Barth Hosp Rep* i:141, 1865; ii:211, 1866.

Ehrlich D, Morgan IG: Kainic acid destroys displaced amacrine cells in post-hatch chicken retina. *Neurosci Lett* 17:43–48, 1980.

Ehrlich P: Uber den jetzigen stand der Chemotherapie. *Ber Dtsch Chem Ges* 42:17–47, 1909.

Elbrink J, Bihler I: Membrane transport of sugars in the rat lens. *Can J Ophthalmol* 7:96–101, 1972.

Elliott TR: The action of adrenalin. *J Physiol* 32:401–467, 1905.

Fett DR, Silverman CA, Yoshizumi MO: Moxolactan retinal toxicity. *Arch Ophthalmol* 102:435–438, 1984.

Figueroa R, Weiss H, Smith JC Jr, et al: Effect of ethambutol on the ocular zinc concentration of dogs. *Am Rev Respir Dis* 104:592–594, 1971.

Flower RW, Patz A: Oxygen studies in retrolental fibroplasia: IV. The effects of elevated oxygen tension in retinal vascular dynamics in the kitten. *Arch Ophthalmol* 85:197–203, 1971.

Forbes M, Kuck NA, Peets EA: Effect of ethambutol on nucleic acid metabolism in mycobacterium smeginatis and its reversal by polyamines and divalent cations. *J Bacteriol* 89:1299–1305, 1965.

François J: Glaucome apparement simple, secondaire à la cortisonothérapie locale *Ophthalmologica* (Suppl) 142:517–523, 1961.

François J, Jönsas C, de Rouck A: Étude expérimentale sur l'effect de l'iodo-acétate de soude sur l'électro-rétinogramme et l'électro-oculogramme du lapin. *Ann Ocul (Paris)* 202:637–642, 1969a.

François J: Experimental studies on the effect of dithizone on the electro-retinogram and the electro-oculogram in rabbits. *Ophthalmologica* 159:472–477, 1969b.

François J, Maudgal MC: Experimentally induced chloroquine retinopathy in rabbits. *Am J Ophthalmol* 64:886–893, 1967.

François J, Verriest G, DeRouck A: Etude des fonctions visuelles dans deux cas d'intoxication par la quine. *Ophthalmologica* 153:324–335, 1967.

Fraser TR: On the characters, actions and therapeutical uses of the ordeal bean of Calabar. *Edinburgh Med J* 9:36–56, 123–132, 235–248, 1863.

Fraunfelder FT: *Drug Induced Ocular Side Effects and Drug Interactions*, 3d ed. Philadelphia: Lea & Febiger, 1989.

Freedman JK, Potts AM: Repression of glutaminase I in the rat retina by administration of sodium-1-glutamate. *Invest Ophthalmol* 1:118–121, 1962.

Friedenwald JS, Hughes WF, Herrmann H: Acid-base tolerance of the cornea. *Arch Ophthalmol* 31:279–283, 1944.

Friedenwald JS: Acid burns of the eye. *Arch Ophthalmol* 35:98–108, 1946.

Friedman L, O'Keefe D, Patel M, Tchang S: Computed tomography findings in methanol intoxication. *S Afr Med J* 71:800, 1987.

Galezowski X: *Des Amlyopies et des Amauroses Toxiques*. Paris: P. Assaebin, 1878.

Gangitano JL, Keltner JL: Abnormalities of the pupil and visual-evoked potential in quinine amblyopia, *Am J Ophthalmol* 89:425–430, 1980.

Garner A, Rahi AHS: Practolol and ocular toxicity. *Br J Ophthalmol* 60:684–686, 1976.

Gates M, Renshaw B: Chemical warfare agents and related chemical problems. *Sum Tech Rep Div 9*. Washington, D.C.: NDRC, 1946.

Gehring PJ, Buerge JF: The cataractogenic activity of 2,4-dinitrophenol in ducks and rabbits. *Toxicol Appl Pharmacol* 14:475–486, 1969a.

Gehring PJ: The distribution of 2,4-dinitrophenol relative to its cataractogenic activity in ducklings and rabbits. *Toxicol Appl Pharmacol* 15:574–592, 1969b.

Gehring PJ, Hammond PB: The interrelationship between thallium and potassium in animals. *J Pharmacol Exp Ther* 155:187–201, 1967.

Gilger AP, Potts AM: Studies on the visual toxicity of methanol: V. The role of acidosis in experimental methanol poisoning. *Am J Ophthalmol* 39:63–86, 1955.

Gilger AP, Potts AM, Farkas I: Studies on the visual toxicity of methanol: IX. The effect of ethanol on methanol poisoning in the rhesus monkey. *Am J Ophthalmol* 42:244–252, 1956.

Goldey JA, Dick DA, Porter WL: Cornpicker's pupil: A clinical note regarding mydriasis from Jimson weed dust (Stramonium). *Ohio State Med J* 62:921, 1966.

Goldmann H: Cortisone glaucoma. *Arch Ophthalmol* 68:621–626, 1962.

Gonda A, Gault H, Churchill D, Hollomby D: Hemodialysis for methanol intoxication. *Am J Med* 64:749–758, 1978.

Gonsaun LM, Potts AM: Possible mechanism of chloroquine induced retinopathy. Presented at the Fifth International Congress on Pharmacology. San Francisco, California, July 23–28, 1972.

Grant WM: *Toxicology of the Eye*, 3d ed. Sprngfield, Ill: Charles C Thomas Pub., 1986.

Graymore CN: Biochemistry of the retina. In Graymore CN (ed): *Biochemistry of the Eye*. New York: Academic Press, 1970.

Graymore CN, Tansley K: Iodoacetate poisoning of the rat retina: I. Production of retinal degeneration. *Br J Ophthalmol* 43:177–185, 1959.

Green J, Ellison T: Uptake and distribution of chlorpromazine in animal eyes. *Exp Eye Res* 5:191–197, 1966.

Greiner AC, Berry K: Skin pigmentation and corneal and lens opacities with prolonged chlorpromazine therapy. *Can Med Assoc J* 90:663–665, 1964.

Grignolo A, Butturini U, Baronchelli A: Richerchi preliminari sul diabete sperimentale da ditizone. III. Manifestazioni oculari. *Boll Soc Ital Biol Sper* 28:1416–1418, 1952.

Grimes P, von Sallmann L: Interference with cell proliferation and induction of polyploidy in rat lens epithelium during prolonged myleran treatment. *Exp Cell Res* 42:265–273, 1966.

Grimes P, von Sallmann L, Frichette A: Influence of myleran on cell proliferation in the lens epithelium. *Invest Ophthalmol* 3:566–576, 1964.

Grisolano J Jr, Peynan GA: Retinal toxicity study of intravitreal cyclosporia. *Ophthalmic Surg* 17:155–156, 1986.

Guillaume C, Perrot D, Bouffard Y, et al: L'intoxication methanolique. *Ann Fr Anesth Reanim* 6:17–21, 1987.

Gupta KC, Chambers WA, Green S, et al: An eye irritation test protocol and an evaluation and classification system. *Food Chem Toxicol* 31(2):117–121, 1993.

Guth PS, Spirtes MA: The phenothiazine tranquilizers: Biochemical and biophysical actions. *Int Rev Neurobiol* 7:231–278, 1964.

Hakim SAE: Argemone oil, sanguinarine, and epidemic-dropsy glaucoma. *Br J Ophthalmol* 38:193–216, 1954.

Hamming NA, Apple DJ, Goldberg MF: Histopathology and ultrastructure of busulfan-induced cataract. *Graefes Arch Ophthalmol* 200:139–147, 1976.

Harding CV, Reddan JR, Unakar NJ, Bagchi M: The control of cell division in the ocular lens. *Int Rev Cytol* 31:215–300, 1971.

Harris JE, Gruber L: The electrolyte and water balance of the lens. *Exp Eye Res* 1:372–384, 1962.

Harris JE: The reversal of triparanol induced cataracts in the rat. *Doc Ophthalmol* 26:324–333, 1969.

Harris JE: Reversal of triparanol-induced cataracts in the rat: II. Exchange of $^{22}Na$, $^{42}K$, $^{86}Rb$ in cataractous and clearing lenses. *Invest Ophthalmol* 11:608–616, 1972.

Haugaard N: Poisoning of cellular reactions by oxygen. *Ann NY Acad Sci* 117, Art. 2:736–744, 1965.

Haugaard N: Cellular mechanisms of oxygen toxicity. *Physiol Rev* 48:311–372, 1968.

Heier JS, Dragoo RA, Enzenauer RW, Waterhouse WJ: Screening for ocular toxicity in asymptomatic patients treated with tamoxifen. *Am J Ophthalmol* 117:772–775, 1994.

Henkes HE, van Lith GHM: Retinopathy due to indomethacin. *Ophthalmologica* 164:385–386, 1972.

Henkes HE, van Lith GHM, Canta LR: Indomethacin retinopathy. *Am J Ophthalmol* 73:846–856, 1972.

Henrichsen J: Tryparsamide in the treatment of syphilis—a review of the literature. *Venereal Dis Inform* 20:293–322, 1939.

Henze T, Scheidt P, Prange HW: Die Methanol-Intoxikation. *Nervenartzt* 57:658–661, 1986.

Heppel LA, Neal PA, Endicott KM, Porterfield VT: Toxicology of dichloroethane: I. Effect on the cornea. *Arch Ophthalmol* 32:391–394, 1944.

Herman MM, Bensch KG: Light and electron microscopic studies of acute and chronic thallium intoxication in rats. *Toxicol Appl Pharmacol* 10:199–222, 1967.

Herzinger T, Korting HC, Maibach HI: Assessment of cutaneous and ocular irritancy: A decade of research on alternatives to animal experimentation. *Fundam Appl Toxicol* 24:29–41, 1995.

Heyroth FF: Thallium, a review and summary of medical literature. *Public Health Service Reports (Suppl)*. Washington, D.C.: U.S. Government Printing Office, 1947.

Hines J, Vinores SA, Campochiaro PA: Evolution of morphologic changes after intravitreous injection of gentamycin. *Curr Eye Res* 12(6):521–529, 1993.

Hirst LW, Sanborn G, Green WR, et al: Amodiaquine ocular changes. *Arch Ophthalmol* 100:1300–1304, 1982.

Hjelmeland LM, Li JW, Toth CA, Landers MB III: Antifibrotic and uveitogenic properties of gamma interferon in the rabbit eye. *Graefes Arch Clin Exp Ophthalmol* 230(1):84–90, 1992.

Hobbs HE, Sorsby A, Friedman A: Retinopathy following chloroquine therapy. *Lancet* 2:478–480, 1959.

Horner WD: Dinitrophenol and its relation to formation of cataract. *Arch Ophthalmol* 27:1097–1121, 1942.

Hübner U, Emmerlich P, Heidenbluth I: Kandidose bei Explosionsverbrennnung und Verätzung durch Trichlorsilan. *Dermatol Monatsschr* 165:795–798, 1979.

Hughes WF: Alkali burns of the eye: I. Review of the literature and summary of present knowledge. *Arch Ophthalmol* 35:423–449, 1946a.

Hughes WF: Alkali burns of the eye: II. Clinical and pathological course. *Arch Ophthalmol* 36:189–214, 1946b.

Hunter D, Bomford RR, Russell DS: Poisoning by methyl mercury compounds. *Q J Med NS* 9:192–219, 1940.

Ide T: Histopathological studies on retina, optic nerve and arachnoidal membrane of mouse exposed to carbon disulfide poisoning. *Acta Soc Ophthalmol Jap* 62A:85–108, 1958.

Ignarro LJ: Lysosome membrane stabilization in vivo. Effects of steroidal and nonsteroidal antiinflammatory drugs on the integrity of rat liver lysosomes. *J Pharmacol Exp Ther* 182:179–188, 1972.

Ikemoto K: Effects of cataractogenic compounds, fatty acids and related compounds on cation transport of incubated lens. *Osaka City Med J* 71:1–18, 1971.

Inturrisi CE: Thallium activation of $K^+$-activated phosphatases from beef brain. *Biochem Biophys Acta* 173:567–569, 1969a.

Inturrisi CE: Thallium-induced dephosphorylation of a phosphorylated intermediate of the (sodium and thallium-activated) ATPase. *Biochim Biophys Acta* 178:630–633, 1969b.

Ishikawa Y, Mine S: Aminoadipic acid toxic effects on retinal glial cells. *Jpn J Ophthalmol* 27:107–118, 1983.

Jachuck SJ, Stephenson J, Bird T, et al: Practolol induced autoantibodies and their relation to oculocutaneous complications. *Postgrad Med J* 53:75–77, 1977.

Jacobs MB: *War Gases*. New York: Interscience, 1942.

Jacobs WA, Heidelberger M: Aromatic arsenic compounds: II. The amides and alkyl amides of *N*-arylglycine arsonic acids. *J Am Chem Soc* 44:1587–1600, 1919.

Jacobson MA, et al: Randomized phase I trial of two different combinations of foscarnet and gancyclovir chronic maintenance therapy regimens for AIDS patients with cytomegalovirus retinitis: AIDS clinical Trials Group Protocol 151. *J Infect Dis* 170(1):189–193, 1994.

Jaffe LS: Photochemical air pollutants and their effect on men and animals: I. General characteristics and community concentrations. *Arch Environ Health* 15:782–791, 1967.

Jay WM, Fishman P, Aziz M, Shockey RK: Intravitreal ceftazidine in a rabbit model: Dose- and time-dependent toxicity and pharmacokinetic analysis. *J Ocul Pharmacol* 3:257–262, 1987.

Kadota I: Studies on experimental diabetes mellitus, as produced by organic reagents. Oxine diabetes and dithizone diabetes. *J Lab Clin Med* 35:568–591, 1950.

Kaiser-Kupfer MI, Lippman ME: Tamoxifen retinopathy. *Cancer Treat Res* 62:315–320, 1978.

Kao GW, Peyman GA, Fiscella R, House B: Retinal toxicity of gancyclovir in vitrectomy infusion solution. *Retina* 7:80–83, 1987.

Kaplan LJ, Cappaert WE: Amiodarone keratopathy: Correlation to dosage and duration. *Arch Ophthalmol* 100:601–602, 1982.

Karacorlu S, Peyman GA, Karacorlu M, et al: Retinal toxicity of 6-methoxypurine arabinoside (ara-M). A new selective and potent inhibitor of varicella-zoster virus. *Retina* 12(3):261–264, 1992.

Karli P: Les dégénérescences rétiniennes spontanées et expérimentales chez l'animal. *Progr Ophthalmol* 14:51–89, 1963.

Kaufman PL, Axelsson U, Bárány EH: Induction of subcapsular cataracts in cynomolgus monkeys by echothiophate. *Arch Ophthalmol* 95:499–504, 1977a.

Kaufman PL: Atropine inhibition of echothiophate cataractogenesis in monkeys. *Arch Ophthalmol* 95:1262–1268, 1977b.

Kayne FJ: Thallium (I) activation of pyruvate kinase. *Arch Biochem Biophys* 143:232–239, 1971.

Keyvan-Larijarni H, Tannenberg AM: Methanol intoxication, comparison of peritoneal dialysis and hemodialysis treatment. *Arch Intern Med* 134:293–296. 1974.

Kini MM, Cooper JR: Biochemistry of methanol poisoning: III. The enzymatic pathway for the conversion of methanol to formaldehyde. *Biochem Pharmacol* 8:207–217, 1961.

Kinoshita JH: Cataracts in galactosemia. *Invest Ophthalmol* 4:786–799, 1965.

Kinross-Wright V: Clinical trial of a new phenothiazine compound NP-207. *Psychiatr Res Rep Am Psychiatr Assoc* 489–94, 1956.

Kinsey VE, McLean IW, Parker J: Studies on the crystalline lens: XVIII. Kinetics of thallium ($Tl^+$) transport in relation to that of the alkali metal cations. *Invest Ophthalmol* 10:932–942, 1971.

Kirby TJ, Achor RWP, Perry HO, Winkelmann RK: Cataract formation after triparanol therapy. *Arch Ophthalmol* 68:486–489, 1962.

Kirmani M, Santana M, Sorgente N, et al: Antiproliferative drugs in the treatment of experimental proliferative retinopathy. *Retina* 3:269–272, 1983.

Klinghardt GW, Fredman P, Svennerholm L: Chloroquine intoxication induces ganglioside storage in nervous tissue: A chemical and histopathological study of brain, spinal cord, dorsal root ganglia, and retina in the miniature pig. *J Neurochem* 37:897–908, 1981.

Koelle GB: Pharmacology of organophosphates. [Review.] *J Appl Toxicol* 14(2):105–109, 1994.

Kolb H, Rosenthal AR, Juxsoll D, Bergsma D: Preliminary results on chloroquine induced damage to retina of rhesus monkey. Presented at Association for Research in Vision and Ophthalmology, Sarasota, Fla., Spring 1972.

Kolker AE, Becker B: Epinephrine maculopathy. *Arch Ophthalmol* 79:552–562, 1968.

Koopmans RA, Li DK, Paty DW: *J Comput Assist Tomogr* 12:168–169, 1988.

Krill AE, Potts AM, Johanson CE: Chloroquine retinopathy. Investigation of discrepancy between dark adaptation and electroretinographic findings in advanced stages. *Am J Ophthalmol* 71:530–543, 1971.

Kuck JFR Jr: Chemical constituents of the lens, in Graymore CN (ed): *Biochemistry of the Eye*. New York: Academic Press, 1970a.

Kuck JFR Jr: Metabolism of the lens. In Graymore CN (ed): *Biochemistry of the Eye*. New York: Academic Press, 1970b.

Kuck JFR Jr: Cataract formation, in Graymore CN (ed): *Biochemistry of the Eye*. New York: Academic Press, 1970c.

Lamping KA, Belkin JK: 5-fluorouracil and mitomycin-C in pseudophakic patients. *Ophthalmology* 102:70–75, 1995.

Lasansky A, de Robertis E: Submicroscopic changes in visual cells of the rabbit induced by iodoacetate. *J Biophys Biochem Cytol* 5:245–250, 1959.

Laughlin RC, Carey TF: Cataracts in patients treated with triparanol *JAMA* 181:339–340, 1962.

Lawwill T, Appleton B, Altstatt L: Chloroquine accumulation in human eyes. *Am J Ophthalmol* 65:530–532, 1968.

Ledet AE: Clinical, toxicological and pathological aspects of arsanilic acid poisoning in swine. Ph.D. thesis, Iowa State University, Ames, Iowa, 1970; University Microfilms, Ann Arbor, Mich., 1979.

Leibold JE: The ocular toxicity of ethambutol and its relation to dose. *Ann NY Acad Sci* 135:904–909, 1977.

Levine RA, Stahl CJ: Eye injury caused by tear-gas weapons. *Am J Ophthalmol* 65:497–508, 1968.

Levinson RA, Paterson CA, Pfister RR: Ascorbic acid prevents corneal ulceration and perforation following experimental alkali burns. *Invest Ophthalmol Visual Sci* 15:986–993, 1976.
Levy NS, Krill AE, Beutler E: Galactokinase deficiency and cataracts. *Am J Ophthalmol* 74:41–48, 1972.
Lewin L, Guillery H: *Die Wirkung von Arzneimitteln und Giften auf das Auge*. Berlin: A. Hirschwald, vols 1 and 2, 1913.
Lieberman TW: Prolonged pharmacology and the eye. Ocular effects of prolonged systemic drug administration. *Dis Nerv Syst* 29 (Suppl):44–50, 1968.
Loredo A, Rodriguez RS, Murillo L: Cataracts after short-term corticosteroid treatment. *N Engl J Med* 286:160, 1972.
Lowry OH, Roberts NR, Lewis C: The quantitative histochemistry of the retina. *J Biol Chem* 220:879–892, 1956.
Lowry OH, Roberts NR, Schulz DW, et al: Quantitative histochemistry of retina: II. Enzymes of glucose metabolism. *J Biol Chem* 236:2813–2820, 1961.
Lubkin VL: Steroid cataract—a review and a conclusion. *J Asthma Res* 14:55–59, 1977.
Lucas DR, Newhouse JP: The toxic effect of sodium 1-glutamate on the inner layers of the retina. *Arch Ophthalmol* 58:193–201, 1957.
Mackenzie AH: An appraisal of chloroquine. *Arthritis Rheum* 13:280–291, 1970.
Maeno T, Maeda N, Ikeda T, Tano Y: Tissue plasminogen activator treatment of postvitrectomy pupillary fibrin membrane [Japanese]. [Medline English Abstract.] *Nippon Ganka Gakkai Zasshi* 95(11):1124–1128, 1991.
Mailer CM: Paradoxical differences in retinal vessel diameters and the effect of inspired oxygen. *Can J Ophthalmol* 5:163–168, 1970.
Manske RHF: $\alpha$-Napthaphenanthredine alkaloids, in Manske RHF, Holmes HL (ed): *The Alkaloids, Chemistry and Physiology*. New York: Academic Press, 1954, vol 4, pp 253–263.
Marchese AL, Slana VS, Holmes EW, Jay WM: Toxicity and pharmokinetics of ciprofloxacin. *J Ocul Pharmacol* 9(1):69–76, 1993.
Martin-Amat G, McMartin KE, Hayreh SS, et al: Methanol poisoning: Ocular toxicity produced by formate. *Toxicol Appl Pharmacol* 45:201–208, 1978.
Maslova MN, Natochin YV, Skulsky IA: Inhitibiton of active sodium transport and activation of $Na^+$-$K^+$-ATPase by ions $Tl^+$ in frog skin. *Biokhimiia* 36:867–869, 1971.
Matthiolus PA: *Commentarius in sex libros super Dioscorides*. N. Baseus, 1598.
Maurice DM: The cornea and the sclera, in Davson H (ed): *The Eye*, 2d ed. New York: Academic Press, 1969, vol 1.
Maynard FP: Preliminary note on increased intraocular tension met within cases of epidemic dropsy. *Indian Med Gaz* 44:373–374, 1909.
Mazue G, Bertolero F, Jacob C, et al: Preclinical and clinical studies with recombinant human basic fibroblast growth factor. *Ann NY Acad Sci* 638:329–340, 1991.
McChesney EW, Banks WF Jr, Fabian RJ: Tissue distribution of chloroquine, hydroxychloroquine and desethychloroquine in the rat. *Toxicol Appl Pharmacol* 10:501–513, 1967.
McChesney EW, Banks WF Jr, Sullivan DJ: Metabolism of chloroquine and hydroxychloroquine in albino and pigmented rats. *Toxicol Appl Pharmacol* 7:627–636, 1965.
McCrea FD, Eadie GS, Morgan JE: The mechanism of morphine miosis. *J Pharmacol Exp Ther* 74:239–246, 1942.
McFarlane JR, Yanoff M, Scheie HG: Toxic retinopathy following sparsomycin therapy. *Arch Ophthalmol* 76:532–540, 1966.
Meier-Ruge W: Die Morphologie der experimentellen Chlorochinretinopathie des Kaninchens. *Ophthalmologica* 150:127–137, 1965a.
Meier-Ruge W: The pathophysiological morphology of the pigment epithelium and its importance for retinal structure and function. *Med Probl Ophthalmol* 8:32–48, 1968.
Meier-Ruge W: Experimental investigation of the morphogenesis of chloroquine retinopathy. *Arch Ophthalmol* 73:540–544, 1965b.
Meier-Ruge W, Cerletti A: Zur experimentellen Pathologie der Phenothiazin-Retinopathie. *Ophthalmologica* 151:512–533, 1966.
Menzel DB: Toxicity of ozone, oxygen, and radiation *Annu Rev Pharmacol* 10:379–394, 1970.
Meyniel G, Doly M, Millerin M, Braquet P: Implication du PAF (Platelet-Activating Factor) dans le retinopathie a la chloroquine. *C.R. Acad des Sciences Serie iiii, Sciences de la Vie* 314(2):61–65, 1992.
Mochizuki K, Torisaki M, Wakabayashi K: Effects of vancomycin and ofloxacin on rabbit ERG in vitro. *Jap J Ophthalmol* 35(4):435–445, 1991.
Mohammed-Ali H: Spatschaden der Giftgaswirkung bei den Uberlebenden des irakischen Giftgaskrieges gegen das kurdische Volk. *Wien Med Wochschr* 142(1):8–15, 1992.
Monteleone JA, Beutler E, Monteleone PL, et al: Cataracts, galactosuria and hypergalactosemia due to galactokinase deficiency in a child. *Am J Med* 50:403–407, 1971.
Moon J, Chung S, Myong Y, et al: Treatment of postcataract fibrinous membranes with tissue plasminogen activator. *Ophthalmology* 99(8):1256–1259, 1992.
Moritera T, Ogura Y, Yoshimura N, et al: Biodegradable microspheres containing adriamycin in the treatment of proliferative vitreoretinopathy. *Invest Ophthalmol* 33(11):3125–3130, 1992.
Nakajima A: The effect of amino-phenoxy-alkanes on rabbit ERG. *Ophthalmologica* 136:332–344, 1958.
Nakamura K, Refojo MF, Crabtree DV, et al: Ocular toxicity of low molecular weight components of silicone and fluorosilicone oils. *Invest Ophthalmol Vis Sci* 32(12):3007–3020, 1991.
Nemeyer VR, Tephly TR: Detection and quantification of 10-formyltetrahydrofolate dehydrogenase (10-FTHFDH) in rat retina, optic nerve, and brain. *Life Sci* 54(22):PL395–399, 1994.
Neujean G, Weyts E, Bacq ZM: Action du B.A.L. sur les accidents ophthalmologiques de la thérapeutique à la tryparsamide. *Bull Acad R Med Belg* 13:341–350, 1948.
Nichols CW, Lambertsen CJ: Effects of high oxygen pressures on the eye. *N Engl J Med* 281:25–30, 1969.
Nieuwveld RW, Halkett JA, Spracklen FHN: Drug resistant malaria in Africa: A case report and review of the problem and treatment. *South Afr Med J* 62:173–175, 1982.
Nirankari VS, Varma SD, Lakhanpal V, Richards RD: Superoxide radical scavenging agents in treatment of alkali burns. *Arch Ophthalmol* 99:886–887, 1981.
Noell WK: The impairment of visual cell structure by iodoacetate. *J Cell Comp Physiol* 40:25–45, 1952.
Nordmann J: L'oculiste et la detection preventive systematique de la galactosemie. *Ophthalmologica* 163:129–135, 1971.
Northover BJ: Mechanism of the inhibitory action of indomethacin on smooth muscle. *Br J Pharmacol* 41:540–551, 1971.
Northover BJ: The effects of indomethacin in calcium, sodium, potassium and magnesium fluxes in various tissues of the guinea pig. *Br J Pharmacol* 45:651–659, 1972.
Nussenblatt R: The expanding use of immunosuppression in the treatment of non-infectious ocular disease. [Review.] *J Autoimmun* 5 Suppl A:247–257, 1992.
Nylander U: Ocular damage in chloroquine therapy. *Acta Ophthalmol* 92 (Suppl):1–71, 1967.
Obstbaum SA, Galin MA, Poole TA: Topical epinephrine and cystoid macular edema. *Ann Ophthalmol* 8:455–458, 1976.
Oglesby RB, Black RL, von Sallmann L, Bunim JJ: Cataracts in patients with rheumatic diseases treated with corticosteroids. *Arch Ophthalmol* 66:625–630, 1961a.
O'Hara MA, Bode DD, Kincaid MC, Perkins MC: Retinal toxicity of intravitreal cefoperazone. *J Ocul Pharmacol* 2:177–184, 1986.
Ohira A, Wilson CA, deJuan E Jr, et al: Experimental retinal tolerance to emulsified silicone oil. *Retina* 11(2):259–265, 1991.
Okamoto K: Experimental pathology of diabetes melitus. (Report II) I. Experimental studies on production and progress of diabetes mellitus by zinc reagents. *Tohoku J Exp Med* 61 (Suppl III):1–35, 1955.

Okun E, Gouras P, Bernstein H, von Sallmann L: Chloroquine retinopathy. *Arch Ophthalmol* 69:59–71, 1963.

Olney JW: The toxic effects of glutamate and related compounds in the retina and the brain. *Retina* 2:341–359, 1982.

Ono S, Hirano H, Obara KO: Absorption of cortisol-4-$^{14}C$ into rat lens. *Jpn J Exp Med* 41:485–487, 1971.

Ono S: Presence of cortisol-binding protein in the lens. *Ophthalmic Res* 3:233–240, 1972a.

Ono S: Study on the conjugation of cortisol in the lens. *Ophthalmic Res* 3:307–310, 1972b.

Orr G, Tervaert DC, Lean JS: Aqueous concentrations of fluorouracil after intravitreal injection. Normal, vitrectomized, and silicone-filled eyes. *Arch Ophthalmol* 104:431–434, 1986.

Orthner H: *Methanol Poisoning*. Berlin: Springer, 1950.

Osgood TB, Ubels JL, Smith GA, Dick CE: Evaluation of ocular irritancy of hair care products. *J Toxicol—Cutan Ocular Toxicol* 9(1):37–51, 1990.

Otto HF: Tierexperimentelle Untersuchungen zur Hepato-Toxizität von Triparanol. *Beitr Pathol* 142:177–193, 1971.

Oum BS, D'Amico DJ, Kwak HW, Wong KW: Intravitreal antibiotic therapy with vancomycin and aminoglycoside: Examination of the retinal toxicity of repetitive injections after vitreous and lens surgery. *Graefe's Arch Clin Exp Ophthalmol* 230(1):56–61, 1992.

Palimeris G, Koliopoulos J, Velissaropoulos P: Ocular side effects of indomethacin. *Ophthalmologica* 164:339–353, 1972.

Pang MP, Branchflower RV, Chang AT, et al: Half-life and vitreous clearance of trifluorothymidine after intravitreal injection in the rabbit eye. *Can J Ophthalmol* 27(1):6–9, 1992.

Pang MP, Peyman GA, Nikoleit J, et al: Intravitreal trifluorothymidine and retinal toxicity. *Retina* 6:260–263, 1986.

Paterson CA: Distribution and movement of ions in the ocular lens. *Doc Ophthalmol* 31:1–28, 1972.

Patz A: Retrolental fibroplasia. *Surv Ophthalmol* 14:1–29, 1969–70.

Pavlidis NA, Petris C, Briassoulis E, et al: Clear evidence that long-term, low-dose tamoxifen treatment can induce ocular toxicity. A prospective study of 63 patients. [Review.] *Cancer* 69(12):2961–2964, 1992.

Pearce L: Studies on the treatment of human tyrpanosomiasis with tryparsamide (the sodium salt of *N*-phenylglycineamide-*p*-arsonic acid). *J Exp Med* 34 (Suppl. 1):1–104, 1921.

Pedersen OO, Karlsen RL: Destruction of Müller cells in the adult rat by intravitreal injection of D,L-alpha-aminoadipic acid. An electron microscopic study. *Exp Eye Res* 28:569–575, 1979.

Peyman GH, Conway MD, Karacorlu M, et al: Evaluation of silicone gel as a long term vitreous substitute in non-human primates. *Ophthalmic Surg* 23(12):811–817, 1992.

Pfister RR, Burstein N: The alkali burned cornea: I. Epithelial and stromal repair. *Exp Eye Res* 23:519–535, 1976.

Pfister RR, Haddox JL, Lank KM: Citrate or ascorbate/citrate treatment of established corneal ulcers in the alkali-injured rabbit eye. *Invest Ophthalmol Visual Sci* 29:1110–1115, 1988.

Pfister RR, Koski J: Alkali burns of the eye: Pathophysiology and treatment. *South Med J* 75:417–422, 1982.

Pfister RR, Paterson CA: Ascorbic acid in the treatment of alkali burns of the eye. *Invest Ophthalmol Visual Sci* 16:1050–1057, 1977.

Pfister RR, Paterson CA, Hayes SA: Topical ascorbate decreases the incidence of corneal ulceration after experimental alkali burns. *Invest Ophthalmol Visual Sci* 17:1019–1024, 1978.

Pflugfelder SC, Hernandez E, Fliesler SJ, et al: Intravitreal vancomycin. Retinal toxicity, clearance, and interaction with gentamycin. *Arch Ophthalmol* 105:831–837, 1987.

Phang PT, Passerini L, Mielke B, et al: Brain hemorrhage associated with methanol poisoning. *Crit Care Med* 16:137–140, 1988.

Place VA, Peets EA, Buyske DA, Little RR: Metabolic and special studies of ethambutol in normal volunteers and tuberculous patients. *Ann NY Acad Sci* 135:775–795, 1966.

Place VA, Thomas JP: Clinical pharmacology of ethambutol. *Am Rev Respir Dis* 87:901–904, 1963.

Podos SM, Canellos GP: Lens changes in chronic granulocytic leukemia. *Am J Ophthalmol* 68:500–504, 1969.

Polyak S: *The Retina*. Chicago: University of Chicago Press, 1941.

Potts AM: Methyl alcohol poisoning. *ONR Res Rev* pp 4–9, Nov. 1952.

Potts AM: The concentration of phenothiazines in the eyes of experimental animals. *Invest Ophthalmol* 1:522–530, 1962a.

Potts AM: Uveal pigment and phenothiazine compounds. *Trans Am Ophthalmol Soc* 60:517–552, 1962b.

Potts AM: Further studies concerning the accumulation of polycyclic compounds on uveal melanin. *Invest Ophthalmol* 3:399–404, 1964a.

Potts AM: The reaction of uveal pigment *in vitro* with polycyclic compounds. *Invest Ophthalmol* 3:405–416, 1964b.

Potts AM: Agents which cause pigmentary retinopathy. *Dis Nerv Syst* 29(Suppl.):16–18, 1968.

Potts AM: Tobacco amblyopia. *Survey Ophthal* 17(5):313–339, 1973.

Potts AM, Au PC: Thallous ion and the eye. *Invest Ophthalmol* 10:925–931, 1971.

Potts AM, Hodges D, Shelman CB, et al: Morphology of the primate optic nerve: III. Fiber characteristics of the foveal outflow. *Invest Ophthalmol* 11:1004–1016, 1972.

Potts AM, Praglin J, Farkas I, et al: Studies on the visual toxicity of methanol: VIII. Additional observations on methanol poisoning in the primate test object. *Am J Ophthalmol* 40:76–82, 1955.

Prick JJG, Sillevis-Smitt WG, Muller L: *Thallium Poisoning*. New York: Elsevier, 1955.

Pulido JS, Palacio W, Peyman GA, et al: Toxicity of intravitreal antiviral drugs. *Ophthalmic Surg* 15:666–669, 1984.

Pulido J, Peyman GA, Lesar T, Vernot J: Intravitreal toxicity of hydroxyacyclovir (BW-B7590), a new antiviral agent. *Arch Ophthalmol* 103:840–841, 1985.

Raitta C, Tolonen M: Microcirculation of the eye in workers exposed to carbon disulfide, in Merrigan WH, Weiss B (eds): *Neurotoxicity of the Visual System*. New York: Raven Press, 1980.

Ravindranathan MP, Paul VJ, Kuriakose ET: Cataract after busulphan treatment. *Br Med J* 1:218–219, 1972.

Rawlins FA, Uzmana BG: Retardation of peripheral nerve myelination in mice treated with inhibitors of cholesterol biosynthesis. A quantitative electron microscopic study. *J Cell Biol* 216:505–517, 1970.

Reading HW, Sorsby A: Retinal toxicity and tissue—SH levels. *Biochem Pharmacol* 15:1389–1393, 1966.

Reim M, Schmidt-Martens FW: Behandlung von Veratzungen. *Klin Monatsbl Augenheilkd* 181:1–9, 1982.

Reim M, Bahrke C, Kuckelhorn R, Kuwert T: Investigation of enzyme activities in severe burns of the anterior eye segment. *Graefes Arch Clin Exp Ophthalmol* 231(5):308–312, 1993.

Riehm W: Ueber Presojod-Schädigung des Auges. *Klin Monatsbl Augenheilkd* 78:87, 1927.

Riehm W: Akute Pigmentdegeneration der Netzhaut nach Intoxikation mit Septojod. *Arch Augenheilkd* 100–101:872–882, 1929.

Rootman DS, Savage P, Hassany SM, et al: Toxicity and pharmacokinetics of intravitreally injected ciprofloxin in rabbit eyes. *Can J Ophthalmol* 27(6):277–282, 1992.

Rosenberg NL: Methyl malonic acid, methanol, metabolic acidosis, and lesions of the basal ganglia. *Ann Neurol* 22:96–97, 1987.

Rubsamen PE, Davis PA, Hernandez E, et al: Prevention of experimental vitreoretinopathy with a biodegradable intravitreal implant for the sustained release of fluorouracil. *Arch Ophthalmol* 112(3):407–413, 1994.

Sadun AA, Martone JF, Muci-Mendoza R, et al: Epidemic neuropathy in Cuba. Eye findings. (Review.) *Arch Ophthalmol* 112(5):661–669, 1994.

Sebelaish S, Hilmi G: Ocular manifestations of mercury poisoning. *WHO Reports* 53 (Suppl):83–86, 1976.

Sarkar SL: Katakar oil poisoning. *Indian Med Gaz* 61:62–63, 1926.
Sarkar SN: Isolation from argemone oil of dihydrosanguinarine and sanguinarine: Toxicity of sanguinarine. *Nature (Lond)* 162:265–266, 1948.
Sarraf D, Equi RA, Holland GN, et al: Transscleral iontophoresis of foscarnet. *Am J Ophthalmol* 115(6):748–754, 1993.
Sassaman FW, Cassidy JJ, Alpern M, Maaseidvaag F: Electroretinography in patients with connective tissue diseases treated with hydroxychloroquine. *Am J Ophthalmol* 70:515–523, 1970.
Schachar RA, Cudmore DP, Black TD: Experimental support for Schachar's hypothesis of accommodation. *Ann Ophthalmol* 25:404–409, 1993.
Scherbel AL, Mackenzie AH, Nousek JE, Atdjian M: Ocular lesions in rheumatoid arthritis and related disorders with particular reference to retinopathy. A study of 741 patients treated with and without chloroquinine drugs. *N Engl J Med* 273:360–366, 1965.
Schmidt IG: Central nervous system effects of ethambutol in monkeys. *Ann NY Acad Sci* 135:759–774, 1966.
Schubert G, Bornschein H: Spezifische Schädigung von Netzhautelementen durch Jodazetat. *Experientia* 7:461–462, 1951.
Schulman JA, Peyman GA, Fiscella R, et al: Toxicity of intravitreal injection of fluconazole in the rabbit. *Can J Ophthalmol* 22:304–306, 1987.
Schutta HS, Neville HE: Effects of cholesterol synthesis inhibitors on the nervous system. A light and electron microscopic study. *Lab Invest* 19:487–493, 1968.
Shaffer RN, Hetherington J: Anticholinesterase drugs and cataracts. *Am J Ophthalmol* 62:613–628, 1966.
Shaffer RN, Ridgway WL: Furmethide iodide in the production of dacryostenosis. *Am J Ophthalmol* 34:718–720, 1951.
Shakiba S, Assil K, Listhaus AD, et al: Evaluation of retinal toxicity and liposome encapsulation of the anti-CMV drug 2′-nor-cyclic GMP. *Invest Ophthalmol Vis Sci* 34(10):2903–2910, 1993.
Shaw C-M, Mottet NK, Body RL, Luschei ES: Variability of neuropathologic lesions in experimental methylmercurial encephalopathy in primates. *Am J Pathol* 80:451–470, 1975.
Shearer RV, Dubois EL: Ocular changes induced by long-term hydroxychloroquine (Plaquenil) therapy. *Am J Ophthalmol* 64:245–252, 1967.
Shigematsu I: Subacute myelo-optico-neuropathy (SMON) and clioquinol. *Jpn J Med Sci Biol* 28(Suppl.):35–55, 1975.
Shockley RK, Jay WM, Friberg TR, et al: Intravitreal ceftriaxone in a rabbit model. Dose- and time-dependent toxic effects and pharmacokinetic analysis. *Arch Ophthalmol* 102:1236–1238, 1984.
Shulman NR: Immunoreactions involving platelets. *J Exp Med* 107:665–729, 1958.
Siddall JR: The ocular toxic findings with prolonged and high dosage chlorpromazine intake. *Arch Ophthalmol* 74:460–464, 1965.
Siddall JR: Ocular toxic changes associated with chlorpromazine and thioridazine. *Can J Ophthalmol* 1:190–198, 1966.
Siddall JR: Ocular complications related to phenothiazines. *Dis Nerv Syst* 29 (Suppl):10–13, 1968.
Siegrist A: Konzentrierte Alkali-und Säurewirkung auf das Auge. *Z Augenheilkd* 43:176–194, 1920.
Slansky HH, Freeman MI, Itoi M: Collagenolytic activity in bovine corneal epithelium. *Arch Ophthalmol* 80:496–498, 1968.
Small GH, Peyman GA, Srinivasan A, et al: Retinal toxicity of combination antiviral drugs in an animal model. *Can J Ophthalmol* 22:300–303, 1987.
Sobue I, Ando K: Myeloneuropathy with abdominal symptoms—5 clinical features and diagnostic criteria. *Clin Neurol* 11:244–248, 1971.
Solomon C, Light AE, De Beer EJ: Cataracts produced in rats by 1,4-dimethanesulfonoxybutane (myleran). *Arch Ophthalmol* 54:850–852, 1955.
Sorsby A: The nature of experimental degeneration of the retina. *Br J Ophthalmol* 25:62–65, 1941.
Sorsby A, Harding R: Protective effect of cysteine against retinal degeneration induced by iodate and iodoacetate. *Nature (Lond)* 187:608–609, 1960.
Sorsby A, Harding R: Experimental degeneration of the retina: VIII. Dithizone retinopathy: Its independence of the diabetogenic effect. *Vision Res* 2:149–155, 1962.
Sorsby A, Nakajima A: Experimental degeneration of the retina: IV. Diaminodiphenoxyalkanes as inducing agents. *Br J Ophthalmol* 42:563–571, 1958.
Steinberg D, Avigan J: Studies on cholesterol biosynthesis: II. The role of desmosterol in the biosynthesis of cholesterol. *J Biol Chem* 235:3127–3129, 1960.
Steinhorst UH, Chen EP, Machemer R, Hatchell DL: N,N-dimethyl adriamycin for treatment of experimental proliferative vitreoretinopathy efficacy and toxicity in the rabbit retina. *Exp Eye Res* 56(4):489–495, 1993a.
Steinhorst UH, Hatchell DL, Chen EP, Machemer R: Ocular toxicity of daunomycin: Effects of subdivided doses on the rabbit retina after vitreous gas compression. *Graefes Arch Clin Exp Ophthalmol* 231(10):591–594, 1993b.
Stern WN, Guerin CJ, Lewis GP, et al: Ocular toxicity of fluorouracil after vitrectomy. *Am J Ophthalmol* 96:43–51, 1983.
Straus DJ, Mausolf FA, Ellerby RA, McCracken JD: Cicatrical ectropion secondary to 5-fluorouracil therapy. *Med Pediatr Oncol* 3:15–19, 1977.
Sugimoto K, Goto S: Retinopathy in chronic carbon disulfide exposure, in Merrigan WH, Weiss B (eds): *Neurotoxicity of the Visual System*. New York: Raven Press, 1980.
Sunalp MA, Wiedemann P, Sorgente N, Ryan SJ: Effect of adriamycin on experimental proliferative retinopathy in the rabbit. *Exp Eye Res* 41:105–115, 1985.
Tanji TM, Peyman GA, Mehta NJ, Millsap CM: Perfluoroperhydrophenanthrene (Vitreon) as a short term vitreous substitute after complex vitreous surgery. *Ophthalmic Surg* 24(10):661–665, 1993.
Tarkkanen A, Esila R, Liesmaa M: Experimental cataracts following long-term administration of corticosteroids. *Acta Ophthalmol* 44:665–668, 1966.
Tateishi J, Otsuki S: Experimental reproduction of SMON in animals by prolonged administration of clioquinol: Clinico-pathological findings. *Jpn J Med Sci Biol* 28 (Suppl.):165–186, 1975.
Tephly TR, Parks RE Jr, Mannering GJ: Methanol metabolism in the rat. *J Pharmacol Exp Ther* 143:292–300, 1963.
Thatcher DB, Blaug SM, Hyndiuk RA, Watzke RC: Ocular effects of chemical Mace in the rabbit. *Clin Med* 78:11–13, 1971.
Thomas HW: Some experiments in the treatment of trypanosomiasis. *Br Med J* 1:1140–1143, 1905.
Thomas JP, Baughn CO, Wilkinson RG, Shepard RG: A new synthetic compound with antituberculous activity in mice: Ethambutol dextro 2,2′ ethylenediimino di-1-butanol. *Am Rev Respir Dis* 83:891–893, 1961.
Trayhurn P, van Heyningen R: Aerobic metabolism in the bovine lens. *Exp Eye Res* 12:315–327, 1971a.
Trayhurn P: The metabolism of glutamate, aspartate and alanine in the bovine lens. *Biochem J* 124:72P–73P, 1971b.
Trumbull GC, Sbarbaro JA, Iseman M: (Correspondence.) High dose ethambutol. *Am Rev Respir Dis* 115:889–890, 1977.
Tsubaki T, Irukayama K (eds): *Minamata Disease*. Kodansha Ltd., Tokyo, Amsterdam: Elsevier, 1977.
Tucker K, Hedges TR: Food shortages and an epidemic of optic and peripheral neuropathy in Cuba. *Nutr Rev* 51(12):349–357, 1993.
Turrini B, Tognon MS, DeCaro G, Secchi AG: Intravitreal use of foscarnet: Retinotoxicity of repeated injections in the rabbit eye. *Ophthalmol Res* 26(2):110–115, 1994.
Uhthoff W: Die Augenstörungen bei Vergiftungen, in Graefe-Saemisch *Handbunch der Gesamten Augenheilkunde* 11:1–180, Leipzig: Engelmann, 1911.
van Haeringen NJ, Oosterhuis JA, van Delft JL: A comparison of the

effects of non-steroidal compounds on the disruption of the blood-aqueous barrier. *Exp Eye Res* 35:271–277, 1982.

van Heyningen R: The lens: Metabolism and cataract, in Davson H (ed): *The Eye, Vegetative Physiology and Biochemistry*, 2d ed. New York: Academic Press, 1969, vol 1.

van Heyningen R: Ascorbic acid in the lens of the naphthalene-fed rabbit. *Exp Eye Res* 9:38–48, 1970a.

van Heyningen R: Effect of some cyclic hydroxy compounds on the accumulation of ascorbic acid by the rabbit lens *in vitro*. *Exp Eye Res* 9:49–56, 1970b.

van Heyningen R: Galactose cataract: A review. *Exp Eye Res* 11:415–428, 1971.

van Heyningen R, Pirie A: The metabolism of naphthalene and its toxic effect on the eye. *Biochem J* 102:842–852, 1967.

Van Joost TH, Crone RA, Overdijk AD: Ocular cicatricial pemphigoid associated with practolol therapy. *Br J Dermatol* 94:447–50, 1976.

Varma DR, Guest I: The Bhopal accident and methyl isocyanate toxicity. (Review.) *J Toxicol Environ Health* 40(4):513–529, 1993.

Velhagen K: Zur Hornhautargyrose. *Klin Monatsbl Augenheilkd* 122:36–42, 1953.

Vinding T, Nielsen NV: Retinopathy caused by treatment with tamoxifen in low dosage. *Acta Ophthalmol* 61:45–50, 1983.

Vito P: Contributo allo studio della degenerazione pigmentaria della retina indotta dalla soluzione iodica di Pregl. *Boll Ocul* 14:945–957, 1935.

von Sallmann L: The lens epithelium in the pathogenesis of cataract. *Am J Ophthalmol* 44:159–170, 1957.

von Sallmann L, Grimes P, Collins E: Triparanol induced cataract in rats. *Arch Ophthalmol* 70:522–530, 1963.

Wagner A: CT-forandringer i cerebrum ved akut metanolforgiftning. *Ugeskr Laeger* 148:178–179, 1986.

Waley SG: The lens: Function and macromolecular composition, in Davson H (ed): *The Eye*, 2d ed. New York: Academic, 1969, vol 1.

Wang Y, Wu L, Wu DZ, et al: Visual functions and trace element metabolism in tobacco-toxic optic neuropathy. *Yen Ko Huseh Pao* 8(3):131–137, 1992.

Warburg O: *Über den Stoffwechsel der Tumoren*. Berlin: Springer, 1926, p 138.

Weber U, Goerz G, Michaelis L, Melnik B: Disorders of retinal function in long-term therapy with retinoid etretinate. *Klin Monatsbl Augenheilkd* 192:706–711, 1988.

Weekley RD, Potts AM, Reboton J, May RH: Pigmentary retinopathy in patients receiving high doses of a new phenothiazine. *Arch Ophthalmol* 64:65–74, 1960.

Weitzel G, Strecker FJ, Roester U, et al: Zinc im tapetum lucidum. *Hoppe Seylers Z Physiol Chem* 296:19–30, 1954.

Weleber RG, Denman ST, Hanifin JM, Cunningham WJ: Abnormal retinal function associated with isoretinoin therapy for acne. *Arch Ophthalmol* 104:831–837, 1986.

Wetterholm DH, Winter FC: Histopathology of chloroquine retinal toxicity. *Arch Ophthalmol* 71:82–87, 1964.

Wheeler MC: Discoloration of the eyelids from prolonged use of ointments containing mercury. *Trans Am Ophthalmol Soc* 45:74–80, 1947.

Wilkes JW: Argyrosis of cornea and conjunctiva. *J Tenn Med Assoc* 46:11–13, 1953.

Williamson J: A new look at the ocular side-effects of long-term systemic corticosteroid and adenocorticotrophic therapy. *Proc R Soc Med* 63:791–792, 1970.

Williamson J, Paterson RWW, McGavin DDN, et al: Posterior subcapsular cataracts and glaucoma associated with long-term oral corticosteroid therapy in patients with rheumatoid arthritis and related conditions. *Br J Ophthalmol* 53:361–372, 1969.

Wilson FM II, Schmitt TE, Grayson M: Amiodarone-induced cornea verticillata. *Ann Ophthalmol* June 1980, pp. 657–660.

Wirth A, Quaranta CA, Chistoni G: The effect of dithizone on the electroretinogram of the rabbit. *Bibl Ophthalmol* 48:66–73, 1957.

Wood CA, Buller F: Poisoning by wood alcohol. Cases of death and blindness from Columbian spirits and other methylated preparations. *JAMA* 43:972–977; 1058–1062; 1117–1123; 1213–1221; 1289–1296, 1904.

Wood DC, Contaxis I, Sweet D, et al: Response of rabbits to corticosteroids: I. Influence on growth, intraocular pressure and lens transparency. *Am J Ophthalmol* 63:841–849, 1967.

Yoshizumi MO, Niizawa JM, Meyers-elliott R: Ocular toxicity of intravitreal vidarbine solubilized in dimethylsulfoxide. *Arch Ophthalmol* 104:426–430, 1986.

Yoshizumi MO, Silverman C: Experimental intravitreal 5-fluorocytosine. *Ann Ophthalmol* 58–61, 1985.

Zemel E, Loewenstein A, Lazar M, Perlman I: The effects of myristyl gamma-picolinium chloride on the rabbit retina: Morphologic observations. *Invest Ophthalmol Vis Sci* 34(7): 2360–2366, 1993.

# CHAPTER 21

# TOXIC RESPONSES OF THE ENDOCRINE SYSTEM

*Charles C. Capen*

Endocrine glands are collections of specialized cells that synthesize, store, and release their secretions directly into the bloodstream. They are sensing and signaling devices located in the extracellular fluid compartment and are capable of responding to changes in the internal and external environments to coordinate a multiplicity of activities that maintain homeostasis.

Endocrine cells that produce polypeptide hormones have a well-developed rough endoplasmic reticulum that assembles hormone and a prominent Golgi apparatus for packaging hormone into granules for intracellular storage and transport. Secretory granules are unique to polypeptide hormone- and catecholamine-secreting endocrine cells and provide a mechanism for intracellular storage of substantial amounts of preformed active hormone. When the cell receives a signal for hormone secretion, secretory granules are directed to the periphery of the endocrine cell, probably by the contraction of microfilaments.

Steroid hormone-secreting cells are characterized by large cytoplasmic lipid bodies that contain cholesterol and other precursor molecules. The lipid bodies are in close proximity to an extensive tubular network of smooth endoplasmic reticulum and large mitochondria which contain hydroxylase and dehydrogenase enzyme systems. These enzyme systems function to attach various side chains to the basic steroid nucleus. Steroid-producing cells lack secretory granules and do not store significant amounts of preformed hormone. They are dependent on continued biosynthesis to maintain the normal secretory rate for a particular hormone.

Many diseases of the endocrine system are characterized by dramatic functional disturbances and characteristic clinicopathological alterations affecting one or several body systems. The affected animal or human patient may have clinical signs that primarily involve the skin (hair loss caused by hypothyroidism), nervous system (seizures caused by hyperinsulinism), urinary system (polyuria caused by diabetes mellitus, diabetes insipidus, and hyperadrenocorticism), or skeletal system (fractures induced by hyperparathyroidism).

The literature suggests that chemically induced lesions of the endocrine organs are most commonly encountered in the adrenal glands, followed in descending order by the thyroid, pancreas, pituitary, and parathyroid glands. In the adrenal glands, chemically induced lesions are most frequently found in the zona fasciculata/zona reticularis and to a lesser extent in either the zona glomerulosa or medulla. In a recent survey, conducted by the Pharmaceutical Manufacturers Association, of tumor types developing in carcinogenicity studies, endocrine tumors developed frequently in rats, with the thyroid gland third in frequency (behind the liver and mammary gland), followed by the pituitary gland (fourth), and adrenal gland (fifth). Selected examples of commonly encountered toxic endpoints involving endocrine organs in laboratory animals are discussed in this chapter. Mechanistic data is included whenever possible to aid in the interpretation of findings in animal toxicology studies and to determine their significance in risk assessment.

## THYROID GLAND

### Goitrogenic Chemicals and Thyroid Tumors in Rodents

Numerous studies have reported that chronic treatment of rodents with goitrogenic compounds results in the development of follicular cell adenomas. Thiouracil and its derivatives have this effect in rats (Napolkov, 1976) and mice (Morris, 1955). This phenomenon also has been observed in rats that consumed brassica seeds (Kennedy and Purves, 1941), erythrosine (FD&C Red No. 3) (Capen and Martin, 1989; Borzelleca et al., 1987), sulfonamides (Swarm et al., 1973), and many other compounds (Hill et al., 1989; Paynter et al., 1988). The pathogenetic mechanism of this phenomenon has been understood for some time (Furth, 1954) and are widely accepted by the scientific community. These goitrogenic agents either directly interfere with thyroid hormone synthesis or secretion in the thyroid gland, increase thyroid hormone catabolism and subsequent excretion into the bile, or disrupt the peripheral conversion of thyroxine ($T_4$) to tri-iodothyronine ($T_3$). The ensuing decrease in circulating thyroid hormone levels results in a compensatory increased secretion of pituitary thyroid stimulating hormone (TSH). The receptor-mediated TSH stimulation of the thyroid gland leads to proliferative changes of follicular cells that include hypertrophy, hyperplasia, and ultimately, neoplasia in rodents.

Excessive secretion of TSH alone (i.e., in the absence of any chemical exposure) also has been reported to produce a high incidence of thyroid tumors in rodents (Ohshima and Ward, 1984, 1986). This has been observed in rats fed an iodine-deficient diet (Axelrod and Leblond, 1955) and in mice that received TSH-secreting pituitary tumor transplants (Furth, 1954). The pathogenetic mechanism of thyroid follicular cell tumor development in rodents involves a sustained excessive stimulation of the thyroid gland by TSH.

### Secondary Mechanisms of Thyroid Oncogenesis

Understanding the mechanism of action of xenobiotics on the thyroid gland provides a rational basis for extrapolation findings from long-term rodent studies to the assessment of a particular compound's safety for humans. Many chemicals and drugs disrupt one or more steps in the synthesis and secretion of thyroid hormones, resulting in subnormal levels of $T_4$ and

$T_3$, associated with a compensatory increased secretion of pituitary TSH (Fig. 21-1). When tested in highly sensitive species, such as rats and mice, early on these compounds resulted in follicular cell hypertrophy/hyperplasia and increased thyroid weights, and in long-term studies they produced an increased incidence of thyroid tumors by a secondary (indirect) mechanism associated with hormonal inbalances.

In the secondary mechanism of thyroid oncogenesis in rodents, the specific xenobiotic chemical or physiological perturbation evokes another stimulus (e.g., chronic hypersecretion of TSH) that promotes the development of nodular proliferative lesions (initially hypertrophy, followed by hyperplasia, subsequently adenomas, infrequently carcinomas) derived from follicular cells. Thresholds for "no effect" on the thyroid gland can be established by determining the dose of xenobiotic that fails to elicit an elevation in the circulating level of TSH. Compounds acting by this indirect (secondary) mechanism with hormonal imbalances usually show little or no evidence for mutagenicity or for producing DNA damage.

In human patients who have marked changes in thyroid function and elevated TSH levels, as is common in areas with a high incidence of endemic goiter due to iodine deficiency, there is little if any increase in the incidence of thyroid cancer (Doniach, 1970; Curran and DeGroot, 1991). The relative resistance to the development of thyroid cancer in humans with elevated plasma TSH levels is in marked contrast to the response of the thyroid gland to chronic TSH stimulation in rats and mice. The human thyroid is much less sensitive to this pathogenetic phenomenon than rodents (McClain, 1989).

Human patients with congenital defects in thyroid hormone synthesis (dyshormonogenetic goiter) and markedly increased circulating TSH levels have been reported to have an increased incidence of thyroid carcinomas (Cooper et al., 1981; McGirr et al., 1959). Likewise, thyrotoxic patients with Grave's disease, in which follicular cells are autonomously stimulated by an immunoglobulin (long-acting thyroid stimulator, or LATS) also appear to be at greater risk of developing thyroid tumors (Pendergrast et al., 1961; Clements, 1954). Therefore, the literature suggests that prolonged stimulation of the human thyroid by TSH will induce neoplasia only in exceptional circumstances, possibly by acting together with some other metabolic or immunologic abnormality (Curran and DeGroot, 1991).

## Chemicals That Directly Disrupt Thyroid Hormone Synthesis and Secretion

### Inhibitors of Thyroid Hormone Synthesis

***Blockage of Iodine Uptake.*** The initial step in the biosynthesis of thyroid hormones is the uptake of iodide from the circulation and transport against a gradient across follicular cells to the lumen of the follicle. A number of anions act as competitive inhibitors of iodide transport in the thyroid, including perchlorate ($ClO_4^-$), thiocyanate ($SCN^-$), and pertechnetate (Fig. 21-2). Thiocyanate is a potent inhibitor of

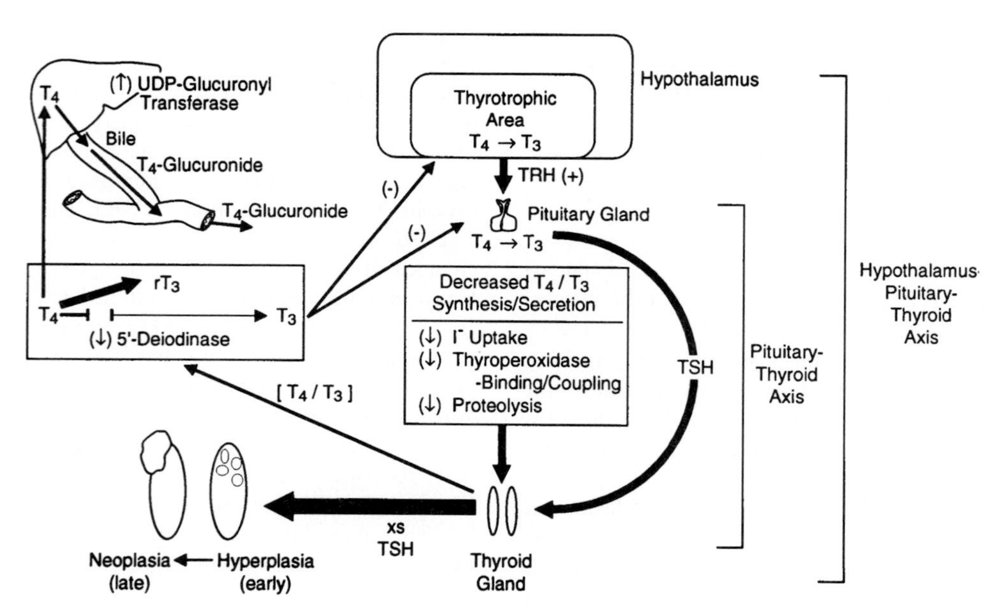


***Figure 21–1. Multiple sites of disruption of the hypothalamic-pituitary-thyroid triad by xenobiotic chemicals.***

Chemicals can exert direct effects by disrupting thyroid hormone synthesis or secretion and indirectly influence the thyroid through an inhibition of 5′-deiodinase or by inducing hepatic microsomal enzymes (e.g., $T_4$-UDP glucuronyl transferase). All of these mechanisms can lower circulating levels of thyroid hormones ($T_4$ and $T_3$), resulting in a release from negative-feedback inhibition and increased secretion of thyroid-stimulating hormone by the pituitary gland. The chronic hypersecretion of TSH predisposes the sensitive rodent thyroid gland to develop an increased incidence of focal hyperplastic and neoplastic lesions (adenomas) by a secondary (epigenetic) mechanism.

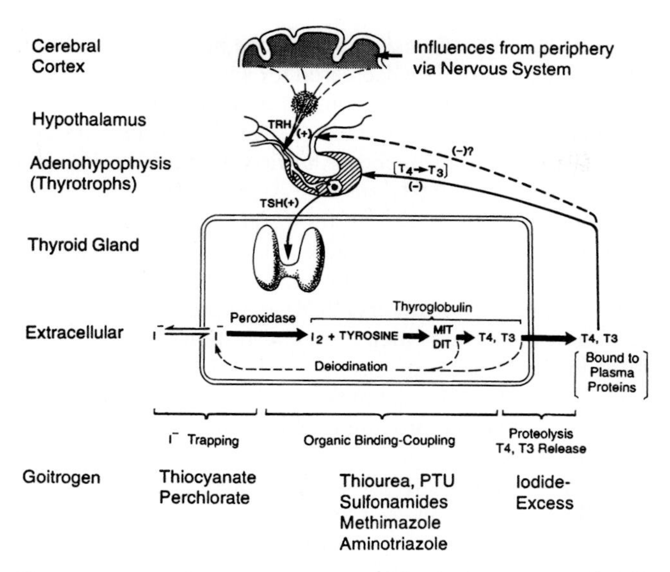


***Figure 21-2. Mechanism of action of goitrogens on thyroid hormone synthesis and secretion. [From Capen and Martin (1989).]***

iodide transport and is a competitive substrate for the thyroid peroxidase but it does not appear to be concentrated in the thyroid. Blockage of the iodide trapping mechanism has a disruptive effect on the thyroid-pituitary axis, similar to iodine deficiency. The blood levels of $T_4$ and $T_3$ decrease, resulting in a compensatory increase in the secretion of TSH by the pituitary gland. The hypertrophy and hyperplasia of follicular cells following sustained exposure results in an increased thyroid weight and the development of goiter.

***Organification Defect: Inhibition of Thyroid Peroxidase.*** A wide variety of chemicals, drugs, and other xenobiotics affect the second step in thyroid hormone biosynthesis (Fig. 21-1). The stepwise binding of iodide to the tyrosyl residues in thyroglobulin requires oxidation of inorganic iodide ($I^-$) to molecular (reactive) iodine ($I_2$) by the thyroid peroxidase present in the luminal aspect (microvillar membranes) of follicular cells and adjacent colloid. Classes of chemicals that inhibit the organification of thyroglobulin include (1) the thionamides (such as thiourea, thiouracil, propylthiouracil, methimazole, carbimazole, and goitrin); (2) aniline derivatives and related compounds (e.g., sulfonamides, paraaminobenzoic acid, paraaminosalicylic acid, and amphenone); (3) substituted phenols (such as resorcinol, phloroglucinol, and 2,4-dihydroxybenzoic acid); and (4) miscellaneous inhibitors (e.g., aminotriazole, tricyanoaminopropene, antipyrine, and its iodinated derivative [iodopyrine]).

Many of these chemicals exert their action by inhibiting the thyroid peroxidase which results in a disruption both of the iodination of tyrosyl residues in thyroglobulin and also the coupling reaction of iodotyrosines [(e.g., monoiodothyronine (MIT) and di-iodothyronine (DIT)] to form iodothyronines ($T_3$ and $T_4$). Propylthiouracil (PTU) has been shown to affect each step in thyroid hormone synthesis beyond iodide transport in rats. The order of susceptibility to the inhibition by PTU is the coupling reaction (most susceptible), iodination of MIT to form DIT, and iodination of tyrosyl residues to form MIT (least susceptible). Thiourea differs from PTU and other thioamides in that it neither inhibits guaiacol oxidation (the standard assay for peroxidase) nor inactivates the thyroid peroxidase in the absence of iodine. Its ability to inhibit organic iodinations is due primarily to the reversible reduction of active $I_2$ to $2I^-$.

The goitrogenic effects of sulfonamides have been known for approximately 50 years, since the reports of the action of sulfaguanidine on the rat thyroid. Sulfamethoxazole and trimethroprim exert a potent goitrogenic effect in rats, resulting in marked decreases in circulating $T_3$ and $T_4$, a substantial compensatory increase in TSH, and increased thyroid weights due to follicular cell hyperplasia. The dog also is a species sensitive to the effects of sulfonamides, resulting in markedly decreased serum $T_4$ and $T_3$ levels, hyperplasia of thyrotrophic basophils in the pituitary gland, and increased thyroid weights.

By comparison, the thyroids of monkeys and human beings are resistant to the development of changes that sulfonamides produce in rodents (rats and mice) and the dog. Rhesus monkeys treated for 52 weeks with sulfamethoxazole (doses up to 300 mg/kg/day) with and without trimethroprim had no changes in thyroid weights and the thyroid histology was normal. Takayama and coworkers (1986) compared the effects of PTU and a goitrogenic sulfonamide (sulfamonomethoxine) on the activity of thyroid peroxidase in the rat and monkey using the guaiacol peroxidation assay. The concentration required for a 50 percent inhibition of the peroxidase enzyme was designated as the inhibition constant$_{50}$ ($IC_{50}$). When the $IC_{50}$ for PTU was set at 1 for rats it took 50 times the concentration of PTU to produce a comparable inhibition in the monkey. Sulfamonomethoxine was almost as potent as PTU in inhibiting the peroxidase in rats. However, it required about 500 times the concentration of sulfonamide to inhibit the peroxidase in the monkey compared to the rat. Studies such as these with sulfonamides demonstrate distinct species differences between rodents and primates in the response of the thyroid to chemical inhibition of hormone synthesis. It is not surprising that the sensitive species (e.g., rats, mice, and dogs) are much more likely to develop follicular cell hyperplasia and thyroid nodules after long-term exposure to sulfonamides than the resistant species (e.g., subhuman primates, human beings, guinea pigs, and chickens).

**Inhibitors of Thyroid Hormone Secretion**

***Blockage of Thyroid Hormone Release by Excess Iodide and Lithium.*** Relatively few chemicals selectively inhibit the secretion of thyroid hormone from the thyroid gland (Fig. 21-1). An excess of iodine has been known for years to inhibit secretion of thyroid hormone and occasionally can result in goiter and subnormal function (hypothyroidism) in animals and human patients. High doses of iodide have been used therapeutically in the treatment of patients with Grave's disease and hyperthyroidism to lower circulating levels of thyroid hormones. Several mechanisms have been suggested for this effect of high iodide levels on thyroid hormone secretion, including a decrease in lysosomal protease activity (in human glands), inhibition of colloid droplet formation (in mice and rats), and inhibition of TSH-mediated increase in cAMP (in dog thyroid slices). Studies in my laboratory demonstrated that rats fed an iodide-excessive diet had a hypertrophy of the cytoplasmic area of follicular cells with an accumulation of numerous colloid droplets and lysosomal bodies (Collins and Capen, 1980). However, there was limited evidence ultrastructurally of the fusion of the membranes of these organelles and of the degradation of the colloid necessary for the release of active thyroid hormones ($T_4$ and $T_3$) from the thyroglobulin. Circulating levels of $T_4$, $T_3$, and $rT_3$ all would be decreased by an iodide-excess in rats.

Lithium also has been reported to have a striking inhibitory effect on thyroid hormone release (Fig. 21-1). The widespread use of lithium carbonate in the treatment of manic states occasionally results in the development of goiter with either euthyroidism or occasionally hypothyroidism in human patients. Lithium inhibits colloid droplet formation stimulated by cAMP in vitro and inhibits the release of thyroid hormones.

## Hepatic Microsomal Enzyme Induction and Thyroid Tumors

Hepatic microsomal enzymes play an important role in thyroid hormone economy because glucuronidation is the rate-limiting step in the biliary excretion of $T_4$ and sulfation by phenol sulfotransferase for the excretion of $T_3$. Long-term exposure of rats to a wide variety of different chemicals may induce these enzyme pathways and result in chronic stimulation of the thyroid by disrupting the hypothalamic-pituitary-thyroid axis (Curran and DeGroot, 1991). The resulting chronic stimulation of the thyroid by increased circulating levels of TSH often results in a greater risk of developing tumors derived from follicular cells in 2-year or lifetime chronic toxicity/carcinogenicity studies with these compounds in rats.

Xenobiotics that induce liver microsomal enzymes and disrupt thyroid function in rats include CNS-acting drugs (e.g., phenobarbital, benzodiazepines); calcium channel blockers (e.g., nicardipine, bepridil); steroids (spironolactone); retinoids; chlorinated hydrocarbons (e.g., chlordane, DDT, TCDD), polyhalogenated biphenyls (PCB, PBB), among others. Most of the hepatic microsomal enzyme inducers have no apparent intrinsic carcinogenic activity and produce little or no mutagenicity or DNA damage. Their promoting effect on thyroid tumors usually is greater in rats than in mice, with males more often developing a higher incidence of tumors than females. In certain strains of mice these compounds alter liver cell turnover and promote the development of hepatic tumors from spontaneously initiated hepatocytes.

Phenobarbital has been studied extensively as the prototype for hepatic microsomal inducers that increase a spectrum of cytochrome P-450 isoenzymes (McClain et al., 1988). McClain and associates (1989) reported that the activity of uridine diphosphate glucuronyltransferase (UDP-GT), the rate limiting enzyme in $T_4$ metabolism, is increased in purified hepatic microsomes of male rats when expressed as picomoles/min/mg microsomal protein (1.3-fold) or as total hepatic activity (3-fold). This resulted in a significantly higher cumulative (4-h) biliary excretion of $^{125}I$-$T_4$ and bile flow than in controls.

Phenobarbital-treated rats develop a characteristic pattern of changes in circulating thyroid hormone levels (McClain et al., 1988, 1989). Plasma $T_3$ and $T_4$ are markedly decreased after 1 week and remain decreased for 4 weeks. By 8 weeks $T_3$ levels return to near normal due to compensation by the hypothalamic-pituitary-thyroid axis. Serum TSH values are elevated significantly throughout the first month but often decline after a new steady state is attained. Thyroid weights increase significantly after 2 to 4 weeks of phenobarbital, reach a maximum increase of 40 to 50 percent by 8 weeks, and remain elevated throughout the period of treatment.

McClain and coworkers (1988) in a series of experiments have shown that supplemental administration of thyroxine (at doses that returned the plasma level of TSH to the normal range) blocked the thyroid tumor-promoting effects of phenobarbital and that the promoting effects were directly proportional to the level of plasma TSH in rats. The sustained increase in circulating TSH levels results initially in hypertrophy of follicular cells, followed by hyperplasia, and ultimately places the rat thyroid at greater risk to develop an increased incidence of benign tumors.

Phenobarbital has been reported to be a thyroid gland tumor promoter in a rat initiation-promotion model. Treatment with a nitrosamine followed by phenobarbital has been shown to increase serum TSH concentrations, thyroid gland weights, and the incidence of follicular cell tumors in the thyroid gland (McClain 1988; McClain et al., 1989). These effects could be decreased in a dose-related manner by simultaneous treatment with increasing doses of exogenous thyroxine. McClain et al. (1989) have demonstrated that rats treated with phenobarbital have a significantly higher cumulative biliary excretion of $^{125}I$-thyroxine than controls. Most of the increase in biliary excretion was accounted for by an increase in $T_4$-glucuronide due to an increased metabolism of thyroxine in phenobarbital-treated rats. This is consistent with enzymatic activity measurements which result in increased hepatic $T_4$-UDP-glucuronyl transferase activity in phenobarbital-treated rats. Results from these experiments are consistent with the hypothesis that the promotion of thyroid tumors in rats was not a direct effect of phenobarbital on the thyroid gland but rather an indirect effect mediated by TSH secretion from the pituitary secondary to the hepatic microsomal enzyme-induced increase of $T_4$ excretion in the bile.

The activation of the thyroid gland during the treatment of rodents with substances that stimulate thyroxine catabolism is a well-known phenomenon and has been investigated extensively with phenobarbital and many other compounds (Curran and DeGroot, 1991). It occurs particularly with rodents, first because UDP-glucuronyl transferase can easily be induced in rodent species, and second because thyroxine metabolism takes place very rapidly in rats in the absence of thyroxine-binding globulin. In humans a lowering of the circulating $T_4$ level but no change in TSH and $T_3$ concentrations has been observed only with high doses of very powerful enzyme-inducing compounds, such as rifampicin with and without antipyrine.

Although phenobarbital is the only UDP-glucuronyl transferase (UDP-GT) inducer that has been investigated in detail to act as a thyroid tumor promoter, the effects of other well-known UDP-GT inducers on the disruption of serum $T_4$ TSH and thyroid gland have been investigated. For example, pregnenolone-16α-carbonitrile (PCN), 3-methylcholanthrene (3MC) and aroclor 1254 (PCB) induce hepatic microsomal

UDP-GT activity towards $T_4$ (Barter and Klaassen, 1992a). These UDP-GT inducers reduce serum $T_4$ levels in both control as well as in thyroidectomized rats that are infused with $T_4$, indicating that reductions in serum $T_4$ levels are not due to a direct effect of the inducers on the thyroid gland (Barter and Klaassen, 1992b; 1994). However, serum TSH levels and thyroid response to reductions in serum $T_4$ levels by UDP-GT inducers is not always predictable. While PCN increases serum TSH and thyroid follicular cell hyperplasia, similar to that observed with phenobarbital, 3MC and PCB do not increase serum TSH levels or produce thyroid follicular cell hyperplasia (Liu et al., 1995; Hood et al., 1995). These findings support the overall hypothesis that UDP-GT inducers can adversely affect the thyroid gland by a secondary mechanism, but this applies only to those UDP-GT inducers that increase serum TSH in addition to reducing serum $T_4$.

There is no convincing evidence that humans treated with drugs or exposed to chemicals that induce hepatic microsomal enzymes are at increased risk for the development of thyroid cancer (Curran and DeGroot, 1991). In a study on the effects of microsomal enzyme-inducing compounds on thyroid hormone metabolism in normal healthy adults, phenobarbital (100 mg daily for 14 days) did not affect the serum $T_4$, $T_3$, or TSH levels (Ohnhaus et al., 1981). A decrease in serum $T_4$ levels was observed after treatment with either a combination of phenobarbital plus rifampicin or a combination of phenobarbital plus antipyrine; however, these treatments had no effect on serum $T_3$ or TSH levels (Ohnhaus and Studer, 1983). Epidemiological studies of patients treated with therapeutic doses of phenobarbital have reported no increase in risk for the development of thyroid neoplasia (Clemmesen et al., 1974; Clemmesen and Hualgrim-Jensen, 1977, 1978, 1981; White et al., 1979; Friedman, 1981; Shirts et al., 1986; Olsen et al., 1989). Highly sensitive assays for thyroid and pituitary hormones are readily available in a clinical setting, to monitor circulating hormone levels in patients exposed to chemicals potentially disruptive of pituitary-thyroid axis homeostasis.

Likewise, there is no substantive evidence that humans treated with drugs or exposed to chemicals that induce hepatic microsomal enzymes are at increased risk for the development of liver cancer. This is best exemplified by the extensive epidemiological information on the clinical use of phenobarbital. Phenobarbital has been used clinically as an anticonvulsant for more than 80 years. Relatively high microsomal enzyme-inducing doses have been used chronically, sometimes for lifetime exposures, to control seizure activity in human beings. A study of over 8000 patients admitted to a Danish epilepsy center from 1933 to 1962 revealed no evidence for an increased incidence of hepatic tumors in phenobarbital-treated humans when patients receiving thorotrast, a known human liver carcinogen, were excluded (Clemmesen and Hjalgrim-Jensen, 1978). A more recent follow-up report on this patient population confirmed and extended this observation (Clemmesen and Hjalgrim-Jensen, 1981; Olsen et al., 1989). The results of two other smaller studies (2099 epileptics and 959 epileptics) also revealed no hepatic tumors in patients treated with phenobarbital (White et al., 1979).

## Chemical Inhibition of 5′-Monodeiodinase and Thyroid Tumors

FD&C Red No. 3 (erythrosine) is an example of a well-characterized xenobiotic that results in perturbations of thyroid function in rodents and in long-term studies is associated with an increased incidence of benign thyroid tumors. Red No. 3 is a widely used color additive in foods, cosmetics, and pharmaceuticals. A chronic toxicity/carcinogenicity study revealed that male Sprague-Dawley rats fed a 4 percent dietary concentration of Red No. 3 beginning *in utero* and extending over their lifetime (30 months) developed a 22 percent incidence of thyroid adenomas derived from follicular cells compared to 1.5 percent in control rats and a historical incidence of 1.8 percent for this strain (Borzelleca et al., 1987; Capen, 1989) (Fig. 21-3). There was no significant increase in follicular cell adenomas in the lower dose groups of male rats or an increase in malignant thyroid follicular cell tumors. Female rats fed similar amounts of the color did not develop a significant

Histopathologic Evaluation of Thyroid Follicular Cells (FC) from Male Sprague-Dawley Rats Fed FD&C Red No. 3

| | Original Study | | | | | High-Dose Study | |
|---|---|---|---|---|---|---|---|
| Groups | $I_A$ | $I_B$ | II | III | IV | $I_C$ | V |
| Red No. 3 (%) (mg/kg/day) | 0 — | 0 — | 0.1 (49) | 0.5 (251) | 1.0 (507) | 0 — | 4.0 (2.464) |
| F.C. Adenoma (%) | 0 | 0 | 0 | 2.9 | 1.5 | 1.5 | 21.8 |
| F.C. Carcinoma (%) | 0 | 0 | 4.5 | 1.5 | 4.4 | 2.9 | 4.4 |
| Cystic follicular hyperplasia (%) | 2.9 | 1.5 | 12 | 16.2 | 7.3 | 0 | 23.2 |
| Diffuse or focal F.C. hyperplasia (%) | 1.4 | 0 | 7.5 | 7.4 | 26.1 | 5.8 | 87.0 |
| Follicular cysts (%) | 10 | 14.5 | 9.0 | 11.8 | 11.6 | 2.9 | 14.5 |

***Figure 21–3.*** ***Thyroid lesions in male Sprague-Dawley rats fed varying doses of FD&C Red No. 3 beginning*** **in utero** ***and for a lifetime of 30 months. [From Borzelleca et al. (1987).]***

increase in either benign or malignant thyroid tumors. Feeding of the color at the high dose (4 percent) level provided male rats with 2464 mg/kg of Red No. 3 daily; by comparison human consumption in the United States is estimated to be 0.023 mg/kg/day.

The results of mechanistic studies with FD&C Red No. 3 have suggested that a primary (direct) action on the thyroid is unlikely to result from: (1) failure of the color ($^{14}C$-labeled) to accumulate in the gland, (2) negative genotoxicity and mutagenicity assays, (3) lack of an oncogenic response in mice and gerbils, (4) a failure to promote thyroid tumor development at dietary concentrations of 1.0 percent or less in male and female rats (Capen, 1989), and (5) no increased tumor development in other organs. Investigations with radiolabeled compound have demonstrated that the color does not accumulate in the thyroid glands of rats following the feeding of either 0.5 percent or 4.0 percent FD&C Red No. 3 for 1 week prior to the oral dose of $^{14}C$-labeled material.

Mechanistic investigations with FD&C Red No. 3 included, among others, a 60-day study of male Sprague-Dawley rats fed either 4 percent (high dose) or 0.25 percent (low dose) Red No. 3 compared to controls, whose food was without the color, in order to determine the effects of the color on thyroid hormone economy. The experimental design of the study was to sacrifice groups of rats (n = 20 rats/interval and dose) fed Red No. 3 and their control groups after 0, 3, 7, 10, 14, 21, 30, and 60 days.

A consistent effect of Red No. 3 on thyroid hormone economy was the striking increase in serum reverse $T_3$ (Fig. 21-4). In the rats fed high doses, reverse $T_3$ was increased at all intervals compared to controls and this also held for rats killed at 10, 14, and 21 days in the low-dose group. The mechanisms responsible for the increased serum reverse $T_3$ appear to be, first, substrate ($T_4$) accumulation due to 5′-monodeiodinase inhibition with subsequent conversion to reverse $T_3$ rather than active $T_3$; and,

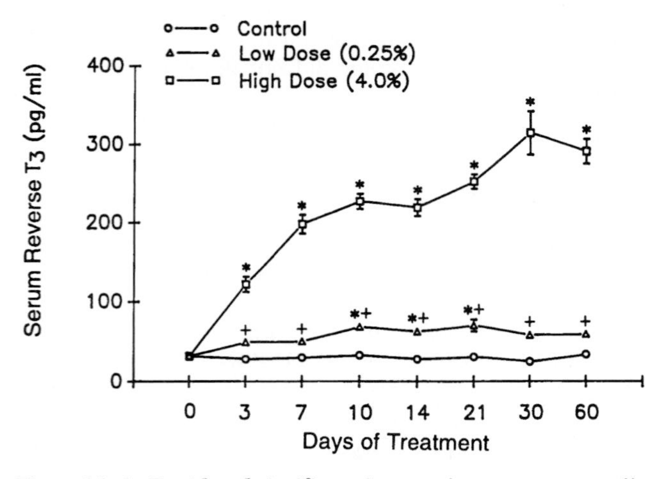


*Figure 21–4. Rapid and significant increase in serum reverse triiodothyronine (rT₃) levels in Sprague-Dawley rats (N = 20 per group and interval) administered a high (4%) and low (0.25%) dose of FD&C Red No. 3.*

The significant increase in $rT_3$ was detected at the initial interval of 3 days and persisted during the 60-day experiment in the high-dose group. (Courtesy of the Certified Color Manufacturers Association, Inc., and Dr. L.E. Braverman and Dr. W.J. DeVito, University of Massachusetts Medical School.)

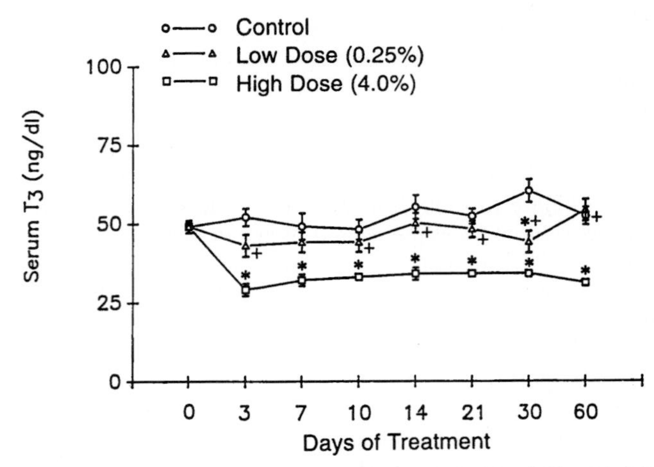


*Figure 21–5. Changes in serum triiodothyronine ($T_3$) following administration of a high (4%) and low (0.25%) dose of FD&C Red No. 3 in the diet to Sprague-Dawley rats. (Courtesy of the Certified Color Manufacturers Association, Inc., and Dr. L.E. Braverman and Dr. W.J. DeVito, University of Massachusetts Medical School.)*

second, reverse $T_3$ accumulation due to 5′-monodeiodinase inhibition resulting in an inability to degrade reverse $T_3$ further to di-iodothyronine ($T_2$). Serum tri-iodothyronine ($T_3$) was decreased significantly at all intervals in rats of the high-dose group compared to interval controls (Fig. 21-5). The mechanism responsible for the reduced serum $T_3$ following feeding of Red No. 3 was decreased monodeiodination of $T_4$ due to an inhibition of the 5′-monodeiodinase by the color.

Serum TSH was increased significantly at all intervals in rats of the high-dose (4 percent) group compared to controls. Rats fed 0.25% Red No. 3 had increased serum TSH only at days 21, 30, and 60 (Fig. 21-6). The mechanism responsible for the increased serum TSH following ingestion of Red No. 3 was a compensatory response by the pituitary gland to the low circulating levels of $T_3$ that resulted from an inhibition of the 5′-monodeiodinase. Serum $T_4$ also was increased significantly at all intervals in rats fed 4% Red No. 3 compared to controls

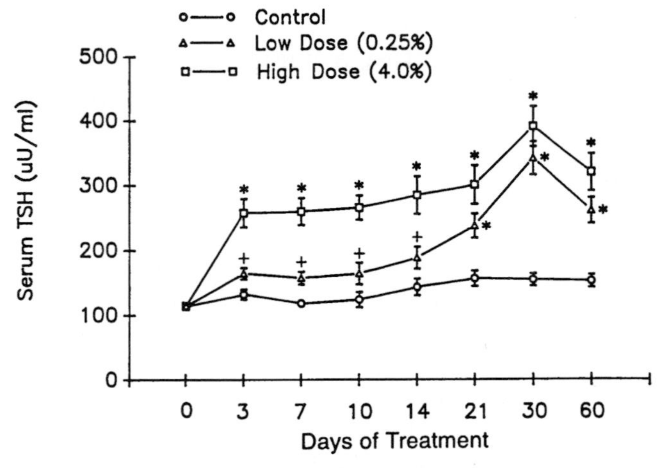


*Figure 21–6. Changes in serum thyroid stimulating hormone (TSH) following administration of a high (4%) and low (0.25%) dose of FD&C Red No. 3 in the diet to Sprague-Dawley rats. (Courtesy of the Certified Color Manufacturers Association, Inc., and Dr. L.E. Braverman and Dr. W.J. DeVito, University of Massachusetts Medical School.)*

(Fig. 21-7). The mechanism responsible for the increased serum $T_4$ was, first, accumulation due to an inability to monodeiodinate $T_4$ to $T_3$ in the liver and kidney from the inhibition of 5′-monodeiodinase by the color; and, second, TSH stimulation of increased $T_4$ production by the thyroid gland.

$^{125}$I-labeled $T_4$ metabolism was significantly altered in liver homogenates prepared from rats fed 4% FD&C Red No. 3. Degradation of labeled $T_4$ was decreased to approximately 40 percent of the values in control homogenates (Fig. 21-8). This was associated with a 75 percent decrease in percent generation of $^{125}$I and an approximately 80 percent decrease in percent generation of $^{125}$I-labeled $T_3$ from radiolabeled $T_4$ substrate. These mechanistic investigations suggested that the color results in a perturbation of thyroid hormone economy in rodents by inhibiting the 5′-monodeiodinase in the liver, resulting in long-term stimulation of follicular cells by TSH, which over their lifetime predisposed to an increased incidence of thyroid tumors (Capen and Martin, 1989; Borzelleca et al., 1987). The color tested negative in standard genotoxic and mutagenic assays, and it did not increase the incidence of tumors in other organs.

Morphometric evaluation was performed on thyroid glands from all rats at each interval during the 60-day study. Four levels of exposure of rat thyroid to Red No. 3 were evaluated, with 25 measurements from each rat. The direct measurements included the diameter of thyroid follicles, area of follicular colloid, and height of follicular cells. Thyroid follicular diameter was decreased significantly in both low- and high-dose groups at 3, 7, 10, and 14 days compared to interval controls. The area of follicular colloid generally reflected the decrease in thyroid follicular diameter and was decreased significantly at days 3 and 10 in high-dose rats and days 7 and 10 in the low-dose group compared to interval controls. These reductions in thyroid follicular diameter and colloid area were consistent with morphological changes expected in response to an increased serum TSH concentration.

Thyroid follicular height was increased significantly only after feeding FD&C Red No. 3 for 60 days in both the high- and low-dose groups compared to interval controls. The ab-

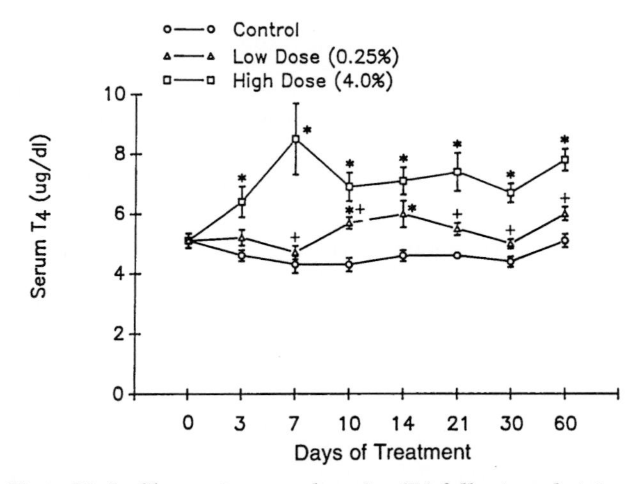


*Figure 21–7. Changes in serum thyroxine ($T_4$) following administration of a high (4%) and low (0.25%) dose of FD&C Red No. 3 in the diet to Sprague-Dawley rats. (Courtesy of the Certified Color Manufacturers Association, Inc., and Dr. L.E. Braverman and Dr. W.J. DeVito, University of Massachusetts Medical School.)*

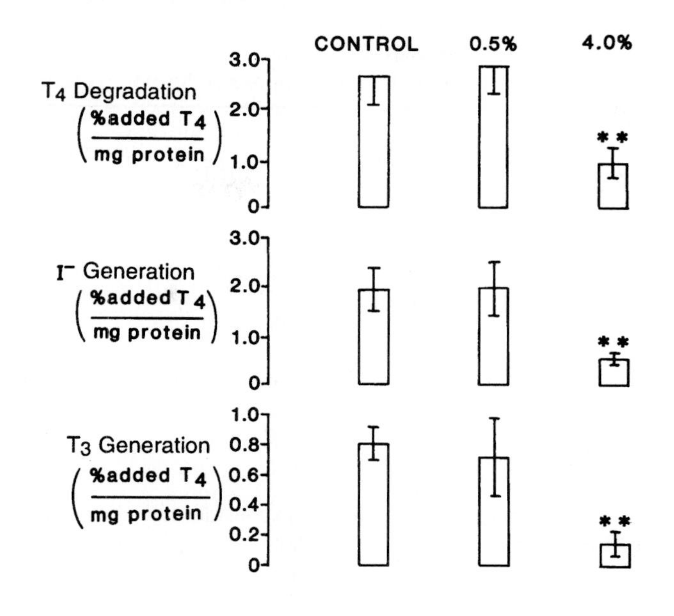


*Figure 21–8. Effects of dietary FD&C Red No. 3 on the hepatic metabolism of $^{125}$I-labeled thyroxine in male Sprague-Dawley rats fed diets containing 0.5 and 4.0% color compared to controls. (Courtesy of the Certified Color Manufacturers Association, Inc., and the late Sidney H. Ingbar, M.D.)*

sence of morphometric evidence of follicular cell hypertrophy at the shorter intervals was consistent with the modest increase (+5.8 percent) in thyroid gland:body weight ratio after this relatively short exposure to the color. The lack of follicular cell hypertrophy at the shorter intervals of feeding Red No. 3 in rats with severalfold elevations in serum TSH levels may be related, in part, to the high iodine content (58 percent of molecular weight) interfering with the receptor-mediated response of thyroid follicular cells to TSH. The thyroid responsiveness to TSH is known to vary inversely with iodine content (Ingbar, 1972; Lamas and Ingbar, 1978). Thyroid glands of rats fed FD&C Red No. 3 would be exposed to an increased iodine concentration primarily from sodium iodide contamination of the color and, to a lesser extent, from metabolism of the compound and release of iodide.

## Species Differences in Thyroid Hormone Economy

Long-term perturbations of the pituitary-thyroid axis by various xenobiotics or physiological alterations (e.g., iodine deficiency, partial thyroidectomy, and natural goitrogens in food) are more likely to predispose the laboratory rat to a higher incidence of proliferative lesions (e.g., hyperplasia and benign tumors [adenomas] of follicular cells) in response to chronic TSH stimulation than in the human thyroid (Capen and Martin, 1989; Curran and DeGroot, 1991). This is particularly true in the male rat which has higher circulating levels of TSH than in females. The greater sensitivity of the rodent thyroid to derangement by drugs, chemicals, and physiological perturbations also is related to the shorter plasma half-life of thyroxine $T_4$ in rats than in humans due to the considerable differences in the transport proteins for thyroid hormones between these species (Döhler et al., 1979).

**Table 21–1**
**Thyroxine ($T_4$) Binding to Serum Proteins in Selected Vertebrate Species**

| SPECIES | $T_4$-BINDING GLOBULIN | POSTALBUMIN | ALBUMIN | PREALBUMIN |
|---|---|---|---|---|
| Human being | ++* | — | ++ | + |
| Monkey | ++ | — | ++ | + |
| Dog | +* | — | ++ | — |
| Mouse | —* | ++ | ++ | — |
| Rat | — | + | ++ | + |
| Chicken | — | — | ++ | — |

* +, ++, Degree of $T_4$ binding to serum proteins; —, Absence of binding of $T_4$ to serum proteins.
From Döhler et al. (1979).

The plasma $T_4$ half-life in rats is considerably shorter (12 to 24 h) than in humans (5 to 9 days). In human beings and monkeys circulating $T_4$ is bound primarily to thyroxine-binding globulin (TBG), but this high-affinity binding protein is not present in rodents, birds, amphibians or fish (Table 21-1).

The binding affinity of TBG for $T_4$ is approximately one thousand times higher than for prealbumin. The percent of unbound active $T_4$ is lower in species with high levels of TBG than in animals in which $T_4$ binding is limited to albumin and prealbumin. Therefore, a rat without a functional thyroid requires about 10 times more $T_4$ (20 $\mu$g/kg body weight) for full substitution than an adult human (2.2 $\mu$g/kg body weight). Tri-iodothyronine ($T_3$) is transported bound to TBG and albumin in human beings, monkey, and dog but only to albumin in mouse, rat, and chicken (Table 21-2). In general, $T_3$ is bound less avidly to transport proteins than $T_4$, resulting in a faster turnover and shorter plasma half-life in most species. These differences in plasma half-life of thyroid hormones and binding to transport proteins between rats and human beings may be one factor in the greater sensitivity of the rat thyroid to developing hyperplastic and/or neoplastic nodules in response to chronic TSH stimulation.

Thyroid-stimulating hormone levels are higher in male than female rats and castration decreases both the baseline serum TSH and response to thyrotropin-releasing hormone (TRH) injection. Follicular cell height often is higher in male than in female rats in response to the greater circulating TSH levels. The administration of exogenous testosterone to castrated male rats restores the TSH level to that of intact rats. Malignant thyroid tumors (carcinomas or "cancer") develop at a higher incidence following irradiation in males than females (2:1) and castration of irradiated male rats decreases the incidence to that of intact irradiated female rats. Testosterone replacement to castrated male rats restores the incidence of irradiation-induced thyroid carcinomas in proportion to the dose of testosterone and, similarly, serum TSH levels increase proportionally to the dose of replacement hormone. Likewise, higher incidence of follicular cell hyperplasia and neoplasia has been reported in males compared to female rats following the administration of a wide variety of drugs and chemicals in chronic toxicity/carcinogenicity testing.

There also are marked species differences in the sensitivity of the functionally important peroxidase enzyme to inhibition by xenobiotics. Thioamides (e.g., sulfonamides) and other chemicals can selectively inhibit the thyroperoxidase and significantly interfere with the iodination of tyrosyl residues incorporated in the thyroglobulin molecule, thereby, disrupting the orderly synthesis of $T_4$ and $T_3$. A number of studies have shown that the long-term administration of sulfonamides results in the development of thyroid nodules frequently in the sensitive species (such as the rat, dog, and mouse) but not in species resistant (e.g., monkey, guinea pig, chicken, and human beings) to the inhibition of peroxidase in follicular cells.

## THE TESTIS

Leydig (interstitial) cell tumors are one of the more frequently occurring endocrine tumors in rodents in chronic toxicity/car-

**Table 21–2**
**Triiodothyronine ($T_3$) Binding to Serum Proteins in Selected Vertebrate Species**

| SPECIES | $T_4$-BINDING GLOBULIN | POSTALBUMIN | ALBUMIN | PREALBUMIN |
|---|---|---|---|---|
| Human being | +* | — | + | — |
| Monkey | + | — | + | — |
| Dog | + | — | + | — |
| Mouse | —* | + | + | — |
| Rat | — | — | + | — |
| Chicken | — | — | + | — |

+, ++, Degree of $T_3$ binding to serum proteins; —, Absence of binding of $T_3$ to serum proteins.
From Döhler et al. (1979).

cinogenicity studies, and a great deal of research has been published in the literature investigating their pathogenesis and implications for safety assessment. Rodent testicular tumors are classified into five general categories including tumors derived from cells of the gonadal stroma, neoplasms of germ cell origin, tumors derived from adnexal structures or serous membranes, and, lastly, a group of tumors derived from the supporting connective tissues and vessels of the testis.

Neoplasms of the gonadal stroma include benign and malignant tumors derived from Leydig (interstitial) cells, Sertoli cells of the seminiferous tubules, as well as a rare mixed tumor with an admixture of both cell types. The Leydig cell tumor is easily the most common tumor developing in the rodent testis and frequently presents a problem in separating between focal hyperplasia and early neoplastic growth (i.e., adenoma formation).

The incidence of Leydig cell tumors in old rats varies considerably depending upon the strain. In general, Sprague-Dawley, Osborne-Mendel, and Brown-Norway strains have a much lower incidence than other strains frequently used in chronic toxicity/carcinogenicity studies, including the Fischer 344 and Wistar strains. The spontaneous incidence of Leydig cell tumors in three different strains of rats is illustrated in Fig. 21-9 (Bär, 1992). The actual incidence of Leydig cell tumors in old rats is lowest in Sprague-Dawley, highly variable in Wistar rats, and highest in Fischer rats (in which the incidence at 2 years of age often approaches 100 percent). The specific numerical incidence of benign Leydig cell tumors in rats also will vary considerably depending upon the histological criteria

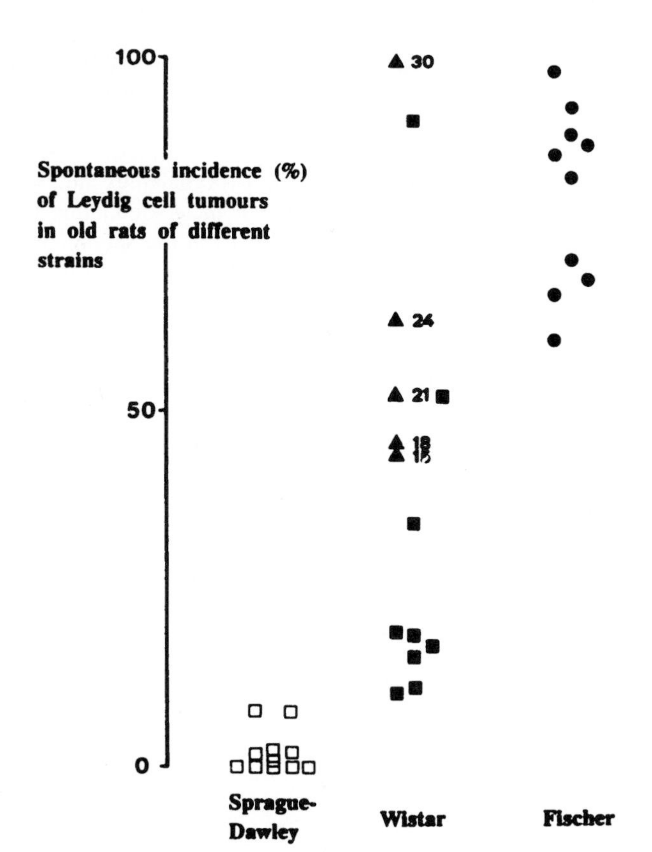


*Figure 21–9. Spontaneous incidence of Leydig cell tumors of the testis in Sprague-Dawley, Wistar, and Fischer rats. [From Bär (1992).]*

used by the pathologist in the separation of focal hyperplasia from adenomas.

In comparison to rodents, the incidence of Leydig cell tumors in human patients is extremely rare, something on the order of one in five million with age peaks at approximately 30 and 60 years. Ninety or more percent of Leydig cell tumors in humans are benign and some appear to be endocrinologically active and associated clinically with gynecomastia.

## Pathology of Leydig (Interstitial) Cell Tumors

Before summarizing the pathology of focal proliferative lesions of Leydig cells, a few points should be made about the importance of standardized sectioning methods for the complete evaluation of the rodent testis. It is not unusual to have less than optimal sections to evaluate, due either to a lack of a consistent plane of section or to inadequate fixation. The goal should be to include the largest testicular area containing all anatomic features on a mid-sagittal section along the long axis of the testis to include spermatic vessels, attachment sites of the epididymis, tubulus rectus, and intratesticular rete testis. It is also important to emphasize the need to cut the thick outer covering, or tunica albuginea, of the testis at several points prior to immersion in the fixative, in order to permit more rapid penetration of the formalin or other fixing solution.

The major issue in the pathology of focal proliferative lesions of Leydig cells in the rodent testis is the accurate and consistent separation of focal hyperplasia from benign tumors (adenomas) that possess autonomous growth. Most pathologists agree that the separation of focal hyperplasia from adenomas derived from Leydig cells is arbitrary and often based primarily on the size of the focal lesion, since cytologic features usually are similar between focal hyperplastic and benign neoplastic lesions derived from Leydig cells.

In the multistage model of carcinogenesis, proliferative lesions are designated as beginning with hyperplasia, often progressing to benign tumors (adenomas), and infrequently a few assume malignant potential and form carcinomas ("cancer") (Fig. 21-10). Although we often apply this terminology to focal proliferative lesions in rodent endocrine tissues for convenience and standardization, it is important to understand that the separation, especially between focal hyperplasia and adenoma, is less than precise. It is important to emphasize that focal proliferative lesions in rodent endocrine tissues, includ-

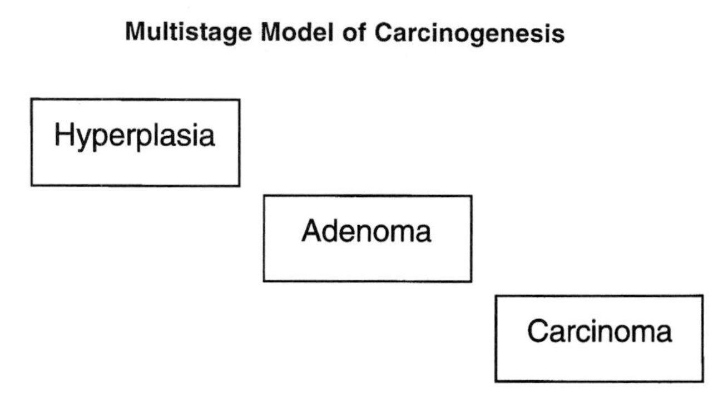


*Figure 21–10. Multistage model of carcinogenesis of proliferative lesions in endocrine tissues of rodents.*

ing Leydig cells, adrenal medullary cells, thyroid follicular and C-cells, among others, represent a morphological continuum that begins with hyperplasia and progresses often but not always to the formation of adenomas that grow autonomously and only occasionally undergo a malignant transformation to form carcinomas ("cancer") (Fig. 21-11).

The National Toxicology Program (NTP), in an attempt to standardize the classification of focal proliferative lesions of Leydig cells between studies with different xenobiotic chemicals and different testing laboratories, established the following diagnostic criteria (Boorman, 1987): (1) Hyperplasia was defined as a focal collection of Leydig cells with little atypia and a diameter of less than 1 seminiferous tubule. (2) An adenoma was defined as a mass of Leydig cells larger in diameter than 1 seminiferous tubule with some cellular atypia and compression of adjacent tubules. (3) It was recognized that the separation was arbitrary since at that time little was known about the biological behavior of these lesions in rodents.

A more contemporary set of diagnostic criteria for focal proliferative lesions of Leydig cells has been published recently by the Society of Toxicologic Pathologists (STP). Recognizing that many small focal proliferative lesions of Leydig cells (i.e., between 1–3 tubule diameters) will regress following removal of the inciting stimulus, they recommend the diagnosis of Leydig cell adenoma be used for a mass of interstitial cells equal to or greater than the diameter of three adjacent seminiferous tubules plus one or more of the following criteria: symmetrical peripheral compression of adjacent tubules, evidence of cellular pleomorphism or an increase in the nuclear:cytoplasmic ratio, an endocrine sinusoidal vascular network, increased mitotic activity, or coalescence of adjacent cell masses.

Leydig cell neoplasms in laboratory rats rarely undergo malignant transformation with progression to the development of carcinomas ("cancer"). Histological features of malignancy include invasion into the epididymus, spermatic cord, or tunica albuginea. The most definitive criteria of malignancy is the demonstration of metastases in extratesticular sites. Leydig cell carinomas are large and often distort the overall contour of the affected testis with extensive areas of both hemorrhage and necrosis. The cytology of Leydig cell carcinomas usually is more pleomorphic than with adenomas consisting of an admixture of poorly differentiated cells with an increased nuclear:cytoplasmic ratio and larger, more differentiated cells with an abundant vacuolated eosinophilic cytoplasmic area. The frequency of mitotic figures may be increased either in focal areas or throughout the Leydig cell carcinomas. The most convincing evidence of malignancy in carcinomas is the establishment of foci of growth outside of the testis, such as multiple foci of tumor cell emboli growing within and distending vessels of the lung.

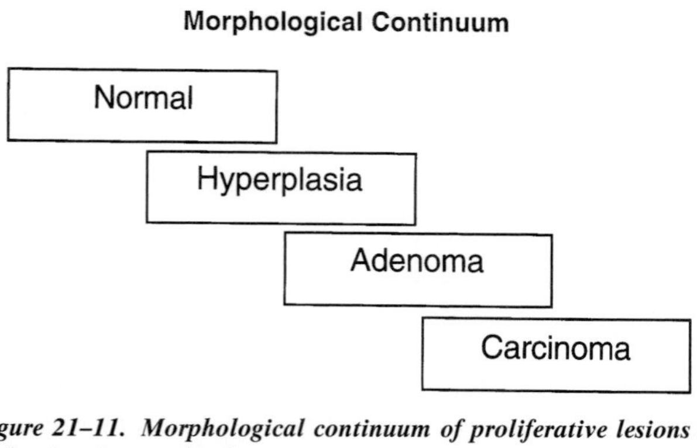

Morphological Continuum

Normal

Hyperplasia

Adenoma

Carcinoma

*Figure 21–11. Morphological continuum of proliferative lesions in endocrine tissues of rodents.*

## Structure and Endocrinologic Regulation of Leydig (Interstitial) Cells

Although the numbers of Leydig cells vary somewhat among different animal species and humans, the basic structural arrangement is similar. In the rat, there are small groups of Leydig cells clustered around blood vessels in the interstitium, between seminiferous tubules with an incomplete layer of endothelial cells around the groups of Leydig cells. In humans, the Leydig cells are present as small groups in the interstitium near blood vessels or in loose connective tissue but without the surrounding layer of endothelial cells. Leydig cells are much more numerous in some animal species, such as the domestic pig. Microscopic evaluation of the normal rat testis reveals the inconspicuous clusters of Leydig cells in the interstitium between the much larger seminiferous tubules composed of spermatogonia and Sertoli cells. The close anatomic association of Leydig cells and interstitial blood vessels permits the rapid exchange of materials between this endocrine cell population and the systemic circulation.

The endocrinological regulation of Leydig cells involves the coordinated activity of the hypothalamus and adenohypophysis (anterior pituitary) with negative feedback control exerted by the blood concentration of gonadal steroids (Fig. 21-12). Hypothalamic gonadotrophin-releasing hormone (GnRH) stimulates the pulsatile release of both luteinizing hormone (LH) and follicle-stimulating hormone (FSH) from gonadotrophs in the adenohypophysis. Luteinizing hormone is the major trophic factor controlling the activity of Leydig cells and the synthesis of testosterone. The blood levels of testosterone exert negative feedback on the hypothalamus and, to a lesser extent, on the adenohypophysis. Follicle-stimulating hormone binds to receptors on Sertoli cells in the seminiferous tubules and, along with the local concentration of testosterone, plays a critical role in spermatogenesis. Testosterone, by controlling GnRH release, is one important regulator of FSH secretion by the pituitary gland. The seminiferous tubules also produce a glycopeptide, designated as inhibin, that exerts negative feedback on the release of FSH by the gonadotrophs.

Leydig cells have a similar ultrastructural appearance as other endocrine cells that synthesize and release steroid hormones. The abundant cytoplasmic area contains numerous mitochondria, abundant profiles of smooth endoplasmic reticulum, prominent Golgi apparatuses associated with lysosomal bodies, and occasional lipofucsin inclusions. However, they lack the hormone-containing secretory granules that are found characteristically in peptide-hormone-secreting endocrine cells.

The hormonal control of testicular function is largely the result of the coordinated activities of LH and FSH from the pituitary gland. LH binds to high-affinity, low-capacity receptors on the surface of Leydig cells and activates adenylate cyclase in the plasma membrane resulting in the generation of an intracellular messenger, cyclic AMP (Fig. 21-13). The cyclic AMP binds to a protein kinase, resulting in the phosphorylation of a specific set of proteins in the cytosol, which increases

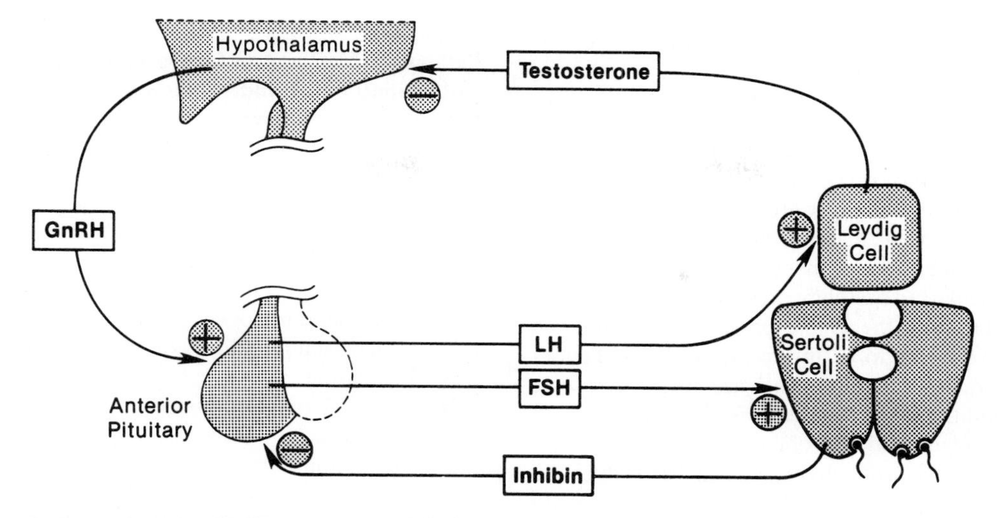


*Figure 21–12. Hypothalamus-anterior pituitary gland-gonad axis in the endocrine control of Leydig and Sertoli cells by luteinizing hormone (LH) and follicle stimulating hormone (FSH). [From Hedge GA, et al:* **Clinical Endocrine Physiology.** *Philadelphia, Saunders (1987, p 25).]*

the conversion of cholesterol to pregnenolone by making more substrate available and increasing the activity of an enzyme that cleaves the side chain of cholesterol. The pregnenolone in Leydig cells is rapidly converted to testosterone, which is released into interstitial blood vessels or taken up by adjacent Sertoli cells. Testosterone in Sertoli's cells binds to nuclear receptors where it increases genomic expression and transcription of mRNAs that direct the synthesis of proteins (e.g., androgen-binding protein and others) involved in spermatogenesis. In the rat, the mitotic phase of gametogenesis can occur without hormonal stimulation but testosterone is necessary for meiosis of spermatocytes to spermatids. FSH is required for the later stages for spermatid maturation to spermatazoa (Fig. 21-13). Once FSH and testosterone initiate spermatogenesis at puberty in the rat, testosterone alone is sufficient to maintain sperm production.

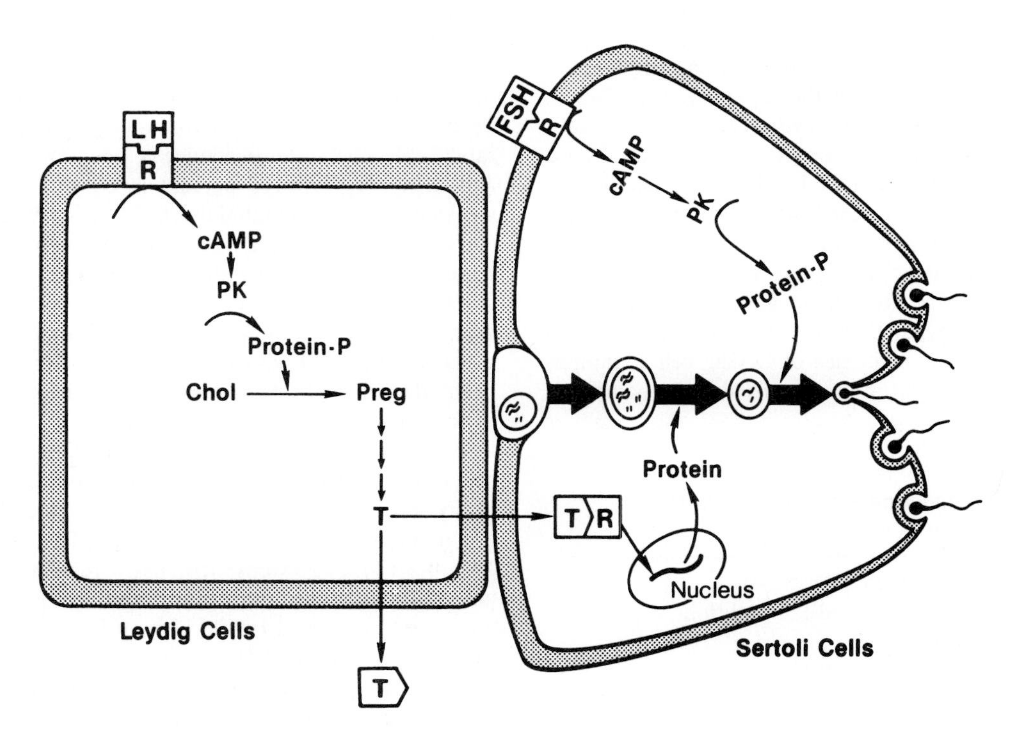


*Figure 21–13. Hormonal control of testicular function.*

Luteinizing hormone (LH) stimulates testosterone (T) release by binding to its receptor (R) and increasing the conversion of cholesterol (chol) to pregnenolone (preg) via a cAMP-protein kinase (PK) cascade. Spermatogenesis (bold arrows) is controlled by both FSH and testosterone acting via Sertoli cells. [From Hedge GA et al: *Clinical Endocrine Physiology*. Philadelphia, Saunders (1987, p 25).]

## Mechanisms of Leydig (Interstitial) Cell Tumor Development

Endocrine organs of rodents, including the testis, pituitary gland, thyroid follicular and C cells, and adrenal medulla among others, frequently undergo proliferative changes with advancing age and following chronic exposure to large doses of xenobiotic chemicals. In addition, it should be emphasized that the "sensitivity" of rodent endocrine tissues appears to be increasing over time, particularly if one compares data generated in the 1970s to that gathered in the 1990s, for the same compound (Table 21-3). This appears to be the result of several factors, including (1) animal husbandry practices, such as specific pathogen-free conditions, that result in a greater survival for 2 years, high body weight, and immobility; and (2) the genetic selection process for high productivity and rapid growth.

Pathogenic mechanisms reported in the literature to be important in the development of proliferative lesions of Leydig cells include irradiation, the species and strain differences mentioned previously, and exposure to certain chemicals such as cadmium salts and 2-acetoaminofluorene (Prentice and Meikle, 1995) (Table 21-4). Other pathogenic mechanisms include physiological perturbations such as cryptorchidism, a compromised blood supply to the testis, or heterotransplantation into the spleen. Hormonal imbalances also are important factors in the development of focal proliferative lesions of Leydig cells, including increased estrogenic steroids in mice and hamsters and elevated pituitary gonadotrophins, especially LH in rats (Table 21-4). Chronic exposure to chemicals with antiandrogenic activity, such as procymidone due to binding to the androgen receptor, increases circulating levels of LH and results in stimulation of Leydig cells leading to an increased incidence of hyperplasia and adenomas in rats (Murakami et al., 1995).

Data from several studies in the recent literature emphasize the importance of several of these pathogenetic factors in the frequent development of Leydig cell tumors in rats. Thurman and colleagues (1994) reported the effects of food restriction on the development of Leydig cell adenomas in the high incidence strain of Fischer 344 rats (Table 21-5). Beginning at 13 weeks of age, rats were either continued on an ad libitum feeding or they were food-restricted 40 percent (NIH-31 diet with 1.67× fat soluble and B vitamins) over their lifetime until they died or became moribund due to spontaneous disease. The incidence of Leydig cell adenomas was decreased to 19 percent in food-restricted rats compared

**Table 21–3**
**Changes in Rodent Endocrine Sensitivity Over Time (1970s–1990s)**

1. Animal husbandry practices
   - Specific pathogen-free (SPF) conditions
     —greater survival to 2 years+
   - High body weight (obesity)
   - Immobility
2. Genetic selection process
   - High productivity
     —Large litters
     —High lactation yield
   - Rapid growth

**Table 21–4**
**Pathogenic Mechanisms for Development of Leydig (Interstitial) Cell Proliferative Lesions in Rodents**

- Physiological Perturbations
  - Cryptorchidism
  - Compromised blood supply
  - Heterotransplantation (spleen)
- Hormonal Imbalances
  - Decreased testosterone
  - Increased estrogens (mice, hamsters)
  - Increased pituitatry gonadotropins (e.g., LH)
- Irradiation
- Species/Strain Differences
- Chemicals
  - Cadmium salts
  - 2-Acetoaminofluorene

to 49 percent in the ad-libitum-fed group (Table 21-5). In another group from the food restriction study reported by Thurman and coworkers (1994), rats were periodically removed for serial sacrifice at 6-month intervals. Food restriction resulted in a similar marked reduction in Leydig cell adenomas (23 percent compared to 60 percent in ad-libitum-fed rats) (Table 21-6). Examination of the serially sacrificed F344 rats in this study also demonstrated that feed restriction delayed the onset of development, as well as decreasing the incidence of Leydig cell adenomas compared to the ad-libitum-fed group (Table 21-7). For example, at the 30-month sacrifice, only 17 percent of feed-restricted F344 rats had developed Leydig cell adenomas compared to 100 percent in the ad libitum group.

Investigations reported by Chatani and associates (1990) documented the importance of hormonal imbalances on the incidence of Leydig cell adenomas and hyperplasia in Fischer rats (Table 21-8). The incidence of adenomas was 70 percent and of hyperplasia 100 percent in control rats killed at 70 weeks of age. In rats administered testosterone for 28 weeks (by silastic tubes implanted subcutaneously at 42 weeks of age), the incidence of Leydig cell adenomas and hyperplasias was decreased to 0 percent for both at 70 weeks of age. This dramatic reduction in the incidence of focal proliferative lesions of Leydig cells was associated with a significant lowering in circulating levels of LH, through negative feedback exerted by testosterone on the pituitary gland.

The important studies reported by Chatani and coworkers (1990) also demonstrated that hormones other than testosterone could markedly decrease the development of Leydig cell adenomas in F344 rats (Table 21-9). The administration of estradiol-17$\beta$ for 28 weeks (by silastic tubes implanted subcutaneously) decreased the incidence of Leydig cell adenomas to 0 percent (compared to 100 percent in controls) and significantly reduced serum LH, due to negative feedback control on the pituitary gland. An LH-releasing hormone agonist administered continuously for 28 weeks (injection of microcapsules every 4 weeks at a dose of 5 mg/2 ml/kg/4 weeks) also decreased the incidence of Leydig cell adenomas to 0 percent and significantly decreased circulating LH levels, most likely a result of the known-down regulation of LH-RH receptors on pituitary gonadotrophs (Table 21-9).

**Table 21–5**
**Effect of Food Restriction on the Development of Interstitial (Leydig) Cell Adenomas in F344 Rats***

| | | INTERSTITIAL CELL ADENOMAS | |
|---|---|---|---|
| FEEDING | RATS (NO.)* | NO. | % |
| Ad libitum | 49 | 24 | 49 |
| Food restricted (40%) | 52 | 10 | 19 |

* Lifetime study without periodic sacrifice removals (died from spontaneous disease).
From Thurman et al. (1994).

**Table 21–6**
**Effect of Food Restriction on the Development of Interstitial (Leydig) Cell Adenomas in F344 Rats***

| | | INTERSTITIAL CELL ADENOMAS | |
|---|---|---|---|
| FEEDING | RATS (NO.)* | NO. | % |
| Ad libitum | 98 | 59 | 60 |
| Food restricted (40%) | 112 | 26 | 23 |

* Lifetime study with periodic removal of serially sacrificed rats (died from spontaneous disease).
From Thurman et al. (1994).

The studies of Bartke and colleagues (1985) demonstrated that hyperprolactinemia also markedly decreased the incidence of Leydig cell adenomas in Fischer rats (Table 21-10). Pituitaries transplanted beneath the renal capsule (four per rat) resulted in a chronic elevation of circulating prolactin levels, owing, most likely, to the lack of dopamine inhibition of prolactin secretion, which occurs when the pituitary gland is in its normal anatomic location in close proximity to the hypothalamus. In this interesting experiment, 83 percent of sham-operated rats developed Leydig cell adenomas at 21 to 24 months of age, whereas 0 percent of rats developed tumors in animals with ectopic pituitaries and elevated serum prolactin levels.

The administration of a calcium-channel blocker (SVZ 200-110) at high doses (62.5 mg/kg/day for 2 years) significantly increased the incidence of Leydig cell adenomas in Sprague-Dawley rats. Endocrinological studies demonstrated that increased serum levels of LH and FSH were present only after 52 and 66 weeks, respectively, and persisted to week 104 for LH. This compound is unusual in that most xenobiotic chemicals that cause hormonal imbalances result in earlier significant changes in circulating hormone levels.

**Table 21–7**
**Effects of Food Restriction on the Development of Interstitial (Leydig) Cell Adenoma (ICA) in F344 Rats at Different Ages**

| | ICA [TUMORS/NO. RATS (%)] | |
|---|---|---|
| AGE AT SACRIFICE (MOS.) | AD LIBITUM | FEED-RESTRICTED (40%) |
| 12 | 0/12 (0) | 0/12 (0) |
| 18 | 5/12 (42) | 0/12 (0) |
| 24 | 10/12 (83) | 1/12 (8) |
| 30 | 9/9 (100) | 2/12 (17) |
| 36 | — | 4/9 (44) |

From Thurman et al. (1994).

Another important mechanism by which xenobiotic chemicals increase the incidence of Leydig cell tumors in rats is by inhibition of testosterone synthesis by cells in the testis. For example, lansoprazole is a substituted benzimidzole which inhibits the hydrogen-potassuim ATPase (proton pump) responsible for acid secretion by the parietal cells in the fundic mucosa of the stomach (Fort et al., 1995). The presence of the imidazole moiety in lansoprazole was suggestive of an effect on testosterone synthesis since several imidazole compounds (eg. ketoconazole and miconazole) are known to inhibit testosterone synthesis. Lansoprazole resulted in decreased circulating levels of testosterone, increased levels of LH, and an increased incidence of Leydig cell hyperplasia and benign neoplasia (adenomas) in chronic studies in rats (Fort et al., 1995). The most sensitive site for inhibition of testosterone synthesis by lansoprazole was the transport of cholesterol to the cholesterol side chain cleavage enzyme.

Although several hormonal imbalances result in an increased incidence of Leydig cell tumors in rodents, in human patients several disease conditions associated with chronic elevations in serum LH (including Klinefelter's syndrome and gonadotroph adenomas of the pituitary gland) have not been associated with an increased development of this type of rare testicular tumor.

There are a number of reports in the literature of xenobiotic chemicals (many of which are marketed drugs) that increase the incidence of proliferative lesions of Leydig cells in

**Table 21–8**
**Effect of Aging and Testosterone on the Incidence of Interstitial Cell Adenomas (ICA) and Hyperplasia (ICH) in Fischer 344 Rats**

| TREATMENT (23 WEEKS) | TERMINAL AGE (WEEKS) | ICA % (NO./NO. TESTES) | ICH % TESTES | ICH† (NODULES/ TESTES) | SERUM LH (ng/ml)† |
|---|---|---|---|---|---|
| 0 | 42 | 0 (0/20) | 10 | 0.3 ± 0.8 | 20.9 ± 19.5 |
| 0 | 50 | 0 (0/20) | 95 | 5.0 ± 2.3 | N.D. |
| 0 | 60 | 0 (0/10) | 90 | 8.3 ± 7.0 | 48.7 ± 16.7 |
| 0 | 70 | 70 (14/20) | 100 | 11.1 ± 6.2 | 22.1 ± 8.4 |
| Testosterone+ | 70 | 0 (0/10)* | 0* | 0.0 ± 0.0* | 8.4 ± 8.8* |

† Mean ± S.D.
* $P < 0.05$ compared to controls.
+ Silastic tubes implanted subcutaneously at 42 weeks.
NTP Criteria: ICA greater and ICH less than one normal seminiferous tubule diameter; from Chatani et al. (1990).

**Table 21–9**
**Effect of Testosterone, Estradiol, and LH-RH Agonist on Incidence of Interstitial Cell Adenoma (ICA) in F344 Rats**

| TREATMENT (28 WEEKS) | TERMINAL AGE (WEEKS) | ICA % (NO./NO. TESTES) | SERUM LH (ng/ml)† |
|---|---|---|---|
| Control | 88 | 100 (18/18) | 12.9 ± 11.7 |
| Testosterone+ | 88 | 0 (0/18)* | 1.7 ± 1.6* |
| Estradiol-17$\beta$+ | 88 | 0 (0/18)* | 4.7 ± 2.4* |
| LH-RH Agonist‡ | 88 | 0 (0/16)* | 4.9 ± 3.5* |

† Mean ± SD.
* $P < 0.05$ compared to controls.
+ Silastic tubes implanted subcutaneously.
‡ Injected subcutaneously at 60 weeks of age.
NTP criteria: ICA greater than one normal seminiferous tubule diameter. From Chatani et al. (1990).

**Table 21–10**
**Effect of Hyperprolactinemia from Ectopic Pituitary Transplants on the Incidence of Interstitial Cell Adenoma (ICA) and Testicular/Seminal Vesicle Weights in Fischer 344 Rats**

| RAT GROUP | ICA % (NO./NO. RATS) | TESTES' WEIGHT (gm)‡ | SEMINAL VESICLES' WEIGHT (gm)‡ |
|---|---|---|---|
| Sham-operated | | | |
| With tumors | 83 (20/24) | 4.88 ± 0.22* | 0.55 ± 0.08* |
| Without tumors | 17 (4/24) | 2.66 ± 0.48 | 1.35 ± 0.14 |
| Pituitary-grafted† | | | |
| With tumors | 0 (0/0) | — | — |
| Without tumors | 100 (24/24) | 2.79 ± 0.05 | 1.26 ± 0.07 |

† Pituitary transplants (4/rat) beneath renal capsule or sham-operated at 2–5 mos. of age; terminated at 21–24 mos. of age.
‡ Mean ± SE.
* $P < 0.05$ compared to other two groups.
From Bartke et al. (1985).

**Table 21–11**
**Drugs That Increase the Incidence of Proliferative Lesions of Leydig Cells in Chronic Exposure Studies in Rats**

| NAME | CLINICAL INDICATION | REFERENCE |
|---|---|---|
| Indomethacin | Anti-inflammatory | Roberts et al. (1989) |
| Lactitol | Laxative | Bär (1992) |
| Metronidazole | Antibacterial | Rustia and Shubik (1979) |
| Muselergine | Parkinson's disease | Prentice et al. (1992) |
| Buserelin | Prostatic and breast carcinoma, endometriosis | Donaubauer et al. (1989) |
| Cimetidine | Reduction of gastric acid secretion | PDR (1992) |
| Flutamide | Prostatic carcinoma | PDR (1992) |
| Gemfibrozil | Hypolipidemia | Fitzgerald et al. (1981) |

**Table 21–12**
**Flutamide: Incidence of Interstitial Cell (IC) Adenoma in Sprague-Dawley Rats After Various Dosing Intervals**

| | 1-YEAR DOSING | | | | 1-YEAR DOSING+ 1-YEAR POSTDOSE | | | | 2-YEAR DOSING | | | |
|---|---|---|---|---|---|---|---|---|---|---|---|---|
| DOSE | 0 | 10 | 30 | 50 | 0 | 10 | 30 | 50 | 0 | 10 | 30 | 50 |
| Number/Group | 58 | 57 | 57 | 57 | 52 | 53 | 53 | 53 | 55 | 55 | 55 | 55 |
| IC Adenoma (>1 Tubule) | 0 | 28 | 43 | 40 | 6 | 25 | 23 | 25 | 6 | 50 | 52 | 52 |
| IC Hyperplasia (<1 Tubule) | 6 | 39 | 44 | 48 | 8 | 7 | 10 | 17 | 5 | 12 | 9 | 12 |

Courtesy of Schering Plough Research Institute, Department of Drug Safety and Metabolism, Lafayette, New Jersey.

chronic toxicology/carcinogenicity in rats. These include indomethacin, lactitol, muselergine, cimetidine, gemfibrozil, and flutamide, among several others (Table 21-11).

Flutamide is a potent nonsteroidal, antiandrogen compound that displaces testosterone from specific receptors in target cells and decreases negative feedback on the hypothalamus-pituitary gland, resulting in elevated circulating levels of LH and FSH. The chronic administration of flutamide is known to result in a striking increase in the incidence of Leydig cell adenomas in rats. The Schering-Plough Research Institute's Department of Drug Safety and Metabolism completed an important reversibility study in which Sprague-Dawley rats were administered flutamide daily either for 1 year, 1 year followed by a 1-year recovery period, or continuously for 2 years (Table 21-12). This important study emphasizes the lack of autonomy of many focal proliferative lesions of Leydig cells in rats and their continued dependence upon compound administration for stimulation of growth. There was a reduction in the incidence of Leydig cell adenomas (using the conservative NTP criteria of greater than 1 tubule diameter) in rats administered 3 dose levels of flutamide daily for 1 year followed by a 1-year recovery prior to termination, compared to rats given flutamide for 1 year and immediately evaluated (Table 21-12). Conversely, in rats administered flutamide for 2 years the numbers of adenomas continued to increase until 95 percent of animals in the mid- and high-dose groups (30 and 50 $\mu$g/kg, respectively) had developed Leydig cell tumors. There also was a marked reduction in the incidence of focal hyperplasia (focus less than 1 tubule diameter) after 1 year of recovery, compared to rats terminated immediately following 1 year of flutamide administration, a finding that emphasizes the frequent reversibility of these small proliferative lesions of Leydig cells.

Although a number of xenobiotic chemicals have been reported to increase the incidence of Leydig cell adenomas in chronic studies in rats, similar compounds such as cimetidine, ketoconizole, and certain calcium channel blocking agents have not resulted in an increased incidence of Leydig cell neoplasia in man. In summary, Leydig cell tumors are a frequently occurring tumor in rats, often associated mechanistically with hormonal imbalances; however, they are not an appropriate model for assessing the potential risk to human males of developing this rare testicular tumor.

# THE OVARY

## Ovarian Tumors in Rodents

Ovarian tumors in rodents can be subdivided into five broad categories including epithelial tumors, sex cord-stromal tumors, germ cell tumors, tumors derived from nonspecialized soft tissues of the ovary, and tumors metastatic to the ovary from distant sites. The epithelial tumors of the ovary include cystadenomas and cystadenocarcinomas, tubulostromal adenomas, and mesothelioma. The tubular (or tubulostromal) adenomas are the most important of the ovarian tumors in mice, and they are the tumors whose incidence often is increased by various endocrine perturbations associated with exposure to xenobiotics, senescence, or inherited genic deletion (Murphy and Beamer, 1973). Tubular adenomas are a unique lesion that develops frequently in the mouse ovary, accounting for approximately 25 percent of naturally occurring ovarian tumors in this species (Alison and Morgan, 1987; Rehm et al., 1984). They are uncommon in rats, rare in other animal species, and not recognized in the ovaries of women. In some ovarian tumors of this type in mice, there is an intense proliferation of stromal (interstitial) cells of sex cord origin. These tumors often are designated tubulostromal adenomas or carcinomas to reflect the bimorphic appearance.

The tubulostromal adenomas in mice are composed of numerous tubular profiles derived from the surface epithelium, plus abundant large luteinized stromal cells from the ovarian interstitium. The differences in histological appearance of this type of unique ovarian tumor in mice are interpreted to represent a morphological spectrum with variable contributions from the surface epithelium and sex cord-derived ovarian interstitium rather than being two distinct types of ovarian tumors. The histogenic origin of this unique ovarian tumor in mice has been a controversial topic in the literature but most investigators currently agree that it is derived from the ovarian surface epithelium, with varying contributions from stromal cells of the ovarian interstitium. However, some early reports suggested an origin from the rete ovarii or thecal/granulosal cells of the ovary.

Another important group of ovarian tumors are those derived from the sex cords and/or ovarian stroma. These include the granulosal cell tumors, luteoma, thecoma, Sertoli cell tumor, tubular adenoma (with contributions from ovarian stroma), and undifferentiated sex cord-stromal tumors. The granulosal cell tumor is the most common of this group which, according to Alison and Morgan (1987), accounts for 27 percent of naturally occurring ovarian tumors in mice. Granulosal cell tumors may develop within certain tubular or tubulostromal adenomas following a long-term perturbation of endocrine function associated with genic deletion, irradiation, oocytotoxic chemicals, and neonatal thymectomy (Frith et al., 1981; Li and Gardner, 1949; Hummel, 1954).

## Model Systems for Ovarian Tumorigenesis

Five model systems of ovarian tumorigenesis in mice have been reported in the literature. The first model system identified was the production of ovarian neoplasms by radiation (Furth and Boon, 1947; Gardner, 1950). After acute radiation exposure, the initial change was a rapid loss of oocytes and a destruction of graafian follicles. There was proliferation and down-growth of the ovarian epithelium into the stroma within 10 weeks after radiation exposure. The first ovarian tumors developed approximately 1 year after exposure. The tubular adenomas that develop following radiation often were bilateral, endocrinologically inactive, and not lethal unless they reached a very large size. Some irradiated mice also developed endocrinologically active granulosal cell tumors, which transplantation experiments have shown to be different from the tubular adenomas. Granulosal cell tumors were transplantable into the spleen and often grew rapidly, whereas tubular adenomas grew slowly after transplantation, most successfully in castrated animals.

The second model of ovarian tumorigenesis arose out of the work published by Biskind and Biskind (1944). They transplanted ovaries into the spleen of castrated rats to prevent negative feedback by circulating sex hormones on the hypothalamus and pituitary gland because estrogen is degraded as it circulates through the liver. Transplantation resulted in a rapid loss of ovarian follicles as well as an interference with estrogen feedback on the hypothalamus. Following the loss of graafian follicles, the epithelial covering of the ovary began to proliferate and invaginate into the ovary, with an accompanying increase in stromal tissue that ultimately resulted in the formation of tubular adenomas and, occasionally, granulosal cell tumors (Guthrie, 1957). The presence of a single functioning gonad prevented the development of the proliferative lesions in the ovary, suggesting that the lack of negative feedback from estrogen was necessary for the changes to develop. Administration of exogenous estrogen or testosterone after transplantation completely suppressed development of the proliferative changes in the ovarian cortex.

The third model of ovarian tumorigenesis was described by Marchant (1957, 1960), who reported that ovarian tumors developed in mice exposed to dimethylbenzanthracene. This chemical is a reproductive toxicant that is cytotoxic to oocytes, resulting in the loss of graafian follicles from the ovary. This was followed by a proliferation of the interstitial (stromal) tissue, invaginations of the surface epithelium, and subsequent development of tubular adenomas and occasionally granulosal cell tumors of the ovary (Taguchi et al., 1988). Support for an endocrinological mechanism of hormonal imbalance included the observation that the xenobiotic chemical first must cause sterility, because the presence of a single normal gonad prevented the development of the hyperplastic lesions and tumors of the ovary. The administration of estrogen prevented tumor formation even in sterile mice, and hypophysectomy also prevented the development of ovarian tumors.

The fourth model of ovarian tumorigenesis was described by Nishizuki and associates (1979). They reported that removal of the thymus from neonatal mice resulted in ovarian dysgenesis and the development of ovarian tumors. Thymectomy prior to 7 days of age resulted in an immune-mediated destruction of follicles in the ovary. Because estrogen was not produced by the follicles, these mice also developed hormone-mediated proliferative lesions and ovarian tumors identical to those in the previously described models. After the immune-mediated destruction of follicles, there was a proliferation of the interstitial (stromal) and surface epithelial cells of the ovary, resulting in the formation of tubular adenomas. If the mice survived for longer periods, some animals developed granulosal cell tumors and luteomas in the ovary. Because this model also did not involve exposure to any carcinogen, it is another indication that the prerequisite for ovarian tumor response in mice is the production of sterility, which results in hormonal imbalances that lead to stimulation of the sensitive populations of target cells (Michael et al., 1981).

**Table 21–13**
**NTP Nitrofurantoin Study of Treatment-Related Ovarian Lesions in $B_6C_3F_1$ Mice (50/Group Exposed for 2 Years in Feed)**

| LESION | CONTROL | LOW DOSE (0.13%) | HIGH DOSE (0.25%) |
|---|---|---|---|
| Tubular adenoma | 0 | 0 | 5* |
| Tubulostromal adenoma | 0 | 0 | 4† |
| Benign GCT | 0 | 3 | 2 |
| Malignant GCT | 0 | 0 | 1 |
| Cystadenoma | 2 | 1 | 1 |
| Cysts | 14 | 15 | 10 |
| Abscess | 18 | 0 | 0 |
| Ovarian atrophy | 0 | 49 | 48 |
| Survival at 2 Years | 19 | 37 | 37 |

NTP, National Toxicology Program; GCT, Granulosal cell tumor.
* Trend test positive (P ≤ 0.05).
† Fischer exact test positive (P ≤ 0.05).

## Ovarian Tumors Associated with Feeding Nitrofurantoin

Nitrofurantoin is an example of a chemical that, when fed at high doses to mice for 2 years in a NTP study, increased the incidence of ovarian tumors of the tubular or tubulostromal type (Table 21-13). Nitrofurantoin fed at both low (1300 ppm) and high (2500 ppm) doses to B6C3F1 mice caused sterility due to the destruction of ovarian follicles, leading to hormonal imbalances, which resulted in the development of an increased incidence of this unique type of ovarian tumor.

Mice administered nitrofurantoin had a consistent change in the ovarian cortex, termed *ovarian atrophy*. This lesion was characterized by an absence of graafian follicles, developing ova, and corpora lutea; by focal or diffuse hyperplasia with localized or diffuse down-growth of surface epithelium into the ovary; and by varying numbers of polygonal, often vacuolated, sex cord-derived stromal (interstitial) cells between the tubular profiles. The ovaries were small, had irregular surfaces due to the tubular down-growths into the cortex, and had scattered eosinophilic stromal cells between tubular profiles. In addition, there was a lack of graafian follicles and corpora lutea throughout the ovarian cortex.

The benign ovarian tumors in this study were classified either as tubular adenomas (5 of 50 mice) or as tubulostromal tumors (4 of 50 mice) (Table 21-13). In tubulostromal adenomas, the proliferating stromal (interstitial) cells between the tubules were considered to represent a significant component of the lesion. However, the separation between these two types of proliferating ovarian lesions in mice was not distinct and both appeared to be part of a continuous morphological spectrum. Because all treated mice in the NTP nitrofurantoin feeding study were sterile due to ovarian atrophy, an indirect mechanism secondary to a disruption of endocrine function leading to hormonal imbalances was suggested to explain the development of the ovarian tubular adenomas.

The results of an investigative study demonstrated that nitrofurantoin had an effect on graafian follicles in the ovary of B6C3F1 mice. Female mice of the same strain were fed 350 or 500 mg/kg/day of nitrofurantoin beginning at 7 weeks of age. These levels approximate the low (1300 ppm) and high (2500 ppm) doses used in the NTP study with nitrofurantoin. Ten female mice per group were sacrificed at 4, 8, 13, 17, 43, and 64 weeks of feeding nitrofurantoin. The numbers of follicles were quantified from nitrofurantoin-treated and control mice on serial sections of the ovary. The morphometric data revealed that the numbers of small, medium, and large follicles in nitrofurantoin-treated mice were numerically decreased at 17 weeks compared with controls and were significantly decreased in rats fed 350 and 500 mg/kg/day nitrofurantoin after 43 and 64 weeks (Fig. 21-14). All mice in the treated groups were sterile by 43 weeks of feeding nitrofurantoin.

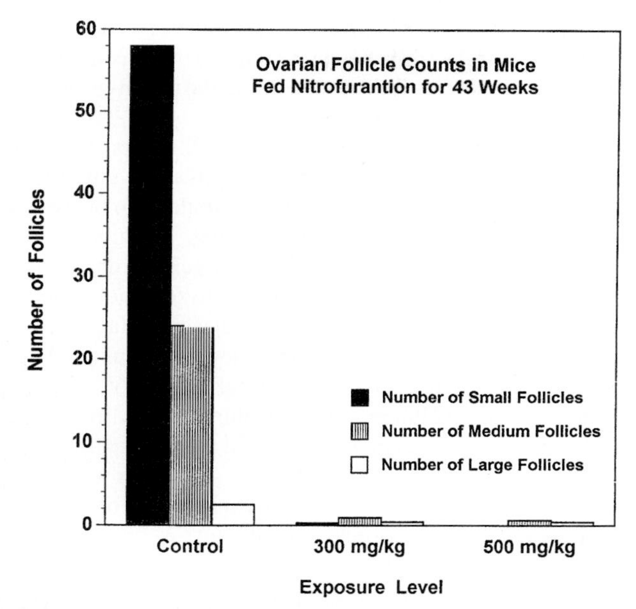


***Figure 21–14. Morphometric evaluation of ovaries of mice following the administration of 350 and 500 mg/kg/day of nitrofurantoin.***

The numbers of small, medium, and large ovarian follicles were numerically decreased after 17 weeks and significantly decreased after 43 and 64 weeks due to a direct action of the nitrofurantoin.

## Ovarian Tumors in Mutant Strains of Mice

**$W^x/W^v$ Strain with Genetic Deletion of Germ Cells in Ovarian Cortex.** In an attempt to arrive at further mechanistic explanations for the development of tubular adenomas in B6C3F1 mice fed high doses of nitrofurantoin, ovaries were evaluated from several mutant mouse strains not exposed to any xenobiotic chemicals but that are known to develop ovarian tumors. In this mutant mouse strain, referred to as $W^x/W^v$, few germ cells migrate into the ovary during development. Murphy (1972) reported that less than 1 percent of the normal complement of oocytes were present in the ovary at 1 day of age and the numbers of graafian follicles decrease progressively until none were present at 13 weeks of age. In this mutant mouse strain ($W^x/W^v$), a mutant allele at the C-kit locus encodes for a defective protein kinase receptor, resulting in an inability to respond to stem cell growth factor encoded by the Steel locus (Witte, 1990; Majumder et al., 1988). A failure of proliferation of primordial germ cells during gonadogenesis leads to the marked reduction of graafian follicles in the ovarian cortex.

Ovaries from mutant mice at age 13 weeks were small, had an irregular surface, were devoid of graafian follicles, and had numerous hyperplastic tubules growing into the cortex. These tubules were lined by a hyperplastic cuboidal epithelium similar to that on the surface of the ovary. Interspersed between the tubular profiles were luteinized stromal cells of the ovarian interstitium with a lightly eosinophilic, often vacuolated, cytoplasm. The proliferative changes observed in the ovary of these mutant ($W^x/W^v$) mice at 13 weeks of age were similar morphologically to the ovarian atrophy lesions in the NTP nitrofurantoin study.

The ovaries of heterozygous controls (+/+) of this strain were larger than in the mutant mice and had a histological appearance similar to normal mouse ovaries. The ovarian cortex in control mice had plentiful graafian follicles with developing ova. The surface epithelium covering the ovary consisted of a single layer of cuboidal cells without the down-growth of tubules into the underlying cortex.

The ovaries of mutant ($W^x/W^v$) mice at 22 weeks of age had a more intense proliferation of surface epithelium either with extensive down-growths of hyperplastic tubules into the cortex or the formation of small tubular adenomas. The tubular adenomas in the mutant ($W^x/W^v$) mice with genetic deletion of graafian follicles but without any exposure to xenobiotic chemicals were composed of proliferating tubules of surface epithelium that replaced much of the ovary. They were similar microscopically to the smaller tubular adenomas in the B6C3F1 mice fed the high dose (2500 ppm) of nitrofurantoin in the 2-year NTP feeding study. Interspersed between the hyperplastic profiles of surface epithelium in the tubular adenomas were scattered luteinized stromal cells with varying degrees of vacuolation of the eosinophilic cytoplasm. In mutant ($W^x/W^v$) mice, age 22 weeks, whose ovaries had been under long-term intense gonadotrophin stimulation, there appeared to be a morphological continuum between ovarian atrophy and tubular adenomas.

At age 20 months, ovaries of the mutant ($W^x/W^v$) mice without any exposure to xenobiotic chemicals consistently had large tubular adenomas that incorporated all of the ovarian parenchyma and greatly enlarged the ovary. These neoplasms were similar histologically to the larger tubular adenomas in the high-dose (2500 ppm) mice of the NTP study. Several of the larger ovarian neoplasms of the 20-month-old mutant mice had evidence of malignancy with invasion of tumor cells through the ovarian capsule into the periovarian tissues, often accompanied by a localized desmoplastic response. Histopathologic evidence of malignancy was not observed in the ovarian tubular adenomas from the high-dose (2500 ppm) female mice in the NTP study. An occasional mutant mouse at 20 months of age also had developed focal areas of hyperplasia of granulosal cells or small granulosal cell tumors.

**Hypogonadal (hpg/hpg) Mice Unable to Synthesize Hypothalamic Gonadotrophin-Releasing Hormone (GnRH).** Mutant hypogonadal mice, designated hpg/hpg, are unable to synthesize normal amounts of hypothalamic GnRH (Tennent and Beamer, 1986). They have low circulating levels of pituitary gonadotrophins, and boast FSH and LH; however, these hypogonadal mice have a normal complement of ovarian follicles (Cattanach et al., 1977).

In the studies of Tennent and Beamer (1986), both genetically normal littermates and hypogonadal (hpg/hpg) mice were irradiated at age 30 days to destroy the oocytes. The irradiated control mice of this strain produced normal amounts of pituitary gonadotrophic hormones and developed ovarian tubular adenomas at age 10 to 15 months. The tumors that developed in the absence of any exposure to xenobiotic chemicals had similar histological characteristics as tubular adenomas in the high-dose (2500 ppm) females of the nitrofurantoin study. They either were small nodules involving only a portion of the ovary or large masses that completely incorporated the affected gonad. They were composed predominantly of tubular profiles, some of which were dilated, with interspersed stromal cells.

The irradiated hypogonadal (hpg/hpg) mice failed to develop tubular adenomas or to have intense hyperplasia of the ovarian surface epithelium and interstitial (stromal) cells, in the absence of GnRH and with low circulating levels of pituitary gonadotrophins. The ovaries of irradiated hypogonadal mice were small and had single- or multiple-layered follicles, without oocytes, scattered throughout the ovary. There also was an absence of stromal cell hypertrophy and hyperplasia, a change frequently observed in ovaries of the irradiated normal littermates.

The experiments reported by Tennent and Beamer (1986) demonstrated that a normal secretion of hypothalamic GnRH and pituitary gonadotrophins was necessary for the intense proliferation of ovarian surface epithelium and stromal cells, leading to the formation of tubular adenomas in mice, which develop subsequent to irradiation-induced loss of ovarian follicles and decreased ability to produce gonadal steroids (especially estradiol-17$\beta$).

A review of studies on mutant mice and the NTP study of nitrofurantoin support an interpretation that the unique intense hyperplasia of ovarian surface epithelium and stromal cells, leading eventually to an increased incidence of tubular adenomas, develops secondary to chronic pituitary gonadotrophic hormone stimulation. Factors that destroy or greatly diminish the numbers of ovarian follicles, such as senescence, genetic deletion of follicles, X-irradiation, drugs and chemicals such as nitrofurantoin, and early thymectomy with the development of autoantibodies to oocytes, are known to diminish sex steroid hormone secretion by the ovary. This results in elevated circulating levels of gonadotrophins, especially LH, due to decreased negative feedback on the hypothalamic-pituitary axis by estrogens and possibly other humoral factors produced by the graafian follicles (Carson et al., 1989). The long-term stimulation of stromal (interstitial) cells, which have receptors for LH (Beamer and Tennent, 1986), and, indirectly, the ovarian surface epithelium appears to place the mouse ovary at increased risk for developing the unique tubular or tubulostromal adenomas.

The finding of similar tubular adenomas in the ovaries of the xenobiotic-treated and genetically sterile mice not exposed to exogenous chemicals supports the concept of a secondary (hormonally mediated) mechanism of ovarian oncogenesis associated with hormonal imbalances. The ovarian tumors developed only in sterile mice in which the pituitary-hypothalamic axis was intact; administration of exogenous estrogen early in the course will prevent ovarian tumor development. The intense proliferation of ovarian surface epithelium and stromal (interstitial) cells with the development of unique tubular adenomas in response to sterility does not appear to have a counterpart in the ovaries of human adult females.

### Summary: Ovarian Tumoringenesis in Rodents

Experimental ovarian carcinogenesis has been investigated in inbred and hybrid strains of mice and induced by a diversity of mechanisms, including X-irradiation, oocytotoxic xenobiotic chemicals, ovarian grafting to ectopic or orthotopic sites, neonatal thymectomy, mutant genes reducing germ cell populations, and aging (Fig. 21-15). Disruptions in the function of graafian follicles by a variety of mechanisms results in a spectrum of ovarian proliferative lesions, including tumors. The findings in mutant mice support the concept of a secondary (hormonally mediated) mechanism of ovarian carcinogenesis in mice, associated with sterility. Multiple pathogenetic factors that either destroy or diminish the numbers of graafian follicles in the ovary result in decreased sex hormone secretion (especially estradiol-17$\beta$), leading to a compensatory overproduction of pituitary gonadotrophins (particularly LH) (Fig. 21-15), which places the mouse ovary at an increased risk for developing tumors (Fig. 21-16). The intense proliferation of ovarian surface epithelium and stromal (interstitial) cells with the development of unique tubular adenomas in response to sterility does not appear to have a counterpart in the ovaries of human adult females.

## PARATHYROID GLAND

Calcium plays a key role as an essential structural component of the skeleton and also in many fundamental biological processes. These processes include neuromuscular excitability, membrane permeability, muscle contraction, enzyme activity, hormone release, and blood coagulation, among others. The precise control of calcium in extracellular fluids is vital to health. To maintain a constant concentration of calcium, despite marked variations in intake and excretion, endocrine control mechanisms have evolved that primarily consist of the interactions of three major hormones—parathyroid hormone (PTH), calcitonin (CT), and cholecalciferol (vitamin D).

### Biosynthesis of Parathyroid Hormone by Chief Cells

Parathyroid chief cells in humans and many animal species store relatively small amounts of preformed hormone but they respond quickly to variations in the need for hormone by changing the rate of hormone synthesis. Parathyroid hormone, like many peptide hormones, is first synthesized as a

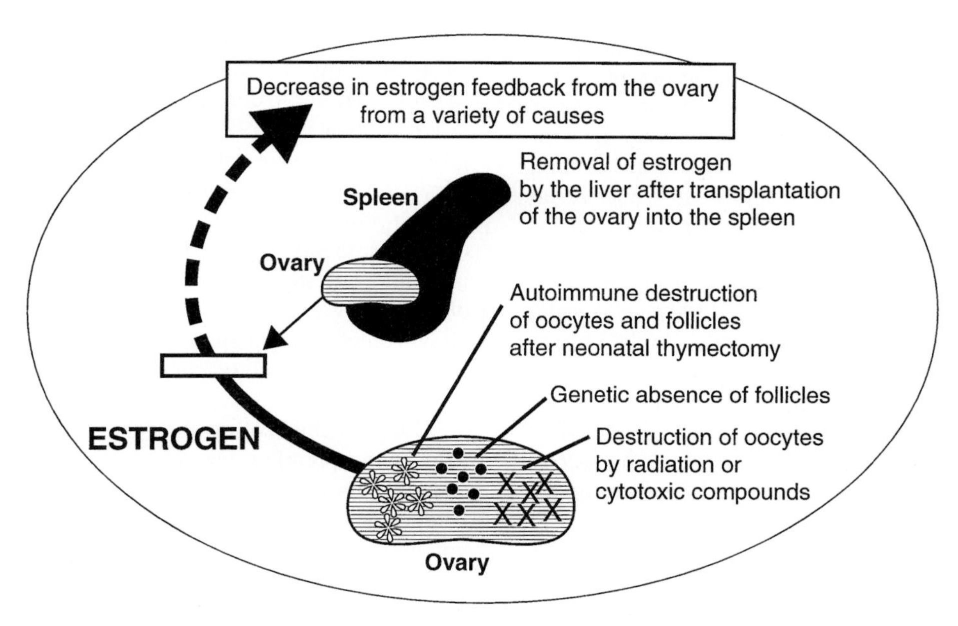


*Figure 21–15. Multiple pathogenic mechanisms in ovarian tumorigenesis of mice resulting in decreased negative feedback by diminished levels of gonadal steroids (estrogen).*

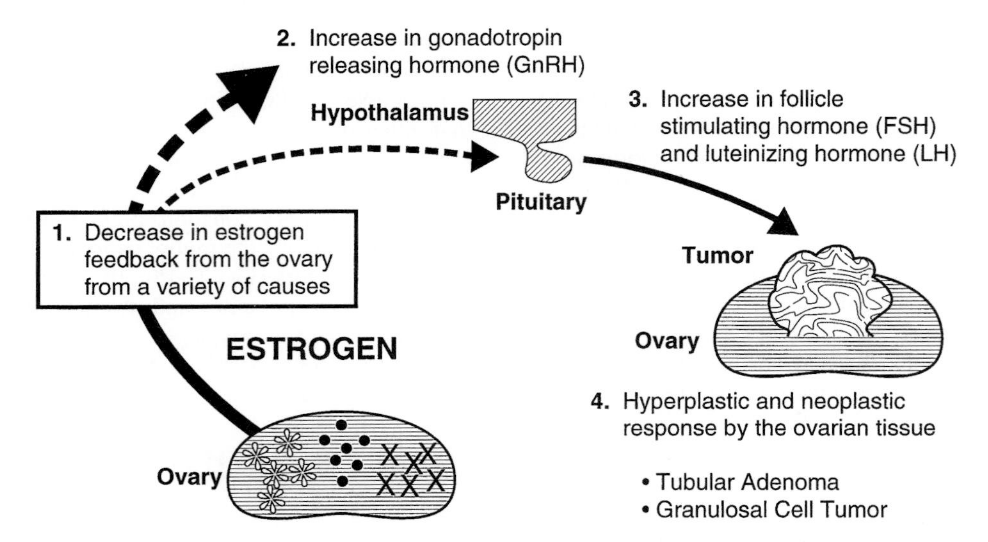


***Figure 21–16. Decreased circulating estrogens release the hypothalamus-pituitary gland from negative feedback inhibition.***

The increased gonadotrophin levels (LH and FSH) result in the mouse ovary being at greater risk of developing tubular adenomas.

larger biosynthetic precursor molecule that undergoes posttranslational processing in chief cells. Preproparathyroid hormone (preproPTH) is the initial translation product synthesized on ribosomes of the rough endoplasmic reticulum in chief cells. It is composed of 115 amino acids and contains a hydrophobic signal or leader sequence of 25 amino acid residues that facilitates the penetration and subsequent vectorial discharge of the nascent peptide into the cisternal space of the rough endoplasmic reticulum (Kronenberg et al., 1986). PreproPTH is rapidly converted within 1 min or less of its synthesis to proparathyroid hormone (ProPTH) by the proteolytic cleavage of 25 amino acids from the $NH_2$-terminal end of the molecule (Habener, 1981). The intermediate precursor, proPTH, is composed of 90 amino acids and moves within membranous channels of the rough endoplasmic reticulum to the Golgi apparatus (Fig. 21-17). Enzymes within membranes of the Golgi apparatus cleave a hexapeptide from the $NH_2$-terminal (biologically active) end of the molecule forming active PTH (Fig. 21-17). Active PTH is packaged into membrane-limited, macromolecular aggregates in the Golgi apparatus for subsequent storage in chief cells. Under certain conditions of increased demand (e.g., a low calcium ion concentration in the extracellular fluid compartment), PTH may be released directly from chief cells without being packaged into secretion granules by a process termed *bypass secretion*.

Although the principal form of active PTH secreted from chief cells is a straight chain peptide of 84 amino acids (molecular weight 9500), the molecule is rapidly cleaved into amino- and carboxy-terminal fragments in the peripheral circulation and especially in the liver. The purpose of this fragmentation is uncertain because the biologically active amino-terminal fragment is no more active than the entire PTH molecule (amino acids 1–84). The plasma half-life of the N-terminal fragment is considerably shorter than that of the biologically inactive carboxy-terminal fragment of parathyroid hormone. The C-terminal and other portions of the PTH molecule are degraded primarily in the kidney and tend to accumulate with chronic renal disease. The immunoheterogeneity caused by the multiple circulating fragments of PTH created significant problems in the development and application of highly specific radioimmunoassays to diagnostic problems in human patients and experimental animals (Goltzman et al., 1986).

## Xenobiotic-Induced Toxic Injury of Parathyroids

**Ozone.** Inhalation of a single dose of ozone (0.75 ppm) for 4 to 8 h has been reported to produce light and electron microscopic changes in parathyroid glands (Atwal and Wilson, 1974). Subsequent studies have utilized longer (48-h) exposure to ozone in order to define the pathogenesis of the parathyroid lesions (Atwal et al., 1975; Atwal, 1979). Initially (1 to 5 days post-ozone exposure), many chief cells undergo compensatory hypertrophy and hyperplasia with areas of capillary endothelial cell proliferation, interstitial edema, degeneration of vascular endothelium, formation of platelet thrombi, leukocyte infiltration of the walls of larger vessels in the gland, and disruption of basement membranes. Chief cells had prominent Golgi complexes and endoplasmic reticulum, aggregations of free ribosomes, and swelling of mitochondria (Atwal and Pemsingh, 1981).

Inactive chief cells with few secretory granules predominate in the parathyroids in the later stages of exposure to ozone. There was evidence of parathyroid atrophy from 12 to 20 days post-ozone exposure with mononuclear cell infiltration and necrosis of chief cells. The reduced cytoplasmic area contained vacuolated endoplasmic reticulum, a small Golgi apparatus, and numerous lysosomal bodies. Plasma membranes of adjacent chief cells were disrupted resulting in coalescence of the cytoplasmic area. Fibroblasts with associated

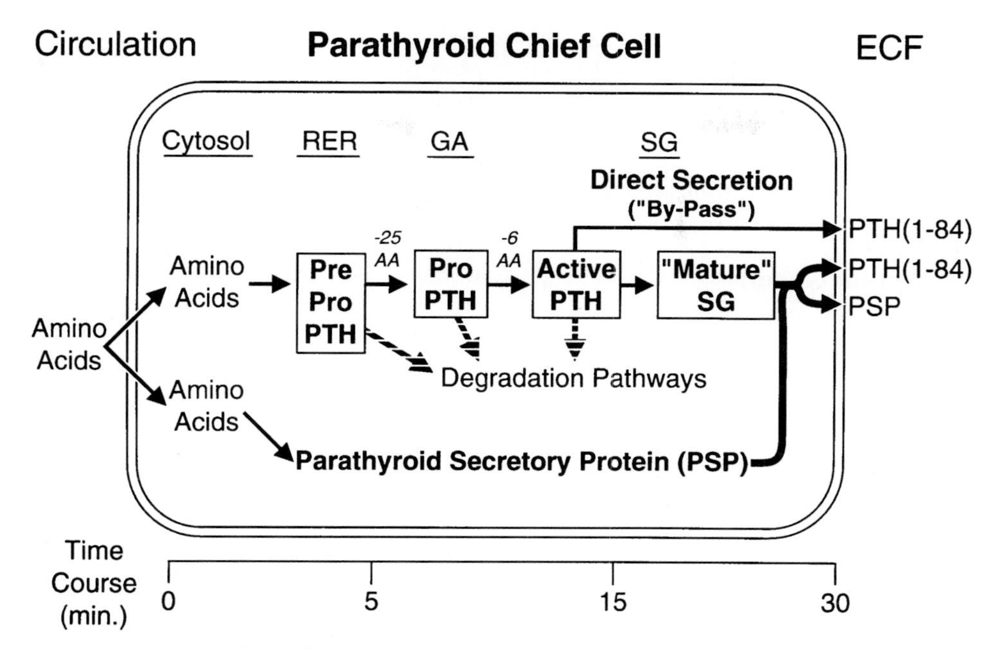


***Figure 21–17. Biosynthesis of parathyroid hormone (PTH) and parathyroid secretory protein (PSP) by parathyroid chief cells.***

Active PTH is synthesized as a larger biosynthetic precursor molecule (preproPTH) that undergoes rapid posttranslational processing to proPTH prior to secretion from chief cells as active PTH (amino acids 1–84).

collagen bundles were prominent in the interstitium and the basal lamina of the numerous capillaries often was duplicated.

The parathyroid lesions in ozone-exposed animals are similar to isoimmune parathyroiditis in other species (Lupulescu et al., 1968). Antibody against parathyroid tissue was localized near the periphery of chief cells by indirect immunofluorescence, especially 14 days following ozone injury (Atwal et al., 1975).

**Aluminum.** Evidence for a direct effect of aluminum on the parathyroid was suggested from studies of patients with chronic renal failure treated by hemodialysis with aluminum-containing fluids or orally administered drugs containing aluminum. These patients often had normal or minimal elevations of immunoreactive parathyroid hormone (iPTH), little histological evidence of osteitis fibrosa in bone, and a depressed response by the parathyroid gland to acute hypocalcemia (Bourdeau et al., 1987). Studies by Morrissey and coworkers (1983) have reported that an increase in aluminum concentration in vitro over a range of 0.5–2.0 mM in a low calcium medium (0.5 mM) progressively inhibited the secretion of PTH. At 2.0 mM aluminum, PTH secretion was inhibited by 68 percent while high calcium-containing medium (2.0 mM) without aluminum maximally inhibited PTH secretion only 39 percent. The inhibition of PTH secretion by aluminum does not appear to be related to an irreversible toxic effect because normal secretion was restored when parathyroid cells were returned to 0.5 mM calcium medium without aluminum. The incorporation of [$^3$H] leucine into total cell protein, parathyroid secretory protein, proparathyroid hormone, or PTH was not affected by aluminum; however, the secretion of radiolabeled protein by dispersed parathyroid cells was inhibited by aluminum (Morrissey et al., 1983).

The molecular mechanism by which aluminum inhibits PTH secretion, reducing diglyceride levels in chief cells (Morrissey and Slatopolsky, 1986), appears to be similar to that of the calcium ion. Aluminum appears to decrease diglyceride synthesis, which is reflected in a corresponding decrease in synthesis of phosphatidylcholine and possible triglyceride; however, phosphatidylinositol synthesis was not affected by aluminum. The mechanism by which aluminum decreases diglycerides and maintains phosphatidylinositol synthesis in parathyroid cells is not known.

**L-Asparaginase.** Tettenborn and colleagues (1970) and Chisari and associates (1972) reported that rabbits administered L-asparaginase develop severe hypocalcemia and tetany characterized by muscle tremors, opisthotonos, carpopedal spasms, paralysis, and coma. This drug was of interest in cancer chemotherapy because of the beneficial effects of guinea pig serum against lymphosarcoma in mice.

Parathyroid chief cells appeared to be selectively destroyed by L-asparaginase (Young et al., 1973). Chief cells were predominately inactive and degranulated, with large autophagic vacuoles present in the cytoplasm of degenerating cells. Cytoplasmic organelles concerned with synthesis and packaging of secretory products were poorly developed in chief cells. Rabbits developed hyperphosphatemia, hypomagnesemia, hyperkalemia, and azotemia in addition to acute hypocalcemia. Rabbits with clinical hypocalcemic tetany did not recover spontaneously; however, administration of parathyroid extract prior to or during treatment with L-asparaginase decreased the incidence of hypocalcemic tetany.

The development of hypocalcemia and tetany have not been observed in other experimental animals administered L-asparaginase (Oettgen et al., 1970). However, this response may not be limited to the rabbit because some human patients receiving the drug also have developed hypocalcemia (Jaffe et al., 1972). The L-asparaginase-induced hypoparathyroidism in rabbits is a valuable model for investigating drug-endocrine cell interactions, somewhat analogous to the selective destruction of pancreatic beta cells by alloxan with production of experimental diabetes mellitus.

## Neoplasms of Parathyroid Gland: Chief Cell Adenoma

Parathyroid adenomas in adult-aged rats vary in size from microscopic to unilateral nodules several millimeters in diameter, located in the cervical region by the thyroids or infrequently in the thoracic cavity near the base of the heart. Parathyroid neoplasms in the precardiac mediastinum are derived from ectopic parathyroid tissue displaced into the thorax with the expanding thymus during embryonic development. Tumors of parathyroid chief cells do not appear to be a sequela of long-standing secondary hyperparathyroidism of either renal or nutritional origin. The unaffected parathyroid glands may be atrophic if the adenoma is functional, normal if the adenoma is nonfunctional, or enlarged if there is concomitant hyperplasia. In functional adenomas the normal mechanism by which PTH secretion is controlled, changes in the concentration of blood calcium, is lost and hormone secretion is excessive in spite of an increased level of blood calcium.

Adenomas are solitary nodules that are sharply demarcated from adjacent parathyroid parenchyma. Because the adenoma compresses the rim of surrounding parathyroid to varying degrees depending upon its size, there may be a partial fibrous capsule, resulting either from compression of existing stroma or from proliferation of fibrous connective tissue.

Adenomas are usually nonfunctional (endocrinologically inactive) in adult-aged rats from chronic toxicity/carcinogenicity studies. Chief cells in nonfunctional adenomas are cuboidal or polyhedral and arranged either in a diffuse sheet, lobules, or acini with or without lumens. Chief cells from functional adenomas often are closely packed into small groups by fine connective tissue septae. The cytoplasmic area varies from normal size to an expanded area. There is a much lower density of cells in functional parathyroid adenoma compared to the adjacent rim with atrophic chief cells.

Larger parathyroid adenomas, such as those that are detected macroscopically, often nearly incorporate the entire affected gland. A narrow rim of compressed parenchyma may be detected at one side of the gland or the affected parathyroid may be completely incorporated by the adenoma. Chief cells in this rim often are compressed and atrophic due to pressure and the persistent hypercalcemia. Peripherally situated follicles in the adjacent thyroid lobe may be compressed to a limited extent by larger parathyroid adenomas. The parathyroid glands that do not contain a functional adenoma also undergo trophic atrophy in response to the hypercalcemia and become smaller.

**Influence of Age on Parathyroid Tumors.** There are relatively few chemicals or experimental manipulations reported in the literature that significantly increase the incidence of parathyroid tumors. Long-standing renal failure with intense diffuse hyperplasia does not appear to increase the development of chief cell tumors in rats. The historical incidence of parathyroid adenomas in untreated control male F344 rats in studies conducted by the NTP was 4/1315 (0.3 percent), and for female F344 rats it was 2/1330 (0.15 percent). However, parathyroid adenomas are an example of a neoplasm in F344 rats whose incidence increases dramatically when lifespan data are compared to 2-year studies. Solleveld and coworkers (1984) reported that the incidence of parathyroid adenomas increased in males from 0.1 percent at 2 years to 3.1 percent in lifetime studies. Corresponding data for female F344 rats was 0.1 percent at 2 years and 0.6 percent in lifetime studies.

**Influence of Gonadectomy on Parathyroid Tumors.** Oslapas and colleagues (1982) reported an increased incidence of parathyroid adenomas in female (34 percent) and male (27 percent) rats of the Long-Evans strain administered 40 $\mu$Ci sodium $^{131}$I and saline at 8 weeks of age. There were no significant changes in serum calcium, phosphorus, and parathyroid hormone compared to controls. Gonadectomy performed at 7 weeks of age decreased the incidence of parathyroid adenomas in irradiated rats (7.4 percent in gonadectomy vs. 27 percent in intact controls) but there was little change in the incidence of parathyroid adenomas in irradiated females. X-irradiation of the thyroid-parathyroid region also increased the incidence of parathyroid adenomas. When female Sprague-Dawley rats received a single absorbed dose of x-rays at 4 weeks of age, they subsequently developed a 24 percent incidence of parathyroid adenomas after 14 months (Oslapas et al., 1981).

**Influence of Xenobiotics on Parathyroid Tumors.** Parathyroid adenomas have been encountered infrequently following the administration of a variety of chemicals in 2-year bioassay studies in Fischer rats. In a study with the pesticide Rotenone in F344 rats, there appeared to be an increased incidence of parathyroid adenomas in high-dose (75 ppm) males (4 of 44 rats) compared to either low-dose (38 ppm) males, control males (1 of 44 rats) or NTP historical controls (0.3 percent) (Abdo et al., 1988). It was uncertain whether the increased incidence of this uncommon tumor was a direct effect of Rotenone feeding or the increased survival in high-dose males. Chief cell hyperplasia was not present in parathyroids that developed adenomas.

**Influence of Irradiation and Hypercalcemia Induced by Vitamin D on Parathyroid Tumors.** Wynford-Thomas and associates (1982) reported that irradiation significantly increases the incidence of parathyroid adenomas in inbred Wistar albino rats and that the incidence could be modified by feeding diets with variable amounts of vitamin D. Neonatal Wistar rats were given either 5 or 10 $\mu$Ci radioiodine ($^{131}$I) within 24 h of birth. In rats 12 months of age and older, parathyroid adenomas were found in 33 percent of rats administered 5 $\mu$Ci $^{131}$I and in 37 percent of rats given 10 $\mu$Ci $^{131}$I compared to 0 percent in unirradiated controls. The incidence of parathyroid adenomas was highest (55 percent) in normocalcemic rats fed a low vitamin D diet and lowest (20 percent) in irradiated rats fed a high vitamin D diet (40,000 IU/kg) that had a significant elevation in plasma calcium.

# REFERENCES


Abdo KM, Eustis SL, Haseman J, et al: Toxicity and carcinogenicity of rotenone given in the feed to F344/N rats and B6C3F1 mice for up to two years. *Drug Chem Toxicol* 11:225–235, 1988.

Alison RH, Morgan KT: Ovarian neoplasms in F344 rats and B6C3F1 mice. *Environ Health Perspect* 73:91–106, 1987.

Atwal OS, Wilson T: Parathyroid gland changes following oxone inhalation. A morphologic study. *Arch Environ Health* 28:91–100, 1974.

Atwal OS, Samagh BS, Bhatnagar MK: A possible autoimmune parathyroiditis following ozone inhalation. II. A histopathologic, ultrastructural, and immunofluorescent study. *Am J Pathol* 80:53–68, 1975.

Atwal OS: Ultrastructural pathology of ozone-induced experimental parathyroiditis. IV. Biphasic activity in the chief cells of regenerating parathyroid glands. *Am J Pathol* 95:611–632, 1979.

Atwal OS, Pemsingh RS: Morphology of microvascular changes and endothelial regeneration in experimental ozone-induced parathyroiditis. III. Some pathologic considerations. *Am J Pathol* 102:297–307, 1981.

Axelrod AA, Leblond CP: Induction of thyroid tumors in rats by low iodine diet. *Cancer* 8:339–367, 1955.

Bär A: Significance of Leydig cell neoplasia in rats fed lactitol or lactose. *J Am Coll Toxicol* 11:189–207, 1992.

Barter RA, Klaassen CD: Reduction of thyroid hormone levels and alteration of thyroid function by four representation UDP-glucuronosyltransferase inducers in rats. *Toxicol Appl Pharmacol* 128:9–17, 1994.

Barter RA, Klaassen CD: Rat liver microsomal UDP-glucuronosyltransferase activity toward thyroxine: Characterization, induction, and form specificity. *Toxicol Appl Pharmacol* 115:261–267, 1992a.

Barter RA, Klaassen CD: UDP-glucuronosyltransferase inducers reduce thyroid hormone levels in rats by an extrathyroidal mechanism. *Toxicol Appl Pharmacol* 113:36–42, 1992b.

Bartke A, Sweeney CA, Johnson L, et al: Hyperprolactinemia inhibits development of Leydig cell tumors in aging Fischer rats. *Exp Aging Res* 11:123–128, 1985.

Biskind MS, Biskind JR: Development of tumors in the rat ovary after transplantation into the spleen. *Proc Soc Exp Biol Med* 55:176–179, 1944.

Boorman GA, Hamlin MH, Eustis SL: Focal interstitial cell hyperplasia, testis, rat, in Jones TC, Möhr U, Hunt RD (eds): *Monographs on Pathology of Laboratory Animals*. Berlin: Springer-Verlag, 1987, pp 200–220.

Borzelleca JF, Capen CC, Hallagan JB: Lifetime toxicity carcinogenicity study of FC&C Red No. 3 (erythrosine) in rats. *Food Chem Toxicol* 25:723–733, 1987.

Bourdeau AM, Plachot JJ, Cournot-Witmer G, et al: Parathyroid response to aluminum in vitro: Ultrastructural changes and PTH release. *Kidney Int* 31:15–24, 1987.

Capen CC: Mechanistic considerations for thyroid gland neoplasia with FD&C Red No. 3 (erythrosine), in: *The Toxicology Forum*. Proceedings of the 1989 Annual Winter Meeting, Washington, DC, 1989, pp 113–130.

Capen CC, Martin SL: The effects of xenobiotics on the structure and function of thyroid follicles and C-cells. *Toxicol Pathol* 17:266–293, 1989.

Carson RS, Zhang Z, Hutchinson LA, et al: Growth factors in ovarian function. *J Reprod Fert* 85:735–746, 1989.

Cattanach BM, Iddon A, Charlton HM, et al: Gonadotropin releasing hormone deficiency in a mutant mouse with hypogonadism. *Nature* 269:238–240, 1977.

Chatani F, Nonoyama T, Katsuichi S, et al: Stimulatory effect of luteinizing hormone on the development and maintenance of 5α-reduced steroid-producing testicular interstitial cell tumors in Fischer 344 rats. *Anticancer Res* 10:337–342, 1990.

Chisari FV, Hochstein HD, Kirschstein RL: Parathyroid necrosis and hypocalcemic tetany induced in rabbits by L-asparaginase. *Am J Pathol* 69:461–476, 1972.

Clements FW: Relationship of thyrotoxicosis and carcinoma of thyroid to endemic goiter. *Med J Aust* 2:894–899, 1954.

Clemmesen J, Fuglsang-Frederiksen V, Plum CM: Are anticonvulsants oncogenic? *Lancet* 1:705–707, 1974.

Clemmesen J, Hjalgrim-Jensen S: On the absence of carcinogenicity to man of phenobarbital, in: *Statistical Studies in the Aetiology of Malignant Neoplasms. Acta Pathol Microb Scand* 261(Suppl):38–50, 1977.

Clemmesen J, Hjalgrim-Jensen S: Is phenobarbital carcinogenic? A follow-up of 8078 epileptics. *Ecotoxicol Environ Safety* 1:255–260, 1978.

Clemmesen J, Hjalgrim-Jensen S: Does phenobarbital cause intracranial tumors? A follow-up through 35 years. *Ecotoxicol Environ Safety* 5:255–260, 1981.

Collins WT Jr, Capen CC: Ultrastructural and functional alterations in thyroid glands of rats produced by polychlorinated biphenyls compared with the effects of iodide excess and deficiency, and thyrotropin and thyroxine administration. *Virchows Arch B Cell Pathol* 33:213–231, 1980.

Cooper DS, Axelrod L, DeGroot LJ, et al: Congenital goiter and the development of metastatic follicular carcinoma with evidence for a leak of non-hormonal iodide: Clinical, pathological, kinetic, and biochemical studies and a review of the literature. *J Clin Endocrinol Metab* 52:294–306, 1981.

Curran PG, DeGroot LJ: The effect of hepatic enzyme-inducing drugs on thyroid hormones and the thyroid gland. *Endocr Rev* 12:135–150, 1991.

Döhler K-D, Wong CC, von zut Mühlen A: The rat as model for the study of drug effects on thyroid function: consideration of methodological problems. *Pharmacol Ther* 5:305–313, 1979.

Doniach I: Aetiological consideration of thyroid carcinoma, in Smithers D (ed): *Tumors of the Thyroid Gland*. London: E & S Livingstone, 1970, pp 55–72.

Fort FL, Miyajima H, Ando T, et al: Mechansim for species-specific induction of Leydig cell tumors in rats by lansoprazole. *Fundam Appl Toxicol* 26:191–202, 1995.

Friedman GD: Barbiturates and lung cancer in humans. *JNCI* 67:291–295, 1981.

Frith CH, Zuna RF, Morgan K: A morphologic classification and incidence of spontaneous ovarian neoplasms in three strains of mice. *JNCI* 67:693–702, 1981.

Furth J: Morphologic changes associated with thyrotropin-secreting pituitary tumors. *Am J Pathol* 30:421–463, 1954.

Furth J, Boon MC: Induction of ovarian tumors in mice by X-rays. *Cancer Res* 7:241–245, 1947.

Gardner WU: Ovarian and lymphoid tumors in female mice subsequent to Roentgen-Ray irradiation and hormone treatment. *Proc Soc Exper Biol Med* 75:434–436, 1950.

Goltzman D, Bennett HPJ, Koutsilieris M, et al: Studies of the multiple molecular forms of bioactive parathyroid hormone and parathyroid hormone2Dlike substances. *Recent Prog Horm Res* 42:665–703, 1986.

Guthrie MJ: Tumorigenesis in intrasplenic ovaries in mice. *Cancer* 10:190–203, 1957.

Habener JF: Recent advances in parathyroid hormone research. *Clin Biochem* 14:223–229, 1981.

Hill RN, Erdreich LS, Paynter O, et al: Thyroid follicular cell carcinogenesis. *Fundam Appl Toxicol* 12:629–697, 1989.

Hood A, Harstad E, Klaassen CD: Effects of UDP-glucuronosyltransferase (UDP-GT) inducers on thyroid cell proliferation. *Toxicologist* 15:229, 1995.

Hummel KP: Induced ovarian tumors. *JNCI* 15:711–715, 1954.

Ingbar SH: Autoregulation of the thyroid. Response to iodide excess and depletion. *Mayo Clin Proc* 47:814, 1972.

Jaffe N, Traggis D, Lakshmi D, et al: Comparison of daily and twice-weekly schedule of L-asparaginase in childhood leukemia. *Pediatrics* 49:590–595, 1972.

Kennedy TH, Purves HD: Studies on experimental goiter: Effect of *Brassica* seed diets on rats. *Br J Exp Pathol* 22:241–244, 1941.

Kronenberg HM, Igarashi T, Freeman MW, et al: Structure and expression of the human parathyroid hormone gene. *Recent Prog Horm Res* 42:641–663, 1986.

Lamas L, Ingbar SH: The effect of varying iodine content on the susceptibility of thyroglobulin to hydrolysis by thyroid acid protease. *Endocrinology* 102:188–197, 1978.

Li MH, Gardner WU: Further studies on the pathogenesis of ovarian tumors in mice. *Cancer Res* 9:35–44, 1949.

Liu YP, Liu J, Barter RA, Klassen CD: Alteration of thyroid function by UDP-Glucuronosyltransferase (UDP-GT) inducers in rats: A dose-response study. *J Pharmacol Exp Ther* 273:977–985, 1995.

Lupulescu A, Potorac E, Pop A: Experimental investigation on immunology of the parathyroid gland. *Immunology* 14:475–482, 1968.

Majumder S, Brown K, Qiu F-H, Besmer P: *c-kit* Protein, a transmembrane kinase: Identification in tissues and characterization. *Mol Cell Biol* 8:4896–4903, 1988.

Marchant J: The chemical induction of ovarian tumours in mice. *Br J Cancer* 11:452–464, 1957.

Marchant J: The development of ovarian tumors in ovaries grafted from mice treated with dimethylbenzanthracene. Inhibition by the presence of normal ovarian tissue. *Br J Cancer* 14:514–519, 1960.

McClain RM, Posch RC, Bosakowski T, Armstrong JM: Studies on the mode of action for thyroid gland tumor promotion in rats by phenobarbital. *Toxicol Appl Pharmacol* 94:254–265, 1988.

McClain RM, Levin AA, Posch R, Downing JC: The effects of phenobarbital on the metabolism and excretion of thyroxine in rats. *Toxicol Appl Pharmacol* 99:216–228, 1989.

McGirr EM, Clement WE, Currie AR, Kennedy JS: Impaired dehalogenase activity as a cause of goiter with malignant changes. *Scott Med J* 4:232–242, 1959.

Michael SD, Taguchi O, Nishizuka Y: Changes in hypophyseal hormones associated with accelerated aging and tumorigenesis of the ovaries in neonatally thymectomized mice. *Endocrinology* 108:2375–2380, 1981.

Morris HP: The experimental development and metabolism of thyroid gland tumors. *Adv Cancer Res* 3:51–115, 1955.

Morrissey J, Rothstein M, Mayor G, Slatopolsky E: Suppression of parathryoid hormone secretion by aluminum. *Kidney Int* 23:699–704, 1983.

Morrissey J, Slatopolsky E: Effect of aluminum on parathryoid hormone secretion. *Kidney Int* 29:S41–S44, 1986.

Murakami M, Hosokawa S, Yamada T, et al: Species-specific mechanism in rat Leydig cell tumorigenesis by procymidone. *Toxicol Appl Pharmacol* 131:244–252, 1995.

Murphy ED: Hyperplastic and early neoplastic changes in the ovaries of mice after genic deletion of germ cells. *JNCI* 48:1283–1295, 1972.

Murphy ED, Beamer WG: Plasma gonadotropin levels during early stages of ovarian tumorigenesis in mice of the $W^x/W^v$ genotype. *Cancer Res* 33:721–723, 1973.

Napalkov NP: Tumours of the thyroid gland, in Turusov VS (ed): *Pathology of Tumors in Laboratory Animals. Part 2. Tumors of the Rat.* Lyons, France: IARC Scientific Publication No. 6, 1976, vol 1, pp 239–272.

Nishizuki Y, Sakakura T, Taguchi O: Mechanism of ovarian tumorigenesis in mice after neonatal thymectomy. *JNCI Monogr* 51:89–96, 1979.

Oettgen HF, Old LJ, Boyse EA, et al: Toxicity of *E. coli* L-asparaginase in man. *Cancer* 25:253–278, 1970.

Ohnhaus EE, Burgi H, Burger A, Studer H: The effect of antipyrine, phenobarbital, and rifampicin on the thyroid hormone metabolism in man. *Eur J Clin Invest* 11:381–387, 1981.

Ohnhaus EE, Studer H: A link between liver microsomal enzyme activity and thyroid hormone metabolism in man. *Br J Clin Pharmacol* 15:71–76, 1983.

Ohshima M, Ward JM: Promotion of N-methyl-N-nitrosourea-induced thyroid tumors by iodine deficiency in F344/NCr rats. *JNCI* 73:289–296, 1984.

Ohshima M, Ward JM: Dietary iodine deficiency as a tumor promoter and carcinogen in male F344/NCr rats. *Cancer Res* 46:877–883, 1986.

Olsen JH, Boice JD, Jensen JP, Fraumeni JF Jr: Cancer among epileptic patients exposed to anticonvulsant drugs. *JNCI* 81:803–808, 1989.

Oslapas R, Prinz R, Ernst K, et al: Incidence of radiation-induced parathyroid tumors in male and female rats. *Clin Res* 29:734A, 1981.

Oslapas R, Shah KH, Hoffman, et al: Effect of gonadectomy on the incidence of radiation-induced parathyroid tumors in male and female rats. *Clin Res* 30:401A, 1982.

Paynter OH, Burin GJ, Jaeger RB, Gregorio CA: Goitrogens and thyroid follicular cell neoplasmia: Evidence for a threshold process. *Reg Toxicol Pharmacol* 8:102–119, 1988.

Pendergrast WJ, Milmore BK, Marcus SC: Thyroid cancer and toxicosis in the United States: Their relation to endemic goiter. *J Chronic Dis* 13:22–38, 1961.

Prentice DE, Meikle AW: A review of drug-induced Leydig cell hyperplasia and neoplasia in the rat and some comparisons with man. *Hum Exp Toxicol* 14:562–572, 1995.

Rehm S, Dierksen D, Deerberg F: Spontaneous ovarian tumors in Han:NMRI mice: Histologic classification, incidence, and influence of food restriction. *JNCI* 72:1383–1395, 1984.

Shirts SB, Annegers JF, Hauser WA, Kurland LT: Cancer incidence in a cohort of patients with seizure disorders. *JNCI* 77:83–87, 1986.

Solleveld HA, Haseman JK, McConnell EE: National history of body weight gain, survival and neoplasia in the F344 rat. *JNCI* 72:929–940, 1984.

Swarm RL, Roberts GKS, Levy AC: Observations on the thyroid gland in rats following the administration of sulfamethoxazole and trimethoprim. *Toxicol Appl Pharmacol* 24:351–363, 1973.

Taguchi O, Michael SD, Nishizuka Y: Rapid induction of ovarian granulosa cell tumors by 7,12-dimethylbenz[a]anthracene in neonatally estrogenized mice. *Cancer Res* 48:425–429, 1988.

Takayama S, Aihara K, Onodera T, Akimoto T: Antithyroid effects of propylthiouracil and sulfamonomethoxine in rats and monkeys. *Toxicol Appl Pharmacol* 82:191–199, 1986.

Tennent BJ, Beamer WG: Ovarian tumors not induced by irradiation and gonadotropins in hypogonadal (*hpg*) mice. *Biol Reprod* 34:751–760, 1986.

Tettenborn D, Hobik HP, Luckhaus G: Hypoparathyroidismus beim Kaninchen nach Verabreichung von L-asparaginase. *Arzneimittelforschung* 20:1753–1755, 1970.

Thurman JD, Bucci TJ, Hart RW, Turturro A: Survival, body weight, and spontaneous neoplasms in ad libitum-fed and food-restricted Fischer-344 rats. *Toxicol Pathol* 22:1–9, 1994.

White SJ, McLean AEM, Howland C: Anticonvulsant drugs and cancer. A cohort study in patients with severe epilepsy. *Lancet* 2:458–461, 1979.

Witte ON: Steel locus defines new multipotent growth factor. *Cell* 63:5–6, 1990.

Wynford-Thomas V, Wynford-Thomas D, Williams ED: Experimental induction of parathyroid adenomas in the rat. *JNCI* 70:127–134, 1982.

Young DM, Olson HM, Prieur DJ, et al: Clinicopathologic and ultrastructural studies of L-asparaginase-induced hypocalcemia in rabbits An experimental animal model of acute hypoparathyroidism. *Lab Invest* 29:374–386, 1973.

# UNIT 5

# TOXIC AGENTS

# CHAPTER 22

# TOXIC EFFECTS OF PESTICIDES

*Donald J. Ecobichon*

The United States Environmental Protection Agency (U.S. EPA) defines *pesticide* as any substance or mixture of substances intended for preventing, destroying, repelling, or mitigating any pest. Pesticides may also be described as any physical, chemical, or biological agent that will kill an undesirable plant or animal pest. The term *pest* includes harmful, destructive, or troublesome animals, plants, or microorganisms. *Pesticide* is a generic name for a variety of agents that are classified more specifically on the basis of the pattern of use and organism killed. In addition to the major agricultural classes that encompass insecticides, herbicides, and fungicides, one finds pest control agents grouped as acaricides, larvacides, miticides, molluscides, pediculicides, rodenticides, scabicides, plus attractants (pheromones), defoliants, desiccants, plant growth regulators, and repellants.

Over the centuries, humans have developed many ingenious methods in their attempts to control the invertebrates, vertebrates, and microorganisms that constantly threatened the supply of food and fiber, as well as posing a threat to health. The historical literature is replete with descriptions of plant diseases and insect plagues and the measures taken to control them. Sulfur was used as a fumigant by the Chinese before 1000 B.C. and as a fungicide in the 1800s in Europe against powdery mildew on fruit; it is still the major pesticide used in California today. In sixteenth-century Japan, poor quality rendered whale oil was mixed with vinegar and sprayed on paddies and fields to prevent the development of insect larvae by weakening the cuticle. The Chinese applied moderate amounts of arsenic-containing compounds as insecticides in the sixteenth century. As early as 1690, water extracts of tobacco leaves (*Nicotiana tabacum*) were sprayed on plants as insecticides, and nux vomica, the seed of *Strychnos nux-vomica* (strychnine), was introduced to kill rodents. In the mid-1800s, the pulverized root of *Derris eliptica*, containing rotenone, was used as an insecticide, as was pyrethrum extracted from the flowers of chrysanthemums (*Chrysanthemum cinerariaefolium*). In the late 1800s, arsenic trioxide was used as a weed killer, particularly for dandelions. Bordeaux mixture (copper sulfate, lime [$Ca(OH)_2$, water]) was introduced in 1882 to combat vine downy mildew (*Plasmopara viticola*), a disease introduced into France from the United States when phylloxera-resistant vine rootstocks were imported. Sulfuric acid, at a concentration of 10 percent v/v, was used in the early 1900s to destroy dicotyledonous weeds that would absorb the acid, whereas cereal grains and cultivates, having a smooth and waxy monocotyledon, were protected. Paris Green (copper arsenite) was introduced for the control of Colorado beetle in the late 1800s; calcium arsenate replaced Paris Green and lead arsenate was a major cornerstone in the agriculturalist's armamentarium against insect pests in the early 1900s. By the 1920s, the widespread use of arsenical pesticides caused considerable public concern because some treated fruits and vegetables were found to have toxic residues. It can be appreciated that although some of these early pesticides caused only minimal harm to the humans exposed, other agents were exceedingly toxic and the medical literature of the era is sprinkled with anecdotal reports of poisonings. Looking back over the early years of pesticide development before the 1930s, it is somewhat surprising to realize just how few pesticides were available (Cremlyn, 1978).

The 1930s ushered in the era of modern synthetic chemistry including the development of a variety of agents such as alkyl thiocyanate insecticides, dithiocarbamate fungicides, and ethylene dibromide, methyl bromide, ethylene oxide, and carbon disulfide as fumigants (Cremlyn, 1978). By the beginning of World War II, there were a number of pesticides including dichlorodiphenyltrichloroethane (DDT), dinitrocresol, 4-chloro-2-methyloxyacetic acid (MCPA), and 2,4-dichlorophenoxyacetic acid (2,4-D) under experimental investigation, much of this activity being kept under wraps during the war (Kirby, 1980). In the postwar era, there was rapid development in the agrochemical field, with a plethora of insecticides, fungicides, herbicides, and other chemical agents being introduced. In no other field of synthetic organic chemistry has there been such a diversity of structures arising from the application of the principles of chemistry to the mechanism(s) of action in pests to develop selectivity and specificity in agents toward certain species while reducing toxicity to other forms of life.

It is important to appreciate that, despite the modern day development of second- and third-generation derivatives of the early chemical pesticides, all pesticides possess an inherent degree of toxicity to some living organism; otherwise they would be of no practical use. Unfortunately, the target species selectivity of pesticides is not as well developed as might be hoped for, and nontarget species frequently are affected because they possess physiological and/or biochemical systems similar to those of the target organisms. There is no such thing as a completely safe pesticide. There are, however, pesticides that can be used safely and/or present a low level of risk to human health when applied with proper attention to the label's instructions. Despite the current conflagration over pesticide use and the presence of low levels of residues in food, groundwater, and air, these agents comprise integral components of our crop and health protection programs. As long as they continue to be used, accidental and/or intentional poisoning of wildlife, domestic stock, and humans can be anticipated and will require treatment.

On a worldwide basis, intoxications attributed to pesticides have been estimated to be as high as 3 million cases of

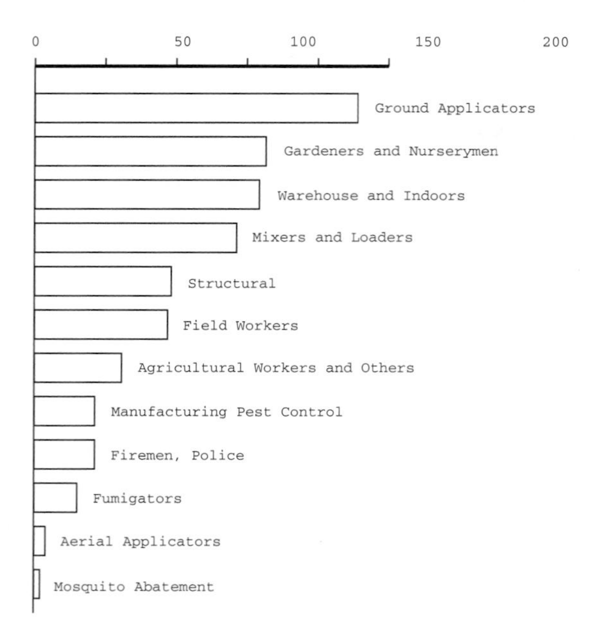


***Figure 22–1. Frequency of pesticide poisoning related to occupational and potential for exposure. [From the records of the California Department of Public Health (Kilgore, 1988).]***

acute, severe poisoning annually, with as many or more unreported cases and some 220,000 deaths (WHO, 1990). These estimates suffer from inadequate reporting of data for developing countries but they may not be too far off the mark. From estimations based on California data, a total of some 25,000 cases of pesticide-related illness occur annually among agricultural workers in that state, with the national estimate for the United States as a whole being on the order of 80,000 cases per year (Coye et al., 1986). Recent results from California, a state that uses a vast amount of chemical pesticides, revealed that 1087 occupationally related exposures occurred in 1978. A breakdown of these poisonings by job category, as shown in Fig. 22-1, revealed that ground applicators were at greatest risk, whereas aerial applicators and workers involved in mosquito abatement programs had the least pesticide-related illness (Kilgore, 1980, 1988). Of 1211 cases of pesticide-related illness reported to California physicians in 1986, 1065 were occupational in nature (Edmiston and Maddy, 1987). However, in other countries, the incidence of poisoning is very low: for example, in the United Kingdom there are fewer than 20 agricultural incidents with organophosphates reported each year (Weir et al., 1992). Such data are not representative of the rest of the agricultural world. The incidence of poisoning is 13 times higher in developing countries than in highly industrialized nations which consume 85 percent of world pesticide production (Forget, 1989). In 1983, the Labor Compensation Fund of Thailand reported only 117 pesticide poisoning cases per 100,000 agricultural workers with 0.8 deaths per 100,000 workers (Boon-Long et al., 1986). However, a survey of hospital admissions/deaths due to pesticides conducted by the Ministry of Public Health of Thailand in the same year estimated a total of 8268 pesticide poisonings within an agricultural community of 100,000 workers. The differences between these two national estimates of pesticide-related toxicity can be explained by the fact that only companies having more than 20 employees must submit claims, whereas a large number of pesticide applicators are individual farmers, members of cooperatives, or those working for small companies. These totals, of course, do not include individuals who were affected but not seriously enough to seek medical attention. In Sri Lanka, approximately 10,000 persons were admitted to hospitals for acute pesticide poisoning annually, with almost 1,000 deaths (Jeyaratram, 1993). A recently published proceedings gives a good overview of the situations found in developing nations where there are few regulations controlling the registration and sale of pesticides (Forget et al., 1993).

No one can doubt the efficacy of pesticides for the protection of crops in the field, thereby providing us with abundant, inexpensive, wholesome, and attractive fruits and vegetables. It has been estimated that in 1830 it took 58 manhours to tend and harvest an acre of grain, whereas today it takes approximately 2 manhours (Kirby, 1980). Over this time period, the price of cereal grain has not risen proportionally to the costs of the labor to produce it. Along with improved strains of crops, insecticides, fungicides, and herbicides have played an important role in crop improvements and yields. Even with such advances, it is estimated that up to 50 percent of harvested crops can be damaged by postharvest infestation by insects, fungi, rodents, and the like (Table 22-1).

The medical miracles accomplished by pesticides have been documented: the suppression of a typhus epidemic in Naples, Italy, by DDT in the winter of 1943–1944 (Brooks, 1974); the control of river blindness (onchocerciasis) in West

**Table 22–1**
**Worldwide Harvest Losses in Five Important Crops**

| CROP | POTENTIAL HARVEST (1000t) | HARVEST 1978 (1000t) | LOSSES THROUGH *Weeds* (%) | LOSSES THROUGH *Diseases* (%) | LOSSES THROUGH *Insects* (%) |
|---|---|---|---|---|---|
| Rice | 715,800 | 378,645 | 10.6 | 9.0 | 27.5 |
| Maize | 563,016 | 362,582 | 13.0 | 9.6 | 13.0 |
| Wheat | 578,400 | 437,236 | 9.8 | 9.5 | 5.1 |
| Sugarcane | 1,603,200 | 737,483 | 15.1 | 19.4 | 19.5 |
| Cotton | 63,172 | 41,757 | 5.8 | 12.1 | 16.0 |

SOURCE: From *GIFAP Bulletin*, March/April, 1986, vol 12. Brussels, Belgium: GIFAP, International Group of National Associations of Agrochemical Manufacturers.

Africa by killing the insect vector (black fly) carrying the filaria for this disease with temephos (Abate) (Walsh, 1986); and the control of malaria in Africa, the Middle East, and Asia by eliminating the plasmodia-bearing mosquito populations with a variety of insecticides (Matsumura, 1985). There is still a great need for advancement in disease vector control by pesticides: 600 million people are at risk from schistosomiasis in the Middle East and Asia; 200 million suffer from filariasis in tropical Africa, Asia, Indonesia, and the Caribbean region; 20 million people in tropical Africa, the Middle East, Mexico, and Guatemala are infected by the filarium causing onchocerciasis; and 1000 million people worldwide harbor pathological intestinal worm infestations (Albert, 1987). Although the benefits of pesticides are recognized by those who require them, certain parts of the world are experiencing an environmentalist- and media-evoked backlash toward all pesticide use because of the carelessness, misuse, and/or abuse of some agents by a relatively few individuals in a limited number of well-publicized incidents. Without bearing any direct responsibility for planning or involvement in health care or food or fiber production, some environmental and consumer advocacy groups propose a total ban on pesticide use. Between the two extremes of overwhelming use and total ban lies a position advocating the careful and rational use of these beneficial chemicals.

The widespread use and misuse of the early, toxic pesticides created an awareness of the potential health hazards and the need to protect the consumer from residues in foods. It was not until 1906 that the Wiley or Sherman Act was passed, creating the first Federal Food and Drugs Act. This was replaced by the Federal Food, Drug and Cosmetic Act (FDCA) in 1938, with specific pesticide amendments being passed in 1954 and 1958 which required that pesticide tolerances be established for all agricultural commodities. The 1958 amendment contained the famous Delaney Clause (Section 409), which states that "no additive shall be deemed safe if it is found to induce cancer when ingested by man or animal or, if it is found, after tests which are appropriate for the evaluation of the safety of food additives, to induce cancer in man or animals" (National Academy of Sciences, 1987). It should be noted that the Delaney Clause does not require proof of carcinogenicity in humans. Pesticides fall under this "additive" legislation.

The Federal Insecticide, Fungicide, and Rodenticide Act (FIFRA) was originally passed by Congress in 1947 as a labeling statute that would group all pest control products, initially only insecticides, fungicides, rodenticides, and herbicides, under one law to be administered by the U.S. Department of Agriculture (USDA). Amendments in 1959 and 1961 added nematicides, plant growth regulators, defoliants, and desiccants to FIFRA jurisdiction plus the authorization to deny, suspend, or cancel registrations of products, although it assured the registrant's right to appeal. In 1972, FIFRA was reorganized and the administrative authority was turned over to the newly formed Environmental Protection Agency (EPA). The new Act, along with subsequent amendments in 1975, 1978, 1980, and 1984, defines the registration requirements and appropriate chemical, toxicological, and environmental impact studies, label specifications, use restrictions, the establishment of tolerances for pesticide residues on raw agricultural products, and the responsibility to monitor pesticide residue levels in foods. However, FIFRA is not all-encompassing because the Food and Drug Administration retains the basic responsibility for both monitoring residue levels and for seizure of foods not in compliance with the regulations; what is more, the USDA continues to be the authority responsible for the monitoring of meat and poultry for pesticides as well as for other chemicals.

FIFRA regulations set out the requirements essential before an EPA–Office of Pesticide Programs review of any pesticide and/or formulated product can occur, for registration purposes. This information base includes product and residue chemistry, environmental fate, toxicology, biotransformation/degradation, occupational exposure and reentry protection, spray drift, environmental impact on nontarget species, and product performance and efficacy. Depending on the proposed use pattern of the pesticide, results from different "groups" of toxicological studies are required to support the registration. The typical spectrum of basic pesticide toxicity data required under FIFRA regulations is summarized in Table 22-2. Extensive ancillary studies of environmental impact on birds, mammals, aquatic organisms, plants, soils, environmental persistence, and bioaccumulation are also required. A schematic diagram showing the "information package" required in support of a registration and the appropriate time span required to develop this database from the point of patenting the newly synthesized chemical until its registration, production, marketing, and user acceptability is shown in Fig. 22-2. Although the ultimate uses of the particular chemical will govern the extent of the information base required prior to registration, estimates of average development costs on the order of $30 to $50 million are not unrealistic.

**Table 22–2**
**Basic Requirements Regarding Toxicity Data for New Pesticide Registrations**

| | |
|---|---|
| Acute | |
| Oral (rat) | |
| Dermal (rabbit) | |
| Inhalation (usually rat) | |
| Irritation studies | |
| Eye (rabbit) | |
| Skin (rabbit, guinea pig) | |
| Dermal sensitization (guinea pig) | |
| Delayed neurotoxicity (hen) | |
| Subchronic | |
| 90-Day feeding study | |
| Rodent (rat, mouse) | |
| Nonrodent (dog) | |
| Dermal | Dependent upon use pattern |
| Inhalation | and potential for occupational |
| Neurotoxicity | exposure |
| Chronic | |
| One- or two-year oral study | |
| Rodent (usually rat) | |
| Nonrodent (dog) | |
| Oncogenicity study (rat or mouse) | |
| Reproductive | |
| In vitro mutagenicity (microorganisms, etc.) | |
| Fertility/reproduction (rat, mouse, rabbit) | |
| Teratogenicity (rat, mouse, rabbit) | |

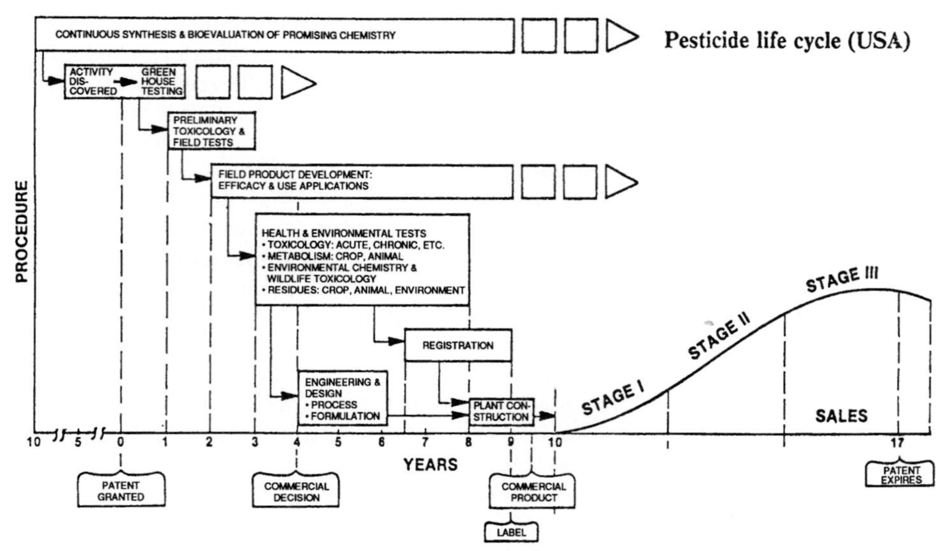


***Figure 22–2.** A schematic diagram depicting the generation of an appropriate toxicity data base, the time frame for data acquisition, and the significant milestones in the life cycle of a pesticide in the United States. (GIFAP Bulletin, Sept. 1983, with permission.)*

Other nations including Canada, the United Kingdom, Japan and, more recently, the European Economic Community (EEC) have promulgated legislation similar to that of the United States as safeguards in human exposure to pesticides in food commodities. Some developing nations, with a shortage of trained technical, scientific, and legal professionals to develop their own legislation, have adopted the regulatory framework of one or another of the industrialized nations, permitting the sale and use of pesticides registered under the legislation of that country but prohibiting the use of agents unable to meet the stringent requirements. In still other countries, almost any pesticide ever manufactured is available, no legislation having been introduced to curb adverse effects to the environment and human health.

## Exposure

The evaluation of the hazards of pesticides to human health begins with the development of a dose-effect relationship based on documented and anecdotal information on human exposure (Fig. 22-3). Several populations of individuals may be identified as having exposure to a range of concentrations of a particular agent including: (1) accidental and/or suicidal poisonings that no amount of legislation or study can prevent; (2) occupational (manufacturing, mixing/loading, application, harvesting, and handling of crops) exposure (Albertson and Cross, 1993; Edmiston and Maddy, 1987); (3) bystander exposure to off-target drift from spraying operations with, in some cases, the development of hypersensitivity (Bartle, 1991); (4) the general public who consume food items containing pesticide residues as a consequence of the illegal use of an agent (aldicarb on melons and cucumbers) or its misuse, in terms of an incorrect application rate or picking and shipping a crop too soon after pesticide application, resulting in residue concentrations above the established tolerance levels. The media is replete with documented incidents of environmental contamination by pesticides: (1) of surface and/or groundwater essential as sources of potable drinking water; (2) of commercial fish stock as well as sporting fish; (3) of wildlife upon which native peoples depend as a major source of dietary protein; and (4) of long-distance aerial transport of undeposited and/or revolatilized pesticide.

The shape of the dose-effect curve is dependent on a detailed knowledge of the amount of exposure received by each of these groups. Within each group, variability will be considerable. Frequently, exposure evaluations begin at the top of the relationship where exposure is greatest, more easily estimated, and, in most cases, the acute biological effects are clearly observed and may be associated with a specific agent or a class of chemicals over a relatively narrow dosage range. If no discernible adverse health effects are seen at high levels of exposure, it is unlikely that anything will be observed at lower levels of exposure. Although this hypothesis may be true for acute systemic effects, it is not applicable to chronic effects (changes in organ function, mutagenicity, teratogenicity, carcinogenicity) that may develop after some latent period following either a single high-level exposure, repeated moderate or high-level exposures, or annual exposure to low levels of the agents for decades.

There is sufficiently detailed documentation on many pesticidal poisonings to permit an estimation of exposure (Hayes, 1982). In some 48 suicide attempts by ingestion of the herbicide glyphosate, the average volume of product (concentrate containing active ingredient and a surfactant) ingested was 120 ml [range of 104 ml (nonfatal) to 206 ml (fatal)] (Sawada et al., 1988). In other cases, such as one involving the insecticide fenitrothion, where the individual was exposed by dermal contact to a 7.5 percent solution of the agent in corn oil wiped up with facial tissues by a bare hand, exposure was more difficult to assess (Ecobichon et al., 1977). It is impera-

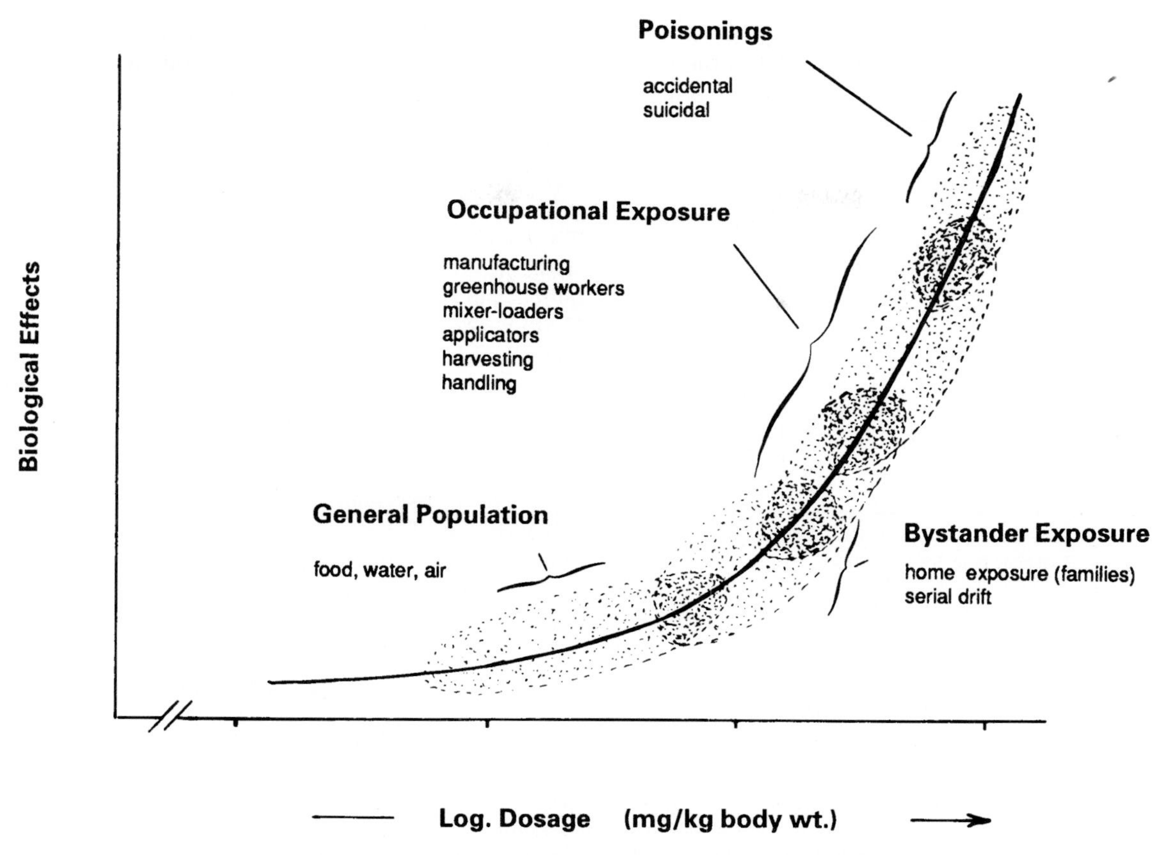


*Figure 22–3. A theoretical dose-effect relationship for acute toxicity comparing the potential for exposure in terms of occupation, level of exposure, and possible biological effects.*

tive that forensic and clinical toxicologists and emergency service personnel attempt to ascertain how much of the material was involved in the poisoning.

Worker exposure can be estimated within reason by considering the various job functions performed (e.g., diluting concentrated formulations, loading diluted end-use formulations into tanks, spray application, harvesting sprayed crops, postharvest handling of sprayed crops, etc.). The potential level(s) of pesticide encountered in each job category and the route(s) of exposure can be estimated. The majority of occupational illnesses arising from pesticides involve dermal exposure enhanced, in certain job categories, by acquisition of a portion of the dosage by the inhalation of the aerosolized spray. Many exposures appear to be entirely dermal in character. The surface area of the unclothed parts of the body of a casually dressed, unprotected worker is shown in Table 22-3, the values having been determined by Batchelor and Walker (1954) using the method of Berkow (1931). Data for the entire surface area of a "50 percentile man," as determined by Spear and coworkers (1977), are shown in Table 22-4. With surface patch (gauze, fabric) testing on various parts of the body, accurate estimates of dermal exposure can be obtained. The reader is referred to the following studies for details: Wolfe and colleagues (1967, 1972), Wojeck and coworkers (1981), and Franklin and coworkers (1981). Where inhalation can be considered to contribute significantly to the total exposure, as in greenhouse and other structural spraying operations in enclosed environments, drivers in tractor cabs, operators of rotary fan mist sprayers, and other operations, measurements of aerial concentrations in the working environment can be made and related to respiratory rates and length of time spent in that environment. Assessment of the inhalation component of an exposure can be obtained with personal air sampling monitors worn during the day (Turnbull et al., 1985; Grover et al., 1986). More direct estimates of total exposure can be made by measuring excretory products (parent chemical, degradation products) in urine and feces over a suitable postexposure time interval (Durham et al., 1972; Kolmodin-Hedman et al., 1983; Frank et al., 1985; Grover et al., 1986).

Minimal protection of certain parts of the body can markedly reduce exposure to an agent. Protection of the hands (5.6

**Table 22–3**
**Estimated Surface Area of Exposed Portions of a Body of a Casually Dressed Individual**

| UNCLOTHED SURFACE | SURFACE AREA (SQ FT) | PERCENT OF TOTAL |
|---|---|---|
| Face | 0.70 | 22.0 |
| Hands | 0.87 | 27.6 |
| Forearms | 1.30 | 41.3 |
| Back of neck | 0.12 | 3.8 |
| Front of neck and "v" of chest | 0.16 | 5.1 |

SOURCE: From Batchelor and Walker, 1954.

**Table 22–4**
**Percent of Total Body Surface Area Represented by Body Regions***

| BODY REGION | SURFACE AREA (% OF TOTAL) |
|---|---|
| Head | 5.60 |
| Neck | 1.20 |
| Upper arms | 9.70 |
| Forearms | 6.70 |
| Hands | 6.90 |
| Chest, back, shoulders | 22.80 |
| Hips | 9.10 |
| Thighs | 18.00 |
| Calves | 13.50 |
| Feet | 6.40 |

*Estimated proportions from the "50 percentile man" having a surface area of 1.92 $m^2$, height of 175 cm, and body weight of 78 kg.
SOURCE: From Spear et al, 1977.

percent of body surface) by appropriate chemical-resistant gloves may reduce contamination by 33 percent (in forest spraying with a knapsack sprayer having a single nozzle lance), by 66 percent (weed control using tractor-mounted booms equipped with hydraulic nozzles), or by 86 percent (filling tanks on tractor-powered sprayers) (Bonsall, 1985). Studies monitoring the absorption of pesticides applied to the skin of different areas of the human body have revealed marked regional variations in percutaneous absorption, with the greatest uptake being in the scrotal region, followed by the axilla, forehead, face, scalp, the dorsal aspect of the hand, the palm of the hand, and the forearm in decreasing order (Feldman and Maiback, 1974).

The exposure of a bystander, an individual accidentally but directly sprayed or exposed to aerial off-target drifting aerosol, is considerably more difficult to assess. The levels encountered may be severalfold lower than those in the occupational setting, making the analysis of residue and the detection of meaningful biological changes more difficult. Greater variation in exposure estimates and biological effects can be anticipated. The adverse health effects may be subtle in appearance and nonspecific, reflecting a slow deterioration of physiological function clouded by the individual's adjustment or adaptation to the changes, taking many years to develop to the point of detection. In a similar fashion, the identification of pesticide-related adverse health effects in the general population, who inadvertently acquire low levels of pesticides daily via food and water, is extremely difficult. The residue levels in these media are often orders of magnitude lower than those encountered in occupational or bystander exposure and are at or near the limits of analytical detection by sophisticated techniques. Any biological effects resulting from such low-level exposure are unlikely to be distinctive and any causal association with a particular chemical or class of agents is likely to be tenuous and confounded by many other factors of a lifestyle.

Many of the public concerns about pesticides are related to "older" chemicals, these having entered the market in the 1950s and 1960s without the benefit of the extensive toxicity and environmental impact studies demanded prior to the registration of chemicals today. It must also be pointed out that many of these older pesticides have received little reassessment using the more definitive techniques and protocols required today. Although government agencies and industry have been slow in their reevaluation of a vast array of pesticides in use, reassessment often comes in the wake of or concomitant with some recently disclosed adverse environmental or health effect. Given the above-mentioned costs of conducting a full range of studies (introductory section, this chapter), the time frame required, and the limited market for some of these chemicals in North America or even worldwide, the registration of many of these pesticides will be withdrawn voluntarily by industry, and the answers to some of the public's concerns will never be obtained. Hazardous chemicals will be removed from use but, unfortunately, it is possible that some very beneficial and essential pesticides will be lost. The problems of today's situation, created by the last generation and inherited by the present one, still must be dealt with. It is imperative that one has a thorough understanding of the toxicity associated with pesticides and, whenever possible, an in-depth knowledge of the basic mechanisms of action of these chemicals.

## INSECTICIDES

The literature pertaining to the chemistry and development of the various classes of insecticides over the past 45 years is extensive and the reader is referred to the monographs of O'Brien (1960, 1967), Melnikov (1971), Fest and Schmidt (1973), Brooks (1974), Eto (1974), Hayes (1982), Kuhr and Dorough (1976), Buchel (1983), Leahey (1985), Chambers and Levi (1992), and Ecobichon and Joy (1994) for detailed discussions of the chemistry, nomenclature (chemical, common, and trade names), biotransformation and degradation, environmental effects, as well as target and nontarget species toxicity. Compilations of $LD_{50}$ values in the laboratory rat may be found in Gaines (1969), Frear (1969), and Worthing (1987). Acute toxicity data for laboratory animals, fish, and wildlife are recorded in a number of reports (Pickering et al., 1962; Tucker and Crabtree, 1970; Worthing, 1987). Only selected examples of the classes of insecticides will be discussed in this chapter, with emphasis on their toxicity to humans.

All of the chemical insecticides in use today are neurotoxicants and act by poisoning the nervous systems of the target organisms. The central nervous system (CNS) of insects is highly developed and not unlike that of the mammal (O'Brien, 1960). While the peripheral nervous system (PNS) of insects is not as complex as that of mammals, there are striking similarities (O'Brien, 1960). The development of insecticides has been based on specific structure-activity relationships requiring the manipulation of a basic chemical structure to obtain an optimal shape and configuration for specificity toward a unique biochemical or physiological feature of the nervous system. Given the fact that insecticides are not selective and affect nontarget species as readily as target organisms, it is not surprising that a chemical that acts on the insect nervous system will elicit similar effects in higher forms of life. The target sites and/or mechanism(s) of action may be similar in all species; only the dosage (level of exposure and duration) will dictate the intensity of biological effects. It is sufficient at this stage to indicate the potential sites of action of the insecticide classes (Fig. 22-4) and their interference with

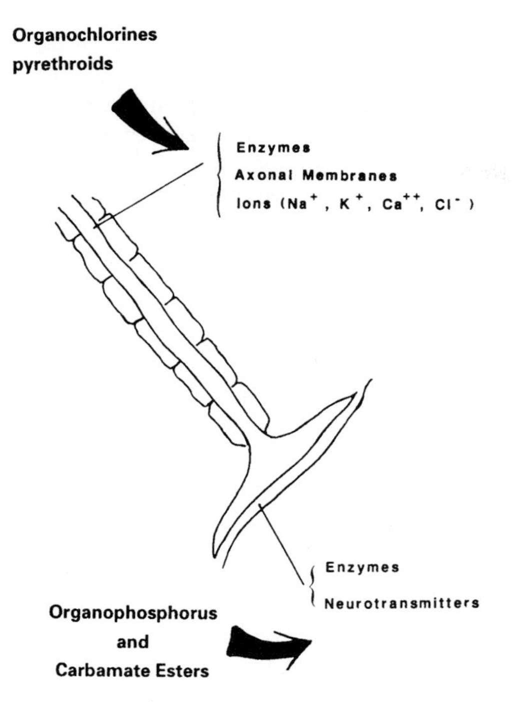


*Figure 22–4. Potential sites of action of classes of insecticides on the axon and the terminal portions of the nerve.*

the membrane transport of sodium, potassium, calcium, or chloride ions; inhibition of selective enzymatic activities; or contribution to the release and/or the persistence of chemical transmitters at nerve endings.

## Organochlorine Insecticides

Although DDT was first synthesized by Zeidler in 1874, it remained for Paul Müller, a Swiss chemist working for J. R. Geigy AG, to rediscover DDT in 1939 while searching for a contact poison against clothes moths and carpet beetles. The effectiveness of DDT against a variety of household and crop insect pests was quickly demonstrated, earning Müller a Nobel Prize in 1948 for his research. Before the end of World War II, DDT was available to the Allies and saw its first medical use in the suppression of a typhus epidemic in Naples, Italy, during the winter of 1943–1944 when it was applied directly to humans to control lice (Brooks, 1974). The discovery of the insecticidal properties of other organochlorine compounds including aldrin, dieldrin, endrin, chlordane, and benzene hexachloride before 1945 had immediate consequences and introduced the era of the synthetic chemical insecticides and their remarkable impact on food production and human health (Metcalf, 1972, 1973; Brooks, 1974).

The organochlorine (chlorinated hydrocarbon) insecticides are a diverse group of agents belonging to three distinct chemical classes including the dichlorodiphenylethane-, the chlorinated cyclodiene-, and the chlorinated benzene- and cyclohexane-related structures (Table 22-5). From the mid-1940s to the mid-1960s, these agents were used extensively in all aspects of agriculture and forestry, in building and structural protection, and in human situations to control a wide variety of insect pests. The properties (low volatility, chemical stability, lipid solubility, slow rate of biotransformation and degradation) that made these chemicals such effective insecticides also brought about their demise because of their persistence in the environment, bioconcentration, and biomagnification within various food chains. The acquisition of biologically active body burdens in many wildlife species that, if not lethal, certainly interfered with the reproductive success of the species became recognized, and Rachel Carson's book, *Silent Spring*, did much to draw attention to the plight of wildlife, particularly avian species such as grebes, pelicans, falcons, and eagles, that occupied the top trophic level of their respective food chains (Carson, 1962).

Definitive studies both in wildlife and laboratory species have demonstrated potent estrogenic and enzyme-inducing properties of the organochlorine insecticides, which interfered directly or indirectly with fertility and reproduction (Stickel, 1968; McFarland and Lacy, 1969; Longcore et al., 1971; McBlain et al., 1977; Crum et al., 1993). In avian species, such interference is related to steroid metabolism and the inability of the bird to mobilize sufficient calcium to produce a strong enough

**Table 22–5**
**Structural Classification of Organochlorine Insecticides**

| Class | Examples |
|---|---|
| Dichlorodiphenylethanes | DDT, DDD<br>Dicofol<br>Perthane<br>Methoxychlor<br>Methlochlor |
| Cyclodienes | Aldrin, Dieldrin<br>Heptachlor<br>Chlordane<br>Endosulfan |
| Chlorinated Benzenes<br>Cyclohexanes | HCB, HCH<br>Lindane ($\alpha$-BHC) |

eggshell to withstand the rigors of being buffeted around in a nest; the resultant cracking allows the entry of bacteria, which causes the developing embryo to die (Carson, 1962; Peakall, 1970). Reproduction in fish is adversely affected by the bioconcentration of these agents in the yolk sac of the fry. Many studies have demonstrated the gradual accumulation of residues of these chemicals and their metabolites in body tissues as well as the slow elimination from the system. Despite the ban on their use in North America and Europe, organochlorine insecticides are used extensively in developing nations because they are inexpensive to manufacture, highly effective, and relatively safe; few substitutes are available and the risk-benefit ratio is highly weighted in favor of their continued use for the control of insects causing devastation to crops and human health. These insecticides are still important toxicologically.

**Signs and Symptoms of Poisoning.** Given the diversity of chemical structures, it is not surprising that the signs and symptoms of toxicity and the mechanisms of action are somewhat different (Table 22-6).

Exposure of humans and animals to high oral doses of DDT results in paresthesia of the tongue, lips, and face; apprehension, hypersusceptibility to external (light, touch, sound) stimuli; irritability; dizziness, vertigo; tremor; and tonic and clonic convulsions. Motor unrest and fine tremors associated with voluntary movements progress to coarse tremors without interruption in moderate to severe poisonings. Symptoms generally appear several hours (6 to 24 h) after exposure to large doses. Little toxicity is seen following the dermal exposure to DDT, presumably because the agent is poorly absorbed through the skin, a physiological phenomenon that has contributed to the fairly good safety record of DDT, despite careless handling by applicators and formulators (Hayes, 1971). It has been estimated that a dose of 10 mg/kg will cause signs of poisoning in humans. Chronic exposure to moderate concentrations of DDT causes somewhat milder signs of toxicity, as listed in Table 22-6.

Although the functional injury of DDT poisoning can be associated with effects on the CNS in humans, few pathological changes can be demonstrated in that tissue in animals.

**Table 22–6**
**Signs and Symptoms of Acute and Chronic Toxicity Following Exposure to Organochlorine Insecticides**

| INSECTICIDE CLASS | ACUTE SIGNS | CHRONIC SIGNS |
|---|---|---|
| Dichlorodiphenylethanes<br>DDT<br>DDD (Rothane)<br>DMC (Dimite)<br>Dicofol (Kelthane)<br>Methoxychlor<br>Methiochlor<br>Chlorbenzylate<br>Hexachlorocyclohexanes<br>Lindane ($\gamma$-isomer)<br>Benzene hexachloride (mixed isomers) | Parathesia (oral ingestion)<br>Ataxia, abnormal stepping<br>Dizziness, confusion, headache<br>Nausea, vomiting<br>Fatigue, lethargy<br>Tremor (peripheral) | Loss of weight, anorexia<br>Mild anemia<br>Tremors<br>Muscular weakness<br>EEG pattern changes<br>Hyperexcitability, anxiety<br>Nervous tension |
| Cyclodienes<br>Endrin<br>Telodrin<br>Isodrin<br>Endosulfan<br>Heptachlor<br>Aldrin<br>Dieldrin<br>Chlordane<br>Toxaphene | Dizziness, headache<br>Nausea, vomiting<br>Motor hyperexcitability<br>Hyperreflexia<br>Myoclonic jerking<br>General malaise<br>Convulsive seizures<br>Generalized convulsions | Headache, dizziness, hyperexcitability<br>Intermittent muscle twitching and myoclonic jerking<br>Psychological disorders including insomnia, anxiety, irritability<br>EEG pattern changes<br>Loss of consciousness<br>Epileptiform convulsions |
| Chlordecone (Kepone)<br>Mirex | | Chest pains, arthralgia<br>Skin rashes<br>Ataxia, incoordination, slurred speech, opsoclonus<br>Visual difficulty, inability to focus and fixate<br>Nervousness, irritability, depression<br>Loss of recent memory<br>Muscle weakness, tremors of hands<br>Severe impairment of spermatogenesis |

However, following exposure to moderate or high nonfatal doses or subsequent to subacute or chronic feeding, major pathological changes are observed in the liver and reproductive organs. Morphological changes in mammalian liver include hypertrophy of hepatocytes and subcellular organelles such as mitochondria, proliferation of smooth endoplasmic reticulum and the formation of inclusion bodies, centrolobular necrosis following exposure to high concentrations, and an increase in the incidence of hepatic tumors (Hayes, 1959; Hansell and Ecobichon, 1974; IARC, 1974). However, there has been no epidemiological evidence linking DDT to carcinogenicity in humans (Hayes, 1975, 1982). When technical DDT (20 percent *o,p'*-DDT plus 80 percent *p,p'*-DDT) was administered to male cockerels or rats, reduced testicular size was observed and, in female rats, the estrogenic effects of the *o,p'*-isomer were observed in the edematous, blood-engorged uteri (Hayes, 1959; Ecobichon and MacKenzie, 1974). The *o,p'*-isomer has been shown to compete with estradiol for binding the estrogen receptors in rat uterine cytosol (Kupfer and Bulger, 1976).

Dicofol (*p-p'*-dichlorodiphenyl-2,2,2-trichloroethanol), an analog of DDT still registered as an agricultural miticide for cotton, beans, citrus, and grapes, has been associated with acute toxicity (nausea, dizziness, double vision, ataxia, confusion, disorientation) in a 12-year-old male whose clothing became saturated in an accident (Lessenger and Riley, 1991). These acute effects progressed to chronic signs (headaches, blurred vision, horizontal nystagmus, numbness/tingling in legs with shooting pains, clumsiness, memory loss and decreasing academic performance, impulsive behavior, restlessness, fatigue) which persisted in some fashion for up to 4 months. Continuing emotional and academic difficulties, impairment of certain cognitive skills, poor self-esteem and depression, all of which were subtle cognitive and psychological changes, persisted for over 18 months. Dicofol is known to be contaminated by a small percentage of *p,p'*-DDT.

Unlike the situation with DDT, in which there have been few recorded fatalities following poisoning, there have been a number of fatalities following poisoning by the cyclodiene- and hexachlorocyclohexane-type insecticides. The chlorinated cyclodiene insecticides are among the most toxic and environmentally persistent pesticides known (Hayes, 1982). One recent study of two patients, one with a history of chronic exposure to aldrin and the other with a chronic exposure to lindane/heptachlor, reported death within 2 years of developing clinical and electromyographic signs and symptoms of chronic motor disease with aggravation of dysphagia and weight loss resulting in the mobilization of adipose tissue and stored insecticide to enhance the neuronal toxicity (Fonseca et al., 1993). Even at low doses, these chemicals tend to induce convulsions before less serious signs of illness occur. Although the sequence of signs generally follows the appearance of headaches, nausea, vertigo and mild clonic jerking, motor hyperexcitability, and hyperreflexia, some patients have convulsions without warning symptoms (Hayes, 1971). An important difference between DDT and the chlorinated cyclodienes is that the latter are efficiently absorbed through the skin and, therefore, pose an appreciable hazard to occupationally exposed individuals. Chronic exposure to low or moderate concentrations of these agents elicits a spectrum of signs and symptoms, including both sensory and motor components of the CNS (Table 22-6). In addition to the recognized neurotoxicity, aldrin and dieldrin interfere with reproduction, increased pup losses (vitality, viability) reported in studies in rats and dogs (Kitselman, 1953; Treon and Cleveland, 1955). Treatment with dieldrin during pregnancy caused a reduction in fertility and increased pup mortality (Treon and Cleveland, 1955). The treatment of pregnant mice with dieldrin resulted in teratological effects (delayed ossification, increases in supernumerary ribs) (Chernoff et al., 1975).

Exposure to lindane (the $\gamma$-isomer of hexachlorocyclohexane, HCH) produces signs of poisoning that resemble those caused by DDT (e.g., tremors, ataxia, convulsions, stimulated respiration, and prostration). In severe cases of acute poisoning, violent tonic and clonic convulsions occur and degenerative changes in the liver and in renal tubules have been noted. Technical grade HCH used in insecticidal preparations contains a mixture of isomers: the $\gamma$- and $\alpha$-isomers are convulsant poisons; the $\beta$- and $\delta$-isomers are CNS depressants. The mechanisms of action remain unknown. Lifetime feeding studies in mice have revealed that technical HCH and some of the isomers caused an increase in hepatocellular tumors (IARC, 1974). Only the $\gamma$-isomer (lindane) sees any medicinal use today, as a component of a pediculicide shampoo for head lice. One undocumented case of lindane toxicity, known to the author, resulted in mild tremors in a child on whose head the shampoo was used vigorously and repeatedly for more than a week. The symptoms disappeared rapidly when the treatment was terminated.

Industrial carelessness during the manufacture of an organochlorine compound chlordecone (Kepone) brought this agent and the closely related insecticide, mirex, to the attention of toxicologists in 1975 when 76 of 148 workers in a factory in Hopewell, Virginia, developed a severe neurological syndrome (Cannon et al., 1978; Taylor et al., 1978; Guzelian, 1982). This condition, known as the "Kepone shakes," was characterized by tremors, altered gait, behavioral changes, ocular flutter (opsoclonus), arthralgia, headache, chest pains, weight loss, hepatomegaly, splenomegaly, and impotence, the onset of symptoms generally occurring with a latency of approximately 30 days from the initiation of exposure and persisting for many months after the termination of exposure (Joy, 1994a). Laboratory tests showed a reduced sperm count and reduced sperm motility. Routine neurological studies revealed nothing untoward, but microscopic examination of biopsies of the sural nerve revealed relative decreases in the populations of small myelinated and unmyelinated axons. With electron microscopy, a number of abnormalities were visible and the significant findings included damage to Schwann cells (membranous inclusions, cytoplasmic folds), prominent endoneural collagen pockets, vacuolization of unmyelinated fibers, focal degeneration of axons with condensation of neurofilaments and neurotubules, focal interlamellar splitting of myelin sheaths, and the formation of myelin bodies and a complex infolding of inner mesaxonal membranes into axoplasm (Martinez et al., 1977). The involvement of unmyelinated fibers and small myelinated fibers may partially explain the clinical picture. It has been suggested that chlordecone may interfere with metabolic processes in Schwann cells. However, it should be noted that all of these degenerative changes are nonspecific in nature and are commonly seen in other toxic polyneuropathies. Many of the toxic manifestations of chlordecone poisoning in these workers have been confirmed in animal studies, the major target organs being the CNS, the liver, the adrenals, and the testes, as summarized by Joy (1994a). As with other organochlorine insecticides, chlordecone is an excellent inducer of hepatic microsomal monooxygenase enzymes and, in rats and mice, has been associated with the formation of hepatomas and malignant tumors in organs other than the liver, female animals being more susceptible than male (Guzelian, 1982). In many ways, mirex behaves like chlordecone and there is evidence for the oxidative biotransformation of mirex to chlordecone in vivo. Mirex causes hepatomegaly and a dose-dependent increase in neoplastic nodules and hepatocellular carcinomas, particularly in male animals (Innes et al., 1969; Waters et al., 1977).

**Site and Mechanism of Toxic Actions.** Essential to the action of organochlorine insecticides is an intact reflex arc consisting of afferent (sensory) peripheral neurons impinging on interneurons in the spinal cord, with accompanying ramifications and interconnections up and down the CNS and interactions with efferent, motor neurons as shown schematically in Fig. 22-5. Examining the mechanism of action of the DDT-type insecticides, the most striking observation in a poisoned insect or mammal is the display of periodic sequences of persistent tremoring and/or convulsive seizures suggestive of repetitive discharges in neurons. These characteristic episodes of hyperactivity interspersed with normal function were recognized as early as 1946. The second most striking observation is that these repetitive tremors, seizures, and electrical activity can be initiated by tactile and auditory stimuli, suggesting that the sensory nervous system appears to be much more responsive to stimuli. An examination of the sequence of electrical events in normal and DDT-poisoned nerves reveals that, in the latter, a characteristic prolongation of the falling phase of the action potential (the negative afterpotential) occurs (Fig. 22-6). The nerve membrane remains in a partially depolarized and partially repolarized state and is extremely sensitive to complete depolarization again by very small stimuli (Joy, 1994a). Thus, following exposure to DDT, the repetitive stimulation of the peripheral sensory nerves by touch or sound is magnified in the CNS, causing generalized tremoring throughout the body.

How does DDT elicit this effect? There are at least four mechanisms, possibly all functioning simultaneously (Matsumura, 1985) as seen in Fig. 22-7. At the level of the neuronal membrane, DDT affects the permeability to potassium ions, reducing potassium transport across the membrane. DDT alters the porous channels through which sodium ions pass—these channels activate (open) normally but, once open, are inactivated (closed) slowly, thereby interfering with the active transport of sodium out of the nerve axon during repolarization. DDT inhibits neuronal adenosine triphosphatase (ATPase), particularly the $Na^+$,$K^+$-ATPase and $Ca^{2+}$-ATPase that play vital roles in neuronal repolarization. DDT also inhibits

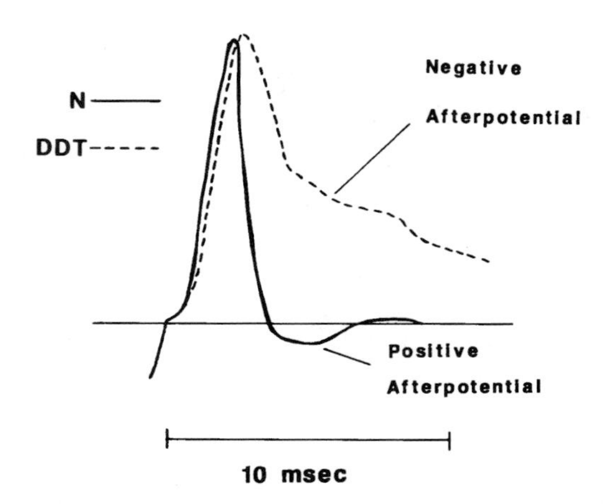


*Figure 22–6. A schematic diagram of an oscilloscope recording of the depolarization and repolarization of a normal neuron (——) and one from a DDT-treated animal (- - - -), showing the prolongation of the negative afterpotential (NAP).*

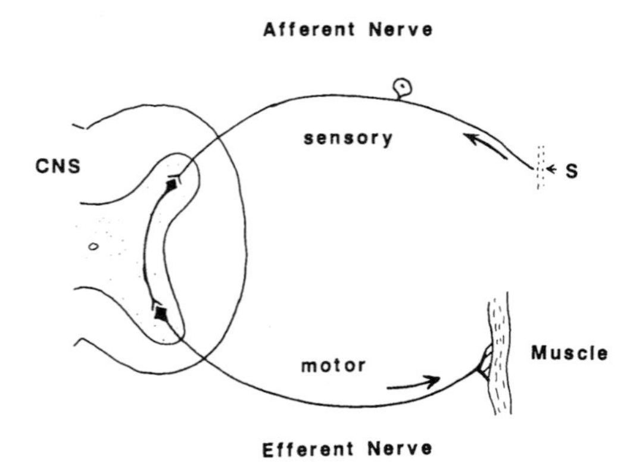


*Figure 22–5. A simple, intact reflex arc involving a peripheral, afferent (sensory) neuron, interneurons in the CNS, and a peripheral, efferent (motor) neuron that innervates a muscle.*

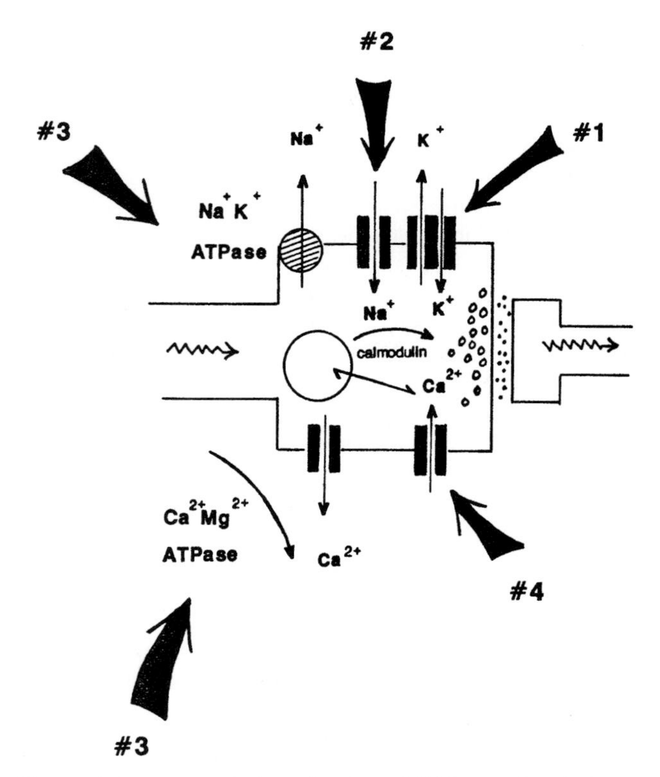


*Figure 22–7. Proposed sites of action of DDT on (1) reducing potassium transport through pores; (2) inactivating sodium channel closure; (3) inhibiting sodium-potassium and calcium-magnesium ATPases; and (4) calmodulin-calcium binding with release of neurotransmitter.*

the ability of calmodulin, a calcium mediator in nerves, to transport calcium ions essential for the intraneuronal release of neurotransmitters. All of these inhibited functions reduce the rate at which repolarization occurs and increase the sensitivity of the neurons to small stimuli that would not elicit a response in a fully repolarized neuron.

The chlorinated cyclodiene-, benzene-, and cyclohexane-type insecticides are different from DDT in many respects, both in the appearance of the intoxicated individual and possibly also in the mechanism(s), which appear to be localized more in the CNS than in the sensory division of the PNS (Table 22-6). The overall appearance of the intoxicated individual is one of CNS stimulation. As is shown in Fig. 22-8, the cyclodiene compounds mimic the action of the chemical picrotoxin, a nerve excitant and antagonist of the neurotransmitter $\gamma$-aminobutyric acid (GABA) found in the CNS (Eldefrawi et al., 1985; Matsumura, 1985). GABA induces the uptake of chloride ions by neurons. The blockage of this activity by picrotoxin, picrotoxinin, or cyclodiene insecticides results in only partial repolarization of the neuron and a state of uncontrolled excitation. The cyclodiene insecticides are also potent inhibitors of $Na^+$, $K^+$-ATPase and, more importantly, of the enzyme $Ca^{2+}$, $Mg^{2+}$-ATPase that is essential for the transport (uptake and release) of calcium across membranes (Matsumura, 1985; Wafford et al., 1989). The inhibition of $Ca^{2+}$, $Mg^{2+}$-ATPase, located in the terminal ends of neurons in synaptic membranes, results in an accumulation of intracellular free calcium ions with the promotion of calcium-induced release of neurotransmitters from storage vesicles and the subsequent depolarization of adjacent neurons and the propagation of stimuli throughout the CNS.

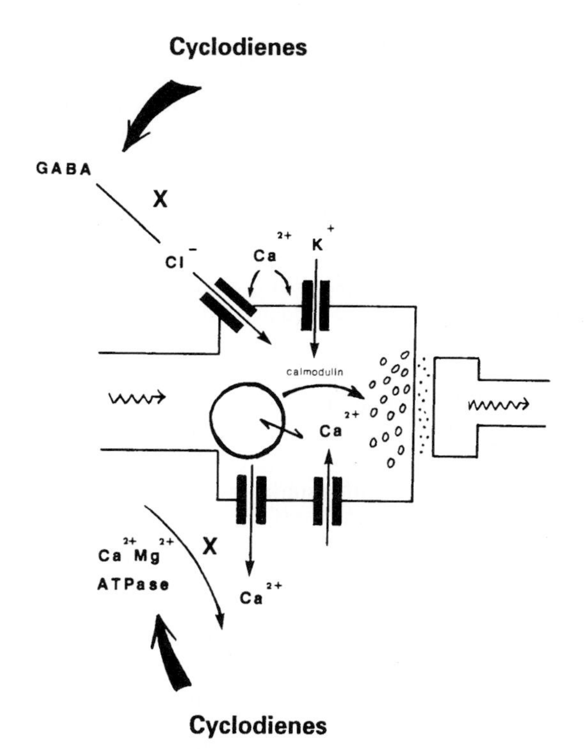


*Figure 22–8. Proposed sites of action of cyclodiene-type organochlorine insecticides on chloride ion transport by antagonizing GABA receptors in the chloride channel as well as inhibition of $Ca^{2+}$, $Mg^{2+}$-ATPase.*

**Biotransformation, Distribution, and Storage.** The phenomenon of bioconcentration and biomagnification of the organochlorine insecticides in food chains has been mentioned. Once acquired, biotransformation proceeds at an exceptionally slow rate due, in part, to the complex aromatic ring structures and the extent of chlorination, because these ring substituents are exceedingly difficult to remove by the enzymatic processes available in body tissues. DDT undergoes slow but extensive biotransformation in mammals—one major metabolite, DDE, is formed nonenzymatically as well as by enzymatic dechlorination (Fig. 22-9) (Ecobichon and Saschenbrecker, 1968). Other degradation products such as DDD and DDA are formed by a series of reductive dechlorination and oxidative reactions, only the latter agent being sufficiently water soluble to be readily excreted (Ecobichon and Saschenbrecker, 1968). Not surprisingly, analysis of body tissues yields a mixture of DDT and various metabolites, all of which possess a relatively high degree of lipid solubility. The results of such analyses are frequently presented in terms of total DDT-derived material. In contrast, the biotransformation of the cyclodiene-type insecticides is extremely slow; aldrin and heptachlor are converted by oxidative reactions to dieldrin and heptachlor epoxide, respectively, without altering significantly either the lipid solubility characteristics or their toxicological properties (Keane and Zavon, 1969; Matthews and Matsumura, 1969). Although the $\alpha$-, $\beta$, and $\gamma$-isomers of hexachlorocyclohexane are biotransformed at significantly different rates in vivo by dehydrochlorination, glutathione conjugation, and aromatic ring hydroxylation to produce a variety of excretable phenolic products, the $\beta$-isomer is much more slowly metabolized and is found as the predominant tissue residue (Egan et al., 1965; O'Brien, 1967; Abbott et al., 1968). Toxophene, a complex mixture of chlorinated comphenes (chlorobornanes) possessing widely varying biological activities, is extensively biotransformed by both oxidative and reductive cytochrome P-450 monooxygenases (Saleh et al., 1977; Turner et al., 1977). Considering the complex cage-structured chlordecone and mirex, there is little evidence of any biotransformation of these chemicals in vivo other than the oxidative conversion of mirex into the ketone chlordecone, prior to either slow excretion in the feces or storage in body fat.

The highly lipid-soluble nature of the organochlorine insecticides, characterized by large fat : water partition coefficients, guarantees that these chemicals will be sequestered in body tissues (liver, kidneys, nervous system, adipose tissue) having a high lipid content, in which the residues either elicit some biological effect or, as in the case of adipose tissue, remain stored and undisturbed (Dale and Quinby, 1963; Davies et al., 1972). Studies in both humans and laboratory animals have demonstrated that there was a log-log relationship between the daily intake of DDT and adipose residues, with a state of equilibrium attained between intake and elimination from the body and plateau residue concentrations related to the amount of agent acquired daily. Following the termination of exposure, the organochlorine insecticides are slowly eliminated from the storage sites in vivo. The elimination of DDT from the body occurs at a rate of approximately 1.0 percent of the stored quantity per day (Hayes, 1971). The elimination rates from animals are exceedingly slow; biological half-lives of DDT in exposed cattle are on the order of 335 days (Laben et al., 1965). The elimination rate and depletion of body storage sites may be enhanced by fasting, which results

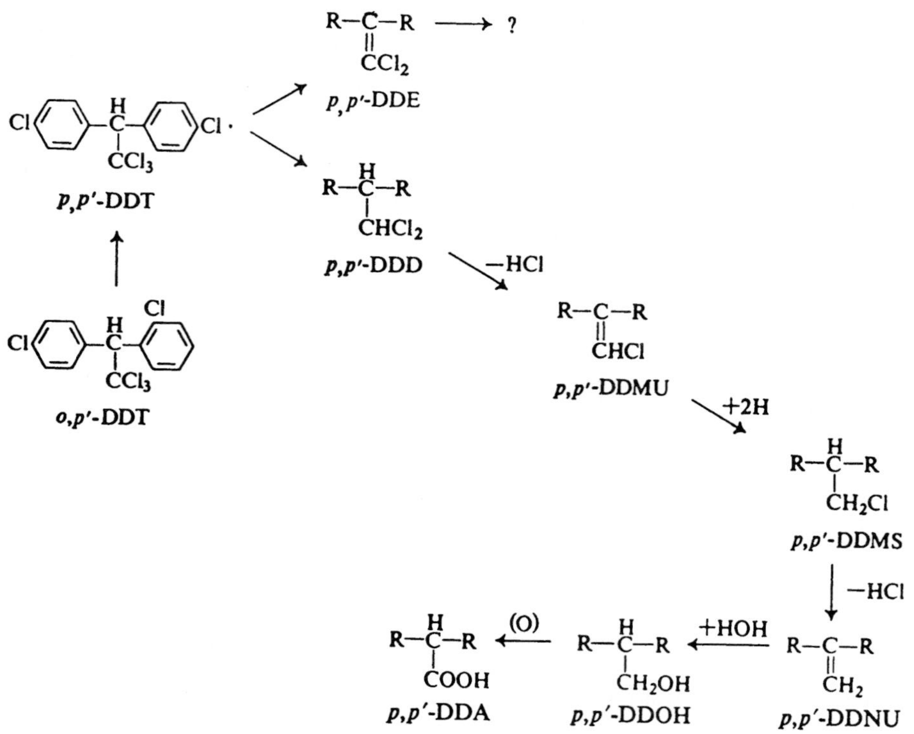

*Figure 22–9. Degradation of DDT by mammalian and avian tissues.*

*Abbreviations:* DDD, 1,1-dichloro-2,2-bis(*p*-chlorophenyl)ethane; DDE, 1,1-dichloro-2,2-bis(*p*-chlorophenyl)ethylene; DDMU, 1-chloro-2,2-bis(*p*-chlorophenyl)ethylene; DDMS, 1-chloro-2,2-(*p*-chlorophenyl)ethane; DDNU, unsym-bis(*p*-chlorophenyl)ethylene; DDOH, 2,2-bis(*p*-chlorophenyl)ethanol; DDA, bis(*p*-chlorophenyl)acetic acid. [From Ecobichon and Saschenbrecker (1968).]

in the mobilization of adipose tissue and the insecticide contained therein (Ecobichon and Saschenbrecker, 1969). However, with a high body burden of toxicant, there is the possibility of enhanced toxicity from the circulating agent being redistributed to target organs, as was seen in a study in cockerels (Ecobichon and Saschenbrecker, 1969). In animals with a body burden of DDT, treatment with phenobarbital has resulted in an enhanced elimination of the agent and metabolites as measured by residue levels in biological fluids and tissues (Alary et al., 1971; Lambert and Brodeur, 1976).

Given the physicochemical properties of the organochlorine insecticides, it is not surprising that humans acquired body burdens of these chemicals during the 1950s and 1960s when they were used on almost all food crops. Depending on the region of the world, the intensity of use, the extent of occupational and accidental exposure, and dietary habits, the bioconcentration and bioaccumulation of DDT in human adipose tissue resulted in levels on the order of 5 ppm DDT and approximately 15 ppm of total DDT-derived material (Quinby et al., 1965; Fiserova-Bergerova et al., 1967; Abbott et al., 1968; Morgan and Roan, 1970). The levels of other organochlorine insecticides sequestered in body fat were never as high as that of DDT. With declining use and the eventual ban of this class of insecticides from the North American market, body burdens of these insecticides declined slowly. By the late 1960s adipose levels of 2 ppm DDT (9 ppm of total DDT-derived material) were detectable. Whereas the daily intake of DDT in the United States was approximately 0.2 mg/day in 1958, this had decreased to about 0.04 mg/day by 1970 (Hayes, 1971). Today, only trace levels of DDT, less than 2.0 ppm of total DDT-derived material, are detectable in human adipose tissue (Mes et al., 1982; Redetzke and Applegate, 1993; Stevens et al., 1993). Currently, major concerns are centered on the Inuit living in Arctic regions where the sources of dietary protein (fish, seals, walruses, whales, etc.) have proven to be major depositories of organochlorine insecticides and other chlorinated hydrocarbons (PCBs, PCDDs, PCDFs). As the ripple effect of global pollution spreads to these distant regions, the resident animal species, possessing significant adipose tissue depots, have acquired body burdens of these chemicals and the human occupies the top position in these food chains.

**Treatment of Poisoning.** The life-threatening situation in organochlorine insecticide poisoning is associated with the tremors, the motor seizures, and the interference with respiratory function (hypoxemia and resulting acidosis) arising from repetitive stimulation of the CNS. In addition to the general decontamination and supportive treatment, diazepam (0.3 mg/kg IV; maximum dose of 10 mg) or phenobarbital (15 mg/kg IV; maximum dose of 1.0 g) may be administered by slow injection to control the convulsions. It may be necessary to repeat the treatment.

Although such treatment was not available when the organochlorine insecticides were at their peak of use, recent experience with chlordecone intoxications introduced a regimen of therapy to enhance the rate of excretion of stored chlordecone from the body. The oral administration of the anion-exchange resin, cholestyramine, to intoxicated patients resulted in a 3- to 18-fold enhanced fecal excretion of chlordecone, significantly reduced the biological half-life of stored chlordecone, and enhanced the rate of recovery from toxic manifestations (Cohn et al., 1978). The rationale for the use of cholestyramine rests on the biliary-enterohepatic circulation of chlordecone, the anion-exchange resin binding the secreted insecticide, reducing reabsorption and retaining the bound agent in the lumen of the intestinal tract for fecal excretion. Indirectly, cholestyramine may reduce chlordecone reabsorption by binding bile salts and thereby reducing the formation of emulsions and the uptake of this lipid-soluble agent. Whether or not such therapy would be suitable for other organochlorine insecticides would be dependent on the extent of biliary secretion of the agents and/or their metabolites. It is possible that cholestyramine might prove efficacious in treating organochlorine insecticide intoxications.

## Anticholinesterase Insecticides

The agents comprising this type of insecticide have a common mechanism of action but arise from two distinctly different chemical classes, the esters of phosphoric or phosphorothioic acid and those of carbamic acid (Fig. 22-10). The anticholinesterase insecticides are represented by a vast array of structures that have demonstrated the ultimate in structure-activity relationships in attempts to produce potent and selective insect toxicity while minimizing the toxicity toward nontarget species. Today, there are some 200 different organophosphorus ester insecticides and approximately 25 carbamic acid ester insecticides in the marketplace, formulated into literally thousands of products. For detailed discussions on nomenclature, chemistry, and development of these insecticides, the reader is referred to the books of O'Brien (1960), Heath (1961), Melnikov (1971), Fest and Schmidt (1973), Eto (1974), Kuhr and Dorough (1976), Ecobichon and Joy (1994), Matsumura (1985), and a review by Holmstedt (1959).

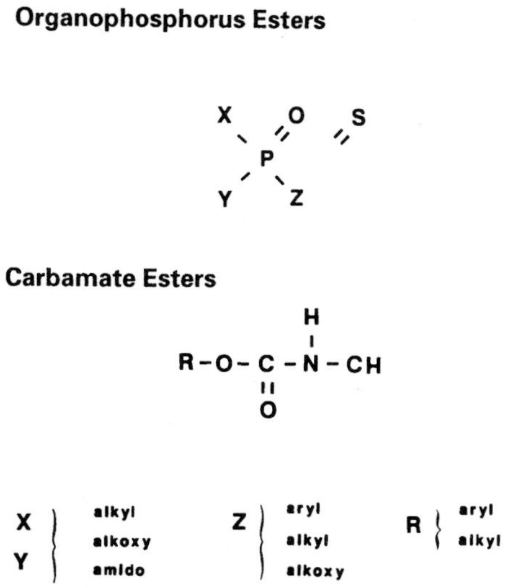

**Organophosphorus Esters**

X, Y, Z attached to P; P=O or P=S

**Carbamate Esters**

R-O-C(=O)-N(H)-CH

X, Y: alkyl, alkoxy, amido

Z: aryl, alkyl, alkoxy

R: aryl, alkyl

*Figure 22–10. The basic backbone structures of the two types of anticholinesterase class insecticides, the organophosphorus and the carbamate esters.*

With the organophosphorus compounds the esters may be of phosphoric acid (P = O) or of phosphorothioic (P = S) acids. The substituents X, Y, Z, and R denote the variety of groups attached directly to or through an oxygen to the phosphorus.

The organophosphorus ester insecticides were first synthesized in 1937 by a group of German chemists led by Gerhard Schrader at Farbenfabriken Bayer AG (Schrader and Kukenthal, 1937). Many of their trial compounds proved to be exceedingly toxic and, unfortunately, under the management of the Nazis in World War II, some were developed as potential chemical warfare agents. It is unwise to dismiss the chemical warfare nerve gases completely as the weapons of a past, more barbaric era, because it is known that at least one country has stocks of a number of these agents (Fig. 22-11) (Clement, 1994; Gee, 1992). Indeed, sarin (*O*-isopropyl methylphosphonofluoridate) was used by Iraq against Kurdish villages in northern Iraq in 1988, and residues of isopropyl methylphosphonic acid were found in soil samples along with minute traces of sarin (Webb, 1993). The physicochemical and toxicological properties of these agents have been reviewed recently (Sidell, 1992; Somani et al., 1992). Although it is true that all of the organophosphorus esters were derived from "nerve gases" (chemicals such as soman, sarin, and tabun), a fact that the media continually emphasizes, the insecticides used today are at least four generations of development away from those highly toxic chemicals. The first organophosphorus ester insecticide to be used commercially was tetraethylpyrophosphate (TEPP) and, although effective, it was extremely toxic to all forms of life and chemical stability was a major problem in that TEPP hydrolyzed readily in the presence of moisture. Further development was directed toward the synthesis of more stable chemicals having moderate environmental persistence, giving rise to parathion (*O,O*-diethyl-*O-p*-nitrophenyl phosphorothioate, E-605) in 1944 and the oxygen analog, paraoxon (*O,O*-diethyl-*O-p*-nitrophenyl phosphate) at a later date. Although these two chemicals had the properties desired in an insecticide (low volatility, chemical stability in sunlight and in the presence of water, environmental persistence for efficacy), they both exhibited a marked mammalian toxicity and were unselective with respect to target and nontarget species. The replacement of DDT with parathion in the 1950s resulted in a series of fatal poisonings and bizarre accidents arising from the fact that workers did not appreciate that this agent was far different from the relatively innocuous organochlorine insecticides with which they were familiar (Ecobichon, 1994a). The number of severe poisonings attributed to parathion provided the stimulus for a search for analogs more selective in their toxicity to target species and less toxic to nontarget organisms, including wildlife, domestic stock, and humans.

The first pesticidal carbamic acid esters were synthesized in the 1930s and were marketed as fungicides. Since these aliphatic esters possessed poor insecticidal activity, interest lay dormant until the mid-1950s when renewed interest in insecticides having anticholinesterase activity but reduced mammalian toxicity led to the synthesis of several potent aryl esters of methylcarbamic acid. The insecticidal carbamates were synthesized on purely chemical grounds as analogs of the drug physostigmine, a toxic anticholinesterase alkaloid extracted from the seeds of the plant *Physostigma venenosum*, the Calabar bean.

**Signs and Symptoms of Poisoning.** Although the structures are diverse in nature, the mechanism by which the organo-

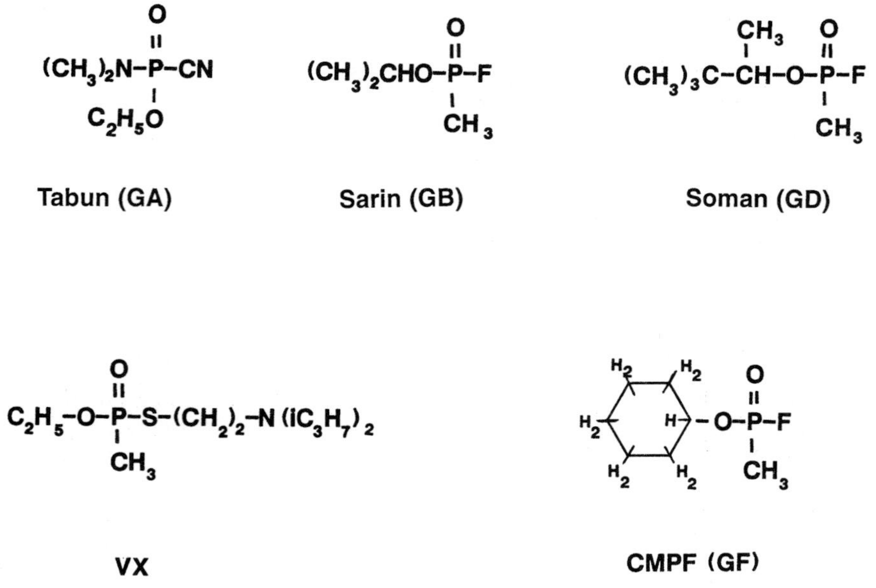

Tabun (GA)

Sarin (GB)

Soman (GD)

VX

CMPF (GF)

*Figure 22–11. Structures of the organophosphorus ester chemical warfare nerve gases, forerunners of the organophosphorus ester insecticides.*

phosphorus and carbamate ester insecticides elicit their toxicity is identical and is associated with the inhibition of the nervous tissue acetylcholinesterase (AChE), the enzyme responsible for the destruction and termination of the biological activity of the neurotransmitter acetylcholine (ACh). With the accumulation of free, unbound ACh at the nerve endings of all cholinergic nerves, there is continual stimulation of electrical activity. The signs of toxicity include those resulting from stimulation of the muscarinic receptors of the parasympathetic autonomic nervous system (increased secretions, bronchoconstriction, miosis, gastrointestinal cramps, diarrhea, urination, bradycardia); those resulting from the stimulation and subsequent blockade of nicotinic receptors, including the ganglia of the sympathetic and parasympathetic divisions of the autonomic nervous system as well as the junctions between nerves and muscles (causing tachycardia, hypertension, muscle fasciculations, tremors, muscle weakness, and/or flaccid paralysis); and those resulting from effects on the CNS (restlessness, emotional lability, ataxia, lethargy, mental confusion, loss of memory, generalized weakness, convulsion, cyanosis, coma) (Table 22-7).

The classic picture of anticholinesterase insecticide intoxication, first described by DuBois (DuBois, 1948; DuBois et al., 1949), has become more complicated in recent years by the recognition of additional and persistent signs of neurotoxicity not previously associated with these chemicals. First, and frequently associated with exposure to high concentrations of the insecticides (resulting from suicide attempts or drenching with dilute or concentrated chemicals) are effects that may persist for several months following exposure and involve neurobehavioral, cognitive, and neuromuscular functions (Ecobichon, 1994a; Marrs, 1993). The first evidence of this type of syndrome, delayed psychopathologic-neurological lesions, was reported by Spiegelberg (1963), who had been studying workers involved in the production and handling of the highly toxic nerve gases in Germany during World War II. The characteristic symptomatology subdivided these patients into two distinct groups. The first and largest group was characterized by persistently lowered vitality and ambition; defective autonomic regulation leading to cephalagia and to gastrointestinal and cardiovascular symptoms; premature decline in potency and libido; intolerance to alcohol, nicotine, and various medicines; and an impression of premature aging. The second group, in addition to the above symptoms, showed one or more of the following: depressive or subdepressive disorders of vital function; cerebral vegetative (syncopal) attacks; slight or moderate amnestic or demential effects; and slight organoneurologic defects. These symptoms developed and persisted for some 5 to 10 years following exposure to these most toxic organophosphorus esters during the war years. The controversial paper of Gershon and Shaw (1961), a study of 16 cases of pesticide applicators exposed primarily to organophosphorus ester insecticides for 10 to 15 years, reported a wide range of persistent signs of toxicity, including tinnitus, nystagmus, pyrexia, ataxia, tremor, paresthesia, polyneuritis, paralysis, speech difficulty (slurring), loss of memory, insomnia, somnambulism, excessive dreaming, drowsiness, lassitude, generalized weakness, emotional lability, mental confusion, difficulty in concentration, restlessness, anxiety, depression, dissociation, and schizophrenic reactions. Although the results of other studies have been equivocal in their support of such an array of long-term signs and symptoms, there is a persistent recurrence of the symptomatology in a number of anecdotal and documented reports (Ecobichon, 1994a; Marrs, 1993). The literature on potential, suspected, and established sequelae of organophosphorus ester insecticide intoxications does not confirm the frequently seen statement that clinical recovery from nonfatal poisoning is always complete in a few days. Continuous and close observation of the acutely intoxicated patients for some weeks following their recovery from the initial toxicity and treatment thereof would be necessary to identify the subtle changes indicated above. The emergency

**Table 22–7**
**Signs and Symptoms of Anticholinesterase Insecticide Poisoning**

| NERVOUS TISSUE AND RECEPTORS AFFECTED | SITE AFFECTED | MANIFESTATIONS |
|---|---|---|
| Parasympatheic autonomic (muscarinic receptors) postganglionic nerve fibers | Exocrine glands | Increased salivation, lacrimation, perspiration |
| | Eyes | Miosis (pinpoint and nonreactive), ptosis, blurring of vision, conjunctival injection, "bloody tears" |
| | Gastrointestinal tract | Nausea, vomiting, abdominal tightness, swelling and carmps, diarrhea, tenesmus, fecal incontinence |
| | Respiratory tract | Excessive bronchial secretions, rhinorrhea, wheezing, edema, tightness in chest, bronchospasms, broncho-constriction, cough, bradypnea, dyspnea |
| | Cardiovascular system | Bradycardia, decrease in blood pressure |
| | Bladder | Urinary frequency and incontinence |
| Parasympathetic and sympathetic autonomic fibers (nicotinic receptors) | Cardiovascular system | Tachycardia, pallor, increase in blood pressure |
| Somatic motor nerve fibers (nicotine receptors) | Skeletal muscles | Muscle fasciculations (eyelids, fine facial muscles), cramps, diminished tendon reflexes, generalized muscle weakness in peripheral and respiratory muscles, paralysis, flaccid or rigid tone |
| | | Restlessness, generalized motor activity, reaction to acoustic stimuli, tremulousness, emotional lability, ataxia |
| Brain (acetylcholine receptors) | Central nervous system | Drowsiness, lethargy, fatigue, mental confusion, inability to concentrate, headache, pressure in head, generalized weakness |
| | | Coma with absence of reflexes, tremors, Cheyne-Stokes respiration, dyspnea, convulsions, depression of respiratory centers, cyanosis |

SOURCE: From Ecobichon and Joy, 1982.

service physician rarely sees the patient following stabilization and initial "recovery." Definitive examples in which such observation has been possible are few but one such fortuitous case illustrates what can be achieved if there is close follow-up (Ecobichon et al., 1977).

A 33-year-old female technician was exposed dermally to an unknown amount of a 7.5 percent v/v solution of fenitrithion [*O,O*-dimethyl-*O*-(4-nitro-*m*-tolyl) phosphorothioate] prepared in corn oil, which had spilled. She had wiped up the spilled material with facial tissues and bare hands. Distinctive symptoms (memory loss, tremors, fatigue) were observed 2 days after exposure accompanied by a 45 percent reduction in plasma cholinesterase activity but only minimal change in erythrocyte AChE activity. She was hospitalized for treatment and the signs and symptoms became more intense, being characteristic of those associated with intoxication by organophosphorus esters (see Table 22-7). The patient responded to repeated antidotal (pralidoxime) treatment (see "Treatment of Poisoning," below). Although the plasma cholinesterate activity returned to normal levels some 15 to 20 days after exposure, moderate neuromuscular (fasciculations, generalized muscle weakness) and psychiatric (emotional lability, decreased ability to concentrate on tasks, memory impairment, lethargy) sequelae persisted for upwards of 4 months after exposure, although recovery was complete within 9 months of the incident.

While most clinical manifestations of acute poisoning are resolved within days to weeks, some symptoms, particularly those of a neuropsychological nature, appear to persist for months or longer. A very complete review of this aspect has been published recently (Ecobichon, 1994a). A 4-month surveillance of 19 acutely poisoned farm workers revealed many subjective signs and symptoms (blurred vision, muscle weakness, nausea, headaches, night sweats) to persist through the study period, accompanied by a slow recovery of plasma and erythrocytic cholinesterases (Whorton and Obrinsky, 1983). Rosenstock and coworkers (1991) described the neuropsychological testing of 36 poisoned Nicaraguan agricultural workers some 2 years postexposure, reporting that the poisoned group did much worse than controls on all subtests, with significantly worse performance on five of six subtests in the World Health Organization (WHO) neuropsychological test battery and on three of six additional tests that assessed verbal and visual attention, visual memory, visuomotor speed, sequencing and problem solving, motor steadiness, and dexterity. In the past 30 years, such reported effects have progressed from the anecdotal stage to a testable basis. Refined test parameters will be necessary to reveal subtle but distinct changes in memory, academic and motor skills, abstraction, and flexibility in thinking.

A second distinct manifestation of exposure to organophosphorus ester insecticides recently has been described by clinicians in Sri Lanka involved in the treatment of suicide attempts (Senanayake and Karalliede, 1987). This paralytic condition, called the *intermediate syndrome*, consisted of a sequence of neurological signs that appeared some 24 to 96 h after the acute cholinergic crisis but before the expected onset of delayed neuropathy, the major effect being muscle weakness, primarily affecting muscles innervated by the cranial nerves (neck flexors, muscles of respiration) as well as those of the limbs. Cranial nerve palsies were common. There was a distinct risk of death during this time interval because of respiratory depression and distress which required urgent ventilatory support and was not responsive to atropine or to oximes. The chemicals involved in these distinctive intoxications included fenthion, dimethoate, monocrotophos, and methamidophos. There were no obvious clinical differences during the acute intoxication phase in those patients who developed the intermediate syndrome and others who did not, and all patients were treated in the same manner.

A third syndrome, that of organophosphate-induced delayed neurotoxicity (OPIDN), is caused by some phosphate, phosphonate, and phosphoramidate esters, only a few of which have ever been used as insecticides (Fig. 22-12). Historically, this syndrome has been known for almost 100 years and has been associated with the chemical tri-*o*-tolyl phosphate (TOTP) (Ecobichon, 1994a). The first major epidemic of OPIDN occurred during the prohibition years in the United States, resulting from the consumption of a particular brand of alcoholic extract of Jamaican ginger contaminated or adulterated with mixed tolyl phosphate esters. The syndrome, affecting some 20,000 individuals to varying degrees, was known as *ginger jake paralysis* or *jake leg* and was studied in detail by Maurice Smith of the U.S. Public Health Service. He not only confirmed that the condition could be reproduced in animals (e.g., rabbits, dogs, monkeys, calves) but also demonstrated that only one of the three isomers found in commercial tri-tolyl phosphate, the *ortho*-isomer, was responsible for the toxicity (Smith and Lillie, 1931). The initial flaccidity, characterized by muscle weakness in the arms and legs giving rise to a clumsy, shuffling gait, was replaced by spasticity, hypertonicity, hyperreflexia, clonus, and abnormal reflexes, indicative of damage to the pyramidal tracts and a permanent upper motor neuron syndrome (Ecobichon, 1994a). In many patients, recovery was limited to the arms and hands and damage to the lower extremities (foot drop, spasticity, and hyperactive reflexes) was permanent, suggesting damage to the spinal cord (Morgan and Penovich, 1978). A similar neuropathy occurred with an experimental organophosphorus ester insecticide, mipafox, following an accident in a manufacturing pilot plant. Details of the effects on two of the workers were described by Bidstrup and coworkers (1953) and Ecobichon (1994a). The poisoning of water buffalo in the early 1970s in Egypt by a phosphonate insecticide, leptophos, revealed a neurological syndrome similar to that observed following exposure to TOTP (Abou-Donia, 1981). There was also evidence of leptophos-induced neuropathies among workers in a manufacturing plant in the United States, but the controversial observations were obscured by concomitant exposure of the workers to *n*-hexane, another neurotoxic chemical (Xintaris et al., 1978).

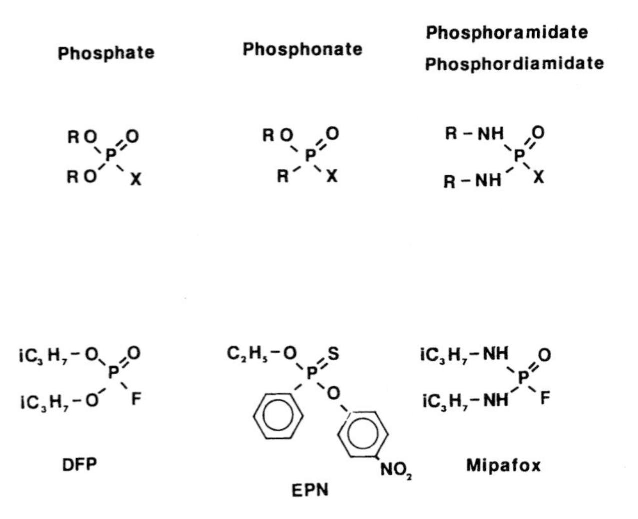


***Figure 22–12. The basic structures and nomenclature of organophosphorus esters, with examples, capable of causing organophosphate-induced delayed neurotoxicity (OPIDN).***

A number of organophosphorus insecticides, including omethoate, trichloronate, trichlorfon, parathion, methamidophos, fenthion, and chlorpyrifos, have been implicated in causing OPIDN in humans (Abou-Donia and Lapadula, 1990). However, it should be emphasized that these incidents all involved accidental or suicidal exposure to excessively high levels. Concern that many of the over 200 organophosphorus ester insecticides in use might cause this unique neuropathy has resulted in an intensive study of the syndrome, the identification of the most susceptible species (the hen and the cat), the development of standard protocols to test all insecticides, and at least a partial elucidation of the mechanisms by which agents elicit this condition. Histological examination of the nervous systems of hens treated with a suitable agent [e.g., TOTP, *0,0*-diisopropyl phosphorofluoridate (DFP), mipafox, leptophos] has revealed a wallerian, "dying-back" degeneration of large diameter axons and their myelinic sheaths in distal parts of the peripheral nerves and of long spinal cord tracts—the rostral ends of ascending tracts and the distal ends of descending tracts (Cavanagh, 1954; Sprague and Bickford, 1981). Biochemical studies have demonstrated that the above-mentioned agents inhibit a neuronal, nonspecific carboxylesterase, neuropathic target esterase (NTE), which appears to have some, as yet unknown, role in lipid metabolism in neurons (Johnson, 1982). If acute exposure to an appropriate organophosphorus ester results in >70 percent inhibition of NTE, the characteristic OPIDN usually follows, with ataxia being observed some 7 to 14 days following treatment and progression to moderate to severe muscular weakness and paralysis with concomitant changes in neuronal morphology (Johnson, 1982; Slott and Ecobichon, 1984). It is the considered opinion of many investigators that many of the commonly used phosphate and phosphorothioate ester insecticides might be capable of causing this syndrome if only sufficient concentrations of the agents could be attained in vivo. However, taking paraoxon as an example of such a phosphate ester, the animal(s) would either die as a consequence of other acute toxic effects or would rapidly detoxify the agent, thereby preventing the acquisition of sufficient paraoxon to inhibit NTE. There also appear to be subtle structure-activity relationships between organophosphorus esters and the active site on the NTE protein because many phosphate esters are not good inhibitors of NTE (Ohkawa et al., 1980; Abou-Donia, 1981). Conversely, while the nerve gases cause a marked inhibition of NTE, the exposed animals do not develop OPIDN, suggesting that NTE inhibition may not be obligatory (Johnson et al., 1985; Lotti, 1992; Marrs, 1993). It should be emphasized that, although NTE inhibition remains a useful function for monitoring the potential of organophosphorus esters to induce OPIDN, the role of this enzyme in the initiation of the syndrome remains unknown and histopathologic evidence is a requirement of the U.S. EPA protocol. Two noninsecticidal organophosphorus esters, the tri-*S*-alkyl defoliant *S,S,S*-tributyl phosphorotrithioite (Merphos) and its oxidation product, *S,S,S*-tributyl phosphorotrithioate (DEF), have been implicated in producing OPIDN in at least one agricultural worker and cause a characteristic delayed neurotoxicity in hens (Abou-Donia and Lapadula, 1990).

The signs and symptoms of acute intoxication by carbamate insecticides are similar to those described for organophosphorus compounds, differing only in the duration and intensity of the toxicity. The most apparent reasons for the relatively short duration of action and the mild to moderate severity of signs are that (1) carbamate insecticides are reversible inhibitors of nervous tissue AChE, unlike most of the organophosphorus esters (see below, "The Site and Mechanism of Toxic Action") and (2) they are rapidly biotransformed in vivo. Despite the extensive toxicological research demonstrating that the pesticidal carbamate esters are "relatively safe" chemicals producing only transient, short-term toxicity following acute administration, carbamate insecticide toxicity has been reported in humans and fatalities have occurred (Ecobichon, 1994b; Hayes, 1982). Invariably, these serious poisonings have involved carbaryl and have occurred as a consequence of accidental or purposeful (suicidal) exposure to high concentrations (Hayes, 1982; Cranmer, 1986). Information on the incidences of human intoxication by carbaryl can be found in the Carbaryl Decision Document (EPA, 1980). For the period 1966–1980, 195 human intoxication cases were reported (3 fatalities, 16 hospitalizations, and 176 cases receiving medical attention). A single oral dose of 250 mg of carbaryl (2.8 mg/kg body weight) is sufficient to elicit moderately severe poisoning in an adult man (Cranmer, 1986). Moderate but transient toxicity has also been observed following exposure to a few of the more potent carbamate ester insecticides such as methomyl (Lannate) and propoxur (Baygon) (Vandekar et al., 1968, 1971; Liddle et al., 1979). More recently, the illegal use of aldicarb (Temik), a very acutely toxic carbamate ester, on watermelons in California and on English cucumbers in British Columbia, Canada, resulted in moderate to severe toxicity in consumers of these products, with signs and symptoms including nausea, vomiting, gastrointestinal cramps, and diarrhea (Goldman et al., 1990a,b).

While there is little evidence of prolonged neurotoxicity after exposure to carbamate ester insecticides, this statement should be made cautiously because the signal danger appears to involve acute single exposures to massive doses or at least repeated exposures to large doses. Anecdotal cases exist that are contrary to everything that we know about carbamates. One case involved a farmer who hand-sprayed a vegetable garden with a water-wettable formulation of carbaryl, drenching himself in the process, who later developed a chronic polyneuropathy which included signs of persistent photophobia, mild and persistent paresthesia, recent memory loss, muscular weakness, fatigue, and lassitude (Ecobichon, 1994b). Another case involved continuous exposure over 8 to 10 months to a fine dust of carbaryl (10 percent dust) in the home (Branch and Jacqz, 1986). Initial influenzalike symptoms were experienced by all family members. However, the signs and symptoms of the elderly male became progressively worse: increasing dyspepsia, headache with severe pressure, tinnitus, vertigo, mental confusion, weakness in major skeletal muscle groups with fasciculations, a persistent stocking-and-glove peripheral neuropathy, and a cerebral atrophy. The patient's well-being improved upon removal from the home, but symptoms returned rapidly upon reentry, accompanied by decreases in both plasma and erythrocytic cholinesterases, with a slow recovery over a period of 2 months. This bizarre reaction to carbaryl may have been enhanced by slow biotransformation due, in part, to the patient's advanced age and perhaps related to the concomitant administration of cimetidine, an agent known to inhibit carbaryl metabolism in the isolated perfused rat liver.

There is evidence in animal studies, albeit at near toxic doses, of a Wallerian-type degeneration of spinal cord tracts in rabbits and hens following treatment with sodium diethyldithiocarbamate (Edington and Howell, 1969). Carbaryl, when fed to hogs (150 mg/kg per day for 72 or 83 days), caused a rear leg paralysis, minimal at rest but, when the animals were forced to move, resulting in marked incoordination, ataxia, tremors, clonic muscle contractions, and prostration, with histological evidence of lesions in the CNS and in skeletal muscle (Smalley et al., 1969). Carbamate ester insecticides do not inhibit NTE or elicit OPIDN-type neurotoxicity. Behavioral changes have been noted in a number of animal studies following the subchronic or chronic administration of different carbamate insecticides (Santalucito and Morrison, 1971; Desi et al., 1974).

**The Site and Mechanism of Toxic Action.** Although the anticholinesterase-type insecticides have a common mode of action, there are significant differences between organophosphorus and carbamate esters. The reaction between an organophosphorus ester and the active site in the AChE protein (a serine hydroxyl group) results in the formation of a transient intermediate complex that partially hydrolyzes with the loss of the "Z" substituent group, leaving a stable, phosphorylated, and largely unreactive inhibited enzyme that, under normal circumstances, can be reactivated only at a very slow rate (Fig. 22-13). With many organophosphorus ester insecticides, an irreversibly inhibited enzyme is formed, and the signs and symptoms of intoxication are prolonged and persistent, requiring vigorous medical intervention, including the reactivation of the enzyme with specific chemical antidotes (see "Treatment of Poisoning," below, this section). Without intervention, the toxicity will persist until sufficient quantities of "new" AChE are synthesized in 20 to 30 days to destroy efficiently the excess neurotransmitter. The nature of the substituent groups at "X," "Y," and "Z" plays an important role in the specificity for the enzyme, the tenacity of binding to the active site, and the rate at which the phosphorylated enzyme dissociates to produce free enzyme. More recently introduced organophosphorus esters (acephate, temephos, dichlorvos, trichlorfon) are less tenacious inhibitors of nervous tissue

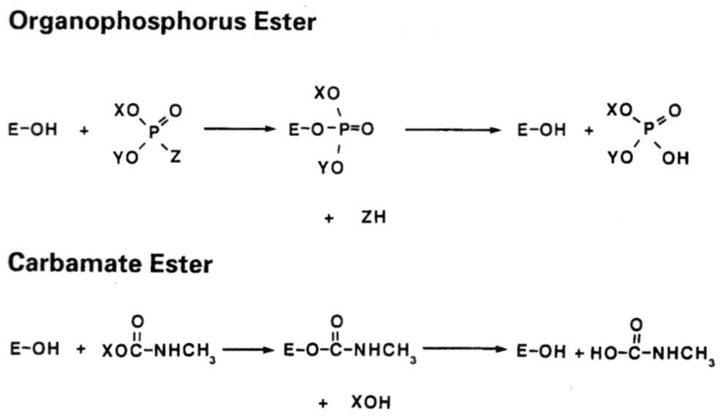

**Organophosphorus Ester**

E–OH + (XO)(YO)P(=O)Z ⟶ E–O–P(=O)(XO)(YO) + ZH ⟶ E–OH + (XO)(YO)P(=O)OH

**Carbamate Ester**

E–OH + XOC(=O)–NHCH$_3$ ⟶ E–O–C(=O)–NHCH$_3$ + XOH ⟶ E–OH + HO–C(=O)–NHCH$_3$

*Figure 22–13. The interaction between an organophosphorus or carbamate ester with the serine hydroxyl group in the active site of the enzyme acetylcholinesterase (E-OH).*

The intermediate, unstable complexes formed before the release of the "leaving" groups (ZH and XOH) are not shown. The dephosphorylation or decarbamoylation of the inhibited enzyme is the rate-limiting step to forming free enzyme.

AChE, the phosphorylated enzyme being more readily and spontaneously dissociated.

In contrast, carbamic acid esters, which attach to the reactive site of the AChE, undergo hydrolysis in two stages: the first stage is the removal of the "X" substituent (an aryl or alkyl group) with the formation of a carbamylated enzyme; the second stage is the decarbamylation of the inhibited enzyme with the generation of free, active enzyme (Fig. 22-13). Carbamic acid esters are nothing more than poor substrates for the cholinesterase-type enzymes.

When the concept of the interaction between organophosphorus and carbamic esters with AChE is presented in another manner (Table 22-8), one can see that the only distinctive difference between the two anticholinesterase-type insecticides lies in the rate at which the dephosphorylation or decarbamoylation takes place. The rate is exceedingly slow for organophosphorus esters, so much so that the enzyme is frequently considered to be irreversibly inhibited. The rate of decarbamoylation is sufficiently rapid that these esters are often considered to be reversible inhibitors with low turnover rates. The characteristics of the various rate constants for the natural substrate (ACh), organophosphorus, and carbamate esters are shown in Table 22-8. It is important to appreciate that the rate at which step 3 proceeds is thousands of times slower with carbamate esters than with ACh, whereas with organophosphorus esters, it is several orders of magnitude slower (Ecobichon, 1979). This subject has been extensively reviewed by Aldridge and Reiner (1972).

A number of organophosphorus (phosphate, phosphonate, and phosphoramidate) esters (Fig. 22-12), the chemical warfare agents sarin, soman, and tabun and a few other compounds such as DFP, mipafox, and leptophos, have the ability to bind tenaciously to the active site of AChE and of NTE to produce an irreversibly inhibited enzyme, by a mechanism known as *aging*. The aging process is dependent on the size and configuration of the alkyl (R) substituent, with the potency of the ester increasing in the order of diethyl, dipropyl, and dibutyl for such analogs as DFP and mipafox (Aldridge and Johnson, 1971). The aging process is generally accepted as being caused by the dealkylation of the intermediate dialkylphosphorylated enzymes by one of two possible mechanisms (Fig. 22-14). The first involves the hydrolysis of a P-O bond following a nucleophile (base) attack on the phosphorus atom. The second mechanism involves the hydrolysis of an O-C bond by an acid catalysis, resulting in the formation of a carbonium ion as the leaving group (O'Brien, 1960; Eto, 1974; Johnson, 1982). The aging process is believed to fix an extra charge to the protein, causing some perturbation to the active site, thereby preventing dephosphorylation. While the exact nature of this reaction has not been demonstrated for AChE and NTE, evidence from experiments with saligenin cyclic phosphorus esters (derivatives of TOTP) and $\alpha$-chymotrypsin points to the possibility of two stabilized forms of "aged" enzyme (Toia and Casida, 1979). As is shown in Fig. 22-15, both of the reactions utilize the imidazole group of a neighboring histidine. In one reaction, the hydroxylated substituent is released and the phosphorylated enzyme is stabilized by a hydrogen on the imidazole group. In the other reaction, the leaving substituent becomes attached to the imidazole, yielding a N-C-hydroxylated derivative of the phosphorylated enzyme. Johnson (1982) proposed that, in the case of NTE, if one or two of the P-R bonds were P-O-C (as in phosphates and phosphonates), aging would occur rapidly, whereas if the P-R bonds were P-C (as in phosphinates), aging would not be possible.

**Biotransformation, Distribution, and Storage.** Both the organophosphorus and carbamate ester insecticides undergo ex-

**Table 22–8**
**Kinetics of Ester Hydrolysis**

| ESTERS | COMPLEX FORMATION ($K_A = k_{-1}/k_{+1}$) | ACYLATION ($k_2$) | DEACYLATION ($k_3$) |
|---|---|---|---|
| | EH + AB ⇄ EHAB → BH + EA → EH + AOH | | |
| Substrates | Small | Extremely fast | Extremely fast |
| Organophosphorus esters | Small | Moderately fast | Slow or extremely slow |
| Carbamate esters | Small | Slow | Slow |

SOURCE: From Ecobichon, 1979.

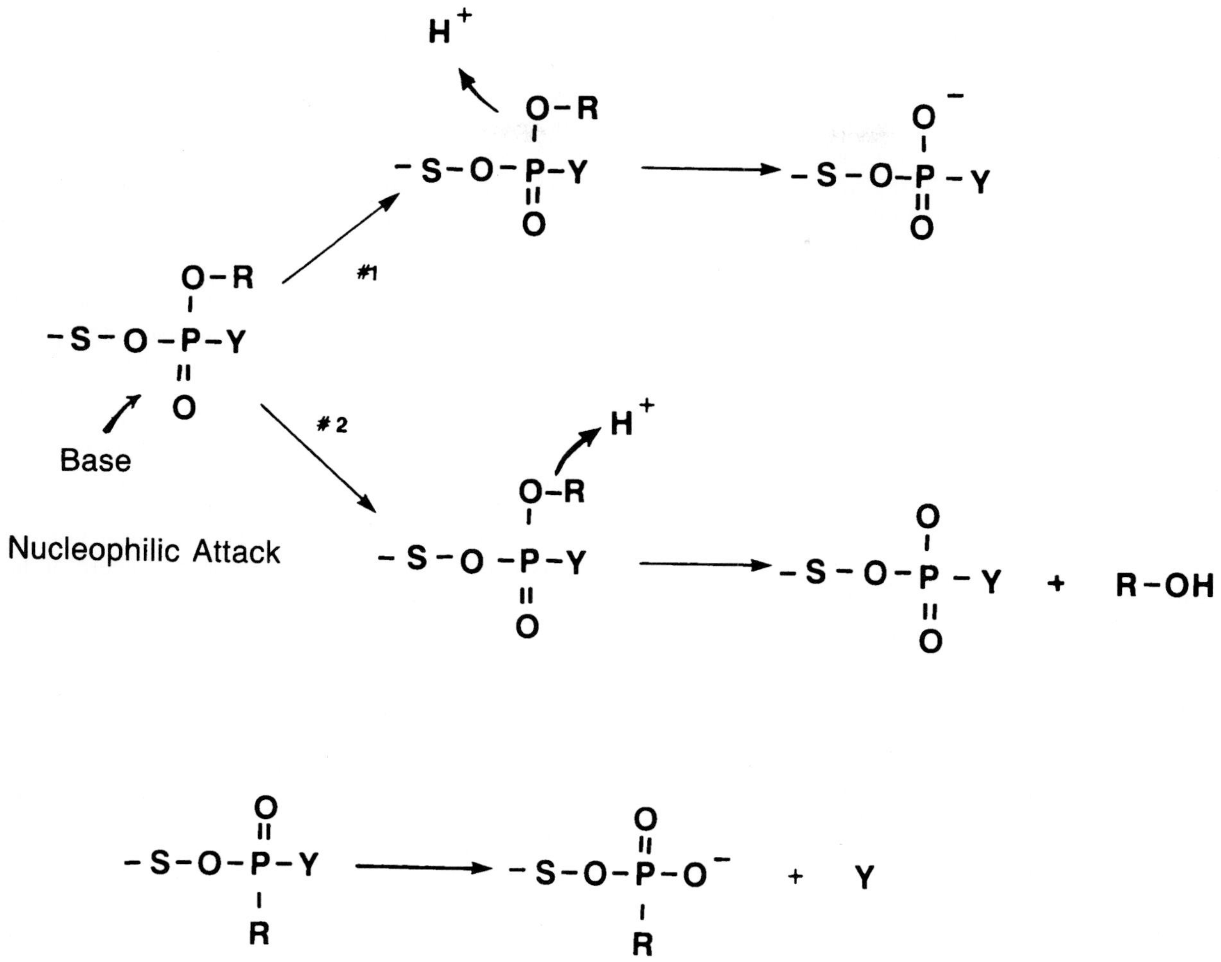

***Figure 22–14.** A schematic diagram illustrating two mechanisms by which the "aging" of organophosphorus ester-inhibited acetylcholinesterase may occur.*

See text for details.

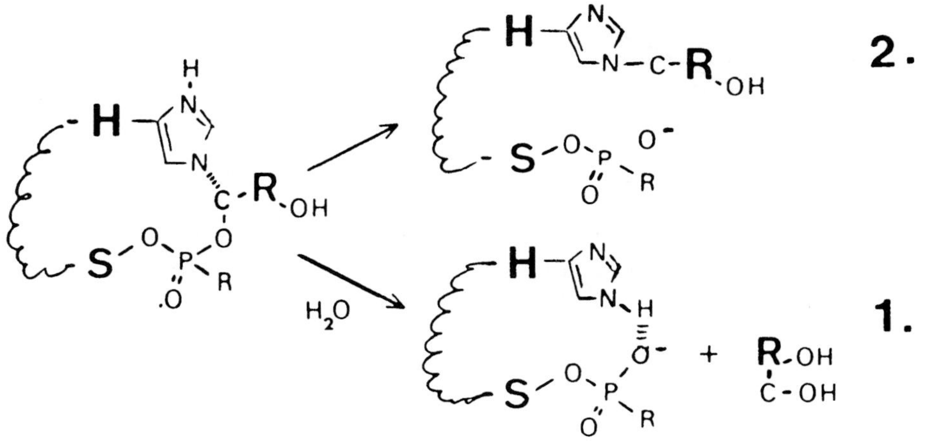

***Figure 22–15.** The phosphorylation, aging, and possible alkylation reactions of saligenin cyclic phosphorus esters with α-chymotrypsin to yield two possible stabilized forms of the aged enzyme, both utilizing an imidazole group of a neighboring histidine in close proximity to the active center of the enzyme. [From Toia and Casida (1979).]*

tensive biotransformation in all forms of life. Both the route(s) and the rate(s) of metabolism are highly species-specific and dependent on the substituent chemical groups attached to the basic "backbone" structure of these esters (Fig. 22-10). Tissue enzymes of both phase I (oxidative, reductive, hydrolytic) and phase II (transfer or conjugative reactions with glutathione, glucuronic acid, glycine, and so forth) types are found in a widespread pattern in plant, invertebrate, and vertebrate species and, indeed, are responsible for some aspects of the species sensitivity and/or both natural and acquired resistance to many of these insecticides. The phase I detoxification processes usually form reactive metabolites whereas phase II processes conjugate the polar phase I metabolites with some natural body substituent to form a product with enhanced water solubility and excretability. The biotransformation of anticholinesterase-type insecticides has been extensively reviewed in the literature and the reader is referred to such sources as O'Brien (1967), Menzie (1969), Eto (1974), Kulkarni and Hodgson (1984), and Matsumura (1985) for details on the various mechanisms involved.

Organophosphorus esters may undergo simultaneous enzymatic attack at a number of different points in the molecule (Fig. 22-16). Only one reaction, that of the oxidative desulfuration of phosphorothioate esters (mechanism 1), results in a significant increase in the toxicity of the biotransformation product, an oxygen analog. In phosphorothioate (parathion, methyl parathion, fenitrothion, etc.) or phosphorodithioate (azinophosmethyl, malathion) esters, the presence of this thiono group reduces the AChE-inhibiting properties of the ester, confers greater chemical stability (nonenzymatic hydrolysis) on the molecule, and also confers species selectivity. While oxidative desulfuration in insects and mammals results in the formation of a more toxic oxygen analog, this intermediate can be readily hydrolyzed by aryl and aliphatic hydrolases found in mammalian tissues, whereas insect species are frequently deficient in these enzymes, making insects more susceptible to such agents (mechanism 8).

Oxidative dealkylation and dearylation reactions (mechanisms 2 and 3) involve enzymes that utilize the coenzyme reduced nicotinamide adenine dinucleotide phosphate (NADPH), the ubiquitously distributed cytochrome P-450 system, and an NADPH-regenerating system to provide the necessary oxygen and electrons to produce polar metabolites. Demethylation, with the formation of an aldehyde, occurs readily, but this reaction pathway does not function efficiently when the alkyl group becomes longer (i.e., ethyl, propyl) (mechanism 2). Dearylation occurs in a similar fashion with the formation of a phenol and a dialkylphosphoric or dialkylphosphorothioic acid (mechanism 3). The monooxygenase system can also catalyze a number of reactions involving substitutents on side groups resulting in (1) aromatic ring hydroxylation (mechanism 4); (2) thioether oxidation (mechanism 5); (3) deamination; (4) alkyl and *N*-hydroxylation; (5) *N*-oxide formation; and (6) *N*-dealkylation. A number of transferases use glutathione (γ-glutamyl-L-cysteinyl glycine, GSH) as a cofactor and acceptor for *O*-alkyl and *O*-aryl

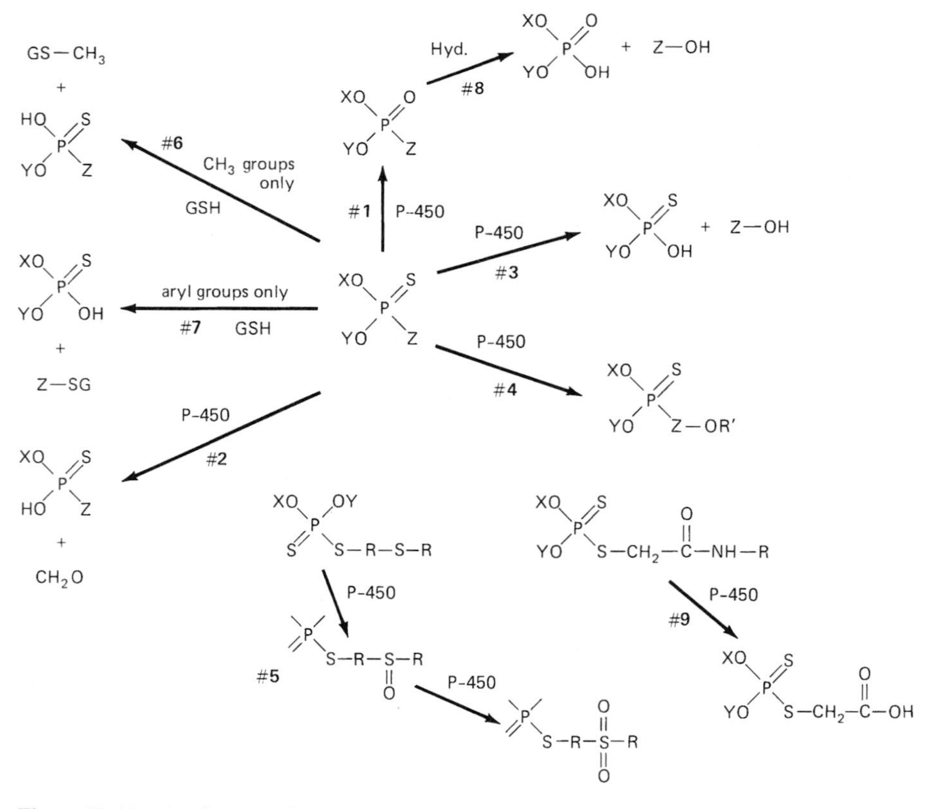


**Figure 22–16.** ***A schematic diagram depicting the various phase I and II biotransformation pathways of an organophosphorus ester and the nature of the products formed as a consequence of oxidative, hydrolytic, GSH-mediated transfer and conjugation of intermediate metabolites in mammals.***

See text for details.

groups (mechanisms 6 and 7) to yield monodesmethyl products plus *S*-methylglutathione or dialkylphosphoric or dialkylphosphorothioic acids plus aryl-glutathione derivatives, respectively.

Hydrolysis of phosphoric and phosphorothioic acid esters occurs via a number of different tissue hydrolases (nonspecific carboxylesterases, arylesterases, phosphorylphosphatases, phosphotriesterases, carboxyamidases) scattered ubiquitously throughout the plant and animal kingdoms, with activity being highly dependent on the nature of the substituents (Ecobichon, 1979). Slight structural modifications to substituents on the insecticide molecule can dramatically alter the specificity of these enzymes toward an agent and affect species selectivity. The arylesterases [aromatic or A-esterases (ArE), EC 3.1.1.2] preferentially hydrolyze aryl (phenol, naphthol, indole) esters of short-chain aliphatic or phosphorus acids, particularly if there is a double bond present in the alcohol moiety in position $\alpha$ with respect to the ester bond (mechanism 8). Carboxylesterases [carboxylic acid ester hydrolases (CE), EC 3.1.1.1] are capable of hydrolyzing a variety of aliphatic and aryl esters of short-chain fatty acids. The most important example of this reaction involving organophosphorus ester insecticides is with malathion [*O,O*-dimethyl-*S*-(1,2-dicarbethoxyethyl) phosphorodithioate], in which one of the two available ethylated carboxylic ester groups is hydrolyzed to yield malathion (or malaoxon) $\alpha$-monoacids that are biologically inactive (Dauterman and Main, 1966). This CE-catalyzed reaction is an important feature of resistance to this insecticide in insects and to tolerance in mammals. Potentiation of anticholinergic effects can be produced by the combined administration of certain pairs of organophosphate ester insecticides, such as EPN (*O*-ethyl-*O*-*p*-nitrophenylbenzenethiophosphonate) and malathion (Frawley et al., 1957). The mechanism for this effect involves the inhibition of carboxyesterases by EPN (Murphy, 1969, 1972, 1980). Carboxyamidases (acylamide amidohydrolase, EC 3.5.1.4), found extensively in plant, insect, and vertebrate tissues, are of limited current interest in the degradation of insecticides; dimethoate [*O,O*-dimethyl-*S*-(*N*-methylcarbamoylmethyl) phosphorodithioate] is the only organophosphorus ester insecticide shown to be hydrolyzed by mammalian tissue amidases (mechanism 9). Phosphorylphosphatases and phosphotriesterases have limited involvement in the biotransformation of organophosphorus ester insecticides but play a role in the detoxification of some of the chemical warfare agents.

Phase II conjugative reactions are of limited use in the biotransformation of organophosphorus ester insecticides, and they are usually relegated to the task of glucuronidating or sulfating the aromatic phenols, cresols, and other substances hydrolyzed from the ester (Yang, 1976). However, one must be wary of these enzyme systems because metabolism studies of chlorfenvinphos [2-chloro-1-(2′,4′-dichlorophenyl)-vinyl diethylphosphate] revealed the presence of glucuronide and glycine conjugates of several products, whereas studies with trichlorfon (*O,O*-dimethyl-1-hydroxy-2,2,2-trichloroethyl phosphonate) revealed direct glucuronidation of the insecticide without prior biotransformation (Hutson et al., 1967; Bull, 1972).

In a similar fashion, carbamate ester insecticides can undergo simultaneous attack at several points in the molecule, depending on the nature of the substituents attached to the basic structure (Fig. 22-17). In addition to the hydrolysis of the carbamate ester group by tissue CE and the release of a substituted phenol, carbon dioxide, and methylamine (mechanism 1), several oxidative and reductive reactions involving cytochrome P-450 related monooxygenases can proceed, the ultimate products being considerably more polar than the parent insecticide. The extent of hydrolysis of carbamate ester insecticides varies greatly between species, ranging from 30 to 95 percent hydrolysis. The type of oxidative reactions observed with carbamate esters can be simplified into two main groups: (1) direct ring hydroxylation (mechanism 2) and (2) oxidation of appropriate side chains as is shown for this "mythical" methylcarbamate, resulting in the hydroxylation of *N*-methyl groups or methyl groups to form hydroxymethyl groups (mechanism 3), *N*-demethylation of secondary and tertiary amines (mechanism 4), *O*-dealkylation of alkoxy side chains (mechanism 5), thioether oxidation (mechanism 6), and so forth. Phase II conjugative reactions can occur at any free, reactive grouping with glucuronide and sulfate derivatives (mechanism 7), and GSH conjugates (mercapturates) may be formed (mechanism 8). For a comprehensive understanding of the various mechanisms involved, the reader is referred to those reviews mentioned above, this section, as well as to pertinent articles by Ryan (1971), Fukuto (1972), and Kuhr and Dorough (1976).

**Treatment of Poisoning.** Despite the qualitative and quantitative differences between organophosphorus and carbamate insecticide intoxications, all cases of anticholinesterase poisoning should be treated as serious medical emergencies and the patient should be hospitalized as quickly as possible. The status of the patient should be monitored by repeated analysis of the plasma (serum) cholinesterase and the erythrocyte AChE; the inhibition of the activities of these two enzymes is a good indicator of the severity of organophosphorus ester poisoning, because only the erythrocytic AChE is inhibited by carbamate esters (except at excessively high levels of exposure). As a consequence of the extensive involvement of the entire nervous system, the life-threatening signs (respiratory depression, bronchospasm, bronchial secretions, pulmonary edema, muscular weakness) resulting in hypoxemia will require immediate artificial respiration and suctioning via an endotracheal tube to maintain a patent airway. Arterial blood gases and cardiac function should be monitored.

The regimen for the treatment of organophosphorus ester insecticide intoxication, based on the analysis of serum pseudocholinesterase, is described in Table 22-9 (Namba et al., 1971; Ecobichon et al., 1977; Marrs, 1993). Atropine is used to counteract the initial muscarinic effects of the accumulating neurotransmitter. However, atropine is a highly toxic antidote and great care must be taken. Frequent small doses of atropine (subcutaneously or intravenously) are indicated for mild signs and symptoms following a brief, intense exposure. Relatively large, cumulative doses of atropine, up to 50 mg daily, may be essential to control severe muscarinic symptoms. The status of the patient must be monitored continuously by examining for the disappearance of secretions (dry mouth and nose) and sweating, facial flushing, and mydriasis (dilatation of pupils).

Supplementary treatment to offset moderate to severe nicotinic and CNS signs and symptoms usually takes the form of one of the specific antidotal chemicals, the oximes (pralidoxime chloride or 2-PAM, pralidoxime methanesulfonate or

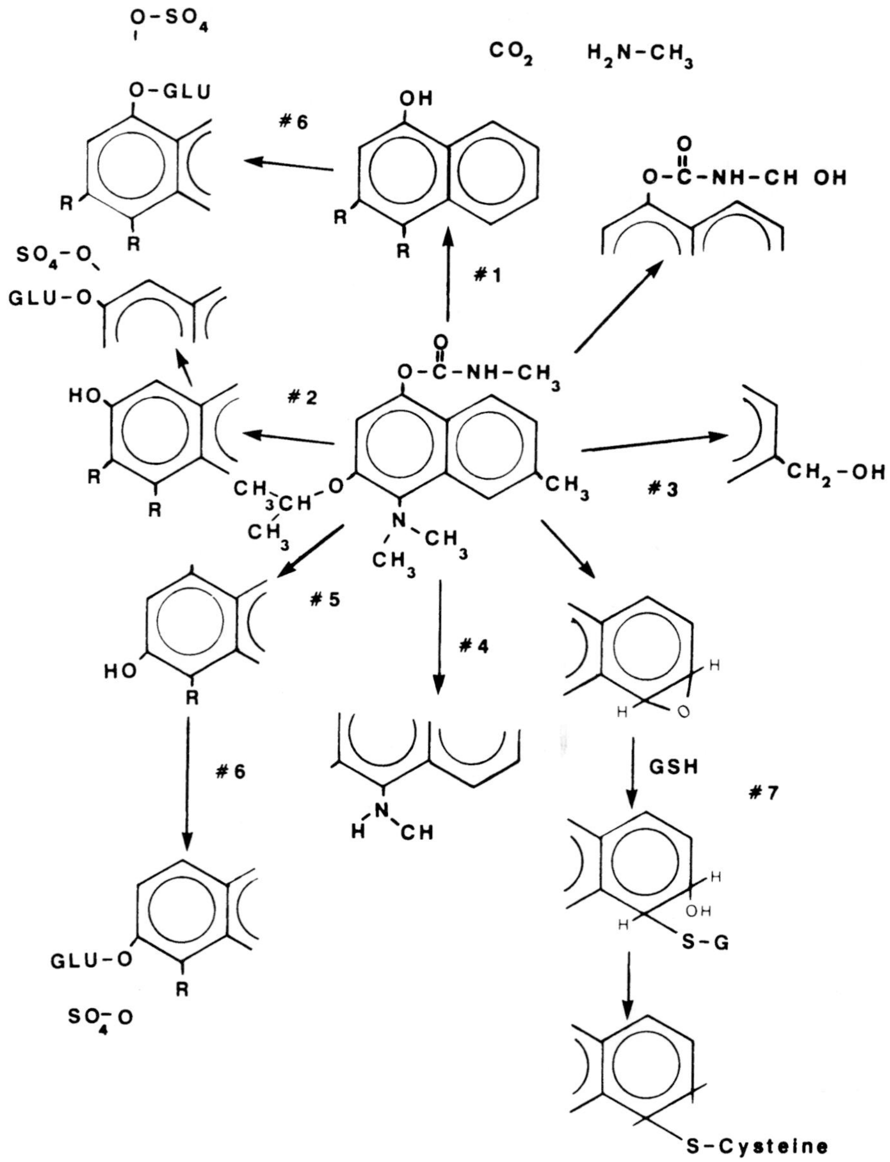

***Figure 22–17. A schematic diagram showing the various mammalian phase I and II biotransformation pathways of a "mythical" carbamate ester and the nature of the products formed and excreted.***

See text for details on the pathways.

P2S), administered intravenously to reactivate the inhibited nervous tissue AChE. The use of pralidoxime may not be necessary for cases of mild intoxication and should be reserved for moderate to severe poisonings. Treatment by slow intravenous infusion of doses of 1.0 g should be initiated as soon as possible, because the longer the interval between exposure and treatment the less effective the oxime will be. In many poisonings, a single treatment with pralidoxime will be sufficient to elicit a reversal of the signs and symptoms and to reduce the amount of atropine needed. In severe poisoning cases, a prodigious amount of pralidoxime may be needed. If absorption, distribution, and/or metabolism of the organophosphorus ester is delayed in the body, pralidoxime may be administered repeatedly over several days after the initial treatment. Care should be taken with repeated dosing because pralidoxime effectively binds calcium ions and causes muscle spasms not unlike those elicited by the organophosphorus esters. Severe muscle cramping, particularly in the extremities, may be alleviated by oral or intravenous calcium solutions (Ecobichon et al., 1977).

The therapeutic action of the oxime compounds resides in their capacity to reactivate AChE without contributing markedly toxic actions of their own. Those organophosphorus esters that possess good "leaving groups" (i.e., the "X" moiety) phosphorylate the nervous tissue AChE by a mechanism similar to that of acetylation by the substrate ACh. These esters are frequently called irreversible inhibitors because the hydrolysis of the phosphorylated enzyme by water is exceedingly slow

**Table 22–9**
**Classification and Treatment of Organophosphorus Insecticide Poisoning Based on Plasma Pseudocholinesterase Activity Measurements**

| CLASSIFICATION OF POISONING | ENZYME ACTIVITY (% OF NORMAL) | TREATMENT | |
|---|---|---|---|
| | | ATROPINE | PRALIDOXIME |
| Mild | 20–50 | 1.0 mg SC | 1.0 g IV over 20 to 30 min |
| Moderate | 10–20 | 1.0 mg IV every 20 to 30 min until sweating and salivation disappear and slight flush and mydriasis appear | |
| Severe | 10 | 5.0 mg IV every 20 to 30 min until sweating and salivation disappear and slight flush and mydriasis appear | 1.0 g IV as above. If no improvement, administer another 1.0 g IV. If no improvement, start IV infusion at 0.5 g/h |

SOURCE: From Ecobichon et al., 1977.

(Table 22-8). However, various nucleophilic agents containing a substituted ammonium group will dephosphorylate the phosphorylated enzyme at a much more rapid rate than water. The basic requirements for a reactivating molecule consist of a rigid structure containing a quaternary ammonium group and an acidic nucleophile that would be complementary with the phosphorylated enzyme, in such a way that the nucleophilic oxygen would be positioned close to the electrophilic phosphorus atom. These structure-activity requirements led to the development of the pralidoxime compounds, with the *syn*-isomer of 2-PAM (2-formyl-*N*-methylpyridinium chloride oxime) being particularly active (Childs et al., 1955; Askew, 1956; Kewitz and Wilson, 1956; Namba and Hiraki, 1958). The reaction of 2-PAM with the phosphorylated enzyme proceeds as shown in Fig. 22-18.

The reactivation is an equilibrium reaction, the oxime reacting either with the phosphorylated enzyme or with free, unbound organophosphorus ester, and the product is a phosphorylated oxime which, in itself, can be a potent cholinesterase inhibitor if it is stable in an aqueous medium (Schoene, 1972). In general, the phosphorylated oxime degrades quickly in water.

A practical limitation on the usefulness of oxime reactivators lies in the inability of these agents to reactivate "aged" AChE, that enzyme in which the phosphorylated enzyme has been further dealkylated and the phosphoryl group becomes tightly bound to the reactive site (see Fig. 22-14). Success with the pyridinium analogs led to an intensive search for more effective oximes and the discovery of the bispyridinium compounds, toxogonin or obidoxime [bis(4-formyl-*N*-methylpyridinium oxime) ether dichloride], TMB-4 [*N,N*-trimethylene bis(pyridine-4-aldoxime) bromide], and, more recently, the H-series compounds. However, these agents are not without toxicity and only pralidoxime and toxogonin have seen extensive antidotal use (Engelhard and Erdmann, 1964; Steinberg et al., 1977). With the apparent availability of organophosphorus nerve gases and their known ability to form rapidly aging complexes with AChE, the relative ineffectiveness of atropine and pralidoxime in such poisonings must be taken into account when the treatment of individuals exposed to these agents is confronted (Koplovitz et al., 1992; Webb, 1993; Clement, 1994). Toxogonin (obidoxime chloride) appears to be effective in tabun poisoning while, of the H-series of bis-pyridinium monooximes, HI-6 appears to be efficacious in soman and cyclohexylmethyl phosphoro-fluoridate (CMPF, or CF) poisonings. However, despite striking therapeutic effects, the issue is clouded by the fact that little reactivation of erythrocytic or brain AChE occurs (Kusic et al., 1991; Shih, 1993).

The clinical treatment of carbamate toxicity is similar to that for organophosphorus ester insecticide intoxication with

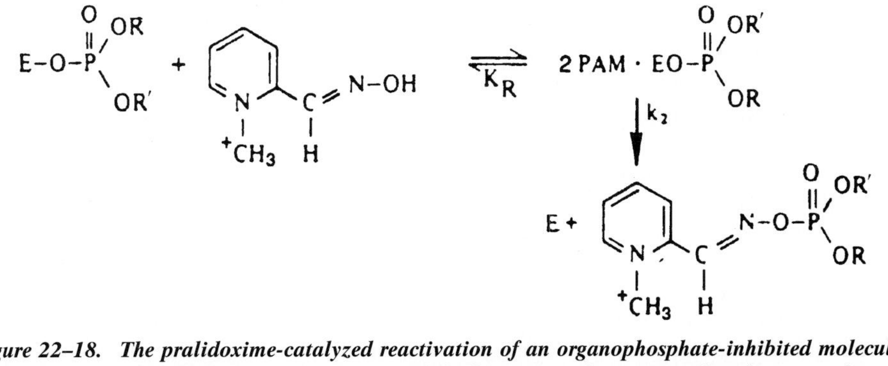

***Figure 22–18.*** ***The pralidoxime-catalyzed reactivation of an organophosphate-inhibited molecule of AChE, showing the release of active enzyme and the formation of an oxime-phosphate complex.***

the exception that the use of oximes is contraindicated. Early reports, in which pralidoxime or toxogonin was used in treating carbaryl intoxications, revealed that the oxime enhanced the carbaryl-induced toxicity (Sterri et al., 1979; Ecobichon and Joy, 1994). With other carbamate esters, pralidoxime had no obvious beneficial effect. Pralidoxime is not an effective antidote in carbamate intoxication because it does not interact with the carbamylated AChE in the same manner as with phosphorylated AChE.

Diazepam (10 mg SC or IV) may be included in the treatment regimen of all but the mildest cases of organophosphorus and/or carbamate intoxications. In addition to relieving any mental anxiety associated with the exposure, diazepam counteracts some aspects of the CNS and neuromuscular signs that are not affected by atropine. Doses of 10 mg (SC or IV) are appropriate and may be repeated. Other centrally acting drugs that may depress respiration are not recommended in the absence of artificial respiration.

It is important to appreciate that vigorous treatment of anticholinesterase-type insecticide intoxications does not offer protection against the possibility of delayed-onset neurotoxicity or the persistent sensory, cognitive, and motor defects discussed earlier. These deficits, albeit reversible over a long time interval, appear consistently in intoxications and are caused by mechanisms as yet unknown. Certain evidence points to severe damage to the neuromuscular junctions in skeletal muscle resulting in a persistent, peripheral muscular weakness (Wecker et al., 1978).

## Pyrethroid Insecticides

The newest major class of insecticides is the synthetic pyrethroids, a group of chemicals entering the marketplace in 1980 but, by 1982, accounting for approximately 30 percent of the worldwide insecticide usage (Anon., 1977; Vijverberg and van den Bercken, 1982). However, these synthetics arise from a much older class of botanical insecticides, pyrethrum, a mixture of six insecticidal esters (pyrethrins, cinerins, and jasmolins) extracted from dried pyrethrum or chrysanthemum flowers (*Chrysanthemum cinerariaefolium, C. coccineum*) (Hartley and West, 1969). Although it is believed that the natural pyrethroids were discovered by the Chinese in the first century A.D., the first written accounts of these agents are found in the seventeenth century literature and commercial preparations made their appearance in the mid-1800s (Neumann and Peter, 1987). Japanese woodblock prints from the early 1800s exist in which one can see smouldering insecticide coils of pressed pyrethrum powder not unlike those manufactured and used today.

In 1965, the world output of pyrethrum was approximately 20,000 tons, with Kenya alone producing some 10,000 tons (Cremlyn, 1978). The ever-increasing demand for this product has far exceeded the limited world production, leading chemists to focus attention on the synthesis of new analogs, hopefully with better stability in light and air, better persistence, more selectivity in target species, and low mammalian toxicity. In addition to extensive agricultural use, the synthetic pyrethroids are components of household sprays, flea preparations for pets, plant sprays for home and greenhouse use, and other applications. For an in-depth discussion of the development of the pyrethroid ester insecticides, their chemistry, and their biological activity, the reader is referred to Elliott (1976), Cremlyn (1978), Casida et al. (1983), Leahey (1985), Matsumura (1985), Narahashi (1985), Narahashi et al. (1985), and Joy (1994b).

The major active principles in pyrethrum are pyrethrin I, esters of chrysanthemic acid (pyrethrin I, cinerin I, and jasmolin I), and pyrethrin II which are esters of pyrethric acid (pyrethrin II, cinerin II, and jasmolin II) (Fig. 22-19). Pyrethrin I is the most active ingredient for lethality, and pyrethrin II possesses remarkable knockdown properties for a wide range of household, veterinary, and postharvest storage insects. The natural pyrethrins and early synthetic chrysanthemic acid derivatives are more active as contact poisons than as stomach poisons, in contrast to the more recent synthetic agents, which show particular potency when ingested and are less susceptible to biotransformation by insects and mammals. Several of the pyrethroid esters exist in isomeric forms which have distinctively different toxicities and potencies (Casida et al., 1983). Distinct molecular structures convey selectivity toward certain insect species and, in certain cases, to toxicity in mammals.

**Signs and Symptoms of Poisoning.** Based on the symptoms produced in animals receiving acute toxic doses, the pyrethroids fall into two distinct classes of chemicals (Table 22-10). The type I poisoning syndrome or *T syndrome* is produced by esters lacking the $\alpha$-cyano substituent and is characterized by restlessness, incoordination, prostration, and paralysis in the cockroach, as compared with the rat, which exhibits such signs as sparring and aggressive behavior, enhanced startle response, whole body tremor, and prostration. The type II syndrome, also known as the *CS syndrome*, is produced by those esters containing the $\alpha$-cyano substituent and elicits intense hyperactivity, incoordination, and convulsions in cockroaches, in contrast to rats, which display burrowing behavior, coarse tremors, clonic seizures, sinuous writhing (choreoathetosis), and profuse salivation without lacrimation; hence the term CS (choreoathetosis/salivation) syndrome. A few of these agents, fenpropanthrin, for example, cause a mixture of type I and II effects, depending on the species (rat or mouse) treated and possibly on the route of administration (Verschoyle and Aldridge, 1980; Gammon et al., 1981; Lawrence and Casida, 1982). The bulk of evidence points to the fact that the type II syndrome involves primarily an action in the mammalian CNS, whereas with the type I syndrome, peripheral nerves are also involved. This hypothesis was based initially on the observed symptomatology, but more recent evidence has revealed a correlation between the severity of type II responses and brain concentrations of deltamethrin in mice, regardless of the route of administration (Barnes and Verschoyle, 1974; Ruzo et al., 1979). Agents eliciting the type II syndrome have greater potency when injected intracerebrally, relative to intraperitoneal injection, than those causing type I syndrome effects (Lawrence and Casida, 1982). There is no indication of a fundamental difference between the mode of action of pyrethroids on neurons of target and nontarget species, and the neurotoxicologic responses depend on a combination of physicochemical properties of the particular pyrethroid ester, the dose applied, the time interval after treatment, and the physiological properties of the particular model used (Leake et al., 1985).

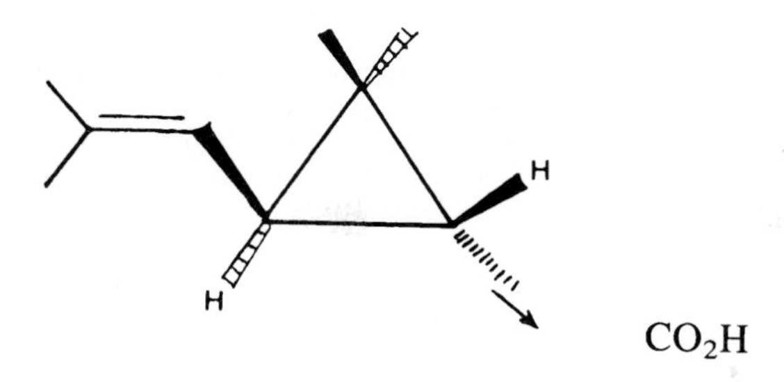


Chrysanthemic Acid

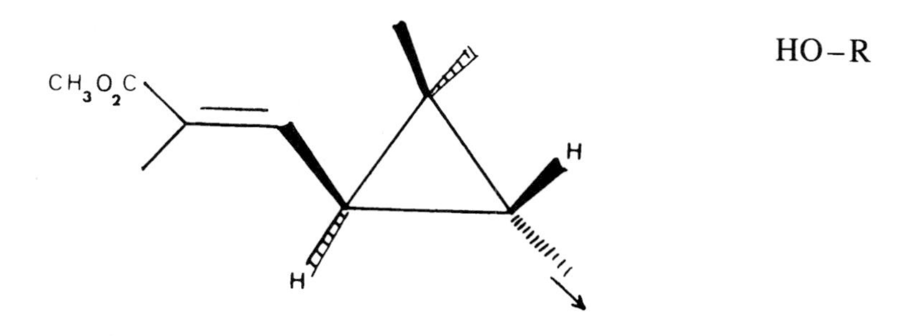


Pyrethric Acid

***Figure 22–19.*** ***The basic structures of the pyrethroid ester insecticides, showing the two characteristic acidic portions, chrysanthemic and pyrethric acids.***

Variations in the alcoholic (HO-R) moieties include alkyl- and aryl-ether chains of complex structure.

Although these insecticides cannot be considered to be highly toxic to mammals, their use indoors in enclosed and poorly ventilated spaces has resulted in some interesting signs and symptoms of toxicity to humans. Exposure to the natural pyrethrum mixture is known to cause contact dermatitis, and descriptions of the effects range from localized erythema to a severe vesicular eruption (McCord et al., 1921). The allergenic nature of this natural product is not surprising, with asthmalike attacks and anaphylactic reactions with peripheral vascular collapse among the responses observed. Human toxicity associated with the natural pyrethrins stems from their allergenic properties rather than from direct neurotoxicity. There has been little evidence of the allergic-type reactions in humans exposed to synthetic pyrethroid esters.

One notable form of toxicity associated with synthetic pyrethroids has been a cutaneous paresthesia observed in workers spraying esters containing an $\alpha$-cyano substituent (deltamethrin, cypermethrin, fenvalerate). The paresthesia developed several hours following exposure, described as a stinging or burning sensation on the skin which, in some cases, progressed to a tingling and numbness, the effects lasting some 12 to 18 h (LeQuesne et al., 1980; Tucker and Flannigan, 1983).

Recent reports have appeared in the literature from the People's Republic of China, where synthetic pyrethroids have been used on a large scale on cotton crops since 1982 (Stuart-Harle, 1988; He et al., 1988, 1989). Associated with the sloppy handling of deltamethrin and fenvalerate, both of which are type II compounds, some 573 cases of acute poisoning have occurred with some 229 cases of occupational exposure. Some 45 cases of intoxication involved cypermethrin. Occupational exposure resulted in some dizziness plus a burning, itching, or tingling sensation of the exposed skin which was exacerbated by sweating and washing with warm water. The signs and symptoms disappeared by 24 h after exposure. Spilling these agents on the head, face, and eyes resulted in pain, lacrimation, photophobia, congestion, and edema of the conjunctiva and eyelids. Ingestion of pyrethroid esters caused epigastric pain, nausea and vomiting, headache, dizziness, anorexia, fatigue, tightness in the chest, blurred vision, paresthesia, palpitations, coarse muscular fasciculations in the large muscles of the extremities, and disturbances of consciousness. In severe poisonings, convulsive attacks persisting from 30 to 120 seconds were accompanied by flexion of the upper limbs and extension of the lower limbs with opisthotonos and loss of consciousness. The frequency of these seizures was on the order of 10 to 30 times a day in the first week after exposure, gradually decreasing in incidence, with recovery within 2 to 3 weeks (He et al., 1989). The signs and symptoms of acute intoxication appear to be reversible and no chronic toxicity has been reported to date.

**Site and Mechanism of Toxicity.** Most of the research to investigate the mechanism(s) by which the pyrethroid esters elicit their effects has been conducted in vitro using cockroach, crayfish, or squid giant axon preparations (Narahashi, 1971, 1976, 1985; Casida et al., 1983). In contrast, as a consequence

**Table 22–10**
**Classification of Pyrethroid Ester Insecticides on the Basis of Chemical Structure and Observed Biological Activity**

| | | SIGNS AND SYMPTOMS | | |
|---|---|---|---|---|
| | STRUCTURE | COCKROACH | RAT | CHEMICALS |
| Type I syndrome ("T" syndrome) | $R-C(=O)-O-R$ | Restlessness<br>Incoordination<br>Prostration<br>Paralysis | Hyperexcitation<br>Sparring<br>Aggressiveness<br>Enhanced startle response<br>Whole body tremor<br>Prostration | Pyrethrin I<br>Allethrin<br>Tetramethrin<br>Kadethrin<br>Resmethrin<br>Phenothrin<br>Permethrin |
| Type II syndrome ("CS" syndrome) | $R-C(=O)-O-C(CN)-R$ | Hyperactivity<br>Incoordination<br>Convulsions | Burrowing<br>Dermal tingling<br>Clonic seizures<br>Sinuous writhing<br>Profuse salivation | Cypermethrin<br>Fenpropanthrin<br>Deltamethrin<br>Cyphenothrin<br>Fenvalerate<br>Fluvalinate |

of the complexity of the mammalian nervous system, studies on intact animals have not yielded conclusive, fundamental information concerning the mechanism of action of these agents. Type I pyrethroid esters affect sodium channels in nerve membranes, causing repetitive (sensory, motor) neuronal discharge and a prolonged negative afterpotential, the effects being quite similar to those produced by DDT. Type I pyrethroids produce slight increases in the time constant for sodium current inactivation (Joy, 1994b). Although the repetitive discharges could occur in any region of the nervous system, those at presynaptic nerve terminals would have the most dramatic effect on synaptic transmission (i.e., the CNS and peripheral ganglia) giving rise to the signs documented in Table 22-10. These changes are not accompanied by a large membrane depolarization so that no blockage of impulse conduction occurs (Narahashi, 1985). Type II pyrethroids extend the time constant for inactivation by hundreds of milliseconds to seconds, causing a persistent depolarization and a frequency-dependent conduction block in sensory and motor axons, and prolonged repetitive firing of sensory end organs and muscle fibers (Joy, 1994b). The depolarizing action would have a dramatic effect on the sensory nervous system because such neurons tend to discharge when depolarized even slightly, resulting in an increase in the number of discharges (van den Bercken and Vijverberg, 1983). This alone could account for the tingling and/or burning sensation felt on exposed skin. In addition, a slight depolarization at presynaptic nerve terminals would result in increased release of neurotransmitter, serious disturbance of synaptic transmission, and the generation of the symptomatology associated with type II esters.

Other sites of action have been noted for pyrethroid esters (Fig. 22-20). Several agents (permethrin, cypermethrin, deltamethrin) inhibit $Ca^{2+}$, $Mg^{2+}$-ATPase, the effect of which would result in increased intracellular calcium levels accompanied by increased neurotransmitter release and postsynaptic depolarization (Clark and Matsumura, 1982). While deltamethrin had an inhibitory action on the GABA-receptor–chloride channel complex, the action of other pyrethroids is unclear and the mechanism of action may be of little importance compared to the effects on sodium channels (Joy, 1994b). Deltamethrin, a type II ester, produced an apparent decrease

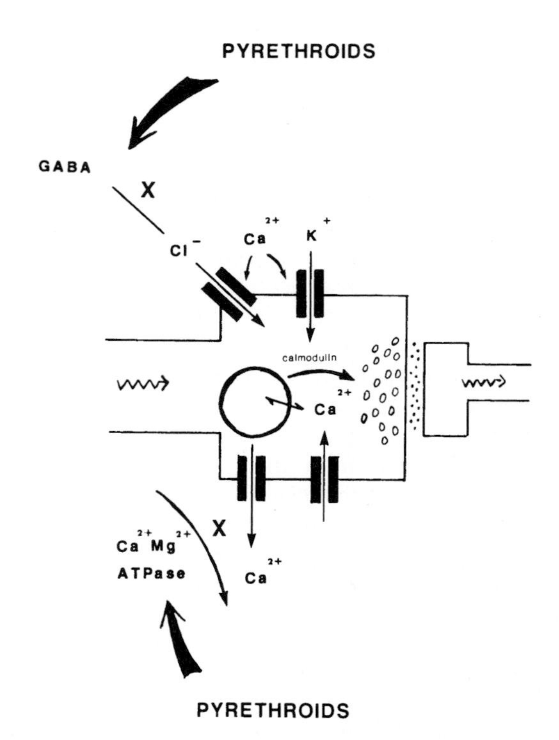


***Figure 22–20. Proposed cellular mechanisms by which pyrethroid esters interfere with neuronal function.***

These are (1) by inhibition of $Ca^{2+}$, $Mg^{2+}$-ATPase, thereby interfering with calcium removal from the ending; (2) questionable binding to GABA receptors in the chloride channel; (3) inhibition of calmodulin that binds calcium ions, thereby increasing the levels of free calcium in the nerve ending to act on neurotransmitter release.

in resting chloride permeability in muscle and unmyelinated vagal C fibers at levels lower than those initiating sodium channel inactivation, while cismethrin, a type I ester, was without effect (Joy, 1994b).

**Biotransformation, Distribution, and Storage.** Evidence to date suggests that pyrethroid esters elicit little chronic toxicity either in animals or the human. Chronic animal feeding studies yield high "no-effect" levels, suggesting that there is little storage or accumulation of a body burden of these agents and, perhaps, an efficient detoxification of the chemicals.

Two ester linkages exist in pyrethroid esters, a terminal methyl ester (pyrethrin II) and one more centrally located ester adjacent to the cyclopropane moiety (allethrin, tetramethrin, phenothrin, deltamethrin) and/or the $\alpha$-cyano substituent (deltamethrin, cypermethrin, fenvalerate, cyphenothrin). Pyrethroid esters are susceptible to degradation by hydrolytic enzymes, possibly by nonspecific carboxylesterases found associated with the microsomal fraction of tissue homogenates in various species (Ecobichon, 1979; Casida et al., 1983). Hydrolysis of the methoxycarbonyl group in pyrethrin II by an esterase in rat liver has been reported, but the major site of hydrolytic activity would appear to be at the central ester linkage (Elliott et al., 1972; Shono et al., 1979; Glickman and Casida, 1982). The importance of ester hydrolysis as a route of detoxification is verified by the fact that many organophosphorus esters, which are capable of inhibiting tissue esterases, potentiate pyrethroid ester toxicity in a variety of species (Casida et al., 1983). Species susceptibility to pyrethroid ester toxicity would appear to be highly dependent on the nature of the tissue esterase, the level of activity detected, the substrate specificity, and rate of hydrolysis encountered in target and nontarget species.

The microsomal monooxygenase system, found in the tissues of almost all species, is extensively involved in the detoxification of every pyrethroid ester in mammals and of some of these agents in insect and fish species. Much of the research in this field has been summarized by Shono et al. (1979), Kulkarni and Hodgson (1984), and Casida et al. (1983). The importance of the oxidative mechanisms in detoxification is demonstrated by the inclusion of the synergist, piperonyl butoxide, a classic monooxygenase inhibitor, in preparations toxic to houseflies and other insects, to enhance the potency of pyrethroid esters in the 10- to 300-fold range (Casida et al., 1983; Matsumura, 1985).

**Treatment of Poisoning.** Limited experience with intoxications by pyrethroid esters has restricted the development of any protocols for treating such poisonings. No specific treatment has been reported other than symptomatic and supportive therapies (He et al., 1989).

## Botanical Insecticides

A number of naturally occurring agents of plant origin have been used to control insect pests. These chemicals ranged from highly toxic agents (to both target and nontarget species), such as nicotine, to relatively innocuous substances, such as derris root. Interestingly, despite the overwhelming number of synthetic insecticide formulations on the market, the two above mentioned agents can still be purchased and are still considered effective insecticides.

**Nicotine.** Nicotine, first used as an insecticide in 1763, has been used as a contact insecticide, stomach poison, and fumigant in the form of nicotine alkaloid, the sulfate salt, or in the form of other derivatives. Commercially, nicotine is extracted from the leaves of *Nicotiana tabacum* and *Nicotiana rustica* by alkali treatment and steam distillation or by extraction with benzene, trichloroethylene, or diethyl ether. Nicotine comprises some 97 percent of the alkaloid content of commercial tobacco. It is marketed under the trade name of Black Leaf 40, an aqueous solution of the sulfate salt of nicotine, containing 40 percent nicotine.

Nicotine is extremely toxic, the acute oral $LD_{50}$ in rats being on the order of 50 to 60 mg/kg. It is readily absorbed through the skin, and any contact with nicotine solutions should be washed off immediately. Anecdotal accounts of experiences by people who sprayed this chemical as an agricultural insecticide make an interesting collection of stories, all pointing to the fact that nicotine mimics the action of acetylcholine at all ganglionic synapses and at neuromuscular junctions, causing muscular fasciculations, convulsions, and death from paralysis of the respiratory muscles via blockade of the neuromuscular junctions (see Table 22-7). It functions as an insecticide in much the same manner, causing a blockade of synapses associated with motor nerves in insects.

**Rotenoids.** Six rotenoid esters occur naturally and are isolated from the plant *Derris eliptica* found in Southeast Asia or from the plant *Lonchocarpus utilis* or *L. urucu* native to South America. Rotenone, one of the alkaloids, is the most potent and can be purified by solvent extraction and recrystallization. It can be used either as a contact or a stomach poison. However, it is unstable in light and heat and almost all toxicity can be lost after 2 to 3 days during the summer.

Rotenone is very toxic to fish, and one of its main uses by native people over the centuries was to paralyze fish for capture and consumption. The mammalian toxicity varies greatly with the species exposed, the method of administration, and the type of formulation. Crystalline rotenone has an acute oral $LD_{50}$ of 60, 132, and 3000 mg/kg for guinea pigs, rats, and rabbits, respectively (Matsumura, 1985). Because the toxicity of derris powders exceeds that of the equivalent content of rotenone, it is obvious that the other esters in crude preparations have significant biological activity. Acute poisoning in animals is characterized by an initial respiratory stimulation followed by respiratory depression, ataxia, convulsions, and death by respiratory arrest (Shimkin and Anderson, 1936). The anestheticlike action on nerves appears to be related to the ability of rotenone to block electron transport in mitochondria by inhibiting oxidation linked to $NADH_2$, this resulting in nerve conduction blockade (O'Brien, 1967; Corbett, 1974). Although toxicity in laboratory and domestic animals has been reported with acute $LD_{50}$ values of 10 to 30 mg/kg reported, human intoxications are rare. The estimated fatal oral dose for a 70-kg man is of the order of 10 to 100 g. Rotenone has been used topically for treatment of head lice, scabies, and other ectoparasites, but the dust is highly irritating to the eyes (potentially causing conjunctivitis), the skin (causing contact dermatitis), and to the upper respiratory tract (causing rhinitis) and throat (linked with pharyngitis).

## HERBICIDES

A herbicide, in the broadest definition, is any compound that is capable of either killing or severely injuring plants and may be used for the elimination of plant growth or the killing off of plant parts (Jager, 1983). Many of the early chemicals, such as sulfuric acid, sodium chlorate, arsenic trioxide, sodium arsenite, petroleum oils, iron and copper sulfate, or sodium borate were frequently hard to handle and/or were very toxic, were relatively nonspecific, or were phytotoxic to the crop as well as the unwanted plant life if not applied at exactly the proper time. In the late 1930s, many studies were initiated to find agents that would selectively destroy certain plant species. Many of these early chemicals were more effective but still possessed considerable mammalian toxicity. However, a few compounds served as prototype chemicals for further development. Summaries of the early days of herbicide development are presented by Cremlyn (1978) and by Kirby (1980).

In the past two decades, the herbicides have represented the most rapidly growing section of the agrochemical pesticide business due in part to (1) movement into monocultural practices where the risk of weed infestation has increased because fallowing and crop rotation which would change weed species are no longer in vogue; and (2) mechanization of agricultural practices (planting, tending, harvesting) because of increased labor costs. The annual rate of growth of herbicide production on a worldwide basis between 1980 and 1985 was 1.9 percent per year, more than double the rate of growth for insecticides during the same period (Marquis, 1986). The result has been a plethora of chemically diverse structures rivalling the innovative chemistry of the insecticides, the aim being to protect desirable crops and to obtain high yields by selectively eliminating unwanted plant species, thereby reducing the competition for nutrients. For a more complete discussion of the development of herbicides, the reader is referred to Cremlyn (1978), McEwen and Stephenson (1979), and Jager (1983).

Herbicides may be classified in a number of ways. The first classification is by chemical structure, although this is not very enlightening, because of overlapping biological effects for a variety of chemical structures. The second method of classification pertains to how and when the agents are applied. *Preplanting* herbicides are applied to the soil before a crop is seeded. *Preemergent* herbicides are applied to the soil before the usual time of appearance of the unwanted vegetation. *Postemergent* herbicides are applied to the soil or foliage after the germination of the crop and/or weeds. Plant biochemists classify herbicides according to their mechanism of toxicity in plants; their action is referred to as *selective* (toxic to some species), *contact* (act when impinging on the plant foliage), or *translocated* (being absorbed via the soil or through the foliage into the plant xylem and phloem). In this chapter, herbicides will be classified by their ability to interfere with specific biochemical processes essential for normal growth and development, interactions that result in severe injury to and the eventual death of the plant. In Table 22-11, the various mechanisms by which herbicides exert their biological effects are shown

**Table 22–11**
**Mechanisms of Action of Herbicides**

| MECHANISM(S) | CHEMICAL CLASSES |
|---|---|
| Inhibition of photosynthesis by disruption of light reactions and blockade of electron transport | Ureas, 1,3,5-triazines, 1,4-triazines, uracils, pyridazones, 4-hydroxybenzonitriles, *N*-arylcarbamates, acylanilides (some) |
| Inhibition of respiration by blockade of electron transfer from NADH or blocking the coupling of electron transfer to ADP to form ATP. | Dinitrophenols<br>Halophenols |
| Growth stimulants, "auxins" | Aryloxyalkylcarboxylic acids<br>Benzoic acids |
| Inhibitors of cell and nucleus division | Alkyl *N*-arylcarbamates |
| Inhibition of protein synthesis | Dinitroanilines |
| Inhibition of carotenoid synthesis, protective pigments in chloroplasts to prevent chlorophyll from being destroyed by oxidative reactions | Chloracetamide<br>*O*-substituted diphenyl ethers<br>Hydrazines |
| Inhibition of lipid synthesis | S-alkyl dialkylcarbamodithioates<br>Aliphatic chlorocarboxylic acids |
| Unknown mechanisms, nonselective chemicals | Inorganic agents (copper sulfate, sulfuric acid, sodium chlorate, sodium borate)<br>Organic agents (dichlobenil, chlorthiamid, bentazone, diphenamid, benzoylpropethyl) |

SOURCE: From Jager, 1983.

along with the generic and chemical names of the classes of herbicides and some examples of each class. The claim has been made that, because the modes of action involve biochemical phytoprocesses having no counterparts in mammalian systems, there is no risk of mammalian toxicity associated with these chemicals. With the exception of a few chemicals, the herbicides have demonstrated low toxicity in mammals. However, the current controversy around these chemicals centers on demonstrated or suspected mutagenicity, teratogenicity, and/or carcinogenicity associated either with the agent(s) or with contaminants and by-products of manufacture found in trace amounts in technical grade material. The presence of some of these contaminants has been largely ignored without realizing that the toxicities associated with them are both different from those observed with the herbicidal chemical and frequently occur at far lower dosages.

In terms of general toxicity, because the major route of exposure to herbicides is dermal and because these agents tend to be strong acids, amines, esters, and phenols, they are dermal irritants, causing skin rashes and contact dermatitis even when exposure involves diluted formulations. There appear to be subpopulations of individuals who are hypersensitive to dermal contact with solutions or aerosolized mists of certain types of herbicides, and moderate to severe urticaria has been observed to persist for 5 to 10 days following exposure. Certain individuals, particularly those prone to allergic reactions, may experience severe contact dermatitis, asthmalike attacks, and even anaphylactic reactions, following dermal or inhalation contact with formulated herbicides. Whether these effects are chemical-specific for the herbicide or for emulsifiers, cosolvents, and so-called inerts found in formulations has not been established. Although skin patch testing of herbicidal chemicals has usually proven to be negative, it is possible that the patients' responses may be associated with a generalized, nonspecific irritant effect of the formulation. Many of these dermal and pulmonary reactions respond satisfactorily to treatment with antihistaminic agents.

In contrast, there are other herbicides that can elicit a range of acute and chronic effects following exposure, and it is on these chemicals that attention will be focused.

## Chlorophenoxy Compounds

During World War II, considerable effort was directed toward the development of effective, broad-spectrum herbicides in both the United States and the United Kingdom with a view to both increasing food production and to finding potential chemical warfare agents (Kirby, 1980). The chlorophenoxy compounds (Fig. 22-21), including the acids, salts, amines, and esters, were the first commercially available products evolving from this research in 1946. This class of herbicides has seen continuous, extensive, and uninterrupted use since 1947 in agriculture for broad-leafed weeds and in the control of woody plants along roadside, railway, and utilities' rights of way and in reforestation programs. In plants, these chemicals mimic the action of auxins, hormones chemically related to indoleacetic acid that stimulate growth. No hormonal activity is observed in mammals and other species, and beyond target organ toxicity that can be associated with the pharmacokinetics, biotransformation, and/or elimination of these chemicals, their mechanisms of toxic action are poorly understood.

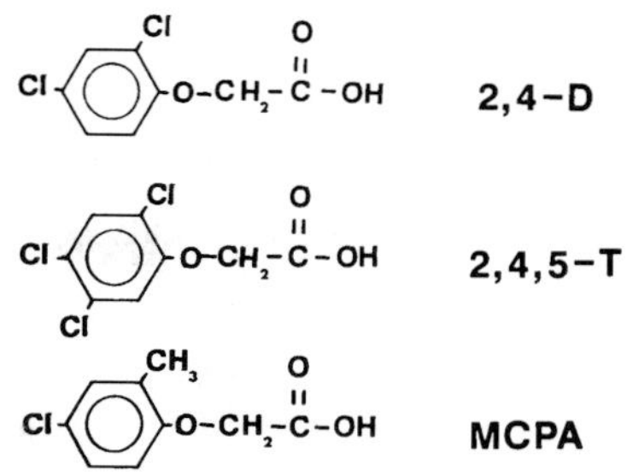

***Figure 22-21. The molecular structure of the three most common chlorophenoxyacetic acid herbicides: 2,4-D, 2,4-dichlorophenoxyacetic acid; 2,4,5-T, 2,4,5-trichlorophenoxyacetic acid; and MCPA, 4-chloro-o-toloxyacetic acid.***

In addition to the salts of the acids, ester and amine derivatives are also marketed.

A tremendous volume of mammalian toxicity data has been collected over the past 42 years from both animal studies and incidents of human exposure (Hayes, 1982; Stevens and Sumner, 1991). It is of interest to note that, in a recent toxicological reevaluation of 2,4-D for the purposes of providing the U.S. EPA with a new toxicity database for the chemical, an industry task force discovered nothing of toxicological significance that was not already known about the chemical, with one exception (Mullison, 1986). The exceptional finding was the appearance of astrocytomas in the brains of male Fischer 344 strain rats exposed to the highest (45 mg/kg per day) dosage. A subsequent review of the findings suggested that this tumor incidence was not treatment related (Koestner, 1986; Solleveld et al., 1984). The acute toxicity elicited by chlorophenoxy herbicides has been described by Hayes (1982). The oral $LD_{50}$ values ranged from 300 to >1000 mg/kg in different animal species, and only the dog appeared to be particularly sensitive, possibly on the basis that it has considerable difficulty in the renal elimination of such organic acids (Gehring et al., 1976). Animals will tolerate repeated oral exposure to doses of chlorophenoxy herbicides marginally below the single, toxic oral dose without showing significant signs of toxicity, an observation suggesting that there is little cumulative effect on target organs. At dosages causing toxicity, few specific signs other than muscular and neuromuscular involvement were observed in animals although tenseness, stiffness in extremities, muscular weakness, ataxia, and paralysis have been reported. Hepatic and renal injury in addition to irritation of the gastrointestinal mucosa have been observed in acute lethality studies in animals.

The case of accidental and/or occupational intoxications by chlorophenoxy herbicides have been reviewed by Hayes (1982). Most patients complained of headache, dizziness, nausea, vomiting, abdominal pains, diarrhea, respiratory complications, aching and tender muscles, myotonia, weakness, and fatigue. Clinically, there is some evidence of renal dysfunction, and transient albuminuria has been observed in some cases. There is little documented evidence of neurotoxicity associated with chlorophenoxy herbicides with the exception of one study in which decreased peripheral nerve conduction velocities were observed in workers employed in manufacturing 2,4-D and 2,4,5-T (Singer et al., 1982). A wide range of human lethal dosages of 2,4-D has been reported, and the average lethal dose is in excess of 300 mg/kg. The oral dose required to elicit symptoms is of the order of 50 to 60 mg/kg. In one poisoning, death occurred in a 75-kg male following the intentional ingestion of 6 g (80 mg/kg), although the actual dose may have been much higher because the individual had vomitted (Nielsen et al., 1965). In another case, the daily ingestion of 500 mg of 2,4-D over a 3-week period elicited no symptoms (Berwick, 1970). The clinical course of one patient who intentionally ingested a sizable volume of a mixture of the butyl esters of 2,4-D and 2,4,5-T was characterized by increased body temperature, increased pulse and respiratory rates, decreased blood pressure, respiratory alkalosis, profuse sweating, oliguria, hemoconcentration, increased blood urea nitrogen, and a deepening coma. At autopsy, focal submucosal hemorrhage, moderate congestion, and edema of the intestine were seen along with congestion in the lungs. Necrosis of the intestinal mucosa as well as necrosis and fatty infiltration of the liver were observed. Pneumonitis and inflammation of terminal bronchioles was observed and renal damage included degeneration of the convoluted tubules, fatty infiltration, and the presence of proteinaceous material in the glomerular spaces (Hayes, 1982). Earlier literature reported significant peripheral neuropathies in three people acquiring toxic concentrations via percutaneous absorption while spraying 2,4-D ester for weeds (Goldstein et al., 1959). In each case, the signs and symptoms began several hours after exposure and progressed until pain, paresthesia, and paralysis were severe. The diagnosis of peripheral neuropathy was supported by electromyographic analysis and recovery was incomplete even after a lapse of some years. In a more recent report of a suicidal ingestion of a 2,4-D concentrate, the morphological examination of nervous tissue revealed extensive plaques of acute demyelination in all parts of the brain that resembled those observed in acute multiple sclerosis (Dudley and Thapar, 1972).

Immediately following the industrial accident that occurred at the Monsanto plant in Nitro, West Virginia, on March 8, 1949 where 2,4,5-T was being synthesized, acute symptoms of exposure to the reaction products included skin, eye, and respiratory tract irritation; headache; dizziness; nausea; acneiform eruptions; severe pain in the muscles of the thorax, shoulders, and extremities; fatigue; nervousness; irritability; dyspnea; complaint of decreased libido; and intolerance to cold (Ashe and Suskind, 1953). In a 1984 epidemiological study of active and retired employees from this plant, clinical evidence of chloracne persisted in some 55.7 percent of those exposed (113 out of 204) and an association was found between the persistence of chloracne and the presence and severity of actinic elastosis of the skin (Suskind and Hertzberg, 1984). Although there was some evidence of exposure and a history of gastrointestinal tract ulcers, there was no evidence of increased risk for cardiovascular, hepatic, or renal disease or of central or peripheral nervous tissue damage.

Serious reservations have been raised about the toxic properties of the chlorophenoxy herbicides because such neuropathies have not been observed in recent years with occupational and/or accidental exposure to high concentrations of these agents. In earlier times, before the method of synthesis was altered, workers involved in the manufacture of this class of herbicides, particularly 2,4,5-T, experienced a severe type of contact dermatitis called "chemical worker chloracne" (Schultz, 1968; Poland et al., 1971). Herbicide sprayers of a few decades ago developed a persistent condition known as "weed bumps" following daily and seasonal exposure to chlorophenoxy herbicides. Chloracne, however, is not a unique condition associated only with chlorophenoxy herbicides and can be caused by a number of chlorinated aromatic compounds including polychlorinated biphenyls, dibenzo-*p*-dioxins, dibenzofurans, and chlorinated naphthalenes (Schultz, 1968). The true culprit was unmasked when teratological studies revealed that commercial 2,4,5-T caused cleft palate and renal malformations in mice and renal anomalies in rats (Courtney et al., 1970). Today, the evidence is conclusive that many of these biological effects were not related to the herbicide but to a contaminant, 2,3,7,8-tetrachloro-dibenzo-*p*-dioxin (TCDD or the news media's dioxin), a by-product formed during synthesis if the temperature is not rigidly controlled. Levels of TCDD of the order of 30 to 50 $\mu$g/g have been estimated to have occurred in commercial 2,4,5-T. The sample of 2,4,5-T used in the teratological studies was found to contain 30 $\mu$g TCDD/g (Courtney and Moore, 1971). More recent teratological studies, conducted with "clean" (i.e., $<0.5$ ppm TCDD) 2,4,5-T have demonstrated that dosages on the order of 15 to 100 mg/kg per day during organogenesis were required to elicit birth defects (cleft palate, cystic kidney) and fetotoxic effects in mice and hamsters, whereas rats and monkeys appeared to be resistant to 2,4,5,-T-induced teratogenicity (Hayes, 1982). The carcinogenicity of 2,4-D and 2,4,5-T in laboratory rodents has not been conclusively demonstrated, but TCDD has caused an increased incidence of tumors at multiple sites when fed in the diet at low (ng or pg/g) concentrations (Van Miller et al., 1977; Kociba et al., 1978). Currently, levels of TCDD detectable in commercial 2,4,5-T are below 0.005 $\mu$g/g, thereby presenting one possible explanation for the absence of present-day toxicity observed with this chemical.

Tetrachlorodibenzo-*p*-dioxin has been shown to be extremely toxic to a number of animal species. The acute oral $LD_{50}$ values ranged from 0.0006 to 0.283 mg/kg, with the guinea pig shown to be the most susceptible species (Schwetz et al., 1973; Moore et al., 1979). However, it should be emphasized that mortality does not occur immediately, the animals undergoing a slow but progressive decline into a moribund state associated with an increased incidence of infections and the eventual death some 14 to 28 days after treatment. It appears that the animals' environment suddenly becomes toxic to them, leading investigators to examine the immune response and the discovery that TCDD and related compounds caused a marked atrophy of the thymus gland, the source of the T-cell components of the immune response (Vos et al., 1983). Although a complete discussion of the toxicity of chlorinated dioxins and furans is beyond the scope of this chapter, the TCDD story emphasizes the toxicological importance of minor contaminants found in pesticides, the necessity for testing technical products/formulations and for cautious interpretation of results from animal experiments in relation to effects in the human. Rather than stress the reader with the voluminous literature on the subject of associations of dioxins, 2,4-D, and 2,4,5-T with adverse health effects (neuropathies, birth defects, cancer, etc.), a perusal of cogent and responsible reviews such as those of Hay (1982), Tucker et al. (1983), Whelan (1985), Gough (1986), and Tschirley (1986) is recommended for an overview of the dioxin literature.

The extensive use of Agent Orange, a 50:50 mixture of the *n*-butyl esters of 2,4-D and 2,4,5-T, as a defoliant during the Vietnam conflict raised the spectre of possible adverse health effects among service personnel handling and spraying the material (e.g., Operation Ranchhand) as well as among soldiers during field operations and civilians who might have acquired body burdens by dermal exposure or ingestion of contaminated drinking water. The facts that: (1) some 11.5 million gallons of Agent Orange were used up to 1971; (2) contamination by TCDD occurred to a maximum of 47 $\mu$g/g; and (3) birth defects and cancers were produced in animals did nothing to reduce the concerns of both those potentially exposed individuals and government departments. Unfortunately, despite many claims of adverse health effects of diverse nature among veterans of this war, various epidemiological studies conducted in Australia, New Zealand, and the United States have provided inconclusive evidence that exposure was high enough to have elicited such effects (Buckingham, 1982; Hay, 1982; Walsh, 1983; Greenwald et al., 1984; Gough, 1986; CDC, 1988; Gochfeld, 1988; Stellman et al., 1988; Tamburro, 1992).

The inability to demonstrate distinct adverse health effects in military personnel and civilians exposed to TCDD-contaminated Agent Orange in Vietnam led investigators to examine larger populations of individuals potentially exposed to chlorophenoxy herbicides, including workers in agriculture and forestry and herbicide manufacturing and formulating who have used 2,4,5-T and/or 2,4-D extensively and, in some cases, almost exclusively since the introduction of these chemicals in 1947. However, the results of a number of studies that focussed on the incidence of carcinogenicity have not resolved the issue. Early studies in Sweden suggested that exposure to chlorophenoxy herbicides and chlorophenols produced a sixfold increase in soft tissue sarcomas, Hodgkin's lymphoma (HL), and non-Hodgkin's lymphoma (NHL), whether or not the chemicals were contaminated by polychlorinated dibenzodioxins and dibenzofurans (Hardell and Sandstrom, 1979; Eriksson et al., 1981; Hardell et al., 1981; Schumacher, 1985). Some studies confirmed the Swedish results but, because of small sample sizes, incidence rates, and the like, they lacked significant statistical power (Axelson et al., 1980; Cantor, 1982; Thiess et al., 1982). Other studies have failed to confirm these results (Ott et al., 1980; Lynge, 1985; Pearce et al., 1986; Wiklund et al., 1988; Bond et al., 1988). A study conducted in Kansas demonstrated an association between farm herbicidal use and NHL, the incidence of which appeared to increase with the number of days exposure per year (Hoar et al., 1986). In the opinion of some, this study went one step too far in associating the blame with 2,4-D even though this chemical was the dominant herbicide used on corn. It is obvious, however, that within the agricultural workforce, there is a higher incidence of certain types of cancer (Cantor, 1982; Woods et al., 1980; Council on Scientific Affairs, 1988; Wiklund et al., 1988). A study of prairie wheat farmers in Saskatchewan, Canada, has revealed no increase in NHL above the incidence observed in the nonfarming population (Wigle et al., 1990). In relation to the general population of Saskatchewan, where 2,4-D has seen the highest and most consistent use since 1947 (60 percent of the national total), farmers had lower overall mortality and cancer rates than expected. One review of the literature presented reasonable evidence that occupational exposure to phenoxy herbicides resulted in an increased risk of developing NHL (Morrison et al., 1992). However, a study of cancer mortality in chlorophenoxy herbicide-exposed workers, using an international database set up by IARC/NIEHS, revealed no clearly detectable excess for NHL or HL but a sixfold excess of soft tissue sarcomas in the cohort and a ninefold excess among sprayers (Saracci et al., 1991). More recent investigations of the toxicity database of chlorophenoxy herbicides concluded that their impact on the incidence of human cancer has been negligible, and the results of these studies are inconsistent and inconclusive (Munro et al., 1992; Bond and Rossbacher, 1993). Lacking the ideal "definitive, clean" cancer study, this controversy will continue in the scientific literature.

## Bipyridyl Derivatives

One chemical class of herbicides deserving of particular attention is the bipyridyl group, specifically paraquat (1,1′-dimethyl-4-,4′-bipyridylium dichloride, methyl viologen) and diquat (1,1′-ethylene-2,2′-bipyridylium dibromide) (Fig. 22-22). Paraquat was first synthesized in 1882, but its pesticidal properties were not discovered until 1959 (Haley, 1979). This agent, a nonselective contact herbicide, is one of the most specific pulmonary toxicants known and has been the subject of intensive investigation because of the startling toxicity observed in humans. A high mortality rate is encountered in poisoning cases. Many countries have banned or severely restricted the use of paraquat because of the debilitating or life-threatening hazards from occupational exposure and the large number of reported accidental and suicidal fatalities (Campbell, 1968; Davies et al., 1977; Haley, 1979; Tinoco et al., 1993). The analog, diquat, is considerably less potent than paraquat, but nonetheless can cause severe acute and chronic poisoning.

In animals, paraquat shows moderate acute toxicity, the oral $LD_{50}$ values for various species ranging from 22 to 262 mg/kg. Intoxication involves a combination of signs and symptoms that include lethargy, hypoxia, dyspnea, tachycardia, hyperapnea, adipsia, diarrhea, ataxia, hyperexcitability, and convulsions, depending on the dosage and the species studied (Smith and Heath, 1976; Haley, 1979). Necropsy reveals hemorrhagic and edematous lungs, intraalveolar hemorrhage, congestion and pulmonary fibrosis, centrilobular hepatic necrosis, and renal tubular necrosis. Lung weights of intoxicated ani-

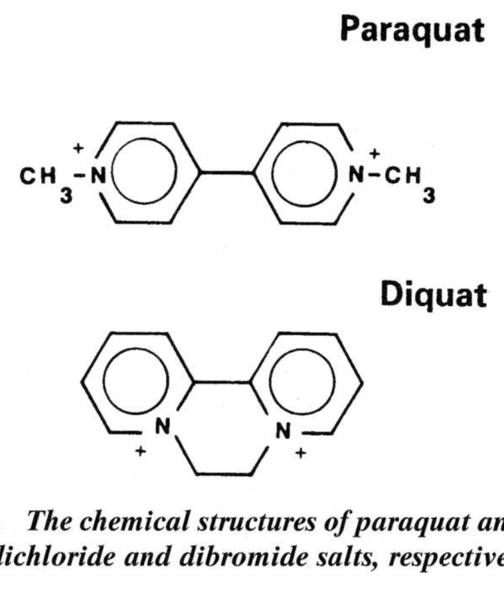

***Figure 22–22. The chemical structures of paraquat and diquat, marketed as the dichloride and dibromide salts, respectively.***

mals increase significantly despite marked losses in body weight. From a catalog of all the signs and symptoms, it is obvious that the lung is the most susceptible target organ, and the same histopathologic picture of pulmonary lesions is observed in mice, rats, dogs, and humans (Clark et al., 1966). In poisonings, immediate effects are usually not seen in animals but, within 10 to 14 days, respiration becomes impaired, rapid, and shallow and the morphological changes seen include degeneration and vacuolization of pneumocytes, damage to type I and type II alveolar epithelial cells, destruction of the epithelial membranes, and the proliferation of fibrotic cells.

Paraquat, a highly polar compound, is poorly absorbed from the gastrointestinal tract, and experiments in rats demonstrate that 52 percent of the administered dose was still localized in the intestinal tract some 32 h after administration (Murray and Gibson, 1974). Approximately 5 to 10 percent of an ingested dose is absorbed (Haley, 1979). In human intoxications by formulation concentrates, it has been suggested that the presence of emulsifiers and/or cosolvents may well enhance absorption. It is the consensus of opinion that paraquat is not extensively metabolized in vivo although intestinal microflora may be responsible for some 30 percent of the excreted, unidentifiable metabolites in animal studies (Daniel and Gage, 1966). The high levels of paraquat found in the renal tissue of intoxicated animals points to the role of this organ in excreting the unchanged herbicide (Rose et al., 1976). Measurable amounts of paraquat were found in urine for up to 21 days posttreatment in rats and monkeys, even though some 45 percent of the dose administered had been excreted in the urine and feces within 48 h of treatment (Murray and Gibson, 1974).

Lung tissue acquires much higher concentrations of paraquat than do most tissues of the body, with the exception of the kidney, and over a 30-h posttreatment period pulmonary concentrations increase disproportionately to those levels found in other tissues (Sharp et al., 1972; Rose et al., 1976). The same phenomenon is observed in vitro, where pulmonary tissue slices acquire relatively high concentrations of unbound (free) paraquat whereas tissue slices from other organs were unable to accumulate paraquat (Rose et al., 1976). Biochemical studies revealed that paraquat is actively acquired by alveolar cells by a diamine/polyamine transport system where it undergoes NADPH-dependent, one-electron reduction to form a free radical capable of reacting with molecular oxygen (in abundant supply) to reform the cation paraquat plus a reactive oxygen (superoxide anion, $O_2^-$). This superoxide anion is converted into hydrogen peroxide by the enzyme superoxide dismutase. The hydrogen peroxide and superoxide anion can attack polyunsaturated lipids present in cell membranes to produce lipid hydroperoxides which, in turn, can react with other unsaturated lipids to form more lipid-free radicals, thereby perpetuating the system (Smith, 1987). The resulting cellular membrane damage reduces the functional integrity of the cell, affects efficient gas transport and exchange, and induces respiratory impairment. The severity of the cellular effects can be modulated by the availability of oxygen, and animals kept in air with only 10% oxygen fare better than those kept in room air (Rhodes, 1974). In paraquat poisonings, even though the patients may suffer from hypoxia and respiratory insufficiency, hyperbaric oxygen is contraindicated because it appears to promote cellular toxicity.

Cases of paraquat poisonings, of both children and adults, have been described in detail in the literature (Almog and Tal, 1967; Davies et al., 1977; Haley, 1979; Hayes, 1982; Tinoco et al., 1993). The ingestion of commercial paraquat formulations, concentrates containing up to 20% active ingredient, is invariably fatal and runs a time course of 3 to 4 weeks. The initial irritation and burning of the mouth and throat, the necrosis and sloughing of the oral mucosa, severe gastroenteritis with esophageal and gastric lesions, abdominal and substernal chest pains, and bloody stools give way to the characteristic and dominant pulmonary symptoms, including dyspnea, anoxia, opacity in the lungs as seen by chest X-ray, coma, and death. Paraquat induces multiorgan toxicity with necrotic damage to the liver, kidneys, and myocardial muscle plus extensive hemorrhagic incidents throughout the body. Although most of the paraquat intoxications involve the ingestion of the compound, there are reports of toxicity following dermal exposure, with blistering and erythema. Swan (1969) found no detectable lung changes in workers exposed to sprays 6 days per week for 12 weeks and Senanayake et al. (1993) showed no changes in lung function tests in Sri Lankan tea plantation workers with chronic occupational exposure to paraquat aerosols.

Treatment of paraquat poisoning should be vigorous and initiated as quickly as possible. Gastric lavage should be followed by the administration of mineral adsorbents such as Fuller's earth (kaolin), bentonite clay, or activated charcoal to bind any unabsorbed paraquat remaining in the gastrointestinal tract. Purgatives may be given. Absorbed paraquat may be removed from the bloodstream by aggressive, lengthy hemoperfusion through charcoal or by hemodialysis. To avoid excessive pulmonary damage, supplemental oxygen should be reduced to a level just sufficient to maintain acceptable arterial oxygen tension (>40 to 50 mmHg) (Haley, 1979; Hayes, 1982).

Diquat is a rapidly acting contact herbicide used as a desiccant, for the control of aquatic weeds and to destroy potato halums before harvesting. Diquat is slightly less toxic than paraquat, the oral $LD_{50}$ values in various species are on the order of 100 to 400 mg/kg. Part of the reduced toxicity may be related to the fact that it is poorly absorbed from the gastrointestinal tract; only 6 percent of an ingested dose is excreted in the urine, whereas following subcutaneous administration, 90 to 98 percent of the dose is eliminated via the urine (Daniel and Gage, 1966). A latency period of 24 h is seen prior to visible toxic effects.

Following acute, high-dose exposure or chronic exposure of animals to diquat, the major target organs were the gastrointestinal tract, the liver, and the kidneys (Hayes, 1982; Morgan, 1982). Chronic feeding studies resulted in an increased incidence of cataracts in both dogs and rats (Clark and Hurst, 1970). It is considered that diquat can form free radicals, and that the tissue necrosis is associated with the same mechanism(s) of superoxide-induced peroxidation as observed with paraquat. However, unlike paraquat, diquat shows no special affinity for the lung and does not appear to bear the same mechanism that selectively concentrates paraquat in the lung (Rose and Smith, 1977).

Few diquat-related human intoxications have been reported to date (Schonborn et al., 1971; Narita et al., 1978; Hayes, 1982). In the few cases of suicidal intent described, ulceration of mucosal membranes, gastrointestinal symptoms, acute renal failure, hepatic damage, and respiratory difficulties were observed. CNS effects were more severe. Interestingly, no fibrosis was evident in the lungs. One individual died of cardiac arrest.

A variety of herbicides representative of several chemical classifications and diverse structures have been introduced over the years into agricultural practices (Table 22-12). In general, these chemicals have relatively low acute toxicity, the oral $LD_{50}$ values in rats being on the order of 100 to 10,000 mg/kg. Large doses can be administered in subchronic and chronic toxicity studies without eliciting significant biological effects. Poisonings in humans have usually been associated with occupational exposure to high concentrations during the manufacturing or mixing/loading phases of application or with a few, atypical but sometimes well publicized incidents (Stevens and Sumner, 1991). However, as was encountered with the chlorophenoxy herbicides, many of these chemicals are old and were registered at a time when the protocols and quality of the toxicological assessment were not as stringent as those required today by regulatory agencies.

In reexamining these chemicals by the state-of-the-art techniques in vogue today, the chemicals themselves or minor contaminant by-products of synthesis have elicited mutagenic, teratogenic, or carcinogenic potential not detected before. In addition, the application of sophisticated analytical techniques to residue analysis of groundwater, food, and air has revealed the presence of low concentrations of many of these agents in media to which the general public is exposed. This has necessitated closer scrutiny of the chemicals and testing procedures and changes in registration and has heightened concerns among consumer groups, to the point where they have lost faith in the system of registration. The task of retesting and reevaluating these chemicals is a tedious and costly endeavor. The dilemma faced by manufacturers and regulators alike is that such reevaluation must be done for all chemical pesticides, because a number of untoward adverse biological effects have been identified among chemicals presently undergoing reassessment.

One good example of the problems encountered is that observed with alachlor (Lasso) and the closely related analog, metolachlor (Dual, Primextra) (Fig. 22-23). Alachlor was registered in the mid-to-late 1960s, and the application was supported by toxicity studies carried out on behalf of the manufacturer by the Industrial Biotest Laboratories (IBT). During the investigations carried out by the United States and Canadian committees on IBT practices, some alachlor studies were deemed to be invalid or inadequate, and the manufacturer was requested to provide replacement studies on long-term effects to support the continued registration of the product. A major controversy arose following the submission of the studies in the early 1980s, reporting the incidence of adenocarcinomas in the stomachs and nasal turbinates of Long-Evans rats and in the lungs of CD-1 mice receiving the highest dosages of 126 mg/kg per day (rats) and 260 mg/kg per day (mice) (Alachlor Review Board, 1987). Using the IARC classification system, alachlor was considered to be a category 2B carcinogen, a probable human carcinogen. There were concerns about potentially hazardous exposure of agricultural workers to the chemical during mixing and loading, with levels ranging from

**Table 22–12**
**Herbicidal Chemicals: Classes, Common Names, and Acute Toxicity**

| CHEMICAL CLASS | GENERIC NAME | TRADE NAME | ORAL $LD_{50}$ (mg/kg) |
|---|---|---|---|
| Acetanilides | | Alachlor | 1,200 |
| | | Metolachlor | 2,780 |
| Amides | 3,4-Dichloropropionanilide | Propanil | |
| Arylaliphatic Acids | 2-Methoxy-3,6-dichlorobenzoic acid | Dicamba | 3,500 |
| | 3-Amino-2,5-dichlorobenzoic acid | Chloramben | 5,000 |
| Carbamates | Isopropyl carbanilate | Propham | 5,000 |
| | 4-Chloro-2-butynyl-*m*-chlorocarbanilate | Barban | 600 |
| Dinitroanilines | *a,a,a*-Trifluoro-2,6-dinitro-*N*,*N*-dipropyl-*p*-toluidine | Trifluralin | 10,000 |
| Nitriles | 2,6-Dichlorobenzonitrile | Dichlobenil | 270 |
| | 4-Hydroxy-3,5-diidobenzonitrile | Ioxynil | 110 |
| Substituted ureas | 3-(*p*-chlorophenyl)-1,1-dimethylurea | Monuron | 3,000 |
| | 3-(3,4-Dichlorophenyl)1,1-dimethylurea | Diuron | |
| Tfiazines | 2-Chloro-4-(ethylamino)-6-(isopropylamino)-*S*-triazine | Atrazine | 1,000 |
| | 2-Chloro-4,6-bis (ethylamino)-*S*-triazine | Simazine | 1,000 |

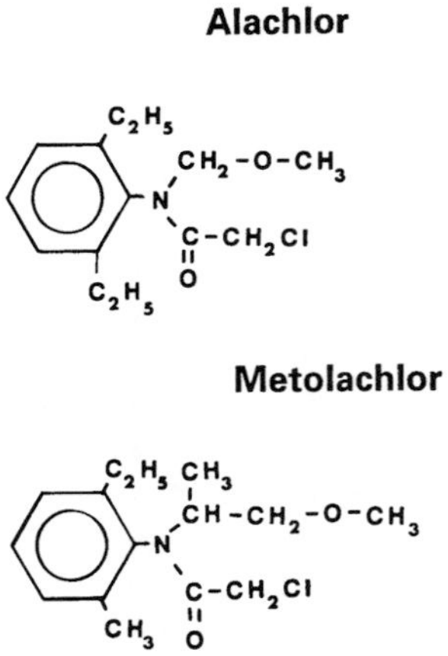

Alachlor

Metolachlor

*Figure 22–23. The chemical structures of alachlor (2-chloro-2′,6′-diethyl-N-(methoxymethyl)acetanilide) and metolachlor (2-chloro-6′-ethyl-N-(2-methoxy-1-methylethyl)acet-o-toluidide.*

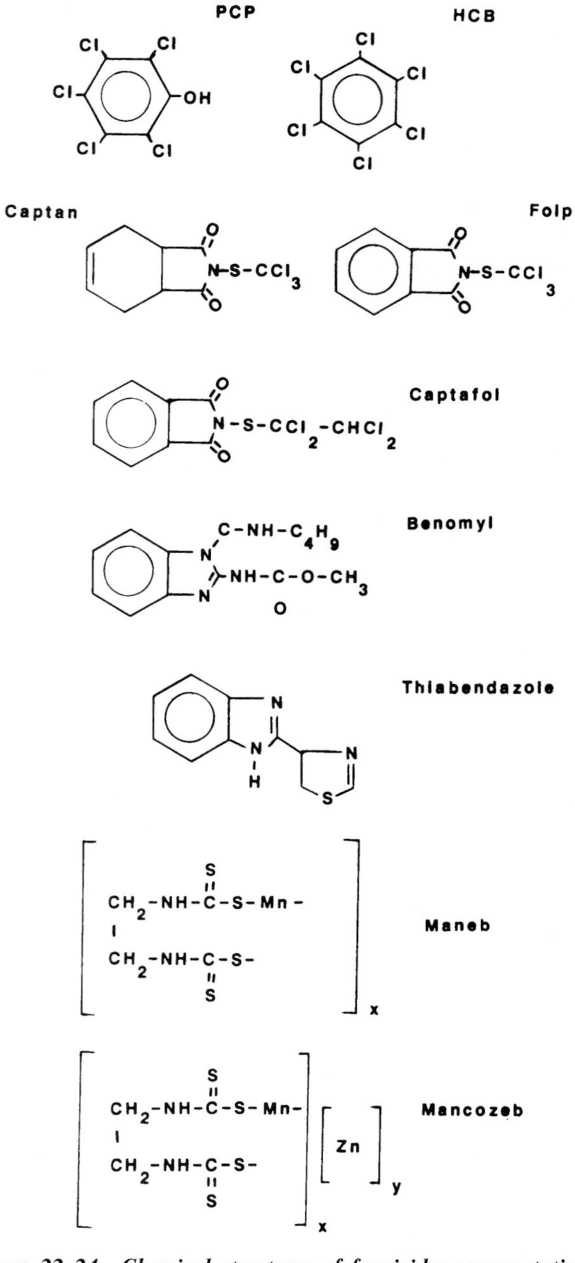

0.00038 to 2.7 mg/kg per day, depending on the exposure model used and whether or not protective clothing was worn. The analysis of selected well water samples revealed contamination by alachlor at 0.10 to 2.11 μg/liter with one sample showing 9.1 μg/liter. Identified carcinogenicity in two species plus the presence of alachlor in the environment in a medium from which the general populace could acquire residues resulted in the cancellation of alachlor's registration in Canada in February 1985.

Unfortunately, during the assessment of alachlor, a competitor's product, another chloroacetanilide substitute for alachlor, was dragged into the discussion, and evidence pointed to the fact that metolachlor caused significant increases in hepatocellular carcinomas and adenocarcinomas in nasal turbinates of female and male Sprague-Dawley rats, respectively. A detailed study of well water in a region where both herbicides were used revealed contamination by either one or the other compound in a number of samples, the mean concentration of metolachlor being between one and two orders of magnitude higher than that observed for alachlor, even though most positive samples were below the IMAC values for alachlor (5.0 μg/liter) and metolachlor (105 μg/liter). Despite the fact that the Canadian federal regulatory agency was of the opinion that metolachlor was much safer, the Alachlor Review Board concluded that there was no difference between the safety of alachlor and metolachlor to humans, because both analogs are animal carcinogens.

## FUNGICIDES

Fungicidal chemicals are derived from a variety of structures ranging from simple inorganic compounds, such as sulfur and copper sulfate, through the aryl- and alkyl-mercurial compounds and chlorinated phenols to metal-containing derivatives of thiocarbamic acid (Fig. 22-24). The chemistry of fungicides and their properties have been discussed by Cremlyn (1978) and by Kramer (1983). *Foliar fungicides* are applied as liquids or powders to the aerial green parts of plants, producing a protective barrier on the cuticular surface and producing systemic toxicity in the developing fungus. *Soil fungicides* are

PCP HCB

Captan Folpet

Captafol

Benomyl

Thiabendazole

Maneb

Mancozeb

*Figure 22–24. Chemical structures of fungicides representative of various chemical classifications.*

applied as liquids, dry powders, or granules, acting either through the vapor phase or by systemic properties. *Dressing fungicides* are applied to the postharvest crop (cereal grains, tubers, corms, etc.) as liquids or dry powders to prevent fungal infestation of the crop, particularly if it may be stored under less than optimum conditions of temperature and humidity. The postharvest loss of food crops to disease is a serious worldwide problem (Table 22-1).

Fungicides may be described as protective, curative, or eradicative according to their mode of action. *Protective fungicides*, applied to the plant before the appearance of any phytopathic fungi, prevent infection by either sporicidal activity or by changing the physiological environment on the leaf surface. *Curative fungicides* are used when an infestation has already begun to invade the plant, and these chemicals function by penetrating the plant cuticle and destroying the young fungal mycelium (the hyphae) growing in the epidermis of the plant, preventing further development. *Eradicative fungicides* control fungal development following the appearance of symptoms, usually after sporulation, by killing both the new spores and the mycelium and by penetrating the cuticle of the plant to the subdermal level (Kramer, 1983).

To be an effective fungicide, a chemical must possess the following properties: (1) low toxicity to the plant but high toxicity to the particular fungus; (2) active per se or capable of conversion (by plant or fungal enzymes) into a toxic intermediate; (3) the ability to penetrate fungal spores or the developing mycelium to reach a site of action; and (4) forms a protective, tenacious deposit on the plant surface that will be resistant to weathering by sunlight, rain, and wind (Cremlyn, 1978). As might be expected, this list of properties is never fulfilled entirely by any single fungicide, and all commercially available compounds show some phytotoxicity, lack of persistence due to environmental degradation, and so forth. Thus, the timing of the application is critical in terms of the development of the plant as well as the fungus.

The topic of fungicidal toxicity has been extensively reviewed by Hayes (1982; Edwards et al., 1991). With a few exceptions, most of these chemicals have a low order of toxicity to mammals, the oral $LD_{50}$ values in the rat being on the order of 800 to 10,000 mg/kg. However, all fungicides are cytotoxic and most produce positive results in the usual in vitro microbial mutagenicity test systems. Such results are not surprising because the microorganisms (salmonella, coliforms, yeasts, and fungi) used in these test systems are not dissimilar from those cell systems for which fungicides were designed to kill, either through a direct lethal effect or via lethal genetic mutations (Lukens, 1971). A safe fungicide (nonmutagenic in test cell systems) would be useless for the protection of food and health. Public concern has been focussed on the positive mutagenicity tests obtained with many fungicides and the predictive possibility of both teratogenic and carcinogenic potential. The fact that nearly 90 percent of all agricultural fungicides are carcinogenic in animal models has not reassured the public, especially when this is translated into the fact that some 75 million pounds of the fungicides used annually fall into this category (NAS, 1987). An evaluation of 11 fungicides concluded that, although the area treated with these chemicals represented only 10 percent of the acreage treated annually with pesticides, they could account for 60 percent of the total estimated dietary carcinogenic risk. Although tolerances have been set for such agents as captan, mancozeb, and benomyl on a few specific crops, no oncogenic fungicides other than benomyl have any Section 409 (Delaney clause) tolerances, making regulation of carcinogenic risk a complex and delicate task.

The entire discipline of fungicidal chemistry and use is in a state of flux. Many older agents, mentioned briefly below, have been deregistered because of overt toxicity encountered during their use. However, they are still being used in other, less regulated parts of the world. Some chemicals are being removed from the market because of perceived potential hazards to health. Other fungicides are undergoing reinvestigation and reevaluation because of suspicions of possible toxicity or incomplete toxicity data, particularly in the area of teratogenicity and carcinogenicity.

## Hexachlorobenzene

The mammalian toxicity of hexachlorobenzene (HCB), not to be confused with the insecticide hexachlorocyclohexane (lindane, HCH), has been reviewed by Hayes (1982). From the late 1940s through the 1950s, HCB saw extensive use as fungicidal dressing applied to seed grain as a dry powder. Between 1955 and 1959, a spectacular epidemic of HCB poisoning, ultimately involving some 4000 patients, occurred in Turkey where people consumed treated grain during times of crop failure. The syndrome was called the *new disease* or *black sore* and was characterized by dermal blistering and epidemolysis, infection with pigmented scars on healing, and alopecia (Schmid, 1960; Wray et al., 1962). The skin was photosensitive, with pigmentation of exposed as well as covered parts of the body seen. The initial diagnosis of the condition was congenital porphyria cutanea tarda but, since it appeared so suddenly, physicians looked for other causes and symptoms. More severe cases developed a suppurative arthritis, osteomyelitis, and osteoporosis of the bones of the hands (Cam and Nigogosyan, 1963). Hepatomegaly was observed in most hospitalized patients and some 30 percent of the cases showed enlarged thyroid glands, although functional changes were not observed. The disease was seen predominantly within families, in males (76 percent) and in children 4 to 14 years of age (81 percent). Young children were particularly at risk, and nursing infants developed a lesion known as *pink sore* that was associated with a 95 percent mortality rate and was related to transplacental and milk acquisition of HCB from women who had consumed contaminated grain. The causative agent was identified in 1958 and the Turkish government stopped the practice of using HCB in 1959, with a gradual disappearance of new cases by 1963.

Like the organochlorine insecticides, HCB possesses all of the properties of chemical stability and environmental persistence, a slow rate of degradation, slow metabolism, bioaccumulation in adipose tissue and other organs having a high content of lipid membranes, and the ability to induce tissue microsomal monooxygenase enzymes. Chronic exposure of animals resulted in hepatomegaly and porphyria, and focal alopecia with dermal itching and eruptions followed by pigmented scars, anorexia, and neurotoxicity expressed as increased irritability, ataxia, and tremors. Immunosuppression was observed in both mice and rats. A dose-dependent increase in hepatic and thyroid tumors was observed in hamsters during a chronic (70-week) study (Lambrecht et al., 1982). Although HCB was not mutagenic in microbial test systems and was negative in dominant lethal mutation tests, it did cause terata in mice (renal and palate malformations) and in rats (increased incidence of 14th rib). It would appear that there are considerable differences among laboratory rat strains in susceptibility to teratogenicity. Hexachlorobenzene was particularly toxic to developing perinatal animals, with transplacental acquisition and, more importantly, acquisition via the milk causing enlarged kidneys, hydronephrosis, hepatomegaly, and possible effects on the immune system.

## Organomercurials

In the past, alkyl-, alkoxyalkyl-, and aryl-mercurial compounds such as methyl- or methoxyethyl-mercuric chloride and dicyandiamide, phenylmercuric acetate, tolylmercuric acetate, ethylmercuric *p*-toluene sulfanilide, and similar agents were used extensively as dressing fungicides for the prevention of seed-borne diseases of cereal grains, vegetables, cotton, soybeans, and sugar beets. Despite the recognized neurotoxicity of these chemicals, their use continued up until the early 1970s, when tragic individual poisonings as well as a large-scale poisoning epidemic, resulted in decisions to ban their use. Once again, the problem was generally associated with either the ingestion of fungicide-treated grain as in the Iraq epidemic or, as in the New Mexico incident, the consumption of meat from animals (hogs) to whom treated grain had been fed (Curley et al., 1971; Bakir et al., 1973).

The toxicology of the mercurial fungicides has been reviewed and the incidents of human poisoning have been described in detail (Ecobichon, 1994c; Edwards et al., 1991). Following acute intoxication, the signs and symptoms arise generally from the mercuric cation and the classic picture emerges of effects primarily in two organ systems, the gastrointestinal tract and the kidney (Koos and Longo, 1976). In contrast, chronic poisoning is generally slow, insidious in onset, and eventually will involve most organ systems. However, the major effects will be associated with the debilitation of the peripheral sensory and motor nerves and the CNS. The perinatal individual is particularly vulnerable to organomercurial poisoning as will be recalled from the Minamata incident following the prolonged consumption of methylmercury-contaminated seafood. While the pregnant mothers were usually asymptomatic, the fetuses acquired most of the methylmercury with such disastrous effects on the developing CNS that postnatal brain development virtually ceased (Matsumoto et al., 1965; Chang et al., 1977; Tsubaki et al., 1978).

Unfortunately, while these chemicals are banned in many countries, they are still in use in developing countries and still present a health hazard.

## Pentachlorophenol

Once used in tremendous volumes as a biocide in leather-tanning, wood preservation, the paper and cellulose industry, and in paints, this chemical has been phased out of use because of the discovery that many commercial products were contaminated by polychlorinated dibenzodioxins and dibenzofurans, predominantly by hexachlorinated, heptachlorinated, and octachlorinated congeners. While these congeners are considerably less toxic than TCDD, evidence from animal studies has pointed to the fact that the contaminants in commercial or technical pentachlorophenol (PCP) were responsible for the toxicity observed. Technical grade PCP fed to rats caused altered plasma enzymes, increased hepatic and renal weights, and hepatocellular degeneration, in addition to changes in blood biochemistry (decreased erythrocyte count, decreased hemoglobin, and serum albumin). The administration of purified PCP resulted only in increased liver and kidney weight. Prolonged treatment of female rats with technical PCP caused hepatic porphyria, increased microsomal monooxygenase activity, and increased liver weight, whereas purified PCP caused no changes over the dosage range studied (Goldstein et al., 1977). Pentachlorophenol was not teratogenic in rats and is not considered to be carcinogenic in mice or rats (Innes et al., 1969; Johnson et al., 1973; Schwetz et al., 1977). A number of environmental problems have been associated with PCP (Eisler, 1989).

Human poisoning by commercial PCP has occurred, usually associated with occupational exposure and instances of sloppy handling and neglect of hygienic principles (Jorens and Schepens, 1993). The chemical is absorbed readily through the skin, the most usual route of acquisition, with several products, including PCP, detected in the urine. High-level exposure can result in death preceded by an elevated body temperature (42°C or 108°F), profuse sweating and dehydration, marked loss of appetite, decrease in body weight, tightness in the chest, dyspnea following exercise, rapid pulse, nausea and vomiting, headache, incoordination, generalized weakness, and early coma (Hayes, 1982). Pentachlorophenol acts cellularly to uncouple oxidative phosphorylation, the target enzyme being $Na^+, K^+$-ATPase (Desaiah, 1977). Survivors frequently display dermal irritation and exfoliation, irritation of the upper respiratory tract, and possible impairment of autonomic function and circulation.

## Phthalimides

Of the three chemicals belonging to this classification, only folpet and captofol are true phthalimides, the prototype chemical, captan, being structurally different with a cyclohexene ring (Fig. 22-24). To study these agents, one must study captan because it is the oldest chemical, the most effective of the class, and it has been embroiled in a prolonged controversy concerning teratogenicity and carcinogenicity.

As early as 1951, compounds containing an *N*-trichloromethylthio group were recognized as being potent surface fungicides. Captan was an effective, persistent foliar fungicide, particularly for Botrytis mold on soft fruit, apple, and pear scab; black spot on roses; and as a seed dressing (Cremlyn, 1978). Captafol and folpet were subsequently developed as foliar fungicides. All three chemicals have oral $LD_{50}$ values of approximately 10,000 mg/kg in the rat. Unfortunately, these chemicals became embroiled in a testing laboratory controversy and, because the structures were similar to that of the drug thalidomide, concerns were raised over potential teratogenicity. At daily doses of 500 mg/kg on days 7 and 8 of gestation in the hamster, teratogenicity was reported. Studies in other species either failed to confirm this effect or produced equivocal results open to speculative interpretation. Mutagenicity associated with these chemicals was confirmed and more recent long-term studies, conducted to support continued registration, revealed that captan caused duodenal tumors in the animal model (rat) being used (Anon., 1982). Studies were to be repeated to ascertain a no-observable-effect level because tumors were observed at all captan concentrations fed in the diet in the replacement studies. These replacement studies have never been published. In initiation-promotion studies of dermal cancers in mice receiving single or multiple dermal applications of commercial captan (purity not reported), Antony et al. (1994) reported that captan showed no promoting activity but was a weak initiator of benign squamous cell papillomas.

Although the mechanism(s) by which captan and its analogs exert their cellular toxicity is not known, it has been demonstrated that captan reacts with cellular thiols to produce thiophosgene, a potent unstable chemical. Thiophosgene could poison cells by interacting with sulfhydryl-, amino-, or hydroxyl-containing enzymes, a hypothesis that is supported by the fact that the fungitoxicity of these three chemicals can be nullified by the addition of thiols (Cremlyn, 1978). Other investigators state that the entire molecule is required to react with thiol groups in fungal cells. It is possible that there are several mechanisms by which these chemicals can induce cellular toxicity. Experiments have shown that a volatile breakdown product of captan was responsible for the mutagenic activity and that the volatile mutagen was short-lived and formed at much higher levels at an alkaline pH, possibly related to hydrolysis of the molecule. There is also a diffusable mutagen causing biological activity distinct from that produced by the volatile component (Bridges et al., 1972). Interestingly, fungal resistance has never developed to captan, whereas fungi have become resistant to both folpet and captofol.

### Dithiocarbamates

Dimethyl- and ethylene-bisdithiocarbamate (EBDC) compounds have been employed since the early 1950s as fungicides, and the EBDC chemicals saw widespread use on a large variety of small fruits and vegetables. The nomenclature of these agents arises from the metal cations with which they are associated; for instance, dimethyldithio-carbamic acid bound to iron or zinc are ferbam and ziram, respectively, whereas EBDC compounds associated with sodium, manganese, or zinc are nabam, maneb, and zineb, respectively. As is shown in Fig. 22-24, these chemicals are polymeric structures which possess environmental stability and yield good foliar protection as well as a low order of acute toxicity, with $LD_{50}$ values in excess of 6000 mg/kg with the exception of nabam (395 mg/kg). Mancozeb is a polymeric mixture of a zinc salt and the chemical maneb.

Although toxicity is negligible in animal feeding trials even at high doses, acceptance of these agents has been marred by reported adverse health effects. Maneb, nabam, and zineb have been reported to be teratogenic (Petrova-Vergieva and Ivanova-Chemischanka, 1973). Mancozeb has not been demonstrated to be teratogenic in the rat but has been associated with abnormally shaped sperm (Hemavathi and Ratiman, 1993). Maneb has been associated with adverse reproductive outcomes (embryotoxicity; changes in usual number of offspring per litter, pregnancy rate, estrous cycle, fetal development) (Lu and Kennedy, 1986). Maneb caused pulmonary tumors in mice but studies in the rat have been equivocal (IARC, 1976). Environmental and mammalian degradation of the EBDC compounds into ethylene thiourea (ETU), a known mutagen, teratogen, and carcinogen, as well as an antithyroid compound, has raised suspicions about these agents and fostered requests for more in-depth studies (IARC, 1976). There is also evidence that ETU may be formed while processing and cooking EBDC-contaminated products. Few additional, definitive, and more recent studies have yielded any evidence of consequence concerning health hazards.

Neurotoxicity has not been attributed to EBDC fungicides in either experimental animals or humans except at excessively high doses (Ecobichon, 1994c). A double (within 2 weeks) acute occupational, dermal exposure to Mandizan (mixture of maneb and zineb) resulted in initial complaints of muscle weakness, dizziness, and fatigue, with disorientation, slurred speech, muscle incoordination, loss of consciousness and tonic/clonic convulsions appearing rapidly following the second exposure (Israeli et al., 1983). A recent report from Brazil on two apparent Parkinson patients revealed that, as sprayers, they had experienced significant annual exposure to maneb over 4 to 5 years (Ferraz et al., 1988). Signs and symptoms included inability to walk, difficulty in talking, tremors in hands and feet, a short-stepped gait with cogwheeling, and bradykinesia. An extended study of 50 rural workers, 84 percent of whom admitted to using maneb improperly or carelessly, revealed milder but similar signs and symptoms. It was suggested that the effects might be related to the manganese content, although blood manganese levels were not elevated. Other evidence might point to breakdown products of EBDC, such as carbon disulphide, as the neurotoxicant, although it is hard to accept such a high level of absorption. It is also known that dithiocarbamates can bind various divalent metals to form more lipophilic complexes capable of entering the CNS (Ecobichon, 1994c).

## FUMIGANTS

Such agents are used to kill insects, nematodes, weed seeds, and fungi in soil, as well as in silo-stored cereal grains, fruit, and vegetables, clothes, and other consumables, generally with the treatment carried out in enclosed spaces because of the volatility of most of the products. Fumigants range from acrylonitrile and carbon disulfide to carbon tetrachloride, ethylene dibromide, chloropicrin, and ethylene oxide; their toxicological properties are discussed under other headings because many have other uses. Attention in this section will be directed only to a very few agents, although all of the chemicals mentioned have the potential for inhalation exposure and, for some of them, dermal and ingestion exposure.

Fumigants may be liquids (ethylene dibromide, dibromochloropropane, formaldehyde) that readily vaporize at ambient temperature, solids that can release a toxic gas on reacting with water ($Zn_2P_3$, AlP) or with acid [NaCN, $Ca(CN)_2$], or gases (methylbromide, hydrogen cyanide, ethylene oxide). These chemicals are nonselective, highly reactive, and cytotoxic. The physicochemical properties of these agents and hence their pattern(s) of use vary considerably (Cremlyn, 1978). With proper attention to use and with appropriate safety precautions, there should be little effect other than occasional occupational exposure, because the volatility of the agents is such that when the enclosed space is opened, the gas or vapor escapes readily. However, reports in the literature have indicated the presence of low residual levels of ethylene dibromide, methylbromide, and other chemicals in various samples of foods that have been treated. More extensive descriptions of fumigant toxicity can be found in Hayes (1982) and Morgan (1982).

### Phosphine

Used extensively as a grain fumigant, phosphine ($PH_3$) is released from aluminum phosphide (AlP) by the natural moisture in the grain over a long period of time, giving continual protection during transhipment of the grain. One serious accident with this chemical has been reported, in which this author played a small role in identifying the causative agent, as the problem originated in the port of Montreal, Canada (Wilson et al., 1980). Grain leaving Canada for European destinations is fumigated by adding a certain number of sachets of AlP per ton of grain in the hold of the ship while loading. Phosphine ($PH_3$), being heavier than air, sinks slowly through the grain. The particular ship in question ran into a bad storm off Nova Scotia and began to leak, hastening the breakdown of the AlP to form $PH_3$. The toxicant penetrated the quarters of the crew and officers where 29 out of 31 crew members became acutely ill and two children, family members of one of the officers, were seriously affected, one dying before reaching a hospital in Boston. Symptoms of $PH_3$ intoxication in the adults included shortness of breath, cough and pulmonary irritation, nausea, headache, jaundice, and fatigue. The highest concentrations of $PH_3$ (20 to 30 ppm) were measured in a void space on the main deck near the air intake for the ship's ventilation system. In some of the living quarters, $PH_3$ levels of 0.5 ppm were detected. Although this could be considered a bizarre situation, it does illustrate an apparent problem with the use of this type of agent in an atmosphere of excess moisture.

## Ethylene Dibromide/Dibromochloropropane

When inhaled, at relatively high (>200 ppm) concentrations, ethylene dibromide can cause pulmonary edema and inflammation in the exposed animals. As one might expect, repeated exposures to lower concentrations produced hepatic and renal damage visualized as morphological changes. Centrolobular hepatic necrosis and proximal tubular damage in the kidneys were observed in one fatal poisoning in which the individual ingested 4.5 ml of ethylene dibromide. This chemical, along with 1,2-dibromo-3-chloropropane (DBCP), was found to elicit malignant gastric squamous cell carcinomas in mice and rats (IARC, 1977). DBCP was also found to cause sterility in male animals, and concentrations as low as 5 ppm had an adverse effect on testicular morphology and spermatogenesis. However, these results in animals came to light only when a similar situation was detected in workers who manufactured the agent. Equivocal results have been reported for the mutagenicity of DBCP, the agent that causes base-pair substitution but not a frame-shift mutation in salmonella strains. In animal studies of the dominant lethal assay, DBCP was positive (mutagenic) in rats but not in mice. DBCP was a reproductive toxicant in rabbits and rats but not in mice (IARC, 1977).

## RODENTICIDES

Many vertebrates, including rats, mice, squirrels, bats, rabbits, skunks, monkeys, and even elephants, on occasion can be considered to be pests. Rodents, the most important of which are the black rat (*Rattus rattus*), the brown or Norway rat (*Rattus norvegicus*), and the house mouse (*Mus musculus*), are particularly serious problems because they act as vectors for several human diseases. They can consume large quantities of postharvest, stored food and/or foul or contaminate even greater amounts of foodstuffs with urine, feces, hair, and bacteria that cause diseases.

A rodenticide, to be effective yet safe, must satisfy the following criteria: (1) it must not be unpalatable to the target species and it therefore must be potent; (2) it must not induce bait shyness so that the animal will continue to eat it; (3) death should occur in a manner that does not raise the suspicions of the survivors; (4) it should make the intoxicated animal go out into the open to die (otherwise the rotting corpses create health hazards); and (5) it should be species-specific, with considerably lower toxicity to other animals that might inadvertently consume the bait or eat the poisoned rodent (Cremlyn, 1978). The agents used constitute a diverse range of chemical structures having a variety of mechanisms of action for at least partially successful attempts to attain species selectivity (Fig. 22-25). With some chemicals, advantage has been taken of the physiology and biochemistry unique to rodents. With other rodenticides, the sites of action are common to most mammals but advantage is taken of the habits of the pest animal and/or the dosage, thereby minimizing toxicity to nontarget species.

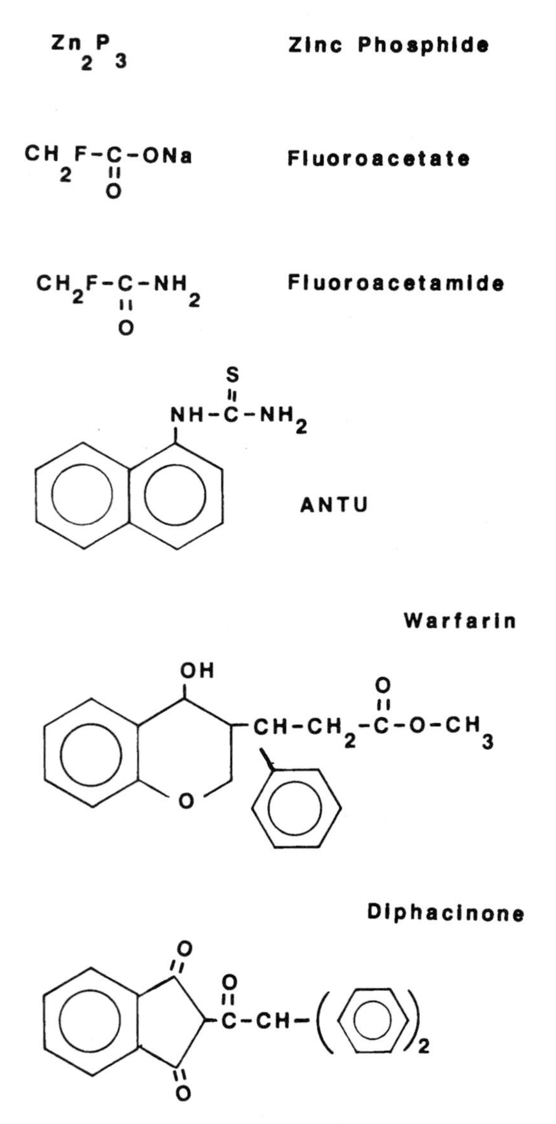


*Figure 22-25. Representative structures of inorganic and organic rodenticides from various chemical classifications.*

Although most rodenticides are formulated in baits that are unpalatable to humans, thereby minimizing the potential hazard, there are surprising numbers of rodenticide intoxications each year. With only a few exceptions, the accidental or intentional ingestion of most rodenticides poses a serious, acute toxicological problem because, invariably, the dosage ingested is high and the signs and symptoms of intoxication are generally well advanced and severe when the patient is seen by a physician. As with other household products, rodenticide poisoning is more frequently seen in children, whose added hazard is a small body weight in relation to the dosage ingested. The toxicology of the various classes of rodenticides has been extensively reviewed and the reader is referred to Hayes (1982) and to Ellenhorn and Barceloux (1988) for in-depth coverage of the subject.

A number of inorganic compounds, including thallium sulfate, arsenious oxide, other arsenic salts, barium carbonate, yellow phosphorus, aluminum phosphide, and zinc phosphide, have been used as rodenticides. A mixture of sodium cyanide with magnesium carbonate and anhydrous magnesium sulfate has been used in rabbit and mole burrows, causing hydrogen cyanide gas to be liberated slowly on contact with moisture. Natural or synthetic organic chemicals including strychnine, red squill (scillaren glycosides), and DDT have been used in the past. All of these agents are nonselective, highly toxic, and hazardous to other forms of life and, with the exception of zinc phosphide, have been abandoned in favor of target-specific, selective chemicals.

## Zinc Phosphide

This agent is used in developing nations because it is both a cheap and an effective rodenticide. The toxicity of the chemical can be accounted for by the phosphine ($PH_3$) formed following a hydrolytic reaction with water in the stomach on ingestion. Phosphine causes widespread cellular toxicity with necrosis of the gastrointestinal tract and injury to other organs, such as the liver and kidneys. Although moist zinc phosphide emits an unpleasant, rotten-fish odor, it is accepted in baits at concentrations of 0.5 or 1.0 percent by rodents.

Accidental poisonings are rare in adults but are a definite problem in children. Hayes (1982) recounts a poisoning attributed to the inhalation of zinc phosphide dust from treated grain, with signs of intoxication that included vomiting, diarrhea, cyanosis, tachycardia, rhales, restlessness, fever, and albuminuria several hours following exposure. It is a favorite chemical in suicides in Egypt (A. Amr, personal communication). The signs and symptoms include nausea, vomiting, headache, lightheadedness, dyspnea, hypertension, pulmonary edema, dysrrhythmias, and convulsions. Doses of the order of 4000 to 5000 mg have been fatal, but other individuals have survived doses of 25,000 to 100,000 mg if early vomiting has occurred. The usual decontamination measures and supportive therapy are often successful if initiated early.

## Fluoroacetic Acid and Derivatives

Sodium fluoroacetate (compound 1080) and fluoroacetamide (compound 1081) are white in color, odorless, and tasteless. The extreme toxicity of these two chemicals has restricted their use to prepared baits. Both agents are well absorbed from the gastrointestinal tract. Acute oral toxicity of fluoroacetate in the rat is of the order of 0.2 mg/kg whereas that of fluoroacetamide is 4 to 15 mg/kg. The mechanism of action involves the incorporation of the fluoroacetate into fluoroacetyl-coenzyme A which condenses with oxaloacetate to form fluorocitrate, the product that inhibits the enzyme aconitase and prevents the conversion of citrate to isocitrate in the tricarboxylic (Krebs) cycle. Inhibition of this system by fluorocitrate results in reduced glucose metabolism and cellular respiration and affects tissue energy stores. These chemicals are uniquely effective in mice and rats because of the high metabolic rate in tissues that are susceptible to inhibition.

Estimates of the lethal dose of fluoroacetate in humans lie in the range of 2 to 10 mg/kg. Gastrointestinal symptoms are seen initially at some 30 to 100 min following ingestion. Initial nausea, vomiting, and abdominal pain are replaced by sinus tachycardia, ventricular tachycardia or fibrillation, hypotension, renal failure, muscle spasms, and such CNS symptoms as agitation, stupor, seizures, and coma. Histopathologic examination of postmortem samples has revealed cerebellar degeneration and atrophy. There are no known antidotes to fluoroacetate intoxication, although glycerol monoacetate proved beneficial in the treatment of poisoned monkeys.

## $\alpha$-Naphthyl Thiourea (ANTU)

Following the discovery that phenylthiourea was lethal to rats but was not toxic to humans, ANTU was introduced as a relatively selective rodenticide (Richter, 1946). A wide range of acute oral $LD_{50}$ values has been reported for different species, the rat being the most sensitive at 3 mg/kg and the monkey the least susceptible at 4 g/kg. The exact mechanism of action is not known, but it is suspected that ANTU must be biotransformed in vivo into a reactive intermediate. Young rats are resistant to the chemical whereas older rats become tolerant to it, evidence which suggests that perhaps microsomal monooxygenases in young rats metabolize the agent too rapidly into nontoxic products, whereas in older rats, either the lower levels of monooxygenases or the inhibition of these enzymes results in less activation and affords protection (Boyd and Neal, 1976). ANTU causes extensive pulmonary edema and pleural effusion as a consequence of action on the pulmonary capillaries. Studies with $^{35}S$- and $^{14}C$-labelled ANTU revealed that covalent binding to macromolecules in the lung and liver occurred following treatment (Boyd and Neal, 1976). Following exposure to ANTU, there are a number of biochemical effects, such as alterations in carbohydrate metabolism, adrenal stimulation, and interaction of the chemical with sulfhydryl groups, but none of these appear to bear any relationship to the observed signs of toxicity.

Although it would appear that the human is very resistant to ANTU intoxication, probably because insufficient quantities are ingested, poisonings have occurred, with tracheobronchial hypersecretion of a white, nonmucous froth containing little protein; pulmonary edema; and respiratory difficulty (Hayes, 1982).

## Anticoagulants

With the discovery that coumadin [3-($\alpha$-acetonylbenzyl)-4-hydroxycoumarin, warfarin), isolated from spoiled sweet clover, acted as an anticoagulant by antagonizing the actions of vitamin K in the synthesis of clotting factors (factors II, VII, IX, and X), it was introduced as a rodenticide. The onset of anticoagulation is delayed 8 to 12 h after the ingestion of warfarin, with this latent period of onset dependent on the half-lives of the various clotting factors (Katona and Wason, 1986). The safety of warfarin as a rodenticide rests with the fact that multiple doses are required before toxicity develops and that single doses have little effect. However, the development of resistance to warfarin in rats in the 1950s prompted research into newer compounds, and the exploration of structure-activity relationships led to the development of the superwarfarins (brodifacoum, bromadiolone, coumachlor, diphencoumarin) and a new class of anticoagulant compounds, the indanediones (diphacinone, chlorophacinone, pindone), which are more water soluble. All of these newer agents differ from one another in terms of acute toxicity, rapidity of action, and acceptance by the rodent. Resistance toward these chemicals has not developed to date.

Human poisonings by these agents are rare because they are dispensed in grain-based baits. However, there are sufficient numbers of suicide attempts, attempted murders, and a famous classic case of the inadvertent consumption of warfarin-laden corn meal bait by an unsuspecting Korean family to provide adequate documentation of the signs and symptoms of poisoning (Lange and Terveer, 1954; Hayes, 1982; Jones, 1984; Lipton, 1984; Katona and Wason, 1986). Following consumption over a period of days, bleeding of the gingiva and nose occurs, with bruising and hematomas developing at the knee and elbow joints and on the buttocks, gastrointestinal bleeding with dark tarry stools, hematuria accompanied by abdominal or low back (flank) pain, epistaxis, and cerebrovascular accidents. The signs and symptoms will persist for many days after cessation of exposure, particularly so in the case of the superwarfarins which have prolonged biological half-lives (e.g., brodifacoun with 156 h compared to 37 h for warfarin) (Katona and Wason, 1986). In the Korean episode, consumption of warfarin was estimated to be on the order of 1 to 2 mg/kg per day for a period of 15 days, and signs and symptoms appeared 7 to 10 days after initial exposure; 2 out of the 14 affected individuals died as a consequence of not receiving any treatment (Lange and Terveer, 1954).

## CONCLUSIONS

With the advent of the chemical pesticides with their diverse nature, structures, and biological activity, the problem of ranking the hazard that each one poses to health has arisen. Should a classification system be based on acute toxicity alone or should some numerical scoring system be used to evaluate other endpoints of toxicity? Should the classification scheme be based on the oral, dermal, or inhalation routes of exposure to the active ingredient or to a formulation concentrate? If one chooses acute toxicity and a definitive endpoint expressed as the $LD_{50}$, one must be cognizant of the fact that the $LD_{50}$ is an estimate, with the range and confidence limits for any particular chemical possibly overlapping a class boundary. To establish a classification system on the basis of other toxicological endpoints would be impossible given the variability of biological effects, the dosages required to attain them, and the significance of such results in terms of human exposure.

In 1972, the WHO Expert Committee on Insecticides recommended the preparation of a classification of pesticides that would serve as a guide for developing countries (WHO, 1973). The classification was to distinguish between the more and the less hazardous forms of each pesticide and should permit formulations to be classified according to the percentage of the active ingredient and its physical state. Only acute hazards to health were considered, meaning those resulting from single or multiple exposures over a relatively short period of time, from handling the product in accordance with the manufacturer's directions. In 1975, the categories of the classification were established and, with only one modification to class III, they are essentially the same as those that appear in Table 22-13. It is important to appreciate that the $LD_{50}$ value quoted for any pesticide is not the median value but the lower confidence limit value for the most sensitive sex, thereby ensuring that a large safety factor has been built into the classification. A recent paper by Copplestone (1988) discusses the advantages and disadvantages of the system and the placement of problem chemicals such as rodenticides (highly toxic to rats but not presenting the same hazard to humans) and paraquat (having a low dermal toxicity but causing fatal effects if ingested).

From experience, the WHO is of the opinion that this classification scheme has worked well in practice, faithfully

**Table 22–13**
**The WHO Recommended Classification of Pesticides by Hazard**

| | | $LD_{50}$ FOR THE RAT (mg/kg BODY WEIGHT) | | | |
|---|---|---|---|---|---|
| | | ORAL | | DERMAL | |
| CLASS | | SOLIDS | LIQUIDS | SOLIDS | LIQUIDS |
| Ia | Extremely hazardous | ≤5 | ≤20 | ≤10 | ≤40 |
| Ib | Highly hazardous | 5–50 | 20–200 | 10–100 | 40–400 |
| II | Moderately hazardous | 50–500 | 200–2000 | 100–1000 | 400–4000 |
| III | Slightly hazardous | >500 | >2000 | >1000 | >4000 |
| III+ | Unlikely to present hazard in normal use | >2000 | >3000 | — | — |

SOURCE: From Copplestone, 1988.

reflecting the toxicity of these chemicals for humans. Only a few changes in classification have been made for chemicals and/or their formulations since the introduction of the scheme, signifying that the system functions effectively. It would appear that acute toxicity is the most effective parameter by which to judge the hazard to human health. With the move away from animal experimentation to in vitro testing, this classification system can be modified to reflect other endpoints of toxicity if they can be quantitated, correlated, and validated to be equivalent to the $LD_{50}$ results. As Dr. Copplestone described it, "the classification has been a meeting point between science and administration and a useful tool in the armamentarium of preventive medicine" (Copplestone, 1988).

# REFERENCES


Abbott DC, Goulding R, Tatton JO'G: Organochlorine pesticide residues in human fat in Great Britain. *Br Med J*, 3:146–149, 1968.

Abou-Donia MB: Organophosphorus ester-induced delayed neurotoxicity. *Annu Rev Pharmacol Toxicol* 21:511–548, 1981.

Abou-Donia MB, Lapadula D: Mechanisms of organophosphorus ester-induced delayed neurotoxicity: Type I and Type II. *Ann Rev Pharmacol Toxicol* 30:405–440, 1990.

Alachlor Review Board: *Report of the Alachlor Review Board*. Ottawa, Canada: Agriculture Canada, Canadian Government Publishing Centre, 1987.

Alary JG, Guay P, Brodeur J: Effect of phenobarbital pretreatment on the metabolism of DDT in the rat and the bovine. *Toxicol Appl Pharmacol* 18:457–468, 1971.

Albert A: *Xenobiosis, Food, Drugs and Poisons in the Human Body*. London: Chapman and Hall, 1987, pp 113–116.

Albertson TE, Cross CE: Pesticides in the workplace: a worldwide issue. *Arch Environ Health* 48:364–365, 1993.

Aldridge WN, Johnson MK: Side effects of organophosphorus compounds: delayed neurotoxicity. *Bull WHO* 44:259–263, 1971.

Aldridge WN, Reiner E: *Enzyme Inhibitors as Substrates*. Amsterdam and New York: North-Holland/American Elsevier, 1972.

Almog C, Tal E: Death from paraquat after subcutaneous injection. *Br Med J* 3:721, 1967.

Anon.: A look at world pesticide markets. *Farm Chem* 141:38–42, 1977.

Anon.: Captan. *A Report by the Consultative Committee on Industrial Bio-Test Pesticides*. Ottawa, Canada: Agriculture Canada, 1982.

Antony M, Shukla Y, Mehrotra NK: Preliminary carcinogenic and cocarcinogenic studies on captan following topical exposure in mice. *Bull Environ Contam Toxicol* 52:203–211, 1994.

Ashe W, Suskind RR: Chloracne cases of the Monsanto Chemical Company, Nitro, West Virginia, in *Reports of the Kettering Laboratory*, University of Cincinnati, October 1949, April 1950, July 1953.

Askew BM: Oximes and hydroxamic acids as antidotes in anticholinesterase poisoning. *Br J Pharmacol Chemother* 11:417–423, 1956.

Axelson O, Sundell L, Andersson K, et al: Herbicide exposure and tumor mortality. *Scand J Work Environ Health* 6:73–79, 1980.

Bakir F, Damluji SF, Amin-Zaki L, et al: Methylmercury poisoning in Iraq. *Science* 181:230–241, 1973.

Barnes JM, Verschoyle RD: Toxicity of new pyrethroid insecticides. *Nature* 248:711, 1974.

Bartle H: Quiet sufferers of the silent spring. *New Scientist* 130:30–35, 1991.

Batchelor GS, Walker KC: Health hazards involved in use of parathion in fruit orchards of north central Washington. *AMA Arch Ind Hyg Occup Health* 10:522–529, 1954.

Berkow SG: Value of surface-area proportions in the prognosis of cutaneous burns and scalds. *Am J Surg* 11:315–320, 1931.

Berwick P: Dichlorophenoxyacetic acid poisoning in man. Some interesting clinical and laboratory findings. *JAMA* 214:1114–1117, 1970.

Bidstrup PL, Bonner JA, Beckett AG: Paralysis following poisoning by a new organic phosphorus insecticide (Mipafox). *Br Med J* 1:1068–1072, 1953.

Bond GG, Rossbacher R: A review of potential human carcinogenicity of the chlorophenoxy herbicides MCPA, MCPP and 2,4-DP. *Br J Ind Med* 50:340–348, 1993.

Bond GG, Wetterstroem NH, Roush GJ, et al: Cause specific mortality among employees engaged in the manufacture, formulation or packaging of 2,4-dichlorophenoxyacetic acid and related salts. *Br J Indust Med* 45:98–105, 1988.

Bonsall JL: Measurement of occupational exposure to pesticides, in Turnbull GS (ed): *Occupational Hazards of Pesticide Use*. London: Francis and Taylor, 1985, pp 13–33.

Boon-Long J, Glinsukon T, Pothisiri P, et al: Toxicological problems in Thailand, in Ruchirawat M, Shank RC (eds): *Environmental Toxicity and Carcinogenesis*. Bangkok: Text and Journal Corp., 1986, pp 283–293.

Boyd MR, Neal RA: Studies on the mechanism of toxicity and of development of tolerance to the pulmonary toxic α-naphthylthiourea (ANTU). *Drug Metab Dispos* 4:314–322, 1976.

Branch RA, Jacqz E: Subacute neurotoxicity following long-term exposure to carbaryl. *Am J Med* 80:741–746, 1986.

Bridges BA, Mottershead RP, Rothwell MA, Green MHL: Repair-deficient bacterial strains suitable for mutagenicity screening: tests with the fungicide captan. *Chem Biol Interact* 5:77–84, 1972.

Brooks GT: *Chlorinated Insecticides. Technology and Application*. Cleveland, Ohio: CRC, 1974, vol 1, pp 12–13.

Büchel KH (ed): *Chemistry of Pesticides*. New York: Wiley, 1983.

Buckingham WA: *Operation Ranch Hand: The Air Force and Herbicides in Southeast Asia, 1961–1971*. U.S. Air Force, Washington, D.C., 1982.

Bull DL: Metabolism of organophosphorus insecticides in animals and plants. *Residue Rev* 43:1–22, 1972.

Cam C, Nigogosyan G: Acquired toxic porphyria cutanea tarda due to hexachlorobenzene. *JAMA* 183:88–91, 1963.

Campbell S: Paraquat poisoning. *Clin Toxicol* 1:245–249, 1968.

Cannon SB, Veasey JM Jr, Jackson RS, et al: Epidemic kepone poisoning in chemical workers. *Am J Epidemiol* 107:529–537, 1978.

Cantor KP: Farming and mortality from non-Hodgkin's lymphoma: a case-control study. *Int J Cancer* 29:239–247, 1982.

Carson R: *Silent Spring*. Boston: Houghton Mifflin, 1962.

Casida JE, Gammon DW, Glockman AH, Lawrence LJ: Mechanisms of selective action of pyrethroid insecticides. *Annu Rev Pharmacol Toxicol* 23:413–438, 1983.

Cavanagh JB: The toxic effects of tri-ortho-cresyl phosphate on the nervous system, an experimental study in hens. *J Neurol Neurosurg Psychiatry* 17:163–172, 1954.

Centers for Disease Control Veterans Health Studies: Serum 2,3,7,8-tetrachlorodibenzo-*p*-dioxin levels in U.S. Army Vietnam-era veterans. *JAMA* 260:1249–1254, 1988.

Chambers JE, Levi PE: Organophosphates. Chemistry, Fate and Effects. New York: Academic Press, 1992.

Chang LW, Reuhl KR, Lee GW: Degenerative changes in the developing nervous system as a result of in utero exposure to methyl mercury. *Environ Res* 14:414–423, 1977.

Chernoff N, Kavlock RJ, Kathrein JR, et al: Prenatal effects of dieldrin and photodieldrin in mice and rats. *Toxicol Appl Pharmacol* 31:302–308, 1975.

Childs AF, Davies DR, Green AL, Rutland JP: The reactivation by oximes and hydroxamic acids of cholinesterase inhibited by organophosphorus compounds. *Br J Pharmacol Chemother* 10:462–465, 1955.

Clark DG, Hurst EW: The toxicity of diquat. *Br J Ind Med* 27:51–55, 1970.

Clark DG, McElligott TF, Hurst EW: The toxicity of paraquat. *Br J Ind Med* 23:126–132, 1966.

Clark JM, Matsumura F: Two different types of inhibitory effects of pyrethroids on nerve Ca and Ca-Mg-ATPase activity in the squid, *Loligo pealei. Pestic Biochem Physiol* 18:180–190, 1982.

Clement JG: Toxicity of the combined nerve agents GB/GF in mice: Efficacy of atropine and various oximes as antidotes. *Arch Toxicol* 68:64–66, 1994.

Cohn WJ, Boylan JJ, Blanke RV, et al: Treatment of chlordecone (Kepone) toxicity with cholestyramine. *N Engl J Med* 298:243–248, 1978.

Committee on Scientific and Regulatory Issues Underlying Pesticide Use Patterns and Agricultural Innovation: *Regulating Pesticides in Food*. Washington, DC: National Academy Press, 1987.

Copplestone JF: The development of the WHO Recommended Classification of Pesticides by Hazard. *Bull WHO* 66:545–551, 1988.

Corbett JR: *The Biochemical Mode of Action of Pesticides*. New York: Academic Press, 1974.

Council on Scientific Affairs: Cancer risk of pesticides in agricultural workers. *JAMA* 260:959–966, 1988.

Courtney KD, Gaylor DW, Hogan MD, et al: Teratogenic evaluation of 2,4,5-T. *Science* 168:864–866, 1970.

Courtney KD, Moore JA: Teratology studies with 2,4,5-trichlorophenoxyacetic acid and 2,3,7,8-tetra-chlorodibenzo-dioxin. *Toxicol Appl Pharmacol* 20:396–403, 1971.

Coye MJ, Lowe JA, Maddy KT: Biological monitoring of agricultural workers exposed to pesticides. I. Cholinesterase activity determinators. *J Occup Med* 28:619–627, 1986.

Cranmer MF: Carbaryl. A toxicological review and risk analysis. *Neurotoxicology* 1:247–332, 1986.

Cremlyn R: *Pesticides. Preparation and Mode of Action*. New York: Wiley, 1978.

Crum JA, Bursian SJ, Aulerich RJ, Brazelton WE: The reproductive effects of dietary heptachlor in mink (Mustela vison). *Arch Environ Contam Toxicol* 24:156–164, 1993.

Curley A, Sedlak VA, Girling EF, et al: Organic mercury identified as the cause of poisoning in humans and hogs. *Science* 172:65–67, 1971.

Dale WE, Quinby GE: Chlorinated insecticides in the body fat of people in the United States. *Science* 142:593–595, 1963.

Daniel JW, Gage JC: Absorption and excretion of diquat and paraquat in rats. *Br J Ind Med* 23:133–136, 1966.

Dauterman WC, Main AR: Relationship between acute toxicity and in vitro inhibition and hydrolysis of a series of homologs of malathion. *Toxicol Appl Pharmacol* 9:408–418, 1966.

Davies JE, Edmundson WF, Schneider NJ, Cassady JC: Problems of prevalence of pesticide residues in humans, in Davies JE, Edmundson WF (eds): *Epidemiology of DDT*. Mount Kisco, NY: Futura, 1972, pp 27–37.

Davies DS, Hawksworth GM, Bennett PN: Paraquat poisoning. *Proc Eur Soc Toxicol* 18:21–26, 1977.

Desaiah D: Effects of pentachlorophenol on the ATPases in rat tissue, in Rao KR (ed): *Pentachlorophenol*. New York: Plenum, 1977, pp 277–283.

Desi I, Gonczi L, Simon G, et al: Neurotoxicologic studies of two carbamate pesticides in subacute animal experiments. *Toxicol Appl Pharmacol* 27:465–476, 1974.

DuBois KP: New rodenticidal compounds, *J Am Pharm Assoc* 37:307–310, 1948.

DuBois KP, Doull J, Salerno PR, Coon JM: Studies on the toxicity and mechanisms of action of *p*-nitrophenyl-diethyl-thionophosphate (Parathion): *J Pharmacol Exp Ther* 95:75–91, 1949.

Dudley AW Jr, Thapar NT: Fatal human ingestion of 2,4-D, a common herbicide. *Arch Pathol* 94:270–275, 1972.

Durham WF, Wolfe HR, Elliott JW: Absorption and excretion of parathion by spraymen. *Arch Environ Health* 24:381–387, 1972.

Ecobichon DJ: Hydrolytic mechanisms of pesticide degradation, in Geissbuhler H (ed): *Advances in Pesticide Science. Biochemistry of Pests and Mode of Action of Pesticides, Pesticide Degradation, Pesticide Residues and Formulation Chemistry*. New York: Pergamon, 1979, part 3, pp 516–524.

Ecobichon DJ: Organophosphorus ester insecticides, in Ecobichon DJ, Joy RM: *Pesticides and Neurological Diseases*, 2d ed. Boca Raton, FL: CRC, 1994a, pp 171–249.

Ecobichon DJ: Carbamic acid ester insecticides, in Ecobichon DJ, Joy RM: *Pesticides and Neurological Diseases*, 2d ed. Boca Raton, FL: CRC, 1994b, pp 251–289.

Ecobichon DJ: Fungicides, in Ecobichon DJ, Joy RM: *Pesticides and Neurological Diseases*, 2d ed. Boca Raton, FL: CRC, 1994c, pp 313–351.

Ecobichon DJ, Joy RM: *Pesticides and Neurological Diseases*, 2d ed. Boca Raton, FL: CRC, 1994.

Ecobichon DJ, MacKenzie DO: The uterotropic activity of commercial and isomerically pure chlorobiphenyls in the rat. *Res Commun Chem Pathol Pharmacol* 9:85–95, 1974.

Ecobichon DJ, Saschenbrecker PW: Pharmacodynamic study of DDT in cockerels. *Can J Physiol Pharmacol* 46:785–794, 1968.

Ecobichon DJ, Saschenbrecker PW: The redistribution of stored DDT in cockerels under the influence of food deprivation. *Toxicol Appl Pharmacol* 5:420–432, 1969.

Ecobichon DJ, Ozere RL, Reid E, Crocker JFS: Acute fenitrothion poisoning. *Can Med Assoc J* 116:377–379, 1977.

Edington N, Howell JM: The neurotoxicity of sodium diethyl-diethiocarbamate in the rabbit. *Acta Neuropathol* 12:339–346, 1969.

Edmiston S, Maddy KT: Summary of illnesses and injuries reported in California by physicians in 1986 as potentially related to pesticides. *Vet Hum Toxicol* 29:391–397, 1987.

Edwards R, Ferry DG, Temple WA: Fungicides and related compounds, in Hayes WJ Jr, Laws ER Jr (eds): *Handbook of Pesticide Toxicology. Classes of Pesticides*. New York: Academic, 1991, vol 3, pp 1409–1470.

Egan H, Goulding R, Toburn J, Tatton JO'G: Organochlorine residues in human fat and human milk. *Br Med J* 2:66–69, 1965.

Eisler R: *Pentachlorophenol Hazards to Fish, Wildlife and Invertebrates: A Synoptic Review*. U.S. Department of the Interior, Fish and Wildlife Service. Biological Report 85 (1.17), April, 1989.

Eldefrawi MES, Sherby SM, Abalis IM, Eldefrawi AT: Interactions of pyrethroid and cyclodiene insecticides with nicotinic acetylcholine and GABA receptors. *Neurotoxicology* 6:47–62, 1985.

Ellenhorn MJ, Barceloux DG: Pesticides, in *Medical Toxicology. Diagnosis and Treatment of Human Poisoning*. New York: Elsevier, 1988, pp 1081–1108.

Elliott M: Future use of natural and synthetic pyrethroids, in Metcalf RL, McKelvey JJ Jr (eds): *The Future for Insecticides: Needs and Prospects*. New York: Wiley, 1976, pp 163–193.

Elliott M, Janes NF, Kimmel EC, Casida JE: Metabolic fate of pyrethrin I, pyrethrin II and allethrin administered orally to rats. *J Agric Food Chem* 20:300–313, 1972.

Englehard H, Erdmann WD: Beziehangen zwischen chemischer struktur und cholinesterase reaktivierendes wirksamkeit bei einen reihe neuer bisquartarer pyridin-4-aldoxime. *Arznem Forsch* 14:870–875, 1964.

EPA: *Carbaryl Decision Document.* U.S. Environmental Protection Agency. Government Printing Office, Washington, D.C., 1980.

Eriksson M, Hardell L, Berg NO, et al: Soft-tissue sarcomas and exposure to chemical substances: a case-referent study. *Br J Indust Med* 38:27–33, 1981.

Eto M: *Organophosphorus Pesticides: Organic and Biological Chemistry.* Cleveland, OH: CRC, 1974.

Feldman RJ, Maiback HI: Percutaneous penetration of some pesticides and herbicides in man. *Toxicol Appl Pharmacol* 28:126–132, 1974.

Ferraz HB, Bertolucci PHF, Pereira JS, et al: Chronic exposure to the fungicide maneb may produce symptoms and signs of CNS manganese intoxication. *Neurology* 38:550–553, 1988.

Fest C, Schmidt K-J: *The Chemistry of Organophosphorus Pesticides.* New York: Springer-Verlag, 1973.

Fiserova-Bergerova V, Radomski JL, Davies JE, Davis JH: Levels of chlorinated hydrocarbon pesticides in human tissues. *Indust Med Surg* 36:65–70, 1967.

Fonseca RG, Resende LAL, Silva MD, Camargo A: Chronic motor neuron disease possibly related to intoxication with organochlorine insecticides. *Acta Neurol Scand* 88:56–58, 1993.

Forget G: Pesticides: necessary but dangerous poisons. *IDRC Rep* 18:4–5, 1989.

Forget G, Goodman T, deVilliers A (eds): *Impact of Pesticide Use on Health in Developing Countries.* Ottawa, Canada: International Development Research Centre, 1993.

Frank R, Campbell RA, Sirons GJ: Forestry workers involved in aerial application of 2,4-dichlorophenoxyacetic acid (2,4-D): exposure and urinary excretion. *Arch Environ Contam Toxicol* 14:427–435, 1985.

Franklin CA, Fenske RA, Greenhalgh R, et al: Correlation of urinary pesticide metabolite excretion with estimated dermal contact in the course of occupational exposure to guthion. *J Toxicol Environ Health* 7:715–731, 1981.

Frawley JP, Fuyat HN, Hagan EC, et al: Marked potentiation in mammalian toxicity from simultaneous administration of two anticholinesterase compounds. *J Pharmacol Exp Ther* 121:96–106, 1957.

Frear DEH: *Pesticide Index*, 4th ed. State College, PA: College Science, 1969.

Fukuto TR: Metabolism of carbamate insecticides. *Drug Metab Rev* 1:117–147, 1972.

Gaines TB: Acute toxicity of pesticides. *Toxicol Appl Pharmacol* 14:515–534, 1969.

Gammon DW, Brown MA, Casida JE: Two classes of pyrethroid action in the cockroach. *Pestic Biochem Physiol* 15:181–191, 1981.

Gee J: Iraqui declarations of chemical weapons: How much did they really have and what is it? Fourth International Symposium on Protection Against Chemical Warfare Agents, Stockholm, June 8–12, 1992.

Gehring PJ, Watanabe PG, Blau GE: Pharmacokinetic studies in evaluation of the toxicological and environmental hazard of chemicals, in Mehlman MA, Shapiro RE, Blumenthal H (eds): *New Concepts in Safety Evaluation.* New York: Wiley, 1976, pp 195–270.

Gershon S, Shaw FH: Psychiatric sequelae of chronic exposure to organophosphorus insecticides. *Lancet* i:1371–1374, 1961.

Glickman AH, Casida JE: Species and structural variations affecting pyrethroid neurotoxicity. *Neurobehav Toxicol Teratol* 4:793–799, 1982.

Gochfeld M: New light on the health of Vietnam veterans. *Environ Res* 47:109–111, 1988.

Goldman LR, Beller M, Jackson RJ: Aldicarb food poisonings in California, 1985–1988: Toxicity estimates for humans. *Arch Environ Health* 45:141–148, 1990a.

Goldman LR, Smith DF, Neutra RR, et al: Pesticide food poisoning from contaminated watermelons in California, 1985. *Arch Environ Health* 45:229–236, 1990b.

Goldstein NP, Jones PH, Brown JR: Peripheral neuropathy after exposure to an ester of dichlorophenoxyacetic acid. *JAMA* 171:1306–1309, 1959.

Goldstein JA, Fridsen M, Linder RE, et al: Effects of pentachlorophenol on hepatic drug-metabolizing enzymes and porphyria related to contamination with chlorinated dibenzo-*p*-dioxins and dibenzofurans. *Biochem Pharmacol* 26:1549–1557, 1977.

Gough M: *Dioxin, Agent Orange. The Facts.* New York: Plenum, 1986.

Greenwald W, Kovasznay B, Collins DN, Therriault G: Sarcomas of soft tissues after Vietnam service. *J Natl Cancer Inst* 73:1107–1109, 1984.

Grover R, Cessna AJ, Muir NI, et al: Factors affecting the exposure of ground-rig applicators to 2,4-dimethylamine salt. *Arch Environ Contam Toxicol* 15:677–686, 1986.

Guzelian PS: Comparative toxicology of chlordecone (kepone) in humans and experimental animals. *Annu Rev Pharmacol Toxicol* 22:89–113, 1982.

Haley TJ: Review of the toxicology of paraquat (1,1′-dimethyl-4,4′-bipyridinium chloride). *Clin Toxicol* 14:1–46, 1979.

Hansell MM, Ecobichon DJ: Effects of chemically pure chlorobiphenyls on the morphology of rat liver. *Toxicol Appl Pharmacol* 28:418–427, 1974.

Hardell L, Eriksson M, Lenner P, Lundgren E: Malignant lymphoma and exposure to chemicals, especially organic solvents, chlorophenols and phenoxy acids: a case-control study. *Br J Cancer* 43:169–176, 1981.

Hardell L, Sandstrom A: Case-control study: soft-tissue sarcomas and exposure to phenoxyacetic acids or chlorophenols. *Br J Cancer* 39:711–717, 1979.

Hartley GS, West TF: *Chemicals for Pest Control.* Oxford, England: Pergamon, 1969, p 26.

Hay A: *The Chemical Scythe. Lessons of 2,4,5,-T and Dioxin.* New York: Plenum, 1982.

Hayes WJ Jr: The pharmacology and toxicology of DDT, in Muller P (ed): *The Insecticide DDT and Its Importance.* Basel: Birkhauser Verlag, 1959, vol 2, pp 9–247.

Hayes WJ Jr: Insecticides, rodenticides and other economic poisons, in DiPalma JR (ed): *Drill's Pharmacology in Medicine*, 4th ed. New York: McGraw-Hill, 1971, pp 1256–1276.

Hayes WJ Jr: *Pesticides Studied in Man.* Baltimore: Williams & Wilkins, 1982.

Hayes WJ Jr, Dale WE, Pirkle CI: Evidence of the safety of long-term, high, oral doses of DDT for man. *Arch Environ Health* 22:19–35, 1971.

He F, Sun J, Han K, et al: Effects of pyrethroid insecticides on subjects engaged in packaging pyrethroids. *Br J Indust Med* 45:548–551, 1988.

He F, Wang S, Liu L, et al: Clinical manifestations and diagnosis of acute pyrethroid poisoning. *Arch Toxicol* 63:54–58, 1989.

Heath DF: *Organophosphorus Poisons. Anticholinesterases and Related Compounds.* London: Pergamon, 1961.

Hemavathi E, Rahiman MA: Toxicological effects of ziram, thiram and Dithane M-45 assessed by sperm shape abnormalities in mice. *J Toxicol Environ Health* 38:393–398, 1993.

Hoar SK, Blair A, Holmes FF, et al: Agricultural herbicide use and risk of lymphoma and soft-tissue sarcoma. *JAMA* 256:1141–1147, 1986.

Holmstedt B: Pharmacology of organophosphorus cholinesterase inhibitors. *Pharmacol Rev* 11:567–688, 1959.

Hutson DH, Akintonwa DAA, Hathway DE: The metabolism of 2,chloro-1-(2′,4′,dichlorophenyl) vinyl diethylphosphate (chlorfenvinphos) in the dog and rat. *Biochem J* 102:133–142, 1967.

IARC: *Monograph on the Evaluation of Carcinogenic Risk of Chemicals to Man. Some Organochlorine Pesticides.* Lyons, France: International Agency for Research on Cancer, 1974, vol 5.

IARC: *Monographs on the Evaluation of Carcinogenic Risk of Chemicals to Man. Some Carbamates, Thiocarbamates and Carbazines.*

Lyons, France: International Agency for Research on Cancer, 1976, vol 12.

IARC: *Monographs on the Evaluation of Carcinogenic Risk of Chemicals to Man. Some Fumigants, the Herbicides 2,4-D and 2,4,5-T, Chlorinated Dibenzodioxins and Miscellaneous Industrial Chemicals*. Lyons, France: International Agency for Research on Cancer, 1977, vol 15.

Innes JRM, Ulland BM, Valerio MG, et al: Bioassay of pesticides and industrial chemicals for tumorigenicity in mice: a preliminary note. *J Natl Cancer Inst* 42:1101–1114, 1969.

Israeli R, Sculsky M, Tiberin P: Acute intoxication due to exposure to maneb and zineb. A case with behavioral and central nervous system changes. *Scand J Work Environ Health* 9:47–51, 1983.

Jager G: Herbicides, in Buchel KH (ed): *Chemistry of Pesticides*. New York: Wiley, 1983, pp 322–392.

Jeyaratnam J: Occupational health issues in developing countries. *Environ Res* 60:207–212, 1993.

Johnson MK: The target for initiation of delayed neurotoxicity by organophosphorus esters: Biochemical studies and toxicological applications, in Hodgson E, Bend JR, Philpot RM (eds): *Reviews of Biochemical Toxicology*. New York: Elsevier, 1982, vol 4, pp 141–212.

Johnson MK, Willems JL, DeBisschop HC, et al: Can soman cause delayed neuropathy? *Fundam Appl Toxicol* 5:S180–S181, 1985.

Johnson RL, Gehring PJ, Kociba RJ, Schwetz BA: Chlorinated dibenzodioxins and pentachlorophenol. *Environ Health Perspect* 5:171–175, 1973.

Jones EC, Growe GH, Naiman SC: Prolonged anticoagulation in rat poisoning. *JAMA* 252:3005–3007, 1984.

Jorens PG, Schepens PJC: Human pentachlorophenol poisoning. *Hum Exp Toxicol* 12:479–495, 1993.

Joy RM: Chlorinated hydrocarbon insecticides, in Ecobichon DJ, Joy RM: *Pesticides and Neurological Diseases*, 2d ed. Boca Raton, FL: CRC, 1994a, pp 81–170.

Joy RM: Pyrethrins and pyrethroid insecticides, in Ecobichon DJ, Joy RM: *Pesticides and Neurological Diseases*, 2d ed. Boca Raton, FL: CRC, 1994b, pp 291–312.

Katona B, Wason S: Anticoagulant rodenticides. *Clin Toxicol Rev* 8:1–2, 1986.

Keane WT, Zavon MR: The total body burden of dieldrin. *Bull Environ Contam Toxicol* 4:1–16, 1969.

Kewitz H, Wilson IB: A specific antidote against lethal alkylphosphate intoxication. *Arch Biochem Biophys* 60:261–263, 1956.

Kilgore W: Human exposure to pesticides, in Newberne PM, Shank RC, Ruchirawat M (eds): *International Toxicology Seminar: Environmental Toxicology*. Bangkok: Chulabhorn Research Institute and Mahidol University, 1988.

Kilgore WW, Akesson NB: Minimizing occupational exposure to pesticides; populations at exposure risk. *Residue Rev* 75:21–31, 1980.

Kirby C: *The Hormone Weedkillers*. Croydon, UK: BCPC Publ., 1980.

Kitselman CH: Long-term studies on dogs fed aldrin and dieldrin in sublethal dosages with reference to the histopathological findings and reproduction. *J Am Vet Med Assoc* 123:28–36, 1953.

Kociba RI, Keyes DG, Beyer JE: Results of a two year chronic toxicity and oncogenicity study of 2,3,7,8-tetrechlorodibenzo-*p*-dioxin in rats. *Toxicol Appl Pharmacol* 46:279–303, 1978.

Koestner A: The brain-tumor issue in long-term toxicity studies in rats. *Food Chem Toxicol* 24:139–143, 1986.

Kolmodin-Hedman B, Hoglund S, Akerblom M: Studies on phenoxy acid herbicides. I. Field Study. Occupational exposure to phenoxy acid herbicides (MCPA, dichlorprop, mecoprop and 2,4-D) in agriculture. *Arch Toxicol* 54:257–275, 1983.

Koos BJ, Longo LD: Mercury toxicity in the pregnant woman, fetus and newborn infant. *Am J Obstet Gynecol* 126:390–409, 1976.

Koplovitz I, Gresham VC, Dochterman LW, et al: Evaluation of the toxicity, pathology and treatment of cyclohexylmethylphosphonofluoridate (CMPF) poisoning in rhesus monkeys. *Arch Toxicol* 66:622–628, 1992.

Kramer W: Fungicides and bacteriocides, in Buchel KH (ed): *Chemistry of Pesticides*. New York: Wiley, 1983, pp 227–321.

Kuhr RJ, Dorough HW: *Carbamate Insecticides: Chemistry, Biochemistry and Toxicology*. Boca Raton, FL: CRC, 1976.

Kulkarni AP, Hodgson E: The metabolism of insecticides: the role of monooxygenase enzymes. *Annu Rev Pharmacol* 24:19–42, 1984.

Kupfer D, Bulger WH: Studies on the mechanism of estrogenic actions of *o,p*-DDT: interactions with the estrogen receptor. *Pestic Biochem Physiol* 6:461–470, 1976.

Kusic R, Jovanovic D, Randjelovic S, et al: HI-6 in man: Efficacy of the oxime in poisoning by organophosphorus insecticides. *Human Exp Toxicol* 10:113–118, 1991.

Laben RC, Archer TE, Crosby DG, Peoples SA: Lactational output of DDT fed postpartum to dairy cattle. *J Dairy Sci* 48:701–708, 1965.

Lambert G, Brodeur J: Influence de certains inducteurs ou de certaines combinaisons d'inducteurs enzymatiques sur l'elimination des residus du DDT chez le rat. *Rev Can Biol* 35:33–39, 1976.

Lambrecht RW, Erturk E, Grunden E, et al: Hepatotoxicity and tumorigenicity of hexachlorobenzene (HCB) in Syrian golden hamsters after subchronic administration. *Fed Proc* 41:329, 1982.

Lange PF, Terveer J: Warfarin poisoning. *US Armed Forces J* 5:872–877, 1954.

Lawrence LJ, Casida JE: Pyrethroid toxicology: mouse intracerebral structure-toxicity relationships. *Pestic Biochem Physiol* 18:9–14, 1982.

Leahey JP: *The Pyrethroid Insecticides*. London: Taylor and Francis, 1985.

Leake LD, Buckley DS, Ford MG, Salt DW: Comparative effects of pyrethroids on neurones of target and non-target organisms. *Neurotoxicology* 6:99–116, 1985.

LeQuesne PM, Maxwell IC, Butterworth ST: Transient facial sensory symptoms following exposure to synthetic pyrethroids: a clinical and electrophysiological assessment. *Neurotoxicology* 2:1–11, 1980.

Lessenger JE, Riley N: Neurotoxicities and behavioral changes in a 12-year-old male exposed to dicofol, an organochlorine pesticide. *J Toxicol Environ Health* 33:255–261, 1991.

Liddle JA, Kimbrough RD, Needham LL, et al: A fatal episode of accidental methomyl poisoning. *Clin Toxicol* 15:159–167, 1979.

Lipton RA, Klass EM: Human ingestion of a "superwarfarin" rodenticide resulting in prolonged anticoagulant effect. *JAMA* 252: 3004–3005, 1984.

Longcore JR, Samson FB, Whittendale TW Jr: DDE thins eggshells and lowers reproductive success of captive black ducks. *Bull Environ Contam Toxicol* 6:485–490, 1971.

Lotti M: The pathogenesis of organophosphate polyneuropathy. *Crit Rev Toxicol* 21:465–487, 1992.

Lu M-H, Kennedy GL Jr: Teratogenic evaluation of mancozeb in the rat following inhalation exposure. *Toxicol Appl Pharmacol* 84:355–368, 1986.

Lukens RJ: *Chemistry of Fungicidal Action*. New York: Springer-Verlag, 1971.

Lynge E: A follow-up study of cancer incidence among workers in manufacture of phenoxy herbicides in Denmark. *Br J Cancer* 52:259–270, 1985.

Marquis JK: *Contemporary Issues in Pesticide Toxicology and Pharmacology*. Basel: S Karger AG, 1982, pp 87–95.

Marrs TC: Organophosphate poisoning. *Pharmacol Ther* 58:51–66, 1993.

Martinez AJ, Taylor JR, Houff SA, Isaacs ER: Kepone poisoning: cliniconeuropathological study, in Roizin L, Shiraki H, Greevic N (eds): *Neurotoxicology*. New York: Raven, 1977, pp 443–456.

Matsumoto H, Koya G, Takeuchi T: Fetal Minamata disease. A study of two cases of intrauterine intoxication by a methyl mercury compound. *J Neuropathol Exp Neurol* 24:563–574, 1965.

Matsumura F: *Toxicology of Insecticides*. New York: Plenum, 1985, pp 122–128.

Matthews HB, Matsumura F: Metabolic fate of dieldrin in the rat. *J Agric Food Chem* 17:845–852, 1969.

McBlain WA, Lewin V, Wolfe FH: Estrogenic effects of the enantiomers of *o,p′*-DDT in Japanese quail. *Can J Zool* 55:562–568, 1977.

McCord CP, Kilker CH, Minster DK: Pyrethrum dermatitis: A record of the occurrence of occupational dermatoses among workers in the pyrethrum industry. *JAMA* 77:448–449, 1921.

McEwen FL, Stephenson GR: *The Use and Significance of Pesticides in the Environment*. New York: Wiley, 1979, pp 91–154.

McFarland LZ, Lacy PB: Physiologic and endocrinologic effects of the insecticide kepone in the Japanese quail. *Toxicol Appl Pharmacol* 15:441–450, 1969.

Melnikov NN: Chemistry of pesticides. *Residue Rev* 36:1–480, 1971.

Menzie CM: *Metabolism of Pesticides*. Washington, DC: Bureau of Sport Fisheries and Wildlife. Special Scientific Report. Wildlife No. 127, 1969.

Mes J, Davies DJ, Turton D: Polychlorinated biphenyl and other chlorinated hydrocarbon residues in adipose tissue of Canadians. *Bull Environ Contam Toxicol* 28:97–104, 1982.

Metcalfe RL: Development of selective and biodegradable pesticides, in *Pest Control Strategies for the Future*. Washington, DC: Agriculture Board, Division of Biology and Agriculture, National Research Council, National Academy of Science, 1972, pp 137–156.

Metcalfe RL: A century of DDT. *J Agric Food Chem* 21:511–519, 1973.

Moore JA, McConnell EE, Dalgard DW, Harris MW: Comparative toxicity of three halogenated dibenzofurans in guinea pigs, mice and rhesus monkeys. *Ann NY Acad Sci* 320:151–163, 1979.

Morgan DP: *Recognition and Management of Pesticide Poisonings*, 3d ed. Publication EPA-540/9-80-005, Washington, DC: U.S. Environmental Protection Agency, 1982.

Morgan DP, Roan CC: Chlorinated hydrocarbon pesticide residue in human tissues. *Arch Environ Health* 20:452–457, 1970.

Morgan JP, Penovich P: Jamaica ginger paralysis. Forty-seven year follow-up. *Arch Neurol* 35:530–532, 1978.

Morrison HI, Wilkins K, Semenciw R, et al: Herbicides and cancer. *J Natl Cancer Inst* 84:1866–1874, 1992.

Mullison WR: An Interim Report Summarizing 2,4-D Toxicological Research Sponsored by the Industry Task Force on 2,4-D Research Data and a Brief Review of 2,4-D Environmental Effects. Technical and Toxicology Committees of the Industry Task Force on 2,4-D Research Data, 1986.

Munro IC, Carlo GL, Orr JC, et al: A comprehensive, integrated review and evaluation of the scientific evidence relating to the safety of the herbicide 2,4-D. *J Amer College Toxicol* 11:559–664, 1992.

Murphy SD: Mechanisms of pesticide interactions in vertebrates. *Residue Rev* 25:201–221, 1969.

Murphy SD: The toxicity of pesticides and their metabolites, in *Degradation of Synthetic Organic Molecules in the Biosphere*. Proceedings of a Conference. Washington, DC: National Academy of Sciences, 1972, pp 313–335.

Murphy SD: Toxic interactions with dermal exposure to organophosphate insecticides, in Holmstedt B, Lauwerys R, Mercier M, Roberfroid M (eds): *Mechanisms of Toxicity and Hazard Evaluation*. Amsterdam: Elsevier/North Holland Biomedical, 1980, pp 615–621.

Murray RE, Gibson JE: Paraquat disposition in rats, guinea pigs and monkeys. *Toxicol Appl Pharmacol* 27:283–291, 1974.

Namba T, Hiraki K: PAM (pyridine-2-aldoxime methiodide) therapy for alkylphosphate poisoning. *JAMA* 166:1834–1839, 1958.

Namba T, Nolte CT, Jackrel J, Grob D: Poisoning due to organophosphate insecticides. *Am J Med* 50:475–492, 1971.

Narahashi T: Mode of action of pyrethroids. *Bull WHO* 44:337–345, 1971.

Narahashi T: Effect of insecticides on nervous conduction and synaptic transmission, in Wilkinson CF (ed): *Insecticide Biochemistry and Physiology*. New York: Plenum, 1976, pp 327–352.

Narahashi T: Nerve membrane ionic channels as the primary target of pyrethroids. *Neurotoxicology* 2:3–22, 1985.

Narahashi T, Cranmer JM, Wooley DE (eds): Pyrethroids and neuroactive pesticides. *Proceedings of the Third International Conference on Neurotoxicology of Selected Chemicals*, Sept. 9–12, 1984. *Neurotoxicology* 6:1985.

Narita S, Motojuku H, Sato J, Mori H: Autopsy in acute suicidal poisoning with diquat dibromide. *Jpn J Rural Med* 27:454–455, 1978.

National Academy of Sciences: Regulating Pesticides in Food. *The Delaney Paradox. Report of Committee on Scientific and Regulatory Issues Underlying Pesticide Use Patterns and Agricultural Innovation*. Washington, DC: National Academy, 1987.

Neumann R, Peter HN: Insecticidal organophosphates: nature made them first. *Experientia* 43:1235–1237, 1987.

Nielsen K, Kaempe B, Jensen-Holm J: Fatal poisoning in man by 2,4-dichlorophenoxyacetic acid (2,4-D). Determination of the agent in forensic materials. *Acta Pharmacol Toxicol* 22:224–234, 1965.

O'Brien RD: *Toxic Phosphorus Esters. Chemistry, Metabolism and Biological Effects*. New York: Academic, 1960.

O'Brien RD: *Insecticides, Action and Metabolism*. New York: Academic, 1967.

Ohkawa N, Oshita H, Miyamoto J: Comparison of inhibitory activity of various organophosphorus compounds against acetylcholinesterase and neurotoxic esterase of hens with respect to delayed neurotoxicity. *Biochem Pharmacol* 29:2721–2727, 1980.

Ott MG, Holder BB, Olson RD: A mortality analysis of employees engaged in the manufacture of 2,4,5-trichlorophenoxyacetic acid. *J Occup Med* 22:47–50, 1980.

Peakall DB: Pesticides and the reproduction of birds. *Sci Am* 222:72–78, 1970.

Pearce NE, Smith AH, Howard JK, et al: Non-Hodgkin's lymphoma and exposure to phenoxyherbicides, chlorophenols, fencing work and meat works employment: A case-control study. *Br J Indust Med* 43:75–83, 1986.

Petrova-Vergieva T, Ivanova-Chemishanska L: Assessment of the teratogenic activity of dithiocarbamate fungicides. *Food Cosmet Toxicol* 11:239–244, 1973.

Pickering QH, Henderson C, Lemke AE: The toxicity of organic phosphorus insecticides to different species of warmwater fishes. *Trans Am Fish Soc* 91:175–184, 1962.

Poland AP, Smith D, Metter G, Possick P: A health survey of workers in a 2,4-D and 2,4,5-T plant with special attention to chloracne, porphyria cutanea tarda and psychologic parameters. *Arch Environ Health* 22:316–327, 1971.

Quinby GE, Hayes WJ Jr, Armstrong JF, Durham WF: DDT storage in the U.S. population. *JAMA* 191:175–179, 1965.

Redetzke KA, Applegate HG: Organochlorine pesticides in adipose tissue of persons from El Paso, Texas. *J Environ Health* 56(3):25–27, 1993.

Rhodes ML: Hypoxic protection in paraquat poisoning. A model for respiratory distress syndrome. *Chest* 66:341–342, 1974.

Richter CP: Biological factors involved in poisoning rats with alphanaphthylthiourea (ANTU). *Proc Soc Exp Biol Med* 63:364–372, 1946.

Rose MS, Lock EA, Smith LL, Wyatt I: Paraquat accumulation: tissue and species specificity. *Biochem Pharmacol* 25:429–423, 1976.

Rose MS, Smith LL: Tissue uptake of paraquat and diquat. *Gen Pharmacol* 8:173–176, 1977.

Rosenstock L, Keifer M, Daniell WE, et al: Chronic central nervous system effects of acute organophosphate pesticide intoxication. *Lancet* 338:223–227, 1991.

Ruzo LO, Engel JL, Casida JE: Decamethrin metabolites from oxidative, hydrolytic and conjugative reactions in mice. *J Agric Food Chem* 27:725–731, 1979.

Ryan AJ: The metabolism of pesticidal carbamates. *CRC Crit Rev Toxicol* 1:33–54, 1974.

Saleh MA, Turner WA, Casida JE: Polychlorobornane components of toxaphene: structure-toxicity relations and metabolic reductive dechlorination. *Science* 198:1256–1258, 1977.

Santalucito JA, Morrison G: EEG of Rhesus monkeys following prolonged low-level feeding of pesticides. *Toxicol Appl Pharmacol* 19:147–154, 1971.

Saracci R, Kogvinas M, Bertazzi PA, et al: Cancer mortality in workers exposed to chlorophenoxy herbicides and chlorophenols. *Lancet* 338:1027–1032, 1991.

Sawada V, Nagai Y, Ueyama M, Yamamoto I: Probable toxicity of surface-active agent in commercial herbicide containing glyphosate. *Lancet* i:299, 1988.

Schmid R: Cutaneous porphyria in Turkey. *N Engl J Med* 263:397–398, 1960.

Schoene K: Reaktivierung von *O,O*-diathylphosphorylacetylcholinesterase. Reaktivierungs-re-phosphorylierungs gleichgewicht. *Biochem Pharmacol* 21:163–170, 1972.

Schonborn H, Schuster HP, Koessling FK: Klinik und morphologie der akuten peroralen diquatintoxikation (re-lone). *Arch Toxicol* 27:204–216, 1971.

Schrader G, Kukenthal H: Farbenfabriken Bayer AG: DBP 767153 and 767723, 1937.

Schultz KN: Clinical picture and etiology of chloracne. *Arb Med Sozialmed Areitshyg* 3:25–29, 1968.

Schumacher MC: Farming occupations and mortality from non-Hodgkin's lymphoma in Utah. *J Occup Med* 27:580–584, 1985.

Schwetz BA, Norris JM, Sparschu GL, et al: Toxicology of chlorinated dioxins. *Adv Chem* 120:55–69, 1973.

Schwetz BA, Quast JF, Keeler PA: Results of two-year toxicity and reproduction studies on pentachlorophenol in rats, in Rao KR (ed): *Pentachlorophenol*. New York: Plenum, 1977, pp 301–315.

Senanayake N, Gurunathan G, Hart TB, et al: An epidemiological study of the health of Sri Lankan tea plantation workers associated with long-term exposure to paraquat. *Br J Ind Med* 50:257–263, 1993.

Senanayake N, Karalliedde L: Neurotoxic effects of organophosphorus insecticides. *N Engl J Med* 316:761–763, 1987.

Sharp CWM, Ottolenghi A, Posner HS: Correlation of paraquat toxicity with tissue concentrations and weight loss of the rat. *Toxicol Appl Pharmacol* 22:241–251, 1972.

Shih T-M: Comparison of several oximes on reactivation of soman-inhibited blood, brain and tissue cholinesterase activity in rats. *Arch Toxicol* 67:637–646, 1993.

Shimkin MB, Anderson NN: Acute toxicities of rotenone and mixed pyrethrins in mammals. *Proc Soc Exp Biol Med* 34:135–138, 1936.

Shono T, Ohsawa K, Casida JE: Metabolism of *trans*- and *cis*-permethrin, *trans*- and *cis*-cypermethrin and decamethrin by microsomal enzymes. *J Agric Food Chem* 27:316–325, 1979.

Sidell FR: Clinical considerations in nerve agent intoxication, in Somani SM (ed): *Chemical Warfare Agents*. New York: Academic, 1992, pp 155–194.

Singer R, Moses M, Valciukas J, et al: Nerve conduction velocity studies of workers employed in the manufacture of phenoxy herbicides. *Environ Res* 29:297–311, 1982.

Slott V, Ecobichon DJ: An acute and subacute neurotoxicity assessment of trichlorfon. *Can J Physiol Pharmacol* 62:513–518, 1984.

Smalley HE, O'Hara PJ, Bridges CH, Radeleff RD: The effects of chronic carboryl administration on the neuromuscular system of swine. *Toxicol Appl Pharmacol* 14:409–419, 1969.

Smith LL: The mechanisms of paraquat toxicity in the lung. *Rev Biochem Toxicol* 8:37–71, 1987.

Smith MI, Lillie RD: The histopathology of triorthocresyl phosphate poisoning. The etiology of so-called ginger paralysis (third report). *Arch Neurol Psychiatry* 26:976–992, 1931.

Smith P, Heath D: Paraquat. *Crit Rev Toxicol* 4:411–445, 1976.

Solleveld HA, Haseman JK, McConnell EE: Natural history of body weight gain, survival and neoplasia in the F344 rat. *J Natl Can Inst* 72:929–940, 1984.

Somani SM, Solana RP, Dube SN: Toxicodynamics of nerve agents, in Somani SM (ed): *Chemical Warfare Agents*. New York: Academic, 1992, pp 67–123.

Spear RC, Popendorf WJ, Leffingwell JT, et al: Field workers' response to weathered residues of parathion. *J Occup Med* 19:406–410, 1977.

Spiegelberg U: Psychopathologisch-neurologische spat und dauerschaden nach gewerblicher intoxikation durch phosphorsaureester (alkylphosphate). *Proc 14th Int Cong Occup Health Excerpta Med Found Int Congr Ser* 62, 1778–1780, 1963.

Sprague GL, Bickford AA: Effect of multiple diisopropylfluorophosphate injections in hens: behavioral, biochemical and histological investigation. *J Toxicol Environ Health* 8:973–988, 1981.

Steinberg GM, Cranmer J, Ash AB: New reactivators of phosphonylated acetylcholinesterase. *Biochem Pharmacol* 26:439–441, 1977.

Stellman SD, Stellman JM, Sommer JF: Health and reproductive outcomes among American legionnaires in relation to combat and herbicide exposure in Vietnam. *Environ Res* 47:150–174, 1988.

Sterri SH, Rognerud B, Fiskum SE, Lyngaas S: Effect of toxogonin and P2S on the toxicity of carbamates and organophosphorus compounds. *Acta Pharmacol Toxicol* 45:9–15, 1979.

Stevens JT, Sumner DD: Herbicides, in Hayes WJ Jr, Laws ER Jr (eds): *Handbook of Pesticide Toxicology. Classes of Pesticides*. New York: Academic, 1991, vol 3, pp 1317–1408.

Stevens MF, Ebell GF, Psaila-Savona P: Organochlorine pesticides in Western Australia nursing mothers. *Med J Aust* 158:238–241, 1993.

Stickel LF: Organochlorine Pesticides in the Environment. Washington, DC: United States Department of the Interior, Fish and Wildlife Service. Special Scientific Report-Wildlife No. 119, 1968.

Stuart-Harle M: "Safe" pesticides found toxic. *Biotechnology* 3:16, 1988.

Suskind RR, Hertzberg VS: Human health effects of 2,4,5-T and its toxic contaminants. *JAMA* 251:2372–2380, 1984.

Swan AAB: Exposure of spray operators to paraquat. *Br J Ind Med* 26:322–329, 1969.

Tamburro CH: Chronic liver injury in phenoxy herbicide-exposed Vietnam veterans. *Environ Res* 59:175–188, 1992.

Taylor JR, Selhorst JB, Houff SA, Martinez AJ: Chlordecone intoxication in man. I. Clinical observations. *Neurology* 28:626–630, 1978.

Thiess AM, Frentzel-Beyme R, Link R: Mortality study of persons exposed to dioxin in a trichlorophenol process accident that occurred in the BASF AG on November 17, 1953. *Am J Indust Med* 3:179–189, 1982.

Tinoco R, Halperin D, Tinoco R, Parsonhet J: Paraquat poisoning in southern Mexico: A report of 25 cases. *Arch Environ Health* 48:78–80, 1993.

Toia RF, Casida JE: Phosphorylation, "aging" and possible alkylation reactions of saligenin cyclic phosphorus esters with α-chymotrypsin. *Biochem Pharmacol* 28:211–216, 1979.

Treon JF, Cleveland FP: Toxicity of certain chlorinated hydrocarbon insecticides for laboratory animals with special reference to aldrin and dieldrin. *J Agric Food Chem* 3:402–408, 1955.

Tschirley FH: Dioxin. *Sci Am* 254:29–35, 1986.

Tsubaki T, Hirota K, Shirakawa K, et al: Clinical, epidemiological and toxicological studies of methylmercury poisoning, in Plaa GL, Duncan, WAM (eds): *Proceedings of the First International Congress of Toxicology. Toxicology as a Predictive Science*. New York: Academic, 1978, pp 339–357.

Tucker RE, Young AL, Gray AP (eds): *Human and Environmental Risks of Chlorinated Dioxins and Related Compounds*. New York: Plenum, 1983.

Tucker RK, Crabtree DG: *Handbook of Toxicity of Pesticides to Wildlife*. Washington, DC: US Department of Interior, Fish and Wildlife Service. Resource Publication No. 84. United States Printing Office, 1970.

Tucker SB, Flannigan SA: Cutaneous effects from occupational exposure to fenvalerate. *Arch Toxicol* 54:195–202, 1983.

Turnbull GJ, Sanderson DM, Crome SJ: Exposure to pesticides during application, in Turnbull GJ (ed): *Occupational Hazards of Pesticide Use*. London: Taylor and Francis, 1985, pp 35–49.

Turner WA, Engel JL, Casida JE: Toxaphene components and related compounds: Preparation and toxicity of some hepta-, octa- and nonachlorobornanes, hexa- and heptachlorobornenes and a hexachlorobornadiene. *J Agric Food Chem* 25:1394–1401, 1977.

Vandekar M, Heyadat S, Plestina R, Ahmady G: A study of the safety of *o*-isopropoxyphenylmethylcarbamate in an operational field-trial in Iran. *Bull World Health Organ* 38:609–623, 1968.

Vandekar M, Plestina R, Wilhelm K: Toxicity of carbamates for mammals. *Bull World Health Organ* 44:241–248, 1971.

Van den Bercken J, Vijverberg HPM: Interaction of pyrethroids and DDT-like compounds with the sodium channels in the nerve membrane, in Miyamoto J, Kearney PC (eds): *Pesticide Chemistry. Human Welfare and the Environment. Mode of Action, Metabolism and Toxicology*. Oxford, England: Pergamon, 1983, vol 3, pp 115–121.

Van Miller JP, Lalich JJ, Allen JR: Increased incidence of neoplasm in rats exposed to low levels of 2,3,7,8-tetrachlorodibenzo-*p*-dioxin. *Chemosphere* 6:537–544, 1977.

Verschoyle RD, Aldridge WN: Structure-activity relationships of some pyrethroids in rats. *Arch Toxicol* 45:325–329, 1980.

Vijverberg HPM, Van den Bercken J: Structure related effects of pyrethroid insecticides on the lateral line sense organ and on peripheral nerves of the clawed frog, *Xenopus laerus. Pestic Biochem Physiol* 18:315–324, 1982.

Vos JG, Krajnc EI, Beekhof PK, van Looten MJ: Methods for testing immune effects of toxic chemicals: evaluation of the immunotoxicity of various pesticides in the rat, in Miyamoto J, Kearney PC (eds): *Pesticide Chemistry. Human Welfare and the Environment. Mode of Action, Metabolism and Toxicology*. Oxford, England: Pergamon, 1983, vol 3, pp 497–504.

Wafford KA, Sattelle DB, Gant DB, et al: Non competitive inhibition of GABA receptors in insect and vertebrate CNS by endrin and lindane. *Pestic Biochem Physiol* 33:213–219, 1989.

Walsh J: River blindness: a gamble pays off. *Science* 232:922–925, 1986.

Walsh RJ (chairman): Case-Control Study of Congenital Anomalies and Vietnam Service (Birth Defects Study). Report to the Minister for Veterans' Affairs. Jan 1983. Canberra: Australian Government Publishing Service, 1983.

Waters EM, Huff JE, Gerstner HB: Mirex. An overview. *Environ Res* 14:212–222, 1977.

Webb J: Iraq caught out over nerve gas attack. *New Scientist* 138: May 1, p 4, 1993.

Wecker L, Kiauta T, Dettbarn W-D: Relationship between acetylcholinesterase inhibition and the development of a myopathy. *J Pharmacol Exp Ther* 206:97–104, 1978.

Weir S, Minton N, Murray V: Organophosphate poisoning: The UK National Poisons Unit experience during 1984–1987, in Ballantyne B, Barrs TC (eds): *Clinical and Experimental Toxicology of Organophosphates and Carbamates*. Oxford: Butterworth-Heinemann, 1992, pp 463–470.

Whelan E: *Toxic Terror*. Ottawa, IL: Jameson Books, 1985.

Whorton MD, Obrinsky DL: Persistence of symptoms after mild to moderate acute organophosphate poisoning among 19 farm field workers. *J Toxicol Environ Health* 11:347–354, 1983.

Wigle DT, Semenciw RM, Wilkins K, et al: Mortality study of Canadian male farm operators: Non-Hodgkin's lymphoma mortality and agricultural practices in Saskatchewan. *J Nat Cancer Inst* 82:575–582. 1990.

Wiklund K, Lindefors B-M, Holm L-E: Risk of malignant lymphoma in Swedish agricultural and forestry workers. *Br J Indust Med* 45:19–24, 1988.

Wilson R, Lovejoy FH, Jaeger RJ, Landrigan PL: Acute phosphine poisoning aboard a grain freighter. *JAMA* 244:148–150, 1980.

Wojeck GA, Nigg HN, Stamper JH, Bradway DE: Worker exposure to ethion in Florida citrus. *Arch Environ Contam Toxicol* 10:725–735, 1981.

Wolfe HR, Durham WF, Armstrong JF: Exposure of workers to pesticides. *Arch Environ Health* 14:622–633, 1967.

Wolfe HR, Armstrong JF, Staiff DC, Comer SW: Exposure of spraymen to pesticides. *Arch Environ Health* 25:29–31, 1972.

Woods J, Polissar L, Severson R, Heuser L: Phenoxy herbicides and chlorophenols as risk factors for soft tissue sarcoma and non-Hodgkin's lymphoma. *Am J Epidemiol* 124:529, 1980.

World Health Organization: *WHO Technical Report Series 513* (Safe use of pesticides: twentieth report of the WHO Expert Committee on Insecticides). Geneva, Switzerland: WHO, 1973, pp 43–44.

World Health Organization (WHO): Public Health Impact of Pesticides Used in Agriculture. WHO, Geneva, 1990.

Worthing CR (ed): *The Pesticide Manual. A World Compendium*, 8th ed, British Crop Protection Council. Lavenham, UK: Lavenham Press, 1987.

Wray JE, Muftu Y, Dogramaci I: Hexachlorobenzene as a cause of porphyria turcica. *Turk J Pediatr* 4:132–137, 1962.

Xintaris C, Burg JR, Tanaka S, et al: *Occupational Exposure to Leptophos and Other Chemicals*. Washington, DC: DHEW (NIOSH) Publication No. 78-136. US Government Printing Office, 1978.

Yang RSH: Enzymatic conjugation and insecticide metabolism, in Wilkinson CF (ed): *Insecticide Biochemistry and Physiology*. New York: Plenum, 1976, pp 177–225.

# CHAPTER 23

# TOXIC EFFECTS OF METALS

*Robert A. Goyer*

Metals differ from other toxic substances in that they are neither created nor destroyed by humans. Nevertheless, their utilization by humans influences the potential for health effects in at least two major ways: first, by environmental transport, that is, by human or anthropogenic contributions to air, water, soil, and food, and second, by altering the speciation or biochemical form of the element (Beijer and Jernelov, 1986).

Metals are probably the oldest toxins known to humans. Lead usage may have begun prior to 2000 B.C. when abundant supplies were obtained from ores as a byproduct of smelting silver. Hippocrates is credited in 370 B.C. with the first description of abdominal colic in a man who extracted metals. Arsenic and mercury are cited by Theophrastus of Erebus (370–287 B.C.) and Pliny the Elder (A.D. 23–79). Arsenic was obtained during the melting of copper and tin, and an early use was for decoration in Egyptian tombs. In contrast, many of the metals of toxicologic concern today are only recently known to humans. Cadmium was first recognized in ores containing zinc carbonate in 1817. About 80 of the 105 elements in the periodic table are regarded as metals, but less than 30 have been reported to produce toxicity in humans. The importance of some of the rarer or lesser known metals such as indium or galium might increase with new applications in microelectronics, antitumor therapy, or other new technologies.

Metals are redistributed naturally in the environment by both geologic and biologic cycles (Fig. 23-1). Rainwater dissolves rocks and ores and physically transports material to streams and rivers, depositing and stripping materials from adjacent soil, and eventually transporting these substances to the ocean to be precipitated as sediment or taken up in rainwater to be relocated elsewhere on earth. The biological cycles include bioconcentration by plants and animals and incorporation into food cycles. These natural cycles may exceed the anthropogenic cycle, as is the case for mercury. Human industrial activity, however, may greatly shorten the residence time of metals in ore, may form new compounds, and may greatly enhance worldwide distribution. The role of human activity in the redistribution of metals is demonstrated by the 200-fold increase in lead content of Greenland ice beginning with a "natural" low level (about 800 B.C.) and a gradual rise in lead content of ice through the evolution of the industrial age, followed by a nearly precipitous rise in lead corresponding to the period when lead was added to gasoline in the 1920s (Ng and Patterson, 1981). Metal contamination of the environment therefore reflects both natural sources and a contribution from industrial activity.

The conceptual boundaries of what is regarded as the toxicology of metals continues to broaden. Historically, metal toxicology largely concerned acute or overt effects, such as abdominal colic from lead toxicity or the bloody diarrhea and suppression of urine formation from ingestion of corrosive (mercury) sublimate. There must continue to be knowledge and understanding of such effects, but they are uncommon with present-day occupational and environmental standards. There is, however, growing interest in, and inquiry into, subtle, chronic, or long-term effects in which cause and-effect relationships are not obvious or may be subclinical. These might include a level of effect that causes a change in an important index of affected individuals performance, that is, lower than expected IQs due to childhood lead exposure. Assigning responsibility for such toxicologic effects is extremely difficult and sometimes impossible, particularly when the endpoint in question lacks specificity, in that it may be caused by a number of agents or even combinations of substances. The challenges, therefore, for the toxicologist are many. The major ones include the need for quantitative information regarding dose and tissue levels, greater understanding of the metabolism of metals, particularly at the tissue and cellular levels where specific effects may occur. Most metals affect multiple organ systems, but each metal has a critical effect seen in a specific organ or tissue.

Knowledge of the critical or specific organ effects of metals provides insight into which metal may be responsible for a specific effect. There is increasing emphasis on the use of biological indicators of toxicity that are directed to specific organ effects, such as heme enzymes in lead toxicity, renal tubular dysfunction in cadmium exposure, and neurological effects in lead and mercury toxicity. Use of such indicators along with measures of exposure provide guidelines for preventive measures or therapeutic intervention.

## DOSE–EFFECT RELATIONSHIPS

Estimates of the relationship of dose or level of exposure to a critical effect for a particular metal are, in many ways, a measure of the dose–response relationships discussed in greater detail in Chap. 2. Background for this topic is also considered elsewhere

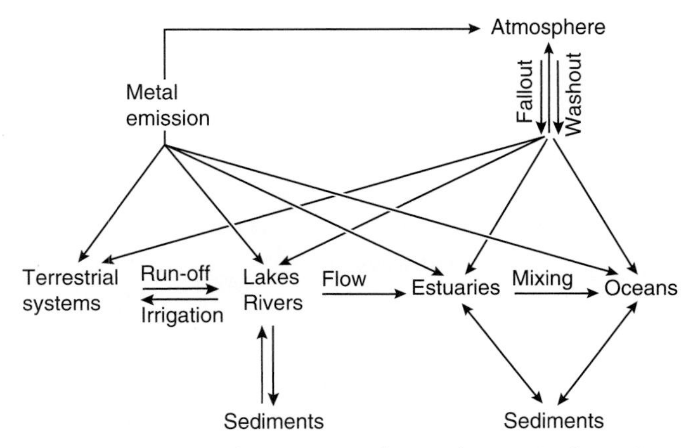


***Figure 23–1. Routes for transport of trace elements in the environment. [From Beijer and Jernelöv (1986)].***

(Friberg et al., 1986, Elinder et al., 1994). Relationships between sources of exposure, transport, and distribution to various organs and excretory pathways are shown in Fig. 23-2. The dose or estimate of exposure to a metal may be a multidimensional concept and is a function of time as well as the concentration of metal. The most precise definition of dose is the amount of metal within cells of organs manifesting a toxicological effect. Results from single measurements may reflect recent exposure or longer-term or past exposure, depending on retention time in the particular tissue. A critical determinant of the metabolism and toxic behavior of a metal is its biological half-time, that is, the time it takes for the body to excrete half of an accumulated amount. The biological half-times of cadmium and lead are 20 to 30 years, whereas for some metals such as arsenic, cobalt, and chromium they are only a few hours or days. For inorganic mercury the half-time is a few days for blood but a few months for the body as a whole.

Cellular targets for toxicity are specific biochemical processes (enzymes) and/or membranes of cells and organelles. The toxic effect of the metal usually involves an interaction between the free metal ion and the toxicological target. Toxicity is determined by dose at the cellular level, and such factors as chemical form or species and ligand binding become critical factors. Alkyl compounds are lipid soluble and pass readily across biological membranes unaltered by their surrounding medium. They are only slowly dealkylated or transformed to inorganic salts. Hence, their excretion tends to be slower than inorganic forms, and the pattern of toxicity of organic forms tends to differ from inorganic forms. For example, alkyl mercury is primarily a neurotoxin, whereas mercuric chloride is toxic to the kidneys. Metals that have strong affinity for osseous tissue like lead and radium have a long retention time and tend to accumulate with age.

Blood, urine, and hair are the most accessible tissues in which to measure an exposure or dose, and they are sometimes referred to as indicator tissues. In vivo, the quantitation of metals within organs is not yet possible, although techniques such as neutron activation and x-ray fluorescence spectroscopy are emerging technologies. Indirect estimates of quantities of toxic metals in specific organs may be calculated from metabolic models derived from autopsy data. Blood and urine concentrations usually reflect recent exposure and correlate best with acute effects. An exception is urinary cadmium, which may reflect renal damage related to an accumulation of cadmium in the kidney. Partitioning of metal between cells and plasma and between filterable and nonfilterable components of plasma should provide more precise information regarding the presence of biologically active forms of a particular metal. Such partitioning is now standard laboratory practice for blood calcium; ionic calcium is by far the most active form of the metal. Speciation of toxic metals in urine may also provide diagnostic insights. For example, cadmium metallothionein in plasma or urine may be of greater toxicological significance than total cadmium.

Hair might be useful in assessing variations in exposure to metals over the long term. Analyses may be performed on segments of the hair so that metal content of the newest growth can be compared with past exposures. Hair levels of

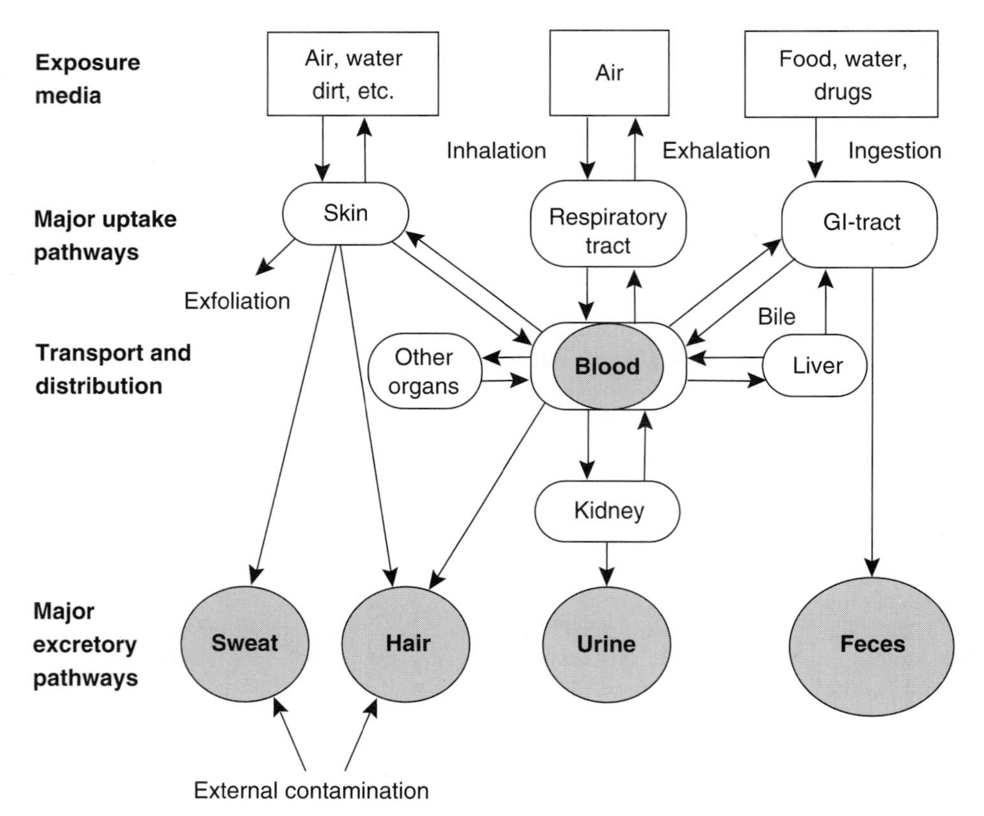


***Figure 23–2. Metabolism after exposure to metals via skin absorption, inhalation, and ingestion.***

The arrows indicate how the metals are transported and distributed. Tissues that are particularly useful for biological monitoring are identified in shaded areas. [From Elinder et al. (1994), with permission.]

mercury have been found to be a reliable measure of exposure to alkyl or methyl mercury. For most other metals, however, hair is not a reliable tissue for measuring exposure because of metal deposits from external contamination that complicate analyses, in spite of washing.

## FACTORS INFLUENCING THE TOXICITY OF METALS

Recognition of factors that influence toxicity of a particular level of exposure to a toxic metal are important in determining the risk of toxicity, particularly in susceptible populations. A number of factors influencing the toxicity of metals are shown in Table 23-1. The interaction of toxic with essential metals occurs when the metabolism of a toxic metal is similar to that of the essential element (Goyer, 1995). Absorption of toxic metals from the lung or gastrointestinal tract may be influenced by an essential metal particularly if the toxic metal shares or influences a homeostatic mechanism, such as occurs for lead and calcium and iron, and for cadmium and iron. There is an inverse relationship between the protein content of the diet and cadmium and lead toxicity. Vitamin C reduces lead and cadmium absorption, probably because of increased absorption of ferrous ion. Toxic metals may influence the role of essential metals as cofactors for enzymes or other metabolic processes (e.g., lead interferes with the calcium-dependent release of neurotransmitters). Lead, calcium, and vitamin D have a complex relationship affecting mineralization of bone and they have a more direct one involving impairment of 1-25-dihydroxy vitamin D synthesis in the kidney.

Metal–protein complexes involved in detoxification or protection from toxicity have now been described for a few metals (Goyer, 1984). Morphologically discernible cellular inclusion bodies are present with exposures to lead, bismuth, and a mercury-selenate mixture. Metallothioneins form complexes with cadmium, zinc, copper, and other metals, and ferritin and hemosiderin are intracellular iron–protein complexes. None of these proteins or metal–protein complexes have any known enzymatic activity. The nature and influences of these complexes are discussed below (this chapter) in the discussion of the toxicology of the particular metals involved.

Persons at either end of the lifespan, whether they are young children or elderly people, are believed to be more susceptible to toxicity from exposure to a particular level of metal than most adults (NRC, 1993). The major pathway of exposure to many toxic metals in children is food, and children consume more calories per pound of body weight than adults. Moreover, children have higher gastrointestinal absorption of metals, particularly lead. Experimental studies have extended these observations to many metals, and a milk diet, probably because of its lipid content, seems to increase metal absorption. The rapid growth and rapid cell division that children's bodies experience represent opportunities for genotoxic effects. Intrauterine toxicity to methyl mercury is well documented. There is no impediment to the transplacental transport of lead, so that fetal blood lead levels are similar to maternal levels.

**Table 23–1**
**Factors Influencing Toxicity of Metals**

| |
|---|
| Interactions with essential metals |
| Formation of metal–protein complexes |
| Age and stage of development |
| Lifestyle factors |
| Chemical form or speciation |
| Immune status of host |

Lifestyle factors such as smoking or alcohol ingestion may have indirect influences on toxicity. Cigarette smoke by itself contains some toxic metals such as cadmium, and cigarette smoking may also influence pulmonary effects. Alcohol ingestion may influence toxicity indirectly by altering diet and reducing essential mineral intake.

Chemical form or speciation of the metal may be an important factor, not only for pulmonary and gastrointestinal absorption but in terms of distribution throughout the body and toxic effects. Dietary phosphate generally forms less soluble salts with metals than with other anions. Alkyl compounds, such as tetraethyl lead and methyl mercury, are lipid soluble and they are more soluble in myelin than the inorganic salts of these metals.

For metals that produce hypersensitivity reactions, the immune status of an individual becomes an additional toxicological variable. Metals that provoke immune reactions include mercury, gold, platinum, beryllium, chromium, and nickel. Clinical effects are varied but usually involve any of four types of immune responses. In anaphylactic or immediate hypersensitivity reactions the antibody, IgE, reacts with the antigen on the surface of mast cells releasing vasoreactive amines. Clinical reactions include conjunctivitis, asthma, urticaria, or even systemic anaphylaxis. Cutaneous, mucosal, and bronchial reactions to platinum have been attributed to this type of hypersensitivity reaction. Cytotoxic hypersensitivity is the result of a complement-fixing reaction of IgG immunoglobulin with antigen or hapten bound to the cell surface. The thrombocytopenia sometimes occurring with exposure to organic gold salts may be brought about in this manner. Immune complex hypersensitivity occurs when soluble immune complex forms deposits (antigen, antibody, and complement) within tissues producing an acute inflammatory reaction. Immune complexes are typically deposited on the epithelial (subepithelial) side of glomerular basement membrane, resulting in proteinuria following exposure to mercury vapor or gold therapy. Cell-mediated hypersensitivity, also known as the *delayed hypersensitivity reaction*, is mediated by thymus-dependent lymphocytes and usually occurs 24 to 48 h after exposure. The histologic reaction consists of mononuclear cells and is the typical reaction seen in the contact dermatitis following exposure to chromium or nickel. The granuloma formation occurring with beryllium and zirconium exposure may be a form of cell-mediated immune response.

## CARCINOGENESIS

Metals regarded as carcinogens by the International Agency of Research on Cancer are listed in Table 23-2 (IARC, 1987, 1994). Specific details pertaining to the carcinogenicity of each metal is discussed later in the chapter along with other toxicologic effects. Given the long history of human exposure to metals, knowledge of the potential carcinogenicity of metal

**Table 23–2**
**Metals Determined to be Carcinogenic**

| METAL | EVIDENCE FOR CARCINOGENESIS | |
|---|---|---|
| | HUMANS | ANIMALS |
| Arsenic | Sufficient | Limited |
| Beryllium | Sufficient | Sufficient |
| Cadmium | Sufficient | Sufficient |
| Chromium | | |
| Trivalent | Insufficient | Insufficient |
| Hexavalent | Sufficient | Sufficient |
| Cisplatin | Insufficient | Sufficient |
| Iron complexes | | |
| Dextran | Insufficient | Sufficient |
| Dextrin | No data | Limited |
| Lead | | |
| Inorganic | Insufficient | Sufficient |
| Mercury | | |
| Inorganic | Inadequate | Limited for chloride |
| Nickel | | |
| Metallic | Insufficient | Sufficient |
| Compounds | Sufficient | Sufficient |
| Selenium | Insufficient | Insufficient |

compounds has evolved slowly, and most of this information has only been obtained in recent years. Table 23-2 provides an overview or summary of the carcinogenicity of metals. The nature of the evidence for specific metals is variable. Human case reports of skin cancer due to arsenic exposure were recognized in the nineteenth century, but epidemiological support from case study observations did not occur until over 50 years later, and there has not yet been confirmation in experimental animals. The reverse is true with lead, the only metal shown to be carcinogenic in animal models by oral administration yet whose evidence for toxicity in humans is limited to case reports. How much of what kind of evidence, animal and/or human, is required to label a metal as a carcinogen must be decided for each metal. The appellations *sufficient, limited*, and *insufficient* are the terms recommended by IARC panels. Animal studies that use routes of administration different from those by which humans may be exposed, such as injection, have limitations for extrapolation to humans.

This is an exceedingly important topic because of the ubiquitousness of metals, their widespread industrial use, and their persistence in the environment. Identification of metal carcinogens in industry is made even more perplexing because seldom are humans exposed only to a single metal: exposures usually involve mixtures. Then there is the additional question of the role of metals as promoters or cocarcinogens with organic carcinogens because of their persistence in tissues, as may be the case for lead. As a general rule, it is the ionic form of the metal that is believed to be responsible for carcinogenic effects. For example, if any form of cadmium or nickel is carcinogenic, the metal should be regarded as a carcinogen. However, some chemical forms of a metal may have more potency for carcinogenesis than others and evidence for carcinogenicity in humans or animals may be adequate for only some forms or compounds of the metal. For example, nickel subsulfide ($Ni_3S_2$) is more carcinogenic than soluble salts of nickel such as nickel sulfate, but such differences may be explained on the basis of cell uptake rates or solubility. Predictive in vitro test methods using nonmammalian systems, such as the Ames test, do not seem to be as responsive as for organic compounds. However, newer methods of evaluation, such as metal–DNA cross-linking, are presently under study (Costa et al., 1993, Zhuang and Costa, 1995).

## CHELATION

Treatment of exposure to toxic metals by chelating agents or antagonists is sometimes warranted to prevent or reverse toxicity and therefore remains an important topic, particularly for those metals that are cumulative and persistent (e.g., lead). It must be emphasized, however, that chelation is only a secondary alternative to reduction or prevention of exposures to toxic metals.

Chelation is the formation of a metal ion complex in which the metal ion is associated with a charged or uncharged electron donor, referred to as a ligand. The ligand may be monodentate, bidentate, or multidentate; that is, it may attach or coordinate using one or two or more donor atoms. Bidentate ligands form ring structures that include the metal ion and the two ligand atoms attached to the metal (Williams and Halstead, 1982). Metals may react with O−, S−, and N− containing ligands present in the form of −OH, −COOH, >C=O, −S−S−, −NH2, and >NH. A resultant metal complex is formed by a coordinate bond (coordination compound), in which both electrons are contributed by the ligand (Klaassen, 1990).

Chelating agents (drugs) vary in their specificity for toxic metals. Ideal chelating agents should be water soluble, resistant to biotransformation, able to reach sites of metal storage, capable of forming nontoxic complexes with toxic metals and of being excreted from the body, and should have a low affinity for essential metals, particularly calcium and zinc (Klaassen, 1990). The challenge in the development of safer and more effective chelating agents is to design all of the desirable chemical, physiological, and pharmacological properties into the drug (Jones, 1992).

The general properties of chelating agents that are of current interest are briefly described. Additional details and comments are provided later in the chapter with discussions of specific metals.

### BAL/British Anti-Lewisite

BAL (2,3-dimercaptopropanol) was the first clinically useful chelating agent. It was developed during World War II as a specific antagonist to vesicant arsenical war gases, based on the observation that arsenic has an affinity for sulfhydryl-containing substances. BAL, a dithiol compound with two sulfur atoms on adjacent carbon atoms, competes with the critical binding sites responsible for the toxic effects. These observations led to the prediction that the "biochemical lesion" of arsenic poisoning would prove to be a thiol with sulfhydryl groups separated by one or more intervening carbon atoms. This prediction was borne out a few years later with the discovery that arsenic interferes with the function of 6,8-dithiooctanoic acid in biologic oxidation (Gunsalus, 1953).

BAL has been found to form stable chelates in vivo with many toxic metals including inorganic mercury, antimony, bismuth, cadmium, chromium, cobalt, gold, and nickel. However, it is not necessarily the treatment of choice for toxicity to these metals. BAL has been used as an adjunct in the treatment of the acute encephalopathy of lead toxicity. It is a potentially toxic drug, and its use may be accompanied by multiple side effects. Although treatment with BAL will increase the excretion of cadmium, there is a concomitant increase in renal cadmium concentration, so that its use in case of cadmium toxicity is to be avoided. It does, however, remove inorganic mercury from the kidneys; but is not useful in the treatment of alkyl mercury or phenyl mercury toxicity. BAL also enhances the toxicity of selenium and tellurium, so it is not to be used to remove these metals from the body.

## DMPS

DMPS (2,3-dimercapto-1-propanesulfonic acid) is a water-soluble derivative of BAL developed in response to BAL's toxicity and unpleasant side effects. DMPS has been shown to reduce blood lead levels in children (Chisholm and Thomas, 1985). It has the advantage over *ethylene diamine tetraacetic acid* (EDTA) in that it is administered orally and does not appear to have toxic side effects. It has been widely used in the former Union of Soviet Socialist Republics (U.S.S.R.) to treat many different metal intoxications. It has even been used to treat atherosclerosis by the adherents of the notion that this degenerative disorder of blood vessels is due to metal–ion accumulations in the blood vessel wall leading to inhibition of enzyme metabolism.

DMPS has been used experimentally to estimate the renal burden of lead (Twarog and Cherian, 1984) and inorganic mercury (Cherian et al., 1988) It increases the urinary excretion of mercury in persons with an increased body burden from industrial exposure, from dentists and dental technicians, and from persons with dental amalgams (Aposhian et al., 1992).

## EDTA

Calcium EDTA is the calcium disodium salt of EDTA. The calcium salt must be used for clinical purposes because the sodium salt has greater affinity for calcium and will produce hypocalcemic tetany. However, the calcium salt will bind lead, with displacement of calcium from the chelate. EDTA is poorly absorbed from the gastrointestinal tract so it must be given parenterally, which distributes it rapidly throughout the body. It has long been the method of choice for the treatment of lead toxicity. The peak excretion point is within the first 24 h and represents the excretion of lead from soft tissues. Removal of lead from the skeletal system occurs more slowly with the restoration of equilibrium with soft tissue compartments. Calcium EDTA does have the potential for nephrotoxicity, so it should be administered only when indicated clinically (EPA, 1986).

## DMSA

DMSA (meso-2.3.-Dimercatosuccinic acid; Succimer), like DMPS, is a chemical analog of BAL. More than 90 percent of DMSA is in the form of a mixed disulfide in which each of the sulfur atoms is in disulfide linkage with a cysteine molecule (Aposhian and Aposhian, 1992). The drug is of current interest clinically because of its ability to lower blood lead levels. It has advantages over EDTA because it is given orally and has greater specificity for lead. It may be safer than EDTA in that it does not enhance excretion of calcium and zinc to the same degree. Studies in rodents showed that a single dose of DMSA primarily removes lead from soft tissues (Smith and Flegal, 1992).

The drug has been licensed recently by the U.S. Food and Drug Administration specifically for the treatment of lead poisoning in children whose blood lead levels are $>45\ \mu g/dl$, and it has been used in Europe. While Succimer has been shown to be effective in lowering blood lead, its effectiveness in removal of lead from the brain and in the reversal of some of the toxic outcomes of lead poisoning, such as negative effects on cognitive and behavioral development, have not been demonstrated.

### Penicillamine

Penicillamine ($\beta,\beta$-dimethylcysteine), a hydrolytic product of penicillin, has been used for the removal of copper in persons with Wilson's disease, and for the removal of lead, mercury, and iron (Walshe, 1964). It is also important to note that penicillamine removes other physiologically essential metals, including zinc, cobalt, and manganese. Attached to its use is the risk of inducing a hypersensitivity reaction with a wide spectrum of undesirable immunologic effects, including skin rash, blood dyscrasia, and possibly proteinuria and nephrotic syndrome. It has cross-sensitivity with penicillin so it should be avoided by persons with penicillin hypersensitivity. For persons who have developed a sensitivity to penicillamine, an orally active chelating agent, triethylene tetramine 2HCl (Trien), is an alternative (Walshe, 1983).

## DTPA

DTPA or diethylenetriaminepentaacetic acid has chelating properties similar to those of EDTA. The calcium salt ($CaNa_2$ DPTA) must be used clinically because of DPTA's high affinity for calcium. It has been used for chelation of plutonium and other actinide elements but with mixed success. Experimental studies have shown that various polydentate ligands are more effective than $CaNa_2$DPTA for promoting excretion of Pu and other actinides (Durbin et al., 1994).

### Desferrioxamine

Desferrioxamine is a hydroxylamine isolated as the iron chelate of *Streptomyces pilosus* and is used clinically in the metal-free form (Keberle, 1964). It has a remarkable affinity for ferric iron and a low affinity for calcium, and it competes effectively for iron in ferritin and hemosiderin but not in transferrin, and not for the iron in hemoglobin or heme-containing enzymes. It is poorly absorbed from the gastrointestinal tract so it must be given parenterally. Clinical usefulness is limited by a variety of toxic effects including hypotension, skin rashes, and, possibly, cataract formation. It seems to be more effective in hemosiderosis due to blood transfusion but is less effective in treatment of hemochromatosis.

## Dithiocarbamate (DTC)

Dithiocarb (diethyldithiocarbanate), or DDC, has been recommended as the drug of choice in the treatment of acute nickel carbonyl poisoning. The drug may be administered orally for mild toxicity and parenterally for acute or severe poisoning (Sunderman, 1979). It has also been used experimentally for removal of cadmium bound to metallothionein (Kojima et al., 1990). A number of DTC compounds with various substitutions of nonpolar, nonionizing groups have been synthesized by Jones and Cherian (1990). Sodium, *N*-(4-methoxybenzyl)-D-glucamine dithiocarbamate (MeOBGDTC) is one of the most effective in removal of cadmium from tissues. The Cd–MeOBGDTC complex is excreted in the bile rather than in the kidney, avoiding the nephrotoxicity characteristic of cadmium chelates. To date the use of this compound has been limited to experimental studies in rodents.

# MAJOR TOXIC METALS WITH MULTIPLE EFFECTS

## Arsenic

Arsenic is particularly difficult to characterize as a single element because its chemistry is so complex and there are many different arsenic compounds. It may be trivalent or pentavalent and is widely distributed in nature. The most common inorganic trivalent arsenic compounds are arsenic trioxide, sodium arsenite, and arsenic trichloride. Pentavalent inorganic compounds are arsenic pentoxide, arsenic acid, and arsenates, such as lead arsenate and calcium arsenate. Organic compounds may also be trivalent or pentavalent, such as arsanilic acid, or may even occur in methylated forms as a consequence of biomethylation by organisms in soil, fresh water, and seawater. A summary of environmental sources of arsenic as well as their potential health effects is contained in the U.S. EPA document on arsenic (EPA, 1987b).

Inorganic arsenic is released into the environment from a number of anthropogenic sources which include primary copper, zinc, and lead smelters, glass manufacturers that add arsenic to raw materials, and chemical manufacturers. The National Air Sampling Network tests conducted by the U.S. EPA indicate that in areas not influenced by copper smelters, maximum 24-h concentrations do not exceed 0.1 $\mu g/m^3$. In near point emissions (copper smelters), concentrations may exceed 1 $\mu g/m^3$. Drinking water usually contains a few micrograms per liter or less. Most major U.S. drinking water supplies contain levels lower than 5 $\mu$g per liter. It has been estimated that about 350,000 people might drink water containing more than 50 $\mu$g per liter (Smith et al., 1992). Levels exceeding 50 $\mu$g per liter have been found in Nova Scotia where the arsenic content of bedrock is high. Even higher concentrations, exceeding the 50 $\mu$g per liter standard have also been reported from various mineral springs (e.g., in Japan, 1.7 mg As/liter; in Cordoba, Argentina, 3.4 mg per liter; in Taiwan, from artesian well water, 1.8 mg per liter). Most foods (meat and vegetables) contain some level of arsenic, but the daily diet in the United States generally contains below 0.04 mg; however, it may contain 0.2 mg per day if the diet contains seafood. Dietary arsenic notwithstanding, the total daily intake of arsenic by humans without industrial exposure is usually less than 0.3 mg per day.

The major source of occupational exposure to arsenic in the United States is in the manufacture of pesticides, herbicides, and other agricultural products. High exposure to arsenic fumes and dust may occur in the smelting industries; the highest concentrations most likely occur among roaster workers.

**Toxicokinetics.** Airborne arsenic is largely trivalent arsenic oxide, but deposition in airways and absorption from lungs is dependent on particle size and chemical form. Six to nine percent of orally administered $^{74}$As-labeled trivalent or pentavalent arsenic is eliminated in the feces of mice, indicating almost complete absorption from the gastrointestinal tract. Limited data also suggest nearly complete absorption of soluble forms of trivalent and pentavalent arsenic. Excretion of absorbed arsenic is mainly via urine. The biological half-life of ingested inorganic arsenic is about 10 h and 50 to 80 percent is excreted in about 3 days. The biological half-life of methylated arsenic is about 30 h.

Arsenic has a predilection for skin and is excreted by desquamation of skin and in sweat, particularly during periods of profuse sweating. It also concentrates in nails and hair. Arsenic in nails produces Mee's lines (transverse white bands across fingernails), which appear about 6 weeks after the onset of symptoms of toxicity. The time of exposure may be estimated from measuring the distance of the line from the base of the nail and the rate of nail growth, which is about 0.3 cm per month or 0.1 mm per day. Arsenic in hair may also reflect past exposure, but intrinsic or systematically absorbed arsenic in hair must be distinguished from arsenic that is deposited from external sources. Human milk contains about 3 $\mu$g per liter of arsenic.

Placental transfer of arsenic has been shown in hamsters injected intravenously with high doses (20 mg/kg body weight) of sodium arsenate, and studies of tissue levels of arsenic in fetuses and newborn babies in Japan show that the total amount of arsenic in the fetus tends to increase during gestation, indicating placental transfer. A study of pregnant women in the United States found cord blood levels of arsenic to be similar to maternal blood levels (Kagey et al., 1977).

**Biotransformation of Arsenic In Vivo.** The metabolism and potential for toxicity of arsenic is further complicated by in vivo transformation of inorganic forms by methylation to monomethyl and dimethyl arsenic. Current knowledge of this process has been summarized by Styblo and colleagues (1995). Dimethyl arsenic is the principal transformation product. This is presumed to be a process of detoxification of the more toxic inorganic forms, and dimethyl arsenic appears to be a terminal metabolite which is rapidly formed and rapidly excreted. However, exposure to inorganic arsenic may exceed the rate of its transformation, resulting in toxicity from the inorganic form, so that consideration of toxic dose–responses to inorganic arsenic must be assessed in the light of what is known about metabolic transformation. Ingestion of arsenic-containing seafood does not result in the increased excretion of inorganic arsenic and methylarsinic and dimethylarsinic acid, but rather it results in large increases in excretion of cacodylic acid (Buchet et al., 1980).

**Oxidation and Reduction Reactions of Inorganic Arsenic.** A number of experiments in animals suggest that reduction of pentavalent arsenic to arsenic trioxide occurs in vivo. The biochemical mechanism for in vivo methylation of inorganic arsenic is a reductive process, and it is presently presumed that reduction of arsenic in vivo is related to biomethylation. Lerman and coworkers (1983) found, using in vitro techniques, that in the rat isolated hepatocytes readily methylate trivalent arsenic while there is virtually no methylation of pentavalent arsenic. These studies suggest that pentavalent arsenic must first be converted to arsenite prior to methylation. Trivalent inorganic arsenic undergoes extensive oxidation in aerated water. The pH of aqueous solutions appears to be a major factor in the relative stability of either valency form. Trivalent arsenic in alkaline solutions is more rapidly oxidized than at acidic pH. Pentavalent inorganic arsenic is, by contrast, relatively stable at neutral or alkaline pH but undergoes reduction with decreasing pH.

**Cellular Effects.** It has been known for some years that trivalent compounds of arsenic are the principal toxic forms, and pentavalent arsenic compounds have little effect on enzyme activity. A number of sulfhydryl-containing proteins and enzyme systems have been found to be altered by exposure to arsenic. Some of these can be reversed by addition of an excess of a monothiol such as glutathione. Effects on enzymes containing two thiol groups can be reversed by dithiols such as 2,3-dimercaptopropanol (BAL) but not by monothiols.

Arsenic affects mitochondrial enzymes and impairs tissue respiration (Brown et al., 1976), which seems to be related to the cellular toxicity of arsenic. Mitochondria accumulate arsenic, and respiration mediated by NAD-linked substrates is particularly sensitive to arsenic and is thought to result from a reaction between the arsenite ion and the dihydrolipoic acid cofactor, which is necessary for oxidation of the substrate (Fluharty and Sanadi, 1961). Arsenite also inhibits succinic dehydrogenase activity and uncouples oxidative phosphorylation, which results in stimulation of mitochondrial ATPase activity. Mitchell et al. (1971) proposed that arsenic inhibits energy-linked functions of mitochondria in two ways: competition with phosphate during oxidative phosphorylation and inhibition of energy-linked reduction of NAD.

Arsenic compounds are inducers of metallothionein in vivo. Potency is dependent on the chemical form of arsenic. As(III) is most potent, followed by As(V), monomethylarsenate, and dimethylarsenate (Kreppel et al., 1993).

Information from experimental studies with rats, chicks, minipigs and goats have shown that arsenic in its inorganic form may be an essential nutrient, but the nutritional essentiality for humans has not been established (EPA, 1987b).

**Toxicology.** Ingestion of large doses (70 to 180 mg) of arsenic may be fatal. Symptoms of acute illness, possibly leading to death, consist of fever, anorexia, hepatomegaly, melanosis, and cardiac arrhythmia with changes in electrocardiograph results that may be the prodroma of eventual cardiovascular failure. Other features include upper-respiratory-tract symptoms, peripheral neuropathy, and gastrointestinal, cardiovascular, and hematopoietic effects. Acute ingestion may be suspected from damage to mucous membranes such as irritation, vesicle formation, and even sloughing. Sensory loss in the peripheral nervous system is the most common neurological effect, appearing 1 or 2 weeks after large exposures and consisting of Wallerian degeneration of axons, a condition that is reversible if exposure is stopped. Anemia and leukopenia, particularly granulocytopenia, occur a few days following exposure and are reversible.

Chronic exposure to inorganic arsenic compounds may lead to neurotoxicity of both the peripheral and central nervous systems. Neurotoxicity usually begins with sensory changes, paresthesia, and muscle tenderness followed by weakness, progressing from proximal to distal muscle groups. Peripheral neuropathy may be progressive involving both sensory and motor neurones leading to demyelination of long axon nerve fibers, but effects are dose related. Acute exposure to a single high dose can produce the onset of paresthesia and motor dysfunction within 10 days. More chronic occupational exposures producing more gradual, insidious effects may occur over a period of years, and it has been difficult to establish dose–response relationships.

Liver injury, characteristic of longer-term or chronic exposure, manifests itself initially in jaundice and may progress to cirrhosis and ascites. Toxic effects on hepatic parenchymal cells result in the elevation of liver enzymes in the blood, and studies in experimental animals show granules and alterations in the ultrastructure of mitochondria, nonspecific manifestations of cell injury including loss of glycogen.

Peripheral vascular disease has been observed in persons with chronic exposure to arsenic in drinking water in Taiwan and Chile; it is manifested by acrocyanosis and Raynaud's phenomenon and may progress to endarteritis obliterans and gangrene of the lower extremities (blackfoot disease). This specific effect seems to be related to the cumulative dose of arsenic, but the prevalence is uncertain because of difficulties in separating arsenic-induced peripheral vascular disease from other causes of gangrene. Recently, Engel and Smith (1994) found an increase in mortality from vascular disease for U.S. counties where arsenic in drinking water exceeded 20 $\mu$g/dl but the authors recognize that the relationship may be spurious.

**Carcinogenicity.** The EPA (1987b) and IARC (1987) classify arsenic as a carcinogen for which there is sufficient evidence from epidemiological studies to support a causal association between exposure and skin cancer. In humans, chronic exposure to arsenic induces a series of characteristic changes in skin epithelium, proceeding from hyperpigmentation to hyperkeratosis. The hyperkeratosis has been described histologically as showing hematin proliferation of a verrucose nature with derangement of the squamous portions of the epithelium or squamous cell carcinoma in some cases. There may actually be two cell types of arsenic-induced skin cancer, basal cell carcinomas and squamous cell carcinomas arising in keratotic areas. The basal cell cancers are usually only locally invasive but squamous cell carcinomas may have distant metastases. The skin cancers related to arsenic differ from ultraviolet-light–induced tumors in that they generally occur on areas of the body not exposed to sunlight (e.g., on palms and soles) and they occur as multiple lesions.

Occupational exposure to airborne arsenic may also be associated with lung cancer, usually a poorly differentiated form of epidermoid bronchogenic carcinoma. The time period between initiation of exposure and occurrence of arsenic-associated lung cancer has been found to be in the order of 35 to 45 years. Enterline and Marsh (1980) report a latency period of 20 years in their study of copper smelter workers in Tacoma, Washington.

Other visceral tumors that have been associated with arsenic exposure include hemangiosarcoma of the liver. Other cancers noted in arsenic-exposed subjects include lymphomas, leukemia, and nasopharyngeal, kidney and bladder cancers. Smith et al. (1992) estimate that the lifetime risk of dying from cancers of the liver, lung, kidney or bladder could be as high as 13 per 1000 for persons drinking 1 liter per day of water containing more than 50 $\mu$g of arsenic per liter.

In contrast to most other human carcinogens, it has been difficult to confirm the carcinogenicity of arsenic in experimental animals. Intratracheal instillations of arsenic trioxide produced an increased incidence of pulmonary adenomas, papillomas, and adenomatoid lesions, suggesting that arsenic trioxide can induce lung carcinomas (Pershagan et al., 1984), but other studies testing As(III) and As(V) compounds by oral administration or skin application have not shown potential for either promotion or initiation of carcinogenicity. Similarly, experimental studies for carcinogenicity of organic arsenic compounds have been negative.

Studies on mutagenic effects of arsenic have been generally negative. Arsenic does not induce gene mutations in bacteria and was found to be inactive in inducing reverse mutation and mitotic gene conversion in yeast. Arsenate was found not to increase forward mutations at the thymidine kinase locus in mouse L51784 cells whereas other known or suggested mutagenic metals (cadmium, nickel, and trans-platinum) showed such activity.

Several studies suggest that both As(III) and As(V) compounds are capable of producing chromosome breaks and chromosome aberrations in human peripheral lymphocyte and human skin cultures. The majority of studies indicate, however, that people with workplace or pharmaceutical exposure to arsenic have increased levels of chromosomal aberrations and sister chromosome exchanges in peripheral lymphocytes, although the scientific rigidity of some of these studies has been questioned (EPA, 1987).

**Reproductive Effects and Teratogenicity.** High doses of inorganic arsenic compounds given to pregnant experimental animals produced various malformations in fetuses and offspring that were somewhat dependent on time and route of administration. However, no such effects have been noted in humans with excessive occupational exposures to arsenic compounds.

**Arsine.** Arsine gas is formed by the reaction of hydrogen with arsenic and is generated as a by-product in the refining of nonferrous metals. Arsine is a potent hemolytic agent, producing acute symptoms of nausea, vomiting, shortness of breath, and headache accompanying the hemolytic reaction. Exposure may be fatal and may be accompanied by hemoglobinuria and renal failure, and even jaundice and anemia in nonfatal cases when exposure persists (Fowler and Weissberg, 1974).

**Biological Indicators.** Biological indicators of arsenic exposure are blood, urine, and hair (Table 23-3). Because of the short half-life of arsenic, blood levels are only useful within a few days of acute exposure but are not useful in assessing chronic exposure. Urinary arsenic is the best indicator of current on recent exposure and has been noted to be several hundred micrograms per liter with occupational exposure. However, some marine organisms may contain very high concentrations of organoarsenicals which do not have significant toxicity and are rapidly excreted in urine without transformation (Lauwerys, 1983). Workers should be advised not to ingest seafood for a day or two before testing. Hair or even fingernail concentrations of arsenic may be helpful in evaluating past exposures, but interpretation is made difficult because of the problem of differentiating external contamination.

There are no specific biochemical parameters that reflect arsenic toxicity, but evaluation of clinical effects must be interpreted with a knowledge of exposure history.

**Treatment.** BAL is used to treat acute dermatitis and the pulmonary symptoms of excess arsenic exposure. BAL has also been used for the treatment of chronic arsenic poisoning, but there are no established biological criteria or measures of effectiveness. BAL has been used most often in cases of dermatitis, but there is usually no change in the keratotic lesions or influence on the progression to skin cancer.

Arsine toxicity is best treated symptomatically. BAL is not considered helpful (Fowler and Weissberg, 1974).

## Beryllium

Beryllium is an uncommon metal with a few specific industrial uses. Environmental sources and toxicological effects of beryllium are reviewed in detail in an EPA Health Criteria Document (EPA, 1987a; WHO, 1990a). Beryllium in the environment largely results from coal combustion. Illinois and Appalachian coal contains an average of about 2.5 ppm; oil contains about 0.08 ppm. The combustion of coal and oil contributes about 1250 or more tons of beryllium to the environment each year (mostly from coal), which is about five times the annual production for industrial use. The major industrial processes that release beryllium into the environment are beryllium extraction plants, ceramic plants, and beryllium alloy manufacturers. These industries also provide the greatest potential for occupational exposure. Currently, the major use for beryllium is as an alloy, but about 20 percent of world production is for applications utilizing the free metal in nuclear reactions, x-ray windows, and other special applications related to space optics, missile fuel, and space vehicles.

**Table 23–3**
**Biological Indicators of Arsenic Exposure**

| | NORMAL | EXCESSIVE EXPOSURE |
|---|---|---|
| Whole blood | 1–4 $\mu$g/L | Up to 50 $\mu$g/L |
| Urine* | $< 10$ $\mu$g/L | $> 100$ $\mu$g/L |
| Hair | $< 1$ $\mu$g/kg | |

* Best indicator of current or recent exposure.

**Toxicokinetics.** Knowledge of the toxicokinetics of beryllium has largely been obtained from experimental animals, particularly the rat. Clearance of inhaled beryllium is multiphasic; half is cleared in about 2 weeks; the remainder is removed slowly, and a residuum becomes fixed in the tissues probably within fibrotic granulomata. Gastrointestinal absorption of ingested beryllium probably only occurs in the acidic milieu of the stomach, where it is in the ionized form, but passes through the intestinal tract as precipitated phosphate. Removal of radiolabeled beryllium chloride from rat blood is rapid, having a half-life of about 3 h. It is distributed to all tissues, but most goes to the skeleton. High doses go predominantly to the liver, but it is gradually transferred to the bone. The half-life in tissues is relatively short, except in the lungs, and a variable fraction of an administered dose is excreted in the urine where it has a long biological half-life. Normal beryllium excretion is on the order of a few nanograms per liter.

**Skin Effects.** Contact dermatitis is the commonest beryllium-related toxic effect. Exposure to soluble beryllium compounds may result in papulovesicular lesions on the skin, which it is a delayed-type hypersensitivity reaction. The hypersensitivity is cell mediated, and passive transfer with lymphoid cells has been accomplished in guinea pigs. If contact is made with an insoluble beryllium compound, a chronic granulomatous lesion develops, which may be necrotizing or ulcerative. If insoluble beryllium-containing material becomes embedded under the skin, the lesion will not heal and may progress in severity. Use of a beryllium patch test to identify beryllium-sensitive individuals may in itself be sensitizing, so any use of this procedure as a diagnostic test is discouraged.

**Pulmonary Effects.** ***Acute Chemical Pneumonitis.*** Acute pulmonary disease from inhalation of beryllium is a fulminating inflammatory reaction of the entire respiratory tract, involving the nasal passages, pharynx, tracheobronchial airways, and the alveoli, and in the most severe cases it produces an acute fulminating pneumonitis. This occurs almost immediately following inhalation of aerosols of soluble beryllium compounds, particularly fluoride, an intermediate in the ore extraction process. Severity is dose related. Fatalities have occurred, although recovery is generally complete after a period of several weeks or even months.

***Chronic Granulomatous Disease, Berylliosis.*** This syndrome was first described among fluorescent lamp workers exposed to insoluble beryllium compounds, particularly beryllium oxide. The major symptom is shortness of breath, which in severe cases may be accompanied by cyanosis and clubbing of fingers (hypertrophic osteoarthropathy, a characteristic manifestation of chronic pulmonary disease). Chest x-rays show miliary mottling. Histologically, the alveoli contain small interstitial granulomata, which resemble those seen in sarcoidosis. In the early stages, the lesions are composed of fluid, lymphocytes, and plasma cells. Multinucleated giant cells are common. Later, the granulomas become organized with proliferation of fibrosis tissue, eventually forming small, fibrous nodules. As the lesions progress, interstitial fibrosis increases with loss of functioning alveoli, impairment of effective air–capillary gas exchange, and increasing respiratory dysfunction.

**Carcinogenicity.** Evidence for carcinogenicity of beryllium was first observed in experimental studies beginning in 1946, before the establishment of carcinogenicity in humans. Epidemiologic confirmation in humans has been evolving so that there is increasing acceptance that beryllium is in fact a human carcinogen. Studies of humans with occupational exposure to beryllium prior to 1970 were negative. However, reports of two worker populations and a registry of berylliosis cases studied earlier show a small excess of lung cancer, although the total number of cases is small. The IARC (1994) states there is sufficient evidence in humans and animals for the carcinogenicity of beryllium and its compounds.

In vitro studies of genotoxicity have shown that beryllium will induce morphological transformation in mammalian cells (Dipaolo and Casto, 1979). Beryllium will also decrease the fidelity of DNA synthesis but is negative when tested as a mutagen in bacterial systems.

## Cadmium

Cadmium is a modern toxic metal. It was only discovered as an element in 1817, and industrial use was minor until about 50 years ago. But now it is a very important metal with many applications. Its main use is in electroplating or galvanizing because of its noncorrosive properties. It is also used as a color pigment for paints and plastics, and as a cathode material for nickel-cadmium batteries. Cadmium is a by-product of zinc and lead mining and smelting, which are important sources of environmental pollution. The toxicology of cadmium is extensively reviewed by Friberg et al. (1986a) and the WHO (1992).

**Exposure.** Airborne cadmium in the present-day workplace environment is generally 0.05 or $\mu g/m^3$ or less. Air from uncontaminated areas contains less than 0.1 $\mu g/m^3$. Meat, fish, and fruit contain 1 to 50 $\mu g/kg$, grains contain 10 to 150 $\mu g/kg$, and the greatest concentrations are in the liver and kidney of animals. Shellfish, such as mussels, scallops, and oysters, may be a major source of dietary cadmium and contain 100 to 1000 $\mu g/kg$. Shellfish accumulate cadmium from the water and then bind to cadmium-binding peptides. Total daily intake from food, water and air in North America and Europe varies considerably but is estimated to be about 10 to 40 $\mu g$ per day.

Cadmium is more readily taken up by plants than other metals, such as lead. Factors contributing to cadmium's presence in soil are fallout from the air, cadmium-containing water used for irrigation, and cadmium added to fertilizers. Commercial phosphate fertilizers usually contain less than 20 mg/kg. Another source of concern about potential sources of cadmium toxicity is the use of commercial sludge to fertilize agricultural fields. Commercial sludge may contain up to 1500 mg of cadmium per kilogram of dry material (Anderson and Hahlin, 1981).

Respiratory absorption of cadmium is about 15 to 30 percent. Workplace exposure to cadmium is particularly hazardous where there are cadmium fumes or airborne cadmium. Most airborne cadmium is respirable. A major nonoccupational source of respirable cadmium is cigarettes. One cigarette contains 1 to 2 $\mu g$ cadmium, and 10 percent of the cadmium in a cigarette is inhaled (0.1 to 0.2 $\mu g$). Smoking one or more packs of cigarettes a day may double the daily absorbed burden of cadmium.

**Toxicokinetics.** Gastrointestinal absorption is less than respiratory absorption and is about 5 to 8 percent. Absorption is enhanced by dietary deficiencies of calcium and iron and by diets low in protein. Low dietary calcium stimulates synthesis of calcium-binding protein, which enhances cadmium absorption. Women with low serum ferritin levels have been shown to have twice the normal absorption of cadmium (Flanagan et al., 1978). Zinc decreases cadmium absorption, probably by stimulating production of metallothionein.

Cadmium is transported in blood by binding to red blood cells and large-molecular-weight proteins in plasma, particularly albumin. A small fraction of blood cadmium may be transported by metallotheionein. Blood cadmium levels in adults without excessive exposure is usually less than 1 μg/dL. Newborns have a low body content of cadmium, usually less than 1 mg total body burden. The placenta synthesizes metallothionein and may serve as a barrier to maternal cadmium, but the fetus may be exposed with increased maternal exposure. Human breast milk and cow's milk are low in cadmium, with less than 1 μg/kg of milk. About 50 to 75 percent of the body burden of cadmium is in the liver and kidneys; its half-life in the body is not known exactly, but it is many years and may be as long as 30 years. With continued retention, there is progressive accumulation in the soft tissues, particularly in the kidneys, through ages 50 to 60, when the cadmium burden in in soft tissues begins to decline slowly. Because of the potential for accumulation in the kidneys, there is considerable concern about the levels of dietary cadmium intake for the general population. Studies from Sweden have shown a slow but steady increase in the cadmium content of vegetables over the years. The increase in body burden has been determined from an historic autopsy study (Friberg et al., 1986).

**Toxicity.** ***Acute Toxicity.*** Acute toxicity may result from the ingestion of relatively high concentrations of cadmium, as may occur in contaminated beverages or food. Nordberg (1972) relates an instance in which nausea, vomiting, and abdominal pain occurred from consumption of drinks containing approximately 16 mg per liter of cadmium. Recovery was rapid without apparent long-term effects. Inhalation of cadmium fumes or other heated cadmium-containing materials may produce an acute chemical pneumonitis and pulmonary edema.

***Chronic Toxicity.*** The principal long-term effects of low-level exposure to cadmium are chronic obstructive pulmonary disease and emphysema and chronic renal tubular disease. There may also be effects on the cardiovascular and skeletal systems (Friberg et al., 1986).

***Chronic Pulmonary Disease.*** Toxicity to the respiratory system is proportional to the time and level of exposure. Obstructive lung disease results from chronic bronchitis, progressive fibrosis of the lower airways, and accompanying alveolar damage leading to emphysema. The lung disease is manifested by dyspnea, reduced vital capacity, and increased residual volume. The pathogenesis of the lung lesion is the turnover and necrosis of alveolar macrophages. Released enzymes produce irreversible damage to alveolar basement membranes, including the rupture of septa and interstitial fibrosis. It has been found that cadmium reduces $\alpha$-1-antitrypsin activity, perhaps enhancing pulmonary toxicity. However, no difference in plasma $\alpha$-1-antitrypsin activity could be found between cadmium-exposed workers with and without emphysema (Lauwerys et al., 1979).

***Cadmium Nephrotoxicity.*** The primary renal toxicity of cadmium affects proximal renal tubular function and is manifested by increased cadmium in the urine, proteinuria, aminoaciduria, glucosuria, and decreased renal tubular reabsorption of phosphate. Morphologic changes are nonspecific and consist of tubular cell degeneration in the initial stages, progressing to an interstitial inflammatory reaction and fibrosis. Analysis of kidney cadmium levels by in vivo neutron activation analysis and x-ray fluorescence has made it possible to study the relationship between renal cadmium levels and the occurrence of effects (Skerfving et al., 1987). The critical concentration of cadmium in the renal cortex that produces tubular dysfunction in 10 percent of the population is about 200 μg/g and is about 300 μg/g for 50 percent of the population. There is a pattern of liver and kidney cadmium levels increasing simultaneously until the average renal cortex cadmium concentration is about 300 μg/g and the average liver level is about 60 μg/g. At higher cadmium liver levels, the level in the renal cortex is disproportionately low, as cadmium is lost from the kidney (Ellis et al., 1984). Daily intake in food of 140–260 μg cadmium per day for more than 50 years or workroom air exposures of 50 μg/m$^3$ for more than 10 years have produced renal dysfunction (Thun et al., 1989; WHO, 1992). An epidemiological study of the dose–response relationship of cadmium intake from eating rice, using historical data, and $\beta_2$-microglobulinuria as an index of renal tubular dysfunction found that the total cadmium intake over a lifetime that produced an adverse health effect was 2000 mg for both men and women (Nogawa et al., 1989).

The proteinuria is principally tubular, consisting of low-molecular-weight proteins whose tubular reabsorption has been impaired by cadmium injury to proximal tubular lining cells. The predominant protein is a $\beta_2$-microglobulin, but a number of other low-molecular-weight proteins have been identified in the urine of workers with excessive cadmium exposure, such as retinol-binding protein, lysozyme, ribonuclease, and immunoglobulin light chains (Lauwerys et al., 1979). The presence of high-molecular-weight proteins in the urine, such as albumin and transferin, indicates that some workers may actually have a mixed proteinuria and suggests a glomerular effect as well. The pathogenesis of the glomerular lesion in cadmium nephropathy is not presently understood.

***The Role of Metallothionein in Cadmium Toxicity.*** The accumulation of cadmium in the kidneys without apparent toxic effect is possible because of the formation of cadmium-thionein or metallothionein, a metal–protein complex with a low molecular weight (~ 6500) (Suzuki, 1982).

The amino acid composition of metallothionein is characterized by approximately 30 percent cysteine and the absence of aromatic amino acids. Specific optical absorption is due to the existence of metal–thiolate complexes in the protein. Metallothionein contains 61 amino acids and 20 are cysteine. Structural studies using nuclear magnetic resonance spectroscopy and electron spin resonance spectroscopy have identified two distinct metal clusters in mammalian metallothionein. The clusters seem to have significant differences in their affinity for different metal ions; one of the clusters has a high level of specificity for zinc. Metal binding is by trimercaptide bridges (Boulanger et al., 1983). Metallothionein is primarily a tissue protein and is ubiquitous in most organs but it exists in the highest concentration in the liver, particularly following recent exposure, and in the kidneys, where it accumulates with age in proportion to cadmium concentration.

Cadmium bound to metallothionein within tissues is thought to be nontoxic; however, when the levels of cadmium exceed the critical concentration, it becomes toxic. The factors that determine the level of cadmium or of cadmium–metallothionein complex that is toxic are not clear, but experimental studies have shown that repeated injections of low levels of cadmium–metallothionein over several weeks results in a chronic and irreversible nephrotoxicity. Renal accumulations of cadmium were only 40 $\mu$g/g, less than the 200 $\mu$g/g suggested as the critical level in humans (Wang et al., 1993). Also, renal tubular necrosis occurs in non-cadmium exposed rats following transplantation of livers from cadmium toxic animals (Chan et al., 1993). These studies suggest that cadmium nephrotoxicity follows the slow release and renal excretion of cadmium–metallothionein from liver and other soft tissues. Cadmium–metallothionein is toxic when taken up by the proximal tubular cells complex whereas cadmium chloride at even greater concentrations in proximal tubular cells is not toxic (Dorian et al., 1995).

***The Reversibility of Renal Effects.*** Follow-up studies of persons with renal tubular dysfunction ($\beta_2$-microglobulinuria) from occupational exposure to cadmium have shown that the proteinuria is irreversible and that there is a significant increase of creatinine in serum with time, suggesting a progressive glomerulopathy (Roels et al., 1989). Also, persons with renal tubular dysfunction from excess dietary ingestion of cadmium (cadmium-polluted rice) do not have a reversal of the defect as long as 10 years after reduced exposure in cases when the $\beta_2$-microglobulinuria exceeds 1000 $\mu$g per gram of creatinine (Kido et al., 1988). Ellis (1985) has shown, however, that liver cadmium in workers no longer exposed to cadmium gradually declines. Persistence of renal tubular dysfunction after cessation of exposure may reflect the level of body burden and the shifting of cadmium from liver to kidney.

***The Skeletal System.*** Cadmium toxicity affects calcium metabolism, and individuals with severe cadmium nephropathy may have renal calculi and excess excretion of calcium, probably related to increased urinary loss, but with chronic exposure, urinary calcium may be less than normal. Associated skeletal changes are probably related to calcium loss and include bone pain, osteomalacia, and/or osteoporosis. Bone changes are part of a syndrome, Itai-Itai disease, recognized in postmenopausal multiparous women living in the Fuchu area of Japan prior to and during World War II. The syndrome consists of severe bone deformities and chronic renal disease. Excess cadmium exposure has been implicated in the pathogenesis of the syndrome, but vitamin D and perhaps other nutritional deficiencies are thought to be cofactors. Itai-Itai translates to "ouch-ouch," reflecting the accompanying bone pain. Also cadmium can affect calcium, phosphorous, and bone metabolism in both industrial workers and in people exposed in the general environment. These effects may be secondary to the cadmium effects on the kidneys, but there has been little study of calcium metabolism in people with excess exposure to cadmium. The increased prevalence of renal stones reported from certain industries is probably one manifestation of the cadmium-induced kidney effects. It is not known if certain factors other than cadmium may play a role.

Osteomalacia has been reported in a few heavily exposed industrial workers and in people with Itai-Itai disease. The industrial cases were mainly male, whereas Itai-Itai cases were almost exclusively female. However, the clinical features and biochemical findings are similar except that Itai-Itai patients may have osteoporosis as well.

Nogawa and colleagues (1987) reported that serum 1,25(OH)$_2$ vitamin D levels were lower in Itai-Itai disease patients and in cadmium-exposed subjects with renal damage than in nonexposed subjects. A decrease in serum 1,25(OH)$_2$ vitamin D levels was closely related to serum concentrations of parathyroid hormone. $\beta_2$-microglobulin and the percentage of tubular reabsorption suggest that cadmium-induced bone effects were mainly due to a disturbance in vitamin D and parathyroid hormone metabolism. Friberg and coworkers (1986) suggest that cadmium in the proximal tubular cells depresses cellular functions, which may be followed by the depressed conversion of 25(OH) vitamin D to 1,25(OH)$_2$ vitamin D. This is likely to lead to a decreased calcium absorption and a decreased mineralization of bone, which in turn may lead to osteomalacia. Bhattacharyya and coworkers (1988) found, in studies of mice, that multiparity enhanced cadmium's toxicity to bone.

***Hypertension and Cardiovascular Effects.*** Epidemiology studies suggest that cadmium is an etiological agent for essential hypertension. A recent study found an increase in systolic and diastolic blood pressures in cadmium workers. Only systolic, but not diastolic blood pressure, was significantly associated with cadmium dose in multivarate analyses (Thun et al., 1989). Studies from Japan have found a twice-as-high cerebrovascular disease mortality rate among people who had cadmium-induced renal tubular proteinuria as among people in cadmium-polluted areas without proteinuria (Nogawa et al., 1979).

Rats exposed to cadmium in drinking water (Kopp et al., 1983) developed electrocardiographic and biochemical changes in the myocardium and impairment of the functional status of the myocardium. These effects may be related to (1) decreased high-energy phosphate stored in the myocardium, (2) reduced myocardial contractility, and (3) diminished excitability of the cardiac conduction system. Jamall and Sprowls (1987) found that rats whose diets were supplemented with copper, selenium, and cadmium had a marked reduction in heart cytosolic glutathione peroxidase, superoxide dismutase, and catalase. They suggested that heart mitochondria are the site of the cadmium-induced biochemical lesion in the myocardium.

***Carcinogenicity.*** There have been a number of epidemiological studies intended to determine a relationship between occupational (respiratory) exposure to cadmium and lung cancer and prostatic cancer. A follow-up study of cadmium-nickel battery workers in Britain (Sorahan and Waterhouse, 1983) and in Sweden (Kjellström et al., 1979) found increased risks to lung and prostate cancer. An increase in respiratory cancers as also found in a re-study of a cohort in a U.S. cadmium recovery plant (Thun et al., 1985). Cadmium has recently been accepted by the International Agency for Research on Cancer as a Category 1 (human) carcinogen based primarily on its relationship to pulmonary tumors (IARC, 1994).

Animal studies have provided considerable support for the carcinogenic potential of cadmium. Cadmium chloride, oxide, sulphate, and sulphide produced local sarcomas in rats after their subcutaneous injection, and cadmium powder and cadmium sulphide produced local sarcomas in rats following their intramuscular administration. Cadmium chloride produced a dose-dependent increase in the incidence of lung carcinomas in rats after exposure by inhalation and a low incidence (5/100) of prostatic carcinomas after injection into the ventral prostate (Takenaka et al., 1983). While the evidence for a relationship between cadmium and cancer of the prostate in humans is debatable, more recent studies in rats have demonstrated carcinogenicity through the induction of cancer in the ventral prostate by oral or parenteral exposures, as well as by direct injection (Waalkes and Rehm, 1994).

***Biological Indicators.*** The most important measure of excessive cadmium exposure is increased cadmium excretion in urine. In persons in the general population without excessive cadmium exposure, urinary cadmium excretion is both small and constant. That is, it is usually on the order of only 1 or 2 $\mu$g/day, or less than 1 $\mu$g/g creatinine. With excessive exposure to cadmium, as might occur in workers, an increase in urinary cadmium may not occur until all of the available cadmium binding sites are saturated. However, when the available binding sites (e.g., metallothionein) are saturated, increased urinary cadmium reflects recent exposure, body burden, and renal cadmium concentration, so that urinary cadmium measurement does provide a good index of excessive cadmium exposure. Nogawa et al. (1979) determined the urinary concentration of cadmium corresponding to a 1 percent prevalence rate of a number of abnormal urinary findings (Table 23-4). Tubular proteinuria, as indicated by measurable excretion of $\beta_2$-microglobulin, occurred at the 1 percent prevalence rate with a urinary cadmium concentration of 3.2 $\mu$g/g of creatinine. This was at a slightly lower urinary cadmium level than other signs of renal tubular dysfunction. Retinol binding protein may be a more practical and reliable test of proximal tubular function than $\beta_2$-microglobulin because sensitive immunological analytic methods are now available, and it is more stable in urine (Lauwerys et al., 1984). Changes in urinary excretion of low-molecular-weight proteins were consistently observed in workers excreting more than 10 $\mu$g cadmium per gram of creatinine (Buchet et al., 1980). Urinary excretion of *N*-acetyl-$\beta$-D-glucosaminidase (NAG) activity may be a sensitive indicator of cadmium-induced renal tubular dysfunction (Kawada et al., 1989), but a dose–response relationship has not been established.

Most of the cadmium in urine is bound to metallothionein, and there is good correlation between metallothionein and cadmium in urine in cadmium workers with normal or abnormal renal function. Therefore, the measurement of metallothionein in urine provides the same toxicological information as the measurement of cadmium and it does not have the problem of external contamination. Radioimmunoassay techniques for measurement of metallothionein are available (Chang et al., 1980).

**Table 23–4**
**Urinary Cadmium Concentration Corresponding to 1 Percent Prevalence rate for Parameters of Renal Dysfunction**

| URINARY FINDING | URINARY CADMIUM $\mu$g/g CREATININE | |
|---|---|---|
| | *Male* | *Female* |
| Tubular proteinuria | | |
| $\beta_2$-Microglobin | 3.2 | 5.2 |
| Retinal binding protein | 4.4 | 7.4 |
| Aminoaciduria (proline) | 10.4 | 5.1 |
| Proteinuria with glucosuria | 7.4 | 7.4 |

SOURCE: Nogawa et al, 1979.

***Treatment.*** Susceptibility to cadmium-induced toxicity is influenced by a number of factors, particularly the ability of the body to provide binding sites on metallothionein. Protection may be provided by induction of metallothionein by dietary zinc, cobalt, or selenium, but the only effective treatment for cadmium toxicity is to eliminate the exposure.

## Chromium

Chromium is a generally abundant element in the earth's crust and occurs in oxidation states ranging from $Cr^{2+}$ to $Cr^{6+}$, but only trivalent and hexavalent forms are of biological significance. The trivalent is the more common form. However, hexavalent forms of chromate compounds are of greater industrial importance. Sodium chromate and dichromate are the principal substances for the production of all chromium chemicals. Sodium dichromate is produced industrially by the reaction of sulfuric acid on sodium chromate. The major source of chromium is from chromite ore. Metallurgic-grade chromite is usually converted into one of several types of ferrochromium or other chromium alloys containing cobalt or nickel. Ferrochrome is used for the production of stainless steel. Chromates are produced by a smelting, roasting, and extraction process. The major uses of sodium dichromate are for the production of chrome pigments, for the production of chrome salts used for tanning leather, mordant dying, wood preservatives, and as an anticorrosive in cooking systems, boilers, and oil drilling muds. Overviews of chromium exposures and health effect have been reviewed (Fishbein, 1981; WHO, 1988; O'Flaherty, 1995).

Chromium in ambient air originates from industrial sources, particularly ferrochrome production, ore refining, chemical and refractory processing, and combustion of fossil fuels. In rural areas, chromium in air is usually less than 0.1

$\mu g/m^3$ and in industrial cities it ranges from 0.01 to 0.03 $\mu g/m^3$. Particulates from coal-fired power plants may contain from 2.3 to 31 ppm, but this is reduced to 0.19 to 6.6 ppm by fly-ash collection. Cement-producing plants are another important potential source of atmospheric chromium. Chromium precipitates and fallout are deposited on land and water; land fallout is eventually carried to water by runoff, where it is deposited in sediments. A controllable source of chromium is waste water from chrome-plating and metal-finishing industries, textile plants, and tanneries. The chromium content in food is low; estimates of daily intake by humans are under 100 $\mu g$, mostly from food, with trivial quantities from most water supplies and ambient air.

Trivalent chromium is the most common form found in nature, and chromium in biological materials is probably always trivalent. There is no evidence that trivalent chromium is converted to hexavalent forms in biological systems. However, hexavalent chromium readily crosses cell membranes and is reduced intracellularly to trivalent chromium.

**Essentiality.** Chromium(III) is considered an essential trace nutrient serving as a component of the "glucose tolerance factor" (Mertz, 1969). It is a cofactor for insulin action and has a role in the peripheral activities of this hormone by forming a ternary complex with insulin receptors, facilitating the attachment of insulin to these sites. The most biologically active form of insulin appears to be a naturally occurring complex containing niacin as well as glycine, glutamic acid, and cysteine.

Human chromium deficiency may occur in infants suffering from protein-caloric malnutrition and in elderly people with impaired glucose tolerance, but this is not well documented. Prolonged use of a synthetic diet without chromium supplementation may lead to chromium deficiency, impaired glucose metabolism, and possibly effects on growth and on lipid and protein metabolism. The half-time for elimination of chromium from rats is 0.5, 5.9, and 83.4 days, according to a three-compartment model (Mertz, 1969).

**Toxicity.** Systemic toxicity to chromium compounds occurs largely from accidental exposures, occasional attempts to use chromium as a suicidal agent, and from previous therapeutic uses. The major effect from ingestion of high levels of chromium is acute tubular and glomerular damage. Evidence of kidney damage from lower level chronic exposure is equivocal. Animal studies of chronic exposure to Cr(VI) have not shown evidence of toxicity (O'Flaherty, 1995). Hexavalent chromium is corrosive and causes chronic ulceration and perforation of the nasal septum. It also causes chronic ulceration of other skin surfaces, which is independent of hypersensitivity reactions on skin. Allergic chromium skin reactions readily occur with exposure and are independent of dose. The known harmful effects of chromium in humans have been attributed to the hexavalent form, and it has been speculated that the biological effects of hexavalent chromium may be related to the reduction to trivalent chromium and the formation of complexes with intracellular macromolecules. Trivalent chromium compounds are considerably less toxic than the hexavalent compounds and are neither irritating nor corrosive. Nevertheless, nearly all industrial workers are exposed to both forms of chromium compounds, and at present there is no information as to whether there is a gradient of risk from predominant exposure to hexavalent or insoluble forms of chromium to exposure to soluble trivalent forms.

**Carcinogenicity.** Exposure to chromium, particularly in the chrome production and chrome pigment industries, is associated with cancer of the respiratory tract (Langard and Norseth, 1986). The mechanism of Cr(VI) carcinogenicity in the lung is believed to be its reduction to Cr(III) and its generation of reactive intermediates.

Animal studies support the notion that the most potent carcinogenic chromium compounds are the slightly soluble hexavalent compounds. Studies on in vitro bacterial systems, however, show no difference between soluble and slightly soluble compounds. Trivalent chromium salts have little or no mutagenic activity in bacterial systems. Because there is preferred uptake of the hexavalent form by cells and it is the trivalent form that is metabolically active and binds with nucleic acids within the cell, it has been suggested that the causative agent in chromium mutagenesis is trivalent chromium bound to genetic material after reduction of the hexavalent form. Costa and coworkers (1993) have shown that detection of DNA–Protein complexes may serve as a biomarker of exposure and of carcinogenic potential from occupational exposure to chromium. The possibility that chromium compounds cause cancer at sites other than the respiratory tract has been suggested but is not certain.

**Human Body Burden.** Tissue concentrations of chromium in the general population have considerable geographic variation—concentrations as high as 7 $\mu g/kg$ occur in the lungs of persons in New York or Chicago, with lower concentrations in liver and kidney. In persons without excess exposure, blood chromium concentration is between 20 and 30 $\mu g$ per liter and is evenly distributed between erythrocytes and plasma. With occupational exposure, an increase in blood chromium is related to increased chromium in red blood cells. Urinary excretion is independent of oxidation state of chromium administered to animals and is less than 10 $\mu g$/day for humans in the absence of excess exposure.

## Lead

If we were to judge of the interest excited by any medical subject by the number of writings to which it has given birth, we could not but regard the poisoning by lead as the most important to be known of all those that have been treated of, up to the present time.

*Orfila,* 1817

Lead is the most ubiquitous toxic metal and is detectable in practically all phases of the inert environment and in all biological systems. Because it is toxic to most living things at high exposures and there is no demonstrated biological need for it, the major issue regarding lead is determining the dose at which it becomes toxic. Specific concerns vary with the age and circumstances of the host, and the major risk is toxicity to the nervous system. The most susceptible populations are children, particularly toddlers, infants in the neonatal period, and the fetus. Several reviews and multiauthored books on the toxicology of lead are available (Goyer and Rhyne, 1973; Mahaffey, 1985; EPA, 1986, 1989a; Goyer, 1993; NRC, 1993).

**Exposure.** The principal route of exposure for people in the general population is food, and sources that produce excess exposure and toxic effects are usually environmental and presumably controllable. These sources include lead-based indoor paint in old dwellings, lead in dust from environmental sources, lead in contaminated drinking water, lead in air from combustion of lead-containing industrial emissions, hand-to-mouth activities of young children living in polluted environments, lead-glazed pottery and, less commonly, lead dust brought home by industrial workers on their clothes and shoes.

Dietary intake of lead has decreased since the 1940s when estimates of intake were 400–500 μg per day for U.S. populations to present levels of under 20 μg per day. One factor reducing the lead content of food has been a reduction in the use of lead-soldered cans for food and beverages (EPA, 1986).

Most municipal water supplies measured at the tap contain less than 0.05 μg/mL, so that daily intake from water is usually about 10 μg, and it is unlikely to be more than 20 μg. Corrosive water (pH 6.4) will leach lead from soldered joints and lead-containing brass fittings (NRC, 1993).

**Toxicokinetics.** Adults absorb 5 to 15 percent of ingested lead and usually retain less than 5 percent of what is absorbed. Children are known to have a greater absorption of lead than adults; one study found an average net absorption of 41.5 percent and 31.8 percent net retention in infants on regular diets. Concentrations of lead in air vary due to point source emissions but are now usually less than 1.0 $\mu g/m^3$. Since the introduction of lead-free gasoline in the U.S., airborne lead is only a minor component of total daily lead exposure. Lead in the atmosphere exists either in solid forms, dust or particulates of lead dioxide, or in the form of vapors. Lead absorption by the lungs also depends on a number of factors in addition to concentration. These include volume of air respired per day, whether the lead is in particle or vapor form, and size distribution of lead-containing particles. Only a very minor fraction of particles over 0.5 μm in mean maximal external diameter are retained in the lung but are then cleared from the respiratory track and swallowed. However, the percentage of particles less than 0.5 μm retained in the lung increases with reduction in particle size. About 90 percent of lead particles in ambient air that are deposited in the lungs are small enough to be retained. Absorption of retained lead through alveoli is relatively efficient and complete.

More than 90 percent of the lead in blood is in red blood cells. There seem to be at least two major compartments for lead in the red blood cell, one associated with the membrane and the other with hemoglobin. Small fractions may be related to other red blood cell components. Plasma ligands are not well defined, but it has been suggested that plasma and serum may contain diffusible fractions of lead in equilibrium with soft tissue or end-organ binding sites for lead. This fraction is difficult to measure accurately, but there is an equilibrium between red cell and plasma lead.

Phase I of the third National Health and Nutrition Examination Surveys (NHANES III), for the period of time from 1988 to 1991, has shown a drop in blood lead for persons ages 1 to 74 from 12.8 to 2.8 μg/dL. This is a remarkable difference from NHANES II results as shown in Fig. 23-3. The decline is attributable in large part to the introduction of lead-free gasoline and to the awareness of indoor leaded paint in housing

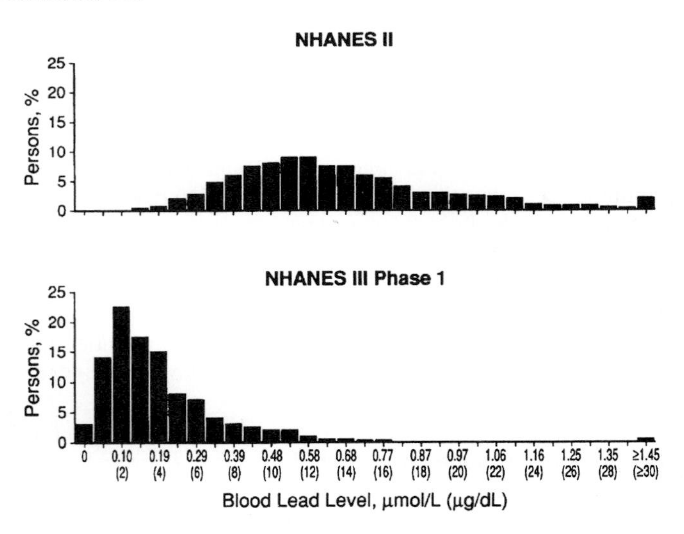


***Figure 23–3.*** ***Blood lead levels for persons aged 1 to 74: U.S., Second National Health and Nutrition Examination Survey (1976 to 1980, top) and phase 1 of the Third National Health and Nutrition Examination Survey (1988 to 1991, bottom). [From Pirkle, et al. (1994), with permission.]***

built prior to 1977. However, the geometric mean blood lead level of nonhispanic black children living in central portions of cities with more than one million people is 13.9 μg/dL, and about 35 percent of these children have blood lead levels greater than 10 μg/dL, above the guideline recommended by the Federal Centers for Disease Control (CDC) to prevent impairment of cognitive and behavioral development. These children have a greater number of the major risk factors for excessive exposure to lead, including lead-based paint in the home, exposure to urban dust, and nutritional problems such as low dietary iron and calcium which enhance lead absorption.

The total body burden of lead may be divided into at least two kinetic pools, which have different rates of turnover. The largest and kinetically slowest pool is the skeleton, with a half-life of more than 20 years, and a much more labile soft tissue pool. Lead in trabecular bone is more labile than cortical bone and trabecular bone has a shorter turnover time. Lead in bone may contribute as much as 50 percent of blood lead, so that it may be a significant source of internal exposure to lead. Mobilization of lead from maternal bone is of particular concern during pregnancy and lactation and may be mobilized in later years in persons with osteoporosis (Silbergeld et al., 1988). The fraction of lead in bone increases with age from about 70 percent of body lead in childhood to as much as 95 percent of the body burden with advancing years. The total lifetime accumulation of lead may be as much as 200 mg to over 500 mg for a worker with heavy occupational exposure.

Lead in the central nervous system tends to concentrate in gray matter and certain nuclei. The highest concentrations are in the hippocampus, followed by the cerebellum, cerebral cortex, and medulla. Cortical white matter seems to contain the least amount, but these comments are based on only a few reported human and animal studies.

Renal excretion of lead is usually with glomerular filtrate with some renal tubular resorption. With elevated blood lead levels, excretion may be augmented by transtubular transport.

Lead crosses the placenta, so that cord blood lead levels generally correlate with maternal blood lead levels but are slightly lower. Maternal blood lead decreases slightly during pregnancy probably due to hemodilution. Lead accumulation in fetal tissues, including brain, is proportional to maternal blood lead levels (Goyer, 1990b).

**Toxicity.** The toxic effects of lead and the minimum blood lead level at which the effect is likely to be observed are shown in Table 23-5. The toxic effects from lead form a continuum from clinical or overt effects to subtle or biochemical effects (Goyer, 1990a). These effects involve several organ systems and biochemical activities. The critical effects or most sensitive effects in infants and children involve the nervous system (EPA, 1989b; Needleman et al., 1990; NRC, 1993). For adults with excess occupational exposure, or even accidental exposure, the concerns are peripheral neuropathy and/or chronic nephropathy. However, the critical effect or most sensitive effect for adults in the general population may be hypertension (EPA, 1989b). Effects on the heme system provide biochemical indicators of lead exposure in the absence of chemically detectable effects, but anemia due to lead exposure is uncommon without other detectable effects or other synergistic factors. Other target organs are the gastrointestinal and reproductive systems.

Nearly all environmental exposure to lead is to inorganic compounds, even lead in food. Lead from mining wastes added to diets of experimental animals is less bioavailable than lead acetate (Freeman et al., 1994). Organolead exposures, including tetraethyl lead, have unique toxicologic patterns (Grandjean and Grandjean, 1984).

***Neurological, Neurobehavioral, and Developmental Effects in Children.*** Clinically overt lead encephalopathy may occur in children with high exposure to lead, probably at blood lead levels of 80 μg/dL or higher. Symptoms of lead encephalopathy begin with lethargy, vomiting, irritability, loss of appetite, and dizziness, progressing to obvious ataxia, a reduced level of consciousness which may progress to coma and death. The pathological findings at autopsy are severe edema of the brain due to extravasation of fluid from capillaries in the brain. This is accompanied by the loss of neuronal cells and an increase in glial cells. Recovery is often accompanied by sequelae including epilepsy, mental retardation, and, in some cases, optic neuropathy and blindness (Perlstein and Attala, 1966).

**Table 23–5**
**Lowest Observed Effect Levels for Lead-Related Health Effects**

| EFFECT | BLOOD LEAD CONCENTRATION (μg/dL) CHILDREN | ADULTS |
|---|---|---|
| Neurological | | |
| Encephalopathy (overt) | 80–100 | 100–12 |
| Hearing deficit | 20 | |
| IQ deficits | 10-15 | – |
| *In-utero* effects | 10–15 | – |
| Peripheral neuropathy | 40 | 40 |
| Hematological | | |
| Anemia | 80-100 | 80-100 |
| U-ALA | 40 | 40 |
| B-EPP | 15 | 15 |
| ALA inhibition | 10 | 10 |
| Py-5-N inhibition | 10 | – |
| Renal | | |
| Nephropathy | 40 | |
| Vitamin D metabolism | <30 | |
| Blood pressure (males) | – | 30 |
| Reproduction | | 40 |

SOURCE:

Over the past 20 or more years there have been a number of cross-sectional and prospective epidemiological studies relating blood lead levels at the time of birth, during infancy, and through early childhood with measures of psychomoter, cognitive, and behavioral outcomes. These studies have been summarized in overviews by Grant and Davis (1989) and NRC (1993). Despite differences in the ranges of blood lead represented in a cohort, most studies report a 2- to 4-point IQ deficit for each μg/dL increase in blood lead within the range of 5–35 μg/dL. A threshold is not evident from these studies.

It has been difficult to discern whether there are specific neuropsychological deficits associated with increased lead exposures. To date there are no specific indicators of the neurological effects of lead. The most sensitive indicators of adverse neurological outcomes are psychomotor tests or mental development indices, such as the Bayley Scales for infants, and broad measures of IQ, such as full-scale WISC-R IQ scores for older children. Blood lead levels at 2 years of age are more predictive of a longer term adverse neurological outcome than umbilical cord blood lead concentration. Children in the lower socioeconomic strata may begin to manifest language deficits by the second year of life which may be prevented in children with greater academic advantages. Increased blood lead levels in infancy and early childhood may be manifested in older children and adolescents as decreased attention span, reading disabilities, and failure to graduate from high school (Needleman et al., 1990).

The public health significance of small deficits in IQ may be considerable. When the actual cumulative frequency distribution of IQ between high- and low-lead subjects are plotted and compared, there is an increase in the number of children with a severe deficit, that is, IQ scores below 80. Also, the same shift truncates the upper end of the curve where there is a 5 percent reduction in children with superior function (IQ 125 or greater). There is presently no estimate of the cost of this effect at the high end of the curve but it may be of considerable importance to both society and to the individual. Small changes in IQ have been associated with differences in measures of socioeconomic status, such as income and educational achievement (Needleman, 1989).

An increase in the maternal blood lead level may also contribute to reducing gestational duration and birthweight (Moore et al., 1989; McMichael et al., 1988; Borschein et al., 1989).

An association between hearing thresholds and blood lead greater than 20 μg/dL has been found in teenagers (Schwartz et al., 1991).

***Mechanisms of Neurotoxicity.*** Neurodevelopment is highly complex and there are numerous opportunities for lead to interfere with normal development. Silbergeld (1992) has divided the intrauterine neurological developmental effects of lead into two broad categories, morphological effects and pharmacological effects. A highly significant morphological effect is the result of lead impairment of the timed programming of cell-to-cell connections, resulting in the modification of neuronal circuitry. Cookman et al. (1988) found that lead induces precocious differentiation of the glia upon which cells migrate to their eventual positions during structuring of the central nervous system.

Lead functions pharmacologically by interfering with synaptic mechanisms of transmitter release. It is suggested that lead can substitute for calcium and possibly for zinc in ion-dependent events at the synapse and is responsible for the observed impairment of various neurotransmitter systems (e.g., cholinergic, noradrenergic, GABergic, and dopaminergic). Markovac and Goldstein (1988) found that micromolecular concentrations of lead activate protein kinase C in brain microvessels. This is a calcium-dependent kinase which acts as a second messenger in the regulation of cellular metabolism. Impairment results in breakdown of the normally tight blood–brain barrier.

Lead may replace calcium in calmodulin-dependent reactions, and it may inhibit membrane-bound Na,K-ATPase, and interfere with the mitochondrial release of calcium and with energy metabolism (Simons, 1986). These effects are potentially reversible if lead can be removed from active sites. At present, there is no information as to whether reduction of blood lead levels, either by removal from exposure or by chelation therapy, removes lead from these sensitive molecular sites.

The fetal brain may be particularly sensitive to the toxic effects of lead because of the immaturity of the blood–brain barrier in the fetus. Rossouw et al. (1987) found a greater uptake of lead by the fetal rat brain during gestation than occurred after birth. Experimental studies suggest that the immature endothelial cells forming capillaries of the developing brain are less resistant to the effects of lead than capillaries from mature brains, and they permit fluid and cations including lead to reach newly formed components of the brain, including astrocytes and neurons.

***Peripheral Neuropathy.*** Peripheral neuropathy is a classic manifestation of lead toxicity, particularly the footdrop and wristdrop that characterized the house painter and other workers with excessive occupational exposure to lead more than a half-century ago. Segmental demyelination and possibly axonal degeneration follow lead-induced Schwann cell degeneration. Wallerian degeneration of the posterior roots of sciatic and tibial nerves is possible, but sensory nerves are less sensitive to lead than motor nerve structure and function. Motor nerve dysfunction, assessed clinically by electrophysiological measurement of nerve conduction velocities, has been shown to occur with blood lead levels as low as 40 $\mu$g/dL (EPA, 1986).

***Hematological Effects.*** Lead has multiple hematologic effects. In lead-induced anemia, the red blood cells are microcytic and hypochromic, as in iron deficiency, and usually there are increased numbers of reticulocytes with basophilic stippling, which results from inhibition of the enzyme pyrimidine-5-nucleosidase (Py-5-N) (Paglia et al., 1975). There is an inverse relationship between Py-5-N inhibition and blood lead concentration. A threshold for Py-5-N inhibition has been found to be 44 $\mu$g/dL or higher, but a study of 21 children aged 2 to 5 found no threshold of effects of lead on the activity of this enzyme or on cell nucleotide contents even below 10 $\mu$g/dL. There was also a significant positive correlation of pyrimidine accumulation and the accumulation of zinc protoporphyrin (ZPP). Inhibition of Py-5-N activity and nucleotide accumulation with lead exposure affects erythrocyte membrane stability and survival by altering cell energy metabolism.

The anemia that occurs in lead poisoning results from two basic defects: shortened erythrocyte lifespan and impairment of heme synthesis. Shortened lifespan of the red blood cell is thought to be due to increased mechanical fragility of the cell membrane. The biochemical basis for this effect is not known but the effect is accompanied by inhibition of sodium- and potassium-dependent ATPase's (EPA, 1986).

A schematic presentation of the effects of lead on heme synthesis is shown in Fig. 23-4. Probably the sensitive effect is inhibition of $\delta$-aminolevulinic acid dehydratase (ALA-D), resulting in a negative exponential relationship between ALA-D and blood lead. There is also depression of coproporphyrinogen oxidase, resulting in increased coproporphyrin activity. Lead also decreases ferrochelatase activity. This enzyme catalyzes the incorporation of the ferrous ion into the porphyrin ring structure. Bessis and Jensen (1965) have shown that iron in the form of apoferritin and ferruginous micelles may accumulate in mitochondria of bone marrow reticulocytes from lead-poisoned rats. Failure to insert iron into protoporphyrin results in depressed heme formation. The excess protoporphyrin takes the place of heme in the hemoglobin molecule and, as the red blood cells containing protoporphyrin circulate, zinc is chelated at the center of the molecule at the site usually occupied by iron. Red blood cells containing zinc-protoporphyrin are intensely fluorescent and may be used to diagnose lead toxicity. Depressed heme synthesis is thought to be the stimulus for increasing the rate of activity of the first step in the heme synthetic pathway. Delta-aminolevulinic acid synthetase, by virtue of negative feedback control. As a consequence, the increased production of $\delta$-aminolevulinic acid (ALA) and decreased activity of ALA-D result in a marked increase in circulating blood levels and urinary excretion of $\delta$-ALA. Prefeeding of lead to experimental animals also raises heme oxygenase activity, resulting in some increase in bilirubin

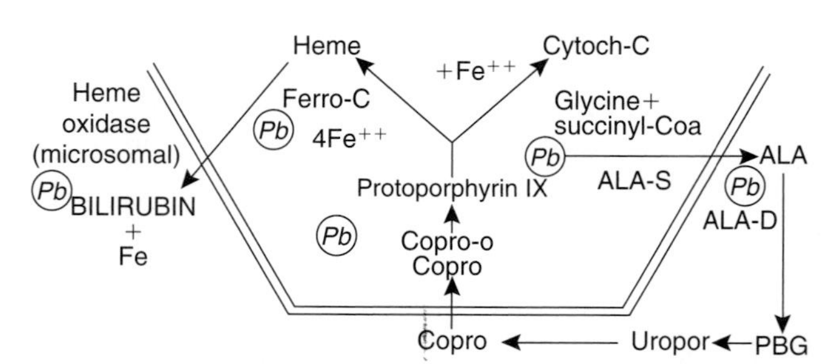


***Figure 23–4. Scheme of heme synthesis showing sites where lead has an effect.***

*CoA*, coenzyme A; *ALA-S*, aminolevulinic acid synthetase; *ALA*, $\delta$-aminolevulinic acid; *ALA-D*, aminolevulinic acid dehydratase; *PBG*, porphobilinogen; *Uropor*, uroporphyrinogen; *Copro*, coproporphyrinogen; *Copro-O*, coproporphyrinogen oxidase; *Ferro-C*, ferrochelatase; *Cytoch-C*, cytochrome c; *Pb*, site for lead effect.

formation. The change in rates of activity of these enzymes by lead produces a dose-related alteration in activity of affected enzymes, but anemia only occurs in very marked lead toxicity. The changes in enzyme activities, particularly ALA-D in peripheral blood and excretion of ALA in urine, correlate very closely with actual blood lead levels and serve as early biochemical indices of lead exposure (EPA, 1986).

The sensitivity of specific individuals to lead's effect on heme metabolism may be related to genetic polymorphisms of heme among people in the general population (EPA, 1986). The ALA-D gene has two common alleles, ALA-$D^1$ and ALA-$D^2$, which results in a polymorphic enzyme system with three distinct isozyme phenotypes, identified as ALA-D1-1, ALA-D1-2, and ALA-D2-2. Frequency of the isoenzyme phenotypes determined in an Italian population are 1-1, (81%), 2-1 (17%), 2-2 (2%), whereas expression of ALA-D2 was not observed in blacks in Liberia. At the biochemical level no differences in reactivation of the isoenzymes has been reported. It has been suggested that individuals with 22-2 phenotype may lead to increased lead accumulation and associated physiological effects (Ziemsen et al., 1986). The $D^2$ allele may provide a basis for increased sensitivity to lead (Astrin et al., 1987).

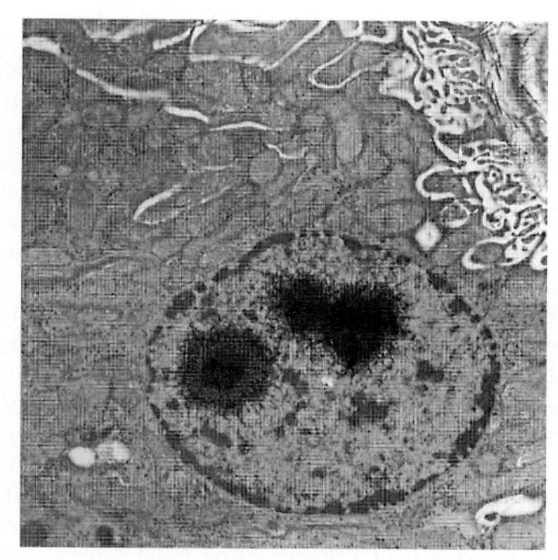

***Figure 23–5. Lead-induced inclusion bodies in nucleus of renal tubular lining cell.***

***Renal Effects.*** Lead nephropathy is one of the oldest recognized health effects of lead (Oliver, 1902). It has been a major hazard from industrial exposure. However, with progressive reduction of exposure in the workplace and more sensitive biological indicators of renal toxicity, lead nephropathy should be a vanishing disease. The pathogenesis of lead nephropathy is described in stages, or as acute (reversible) or chronic (irreversible). Lead is a renal carcinogen in rodents but whether it is carcinogenic to people is unclear.

Acute lead nephrotoxicity is limited to functional and morphologic changes in proximal tubular cells (Goyer and Rhyne, 1973). It is manifested clinically by decrease in energy-dependent transport functions, including aminoaciduria, glycosuria, and ion transport. The functional changes are thought to be related to a lead effect on mitochondrial respiration and phosphorylation. In experimental models and in biopsies from children with lead toxicity there are ultrastructural changes in mitochondria consisting of swelling with distorted cristae. Mitochondria isolated from lead-poisoned rats show decreased state III respiration. These changes are reversible by treatment with a chelating agent.

A characteristic microscopic change is the formation of a lead–protein complex which appears in renal tubular cells as inclusion bodies. By light microscopy the inclusions are dense, homogeneous, eosinophilic bodies. They are acid-fast when stained with carbolfuchsin. Ultrastructurally, the bodies have a dense central core as shown in Fig. 23-5. The bodies are composed of a lead–protein complex (Goyer et al., 1970). The protein is acidic and contains large amounts of aspartic and glutamic acids and little cystine. It is suggested that lead binds loosely to the carboxyl groups of the acidic amino acids (Moore et al., 1973). Treatment of lead-exposed animals with chelating agents such as EDTA is accompanied by a sudden increase of urinary lead, which is at a maximum 12 to 24 h after treatment (Goyer and Wilson, 1975). Also, no inclusion bodies are found in people after treatment with EDTA. The bodies may be found intact in the urinary sediment of workmen with heavy exposure to lead. The inclusion bodies account for the major fraction of intracellular lead and may provide a major pathway for the cellular excretion of lead (Goyer, 1971b). The origin of the protein forming the inclusion bodies is uncertain. Egle and Shelton (1986) have shown that a nuclear matrix protein termed *p32/6.3* is the most abundant protein component of the inclusion bodies. Lead will form inclusion bodies in the cytoplasm of kidney cells grown in culture and tends to migrate into nuclei secondarily (McLaughlin et al., 1980).

Renal biopsies from a group of shipwreckers with heavy exposure to lead have shown that the histologic features of early and chronic exposure to lead are similar in experimental animals and humans, suggesting similar pathogenetic mechanisms. Nuclear inclusion bodies become less common as renal tubules atrophy and as interstitial fibrosis increases in severity. Proximal tubular dysfunction is usually not demonstrable in the chronic phase of lead nephropathy, but interstitial fibrosis is usually associated with asymptomatic renal azotemia and reduced glomerular filtration rate. In workers without azotemia but with decreased inulin clearance, there is decreased maximum re-absorption of glucose. Although progression from acute reversible to chronic, irreversible lead nephropathy has not been clearly shown to occur in humans, this progression has been demonstrated in rodent models (Goyer, 1971a).

There is not a specific biomarker for lead-induced renal disease. Lead may produce a chronic interstitial nephropathy, most commonly with blood lead levels greater than 60 $\mu$g/dL. Steenland et al. (1992) reviewed the patterns of death for a cohort of 1987 male smelter workers employed between 1940 and 1965. Although overall mortality was similar to that of the U.S. white male population, there was an excess mortality from chronic renal disease. The study showed that the risk of death from renal disease increased with increasing duration of employment. In a mortality study of 4519 battery plant workers and 2300 lead production workers by Cooper and coworkers (1985), there was excess mortality from chronic nephritis. The mean blood concentration of 1326 of the battery workers in this study with three or more analyses was

62.7 $\mu$g/100 g. For the lead production workers in four plants the mean for 537 men was 79.7 $\mu$g/100 g. Gennart and colleagues (1992) found that none of the indicators of renal function, including red blood-plasma (RBP), $\beta_2$-microglobin, albumin and NAG in urine, and creatinine in serum did not differ from controls, and did not correlate with blood lead levels (mean 51 $\mu$g/dL, range 40–75) or duration of exposure. This finding is consistent with the observation of Buchet and coworkers (1980) that workers who do not have recorded blood lead levels over 62 or 63 $\mu$g/dL for up to 12 years do not have lead nephropathy. However, depressed glomerular filtration rates have been reported in a group of lead-exposed workers whose blood lead levels were as low as 40 $\mu$g/dL. Some studies report correlations of blood lead levels as low as 30 $\mu$g/dL with urinary levels of NAG and urinary and serum $\beta_2$-microglobulin, but these findings are not confirmed by others (Buchet et al., 1980; Gennart et al., 1992). Increase in urinary $\beta_2$-microglobulin is not a characteristic finding in lead-induced nephropathy and there is no meaningful correlation with blood lead levels (Bernard and Lauwerys, 1989). Also, Ong et al. (1987) were not able to find a dose–response relationship between blood lead levels and urinary excretion of NAG. Urinary excretion of NAG might occur at an early stage of lead nephropathy, perhaps reflecting increased urinary leakage from damaged renal tubular epithelium.

Cardenas et al. (1993) compared a battery of more than 20 potential indicators in lead- exposed workers with an average blood lead level of 48 $\mu$g/dL with nonlead-exposed controls. The battery of tests included parameters capable of detecting functional deficits (high and low molecular weight urinary proteins), biochemical alterations (e.g., urinary eicosanoids, glycoaminoglycans, and sialic acid) and indicators of cell damage (e.g., urinary tubular antigens and enzymes). The most outstanding effect in workers exposed to lead was an interference with renal synthesis of eicosanoids resulting in lower urinary excretion of 6-keto-prostaglandin F1 and an enhanced excretion of thromboxane (TXB1). These changes were not associated with any sign of renal dysfunction and the health significance of these changes is unknown. They are most likely reversible biochemical effects and need further study. Increased excretion of tubular cell antigens was positively associated with duration of exposure. There was also increased excretion of sialic acid. However, there was no significant change in urinary excretion of kallikrein. Decrease in urinary excretion of this enzyme, which mediates vasodilation, has been found in exposed workers with blood lead levels higher than were present in workers in this study and has been suggested as a possible factor in lead-related hypertension (Boscolo et al., 1981).

Other studies have shown subtle effects of lead on heme-containing enzyme systems, such as the synthesis of cytochrome b and decreased vitamin D metabolism. Vitamin D synthesis requires a heme-containing hydroxylase enzyme in the kidney for the hydroxylation of 25-hydroxyvitamin D to 1,25-dehydroxy-vitamin D, which is important in the gastrointestinal absorption of calcium. These effects may occur below the levels of lead that alter other biomarkers for nephrotoxicity (Goyer, 1990a).

The relationship between chronic lead exposure and gouty nephropathy, suggested more than a hundred years ago by the English physician Garrod, has received recent support from studies showing that gout patients with renal disease have a greater chelate-provoked lead excretion than do renal patients without gout. Lead reduces uric acid excretion. Elevated blood uric acid has been demonstrated in rats with chronic lead nephropathy (Goyer, 1971a).

***Blood Pressure Effects.*** An increase in blood pressure is probably the most sensitive adverse health effect from lead exposure occurring in the adult population. The Addendum to the 1986 EPA Air Quality Criteria for Lead Document (EPA, 1989b) noted that a number of epidemiological studies provided generally consistent evidence for the association between increased blood pressure and an elevated body burden of lead in adults.

The largest study populations have been the second National Health and Nutrition Examination Survey (NHANES II) for the U.S. population, performed during the years 1976 to 1980, and the British Regional Heart Study, an ongoing evaluation of men aged 40–59 from 24 British towns. The data collectively provides highly convincing evidence demonstrating small but statistically significant associations between blood lead levels and increased blood pressure in adult men, and it shows the strongest association for males aged 40–59 and for systolic somewhat more than for diastolic blood pressure. Virtually all of the analyses demonstrate positive associations for the 40- to 59-year-old group which remain or become significant (at $p < 0.05$) when adjustments are made for geographic site. Quantitatively, the relationship appears to hold across a wide range of blood lead values extending down to as low as 7 $\mu$g/dL for middle-aged men. An estimated increase of about 1.5–3.0 mmHg in systolic blood pressure occurs for every doubling of blood lead concentration in adult males, but for the same blood lead levels the estimated increase is less than 1.0–2.0 mmHg for adult females (Tyroler et al., 1988).

Lead may affect blood pressure by altering sensitivity of vascular smooth muscle to vasoactive stimuli, or indirectly by altering neuroendocrine input to vascular smooth muscle. Lead-exposed persons may have higher plasma renin activity than normal during periods of modest exposure, but during more chronic severe exposures they may show normal or depressed plasma renin activity (Vander, 1988). Boscolo et al. (1981) found a slight but significant relationship between plasma renin and urinary kallikrein in men with occupational exposure to lead. Lead exposure may alter calcium-activated functions of vascular smooth muscle cells including contractility by decreasing $Na^+/K^+$-ATPase activity and stimulation of the Na/Ca exchange pump.

***Reproductive Effects.*** Overt or clinically apparent lead toxicity has long been associated with sterility and neonatal deaths in man. Gametotoxic effects have been demonstrated in both male and female animals (Stowe and Goyer, 1971). A few clinical studies have found increased chromosomal defects in workers with blood lead levels above 60 $\mu$g/dL. More recently, Assenato and coworkers reported reduction in sperm counts and abnormal sperm motility and morphology in lead battery workers down to blood lead levels of 40 $\mu$g/dL (Assenato et al., 1986). Decreases in testicular endocrine function were found to be related to duration of lead exposure of smelter workers with mean blood lead level of 60 $\mu$g/dL (Rodamilans et al., 1988).

***Carcinogenicity.*** Lead is classified as a 2B carcinogen by the IARC (1987) (Table 23-2). A study of workmen in England many years ago with occupational exposure to lead did not show an increased incidence of cancer (Dingwall-Fordyce and Lane, 1963). Causes of mortality in 7000 lead workers in the United States showed a slight excess of deaths from cancer (Cooper and Gaffey, 1975), but the statistical significance of these findings has been debated (Kang et al., 1980; Cooper, 1980). The most common tumors found were of the respiratory and digestive systems, not the kidney. However, case reports of renal adenocarcinoma in workmen with prolonged occupational exposure to lead have appeared (Baker et al., 1980; Lilis, 1981).

Lead compounds stimulate the proliferation of renal tubular epithelial cells (Choie and Richter, 1980) and similar effects have been noted in the livers of rats (Columbano et al., 1983). Lead compounds induce cell transformation in Syrian hamster embryo cells (DiPaolo and Casto, 1979; Zelikoff et al., 1988).

Lead induction of renal adenocarcinoma in rats and mice is dose related and has not been reported at levels below that which produces nephrotoxicity (EPA, 1989b). The pathogenesis of lead-related renal tumors may be a related direct genetic effect on renal tubular cells, but it may also be a nonspecific response to epithelial hyperplasia as has been noted in other experimental nephropathies and human diseases where renal tubular cysts and hyperplasia occur (Bernstein et al., 1987).

***Other Effects.*** Lead lines (Burton's lines) or purple-blue discoloration of gingiva is a classical feature of severe lead toxicity in children with lead encephalopathy. However, this feature of lead toxicity as well as the presence of lead lines at the epiphyseal margins of long bones seen on x-rays of children with severe lead exposure are uncommon today.

***Treatment.*** Foremost in the treatment of increased blood lead levels and lead toxicity is removal of the subject from source(s) of exposure. At what blood lead levels should treatment with chelating drugs begin is debatable. Certainly, chelation usually has a role in the treatment of the symptomatic worker or child. Institution of chelation therapy is probably warranted in workmen with blood lead levels over 60 $\mu$g/100 mL, but this determination must be made after an assessment of exposure factors, including biological estimates of clinical and biochemical parameters of toxicity. For children, criteria have been established that may serve as guidelines to assist in evaluating the individual case (CDC, 1991). For children with severe lead poisoning, including encephalopathy, chelation therapy is standard practice. Even then, the mortality rate may be 25 to 38 percent when EDTA or BAL is used singly whereas combination therapy of EDTA and BAL has been shown to be effective in reducing mortality. The oral chelating agent Succimer (DMSA) has been licensed recently by the U.S. Food and Drug Administration for reduction of blood lead levels of 45 $\mu$g or greater. As stated above in a previous section of this chapter, it is not known what effect reduction of blood lead levels has on the removal of lead from the nervous system or on the reversal of neurological effects of lead.

## Mercury

No other metal better illustrates the diversity of effects caused by different chemical species than does mercury (WHO, 1990b; WHO, 1991). On the basis of chemical speciation, there are three forms of mercury: elemental, inorganic, and organic compounds, each of which has characteristic toxicokinetics and health effects.

**Exposure.** The major source of mercury is the natural degassing of the earth's crust, including land areas, rivers, and the ocean, and this source is estimated to produce on the order of 2700 to 6000 tons per year. About 10,000 tons of mercury per year are mined but there is considerable year-to-year variation. The total man-made release into the atmosphere is about 2000 to 3000 tons, and it is difficult to assess what quantities of mercury come from human activities and what quantities from natural sources. Run-off into natural bodies of water may contain mercury from both anthropogenic and natural sources, so it is difficult to assess how much released into the atmosphere is from man-made or natural sources. Nevertheless, mining, smelting, and industrial discharge have been factors in environmental contamination in the past. For instance, it is estimated that loss in water effluent from chloralkali plants, one of the largest users of mercury, has been reduced to 99 percent in recent years. Also, the use of mercury in the paper pulp industries has been reduced dramatically and has been banned in Sweden since 1966. Industrial activities not directly employing mercury or mercury products give rise to substantial quantities of this metal. Fossil fuel may contain as much as 1 ppm of mercury, and it is estimated that about 5000 tons of mercury per year may be emitted from burning coal, natural gas, and from the refining of petroleum products. Calculations based on the mercury content of the Greenland ice cap show an increase from the year 1900 to the present and suggest that the increment is related both to an increase in background levels of mercury in rainwater and to man-made release. Metallic mercury in the atmosphere represents the major pathway of global transport of mercury. Regardless of source, both organic and inorganic forms of mercury may undergo environmental transformation. Metallic mercury may be oxidized to inorganic divalent mercury, particularly in the presence of organic material such as in the aquatic environment. Divalent inorganic mercury may, in turn, be reduced to metallic mercury when conditions are appropriate for reducing reactions to occur. This is an important conversion in terms of the global cycle of mercury and a potential source of mercury vapor that may be released to the earth's atmosphere. A second potential source of alkylation of divalent mercury is methylation to dimethyl mercury by anaerobic bacteria. Methyl mercury is of major toxicological significance. If it is taken up into the food chain by fish, it may eventually cycle through humans or it may diffuse into the atmosphere and return to the earth's crust or to bodies of water as methyl mercury in rainfall.

**Toxicokinetics.** The toxicity of various forms or salts of mercury is related to cationic mercury per se whereas solubility, biotransformation, and tissue distribution are influenced by the valence state and an anionic component (Berlin, 1986).

Metallic or elemental mercury volatilizes to mercury vapor at ambient air temperatures, and most human exposure is by inhalation. Mercury vapor readily diffuses across the alveolar membrane and is lipid soluble so that it has an affinity for red blood cells and the central nervous system. Metallic mercury, such as may be swallowed from a broken thermometer, is only slowly absorbed by the gastrointestinal tract (0.01 percent) at a rate related to the vaporization of the elemental mercury and is generally thought to be of no toxicological consequence.

Inorganic mercury salts may be divalent (mercuric) or monovalent (mercurous). Gastrointestinal absorption of inorganic salts of mercury from food is less than 15 percent in mice and about 7 percent in a study of human volunteers, whereas absorption of methyl mercury is on the order of 90 to 95 percent. Distribution between red blood cells and plasma also differs. For inorganic mercury salts the cell : plasma ratio ranges from a high of two with high exposure to less than one, but for methyl mercury it is about ten. The distribution ratio of the two forms of mercury between hair and blood also differs; for organic mercury it is about 250.

Kidneys contain the greatest concentrations of mercury following exposure to inorganic salts of mercury and mercury vapor, whereas organic mercury has a greater affinity for the brain, particularly the posterior cortex. However, mercury vapor has a greater predilection for the central nervous system than do inorganic mercury salts, but less than organic forms of mercury. Excretion of mercury from the body is by way of urine and feces, again differing with the form of mercury, size of the dose, and time after exposure. Exposure to mercury vapor is followed by exhalation of a small fraction, but fecal excretion is the major and predominant route of excretion initially, after exposure to inorganic mercury. Renal excretion increases with time. About 90 percent of methyl mercury is excreted in feces after acute or chronic exposure and does not change with time (Miettinen, 1973).

All forms of mercury cross the placenta to the fetus, but most of what is known has been learned from experimental animals. Fetal uptake of elemental mercury in rats, probably because of lipid solubility, has been shown to be 10 to 40 times higher than uptake after exposure to inorganic salts. Concentrations of mercury in the fetus after exposure to alkylmercuric compounds are twice those found in maternal tissues, and methyl mercury levels in fetal red blood cells are 30 percent higher than in maternal red cells. The positive fetal–maternal gradient and increased concentration of mercury in fetal red blood cells enhance fetal toxicity to mercury, particularly following exposure to alkyl mercury. Although maternal milk may contain only 5 percent of the mercury concentration of maternal blood, neonatal exposure to mercury may be increased by nursing (Grandjean et al., 1994).

***Metabolic Transformation and Excretion.*** Elemental or metallic mercury is oxidized to divalent mercury after absorption to tissues in the body and is probably mediated by catalases. Inhaled mercury vapor absorbed into red blood cells is transformed to divalent mercury, but a portion is also transported as metallic mercury to more distal tissues, particularly the brain, where biotransformation may occur. Methyl mercury undergoes biotransformation to divalent mercury compounds in tissues by cleavage of the carbon–mercury bond. There is no evidence of formation of any organic form of mercury in mammalian tissues. The aryl (phenyl) compounds are converted to inorganic mercury more rapidly than the shorter-chain alkyl (methyl) compounds. The relationship of these differences in rate of biotransformation versus rate of excretion and toxicity is not well understood. In those instances where the organomercurial is more rapidly excreted than inorganic mercury, increasing the rate of biotransformation will decrease the rate of excretion. Phenyl and methoxyethyl mercury are excreted at about the same rate as inorganic mercury whereas methyl mercury excretion is slower (Berlin, 1986).

Biological half-times are available for a limited number of mercury compounds. Biological half-time for methyl mercury is about 70 days and is virtually linear, whereas the half-time for salts of inorganic mercury is about 40 days. There are few studies on biological half-times for elemental mercury or mercury vapor, but it also appears to be linear with a range of values from 35 to 90 days.

***Cellular Metabolism.*** Within cells, mercury may bind to a variety of enzyme systems including those of microsomes and mitochondria, producing nonspecific cell injury or cell death. It has a particular affinity for ligands containing sulfhydryl groups. In liver cells, methyl mercury forms soluble complexes with cysteine and glutathione, which are secreted in bile and reabsorbed from the gastrointestinal tract. Organomercurial diuretics are thought to be absorbed in the proximal-tubule-binding specific receptor sites that inhibit sodium transport. In general, however, organomercury compounds undergo cleavage of the carbon–mercury bond releasing ionic inorganic mercury.

Mercuric mercury, but not methyl mercury, induces synthesis of metallothionein probably only in kidney cells, but unlike cadmium-metallothionein it does not have a long biological half-life. Mercury within renal cells becomes localized in lysosomes (Madsen and Christensen, 1978).

**Toxicology.** ***Mercury Vapor.*** Inhalation of mercury vapor (elemental mercury) may produce an acute, corrosive bronchitis and interstitial pneumonitis and, if not fatal, may be associated with symptoms of central nervous system effects such as tremor or increased excitability. With chronic exposure to mercury vapor the major effects are on the central nervous system. Early signs are nonspecific and have been termed the "asthenic-vegetative syndrome" or "micromercurialism." Identification of the syndrome requires neurasthenic symptoms and three or more of the following clinical findings: tremor, enlargement of the thyroid, increased uptake of radioiodine in the thyroid, labile pulse, tachycardia, dermographism, gingivitis, hematologic changes, or increased excretion of mercury in urine. With increasing exposure the symptoms become more characteristic, beginning with intentional tremors of muscles that perform fine-motor functions (highly innervated), such as fingers, eyelids, and lips, and may progress to generalized trembling of the entire body and violent chronic spasms of the extremities. This is accompanied by changes in personality and behavior, with loss of memory, increased excitability (erethism), severe depression, and even delirium and hallucination. Another characteristic feature of mercury toxicity is severe salivation and gingivitis.

The triad of increased excitability, tremors, and gingivitis has been recognized historically as the major manifestation of mercury poisoning from inhalation of mercury vapor and exposure to mercury nitrate in the fur, felt, and hat industry (Goldwater, 1972).

Sporadic instances of proteinuria and even nephrotic syndrome may occur in persons with exposure to mercury vapor, particularly with chronic occupational exposure. The pathogenesis is probably immunologically similar to that which may occur following exposure to inorganic mercury. There is growing concern that the toxic potential of mercury vapor released from dental amalgams may cause various health effects. Estimates of absorption of mercury by an adult with the average number of amalgams (8 per adult) is 30 to 40 percent of the total mercury exposure of 5 to 6 $\mu$g per day (Richardson et al., 1995). An increase in urinary mercury and accumulation in several organs including the central nervous system and kidneys has been related to the release of mercury from dental amalgams (Clarkson et al., 1988; Langworth et al., 1988). Aposhian and coworkers (1992) found a highly positive correlation between mercury excreted in urine following the administration of DMPS and numbers of dental amalgams. However, this level of mercury exposure is believed to be below that which will produce any discernible health effect except for highly sensitive people.

***Mercuric Salts.*** Mercuric compounds of mercury or bichloride of mercury (corrosive sublimate) is the best-known inorganic salt of mercury, and the trivial name suggests its most apparent toxicological effect when ingested in concentrations greater than 10 percent. A reference from the Middle Ages in Goldwater's book on mercury describes oral ingestion of mercury as causing severe abdominal cramps, bloody diarrhea, and suppression of urine (Goldwater, 1972). This is an accurate report of the effects following accidental or suicidal ingestion of mercuric chloride or other mercuric salts. Corrosive ulceration, bleeding, and necrosis of the gastrointestinal tract are usually accompanied by shock and circulatory collapse. If the patient survives the gastrointestinal damage, renal failure occurs within 24 h owing to necrosis of the proximal tubular epithelium followed by oliguria, anuria, and uremia. If the patient can be maintained by dialysis, regeneration of the tubular lining cells is possible. These changes may be followed by ultrastructural changes consistent with irreversible cell injury, including actual disruption of mitochondria, release of lysosomal enzymes, and rupture of cell membranes.

Injection of mercuric chloride produces necrosis of the epithelium of the pars recta kidney (Gritzka and Trump, 1968). Cellular changes include fragmentation and disruption of the plasma membrane and its appendages, vesiculation and disruption of the endoplasmic reticulum and other cytoplasmic membranes, dissociation of polysomes and loss of ribosomes, mitochondrial swelling with appearance of amorphous intramatrical deposits, and condensation of nuclear chromatin. These changes are common to renal cell necrosis due to various causes. Slight tubular cell injury may occur in workers with low-level exposure to metallic mercury vapor manifested by enzymuria and low molecular weight proteinuria (Roels et al., 1985).

Although exposure to a high dose of mercuric chloride is directly toxic to renal tubular lining cells, chronic low-dose exposure to mercuric salts or even elemental mercury vapor levels may induce an immunological glomerular disease. This form of chronic mercury injury to the kidney is clinically the most common form of mercury-induced nephropathy. Exposed persons may develop a proteinuria that is reversible after workers are removed from exposure.

Experimental studies have shown that the pathogenesis of chronic mercury nephropathy has two phases: an early phase characterized by an antibasement membrane glomerulonephritis followed by a superimposed immune-complex glomerulonephritis with transiently raised concentrations of circulating immune complexes (Henry et al., 1988). The pathogenesis of the nephropathy in humans appears similar, although antigens have not been characterized. Also, the early glomerular nephritis may progress in humans to an interstitial immune complex nephritis (Pelletier and Druet, 1995).

***Mercurous Mercury.*** Mercurous compounds of mercury are less corrosive and less toxic than mercuric salts, presumably because they are less soluble. Calomel, a powder containing mercurous chloride, has a long history of use in medicine. Perhaps the most notable modern usage has been as teething powder for children and is now known to be responsible for acrodynia or "pink disease." This is most likely a hypersensitivity response to the mercury salts in skin producing vasodilation, hyperkeratosis, and hypersecretion of sweat glands. Children develop fever, a pink-colored rash, swelling of the spleen and lymph nodes, and hyperkeratosis and swelling of fingers. The effects are independent of dose and are thought to be a hypersensitivity reaction (Matheson et al., 1980).

***Methyl Mercury.*** Methyl mercury is the most important form of mercury in terms of toxicity and health effects from environmental exposures. Many of the effects produced by short-term alkyls are unique in terms of mercury toxicity but nonspecific in that they may be found in other disease states. Most of what is known about the clinical signs and symptoms and neuropathology of high-level or overt methyl mercury toxicity has been learned from studies of epidemics in Japan and Iraq (WHO, 1990b; Berlin, 1986), from studies of populations eating mercury-contaminated fish (Skerving, 1974), and from published reports of occupational exposures (Eyssen et al., 1983). Observations of changes in nonhuman primates studied experimentally are consistent with findings in humans and therefore provide additional information about time, dose, and tissue burden relationship, particularly for subclinical and subtle, low-level effects (Mottet et al., 1985).

The major human health effects from exposure to methyl mercury are neurotoxic effects in adults (Bakir et al., 1973) and toxicity to the fetuses of mothers exposed to methyl mercury during pregnancy (Cox et al., 1989). The major source of exposure for people in the general population is from the consumption of fish, and in this instance the brain is the critical organ. A genotoxic effect resulting in chromosomal aberrations also has been demonstrated in methyl mercury-exposed populations.

Clinical manifestations of neurotoxic effects are (1) paresthesia, a numbness and tingling sensation around the mouth, lips, and extremities, particularly the fingers and toes; (2) ataxia, a clumsy stumbling gait, difficulty in swallowing and articulating words; (3) neurasthenia, a generalized sensation of weakness, fatigue, and inability to concentrate; (4) vision and hearing loss; (5) spasticity and tremor; and, finally, (6) coma and death.

Neuropathological observations have shown the cortex of the cerebrum and cerebellum are selectively involved with focal necrosis of neurons, with lysis and phagocytosis and replacement by supporting glial cells. These changes are most prominent in the deeper fissures (sulci) such as in the visual cortex and insula. The overall acute effect is cerebral edema but with prolonged destruction of grey matter and subsequent gliosis. Cerebral atrophy results (Takeuchi, 1977).

***Mechanisms of Neurotoxicity of Methyl Mercury.*** Experimental studies on the mechanisms of methyl mercury toxicity provide some insight into the basis for the clinical observations as well as the greater sensitivity of the developing brain (Clarkson, 1983).

Exposure of the fetus *in utero* to high levels of mercury results in abnormal neuronal migration and deranged organization of brain nuclei (clusters of neurons) and layering of neurons in the cortex. Methyl mercury interacts with DNA and RNA and binds with sulfhydryl groups, resulting in changes of the secondary structure of DNA and RNA synthesis. Studies in mice have demonstrated an effect of methyl mercury on the microtubules of neurons. These observations may provide the cellular basis for the observed neuropathological changes in the migration pattern of neurons during development and is thought to be the basis for the developmental effects in the central nervous system. Male mice are more sensitive than females, consistent with the findings in humans (Sager et al., 1984; Choie et al., 1978).

***Dose–Response Relationships between Health and Risk and Intake of Methyl Mercury.*** The relationship between health risks and intake of methyl mercury has been developed from toxicological data obtained from studies of epidemics due to accidental poisoning in Minamata and Niigeta, Japan in the 1950s and from studies of the episode in Iraq in 1972 (Berlin, 1986).

The critical or lowest level of observed adverse health effect in adults is paresthesia. By combining the two relationships, body burden versus intake and effect versus body burden, it was possible to calculate the average long-term daily intake associated with health effects in the most susceptible individual. This was estimated to be about 300 $\mu$g/day for an adult or 4300 ngHg/day/kg body weight.

The critical effect from prenatal exposure to methyl mercury is psychomotor retardation. The infant may appear normal at birth but there is a 12-month or more delay in learning to walk and talk and an increased incidence of seizures. The "threshold" or point at which the occurrence of the critical effect exceeds the background occurs at a lower dose for the prenatal effect than with adult exposure. Epidemiological studies relating dose to effects from prenatal exposures have now been conducted in Iraq, Canada, and New Zealand. From information obtained in these studies, Cox et al. (1989) have calculated that the lowest observed adverse effect level for psychomotor retardation occurs when maternal hair concentrations during pregnancy are between 10 to 20 ppm. Assuming that the relationship between intake and body burden of methyl mercury is the same in the pregnant and nonpregnant adult, this hair value would correspond to an intake of 800 to 1700 ngHg/kg/day, with the mother's red blood cell level at 40–80 $\mu$g/L. In more severe cases from higher levels of exposure *in utero*, the child may develop ataxia, motor disturbance, and mental symptoms similar to those occurring in a child with cerebral palsy of unknown etiology. Postnatal poisoning may occur from the transfer of methyl mercury via breast milk (Grandjean, 1994). Symptoms of this type of poisoning in the infant are similar to those in the adult.

The potential for recovery from the neurological effects may be better in cases of acute poisoning compared to prolonged exposure but, generally, neurotoxicity is irreversible.

***Biological Indicators.*** The recommended standard (time–weight average) for permissible exposure limits for inorganic mercury in air in the workplace is 0.05 mg Hg/m$^3$ (DHEW, 1977), and is equivalent to an ambient air level of 0.015 mg/m$^3$ for the general population (24-h exposure) (Table 23-6). The U.S. federal standard for alkyl mercury exposure in the workplace is 0.01 mg/m$^3$ as an 8-h time-weighted average with an acceptable ceiling of 0.04 mg/m$^3$. Although a precise correlation has not been found between exposure levels and mercury content of blood and urine, study of the Iraq epidemic has provided estimates of the body burden of mercury and onset and of the frequency of occurrence of symptoms (Fig. 23-6).

***Treatment.*** Therapy for mercury poisoning should be directed toward lowering the concentration of mercury at the critical organ or site of injury. For the most severe cases, particularly with acute renal failure, hemodialysis may be the first measure along with infusion of chelating agents for mercury such as cysteine or penicillamine. For less severe cases of inorganic mercury poisoning, chelation with BAL may be effective. However, chelation therapy is not very helpful for alkyl mercury exposure. Biliary excretion and reabsorption by the intestine and the enterohepatic cycling of mercury may be interrupted by surgically establishing gallbladder drainage or by the oral administration of a nonabsorbable thiol resin that binds mercury and enhances intestinal excretion (Berlin, 1986).

## Nickel

Nickel is a respiratory tract carcinogen in workers in the nickel-refining industry. Other serious consequences of long-

**Table 23–6**
**The Time-Weighted Average Air Concentrations Associated with the Earliest Effects in the Most Sensitive Adults Following Long-Term Exposure to Elemental Mercury Vapor**

| EQUIVALENT CONTRATIONS* | | | |
|---|---|---|---|
| AIR (mg/m$^3$) | BLOOD ($\mu$g/100 ml) | URINE ($\mu$g/L) | EARLIEST EFFECTS |
| 0.05 | 3.5 | 150 | Nonspecific symptoms |
| 0.1–0.2 | 7–14 | 300–600 | Tremor |

* Blood and urine values may be used only on a group basis owing to gross individual variations. These average values reflect exposure for a year or more. After shorter periods of exposure, air concentrations would be associated with lower concentrations in blood and urine.

SOURCE: WHO, 1976.

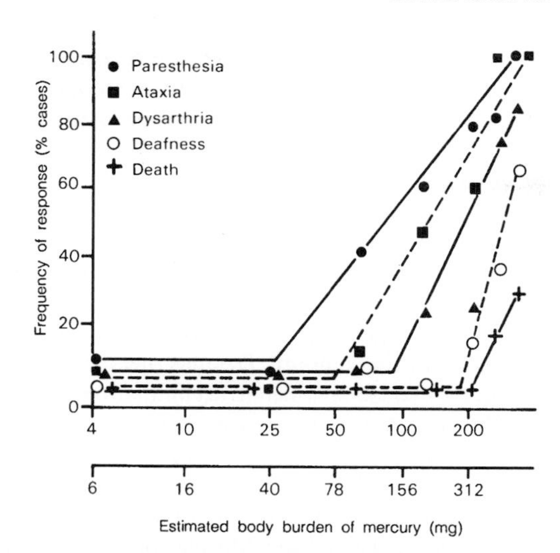


*Figure 23–6. Dose–response relationships for methyl mercury.*

The upper scale of estimated body burden of mercury was based on the author's actual estimate of intake. The lower scale is based on the body burden, which was calculated based on the concentration of mercury in the blood and its relationship to intake derived from radioisotopic studies of methyl mercury kinetics in human volunteers. [From Bakir et al. (1973).]

term exposure to nickel are not apparent, but severe acute and sometimes fatal toxicity may follow nickel carbonyl exposure. Allergic contact dermatitis is common among persons in the general population. A deficiency of nickel alters glucose metabolism and decreases tolerance to glucose. From studies on rats, there is growing evidence that nickel may be an essential trace metal for mammals (Anke et al., 1983).

**Toxicokinetics.** Nickel is only sparsely absorbed from the gastrointestinal tract. It is transported in the plasma bound to serum albumin and multiple small organic ligands, amino acids, or polypeptides. Excretion in the urine is nearly complete in 4 or 5 days. Kinetics have been described in rodents as a two-compartment model.

Serum nickel is influenced by environmental nickel or nickel concentration in the ambient air. Serum nickel measured in persons living in Sudbury, Ontario, which is in the vicinity of a large nickel mine, showed concentrations of 4.6 ± 1.4 $\mu$g/L (range: 2.0 to 7.3) and urinary concentrations were 7.9 ± 3.7 $\mu$g/day (range: 2.3 to 15.7).

Generally, fecal nickel is about 100 times urinary nickel concentration. The nickel content of diets prepared in university or hospital kitchens in the United States (Myron et al., 1978) averaged 165 (S.D. ± 11) $\mu$g/day or 75 ± 10 $\mu$g/1000 calories.

Nickel administered parenterally to animals is rapidly distributed to the kidneys, pituitary, lungs, skin, adrenals, ovaries and testes (Sunderman, 1981). The intracellular distribution and binding of nickel is not well understood. Ultrafilterable ligands seem to be of major importance in the transport in serum and in bile and urinary excretion, as well as in intracellular binding. The ligands are not well characterized, but Sunderman (1981) suggests that cysteine, histidine, and aspartic acid form nickel complexes either singly or as nickel–ligand species. In vivo binding with metallothionein has been demonstrated, but nickel at best induces metallothionein synthesis in liver or kidney only slightly. A nickel-binding metalloprotein has also been identified in plasma with properties suggesting an α-one-glycoprotein complex with serum α-one-macroglobulin complex.

Evidence has accumulated over the past few years indicating that nickel is a nutritionally essential trace metal. Jack-bean urease has been identified as a nickel metalloenzyme, and nickel is required for urea metabolism in cell cultures of soybean. However, a nickel-containing metalloenzyme has not yet been recovered from animal tissues. Nickel deficiency in rats is associated with retarded body growth and anemia, probably secondary to impaired absorption of iron from the gastrointestinal tract. In addition, there is significant reduction in serum glucose concentration. An interaction of nickel with copper and zinc is also suspected because anemia-induced nickel deficiency is only partially corrected with nickel supplementation in rats receiving low dietary copper and zinc (Spears, 1978).

**Toxicity.** ***Carcinogenicity.*** It has been known for 40 years that occupational exposure to nickel predisposes humans to lung and nasal cancer (Doll et al., 1977). Epidemiological studies showed in 1958 that nickel refinery workers in Britain had a fivefold increase in the risk of lung cancer and a 150-fold increase in the risk of nasal cancers compared to people in the general population. More recently, increases in lung cancer among nickel workers have been reported from several different countries, including suggestions of increased risks of laryngeal cancer in nickel refinery workers in Norway (Pedersen et al., 1978) and gastric carcinoma and soft tissue sarcomas from the Soviet Union. Six cases of renal cancer have been reported among Canadian and Norwegian workers employed in the electrolytic refining of nickel (Sunderman, 1981). McEwan (1978) has been able to detect early cytologic changes in the sputum of exposed workers prior to chest x-ray or clinical indicators of respiratory tract cancer.

Because the refining of nickel in the plants that were studied involved the Mond process with the formation of nickel carbonyl, it was believed for some time that nickel carbonyl was the principal carcinogen. However, additional epidemiological studies of workers in refineries that do not use the Mond process also showed an increased risk of respiratory cancer, suggesting that the source of the increased risk is the mixture of nickel sulfides present in molten ore. Indeed, studies with experimental animals have shown that the nickel subsulfide ($Ni_3S_2$) produces local tumors at injection sites and by inhalation in rats, and in vitro mammalian cell tests demonstrate that $Ni_3S_2$ and $NiSO_4$ compounds give rise to mammalian cell transformation. Differences in the carcinogenic activities of nickel compounds may be attributable to variations in their capacities to provide nickel ion at critical sites within target cells, but this has not been established experimentally (Sunderman, 1989). However, the order of lung toxicity corresponds to the water solubility of various compounds, with nickel sulfate being most toxic, followed by nickel subsulfide and nickel oxide (Dunick et al., 1989).

***Nickel Carbonyl Poisoning.*** Metallic nickel combines with carbon monoxide to form nickel carbonyl ($Ni[CO]_4$, which decomposes to pure nickel and carbon monoxide on heating to 200°C (the Mond process). This reaction provides a convenient and efficient method for the refinement of nickel. However, nickel carbonyl is extremely toxic, and many cases of acute toxicity have been reported. The illness begins with headache, nausea, vomiting, and epigastric or chest pain, followed by cough, hyperpnea, cyanosis, gastrointestinal symptoms, and weakness. The symptoms may be accompanied by fever and leucocytosis and the more severe cases progress to pneumonia, respiratory failure, and eventually to cerebral edema and death. Autopsy studies show the largest concentrations of nickel in lungs with lesser amounts in kidneys, liver, and brain (Sunderman 1981).

***Dermatitis.*** Nickel dermatitis is one of the most common forms of allergic contact dermatitis: 4 to 9 percent of persons with contact dermatitis react positively to nickel patch tests. Sensitization might occur from any of the numerous metal products in common use, such as coins and jewelry. The notion that increased ingestion of nickel-containing food increases the probability of external sensitization to nickel is supported by the finding of increased urinary nickel excretion in association with episodes of acute nickel dermatitis (Menne and Thorboe, 1976).

***Indicators of Nickel Toxicity.*** Blood nickel levels immediately following exposure to nickel carbonyl provide a guideline as to the severity of exposure and indication for chelation therapy (Sunderman, 1979). Sodium diethyldithiocarbamate is the preferred drug, but other chelating agents, such as d-penicillamine and DMPS, provide some degree of protection from clinical effects.

## ESSENTIAL METALS WITH POTENTIAL FOR TOXICITY

This group includes eight metals generally accepted as essential: cobalt, copper, iron, magnesium, manganese, molybdenum, selenium, and zinc. Each essential metal has three levels of biological activity: trace levels required for optimum growth and development, homeostatic levels (storage levels), and toxic levels. For these metals, environmental accumulations are generally less important routes of excess exposure than accidents or occupation.

Although chromium and arsenic are regarded as essential to humans and animals, respectively, the toxicological significance of chromium and arsenic warrant their being discussed as major toxic metals in the context of this chapter. Tin and vanadium are also essential to animals but are of less importance toxicologically and are included in the group of minor toxic metals.

### Cobalt

Cobalt is essential as a component of vitamin $B_{12}$ required for the production of red blood cells and prevention of pernicious anemia. There is 0.0434 $\mu$g of cobalt per microgram of vitamin $B_{12}$. If other requirements for cobalt exist, they are not well understood. Deficiency diseases of cattle and sheep, caused by insufficient natural levels of cobalt, are characterized by anemia and loss of weight or retarded growth. The occurrence, metabolism and toxicity of cobalt are reviewed by Elinder and Friberg (1986) and Angerer and Heinrich (1988).

Cobalt is a relatively rare metal produced primarily as a by-product of other metals, chiefly copper. It is used in high-temperature alloys and in permanent magnets. Its salts are useful in paint dryers, as catalysts, and in the production of numerous pigments.

Cobalt salts are generally well absorbed after oral ingestion, probably in the jejunum. Despite this fact, increased levels tend not to cause significant accumulation. About 80 percent of the ingested cobalt is excreted in the urine. Of the remaining portion, about 15 percent is excreted in the feces by an enterohepatic pathway, while the milk and sweat are other secondary routes of excretion. The total body burden has been estimated as 1.1 mg. Muscle contains the largest total fraction, but fat has the highest concentration. The liver, heart, and hair have significantly higher concentrations than other organs, but the concentration in these organs is relatively low. The normal levels in human urine and blood are about 98 and 0.18 $\mu$g/liter, respectively. The blood level is largely associated with the concentration in red cells. Significant species differences have been observed in the excretion of radiocobalt. In rats and cattle, 80 percent is eliminated in the feces.

Polycythemia is the characteristic response of most mammals, including humans, to ingestion of excessive amounts of cobalt. Toxicity resulting from overzealous therapeutic administration has been reported to produce vomiting, diarrhea, and a sensation of warmth. Intravenous administration leads to flushing of the face, increased blood pressure, slowed respiration, giddiness, tinnitus, and deafness due to nerve damage (Browning, 1969).

High levels of chronic oral administration may result in the production of goiter. Epidemiological studies suggest that the incidence of goiter is higher in regions containing increased levels of cobalt in the water and soil. The goitrogenic effect has been elicited by the oral administration of 3 to 4 mg/kg to children in the course of sickle cell anemia therapy.

Cardiomyopathy has been caused by an excessive intake of cobalt, particularly from the drinking of beer to which 1 ppm cobalt was added to enhance its foaming qualities. Why such a low concentration should produce this effect in the absence of any similar change when cobalt is used therapeutically is unknown. The signs and symptoms were those of congestive heart failure. Autopsy findings revealed a tenfold increase in the cardiac levels of cobalt. Ethanol may have potentiated the effect of the cobalt (Morin and Daniel, 1967).

Hyperglycemia due to $\beta$-cell pancreatic damage has been reported after injection of cobalt into rats. Reduction of blood pressure has also been observed in rats after injection and has led to some experimental use in humans (Schroeder et al., 1967).

Occupational inhalation of cobalt-containing dust (0.1 Co/m$^3$ or higher) in the cemented tungsten carbide industry may cause respiratory irritation at air concentrations of 0.002–0.01 mg/m$^3$ and may be a cause of "hard-metal" pneumoconiosis. This may result in interstitial fibrosis. Allergic dermatitis of an erythematous papular type may also occur, and affected persons may have positive skin tests.

Single and repeated subcutaneous or intramuscular injection of cobalt powder and salts in rats may cause sarcomas at the site of injection, but there is no evidence of carcinogenicity from any other route of exposure (Gilman, 1962).

## Copper

Copper is widely distributed in nature and is an essential element. Copper deficiency is characterized by hypochromic, microcytic anemia resulting from defective hemoglobin synthesis. Oxidative enzymes, such as catalase, peroxidase, cytochrome oxides, and others, also require copper. Copper sulfate is used medicinally as an emetic. It has also been used for its astringent and caustic action and as an anthelmintic. Copper sulfate mixed with lime has been used as a fungicide. The potential health effects associated with copper are reviewed by the EPA (1987c).

Gastrointestinal absorption of copper is normally regulated by body stores (Sarkar et al., 1983). It is transported in serum bound initially to albumin and later more firmly bound to ceruloplasmin, where it is exchanged in the cupric form. The normal serum level of copper is 120 to 145 $\mu$g per liter. The bile is the normal excretory pathway and plays a primary role in copper homeostasis. Most copper is stored in liver and bone marrow where it may be bound to metallothionein. The amount of copper in milk is not enough to maintain adequate copper levels in the liver, lungs, and spleen of the newborn. Tissue levels gradually decline up to about ten years of age, remaining relatively constant thereafter. Brain levels, on the other hand, tend to almost double from infancy to adulthood. The ratio of newborn to adult liver copper levels shows considerable species difference: human, 15 : 4; rat, 6 : 4, and rabbit, 1 : 6. Since urinary copper levels may be increased by soft water, under these conditions concentrations of approximately 60 $\mu$g per liter are not uncommon.

Copper is an essential component of several enzymes, including tyrosinase, involved in the formation of melanin pigments, cytochrome oxidase, superoxide dismutase, amine oxidases, and uricase. It is essential for the utilization of iron. Iron deficiency anemia in infancy is sometimes accompanied by copper deficiency. Molybdenum also influences tissue levels of copper.

Copper is not an effective inducer of metallothionein relative to zinc or cadmium. Nevertheless, copper bound to metallothionein is thought to be a normal storage form of copper, particularly in infancy and childhood. Isolated hepatic cells are protected from copper toxicity by prior induction of metallothionein with zinc. Copper-metallothionein accumulates in lysosomes facilitating the biliary excretion of copper (Winge and Mehra, 1990).

Acute poisoning resulting from ingestion of excessive amounts of oral copper salts, most frequently copper sulfate, may produce death. The symptoms are vomiting, sometimes with a blue-green color observed in the vomitus, hematemesis, hypotension, melena, coma, and jaundice. Autopsy findings have revealed centrilobular hepatic necrosis (Chuttani et al., 1965). Few cases of copper intoxication as a result of burn treatment with copper compounds have resulted in hemolytic anemia. Copper poisoning producing hemolytic anemia has also been reported as the result of using copper-containing dialysis equipment (Manzer and Schreiner, 1970). Individuals with glucose-6-phosphate deficiency may be at increased risk to the hematologic effects of copper, but there is uncertainty as to the magnitude of the risk (Goldstein et al., 1985).

The U.S. EPA maximum contaminant level for copper in drinking water, proposed in 1985 (EPA, 1985) and adopted in 1991, is 1.3 mg/liter.

Chronic hepatic copper overload is observed in three conditions, Indian childhood cirrhosis, chronic cholestatic conditions and in inherited disorders of copper metabolism. Indian childhood disorder is thought to be an environmental disorder associated with chronic ingestion of copper-contaminated water, although a genetic component is now suggested. A recent report of copper overload and cirrhosis in four Mexican children suggests that the clinical and laboratory findings, including the findings from liver biopsies and ultrastructure, are not distinguishable from Wilson's disease (Valencia and Gamboa, 1993).

There are two genetically inherited inborn errors of copper metabolism that are in a sense a form of copper toxicity (Sarkar et al., 1983). Wilson's disease is characterized by the excessive accumulation of copper in liver, brain, kidneys, and cornea. Serum ceruloplasmin is low and serum copper, not bound to ceruloplasmin, is elevated. Urinary excretion of copper is high. The disorder is sometimes referred to as hepatolenticular degeneration in reference to the major symptoms. Clinical abnormalities of the nervous system, liver, kidneys, and cornea are related to copper accumulation. Although the etiology of this disorder is genetic, the basic defect at the biochemical level is not known. Increased binding of copper to an abnormal intracellular thionein or altered tissue excretion has been proposed. Cultured fibroblasts from persons with Wilson's disease have increased intracellular copper when cultured in Eagle's minimum essential medium with fetal bovine serum (Chan et al., 1983). Clinical improvement can be achieved by chelation of copper with penicillamine (Walshe, 1964). Trien [triethylene tetramine (2HCl)] is also effective and has been used in patients with Wilson's disease who have toxic reactions to penicillamine (Walshe, 1983).

Menke's disease or Menke's "kinky-hair syndrome" is a sex-linked trait characterized by peculiar hair, failure to thrive, severe mental retardation, neurological impairment, and death before 3 years of age. There is extensive degeneration of the cerebral cortex and of white matter. Again, the basic defect is not known. There are low levels of copper in the liver and brain but high concentrations in other tissues. Even in cells with increased copper concentration there is a relative deficiency in the activities of some copper-dependent enzymes. Some laboratories have reported larger-than-normal quantities of copper-thionein accumulated in fibroblasts, so that the basic defect may be in the regulation of metallothionein synthesis. The finding of increased amounts of other metallothionein-binding metals (zinc, cadmium, and mercury) in the kidneys of patients with the disease supports this hypothesis (Riordan, 1983).

## Iron

The major scientific and medical interest in iron is as an essential metal, but toxicological considerations are important in terms of accidental acute exposures and chronic iron overload, due to idiopathic hemochromatosis or as a consequence of excess dietary iron or frequent blood transfusions. The complex metabolism of iron and mechanisms of toxicity are detailed by Jacobs and Worwood (1981) and Spivey Fox and Rader (1988).

**Toxicokinetics.** The disposition of iron is regulated by a complex mechanism to maintain homeostasis. Generally, about 2 to 15 percent is absorbed from the gastrointestinal tract, whereas elimination of absorbed iron is only about 0.01 percent per day (percent body burden or amount absorbed). During periods of increased iron need (childhood, pregnancy, or blood loss), absorption of iron is greatly increased. Absorption occurs in two steps: absorption of ferrous ions from the intestinal lumen into the mucosal cells, and transfer from the mucosal cell to plasma where it is bound to transferrin for transfer to storage sites. Transferrin is a $\beta_1$-globulin with a molecular weight of 75,000 and is produced in the liver. As ferrous ion is released into plasma, it becomes oxidized by oxygen in the presence of ferroxidase I, which is identical to ceruloplasmin. There are 3 to 5 g of iron in the body. About two-thirds is bound to hemoglobin, 10 percent in myoglobin and iron-containing enzymes, and the remainder is bound to the iron storage proteins ferritin and hemosiderin. Exposure to iron induces synthesis of apoferritin, which then binds ferrous ions. The ferrous ion becomes oxidized, probably by histidine and cysteine residues and carbonyl groups. Iron may be released from ferritin by reducing agents: Ascorbic acid, cysteine, and reduced glutathione release iron slowly. Normally, excess ingested iron is excreted, and some is contained within shed intestinal cells and in bile and urine and in even smaller amounts in sweat, nails, and hair. Total iron excretion is usually on the order of 0.5 mg/day.

With excess exposure to iron or iron overload, there may be a further increase in ferritin synthesis in hepatic parenchymal cells. In fact, the ability of the liver to synthesize ferritin exceeds the rate at which lysosomes can process iron for excretion. Lysosomes convert the protein from ferritin to hemosiderin, which then remains in situ (Trump et al., 1973). The formation of hemosiderin from ferritin is not well understood, but it seems to involve denaturation of the apoferritin molecule. With increasing iron loading, ferritin concentration appears to reach a maximum and a greater portion of iron is found in hemosiderin. Both ferritin and hemosiderin are, in fact, storage sites for intracellular metal and are protective in that they maintain intracellular iron in bound form. A portion of the iron taken up by cells of the reticuloendothelial system enters a labile iron pool available for erythropoiesis and part becomes stored as ferritin.

**Toxicity.** Acute iron toxicity is nearly always due to accidental ingestion of iron-containing medicines and most often occurs in children. As of 1970, there were about 2000 cases in the United States each year, generally among children ages 1 through 5 who eat ferrous sulfate tablets with candylike coatings. A decrease in occurrences of this type followed the use of "childproof" lids on prescription medicines. Severe toxicity occurs after the ingestion of more than 0.5 g of iron or 2.5 g of ferrous sulfate. Toxicity becomes manifest with vomiting 1 to 6 h after ingestion. The vomitus may be bloody owing to ulceration of the gastrointestinal tract; stools may be black. This is followed by signs of shock and metabolic acidosis, liver damage, and coagulation defects within the next couple of days. Late effects may include renal failure and hepatic cirrhosis. The mechanism of the toxicity is thought to begin with acute mucosal cell damage, absorption of ferrous ions directly into the circulation, which cause capillary endothelial cell damage in the liver.

Chronic iron toxicity or iron overload in adults is a more common problem. There are three basic ways in which excessive amounts of iron can accumulate in the body (Muller-Eberhard et al., 1977). The first circumstance is idiopathic hemochromatosis due to abnormal absorption of iron from the intestinal tract. The condition may be genetic. A second possible cause of iron overload is excess dietary iron. The African Bantu who prepares his daily food and brews fermented beverages in iron pots is the classic subject for this form of iron overload. Sporadic other cases occur owing to excessive ingestion of iron-containing tonics or medicines. The third circumstance in which iron overload may occur is from the regular requirement for blood transfusion for some form of refractory anemia and is sometimes referred to as transfusional siderosis.

The pathologic consequences of iron overload are similar regardless of basic cause. The body iron content is increased to between 20 g and 40 g. Most of the extra iron is hemosiderin. The greatest concentrations are in the parenchymal cells of liver and pancreas, as well as in endocrine organs and the heart. Iron in reticuloendothelial cells (in the spleen) is greatest in transfusional siderosis and in the Bantu. Further clinical effects may include disturbances in liver function, diabetes mellitus, and even endocrine disturbances and cardiovascular effects. At the cellular level, increased lipid peroxidation occurs with consequent membrane damage to mitochondria, microsomes, and other cellular organelles (Jacobs, 1977).

Treatment of acute iron poisoning is directed toward removal of the ingested iron from the gastrointestinal tract by inducing vomiting or gastric lavage and providing corrective therapy for systemic effects such as acidosis and shock. Deferrioxamine is the chelating agent of choice for the treatment of iron overload absorbed from acute exposure as well as for removal of tissue iron in hemosiderosis. Repeated phlebotomy can remove as much as 20 g of iron per year. Ascorbic acid will also increase iron excretion by as much as twice normal levels (Brown, 1983).

Inhalation of iron oxide fumes or dust by workers in metal industries may result in deposition of iron particles in lungs, producing an x-ray appearance resembling silicosis. These effects are seen in hematite miners, iron and steel workers, and arc welders. Hematite is the most important iron ore (mainly $Fe_2O_3$). A report on autopsies of hematite miners noted an increase in lung cancer, as well as tuberculosis and interstitial fibrosis (Boyd et al., 1970). The etiology of the lung cancer may be related to concomitant factors such as cigarettes or other workplace carcinogens. Hematite miners are also exposed to silica and other minerals, as well as radioactive materials; other iron workers have exposures to polycyclic hydrocarbons (McLaughlin and Harding, 1956). Dose levels of iron among iron workers developing pneumoconiosis have been reported to exceed 10 mg $Fe/m^3$.

## Magnesium

Magnesium is a cofactor of many enzymes; it is apparently associated with phosphate in these functions. Deficiency may occur in human and animal populations but may be difficult to substantiate. In humans it has been associated with magnesium-losing renal disease, alcoholism, and low-magnesium-induced ischemic heart disease. Deficiency in animals may result from ingestion of grasses grown in magnesium-poor soil. Deficiency causes neuromuscular irritability, calcification, and cardiac and renal damage, which can be prevented by supplementation. The deficiency is called *grass staggers* in cattle and *magnesium tetany* in calves.

Nuts, cereals, seafoods, and meats are high dietary sources of magnesium. The average city water contains about 6.5 ppm but varies considerably, increasing with the hardness of the water (Schroeder et al., 1969). Magnesium citrate, oxide, sulfate, hydroxide, and carbonate are widely taken as antacids or cathartics. Magnesium hydroxide, or milk of magnesia, is one of the constituents of the universal antidote for poisoning. Topically, the sulfate also is used widely to relieve inflammation. Magnesium sulfate may be used as a parenterally administered central depressant. Its most frequent use for this purpose is in the treatment of seizures associated with eclampsia of pregnancy and acute nephritis.

Magnesium also has a number of industrial uses. It is used in lightweight alloys, as an electrical conductive material, and for incendiary devices such as flares.

**Toxicokinetics.** Magnesium salts are poorly absorbed from the intestine. In cases of overload this may be due in part to their dehydrating action. Magnesium is absorbed mainly in the small intestine; the colon also absorbs some. Calcium and magnesium are competitive with respect to their absorptive sites, and excess calcium may partially inhibit the absorption of magnesium.

Magnesium is excreted into the digestive tract by the bile and pancreatic and intestinal juices. A small amount of radiomagnesium given intravenously appears in the gastrointestinal tract. The serum levels are remarkably constant. There is an apparent obligatory urinary loss of magnesium, which amounts to about 12 mg/day, and the urine is the major route of excretion under normal conditions. Magnesium found in the stool is probably not absorbed. Magnesium is filtered by the glomeruli and reabsorbed by the renal tubules. In the blood plasma about 65 percent is in the ionic form, while the remainder is bound to protein. The former is that which appears in the glomerular filtrate. Excretion also occurs in the sweat and milk. Endocrine activity, particularly of the adrenocortical hormones, aldosterone, and parathyroid hormone, has an effect on magnesium levels, although these effects may be related to the interaction of calcium and magnesium.

Tissue distribution studies indicate that of the 20-g body burden, the majority is intracellular in the bone and muscle, but some magnesium is present in every cell of the body. Bone concentration of magnesium decreases as calcium increases. Most of the remaining tissues have higher concentrations than blood, except for fat and omentum.

***Toxicity.*** Freshly generated magnesium oxide can cause metal fume fever if inhaled in sufficient amounts, analogous to the effect caused by zinc oxide. Both zinc and magnesium exposure of animals produced similar effects. It is reported that particles of magnesium in the subcutaneous tissue produce lesions that resist healing. In animals, magnesium subcutaneously or intramuscularly administered produces gas gangrene as a result of interaction with the body fluids and subsequent generation of hydrogen and magnesium hydroxide. The tissue lesion is reversible.

Conjunctivitis, nasal catarrh, and coughing up of discolored sputum results from industrial inhalation exposure. With industrial exposures, increases of serum magnesium up to twice the normal levels failed to produce ill effects but were accompanied by calcium increases. Intoxication occurring after oral administration of magnesium salts is rare but may be present in the face of renal impairment. The symptoms include a sharp drop in blood pressure and respiratory paralysis due to central nervous system depression (Browning, 1969; Birch, 1988).

## Manganese

Manganese is an essential element and is a cofactor for a number of enzymatic reactions, particularly those involved in phosphorylation, cholesterol, and fatty acids synthesis. Manganese is present in all living organisms. While it is present in urban air and in most water supplies, the principal portion of the intake is derived from food. Vegetables, the germinal portions of grains, fruits, nuts, tea, and some spices are rich in manganese (Underwood, 1977; Keen and Leach, 1988).

Daily manganese intake ranges from 2 to 9 mg. Gastrointestinal absorption is less than 5 percent. Manganese is transported in plasma bound to a $\beta_1$-globulin, thought to be transferrin, and is widely distributed in the body. Manganese concentrates in mitochondria so that tissues rich in these organelles have the highest concentrations of manganese, including the pancreas, liver, kidneys, and intestines. Biological half-life in the body is 37 days. Manganese readily crosses the blood–brain barrier and its half-time in the brain is longer than in the whole body.

Manganese is eliminated in the bile and is reabsorbed in the intestine, but the principal route of excretion is with feces. This system apparently involves the liver, auxiliary gastrointestinal mechanisms for excreting excess manganese, and perhaps the adrenal cortex. This regulating mechanism, plus the tendency for extremely large doses of manganese salts to cause gastrointestinal irritation, accounts for the lack of systemic toxicity following oral administration or dermal application.

Manganese and its compounds are used in making steel alloys, dry-cell batteries, electrical coils, ceramics, matches, glass, dyes, in fertilizers, welding rods, as oxidizing agents, and as animal food additives. Industrial toxicity from inhalation exposure, generally to manganese dioxide in mining or manufacturing, is of two types: The first, manganese pneumonitis, is the result of acute exposure. Men working in plants with high concentrations of manganese dust show an incidence of respiratory disease 30-times greater than normal. Pathological changes include epithelial necrosis followed by mononuclear proliferation.

The second and more serious type of disease resulting from chronic inhalation exposure to manganese dioxide, generally over a period of more than 2 years, involves the central nervous system. Chronic manganese poisoning (manganism) produces a neuropsychiatric disorder characterized by irritability, difficulty in walking, speech disturbances, and compulsive behavior that may include running, fighting, and singing. If the condition persists, a masklike face, retropulsion or propulsion, and a Parkinsonlike syndrome develop (Mena et al.,

1967). The outstanding feature of manganese encephalopathy has been classified as severe selective damage to the subthalamic nucleus and pallidum (Pentschew et al., 1963). These symptoms and the pathological lesions, degenerative changes in the basal ganglia, make the analogy to Parkinson's disease feasible. In addition to the central nervous system changes, liver cirrhosis is frequently observed.

Victims of chronic manganese poisoning tend to recover slowly, even when removed from the excessive exposure. Metal-sequestering agents have not produced remarkable recovery; L-dopa, which is used in the treatment of Parkinson's disease, has been more consistently effective in the treatment of chronic manganese poisoning than in Parkinson's disease (Cotzias et al., 1971).

The oral absorption of manganese is increased by iron deficiency which may contribute to variations in individual susceptibility (Mena et al., 1969).

The syndrome of chronic nervous system effects has only been duplicated in squirrel monkeys by inhalation or intraperitoneal injection.

## Molybdenum

Molybdenum is an essential metal that acts as a cofactor for the enzymes xanthine oxidase and aldehyde oxidase. In plants it is necessary for fixing of atmospheric nitrogen by bacteria at the start of protein synthesis. Because of these functions it is ubiquitous in food. Because plankton tend to concentrate molybdenum at a rate 25 times that of seawater, shellfish tend to have high concentrations of molybdenum. Molybdenum is added in trace amounts to fertilizers to stimulate plant growth. The average daily human intake in food is approximately 350 $\mu$g. The concentration of molybdenum in urban air is minimal, but it is present in more than one third of freshwater supplies and in certain areas the concentration may be near 1 $\mu$g per liter. Excess exposure can result in toxicity to animals and humans.

The most important mineral source of molybdenum is molybdenite ($MoS_2$). The United States is the major world producer of molybdenum. The industrial uses of this metal include the manufacture of high-temperature resistant steel alloys for use in gas turbines and jet aircraft engines and in the production of catalysts, lubricants, and dyes.

**Toxicokinetics.** While molybdenum exists in various valence forms, biological differences with respect to valence are not clear. The soluble hexavalent compounds are well absorbed from the gastrointestinal tract into the liver. It is a component of xanthine oxidase, which has a role in purine metabolism and has been shown to be a component of aldehyde oxidase and sulfite oxidase. Increased molybdenum intake in experimental animals has been shown to increase tissue levels of xanthine oxidase. In humans, molybdenum is contained principally in the liver, kidneys, fat, and blood. Of the approximate total of 9 mg in the body, most is concentrated in the liver, kidneys, adrenal, and omentum. More than 50 percent of molybdenum in the liver is contained in a nonprotein cofactor bound to the mitochondrial outer membrane and can be transferred to an apoenzyme transforming it into an active enzyme molecule (Johnson et al., 1977). The molybdenum level is relatively low in the newborn and increases until age 20, declining in concentration thereafter. More than half of the molybdenum excreted is in the urine. The blood level, at least in sheep, is in association with the level in red blood cells. However, molybdenum has been detected in only about 25 percent of the blood samples of the human urban population. The excretion of molybdenum is rapid, mainly as molybdate. Excesses may be excreted also by the bile, particularly the hexavalent forms.

Inhalation of molybdenum by guinea pigs has resulted in increased bone levels. Injected radiomolybdenum increased liver and kidney levels, but the endocrine glands also showed an exceptionally high content.

**Toxicity.** Pastures containing 20 to 100 ppm molybdenum may produce a disease referred to as *teart* in cattle and sheep. It is characterized by anemia, poor growth rate, and diarrhea. Copper or sulfate in the diet prevents the disease, and removal of the animals from pastures containing high levels of molybdenum facilitates their rapid recovery. Prolonged exposure has led to deformities of the joints. Experimental studies have revealed differences in toxicity of molybdenum salts. Molybdenum sulfide was well tolerated in rats at 500 mg/kg/day and was not injurious to guinea pigs at 28 mg/m$^3$. Hexavalent compounds were more toxic. In rats molybdenum trioxide at a dose of 100 mg/kg/day, by inhalation, was irritating to the eyes and mucous membranes and subsequently lethal. After repeated oral administration at sufficient levels, fatty degeneration of the liver and kidney was induced. In comparison with chromium and tungsten salts, sodium molybdate by intraperitoneal injection was less toxic in mice.

Interesting relationships of molybdenum with other metals with respect to toxicity in cattle and sheep have been documented. For example, copper prevents the accumulation of molybdenum in the liver and may antagonize the absorption of molybdenum from food. It is reported that by alternating the intake of copper and molybdenum at weekly intervals, black sheep can be made to grow striped wool. White wool in black sheep is a sign of copper deficiency. The antagonism of copper is dependent on sulfate in the diet. It has been suggested that sulfate may displace molybdate in the body. It may be that the anemia caused by molybdenum is due to the reduction of sulfide oxidase in the liver, resulting in the formation of copper sulfide, thereby inducing a functional copper deficiency. Feeding of tungstate has also been shown to displace molybdate. In addition, it has been reported that molybdenum may promote fluoride retention and thereby decrease dental caries (Underwood, 1977), but the incidence of caries in children living in high-molybdenum areas compared to children living in normal- or low-molybdenum areas does not differ (Curzon et al., 1970).

## Selenium

The availability as well as the toxic potential for selenium and selenium compounds is related to their chemical form and, most importantly, to solubility. Selenium occurs in nature and biological systems as selenate ($Se^{6+}$), selenite ($Se^{4+}$), elemental selenium ($Se^0$), and selenide ($Se^{2-}$), and deficiency leads to a cardiomyopathy in mammals, including humans (NAS,1975; Underwood, 1977; Wilber, 1983; Levander, 1985; WHO, 1986).

Selenium in foodstuffs provides a daily source (NAS, 1975). Seafoods, especially shrimp, and meat, milk products, and grains provide the largest amounts in the diet. River water levels of selenium vary depending on environmental and geological factors; 0.02 ppm has been reported as a representative estimate. Selenium has also been detected in urban air, presumably from sulfur-containing materials.

**Toxicokinetics.** Selenates are relatively soluble compounds, similar to sulfates, and are readily taken up by biological systems, whereas selenites and elemental selenium are virtually insoluble. Because of their insolubility, these forms may be regarded as a form of inert selenium sink. Selenides of heavy metals are also very insoluble compounds; in fact, they are so insoluble that the in vivo formation of mercury selenide by dietary administration of selenite has been proposed as a method for detoxication of methyl mercury-poisoned subjects. Other metallic selenides such as arsenic, cadmium, and copper also have low solubility, affecting the absorption, retention, and distribution within the body of selenium and heavy metals. Elemental selenium is probably not absorbed from the gastrointestinal tract. Absorption of selenite is from the duodenum. Monogastric animals have a higher intestinal absorption than ruminants, probably because selenite is reduced to an insoluble form in rumen. Over 90 percent of milligram doses of sodium selenite may be absorbed by humans and widely distributed in organs, with the highest accumulation initially in the liver and kidneys, but appreciable levels remaining in the blood, brain, myocardium, skeletal muscle, and testes. Selenium is transferred through the placenta to the fetus and it also appears in milk. Levels in milk are dependent on dietary intake. Selenium in red cells is associated with glutathione peroxidase and is about three times more concentrated than in plasma (Burk, 1976).

Selenium compounds may be biotransformed in the body by incorporation into amino acids or proteins or by methylation (Diplock, 1976). Selenium amino acids, Se-cysteine, and Se-methionine are formed in plants and absorbed as free amino acid or from digested protein. Se-methionine can be directly incorporated into proteins in place of methionine (McConnell and Hoffman, 1972). It is also suggested that selenite may be converted to Se-cysteine and incorporated into protein. Dimethyl selenium is an intermediate in the formation of a urinary metabolite, trimethyl selenium. It may be exhaled during acute selenium toxicity when its formation exceeds the rate of further methylation and urinary excretion.

The excretion pattern of a single exposure to selenite appears to have at least two phases: a rapid initial phase with as much as 15 to 40 percent of the absorbed dose excreted in the urine the first week. There is an exponential excretion of the remainder of the dose with a half-life of 103 days. The half-life of Se-methionine is 234 days. In the steady state, urine contains about twice as much as feces and increased urinary levels provide a measure of exposure. Urinary selenium is usually less than 100 $\mu g$ per liter.

Excretory products appear in sweat and expired air. The latter may have a garlicky odor due to dimethyl selenide. Within certain physiological limits, the body appears to have a homeostatic mechanism for retaining trace amounts of selenium and excreting the excess material. Selenium toxicity occurs when the intake exceeds the excretory capacity (Schroeder and Mitchener, 1972).

***Essentiality.*** The biological role of selenium in mammals including humans is attributed to the presence of selenocysteine at each of four catalytic sites of the enzyme glutathione peroxidase (Editorial, 1988; WHO, 1986; Hogberg and Alexander, 1986). This enzyme uses glutathione to reduce peroxides in cells and, in this way, protects membrane lipids and possibly proteins and nucleic acids from damage by oxidants or free radicals. It may be a functional component of hemeoxidase, another enzyme that contains selenium. The requirement for selenium is related to the degree of oxidant activity and the supply of nutrients such as zinc, copper, manganese, iron and vitamin E, so that increased amounts of these elements increase the need for selenium. Large doses of iron and copper in animals may produce myopathies that resemble the effects produced by selenium deficiency per se.

***Selenium Deficiency.*** Deficiency of selenium in lambs and calves produces congenital "white muscle disease," a form of nutritionally induced muscular dystrophy. Deficiency of selenium produces liver necrosis in rats, a bleeding disorder in poultry, and cellular necrosis in the liver, kidneys, and skeletal and heart muscle in mice, resulting in cardiac failure and death (Fishbein, 1977). In each of these entities the health effect is prevented by adding selenium to the diet so that now there are well-defined dietary requirements for selenium for livestock and poultry.

The most extensively documented deficiency of selenium in humans is Keshan disease. This is an endemic cardiomyopathy first discovered in Keshan county in the People's Republic of China in 1935. It occurs most frequently in children under 15 years of age and in women of child-bearing age. The disease is characterized clinically by various degrees of cardiomegaly and cardiac decompensation, and the histopathology of the myocardium consists of the degeneration and necrosis of myocardial fibers and their replacement by fibrosis and scar formation (Yang et al., 1983). Chen et al. (1980) studied the Se status in susceptible populations to determine the etiology of the disease. Occurrence of the disease was invariably associated with a lower selenium diet content of maize and rice than that grown in unaffected areas. The average hair selenium concentration of residents of affected areas was $0.122 \pm 0.010$ ppm versus $0.270 \pm 0.066$ ppm in the hair of people in unaffected areas. Also, low glutathione peroxidase activities of whole blood in the affected population coincided with low blood selenium levels in affected areas. It was suggested that the low blood selenium content and low blood glutathione peroxidase activity might play a role in the myocardial lesions. Administration of sodium selenite greatly reduced the incidence of the disease, a fact that provides additional support for the role of selenium deficiency in the etiology of the disorder.

**Toxicity.** The potential toxicity of selenium was first suspected over 50 years ago and through the years well-defined syndromes of toxicity have been described in animals and humans living in seminiferous areas where the soil content is relatively rich in selenium, contributing to relatively high selenium in vegetation. Plants vary in their ability to accumulate selenium. Grasses, grains and most weeds do not accumulate selenium even when grown in high-selenium areas, so that these plants add very little to the selenium content of livestock feed. But there are several plant species that are classified as "selenium accumulators" and they may contain selenium levels of 100 to 10,000 mg/kg. These plants, however, usually grow in nonagricultural areas and when consumed by livestock may, within a few weeks, cause a disease syndrome described as the *blind staggers*. Early symptoms are impaired vision, depressed appetite, and a tendency to wander in circles. This may progress to various degrees of paralysis and death from respiratory failure (Hogberg and Alexander, 1986).

A more chronic syndrome described in livestock and horses is *alkali disease* and is characterized by the loss of vitality, emaciation, deformity and shedding of hoofs, the loss of long hair, and the erosion of joints of long bones. Similar syndromes have been described in sheep and dogs (Shamberger, 1983).

The areas of the world where human toxicity have been noted include several areas of China, areas of Venezuela, and in the state of South Dakota in the U. S. A study of 70 families living in three counties of South Dakota and in one county of northern Nebraska, from farms where alkali disease in cattle had been recognized, found bad teeth, a yellowish discoloration of the skin, skin eruptions, and diseased nails of the fingers and toes in various family members.

A syndrome now believed to be the result of selenium intoxication was discovered in 1961 to affect about 50 percent of 248 inhabitants of five villages in the Hubei province of China (Yang et al., 1983). There are similarities between this syndrome and the chronic effects in livestock and horses. The main symptoms were brittle hair with intact follicles, brittle nails with spots and streaks, and skin lesions on the backs of hands and feet and on the forearms, legs, and the back of the neck. These areas were red and swollen and contained blisters. In addition, 13 of 22 people in one village had neurological symptoms including peripheral anesthesia, pain, and hyperreflexia. In some individuals these symptoms progressed to numbness, convulsions, paralysis, and altered motor function.

Selenium has produced loss of fertility and congenital defects and is considered embryotoxic and teratogenic on the basis of animal experiments. Selenium sulfide produced an increase in hepatocellular carcinomas and adenomas, but selenium sulfide suspension and Selsun™, an antidandruff shampoo containing 2.5 percent selenium sulfide, applied to the skin of Swiss mice did not produce dermal tumors. Selenium is probably not a human carcinogen (Hogberg and Alexander, 1986).

**Biological Interactions.** There is a growing body of information regarding the biological interactions of selenium. Some of these interactions impact on the toxicity from or deficiency of selenium; some impact on the toxicity of another metal. If the intake of vitamin E is low, susceptibility to selenium toxicity is increased in experimental animals, whereas resistance is increased if vitamin E intake is increased. Selenium also forms insoluble complexes with silver, copper, cadmium, and mercury. Feeding silver to experimental animals results in tissue accumulations of both metals and symptoms of selenium deficiency may occur. Selenium forms complexes with copper, and toxicity to either selenium or copper is influenced by the intake of both metals.

Selenium may prevent the toxic effects of cadmium on rat testicular tissue and dietary selenium can reduce the toxic effects of methyl mercury. Workers in a mercury mine and local inhabitants accumulate equimolar amounts of mercury and selenium in the pituitary and thyroid glands and in the brain. And finally, arsenite increases the biliary excretion of selenium, enhancing selenium excretion in urine. The mechanisms for these interactions are only partially understood but their occurrence certainly influences the determination of safe and toxic levels of selenium for persons in the general population.

**Anticarcinogenicity.** Epidemiological investigations have indicated a decrease in human cancer death rates (age- and sex-adjusted) correlated with an increasing selenium content of forage crops (Shamberger et al., 1983). In addition, experimental evidence supports the antineoplastic effect of selenium with regard to benzo[a]pyrene- and benzanthracene-induced skin tumors in mice, N-2-fluorenylacetamide- and diethylaminoazobenzene-induced hepatic tumors in rats, and spontaneous mammary tumors in mice. A possible mechanism of the protective effects of selenium has been postulated to involve inhibition of the formation of malonaldehyde, a product of peroxidative tissue damage, which is carcinogenic.

In addition to the apparent protective effect against some carcinogenic agents, selenium is an antidote to the toxic effects of other metals, particularly arsenic, cadmium, mercury, copper, and thallium. The mechanism underlying these interactions is unknown.

**Dose–Effect Relations in Humans.** Because of the potential for producing adverse health effects from both selenium excess and from deficiency, risk assessment must include both possible effects. The margin for optimal selenium nutrition and nontoxicity is relatively narrow. The National Research Council's Food and Nutrition Board (NAS, 1980) recommends 200 μg Se per day as the maximum safe upper limit for adult human intake. Metabolic balance studies on North American adults showed that 70 μg Se per day for the standard human (70 kg body weight) appears to be required to maintain Se balance and presumably to satisfy selenium requirements in these subjects. Chinese data indicate that daily intake of less than 20 μg Se can cause Keshan disease. Countries such as New Zealand have areas where daily intake is around 30 μg, but there is no evidence that this has a significant effect on the health of the people living in these areas. The critical level for prevention of deficiency, therefore, is 20 μg Se per day.

## Zinc

Zinc is a nutritionally essential metal, and a deficiency results in severe health consequences. At the other extreme, excessive exposure to zinc is relatively uncommon and requires heavy exposure. Zinc does not accumulate with continued exposure, but body content is modulated by homeostatic mechanisms that act principally on absorption and liver levels (Bertholf, 1986; Walshe et al., 1994).

Zinc is ubiquitous in the environment so that it is present in most foodstuffs, water, and air. Content of substances in contact with galvanized copper or plastic pipes may be increased. Seafoods, meats, whole grains, dairy products, nuts, and legumes are high in zinc content, while vegetables are lower, although zinc applied to soil is taken up by growing vegetables. Atmospheric zinc levels are higher in industrial areas. The average daily intake for Americans is approximately 12 to 15 mg, mostly from food.

**Toxicokinetics.** About 20 to 30 percent of ingested zinc is absorbed. The mechanism is thought to be homeostatically controlled and is probably a carrier-mediated process (Davies, 1980). It is influenced by prostaglandins $E_2$ and $F_2$ and is chelated by picolinic acid, a tryptophan derivative. Deficiency of pyridoxine or tryptophan depresses zinc absorption. Within the mucosal cell, zinc induces metallothionein synthesis and, when saturated, may depress zinc absorption. In the blood, about two-thirds of the zinc is bound to albumin and most of the remainder is complexed with $\beta_2$-macroglobulin. Zinc enters the gastrointestinal tract as a component of metallothionein secreted by the salivary glands, intestinal mucosa, pancreas, and liver. About 2 g of zinc is filtered by the kidneys each day, and about 300 to 600 $\mu$g/day is actually excreted by normal adults. Renal tubular reabsorption is impaired by commonly prescribed drugs, such as thiazide diuretics, and is further influenced by dietary protein. There is a good correlation between dietary zinc and urinary zinc excretion.

Zinc concentration in tissues varies widely. The liver receives up to about 40 percent of a tracer dose, declining to about 25 percent within 5 days. Liver concentration is influenced by humoral factors, including adrenocorticotropic hormone, parathyroid hormone, and endotoxin. In the liver, as well as in other tissues, zinc is bound to metallothionein. The greatest concentration of zinc in the body is in the prostate, probably related to the rich content of zinc-containing enzyme acid phosphatase.

**Deficiency.** More than 200 metalloenzymes require zinc as a cofactor, and deficiency results in a wide spectrum of clinical effects depending on age, stage of development, and deficiencies of related metals.

Zinc deficiency in humans was first characterized by Prasad (1983) in adolescent Egyptian boys with growth failure and delayed sexual maturation and is accompanied by protein-caloric malnutrition, pellegra, iron, and folate deficiency. Zinc deficiency in the newborn may be manifested by dermatitis, loss of hair, impaired healing, susceptibility to infections, and neuropsychological abnormalities. Dietary inadequacies coupled with liver disease from chronic alcoholism may be associated with dermatitis, night blindness, testicular atrophy, impotence, and poor wound healing. Other chronic clinical disorders, such as ulcerative colitis and the malabsorption syndromes, chronic renal disease, and hemolytic anemia, are also prone to zinc deficiency. Many drugs affect zinc homeostasis, particularly metal-chelating agents and some antibiotics, such as penicillin and isoniazid. Less common zinc deficiency may occur with myocardial infarction, arthritis, and even hypertension.

**Biological Indicators of Abnormal Zinc Homeostasis.** The range of normal plasma zinc levels is from 85 to 110 $\mu$g per dL. Severe deficiency may decrease plasma zinc to 40 to 60 $\mu$g per dL, accompanied by increased serum $\beta_2$-globulin and decreased $\alpha$-globulin. Urine zinc excretion may decrease from over 300 $\mu$g per day to less than 100 $\mu$g per day. Zinc deficiency may exacerbate impaired copper nutrition and, of course, zinc interactions with cadmium and lead may modify the toxicity of these metals.

**Toxicity.** Zinc toxicity from excessive ingestion is uncommon, but gastrointestinal distress and diarrhea have been reported following ingestion of beverages standing in galvanized cans or from use of galvanized utensils. However, evidence of hematologic, hepatic, or renal toxicity has not been observed in individuals ingesting as much as 12 g of elemental zinc over a 2-day period.

With regard to industrial exposure, metal fume fever resulting from inhalation of freshly formed fumes of zinc presents the most significant effect. This disorder has been most commonly associated with inhalation of zinc oxide fumes, but it may be seen after inhalation of the fumes of other metals, particularly magnesium, iron, and copper. Attacks usually begin after 4 to 8 h of exposure—chills and fever, profuse sweating, and weakness. Attacks usually last only 24 to 48 h and are most common on Mondays or after holidays. The pathogenesis is not known, but it is thought to be due to endogenous pyrogen released from cell lysis. Extracts prepared from tracheal mucosa and from the lungs of animals with experimentally induced metal fume fever produce similar symptoms when injected into other animals. Other aspects of zinc toxicity are not well established. Experimental animals have been given 100 times their dietary requirements without discernible effects (Goyer et al., 1979).

Exposure of guinea pigs for 3 h per day for 6 consecutive days to 5 mg/m$^3$ freshly formed ultrafine zinc oxide (the recommended threshold limit value) produced decrements in lung volumes and carbon monoxide diffusing capacity that persisted 72 h after exposure. These functional changes were correlated with microscopic evidence of interstitial thickening and cellular infiltrate in alveolar ducts and alveoli (Lam et al., 1985). Testicular tumors have been produced by direct intratesticular injection in rats and chickens. This effect is probably related to the concentration of zinc normally in the gonads and may be hormonally dependent. Zinc salts have not produced carcinogenic effects when administered to animals by other routes (Furst, 1981).

## METALS WITH TOXICITY RELATED TO MEDICAL THERAPY

Metals considered in this group include aluminum, bismuth, gold, lithium, and platinum. Metals at one time were used to treat a number of human ills, particularly heavy metals like mercury and arsenic. Gold salts are still useful for the treatment of forms of rheumatism, and organic bismuth compounds are used to treat gastrointestinal disturbances. Lithium has become an important aid in the treatment of depression. The toxicological hazards from aluminum are not from its use as an antacid but rather from the accumulations that occur in bone and from neurotoxicity in patients with chronic renal failure receiving hemodialysis therapy. A more recent concern regarding the potential neurotoxicity of aluminum involves its relationship to Alzheimer's dementia and its increase in bioavailability from changes in soil and water pH from acid rain. Platinum is receiving attention as an antitumor agent. Barium and gallium are used as radiopaque and radiotracer materials, respectively, and gallium is used for treating hypercalcemia.

## Aluminum

Aluminum is one of the most ubiquitous elements in the environment. It has, until recently, existed predominantly in forms not available to humans and most other species. Acid rain, however, has increased dramatically the amount of aluminum appearing in biological ecosystems, resulting in well-described destructive effects on fish and plant-life species.

**Toxicokinetics.** Daily intake of aluminum for people in the general population has been reported to range from 9 mg per day to 36 mg per day, with an average of about 20 mg per day. Human exposure to aluminum comes from foods and drinking water as well as pharmaceuticals. The biological speciation is thought to be of major importance in the absorption, distribution, and excretion of aluminum in mammals. Absorption from the gut depends largely on pH and the presence of complexing ligands, particularly carboxylic acids, which are absorbable. Uremic animals and humans have higher than normal levels of aluminum in spite of increased urinary clearance. In plasma, 80 to 90 percent of aluminum binds to transferrin, an iron-transport protein for which there are receptors in many body tissues. Based on potentiometric and nuclear magnetic resonance studies it is predicted that the remainder of aluminum in plasma is in the form of small-molecule hydroxy species and small complexes with carboxylic acids, phosphate, and, to a lesser degree, amino acids. These are charged species and probably not available for transport into tissues (DeVoto and Yokel, 1994). Bone and lung have the highest concentrations of aluminum, suggesting that bone may be a "sink" for aluminum. Aluminum does not normally accumulate in blood to any great extent (Ganrot, 1986).

Aluminum compounds can affect absorption of other elements in the gastrointestinal tract and alter intestinal function. Aluminum inhibits fluoride absorption and may decrease the absorption of calcium and iron compounds and possibly the absorption of cholesterol by forming an aluminum–pectin complex that binds fats to nondigestible vegetable fibers (Nagyvary and Bradbury, 1977). The binding of phosphorus in the intestinal tract can lead to phosphate depletion and osteomalacia. Aluminum may alter gastrointestinal tract motility by inhibition of acetylcholine-induced contractions and may be the explanation of why aluminum-containing antacids often produce constipation.

**Experimental Toxicity Studies.** Aluminum has marked differences in its effects on animals at different points in their lifespan and in different species. The normal concentration of aluminum in the mammalian brain is approximately 1 to 2 $\mu$g/g. In certain aluminum-sensitive species, such as cats and rabbits, increasing aluminum by intrathecal infusion, so that brain concentration is greater than 4 $\mu$g/g, induces a characteristic clinical and pathological response. Initially, animals show subtle behavioral changes, including learning and memory deficits and poor motor function. These changes progress to tremor, incoordination, weakness, and ataxia. This is followed by focal seizures and death within 3 or 4 weeks of initial exposure. With lesser doses, there is longer survival but no recovery (Deboni et al., 1976).

The most prominent early pathological change is an accumulation of neurofibrillary tangles (NFT) in cell body, proximal axons, and dendrites of neurones of many brain regions. This is associated with loss of synapsis and atrophy of the dendritic tree. Not all species show this reaction to aluminum, however. The rat fails to develop NFTs or encephalopathy and the monkey develops these only after more than a year following aluminum infusion. NFTs are found primarily in large neurons such as Purkinje cells of the cerebellum and large neurons of the cerebral cortex. There is marked reduction in the numbers of neurotubules and the rate of cytoplasmic transport with impairment of intracellular transport. Aluminum also interacts with neuronal chromatin or DNA and is associated with a decreased rate of DNA synthesis. RNA polymerase activity is also reduced.

Aluminum competes with or alters calcium metabolism in several organ systems including the brain. Brain tissue calcium rises following aluminum exposure. Aluminum also binds to calmodulin and induces changes in its structure, leading to the suggestion that aluminum impairs the function of calmodulin as a calcium regulator. This would have profound effects on central nervous system function and would disrupt neurotubular integrity and transport. While these studies in animals have provided some insights into the mechanisms of the neurotoxicity of aluminum in experimental models, the relationship to human disease is presently uncertain (Siegal and Haug, 1983; Bizzi and Gambetti, 1986; Birchall and Chappel, 1988).

**Human Dementia Syndromes.** ***Dialysis Dementia.*** A progressive, fatal neurological syndrome has also been reported in patients on long-term intermittent hemodialysis treatment for chronic renal failure (Alfrey, 1988). The first symptom in these patients is a speech disorder followed by dementia, convulsions, and myoclonus. The disorder, which typically arises after 3 to 7 years of dialysis treatment, may be due to aluminum intoxication. The aluminum content of brain, muscle, and bone tissues increases in these patients. Sources of the excess aluminum may be from oral aluminum hydroxide commonly given to these patients or from aluminum in dialysis fluid derived from the tap water used to prepare the dialysate fluid. The high serum and aluminum concentrations may be related to increased parathyroid hormone, which is due to the low blood calcium and osteodystrophy common in patients with chronic renal disease. The syndrome may be prevented by avoidance of the use of aluminum-containing oral phosphate binders and by monitoring of aluminum in the dialysate. Chelation of aluminum may be achieved with use of desferrioxamine, and progression of the dementia may be arrested or slowed (Wills and Savory, 1983).

***Amyotrophic Lateral Sclerosis and Parkinsonism-Dementia Syndromes of Guam (Guam ALS-PD Complex).*** The Chamorro peoples of the Mariana Islands in the western Pacific Ocean, particularly Guam and Rota, have an unusually high incidence of neurodegenerative diseases associated with nerve cell loss and neurofibrillary degeneration of the Alzheimer's type. Garruto et al. (1984) noted that the volcanic soils of the regions of Guam with a high incidence of ALS-PD contained high concentrations of aluminum and manganese and were low in calcium and magnesium. They postulated that a low intake of calcium and magnesium induced secondary hyperparathyroidism, resulting in an increase in calcium, aluminum, and other toxic metals, resulting in neuronal injury and death. How and why aluminum enters the brain of these people is unclear. A recent study of mineral content of food did not indicate high exposure to aluminum or low dietary calcium (Crapper-McLachlan et al., 1989). These authors suggest that the diet of the inhabitants of Guam may be the source of the aluminum, particularly through the respiratory tract. Perl and Good (1987) have shown that aluminum may be taken up through nasal-olfactory pathways.

***Alzheimer's Disease.*** Two observations have provided a suspected link between Alzheimer's disease and aluminum. One is that increased amounts of aluminum have been found in the brains of persons dying of Alzheimer's disease. Although brain aluminum content has been found to vary greatly (from 0.4 to 107.9 $\mu$g/g), the overall mean aluminum content is approximately 5 to 10 $\mu$g per g, similar to levels related to encephalopathy in animal models. These levels of aluminum, however, are also found in dialysis patients, even those who are not demented (see section on Dialysis Dementia, above).

The second major finding that relates aluminum encephalopathy to Alzheimer's disease is the finding of NFTs in both conditions (Klatzo et al., 1965). Perl and Brody (1980) developed a sensitive technique using the scanning electron microscope, in conjunction with energy dispersive x-ray spectrometry, for analysis of trace element constituents of the nervous system at the cellular level of resolution. With this technique they were able to identify intraneuronal accumulations of aluminum in association with NFT formation in the hippocampal neurons of brain tissues obtained from patients with Alzheimer's disease. However, it is now clear that the NFTs induced by the two conditions are different both structurally and chemically. Also, NFTs are present in a wide variety of neurological disorders. Using x-ray spectrometry, Perl and Brody (1980) found aluminum in the nuclei of virtually all NFT-containing neurons and in virtually no non-NFT-containing neurons, so that aluminum may be, in some way, a secondary or interactive factor producing a different type of cellular dysfunction in Alzheimer's disease.

The question that has been raised about the increase in aluminum in brains of persons with Alzheimer's disease has not so much to do with exposure to aluminum as with its mode of uptake by the brain. The blood–brain barrier is normally only permeable to small molecules or large molecules by active transport mechanisms. Aluminum–protein complexes are unlikely to cross the blood–brain barrier, although transferrin receptors present in the brain offer a possible mechanism. Nevertheless, the actual mode of uptake of aluminum by the brain has not yet been determined (Perl and Good, 1988; DeVoto and Yokel, 1994).

**Epidemiological Studies of Alzheimer's Disease and Aluminum Exposure.** Studies of the prevalence of dementia have been reviewed by Henderson (1986) and Ineichen (1987). Prevalence rates varied from 2.5 percent in people over age 65 in London to 25 percent in people over age 60 in the former U.S.S.R. Such variation most probably indicates differences in the criteria for ascertaining the diagnosis but it may also reflect differences in environment.

Epidemiological studies relating geographical variation in the rate of Alzheimer's disease and its relation to differences in the population exposure to aluminum are limited. A recent study in England found that where aluminum concentrations in the water supplies were high, daily intake of aluminum by people living in these areas was likely to be increased (Martyn et al., 1989). A Norwegian study reported that mortality from dementia was higher in areas of the country where higher concentrations of aluminum in the water supply was found. In each of these studies, however, there are inconsistencies in the criteria for dementia and in information available from death certificates.

## Bismuth

Bismuth has a long history of use in pharmaceuticals in Europe and North America. Both inorganic and organic salts have been used, depending on the specific application. Trivalent insoluble bismuth salts are used medicinally to control diarrhea and other types of gastrointestinal distress. Various bismuth salts have been used externally for their astringent and slight antiseptic properties. Bismuth salts have also been used as radiocontrast agents. Further potential for exposure comes from the use of insoluble bismuth salts in cosmetics. Injections of soluble and insoluble salts, suspended in oil to maintain adequate blood levels, have been used to treat syphilis. Bismuth sodium thioglycollate, a water-soluble salt, was injected intramuscularly for malaria (*Plasmodium vivax*). Bismuth glycolyarsanilate is one of the few pentavalent salts that have been used medicinally. This material was formerly used for treatment of amebiasis (Fowler and Vouk, 1986). Exposure to various bismuth salts for medicinal use has decreased with the advent of newer therapeutic agents. However, in the 1970s reports appeared from France and Australia of a unique encephalopathy occurring in colostomy and ileostomy patients using bismuth subgallate, bismuth subnitrate, and tripotassium-dicitrate-bismuthate for control of fecal odor and consistency. The symptoms included progressive mental confusion, irregular myoclonic jerks, a distinctive pattern of disordered gait, and a variable degree of dysarthria. The disorder was fatal to patients who continued use of the bismuth compounds, but full recovery was rapid in those in whom therapy was discontinued. The severity of the disorder seemed to be independent of dose and duration of therapy (Thomas et al., 1977).

Most bismuth compounds are insoluble and poorly absorbed from the gastrointestinal tract or when applied to the skin, even if the skin is abraded or burned. Patients taking bismuth subgallate were found to have an elevated median blood bismuth level of 14.6 $\mu$g Bi/dL, while patients with clinical symptoms of bismuth toxicity had a median blood level of 3 $\mu$g/dL, and colostomy patients not on bismuth therapy had a median bismuth blood level of 0.8 $\mu$g/dl. Health laboratory workers had a median bismuth blood level of 1.0 $\mu$g/dL. Binding in blood is thought to be largely to a plasma protein with a molecular weight greater than 50,000. A diffusible equilibrium between tissues, blood, and urine is established. Tissue distribution, omitting injection depots, reveals the kidney as the site of the highest concentration. The liver concentration is considerably lower at therapeutic levels, but with massive doses in experimental animals (dogs), the kidney-to-liver ratio is decreased. Passage of bismuth into the amniotic fluid and into the fetus has been demonstrated. The urine is the major route of excretion. Traces of bismuth can be found in milk and saliva. The total elimination of bismuth after injection is slow and dependent on its mobilization from the injection site.

Acute renal failure can occur following oral administration of such compounds as bismuth sodium triglycocollamate or thioglycollate, particularly in children (Urizar and Vernier, 1966). The tubular epithelium is the primary site of toxicity, producing degeneration of renal tubular cells and nuclear inclusion bodies composed of a bismuth–protein complex analogous to those found in lead toxicity (Fowler and Goyer, 1975).

The symptoms of chronic toxicity in humans consist of decreased appetite, weakness, rheumatic pain, diarrhea, fever, metal line on the gums, foul breath, gingivitis, and dermatitis. Jaundice and conjunctival hemorrhage are rare but have been reported. Bismuth nephropathy with proteinuria may occur.

Recently there has been an increased interest in bismuth to treat peptic ulcer disease. This interest was prompted by the discovery in 1982 of a Gram-negative bacterium from the gastric mucosa of patients suffering from gastritis. The bacterium, *Helicobacter pylori*, is now thought to predispose patients with chronic gastritis to peptic ulcer formation and duodenal ulceration. Antiacids containing bismuth compounds have been effective in promoting healing of peptic ulcers which is now thought to be due to the antibacterial action of bismuth. The compound used clinically is colloidal bismuth subcitrate and is poorly absorbed (Abrams and Murrer, 1993).

Chelation therapy using dimercaprol (BAL) is said to be helpful in the removal of bismuth from children with acute toxicity (Arena, 1974).

## Gallium

Gallium is of interest because of the use of radiogallium as a diagnostic tool for the localization of bone lesions and the use of nonradioactive gallium $Ga(NO_3)_3$ as an antitumor agent. Also, it has been approved recently in the U.S. for the treatment of hypercalcemia. It is obtained as a by-product of copper, zinc, lead, and aluminum refining and is used in high-temperature thermometers, as a substitute for mercury in arc lamps, as a component of metal alloys, and as a seal for vacuum equipment. It is only sparsely absorbed from the gastrointestinal tract, but concentrations of less than 1 ppm can be localized radiographically in bone lesions. Higher doses will allow one to visualize the liver, spleen, and kidney as well (Hayes, 1988). Urine is the major route of excretion.

As an antitumor agent, $Ga(NO_3)_3$ is especially effective as a single agent for treatment of Hodgkin's disease and non-Hodgkin's lymphoma. It has also been noted that patients given continuous infusions of $Ga(NO_3)_3$ became hypocalcemic, suggesting a role for gallium in the treatment of hypercalcemia. The mechanism of action is unclear, but in vitro studies have shown that gallium inhibits calcium loss from bone and increases bone calcium levels (Abrams and Murrer, 1993).

There are no reported adverse effects of gallium following industrial exposure. Therapeutic use of radiogallium produced some adverse effects, mild dermatitis, and gastrointestinal disturbances. Bone marrow depression has been reported and may be due largely to the radioactivity. In animals gallium acts as a neuromuscular poison and causes renal damage. Photophobia, blindness, and paralysis have been reported in rats. Renal damage ranging from cloudy swelling to tubular cell necrosis has been reported. Large doses given to rats causes renal precipitates consisting of gallium, calcium, and phosphate (Newman et al., 1979). Administration of gallium arsenide to experimental animals results in arsenic intoxication (Webb et al., 1984).

## Gold

Gold is widely distributed in small quantities but economically usable deposits occur as the free metal in quartz veins or alluvial gravel. Seawater contains 3 or 4 mg/ton and small amounts, 0.03 to 1 mg percent, have been reported in many foods. Gold has a number of industrial uses because of its electrical and thermal conductivity.

While gold and its salts have been used for a wide variety of medicinal purposes, their present uses are limited to the treatment of rheumatoid arthritis and rare skin diseases such as discoid lupus. Gold salts are poorly absorbed from the gastrointestinal tract. Normal urine and fecal excretions of 0.1 and 1 mg/day, respectively, have been reported. After injection of most of the soluble salts, gold is excreted via the urine, while the feces account for the major portion of insoluble compounds. Gold seems to have a long biological half-life, and detectable blood levels can be demonstrated for 10 months after cessation of treatment.

Dermatitis is the most frequently reported toxic reaction to gold and is sometimes accompanied by stomatitis. Increase in serum IgE has been noted in patients with dermatological side effects.

The use of gold in the form of organic salts to treat rheumatoid arthritis may be complicated by the development of proteinuria and the nephrotic syndrome, which morphologically consists of an immune-complex glomerulonephritis, with granular deposits along the glomerular basement membrane and in the mesangium. The pathogenesis of the immune-complex disease is not certain, but gold may behave as a hapten and generate the production of antibodies with subsequent disposition of gold protein–antibody complexes in the glomerular subepithelium. Another hypothesis is that antibodies are formed against damaged tubular structures, particularly mitochondria, providing immune complexes for the glomerular deposits (Voil et al., 1977).

**Gold Salts.** The pathogenesis of the renal lesions induced by gold therapy also have a direct toxicity to renal tubular cell components. From experimental studies it appears that gold salts have an affinity for mitochondria of proximal tubular lining cells, which is followed by autophagocytosis and accumulation of gold in amorphous phagolysosomes (Stuve and Galle, 1970), and gold particles can be identified in degenerating mitochondria in tubular lining cells and in glomerular epithelial cell by x-ray microanalysis (Ainsworth et al., 1981).

## Lithium

Lithium carbonate is an important aid in the treatment of depression. There must be careful monitoring of usage to provide optimal therapeutic value and to produce toxicity. Lithium is a common metal and present in many plant and animal tissues. Daily intake is about 2 mg. It is readily absorbed from the gastrointestinal tract. Distribution in the human organs is almost uniform. The normal plasma level is about 17 $\mu$g per liter. The red cells contain less. Excretion is chiefly through the kidneys, but some is eliminated in the feces. The greater part of lithium is contained in the cells, perhaps at the expense of potassium. In general, the body distribution of lithium is similar to that of sodium, and it may be competing with sodium at certain sites, for example, in renal tubular reabsorption.

Lithium has some industrial uses, in alloys, as a catalytic agent, and as a lubricant. Lithium hydride produces hydrogen on contact with water and is used in manufacturing electronic tubes, in ceramics, and in chemical synthesis. From the industrial point of view, except for lithium hydride, none of the other salts is hazardous, nor is the metal itself. Lithium hydride is intensely corrosive and may produce burns on the skin because of the formation of hydroxides (Cox and Singer, 1981). The therapeutic use of lithium carbonate may produce unusual toxic responses. These include neuromuscular changes (tremor, muscle hyperirritability, and ataxia), central nervous system changes (blackout spells, epileptic seizures, slurred speech, coma, psychosomatic retardation, and increased thirst), cardiovascular changes (cardiac arrhythmia, hypertension, and circulatory collapse), gastrointestinal changes (anorexia, nausea, and vomiting) and renal damage (albuminuria and glycosuria). The latter is believed to be due to temporary hypokalemic nephritis. These changes appear to be more frequent when the serum levels increase above 1.5 nEq/L, suggesting that careful monitoring of this parameter is needed, rather than reliance on a given dose.

Chronic lithium nephrotoxicity and interstitial nephritis can occur with long-term exposure even when lithium levels remain within the therapeutic range (Singer, 1981). Animal studies have shown a similarity between lithium and sodium handling and that lithium may cause an antidiuretic hormone (ADH)-resistant polyuria and secondary polydipsia. This abnormality appears to be mediated by a central pituitary effect that reduces ADH release. Treatment with lithium salts has also been associated with nephrotic syndrome with minimal glomerular changes.

The cardiovascular and nervous system changes may be due to the competitive relationship between lithium and potassium and may thus produce a disturbance in intracellular metabolism. Thyrotoxic reactions, including goiter formation, have also been suggested (Davis and Fann, 1971). While there has been some indication of adverse effects on fetuses following lithium treatment, none was observed in rats (4.05 mEq/kg), rabbits (1.08 mEq/kg), or primates (0.67 mEq/kg). This dose to rats was sufficient to produce maternal toxicity and effects on the pups of treated, lactating dams.

Lithium overdosage and toxicity may be treated by the administration of diuretics and lowering of blood levels. Acetazolamide, a carbonic anhydrase inhibitor, has been used clinically. Animal studies have shown that urinary excretion of lithium can be further enhanced by the combined administration of acetazolamide and furosemide. Treatment with diuretics must be accompanied by replacement of water and electrolytes (Steele, 1977).

## Platinum

Platinum-group metals include a relatively light triad of ruthenium, rhodium, and palladium and the heavy metals osmium, iridium, and platinum. They are found together in sparsely distributed mineral deposits or as a by-product of refining other metals, chiefly nickel and copper. Osmium and iridium are not important toxicologically. Osmium tetroxide, however, is a powerful eye irritant. The other metals are generally nontoxic in their metallic states but have been noted to have toxic effects in particular circumstances. Platinum is interesting because of its extensive industrial applications and because of the use of certain complexes as antitumor agents.

Toxicological information for ruthenium is limited to references in the literature indicating that fumes may be injurious to eyes and lungs (Browning, 1969).

Palladium chloride is not readily absorbed from subcutaneous injection, and no adverse effects have been reported from industrial exposure. Colloid palladium ($Pd[OH]_2$) is reported to increase body temperature, produce discoloration and necrosis at the site of injection, decrease body weight, and cause slight homolysis.

Platinum metal itself is generally harmless, but an allergic dermatitis can be produced in susceptible individuals. Skin changes are most common between the fingers and in the antecubital fossae. Symptoms of respiratory distress, ranging from irritation to an "asthmatic syndrome," with coughing, wheezing, and shortness of breath, have been reported following exposure to platinum dust. The skin and respiratory changes are termed platinosis. They are mainly confined to persons with a history of industrial exposure to soluble compounds such as sodium chloroplatinate, although cases resulting from wearing platinum jewelry have been reported (WHO, 1991).

**Allergenic Effects of Platinum Salts.** The complex salts of platinum may act as powerful allergens, particularly ammonium hexachloroplatinate and hexachloroplatinic acid. The allergenicity appears to be related to the number of chlorine atoms present in the molecule, but other soluble nonchlorinated platinum compounds may also be allergenic. Major consideration for this group of metals are the potential antitumor and carcinogenic effects of certain neutral complexes of platinum such as cis-dichlorodiammine platinum (II) (or cisplatin), and various analogs (Kazantzis, 1981). They can inhibit cell division and have antibacterial properties as well. These compounds can react selectively with specific chemical sites in proteins such as disulfide bonds and terminal-$NH_2$ groups, with functional groups in amino acids, and in particular with receptor sites in nucleic acids. These compounds also exhibit neuromuscular toxicity and nephrotoxicity.

**Antitumor Effects of Platinum Complexes (Cisplatin).** Platinum complexes, particularly cisplatin, are effective antitumor agents and are used clinically for the treatment of cancers of the head and neck, certain lymphomas, and testicular and ovarian tumors. For antitumor activity, the complexes should be neutral and should have a pair of cis-leaving groups. Other metals in the group give complexes that are inactive or less active than the platinum analog. At dosages that are therapeutically effective (antitumor), these complexes produce severe and persistent inhibition of DNA synthesis and little inhibition of RNA and protein synthesis. DNA polymerase activity and transport of DNA precursors through plasma membranes are not inhibited. The complexes are thought to react directly with DNA in regions that are rich in guanosine and cytosine (Abrams and Murrer, 1993).

**Mutagenic and Carcinogenic Effects of Platinum Complexes.** Cisplatin is a strong mutagen in bacterial systems and has been shown to form both intrastrand interstrand cross-links, probably involving the whole molecule with human DNA in HeLa cell cultures. There is also a correlation between antitumor activity of cisplatin and its ability to bind DNA and induce phage from bacterial cells. It also causes chromosomal aberrations in cultured hamster cells and a dose-dependent increase in sister chromosome exchanges.

Although cisplatin has antitumorigenic activity, it also seems to increase the frequency of lung adenomas and give rise to skin papillomas and carcinomas in mice. These observations are consistent with the activity of other alkylating agents used in cancer chemotherapy. There are no reports of increased risk to cancer from occupational exposure to platinum compounds.

**Nephrotoxicity.** Cisplatin is also a nephrotoxin, which compromises its usefulness as a therapeutic agent. Platinum compounds with antitumor activity produce proximal and distal tubular cell injury, mainly in the corticomedullary region where the concentration of platinum is highest (Madias and Harrington, 1978). Although 90 percent of administered cisplatin becomes tightly bound to plasma proteins, only unbound platinum is rapidly filtered by the glomerulus and has a half-life of only 48 min. Within tissues, platinum is protein bound with the largest concentrations in kidney, liver, and spleen, and it has a half-life of 2 or 3 days. Tubular cell toxicity seems to be directly related to dose, and prolonged weekly injection in rats causes atrophy of the cortical portions of nephrons, cystic dilatation of inner cortical or medullary tubules, and chronic renal failure due to tubulointerstitial nephritis (Choie et al., 1981). Experimental studies suggest that the preadministration of bismuth subnitrate, a potent inducer of metallothionein in the kidney, reduces the nephrotoxicity of cis-platinum without interfering with its anticancer effect (Kondo et al., 1992).

## MINOR TOXIC METALS

### Antimony

Antimony may have a trivalence or pentavalance and it belongs to the same periodic group as arsenic. Antimony is included in alloys in the metals industry and is used for producing fireproofing chemicals, ceramics, glassware, and pigments. Antimony has been used medicinally in the treatment of schistosomiasis and leishmaniasis. The metabolism of antimony resembles that of arsenic. It is absorbed slowly from the gastrointestinal tract, and many antimony compounds are gastrointestinal irritants. Trivalent antimony is concentrated in red blood cells and liver, whereas the penta form is mostly in plasma. Both forms are excreted in feces and urine, but more trivalent antimony is excreted in urine; there is greater gastrointestinal excretion of pentavalent antimony. Antimony is a common air pollutant from industrial emissions, but exposure for the general population is largely from food.

Most information about antimony toxicity has been obtained from industrial experiences. Occupational exposures are usually by inhalation of dust containing antimony compounds, antimony pentachloride and trichloride, trioxide, and trisulfide. Effects may be acute, particularly from the penta and trichloride exposures, producing a rhinitis and even acute pulmonary edema. Chronic exposures by inhalation of other antimony compounds result in rhinitis, pharyngitis, tracheitis, and, over the longer term, bronchitis and eventually pneumoconiosis with obstructive lung disease and emphysema. Antimony does accumulate in lung tissue. Transient skin eruptions, "antimony spots," may occur in workers with chronic exposure (Elinder and Friberg, 1986).

Antimony-containing compounds may also produce alterations in cardiac function and autopsy studies have shown that cardiac toxicity was the cause of death in patients treated with antimonial drugs (Winship, 1987).

Oral feeding of antimony to rats has not produced an excess of tumors. However, increased chromosome defects occur when human lymphocytes are incubated with a soluble antimony salt (Paton and Allison, 1972), and Syrian hamster embryo cells show and undergo neoplastic transformation when treated with antimony acetate.

The metal hydride of antimony, stibine ($H_3S_6$), is a highly toxic gas that can be generated when antimony is exposed to reducing acids or when batteries are overcharged. High-purity stibine is also used in the production of semiconductors. Stibine, like arsine, causes hemolysis.

### Barium

Barium is used in various alloys, in paints, soap, paper, and rubber, and in the manufacture of ceramics and glass. Barium fluorosilicate and carbonate have been used as insecticides. Barium sulfate, an insoluble compound, is used as a radiopaque aid to x-ray diagnosis. Barium is relatively abundant in nature and is found in plants and animal tissue. Plants accumulate barium from the soil. Brazil nuts have very high concentrations (3000 to 4000 ppm). Some water contains barium from natural deposits.

The toxicity of barium compounds depends on their solubility. The soluble compounds of barium are absorbed, and small amounts are accumulated in the skeleton. The lung has an average concentration of 1 ppm (dry weight). The kidney, spleen, muscle, heart, brain, and liver concentrations are 0.10, 0.08, 0.05, and 0.03 ppm, respectively. Although some barium is excreted in urine, it is reabsorbed by the renal tubules. The major route of excretion is the feces. Occupational poisoning to barium is uncommon, but a benign pneumoconiosis (baritosis) may result from inhalation of barium sulfate (barite) dust and barium carbonate. It is not incapacitating and is usually reversible with cessation of exposure. Accidental poisoning from ingestion of soluble barium salts has resulted in gastroenteritis, muscular paralysis, decreased pulse rate, and ventricular fibrillation and extra-systoles. Potassium deficiency occurs in acute poisoning, and treatment with intravenous potassium appears beneficial. The digitalis-like toxicity, muscle stimulation, and central nervous system effects have been confirmed by experimental investigation (Reeves, 1986).

### Indium

Indium is a rare metal whose toxicological importance was related to its use in alloys, solders, and as a hardening agent for bearings. Use in the electronics industry for production of semiconductors and photovoltaic cells may greatly expand worker exposure. It is currently being used in medicine for the scanning of organs and the treatment of tumors. Indium is poorly absorbed from the gastrointestinal tract. It is excreted in the urine and feces. Its tissue distribution is relatively uniform. The kidney, liver, bone, and spleen have relatively high concentrations. Intratracheal injections produce similar concentrations, but the concentration in the tracheobronchial lymph nodes is increased.

There are no meaningful reports of human toxicity to indium. From animal experiments it is apparent that toxicity is related to the chemical form. Indium chloride given intravenously to mice produces renal toxicity and liver necrosis. These effects are accompanied by the induction of P-450-dependent microsomal enzyme activity and by the decreased activity of heme-synthesizing enzymes (Woods et al., 1979). Hydrated indium oxide produces damage to phagocytic cells in liver and the reticuloendothelial system (Fowler, 1982).

## Silver

The principal industrial use of silver is as silver halide in the manufacture of photographic plates. Other uses are for jewelry, coins, and eating utensils. Silver nitrate is used for making indelible inks and for medicinal purposes. The use of silver nitrate for prophylaxis of ophthalmia neonatorum is a legal requirement in some states. Other medicinal uses of silver salts are as a caustic, germicide, antiseptic, and astringent.

Silver does not occur regularly in animal or human tissue. The major effect of excessive absorption of silver is local or generalized impregnation of the tissues where it remains as silver sulfide, which forms an insoluble complex in elastic fibers, resulting in argyria. Silver can be absorbed from the lungs and gastrointestinal tract. Complexes with serum albumin accumulate in the liver from which a fractional amount is excreted. Intravenous injection produces accumulation in the spleen, liver, bone marrow, lungs, muscle, and skin. The major route of excretion is via the gastrointestinal tract. Urinary excretion has not been reported to occur even after intravenous injection.

Industrial argyria, a chronic occupational disease, has two forms, local and generalized. The local form involves the formation of gray-blue patches on the skin or may manifest itself in the conjunctiva of the eye. In generalized argyria, the skin shows widespread pigmentation, often spreading from the face to most uncovered parts of the body. In some cases the skin may become black with a metallic lustre. The eyes may be affected to such a point that the lens and vision are disturbed. The respiratory tract may also be affected in severe cases. Large oral doses of silver nitrate cause severe gastrointestinal irritation due to its caustic action. Lesions of the kidneys and lungs and the possibility of arteriosclerosis have been attributed to both industrial and medicinal exposures. Large doses of colloidal silver administered intravenously to experimental animals produced death due to pulmonary edema and congestion. Hemolysis and resulting bone marrow hyperplasia have been reported. Chronic bronchitis has also been reported to result from medicinal use of colloidal silver (Browning, 1969; Luckey et al., 1975).

## Tellurium

Tellurium is found in various sulfide ores along with selenium and is produced as a by-product of metal refineries. Its industrial uses include applications in the refining of copper and in the manufacture of rubber. Tellurium vapor is used in "daylight" lamps. It is used in various alloys as a catalyst and as a semiconductor.

Condiments, dairy products, nuts, and fish have high concentrations of tellurium. Food packaging contains some tellurium; higher concentrations are found in aluminum cans than in tin cans. Some plants, such as garlic, accumulate tellurium from the soil. Potassium tellurate has been used to reduce sweating.

The average body burden in humans is about 600 mg; the majority is in bone. The kidney has the highest content among the soft tissues. Some data suggest that tellurium also accumulates in the liver (Schroeder and Mitchener, 1972). Soluble tetravalent tellurites, absorbed into the body after oral administration, are reduced to tellurides, partly methylated, and then exhaled as dimethyl telluride. The latter is responsible for the garlic odor in persons exposed to tellurium compounds. Tellurium in the food is probably in the form of tellurates. The urine and bile are the principal routes of excretion. Sweat and milk are secondary routes of excretion.

Tellurates and tellurium are of low toxicity, but tellutites are generally more toxic. Acute inhalation exposure results in decreased sweating, nausea, a metallic taste, and sleeplessness. A typical garlic breath is a reasonable indicator of exposure to tellurium by the dermal, inhalation, or oral route. Serious cases of tellurium intoxication from industrial exposure have not been reported. In rats, chronic exposure to high doses of tellurium dioxide has produced decreased growth and necrosis of the liver and kidney (Cerwenka and Cooper, 1961; Browning, 1969).

Sodium tellurite at 2 ppm in drinking water or potassium tellurate at 2 ppm of tellurium plus $0.16\,\mu g/g$ in the diet of mice for their lifetime produced no effects in the tellurate group. The females of the tellurite (tetravalent) group did not live as long. In rats, 500 ppm in the diet of pregnant females induced hydrocephalus in the offspring. Abnormalities of and reduction in numbers of mitochondria were thought to be possible cellular causes of the transplacental effect.

One of the few serious recorded cases of tellurium toxicity resulted from accidental poisoning by injection of tellurium into the ureters during retrograde pyelography. Two of the three victims died. Stupor, cyanosis, vomiting, garlic breath, and loss of consciousness were observed in this unlikely incident.

Dimercaprol treatment for tellurium toxicity increases the renal damage. While ascorbic acid decreases the characteristic garlic odor, it may also adversely affect the kidneys in the presence of increased amounts of tellurium (Fishbein, 1977).

## Thallium

Thallium is one of the more toxic metals and can cause neural, hepatic, and renal injury. It may also cause deafness and loss of vision. It is obtained as a by-product of the refining of iron, cadmium, and zinc. It is used as a catalyst, in certain alloys, optical lenses, jewelry, low-temperature thermometers, semiconductors, dyes and pigments, and scintillation counters. It has been used medicinally as a depilatory. Thallium compounds, chiefly thallous sulfate, have been used as rat poison and insecticides. This is one of the commonest sources of thallium poisoning.

**Toxicokinetics.** Thallium is not a normal constituent of animal tissues. It is absorbed through the skin and gastrointestinal tract. After parenteral administration a small amount can be identified in the urine within a few hours. The highest concentrations after poisoning are in the kidney and urine. The intestines, thyroids, testes, pancreas, skin, bone, and spleen have lesser amounts. The brain and liver concentrations are still lower. Following the initial exposure, large amounts are excreted in urine during the first 24 h, but after that period excretion is slow and the feces may be an important route of excretion.

**Toxicology.** There are numerous clinical reports of acute thallium poisoning in humans characterized by gastrointestinal irritation, acute ascending paralysis, and psychic disturbances. Acute toxicity studies in rats have indicated that thallium is quite toxic. It has an oral $LD_{50}$ of approximately 30 mg/kg. The estimated lethal dose in humans, however, is 8 to 12 mg/kg. Rat studies also indicate that thallium oxide, while relatively insoluble, is more toxic orally than by the intravenous or intraperitoneal route (Downs et al., 1960). The acute cardiovascular effects of thallium ions probably result from competition with potassium for membrane transport systems, inhibition of mitochondrial oxidative phosphorylation, and disruption of protein synthesis. It also alters heme metabolism.

The signs of subacute or chronic thallium poisoning in rats were hair loss, cataracts, and hindleg paralysis occurring with some delay after the initiation of dosing. Renal lesions were observed at gross necropsy. Histological changes revealed damage of the proximal and distal renal tubules. The central nervous system changes were most severe in the mesencephalon where necrosis was observed. Perivascular cuffing was also reported in several other brain areas. Electron microscope examination indicated that the mitochondria in the kidney may have been the first organelles affected. Liver mitochondria also revealed degenerative changes. The livers of newborn rats whose dams had been treated throughout pregnancy showed these changes. Similar mitochondrial changes were observed in the intestine, brain, seminal vesicle, and pancreas. It has been suggested that thallium may combine with the sulfhydryl groups in the mitochondria and thereby interfere with oxidative phosphorylation. A teratogenic response to thallium salts characterized as achondroplasia (dwarfism) has been described in rats (Nogami and Terashima, 1973).

In humans, fatty infiltration and necrosis of the liver, nephritis, gastroenteritis, pulmonary edema, degenerative changes in the adrenals, degeneration of the peripheral and central nervous system, alopecia, and in some cases death have been reported as a result of long-term systemic thallium intake. These cases usually are caused by the contamination of food or the use of thallium as a depilatory. Industrial poisoning is a special risk in the manufacture of fused halides for the production of lenses and windows. Loss of vision plus the other signs of thallium poisoning have been related to industrial exposures (Browning, 1969; Fowler, 1982).

## Tin

Tin is used in the manufacture of tinplate, in food packaging, and in solder, bronze, and brass. Stannous and stannic chlorides are used in dyeing textiles. Organic tin compounds have been used in fungicides, bactericides, and slimicides, as well as in plastics as stabilizers. The disposition and possible health effects of inorganic and organic tin compounds have been summarized in a WHO report (1980).

**Toxicokinetics.** There is only limited absorption of even soluble tin salts such as sodium stannous tartrate after oral administration. Ninety percent of the tin administered in this manner is recovered in the feces. The small amounts absorbed are reflected by increases in the liver and kidneys. Injected tin is excreted by the kidneys, with smaller amounts in bile. A mean normal urine level of 16.6 $\mu$g/L or 23.4 $\mu$g/day has been reported. The majority of inhaled tin or its salts remains in the lungs, most extracellularly, with some in the macrophages, in the form of $SnO_2$. The organic tins, particularly triethyltin, may be somewhat better absorbed. The tissue distribution of tin from this material shows the highest concentrations in the blood and liver, with smaller amounts in the muscle, spleen, heart, or brain. Tetraethyltin is converted to triethyltin in vivo.

Chronic inhalation of tin in the form of dust or fumes leads to benign pneumoconiosis. Tin hydride ($SnH_4$) is more toxic to mice and guinea pigs than is arsine; however, its effects appear mainly in the central nervous system and no hemolysis is produced. Orally, tin or its inorganic compounds require relatively large doses (500 mg/kg for 14 months) to produce toxicity. The use of tin in food processing seems to demonstrate little hazard. The average U.S. daily intake, mostly from foods as a result of processing, is estimated at 17 mg. Inorganic tin salts given by injection produce diarrhea, muscle paralysis, and twitching.

**Toxicology.** Some organic tin compounds are highly toxic, particularly triethyltin. Trialkyl compounds including triethyltin cause an encephalopathy and cerebral edema. Toxicity declines as the number of carbon atoms in the chain increases. An outbreak of almost epidemic nature took place in France due to the oral ingestion of a preparation (Stalinon) containing diethyltin diodide for the treatment of skin disorders.

Excessive industrial exposure to triethyltin has been reported to produce headaches, visual defects, and electroencephalograph (EEG) changes that were very slowly reversed (Prull and Rompel, 1970). Experimentally, triethyltin produces depression and cerebral edema. The resulting hyperglycemia may be related to the centrally mediated depletion of catecholamines from the adrenals. Acute burns or subacute dermal irritation has been reported among workers as a result of tributyltin. Triphenyltin has been shown to be a potent immunosuppressant (Verschuuren et al., 1970). Inhibition in the hydrolysis of adenosine triphosphate and an uncoupling of the oxidative phosphorylation taking place in the mitochondria have been suggested as the cellular mechanisms of tin toxicity (WHO, 1980).

## Titanium

Most titanium compounds are in the oxidation state +4 (titanic), but oxidation state +3 (titanous) and oxidation state +2 compounds as well as several organometallic compounds do occur. Titanium dioxide, the most widely used compound, is a white pigment used in paints and plastics, as a food additive to whiten flour, dairy products, and confections, and as a whitener in cosmetic products. Because of its resistance to corrosion and inertness it has many metallurgical applications, particularly as a component of surgical implants and prostheses. It occurs widely in the environment; it is present in urban air, rivers, and drinking water and is detectable in many foods.

**Toxicokinetics.** Approximately 3 percent of an oral dose of titanium is absorbed. The majority of that absorbed is excreted in the urine. The normal urinary concentration has been estimated at 10 $\mu$g/L (Schroeder et al., 1963; Kazantzis, 1981). The estimated body burden of titanium is about 15 mg. Most of it is in the lungs, probably as a result of inhalation exposure. Inhaled titanium tends to remain in the lungs for long periods. It has been estimated that about one third of the inhaled titanium is retained in the lungs. The geographic variation in lung burden is to some extent dependent on air concentration. For example, concentrations of 430, 1300, and 91 ppm in ashed lung tissue have been reported for the United States, Delhi, and Hong Kong, respectively. Mean concentrations of 8 and 6 ppm for the liver and kidney, respectively, were reported in the U.S. Newborns have little titanium. Lung burdens tend to increase with age.

**Toxicology.** Occupational exposure to titanium may be heavy, and concentrations in air up to 50 mg/m$^3$ have been recorded. Titanium dioxide has been classified as a nuisance particulate with a TLV of 10 mg/m$^3$. Nevertheless, slight fibrosis of lung tissue has been reported following inhalation exposure to titanium dioxide pigment, but the injury was not disabling. Otherwise, titanium dioxide has been considered physiologically inert by all routes (ingestion, inhalation, dermal, and subcutaneous). The metal and other salts are also relatively nontoxic except for titanic acid, which, as might be expected, will produce irritation (Berlin and Nordman, 1986).

A titanium coordination complex, titanocene, suspended in trioctanoin, administered by intramuscular injection to rats and mice, produced fibrosarcomas at the site of injection and hepatomas and malignant lymphomas (Furst and Haro, 1969). A titanocene is a sandwich arrangement of titanium between two cyclopentadiene molecules. Titanium dioxide was found not to be carcinogenic in a bioassay study in rats and mice (NCI, 1979).

## Uranium

The chief raw material of uranium is pitchblende or carnotite ore. This element is largely limited to use as a nuclear fuel. The uranyl ion is rapidly absorbed from the gastrointestinal tract. About 60 percent is carried as a soluble bicarbonate complex, while the remainder is bound to plasma protein. Sixty percent is excreted in the urine within 24 h. About 25 percent may be fixed in the bone (Chen et al., 1961). Following inhalation of the insoluble salts, retention by the lungs is prolonged. Uranium tetrafluoride and uranyl fluoride can produce a typical toxicity because of hydrolysis to HF. Skin contact (burned skin) uranyl nitrate has resulted in nephritis.

The soluble uranium compound (uranyl ion) and those that solubilize in the body by the formation of a bicarbonate complex produce systemic toxicity in the form of acute renal damage and renal failure, which may be fatal. However, if exposure is not severe enough, the renal tubular epithelium is regenerated and recovery occurs. A study of uranium mill workers suggested that workers long-term low level exposure is associated with $\beta$-2-microglobulinuria and aminoaciduria (Thun et al., 1985). Renal toxicity with the classic signs of impairment, including albuminuria, elevated blood urea nitrogen, and loss of weight, is brought about by filtration of the bicarbonate complex through the glomerulus, reabsorption by the proximal tubule, liberation of uranyl ion, and subsequent damage to the proximal tubular cells. Uranyl ion is most likely concentrated intracellularly in lysosomes (Ghadially et al., 1982).

Inhalation of uranium dioxide dust by rats, dogs, and monkeys at a concentration of 5 mg U/m$^3$ for up to 5 years produced accumulation in the lungs and tracheobronchial lymph nodes that accounted for 90 percent of the body burden. No evidence of toxicity was observed, despite the long duration of observation (Leach et al., 1970).

## Vanadium

Vanadium is a ubiquitous element. It is a by-product of petroleum refining, and vanadium pentoxide is used as a catalyst in the reactions of various chemicals including sulfuric acid. It is used in the hardening of steel, in the manufacture of pigments, in photography, and in insecticides. It is common in many foods; significant amounts are found in milk, seafoods, cereals, and vegetables. Vanadium has a natural affinity for fats and oils; food oils have high concentrations. Municipal water supplies may contain on the average about 1 to 6 ppb. Urban air contains some vanadium, perhaps due to the use of petroleum products or from refineries (Table 23-1), about 30 mg. The largest single compartment is the fat. Bone and teeth stores contribute to the body burden. It has been postulated that some homeostatic mechanism maintains the normal levels of vanadium in the face of excessive intake, because the element, in most forms, is moderately absorbed. The principal route of excretion of vanadium is the urine. The normal serum level is 35 to 48 $\mu$g/100 mL. When excess amounts of vanadium are in the diet, the concentration in the red cells tends to increase. Parenteral administration increases levels in the liver and kidney, but these increased amounts may only be transient. The lung tissue may contain some vanadium, depending on the exposure by that route, but normally the other organs contain negligible amounts.

The toxic action of vanadium is largely confined to the respiratory tract. Bronchitis and bronchopneumonia are more frequent in workers exposed to vanadium compounds. In industrial exposures to vanadium pentoxide dust a greenish-black discoloration of the tongue is characteristic. Irritant activity with respect to skin and eyes has also been ascribed to industrial exposure. Gastrointestinal distress, nausea, vomiting, abdominal pain, cardiac palpitation, tremor, nervous depression, and kidney damage, too, have been linked with industrial vanadium exposure.

Ingestion of vanadium compounds ($V_2O_5$) for medicinal purposes produced gastrointestinal disturbances, slight abnormalities of clinical chemistry related to renal function, and nervous system effects. Acute vanadium poisoning in animals is characterized by marked effects on the nervous system, hemorrhage, paralysis, convulsions, and respiratory depression. Short-term inhalation exposure of experimental animals tends to confirm the effects on the lungs as well as the effect on the kidneys. In addition, experimental investigations have suggested that the liver, adrenals, and bone marrow may be adversely affected by subacute exposure at high levels (Waters, 1977; Wennig and Kirsch, 1988).

# REFERENCES


Abrams M, Murrer BA: Metal compounds in therapy and diagnosis. *Science* 261: 725–730, 1993.

Ainsworth SK, Swain RP, Watabe N, Brackett NC, et al: Gold nephropathy, ultrastructural fluorescent, and energy-dispersive x-ray microanalysis study. *Arch Pathol Lab Med* 105:373–78, 1981.

Alfrey AC: Aluminum and tin, in Bonner F, Coburn JW (eds): *Disorders of Mineral Metabolism*. New York: Academic Press, 1988, pp 353–369.

Anderson A, Hahlin M: Cadmium effects from phosphorus fertilization in field experiments. *Swedish J Agric Res* 11:2, 1981.

Angerer J, Heinrich R: Cobalt, in Seiler HG, Sigel H (eds): *Handbook on Toxicity of Inorganic Compounds*. New York: Marcel Dekker, 1988, pp 251–263.

Anke M, Grun M, Gropped B, Kronemann H: Nutritional requirement of nickel, in Sarkar B (ed): *Biologic Aspect of Metals and Metal-Related Diseases*. New York: Raven Press, 1983, pp 88–105.

Aposhian HV, Aposhian MM: Meao-2,3-dimercaptosuccinic acid: Chemical, pharmacological and toxicological properties of an orally effective metal chelating agent. *Ann Rev Pharmacol Toxicol* 30:279–306, 1992.

Aposhian HV, Bruce DC, Alter W, et al: Urinary mercury after administration of 2,3-dimercaptopropane-1-sulfonic acid: Correlation with dental amalgam score. *FASEB J* 6:2472–2476, 1992.

Araki S, Ushio K: Mechanism of increased osmotic resistance of red cells in workers exposed to lead. *Br J Industr Med* 39:157–60, 1982.

Arena JM: *Poisoning*, 3d ed. Springfield, IL: Charles C. Thomas, 1974.

Assenato G, Paci C, Molinini R, et al: Sperm count suppression without endocrine dysfunction in lead-exposed men. *Arch Environ Health* 41:387–390, 1986.

Astrin KH, Bishop DF, Wetmur JG, et al: Delta-aminolevulinic acid dehydratase isozymes and lead toxicity. *Ann NY Acad Sci* 514: 23–29, 1987.

Baker EL, Goyer RA, Fowler BA, et al: Occupational lead exposure, nephropathy and renal cancer. *Am J Industr Med* 1:139–148, 1980.

Bakir R, Damluji SF, Amin-Zaki L, et al: Methyl mercury poisoning in Iraq. *Science* 181:230–241, 1973.

Beijer K, Jernelov A: Sources, transport and transformation of metals in the environment, in Friberg L, Bordberg GF, Vouk VB (eds): *Handbook on the Toxicology of Metals,* 2d ed. General Aspects. Amsterdam: Elsevier, 1986, vol 1, pp 68–74.

Berlin M: Mercury, in Friberg L, Nordberg GF, Nordman C (eds): *Handbook on the Toxicology of Metals.* 2d ed. Specific Metals. Amsterdam: Elsevier, 1986, vol 2, pp 386–445.

Berlin M, Nordman C: Titanium, in Friberg L, Nordberg GF, Vouk VB (eds): *Handbook on the Toxicology of Metals*. Specific Metals. Amsterdam: Elsevier, 1986, vol 2, pp 594–609.

Bernard A, Lauwerys R: Epidemiological application of early markers of nephrotoxicity. *Toxicol Lett* 46:293–306, 1989.

Bernstein J, Evan AP, Gardner KD: Epithelial hyperplasia in human polycystic kidney disease. Its role in pathogenesis and risk of neoplasia. *Am J Pathology* 129:92–101, 1987.

Bertholf RL: Zinc, in Seiler HG, Sigel H (eds): *Handbook on Toxicity of Inorganic Compounds.* New York: Marcel Dekker, 1986, pp 787–800.

Bessis MD, Jensen WN: Sideroblastic anemia, mitochondria and erythroblastic iron. *Br J Haematol* 11:49–51, 1965.

Bhattacharyya MH, Whelton BD, Peterson DP, et al: Skeletal changes in multiparous mice fed a nutrient-sufficient diet containing cadmium. *Toxicology* 50:193–204, 1988.

Birch NJ: Magnesium, in Seiler HG, Sigel H (eds): *Handbook on Toxicity of Inorganic Compounds*, New York: Marcel Dekker, 1988, pp 397–415.

Birchall J, Chappel J: The chemistry of aluminum and silicon in relation to Alzheimer's disease. *Clin Chem* 34:265–267, 1988.

Bizzi A, Gambetti P: Phosphorylation of neurofilaments is altered in aluminum intoxication. *Acta Neuropath* 71:154–158, 1986.

Borschein RL, Grote J, Mitchell T, et al: Effects of prenatal lead exposure on infant size at birth, in Smith MA, Grant LD, Sors AI (eds): *Lead Exposure and Child Development*. Boston: Kluwer Academic Publishers, 1989, pp 307–319.

Boscolo P, Carmignani M: Neurohumoral blood pressure regulation in lead exposure. *Environ Health Perspect* 78:101–106, 1988.

Boulanger Y, Goodman CM, Forte CP, et al: Model for mammalian metallothionein structure. *Proc Natl Acad Sci USA* 80:1501–1505, 1983.

Boyd JT, Doll R, Foulds JS, Leiper J: Cancer of the lung in iron ore (haematite) miners. *Br J Industr Med* 27:97–103, 1970.

Brown EB: Therapy for disorders of iron excess, in Sarkar B (ed): *Biological Aspects of Metal-Related Diseases.* New York: Raven Press, 1983, pp 263–278.

Brown MM, Rhyne BC, Goyer RA, Fowler BA: Intracellular effects of chronic arsenic administration on renal proximal tubule cells. *J Toxicol Environ Health* 1:505–514, 1976.

Browning E: Toxicity of Industrial Metals, 2d ed. London: Butterworth, 1969.

Buchet J-P, Roels H, Bernard A, Lauwerys R: Assessment of renal function of workers exposed to inorganic lead, cadmium, or mercury vapor. *J Occup Med* 22:741–750, 1980.

Burk RF: Selenium in man, in Prasad AS, Oberleas D (eds): *Trace Elements in Human Health and Disease*. New York: Academic Press, 1976, vol 2, pp 105–234.

Cardenas A, Roels H, Bernard AM, et al: Markers of early renal changes induced by industrial pollutants. II. Application to workers exposed to lead. *Brit J Ind Med* 50:28–36, 1993.

Casto BC, Meyers J, DiPaolo JA: Enhancement of viral transformation for evaluation of the carcinogenic or mutagenic potential of inorganic metal salts. *Cancer Res* 39:193–198, 1979.

CDC: Preventing Lead Poisoning in Young Children—A Statement by the Centers for Disease Control, Atlanta, Ga. U.S. Department of Health and Human Services. No. 99-2230. Washington, DC: U.S. Government Printing Office, 1991, pp 51–64.

Cerwenka EA, Cooper WC: Toxicology of selenium and tellurium and their compounds. *Arch Environ Health* 3:189–200, 1961.

Chan HM, Zhu L-F, Zhong R, et al: Nephrotoxicity in rats following liver transplantation from cadmium-exposed rats. *Toxicol Appl Pharmacol* 123:89–96, 1993.

Chan WY, Tease LA, Liu HC, Rennert OM: Cell culture studies in Wilson's disease, in Sarkar B (ed): *Biological Aspects of Metals and Metal-Related Diseases*. New York: Raven Press, 1983, pp 147–158.

Chang CC, Vander Mallie RJ, Garvey JS: A radioimmunoassay for human metallothionein. *Toxicol Appl Pharmacol* 55:94–102, 1980.

Chen X, Yang G, Chen J, et al: Study on the relationship of selenium and Keshan disease. *Biol Trace Elem Res* 2:91–107, 1980.

Chen PS, Terepka R, Hodge HC: The pharmacology and toxicology of the bone seekers. *Ann Rev Pharmacol* 1:369–393, 1961.

Cherian MG, Miles EF, Clarkson TW, Cox C: Estimation of mercury burdens in rats by chelation with dimercaptopropane sulfonate. *J Pharmacol Exp Ther* 245:479–484, 1988.

Chisholm JJ Jr, Thomas D: Use of 2,3-dimercaptopropane-1-sulfonate in treatment of lead poisoning in children. *J Pharmacol Exp Ther* 235:665–669, 1985.

Choie BH, Lapham LW, Amin-Zaki L, Al-Saleem T: Abnormal neuronal migration, deranged cerebral cortical organization and diffuse white matter astrocytosis of human fetal brain. *J Neuropath Exp Neurol* 37:719–733, 1978.

Choie DD, Longenecker DS, Del Campo AA: Acute and chronic cisplatin nephropathy in rats. *Lab Invest* 44:397–402, 1981.

Choie DD, Richter GW: Effect of lead on the kidney, in Singhal RO, Thomas JA (eds): *Lead Toxicity*. Baltimore: Urban and Schwarzenberg, 1980.

Chuttani HK, Gupti PS, Gultati S: Acute copper sulfate poisoning. *Am J Med* 39:849–854, 1965.

Clarkson TW, Friberg L, Hursh JB, Nylander M: The prediction of intake of mercury vapor from amalgams, in Clarkson TW, Friberg L, Nordberg GF, Sager P (eds): *Biological Monitoring of Metals*. New York: Plenum Press, 1988, pp 247–264.

Clarkson TW: Methylmercury toxicity to the mature and developing nervous system: possible mechanisms, in Sarkar B (ed): *Biological Aspects of Metals and Metal-Related Diseases*. New York: Raven Press, 1983, pp 183–197.

Columbano A, Ledda GM, Siriqu P, et al: Liver cell proliferation induced by a single dose of lead nitrate. *Am J Pathol* 110:83–88, 1983.

Cookman GR, Hemmens SE, Keane GJ, et al: Chronic low level lead exposure precociously induces rat glial development in vitro and in vivo. *Neurosci Lett* 86:33–37, 1988.

Cooper WC: Occupational lead exposure. What are the risks? *Science* 180:129, 1980.

Cooper WC, Gaffey WR: Mortality of lead workers. *J Occup Med* 17:100–107, 1975.

Cooper WC, Wong O, Kheifets L: Mortality among employees of lead battery plants and lead-producing plants, 1947–1980. *Scand J Work Environ Hlth* 11:331–345, 1985.

Costa M, Zhitkovich A, Toniolo P: DNA-protein cross-links in welders: molecular implications. *Cancer Res* 53:460–463, 1993.

Cotzias GC, Papavasiliou PS, Ginos J, et al: Metabolic modification of Parkinson's disease and of chronic manganese poisoning. *Annu Rev Med* 22:305–36, 1971.

Cox C, Clarkson TW, Marsh DO, et al: Dose–response analysis of infants prenatally exposed to methyl mercury: An application of a single compartment model to single-strand hair analysis. *Environ Res* 49:318–332, 1989.

Cox M, Singer I: Lithium, in Bronner F, Coburn JW (eds): *Disorders of Mineral Metabolism*. New York: Academic Press, 1981, pp 369–438.

Crapper-McLachlan DR, McLachlan CD, Krishnan B, et al: Aluminum and calcium in soil and food from Guam, Palau and Jamaica: Implications for amyotropic lateral sclerosis and parkinsonism-dementia syndromes of Guam. *Environ Geochem Health* 11:47–53, 1989.

Curzon ME, Adkins BL, Bibby BG, Losee FL: Combined effect of trace elements and fluorine on caries. *J Dent Res* 49:526–528, 1970.

Davies NT: Studies on the absorption of zinc by rat intestine. *Br J Nutr* 43:189–203, 1980.

Davis JW, Fann WE: Lithium. *Annu Rev Pharmacol* 11:285–298, 1971.

DeBoni U, Otvos A, Scott JW, Crapper DR: Neurofibrillary degeneration induced by system aluminum. *Acta Neuropathol* 35:285–294, 1976.

DHEW: *Occupational Diseases: A Guide to Their Recognition*. Washington, DC: U.S. Department of Health, Education and Welfare, Publication No. 77-1811, 1977, p 305.

DeVoto E, Yokel RA: The biological speciation and toxicokinetics of aluminum. *Environ Health Perspect* 102:940–951, 1994.

Dingwall-Fordyce I, Lane RE: A follow-up study of lead workers. *Br J Ind Med* 20:313–315, 1963.

DiPaolo JA, Casto BC: Quantitative studies of in vitro morphologic transformation of Syrian hamster cells by inorganic metal salts. *Cancer Res* 39:1008–1019, 1979.

Diplock AT: Metabolic aspects of selenium action and toxicity. *Crit. Rev Toxicol* 4:271–329, 1976.

Doll R, Mathews JD, Morgan LG: Cancers of the lung and nasal sinuses in nickel workers: reassessment of the period of risk. *Br J Ind Med* 34:102–106, 1977.

Dorian C, Gattone VH, Klaassen CD: Discrepancy between the nephrotoxic potencies of cadmium-metallothionein and cadmium chloride and renal concentration in the proximal convoluted tubules. *Toxicol Appl Pharmacol* 130:161–168, 1995.

Downs WL, Scott JK, Steadman LT, Maynard EA: Acute and subacute toxicity studies of thallium compounds. *Am Ind Hyg Assoc J* 21:399–406, 1960.

Dunick JK, Elwell MR, Benson JM, et al: Lung toxicity after 13-week inhalation exposure to nickel oxide, nickel subsulfide or nickel sulfate hexahydrate in F344/N rats and B6C3F mice. *Fund Appl Toxicol* 12:584–594, 1989.

Durbin PW, Kullgren B, Xu J, Raymond KN: In vivo chelation of Am(III), Pu(IV), Np(V) and U(VI) in mice by TREN-(Me-3,2-HOPO). *Radiat Prot Dosimetry* 53:305–309, 1994.

Editorial: Selenium perspectives. *Lancet* 1:685, 1988.

Egle PM, Shelton KR: Chronic lead intoxication causes a brain-specific nuclear protein to accumulate in the nuclei of cells lining kidney tubule, *J Biol Chem*. 261: 2294–2298, 1986.

Elinder C-G, Friberg L: Cobalt, in Friberg L, Nordberg GF, Vouk V (eds): *Handbook of the Toxicology of Metals*, 2d ed. Specific Metals. Amsterdam: Elsevier, 1986, vol 2, pp 211–232.

Elinder C-G, Friberg L, Kjellstrom T, et al: *Biological Monitoring of Metals.* Geneva: World Health Organization, 1994.

Ellis KJ, Yuen K, Yasumura S, Cohn SH: Dose–response analysis of cadmium in man: Body burden vs. kidney dysfunction. *Environ Res* 33:216–226, 1984.

Ellis KJ, Cohn SH, Smith T: Cadmium inhalation exposure estimates: Their significance with respect to kidney and liver cadmium burden. *J Toxicol Environ Health* 15:173–187, 1985.

Engel RR, Smith AH: Arsenic in drinking water and mortality from vascular disease: An ecological analysis in 30 counties in the United States. *Arch Environ Health* 49:418–428, 1994.

Enterline PE, Marsh GM: Mortality studies of smelter workers. *Am J Ind Med* 1:251–259, 1980.

EPA: *Health Assessment Document for Cadmium.* EPA 60/8-81/023. Washington, DC: U.S. Environmental Protection Agency, 1981.

EPA: *National Drinking Water Regulations*. 40 CFR Part 141. *Fed Reg* 50:46967, 1985.

EPA: *Air Quality Criteria for Lead,* vol I–IV, EPA-600/8-83/02aF. Washington, DC: U.S. Environmental Protection Agency, 1986.

EPA: *Health Assessment Document for Beryllium.* EPA/600/8-84/026F. Washington, DC: U.S. Environmental Protection Agency, 1987a.

EPA: *Special Report on Ingested Inorganic Arsenic: Skin Cancer and Nutritional Essentiality.* Risk Assessment Form. Washington, DC: U.S. Environmental Protection Agency, 1987b.

EPA: *Summary Review of the Health Effects Associated with Copper.* Health Issue Assessment. EPA/600/8-87/001. Washington, DC: U.S. Environmental Protection Agency, 1987c.

EPA: *Evaluation of the Potential Carcinogenicity of Lead and Lead Compounds.* EPA-600/8-89/045A. Washington, DC: U.S. Environmental Protection Agency, 1989a.

EPA: *Supplement to the 1986 EPA Air Quality Criteria for Lead.* Addendum EPA/600/8-89/049A. Office of Health and Environmental Assessment. Washington, DC: U.S. Environmental Protection Agency, 1989b, vol 1, pp A1–A67.

Eyssen GEM, Reudy J, Neims A: Methylmercury exposure in Northern Quebec: II. Neurological finds in children. *Am J Epidemiol* 118:470–478, 1983.

Fan PL: Safety of amalgam. *CDAJ* September: 34–36, 1987.

Fishbein L: Sources, transport and alteration of metal compounds: an overview. I. Arsenic, beryllium, cadmium, chromium, and nickel. *Environ Health Perspect* 40:43–64, 1981.

Fishbein L: Toxicology of selenium and tellurium, in Goyer RA, Mehlman MA (eds): *Toxicology of Trace Metals.* New York: Wiley, 1977, pp 191–240.

Flanagan PR, McLellan J, Haist J, et al: Increased dietary cadmium absorption in mice and human subject with iron deficiency. *Gastroenterology* 74:841–846, 1978.

Fluharty AL, Sanadi DR: On the mechanism of oxidative phosphorylation. II. Effect of arsenite alone and in combination with 2,3-dimercaptopropanol. *J Biol Chem* 236:2772–2778, 1961.

Fowler BA: Indium and thallium in health, in Rose J (ed): *Trace Metals in Human Health.* London: Butterworth, 1982, pp 74–82.

Fowler BA, Goyer RA: Bismuth localization within nuclear inclusions by x-ray microanalysis. *J Histochem Cytochem* 23:722–726, 1975.

Fowler BA, Weissberg JB: Arsine poisoning. *N Engl J Med* 291:1171–1174, 1974.

Freeman GB, Johnson JD, Liao SC, et al: Absolute bioavailability of lead acetate and mining waste in rats. *Toxicology* 91:151–163, 1994.

Friberg L, Elinder CG, Kjellstrom T, Nordberg G: *Cadmium and Health. A Toxicological and Epidemiological Appraisal. General Aspects. Effects and Response.* Boca Raton, FL: CRC Press, 1986, vols 1, 2.

Friberg L, Lener J: Molybdenum, in Friberg L, Nordberg G, Vouk VB (eds): *Handbook on the Toxicology of Metals,* 2d ed. *Specific Metals.* Amsterdam: Elsevier, 1986, vol 2, pp 446–461.

Furst A: Bioassay of metals for carcinogenesis: whole animals. *Environ Health Perspect* 40:83–91, 1981.

Furst A, Haro RT: A survey of metal carcinogenesis. *Prog Exp Tumour Res* 12:102–133, 1969.

Gabard B: Treatment of methyl mercury poisoning in the rat with sodium 2,3-dimercaptopropane-i-sulfonate: Influence of dose and mode of administration. *Toxicol Appl Pharmacol* 38:415–424, 1976.

Ganrot PO: Metabolism and possible health effects of aluminum. *Environ Health Perspect* 65:363–441, 1986.

Garruto RM, Fukatsu R, Yanaghara R, et al: Imaging of calcium and aluminum in neurofibrillary tangle-bearing neurons in parkinsonism-dementia of Guam. *Proc Nat Acad Sci USA* 81:1875–1879, 1984.

Gennart JP, Bernard A, Lauwerys R: Assessment of thyroid, testis, kidney, and autonomic nervous system function in lead-exposed workers. *Int Arch Occup Health* 64:49–58, 1992.

Ghadially FN, Lalonde JA, Yang-Steppuhn S: Uraniosomes produce in cultured rabbit kidney cells by uranyl acetate. *Virchows Arch (Cell Pathol.)* 39:21–30, 1982.

Gilman W: Metal carcinogenesis. II. Study on the carcinogenicity of cobalt, copper, iron, and nickel compounds. *Cancer Res* 22:158–170, 1962.

Goldstein BD, Amoruso M, Witz G: Erythrocyte glucose-6-phosphate dehydrogenase deficiency does not pose an increased risk for Black Americans exposed to oxidant gases in the workplace or general environment. *Toxicol Ind Health* 1:75–80, 1985.

Goldwater LJ: Mercury: A History of Quicksilver. Baltimore: York Press, 1972, pp 270–277.

Goyer RA: Lead and the kidney. *Curr Topics Pathol* 55:147–176, 1971a.

Goyer RA: Lead Toxicity: A problem in environmental pathology. *Am J Pathol* 64:167–182, 1971b.

Goyer RA: Metal-protein complexes in detoxification process, in Brown SS (ed): *Clinical Chemistry and Clinical Toxicology.* London: Academic Press, 1984, vol 2, pp 199–209.

Goyer RA: Lead toxicity: from overt to subclinical to subtle health effects. *Environ Health Perspect* 86:177–181, 1990a.

Goyer RA: Transplacental transport of lead. *Environ Health Perspect* 89:101–108, 1990b.

Goyer RA: Lead toxicity: current concerns. *Environ Health Perspect* 100:177–187, 1993.

Goyer RA: Nutrition and metal toxicity. *Am J Clin Nutr,* 61 (suppl):646S–650S, 1995.

Goyer RA, Apgar J, Piscator M: Toxicity of zinc, in Henkin RI, et al (eds): *Zinc.* Baltimore: University Park Press, 1979, pp 249–268.

Goyer RA, Leonard DL, Moore JF, et al: Lead dosage and the role of the intranuclear inclusion body. An experimental study. *Arch Environ Health* 20:705–711, 1970.

Goyer RA, Rhyne B: Pathological effects of lead. *Int Rev Exp Pathol* 12:1–77, 1973.

Goyer RA, Wilson MH: Lead-induced inclusion bodies: results of EDTA treatment. *Lab Invest* 32:149–156, 1975.

Grandjean P, Grandjean E (eds): Effects of Organolead Compounds. Boca Raton, FL: CRC Press, 1984.

Grandjean P, Jorgensen PJ, Weihe P: Human milk as a source of methylmercury exposure in infants. *Environ Health Perspect* 102:74–77, 1994.

Grant LD, Davis JM: Effects of low-level lead exposure on paediatric neurobehavioral development: current findings and future directions, in Smith MA, Grant LD, Sors AI (eds): *Lead Exposures and Child Development.* Boston: Kluwer, 1989, pp 49–118.

Gritzka TL, Trump BF: Renal tubular lesions caused by mercuric chloride. *Am J Pathol* 52:1225–1277, 1968.

Gunsalus IC: The chemistry and function of the pyruvate oxidation factor (lipoic acid). *J Cell Comp Physiol* 41 (Suppl 1):113–136, 1953.

Hayes RL: Gallium, in Seiler HG, Sigel N (eds): *Handbook on Toxicity of Inorganic Compounds.* New York: Marcel Dekker, 1988, pp 297–300.

Henderson AS: The epidemiology of Alzheimer's disease. *Br Med Bull* 42:3–10, 1986.

Henry GA, Jarnot BM, Steinhoff MM, Bigazzi PE: Mercury-induced autoimmunity in the MAXX rat. *Clin Immunol Immunopathol* 49:187–203, 1988.

Hogberg J, Alexander J: Selenium, in Friberg L, Nordberg G, Vouk VB (eds): *Handbook on the Toxicology of Metals*, 2d ed. Specific Metals. Amsterdam: Elsevier, 1986, pp 482–512.

IARC: *Monograph on the Evaluation of Carcinogenicity: An Update of IARC Monographs.* Lyons: World Health Organization, International Agency for Research on Cancer, 1987, vols 1–42. Suppl 7.

IARC: *Monograph on the Evaluation of Risks to Humans. Cadmium, Mercury, Beryllium and the Glass Industry.* Lyons: International Agency for Research on Cancer, 1994, vol 58.

Ineichen B: Measuring the rising tide. How many dementia cases will there be by 2001? *Br J Psychiatry* 11:26–35, 1987.

Jacobs A: Iron overload—clinical and pathological aspects. *Semin Hematol* 14:89–113, 1977.

Jacobs A, Worwood M: Iron, in Bronner F, Coburn JW (eds): *Disorders of Mineral Metabolism. Trace Minerals.* New York: Academic Press, 1981, vol 1, pp 2–59

Jamall IS, Sprowls JT: Effects of cadmium and dietary selenium on cytoplasmic and mitochondrial antioxidant defense systems in the heart of rats fed high dietary copper. *Toxicol Appl Pharmacol* 87:102–110, 1987.

Johnson JL, Jones HP, Rajagopalan KV: In vitro reconstitution of demolybdosulfite oxidase by a molydenum cofactor from rat liver and other sources. *J Biol Chem* 252:4994–5003, 1977.

Jones MM: Newer chelating agents for in vivo toxic metal mobilization. *Comments Inorg Chem* 13:91–110, 1992.

Jones MM, Cherian MG: The search for chelate antagonists for chronic cadmium intoxication. *Toxicology* 62:1–25, 1990.

Kagey BT, Bumgarner JE, Creason JP: Arsenic levels in maternal-fetal tissue sets, in Hemphill OD (ed): *Trace Substances in Environmental Health XI.* Columbia: University of Missouri Press, 1977, pp 252–256.

Kang HK, Infante PF, Carra JS: Occupational lead exposure and cancer. *Science* 207:935–936, 1980.

Kawada T, Koyama H, Suzuko S: Cadmium, NAG activity and $\beta_2$-microglobulin in the urine of cadmium pigment workers. *Brit J Ind Med* 46:52–55, 1989.

Kazantzis G: Renal tubular dysfunction and abnormalities of calcium metabolism in cadmium workers. *Environ Health Perspect* 28:155–160, 1979.

Kazantzis G: Role of cobalt, iron, lead, manganese, mercury, platinum, selenium and titanium in carcinogenesis. *Environ Health Perspect* 40:143–161, 1981.

Keberle H: The biochemistry of desferrioxamine and its relation to iron metabolism. *Ann NY Acad Sci* 119:758–768, 1964.

Keen CL, Leach RM: Manganese, in Seiler HG, Sigel H (eds): *Handbook on Toxicity of Inorganic Compounds.* New York: Marcel Dekker, 1988, pp 405–415.

Kido T, Honda R, Tsuritani I, et al: Progress of renal dysfunction in inhabitants environmentally exposed to cadmium. *Arch Environ Health* 43:213–217, 1988.

Kjellström T, Friberg L, Rahnster B: Mortality and cancer morbidity among cadmium-exposed workers. *Environ Health Perspect* 28:199–204, 1979.

Klaassen CD: Heavy metal and heavy-metal antagonists, in Gilman AG, Rall TW, Nies AS, Taylor P (eds): *Goodman and Gilman's The Pharmacological Basis of Therapeutics.* New York: Pergamon Press, 1990, pp 1592-1614.

Kojima S, Ono H, Furukawa A, Kiyozumi M: Effect of N-benzyl-D-glucamine dithiocarbamate on renal toxicity induced by cadmium-metallothionein. *Arch Toxicol* 64:91–96, 1990.

Klatzo I, Wisniewski H, Streicher E: Experimental production of neurofibrillary degenerations I. Light microscopic observations. *J Neuropathol Exp Neurol* 24:187–199, 1965.

Kondo Y, Satoh M, Imura N, Akimoto M: Tissue-specific induction of metallothionein by bismuth as a promising protocol for chemotherapy with repeated administration of cis-diaminedichlorplatinum (II) against bladder cancer. *Anticancer Res* 12:2303–2308, 1992.

Kopp SJ, Perry HM, Perry EF, Erlanger M: Cardiac physiologic and tissue metabolic changes following chronic low-level cadmium and cadmium plus lead ingestion in the rat. *Toxicol Appl Pharmacol* 69:149–160, 1983.

Kreppel H, Bauman JW, Liu J, et al: Induction of metallothionein by arsenicals in mice. *Fund Appl Toxicol* 20:184–189, 1993.

Lam HF, Conner MW, Rogers AE, et al: Functional and morphological changes in the lungs of guinea pigs exposed to freshly generated ultrafine zinc oxide. *Toxicol Appl Pharmacol* 78:29–38, 1985.

Langard S, Norseth T: Chromium, in Friberg L, Nordberg GF, Vouk VB (eds): *Handbook on Toxicology of Metals.* Amsterdam: Elsevier, 1986, vol 2, pp 185–210.

Langworth S, Elinder CG, Akesson A: Mercury exposure from dental fillings. *Swed Dent J* 12:69–70, 1988.

Lauwerys RR: In vivo tests to monitor body burdens of toxic metals in man, in Brown S, Savory J (eds): *Clinical Toxicology and Clinical Chemistry of Metals.* New York: Academic Press, 1983, pp 113–122.

Lauwerys RR, Roels HA, Bernard A, Buchet J-P: Renal response to cadmium in a population living in a nonferrous smelter area in Belgium. *Int Arch Occup Environ Health* 45:271–274, 1980.

Lauwerys RR, Roels HA, Bucket J-P, et al: Investigations on the lung and kidney function in workers exposed to cadmium. *Environ Health Perspect* 28:137–146, 1979.

Leach LJ, Maynard EA, Hodge HC, et al: A five year inhalation study with uranium dioxide ($UO^2$) dust. I. Retention and biologic effect in the monkey, dog and rat. *Health Phys* 18:599–612, 1970.

Lerman SA, Clarkson TW, Gerson RJ: Arsenic uptake and metabolism by liver cells is dependent on arsenic oxidation state. *Chem Biol Interact* 45:401–406, 1983.

Levander OA: Considerations on the assessment of selenium status. *Fed Proc* 44:2579–2583, 1985.

Lilis R: Long-term occupational lead exposure: Chronic nephropathy and renal cancer: A case report. *Am J Ind Med* 2:293–297, 1981.

Madias NE, Harrington JT: Platinum nephrotoxicity. *Am J Med* 65:307–314, 1978.

Madsen KM, Christensen EF: Effects of mercury on lysosomal protein digestion in the kidney proximal tubule. *Lab Invest* 38:165–171, 1978.

Mahaffey KR (ed): *Dietary and Environmental Lead: Human Health Effects.* New York: Elsevier, 1985.

Manzer AD, Schreiner AW: Copper-induced acute hemolytic anemia. A new complication of hemodialysis. *Ann Intern Med* 73:409–412, 1970.

Markovac J, Goldstein GW: Lead activates protein kinase C in immature rat brain microvessel. *Toxicol Appl Pharmacol* 96:14–23, 1988.

Martyn CN, Barber DJ, Osmond C, et al: Geographical relation between Alzheimer's disease and aluminum in drinking watei. *Lancet* 1:59–62, 1989.

Matheson DS, Clarkson TW, Gelfand EW: Mercury toxicity (acrodynia) induced by long-term injection of gamma globulin. *J Pediatr* 97:153–155, 1980.

McConnell KP, Hoffman JG: Methionine selenomethionine parallels in E. coli polypeptide chain initiation and synthesis. *Proc Soc Exp Biol Med* 140:638–641, 1972.

McEwan JC: Five-year review of sputum cytology in workers at a nickel sinter plant. *Ann Clin Lab Sci* 8:503–509, 1978.

McLaughlin JR, Goyer RA, Cherian MG: Formation of lead-induced inclusion bodies in primary rat kidney epithelial cell cultures: effect of actinomycin D and cycloheximide. *Toxicol Appl Pharmacol* 56:418–431, 1980.

McLaughlin AIG, Harding HE: Pneumoconiosis and other causes of death in iron and steel foundry workers. *Arch Ind Health* 14:350–362, 1956.

McMichael AJ, Baghurst PA, Wigg NR, et al: Port Pirie cohort study: environmental exposure to lead and children's abilities at the age of four years. *N Engl J Med* 319:468–475, 1988.

Mena I, Meurin O, Feunzobda S, Cotzias GC: Chronic manganese poisoning. Clinical picture and manganese turnover. *Neurology* 17:128–136, 1967.

Mena I, Kazuko H, Burke K, Cotzias GC: Chronic manganese poisoning, individual susceptibility and absorption of iron. *Neurology* 19:1000–1006, 1969.

Menne T, Thorboe A: Nickel dermatitis—nickel excretion. *Contact Dermatitis* 2:353–354, 1976.

Mertz W: Chromium occurrence and function in biological systems. *Physiol Rev* 49:163–239, 1969.

Miettenen JK: Absorption and elimination of dietary mercury (Hg++) and methyl mercury in man, in Miller MW, Clarkson TW (eds): *Mercury Mercurials and Mercaptans*. Springfield, IL: Charles C. Thomas, 1973, p 233.

Mitchell RA, Change BF, Huang CH, DeMaster EG: Inhibition of mitochondrial energy-linked functions by arsenate. *Biochemistry* 10:2049–2054, 1971.

Moore MR, Bushnell IWR, Goldberg A: A prospective study of the results of changes in environmental lead exposure in children in Glasgow, in Smith MA, Grant LD, Sors AJ (eds): *Lead Exposure and Child Development.* Boston: Kluwer, 1989, pp 371–378.

Morin Y, Daniel P: Quebec beer-drinkers cardiomyopathy: Etiological consideration. *J Can Med Assoc* 97:926–931, 1967.

Mottet NK, Shaw C-M, Burbacher TM: Health risks from increases in methylmercury exposure. *Environ Health Persp* 63:133–140, 1985.

Muller-Eberhard U, Miescher PA, Jaffe ER: *Iron Excess. Aberrations of Iron and Porphyrin Metabolism.* New York: Grune & Stratton, 1977.

Myron DR, Zimmerman TJ, Schuler TR, et al: Intake of nickel and vanadium by humans. A survey of selected diet. *Am J Clin Nutr* 31:527–531, 1978.

Nagyvary J, Bradbury EL: Hypocholesterolemic effects of $Al^{3}+$ complexes. *Biochem Res Commun* 2:592–598, 1977.

NCI: *Bioassay of Titanium Dioxide for Possible Carcinogenicity.* National Cancer Institute Carcinogenesis Technical Report Series No. 97. Washington, DC: Department of Health, Education and Welfare Publication No. (NIH) 79-1347, 1979.

Needleman HL: The persistent threat of lead: A singular opportunity. *Am J Public Health* 79:643–645, 1989.

Needleman HL, Schell A, Bellinger D, et al: Long-term effects of childhood exposure to lead at low dose; an eleven-year follow-up report. *New Engl J Med* 322:83–88, 1990.

Newman RA, Brody AR, Krakoff IH: Gallium nitrate induced toxicity in the rat: A pharmacologic histopathologic and microanalytical investigation. *Cancer* 44:1728–1740, 1979.

Ng A, Patterson C: Natural concentrations of lead in ancient Arctic and Antarctica ice. *Geochim Cosmochim Acta* 45:2109–2121, 1981.

Nogami H, Terashima Y: Thallium-induced achondroplasia in the rat. *Teratology* 8:101–102, 1973.

Nogawa K, Honda R, Kido T, et al: A dose–response analysis of cadmium in the general environment with special reference to total cadmium intake limit. *Environ Res* 48:7–16, 1989.

Nogawa K, Tsuritani I, Kido T, et al: Mechanism for bone disease found in inhabitants environmentally exposed to cadmium: decreased 1,25-dihydroxyvitamin D level. *Int Arch Occupat Environ Health* 59:21–30, 1987.

Nogawa K, Kobayashi E, Honda R: A study of the relationship between cadmium concentrations in urine and renal effects of cadmium. *Environ Health Perspect* 28:161–168, 1979.

Nordberg GF: Cadmium metabolism and toxicity. *Environ Physiol Biochem* 2:7–36, 1972.

NRC: *Measuring Lead Exposure in Infants, Children and Other Sensitive Populations.* Washington, DC: National Academy Press, 1993.

O'Flaherty EJ: Chromium toxicokinetics, in Goyer RA, Cherian MG, (eds): *Toxicology of Metals: Biochemical Aspects.* Heidelberg: Springer-Verlag, 1995, pp 315–228.

Ong CN, Endo G, Chia KS, et al: Evaluation of renal function in workers with low blood lead levels, in Foa V, Emmett EA, Maroni M, Colombi A (eds): *Occupational and Environmental Chemical Hazards: Cellular and Biochemical Indicies for Monitoring Toxicity.* New York: Halsted Press, 1987, pp 327–333.

Orfila MP: *A General System of Toxicology.* Philadelphia: M. Carey, 1817.

Paglia DE, Valentine WN, Dahlgner JG: Effects of low level lead exposure on pyrimidine-5′-nucleotidase and other erythrocyte enzymes. *J Clin Invest* 56:1164–1169, 1975.

Paton FR, Allison AC: Chromosome damage in human cell cultures induced by metal salts. *Mutat Res* 16:332–336, 1972.

Pederson E, Anderson A, Hogetveit A: A second study of the incidence and mortality of cancer of respiratory organs among workers at a nickel refinery. *Ann Clin Lab Sci* 8:503–510, 1978.

Pelletier L, Druet P: Immunotoxicology of metals, in Goyer RA, Cherian MG (eds): *Handbook of Experimental Pharmacology* Heidelberg: Springer-Verlag, 1995, vol 115, pp 77–92.

Pentschew W, Ebner FF, Kovatch RM: Experimental manganese encephalopathy in monkeys. *J Neuropathol Exp Neurol* 22:488–499, 1963.

Perl DP, Good PF: Uptake of aluminum in central nervous system along nasal-olfactory pathways. *Lancet* 1:1087, 1987.

Perl DP, Good PF: Aluminum, environment and central nervous system disease. *Environ Tech Lett* 9:901–906, 1988.

Perl DP, Brody AR: Detection of aluminum by SEM-X-ray spectrometry within neurofibrillary tangle-bearing neurons of Alzheimer's disease. *Neurotoxicology* 1:133–137, 1980.

Perlstein MA, Attala R: Neurologic sequelae of plumbism in children. *Clin Pediatr* 5:292–298, 1966.

Pershagan G, Nordberg G, Bjorklund N-E: Carcinoma of the respiratory tract in hamsters given arsenic trioxide and/or benzoapyrene by the pulmonary route. *Environ Res* 34:227–241, 1984.

Pirkle JL, Brody DJ, Gunter EW, et al: The decline in blood lead levels in the United States. *JAMA* 272:284–291, 1994.

Prasad AS: Human zinc deficiency, in Sarkar B (ed): *Biological Aspects of Metals and Metal-Related Disease.* New York: Raven Press, 1983, pp 107–119.

Prull G, Rompel K: EEG changes in acute poisoning with organic tin compounds. *Electroencephalog Clin Neurophysiol* 29:215–222, 1970.

Reeves AL: Barium, in Friberg L, Nordberg GF, Vouk VB (eds): *Handbook on the Toxicology of Metals,* 2d ed. *Specific Metals.* Amsterdam: Elsevier, 1986, vol 2, pp 84–94.

Richardson M, Mitchell M, Coad S, Raphael R: Exposure to mercury on Canada: A multimedia analysis. *Water, Air, and Soil Pollution*, 1995 (in press).

Riordan JR: Handling of heavy metals by cultured cells from patients with Menke's disease, in Sarkar B (ed): *Biological Aspects of Metals and Metal-Related Diseases*. New York: Raven Press, 1983, pp 159–170.

Rodamilans M, Martinez-Osaba MJ, To-Figueras J, et al: Lead toxicity on endocrine testicular function in an occupationally exposed population. *Hum Toxicol* 7:125–128, 1988.

Roels H, Lauwerys RR, Dardenne AN: The critical level of cadmium in human renal cortex: a re-evaluation. *Toxicol Lett* 15:357–360, 1983.

Roels HA, Lauwerys RR, Buchet JP, et al: Health significance of cadmium induced renal dysfunction: A five-year follow-up. *Br J Ind Med* 46:755–764, 1989.

Roels H, Gennart J-P, Lauwerys R, et al: Surveillance of workers exposed to mercury vapor: validation of a previously proposed biological threshold limit value for mercury concentration in urine. *Am J Ind Med* 7:45–71, 1985.

Rossouw J, Offermeier J, van Rooyen JM: Apparent central neurotransmitter receptor changes induced by low-level lead exposure during different developmental phases in the rat. *Toxicol Appl Pharmacol* 91:132–139, 1987.

Sager PR, Aschner M, Rodier PM: Persistent differential alterations in developing cerebellar cortex of male and female mice after methylmercury exposure. *Dev Brain Res* 12:1–11, 1984.

Sarkar B, Laussac J-P, Lau S: Transport forms of copper in human serum, in Sarkar B (ed): *Biological Aspects of Metals and Metal-Related Diseases*. New York: Raven Press, 1983, pp 23–40.

Schroeder HA, Mitchener M: Selenium and tellurium in mice. *Arch Environ Health* 24:66–71, 1972.

Schroeder HA, Balassa JJ, Tipton IH: Abnormal trace metals in man: titanium. *J Chronic Dis* 16:55–69, 1963.

Schroeder HA, Nason AP, Tipton IH: Essential trace metals in man: Cobalt. *J Chronic Dis* 20:869–890, 1967.

Schroeder HA, Nason AP, Tipton IH: Essential trace metals in man: Magnesium. *J Chronic Dis* 21:815–841, 1969.

Schumann GB, Lerner SI, Weiss MA, et al: Inclusion bearing cells in industrial workers exposed to lead. *Am J Clin Pathol* 74:192–196, 1980.

Schwartz J, Otto D: Lead and minor hearing impairment. *Arch Environ Health* 46:300–306, 1991.

Shamberger RJ: *Biochemistry of Selenium*. New York: Plenum Press, 1983, p 243.

Siegel N, Haug A: Aluminum interaction with calmodulin. Evidence for altered structure and function from optical enzymatic studies. *Biochimica et Biophysica Act* 744:36–45, 1983.

Silbergeld EK: Mechanisms of lead neurotoxicity, or looking beyond the lamppost. *FASEB J* 6:3201–3206, 1992.

Silbergeld EK, Schwartz J, Mahaffey K: Lead and osteoporosis: Mobilization of lead from bone in postmenopausal women. *Environ Res* 47:79–94, 1988.

Simons TJB: Cellular interactions between lead and calcium. *Br Med Bull* 42:431–434, 1986.

Singer I: Lithium and the kidney. *Kidney Int* 19:374–387, 1981.

Skerfving S: Methylmercury exposure, mercury levels in blood and hair, and health status in Swedes consuming contaminated fish. *Toxicology* 2:3–23, 1974.

Skerfving S, Christoffersson J-O, Schutz A, et al: Biological monitoring by in vivo XRF measurement of occupational exposure to lead cadmium and mercury. *Biol Trace Elem Res* 13:241–251, 1987.

Smith AH, Hopenhayn-Rich C, Bates MN, et al: Cancer risks from arsenic in drinking water. *Environ Health Perspect* 97:259–267, 1992.

Smith DR, Flegal AR: Stable isotopic tracers of lead mobilized by DMSA chelation in low lead-exposed rats. *Toxicol Appl Pharmacol* 116:85–91, 1992.

Sorahan T, Waterhouse JAJ: Mortality study of nickel cadmium battery workers by the method of regression models in life tables. *Br J Ind Med* 40:293–300, 1983.

Spears JW, Hatfield EE, Forbes RM, Koenig SE: Studies on the role of nickel in the ruminant. *J Nutr* 108:313–320, 1978.

Spivey Fox MR, Rader JI: Iron, in Seiler HG, Sigel H (eds): *Handbook on Toxicity of Inorganic Compounds*. New York: Marcel Dekker, 1988, pp 346–358.

Steele TN: Treatment of lithium intoxication with diuretics, in Brown SS (ed): *Clinical Chemistry and Chemical Toxicology of Metals*. Amsterdam: Elsevier, 1977, pp 289–292.

Steenland K, Selevan S, Landrigan P: The mortality of leadmelter workers: An update. *Am J Pub Health* 82:1641–1644, 1992.

Stowe HD, Goyer RA: The reproductive ability and progeny of $F_1$ lead-toxic rats. *Fertil Steril* 22:755–760, 1971.

Stuve J, Galle P: Role of mitochondria in the renal handling of gold by the kidney. *J Cell Biol* 44:667–76, 1970.

Styblo M, Delnomdedieu M, Thomas DJ: Biological mechanisms and toxicological consequences of the methylation of arsenic, in Goyer RA, Cherian MG (eds): *Handbook of Experimental Pharmacology, Toxicology of Metals*. Heidelberg: Springer-Verlag, 1995, vol 115, pp 408–433.

Sunderman FW Jr: Nickel, in Bronner F, Coburn JW (eds): *Disorders of Mineral Metabolism*. New York: Academic Press, 1981, vol 1, pp 201–232.

Sunderman FW Jr: Mechanisms of nickel carcinogenesis. *Scand J Work Environ Health* 15:1–12, 1989.

Sunderman FW Sr: Efficacy of sodium diethyldithiocarbamate (dithiocarb) in acute nickel carbonyl poisoning. *Ann Clin Lab Sci* 9:1–10, 1979.

Suzuki KT: Induction and degradation of metallothioneins and their relation to the toxicity of cadmium, in Foulkes EC (ed): *Biological Roles of Metallothionein*. Amsterdam: Elsevier, 1982, pp 215–235.

Takenaka S, Oldiges H, Konig H, et al: Carcinogenicity of cadmium chloride aerosols in W rats. *J Natl Cancer Inst* 70:367–373, 1983.

Takeuchi T: Neuropathology of Minamata disease in Kumamoto: Especially at the chronic stage, in Roizin L, Shiraki H, Grcevic N (eds): *Neurotoxicology*. New York: Raven Press, 1977, pp 235–246.

Tanaka K, Min K-S, Onasaka S, et al: The origin of metallothionein in red blood cells. *Toxicol Appl Pharmacol* 78:63–66, 1985.

Thomas DW, Hartly TF, Sobecki S: Clinical and laboratory investigations of the metabolism of bismuth containing pharmaceuticals by man and dogs, in Brown SS (ed): *Clinical Chemistry and Clinical Toxicology of Metals*. Amsterdam: Elsevier, 1977, pp 293–296.

Thun MJ, Osorio AM, Schober S, et al: Nephropathy in cadmium workers: Assessment of risk from airborne occupational exposure to cadmium. *Br J Ind Med* 46:689–697, 1989.

Thun MJ, Schnorr TM, Smith AB, et al: Mortality among a cohort of U.S. cadmium production workers—An update. *J Natl Cancer Inst* 74:325–333, 1985.

Thun MJ, Baker DB, Steenland K, et al: Renal toxicity in uranium mill workers. *Scand J Work Environ Health* 11:83–90, 1985.

Trump BF, Valigersky JN, Arstila AU, et al: The relationship of intracellular pathways of iron metabolism to cellular iron overload and the iron storage diseases. *Am J Pathol* 72:295–324, 1973.

Tyroler HA: Epidemiology of hypertension as a public health problem: An overview as background for evaluation of blood lead–blood pressure relationship (Symposium). *Environ Health Persp* 78:3–8, 1988.

Underwood EJ: *Trace Elements in Human and Animal Nutrition*, 4th ed. New York: Academic Press, 1977.

Urizar R, Vernier RL: Bismuth nephropathy. *JAMA* 198:187–189, 1966.

Valencia MP, Gamboa MJ: Copper overload and cirrhosis in four Mexican children (abstract). *Lab Invest* 68:10pp, 1993.

Vander AJ: Chronic effects of lead on renin–angiotensin system. *Environ Health Perspect 78:77–83, 1988.*

Verschuuren HG, Ruitenberg EJ, Peetoom F, et al: Influence of triphenyltin acetate on lymphatic tissue and immune response in guinea pigs. *Toxicol Appl Pharmacol* 16:400–410, 1970.

Voil GW, Minielly JA, Bistricki T: Gold nephropathy tissue analysis by x-ray fluorescent spectroscopy. *Arch Pathol Lab Med* 101: 635–640, 1977.

Waalkes M P, Rehm S: Cadmium and prostate cancer. *J Toxicol Environ Health* 43:251–269, 1994.

Walshe CT, Sandstead HH, Prasad AS, et al: Zinc: Health effects and research priorities for the 1990s. *Environ Health Perspect* 102 (Suppl 2):5–46, 1994.

Walshe JM: Endogenous copper clearance in Wilson's disease: A study of the mode of action of penicillamine. *Clin Sci* 26:461–469, 1964.

Walshe JM: Assessment of treatment of Wilson's disease with triethylene tetramine 2HCl (trien 2HCl), in Sarkar B (ed): *Biological Aspects of Metals and Metal Related Diseases*. New York: Raven Press, 1983, pp 243–261.

Wang X-P, Chan HN, Goyer RA, Cherian MG: Nephrotoxicity of repeated injections of cadmium-metallothionein in rats. *Toxicol Appl Pharmacol* 119:11–16, 1993.

Waters MD: Toxicology of vanadium, in Goyer RA, Mehlman MA (eds): *Toxicology of Trace Metals*. New York: Wiley, 1977, pp 147–189.

Webb DR, Sipes IG, Carter DE: In vitro solubility and in vivo toxicity of gallium arsenide. *Toxicol Appl Pharmacol* 76:96–104, 1984.

Wennig R, Kirsch N: Vanadium, in Seiler HG, Sigel H (eds): *Toxicity of Inorganic Compounds*. New York: Marcel Dekker, 1988, pp 749–758.

WHO: *Environmental Health Criteria 125. Platinum*. Geneva: World Health Organization, 1991.

WHO: *Environmental Health Criteria 58. Selenium*. Geneva: World Health Organization, 1986.

WHO: *Environmental Health Criteria 15. Tin and Organotin Compounds: A Preliminary Review*. Geneva: World Health Organization, 1980.

WHO: *Evaluation of Certain Food Additives and Contaminants*. World Health Organization Technical Report, Series 776. Geneva: World Health Organization, 1989.

WHO: *IPCS Environmental Health Criteria 61. Chromium*. Geneva: World Health Organization, 1988.

WHO: *IPCS Environmental Health Criteria 106. Beryllium*. Geneva: World Health Organization, 1990a.

WHO: *IPCS Environmental Health Criteria 101. Methylmercury*. Geneva: World Health Organization, 1990b.

WHO: *IPCS Environmental Health Criteria 118, Inorganic Mercury*. Geneva: World Health Organization, 1991.

WHO *IPCS Environmental Health Criteria 134. Cadmium*. Geneva: World Health Organization, 1992.

Wilber CG: *Selenium: A Potential Environmental Poison and a Necessary Food Constituent*. Springfield, IL: Charles C. Thomas, 1983.

Williams DR, Halstead BW: Chelating agents in medicine. *Clin Toxicol* 19:1081–1115, 1982.

Wills MR, Savory J: Aluminum poisoning: Dialysis encephalopathy, osteomalacia and anemia. *Lancet* 2:29–33, 1983.

Winge DR, Mehra RK: Host defenses against copper toxicity. *Intl Rev Exp Path* 31:47–83, 1990.

Winship KA: Toxicity of antimony and its compounds. *Adv Drug React Acute Pois Rev* 2:67–90,1987.

Winston PW: Molybdenum, in Bonner F, Coburn JW (eds): *Disorders of Mineral Metabolism*. Trace Minerals. New York: Academic Press, 1981, vol 1, pp 295–315.

Woods JS, Carver GT, Fowler BA: Altered regulation of hepatic heme metabolism by indium chloride. *Toxicol Appl Pharmacol* 49:455–461, 1979.

Yang G, Wang S, Zhou R, Sun S: Endemic selenium intoxication of humans in China. *Am J Clin Nutr* 37:872–881, 1983.

Zelikoff JT, Li JH, Hartwig A, et al: Genetic toxicology of lead compounds. *Carcinogenesis* 9:1727–1732, 1988.

Zhuang Z, Costa M: Development of an 125 I-post-labeling assay as a simple, rapid, and sensitive index of DNA-protein cross-links. *Environ Health Perspect* 102 (Suppl 3):301–304, 1995.

Ziemsen B, Angerer J, Lehnert G, et al: Polymorphism of delta-aminolevulinic acid dehydratase in lead-exposed workers. *Int Arch Occup Environ Health* 58:245–247, 1986.

# CHAPTER 24

# TOXIC EFFECTS OF SOLVENTS AND VAPORS

*Robert Snyder and Larry S. Andrews*

Nearly everyone is exposed to solvents. The utility of these fluids as solubilizers, dispersants, or diluents leads to the manufacture and use of billions of pounds each year. Occupational exposures can involve applications ranging from a secretary using correction fluid to a gas station attendant pumping gasoline. A refinery worker may be exposed to solvents on the job and upon returning home may paint a room, change the oil in the family car, or glue together an item in need of repair, thereby extending his exposure to solvents. Although the solvents, which are usually mixtures, have different trade names, they frequently contain similar chemicals. Clearly, exposure should not be equated with toxicity. The fundamental principle of toxicology, which is the dose-response relationship, requires that there be (1) exposure and (2) a toxic effect. Nevertheless, the potential for toxicological interaction increases as exposure increases, and exposure to mixtures leads to the possibility of unpredictable additivity, synergism, or potentiation of effects. In the long run we must learn to understand the interactive effects of solvents because the exposure of human populations in the environment is not usually to a single chemical. Until we have developed that needed body of knowledge we must make use of the database available to us, which is the toxicology of individual solvents and the relationship between the structures of solvents and their toxicity within chemical classes.

## THE PROPERTIES OF SOLVENTS

### Exposure

Many solvents exhibit appreciable volatility under conditions of use, and consequently the worker, or people who use products containing solvents in the home, may be exposed to solvent vapors. The potential hazard posed as a result of exposure to a solvent is a function of the dose-response relationship. The dose, ideally, is the concentration of the toxic form of the chemical at its physiological receptor. Because that information is usually not available, the next best estimate of dose is the blood level of the chemical, and sometimes, by extrapolation, we can derive an accurate estimate of body levels from the concentration in the urine. Concentrations in physiological fluids, such as blood and urine, are often expressed as units of weight/volume (w/v), for example, mg/mL, mg/L and so on. Concentrations of gas mixtures given in w/v units depend on both temperature and pressure, as mass depends on the number of molecules present, but the volume occupied by that mass depends on temperature and pressure and is described by the ideal gas law ($PV = nRT$). For regulatory purposes, and in many experimental situations, vapor concentrations are expressed as parts of vapor per million parts of contaminated air (ppm) by volume at a specified temperature and pressure or as mg solvent/$m^3$ air. Given that respiratory rates and volumes are fairly consistent among people, mg/$m^3$ provides a means of readily estimating exposure to a solvent over a period of time. Examples of methods for interconverting ppm and mg/$m^3$ are shown in the appendix to this chapter.

The volatility of solvents indicates that a major route of exposure will be by the respiratory system. Once vapors enter the lungs they may readily diffuse across a large surface area of respiratory membranes and enter the bloodstream. The ability of solvent vapors to enter the bloodstream and their rate of membrane transport depend upon their lipid solubility, since lipoprotein cell membranes must be traversed. Many solvents are very lipid soluble and will enter the blood with ease. Because diffusion occurs from relatively high concentrations in lung air to low concentrations in blood and tissues, the driving force for the movement is the vapor concentration in inspired air.

Concerns for solvent exposures include both acute and chronic effects. Any situation in which a person may be harmed by exposure to high levels of vapor should be controlled by adequate techniques of safety engineering. In the event of an unexpected release of vapor, emergency operating procedures will require the availability of emergency respiratory equipment and rapid evacuation of the premises. Safety engineering procedures are designed around acceptable exposure standards established by regulatory agencies to protect against both acute and chronic effects of chemicals. Standard setting for solvent exposures often includes recommendations for short-term exposure limits (STEL) to protect against acute toxicity. The establishment of 15-min STEL values for volatile solvents is aimed at determining an air level of vapor below which workers could perform for 15 min without loss of consciousness or loss of the ability to perform the tasks expected of them. The need to remain in an area where there is an unacceptable level of solvent vapor may relate to the need to stabilize a dangerous situation which might otherwise lead to greater danger to the exposed individual or to others in danger of exposure. There are, therefore, two issues. One is loss of consciousness; the second is the potential impairment of ability to perform essential emergency procedures.

In this discussion volatile solvents will initially be examined as if they were anesthetic agents. Organic vapors may produce depression of the central nervous system and, in theory, are capable of producing anesthesia. Anesthetic potency, that is, the dose of each solvent vapor necessary to produce anesthesia, varies widely. As the dose of vapor increases, the relative concentration of oxygen in the inspired air may decrease, with the effect that the vapor acts as an asphyxiant. A number of the more potent vapors, however, have been used to produce surgical anesthesia.

In the parlance of anesthesiology, the maximum allowable concentration (MAC) is the minimum alveolar concentration of an anesthetic, at 1 atmosphere pressure, which produces immobility in 50 percent of patients exposed to a noxious stimulus (Kennedy and Longnecker, 1990). People respond to anesthetics over a very narrow concentration range. Selection of a dose that will ensure that 100 percent of the population of patients will exhibit anesthesia can usually be accomplished by multiplying the MAC value by 1.3, which yields a value about 30 percent higher than the MAC. There is no reason to believe that the dose-response curve for these agents is not symmetrical. Therefore, it is likely that a value that is approximately 30 percent below the MAC would not produce anesthesia.

Considerable efforts in the field of the behavioral toxicology of solvent vapors, some of which will be summarized below, suggest that sufficient neurological impairment to prevent acceptable work activity can be observed at subanesthetic levels. Thus, values below 30 percent of the MAC may cause other signs of vapor intoxication such as unsteadiness, inability to concentrate, impaired motor coordination, or decrements in motor or intellectual function not related to readily observed symptoms. As a result, estimating the STEL based on knowledge of the lower end of the dose-response curve for anesthesia is difficult and requires estimation of additional factors.

For example, in addition to knowing the concentration of vapor necessary to produce anesthesia, it is also important to consider the partition coefficient. The partition coefficient is directly related to the time necessary to establish anesthesia. The partition coefficient of interest here is the blood/gas partition coefficient. The gas is placed in a closed container containing a sample of blood, and the concentration of gas in the blood and in the air is measured once equilibrium has been reached. The ratio of blood gas concentration to air gas concentration is the partition coefficient. Thus, for well-known anesthetics values include 0.41 for cyclopropane, 1.8 for enflurane, 2.3 for halothane, 12.0 for methoxyflurane, and 12.1 for diethyl ether. The higher the partition coefficient, that is, the more soluble the gas is in blood, the slower the onset of anesthesia regardless of the relative potencies of the gases. Information on partition coefficients for solvents can be used to estimate the rate of onset of narcosis in much the same way as for general anesthetics. It is likely that the rate of onset for subanesthetic functional impairments by volatile solvents will also be a function of partition coefficients. It is likely that the rate of onset for subanesthetic functional impairments by volatile solvents will also be a function of partition coefficients.

Many factors including rate and depth of respiration will affect blood solvent concentrations (Astrand, 1975). The rate at which the solvent distributes to the body organs through the blood is controlled by the cardiac output. The rate at which it leaves the blood to enter the organs is a function of the partition coefficient. Agents having a high blood/air partition coefficient, such as diethyl ether, leave the blood and enter the organs at a slow rate, whereas agents such as halothane have a low partition coefficient and therefore distribute more rapidly. It is clear that there is a need for more studies relating the toxicokinetics of these chemicals with measurements of their effects on the central nervous system (CNS).

Decisions on setting exposure standards to protect against the effects of vapors on the CNS will require a better understanding of the dose-response curves for both anesthetic activity and behavioral impairment for each solvent. Although it might be postulated that among these agents there is a demonstrable relationship between their potencies to impair behavior and their potencies to produce anesthesia, that relationship has yet to be explored. In addition to the short-term effects of exposure, it is necessary to determine whether chronic effects occur as well.

A second major potential route of exposure is the skin. The ubiquity of solvents and the casual approach to their use almost assures skin contact. Frequent contact with lipid soluble solvents can lead to a defatting of skin or to skin irritation. Of more importance for systemic toxicity is that some solvents may penetrate skin barriers to absorption (from both liquid and vapor phases) and enter the bloodstream (Rihimaki and Pfaffli, 1978; DiVincenzo et al., 1978; Marzulli and Maibach, 1983). Susten and colleagues (1985) estimated that dermal exposure to benzene in tire building operations could account for 20 to 40 percent of the total dose. These observations have raised the possibility that toxic amounts of solvents may be absorbed through the skin as a result of occupational and consumer exposures. This question has not, as yet, been approached in a systematic fashion. However, it does not seem likely that the percutaneous route will be a major contributor to establishing a body burden for most solvents, because the lung provides a much more efficient transfer of vapors to the bloodstream than does skin, and the area of skin in contact with a liquid solvent must be large for there to be absorption of appreciable amounts. Clearly, abraded or burned skin will be less of a barrier to absorption of solvents and the likelihood of systemic effects from dermal exposure will be increased.

Another aspect of exposure to solvents is the frequency of exposure. Consumers, who generally use small amounts of products, are usually not exposed to large amounts of solvents over long periods of time. Exposure to low background levels with intermittent exposure to much higher levels is a likely exposure scenario in the consumer setting. For example, solvent from an opened can of paint stripper may evaporate into the garage over a period of time, but furniture refinishing is an infrequent activity. In the occupational setting, a similar situation exists, where there may be continuous exposure to low levels of solvents with brief exposure to high concentrations of solvents. It seems axiomatic that toxicity testing of solvents in experimental animals should incorporate these exposure realities into test protocols. However, little information is currently available on effects of intermittent exposure.

The American Conference of Governmental Industrial Hygienists (ACGIH, 1995–1996) recognizes the potential for adverse effects of solvent vapors and has established threshold limit values (TLVs) designed to protect workers from exposure to solvents. ACGIH defines TLVs as airborne concentrations of substances that represent conditions under which it is believed that nearly all workers may be exposed, day after day, without adverse effect. TLVs are based on the best available information from industrial experience, animal tests, and studies in human volunteers. This information is summarized in the appendix of this book and detailed in ACGIH's Documentation of Threshold Limit Values series. The ACGIH develops three categories of TLVs: (1) the time-weighted average (TWA), which is a value for a normal 8-h work day and 40-h work week; (2) the short-term exposure limit (STEL) is a value for a short period of time (usually 15 min); (3) the ceiling

(TLV-C) is a value that should not be exceeded even briefly. The ACGIH meets each year to consider new information and revises TLVs when warranted by new data.

The official United States government body assigned the task of establishing exposure levels in industry is the Occupational Safety and Health Administration (OSHA) of the Department of Labor. Standards are established based largely on information supplied by the National Institute of Occupational Safety and Health and other agencies concerned with the effects of chemicals on human health. Opinions are solicited from all interested parties and decisions made on the basis of the weight of evidence and the intent to act conservatively with respect to the protection of the health of the worker. The availability of the expertise of both agencies is to the advantage of the worker and the health professional charged with assuring the safety of the workplace.

## The Toxic Effects of Solvents

The toxic effects of solvents are both general and specific. The effects observed in studies in experimental animals or in the occupational exposure setting will depend upon many factors, including chemical structure, the inherent toxicity of the chemical, the level and pattern of exposure, coexposure to more than one chemical, and subject sensitivity.

**General.** Factors relating to exposure to solvent vapors were introduced above. An infrequent but typical exposure scenario leading to a toxic effect is the worker who enters a reaction vessel or holding tank without appropriate respiratory equipment. In such a confined space, solvent vapor concentrations may reach many hundreds or thousands of parts per million and workers may be quickly overcome. Of course, the experimental animal analogy to this scenario is the acute inhalation toxicity study ($LC_{50}$).

Workers exposed to solvents under these conditions will typically show signs of CNS disturbance. While there is some variation in signs and symptoms with different solvent structures, results of high-level exposure are very similar. Disorientation, euphoria, giddiness and confusion, progressing to unconsciousness, paralysis, convulsion, and death from respiratory or cardiovascular arrest is typically observed (Browning, 1965). The rapidity of the development of these symptoms almost ensures that the acute narcotic effects of solvents are due to the solvent itself and not to metabolites. In the majority of subjects, recovery from CNS effects is rapid and complete following removal from exposure.

The similarity of the narcosis produced by solvents of diverse structures suggests that these effects result from a physical interaction of a solvent with cells of the CNS. If a purely physical interaction is assumed, then the narcotic effect of the solvent will be dependent only upon the molar concentration of the solvent in the CNS cell. Equimolar concentrations of different solvents will result in narcotic effects of equal intensity. Although an increased emphasis on worker protection has lessened the likelihood of acute high-level exposure to solvents, it is important to retain the concept that solvent-induced behavioral deficits and narcosis remain important aspects of solvent toxicity.

It was suggested above that solvents may demonstrate effects on the CNS at subanesthetic doses. These effects can be examined using behavioral toxicity tests in humans. A list of such tests has been compiled from several reviews and is presented in Table 24-1 (Feldman et al., 1980; Tilson and Cabe, 1978; Buelke-Sam and Kimmel, 1979).

Ideally, behavioral toxicity studies should be performed in animal models first to set the stage for developing tests applicable to humans. Animal models involving birds and apes can detect solvent-induced behavioral impairments. Current methodology permits the use of well-designed experiments that can yield highly reproducible results under conditions of well-controlled exposure to solvent vapors. The results suggest that impairment of the performance of various activities may occur when humans are exposed to similar doses. Efforts by the U.S. Environmental Protection Agency and other regulatory agencies to require screening of chemicals for neurobehavioral effects in acute and repeated exposure animal studies appear to offer an increased potential to identify both doses of solvents which may impair performance as well as materials that exert unique effects on the CNS. It will be essential that direct parallels be established between specific animal tests and the changes in human behavior/performance for which the animal models predict.

It is important, however, that results obtained in these studies be validated. Rebert and Hall (1994) examined the neurotoxicology literature and selected 38 reports relating to chronic exposure of workers to styrene and solvents in the plastics industry published between the mid-1960s and 1993. They established criteria for reviewing these reports and used these criteria to determine whether the experimental design was adequate, appropriate statistics were employed, confounding factors were controlled for, exposures were documented, appropriate endpoints were measured, dose-effect relationships were observed, the experimenter or the subject demonstrated bias, procedures were followed exactly, and whether the results were consistent with other findings. Using

**Table 24–1**
**Symptomatology and Commonly Used Tests for Behavioral Effects**

| SYMPTOMATOLOGY | TEST |
|---|---|
| *Sensory*—paresthesias, visual or auditory deficits | Neurologic, sight, and hearing examinations |
| *Cognitive*—memory (both short-term and long-term), confusion, disorientation | Wechsler memory scale<br>Wechsler Adult Intelligence Scale (WAIS) |
| *Affective*—nervousness, irritability, depression, apathy, compulsive behavior | Eysenck Personality Inventory<br>Rorschach test<br>Digit-symbol substitution task<br>Bourdon-Wiersma vigilance task |
| *Motor*—weakness in hands, incoordination, fatigue, tremor | Neurologic examination<br>Santa Ana dexterity test<br>Finger-tapping test<br>Simple or choice reaction time |

these criteria they concluded that the data did not support the conclusion that workers in the styrene industry developed chemically related neurotoxicity. Reviews of this type provide insight which can lead to improvements in the design of better studies to evaluate the effects of long-term exposure to specific solvents. The results of this review emphasize the need for experimenters and regulatory agencies to guard against the noncritical use of such databases when attempting to establish permissible industrial or environmental exposure limits.

Despite these obvious difficulties in methodology and interpretation there have been a number of claims that frequently used solvents may cause behavioral toxicity. These include carbon disulfide ($CS_2$) (Hanninen et al., 1978; Tolonen et al., 1978; Tuttle, 1977; Lillis, 1974), toluene (Saito and Wada, 1993), trichloroethylene (Lillis et al., 1969; Grandjean et al. 1955), and styrene (Cherry et al., 1980). Reviews include Grasso (1988) and Wood (1994). A number of epidemiological studies on workers exposed to solvent mixtures have also been reported (Elofsson et al., 1980; Linz et al., 1986; Knave et al., 1978; Seppalainen et al., 1980). These studies involved painters, workers occupationally exposed to jet fuel, and workers with a diagnosis of "solvent poisoning," respectively.

The effects that have in the past been described as the general effects of solvents are quite complex and difficult to define and measure in humans. Only through the expansion of research in this area can we anticipate a better understanding of these effects and a more rational approach to the use of the developing literature in the proper control of exposures to solvent vapors.

**Specific.** Distinct from general acute CNS depressant actions of solvents are their specific organ toxicities. Such effects include the hemopoietic toxicity of benzene, the CNS depressant effects of alkylbenzenes, the hepatotoxicity of ethanol and certain chlorinated hydrocarbons, the ocular toxicity of methanol, and the reproductive toxicity of ethylene glycol ethers. Many of these effects are described in this chapter or elsewhere in this volume. It would be helpful, however, to discuss two topics that pertain to solvents in general but relate to their specific effects, namely, exposure and metabolism.

## Exposure

In contrast to the general effects of solvents, specific toxicity usually results from repeated exposure to tolerable levels of solvents rather than from acute exposure to very high levels. A typical exposure scenario is a worker who is exposed to a material daily. Tissue damage caused either by the solvent or a toxic metabolite of the solvent may accumulate until the worker develops a clinically recognizable illness. Good estimates of dose or time required to develop an illness are generally not available for solvents for which specific human toxicities are recognized. The development of personal monitors that measure total exposure of the worker over a given period of time are helping to solve the problem. However, predictive measures of the possible range of variations between individual workers, leading to an appreciation of differences in biological responses to chemicals, are required.

The result has been a sizable effort in many laboratories to develop so-called biomarkers reflective of exposure to a chemical. In the past these often have been measurements of blood or urine levels of chemicals following exposure. Many have not been highly specific. For example, attempts to estimate benzene exposure using blood or urinary phenol levels have been of limited value because phenol enters the body as a result of a variety of exposures exclusive of benzene. Nevertheless, there is a need for the development of several types of biomarkers such as those that can be used to quantify exposure, provide evidence of a health effect, or be used to identify sensitive individuals. These may include characterization and quantitation of unique metabolites in body fluids, measurement of covalent binding of reactive metabolites to proteins, lipids, or nucleic acids, evidence for chemically related and specific forms of chromosome damage, as well as other types of tests currently in development.

Adequate measurements of air levels of solvents in any environment where they may pose a threat to health will continue to be essential despite the development of biomarkers. Concentrations of chemicals in the air can be measured more rapidly than biomarkers and can provide an early warning system when coupled to alarms much before biomarkers can be used. The ideal situation will be to maintain air level monitoring of solvent vapors, personal monitoring of workers, and monitoring of biomarkers on a regular basis to provide warning of both acute exposure and of longer term impacts of exposure to solvents.

## Metabolism

Specific toxicities of solvents, as distinct from general effects discussed above, are often directly related to the metabolism of the solvent. Thus, the hemopoietic toxicity of benzene, the neurotoxicity of n-hexane, and the reproductive toxicity of ethylene glycol ethers have all been attributed to toxic metabolites of these materials. This general phenomenon is known as *bioactivation* and is largely mediated by the family of enzymes termed *cytochrome P450-dependent mixed function oxidases* (Omura and Sato, 1964; Schenkman and Kupffer, 1982; Snyder et al., 1982; Kocsis et al., 1986; Witmer et al., 1991; Lechner, 1994). Of course, not all metabolism of a given solvent need result in bioactivation. Typically one or more cytochrome P450 mixed function oxidases may mediate the conversion of a large percentage of the dose of solvent to a harmless metabolite, a process termed *detoxication*.

Mixed function oxidases are a family of enzymes, consisting primarily of the hemoprotein cytochrome P450, which are located in the smooth endoplasmic reticulum of the liver as well as in most other organs. These enzymes catalyze the oxidation or reduction of a wide variety of chemical structures. A postulated mechanism for mixed function oxidative reactions is visualized in Chap. 6. The chemical is reversibly bound by the oxidized form of cytochrome P450. The resulting chemical complex is next reduced by an electron supplied by NADPH (the reduced form of nicotinamide adenine dinucleotide phosphate)-cytochrome P450 reductase. The reduced chemical P450 complex binds a molecule of oxygen and, upon addition of further reducing equivalents, one atom of oxygen is introduced into the chemical and the other is reduced to water. Upon release of the oxidized product, cytochrome P450, in its oxidized state, is capable of binding another drug molecule. As a result of this process, oxygen is introduced into any chemical that contains a favorably positioned C-H, N-H, S-H, or C-X

(X=halogen) bond. Several aspects of the cytochrome P450 mixed function oxidases are of importance for the conduct and interpretation of toxicity tests for solvents.

**Interactions.** Because some mixed function oxidases have a broad specificity, it is not surprising that one solvent can compete with another for available catalytic sites. Thus, toluene has been shown to be a competitive inhibitor of the metabolism of benzene (Andrews et al., 1977; Sato and Nakajima, 1979). This competitive interaction alleviates the metabolite-mediated toxicity of benzene as discussed in "Enzyme Induction," below.

**Enzyme Induction.** The mixed function oxidase system contains a group of related enzymes, termed epitopes, which go by the common name cytochrome P450. Treatment of animals, and presumably humans, with any of a great number of chemicals leads to increases in the metabolism of these and other chemicals because of elevations in the levels of the cytochromes P450 (Snyder and Remmer, 1979; Gonzalez, 1988; Lechner, 1994). The specificity of the induced enzymes vary. Some chemicals, such as benzene, are capable of increasing their own metabolism and that of some other chemicals (Snyder et al., 1967), whereas drugs like phenobarbital or environmental chemicals such as polychlorinated biphenyls can increase the metabolism of a wide variety of chemicals.

The toxicity of a chemical may be dramatically altered as a result of enzyme induction. If metabolic activation of a solvent to its toxic metabolite is limited by the constitutive concentration of the specific species of cytochrome P450 through which it is metabolized, enzyme induction may lead to greater toxicity. Thus, bromobenzene given to rats at doses that do not produce serious toxicity in noninduced animals yields massive hepatic necrosis in animals pretreated with phenobarbital (Zampaglione et al., 1973). Alternatively, the toxicity of a given dose may be reduced by decreasing the fraction processed by the bioactivation pathway. Thus, treating rats with 3-methylcholanthrene prior to dosing with bromobenzene led to a reduction in expected hepatotoxicity. In this case, an alternative pathway leading to less toxic metabolites was induced, thereby reducing the fraction of the dose that passed through the bioactivation pathway.

The process of enzyme induction is best studied by examining the molecular biology of individual cytochromes P450 (Gonzalez, 1988). Increases in specific cytochromes P450 activity can be detected by increases in the metabolism of specific chemicals, but increases in the specific enzyme can be measured using blotting techniques that identify antibody-responsive sites on specific P450 proteins using the Western blot technique. The formation of specific messenger RNA in response to treatment with chemicals can be detected using the Northern blot method. These and related techniques have led to our understanding that there is a superfamily of cytochrome P450 genes that have played a critical role in many species throughout evolution and that these enzymes are inducible.

**Generation of Biological Reactive Intermediates.** During the course of metabolism, relatively inactive chemicals are often converted to highly reactive metabolites which can be inactivated by glutathione, ascorbic acid, or other cellular antioxidants. If these are not inactivated they can react and covalently bind to cellular macromolecules such as protein, lipid, RNA, or DNA. The result can be inactivation of receptors and specific proteins, damage to cell membranes, or initiation of mutagenic reactions as a result of DNA binding. Although these effects can occur at some level whenever these chemicals undergo metabolism, the likelihood that they will result in cellular damage is increased when the dose of the chemical is high, the specific form of cytochrome P450 that generates the reactive metabolite is increased by enzyme induction, or the cell is deficient in protective detoxication factors.

Implicit in the concept of enzyme-mediated detoxication or bioactivation is the phenomenon of enzymatic saturation. Exposure to massive amounts of a solvent may result in saturation of detoxication pathways, resulting in a spillover into bioactivation pathways. Metabolic saturation has been demonstrated for a number of solvents including n-hexane, vinylidene chloride, methylchloroform, perchloroethylene, and ethylene dichloride (Baker and Rickert, 1981; Reitz et al., 1982; Schumann et al., 1980, 1982; McKenna et al., 1978).

Occurrence of metabolic saturation may be of profound importance for the design and interpretation of safety evaluation studies employing maximum tolerated doses. When considering exposures at or below permissible standards, however, metabolic saturation may be less important in determining ultimate toxicity. Thus, Andersen and colleagues (1980) found that at low vapor concentrations of several solvents, respiration and hepatic perfusion indices were rate limiting factors in metabolism and hence in the production of toxic metabolites.

**Generation of Reactive Oxygen Species.** A variety of mechanisms have been uncovered by which reactive oxygen species may be generated during the metabolism of many solvents. These include the production of free radicals, which can lead to lipid peroxidation and subsequent production of oxygen radicals, or the metal-mediated reduction of oxygen to yield superoxide, hydrogen peroxide, the hydroxyl ion, and so forth. Radical reactive compounds such as glutathione, vitamins C and E, and enzymes such as superoxide dismutase, catalase, and glutathione peroxidase protect against oxidative damage. Reactive oxygen species can attack cellular macromolecules by mechanisms distinct from those of the reactive metabolites. For example, instead of forming covalently bound adducts, reactive oxygen may alter DNA by converting deoxyguanosine residues of DNA to 8-OH-deoxyguanosine.

**Species, Genetics and Age.** Among many factors that can affect cytochrome P450 mixed function oxidase reactions are species, genetics, and age (Gillette, 1976; Schumann, et al., 1980). Such confounding factors can greatly influence the metabolism and toxicity of solvents and are discussed in Chap. 6.

## Benzene

The development of the steel industry and its need for coke led to a readily available source of benzene as a by-product in the nineteenth century, and the later development of the petroleum industry to produce fuels resulted in an abundance of benzene, as both a fuel component and by-product in the twentieth century. Benzene has been used as a solvent for rubber, inks, and other materials and as a starting material in chemical synthesis. Today it remains one of the largest volume chemicals produced and used in the world.

The heavy industrial production and use of benzene has resulted in a plethora of reports relating to its toxic effects in humans and to studies of its toxicity in animals and other nonhuman biological systems (Snyder and Kocsis, 1975; Snyder et al., 1993a) Benzene toxicity in the workplace is most frequently thought to be the result of the inhalation of benzene vapors with some undefined contribution from skin absorption. Current environmental concerns also include the potential effects of benzene found in samples of well water used for drinking.

**Metabolism and Hematopoietic, Leukemogenic, and Clastogenic Effects.** Although acute exposure to high concentrations of benzene may depress the CNS, leading to unconsciousness and death, or cause death by producing fatal cardiac arrhythmias (Snyder and Kocsis, 1975), the major toxic effect of benzene is hematopoietic toxicity, an effect unique to benzene among the simple aromatic hydrocarbons. Chronic exposure of humans to benzene in the workplace leads to bone marrow damage, which may be manifested initially as anemia, leukopenia, or thrombocytopenia. The extent to which each of the cell types is depleted varies with the individual and the degree of exposure to benzene. In both human and animal studies, it appears that benzene-induced bone marrow depression is a dose-dependent phenomenon. Continued exposure may result in pancytopenia resulting from marrow aplasia, an often fatal outcome. Survivors of aplastic anemia frequently exhibit a preleukemic state, termed *myelodysplasia*, and progress to acute myelogenous leukemia (Browning, 1965; Snyder and Kocsis, 1975; Snyder et al., 1977; Snyder et al., 1993a; Snyder and Kalf, 1994.)

Evidence that benzene is a human leukemogen is based on both epidemiological and case studies and is very compelling (IARC, 1982; Snyder et al., 1993a; Snyder and Kalf, 1994). Benzene-induced leukemia has been observed in humans but, unlike bone marrow depression leading to aplastic anemia, no animal model for benzene-induced leukemia exists that mimics the course of the human disease. As a result, it has been difficult to study the etiology and development of benzene-induced leukemia in animal systems. However, solid tumors have been reported in animals exposed to benzene by inhalation or orally (Maltoni, 1983; Huff et al., 1989), suggesting that in mice and rats benzene may produce tumors in nonhematopoietic organs.

The generation of chronic benzene toxicity is dependent upon two separate series of events. One is the physiological disposition of benzene, the generation of a series of biologically reactive intermediates and their ability to interact with cells of the bone marrow to initiate toxicity. The second is the series of events within bone marrow, which results from the interaction of benzene and its metabolites, that leads to bone marrow depression and neoplasia.

To understand the mechanism of benzene toxicity, it is essential to study its disposition. Benzene metabolites that appear in the urine include ethereal sulfates and glucuronides of the phenolic metabolites, muconic acid resulting from ring opening, and mercapturic acids resulting from glutathione conjugation. Medinsky and coworkers (1989) published a model for the simulation of benzene metabolism by mice and rats. They assumed that benzene metabolism follows Michaelis-Menten kinetics, that total benzene metabolism occurs via benzene oxide, and that total benzene metabolism could be accounted for by summing the conjugated phenolic metabolites, mercapturic acids, and muconic acid in urine. The results suggest that formation of toxic metabolites occurs via high-affinity, low-capacity pathways, whereas detoxication is accomplished via low-affinity, high-capacity pathways. These authors infer that at low substrate concentration a significant percentage of the metabolism follows pathways leading to the production of toxic metabolites. These simulations were supported by studies in animals which indicated that detoxication pathways predominated in rats, which are known to be less susceptible to benzene toxicity, but not in more susceptible mice, in which the production of toxic metabolites was a more important factor.

Parke and Williams (1953) suggested that one of benzene's metabolites might be responsible for benzene toxicity and it has been demonstrated that inhibition of benzene metabolism leads to decreases in benzene toxicity (Andrews et al., 1977; Longacre et al., 1981a,b; Sammet et al., 1979). The metabolic pathways for benzene are pictured as a diagram of the fate of benzene oxide (Fig. 24-1). Benzene is converted to benzene oxide by the hepatic microsomal mixed function oxidase. The oxide, which is in equilibrium with its oxepin form, may rearrange nonenzymatically to form phenol; react with glutathione to form a premercapturic acid, which is subsequently converted to phenyl-mercapturic acid; or it may react with epoxide hydrolase, which converts it to benzene 1,2-dihydrodiol, or as recently postulated (Snyder et al., 1993b) to the 1,4-dihydrodiol. The mixed function oxidase and epoxide hydrolase are microsomal enzymes, but the cytosolic dihydrodiol dehydrogenase appears to be responsible for the rearomatization of the ring to yield catechol or hydroquinone (Ayengar et al., 1959). Hydroquinone or catechol may also be formed by the hydroxylation of phenol. 1,2,4-Trihydroxybenzene is thought to arise from the hydroxylation of hydroquinone or catechol.

Another potentially toxic metabolite, muconaldehyde, which may arise via a ring opening at the epoxide stage (Latriano et al., 1986), undergoes a series of reactions (Kirley et al., 1989; Goon et al., 1992; Zhang et al., 1993) that ultimately leads to trans,trans-muconic acid (Figure 24-2), which is one of the urinary end products reported by Parke and Williams (1953). Jerina and Daly (1974) suggested that the hydroxylation involves the intermediate formation of an epoxide, and much of the theory of carcinogenesis by bay region diol-epoxides is founded upon this concept. Benzene oxide has never been isolated and identified during the enzymatic oxidation of benzene. However, Tunek and colleagues (1982) and Snyder and coworkers (1993b) added epoxide hydrolase to in vitro systems actively engaged in benzene metabolism and demonstrated the formation of 1,2-benzene dihydrodiol, an intermediate that could only be formed from the epoxide or the oxepin. Indeed Busby and coworkers (1990) have suggested that benzene oxide and/or the dihydrodiol of benzene oxide may play a role in benzene-induced neoplasia in a mouse model.

Ingelman-Sundberg and Hagbjork (1982) suggested that hydroxylation could occur via the insertion of a hydroxyl free radical (Fig. 24-3). They postulate that the free radicals are generated by an iron-catalyzed cytochrome P450-dependent

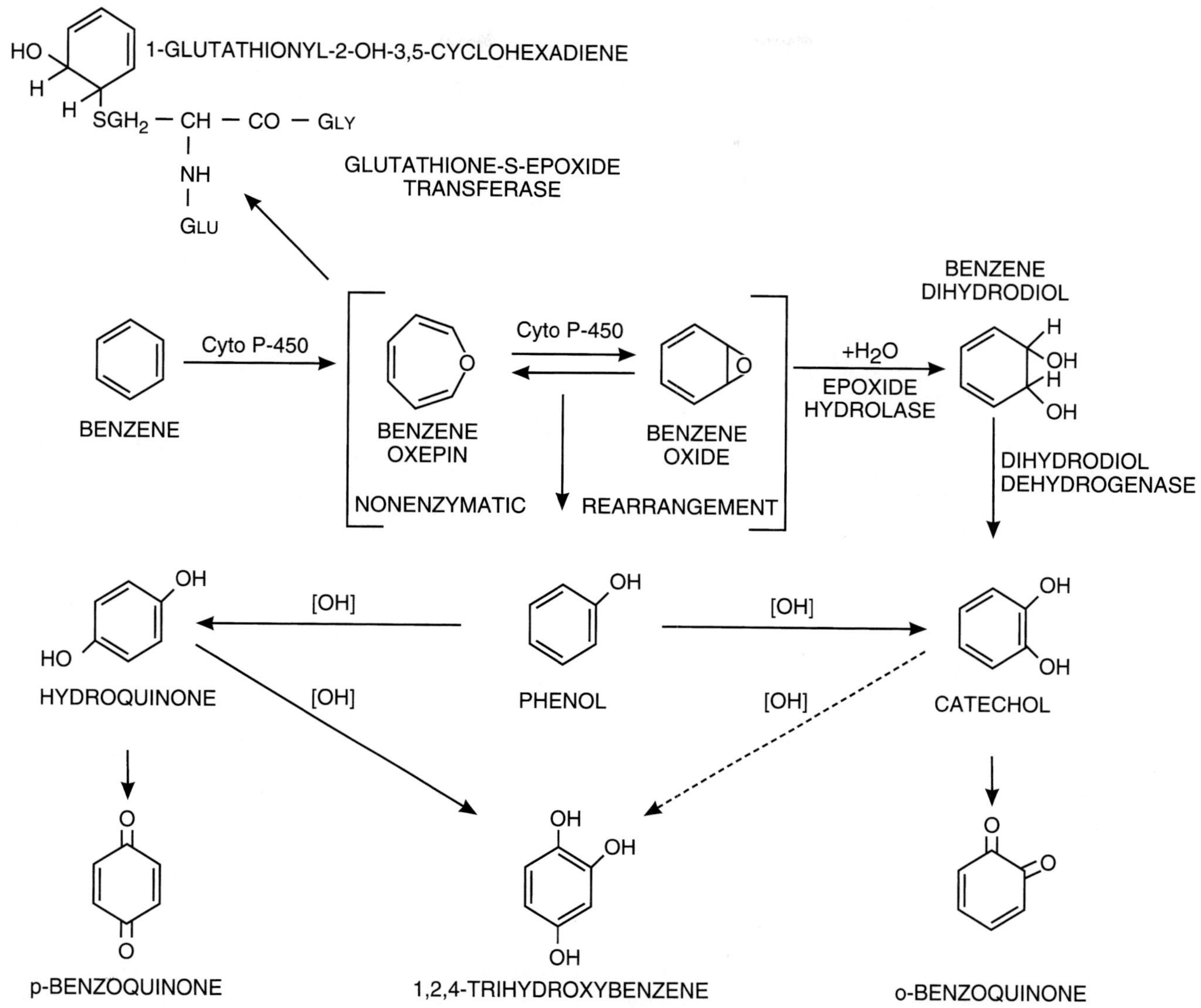

***Figure 24–1. Biotransformation of benzene.***

A question mark leads to trans,trans-muconaldehyde from the oxepin-oxide compartment because the substrate for ring opening has yet to be identified. A question mark leads to the diol epoxide from the diol because that pathway has been postulated but not demonstrated. The dotted lines leading to 1,2,4-trihydroxybenzene indicate that it is not clear what the relative contributions of hydroquinone and catechol are to the formation of the trihydroxylated compound.

Haber-Weiss reaction, and their data are supported by the demonstration that several compounds that prevent free radical formation or act as free radical scavengers can inhibit the hydroxylation of benzene by an isolated, reconstituted rabbit liver microsomal mixed function oxidase. Gorsky and Coon (1985) proposed that a free radical mechanism occurs only at very low substrate concentrations when cytochrome P450 could be uncoupled and yield hydrogen peroxide.

Post and Snyder (1983) demonstrated that there are at least two different rat liver mixed function oxidases active in benzene hydroxylation and these have now been shown to be cytochromes P450 2B1 in rat liver (Snyder et al., 1993b) and 2E1 in rat liver (Snyder et al., 1993b) and rabbit liver (Koop et al., 1989). Kinetic studies of these enzymes suggest that cytochrome P450 2E1 is the predominant form active in benzene metabolism.

The dihydroxylated metabolites, hydroquinone and catechol, may be formed by hydroxylation of phenol by cytochrome P450 or via epoxide hydrolase in liver (Gilmour et al., 1986; Koop et al., 1989; Snyder et al., 1993b), by peroxidase (Sawahata and Neal, 1982), by myeloperoxidase (Eastmond et al., 1987), or by the cyclooxygenase component of prostaglandin H synthetase (Pirozzi et al., 1989). It is likely that the noncytochrome P450 mechanisms play a more significant role in bone marrow than in liver where they can generate semiquinones, or quinones. Nevertheless, initial metabolism in liver appears to be essential for the development of bone marrow toxicity (Sammet et al., 1979).

Given that benzene metabolism occurs largely in liver but benzene toxicity is a function of the bone marrow, it is important to designate the site at which the toxic metabolites are generated. It is likely that if quinones and semiquinones

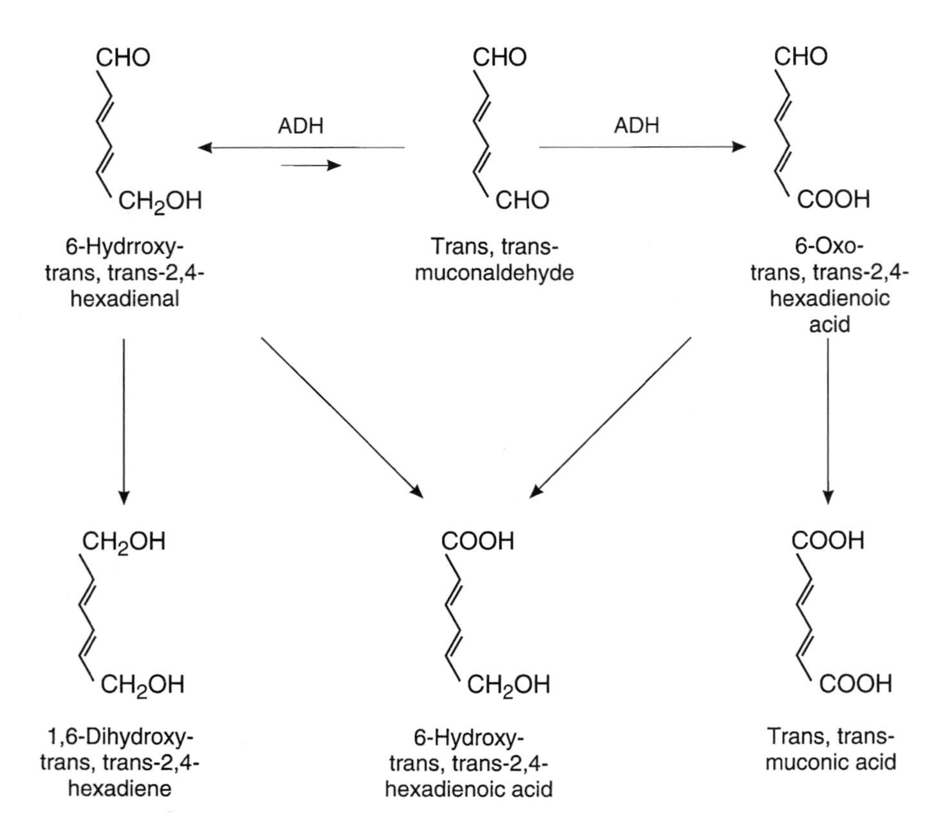


*Figure 24–2. The intermediary metabolism of trans,trans-muconaldehyde.*

are the ultimate toxic metabolites among those with an intact ring and muconaldehyde is the ultimate toxic metabolite among the ring-opened products, they are probably generated in bone marrow because they would otherwise react covalently within the liver and never reach their bone marrow targets. By contrast the transport of phenolic conjugates, their entry into selected target cells, and their hydrolysis and subsequent oxidation suggest a mechanism by which hepatically generated phenolic compounds could have an impact on the bone marrow. By the same token, ring-opened metabolites of muconaldehyde, which are less reactive, might be transported to bone marrow and reoxidized to yield the toxic effects.

If transport of metabolites from liver to bone marrow is an essential feature of the mechanism of toxicity, it is necessary to explain why the administration of individual phenolic metabolites does not reproduce benzene toxicity. The reports of Eastmond and coworkers (1987) and Guy and colleagues (1990, 1991) suggest that although individual compounds may mimic some aspects of benzene toxicity, an array of metabolites are necessary to reproduce the disease. Furthermore, it has been demonstrated that benzene, rather than benzene metabolites, stimulates protein kinase C (daSilva et al., 1989), an event that may play a significant role in benzene toxicity. It is postulated, therefore, that both benzene and a defined mixture of specific benzene metabolites are needed to produce benzene toxicity.

An alternative fate for benzene metabolites is the covalent binding to cellular macromolecules, which many investigators believe is related to the mechanism of benzene toxicity and/or carcinogenicity. In studies in which radiolabeled benzene was used to detect covalent binding Snyder and colleagues (1978) and Longacre and coworkers (1981a, 1981b) reported that benzene metabolites bind to proteins in mouse liver, bone marrow, kidney, spleen, blood, and muscle. Less covalent binding in bone marrow, blood, and spleen was observed in relatively benzene-resistant C57Bl/6 mice than in more benzene-sensitive DBA/2 mice. Irons and coworkers (1980) found covalent binding to protein in perfused bone marrow preparations. The observation of covalent binding demonstrates the chemical reactivity of one or more benzene metabolites. The ultimate significance of covalent binding to proteins will depend on the identification of the proteins, their function, and the degree to which adduct formation modifies protein function.

(a) Jerina and Daly (1974):

O OH

(b) Ingelman-Sundberg and Hagbjork (1982):

\+ OH OH

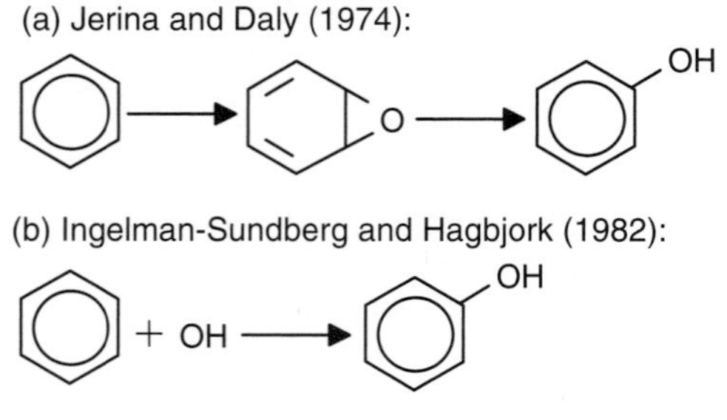

*Figure 24–3. The mechanism of benzene hydroxylation.*

Covalent binding of benzene metabolites to DNA offers a potential mechanism for inhibition of cell replication or for the initiation of leukemia. Lutz and Schlatter (1977) reported that in rats exposed to benzene vapor, liver DNA contained labeled benzene residues. Bauer and coworkers (1989) reported on DNA adduct formation in both nuclei and mitochondria in the liver of rabbits treated with benzene and suggested the presence of several different adducts on the basis of the [$^{32}$P]postlabeling technique (Randerath et al., 1981). In contrast, Reddy and colleagues (1994), using the [$^{32}$P]postlabeling technique, failed to detect binding of benzene metabolites to DNA. However, Creek and coworkers (1994) reported covalent binding of benzene metabolites at extremely low levels of exposure in mice. The occurrence and significance of DNA adduct formation from benzene metabolites requires further examination.

Mitochondria represent an important site of covalent binding for benzene (Gill and Ahmed, 1981). Kalf and colleagues (1982) have demonstrated that the inhibition of RNA synthesis in mitochondria from both liver and bone marrow correlates with covalent binding of benzene metabolites to DNA. It appears that phenol, hydroquinone, catechol, benzoquinone, and 1,2,4-trihydroxybenzene can lead to adduct formation in bone marrow mitochondria. The significance of inhibited RNA synthesis in mitochondria relates to inhibition of the synthesis of critical mitochondrial proteins and the resulting impairment of mitochondrial function. Furthermore, the demonstration by Post and coworkers (1984) that the benzene metabolites hydroquinone and benzoquinone inhibit nuclear mRNA synthesis adds further weight to the significance of the interactions of benzene metabolites and DNA.

The effects of benzene of greatest concern are the production of aplastic anemia, which is frequently fatal, and acute myelogenous leukemia. Exposure of animals to benzene in vivo results in the inhibition of growth and development of the pluripotential bone marrow stem cell as measured by the spleen colony forming unit assay (CFU-S), as well as the growth inhibition of more mature precursors such as myeloid colony forming units (CFU-C) and erythroid colony forming units (CFU-E and BFU-E) (Uyeki et al., 1977; Green et al., 1981; Harigaya et al., 1981; Toft et al., 1982; Baarson et al., 1984; Seidel et al., 1989). Benzene metabolites have been shown to be toxic in most colony forming units when added in vitro. A significant element in the inhibition of bone marrow function by benzene is the demonstration that hydroquinone is capable of inhibiting the activation of preinterleukin-1 (pre-IL-1) to active IL-1 in the stromal macrophage (Renz and Kalf, 1991). IL-1 is critical for bone marrow cell function and this may be an important site of action in the development of aplastic anemia.

The stem and progenitor cells cannot develop normally in marrow without the presence of a functional hematopoietic microenvironment. The stromal cells of the microenvironment form a supporting matrix for the development of cells in the bone marrow. Benzene has been demonstrated to impair mouse bone marrow stromal cells both in vitro and in vivo (Gaido and Wierda, 1984, 1985). Among these cells are lymphocytes and macrophages. Post and colleagues (1985) reported that treatment with benzene or its metabolites, hydroquinone or benzoquinone, inhibited the production of interleukin-2 (IL-2) in T lymphocytes. MacEachern and coworkers (1989) and Robertson and colleagues (1989) reported that treatment of mice with benzene or with a combination of phenol and hydroquinone resulted in the release of elevated levels of hydrogen peroxide, IL-1, and tumor necrosis factor from stromal macrophages. These and other studies suggest that the hematopoietic microenvironment is another target for benzene.

Although benzene-induced aplastic anemia is often fatal, those who survive usually enter a stage in the disease termed preleukemia, or myelodysplasia (Snyder and Kalf, 1994). Myelodysplastic syndrome is a clonal disease with many characteristics of neoplasia. The patients may display anemia, leukopenia, or thrombocytopenia in various combinations. Abnormal looking cells and chromosome damage are observed. Eventually the disease converts to full-blown acute leukemia. A similar series of events has been described in people who have been treated for cancer with a variety of alkylating agents and undergo remission but in the process suffer from bone marrow damage induced by the anticancer drugs. A high percentage eventually demonstrate acute leukemia similar to that caused by benzene (Koeffler and Rowley, 1985).

Benzene-induced leukemia may develop by a mechanism heretofore unrecognized. The erythroid series is more susceptible to benzene than the myeloid series. Paradoxically, short-term exposure of mice to benzene enhances granulopoiesis (Dempster and Snyder, 1990). In both HL-60 promyelocytic leukemia cells and 32D mouse interleukin-3 (IL-3)-dependent myeloid cells, benzene induces granulocytic differentiation (Kalf and O'Connor, 1993). Furthermore, hydroquinone synergized with granulocyte-macrophage colony stimulating factor (GM-CSF) to enhance the growth of granulocyte-macrophage colonies from mouse lineage restricted marrow cells (GM-CFU) (Irons et al., 1992). These cells do not reach full maturity but are arrested at the myelocyte stage. These and other data suggest that benzene may create conditions whereby immature myeloid cells can proliferate in the face of the restricted development of erythroid or other cells. If myelocyte differentiation is impaired and cells acquire neoplastic characteristics, the result is acute myelogenous leukemia. These observations suggest a pathway for studying the mechanism of benzene-induced leukemia.

Mechanistic studies on benzene toxicity/leukemogenesis have uncovered a variety of potential target sites which might be implicated in the etiology of these diseases. While it is tempting to select the most sensitive endpoint as the etiological locus, the reality may be somewhat more complex. Multiple sites have been identified as potential targets for benzene metabolites. Irons and coworkers (1982) and Irons and Neptun (1980) have shown that microtubule assembly, a critical process for cell replication, is inhibited by benzene metabolites. The data cited above demonstrate that benzene metabolites can covalently bind to DNA, RNA, and protein. Benzene metabolites may also inhibit specific enzymes. In each case, an argument can be made that one of these events is responsible for the inhibition of cell replication. However, it may not be necessary to attempt to exclude any of these from consideration as a contributing event. Furthermore, as emphasized above, toxicity may result from the complementary action of more than one metabolite. Thus, a useful approach to further work in this area might be to consider that benzene toxicity is the result of (1) the effects of benzene metabolites on more than one target and (2) the effects of more than one metabolite.

Another area of continuing interest in the study of benzene toxicity is the impact of benzene on chromosome structure and function. Cultured bone marrow cells taken from people suffering with benzene-induced aplastic anemia revealed extensive aneuploidy and fragmented chromosomes (Pollini and Colombi, 1964a, 1964b). In a series of studies Forni and her colleagues (Forni and Moreo, 1967, 1969; Forni et al., 1971a,b) described chromosomal aberrations in benzene-exposed workers. Many reports of chromosomal damage in workers exposed to benzene followed, among the most recent of which was a report on the nonrandom distribution of breakpoints in the karyotypes of workers exposed to benzene in Poland (Sasiadek, 1992).

Studies in animals have revealed gross chromosomal aberrations in micronuclei and they have also shown sister chromatid exchanges by both benzene and some benzene metabolites (Kissling and Speck, 1973; Siou et al., 1981; Styles and Richardson, 1984; Tunek et al., 1982; Hite et al., 1980; Choy et al., 1985; Gad-el-Karim et al., 1986; Anwar et al., 1989; Harper et al., 1984; Ciranni et al., 1988a,b; Adler and Kliesch, 1990; Tice et al., 1980, 1982; Morimoto and Wolf, 1980; Morimoto, 1983; Morimoto et al., 1983; Erexson, et al., 1985; Witz et al., 1990). Nevertheless, benzene has not been demonstrated to be mutagenic using standardized tests. It is possible that these tests failed due to inadequate metabolism of benzene to its metabolites in these systems.

The critical question regarding chromosome damage by benzene and its metabolites is whether the identification of these changes in circulating blood is useful solely as a biomarker of benzene exposure or is a surrogate for the detection of choromosome damage in bone marrow cells, which might be a predictor for eventual leukemia. Chromosome damage that is observed as a change in structure also causes changes in chromosome function. The result may be changes in production of cytokines necessary for proliferation and maturation of bone marrow cells, changes in the production of oncogenes, tumor suppressor genes, or transcription factors. Chromosome damage may be manifested as breaks or translocations, and efforts are currently underway to understand the specific implications of benzene-induced chromosome damage in terms of the development of both aplastic anemia and leukemia.

The literature on benzene toxicity extends back into the last century and to a large degree, of necessity, paralleled the increasing use of benzene as an industrial solvent, the development of our knowledge of bone marrow function, and our appreciation of the role of xenobiotic metabolism as a mechanistic factor in chemically induced diseases. Among the messages to be derived from this extensive and complex story is that benzene offers an example of how metabolic activation, the transport of chemicals between organs and pharmacokinetics, the effects of multiple metabolites on a variety of targets, species differences in both susceptibility and metabolism, and the production of a series of disease entities (syndromes) have to be examined to interpret the effects seen in individual humans and in epidemiological studies.

## Alkylbenzenes

The alkylbenzenes are single-ring aromatic compounds containing one or more saturated aliphatic side chains. The major products of commerce and, therefore, those to which humans are most likely to be exposed include toluene (methylbenzene), ethylbenzene, cumene (isopropylbenzene), and the three xylenes (1,2-, 1,3-, and 1,4-dimethylbenzene) (C&EN, June 26, 1995). These compounds are primarily derived from petroleum distillation and coke oven effluents. The National Academy of Sciences (NRC, 1980) reported that in 1980 the production levels of the alkylbenzenes in the United States, expressed in millions of metric tons, were as follows: toluene, 6.4; xylenes, 3.7; ethylbenzene, 3.9; and cumene, 1.8. It is clear that these compounds are major commodity chemicals and there is a high potential for many workers to be exposed. It also should be recognized that mixtures of these compounds have accounted for levels as high as 38 percent of the content of unleaded gasoline (NRC, 1980). The potential for human exposure, albeit often at low levels, is accordingly expanded beyond industrial workers to gasoline station workers and the general public at large. It is therefore necessary to have a full understanding of the potential effects of these compounds.

The acute toxicity of inhaled alkylbenzenes is best described as CNS depression. The CNS depressant effects of solvents were introduced in "The Toxic Effects of Solvents," above. Inhaled alkylbenzene vapors cause death in animal models at air levels that are relatively similar. Thus, the $LC_{50}$ for toluene in mice is 5320 ppm/8 h, for mixed xylenes in rats the value is 6700 ppm/4 h, for cumene in rats the value is 8000 ppm/4 h, and the lowest dose of ethylbenzene reported to kill rats is 4000 ppm/4 h.

Less information is available regarding long-term exposure to alkylbenzenes. Cragg and coworkers (1989) reported the effects of 4-week exposures (6 h/day, 5 days/week) of mice, rats, and rabbits to ethylbenzene vapors at a variety of doses. Exposures did not increase mortality nor did they adversely affect clinical chemistries or gross/microscopic pathology. At the higher exposure levels, mice and rats exhibited increases in liver weights consistent with microsomal enzyme induction previously reported by Elovaara and colleagues (1985). The significance of this finding in the liver is uncertain. However, Bardodej and Cirek (1988) reported no adverse responses in hematological and liver function tests for workers exposed to ethylbenzene and monitored over 20 years.

Commercial xylenes from petroleum sources typically consist of 20 percent o-xylene, 44 percent m-xylene, 20 percent p-xylene, and up to 15 percent ethylbenzene. Carpenter and coworkers (1975) failed to identify target organs or any significant adverse effects in rats and dogs exposed to either 460 ppm or 810 ppm xylene vapors 6 h/day, 5 days/week for a total of 66 days. Workers repeatedly exposed to xylene vapor concentrations in excess of 100 ppm frequently complain of gastrointestinal disturbances (Browning, 1965; Carpenter et al., 1975). The toxicity of xylenes was reviewed by Low and coworkers (1989).

Epidemiological studies in workers (Matsushita et al., 1975; Benignus, 1981) and in chronic solvent abusers (Morton, 1987) as well as animal studies (Sullivan et al., 1989) have identified the CNS as a target organ for injury following repeated exposure to toluene. Workers exposed repeatedly to 200 to 300 ppm have been observed to have an impaired simple and choice reaction time and impaired speed of perception. The very high levels of toluene encountered by glue sniffers result in cerebellar damage as well as changes in CNS integrative functions.

The neurobehavioral effects of several alkylbenzenes have also been explored. Saito and Wada (1993) reviewed the behavioral toxicology of toluene and concluded that learned responses in rats can be altered as a result of exposure at various concentrations, among which are air levels well below anesthetic concentrations. For example, using a fixed interval schedule, in which a fixed period must pass between rewards for pressing a lever, the control learned to wait the proper period before pressing. Subacute exposure to toluene (4 h/day for 5 days) at 500 ppm produced no effect, 1000 ppm produced an increase in correct responses, and 2000 ppm caused a decrease in correct responses. Using a fixed ratio schedule, in which a reward is obtained after pressing a lever a fixed number of times, 574 ppm decreased the responses and a 50 percent decrease in responses was produced at 1853 ppm. By now there have been a large number of behavioral toxicity studies performed using toluene and the general conclusion is that toluene can alter learned behavior at concentrations below anesthetic levels but, in general, above 1000 ppm.

Nevertheless, Wood (1994) has suggested that the neurobehavioral effects of toluene in particular and solvents in general have not been well studied. He argues the need for a tiered system of examinations to uncover effects on the CNS that might go undetected in safety evaluation studies in the absence of a series of tests designed to detect specific forms of neurobehavioral deficits. Extrapolation from studies of acute or chronic exposure of animals to solvent vapors in which performance is impaired in a variety of tests, ranging from observed changes in simple motor activity to alterations in performance in schedule-controlled operant behavior, can help to prevent "increased accident proneness or impaired self-rescue" in exposed workers. These tests may also uncover unexpected forms of toxicity, such as the observation by Pryor and colleagues (1991) that chronic exposure to toluene produced an irreversible progressive high frequency hearing loss in animals that was dose- and time-dependent.

Studies of genetic toxicity with toluene, xylene, and cumene have shown that they do not produce mutations in the various Salmonella strains used in the Ames test, with or without metabolic activation (NRC, 1980). Toluene and xylene are inactive as mutagens in the *Saccharomyces cerevisiae* D4 test for mitotic gene conversion and in the mouse lymphoma test. Toluene, but not ethylbenzene or xylene isomers, was weakly active in the mouse micronucleus test (Mohtashamipur et al., 1985). Although chromosome aberrations have been observed in rats exposed to toluene, they have not been seen in toluene-exposed humans. Weak or absent activity in genotoxicity tests suggests that alkylbenzenes are not carcinogenic, although they have not been systematically evaluated in animal tests.

Although it is important, with respect to the production of toxicity by most compounds, to ask why they are toxic, in the case of the alkylbenzenes, an important question may be why they are relatively nontoxic except during acute exposure to high concentrations. The toxicity of many chemicals requires metabolic activation to reactive species which then cause adverse effects. In the case of the aklylbenzenes, however, the major metabolic pathways appear to be toward metabolites that have a low order of toxicity and are readily excreted. Thus, toluene is oxidized at the methyl group, and a series of oxidations leads to benzoic acid, which is conjugated with glycine to form hippuric acid, which is then excreted. Hippuric acids are also metabolites of xylene and ethylbenzene. There is no evidence at present to indicate that these metabolic pathways can be saturated, leading to spillover into alternative metabolic pathways and the formation of toxic reactive intermediates and subsequent toxic or mutagenic effects.

# CHLORINATED ALIPHATIC HYDROCARBONS

## Dichloromethane

Dichloromethane (methylene chloride, $CH_2Cl_2$) is a widely used solvent that has been used for removing paint and degreasing, as a solvent for extracting foods (e.g., for the removal of caffeine from coffee), in the manufacture of plastics, and for other purposes. Concern for the ability of dichloromethane to cause CNS depression was confirmed when two deaths were reported following exposure to air concentrations in the range of 168,000 ppm (Manno et al., 1992). Blood concentrations at the time of death were 572 and 601 mg/liter. Metabolism of dichloromethane to carbon monoxide (see below) resulted in carboxyhemoglobin concentrations of 30 percent.

Despite concerns about its potential carcinogenicity, dichloromethane does not appear to pose a threat as a genotoxic agent. Neither rats (Serota et al., 1986a) nor mice (Serota et al., 1986b) displayed neoplastic lesions after the administration of dichloromethane in drinking water at concentrations of 0, 0.15, 0.45, or 1.5 percent for 2 years, although hepatotoxicity was noted at higher doses.

When rats were exposed to dichloromethane vapors (0, 50, 200, or 500 ppm) for 5 days per week for 2 years, the highest dose resulted in hepatocellular vacuolization in both sexes and the females developed benign breast tumors, but there was no increase in the incidence of malignant neoplastic disease, and the no-observed-effect level (NOEL) was set at 200 ppm (Nitschke et al., 1988). However, a separate inhalation study in mice and rats conducted by the National Toxicology Program in 1986 identified tumors in the livers and lungs of male and female mice and mammary tumors in female rats. Accordingly, dichloromethane was banned from use as a component of aerosol cosmetics (Federal Register, 1989).

The hepatotoxic or carcinogenic effects of the halocarbons are thought to require metabolic activation by mixed function oxidases. Pankow and Jagielki (1993) suggested that the specific mixed function oxidase is CYP450 2E1. The breakage of the C-H bond is the rate-limiting step (Ahmed et al., 1980). Metabolism of the dihalomethanes leads to dehalogenation involving a formyl halide intermediate, and the end product is carbon monoxide. As a result, an elevation in carboxyhemoglobin levels may be observed (Nitschke et al., 1988). Andersen and coworkers (1991) described the production and fate of CO during dichloromethane metabolism in rats and humans using a physiologically based pharmacokinetic model.

An alternative metabolic pathway for dichloromethane is a reaction with glutathione mediated by a glutathione transferase (Casanova et al., 1992; Hashmi et al., 1994). The resulting halomethylglutathione undergoes nonenzymatic hydrolytic dehalogenation, leaving hydroxymethylglutathione. The next step in the metabolic sequence results in the release of the hydroxymethyl group as formaldehyde. Casanova and colleagues (1992) reported that dichloromethane-derived formaldehyde can form cross links between DNA and proteins. The activity was greater in mice, where dichloromethane yields tumors, than in hamsters, in which dichloromethane-related tumors were not observed. Bogaards and coworkers (1993) examined the rates of glutathione conjugation with dichloromethane and concluded that they were slower than comparable rates in the rat. Furthermore, the rate of metabolism in humans appears to be closer to the hamster than the mouse (Casanova et al., 1992).

## Chloroform

Chloroform ($CHCl_3$) was one of the earliest anesthetics used in humans. As a result there is extensive information available on both its anesthetic and toxic properties. Concentrations up to about 400 ppm can be endured for 30 min without complaint; 1000 ppm exposure for 7 min can cause dizziness and gastrointestinal upset; 14,000 ppm can cause narcosis.

Exposure to very high levels of $CHCl_3$ can cause liver and kidney damage as well as cardiac arrhythmias apparently due to sensitization of the myocardium to catecholamines. Orth (1965) has emphasized, however, that in human anesthesia, the major effect on the heart is more likely to be cardiac arrest secondary to vagal stimulation. He suggests that ventricular fibrillation occurs only after the heart has stopped, anoxia develops, and carbon dioxide levels are elevated. These effects can be prevented by adequate anticholinergic therapy. Nevertheless, the use of chloroform in anesthesia in this country has been discouraged since 1912 (Pohl, 1979).

In humans who have developed liver failure following anesthesia, symptoms were observed within a few days following surgery (Whipple and Sperry, 1909). Nausea and vomiting are followed by jaundice and coma. Upon autopsy, evidence for centrilobular necrosis extending into periportal areas was seen. The intermediate zones separating healthy and necrotic tissue contained ballooned and vacuolated cells laden with fat.

Repeated exposure to lower, subnarcotic levels of chloroform can also cause liver and kidney toxicity. However, these effects typically have not been seen in workers, despite the extensive and long history of the use of $CHCl_3$. Challen and colleagues (1958) reported on workers exposed in an industrial setting to 21 to 237 ppm $CHCl_3$. Worker complaints were of depression and gastrointestinal distress. Liver function tests did not reveal any evidence of liver damage.

Chloroform-induced liver damage is also well-recognized in experimental animal models. Torkelson and coworkers (1976) exposed rabbits, rats, guinea pigs, and dogs to 25, 50, or 85 ppm $CHCl_3$, 7 h/day, 5 days/week for 6 months. Histopathological evaluation of animals indicated centrilobular necrosis and cloudy swelling of the kidneys. The effects of the 25 ppm dose were characterized as mild and reversible. Following oral administration of chloroform in a National Cancer Institute bioassay, it was concluded that male rats developed an excess of renal epithelial cell tumors and mice developed liver tumors (Pohl, 1979).

Chloroform is metabolized (Pohl, 1979) to reactive metabolites that covalently bind to hepatic proteins of the liver and deplete its glutathione. The postulated toxic metabolite is phosgene. Protection against chloroform-induced nephrotoxicity is afforded by sulfhydryl compounds such as L-cysteine (Bailie et al., 1984) and GSH (Kluwe and Hook, 1981). Alternatively, the inhibition of chloroform metabolism by piperonyl butoxide (Kluwe and Hook, 1981) or by methoxsalen (Letteron et al., 1987) resulted in protection. Dietz and coworkers (1982) suggested that, although reactive metabolites are formed from chloroform, the carcinogenic effect is not related to the formation of a DNA adduct but rather to recurrent cytotoxicity with chronic tissue regeneration.

Smith and colleagues (1983) proposed that hepatotoxic and nephrotoxic effects of chloroform occur independently and are related to the differential metabolism of chloroform in the two organs. Whereas male mice display both hepatotoxicity and nephrotoxicity, only hepatotoxicity was observed in females. The underlying mechanism was postulated to be the conversion of chloroform to a reactive metabolite, probably phosgene, by male-specific cytochrome P450, in male mouse kidney (Smith and Hook, 1984; Smith et al., 1984). A similar phenomenon is observed in male rabbits (Bailie et al., 1984). Chloroform is metabolized by cytochrome P450 2E1 (Brady et al., 1989). Hong and coworkers (1989) reported that in mouse kidney a specific form of cytochrome P450 2E1 was found in males and in testosterone-treated females. The corresponding enzyme in liver was not sex-specific. This enzyme is induced by secondary ketones in both the liver and kidney, which suggests that the potentiation of both hepatotoxicity and nephrotoxicity by chloroform after treating animals with methyl-n-butyl ketone, acetone, 2-butanone, 2-pentanone, 2-hexanone, or 2-heptanone results from increased production of a reactive metabolite (Branchflower and Pohl, 1981).

Attempts to extrapolate from the rodents to humans, as part of the risk assessment process, are hampered when the sites of tumor formation vary with the route or mode of administration. For example, a carcinogenesis bioassay by the National Cancer Institute (NCI, 1976) revealed that when chloroform was administered by gavage in corn oil, B6C3F1 mice of both sexes developed liver tumors and kidney tumors were observed in male Osborne-Mendel rats. Jorgenson and coworkers (1985) conducted a bioassay in which chloroform was administered in drinking water with the result that no liver tumors were observed in mice, but rats again demonstrated kidney tumors. Larson and colleagues (1993) reported that chloroform, administered in corn oil by gavage caused necrosis and regenerative hyperplasia in rat kidney and cytotoxicity and subsequent regenerative hyperplasia in mouse liver. A comparison of the effects of giving the same dose of chloroform, either in a single gavage in corn oil or over the course of a day in drinking water, revealed no liver damage when the chloroform was given in water (Larson et al., 1994a). In a parallel series of studies, chloroform was administered to rats and mice by inhalation. High doses (300 ppm/6 h/day for 7 days) caused significant hepatotoxicity and mild renal toxicity (Larson et al., 1994b). Both hepatotoxicity and renal toxicity were observed in rats. The rats developed a series of nasal lesions involving degeneration of Bowman's glands and osseous hyperplasia (Mery et al., 1994). Despite some increased cell proliferation, no osseous hyperplasia was observed in mice. In these studies the expression of chloroform toxicity was influenced by the dose rate and the vehicle in which chloroform was given, as well as the route of administration. The risk assessor is faced with deciding which model is most appropriate for extrapolation to humans. It is more likely, in our society, that people will be exposed to low levels of chloroform as a contaminant in chlorinated drinking water than that they will drink large amounts of chloroform dissolved in oil. Furthermore, the likelihood of exposure to high concentrations of chloroform in air, except under emergencies in the workplace or the laboratory, is remote.

## Carbon Tetrachloride

The mechanism of carbon tetrachloride-induced hepatic necrosis has been the subject of extensive research. Zimmerman (1978) has thoroughly reviewed the hepatotoxicity of $CCl_4$. In humans, monkeys, rats, mice, rabbits, guinea pigs, hamsters, cats, dogs, sheep, and cattle, $CCl_4$ causes centrilobular necrosis and fat accumulation. The extent of injury may be modified by factors such as species differences, age, and sex. Less sensitive models include birds, fish, amphibians and, among mammals, some types of monkeys, female rats, and newborn rats and dogs. It is likely that the differences in sensitivity are more closely related to the relative ability of the various models to activate $CCl_4$ metabolically to toxic species than to differences in the sensitivity of target sites. This concept is supported by the observation of Recknagel and Glende (1973) that administration of small doses of $CCl_4$ to rats 1 day before administration of a large dose results in protection against the toxicity otherwise produced by the large dose. The apparent reason is that the small dose was sufficient to inactivate the mixed function oxidase and thereby prevent metabolic activation to toxic metabolites. As our understanding of intracellular processes increases, however, we may learn that other events may influence the susceptibility of the hepatocyte to $CCl_4$. For example, low doses cause an increase in liver protein kinase C activity whereas high doses inhibit the enzyme which is degraded by the proteolytic enzymes calpain and calpastatin (Pronzato et al., 1993). The implications of the effects on protein kinase C have yet to be appreciated.

The effects of nutritional alterations have been difficult to interpret, but they suggest that diets sufficiently low in protein to reduce mixed function oxidase activity may be protective because of the reduced ability to yield metabolic activation of $CCl_4$. More prolonged protein deprivation, however, in the presence of residual mixed function oxidase activity, may lead to more severe liver damage because of the loss of protective sulfhydryl compounds, such as glutathione.

The hepatic injury follows a well-studied course. After a single dose of $CCl_4$ given by gavage, or by most other routes, centrilobular necrosis begins to develop, with evidence of the lesion by 12 h and full-blown necrosis by 24 h. However, evidence for the beginning of recovery, as indicated by the appearance of mitotic figures, begins within 24 h, and the liver may be restored to normal within 14 days with removal of the residues of necrotic tissue (Smuckler, 1975). During the initial 48-h period, liver enzymes, such as glutamic oxaloacetic transaminase, glutamic pyruvic transaminase, and lactic dehydrogenase, appear and then recede from the serum and can be used as measures of the extent of liver damage. Lipid accumulation develops early, with the first drops of lipid seen under the electron microscope within the first hour; these become observable under the light microscope within 3 h. Single cell necrosis is observable within 5 to 6 h (Smuckler, 1975). Damage to mitochondria and the Golgi apparatus is evident. Other early signs of cell injury include disassociation of ribosomes from the rough endoplasmic reticulum to scattered sites in the cytoplasm and disarray of the smooth endoplasmic reticulum. This apparent membrane denaturing effect described by Reynolds (1972) is probably reflected in the loss of basophilia seen under the light microscope.

Although $CCl_4$-induced hepatotoxicity is dependent on its metabolism by cytochrome P450 2E1 (Raucy et al., 1993), there is much discussion concerning the precise nature of the reactive metabolite. Biochemically, damage to the endoplasmic reticulum leads to the accumulation of lipid and to depression of protein synthesis and of mixed function oxidase activity. The mechanism of impaired mixed function oxidase activity is thought to be the irreversible binding of a $CCl_4$ metabolite to cytochrome P450, thereby rendering it inactive. Eventually, decreased mitochondrial function is also observed (Recknagel and Glende, 1973). Recknagel and coworkers (1973, 1977) and Slater (1972) have argued that the mechanism of toxicity of $CCl_4$ involves the initial homolytic cleavage of a C-Cl bond by cytochrome P450 to yield trichloromethyl and chlorine free radicals (Fig. 24-4). The trichloromethyl free radical is then thought to attack enoic fatty acids in the membranes of the endoplasmic reticulum, leading to secondary free radicals within the fatty acids. These fatty acids are now subject to attack by oxygen, and the subsequent process, which is termed *lipid peroxidation*, produces damage to membranes and enzymes. Slater (1982) has suggested that the trichloromethyl free radical is less reactive than was once thought and that it is more likely that the reaction of $O_2$ with the trichloromethyl radical leads to a more reactive species, that is, $Cl_3COO\cdot$, the trichloromethylperoxy free radical. This free radical would readily interact with unsaturated membrane lipids to produce lipid peroxidation. The net effect of

(1) Rechnagel and Glende (1973):

$$CCl_4 \longrightarrow CCl_3\cdot + Cl\cdot$$

(2) Slater (1982):

$$CC_3\cdot + O_2 \longrightarrow Cl_3COO\cdot$$

(3) Reiner and Uehleke (1971),

$$CCl_4 \longrightarrow Cl_3C:$$

(carbene)

***Figure 24–4. Proposed reactive metabolites of $CCl_4$.***

lipid peroxidation is to set in motion the series of inevitable cellular degradations, described above, that follow upon this initial insult.

An alternative to the hypothesis of free radical involvement is that covalent binding of $CCl_4$ metabolites to critical cellular macromolecules may lead to cell damage as in the case of acetaminophen and bromobenzene (Jollow and Smith, 1977). The demonstration by Laskin and coworkers (1986a,b) that Kupffer cells in liver contributed to acetaminophen-induced toxicity via the generation of reactive oxygen species which impact on hepatocytes has led to a search for similar mechanisms induced by other hepatotoxic agents. Edwards and colleagues (1993) demonstrated that $CCl_4$ toxicity in rats was reduced after treating the animals with $GdCl_3$, an agent toxic to Kupffer cells. The reactive oxygen species from Kupffer cells can attack lipids and contribute to lipid peroxidation.

Mansuy and coworkers (1974) and Reiner and Uehleke (1971) have studied the splitting of carbon-halogen bonds under anaerobic conditions to yield highly reactive metabolites having the general structure $R_3C$: and called carbenes. Uehleke (1977) reported on the covalent binding of $CCl_4$, $CHCl_3$, and halothane to macromolecules and suggested that under anaerobic conditions covalent binding is probably mediated by carbenes. Sipes and Gandolfi (1982) showed that halothane-induced liver damage produced under relatively anaerobic conditions is probably related to the formation of a carbene intermediate. Thus, it appears that aerobic covalent binding and hepatotoxicity may be accounted for by the trichloromethyl free radical or the trichloromethylperoxy free radical, whereas carbenes may play a more important role when oxygen tension is low (Uehleke, 1977; Sipes and Gandolfi, 1982; Slater, 1982).

LaCagnin and coworkers (1988) have identified another free radical metabolite of carbon tetrachloride, namely, the carbon dioxide anion radical, $CO_2^{-}\cdot$. They have demonstrated the appearance of this radical at the time of onset of LDH release from the liver, which is indicative of the onset of hepatotoxicity. Although the role played by the radical in hepatotoxicity is not yet defined, it appears to be an early marker of cell damage. Several publications have demonstrated that agents that trap free radicals may protect against $CCl_4$-induced hepatotoxicity.

## Other Haloalkanes and Haloalkenes

Many of the haloalkanes and haloalkenes are used as solvents and appear to have related mechanisms of toxic actions. Carbon tetrachloride is the prototype for these compounds and its ability to cause both fatty infiltration and hepatic necrosis serves as the model for comparison.

It should be stressed that, although carbon tetrachloride, chloroform, and 1,1,2-trichloroethane also produce renal toxicity, there is no indication that this is a common property of other haloalkanes or haloalkenes (Plaa and Larson, 1965). Zimmerman (1978) has collected the data on the hepatotoxicity of the haloalkanes and haloalkenes and has classified them according to the severity of the hepatic effects. Thus, methylchloride, methylbromide and methyliodide; dichlorodifluoromethane, trans-1,2-dichloroethylene, ethylchloride, ethylbromide, and ethyliodide, and n-butylchloride produce no liver damage and only slight fat accumulation in the liver. Chlorobromomethane, dichloromethane, cis-1,2-dichloroethylene, tetrachloroethylene, and 2-chlorobutane produce a fatty liver without necrosis. Similarly, biochemical analyses, which attempted to relate both potential carcinogenicity and hepatotoxicity, showed that, with respect to their ability to induce ornithine decarboxylase and serum alanine aminotransferase, on an equimolar basis: carbon tetrachloride > chloroform > dichloromethane (Kitchin and Brown, 1989). The following are characterized by the production of both a fatty liver and necrosis:

Carbon tetrachloride
Carbon tetraiodide
Carbon tetrabromide
Bromotrichloromethane
Chloroform
Iodoform
Bromoform
1,1,2,2,-Tetrachloroethane
1,2-Dichloroethane
1,2,-Dibromoethane
1,1,1-Trichloroethane
Pentamethylethane
1,1,2-Trichloroethylene
2-Chloro-*n*-propane
1,2-Dichloro-*n*-propane

The hepatotoxicity of these agents has been associated with the ease with which a halogen can be removed to produce a reactive metabolite. The factors associated with increasing toxicity are increasing numbers of halogens in the molecule, increasing size (i.e., atomic number or weight of the halogens), and increasing ease of homolytic cleavage. By the same token there is an inverse relationship between the severity of toxicity and the electronegativity of the halogens, or the chain length.

The metabolism of the haloforms (trihalomethanes) also involves the mixed function oxidase. The initial step is the loss of a halide. Subsequent metabolism may lead to CO production. Covalent binding to macromolecules resulting from the metabolism of haloforms has been postulated to occur via the formation of phosgene, in the case of chloroform and its analog, dibromocarbonyl, in the case of bromoform.

The metabolism and the production of reactive intermediates from the haloethylenes appears to proceed by a different mechanism. The first step in the metabolism of vinyl chloride, trichloroethylene, perchloroethylene, vinyl bromide, vinyl fluoride, vinylidene chloride, and vinylidene fluoride has been proposed to involve microsomal oxidation leading to epoxide formation across the double bond (Figure 24-5) (Henschler and Bonse, 1977, 1979; Henschler and Hoos, 1982). These authors have suggested that the resulting oxiranes are highly reactive and, therefore, can covalently bind to nucleic acids.

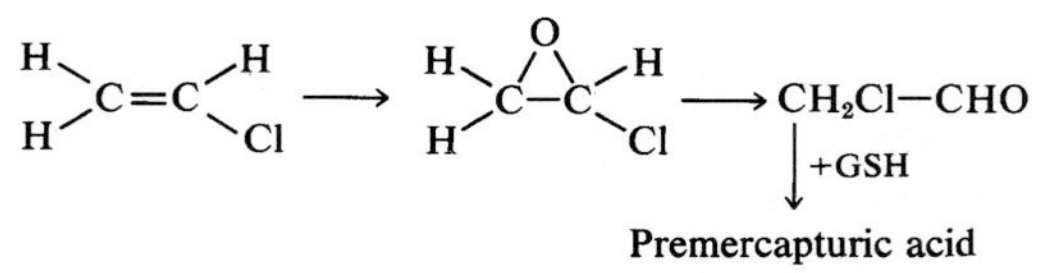

$H_2C{=}CHCl \longrightarrow$ (epoxide, $H_2C{-}O{-}CHCl$) $\longrightarrow CH_2Cl{-}CHO$
+GSH
Premercapturic acid

***Figure 24–5. The biotransformation of vinyl chloride as an example of the metabolism of haloalkenes.***

Bolt and coworkers (1982a,b) collected the data on covalent binding to protein, both in vivo and in vitro, covalent binding to nucleic acids, mutagenicity in bacterial test systems, and carcinogenicity for these compounds. Although not all of these data points were available for each compound, some important comparisons result. Vinyl chloride and vinyl bromide exhibited positive responses in each category studied, whereas trichloroethylene, which displayed some degree of positive response in each of the other categories, was not carcinogenic. Vinylidene chloride, which covalently bound to protein and nucleic acids and displayed mutagenicity, was an equivocal carcinogen. They postulated that, based on carcinogenic potency, the relative carcinogenicity of compounds that produced significant preneoplastic foci in the livers of treated rats in this series was: vinyl chloride > vinyl fluoride > vinyl bromide. Furthermore, a comparison of the monohaloethylenes and the 1,1-dihaloethylenes indicated that monohalo compounds were more carcinogenic.

The chemical reactivity of chlorinated ethylene epoxides was studied by Politzer and coworkers (1981) who compared the ease with which the two C-O bonds could be broken as a function of halogenated substituents on the carbons using ethylene oxide as the standard of reference. They showed that, in a comparison of ethylene oxide, vinyl chloride, and vinylidene chloride, with increasing chlorination of one carbon there is an increase in the bond strength of the chlorinated carbon to the oxygen and a decrease in the bond strength to the other, nonchlorinated carbon. When both carbons are substituted with a single chloride the C-O bonds are equal. When there are two chlorines on one carbon and one on the other again there is weakening of the less chlorinated carbon-to-oxygen bond. These authors suggest that the asymmetrical chloroethylenes are more carcinogenic than those that are symmetrical because the ease of bond breakage potentiates covalent binding to DNA.

While reactivity appears to be a fundamental principle of covalent binding, that is, the toxic or carcinogenic metabolite must indeed be a highly reactive compound, Bolt and colleagues (1982a) suggest that there are limits to the effectiveness of highly reactive species. For example, they postulate that a major reason for the weak activity of vinylidene chloride as a carcinogen may be related to the instability of its putative metabolite, 1,1-dichlorooxirane, which is likely to be largely degraded before it reaches its site of action. Thus, these authors suggest that there is an optimum degree of stability that allows the intermediate to be formed by the mixed function oxidase, reach the DNA, and form the covalent bond. If the reactivity is too low, little covalent binding may result. If the reactivity is too high the intermediate may never reach the target.

In addition to the well-described hepatotoxicity related to the haloalkanes and haloalkenes, several haloalkenes (e.g., tetrafluoroethylene, chlorotrifluoroethylene, 1,1-dichloro-2,2-difluoroethylene, hexafluoropropene, trichloroethylene, tetrachloroethylene, and hexachloro-1,3-butadiene) are nephrotoxic (Dekant et al., 1989). The early demonstration that trichloroethylene-extracted soybean meal yielded S-(dichlorovinyl)-L-cysteine, which produced aplastic anemia in cattle, led to the observation that in rodents this compound caused nephrotoxicity. The mechanism appears to involve the cleavage of the cysteine derivative to 1,2-dichlorovinylthiol by renal cysteine conjugate beta lyase. It has been suggested that those haloalkenes that induce nephrotoxicity act by first undergoing glutathione conjugation in the liver and are then transported to the kidney. There they are metabolized to the cysteine conjugate, which is ultimately acted upon by beta lyase to yield highly reactive episulfonium ions; these covalently bind to proteins and DNA. While the predominant effect is nephrotoxicity, in some cases the end result may be renal carcinogenesis.

Simple aliphatic halocarbons will continue to be an important area of research for some time to come. Some are found in drinking water as a result of chlorination or because they enter groundwater from leachates at chemical dump sites. Although some have been shown to be carcinogenic in long-term bioassays, it will be essential for us to assess the risk of human exposure to these chemicals accurately, at the levels at which they are found in the environment.

## Ethyl Alcohol (Ethanol, Alcohol)

Humans probably experience greater exposure to ethyl alcohol than to any other solvent, with the exception of water. Not only is it used as a solvent in industry but it is heavily consumed by large numbers of people as a component of potentially intoxicating beverages. As a result of calls for oxygenated fuels, plans for reforming gasoline to include alcohols such as ethanol suggest that we may experience universal exposure to ethanol. Nevertheless, historically, occupational exposure has been less important as a cause of injury than the fact that the worker may imbibe alcohol and thereby be rendered less likely to use safety precautions on the job. By the same token, the most important cause of death in auto accidents is driving while under the influence of alcohol. Thus, most instances of death or injury related to ethanol come via the abuse of ethanol as a beverage rather than from occupational exposure.

**Blood Levels.** Our information on the toxicity of ethanol comes from either clinical observations of human drinkers or controlled studies in animals and humans in which ethanol has been administered either orally or parenterally. Although a threshold limit value (TLV) for ethanol has been established, of greater concern has been the dose level likely to cause inebriation. In many states the demonstration that the driver has a blood alcohol level of 100 mg per 100 milliliters of blood (100 mg%) is *prima facie* evidence of "driving under the influence of alcohol." In a 70-kg human it would require approximately 3 oz of pure alcohol to achieve a blood alcohol concentration of 90 to 150 mg%. To achieve the same blood alcohol level by imbibing alcoholic beverages would require the drinking of 6 oz of 100 proof whiskey, 12 oz of fortified wine (e.g., sherry), or eight 12-ounce bottles of beer. Drinking this quantity of alcohol would produce inebriation.

The blood alcohol level and the time necessary for it to be achieved are controlled largely by the quantity of food in the gastrointestinal tract. Once absorbed the alcohol equilibrates with body water, and when a drinking session ceases the blood alcohol level begins to drop to some extent because of the excretion of alcohol in the breath and urine and, more importantly, because it is metabolized in the liver. Ethanol is metabolized at a rate sufficient to reduce the blood alcohol level linearly by approximately 15 to 20 mg% per h until low concentrations are reached, at which time the rate becomes asymptotic. Thus, if a blood alcohol concentration of 120 mg%

were detected it could be assumed that it would require approximately 6 to 8 h for ethanol to reach negligible levels in the blood.

**Central Nervous System (CNS) Effects.** The pharmacological and toxicological effects of alcohol relate to the fact that alcohol acts as both a general anesthetic and as a nutrient. As a general anesthetic, ethanol causes a dose-dependent CNS depression. Although many people appear to be animated under the influence, it is likely that this is a manifestation of the release of inhibitions and resembles a mild form of the stage II excitement and delirium observed during anesthesia with diethyl ether.

The overt display of inebriation occurs at different blood alcohol levels depending upon the extent to which the subject has had previous experience with alcohol. In heavy drinkers tolerance to the low level effects of ethanol can be observed and even social drinkers may not show obvious signs of intoxication at blood alcohol levels that would render novice drinkers clearly "under the influence." There are two reasons for these effects. Heavy drinkers may actually demonstrate a greater rate of ethanol metabolism. More important may be the fact that experienced drinkers have learned not to display their inebriation at the lower blood levels at which inexperienced drinkers overtly respond.

The literature on the biological and medical effects of alcohol is the largest single literature in medical science. Ethanol is distributed with body water and its adverse effects to most organs have been reported. For the purposes of this discussion, some specific areas of the pharmacology and toxicology of ethanol will be discussed. These will include the effects of ethanol on the CNS, the fetal alcohol syndrome, the metabolism of ethanol, and the effects of ethanol on the liver. For additional detailed reports on current trends in alcohol research the student is referred to compendia edited by Avogadro and colleagues (1979), Sherlock (1982a), and Thurman and Hoffman (1983). Among the areas covered are the interaction of ethanol with the endocrine system, interactions with xenobiotics, effects on renal, cardiovascular, and gastrointestinal systems, hematopoietic effects, enzymology, dependence and withdrawal, and other effects which indicate that alcoholism is a disease that encompasses the entire body.

The obvious behavioral effects of alcohol are well known. The loss of inhibitions has been eloquently described through several editions of a noted textbook of pharmacology: "Confidence abounds, the personality becomes expansive and vivacious, and speech may become eloquent and occasionally brilliant" (Ritchie, 1970). Although some reflexes may be enhanced at low blood ethanol concentrations because of the release of higher center control, they soon deteriorate as the blood level increases. It can be demonstrated that, despite outer appearances, objective tests of manual dexterity and simple intellectual challenges demonstrate impairment at relatively low blood alcohol levels.

With increasing blood alcohol levels there is gradual reduction of visual acuity, decreased sense of smell and taste, increased pain threshold, impaired muscular coordination, and possibly nystagmus. A staggering gait becomes apparent. Eventually nausea and vomiting, diplopia, hypothermia, and loss of consciousness ensue. As an anesthetic, ethanol is thought to have a very low therapeutic index and the subject is not far from death when anesthetic concentrations of ethanol are reached. While the level necessary to achieve loss of consciousness is not clearly defined, it is likely that at a blood alcohol level of 350 to 400 mg% most people would be asleep.

The mechanism by which ethanol causes these effects is not known. By the same token it is not known how any of the general anesthetics function. Because the structures of the general anesthetics are so varied, theories of anesthesia have developed that consider generalized interactions with the CNS rather than effects at specific receptors. A number of physicochemical theories have been proposed to explain the mechanism of action of general anesthetics. For example, the Meyer-Overton theory, as described by Meyer (1937), suggested that the potency of a general anesthetic was directly related to its solubility in lipid membranes and was otherwise unrelated to its structure. Ferguson (1939) argued that the chemical potential or thermodynamic activity was more closely related to anesthetic activity, whereas Wulf and Featherstone (1957) argued that the critical property was the van der Waals constant. Pauling (1961) and Miller (1961) built their arguments around the effect of ethanol on water and suggested that clathrate formation in cells of the CNS created a structure for water that was conducive to anesthesia. The observation that the elevation of ambient pressure caused experimental animals to awaken from anesthesia led Miller and coworkers (1973) to formulate a hypothesis suggesting there was a linear relationship that linked the elevation of atmospheric pressure with a decrease in anesthetic potency. It could then be suggested that the gas enters and distorts the membrane, taking up a given volume of space. According to the thermodynamic gas laws, the volume of the gas must decrease as the pressure increases; this suggests that the volume of anesthetic in the membranes of the CNS decreases with increasing pressure, leading to the reversal of anesthesia.

Singer and Nicolson (1972) have visualized the cell membrane as a two-dimensional solution of proteins and lipids. They visualize a bilayer composed largely of phospholipids, in which the polar ends are in contact with water and the lipid ends meet in the membrane. The lipid bilayer is studded with proteins, which are partially embedded in the lipid and partially extend into the aqueous medium. It has been suggested that ethanol interacts with the bilayer to distort and expand the membrane, thereby increasing its fluidity (Seeman, 1972; Hunt, 1975; Hill and Bangham, 1975; Richards et al., 1978; Chin and Goldstein, 1977; Rubin and Rottenberg, 1983). The result is the displacement of critical membrane enzymes and alterations in membrane function. The outward signs of ethanol inebriation and anesthesia would then be a function of the significance of the role of the membranes of various CNS cells in controlling these physiological functions. It has been suggested that ethanol plays a role in depressing the activities of the reticular activating system in the CNS, and thereby releases many functions from integrating control (Kalant, 1961). If that is true, the cell membranes of the reticular activating system may be especially sensitive to ethanol-induced changes in membrane fluidity, or their activity is so critical that small alterations in their function lead rapidly to readily observed changes in behavior.

Several recent observations in vitro may shed further light on the molecular mechanisms underlying the effects of ethanol. Ethanol has been shown to block the N-methyl-D-aspartate

(NMDA) receptor in brain cells (Lovinger et al., 1989) and to inhibit the related production of cyclic guanosine monophosphate (GMP) (Hoffman et al., 1989) at levels in the range that would be expected to produce mild intoxication. These events are associated with a decrease in calcium uptake into cerebellar cells, an event normally stimulated by NMDA. It has been suggested that these effects may help to explain short-term memory loss and impairment of motor function associated with drinking. Among its many functions ATP has been reported to act as an extracellular excitatory mediator. Li and coworkers (1994) have argued that ethanol reacts with a small hydrophobic pocket in an ATP-gated ion channel to inhibit its normal functioning. These suggestions argue that perhaps there is a specific receptor for ethanol, rather than the more generalized receptor previously envisioned, and suggest that more evidence is needed. Reconsideration of the problem of anesthesia in general and the effects of ethanol in particular indicates that perhaps generalized effects on membranes may occur side by side with specific effects on appropriate receptors.

**Fetal Alcohol Syndrome.** One of the more serious consequences of ethanol consumption is the effect on the development of the embryo and fetus in utero (Pratt, 1982). The so-called fetal alcohol syndrome (FAS) is characterized by mental deficiency and microcephaly. The infants are generally small and demonstrate poor muscular coordination. These children also exhibit a characteristic facies recognizable to the specialist. The severity appears to be related to the extent of alcohol consumption by the mother during pregnancy. In addition to the suggestion that ethanol may interfere with membrane function during development, other factors may be related to the cause of FAS. These include the possibility that acetaldehyde may escape the damaged liver of the alcoholic mother and reach the developing fetal brain; changes in the patterns of amino acids in the maternal circulation available to the fetus; and alcohol-induced hypoglycemia. These effects, individually or in concert, could cause damage to the developing brain and lead to FAS.

**Biotransformation.** It is recognized that the toxic effects of alcohol on the liver are directly related to its metabolism and it is, therefore, important to understand the pathways of alcohol metabolism. In the larger sense these have been well worked out over a considerable period of time. In recent years there has been considerable discussion over the relative toxicological significance of the various enzymes capable of mediating the first step in alcohol metabolism, namely, its oxidation to acetaldehyde. Alcohol dehydrogenase is a soluble enzyme found in high concentrations in the liver, which appears to play the major role in alcohol metabolism. Nicotinamide-adenine dinucleotide (NAD) is the coenzyme and the products are acetaldehyde and NADH (the reduced form of NAD). The reverse of this reaction, the conversion of acetaldehyde to ethanol, is favored but during metabolism the products are rapidly removed, thereby preventing the reversal of the reaction.

$$CH_3CH_2OH + NAD \xrightarrow{\text{Alcohol Dehydrogenase}} CH_3CHO + NADH$$

A second enzyme capable of converting ethanol to acetaldehyde is catalase, which by virtue of its peroxidative activity uses hydrogen peroxide to perform the oxidation. However, normally there is very little peroxide available to support the reaction in hepatocytes (Thurman et al., 1975) and it is unlikely that catalase can account for more than 10 percent of ethanol metabolism (Feytmans and Leighton, 1973). This situation could change if peroxide levels in hepatocytes were elevated. For example, Peters (1982) indicated that clofibrate, which stimulates peroxisomal fatty acid oxidation, increases peroxide levels and thereby enhances ethanol oxidation by catalase. Catalase would be expected to play a significant role in ethanol metabolism primarily at high blood alcohol levels (Bradford et al., 1993).

$$CH_3CH_2OH + H_2O_2 \xrightarrow{\text{Catalase}} CH_3CHO + H_2O$$

The third enzyme, termed the microsomal ethanol oxidizing system (MEOS) by Lieber and DiCarli (1970), is located in the smooth endoplastic reticulum; it can be demonstrated that the addition of ethanol to isolated microsomes fortified with NADPH and oxygen results in the oxidation of ethanol to acetaldehyde.

$$CH_3CH_2OH + NADPH + O_2 \xrightarrow{\text{MEOS}} CH_3CHO + NADP + H_2O$$

Ohnishi and Lieber (1977) isolated a cytochrome P450 which mediates this reaction. Coon and Koop (1987) suggested that although this nomenclature was useful in the early days of these investigations it has several drawbacks, including the fact that the enzyme is induced by many chemicals in addition to ethanol and the fact that it metabolizes a wide range of substrates. Its official nomenclature today is cytochrome P450 2E1 (CYP2E1).

The contribution made by each of these enzymes to ethanol metabolism has been estimated by various authorities. Damgaard (1982) and Havre and colleagues (1977) have argued that nonalcohol dehydrogenase-mediated metabolism of ethanol accounts for no more than 10% of total ethanol metabolism. In contrast, Vind and Grunnet (1983) estimate that nonalcohol dehydrogenase metabolism of ethanol may account for as much as 20%, and it may increase to 30% or higher when substrates such as xylitol, which are capable of generating exceedingly high levels of NADH, are added. The argument is that at these high NADH levels electron transfer into the mixed function oxidase pathway via cytochrome b5 is stimulated and, therefore, MEOS activity is enhanced. Nevertheless, regardless of which estimate more accurately reflects the percentage of nonalcohol dehydrogenase-mediated ethanol metabolism, it appears that the major enzyme involved in ethanol oxidation is alcohol dehydrogenase. It is unlikely that catalase plays a significant role in ethanol metabolism at concentrations of peroxide normally present in the liver. The quantitative significance of the role of mixed function oxidases in ethanol metabolism has yet to be established.

The further metabolism of ethanol relates to the metabolism of acetaldehyde. In the past, the fate of acetaldehyde has been linked to several enzymes, located in various parts of the cell. In recent years, however, it has been postulated that acetaldehyde dehydrogenase, an NAD-requiring enzyme, plays the major role in its degradation and this enzyme, although largely mitochondrial in rat liver, is a cytosolic enzyme in humans (Peters, 1982).

$$CH_3HO + NAD \xrightarrow{\text{Acetaldehyde Dehydrogenase}} CH_3COO^- + NADH$$

The resulting acetate is released from the liver and oxidized peripherally (Forsander et al., 1960), probably because during ethanol oxidation there is an increase in the NADH/NAD ratio, which leads to decreased availability of oxaloacetate, decreased pyruvic dehydrogenase activity, and inhibition of citrate synthetase (Forsander et al., 1965) which taken together inhibit the oxidation of acetate in the liver.

**Liver Injury.** The drinking of alcohol remains a leading cause of death due to liver cirrhosis (Sherlock, 1982b). The diagnosis of early alcohol-induced liver disease involves a recognition that the patient drinks alcohol to excess, that the patient may be experiencing social problems indicative of alcoholism, and that these are coupled with the finding of hepatomegaly, elevated serum transaminase, and possibly other clinical signs. At more advanced stages, patients may exhibit acute alcoholic hepatitis following heavy bouts of drinking. Signs include vomiting, diarrhea, jaundice, and psychiatric disturbances. The liver is enlarged and painful to palpation whereas the spleen may be impalpable. The enlarged liver is due to fat accumulation, as well as swelling of liver cells, and to the accumulation of other components, such as proteins that would otherwise be secreted (Sherlock, 1982b). A wide variety of changes in serum enzymes and proteins that reflect the impairment of hepatic function can be determined. Eventually, with continued heavy drinking frank hepatic cirrhosis, not unlike end stage liver disease derived from other causes, will be observed and may be fatal.

The mechanism by which alcohol mediates liver damage has also generated much discussion. For many years there has been debate over whether alcoholic liver disease is the result of a direct toxic effect of ethanol on the liver or is the result of nutritional deficiencies that accompany excessive alcohol consumption. Alcohol provides 7.1 kcal/g. A pint of 100-proof whiskey would provide 1400 kcal, which is a significant portion of total caloric intake for most people. If alcoholics would maintain their normal diet in addition to consuming large quantities of alcohol, they would gain weight at a rapid pace. Since obesity is not a usual corollary to alcoholism, it appears that alcohol replaces other sources of calories in the alcoholic's diet. Because alcohol contains no essential nutrients such as proteins, vitamins, or minerals and it replaces food that would contain these dietary components, it would be expected that alcoholics should develop nutritional deficiencies.

Clinical experience with alcoholics (Morgan, 1981, 1982) suggests that the stage of alcoholism in which the individual is viewed is critical to making nutritional judgments. Early clinical studies of patients with advanced alcohol-induced liver disease, especially involving patients from poor socioeconomic backgrounds, have reported that the patients exhibited weight loss and nutritional deficiencies. However, studies of alcoholics who did not display overt liver disease revealed normal nutrition. In another study in which a segment of the alcoholic study group displayed liver disease and a segment was clinically malnourished, there did not appear to be a relationship between nutritional status and the severity of the disease. Morgan (1982) suggests that although the intake of nutrients in the diet in a controlled experiment may be similar between control and alcoholic groups, the greater percent of calories derived from alcohol led to a significantly different nutritional status. Among the nutritional problems caused by alcohol consumption are decreases in thiamine absorption, decreased enterohepatic circulation of folate, degradation of pyridoxal phosphate, and disturbances in the metabolism of vitamins A and D (Mezey, 1985). Other factors that taken together can be considered as contributing to malabsorption and may contribute to the development of malnourishment, despite adequate intake of essential nutrients, include the effects of alcohol on gastric emptying time and changes in the physiology and morphology of the small intestine, secretion by the pancreas and biliary system, and splanchnic blood and lymph flow.

Lieber (1979) has suggested that alcohol has a direct toxic effect on the liver that is not dependent on nutritional deficiency. The data come from studies in which humans given nutritional supplements while consuming excessive quantities of alcohol developed fatty livers. Furthermore, in a long-term study in which 15 baboons fed alcohol and given nutritional supplements all developed fatty liver, 5 developed hepatitis and 5 were found to have cirrhosis (Lieber et al., 1975). These results were not confirmed, however, by Ainley and coworkers (1988), who performed a similar study in baboons with the aim of determining whether enrichment of the diet with Zn protected against hepatic fibrosis and cirrhosis.

An alternative mechanism for ethanol-induced liver injury derives from the study of liver reperfusion following hepatic transplantation. Livers recovered from accident victims whose death was associated with drinking alcohol are often found to be fatty and following transplant are often nonfunctional. During both chronic alcohol usage and reperfusion, Kupffer cells undergo activation leading to the release of various toxic mediators, including reactive oxygen species, tumor necrosis factor (TNF), and other reactive species which may impinge on and damage hepatocytes (Lemaster and Thurman, 1993). Ethanol is also associated with increased production of endotoxin, another Kupffer's cell activator, by gram negative bacteria of the intestine. Thus, it has been postulated that ethanol-induced hepatic injury may be related to the stimulation of endotoxin production by intestinal bacteria, leading to Kupffer's cell activation and the release of toxic mediators such as free radicals, TNF, and other factors (Adachi et al., 1994). The products of Kupffer's cell activation then lead to hepatocyte damage described as ethanol-induced liver toxicity. Several supporting lines of evidence have been presented. Among these are the demonstration that antibiotics, which inhibit the growth of gram negative bacteria, and the destruction of Kupffer cells by $GdCl_3$ both protect against ethanol-induced liver damage and reduce the appearance of radicals in liver cells otherwise associated with ethanol exposure.

The conclusions that can be drawn at this time are that, given the severe derangement of hepatic metabolism produced by chronic alcohol feeding, the effects of ethanol on the gastrointestinal (GI) tract, and the frequency of malnourishment among alcoholics, it is likely that nutritional factors play a role in the development of alcoholic liver disease. However, if the endotoxin theory is correct, the idea that malnutrition plays a role may have less significance but may still contribute to hepatic damage. The direct toxic effect then may be the impact on the Kupffer cell of ethanol directly or as a result of the stimulation of endotoxin release. The development of a rodent model for hepatic cirrhosis in which the disease can be accurately reproduced would help to settle the question because it would permit the determination of the relative roles of nutritional requirements and the effects of Kupffer cell activation.

**Interaction with Other Chemicals.** The toxicological interaction of ethanol with other hepatotoxic agents is a well-recognized phenomenon (Zimmerman, 1978; Strubelt, 1980). The earliest reported indication of an interaction was between ethanol and $CCl_4$ used as a vermifuge in the treatment of hookworm in humans who drank alcoholic beverages (Smillie and Pessoa, 1923; Moon, 1950; Hyatt and Salmons, 1952). The observation that ethanol potentiates $CCl_4$ toxicity has also been made in several species of laboratory animals (Zimmerman, 1978; Strubelt, 1980; Shibayama, 1988). Ethanol can increase the toxicity of $CCl_4$ as well as a number of other chemicals. Strubelt (1980) reviewed the literature and reported that ethanol also increased the toxicity of chloroform, trichloromethane, trichloroethylene, thioiacetamide, dimethylnitrosamine, paracetamol, aflatoxin $b_1$, and chlorpromazine. As suggested above (Pankow and Jagielki, 1993) the specific mixed function oxidase that is known to metabolically activate several of these compounds is CYP450 2E1. Reinke and coworkers (1988) reported that ethanol stimulated the production of trichloromethyl free radicals from carbon tetrachloride.

Pretreatment with ethanol also increases the hepatotoxicity of chloroform (Kutob and Plaa, 1962), trichloroethane (Klaassen and Plaa, 1966), trichloroethylene (Cornish and Adefuin, 1966), thioacetamide, dimethylnitrosamine (Maling et al., 1975), paracetamol (Strubelt et al., 1978), and aflatoxin $B_1$ (Glinsukon et al., 1978). Ethanol was less effective in increasing the hepatotoxicity of allyl alcohol and galactosamine (Strubelt et al., 1980) and did not alter the effects of bromobenzene, phalloidin, or praseodymium. The toxic effects of $\alpha$-amantadine were reduced by ethanol.

Methanol, 2-propanol, 2-butanol, and 2-methyl-propanol mimicked the effects of ethanol and were more active in potentiating the hepatotoxic effects of other agents (Cornish and Adefuin, 1967; Traiger and Plaa, 1971a,b). Traiger and coworkers (Traiger and Plaa, 1971a,b; 1974; Traiger and Bruckner, 1976) have shown that whereas the ketone metabolites of the secondary alcohols (i.e., acetone and 2-butanone) increase the hepatotoxicity of $CCl_4$ and other halocarbons, acetaldehyde is lacking in this property and the inhibition of ethanol metabolism by pyrazole does not protect against the potentiating effect. The most likely mechanism appears to be the induction of cytochrome P450 2E1 by ethanol, which then increases the production of reactive metabolites of cosubstrates for the enzyme.

**Ethanol as a Carcinogen.** Because of the widespread use of alcoholic beverages there has been understandable concern regarding the role of ethanol in carcinogenesis. IARC convened an expert panel to review all of the literature in this field (IARC, 1988). They concluded that, whereas the evidence for the carcinogenicity of ethanol and alcoholic beverages in animals was inadequate, there is "sufficient evidence" for the carcinogenicity of alcoholic beverages in humans. The panel agreed that the evidence linked tumors of the oral cavity, pharynx, larynx, esophagus, and liver to the consumption of alcoholic beverages. Seitz and Simanowski (1986) suggested that ethanol did not act as an initiator but was more likely to be a cocarcinogen which interacts with other carcinogens to cause tumorigenic responses. Unlike most environmental carcinogens to which people are exposed either infrequently or at a low dose, the consumption of alcoholic beverages is common to millions of people on a relatively frequent basis at dietary dose levels. Further studies are required to accurately define the risk to the general population of users.

## Methanol

Methanol, or wood alcohol, is another potential neurotoxin that finds extensive use in industry as a solvent. The proposal to add methanol to gasoline or to design automobiles that use methanol as a primary fuel will necessarily widen consumer exposure. It has been suggested that no acute toxic health effects would be expected to occur during the normal course of using methanol-containing automotive fuels (Reese and Kimbrough, 1993). Nevertheless, Costantini (1993), while agreeing with this conclusion, suggests that more extensive evaluation of the effects of methanol in humans is needed. Clearly, aspiration pneumonia remains a problem and more attention should be paid to accidental ingestion, especially by children, of methanol-containing fuel.

The target of methanol toxicity is the retina, a fact that has been documented in many case reports of unfortunate individuals who suffered the effects of ingesting large amounts of the solvent (Bennett et al., 1953; Kane et al., 1968). At high doses, methanol can cause reversible or permanent blindness and, in severe cases, death. Intoxication is characterized by initial mild inebriation followed by an asymptomatic period of 12 to 24 h. At this time, a marked metabolic acidosis develops, which if not treated can be fatal. Visual problems include eye pain, blurred vision, constriction of visual fields, and other visual complaints. Permanent blindness can develop within 48 h (Bennett et al., 1953). The pathology of the visual lesion has been described in some detail. A marked optic disk edema and dilated pupils with a greatly reduced reaction to light are observed. Intraaxonal swelling in the areas of the optic disk and anterior optic nerve are observed with light microscopy (Benton and Calhoun, 1952; Roe, 1943, 1946, 1948).

**Biotransformation.** Methanol is rapidly and well absorbed by inhalation, oral, and topical exposure routes (Dutkiewicz et al., 1980; Leaf and Zatman, 1952; Sayers et al., 1944; Egle and Gochberg, 1975). Following absorption, the alcohol is rapidly distributed to organs according to the distribution of body water (Yant and Schrenk, 1937).

There are two pathways available in the mammalian organism for oxidation of methanol: a catalase peroxidative pathway and an alcohol dehydrogenase system. Studies in the rat, guinea pig, and rabbit showed that the major route of methanol oxidation is through a catalase-dependent pathway, whereas an alcohol dehydrogenase system functions in the monkey and human (Makar and Tephly, 1968; Mannering and Parks, 1975). Metabolism to formic acid is rapid. Indeed, in monkeys or humans poisoned with large amounts of methanol, formaldehyde is not detected even in very low levels in tissues at autopsy. Formic acid is further oxidized to carbon dioxide by an enzymatic pathway dependent upon the presence of the cofactor, folic acid. The enzyme is active in both rodents and primates but conversion of formic acid to $CO_2$ appears to be slower in primates than in rodents (Tephly et al., 1979).

**The Mechanism of Visual Impairment.** The monkey was proposed as an appropriate animal model for studying methanol poisoning, because the resulting syndrome closely resembles that seen in humans (McMartin et al., 1975). Indeed, while metabolic acidosis and ocular toxicity are observed in humans and monkeys, rodents, dogs, and cats display only mild CNS depression following dosing with methanol (Tephly, 1977). Using the primate as a model, Tephly and coworkers have elucidated in detail the relationship between methanol metabolism and toxicity (McMartin et al., 1977, 1979, 1980). In rodents, species that are not susceptible to methanol-induced ocular toxicity, methanol is rapidly metabolized to $CO_2$. In contrast, in primates and humans, alcohol dehydrogenase and folate-dependent pathways slowly metabolize methanol to $CO_2$. The kinetics of metabolism and elimination of large doses of methanol in primates are such that formic acid accumulates in tissues including the eye (Tephly et al., 1979; McMartin et al., 1975; 1977; Noker and Tephly, 1980). A metabolic acidosis and the characteristic ocular toxicity of methanol exposure results. It was proposed that ocular toxicity was related to the presence of elevated levels of formic acid in blood (Tephly et al., 1979; McMartin et al., 1975; 1977; Noker and Tephly, 1980).

Lee and colleagues (1994a,b) proposed an alternative model for methanol toxicity. The "folate-reduced rat (FR) model" is derived from an animal that accumulates formate and has the capacity to respond to methanol challenge in a manner similar to humans. Using the FR rat they demonstrated that methanol (3.5 g/kg, orally, or 2000 ppm by inhalation) inhibited the normal functioning of the retino-geniculo-cortical visual pathway and caused a reduction in the beta-wave amplitude of the electroretinogram, in a manner similar to that seen in cases of human methanol poisoning. Although the inhibition of formaldehyde oxidation to formate prevented retinal damage, the administration of formate did not cause retinal toxicity. They suggest (Garner et al., 1995a) that the intraretinal metabolism of methanol, rather than elevated blood formate levels, is required to initiate methanol-induced retinal toxicity. They have postulated that the oxidation of methanol to formate parallels the depletion of retinal ATP and that the Müller cell, which is a retinal glial cell, is the initial target cell leading to retinal damage (Garner et al., 1995b).

**Chronic Exposure.** Much less information is available on the health effects of long-term exposure to low levels of methanol. Office workers exposed to methanol in the vicinity of duplicating machines were studied by Kingsley and Hirsch (1954–1955). The workers complained of frequent and recurrent headaches but of no other symptoms. Methanol exposure levels were reported to range from 15 to 375 ppm, although most measurements fell in the 200 to 375 ppm range. Duplicating fluids were changed in favor of less methanol, but the authors fail to mention if there were any beneficial effects on worker headaches. It is unclear from this study whether headaches were attributable to methanol or to other components of duplicating fluids.

It is of interest that nearly 30 years following the report by Kingsley and Hirsch, NIOSH (1980) performed a health hazard investigation on teacher's aides using spirit duplicating machines. No local exhaust ventilation was available and most measurements exceeded the NIOSH recommended STEL for 15 min (800 ppm). The adverse health effects of blurred vision, headache, nausea, and dizziness reported by teachers on questionnaires appear to refer to the CNS depressant effects of methanol.

Maejima and coworkers (1994) exposed rats to exhaust from an engine that burned methanol containing 15 percent gasoline and contained no catalyst, for 12 weeks. Significant findings were an increase in carboxyhemoglobin and a decrease in the concentration of cytochrome P450 in the lungs. In addition to carbon monoxide, blood levels of formaldehyde, methanol, and nitrogen oxides increased. These results suggest that studies involving longer-term exposures may be warranted.

In the absence of well-designed epidemiological studies and long-term animal studies, one may use pharmacokinetic principles to consider whether or not chronic exposure to low levels of methanol is likely to result in ocular toxicity. In poisoning cases in which humans consumed several ounces of methanol, blood concentrations in the hundreds of mg per 100 ml of blood were established (Kane et al., 1968; Bennett et al., 1953; Gonda et al., 1978). A review of these papers, which have extensively considered methanol concentration in blood and the clinical outcome of poisoning, indicates that an initial blood level in excess of 100 mg per 100 mL would be required for irreversible effects, such as visual disturbances. Additionally, a typical half-life for methanol in the blood was estimated to be in the range of 30 h (Kane et al., 1968). While the half-life of blood methanol is long in poisoning cases, studies in human volunteers who ingested small amounts (1 to 5 mL) of methanol revealed that under these conditions the blood half-life is only about 3 h (Leaf and Zatman, 1952; Dutkiewicz, 1980; Ferry et al., 1980; Sedivec et al., 1981). Thus, peak blood levels were in the range of 10 mg per 100 mL.

If one considers the present ACGIH (1995–1996) TLV of 200 ppm (262 mg/m$^3$) and assumes that there is 100 percent absorption of vapors and a respiratory volume of 10 m$^3$ in an 8-h workday, then a total body burden may be calculated.

$$\text{Body Burden} = 262\ \text{mg/m}^3 \times 10\ \text{m}^3 \times 1.0 = 2620\ \text{mg}$$

If one further assumes that this total body burden is absorbed within the first few minutes of the work shift and that the methanol distributes with total body water, a worst-case peak blood methanol level may be calculated.

$$\text{Peak blood level} = 2620\ \text{mg}/49^{*}\ \text{l} = 53\ \text{mg/l} = 5.3\ \text{mg}/100\ \text{mL}$$

*Assumes a 70 kg person with a 70% water content.

This peak blood level is about 1/20 of a level that would be associated with acute irreversible toxic effects. Because the half-life of blood methanol in this blood concentration range is 3 h, blood methanol concentrations would be at negligible levels by the time the next work shift began 24 h later. Thus, it seems unlikely that vapor exposure to methanol under ACGIH-recommended exposures (ACGIH, 1995–1996) has any possibility of causing ocular toxicity. The possibility of achieving a high enough body burden under dermal exposure conditions seems even more remote.

## GLYCOLS

In addition to their general use as heat exchangers, antifreeze formulations, hydraulic fluids, and chemical intermediates, glycols also have some use as an industrial solvent for nitrocellulose and cellulose acetate and as a solvent for pharmaceuticals, food additives, cosmetics, inks, and lacquers. Due to their low volatility, the glycols in general produce little vapor hazard at ordinary temperatures. However, since they are used in antifreeze mixtures, as hydraulic fluids, and as heat exchangers they may be encountered in the vapor or mist form, particularly where the temperature is markedly elevated, or they may enter groundwater following consumer use and disposal. OSHA has recognized the respiratory irritation potential of ethylene glycol vapors by setting an exposure standard of 50 ppm as a ceiling limit not to be exceeded (OSHA, 1989).

### Ethylene Glycol (1,2-Ethanediol, $HOCH_2CH_2OH$)

When taken orally, ethylene glycol appears to be considerably more toxic to humans than to other animal species. The lethal oral dose in humans is estimated to be 1.4 mL/kg based on poisonings from accidental ingestion or ingestion with suicidal intent. This amount would be equivalent to approximately 100 mL for a 70-kg person. The acute oral $LD_{50}$s reported for rats, guinea pigs, and mice ranged from approximately 5.5 to 13 mL/kg, indicating that, on a weight basis, ethylene glycol appears to be less toxic in these animal species than in humans.

Cats appear to share the primate's susceptibility to poisoning with ethylene glycol. Gessner and coworkers (1961) reported a minimal lethal dose of 1 g/kg for cats and noted that this may be due to an already high baseline excretion of oxalic acid. Ethylene glycol poisoning is a serious and frequently encountered problem for the veterinarian in small animal practice. Exposure typically occurs when pets ingest spilled ethylene glycol-based antifreezes (Rowland, 1987; Mueller, 1982).

While species sensitivity to ethylene glycol varies considerably, the kidney damage resulting from acute or chronic exposure was identified early in the rat and was repeated in several other animal species (Morris et al., 1942; Blood, 1965; Gershoff and Andrus, 1962; Blood et al., 1962; Roberts and Seibold, 1969).

DePass and colleagues (1986) fed rats of both sexes diets containing ethylene glycol for 2 years. Rats were considerably more sensitive than were mice. High-dose male rats exhibited a variety of signs and symptoms. Urinary calcium oxalate crystals and increased kidney weight was noted in all high-dose male rats; effects relevant to the kidney included tubular cell hyperplasia, tubular dilatation, and peritubular nephritis. Ethylene glycol was not carcinogenic in rats and mice. Studies on ethylene glycol toxicity in the monkey were reported by Roberts and Seibold (1969). The renal histopathology, after 6 to 13 days, varied depending on the amount of ethylene glycol consumed. At high dose levels, deposition of calcium oxalate crystals occurred in the proximal renal tubules, and necrotic areas of tubular epithelium occurred adjacent to the crystals. In this study, it appeared that oxalate crystallization did not occur following doses less than 15 mL/kg. However, functional renal changes were present at dose levels above 1 mL/kg, suggesting that renal damage can occur in the absence of oxalate crystal formation.

In acute poisoning in humans, ingestion of ethylene glycol is followed by an asymptomatic period during which it is metabolized to glycolic and eventually oxalic acid. A profound acidosis may develop. Unlike methanol poisonings, in which vision is affected, acidosis is accompanied by disturbances in renal function or even renal failure. The full clinical picture may take up to 72 h to develop. Aggressive management of both ethylene glycols and methanol poisoning is needed, and knowledge of the metabolism of these two solvents forms the basis of treatment. An abbreviated scheme for the metabolism of ethylene glycol is presented below:

$$\begin{array}{ccccc} CH_2OH & & COOH & & COOH \\ | & \rightarrow & | & \rightarrow & | \\ CH_2OH & & CH_2OH & & COOH \\ \text{Ethylene Glycol} & & \text{Glycolic Acid} & & \text{Oxalic Acid} \end{array}$$

Ethylene glycol is oxidized by alcohol dehydrogenase to glycolaldehyde and further to glycolic acid by cytosolic aldehyde oxidase. Glycolic acid is further oxidized via glyoxylic acid to oxalic acid by glycolic acid oxidase (von Wartburg et al., 1964; Liao and Richardson, 1973; Gessner et al., 1960). Thus, both ethylene glycol and methanol are oxidatively metabolized to acids.

Bove (1966) studied the renal pathology in a series of rats given ethylene glycol or its metabolites, including glycolaldehyde, glycolic acid, and glyoxylic acid. In animals given single large doses of ethylene glycol (9 to 12 g/kg body weight), striking oxalate formation was present in renal tubules. Crystals appeared throughout the proximal and distal convoluted tubules and were less numerous in the collecting tubules. In one rat, oxalate crystals were present in the brain. This observation has also been made in humans (Pons and Custer, 1946). Oxalate crystals were also present in the renal tubules of animals receiving glycolaldehyde, glycolic acid, and glyoxylic acid, although the renal oxalosis was less extensive with glycolaldehyde. The three proposed intermediates were all more toxic on an acute basis than was ethylene glycol, as a number of animals died within 8 h of receiving 5 to 6 g/kg of body weight of the metabolites. Renal tubular pathology was not always accompanied by crystal formation, and the author concludes that cytotoxicity rather than simple mechanical obstruction is largely responsible for renal failure.

Von Wartburg and coworkers (1964) demonstrated that human liver alcohol dehydrogenase biotransformed ethylene glycol. Ethanol, which is a much better substrate for alcohol dehydrogenase than is ethylene glycol, is a potent competitive inhibitor of ethylene glycol metabolism and should duly protect against its toxic effects.

Wacker and associates (1965) reported two cases of individuals who had ingested 250 to 1000 mL of ethylene glycol antifreeze. Gastric lavage was not undertaken until admission to the hospital, some 6 to 9 h after the antifreeze was ingested; thus large quantities were presumably absorbed into the general circulation. Both patients were treated with ethanol infusion, which resulted in a prompt disappearance of oxaluria, and adequate urinary output was maintained. These individuals made uneventful recoveries from these rather massive ingestions of ethylene glycol.

The value of ethanol administration in treating methanol poisoning has also been demonstrated (Jacobsen and McMartin, 1986). Administration of 4-methylpyrazole, a noncompetitive inhibitor of alcohol dehydrogenase, is also used in treating ethylene glycol and methanol poisoning. Control of blood pH by the administration of sodium bicarbonate and the use of hemodialysis to remove the parent compound and metabolites are important additional means of treating poisoned individuals (Jacobsen and McMartin, 1986; Wiener and Richardson, 1988; Baud et al., 1988).

Lamb and coworkers (1985) administered ethylene glycol to male and female mice in the drinking water and pairs of animals were mated. After 14 weeks a second generation was selected and evaluated in a similar manner. Ethylene glycol (1.0 percent in drinking water) caused a decrease in the number of litters per fertile pair, in the number of pups per litter, and in live pup weight. These effects were observed without any concurrent effects on body weight, water consumption, or clinical signs of toxicity in the parents. Examination of offspring revealed a pattern of skeletal defects in treated mice including the skull, sternebrae, ribs, and vertebrae. The developmental toxicity of ethylene glycol was confirmed using a conventional teratology protocol in rats and mice (Price et al., 1985).

## Diethylene Glycol ($HOCH_2CH_2OCH_2CH_2OH$)

Diethylene glycol is used in the lacquer industry, in cosmetics, in permanent antifreeze formulations, in lubricants, as a softening agent, and as a plasticizer. It presents little hazard during industrial handling at ordinary temperatures. Where mists are generated or where operations are carried out at high temperatures, industrial hygiene control methods should be followed to eliminate repeated prolonged inhalation. The major hazard from diethylene glycol occurs following the ingestion of relatively large single doses. Impetus for the study of the toxicity of diethylene glycol was provided by 105 fatalities among 353 people who ingested a solution of sulfanilamide in an aqueous mixture containing 72 percent diethylene glycol (Ruprecht and Nelson, 1937; Smyth, 1952). The symptoms included nausea, dizziness, and pain in the kidney region. This was followed in a few days by oliguria and anuria with death resulting from uremic poisoning. Based on these data it has been estimated that the single oral dose lethal for humans is approximately 1 mL/kg. Following an episode of poisoning known as the elixir of sulfanilamide incident, the Food, Drug and Cosmetics Act was subsequently amended in 1938 to require that marketed drugs be proved safe and effective.

A long-term rat-feeding study by Fitzhugh and Nelson (1946) showed that 1 percent diethylene glycol in the diet over a 2-year period resulted in slight growth depression, a few calcium oxalate bladder stones, minimal kidney damage, and occasional liver damage. At the 4 percent dietary level there was increased mortality, a marked depression of the growth rate, bladder stones, severe kidney damage, and moderate liver damage. In addition, bladder tumors appeared frequently. The authors concluded that bladder tumors never developed in the experimental rats without the preceding or concurrent presence of a foreign body. They suggest that diethylene glycol is not a primary carcinogen, but when it is fed in very high concentrations it does result in the formation of calcium oxalate bladder stones and subsequent rare bladder tumors. The toxic effects seen following exposure to diethylene glycol are consistent with its metabolic conversion to ethylene glycol and subsequent acidosis and oxalate crystal formation.

## Propylene Glycol (1,2-Propanediol, $CH_3CHOHCH_2OH$)

Propylene glycol, in sharp distinction to ethylene and diethylene glycol, has a low order of toxicity. Propylene glycol is used in human and pet foods, cosmetics, and pharmaceuticals with no apparent adverse effects. Other major uses of propylene glycol include antifreeze formulations, heat exchangers, and hydraulic fluids. Propylene glycol has a very low order of acute toxicity. The acute oral $LD_{50}$s of propylene glycol in rats, rabbits, and dogs are approximately 30, 18, and 19 g/kg body weight, respectively (Ruddick, 1972). Symptoms of acute propylene glycol intoxication in animals are those of CNS depression or narcosis. No system or organ has been established as a target for the acute oral lethal effects of propylene glycol. In contrast to ethylene glycol, propylene glycol vapors do not appear to be irritating. Neither OSHA nor ACGIH have established exposure limits for propylene glycol vapors.

Because of propylene glycol's use in foods and pharmaceuticals, extensive toxicity data are available. Robertson and coworkers (1947) exposed monkeys and rats to atmospheres saturated with propylene glycol vapor and found no adverse effects in animals after periods of 12 to 18 months. No adverse effects were noted and there were no increases in tumor incidences in rats fed diets containing up to 5 percent propylene glycol for 2 years (Robertson et al., 1947; Gaunt et al., 1972). Furthermore, propylene glycol is used as a carbohydrate source without any adverse effects when fed to dogs at a concentration of 8 percent in the diet for 2 years. This dietary concentration equates to approximately 2 g propylene glycol per kg body weight per day (Weil et al., 1971). Propylene glycol is not mutagenic or teratogenic, nor did propylene glycol adversely affect reproduction when fed at a 7.5 percent dietary concentration to rats for three generations (FDA, 1973, 1974, 1977).

The explanation for the low toxicity of propylene glycol lies in its metabolism. Propylene glycol, in contrast to ethylene glycol, is metabolized by alcohol dehydrogenase to lactic acid and further to pyruvic acid (Ruddick, 1972). These acids are normal constituents of carbohydrate metabolism and are further broken down to carbon dioxide and water. Propylene glycol, like ethanol, has been reported to be an effective antidote for ethylene glycol poisoning (Holman et al., 1979).

Based on a review of existing health effects data for propylene glycol, a select committee of experts convened by the FDA reaffirmed the "generally recognized as safe" (GRAS) status of propylene glycol (FDA, 1977).

## GLYCOL ETHERS

Glycol ethers (Fig. 24-6) find extensive use in industry as solvents in the manufacture of lacquers, varnishes, resins, printing inks, textile dyes, anti-icing additives in brake fluids, and as gasoline additives. In consumer products they are found in latex paints, cleaners, and other household products. Structurally, the glycol ethers are categorized as ethylene glycol ethers, or monopropylene, dipropylene, or tripropylene glycol ethers. The ether function may be bound to methyl, ethyl, n-propyl, n-butyl, or t-butyl groups. In some cases the alcohol groups are bound in the form of their acetate esters. Because of the ease and rapidity of ester hydrolysis in vivo there is no reason to assume that the toxicities of the esters differ from those of the unesterified glycols.

The glycol ethers, as a class of materials, are not acutely hazardous by the oral route. The rabbit appears to be more sensitive than the rat with regard to acute oral toxicity. Tanii and coworkers (1992) studied correlations between acute in vivo and in vitro toxicity and log P (where P is the n-octanol-water partition coefficient) among glycol ethers. Data collected included toxicity to neuroblastoma and glial cells in vitro expressed as $ED_{50}$, $LD_{50}$ in mice pretreated with corn oil or with $CCl_4$, and log P. The data were analyzed by multiple regression analysis and revealed that acute toxicity was probably a function of the parent compound rather than of metabolites and that relative hydrophobicity played a significant role in acute toxicity.

Glycol ethers, particularly the ethylene series, are well-absorbed from the skin. Sabourin and colleagues (1992) reported that 20 to 25 percent of the applied dose of methoxyethanol, ethoxyethanol, or butoxyethanol was absorbed from the shaved skin of F344/N rats regardless of the dose. Indeed, the dermal $LD_{50}$ to oral $LD_{50}$ ratio is approximately 1 for ethylene glycol ethers. High vapor concentrations of the ethylene series are lethal, but saturation levels or levels approaching saturation of the propylene series are not lethal to rodents.

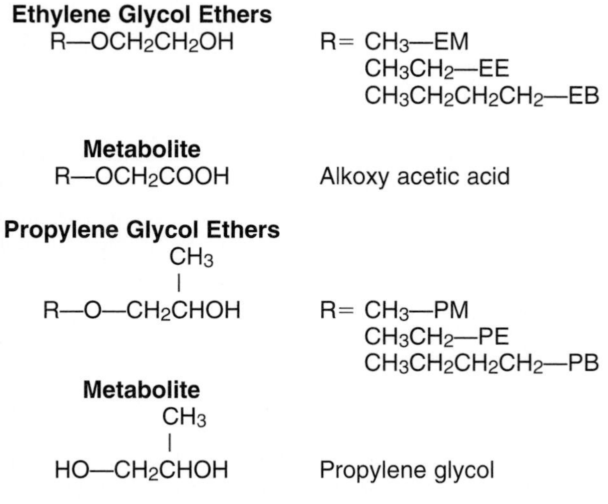

**Ethylene Glycol Ethers**

$R{-}OCH_2CH_2OH$ — R= $CH_3$—EM; $CH_3CH_2$—EE; $CH_3CH_2CH_2CH_2$—EB

**Metabolite**

$R{-}OCH_2COOH$ — Alkoxy acetic acid

**Propylene Glycol Ethers**

$R{-}O{-}CH_2CH(CH_3)OH$ — R= $CH_3$—PM; $CH_3CH_2$—PE; $CH_3CH_2CH_2CH_2$—PB

**Metabolite**

$HO{-}CH_2CH(CH_3)OH$ — Propylene glycol

*Figure 24–6. Glycol ethers and their metabolites.*

It has been known for many years (Wiley et al., 1938; Nagano et al., 1979) that ethylene glycol ethers cause reproductive toxicity. Mice given large amounts of ethylene glycol monomethyl ether (EM), ethylene glycol monoethyl ether (EE), or their respective acetic acid esters for 5 weeks displayed testicular atrophy. Ahmed and coworkers (1994), using whole body autoradiography, demonstrated that treating mice with labeled EE led to accumulation of radioactivity not only in the liver, kidney, and bladder but also in the epididymis and bone marrow. Rabbits and rats exposed to EM vapor exhibited degeneration of the testicular germinal epithelium. At the end of the exposure period male rats were mated to unexposed females and found to be infertile (Miller et al., 1983a; Rao et al., 1983). A second mating at 13 weeks postexposure revealed a partial recovery of fertility. The dose-response relationship demonstrated that the rabbit is the more sensitive of the two species.

Fetotoxic and teratogenic responses were observed in pregnant rabbits and rats exposed by inhalation to either EM or EE (Nelson et al., 1984; Andrew et al., 1981) or to EE applied dermally. The site most commonly affected was the cardiovascular system, but skeletal and other malformations also were observed.

Ethylene glycol monobutyl ether (EB), in contrast to EM and EE, exerts its primary effect upon the red blood cell. Rats exposed to high vapor concentrations (Dodd et al., 1983) or to EB applied to the skin (Bartnik et al., 1987) exhibited a marked degree of hemolysis. Bartnik and coworkers (1987) measured the degree of absorption of EB from the skin and reported that approximately 25 percent of the applied material was absorbed from unoccluded skin within 48 h. EB appears to be an exception to the rule that the inhalation route of exposure is quantitatively more important than skin contact.

Treatment of pregnant mice and rabbits with ethylene glycol diethyl ether (George et al., 1992) resulted in embryo/fetal toxicity. Litters were smaller and malformations increased with increasing doses. Similar results were observed (Schwetz et al., 1992) using diethylene glycol dimethyl ether and triethylene glycol dimethyl ether.

The monopropylene, dipropylene, and tripropylene glycol ethers do not share the potent reproductive toxicity exhibited by the ethylene glycol ethers regardless of whether the route of administration is oral, dermal, or by inhalation (Miller et al., 1984). Whereas some embryo or fetal toxicity may have been observed at the highest doses, no dose produced birth defects, testicular atrophy, or damage to blood or thymic tissues. In a National Toxicology Program bioassay (NTP, 1986) mice were given PM in drinking water at several doses over 14 weeks in a two-generation study of reproductive toxicity. In both generations no effects were observed on fertility, litters per pair, live pups per litter, or sex ratio. Examination of sperm revealed no effects on motility, density, or abnormal sperm frequency. Aberrant observations included decreased pup body weights in the first generation and decreased weights of the right epididymis and prostate gland in the second generation. The latter effects were not seen in both generations and their physiological significance has yet to be determined. Nevertheless it is clear that the propylene glycol ethers exhibit considerably less reproductive toxicity than the ethylene glycol ethers.

These differences in reproductive toxicity between EM and propylene glycol monomethyl ether (PM) are explained by the differences in metabolism of the two materials. Miller and colleagues (1983b) studied the metabolism of orally administered EM or PM, radiolabeled in the glycol carbons, in rats. Most of the administered PM is metabolized, via propylene glycol, to $^{14}CO_2$. In contrast, methoxyacetic acid is the major metabolite of EM. Liver alcohol dehydrogenase can oxidize EM to methoxyacetaldehyde, which can then be oxidized to methoxyacetic acid. It is of interest that methoxyacetaldehyde (Chiewchanwit and Au, 1994) induced mutations in the bacterial *gpt* gene inserted into an autosome of CHO-AS52 cells but not in the *hprt* gene on the X chromosome of CHO-K1-BH4 cells. In both cell lines and in human lymphocytes in culture, methoxyacetaldehyde caused both sister chromatid exchanges and chromosome aberrations. Methoxyacetic acid has been shown to produce the same toxic effects as EM in male rats (Miller et al., 1982; Moss et al., 1985; Sleet et al., 1988).

Administration of 4-methylpyrazole, an inhibitor of alcohol dehydrogenase, significantly reduced EM-induced embryotoxicity, underscoring the importance of this enzyme in the metabolic activation of EM. Because EE, EB, and ethylene glycol monoisopropyl ether (EIP) are metabolized to analogous metabolites (ethoxyacetic, butoxyacetic, and isopropoxyacetic acids, respectively), alkoxyacids are also considered to be toxic metabolites (Jonsson et al., 1982).

Although the primary alcohol function on glycol ethers is easily oxidized by liver alcohol dehydrogenase, propylene glycol ethers have a secondary alcohol function and are relatively poorer substrates for alcohol dehydrogenase (von Wartburg, 1964). They undergo microsomal *o*-dealkylation to propylene glycol, a material that is not a reproductive toxin. However, propylene glycol ethers may exist in either of two isomeric forms termed the alpha and beta forms:

| Major isomer | Minor isomer |
|---|---|
| $CH_3{-}O{-}CH_2{-}CH(OH){-}CH_3$ | $HO{-}CH_2{-}CH(O{-}CH_3){-}CH_3$ |
| 1-methoxy-2-propanol | 2-methoxy-1-propanol |
| secondary alcohol | primary alcohol |
| $\alpha$ isomer | $\beta$ isomer |

Merkle and colleagues (1987) reported that the acetic acid ester of 2-methoxy-1 propranol was capable of inducing malformations in rabbits. Miller and coworkers (1986) showed that the beta isomer of PM is indeed metabolized to methoxypropionic acid. Since commercial PM is more than 95 percent of the alpha-isomer, there is no occupational concern for adverse effects on reproduction from exposure to PM vapors.

Mebus and coworkers (1989) suggested that simple physiological substrates such as serine, acetate, sarcosine, and glycine, given concomitantly with EM, ameliorated developmental toxicity and testicular damage in rats. It is postulated that the toxic metabolite of EM may interfere with the availability of one-carbon units for incorporation into purine and pyrimidine bases. Substrates such as sarcosine or acetate can provide additional one-carbon units needed during differentiation of the developing embryo or for maturation of pachytene spermatocytes. Another protective mechanism was described by Burhan and Chapin (1990), who demonstrated that calcium channel blockers protected against EM-induced testicular toxicity.

An addition to the well-studied reproductive toxicity associated with ethylene glycol ethers is the observation that these compounds can also produce hemolytic anemia. These compounds are taken up into rat erythrocytes over time, the cells swell, and they then hemolyze (Burhan, 1989). Structure-activity studies revealed that in order of effectiveness butoxyacetic acid > propoxyacetic acid > ethoxyacetic acid > methoxyacetic acid. Hemolysis appears to parallel decreases in red cell ATP. The susceptibility of human erythrocytes is less than that of rat erythrocytes (Burhan, 1989).

## CARBON DISULFIDE

Carbon disulfide ($CS_2$) is primarily used in the production of regenerated rayon and cellophane and in the manufacture of carbon tetrachloride. It is also used as a solvent for many applications (Timmerman, 1985). A recent estimate of $CS_2$ production worldwide was one million metric tons.

Adverse effects resulting from prolonged human exposure to high levels of $CS_2$ have been extensively reported and documented. These include organic brain damage, peripheral nervous system decrements, neurobehavioral dysfunction, ocular and auditory effects, and atherosclerosis. Hearing loss to high frequency tones is a common feature of $CS_2$ intoxication (Zenk, 1970). Excellent reviews of these effects are available (Coppack et al., 1981; Beauchamp et al., 1983). Recent studies have also implicated $CS_2$ in alimentary and endocrine defects (Peplonska, 1994). $CS_2$ toxicity is reviewed in Chap. 16.

Exposure to $CS_2$ has been called a contributing factor in coronary heart disease (Tiller et al., 1968). This effect has been confirmed by Finnish epidemiologists studying an occupationally exposed cohort using a 10-year follow-up plan. While advanced age and hypertension were predominant factors in determining coronary heart disease, exposure to $CS_2$ alone contributed a statistically significant relative risk (Tolonen et al., 1975, 1979). Occupational $CS_2$ exposure can be an important contributing factor to the development of coronary heart disease and this issue should continue to be monitored in future epidemiological studies.

Hoffmann and coworkers (Hoffmann and Muller, 1990; Hoffman and Klapperstuck, 1994) examined the effects of acute and subacute exposure to $CS_2$ in rats. Using the urethane-anesthetized rat model, they found that $CS_2$ (1.66 or 3.32 mmol/kg) enhanced the hypertensive effect and decreased the inotropic effects of epinephrine and norepinephrine on the heart. They concluded that $CS_2$ caused a delay in atrioventricular conduction time.

## GASOLINE AND KEROSENE

Gasoline and kerosene are primarily mixtures of hydrocarbons, including not only aliphatic hydrocarbons but, particularly in the case of gasoline, a variety of branched and unsaturated hydrocarbons, as well as aromatic hydrocarbons.

In spite of the widespread use of gasoline and the intermittent vapor exposure encountered by gas station attendants and the home auto mechanic, toxic effects do not normally occur under these conditions. Some gasolines contain a considerable amount of benzene or other additives and could present a hazard that would be difficult to assess in the exposed population.

Extremely high level exposures to gasoline vapor may result in dizziness, coma, collapse, and death. Exposure to high nonlethal levels is usually followed by complete recovery, although cases of permanent brain damage following massive exposure have been reported. Atmospheric concentrations of approximately 2000 ppm are not safe to enter for even a brief time.

Reports of the results of 2-year carcinogenicity studies in mice and rats has raised the issue of the adverse effects of long-term low level exposure to unleaded gasoline vapors. In these studies, male rats but neither female rats nor either sex of mice developed renal tumors and/or a characteristic nephropathy characterized by protein droplet formation in the proximal tubular epithelium (Kitchen, 1984; MacFarland, 1984; Alden, 1986). Because kidney effects were both sex- and species-specific and because unleaded gasoline is not mutagenic (Conaway et al., 1982; Loury et al., 1987; Richardson, et al., 1986), a nongenotoxic mechanism of renal tumor development was postulated.

The observation of these renal effects of unleaded gasoline led to an evaluation of the nephrotoxic properties of many components of this complex mixture and the identification of isoparaffins as nephrotoxic materials specific for the male rat (Halder et al., 1985; Phillips and Egan, 1984; Phillips and Cockrell, 1984). Trimethylpentane is one isoparaffin that is very active in causing protein-droplet (hyaline-droplet) toxicity in the male rat kidney and has been used as a prototype chemical (Short et al., 1986). Treatment of male rats with trimethylpentane or unleaded gasoline leads to a high accumulation of $\alpha$-2$\mu$-globulin protein in renal tubular cells. This protein is not found in humans or immature male or female rats (Kloss et al., 1985; Loury et al., 1987). This syndrome has been termed the *male rat hydrocarbon nephropathy* (Alden, 1986).

It has been shown that exposing male rats to unleaded gasoline or trimethylpentane vapors results in a marked increase in cellular proliferation in the kidneys. Based on this observation it has been postulated that renal tumors develop secondary to tissue damage resulting from $\alpha$-2$\mu$-globulin accumulation in renal tubular cells (Loury et al., 1987). Thus, it may be postulated that the observation of renal tumors in rats is not relevant to possible human health effects from gasoline exposure.

The 1990 Amendments to the Clean Air Act recognized the automobile's contribution to the growing problem of air pollution and mandated that gasoline be reformulated specifically to reduce carbon monoxide and ground level ozone air pollutants.

A cornerstone of reformulated gasoline is the addition of *oxygenates*, oxygen-containing materials that provide added octane and a more complete combustion of fuel. Oxygenates include materials such as methanol, ethanol, methyl tertiary butyl ether (MTBE), ethyl tertiary butyl ether (ETBE) and tertiary amyl methyl ether (TAME). They are added to gasoline at levels up to 15 volume percent. Beginning in 1987, in concert with the EPA manufacturers of MTBE undertook a comprehensive research program to look for potential adverse health effects in experimental animals and human volunteers. While some consumers find the odor of MTBE unpleasant, there are no objective data from human clinical studies to support MTBE's being a cause of headaches, nausea, or other claimed health effects. Chronic studies of MTBE vapors in rats and mice at levels up to 8000 ppm (about one-half of the lower explosive limit) caused elevations in the same types of tumors described for unleaded gasoline itself.

Research is underway to help clarify these health effects issues for MTBE and to expand the health effects database for other alcohols and ethers. This is an important effort so that we can be assured that, while cleaning up the air, the addition of these materials to gasoline does not increase any hazard from gasoline itself.

## CONCLUSIONS

Solvents are a group of chemicals that have only two features in common: (1) They are liquid and, (2) because of their widespread use in commerce, there is a potential for human exposure both during their use and after they have been discarded as chemical wastes.

It is not possible to predict the toxic effects of these chemicals merely because they share the name solvent. Their toxic effects vary as widely as those of other chemicals. While there are groups of structurally related solvents, such as the haloalkanes and the haloalkenes, in which toxic effects may be related, among these substances there are both quantitative and qualitative differences in toxicity. Among single ring aromatic compounds, alkylbenzenes are dramatically different from benzene. Our ability to predict toxicity among solvents and to perform accurate risk assessment depends upon our knowledge not only of descriptive toxicology gained in acute and chronic treatment studies, it also depends on our understanding of the metabolic disposition and mechanism of action of these agents.

The major drawback to most studies on the toxicology of solvents is that actual occupational and environmental exposures is not to the pure compounds used in toxicological research but to commercial mixtures of solvents. The need for the future is to develop strategies for studying the toxicology of mixtures. It is impractical to study the interactions of more than three to four compounds at more than one dose level in a well-controlled study using procedures commonly employed in safety evaluation today. Yet in effluents from chemical waste sites there are frequently as many as one hundred chemicals identified, some of which may be present at concentrations that pose a potential hazard for humans. Methods for studying these interactive effects have yet to be developed. Until that time risk assessment must depend upon knowledge of the toxicity of the most toxic chemicals in the mixture modified with our understanding of the interactions between chemicals in the mixture. For the most part this information is currently insufficient for accurate predictions.

The ability to measure the dose of individual solvents or their reactive metabolites delivered to the target organ or receptor could greatly improve our confidence in models of dose responsiveness. In most cases these data are not available for solvents. However, methods exist to measure the levels of solvents or metabolites in body fluids of both humans and experimental animals. Such data can provide specific information on exposure to active metabolites. In 1989, the National Academy of Sciences published a status report on biomarkers for toxicity to pulmonary and reproductive systems (NAS, 1989a,b). Further development of indices of exposure to solvents and markers of toxicity could lead to more effective medical surveillance programs, the potential for identifying sensitive individuals prior to exposure, and a means of evaluating the validity and predictability of our assessments of hazard and risk.

The potential for exposure to organic solvents in the workplace and the environment at large has led to the establishment of exposure standards which must be maintained by engineering means or by restrictions on the disposal of waste products. Although arguments persist regarding the acceptable levels of human exposure in various media, all control technologies bear a cost which must be paid by one or more of the involved parties—by the industry, the workers, or the exposed or potentially exposed populace. Restricting the escape of chemicals from manufacturing facilities is considerably more cost effective than attempting to clean up the environment after accidental releases. Among the most expensive processes in industry is the disposal of waste solvents. A significant addition to the costs of release are legal remedies for which people apply when they fear that they have been affected by chemicals in the various environments in which exposure may have occurred.

There are several solutions available for dealing with these issues in the future. One is to tightly restrict the exposure of people to solvents in any media. Solvents must be used in enclosed streams. Air handling equipment must be available wherever one may encounter vapors of the solvent. Careful monitoring of workers and of areas where vapors may potentially migrate will be essential. Nevertheless, exposure to solvents at some levels is inevitable. An alternative solution, then, is to the restrict use of the more toxic solvents. Benzene, for example, should never be used as a solvent. Safer and equally effective solvents are already available. New types of solvents should be developed that display less toxicity, are more environmentally friendly, and carry lower costs for disposal. The challenge for the chemist will be to devise solvents that have greater water solubility but retain the ability to dissolve otherwise water-insoluble compounds. The challenge is great, but the rewards of solving the current problems associated with toxic organic solvents are even greater.

## APPENDIX

Convert between ppm and mg/m$^3$ using the following approaches. Combining equations from the Ideal Gas Law and Dalton's Law of Partial Pressures yields an equation for the ready conversion of these units:

Ideal Gas Law $PV = nRT$

Dalton's Law $\frac{P_s}{P_t} = \frac{n_s}{n_t}$

$P_s$ = Partial pressure of solvents (atm)
$P_t$ = Total atmospheric pressure (1 atm)
$n_s$ = Number of moles of solvents
$n_s$ = Weight (wt.) of S/molecular weight (MW) of S

$n_t$ = Total number of moles
$V$ = Volume (m$^3$)
$R$ = Gas constant (0.082 atm/°K mol)
$T$ = Temperature (298°K = 25°C)
$C_s$ = Concentration of S (weight of s/volume)

$$P_sV = n_s RT$$

$$P_s = \frac{n_s RT}{V}$$

$$P_s = \frac{C_s}{\text{MW}_s} 24.45$$

$$\frac{P_s}{P_t} = \frac{n_s}{n_t} (\text{ppm}) = \frac{C_s}{\text{MW}_s} 24.45$$

$$\text{ppm} = \frac{C_s}{\text{MW}_s} 24.45$$

Thus, using benzene (MW = 78) as an example, converting 32 mg/m$^3$ to ppm would involve the following calculation:

$$(\text{ppm}) = \frac{32 \text{ mg/m}^3}{78/\text{g/mol}} (24.45) = 10$$

Thus, 32 mg/m$^3$ is equivalent to 10 ppm.

The following alternative approach is equally useful: We can express the concentration of a gas in a mixture using the following equation and assuming that the weight of 1 ml of gas, $d$, is a function of the molecular weight ($MW$), the molecular volume ($MV_0$), and the temperature and pressure, as shown in the following equation:

$$d = \frac{MW}{MV_o} \cdot \frac{T_o}{T_o + T} \cdot P_{P_o}$$

$$d = \frac{MW}{22.4} \cdot \frac{273}{273 + T} \cdot \frac{P}{760}$$

$$= 0.016 \cdot MW \cdot \frac{P}{273 + T}, \text{ units} = \text{mg/liter}$$

where $MV_o$ = molecular volume (22.4 liters) at standard temperature and pressure ($T_o$ = 273°C; $P_o$ = 760 torr), and $T$ and $P$ are ambient values for temperature and pressure. The coefficient 0.0160 is the reciprocal of the gas constant, $R$.

We can convert the concentration of the gas from ppm to mg/m$^3$. For example, 10 ppm equals 10 ml of gas in 10$^6$ ml of air. Accordingly, we must multiply $d$, from the equation shown above, by 10/10$^3$ or 0.01 and factor in the $MW$. Thus, for benzene at 10 ppm:

$$d = \frac{78}{22.4} \cdot \frac{273}{273 + T} \cdot \frac{P}{760}$$

$$= 0.016 \cdot 78 \cdot \frac{760}{298} = 3.19 \text{ mg/liter}$$

$$10 \text{ ppm} = 0.01 \cdot 3.19 = 0.0319 \text{ mg/liter}$$

To convert mg/liter to mg/m$^3$, multiply by 1000.
The result indicates that 10 ppm of benzene is equivalent to 31.9 mg/m$^3$.

# REFERENCES


ACGIH: *TLVs, Threshold Limit Values for Chemical Substances and Physical Agents and Biological Exposure Indices (BEIs)*. Cincinnati: American Conference of Governmental Industrial Hygienists, 1995–1996, p. 138.

Adachi Y, Bradford BH, Gao W, et al: Inactivation of Kupffer cells prevents early alcohol-induced liver injury. *Hepatology* 20:453–460, 1994.

Adler ID, Kliesch U: Comparison of single and multiple treatment regiments in the mouse bone marrow micronucleus assay for hydroquinone, HQ and cyclophosphamide, CP. *Mut Res* 234:115, 1990.

Ahmed AE, Jacob S, Au WW: Quantitative whole body autoradiographic disposition of glycol ether in mice: Effect of route of administration. *Fund Appl Toxicol* 22:266–276, 1994.

Ahmed AE, Kubic VJ, Stevens JL, Anders MW: Halogenated methanes: metabolism and toxicity. *Fed Proc* 39:3150–3155, 1980.

Ainley CC, Senapati A, Brown IMH, et al: Is alcohol hepatotoxic in the baboon? *Hepatology* 7:85–92, 1988.

Alden CL: A review of unique male rat hydrocarbon nephropathy. *Toxicol Pathol* 14:109–111, 1986.

Andersen ME, Clewell HJ III, Gargas ML, et al: Physiologically based pharmacokinetic modeling with dichloromethane its metabolite, carbon monoxide, and blood carboxyhemoglobin in rats and humans. *Toxicol Appl Pharmacol* 108:14–27, 1991.

Andersen ME, Gargas ML, Jones RA, Jenkins LJ Jr: Determination of the kinetic constants for metabolism of inhaled toxicants *in vivo* using gas uptake measurements. *Toxicol Appl Pharmacol* 54:100–116, 1980.

Andrew FD, Buschbom RL, Cannon WC, et al: *Teratologic Assessment of Ethylbenzene and 2-Ethoxyethanol*. Battelle Pacific Northwest Laboratories Report to NIOSH, 1981.

Andrews LS, Lee EW, Witmer CM, et al: Effects of toluene on metabolism, disposition, and hematopoietic toxicity of ($^3$H) benzene. *Biochem Pharmacol* 26:293–300, 1977.

Anwar WA, Au WW, Legator MS, Sadagopa RVM: Effect of dimethyl sulfoxide on the genotoxicity and metabolism of benzene *in vivo*. *Carcinogenesis* 10:441, 1989.

Astrand I: Uptake of solvents in the blood and tissues of man. *Scand J Work Environ Hlth* 1:199–218, 1975.

Avogadro P, Sirtori CR, Tremoli E (eds): *Metabolic Effects of Ethanol*. Amsterdam: Elsevier, 1979.

Ayengar PK, Hayaishi O, Nakajima M, Tomida I: The enzymatic aromatization of 3,5-cyclohexadiene-1,2-diol. *Biochim Biophys Acta* 33:111–119, 1959.

Baarson K, Snyder CA, Albert RE: Repeated exposures of C57B16 mice to 10 ppm inhaled benzene markedly depressed erythropoietic colony formation. *Toxicol Lett* 20:337–342, 1984.

Bailie MB, Smith JH, Newton JF, Hook JB: Mechanism of chloroform toxicity: IV Phenobarbital potentiation of *in vitro* chloroform metabolism and toxicity in rabbit kidneys. *Toxicol Appl Pharmacol* 74:285–292, 1984.

Baker TS, Rickert DE: Dose-dependent uptake, distribution, and elimination of inhaled n-hexane in the Fischer-344 rat. *Toxicol Appl Pharmacol* 61:414–422, 1981.

Bardodej Z, Cirek A: Long-term study on workers occupationally exposed to ethylbenzene. *J Hyg Epidemiol Microbiol Immunol* 32:1–5, 1988.

Bartnik FG, Reddy AK, Klecak G, et al: Percutaneous absorption, metabolism, and hemolytic activity of n-butoxyethanol *Fund Appl Toxicol* 8:59–70, 1987.

Baud FJ, Galliot M, Astier A, et al: Treatment of ethylene glycol poisoning with intravenous 4-methyl pyrazole. *N Engl J Med* 319:97–100, 1988.

Bauer H, Dimitriadis EA, Snyder R: An *in vivo* study of benzene metabolite DNA adduct formation in liver of male New Zealand rabbits. *Arch Toxicol* 63:209–213, 1989.

Beauchamp RO Jr, Bus JS, Popp JA, et al: A Critical review of the literature on carbon disulfide toxicity. *CRC Crit Rev Toxicol* 11:169–278, 1983.

Benignus VA: Behavioral effects of toluene: A review. *J Neurobehav Toxicol Teratol* 3:407–415, 1981.

Bennett IL, Cary FH, Mitchell GL Jr, Cooper MN: Acute methyl alcohol poisoning: A review based on experiences in an outbreak of 323 cases. *Medicine* 32:431–463, 1953.

Benton CD, Calhoun FP: The ocular effect of methyl alcohol poisoning trans. *Am Acad Ophthalmol Laryngol* 56:874–885, 1952.

Blood FR: Chronic toxicity of ethylene glycol in the rat. *Food Cosmet Toxicol* 3:229–234, 1965.

Blood FR, Elliot GA, Wright MS: Chronic toxicity of ethylene glycol in the monkey. *Toxicol Appl Pharmacol* 4:489–491, 1962.

Bogaards XX: Interindividual differences in the *in vitro* conjugation of methylene chloride with glutathione by cytosolic glutathione S-transferase in 22 human liver samples. *Biochem Pharmacol* 45:2166–2169, 1993.

Bolt HM, Laib RJ, Filser JG: Reactive metabolites and carcinogenicity of halogenated ethylenes. *Biochem Pharmacol* 31:1–4, 1982a.

Bolt HM, Filser JG, Laib RJ: Covalent binding of haloethylenes, in Snyder R, Parke DV, Kocsis JJ, et al (eds): *Biological Reactive Intermediates. Chemical Mechanisms and Biological Effects*. New York: Plenum, 1982, vol 2, pp 667–683.

Bove KE: Ethylene glycol toxicity. *Am J Clin Pathol* 45:46–50, 1966.

Bradford BU, Seed CB, Handler JA, et al: Evidence that catalase is a major pathway of ethanol oxidation *in vivo*: Dose response studies in deer mice using methanol as a selective substrate. *Arch Biochem Biophys* 303:172–176, 1993.

Brady JF, Li D, Ishizaki H, et al: Induction of cytochromes P450IIE1 and P450IIB1 by secondary ketones and the role of P450IIE1 in chloroform metabolism. *Toxicol Appl Pharmacol* 100:342–348, 1989.

Branchflower RV, Pohl LR: Investigation of the mechanism of the potentiation of chloroform-induced hepatotoxicity and nephrotoxicity by methyl n-butyl ketone. *Toxicol Appl Pharmacol* 61:407–413, 1981.

Browning E: *Toxicity and Metabolism of Industrial Solvents*. New York: Elsevier, 1965.

Buelke-Sam J, Kimmel CA: Development and standardization of screening methods for behavioral teratology. *Teratology* 20:17–30, 1979.

Burhan IG: Metabolic and cellular basis of 2-butoxyethanol-induced hemolytic anemia in rats and assessment of human risk *in vitro*. *Biochem Pharmacol* 38(10):1679–1684, 1989.

Burhan IG, Chapin RE: Calcium channel blockers protect against ethylene glycol monomethyl ether (2-methoxyethanol)-induced testicular toxicity. *Exp Mol Pathol* 52:279–290, 1990.

Busby WF Jr, Wang JS, Stevens EK, et al: Lung tumorigenicity of benzene oxide, benzene diohydrodiols, and benzene diolepoxides in the BLU:ha newborn mouse assay. *Carcinogenesis* 11:1473–1478, 1990.

Carpenter CP, Kinkead ER, Geary DL Jr, et al: Petroleum hydrocarbon toxicity studies V Animal and human response to vapors of mixed xylenes. *Toxicol Appl Pharmacol* 33:543–558, 1975.

Casanova M, Devo DF, Heck H D'a: Dichloronethane (Methylene chloride): Metabolism to formaldehyde and formation of DNA-protein cross-links in B6C3F1 mice and Syrian golden hamsters. *Toxicol Appl Pharmacol* 114:162–165, 1992.

Challen PJR, Hickish DE, Bedford J: Chronic chloroform intoxication. *Br J Ind Med* 15:243–249, 1958.

Cherry N, Waldron HA, Wells GC, et al: An investigation of the acute behavioral effects of styrene factory workers. *Br J Ind Med* 37:234–240, 1980.

Chiewchanwit T, Au WW: Cytogenetic effects of 2-methoxyethanol and its metabolite, methoxyacetaldehyde, in mammalian cells *in vitro*. *Mut Res* 320:125–132, 1994.

Chin JH, Goldstein BD: Effects of low concentrations of ethanol on the fluidity of spin-labeled crythrocyte and brain membranes. *J Mol Pharmacol* 13:435–441, 1977.

Choy WN, MacGregor JT, Shelby MD, Maronpot RR: Induction of micronuclei by benzene in B6C3F$_1$ mice, Retrospective analysis of blood smears from NTP carcinogenesis bioassay. *Mut Res* 143:55, 1985.

Ciranni R, Barale R, Ghelardini G, Loprieno N: Benzene and the genotoxicity of its metabolites II The effect of the route of administration on the micronuclei and bone marrow depression in mouse bone marrow cells. *Mut Res*, 209:23, 1988b.

Ciranni R, Barale R, Marrazzini A, Loprieno N: Benzene and the genotoxicity of its metabolites I Transplacental activity in mouse fetuses and in their dams. *Mut Res* 208:61, 1988a.

Conaway CC, Schreiner CA, Cragg ST: Mutagenicity evaluation of petroleum hydrocarbons, in Mehlman MA (ed): *Applied Toxicology of Petroleum Hydrocarbons*. Princeton: Princeton Scientific, 1982, pp 89–108.

Coon MJ, Koop DR: Alcohol-inducible cytochrome P-450 (P-450 ALC). *Arch Toxicol* 60:16–21, 1987.

Costantini MG: Health effects of oxygenated fuels. *Environ Hlth Perspect* 101:6(Suppl):151–160, 1993.

Coppack RW, Buch WB, Mabee RL: Toxicology of carbon disulfide: A review. *J Vet Hum Toxicol* 23:331–336, 1981.

Cornish HH, Adefuin J: Ethanol potentiation of halogenated aliphatic solvent toxicity. *Am J Ind Hyg* 27:57–61, 1966.

Cragg ST, Clarke EA, Daly IW, et al: Subchronic inhalation toxicity of ethylbenzene in mice rats and rabbits. *Fund Appl Toxicol* 13:399–408, 1989.

Creek MR, Vogel JS, Turteltaub KW: Extremely low dose benzene pharmacokinetics and macromolecular binding in B6C3F1 male mice. *The Toxicologist* 14(1):430, 1994.

Damgaard SE: The D(VK) isotope effect of the cytochrome P-450-mediated oxidation of ethanol and its biological applications. *Eur J Biochem* 125:593–603, 1982.

daSilva C, Fan X, Castagna M: Benzene-mediated protein kinase C activation. *Environ Health Perspect* 83:91–95, 1989.

Dekant W, Vamvakas S, Anders MW: Bioactivation of nephrotoxic haloalkenes by glutathione conjugation: Formation of toxic and mutagenic intermediates by cysteine conjugate beta-lyase. *Drug Metab Rev* 20:43–83, 1989.

Dempster AM, Snyder C: Short term benzene exposure provides a growth advantage for granulopoietic progenitor cells over erythroid progenitor cells. *Toxicology* 64:539–544, 1990.

DePass LR, Garman RH, Woodside MD, et al: Chronic toxicity and oncogenicity studies of ethylene glycol in rats and mice. *Fund Appl Toxicol* 7:547–565, 1986.

Dietz FK, Reitz RH, Watanabe PG, Gehring PJ: Translation of pharmacokinetic/biochemical data into risk assessment, in Snyder R, Parke DV, Kocsis JJ, et al (eds): *Biological Reactive Intermediates II: Chemical Mechanisms and Biological Effects*. New York: Plenum, 1982, pp 1399–1424.

DiVincenzo GD, Hamilton ML, Kaplan CJ, et al: Studies on the respiratory uptake and excretion and the skin absorption of methyl n-butyl ketone in humans and dogs. *Toxicol Appl Pharmacol* 44:593–604, 1978.

Dodd DE, Snellings WM, Maronpot RR, Ballantyne B: Ethylene glycol monobutyl ether. Acute 9-day and 90-day vapor inhalation studies in Fischer 344 rats. *Toxicol Appl Pharmacol* 68:405–414, 1983.

Dutkiewicz B, Konczalik J, Karwacki W: Skin absorption and per os administration of methanol. *Int Arch Occup Environ Health* 47:81–88, 1980.

Eastmond DA, Smith MT, Irons RD: An interaction of benzene metabolites reproduces the myelotoxicity observed with benzene exposure. *Toxicol Appl Pharmacol* 91:85–95, 1987.

Edwards MJ, Keller BJ, Kauffman FC, Thurman RG: The involvement of Kupffer cells in carbon tetrachloride toxicity. *Toxicol Appl Pharmacol* 119:275–279, 1993.

Egle JL Jr, Gockberg BJ: Retention of inhaled isoprene and methanol in the dog. *Am Ind Hyg Assoc J* 36:369–373, 1975.

Elofsson SA, Gamberale F, Hindmarsch T, et al: Exposure to organic solvents. *Scand J Work Environ Health* 6:239–273, 1980.

Elovaara E, Engstrom K, Nickles J, et al: Biochemical and morphological effects of long-term inhalation exposure of rats to ethylbenzene. *Xenobiotica* 15:299–308, 1985.

Erexson GL, Wilmer JL, Kligerman AD: Sister chromatid exchange induction in human lymphocytes exposed to benzene and its metabolites *in vitro*. *Cancer Res*, 45:2471, 1985.

FDA: *Mutagenic Evaluation of Compound FDA 71-56 Propylene Glycol*. PB-245450, 1974.

FDA: *Teratologic Evaluation of Compound FDA 71-56 (Propylene Glycol) in Mice, Rats, Hamsters and Rabbits*. PB-223-822, 1973.

FDA: Federal Register 42:30865-66 June 17, 1977.

Federal Register (FR): Cosmetics: Ban on the use of methylene chloride as an ingredient of cosmetic producers, in: *Docket No 85H-05361*. Food and Drug Administration CFR Part 700, Washington, D.C. 1989.

Feldman RG, Ricks NL, Baker EL: Neuropsychological effects of industrial neurotoxins: A review. *Am J Ind Med* 1:211–227, 1980.

Ferguson J: The use of chemical potentials as indices of toxicity. *Proc Royal Soc Lond B Biol Sci* 127:387–404, 1939.

Ferry DG, Temple WA, McQueen EG: Methanol monitoring: Comparison of urinary methanol concentration with formic acid excretion rate as a measure of occupational exposure. *Int Arch Occup Environ Health* 47:155–163, 1980.

Feytmans E, Leighton F: Effects of pyrazole and 3-amino-124-triazole methanol and ethanol metabolism by the rat. *Biochem Pharmacol* 22:349–360, 1973.

Fitzhugh OG, Nelson AA: Comparison of the chronic toxicity of triethyelene glycol with that of diethylene glycol. *J Ind Hyg Toxicol* 28:40–43, 1946.

Forni A, Moreo L: Cytogenetic studies in a case of benzene leukemia. *Eur J Cancer* 3:251, 1967.

Forni A, Moreo L: Chromosome studies in a case of benzene-induced erythroleukemia. *Eur J Cancer* 5:459, 1969.

Forni A, Pacifico E, Limonta A: Chromosome studies in workers exposed to benzene or toluene or both. *Arch Environ Health* 22:373, 1971a.

Forni A, Cappellini A, Pacifico E, Vigliani E: Chromosome changes and their evolution with past exposure to benzene. *Arch Environ Health* 23:385, 1971b.

Forsander OA, Raiha N, Salaspuro M, Maenpaa P: Influence of ethanol on the liver metabolism of fed and starved rats. *Biochem J* 94:259–265, 1965.

Forsander OA, Raiha N, Suomalainen H: Oxydation des Aethylalkohols in isolieter Leber und isolietem Hinterkorper der Ratte. *Z Physiol Chem* 318:1–5, 1960.

Gad-El-Karim MM, Ramanujam S, Legator MS: Correlation between the induction of micronuclei in bone marrow by benzene exposure and the excretion of metabolites in the urine by CD-1 mice. *Toxicol Appl Pharmacol* 85:464, 1986.

Gaido KW, Wierda D: *In vitro* effects of benzene metabolites on mouse bone marrow stromal cells. *Toxicol Appl Pharmacol* 76:45–55, 1984.

Gaido KW, Wierda D: Modulation of stromal cell function in DBA/2J and B6C3F1 mice exposed to benzene or phenol. *Toxicol Appl Pharmacol* 81:469–475, 1985.

Garner CD, Lee EW, Louis-Ferdinand RT: Müller cell involvement in methanol-induced retinal toxicity. *Toxicol Appl Pharmacol* 130:101–107, 1995a.

Garner CD, Lee EW, Terzo TS, Louis-Ferdinand RT: Role of retinal metabolism in methanol-induced retinal toxicity. *Toxicol Environ Hlth* 44:43–56, 1995b.

Gaunt IF, Carpanini FMB, Grasso P, Lansdown ABG: Long-term toxicity of propylene glycol in rats. *Food Cosmet Toxicol* 10:151–162, 1972.

George JD, Price CJ, Marr MC, Kimmel CA: The developmental toxicity of ethylene glycol diethyl ether in mice and rabbits. *Fund Appl Toxicol* 19:15–25, 1992.

Gershoff SN, Andrus SB: Effect of vitamin $B_6$ and magnesium on renal deposition of calcium oxalate by ethylene glycol administration. *Proc Soc Exp Biol Med* 109:99–102, 1962.

Gessner PK, Parke DV, Williams RT: Studies in detoxication. *Biochem J* 74:1–5, 1960.

Gill GF, Ahmed A: Covalent binding of [14C] benzene to cellular organelles and bone marrow nucleic acids. *Biochem Pharmacol* 30:1127–1131, 1981.

Gillette JR: The phenomenon of species variations. Problems and opportunities, in Parke DV, Smith RL (eds): *Drug Metabolism from Microbe to Man*. London: Taylor and Francis, 1976, pp 147–168.

Gilmour S, Kalf GF, Snyder R: Comparison of the metabolism of benzene and its metabolite phenol in rat liver microsomes, in Kocsis JJ, Jollow DJ, Witmer CM, et al (eds): *Biological Reactive Intermediates*. New York: Plenum, 1986, vol 3, pp 223–236.

Glinsukon T, Taycharpipranat S, Tskulkao C: Aflatoxin B1 hepatotoxicity in rats pretreated with ethanol. *Experientia* 34:869–871, 1978.

Gonda A, Bault H, Churchill D, Hollomby D: Hemodialysis for methanol intoxication. *Am J Med* 64:749–758, 1978.

Gonzalez FJ: The molecular biology of cytochrome P-450s. *Pharmacol Rev* 40:243–288, 1988.

Goon D, Cheng X, Ruth J, et al: Metabolism of transtransmuconaldehyde by aldehyde and alcohol dehydrogenase: identification of a novel metabolite. *Toxicol Appl Pharmacol* 114:147–155, 1992.

Gorsky LD, Coon MJ: Evaluation of the role of free hydroxyl radicals in the cytochrome P-450-catalyzed oxydation of benzene and cyclohexanol. *Drug Metab Dispos* 13:169–174, 1985.

Grandjean E, Munchinger R, Turrien V, et al: Investigations into the effects of exposure to trichloroethylene in mechanical engineering. *Br J Ind Med* 12:131–142, 1955.

Grasso P: Neurotoxic and neurobehavioral effects of organic solvents on the nervous system. *State Art Rev Occup Med* 3:525–539, 1988.

Green JD, Snyder CA, Lobue J, et al: Acute and chronic dose/response effects of inhaled benzene on multipotential hemopoietic stem CFU-S and granulocyte/macrophage progenitor GM CFU-C cells in CD-1 mice. *Toxicol Appl Pharmacol* 58:492, 1981.

Guy R, Dimitriadis E, Hu P, et al: Interactive inhibition of erythroid $^{59}$Fe utilization by benzene metabolites in female mice. *Chem-Biol Interact* 74:55–62, 1990.

Guy RL, Hu P, Witz G, et al: Depression of iron uptake into erythrocytes in mice by treatment with the combined benzene metabolites p-benzoquinone muconaldehyde and hydroquinone. *J Appl Toxicol* 11:443–446, 1991.

Halder CA, Holdsworth CE, Cockrell BY, Piccirillo VJ: Hydrocarbon nephropathy in male rats: Identification of the nephrotoxic components of unleaded gasoline. *Toxicol Ind Health* 1:67–87, 1985.

Hanninen H, Nurminen M, Tolonen M, Martelin T: Psychological tests as indicators of excessive exposure to carbon disulfide. *Scand J Work Environ Health* 19:163–174, 1978.

Harigaya K, Miller ME, Cronkite EP, Drew RT: The detection of *in vivo* liquid bone marrow cultures. *J Appl Pharmacol* 60:346, 1981.

Harper BL, Ramanujam VMS, Gad-El-Karim MM, Legator MS: The influence of simple aromatics on benzene clastogenicity. *Mut Res* 128:105, 1984.

Hashmi M, Dechert S, Dekant W, Anders MW: Bioactivation of [$^{13}$C]dichloromethane in mouse, rat and human liver cytosol: $^{13}$C nuclear magnetic resonance spectroscopic studies. *Chem Res Toxicol* 7:291–296, 1994.

Havre P, Abrams MA, Corall RJM, et al: Quantitation of pathways of ethanol metabolism. *Arch Biochem Biophys* 182:14–23, 1977.

Henschler D, Bonse G: Metabolic activation of chlorinated ethylenes: Dependence of mutagenic effect on electrophilic reactivity of the metabolically formed epoxides. *Arch Toxicol* 39:2–12, 1977.

Henschler D, Bonse G: Metabolic activation of chlorinated ethylene derivatives, in Boissier JR, Lechat P, Fichelle J (eds): *Advances in Pharmacology and Therapeutics*. Proceedings of the 7th International Congress of Pharmacology (Paris) 9:123–130, 1979.

Henschler D, Hoos R: Metabolic activation and deactivation mechanisms of di-, tri- and tetrachloroethylenes, in Snyder R, Parke DV, Kocsis JJ, et al (eds): *Biological Reactive Intermediates: Chemical Mechanisms and Biological Effects*. New York: Plenum, 1982, vol 2, pp 659–666.

Hill MW, Bangham AD: General depressant drug dependency: A biophysical hypothesis. *Adv Exp Med Biol* 59:1–9, 1975.

Hite M, Pecharo M, Smith I, Thornton S: The effect of benzene in micronucleus test. *Mut Res* 77:149, 1980.

Hoffmann P, Klapperstuck M: Effects of carbon disulfide on cardiovascular function after acute and subacute exposure of rats. *Biomed Biochim Acta* 49:121–128, 1994.

Hoffmann P, Muller S: Subacute carbon disulfide exposure modifies adrenergic cardiovascular actions in rats. *Biomed Biochim Acta* 49:115–120, 1990.

Hoffmann PL, Rabe CS, Moses F, Tabakoff B: N-Methyl-D-Aspartate receptors and ethanol: inhibition of calcium flux and cyclic GMP production. *J Neurochem* 52:1937–1940, 1989.

Holman NW, Mundy RL, Teague RS: Alkyldiol antidotes to ethylene glycol toxicity in mice. *Toxicol Appl Pharmacol* 49:385–392, 1979.

Hong JY, Pan J, Ning SM, Yang CS: Molecular basis for the sex-related difference in renal N-nitrosodimethylamine demthylase in C3H/HeJ mice. *Cancer Res* 49:2973–2979, 1989.

Huff JE, Haseman JK, DeMartini DM: Multiple site carcinogenicity of benzene in Fischer 344 rats and B6C3F1 mice. *Environ Hlth Perspect* 82:125, 1989.

Hunt WA: The effect of aliphatic alcohols on the biophysical and biochemical correlate or membrane function. *Adv Exp Med Biol* 56:195–210, 1975.

Hyatt AV, Salmons JA: Carbon tetrachloride poisoning. *AMA Arch Ind Hyg* 6:74–82, 1952.

IARC: Benzene, in *IARC Monographs on the Evaluation of the Carcinogenic Risk of Chemicals to Humans: Some Industrial Chemical Dyestuffs*. Lyons, France: International Agency for Research on Cancer, 1982, pp 93–148.

IARC: *IARC Monographs on the Evaluation of Carcinogenic Risks to Humans: Alcohol Drinking*. Lyons, France: International Agency for Research on Cancer, 1988, vol 44.

Ingelman-Sundberg M, Hagbjork AL: On the significance of the cytochrome P-450-dependent hydroxyl radical-mediated oxygenation mechanism. *Xenobiotica* 12:673–686, 1982.

Irons RD, Dent JG, Baker TS, Rickert DE: Benzene is metabolized and covalently bound in bone marrow in situ. *Chem-Biol Interact* 30:241–245, 1980.

Irons RD, Greenlee WF, Wierda D, Bus JS: Relationship between benzene metabolism and toxicity: A proposed mechanism for the formation of reactive intermediates from polyphenol metabolites; in Snyder R, Parke DV, Kocsis JJ, et al (eds): *Biological Reactive Intermediates: Chemical Mechanisms and Biological Effects*. New York: Plenum, 1982, vol 2, pp 229–243.

Irons RD, Neptun DA: Effects of the principle hydroxy metabolites of benzene on microtubule polymerization. *Arch Toxicol* 45:297–305, 1980.

Irons RD, Stillman WS, Colagiovanni DB, Henry VA: Synergistic action of the benzene metabolite hydroquinone on myelopoietic stimulating activity of granulocyte/macrophage colony stimulating factor *in vitro*. *Proc Natl Acad Sci USA* 98:3691–3695, 1992.

Jacobsen D, McMartin KE: Methanol and ethylene glycol poisonings: Mechanism of toxicity clinical course diagnosis and treatment. *Med Toxicol* 1:309–334, 1986.

Jerina D, Daly JW: Arene oxides: A new aspect of drug metabolism. *Science* 185:573–582, 1974.

Jollow DJ, Smith C: Biochemical aspects of toxic metabolites: Formation detoxication and covalent binding, in Jollow DJ, Kocsis JJ, Snyder R, Vainio H (eds): *Biological Reactive Intermediates: Formation Toxicity and Inactivation*. New York: Plenum, 1977, vol 1, pp 42–59.

Jonsson AK, Pederson J, Steen G: Ethoxyacetic acid and N-ethoxyacetylglycine: Metabolites of ethoxyethanol (Ethylcellosolve) in rats. *Acta Pharmacol Toxicol* 50:358–362, 1982.

Jorgenson TA, Meierhenry EF, Rushbrook CJ et al: Carcinogenicity of chloroform in drinking water to male Osborne-Mendel rats and female B6C3F1 mice. *Fund Appl Toxicol* 5:760–769, 1985.

Kalant H: The pharmacology of alcohol intoxication. *Q J Stud Alc* 22(suppl):1–23, 1961.

Kalf GF, Rushmore T, Snyder R: Benzene inhibits RNA synthesis in mitochondria from liver and bone marrow. *Chem Biol Interact* 42:353–370, 1982.

Kalf GF, O'Connor A: The effects of benzene and hydroquinone on myeloid differentiation of HL-60 promyelocytic leukemia cells. *Leuk Lymph* 11:331–338, 1993.

Kane RL, Talbert W, Harlan J, et al: A methanol poisoning outbreak in Kentucky—A clinical epidemiologic study. *Arch Environ Hlth* 17:119–129, 1968.

Kennedy SK, Longnecker DE: History and principles of anesthesiology, in Goodman AG, Rall TW, Nies AS, Taylor P (eds): *Goodman and Gilman's The Pharmacological Basis of Therapeutics*, 8th ed. New York: McGraw-Hill, 1990, pp 269–284.

Kingsley WH, Hirsch FG: Toxicologic considerations in direct process spirit duplicating machines. *Compens Med* 40:7–8, 1954–1955.

Kirley TA, Goldstein BD, Maniara WM, Witz G: Metabolism of trans, transmuconaldehyde a microsomal metabolite of benzene by purified yeast aldehyde dehydrogenase and a mouse liver soluble fraction. *Toxicol Appl Pharmacol* 100:360–367, 1989.

Kissling M, Speck B: Chromosome aberrations in experimental benzene intoxication. *Helv Med Acta* 36:59–66, 1971.

Kitchen DN: Neoplastic renal effects of unleaded gasoline in Fischer 344 rats, in Mehlman MA, Hemstreet CP, Thorpe JJ, et al (eds): *Renal Effects of Petroleum Hydrocarbons. Advances in Modern Environmental Toxicology*. Princeton: Princeton Scientific, 1984, vol 7, pp 65–71.

Kitchin KT, Brown JL: Biochemical effects of three carcinogenic chlorinated methanes in rat liver. *Teratogenesis Carcinog Mutagen* 9:61–69, 1989.

Klaassen CD, Plaa GL: Relative effects of various chlorinated hydrocarbons on liver and kidney function in mice. *Toxicol Appl Pharmacol* 9:139–151, 1966.

Kloss MW, Cox MG, Norton RM, et al: Sex-dependent differences in the disposition of 14C-5-224-trimethylpentane in Fischer 344 rats, in Bach PH, Lock EA (eds): *Renal Heterogeneity and Target Cell Toxicity*. London: John Wiley, 1985, pp 489–492.

Kluwe WM, Hook JB: Potentiation of acute chloroform nephrotoxicity by the glutathione depletor diethyl maleate and protection by the microsomal enzyme inhibitor piperonyl butoxide. *Toxicol Appl Pharmacol* 59:457–466, 1981.

Knave B, Anshelm Olson B, Elofsson S, et al: Long term exposure to jet fuel. *Scand J Work Environ Health* 4:19–45, 1978.

Kocsis JJ, Jollow DJ, Witmer CM, et al (eds): *Biological Reactive Intermediates: Mechanisms of Action in Animal Models and Human Disease*. New York: Plenum, 1986, vol 3.

Koeffler HF, Rowley JD: Therapy-related acute nonlymphocytic leukemia, in Wiernik PH, Canelloe GP, Kyle RA, Schiffer CA (eds): *Neoplastic Diseases of the Blood*. New York: Churchill Livingstone, 1985, p 357.

Koop DR, Laethem CL, Schiner GC: Identification of ethanol-inducible P450 isozyme 3a (p450IIE1) as a benzene and phenol hydroxylase. *Toxicol Appl Pharmacol* 98:278–288, 1989.

Kutob SD, Plaa GL: The effect of acute ethanol intoxication on chloroform induced liver damage. *J Pharmacol Exp Ther* 135:245–251, 1962.

LaCagnin LB, Connor HD, Mason RP, Thurman RG: The carbon dioxide anion radical adduct in the perfused rat liver: Relationship to halocarbon-induced toxicity. *Mol Pharmacol* 33:351–357, 1988.

Lamb JC IV, Maronpot RR, Gulati DK, et al: Reproductive developmental toxicity of ethylene glycol in the mouse. *Toxicol Appl Pharmacol* 81:100–112, 1985.

Larson JL, Wolf DC, Butterworth BE: Acute hepatotoxic and nephrotoxic effects of chloroform in male F-344 rats and female B6C3F1 mice. *Fund Appl Toxicol* 20:302–315, 1993.

Larson JL, Wolf DC, Butterworth BE: Induced cytotoxicity and cell proliferation in the hepatocarcinogenicity of chloroform in female B6C3F1 mice: Comparison of administration by gavage in corn oil vs ad libidum in drinking water. *Fund Appl Toxicol* 22:90–102, 1994a.

Larson JL, Wolf DC, Morgan KT, et al: The toxicity of 1-week exposures to inhaled chloroform in female B6C3F1 and male F-344 rats. *Fund Appl Toxicol* 22:431–446, 1994b.

Laskin DL, Pilaro AM: Potential role of macrophages in acetaminophen hepatotoxicity. I. Isolation and characterization of activated macrophages from rat liver. *Toxicol Appl Pharmacol* 86:204–215, 1986a.

Laskin DL, Pilaro AM, Ji S: Potential role of macrophages in acetaminophen hepatotoxicity. II. Mechanism of macrophage accumulation and activation. *Toxicol Appl Pharmacol* 86:216–226, 1986b.

Latriano L, Goldstein BD, Witz G: Formation of muconaldehyde, an open ring metabolite of benzene in mouse liver microsomes: An additional pathway for toxic metabolites. *Proc Nat Acad Sci USA* 83:8356–8360, 1986.

Leaf G, Zatman LJ: A study of the conditions under which methanol may exert a toxic hazard in industry. *Br J Ind Med* 9:19–31, 1952.

Lechner MC (ed): *Cytochrome P450: Biochemistry Biophysics and Molecular Biology*. Proceedings of the 8th International Conference. London: John Libbey, 1994.

Lee EW, Garner CD, Terzo TS: Animal model for the study of methanol toxicity: Comparison of folate-reduced rat responses with published monkey data. *J Toxicol Environ Hlth* 41:71–82, 1994a.

Lee EW, Garner CD, Tergo TS: A rat model manifesting methanol-induced visual dysfunction suitable for both acute and long-term exposure studies. *Toxicol Appl Pharmacol* 128:199–206, 1994b.

Lemaster JJ, Thurman RG: Hypoxia and reperfusion liver injury. *Prog Liver Dis* 11:85–114, 1993.

Letteron P, Degott C, Labbe G, et al: Methoxsalen decreases the metabolic activation and prevents the hepatotoxicity and nephrotoxicity of chloroform in mice. *Toxicol Appl Pharmacol* 91:266–273, 1987.

Li C, Peoples RW, Weight FF: Alcohol action on a neuronal membrane receptor: Evidence for a direct interaction with the receptor protein. *Proc Natl Acad Sci USA* 91:8200–8240, 1994.

Liao LL, Richardson KE: The inhibition of oxalate biosynthesis in isolated perfused rat liver by DL-phenyllactate and n-heptanoate. *Arch Biochem Biophys* 154:68–75, 1973.

Lieber CS: Pathogenesis and diagnosis of alcoholic liver injury, in Avogadro P, Sirtori CR, Tremoli E (eds): *Metabolic Effects of Alcohol*. Amsterdam: Elsevier, 1979, pp 237–258.

Lieber CS, DeCarli LM, Rubin E: Sequential production of fatty liver hepatitis and cirrhosis in sub-human primates fed ethanol with adequate diets. *Proc Nat Acad Sci USA* 72:437–441, 1975.

Lieber CS, DeCarli LM: Hepatic microsomal ethanol oxidizing system: *In vitro* characteristics and adaptive properties *in vivo*. *J Biol Chem* 245:2505–2512, 1970.

Lillis R, Stanescu D, Muica N, Roventa M: Chronic effects of trichloroethylene exposure. *Med Lav* 60:591–601, 1969.

Lillis R: Behavioral effects of occupational carbon disulfide exposure, in: Behavioral Toxicology: Early Detection of Occupational Hazards. NIOSH Publication 74–126, 1974, pp 51–59.

Linz DH, deGarmo PL, Morton WE, et al: Organic solvent-induced encephalopathy in industrial painters. *J Occup Med* 28:119–125, 1986.

Longacre SL, Kocsis JJ, Witmer CM, et al: Toxicological and biochemical effects of repeated administration of benzene to mice. *J Toxicol Environ Hlth* 7:223–237, 1981a.

Longacre SL, Kocsis JJ, Snyder R: Influence of strain differences in mice on the metabolism and toxicity of benzene. *Toxicol Appl Pharmacol* 60:398–409, 1981b.

Loury DJ, Smith-Oliver T, Butterworth BE: Assessment of unscheduled and replicative DNA synthesis in rat kidney cells exposed *in vitro* and *in vivo* to unleaded gasoline. *Toxicol Appl Pharmacol* 87:127–140, 1987.

Lovinger DM, White G, Weight F: Ethanol inhibits NMDA-activated current in hippocampal neurons. *Science* 243:1721–1724, 1989.

Low LK, Meeks JR, Mackerer CR: Health Effects of the alkylbenzenes. II. Xylenes. *Toxicol Ind Health* 5:86–105, 1989.

Lutz WK, Schlatter C: Mechanism of the carcinogenic action of benzene: Irreversible binding to rat liver DNA. *Chem Biol Interact* 18:241–245, 1977.

MacEachern L, Snyder R, Laskin DL: Enhanced production of tumor necrosis factor (TNF) by stromal macrophages following benzene treatment of mice. *Toxicologist* 9:289, 1989.

MacFarland HN: Xenobiotic induced kidney lesions: Hydrocarbons The 90-day and 2-year gasoline studies, in Mehlman MA, Hemstreet CP, Thorpe JJ, Weaver NK (eds): Renal Effects of Petroleum Hydrocarbons. Advances in Modern Environmental Toxicology. Princeton: Princeton Scientific, 1984, pp 51–56.

Maejima K, Suzuki T, Humata H, Maekawa A: Subchronic (12 week) inhalation toxicity study of methanol-fueled engine exhaust in rats. *J Toxicol Environ Hlth* 41:315–317, 1994.

Makar AB, Tephly TR: Methanol Poisoning. VI. Role of folic acid in the production of methanol poisoning in the rat. *J Toxicol Environ Health* 2:1201–1209, 1977.

Maling HM, Stripp B, Sipes IG, et al: Enhanced hepatotoxicity of carbon tetrachloride thioacetamide and dimethyl nitrosamine by pretreatment of rats with methanol and some comparisons with potentiation by isopropanol. *Toxicol Appl Pharmacol* 33:291–308, 1975.

Maltoni C, Conti B, Cotti G: Benzene: A multipotential carcinogen Results of long-term bioassays performed at the Bologna Institute of Oncology. *Am J Ind Med* 4:589–630, 1983.

Mannering GJ, Parks RE Jr: Inhibition of methanol metabolism with 3-amino-124-triazole. *Science* 126:1241–1242, 1975.

Manno M, Rugge M, Cocheo V: Double fatal inhalation of dichloromethane. *Hum Exp Toxicol* 11:540–545, 1992.

Mansuy D, Nastainczyk W, Ullrich V: The mechanism of halothane binding to microsomal cytochrome P-450. *Naunyn Schmiedebergs Arch Pharmacol* 285:315–324, 1974.

Marzulli FN, Maibach HI: *Dermatotoxicology*. New York: Hemisphere, 1983.

Matsushita T, Arimatsu T, Ueda A, et al: Hematological and neuromuscular response of workers exposed to low concentration of toluene vapor. *Ind Health* 13:115–121, 1975.

McKenna MJ, Zempel JA, Madrid EO, Gehring PJ: The pharmacokinetics of $^{14}C$-vinylidene Chloride in rats following inhalation exposure. *Toxicol Appl Pharmacol* 45:599–610, 1978.

McMartin KE, Ambre JJ, Tephly TR: Methanol poisoning in human subjects—Role for formic acid accumulation in the metabolic acidosis. *Am J Med* 68:414–418, 1980.

McMartin KE, Makar AB, Martin AG, et al: Methanol poisoning. I. The Role of formic acid in the development of metabolic acidosis in the monkey and the reversal by 4-methylpyrazole. *Biochem Med* 13:319–333, 1975.

McMartin KE, Martin-Amat G, Makar AB, Tephly TR: Methanol poisoning V Role of formate metabolism in the monkey. *J Pharmacol Exp Ther* 201:564–572, 1977.

McMartin KE, Martin-Amat G, Noker PE, Tephly TR: Lack of a role for formaldehyde in methanol poisoning in the monkey. *Biochem Pharmacol* 28:645–649, 1979.

Mebus CA, Welsch F, Working PK: Attenuation of 2-methoxyethanol-induced testicular toxicity in the rat by simple physiological compounds. *Toxicol Appl Pharmacol* 99:110–121, 1989.

Medinsky MA, Sabourin PJ, Lucier G, et al: A physiological model for simulation of benzene metabolism by rats and mice. *Toxicol Appl Pharmacol* 99:193–206, 1989.

Merkle J, Klimisch H-J, Jaeck R: Prenatal toxicity of 2-methoxypropylacetate-1 in rats and rabbits. *Fund Appl Toxicol* 8:71–79, 1987.

Mery S, Larson JL, Butterworth BE, et al: Nasal toxicity of chloroform in male F-344 rats and female B6C3F1 mice following a 1-week inhalation exposure. *Toxicol Appl Pharmacol* 125:214–227, 1994.

Meyer KH: Contributions to the theory of narcosis. *Faraday Soc Trans* 33:1062–1064, 1937.

Mezey E: Metabolic effects of alcohol. *Fed Proc* 44:134–138, 1985.

Miller RR, Langvardt PW, Calhoun LL, Yahrmardt MA: Metabolism and disposition of propylene glycol monomethyl ether (PGME) beta isomer in male rats. *Toxicol Appl Pharmacol* 83:170–177, 1986.

Miller KW, Paton WDM, Smith RA, Smith EB: The pressure reversal of general anesthesia and the critical volume hypothesis. *Mol Pharmacol* 9:131–143, 1973.

Miller RR, Carreon RE, Young JT, McKenna MJ: Toxicity of methoxyacetic acid in rats. *Fund Appl Toxicol* 2:158–160, 1982.

Miller RR, Ayres JA, Young JT, McKenna MJ: Ethylene glycol monoethyl ether. I. Subchronic vapor inhalation study with rats and rabbits. *Fund Appl Toxicol* 3:49–54, 1983a.

Miller RR, Hermann EA, Langvardt PW, et al: Comparative metabolism and disposition of ethylene glycol monomethyl ether and propylene glycol monomethyl ether in male rats. *Toxicol Appl Pharmacol* 67:229–237, 1983b.

Miller RR, Hermann EA, Young JT, et al: Ethylene glycol monomethyl ether and propylene glycol monomethyl ether: Metabolism, disposition, and subchronic inhalation toxicity studies. *Environ Health Perspect* 57:233–239, 1984.

Miller SL: A theory of gaseous anesthetics. *Proc Nat Acad Sci USA* 47:1515–1524, 1961.

Mohtashamipur E, Norpoth K, Woelke U, Huber P: Effects of ethylbenzene toluene and xylene on the induction of micronuclei in bone marrow polychromatic erythrocytes of mice. *Arch Toxicol* 58:106–109, 1985.

Moon HD: The pathology of fatal carbon tetrachloride poisoning with special reference to the histogenesis of the hepatic and renal lesions. *Am J Pathol* 26:1041–1058, 1950.

Morgan MY: Alcohol and nutrition. *Br Med Bull* 38:21–29, 1982.

Morgan MY: Enteral nutrition in chronic liver disease. *Acta Chir Scand* 507(suppl):81–90, 1981.

Morimoto K: Induction of sister chromatid exchanges and cell division delays in human lymphocytes by microsomal activation of benzene. *Cancer Res* 43:1330–1334, 1983.

Morimoto K, Wolff S: Increase in sister chromatid exchanges and perturbations of cell division kinetics in human lymphocytes by benzene metabolites. *Cancer Res* 40:1189–1193, 1980.

Morimoto K, Wolff S, Koizumi A: Induction of sister chromatid exchanges in human lymphocytes by microsomal activation of benzene metabolites. *Mut Res* 119:355–360, 1983.

Morris HJ, Nelson AA, Calvery HO: Observations on the chronic toxicities of propylene glycol ethylene glycol diethylene glycol ethylene glycol monoethylether and diethylene glycol monoethylether. *Pharmacol Exp Ther* 74:266–273, 1942.

Morton HG: Occurrence and treatment of solvent abuse in children and adolescents. *Pharmacol Ther* 33:449–469, 1987.

Moss EJ, Thomas LV, Cook MW, et al: The role of metabolism in 2-methoxyethanol-induced testicular toxicity. *Toxicol Appl Pharmacol* 79:480–489, 1985.

Mueller DH: Epidemiologic considerations of ethylene glycol intoxication in small animals. *Vet Hum Toxicol* 24:21–24, 1982.

Nagano K, Nakayama E, Koyano M, et al: Testicular atrophy of mice induced by ethylene glycol monoalkyl ethers. *Jpn J Ind Health* 21:29–35, 1979.

NAS: *Biologic Markers in Reproductive Toxicology*. Washington, DC: National Academy Press, 1989a, pp 1–395.

NAS: *Biologic Markers in Pulmonary Toxicology*. Washington, DC: National Academy Press, 1989b, pp 1–179.

NCI (National Cancer Institute): *Carcinogenesis Bioassay for Chloroform*. Bethesda: National Technical Information Service, PB264018/AS, 1976.

Nelson BK, Setzer JV, Brightwell WS, et al: Comparative inhalation teratogenicity of three glycol ether solvents and an amino derivative in rats. *Environ Health Perspect* 57:261–271, 1984.

NIOSH: Hazard Evaluation and Technical Assistance. Report TA 80-32. Everett School District, Everett, WA, NTIS PB 81-111155, 1980.

Nitschke KD, Burek JD, Bell TJ, et al: Methylene chloride: 2-Year inhalation toxicity and oncogenicity study in rats. *Fund Appl Toxicol* 11:48–59, 1988.

Noker PE, Tephly TR: The role of folates in methanol toxicity. *Adv Exp Med Biol* 132:305–315, 1980.

NRC: The Alkyl Benzenes Committee on Alkyl Benzene Derivatives, Board on Toxicology and Environmental Health Hazards. Assembly of Life Sciences National Research Council, National Academy of Sciences. Washington, DC: National Academy Press, 1980.

NTP (National Toxicology Program): Report on a Continuous Breeding Study on CD-1 Mice Administered Propylene Glycol Methyl Ether in Drinking Water. Report No. NTP-86-062.

Ohnishi K, Lieber CS: Reconstitution of the microsomal ethanol oxidizing system (MEOS): Qualitative and quantitative changes of cytochrome P-450 after chronic ethanol consumption. *J Biol Chem* 252:7124–7131, 1977.

Omura T, Sato R: The carbon monoxide-binding pigment of liver microsomes. I. Evidence for its hemoprotein nature. *J Biol Chem* 239:2370–2378, 1964.

Orth OS: General anesthesia I: Volatile agents, in DiPalma JR (ed): *Drill's Pharmacology in Medicine*. New York: McGraw-Hill, 1965, pp 100–115.

OSHA: Federal Register 54:2462, Jan. 19, 1989.

Pankow D, Jagielki S: Effect of methanol or modifications of hepatic glutathione concentration on the metabolism of dichloromethane to carbon monoxide in rats. *Hum Exp Toxicol* 12:227–231, 1993.

Parke DV, Williams RT: Studies in detoxication. The metabolism of benzene containing $^{14}C$ benzene. *Biochem J* 54:231–238, 1953.

Pauling L: A molecular theory of general anesthesia. *Science* 134:15–21, 1961.

Peplonska B: Epidemiologic evaluation of health effects of occupational and nonoccupational exposure to carbon disulfide. *Med Pr* 45:359–369, 1994.

Peters TJ: Ethanol metabolism. *Br Med Bull* 38:17–20, 1982.

Phillips RD, Cockrell BY: Kidney structural changes in rats following inhalation exposure to $C_{10}$-$C_1{}^1$ isoparafinic solvent. *Toxicology* 33:261–273, 1984.

Phillips RD, Egan GF: Effect of $C_{10}$-$C_{11}$ Isoparaffinic solvent on kidney function in Fischer 344 rats during eight weeks of inhalation. *Toxicol Appl Pharmacol* 73:500–510, 1984.

Pirozzi SJ, Schlosser MJ, Kalf GF: Prevention of benzene-induced myelotoxicity and prostaglandin synthesis in bone marrow of mice by inhibitors of prostaglandin H synthetase. *Immunopharmacology* 18:39–55, 1989.

Plaa GL, Larson RE: Relative nephrotoxic properties of chlorinated methane, ethane, and ethylene derivatives in mice. *Toxicol Appl Pharmacol* 7:37–44, 1965.

Pohl LR: Biochemical toxicology of chloroform, in Hodgson E, Bend JR, Philpot RM (eds): *Reviews in Biochemical Toxicology*. New York: Elsevier North Holland, 1979, vol 1, pp 79–107.

Politzer P, Trfonas P, Politzer IR: Molecular properties of the chlorinated ethylenes and their epoxide metabolites. *Ann NY Acad Sci* 367:478–492, 1981.

Pollini G, Colombi R: Damage to bone marrow chromosomes in benzolic aplastic anemia. *Med Lav* 55:241, 1964a.

Pollini G, Colombi R: Chromosomal damage in lymphocytes during benzene hemopathy. *Med Lav* 55:641, 1964b.

Pons CA, Custer RP: Acute ethylene glycol poisoning. *Am J Med Sci* 211:544–552, 1946.

Post GG, Snyder R: Effects of enzyme induction on microsomal benzene metabolism. *J Toxicol Environ Hlth*, 11:811–825, 1983.

Post G, Snyder R, Kalf GF: Inhibition of mRNA synthesis in rabbit bone marrow nuclei *in vitro* by quinone metabolites of benzene. *Chem Biol Interact* 50:203–211, 1984.

Post G, Snyder R, Kalf GF: Inhibition of RNA synthesis and interleukin-2 production in lymphocytes *in vitro* by benzene and its metabolites hydroquinone and p-benzoquinone. *Toxicol Lett* 29:161–167, 1985.

Pratt OE: Alcohol and the developing fetus. *Br Med Bull* 38:48–53, 1982.

Price CJ, Kimmel CA, Tyl RW, Marr MC: The developmental toxicity of ethylene glycol in rats and mice. *Toxicol Appl Pharmacol* 81:113–127, 1985.

Pronzato MA, Domenicotti C, Bellochio A, et al: Modulation of rat liver protein kinase C during "*in vivo*" $CCl_4$-induced oxidative stress. *Biochem Biophys Res Commun* 194:635–641, 1993.

Pryor G, Rebert C, Kassay K, et al: The hearing loss associated with exposure to toluene is not caused by a metabolite. *Brain Res Bull* 27:109–113, 1991.

Randerath K, Reddy MV, Gupta RC: 32P-postlabeling test for DNA damage. *Proc Nat Acad Sci USA* 87:6162–6169, 1981.

Rao KS, Cobel-Geard SR, Young JT, et al: Ethylene glycol monomethyl ether II. Reproductive and dominant lethal studies in rats. *Fund Appl Toxicol* 3:80–85, 1983.

Raucy JL, Kraner JC, Lasker JM: Bioactivation of halogenated hydrocarbons by cytochrome P4502E1. *Crit Rev Toxicol* 23(1):1–20, 1993.

Rebert CS, Hall SA: The neuroepidemiology of styrene: A critical review of representative literature. *Crit Rev Toxicol* 24:57–106, 1994.

Recknagel RO, Glende EA Jr: Carbon tetrachloride toxicity: An example of lethal cleavage. *CRC Crit Rev Toxicol* 2:263–297, 1973.

Recknagel RO, Glende EA Jr, Hruszkewycz AM: New data supporting an obligatory role for lipid peroxidation in carbon tetrachloride-induced loss of aminopyrine demthylase cytochrome P-450 and glucose-6-phophatase, in Jollow DJ, Kocsis JJ, Snyder R, Vainio H (eds): *Biological Reactive Intermediates: Formation Toxicity and Inactivation*. New York: Plenum, 1977, pp 417–428.

Reddy VJ, Schultz SC, Blackburn GR, Mackerer CR: Lack of DNA adduct formation in mice treated with benzene. *Mut Res* 325:149–155, 1994.

Reese E, Kimbrough RD: Acute toxicity of gasoline and some additives. *Environ Hlth Perspect* 101(Suppl 6):115–131, 1993.

Reiner O, Uehleke H: Bindung von Tetrachlokohlenstoff and reduziertes mikrosomales Cytochrom P-450 und an Haem. *Hoppe-Zeyler's Z Physiol Chem* 352:1048–1052, 1971.

Reinke LA, Lai EK, McCay PB: Ethanol feeding stimulates trichloromethyl radical formation from carbon tetrachloride. *Xenobiotica* 18:1311–1318, 1988.

Reitz RH, Fox TR, Ramsey JC, et al: Pharmacokinetics and macromolecular interactions of ethylene dichloride in rats after inhalation or gavage. *Toxicol Appl Pharmacol* 62:190–204, 1982.

Renz JF, Kalf GF: Role for interleukin-1 (IL-1) in benzene-induced hematotoxicity: Inhibition of conversion of pre-IL-1 to mature cytoline in murine macrophages by hydroquinone and prevention of benzene-induced hematotoxicity in mice by IL-1. *Blood* 78:938–944, 1991.

Reynolds ES: Comparison of early injury to liver endoplasmic reticulum by halomethanes hexachloroethane benzene toluene bromobenzene ethionine thioacetamide and dimethylnitrosamine. *Biochem Pharmacol* 21:2555–2561, 1972.

Richards CD, Martin K, Gregory S, et al: Degenerate perturbations of protein structure as the mechanism of anaesthetic action. *Nature* 276:775–779, 1978.

Richardson KA, Wilmer JL, Smith-Simpson D, Skopek TR: Assessment of the genotoxic potential of unleaded gasoline and 224-trimethylpentane in human lymphoblasts *in vitro*. *Toxicol Appl Pharmacol* 82:316–322, 1986.

Rihimaki V, Pfaffli P: Percutaneous absorption of solvent vapors in man. *Scand J Work Environ Health* 4:73–85, 1978.

Ritchie JM: The aliphatic alcohols, in Goodman LS, Gilman A (eds): *The Pharmacological Basis of Therapeutics*, 4th ed. New York: Macmillan, 1970, p 136.

Roberts JA, Seibold HR: Ethylene glycol toxicity in the monkey. *Toxicol Appl Pharmacol* 15:624–631, 1969.

Robertson FM, MacEachern L, Liesch JB, et al: Potential role of interleukin-1 in benzene-induced bone marrow toxicity. *Toxicologist* 9:289, 1989.

Robertson OH, Loosli CG, Puck TT, et al: Tests for the chronic toxicity of propylene glycol on monkeys and rats by vapor inhalation and oral administration. *J Pharmacol Exp Ther* 91:52–76, 1947.

Roe O: Clinical investigations of methyl alcohol poisoning with special reference to the pathogenesis and treatment of amblyopia. *Acta Med Scand* 113:558–608, 1943.

Roe O: Methanol poisoning. Its clinical course, pathogenesis and treatment. *Acta Med Scand* 126(Suppl 182): 1–253, 1946.

Roe O: The ganglion cells of the retina in cases of methanol poisoning in human beings and experimental animals. *Acta Ophthalmol* 26:169–182, 1948.

Rowland J: Incidence of ethylene glycol intoxication in dogs and cats seen at Colorado State University Teaching Hospital. *Vet Hum Toxicol* 29:41–44, 1987.

Rubin A, Rottenberg H: Ethanol and biological membranes: Injury and adaptation. *Pharmacol Biochem Behav* 18:(Suppl 1):7–13, 1983.

Ruddick JA: Toxicology metabolism and biochemistry of 12-Propanediol. *Toxicol Appl Pharmacol* 21:102–111, 1972.

Ruprecht HA, Nelson IA: Preliminary toxicity reports on diethylene glycol and sulfanilamide. V. Clinical and pathologic observations. *JAMA* 109(2):1537, 1937.

Sabourin PJ, Medinsky MA, Thurmond F, et al: Effect of dose on the disposition of methoxyethanol ethoxyethanol and butoxyethanol administered dermally to male F344/N rats. *Fund Appl Toxicol* 19:124–132, 1992.

Saito K, Wada H: Behavioral approaches to toluene intoxication. *Environ Res* 62:53–62, 1993.

Sammett D, Lee EW, Kocsis JJ, Snyder R: Partial hepatectomy reduces both metabolism and toxicity of benzene. *J Toxicol Environ Health* 5:785–792, 1979.

Sasiadek M: Non-random distribution of breakpoints in the karyotypes of workers occupationally exposed to benzene. *Environ Health Perspect* 97:255, 1992.

Sato A, Nakajima T: Dose-dependent metabolic interaction between benzene and toluene *in vivo* and *in vitro*. *Toxicol Appl Pharmacol* 48:249–256, 1979.

Sawahata T, Neal RA: Horseradish peroxidase-mediated oxidation of phenol. *Biochem Biophys Res Commun* 109:988–994, 1982.

Sayers RR, Yant WP, Schrenk HH, et al: Methanol Poisoning—II. Exposure of dogs for brief periods eight times daily to high concentrations of methanol vapor in air. *J Ind Hyg Toxicol* 26:255–259, 1944.

Schenkman JB, Kupffer D: *Hepatic Cytochrome P-450 Mono-Oxygenase System*. New York: Pergamon, 1982.

Schumann AM, Fox TR, Watanabe PG: $^{14}$C-Methyl chloroform (111-trichloroethane): Pharmacokinetics in rats and mice following inhalation exposure. *Toxicol Appl Pharmacol* 62:390–401, 1982.

Schumann AM, Quast JF, Watanabe PG: The pharmacokinetics and macromolecular interactions of perchloroethylene in mice and rats as related to oncogenicity. *Toxicol Appl Pharmacol* 55:207–219, 1980.

Schwetz BA, Price CJ, George JD, Kimmel CA: The developmental toxicity of diethylene and triethylene glycol dimethyl ethers in rabbits. *Fund Appl Toxicol* 19:238–245, 1992.

Sedivec V, Mraz M, Flek J: Biological monitoring of persons exposed to methanol vapours. *Int Arch Occup Environ Health* 48:257–271, 1981.

Seeman P: The membrane action of anesthetics and tranquilizers. *Pharmacol Rev* 24:583–655, 1972.

Seidel HJ, Barthel E, Zinser D: The hematopoietic stem cell compartments in mice during and after long term inhalation of three doses of benzene. *Exp Hematol* 17:300, 1989.

Seitz HK, Simanowski UA: Ethanol and carcinogenesis of the alimentary tract. *Alcohol Clin Exp Res* 10:33S–40S, 1986.

Seppalainen AM, Lindstrom K, Martelin T: Neurophysiological and psychological picture of solvent poisoning. *Am J Ind Med* 1:31–42, 1980.

Serota DG, Thakur AK, Ulland BM, et al: A two-year drinking-water study of dichloromethane in rodents. I. Rats. *Food Chem Toxicol* 24:951–958, 1986a.

Serota DG, Thakur AK, Ulland BM, et al: A two-year drinking-water study of dichloromethane in rodents. II. Mice. *Food Chem Toxicol* 24:959–963, 1986b.

Sherlock S (ed): Alcohol and Disease. *Br Med Bull* 38:1–113, 1982a.

Sherlock S: Alcohol-related liver disease. *Br Med Bull* 38:67–70, 1982b.

Shibayama Y: Hepatotoxicity of carbon tetrachloride after chronic ethanol consumption. *Exp Mol Pathol* 49:234–242, 1988.

Short BG, Burnett VL, Swenberg JA: Histopathology and cell proliferation induced by 224-trimethylpentane in the male rat kidney. *Toxicol Pathol* 14:194–203, 1986.

Singer SJ, Nicolson GL: The fluid mosaic model of the structure of cell membranes. *Science* 175:720–731, 1972.

Siou G, Conan L, el Haitem M: Evaluation of the clastogenic action of benzene by oral administration with 2 cytogenetic techniques in mouse and Chinese hamster. *Mut Res* 90:273–278, 1981.

Sipes IG, Gandolfi AJ: Role of reactive intermediates in halothane associated liver injury, in Snyder R, Parke DV, Kocsis JJ, et al (eds): *Biological Reactive Intermediates. Chemical Mechanisms and Biological Effects*. New York: Plenum, 1982, vol 2, pp 603–618.

Slater TF: *Free Radical Mechanisms in Tissue Injury*. Bristol, England: J.W. Arrowsmith, 1972, pp 118–163.

Slater TF: Free radicals as reactive intermediates in tissue injury, in Snyder R, Parke DV, Kocsis JJ, et al (eds): *Biological Reactive Intermediates. Chemical Mechanisms and Biological Effects*. New York: Plenum, 1982, vol 2, pp 575–589.

Sleet RB, Greene JA, Welsch F: The relationships of embryotoxicity to disposition of 2-methoxyethanol in mice. *Toxicol Appl Pharmacol* 93:195–207, 1988.

Smillie WG, Pessoa SB: The treatment of hookworm disease with carbon tetrachloride. *Am J Hyg* 3:35–45, 1923.

Smith JH, Hook JB: Mechanism of chloroform toxicity. III. Renal and hepatic microsomal metabolism of chloroform in mice. *Toxicol Appl Pharmacol* 73:511–524, 1984.

Smith JH, Maita K, Sleight SD, Hook JB: Mechanism of chloroform toxicity: I Time course of chloroform toxicity in male and female mice. *Toxicol Appl Pharmacol* 70:467–479, 1983.

Smith JH, Maita K, Sleight SD, Hook JB: Effect of sex hormone status on chloroform nephrotoxicity and renal mixed function oxidases in mice. *Toxicology* 30:305–316, 1984.

Smuckler EA: The molecular basis of acute liver cell injury, in Good RA, Day SB, Yunes JJ (eds): *Molecular Pathology*. Springfield, IL: Charles C. Thomas, 1975, pp 490–510.

Smyth HF Jr: Physiological aspects of glycols and related compounds, in Curme GO Jr, Johnston F (eds): *Glycols*. New York: Reinhold, 1952.

Snyder R, Chepiga T, Yang CS, et al: Benzene metabolism by reconstituted cytochromes P450 2B1 and 2E1 and its modulation by cytochrome $b_5$ microsomal epoxide hydrolase and glutathione transferases: evidence for an important role of microsomal epoxide hydrolase in the formation of hydroquinone. *Toxicol Appl Pharmacol* 122:172–181, 1993b.

Snyder R, Kalf GF: A perspective on benzene leukemogenesis. *Crit Rev Toxicol* 24:177–209, 1994.

Snyder R, Kocsis JJ: Current concepts of chronic benzene toxicity. *CRC Crit Rev Toxicol* 3:265–288, 1975.

Snyder R, Lee EW, Kocsis JJ: Binding of labeled benzene metabolites to mouse liver and bone marrow. *Res Commun Chem Pathol Pharmacol* 20:191–194, 1978.

Snyder R, Lee EW, Kocsis JJ, Witmer CM: Bone marrow depressant and leukemogenic actions of benzene. *Life Sci* 21:1709–1722, 1977.

Snyder R, Parke DV, Kocsis JJ, et al (eds): *Biological Reactive Intermediates. Chemical Mechanisms and Biological Effects*. New York: Plenum, 1982.

Snyder R, Remmer H: Classes of hepatic microsomal mixed function oxidase inducers. *Pharmacol Therap* 7:203–244, 1979.

Snyder R, Uzuki F, Gonasun L, et al: The metabolism of benzene *in vitro*. *Toxicol Appl Pharmacol* 11:346–360, 1967.

Snyder R, Witz G, Goldstein BD: The toxicology of benzene. *Environ Health Perspect* 100:293–306, 1993a.

Strubelt O: Interactions between ethanol and other hepatotoxic agents. *Biochem Pharmacol* 29:1445–1449, 1980.

Styles JA, Richardson CR: Cytogenetic effects of benzene dosimetric studies on rats exposed to benzene vapour. *Mut Res* 135:203–209, 1984.

Sullivan MJ, Rarey KE, Conolly RB: Ototoxicity of toluene in rats. *Neurotoxicol Teratol* 10:525–530, 1989.

Susten AS, Dames BL, Burg JR, Niemeier RW: Percutaneous penetration of benzene in hairless mice: An estimate of dermal absorption during tire-building operations. *Am J Ind Med* 7:323–335, 1985.

Szendzikowski S, Stetkiewicz J, Wronska-Nofer T, Karasek M: Pathomorphology of the experimental lesion of the peripheral nervous system in white rats chronically exposed to carbon disulphide, in Hausmanowa-Petrusewicz I, Vedrzejowska H (eds.): *Structure and Function of Normal and Diseased Muscle and Peripheral Nerve*. Warsaw: Medical Publ, 1974, pp 319–326.

Tanii H, Saito S, Hashimoto K: Structure-toxicity relationship of ethylene glycol ethers. *Arch Toxicol* 66:368–371, 1992.

Tephly TR: Introduction factors in responses to the environment. *Fed Proc* 36:1627–1628, 1977.

Tephly TR, Makar AB, McMartin KE, et al: Methanol—its metabolism and toxicity. *Biochem Pharmacol Methanol* 1:145–164, 1979.

Thurman RG, Hoffman PL (ed): First Congress of the International Society for Biomedical Research on Alcoholism. *Pharmacol Biochem Behav* 518:(Suppl 1)593, 1983.

Thurman RG, McKenna WR, Brenzel HJ, Hesse S: Significant pathways of hepatic ethanol metabolism. *Fed Proc* 34:2075–2081, 1975.

Tice RR, Costa DL, Drew RT: Cytogenetic effects of inhaled benzene in murine bone marrow induction of sister chromatid exchanges chromosomal aberrations and cellular proliferation inhibition in DBA/2 mice. *Proc Natl Acad Sci USA* 77:2148, 1980.

Tice RR, Vogt TF, Costa DL: Cytogenetic effects of inhaled benzene on murine bone marrow, in Tice RR, Costa DL, Schaich KM (eds): *Genotoxic Effects of Airborne Agents*. New York: Plenum, 1982, pp 257–275.

Tiller JR, Schilling RSF, Morris JW: Occupational toxic factor in mortality from coronary heart disease. *Br Med J* 4:407–411, 1968.

Tilson HA, Cabe PA: Strategy for the assessment of neurobehavioural consequences of environmental factors. *Environ Hlth Perspect* 26:287–299, 1978.

Timmerman RW: Carbon disulfide, in: *Kirk-Othmer Encyclopedia of Chemical Technology*, 3d ed., New York: John Wiley, vol 4, 1978, p 742.

Timmerman RW: Carbon disulfide, in Grayson L (ed): *Kirk-Othmer Consise Encyclopedia of Chemical Technology*. New York: John Wiley, 1985, pp 213–214.

Toft K, Oloffson T, Tunek A, Berlin M: Toxic effects on mouse bone marrow caused by inhalation of benzene. *Arch Toxicol* 51:295–302, 1982.

Tolonen M, Hernberg S, Nuriminen M, Tiitola K: A follow-up study of coronary heart disease in viscose rayon workers exposed to carbon disulfide. *Br J Ind Med* 32:1–10, 1975.

Tolonen M, Hanninen H, Nuriminen M: Psychological tests specific to individual carbon disulphide exposure. *Scand J Psychol* 19:241–245, 1978.

Tolonen M, Nurminen M, Hernberg S: Ten-year coronary mortality of workers exposed to carbon disulfide. *Scand J Work Env Health* 5:109–114, 1979.

Torkelson TR, Oyen F, Rowe VK: The toxicity of chloroform as determined by single and repeated exposure of laboratory animals. *Am Ind Hyg Assoc J* 37:697–705, 1976.

Traiger GJ, Bruckner JV: The participation of 2-butanone in 2-butanol-induced potentiation of carbon tetrachloride hepatotoxicity. *J Pharmacol Exp Ther* 196:493–500, 1976.

Traiger GJ, Plaa GL: Differences in the potentiation of carbon tetrachloride in rats by ethanol and isopropanol pretreatment. *Toxicol Appl Pharmacol* 20:105–112, 1971a.

Traiger GJ, Plaa GL: Relationship of alcohol metabolism to the potentiation of $CCl_4$ hepatotoxicity induced by aliphatic alcohols. *J Pharmacol Exp Ther* 183:481–488, 1971b.

Traiger GJ, Plaa GL: Chlorinated hydrocarbon toxicity. Potentiation by isopropyl alcohol and acetone. *AMA Arch Environ Health* 28:276–278, 1974.

Tunek A, Hogstedt B, Oloffson T: Mechanism of benzene toxicity. Effects of benzene and benzene metabolites on bone marrow cellularity number of granulopoietic stem cells and frequency of micronuclei in mice. *Chem Biol Interact* 3:129–138, 1982.

Tuttle TC, Wood GD, Grether CG: Behavioral and neurological evaluation of workers exposed to carbon disulphide ($CS_2$). *NIOSH Publication* No. 77–128, 1977.

Uehleke H: Binding of haloalkanes to liver microsomes, in Jollow DJ, Kocsis JJ, Snyder R, Vainio H (eds): *Biological Reactive Intermediates: Formation Toxicity and Inactivation*. New York: Plenum 1977, pp 431–445.

Uyeki EM, Ashkar AE, Shoeman DW, Bisel TU: Acute toxicity of benzene inhalation to hemopoietic precursor cells. *Toxicol Appl Pharmacol* 40:49–57, 1977.

Vind C, Grunnet N: Interaction of cytoplasmic dehydrogenases: Quantitation of pathways of ethanol metabolism. *Pharmacol Biochem Behav* 18(Suppl 1):209–213, 1983.

von Wartburg JP, Bethuen JL, Vallee BL: Human liver alcohol dehydrogenase Kinetic and physico-chemical properties. *Biochemistry* 3:1775–1782, 1964.

Wacker EC, Haynes H, Druyan R, et al: Treatment of ethylene glycol poisoning with ethyl alcohol. *JAMA* 194:1231–1233, 1965.

Weil CS, Woodside MD, Smith NF Jr, Carpenter CP: Results of feeding propylene glycol in the diet to dogs for two years. *Food Cosmet Toxicol* 9:479–490, 1971.

Whipple GH, Sperry JA: Chloroform poisoning liver necrosis and repair. *Johns Hopkins Hospital-Bull* 222:278, 1909.

Wiener HL, Richardson KE: The metabolism and toxicity of ethylene glycol. *Res Commun Subst Abuse* 9:77–87, 1988.

Wiley FH, Hueper WC, Bergen DS, Blood FR: The formation of oxalic acid from ethylene glycol and related solvents. *J Ind Hyg Toxicol* 20:269–277, 1938.

Witmer CM, Snyder R, Jollow DJ, et al: *Biological Reactive Intermediates. Molecular and Cellular Effects and Their Impact on Human Health*. New York: Plenum, 1991, vol 4.

Witz G, Gad SC, Tice RR, et al: Genetic toxicity of the benzene metabolite transtrans-muconaldehyde in mammalian and bacterial cells. *Mut Res* 240:295, 1990.

Wood R: Toluene: A prototype for the evaluation of the behavior and nervous system toxicity of solvents, in Weiss B, O'Donoghue J (eds): *Neurobehavioral Toxicity: Analysis and Interpretation*. New York: Raven, 1994, pp 367–375.

Wulf BS, Featherstone RM: A correlation of van der Waals constants with anesthetic potency. *Anesthesiology* 18:97–105, 1957.

Yant WP, Schrenk HH: Distribution of methanol in dogs after inhalation and administration by stomach tube and subcutaneously. *J Ind Hyg Toxicol* 19(7):337–345, 1937.

Zampaglione N, Jollow JD, Mitchell JR, et al: Role of detoxifying enzymes in bromobenzene-induced liver necrosis. *J Pharmacol Exp Ther* 187:218–227, 1973.

Zenk H: $CS_2$ effects upon olfactory and auditory functions of employees in the synthetic-fiber industry. *Int Arch Arbeitsmed* 27:210, 1970.

Zhang Z, Kline SA, Kirley TA, Goldstein BD: Pathways of transtrans-muconaldehyde metabolism in mouse liver cytosol: reversibility of monoreductive metabolism and formation of end products. *Arch Toxicol* 67:461–467, 1993.

Zimmerman HJ: *Hepatotoxicity: The Adverse Effects of Drugs and Other Chemicals on the Liver*. New York: Appleton-Century-Crofts, 1978.

# CHAPTER 25

# TOXIC EFFECTS OF RADIATION AND RADIOACTIVE MATERIALS

*Naomi H. Harley*

Among all the branches of toxicology, ionizing radiation provides the most quantitative estimates of health detriments for humans. Five large studies provide data on the health effects of radiation on people. These effects include external x-rays and gamma-ray radiation and internal alpha radioactivity. The studies encompass radium exposures (including radium dial painters), atom bomb survivors, patients irradiated with x-rays for ankylosing spondylitis, children irradiated with x-rays for tinea capitis (ringworm), and uranium miners exposed to radon and its short-lived daughter products. The only health effect subsequent to radiation exposure seen with statistical significance to date is cancer. The various types and the quantitative risks are described in subsequent sections.

All the studies provide a consistent picture of the risk of exposure to ionizing radiation. There are sufficient details in the atom bomb, occupational, and medical exposures to estimate the risk from lifelong low-level environmental exposure. Natural background radiation is substantial, and only within the past 10 to 15 years has the extent of the radiation insult to the global population from natural radiation and radioactivity been appreciated.

## BASIC RADIATION CONCEPTS

There are four main types of radiation: alpha particles, beta particles (negatively charged) and positrons (positively charged), gamma rays, and x-rays. An atom can decay to a product element through the loss of a heavy (mass = 4) charged (+2) alpha particle consisting of two protons and two neutrons. An atom can decay by loss of a negatively or positively charged electron (beta particle or positron). Gamma radiation results when the nucleus releases excess energy, usually after an alpha, beta, or positron transition. X-rays occur whenever an inner-shell orbital electron is removed and rearrangement of the atomic electrons results, with the release of the element's characteristic x-ray energy.

There are several excellent textbooks that describe the details of radiological physics (Evans, 1955; Andrews, 1974; Turner, 1986).

### Energy

Alpha particles and beta rays (or positrons) have kinetic energy as a result of their motion. The energy is equal to

$$E = \tfrac{1}{2} mV^2 \qquad (1)$$

where

$m$ = mass of particle
$V$ = velocity of particle

Alpha particles have a low velocity compared with the speed of light, and calculations of alpha particle energy do not require any corrections for relativity. Most beta particles (or positrons) do have high velocity, and the basic expression must be corrected for their increased relativistic mass (the rest mass of the electron is 0.511 MeV). The total energy is equal to

$$E = \frac{0.511}{(1 - v^2/c^2)^{1/2}} + 0.511 \qquad (2)$$

where

$v$ = velocity of beta particle
$c$ = speed of light

Gamma rays and x-rays are pure electromagnetic radiation with energy equal to

$$E = hv \qquad (3)$$

where

$h$ = Planck's constant ($6.626 \times 10^{-34}$ J s)
$v$ = frequency of radiation

The conventional energy units for ionizing radiation are the electron volt (eV) or multiples of this basic unit, million electron volts (MeV), and kiloelectron volts (keV). The conversion to the international system of units [Systeme Internationale (SI)] is currently taking place in the United States, and the more fundamental energy unit of the Joule (J) is slowly replacing the older unit. The relationship is

$$1 \text{ eV} = 1.6 \times 10^{-19} \text{ J}$$

Authoritative tables of nuclear data such as those of Lederer and associates (1978) and Browne and colleagues (1986) contain the older units.

### Alpha Particles

Alpha particles are helium nuclei (consisting of two protons and two neutrons) with a charge of +2 that are ejected from the nucleus of an atom. When an alpha particle loses energy, slows to the velocity of a gas atom, and acquires two electrons from the vast sea of free electrons present in most media, it becomes part of the normal background helium in the environment.

The formula for alpha decay is

$$^{A}_{Z}X \rightarrow {}^{A-4}_{Z-2}Y + He^{2+} + \text{gamma} + Q_a$$

where

$Z$ = atomic number
$A$ = atomic weight

The energy available in this decay is $Q_a$ and is equal to the mass difference of the parent and the two products. The energy is shared among the particles and the gamma ray if one is present.

An example of alpha decay is given by the natural radionuclide $^{226}Ra$:

$$^{226}_{86}Ra \rightarrow {}^{222}_{84}Rn + \text{alpha (5.2 MeV)}$$

The energy of alpha particles for most emitters lies in the range of 4 to 8 MeV. More energetic alpha particles exist but are seen only in very short-lived emitters such as those formed by reactions occurring in particle accelerators. These particles are not considered in this chapter.

Although there may be several alpha particles with very similar energy emitted by a particular element such as radium, each particular alpha is monoenergetic. No continuous spectrum of energies exists, only discrete energies.

## Beta Particles, Positrons, and Electron Capture

Beta particle decay occurs when a neutron in the nucleus of an element is effectively transformed into a proton and an electron. Subsequent ejection of the electron occurs, and the maximum energy of the beta particle equals the mass difference between the parent and the product nuclei. A gamma ray may also be present to share the energy, $Q_\beta$:

$$^{A}_{Z}X \rightarrow {}_{Z+1}^{A}Y + \text{beta} + Q_\beta$$

An example of beta decay is given by the natural radionuclide $^{210}Pb$:

$$^{210}_{82}Pb \rightarrow {}^{210}_{83}Bi + \text{beta (0.015 MeV)} + \text{0.046 MeV gamma ray}$$

Unlike alpha decay, in which each alpha particle is monoenergetic, beta particles are emitted with a continuous spectrum of energy from zero to the maximum energy available for the transition. The reason for this is that the total available energy is shared in each decay or transition by two particles: the beta particle and an antineutrino. The total energy released in each transition is constant, but the observed beta particles then appear as a spectrum. The residual energy is carried away by the antineutrino, which is a particle with essentially zero mass and charge that cannot be observed without extraordinarily complex instrumentation. The beta particle, by contrast, is readily observed with conventional nuclear counting equipment.

Positron emission is similar to beta particle emission but results from the effective nucleon transformation of a proton to a neutron plus a positively charged electron. The atomic number decreases rather than increases as it does in beta decay.

An example of positron decay is given by the natural radionuclide $^{64}Cu$, which decays by beta emission 41 percent of the time, positron emission 19 percent of the time, and electron capture 40 percent of the time:

$$^{64}_{29}Cu \rightarrow {}^{64}_{28}Ni + \text{positron (0.66 MeV)} \quad \text{19 percent}$$

$$^{64}_{29}Cu \rightarrow {}^{64}_{30}Zn + \text{beta (0.57 MeV)} \quad \text{41 percent}$$

$$^{64}_{29}Cu \rightarrow {}^{64}_{28}Ni \text{ electron capture} \quad \text{40 percent}$$

The energy of the positron appears as a continuous spectrum, similar to that in beta decay, where the total energy available for decay is again shared between the positron and a neutrino. In the case of positron emission, the maximum energy of the emitted particle is the mass difference of the parent and product nuclide minus the energy needed to create two electron masses (1.02 MeV), whereas the maximum energy of the beta particle is the mass difference itself. This happens because in beta decay, the increase in the number of orbital electrons resulting from the increase in atomic number of the product nucleus cancels the mass of the electron lost in emitting the beta particle. This does not happen in positron decay, and there is an orbital electron lost as a result of the decrease in atomic number of the product and the loss of the electron mass in positron emission.

Electron capture competes with positron decay, and the resulting product nucleus is the same. In electron capture, an orbiting electron is acquired by the nucleus and the transformation of a proton plus the electron to form a neutron takes place. In some cases the energy available is released as a gamma-ray photon, but this is not necessary, and a monoenergetic neutrino may be emitted. If the 1.02 MeV required for positron decay is not available, positron decay is not kinetically possible and electron capture is the only mode observed.

## Gamma-Ray (Photon) Emission

Gamma-ray emission is not a primary process except in rare instances but occurs in combination with alpha, beta, or positron emission or electron capture. Whenever the ejected particle does not utilize all the available energy for decay, the nucleus contains the excess energy and is in an excited state. The excess energy is released as photon or gamma-ray emission coincident with the ejection of the particle.

One of the rare instances of pure gamma-ray emission is Tc:

$$^{99m}_{43}Tc \rightarrow {}^{99}_{43}Tc + \text{gamma (0.14 MeV)}$$

In many cases, the photon will not actually be emitted by the nucleus but the excess excitation energy will be transferred to an orbital electron. This electron is then ejected as a monoenergetic particle with energy equal to that of the photon minus the binding energy of the orbital electron. This process is known as internal conversion. In tables of nuclear data such as those of Lederer and associates (1978), the ratio of the conversion process to the photon is given as *e/v*. For example, the *e/v* ratio for $^{99m}Tc$ is 0.11, and therefore the photon is emitted 90 percent of the time and the conversion electron is emitted 10 percent of the time.

## INTERACTION OF RADIATION WITH MATTER

All ionizing radiation loses energy when passing through matter by producing ion pairs (an electron and a positively charged atom residue) or by raising atomic electrons to an excited state. The average energy needed to produce an ion pair is given the notation $W$ and is numerically equal to 33.85 eV. This energy is roughly two times the ionization potential of most gases or other elements because it includes the energy lost in the excitation process. It is not clear what role the excitation plays, for example, in damage to targets in the cellular DNA. Ionization, by contrast, can break bonds in DNA, causing strand breaks and easily understood damage.

All particles and rays interact through their charge or field with atomic or free electrons in the medium through which they are passing. There is no interaction with the atomic nucleus except at energies above about 8 MeV, which is required for interactions that break apart the nucleus (spallation).

Alpha and beta particles and gamma rays lose energy by ionization and excitation in somewhat different ways, as described in the following sections.

### Alpha Particles

The alpha particle is a heavy charged particle with a mass that is 7300 times that of the electrons with which it interacts. A massive particle interacting with a small particle has the interesting property that it can give a maximum velocity during energy transfer to the small particle of only two times the initial velocity of the heavy particle. In terms of the maximum energy that can be transferred per interaction, this is

$$E_{(\text{maximum electron})} = 4/7300\ E_{(\text{alpha particle})} \quad (4)$$

Although alpha particles can lose perhaps 10 to 20 percent of their energy in traveling 10 $\mu$m in tissue (1 cm in air), each interaction can impart only the small energy given in the maximum in equation 4. Thus, alpha particles are characterized by a high energy loss per unit path length and a high ionization density along the track length. This is called a high linear energy transfer (LET).

An exact expression for the energy loss in matter, $dE/dX$ or stopping power, was derived by Hans Bethe (1953), with modifications added by Bloch and others. For alpha energies between 0.2 and 10 MeV, the Bethe-Bloch expression can be simplified to

$$dE/dx = 3.8 \times 10^{-25}\ C\ NZ/E\ \ln\{548\ E/I\}\ \text{MeV}\ \mu\text{m}^{-1} \quad (5)$$

where

$N$ = number of atoms cm$^{-3}$ in medium
$Z$ = atomic number of medium
$I$ = ionization potential of medium
$E$ = energy of alpha particle
$C$ = charge correction for alpha particles with energy below 1.6 MeV

A simple rule of thumb derived by Bloch may be used to estimate the ionization potential of a compound or element,

$$I = 10(Z) \quad (6)$$

or the Bragg additivity rule (Attix et al., 1968) may be used for compounds when the individual values of ionization potential for the elements are available. A tabulation of values of ionization potential is given in ICRU 37 (ICRU, 1984), and the stopping power in all elements has been calculated by Ziegler (1977).

When alpha particles are near the end of their range, the charge is not constant at +2 but can be +1 or even zero as the particle acquires or loses electrons. A correction factor, $C$, is needed for energies between 0.2 and 1.5 MeV to account for this effect. Whaling (1958) published values for the correction factor by which equation 4 should be multiplied. These factors vary from 0.24 at 0.2 MeV, 0.75 at 0.6 MeV, 0.875 at 1.0 MeV, up to 1.0 at 1.6 MeV.

For the case of tissue, equation 5 reduces to

$$dE/dX_{\text{tissue}} = [0.126C/E]\ \ln\{7.99\ E\}\ \text{MeV}\ \mu\text{m}^{-1} \quad (7)$$

***Example 1.*** Find the energy loss (stopping power) of a 0.6 and a 5 MeV alpha particle in tissue.

$$\begin{aligned} dE/dX &= 0.126\ (0.75)/0.6\ \ln\ (7.99 \times 0.6) \\ &= 0.25\ \text{MeV}\ \mu\text{m}^{-1} \\ &= 0.126\ (1.0)/5.0\ \ln\ (7.99 \times 5.0) \\ &= 0.093\ \text{MeV}\ \mu\text{m}^{-1} \end{aligned}$$

### Beta Particles

The equations for beta particle energy loss in matter cannot be simplified as in the case of alpha particles because of three factors:

1. Even at low energies of a few tenths of an MeV, beta particles are traveling near the speed of light and relativistic effects (mass increase) must be considered.
2. Electrons are interacting with particles of the same mass in the medium (free or orbital electrons), and so large energy losses per collision are possible.
3. Radiative or bremsstrahlung energy loss occurs when electrons or positrons are slowing down in matter. Such a loss also occurs with alpha particles, but the magnitude of this energy loss is negligible.

Including the effects of these three factors, the energy loss for electrons and positrons has been well quantitated. Tabulations of energy loss in various media have been prepared with the ionization energy loss and the radiative loss detailed. Ta-

**Table 25–1**
**Stopping Power, Range, and Radiation Yield for Electrons in Air**

| ENERGY, MeV | STOPPING POWER COLLISION, MeV cm$^2$ g$^{-1}$ | RADIATIVE, MeV cm$^2$ g$^{-1}$ | TOTAL, MeV cm$^2$ g$^{-1}$ | CSDA RANGE, g cm$^{-2}$ | RADIATION YIELD |
|---|---|---|---|---|---|
| 0.0100 | 1.975E+01 | 3.897E−03 | 1.976E+01 | 2.883E−04 | 1.082E−04 |
| 0.0125 | 1.663E+01 | 3.921E−03 | 1.663E+01 | 4.269E−04 | 1.299E−04 |
| 0.0150 | 1.445E+01 | 3.937E−03 | 1.445E+01 | 5.886E−04 | 1.506E−04 |
| 0.0175 | 1.283E+01 | 3.946E−03 | 1.283E+01 | 7.726E−04 | 1.706E−04 |
| 0.0200 | 1.157E+01 | 3.954E−03 | 1.158E+01 | 9.781E−04 | 1.898E−04 |
| 0.0250 | 9.753E+00 | 3.966E−03 | 9.757E+00 | 1.451E−03 | 2.267E−04 |
| 0.0300 | 8.492E+00 | 3.976E−03 | 8.496E+00 | 2.001E−03 | 2.618E−04 |
| 0.0350 | 7.563E+00 | 3.986E−03 | 7.567E+00 | 2.626E−03 | 2.955E−04 |
| 0.0400 | 6.848E+00 | 3.998E−03 | 6.852E+00 | 3.322E−03 | 3.280E−04 |
| 0.0450 | 6.281E+00 | 4.011E−03 | 6.285E+00 | 4.085E−03 | 3.594E−04 |
| 0.0500 | 5.819E+00 | 4.025E−03 | 5.823E+00 | 4.912E−03 | 3.900E−04 |
| 0.0550 | 5.435E+00 | 4.040E−03 | 5.439E+00 | 5.801E−03 | 4.197E−04 |
| 0.0600 | 5.111E+00 | 4.057E−03 | 5.115E+00 | 6.750E−03 | 4.488E−04 |
| 0.0700 | 4.593E+00 | 4.093E−03 | 4.597E+00 | 8.817E−03 | 5.049E−04 |
| 0.0800 | 4.198E+00 | 4.133E−03 | 4.202E+00 | 1.110E−02 | 5.590E−04 |
| 0.0900 | 3.886E+00 | 4.175E−03 | 3.890E+00 | 1.357E−02 | 6.112E−04 |
| 0.1000 | 3.633E+00 | 4.222E−03 | 3.637E+00 | 1.623E−02 | 6.618E−04 |
| 0.1250 | 3.172E+00 | 4.348E−03 | 3.177E+00 | 2.362E−02 | 7.826E−04 |
| 0.1500 | 2.861E+00 | 4.485E−03 | 2.865E+00 | 3.193E−02 | 8.968E−04 |
| 0.1750 | 2.637E+00 | 4.633E−03 | 2.642E+00 | 4.103E−02 | 1.006E−03 |
| 0.2000 | 2.470E+00 | 4.789E−03 | 2.474E+00 | 5.082E−02 | 1.111E−03 |
| 0.2500 | 2.236E+00 | 5.126E−03 | 2.242E+00 | 7.212E−02 | 1.311E−03 |
| 0.3000 | 2.084E+00 | 5.495E−03 | 2.089E+00 | 9.527E−02 | 1.502E−03 |
| 0.3500 | 1.978E+00 | 5.890E−03 | 1.984E+00 | 1.199E−01 | 1.688E−03 |
| 0.4000 | 1.902E+00 | 6.311E−03 | 1.908E+00 | 1.456E−01 | 1.869E−03 |
| 0.4500 | 1.845E+00 | 6.757E−03 | 1.852E+00 | 1.722E−01 | 2.048E−03 |
| 0.5000 | 1.802E+00 | 7.223E−03 | 1.809E+00 | 1.995E−01 | 2.225E−03 |
| 0.5500 | 1.769E+00 | 7.708E−03 | 1.776E+00 | 2.274E−01 | 2.401E−03 |
| 0.6000 | 1.743E+00 | 8.210E−03 | 1.751E+00 | 2.558E−01 | 2.577E−03 |
| 0.7000 | 1.706E+00 | 9.258E−03 | 1.715E+00 | 3.135E−01 | 2.929E−03 |
| 0.8000 | 1.683E+00 | 1.036E−02 | 1.694E+00 | 3.722E−01 | 3.283E−03 |
| 0.9000 | 1.669E+00 | 1.151E−02 | 1.681E+00 | 4.315E−01 | 3.638E−03 |
| 1.0000 | 1.661E+00 | 1.271E−02 | 1.674E+00 | 4.912E−01 | 3.997E−03 |
| 1.2500 | 1.655E+00 | 1.588E−02 | 1.671E+00 | 6.408E−01 | 4.906E−03 |
| 1.5000 | 1.661E+00 | 1.927E−02 | 1.680E+00 | 7.900E−01 | 5.836E−03 |
| 1.7500 | 1.672E+00 | 2.284E−02 | 1.694E+00 | 9.382E−01 | 6.784E−03 |
| 2.0000 | 1.684E+00 | 2.656E−02 | 1.711E+00 | 1.085E+00 | 7.748E−03 |
| 2.5000 | 1.712E+00 | 3.437E−02 | 1.747E+00 | 1.374E+00 | 9.716E−03 |
| 3.0000 | 1.740E+00 | 4.260E−02 | 1.783E+00 | 1.658E+00 | 1 173E−02 |
| 3.5000 | 1.766E+00 | 5.115E−02 | 1.817E+00 | 1.935E+00 | 1.377E−02 |

$I$ = 85.7 eV; density = 1.205E−03 g/cm$^3$ (20°C).
SOURCE: ICRU (1984).

bles 25-1 and 25-2 are reproduced from ICRU 37 (1984) to show the energy loss in air and muscle.

***Example 2.*** What is the energy loss in tissue for an electron with an initial energy of 1.75 MeV? What is its range, and what fraction of the initial energy is given up as bremsstrahlung as the electron slows from 1.75 MeV to rest?

From Table 25-2, the stopping power at the initial energy of 1.75 MeV is 1.82 MeV cm$^2$ g$^{-1}$, the range is 0.85 g cm$^{-2}$, and the fraction of the energy given up as bremsstrahlung in slowing to rest is 0.006.

## Gamma Rays

Photons do not have a mass or charge as do alpha and beta particles. The interaction between a photon and matter there-

**Table 25–2**
**Stopping Power, Range, and Radiation Yield for Electrons in Muscle Tissue**

| | STOPPING POWER | | | | |
|---|---|---|---|---|---|
| ENERGY, MeV | COLLISION, MeV cm$^2$ g$^{-1}$ | RADIATIVE, MeV cm$^2$ g$^{-1}$ | TOTAL, MeV cm$^2$ g$^{-1}$ | CSDA RANGE, g cm$^{-2}$ | RADIATION YIELD |
| 0.0100 | 2.231E+01 | 3.835E−03 | 2.231E+01 | 2.543E−04 | 9.366E−05 |
| 0.0125 | 1.876E+01 | 3.863E−03 | 1.877E+01 | 3.771E−04 | 1.127E−04 |
| 0.0150 | 1.628E+01 | 3.880E−03 | 1.629E+01 | 5.205E−04 | 1.310E−04 |
| 0.0175 | 1.445E+01 | 3.892E−03 | 1.445E+01 | 6.838E−04 | 1.485E−04 |
| 0.0200 | 1.303E+01 | 3.901E−03 | 1.303E+01 | 8.662E−04 | 1.655E−04 |
| 0.0250 | 1.097E+01 | 3.913E−03 | 1.098E+01 | 1.286E−03 | 1.980E−04 |
| 0.0300 | 9.547E+00 | 3.924E−03 | 9.551E+00 | 1.776E−03 | 2.290E−04 |
| 0.0350 | 8.498E+00 | 3.934E−03 | 8.502E+00 | 2.332E−03 | 2.587E−04 |
| 0.0400 | 7.692E+00 | 3.946E−03 | 7.696E+00 | 2.951E−03 | 2.874E−04 |
| 0.0450 | 7.052E+00 | 3.959E−03 | 7.056E+00 | 3.631E−03 | 3.151E−04 |
| 0.0500 | 6.531E+00 | 3.973E−03 | 6.535E+00 | 4.368E−03 | 3.421E−04 |
| 0.0550 | 6.099E+00 | 3.988E−03 | 6.102E+00 | 5.160E−03 | 3.683E−04 |
| 0.0600 | 5.733E+00 | 4.004E−03 | 5.737E+00 | 6.006E−03 | 3.939E−04 |
| 0.0700 | 5.151E+00 | 4.040E−03 | 5.155E+00 | 7.848E−03 | 4.435E−04 |
| 0.0800 | 4.706E+00 | 4.079E−03 | 4.710E+00 | 9.881E−03 | 4.912E−04 |
| 0.0900 | 4.355E+00 | 4.122E−03 | 4.359E+00 | 1.209E−02 | 5.373E−04 |
| 0.1000 | 4.071E+00 | 4.168E−03 | 4.075E+00 | 1.447E−02 | 5.821E−04 |
| 0.1250 | 3.552E+00 | 4.294E−03 | 3.557E+00 | 2.106E−02 | 6.889E−04 |
| 0.1500 | 3.203E+00 | 4.431E−03 | 3.207E+00 | 2.848E−02 | 7.899E−04 |
| 0.1750 | 2.951E+00 | 4.579E−03 | 2.956E+00 | 3.662E−02 | 8.865E−04 |
| 0.2000 | 2.763E+00 | 4.734E−03 | 2.768E+00 | 4.537E−02 | 9.795E−04 |
| 0.2500 | 2.501E+00 | 5.070E−03 | 2.506E+00 | 6.442E−02 | 1.157E−03 |
| 0.3000 | 2.329E+00 | 5.438E−03 | 2.335E+00 | 8.513E−02 | 1.327E−03 |
| 0.3500 | 2.211E+00 | 5.832E−03 | 2.216E+00 | 1.071E−01 | 1.492E−03 |
| 0.4000 | 2.125E+00 | 6.252E−03 | 2.131E+00 | 1.302E−01 | 1.653E−03 |
| 0.4500 | 2.061E+00 | 6.694E−03 | 2.068E+00 | 1.540E−01 | 1.812E−03 |
| 0.5000 | 2.012E+00 | 7.158E−03 | 2.019E+00 | 1.785E−01 | 1.970E−03 |
| 0.5500 | 1.972E+00 | 7.642E−03 | 1.980E+00 | 2.035E−01 | 2.128E−03 |
| 0.6000 | 1.941E+00 | 8.141E−03 | 1.949E+00 | 2.290E−0I | 2.285E−03 |
| 0.7000 | 1.895E+00 | 9.186E−03 | 1.904E+00 | 2.809E−01 | 2.602E−03 |
| 0.8000 | 1.863E+00 | 1.028E−02 | 1.874E+00 | 3.339E−01 | 2.921E−03 |
| 0.9000 | 1.842E+00 | 1.143E−02 | 1.853E+00 | 3.876E−01 | 3.244E−03 |
| 1.0000 | 1.827E+00 | 1.262E−02 | 1.839E+00 | 4.418E−01 | 3.571E−03 |
| 1.2500 | 1.806E+00 | 1.578E−02 | 1.822E+00 | 5.784E−01 | 4.408E−03 |
| 1.5000 | 1.799E+00 | 1.916E−02 | 1.818E+00 | 7.158E−01 | 5.272E−03 |
| 1.7500 | 1.799E+00 | 2.271E−02 | 1.821E+00 | 8.532E−01 | 6.162E−03 |
| 2.0000 | 1.801E+00 | 2.642E−02 | 1.828E+00 | 9.903E−01 | 7.074E−03 |
| 2.5000 | 1.812E+00 | 3.421E−02 | 1.846E+00 | 1.263E+00 | 8.956E−03 |
| 3.0000 | 1.824E+00 | 4.241E−02 | 1.866E+00 | 1.532E+00 | 1.090E−02 |
| 3.5000 | 1.836E+00 | 5.095E−02 | 1.887E+00 | 1.798E+00 | 1.289E−02 |

$I = 75.3$ eV; density = 1.040E+00 g/cm$^3$
SOURCE: ICRU (1984).

fore is controlled not by the Coulomb fields but by interaction of the electric and magnetic field of the photon with the electron in the medium.

There are three modes of interaction with the medium.

**The Photoelectric Effect.** The photon interaction with an orbital electron in the medium is complete, and the full energy of the photon is given to the electron.

**The Compton Effect.** Part of the photon energy is transferred to an electron, and the photon scatters (usually at a small angle from its original path) (Evans, 1955) with reduced energy.

The governing expressions are

$$E' = E\,0.511/(1 + 1/a - \cos\Theta) \qquad (8)$$

$$T = E\,a\,(1 - \cos\Theta)/[1 + a(1 - \cos\Theta)]$$

where

$E, E'$ = initial and scattered photon energy in MeV
$T$ = kinetic energy of electron in MeV
$a$ = $E/0.511$
$\Theta$ = angle of photon scatter from its original path

**Pair Production.** Pair production occurs whenever the photon energy is greater than the rest mass of two electrons, 2(0.511 MeV) = 1.02 MeV. The electromagnetic energy of the photon can be converted directly to an electron-positron pair, with any excess energy above 1.02 MeV appearing as kinetic energy given to these particles.

The loss of photons and energy loss from a photon beam as it passes through matter are described by two coefficients. The attenuation coefficient determines the fractional loss of photons per unit distance (usually in normalized units of g/cm$^2$, which is the linear distance times the density of the medium). The mass energy absorption coefficient determines the fractional energy deposition per unit distance traveled. The loss of photons from the beam is given by

$$I/I_0 = \exp(-\mu/\rho\ d) \tag{9}$$

where

$I$ = intensity of photon beam (numbers of photons)
$I_0$ = beam intensity
$\mu/\rho$ = attenuation coefficient in medium for energy considered (in cm$^2$ g$^{-1}$)
$d$ = thickness of medium in g cm$^{-2}$ (thickness in cm $\times$ density)

The energy actually deposited in the medium per unit distance is given by

$$\Delta E = (\mu_{en}/\rho)E_0 \tag{10}$$

where

$\Delta E$ = energy loss in medium per unit distance (in MeV cm$^2$ g$^{-1}$)
$\mu_{en}/\rho$ = mass energy absorption coefficient (cm$^2$ g$^{-1}$)
$E_0$ = initial photon energy

Tables 25-3 and 25-4 give the attenuation coefficients for photons in air and the mass energy absorption coefficients for photons in air and in muscle tissue. Both tables are reproduced from Hubbell (1969).

# ABSORBED DOSE

## Dose and Dose Rate

Absorbed dose is defined as the mean energy, $e$, imparted by ionizing radiation to matter of mass $m$ (ICRU 1980)

$$D = e/m \tag{11}$$

where

$D$ = absorbed dose
$e$ = mean energy deposited in mass
$m$ = mass

The unit for absorbed dose is the Gray (Gy), which is equal to 1 J kg$^{-1}$. The older unit of dose is the rad, which is equal to 100 erg g$^{-1}$. The conversion for these units is 100 rad = 1 Gy.

For uncharged particles (gamma rays and neutrons), kerma is sometimes used. It is the sum of the initial kinetic energies of all the charged ionizing particles liberated in unit mass. The units of kerma are the same as those for dose.

Exposure often is confused with absorbed dose. Exposure is defined only in air for gamma rays or photons and is the charge of the ions of one sign when all electrons liberated by photons are completely stopped in air of mass $m$:

$$X = Q/m \tag{12}$$

where

$X$ = exposure
$Q$ = total charge of one sign
$m$ = mass of air

The unit of exposure is the Coulomb per kilogram of air. The older unit of exposure is the Roentgen, which is equal to $2.58 \times 10^{-4}$ C kg$^{-1}$ of air.

Exposure and dose are used interchangeably in some publications even though this is not correct. The reason is that the older numerical values of dose in rad and exposure in Roentgen are similar. Although they are similar numerically, they are fundamentally different in that exposure is ionization (only in air) and dose is absorbed energy in any specified medium:

1 Roentgen = 0.87 rad (in air)

The SI units are not numerically similar:

1 C kg$^{-1}$ = 33.85 Gy

Dose rate is the dose expressed per unit time interval. The dose rate delivered to the thyroid by $^{99m}$Tc for a nuclear medicine scan, for example, diminishes with time because of the 6.0-h half-life of the nuclide. The total dose is a more pertinent quantity in this case because it can be related directly to risk and compared with the benefit of the thyroid scan.

The dose rate from natural body $^{40}$K in all cells, by contrast, is relatively constant throughout life and usually is expressed as the annual dose rate.

## Equivalent Dose

The linear energy transfer (LET) from alpha and beta particles is much greater than it is for gamma rays. In considering the health or cellular effects of each particle or ray, it is convenient to normalize the various types of radiation. For a particular biological endpoint such as cell death in an experiment with mouse fibroblasts, it is common to calculate a relative biological effectiveness (RBE). This is defined as the ratio of the gamma dose to the dose from radiation under study which yields the same endpoint.

Such refinement in the normalization of endpoints (cancer) in the human is not possible with the available data. An attempt to normalize human health effects is made through the values for LET of the various types of radiation in water. The ratio of the LET for gamma to the radiation in question

**Table 25–3**
**Mass Attenuation Coefficients for Photons in Air**

| | SCATTERING | | | PAIR PRODUCTION | | TOTAL | |
|---|---|---|---|---|---|---|---|
| PHOTON ENERGY, MeV | *With Coherent,* $cm^2/g^{-1}$ | *Without Coherent,* $cm^2/g^{-1}$ | PHOTO ELECTRIC $cm^2/g^{-1}$ | *Nuclear Field,* $cm^2/g^{-1}$ | *Electron Field,* $cm^2/g^{-1}$ | *With Coherent,* $cm^2/g^{-1}$ | *Without Coherent* $cm^2/g^{-1}$ |
| 1.00−02 | 3.64−01 | 1.93−01 | 4.63+00 | | | 4.99+00 | 4.82+00 |
| 1.50−02 | 2.85−01 | 1.89−01 | 1.27+00 | | | 1.55+00 | 1.45+00 |
| 2.00−02 | 2.47−01 | 1.86−01 | 5.05−01 | | | 7.52−01 | 6.91−01 |
| 3.00−02 | 2.11−01 | 1.80−01 | 1.39−01 | | | 3.49−01 | 3.18−01 |
| 4.00−02 | 1.93−01 | 1.74−01 | 5.53−02 | | | 2.48−01 | 2.29−01 |
| 5.00−02 | 1.81−01 | 1.69−01 | 2.70−02 | | | 2.08−01 | 1.96−01 |
| 6.00−02 | 1.73−01 | 1.64−01 | 1.52−02 | | | 1.88−01 | 1.79−01 |
| 8.00−02 | 1.61−01 | 1.56−01 | 6.06−03 | | | 1.67−01 | 1.62−01 |
| 1.00−01 | 1.51−01 | 1.48−01 | 2.94−03 | | | 1.54−01 | 1.51−01 |
| 1.50−01 | 1.35−01 | 1.33−01 | 8.05−04 | | | 1.36−01 | 1.34−01 |
| 2.00−01 | 1.23−01 | 1.22−01 | 3.24−04 | | | 1.23−01 | 1.23−01 |
| 3.00−01 | 1.07−01 | 1.06−01 | 9.30−05 | | | 1.07−01 | 1.06−01 |
| 4.00−01 | 9.53−02 | 9.52−02 | 3.99−05 | | | 9.54−02 | 9.53−02 |
| 5.00−01 | 8.70−02 | 8.70−02 | 2.15−05 | | | 8.70−02 | 8.70−02 |
| 6.00−01 | 8.05−02 | 8.04−02 | 1.34−05 | | | 8.05−02 | 8.05−02 |
| 8.00−01 | | 7.07−02 | 6.79−06 | | | | 7.07−02 |
| 1.00+00 | | 6.36−02 | 4.20−06 | | | | 6.36−02 |
| 1.50+00 | | 5.17−02 | 1.96−06 | 9.89−05 | | | 5.18−02 |
| 2.00+00 | | 4.41−02 | 1.25−06 | 3.94−04 | | | 4.45−02 |
| 3.00+00 | | 3.47−02 | 6.97−07 | 1.13−03 | 1.21−05 | | 3.58−02 |
| 4.00+00 | | 2.89−02 | 4.73−07 | 1.83−03 | 4.97−05 | | 3.08−02 |
| 5.00+00 | | 2.50−02 | 3.61−07 | 2.46−03 | 9.76−05 | | 2.75−02 |
| 6.00+00 | | 2.21−02 | 2.88−07 | 3.01−03 | 1.50−04 | | 2.52−02 |
| 8.00+00 | | 1.81−02 | 2.06−07 | 3.94−03 | 2.57−04 | | 2.23−02 |
| 1.00+01 | | 1.54−02 | 1.61−07 | 4.70−03 | 3.51−04 | | 2.04−02 |
| 1.50+01 | | 1.14−02 | | 6.14−03 | 5.47−04 | | 1.81−02 |
| 2.00+01 | | 9.14−03 | | 7.18−03 | 7.02−04 | | 1.70−02 |
| 3.00+01 | | 6.65−03 | | 8.65−03 | 9.35−04 | | 1.62−02 |
| 4.00+01 | | 5.28−03 | | 9.67−03 | 1.11−03 | | 1.61−02 |
| 5.00+01 | | 4.41−03 | | 1.04−02 | 1.24−03 | | 1.61−02 |
| 6.00+01 | | 3.80−03 | | 1.11−02 | 1.36−03 | | 1.62−02 |
| 8.00+01 | | 3.00−03 | | 1.20−02 | 1.53−03 | | 1.65−02 |
| 1.00+02 | | 2.55−03 | | 1.26−02 | 1.65−03 | | 1.68−02 |
| 1.50+02 | | 1.77−03 | | 1.38−02 | 1.87−03 | | 1.74−02 |
| 2.00+02 | | 1.39−03 | | 1.45−02 | 2.02−03 | | 1.79−02 |
| 3.00+02 | | 9.85−04 | | 1.53−02 | 2.22−03 | | 1.85−02 |
| 4.00+02 | | 7.71−04 | | 1.58−02 | 2.34−03 | | 1.89−02 |
| 5.00+02 | | 6.38−04 | | 1.61−02 | 2.43−03 | | 1.92−02 |
| 6.00+02 | | 5.47−04 | | 1.63−02 | 2.50−03 | | 1.94−02 |
| 8.00+02 | | 4.27−04 | | 1.67−02 | 2.60−03 | | 1.97−02 |
| 1.00+03 | | 3.51−04 | | 1.69−02 | 2.67−03 | | 1.99−02 |
| 1.50+03 | | 2.45−04 | | 1.72−02 | 2.79−03 | | 2.02−02 |
| 2.00+03 | | 1.90−04 | | 1.73−02 | 2.86−03 | | 2.04−02 |
| 3.00+03 | | 1.32−04 | | 1.75−02 | 2.95−03 | | 2.06−02 |
| 4.00+03 | | 1.02−04 | | 1.76−02 | 2.99−03 | | 2.07−02 |
| 5.00+03 | | 8.33−05 | | 1.77−02 | 3.02−03 | | 2.08−02 |

**Table 25–3**
**Mass Attenuation Coefficients for Photons in Air (*Continued*)**

| | SCATTERING | | | PAIR PRODUCTION | | TOTAL | |
|---|---|---|---|---|---|---|---|
| PHOTON ENERGY, MeV | *With Coherent,* $cm^2/g^{-1}$ | *Without Coherent,* $cm^2/g^{-1}$ | PHOTO ELECTRIC $cm^2/g^{-1}$ | *Nuclear Field,* $cm^2/g^{-1}$ | *Electron Field,* $cm^2/g^{-1}$ | *With Coherent,* $cm^2/g^{-1}$ | *Without Coherent* $cm^2/g^{-1}$ |
| 6.00+03 | | 7.07−05 | | 1.77−02 | 3.05−03 | | 2.08−02 |
| 8.00+03 | | 5.44−05 | | 1.78−02 | 3.08−03 | | 2.09−02 |
| 1.00+04 | | 4.44−05 | | 1.78−02 | 3.10−03 | | 2.09−02 |
| 1.50+04 | | 3.07−05 | | 1.78−02 | 3.12−03 | | 2.10−02 |
| 2.00+04 | | 2.36−05 | | 1.79−02 | 3.14−03 | | 2.12−02 |
| 3.00+04 | | 1.63−05 | | 1.79−02 | 3.15−03 | | 2.11−02 |
| 4.00+04 | | 1.25−05 | | 1.79−02 | 3.16−03 | | 2.11−02 |
| 5.00+04 | | 1.02−05 | | 1.79−02 | 3.17−03 | | 2.11−02 |
| 6.00+04 | | 8.60−06 | | 1.79−02 | 3.17−03 | | 2.11−02 |
| 8.00+04 | | 6.60−06 | | 1.79−02 | 3.18−03 | | 2.11−02 |
| 1.00+05 | | 5.37−06 | | 1.79−02 | 3.18−03 | | 2.11−02 |

SOURCE: From Hubbell (1969).

is defined as a radiation weighting factor, $W_r$ (formerly Q), and the normalized dose is called the equivalent dose. The unit for the equivalent dose is the Sievert, and the older unit is the rem:

$$H = DW_r \tag{13}$$

where

$H$ = equivalent dose in Sievert (older unit rem)
$D$ = dose in Gray (older unit rad)
$W_r$ = radiation weighting factor

Table 25-5 is reproduced from NCRP (1987) and ICRP (1990).

***Example 3.*** Find the equivalent dose (in Sievert) for a dose to lung from an internal emitter of 0.01-Gy alpha particles and 0.01 Gy from external gamma-ray radiation.

alpha $H = 0.01\ (20) = 0.20$ Sv
gamma $H = 0.01\ (1) = 0.01$ Sv

**Table 25–4**
**Mass Energy Absorption Coefficients for Air and Water**

| PHOTON ENERGY, MeV | AIR $\mu_{en}/\rho$ $m^2\ kg^{-1}$ | MUSCLE, STRIATED (ICRU) $\mu_{en}/\rho$, $m^2\ kg^{-1}$ |
|---|---|---|
| 0.01 | 0.46 | 0.49 |
| 0.015 | 0.13 | 0.14 |
| 0.02 | 0.052 | 0.055 |
| 0.03 | 0.015 | 0.016 |
| 0.04 | 0.0067 | 0.0070 |
| 0.05 | 0.0040 | 0.0043 |
| 0.06 | 0.0030 | 0.0032 |
| 0.08 | 0.0024 | 0.0026 |
| 0.10 | 0.0023 | 0.0025 |
| 0.15 | 0.0025 | 0.0027 |
| 0.20 | 0.0027 | 0.0029 |
| 0.30 | 0.0029 | 0.0032 |
| 0.40 | 0.0029 | 0.0032 |
| 0.50 | 0.0030 | 0.0033 |
| 0.60 | 0.0030 | 0.0033 |
| 0.80 | 0.0029 | 0.0032 |
| 1.00 | 0.0028 | 0.0031 |
| 1.50 | 0.0025 | 0.0028 |
| 2.00 | 0.0023 | 0.0026 |
| 3.00 | 0.0021 | 0.0023 |

SOURCE: From Hubbell (1982).

## Effective Dose and Cancer Risk

The term "effective dose" (ED) (formerly effective dose equivalent) was introduced formally by ICRP in 1977 to allow one to add or directly compare the cancer and genetic risk from different partial-body or whole-body doses. A partial-body dose to the lung, for example, is thought to give 0.0064 cancers

**Table 25–5**
**Recommended Values of $W_r$ for Various Types of Radiation**

| TYPE OF RADIATION | APPROXIMATE $W_r$ |
|---|---|
| X-rays, gamma rays, beta particles, and electrons | 1 |
| Thermal neutrons | 5 |
| Neutrons (other than thermal >100 kev to 2 Mev), protons, alpha particles, charged particles of unknown energy | 20 |

SOURCE: NCRP (1987) and ICRP (1990).

over a lifetime per Sievert, whereas a whole-body dose would result in 0.056 total cancers and early genetic effects over the same lifetime interval. The ratio 0.0064/0.056 was defined as a tissue weighting factor, $w_t$, for lung and is numerically equal to 0.12.

The effective dose, $H_E$, is defined as

$$H_E = w_t D W_r \tag{14}$$

This concept is useful in the case of occupational exposure because $H_E$ values from different sources can be simply summed to yield a direct estimate of total cancer and genetic risk.

Table 25-6 is taken from ICRP (1990) and gives the values of $w_t$ for various organs.

The occupational guideline for $H_E$ is 20 mSv per annum (NCRP, 1987; ICRP, 1990). This requires that the sum of all $H_E$ be less than or equal to this value:

$$H_E = \Sigma w_t H \leq 20 \text{ mSv} \tag{15}$$

In 1990, the International Commission on Radiation Protection (ICRP) revised its 1977 estimates of risk and adopted and published Publication 60. This document includes new estimates of risk for both fatal and nonfatal cancer and new guidelines for the exposure of workers to external and internal radiation. The risk estimates are based largely on the analysis of Japanese A-bomb survivors. The occupational guidelines for radiation protection developed from the 1990 document are 100 mSv in 5 years (average, 20 mSv per year) with a limit of 50 mSv in any single year. This is compared with the 1977 limit of 50 mSv per year.

**Table 25–6**
**Recommended Values of the Weighting Factors, $w_t$, for Calculating Effective Dose**

| TISSUE OR ORGAN | TISSUE WEIGHTING FACTOR, $w_T$ |
|---|---|
| Gonads | 0.20 |
| Bone marrow (red) | 0.12 |
| Colon | 0.12 |
| Lung | 0.12 |
| Stomach | 0.12 |
| Bladder | 0.05 |
| Breast | 0.05 |
| Liver | 0.05 |
| Esophagus | 0.05 |
| Thyroid | 0.05 |
| Skin | 0.01 |
| Bone surface | 0.01 |
| Remainder | 0.05*† |

*Note*: The values have been developed from a reference population of equal numbers of both sexes and a wide range of ages. In the definition of effective dose they apply to workers, to the whole population, and to either sex.

* For purposes of calculation, the remainder is composed of the following additional tissues and organs: adrenals, brain, upper large intestine, small intestine, kidney, muscle, pancreas, spleen, thymus, and uterus. The list includes organs which are likely to be selectively irradiated. Some organs in the list are known to be susceptible to cancer induction. If other tissues and organs subsequently become identified as having a significant risk of induced cancer, they will then be included either with a specific $w_T$ or in this additional list constituting the remainder. The latter also may include other tissues or organs selectively irradiated.

† In exceptional cases in which a single one of the remainder tissues or organs receives an equivalent dose in excess of the highest dose in any of the 12 organs for which a weighting factor is specified, a weighting factor of 0.025 should be applied to that tissue or organ and a weighting factor of 0.025 should be applied to the average dose in the rest of the remainder as defined above.

The ICRP document (ICRP, 1990) is a response to the increase in cancer risk from ionizing radiation observed in atom bomb survivors. Mental retardation is a recent finding in the atom bomb survivor cohort and is now included in the risk estimates. There are no conclusive data from A-bomb survivors on cancer in the thyroid, bone, liver, and skin from external radiation. Therefore, the risks to these tissues are developed from other epidemiological studies discussed in this chapter.

The overall risk per unit exposure for adult workers and the risk for the whole population given in the draft document are shown in Table 25-7. The risk of fatal cancer is adopted as 0.04 per Sievert (4 percent per Sievert) for adult workers and 0.05 per Sievert (5 percent per Sievert) for the whole adult population.

ICRP had been criticized for excluding the effects of nonfatal cancer in previous documents. An attempt to correct this omission was made in ICRP 60 (1990). An attempt was made to calculate the total detriment and is given the notation "aggregated detriment." The aggregated detriment is the product of four factors: the probability of attributable fatal cancer, the weighted probability of nonfatal cancer, the weighted probability of severe hereditary effects, and the relative length of life lost.

The nominal probability of fatal cancer per Sievert, *F*, and the aggregated detriment are shown in Table 25-7. The computation of the aggregated detriment proceeds as follows. A cancer lethality fraction, *K* (the fraction of total cancer that is lethal), is used as a weighting factor for nonfatal cancers. The total number of cancers (fatal plus nonfatal) $Sv^{-1}$ will be *F/K*. The total number of nonfatal cancers is $(1 - K)F/K$. The total weighted detriment is then

$$F + K(1 - K)F/K = F(2 - K)$$

The aggregated detriment is then the product of $F(2 - K)$ times the relative length of life lost, $l/l_{av}$, for a particular cancer. The average length of life lost, $l_{av}$, is 15 years per cancer. The aggregated detriment is tabulated as 7.3 $Sv^{-1}$ for the whole adult population and 5.6 $Sv^{-1}$ for the working population.

In assessing radiation risk from low-dose, low-dose-rate, low-LET radiation using risk coefficients derived from high-dose, high-dose-rate exposures, a dose rate reduction factor (DREF) needs to be applied. NCRP (1980) and UNSCEAR (1988, 1993) have shown that the human data cover a range for the DREF of 2 to 10. That is, the original risk coefficients derived from the high-dose data are divided by the DREF factor to obtain the best estimate of effects at typical low-dose exposures. ICRP has used 2.5 as the adopted DREF; however, in ICRP (1990) a DREF of 2.0 was used, and this is incorporated in the nominal probability coefficients in Table 25-7. The overall objective of both NCRP and ICRP dose limitation recommendations is to control the lifetime risk to maximally exposed individuals. ICRP (1990) limits the lifetime occupational effective dose to (20 mSv × 50 years) = 1000 mSv. In 1993, NCRP (1993) reduced the U.S. Recommendation for Lifetime Exposure to (age × 10 mSv) or approximately 700 mSv, with an annual limit of 50 mSv.

**Table 25–7**
**Nominal Probability Coefficients for Individual Tissues and Organs**

| | PROBABILITY OF FATAL CANCER, $10^{-2}$ $Sv^{-1}$ | | AGGREGATED DETRIMENT, $10^{-2}$ $Sv^{-1}$ | |
|---|---|---|---|---|
| TISSUE OR ORGAN | WHOLE POPULATION | WORKERS | WHOLE POPULATION | WORKERS |
| Bladder | 0.30 | 0.24 | 0.29 | 0.24 |
| Bone marrow | 0.50 | 0.40 | 1.04 | 0.83 |
| Bone surface | 0.05 | 0.04 | 0.07 | 0.06 |
| Breast | 0.20 | 0.16 | 0.36 | 0.29 |
| Colon | 0.85 | 0.68 | 1.03 | 0.82 |
| Liver | 0.15 | 0.12 | 0.16 | 0.13 |
| Lung | 0.85 | 0.68 | 0.80 | 0.64 |
| Esophagus | 0.30 | 0.24 | 0.24 | 0.19 |
| Ovary | 0.10 | 0.08 | 0.15 | 0.12 |
| Skin | 0.02 | 0.02 | 0.04 | 0.03 |
| Stomach | 1.10 | 0.88 | 1.00 | 0.80 |
| Thyroid | 0.08 | 0.06 | 0.15 | 0.12 |
| Remainder | 0.50 | 0.40 | 0.59 | 0.47 |
| Total | 5.00 | 4.00 | 5.92 | 4.74 |
| | PROBABILITY OF SEVERE HEREDITARY DISORDERS | | | |
| Gonads | 1.00 | 0.6 | 1.33 | 0.80 |
| Grand total (rounded) | | | 7.3 | 5.6 |

*Note*: The values relate to a population of equal numbers of both sexes and a wide range of ages.
SOURCE: ICRP (1990).

## Committed Equivalent Dose

A problem arises with internal emitters in that once they are ingested, there is an irreversible dose that is committed because of the biokinetics of the particular element. The absorbed dose depends on the biological and physical half-times of the element in the body. For this reason, the concepts of committed equivalent dose and committed effective dose were derived to accommodate the potential for dose to be delivered over long periods after incorporation in the body. The committed dose is taken over a 50-year interval after exposure and is equal to

$$H_{T,50} = \int_{t_0}^{t_0+50} H_T dt \qquad (16)$$

where

$H_{T,50}$ = 50-year dose to tissue $T$ for a single intake at time $t_0$
$H_T$ = equivalent dose rate in organ or tissue $T$ at time $t$

NCRP (1987, 1993) recognizes that for radionuclides with half-lives ranging up to about 3 months the committed equivalent dose is equal to the annual dose for the year of intake. For longer-lived nuclides the committed equivalent dose will be greater than the annual equivalent dose and must be calculated on an individual basis. ICRP Publication 30 (ICRP, 1978) provides the details of this calculation for all nuclides.

## Negligible Individual Risk Level

The current radiobiological principle commonly accepted is that of linear, nonthreshold cancer induction from ionizing radiation. Thus, regardless of the magnitude of the dose, a numerical cancer risk can be calculated. For this reason, the National Council on Radiation Protection and Measurements proposed the Negligible Individual Risk Level (NIRL) and defined it as

> a level of annual excess risk of fatal health effects attributable to irradiation below which further effort to reduce radiation exposure to the individual is unwarranted.

NCRP emphasized that the NIRL is not to be confused with an acceptable risk level, a level of significance, or a limit.

The NCRP recommended an annual effective equivalent dose limit for continuous exposure of members of the public of 1 mSv (0.1 rem). This value is in addition to that received from natural background radiation (about 2 mSv). In this context, the NIRL was taken to be 0.01 mSv (1 mrem). In NCRP (1993) the notation used currently is Negligible Individual Dose (NID).

# HUMAN STUDIES OF RADIATION TOXICITY

There have been five major studies of the health detriment resulting from exposure of humans to ionizing radiation.

Other studies of large worker populations exposed to very low levels of radiation and environmental populations exposed to radon are ongoing, but they are not expected to provide new data on the risk estimates from ionizing radiation. These worker or environmental populations are studied to ensure that there is no inconsistency in the radiation risk data in extrapolating from the higher exposures.

The basic studies on which the quantitative risk calculations are founded include radium exposures, atom bomb survivors, underground miners exposed to radon, patients irradiated with x-rays for ankylosing spondylitis, and children irradiated with x-rays for tinea capitis (ringworm).

## Radium Exposures ($^{226,228}Ra$)

Radium was discovered in the early part of the twentieth century. Its unique properties suggested a potential for the healing arts. It was incorporated into a wide variety of nostrums, medicines, and artifacts. The highest exposure occurred in the United States among radium dial painters who ingested from 10s to 1000s of micrograms (microcuries). These exposed groups, including patients, chemists, and dial painters, have been studied for over 60 years to determine the body retention of radium and the health effects of long-term body burdens.

The only late effect of ingestion of $^{226,228}Ra$ seen is osteogenic sarcoma. It is significant that no study has identified a statistically significant excess of leukemia after even massive doses of radium. This implies that the target cells for leukemia residing in bone marrow are outside the short range of the radium series alpha particles (70 $\mu$m).

Several thousand people were exposed to radium salts either as part of the modish therapies using radium in the era from 1900 to 1930 or occupationally in the radium dial-painting industry around 1920. Radium therapy was accepted by the American Medical Association, and in around 1915 advertisements were common for radium treatment of rheumatism and as a general tonic and in the treatment of mental disorders. Solutions were available for drinking containing 2 $\mu$g/60 cm$^3$ as well as ampoules for intravenous injection containing 5 to 100 $\mu$g radium (Woodard, 1980). Luminous paint was developed before World War I, and in 1917 there were many plants in New England and New Jersey painting watch dials, clocks, and military instruments (Woodard, 1980).

The first large studies on osteogenic sarcoma in radium-exposed people were done by Martland (1931) and Aub and associates (1952), who found 30 cases of bone sarcoma; Evans and associates (1969) with 496 cases of sarcoma out of 1064 studied at the Massachusetts Institute of Technology; and Rowland et al. (1978), 61 cases out of 1474 female dial painters (Woodard 1980).

Radium, once ingested, is somewhat similar to calcium in its metabolism and is incorporated on bone surfaces into the mineralized portion of bone. The long half-life of $^{226}Ra$ allows distribution throughout the mineral skeleton over life. The target cells for osteogenic sarcoma reside in marrow on endosteal surfaces at about 10 $\mu$m from the bone surface. At long times after exposure, target cells are beyond the range of alpha particles from radium not on bone surfaces.

The loss of radium from the body by excretion was determined to follow a relatively simple power function (Norris et al., 1955):

$$R = 0.54\, t^{-0.52} \tag{17}$$

where

$R$ = total body retention
$t$ = time in days

Other models to fit the data were developed as more information became available, the most recent being that of Marshall et al. (1972). The entire body of radium data and the various models are shown in Figure 25-1. It can be seen that the Norris function fits the observed data well except at very long times

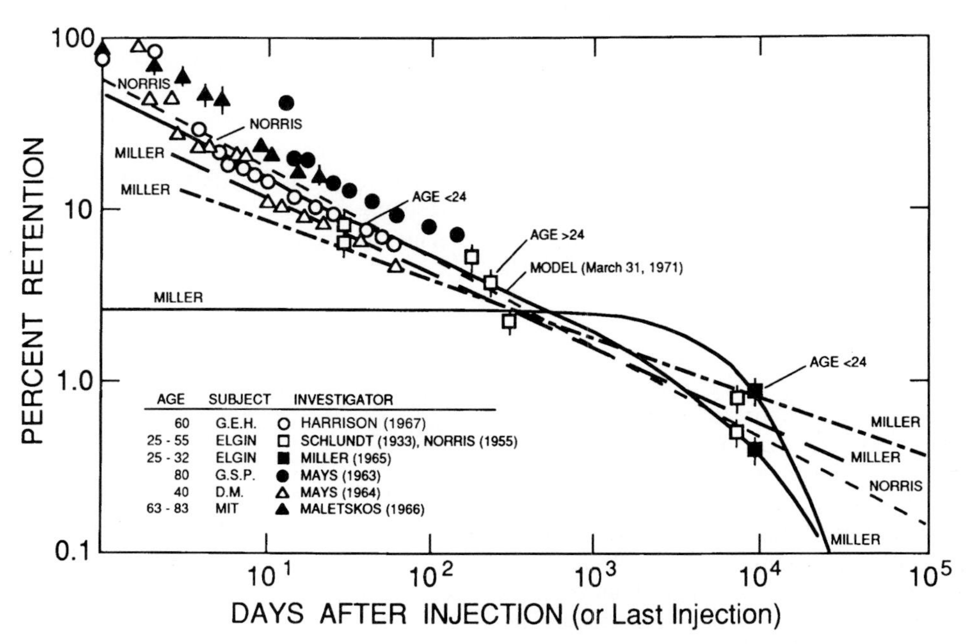


***Figure 25–1.*** *Whole-body radium retention in humans. Summary of all available data for adult humans. [From Marshall et al. (1972).]*

after exposure. A simplified form of the more complex later model of Marshal and associates (1972) which fits the human data over all observed times is

$$R = 0.8t^{-0.5}\,(0.5e^{-\lambda t} + 0.5e^{-4\lambda t}) \tag{18}$$

where

$R$ = whole body retention
$\lambda$ = rate of bone apposition or resorption = 0.0001 day$^{-1}$
$t$ = time in days

For most purposes, the Norris formula is applicable. It can be seen from Figure 25-1 for the Norris equation that even 1 year after exposure, only about 2 percent of the radium is retained in the body but that after 30 years, about 0.5 percent still remains.

The risk of osteogenic bone cancer after radium exposure has been summarized in the National Academy of Sciences Report BEIR IV (NAS, 1988).

Equations were proposed by Rowland and coworkers (1978) for the annual risk of sarcoma (including the natural risk) expressed as a function of either radium intake or dose from $^{226,228}$Ra. Risk per unit intake:

$$I = [0.7 \times 10^{-5} + (7 \times 10^{-8})D^2]\exp[-(1.1 \times 10^{-3})D] \tag{19}$$

where

$I$ = total bone sarcomas per person year at risk
$D$ = total systemic intake of $^{226}$Ra plus 2.5 times total systemic intake of $^{228}$Ra, both in microcuries

Risk per unit dose:

$$I = [10^{-5} + 9.8 \times 10^{-6}D^2]\exp(-1.5 \times 10^{-2}D) \tag{20}$$

where

$I$ = total bone sarcomas per person year at risk
$D$ = total mean skeletal dose in Gray from $^{226}$Ra plus 1.5 times mean skeletal dose from $^{228}$Ra

Raabe and associates (1980) modeled bone sarcoma risk in the human, dog, and mouse and determined that there is a practical threshold dose and dose rate (a dose low enough so that bone cancer will not appear within the human life span). The dose rate is 0.04 Gy per day or a total dose of 0.8 Gy to the skeleton. This practical threshold for bone cancer has useful implications in considering health effects from exposures to environmental radioactivity.

## Radium Exposure ($^{224}$Ra)

In Europe, $^{224}$Ra was used for more than 40 years in the treatment of tuberculosis and ankylosing spondylitis. The treatment of children was abandoned in the 1950s, but the ability to relieve debilitating pain from ankylosing spondylitis in adults has prolonged its use. $^{224}$Ra is different from $^{226}$Ra in that it has a short half-life (3.62 days) and the alpha dose is delivered completely while the radium is still on bone surfaces.

Spiess and Mays (1970) and Mays (1988) studied the health of 900 German patients given $^{224}$Ra therapeutically. The calculated average mean skeletal dose was 4.2 Gy (range, 0.06 to 57.5 Gy) with injection time spans ranging from 1 to 45 months. There were two groups—juveniles and adults—and the bone sarcoma response was not significantly different for the two. There were 54 patients who developed bone sarcoma, the last one in 1983.

In a second cohort, Wick and colleagues (1986) studied 1432 adult patients treated for ankylosing spondylitis with an average skeletal dose of 0.65 Gy. This study was originally started by Otto Hug and Fritz Schales and has been continued since their deaths. Two patients in this group have developed osteogenic sarcoma, with none in the control group.

Spiess and Mays (1973) found that the observed effectiveness of the $^{224}$Ra in their cohort in producing bone sarcomas increased if the time span of the injections was long. Injections were given in 1, 10, or 50 weekly fractions. They developed an empirical expression to estimate the added risk from this protracted injection schedule:

$$I = \{0.003 + 0.014\,[1 - \exp(0.09m)]D \tag{21}$$

where

$I$ = cumulative incidence of bone sarcomas after most tumors have appeared (25 years)
$m$ = span of injections in months
$D$ = average skeletal dose in Gy

Chemelevsky and coworkers (1986) analyzed the Spiess data and developed an equation for the total cumulative sarcoma risk from $^{224}$Ra:

$$R = (0.0085D + 0.0017D^2)\exp(-0.025D) \tag{22}$$

where

$R$ = cumulative risk of bone sarcoma
$D$ = average skeletal dose in Gy

These two equations for risk predict 5.7 and 5.8 bone sarcomas in the second series of (spondylitis) patients, with 2 actually observed.

Chemelevsky and coworkers (1986) also showed that in the Spiess study, linearity (sarcoma response with dose) could be rejected. For example, equation 22 results in a lifetime risk of sarcoma of 0.02 Gy$^{-1}$ at an average skeletal dose of 10 Gy but 0.01 Gy$^{-1}$ at 1 Gy. Also, there was no difference in sarcoma response between juveniles and adults. These data are presented in Figure 25-2.

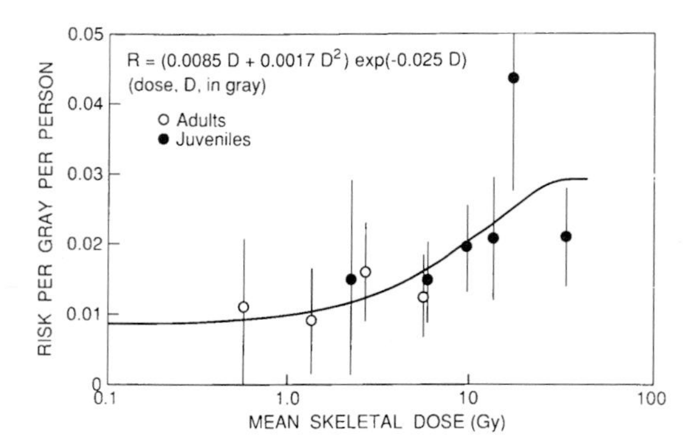


***Figure 25–2. Lifetime risk per Gray versus mean skeletal dose in $^{224}$Ra-exposed subjects. [From Chemelevsky et al. (1986).]***

Again, no excess leukemia was found in either series of $^{224}Ra$ patients.

## Atomic Bomb Survivors

On August 6, 1945, the U.S. military dropped an atomic bomb on the city of Hiroshima, Japan. Three days later a second bomb was dropped on Nagasaki which effectively ended World War II. The weapons were of two different types, the first being $^{235}U$ and the second a $^{239}Pu$ device.

Within 1 km of the explosions in both cities, a total of 64,000 people were killed by the blast and the thermal effects and as a result of the instantaneous gamma and neutron radiation released by the weapons. Others between 1 and 2 km away received radiation doses up to several Gray.

Within a few years it was decided to follow the health of the people in both cities over their lifetime to determine quantitatively the effects of external ionizing radiation.

The study of prospective mortality of atom bomb survivors was initiated by the Atomic Bomb Casualty Commission (ABCC) in 1950 and is ongoing by the Radiation Effects Research Foundation (RERF). The main study, called the Life Span Study (LSS), included 92,228 people within 10,000 m of the hypocenter (the point on earth directly below the detonation point in air) and 26,850 people who were not in either city at the time of bombing (ATB). The most recent report of the RERF (1987) is a follow-up of the cancer mortality of a subcohort (DS86 subcohort) of 75,991 persons over the period 1950–1985.

In 1978, questions arose that the original dose estimates for persons in the LSS might be somewhat in error and that an effort should be made to improve the dose estimates. This study is now complete, and the dosimetry was published in a United States–Japan joint reassessment of dose called DS86—Dosimetry System 1986 (RERF, 1987).

Dose estimation by reconstruction of the event is always problematic, but direct computation of dose to about 18,500 persons in the LSS with detailed shielding information is complete. The remaining DS86 dose values for 57,000 individuals without detailed shielding information are also incorporated into the mortality study by various estimation techniques. Of the 75,991 persons in the DS86 subcohort, 16,207 were within 2000 m of the hypocenter, and these are the individuals who received a substantial exposure.

Previous reports of cancer risk estimates were based on the air dose (gamma ray plus neutron tissue kerma in air) adjusted for shielding by structures or terrain. The 1987 and 1988 reports also include DS86 organ dose estimates, and these are about 80 percent of the shielded kerma (Shimizu et al., 1988).

The dose from fallout at Hiroshima and Nagasaki has not been included in the health effects studies. Fallout was found in certain restricted localities in Nagasaki and Hiroshima. The absorbed dose from gamma rays at Nagasaki for persons continuously in the fallout area from 1 h on ranged from 0.12 to 0.24 Gy. The absorbed doses at Hiroshima ranged from 0.006 to 0.02 Gy. Because the region of fallout was quite limited, it would appear that the total contribution of fallout to survivor dose was probably negligible in Hiroshima but may have been significant for a limited number of survivors in Nagasaki, where an exposure of one-fifth the maximum extends over some 1000 hectares. Estimates of internal dose from ingested $^{137}Cs$ yield about 0.0001 Gy integrated over 40 years (Harley, 1987; RERF, 1987).

Complete mortality data and the dose estimates are reported in RERF Technical Reports 5-88 (RERF, 1988), and so it is possible to calculate the lifetime cancer risk as of the follow-up through 1985. This is done for this chapter in Table 25-8. The dose used in the calculation is the shielded kerma dose so that it is more comparable with the older publications. The organ dose estimates are about 80 percent of the shielded

**Table 25–8**
**Cancer Mortality and Lifetime Cancer Risk at Selected Sites for Atom Bomb Survivors with Average Shielded Kerma of 0.295 Gy**

| SITE | NUMBER OF SUBJECTS* (0.01+) Gy | TOTAL CANCER MORTALITY* | ATTRIBUTABLE RISK, %† | RADIATION CANCERS | LIFETIME‡ RISK ($Gy^{-1}$) |
|---|---|---|---|---|---|
| All sites | 41,719 | 3435 | 10.4 | 357 | 0.029 |
| All sites (except leukemia) | 41,719 | 3291 | 8.0 | 265 | 0.022 |
| Leukemia | 40,701 | 144 | 56.6 | 81 | 0.0067 |
| Multiple myeloma | (40,701)§ | 23 | 32.9 | 8 | 0.0007 |
| Colon | 39,859 | 129 | 15.2 | 20 | 0.0017 |
| Esophagus | (39,859)§ | 93 | 12.8 | 12 | 0.0010 |
| Lung | 40,382 | 385 | 11.6 | 45 | 0.0038 |
| Stomach | 39,961 | 1153 | 6.4 | 74 | 0.0063 |
| Female breast | 25,252 | 98 | 22.4 | 22 | 0.0029 |
| Bladder | 40,060 | 84 | 23.4 | 20 | 0.0017 |
| Ovary | 24,581 | 51 | 18.6 | 9 | 0.0012 |

*Note*: Average organ dose equivalent in Sievert is essentially identical to shielded air dose in Gray. See text.

* From RERF Report TR-12-87 Part 1, Tables 2 and 3 (Shimizu et al., 1987).

† From RERF Report TR-12-87 Part 1, Table 6. Attributable risk is the percentage of cancer deaths caused by radiation.

‡ Lifetime risk $Gy^{-1}$ is calculated as (radiation cancers)/(number of subjects) (average dose).

§ Estimated as the leukemia or colon population.

kerma dose, and so the risk estimates would increase by about 20 percent if organ dose were utilized (Shimizu et al., 1988). However, when the organ dose equivalent is calculated, the organ dose equivalent in Sievert is almost identical to the organ dose in Gray. This is due to the small neutron component in the DS86 dosimetry (about 1 percent of the organ gamma-ray dose). When multiplied by a value of 20 for $Q$, the neutron dose increases the total organ dose equivalent by 20 percent.

No statistically significant excess cancer of the gallbladder, pancreas, uterus, or prostate or of malignant lymphoma has been seen in the LSS to date.

The calculations shown in Table 25-8 indicate that the increase in risk is due to differences between the older dose and the DS86 estimates as well as the added number of cancers observed since the previous update in the mortality studies. The leukemia risk is about a factor of 3 higher than that projected by ICRP in 1977, and the lung cancer risk is about a factor of 2 higher.

It is of interest to consider the effects of smoking as it is the most important factor in assessing lung cancer risk. The analysis performed by Shimuzu and associates (1988) examined the interaction of smoking and radiation in detail. The results showed no interaction indicating that smoking and the atom bomb radiation act independently rather than multiplicatively in lung cancer induction.

It is also possible to model the risk over the full life if a projection model is assumed. RERF has preferred a constant relative risk model (radiation mortality is a constant fraction of the baseline age-specific mortality per Gray) for this purpose. There is evidence in the atom bomb mortality and in several other studies discussed later (ankylosing spondylitis patients, uranium miners) that the constant relative risk model is not appropriate but that the risk coefficient decreases with time subsequent to exposure. In most cases this also means that the absolute excess cancer risk (risk above that expected) declines with time. This is a biologically plausible model suggesting the loss or repair of the damaged stem cell population.

The National Academy of Sciences BEIR V Committee (NAS, 1990) utilized the atom bomb mortality data through 1985 and the DS86 dosimetry to model the lifetime risk of all cancer, leukemia, female breast cancer, respiratory cancer, and digestive cancer. The expressions for respiratory, breast, and digestive cancer all include a term for reduction in relative risk with time since exposure. For example, the model for respiratory cancer is

$$\gamma(d) = \gamma_0 \,[1 + f(d)\, g(\beta)] \tag{23}$$

where

$\gamma(d)$ = an individual's age-specific lung cancer risk for dose $d$
$\gamma_0$ = age-specific background risk of death due to lung cancer
$f(d)$ = 0.636 × (dose in Gray)
$g(\beta)$ = $\exp[-1.437 \ln(T/20) + 0.711\, I(S)]$
$T$ = years after exposure
$I(S)$ = 1 if female, 0 if male

The integration of this model yields a lifetime risk of respiratory cancer in males of 0.002, 0.0124, and 0.039 for exposure to 1 Gray at ages 5, 25, and 55, or a risk of 0.019 for a stationary male population with U.S. mortality rates. Given the existing risk in the Japanese cohort of 0.0038 $Gy^{-1}$, the BEIR V lifetime risk estimate is clearly conservative.

The lifetime risk of cancer from exposure to atom bomb radiation estimated by the National Academy of Sciences BEIR V Committee is 4 times that of the BEIR III Committee values (NAS, 1980). This difference is due partly to more complete follow-up of the population and the difference in the new DS86 dosimetry but primarily to the models used for risk expression after exposure. Given the small number of radiation-induced cancers in the Japanese population studied, the models cannot be derived with a high degree of certainty.

The estimates of lifetime risk of cancer will undoubtedly increase somewhat with time, but given the present age of the population, the final values are unlikely to be higher than the values in Table 25-7 that are based on the models of ICRP (1990).

## Tinea Capitis (Ringworm) Irradiation

During the period 1905–1960, x-ray epilation in the treatment of tinea capitis was performed regularly in children. The treatment was introduced by Sabouraud in 1904 and was standardized by Kienbock (1907) and Adamson (1909). Over the half century it was used, as many as 200,000 children worldwide may have been irradiated (Albert et al., 1986).

No follow-up studies of the long-term effects of irradiation were performed until Albert and Omran (1968) reported on 2200 children irradiated at the Skin and Cancer Unit of New York University Hospital during 1940–1959. Subsequent publications on this group have appeared at regular intervals (Shore et al., 1976, 1984).

Since the New York University (NYU) study, a follow-up of 11,000 children irradiated in Israel was performed (Ron and Modan, 1984).

The mean age of children irradiated in both the New York and Israeli studies was between 7 and 8 years. Dose reconstruction in the NYU series was performed using a head phantom containing the skull of a 7-year-old child covered with tissue-equivalent material (Schulz and Albert, 1963; Harley et al., 1976, 1983). The doses to organs in the head and neck for a typical Adamson-Kienbock five-field treatment of the scalp

**Table 25–9**
**Average Dose to Organs in the Head and Neck from Measurements Performed with a Phantom for a Child's Head**

| ORGAN | AVERAGE DOSE AT 25 CM TREATMENT DISTANCE, rad |
|---|---|
| Scalp | 220–540 |
| Brain | 140 |
| Eye | 16 |
| Internal ear | 71 |
| Cranial marrow | 385 |
| Pituitary | 49 |
| Parotid gland | 39 |
| Thyroid | 6 |
| Skin (eyelid) | 16 |
| Skin (nose) | 11 |
| Skin (midneck) | 9 |

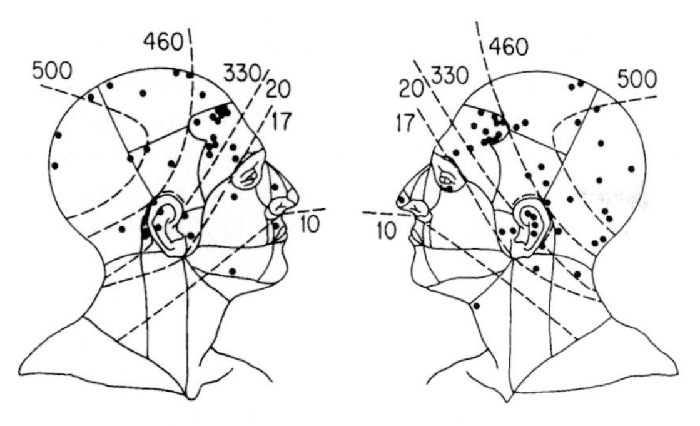


*Figure 25–3. X-ray dose in rads for the Adamson-Kienbock five-field tinea capitis treatment and locations of basal cell lesions. [From Shore et al. (1984).]*

are shown in Table 25-9, and the dose to the skin is shown in Fig. 25-3.

In the NYU series there were eight thyroid adenomas and no thyroid cancers. In the Israeli series there were 29 thyroid cancers. In the NYU series there are 80 skin lesions, predominantly basal cell carcinoma, in 41 persons. Lightness of skin is an important factor in the appearance of skin cancer (Shore et al., 1984). Skin cancer was found only in whites even though 25 percent of the study population consisted of blacks. This and the fact that there appears to be a much lower dose response on the hair-covered scalp than on the face and neck (Harley et al., 1983) suggest that the promotional effects of UV radiation play an important role in skin cancer.

A summary of the tumors of the head and neck and hematopoietic/lymphoietic tumors for the NYU studies is shown in Table 25-10 and for the Israeli studies in Table 25-11. In the Israeli study the estimate of the dose to the thyroid is 0.09 Gy compared with 0.06 Gy in the NYU study.

**Table 25–10**
**Tumors in the New York University Series of Childhood Irradiations for Tinea Capitis**

| TUMOR | IRRADIATED CASES | CONTROL CASES |
|---|---|---|
| Neurogenic | | |
| Brain | 6 | 0 |
| Acoustic neuroma | 2 | 0 |
| Neck | 2 | 0 |
| Parotid | | |
| Skin | 4 | |
| Basal cell | 41 | 3 |
| Cylindroma | 4 | 0 |
| Other | 3 | 2 |
| Bone (skull/jaw) | 4 | 0 |
| Mouth/larynx | | |
| Papilloma | 7 | 2 |
| Thyroid adenoma | | |
| Male | 3 | 0 |
| Female | 5 | 0 |
| Hematopoietic | | |
| Lymphopoietic | | |
| Leukemia | 4 | 1 |
| Hodgkin's disease | 5 | 2 |
| Other lymphoma | 2 | 0 |

**Table 25–11**
**Tumors in the Israeli Study by Sex**

| TUMOR | IRRADIATED CASES | CONTROL CASES |
|---|---|---|
| Leukemia | | |
| Male | 6 | 4 |
| Female | 4 | 1 |
| Thyroid malignancies | | |
| Male | 6 | 1 |
| Female | 23 | 5 |
| CNS (malignant/benign) | | |
| Male | 21 | 3 |
| Female | 9 | 0 |

SOURCE: From Ron and Modan (1984).

Iodine-131 is given medically in three ways. Very large quantities (about 100 mCi or $3.7 \times 10^9$ Bq) are administered to ablate the thyroid in thyroid cancer, lesser quantities (about 10 mCi or $3.7 \times 10^8$ Bq) are given for hyperthyroidism, and the lowest quantity is given (0.1 mCi or $3.7 \times 10^6$) for diagnostic purposes (UNSCEAR, 1993). Individuals have also been exposed to $^{131}$I as a result of nuclear weapons testing, and nuclear power plants have discharged $^{131}$I into the air after accidents.

Very few thyroid cancers have been found subsequent to these exposures, with the exception of the 243 Marshall Island inhabitants who received a large dose from a mixture of radionuclides ($^{131}$I, $^{132}$I, $^{133}$I, $^{134}$I, and $^{135}$I), tellurium, and gamma-ray radiation from the 1954 Bravo thermonuclear test (Conard, 1984). The mean thyroid dose was estimated as 3 to 52 Gy in children and 1.6 to 12 Gy in adults. Over a 32-year follow-up period, 7 of 130 women and 2 of 113 men developed thyroid cancer.

Attempts have been made to relate external gamma-ray radiation and $^{131}$I exposure. The National Council on Radiation Protection and Measurements (NCRP, 1985) estimated from human data that the effectiveness ratio of $^{131}$I/gamma-ray radiation is between 0.1 and 1.0. In a more recent review of the human data, Shore (1992) found 8.3 observed excess cancers derived from all $^{131}$I studies and 37 cases expected on the basis risk of estimates from external exposure. The ratio 8.3/37 yields an estimate for the effectiveness ratio of 0.224. The protracted dose to the thyroid during the decay of $^{131}$I may explain the difference; however, the nonuniform distribution of $^{131}$I in the thyroid also may be a factor (Sinclair et al., 1956).

Iodine-131 can expose large populations after nuclear weapons testing or nuclear accidents. Generally, it is the ingestion pathway that is most significant. Iodine is transferred quickly from surface deposition to the cow, to milk, and to the thyroid. A large body of data exists on the transfer coefficients, $P_{24}$ (intake to the body per unit deposition), $P_{45}$ (effective dose per unit intake), and $P_{25}$ ($P_{25} = P_{24} \times P_{45}$ = effective dose per unit deposition).

UNSCEAR (1993) reported the transfer coefficients for $^{131}$I to be

$P_{24} = 0.07$ Bq per Bq m$^{-2}$
$P_{45} = 61$ nSv per Bq intake (effective dose for the thyroid)
$P_{25} = P_{24} \times P_{45} = 4.2$ nSv per Bq m$^{-2}$ (effective dose for the thyroid)

A risk projection model was used to estimate the lifetime risk of basal cell carcinoma (BCC) for facial skin and for the hair-covered scalp after x-ray epilation in whites. The model used was a cumulative hazard plot which assumes that the BCC appearance rate in the exposed population remains constant over time (Harley et al., 1983). The result of this risk projection for BCC is shown in Table 25-12.

The small numbers of tumors other than skin cancers in the NYU study make it of dubious value in estimating the lifetime risk per Gy although a clear excess is appearing. The tinea capitis studies are prospective, and sound numerical values should be forthcoming as these populations age. These are particularly important studies because children were the exposed group and because only partial body irradiation was involved. The temporal pattern of appearance of these tumors is also important. The dose was delivered over a short time interval (minutes at NYU and 5 days in Israel), and lifetime patterns will be indicative of the underlying carcinogenic mechanisms.

Skin and thyroid cancers are of importance in documenting health effects from ionizing radiation. However, both types of cancer are rarely fatal. NCRP (1985) reported that about 10 percent of thyroid cancer is lethal. It is estimated that the fatality rate of skin cancer is 1 percent (NCRP, 1990). The lifetime risk per Gray derived by NCRP for total thyroid cancer incidence (0.003 for females and 0.0014 for males for external x-ray or gamma radiation for persons under 18 years of age) is about a factor of 10 lower than that reported by Ron and Modan in tinea capitis irradiations. However, the tinea irradiations were given to children with a mean age of about 7 years, and in the Israeli study there is apparently an increased sensitivity resulting from ethnicity.

The effect of ethnicity and sex is also suggested by NCRP (1985) for thyroid cancer. The incidence rates of spontaneous thyroid cancer for persons of Jewish origin in Europe and North America is three to four times that for other racial groups. There is an obvious susceptibility of women for thyroid cancer and adenomas in both the NYU and Israeli tinea capitis studies.

## Ankylosing Spondylitis

About 14,000 persons, mostly men, were treated with x-rays for ankylosing spondylitis at 87 radiotherapy centers in Great Britain and Northern Ireland between 1935 and 1954. Court Brown and Doll (1957) were the first to report that these patients had a leukemia risk substantially in excess of that for the general population. Subsequent publications have developed the time pattern of appearance not only of leukemia but also of solid tumors (Court Brown and Doll, 1959, 1965; Smith and Doll, 1978, 1982; Smith, 1984; Darby et al., 1985, 1987; Weiss et al., 1994).

**Table 25–12**
**Lifetime Risk Estimates for Basal Cell Carcinoma (BCC) and Thyroid Cancer after X-Ray Irradiation for Tinea Capitis**

| | TOTAL INCIDENCE, Risk $Gy^{-1}$ | MORTALITY, Risk $Gy^{-1}$ |
|---|---|---|
| Skin malignancies (NYU study) | | |
| BCC (facial skin) | 0.32 | |
| BCC (hair-covered scalp) | 0.01 | |
| Thyroid malignancies (Israeli study) | | |
| Male | 0.01 | 0.001 |
| Female | 0.04 | 0.004 |

A group was selected consisting of 11,776 men and 2335 women all of whom had been treated with x-rays either once or twice. About half the total group received a second x-ray treatment or treatment with thorium. The reports on the ankylosing spondylitis patients attempt to consider health effects from only the first x-ray treatment. For this reason, an individual receiving a second treatment is included in their follow-up only until 18 months after the second course (a short enough time so that any malignancies in this interval cannot be ascribed to the second x-ray treatment).

The appearance of excess leukemia is now well documented, and solid tumors are also apparent in the population. The part of the body in the direct x-ray beam (spine) received the highest dose, but it is thought that other sites received substantial radiation from scatter or from the beam itself.

The importance of this study lies in the health effects of partial body exposure and in the temporal pattern of appearance of solid tumors in irradiated adults. Smith and Doll (1978, 1982) and Darby et al. (1985, 1987) in the most recent follow-up publications concerning these patients have shown that the excess risk for solid tumors diminishes with time since exposure, with maximum appearance 5 to 20 years after exposure. This has significant implications for risk projection modeling. Many projection models assume a constant rate of appearance either as an absolute number of tumors per person per unit exposure (constant absolute risk) or as a fraction of the baseline age-specific cancer mortality rate (constant relative risk). The emerging pattern is that constant risk models, either absolute or relative, are not correct for certain cancers, such as lung cancer. Thirty-five years after the first treatment, excess lung cancer had completely disappeared.

The dosimetry was redone in 1988 (Lewis et al., 1988), and although better estimates of dose are now available, it is still the dose which is most uncertain for the cohort. No details about the x-ray machines used to deliver the exposures, such as output, kilovoltage, and half-value layer, are reported.

The excess cancers and the estimate of lifetime cancer risk at three sites in the ankylosing spondylitis cohort are shown in Table 25-13. For the purpose of calculating lifetime risks as of the time of follow-up, the number of persons used here as the individuals at risk is the number actually receiving only one x-ray treatment (6158). This assumes that those followed for 18 months after the second treatment do not contribute significantly to the malignancies.

The relatively low risk for leukemia (compared with atom bomb survivors) has been suggested to be due to cell sterilization at the high dose delivered. It is also possible that the low risk is due to partial irradiation of the skeletal red marrow. The volume of bone marrow irradiated in the spine, rib, and pelvis is much less than 50 percent of that in whole body irradiation.

The deaths resulting from causes other than neoplasms in the total cohort are about 30 percent higher than expected.

**Table 25–13**
**Excess Cancer in 6158 Ankylosing Spondylitis Patients Given a Single X-Ray Treatment as of the Last Follow-Up**

| SITE | OBS | EXP | DOSE, Gy* | LIFETIME, Risk $Gy^{-1}$ |
|---|---|---|---|---|
| Leukemia | 31 | 6.5 | 2.9 | 0.0011 |
| Lung† | 101 | 69.5 | 1.8–6.8‡ | 0.0008–0.0028 |
| Esophagus | 28 | 12.7 | 4.2 | 0.0006 |

* The doses are taken from Lewis and colleagues (1988).
† Lung cancer appearing less than 5 years after exposure is not included as this is less than the minimum latency for tumor expression.
‡ The doses to the pulmonary lung and main bronchi were estimated as 1.8 Gy and 6.8 Gy, respectively. The majority of lung cancer is bronchogenic, and the dose estimates for the main bronchi are probably most pertinent.

This higher total mortality is of significance in risk modeling as the premature deaths resulting from competing causes decrease the observed fractional cancer mortality. Thus, the lifetime risk in this population probably underestimates the risk when projecting the effects of exposure in a healthy population.

## Uranium Miners

Radon is ubiquitous on earth. It is found outdoors and in all dwellings as a result of the decay of the parent $^{226}$Ra, which is present in all of earth's minerals.

Although the risk of developing lung cancer from radon exposure among underground miners is firmly documented and quantitative risk estimates are available, the current interest lies in whether this risk carries over into environmental situations. Radon levels in homes that are comparable to those in mines surely confer risks to the residents. The question remains, Can the risks in mines for exposures at higher concentrations over short time periods be used to model risks at lower environmental levels over a lifetime?

**Underground Mines.** There are 11 large studies of underground miners exposed to high concentrations of radon and radon daughters, and the documentation of excess lung cancer is convincing (NCRP, 1984; NAS, 1988; NIH, 1994). The carcinogen in the case of radon is actually the alpha-emitting short-lived daughters of radon, $^{218}$Po and $^{214}$Po. The decay scheme for the entire uranium series, including radon and the daughter species, is shown in Fig. 25-4. The daughters are solids and are deposited on the bronchial airways during inhalation and exhalation according to the laws of diffusion. As the airway lining (bronchial epithelium) is only 40 $\mu$m thick, the alpha particles emitted are able to reach and transfer a significant amount of energy to all the cells implicated in lung cancer induction. Although the daughters are the carcinogen, the term "radon" will be used interchangeably for "radon daughters," because without the parent radon, the daughters could not exist for longer than a few hours. The measurements in mines were usually of the daughter species rather than radon, and the term "working level" (WL) was defined for occupational exposure. It indicated the total potential energy content in 1 liter of air for complete decay of the short-lived daugh-

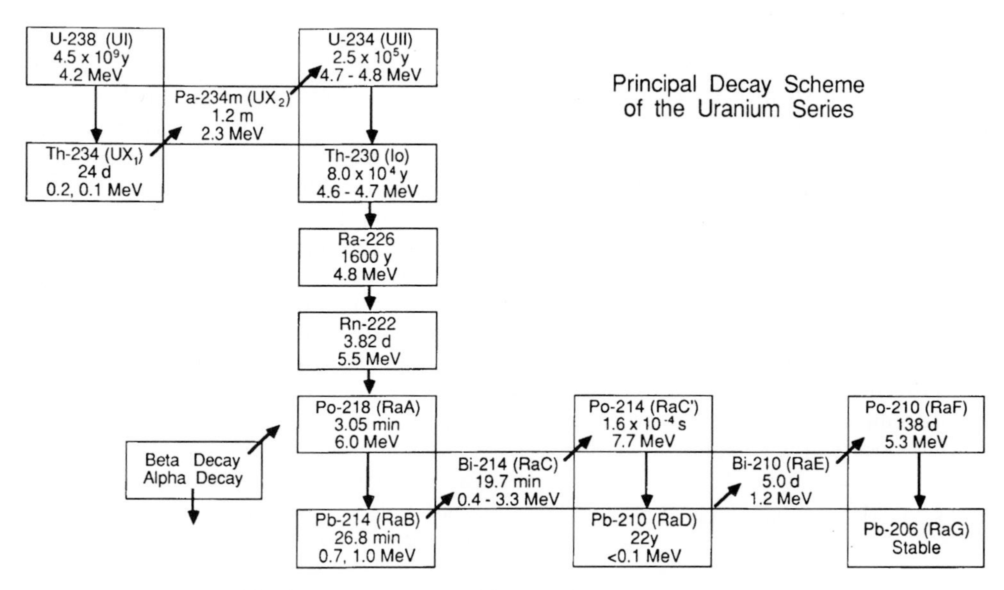


*Figure 25–4. Uranium-238 decay series. [From NCRP (1987).]*

ters.* The exposure attributed to miners was developed in working level months (WLMs), which is the numerical value of WL times the time exposed in multiples of a working month of 170 h (Holaday et al., 1957).

The follow-up studies from 11 large underground mining cohorts in Australia, Canada, Czechoslovakia, France, Sweden, and the United States have all produced data that show that the excess lung cancer risk from exposure to radon is about 1 to 3 per 10,000 persons per WLM exposure (Radford and Renard, 1984; Hornung and Meinhardt, 1987; Sevc et al., 1988; Muller et al., 1989; Howe et al., 1986, 1987; Tirmarche et al., 1993; Woodward et al., 1991; NIH, 1994). Expressed in another way, radon exposure increases the normal age-specific lung cancer risk by about 0.5 percent for each WLM exposure. This way of expressing risk leads to the thought that many epidemiologists prefer, that the lung cancer risk is proportional to the normal baseline risk. This means, for example, that the lifetime excess lung cancer risk from radon is different for smokers and nonsmokers (NAS, 1988; NIH, 1994).

The actual data from the underground studies are not clear-cut with regard to the effect of smoking, and it is apparent from more recent analyses that radon exposure does not simply multiply the baseline risks of the population by a constant factor. This is discussed in the section on risk. The excess lung cancer risk in each of the exposure cohorts for the 11 major mining populations as of the date of the last published follow-up are summarized in Fig. 25-5. It can be seen in the figure that the range of risks for the same exposure varies by about a factor of 3 among the different studies. The differences are probably accounted for by errors in measuring and estimating total exposure. However, the Czech mine atmosphere contained arsenic as well as radon, and the arsenic contributed to the excess lung cancers observed. A maximum value of 50 percent lung cancer risk is the highest value ever observed in a mining population and was reported in mines in Saxony at the turn of the century (Muller, 1989). These mines are thought to have had about 100,000 Bq m$^{-3}$ of radon. It is noteworthy that concentrations this high have been reported in a few homes in the United States. In Fig. 25-5, the lowest (well-documented) exposures were in the Ontario mines, and a mean exposure of 35 WLM has given an excess lung cancer risk of about 1 percent to date.

To date, the most comprehensive epidemiological analysis of underground miners exposed to high concentrations of $^{222}$Rn is a joint analysis of 11 underground mining studies conducted by the National Cancer Institute (NIH, 1994). This study encompassed the Chinese, Czechoslovakian, Colorado, Ontario, Newfoundland, Swedish, New Mexico, Beaverlodge, Port Radium, Radium Hill, and French mining data. Any effect of $^{222}$Rn in the environment is obscured because of the typical lower exposure rate and the large numbers of lung cancers caused by smoking. In mines, the average concentration can be thousands of Bq m$^{-3}$ compared with less than 100 Bq m$^{-3}$ in a typical domestic environment. The occupational exposure in mines is relatively short compared with that in the full life in homes. The cumulative exposure in mines, however, is generally many times that in homes. Thus, some detail can be determined by describing the response to $^{222}$Rn exposure. The Joint Analysis (NIH, 1994) focused on 10 variables:

*One working level is any combination of short-lived daughters in 1 liter of air that will result in 1.3 × 10$^5$ MeV of alpha energy when complete decay occurs. One working level is approximately equal to concentrations of 7400 Bq m$^{-3}$ (200 pCi/liter) of radon in a home and 11000 Bq m$^{-3}$ (300 pCi/liter) in a mine.

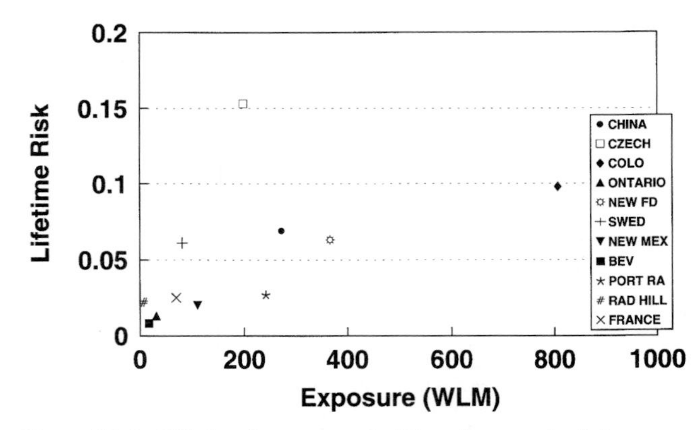


*Figure 25–5. Lifetime lung cancer in 11 underground mining populations as a function of radon exposure in WLM. (Derived from NIH, 1994.)*

1. The estimation of excess relative risk per working level month (ERR/WLM) and the form of the exposure response
2. The variation of ERR/WLM with attained age
3. The variation of ERR/WLM with duration of exposure, considering total exposure as well as exposure rate
4. The variation of ERR/WLM with age at first exposure
5. The variation of ERR/WLM as a function of time after exposure ceased
6. The evaluation of an optimal exposure lag interval, that is, the interval before lung cancer death during which $^{222}$Rn exposure has no effect
7. The consistency among the 11 cohorts
8. The joint effect of smoking and $^{222}$Rn exposure
9. The role of exposure to other airborne contaminants in mines
10. The direct modeling of the relative risk of lung cancer with duration and rate of exposure

Figure 25-6 shows the relative risk of lung cancer for all 11 cohorts combined; Fig. 25-7, for those groups with exposures below 400 WLM.

The pooled cohorts included 2620 lung cancer deaths among 60,570 exposed miners accumulating 1.2 million person years of observation. The excess relative risk of lung cancer is seen in Fig. 25-6 to be linearly related to the cumulative radon decay product exposure in units of WLM. The exception is at the highest exposures, where a clear reduction in excess relative risk is evident. This is often noted as an "inverse dose rate effect." Confusion exists concerning the inverse dose rate effect in that the relative risk is not *higher at lower dose rates* but is *lower at higher dose rates*, suggestive of cell killing and removal of damaged cells from the pool of cells that are potential sites of malignant transformation.

Data on tobacco use were available in six of the cohorts. The ERR/WLM was not found to be related to age at first exposure in this analysis. The joint effect of smoking and $^{222}$Rn exposure did not show a clear pattern except that the risk was consistent with a relationship that was intermediate between additive and multiplicative.

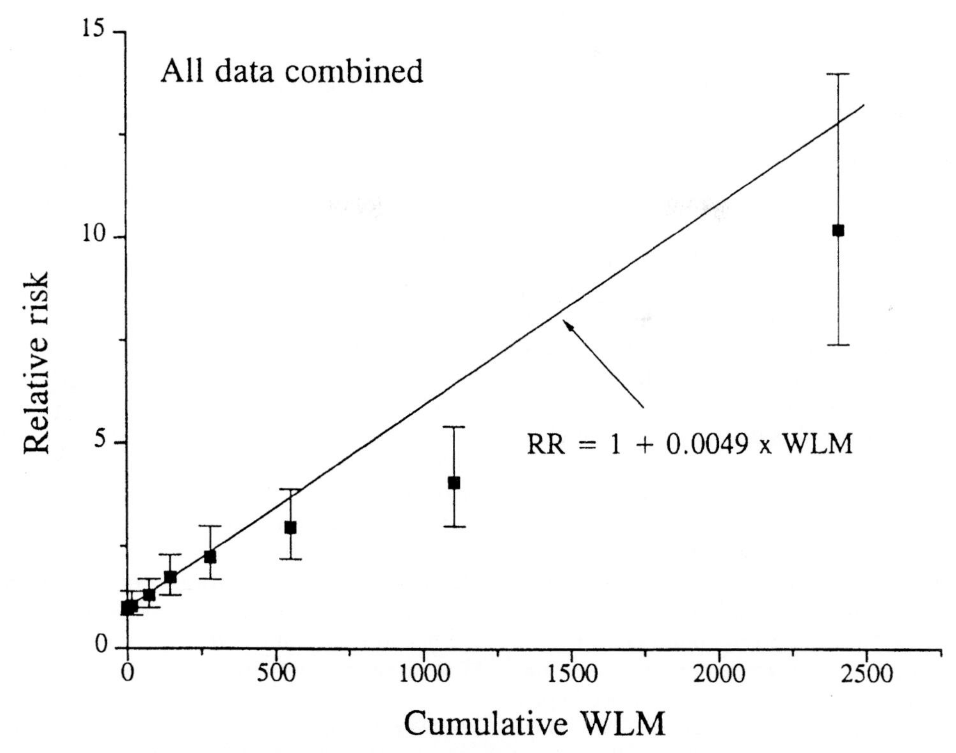


***Figure 25–6. Relative risk (RR) of lung cancer by cumulative WLM and fitted linear excess RR model for each cohort and for all data combined.***

RRs plotted at mean WLM for category. When the referent category for RRs is not zero exposure, a fitted exposure-response line is adjusted to pass through the mean of the referent category. For the China, Ontario, and Beaverlodge cohorts, the excess RR model was fitted with a free intercept. [From NIH (1994).]

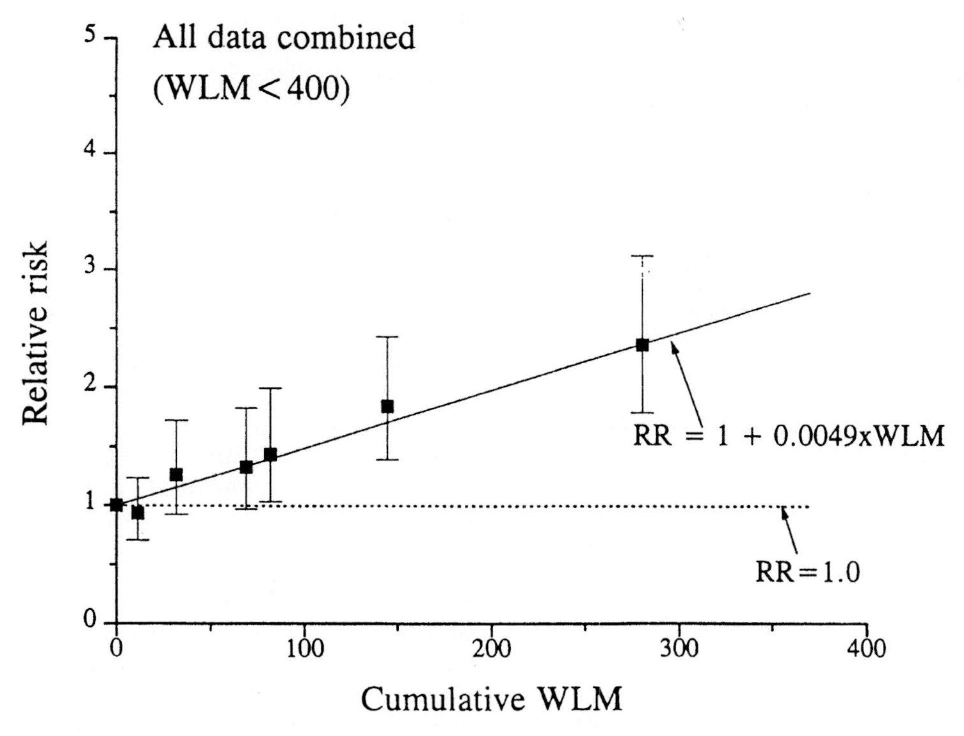


***Figure 25–7. Relative risk (RR) of lung cancer by cumulative WLM and fitted linear excess RR model for each cohort and for all data combined (WLM < 400).***

RRs plotted at mean WLM for category. When the referent category for RRs is not zero exposure, a fitted exposure-response line is adjusted to pass through the mean of the referent category. For the China, Ontario, and Beaverlodge cohorts, the excess RR model was fitted with a free intercept. [From NIH (1994).]

When radon gas decays to its solid decay products, some 8 to 15 percent of the $^{218}Po$ atoms do not attach to the normal aerosol particles. This ultrafine species (unattached fraction) is deposited with 100 percent efficiency on the upper bronchial airways. In mines the unattached fraction is low (4 to 5 percent) because of the normal aerosol loading. The rest of the decay products attach to the ambient aerosol of about 100-nm average diameter (George and Breslin, 1980) and only a few percent of this aerosol is deposited on these airways. Measurements in mines have mostly involved the short-lived radon daughters, as they are the easiest to measure rapidly. The alpha dose from radon gas itself is very low in comparison with that from the daughters, as the daughters deposit and accumulate on the airway surfaces.

The first few branching airways of the bronchial tree are the region where almost all the lung cancers appear. This is true in general, not only for miners exposed to radon daughters.

The alpha dose from radon daughters therefore must be calculated in these airways, not in the pulmonary or gas exchange regions. Although the dose to the pulmonary region should not be neglected, it is about 15 percent of that to the airways. Several calculations regarding the absorbed alpha dose exist for radon daughters (NCRP, 1984; ICRP, 1987; Harley, 1987, 1989; NRC, 1991). The authors make different assumptions about the atmospheric and biological parameters that go into the dose calculation, and this can cause discrepancies among the models. The most significant variables are the particle size of the ambient aerosol, the assumed breathing rate, and the target cells considered.

Very small particles deposit more efficiently in the airways, and so if small particles, such as from open flame burning (Tu and Knutson, 1988), contribute to the atmosphere, the dose delivered to the bronchial epithelium can be higher per unit WLM exposure than is the dose predicted from an average particle size. Conversely, a hygroscopic particle can increase in size in the humid environment of the bronchial airways, and deposition will be diminished. The particle size of the aerosol in mines is somewhat larger than that for environmental conditions (200 to perhaps 600 nm versus 100 nm) (George et al., 1975). Figure 25-8 shows the alpha dose per unit exposure as it is related to the variables (particle size, unattached fraction, breathing rate) known to affect dose.

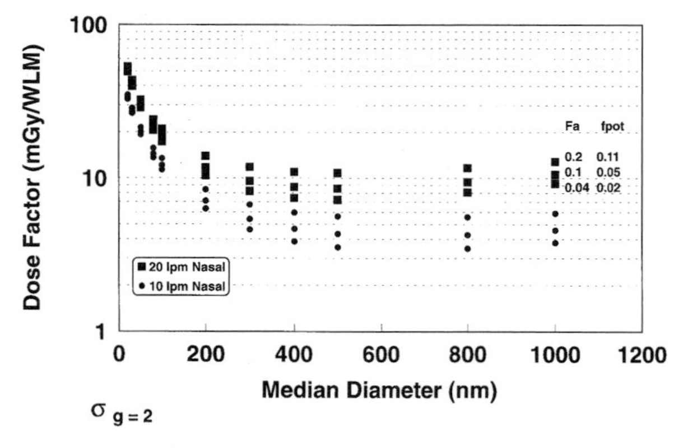


***Figure 25–8. Radon decay product bronchial dose as a function of inhaled aerosol diameter, breathing rate, and unattached fraction. [Breathing rates from Ruzer et al. (1995); target cells from Robbins and Meyers (1995).]***

As carcinogenesis is related to absorbed alpha dose, Fig. 25-8 shows that particle size is an important determinant of risk. The average dose per unit exposure in WLM for miners in Fig. 25-8 is about the same as that for average environmental conditions, assuming 100 nm aerosol in homes and 200 to 600 nm aerosol in mines.

Radon can deliver a greater or lesser carcinogenic potential by about a factor of 2 over the range of realistic indoor conditions (average particle size ranging from 80 to 300 nm). The allowable effective dose for continuous exposure of the population in the United States is 1 mSv/year (100 mrem/year) (NCRP, 1993). This limit would be delivered by exposure to 10 Bq $m^{-3}$ of radon, or one-quarter the actual average measured indoor concentration in most countries where measurements have been made. Thus, the guidelines for exposure cannot be set in the usual way from dosimetric considerations.

**Lifetime Environmental Lung Cancer Risk Projections.** There are at present four sets of publications that provide risk projection calculations for exposure to radon daughters. The following sections describe each in detail.

***National Council on Radiation Protection and Measurements.*** In 1984, the U.S. National Council on Radiation Protection and Measurements (NCRP, 1984) developed a model to project the risk derived from miner studies to whole-life risk in the environment. It is a modified absolute risk model that reduces the risk subsequent to exposure with a half-life of 20 years. Risk is not accumulated until after age 40, the time when lung cancer normally appears in the population. There is no indication that early exposure produces any significant shift to younger ages, even for young miners exposed at significantly higher concentrations. This model was the first to incorporate a time since exposure reduction in risk.

***National Academy of Sciences.*** The National Academy of Sciences report in 1988 (BEIR IV) developed a model based on examination of the raw data from five mining cohorts (NAS, 1988). The data indicated that the highest risk appears from 5 to 15 years after exposure. After 15 years, the risk is one-half that of the 5- to 15-year risk (per unit exposure), and this risk was assumed to persist to the end of life. Again, no significant risk appears before 40, the usual age for the appearance of lung cancer. The NAS model also included a correction for attained age (at age 65, the risk is 0.4 of that for ages 55 to 64). The BEIR IV Committee assumed a relative risk model (risk is proportional to the normal age-specific lung cancer risk per unit radon exposure), but with risk dependent on time from exposure. This was the first modified relative risk model. This means that the risk for smokers and nonsmokers differs because of their different baseline lung cancer values. Although the miners' epidemiology did not support this strictly multiplicative relationship, the NAS chose the relative risk model as a conservative one. Its analysis supported the risk reduction subsequent to exposure by using a two-step risk reduction window.

***ICRP.*** The International Commission on Radiation Protection (ICRP, 1987) developed two risk projection models; one was based on a constant relative risk, and the other was a constant absolute risk model. Although neither risk model is correct because of the temporal reduction pattern of lung cancer subsequent to the cessation of exposure, the numerical values obtained for the lifetime risk of lung cancer from radon exposure are not significantly different from those in other models. Later follow-up of the Czechoslovakian underground uranium miners presented by Kunz and Sevc (1988) indicates that the excess lung cancer risk may actually be reduced to zero 35 years after exposure. If this factor were included in the NAS model (zero risk after 35 years), it would reduce those values by about a factor of 2. The risk values obtained from the three models are shown in Table 25-14. In 1993, ICRP simply adopted a lifetime lung cancer fatality coefficient of $3 \times 10^{-4}$ per WLM.

***Joint Analysis of 11 Underground Mining Cohorts.*** The pooled analysis from the 11 underground mining cohorts was used to develop two models for full life risk projection. The models are similar to the model used by the NAS (1988), utilizing time since exposure reduction and reduction with attained age. Three time windows for reduction of risk with time since exposure are used instead of two. Also, an additional parameter is incorporated; one model decreases the risk with increasing exposure rate, and the other decreases the risk with decreasing exposure duration. The lifetime domestic risk for lifetime exposure to unit concentration was not reported. However, the ratio of the relative risk of lung cancer for the BEIR IV and Joint Analysis model was given as 0.9 for continuous exposure to 4 pCi $l^{-1}$ (1 WLM/year) for the model incorporating exposure duration as a parameter. The Joint Analysis estimated that there are 15,000 lung cancer deaths in the United States attributable to $^{222}$Rn: 10,000 in smokers and 5000 in those who have never smoked.

**Environmental Epidemiology.** There are at least 22 published studies that attempt to define or detect the effect of radon exposure in the environment. They have been summarized by Borak and Johnson (1988), Neuberger (1989, 1992), and Samet and associates (1991). One recent study in the United States was performed in 1989 by the New Jersey Department of Health (NJDOH) (Schoenberg and Klotz, 1989; Schoenberg et al., 1990). This is a case-control study of women, 433 lung cancer cases and 402 controls with yearlong measurements of radon in the homes where the individuals lived for 10 or more years. This study devoted considerable effort to quality control concerning the exposure measurements. The results of this study are slightly positive, suggesting an association of radon and lung cancer even at concentrations of 80 Bq $m^{-3}$, but the results are not statistically significant. A case-control study of 538 nonsmoking women (1183 controls) in Missouri with an average exposure of 70 Bq $m^{-3}$ also showed no statistically significant increase in lung cancer (Alavanja et al., 1994).

The largest case-control study to date concerning the effects of residential $^{222}$Rn exposure was conducted nationwide in 109 municipalities in Sweden. It included all subjects 35 to 74 years old who had lived in one of the 109 municipalities at some time between January 1980 and December 31, 1984, and who had been living in Sweden on January 1, 1947. Fifty-six of the municipalities were known to have elevated $^{222}$Rn concentrations on the basis of earlier measurements.

Thus, an attempt was made to study a large group of persons living in a known area of greater than average $^{222}$Rn and to estimate their exposure over a large fraction of life (34 years). The primary aim of the study was to narrow the uncertainty in the estimation of lung cancer risk.

The environmental epidemiological studies conducted before this study suffered from the small numbers of persons observed and relatively low $^{222}$Rn exposures. For this reason, although the risk in underground miners was clearly seen, the outcome regarding the lung cancer risk from residential exposure has been ambiguous. All the existing domestic studies, including the measurement protocols, have been reviewed (Neuberger, 1992, 1994; Samet, 1989; Samet et al., 1991, 1989; Lubin et al., 1990).

Pershagen and coworkers (1994) included 586 women and 774 men with lung cancer diagnosed between 1980 and 1984. For a comparison control population, 1380 women and 1467 men were studied.

The $^{222}$Rn concentration in 8992 homes was measured for 3 months during the heating season. The geometric and arithmetic mean concentrations were 1.6 and 2.9 pCi $L^{-1}$ (60 and 106 Bq $m^{-3}$). The cumulative exposure since 1947 was estimated for each subject by the addition of the products of concentration by the length of time the subject lived in each residence.

The data were reported in terms of the relative risk (RR) of lung cancer (ratio of observed to expected lung cancer) normalized to a relative risk of 1.0 for persons who never smoked and who had radon exposure below 50 Bq $m^{-3}$. The excess risk due to smoking could be seen easily. Smokers smoking less than or more than 10 cigarettes per day with a radon concentration of <50 Bq $m^{-3}$ had RR of 6.2 (with a confidence interval from 4.2 to 9.2) and 12.6 (C.I. from 8.7 to 18.4), respectively.

The only statistically significant lung cancer excess resulting from $^{222}$Rn was seen in those who smoked fewer than 10 cigarettes per day and had a time-weighted mean $^{222}$Rn con-

**Table 25–14**
**Lung Cancer Risk for Continuous Exposure to 1 WLM Year$^{-1}$ (150 Bq m$^{-3}$ or 4 pCi Liter$^{-1}$) as Predicted by Various Models**

| | LIFETIME RISK, % | MODEL TYPE | COMMENT |
|---|---|---|---|
| NCRP | 0.9 | Modified absolute | Risk decreases with time from exposure |
| ICRP | 1.6 | Constant relative | No reduction in risk with time from exposure for either model |
| | 1.1 | Constant absolute | |
| BEIR IV | 3.4 (2.2)* men<br>1.4 (0.9)* women | Modified relative | Risk decreases with time from exposure |

* Beir IV values are modified to express risk for 35 years after exposure rather than for the entire lifetime.

centration >400 Bq $m^{-3}$. Their relative risk was 25.1 (C.I. 7.7 to 82.4). For those smoking more than 10 cigarettes per day, the relative risk compared with those who had never smoked and had $^{222}Rn$ concentrations <50 Bq $m^{-3}$ was 32.5 (C.I. 10.3 to 23.7). Although this relative risk appears higher than that for those smoking <10 cigarettes per day, the result is not statistically significant. If the effect of $^{222}Rn$ alone is examined by comparing the risk only among smokers, that is, those with <50 Bq $m^{-3}$ against smokers having >400 Bq $m^{-3}$, the relative risk due to $^{222}Rn$ alone is 3.7 (C.I. 1.1 to 11.7) for those smoking less than 10 cigarettes per day and 2.5 (C.I. 0.8 to 7.9) for those smoking more than 10 cigarettes per day (Pershagen et al., 1993). Because the confidence interval includes 1.0, it cannot be stated with statistical certainty that there was increased lung cancer caused by $^{222}Rn$ exposure although the point estimate RR = 2.5 suggests at least an upper bound of risk.

The analysis was done for the combined group of men and women (Pershagen et al., 1994). There were no details given concerning lung cancer and sex difference. However, the preliminary report (Pershagen et al., 1994) suggested that women may indeed have had less lung cancer than men for the same exposure conditions.

Also of interest in the study of Pershagen and associates (1994) was the relative risk of lung cancer by histological type. In the >400 Bq $m^{-3}$ group, only small cell carcinoma and adenocarcinoma had a statistically significant increased risk.

The pattern emerging from the domestic studies indicates that the lung cancer risk from $^{222}Rn$ exposure is difficult to determine with accuracy or precision. This is mostly due to the high background lung cancer mortality caused by smoking.

Among the 22 published domestic studies, 13 are ecological and 9 are case-control (Neuberger 1989). Ecological studies depend on relating the disease response of a population to some measure of a suspected causative agent. There usually are not enough data on all the variables involved in the disease to infer any reliable associations. Ecological studies are the weakest type of epidemiological exploration. Unless a biological marker for radon-induced lung cancer is found, it is unlikely that environmental epidemiology will be effective. The effects of radon in the environment are subtle compared with the overwhelming lung cancer mortality that results from smoking.

Four concepts have emerged from the radon research so far:

1. The mining epidemiology indicates that short exposure to high levels of radon and daughters produces a clear excess of lung cancer.
2. Particle size can change the actual dose delivered by radon to bronchial tissue, with small particles giving a substantially higher dose per unit exposure. The use of open flames, electric motors, and the like indoors produces a higher dose per unit exposure.
3. Smokers are at higher risk from radon per unit exposure than are nonsmokers. The relative risk for nonsmokers is about 3 times that for smokers, but their age-specific lung cancer mortality is about 10 times lower than that for smokers. Thus, the overall lifetime lung cancer risk is 3 times higher for smokers.
4. Urban areas almost universally have low radon, and apartment dwellers removed from the ground source have particularly low radon exposure at home.

The miners' data show clearly that there is a risk of lung cancer from exposure to high concentrations of radon delivered over short periods. Comparable exposures delivered over a lifetime in the home have not produced statistically significant increases in lung cancer mortality except among smokers in one large study in Sweden. The risk can still exist, but the confounding effects of other carcinogens, such as smoking and urbanization, make it impossible to extract the more subtle impact of radon in existing studies.

## Natural Radioactivity and Radiation Background

The occupational, accidental, and wartime experiences detailed in the preceding sections have provided the bases for all the current radiation risk estimates. For many years, the radioisotopes deposited internally were compared with $^{226}Ra$ to evaluate the maximum permissible body burden for a particular emitter. The present limits for external and internal radiation are based on dose estimates which in turn can be related to cancer risks. One standard of comparison has always been the exposure from natural background, and this source is assessed here.

Background radiation from all sources is described in detail in NCRP report 94 (1987b), and some of the information is summarized here.

The risk estimates in the previous sections must be placed in context with the radiation dose received by all humans from natural background radiation. A substantial dose is received annually from cosmic radiation and from external terrestrial radiation present from uranium, thorium, and potassium in the earth's crust. Internal emitters are present in the body as a consequence of dietary consumption and inhalation. For example, potassium is a necessary element in the body and is homeostatically controlled. Radioactive $^{40}K$ constitutes a constant fraction of all natural potassium. Potassium delivers the largest internal dose from the diet of 0.15 mSv per year. However, the data are scanty on the dietary intake of other radionuclides in the U.S. population. Given the usual distribution of intakes across a large population, it is probable that other emitters, notably $^{210}Pb$, could deliver a significant dose to a fraction of the population.

The largest dose received by the population is from the inhaled short-lived daughters of radon. These are present in all atmospheres because radon is released rather efficiently from the $^{226}Ra$ in rock and soil. The short-lived daughters $^{218}Po$, $^{214}Pb$, $^{214}Bi$-$^{214}Po$, have an effective half-life of 30 min, but the 3.8-day parent radon supports their presence in the atmosphere. Figure 25-4 shows the entire uranium series decay.

Average outdoor concentrations in the United States have been measured as 7 Bq $m^{-3}$; those indoors, as 40 to 80 Bq $m^{-3}$. A structure such as a house prevents the rapid upward distribution of radon into the atmosphere, and substantial levels can be built up indoors. The source of radon is the ground, and so levels in living areas above the ground are generally one-third to one-fifth the concentrations measured in basements. An effective barrier across the soil-building interface also inhibits the entry of radon to buildings. Ventilation with outdoor air reduces indoor radon. For this reason, industrial buildings with more substantial foundations and higher ventilation rates tend to have lower radon concentrations than do

**Table 25–15**
**Equivalent Dose Rates to Various Tissues from Natural Radionuclides Contained in the Body**

| RADIONUCLIDE | EQUIVALENT DOSE RATE, mSv yr$^{-1}$ | | | |
|---|---|---|---|---|
| | *Bronchial Epithelium* | *Soft Tissue* | *Bone Surfaces* | *Bone Marrow* |
| $^{14}C$ | — | 0.10 | 0.08 | 0.30 |
| $^{40}K$ | — | 1.80 | 1.40 | 2.70 |
| $^{87}Rb$ | — | 0.03 | 0.14 | 0.07 |
| $^{238}U$-$^{234}Th$ | — | 0.046 | 0.03 | 0.004 |
| $^{230}Th$ | — | 0.001 | 0.06 | 0.001 |
| $^{226}Ra$ | — | 0.03 | 0.90 | 0.15 |
| $^{222}Rn$ | — | 0.07 | 0.14 | 0.14 |
| $^{222}Rn$ daughters | 24 | — | — | — |
| $^{210}Pb$-$^{210}Po$ | — | 1.40 | 7.00 | 1.40 |
| $^{232}Th$ | — | 0.001 | 0.02 | 0.004 |
| $^{228}Ra$-$^{224}Ra$ | — | 0.0015 | 1.20 | 0.22 |
| $^{220}Rn$ | — | 0.001 | — | — |
| Total | 24 | 3.50 | 11.00 | 5.00 |

single-family (or detached) houses. Apartments above ground level have radon concentrations about half the average of those in single-family dwellings.

It is of significance that an average radon concentration indoors of 40 Bq m$^{-3}$ results in an equivalent dose to bronchial epithelium of 24 mSv/year or an effective dose of 2 mSv per year.

The equivalent doses for the major natural internal emitters are shown in Table 25-15. These are reproduced from NCRP (1987).

The annual effective dose equivalents for all the external and internal emitters from natural background are summarized in NCRP Report 94 (1987) and are shown in Table 25-16.

The lifetime dose from natural emitters is shown in Table 25-17, assuming an average exposure from birth to a full life of 85 years. It should be recognized that the actual dose accumulated by an individual depends on dietary habits, location (Denver, for example, at an altitude of 1.6 kilometers, has double the average cosmic ray exposure), and the dwelling. An apartment dweller would accumulate approximately half the dose from inhaled radon daughters as would a person living in a single-family dwelling.

Table 25-17 is informative in considering the effects of radiation exposure from sources other than natural sources. For example, in assessing an occupational dose, which might add, say, 10 mSv effective dose equivalent, natural background would be a strong confounder. Any health detriment would have to be calculated rather than observed directly. No study would be able to detect an increase in health effects from 10 mSv above the average whole-life natural background of 260 mSv.

## Environmental Releases

Large-scale accidents will undoubtedly occur that release substantial radioactivity into the environment. The accident at the

**Table 25–16**
**Estimated Total Effective Dose Rate for a Member of the Population in the United States and Canada from Various Sources of Background Radiation**

| SOURCE | | TOTAL EFFECTIVE DOSE RATE, mSv yr$^{-1}$ | | | | | |
|---|---|---|---|---|---|---|---|
| | | *Lung* | *Gonads* | *Bone Surf* | *Bone Marrow* | *Other Tissues* | *Total* |
| | $W_t$ | 0.12 | 0.25 | 0.03 | 0.12 | 0.48 | 1.0 |
| Cosmic | | 0.03 | 0.07 | 0.008 | 0.03 | 0.13 | 0.27 |
| Cosmogenic | | 0.001 | 0.002 | — | 0.004 | 0.003 | 0.01 |
| Terrestrial | | 0.03 | 0.07 | 0.008 | 0.03 | 0.14 | 0.28 |
| Inhaled | | 2.0 | — | — | — | — | 2.0 |
| In body | | 0.04 | 0.09 | 0.03 | 0.06 | 0.17 | 0.40 |
| Total | | 2.1 | 0.23 | 0.05 | 0.12 | 0.44 | 3.0 |

SOURCE: From NCRP (1987).

Windscale nuclear power reactor in 1957 was a local incident in Great Britain. The nearby population has been studied for over 30 years without the appearance of significant health effects.

The accident at the Chernobyl nuclear power plant was another such occasion, but in this case the radioactivity was widespread over Europe. The United Nations Scientific Committee on the Effects of Atomic Radiation (UNSCEAR, 1988, 1993) has summarized the committed dose from measurements made in the affected countries, and these are shown in

**Table 25–17**
**Lifetime Effective Dose (in mSv from Birth to Age 85) from Natural Radionuclide Exposure**

| | LUNG | BONE MARROW | WHOLE BODY |
|---|---|---|---|
| Effective Dose | 180 | 10 | 260 |

SOURCE: From NCRP (1987).

**Table 25–18**
**Estimates of Radionuclide Released and Collective Effective Dose From Human-Made Environmental Sources of Radiation**

| | RELEASE, PBq | | | | | | COLLECTIVE EFFECTIVE DOSE*, HUMAN SV | |
|---|---|---|---|---|---|---|---|---|
| SOURCE | $^{3}H$ | $^{14}C$ | NOBLE GASES | $^{90}Sr$ | $^{131}I$ | $^{137}Cs$ | LOCAL AND REGIONAL | GLOBAL |
| Atmospheric nuclear testing | | | | | | | | |
| Global | 240000 | 220 | | 604 | 650,000 | 910 | | 2,230,000 |
| Local | | | | | | | | |
| Semipalatinsk | | | | | | | 4600 | |
| Nevada | | | | | | | 500† | |
| Australia | | | | | | | 700 | |
| Pacific test site | | | | | | | 160† | |
| Underground nuclear testing | | | 50 | | 15 | | 200 | |
| Nuclear weapons fabrication | | | | | | | | |
| Early practice | | | | | | | | |
| Hanford | | | | | | | 8000‡ | |
| Chelyabinsk | | | | | | | 15,000§ | |
| Later practice | | | | | | | 1000 | 10,000 |
| | | | | | | | 30,000# | |
| Nuclear power production | | | | | | | | |
| Milling and mining | | | | | | | 2700 | |
| Reactor operation | 140 | 1.1 | 3200 | | 0.04 | | 3700 | |
| Fuel reprocessing | 57 | 0.3 | 1200 | 6.9 | 0.004 | 40 | 4600 | |
| Fuel cycle | | | | | | | 300,000# | 100,000 |
| Radioisotope production and use | 2.6 | 1.0 | 52 | | 6.0 | | 2000 | 80,000 |
| Accidents | | | | | | | | |
| Three Mile Island | | | 370 | | 0.0006 | | 40 | |
| Chernobyl | | | | | 630 | 70 | | 600,000 |
| Kyshtym | | | | 5.4 | | 0.04 | 2500 | |
| Windscale | | | 1.2 | | 0.7 | 0.02 | 2000 | |
| Palomares | | | | | | | 3 | |
| Thule | | | | | | | 0 | |
| SNAP 9A | | | | | | | | 2100 |
| Cosmos 954 | | | | 0.003 | 0.2 | 0.003 | | 20 |
| Ciudad Juarez | | | | | | | 150 | |
| Mohammedia | | | | | | | 80 | |
| Goiania | | | | | | 0.05 | 60 | |
| Total | | | | | | | 380,000 | 23,100,000 |
| Total collective effective dose (human Sv) | | | | | | | 23,500,000 | |

* Truncated at 10,000 years.
† External dose only.
‡ From release of $^{131}I$ to the atmosphere.
§ From releases of radionuclides into the Techa River.
\# Long-term collective dose from release of $^{222}Rn$ from tailings.
SOURCE: UNSCEAR (1993).

**Table 25–19**
**Lifetime Cancer Mortality per Gray from Five Major Epidemiological Studies (in parentheses, risk per Sievert for alpha emitters)**

| STUDY | ALL SITES | LEUKEMIA | LUNG | FEMALE BREAST | BONE | THYROID | SKIN |
|---|---|---|---|---|---|---|---|
| Atom bomb whole-body gamma | 0.029 | 0.0067 | 0.0038 | 0.0029 | | | |
| Uranium miner bronchial epithelium alpha | | | (0.04) 0.0020 | | | | |
| Ankylosing spondylitis spine x-ray | | 0.0011 | 0.0008–0.0028 | 0.0015 | | | |
| Tinea capitis head x-ray | | | | | | 0.0010§ 0.0040‖ | 0.0030‡ |
| Radium ingestion bone alpha ($^{226}$Ra) | | | | | (0.0040*) 0.0002 | | |
| Radium ingestion bone alpha ($^{224}$Ra) | | | | | (0.02†) 0.0010 | | |

* The lifetime risk is calculated for an average skeletal dose of 10 Gy, assuming that the risk persists for 50 years and using equation 20 The risk is nonlinear and is about 0.01 $Gy^{-1}$ at 100 Gy, for example.
† The lifetime risk is calculated for an average skeletal dose of 10 Gy using equation 22. The risk is nonlinear and is about 0.01 $Gy^{-1}$ for a skeletal dose of 1 Gy.
‡ The mortality for skin cancer is estimated as 1 percent of the incidence; see text.
§ Thyroid mortality for males. Estimated as 10 percent of incidence.
‖ Thyroid mortality for females. Estimated as 10 percent of incidence.

Table 25-18. Table 25-18 includes environmental releases from all sources.

There are plans to follow up on the health results in the local population affected by Chernobyl.

## SUMMARY OF HUMAN CANCER RISKS FROM RADIATION

The details of the five major studies have been given in the preceding sections. The data are summarized in Table 25-19. This table shows the lifetime cancer risks which are significant. The risks are given in units of per Gray (or per Sievert where appropriate for alpha emitters).

Within the table, leukemia and cancers of the lung and female breast are the most critical. Osteogenic sarcoma is seen in the radium exposures. There is no clear linear dose response for $^{224,226}$Ra. This has been attributed to the existence of an apparent threshold.

The cancer risk to individual organs from different study groups is in general agreement regardless of radiation type or whole or partial body exposure.

## ACKNOWLEDGMENT

The author would like to thank Dr. John H. Harley for many helpful suggestions in the preparation of this manuscript.

# REFERENCES

Adamson HG: A simplified method of x-ray application for the cure of ringworm of the scalp; Kienbock's method, *Lancet* i:1378–1380, 1909.

Alavanja MCR, Brownson RC, Lubin JH, et al: Residential radon exposure and lung cancer among nonsmoking women. *JNCI* 86:1829–1837, 1994.

Albert RE, Omran A: A follow-up study of patients treated by X-ray epilation for tinea capitis: I Population characteristics, posttreatment illnesses, and mortality experience. *Arch Environ Health* 17:899–918, 1968.

Albert RE, Shore RE, Harley NH, Omran A: Follow-up studies of patients treated by X-ray epilation for tinea capitis, in Burns F, Upton AC, Silini G (eds): *Radiation Carcinogenesis and DNA Alterations*. New York: Plenum Press, 1986, pp 1–25.

Andrews HL: *Radiation Biophysics*. Englewood Cliffs, NJ: Prentice-Hall, 1974.

Attix FH, Roesch WC, Tochilin E: *Radiation Dosimetry*, vol I, New York: Academic Press, 1968.

Aub JC, Evans RD, Hempelmann LH, Martland HS: The late effects of internally deposited radioactive materials in man. *Medicine (Baltimore)* 31:221–329, 1952.

Bethe HA, Ashkin J: Passage of radiations through matter, in Segre E (ed): *Experimental Nuclear Physics*. New York: Wiley, 1953, pp 166–357.

Borak TB, Johnson JA: *Estimating the Risk of Lung Cancer from Inhalation of Radon Daughters Indoors: Review and Evaluation*. Environmental Protection Agency Report EPA 600/6-88/008, Environmental Monitoring Systems Laboratory. Las Vegas, NV: EPA, 1988.

Brown E, Firestone RB, Shirley VS: *Table of Radioactive Isotopes*. New York: Wiley, 1986.

Chemelevsky D, Kellerer AM, Spiess H, Mays CW: A proportional hazards analysis of bone sarcoma rates in German radium-224 patients, in Gossner W, Gerber GB (eds): *The Radiobiology of Radium and Thorotrast*. Munich: Urban and Schwarzenberg, 1986.

Conard RA, Boice JD, Fravwenie JF Jr (eds): Late radiation effects in Marshall Islanders exposed to fallout 28 years ago, in Boice JD, Fraumeni JF Jr (eds): *Radiation Carcinogenesis: Epidemiology and Biological Significance*. New York: Raven Press, 1984, pp 57–71.

Court Brown WM, Doll R: *Leukemia and Aplastic Anemia in Patients Treated for Ankylosing Spondylitis*. London: HMSO, 1957.

———: Adult leukemia. Trends in mortality in relation to aetiology. *Br Med J* 1:1063, 1959.

———: Mortality from cancer and other causes after radiotherapy for ankylosing spondylitis. *Br Med J* 2:1327, 1965.

Darby SC, Doll R, Smith PG: Long term mortality after a single treatment course with X-rays in patients treated for ankylosing spondylitis. *Br J Cancer* 55:179–190, 1987.

Darby SC, Nakashima E, Kato H: A parallel analysis of cancer mortality among atomic bomb survivors and patients with ankylosing spondylitis given x-ray therapy. *JNCI* 72:1, 1985.

Evans RD: *The Atomic Nucleus*. New York: McGraw-Hill, 1955.

Evans RD, Keane AT, Kolenkow RJ, et al: Radiogenic tumors in the radium cases studied at M.I.T., in Mays CW, Jee WSS, Lloyd RD, et al (eds): *Delayed Effects of Bone Seeking Radionuclides*. Salt Lake City: University of Utah Press, 1969, pp 157–194.

George AC, Breslin AJ: The distribution of ambient radon and radon daughters in residential buildings in the New Jersey–New York area, in Gesell TF, Lowder WM (eds): *Natural Radiation Environment III CONF-780422*. Washington, DC: USDOE, 1980, pp 1272–1292.

George AC, Hinchliffe L, Sladowski R: Size distribution of radon daughter particles in uranium mine atmospheres. *Am Ind Hyg Assoc J* 36:4884, 1975.

Harley JH: Dose from residual radioactivity at Hiroshima and Nagasaki, in *New Dosimetry at Hiroshima and Nagasaki and Its Implications for Risk Estimates. Proc. Number 9 National Council on Radiation Protection*. Bethesda: NCRP, 1987.

Harley NH: *Lung Cancer Risk from Exposure to Environmental Radon*. Presented at the 3rd International Conference on Anticarcinogenesis and Radiation Protection, Dubrovnik, 1989.

Harley NH, Albert RE, Shore RE, Pasternack BS: Follow-up study of patients treated by X-ray epilation for tinea capitis: Estimation of the dose to the thyroid and pituitary glands and other structures of the head and neck. *Phys Med Biol* 21:631–642, 1976.

Harley NH, Cohen BS: Updating radon daughter dosimetry, in Hopke PK (ed): *American Chemical Society Symposium on Radon and Its Decay Products*. Washington, DC: ACS, 1987, pp 419–429.

Harley NH, Kolber AB, Shore RE, et al: The skin dose and response for the head and neck in patients irradiated with X-ray for tinea capitis: Implications for environmental radioactivity, in *Proceedings in Health Physics Society Mid-Year Symposium*. Albuquerque: Health Physics Society, 1983, pp 125–142.

Holaday DA, Rushing DE, Coleman RD, et al: *Control of Radon and Daughters in Uranium Mines and Calculations on Biologic Effects*. U.S. PHS Report 494. Washington, DC: U.S. Government Printing Office, 1957.

Hornung RW, Meinhardt TJ: Quantitative risk assessment of lung cancer in U.S. uranium miners. *Health Phys* 52:417–430, 1987.

Howe GR, Nair RC, Newcombe HB, et al: Lung cancer mortality (1950–80) in relation to radon daughter exposure in a cohort of workers at the Eldorado Beaverlodge Uranium Mine. *JNCI* 77:357–362, 1986.

Howe GR, Nair RC, Newcombe HB, et al: Lung cancer mortality (1950–80) in relation to radon daughter exposure in a cohort of workers at the Eldorado Port Radium Mine: Possible modification of risk by exposure rate. *JNCI* 79:1255–1260, 1987.

Hubbell JH: *Photon Cross Sections, Attenuation Coefficients, and Energy Absorption Coefficients from 10 keV to 100 GeV*. U.S. Department of Commerce, National Bureau of Standards Report NSRDS-NBS 29. Washington, DC: U.S. Government Printing Office, 1969.

———: Photon mass attenuation and energy-absorption coefficients from 1 keV to 20 MeV. *Int J Appl Radiat Isotop* 33:1269–1290, 1982.

ICRP: *Recommendations of the International Commission on Radiological Protection. International Commission on Radiation Protection Publication 26*. New York: Pergamon, 1977.

———: *Limits for Intakes of Radionuclides by Workers. International Commission on Radiological Protection Publication 30 Part I*. New York: Pergamon, 1978.

———: *Limits for Inhalation of Radon Daughters by Workers. International Commission on Radiological Protection Publication 32*. New York: Pergamon, 1981.

———: *Lung Cancer Risk from Indoor Exposures to Radon Daughters. International Commission on Radiological Protection Publication 50*. Oxford: Pergamon, 1987.

ICRP: *1990 Recommendations of the International Commission on Radiological Protection*. Annals of the ICRP Publication 60. New York: Pergamon, 1990.

ICRP: *Protection against Radon-222 at Home and at Work*. Publication 65, New York: Pergamon, 1993.

ICRU: *Radiation Quantities and Units. International Commission on Radiation Units and Measurements, Report Number 33*. Bethesda: ICRU, 1980.

———: *Stopping Powers for Electrons and Positrons. International Commission on Radiation Units and Measurements Report Number 37*. Bethesda: ICRU, 1984.

Kienbock R: Über Radiotherapie und Harrerkrankungen. *Arch Derm Syph Wien* 83:77–111, 1907.

Kunz E, Sevc J: Radiation risks to underground miners in the light of Czechoslovak epidemiological studies, in Kvasnicka J (ed): *Proceedings of the International Workshop on Radiological Protection in Mining, Darwin, Australia*, 1988.

Lederer CM, Shirley VS, Browne E, et al: *Table of Isotopes*. New York: Wiley, 1978.

Lewis CA, Smith PG, Stratton M, et al: Estimated radiation doses to different organs among patients treated for ankylosing spondylitis with a single course of X-rays. *Br J Radiol* 61:212–220, 1988.

Lubin JH, Samet JM, Weinberg C: Design issues in studies of indoor exposure to radon and risk of lung cancer. *Health Phys* 59:807–817, 1990.

Marshall JH, Lloyd EL, Rundo J, et al: *Alkaline Earth Metabolism in Adult Man ICRP Report Number 20*. Elmsford, NY: Pergamon, 1972.

Martland HS: The occurrence of malignancy in radioactive persons. *Am J Cancer* 15:2435–2516, 1931.

Mays CW: Alpha particle induced cancer in humans. *Health Phys* 55:637–652, 1988.

Muller J, Kusiak R, Ritchie AC: *Factors Modifying Lung Cancer Risk in Ontario Uranium Miners, 1955–1981*. Ontario Ministry of Labour Report. Toronto: Ministry of Labour, 1989.

NAS: *The Effects on Populations of Exposure to Low Levels of Ionizing Radiation. National Academy of Sciences Report, BEIR III*. Washington, DC: National Academy Press, 1980.

———: *Health Risks of Radon and Other Internally Deposited Alpha Emitters Committee on the Biological Effects of Ionizing Radiation BEIR IV National Research Council*. Washington, DC: National Academy Press, 1988.

———: *Health Effects of Exposure to Low Levels of Ionizing Radiation. National Academy of Sciences Report BEIR V*. Washington, DC: National Academy Press, 1990.

NCRP: *Influence of Dose and Its Distribution in Time on Dose-Response Relationships of Low-LET Radiations. National Council on Radiation Protection and Measurements Report Number 64*. Bethesda: NCRP, 1980.

———: *Evaluation of Occupational and Environmental Exposures to Radon and Radon Daughters in the United States National Council on Radiation Protection Report No. 78*. Bethesda: NCRP, 1984.

———: *Induction of Thyroid Cancer by Ionizing Radiation. Report Number 80. National Council on Radiation Protection and Measurements*. Bethesda: NCRP, 1985.

NCRP: Induction of thyroid cancer by ionizing radiation. NCRP Report No. 80, 1985.

NCRP: *Limitation of Exposure to Ionizing Radiation. Report Number 116*. March 31 1993. National Council on Radiation Protection and Measurements, Bethesda: 1993.

———: *Recommendations on Limits for Exposure to Ionizing Radiation. National Council on Radiation Protection and Measurements, Report Number 91*. Bethesda: NCRP, 1987a.

———: *Exposure of the Population in the United States and Canada from Natural Background Radiation. National Council on Radiation Protection and Measurements Report Number 94*. Bethesda: NCRP, 1987b.

———: *Recommendation on Limits of Exposure to Hot Particles on the Skin. National Council on Radiation Protection and Measurements Report Number 106*. Bethesda: NCRP, 1990.

Neuberger JS: *Worldwide Studies of Household Radon Exposure and Lung Cancer. Final Report to the U.S. Department of Energy, Office of Health and Environmental Research*. Washington, DC: USDOE, 1989.

Neuberger JS: Residential radon exposure and lung cancer. *Health Phys* 63:503–509, 1992.

Neuberger JS: Residential radon exposure and lung cancer (letter). *N Engl J Med* 330:1685, 1994.

NIH: *Radon and Lung Cancer Risk: A Joint Analysis of 11 Underground Miner Studies*. U.S. Department of Health and Human Services, National Institutes of Health, NIH Publication 94-3644, Bethesda: 1994.

Norris WP, Speckman TW, Gustafson PF: Studies of metabolism of radium in man. *AJR* 73:785–802, 1955.

Norris WP, Tyler SA, Brues AM: Retention of radioactive bone seekers. *Science* 128:456, 1958.

NRC: *Comparative Dosimetry of Radon in Mines and Homes*. Washington, DC: National Academy Press, 1991.

Pershagen G, Ackerblow G, Axelson O, et al: IMM Report 2/93 Radon i bostader och lungcancer (in Swedish). Stockholm: Institute for Miljomedicin, Karolinska Institute, 1993.

Pershagen G, Ackerblom G, Axelson O, et al: Residential radon exposure and lung cancer in Sweden. *N Engl J Med* 330:159–164, 1994.

Raabe OG, Book SA, Parks NJ: Bone cancer from radium: Canine dose response explains data for mice and humans. *Science* 208:61–64, 1980.

Radford EP, Renard KGS: Lung cancer in Swedish iron miners exposed to low doses of radon daughters. *N Engl J Med* 310:1485–1494, 1984.

RERF: *US–Japan Joint Reassessment of Atomic Bomb Radiation Dosimetry in Hiroshima and Nagasaki. Final Report DS86*. Hiroshima, Japan: RERF, 1987.

RERF: *US–Japan Joint Reassessment of Atomic Bomb Radiation Dosimetry in Hiroshima and Nagasaki*. Final Report. Radiation Effects Research Foundation Vol I, Roesch WC (ed). Hiroshima, Japan, 1987.

Robbins ES, Meyers O: Cycling cells of human and dog tracheobronchial mucosa: Normal and repairing epithelia. *Technol J Franklin Inst* 332A:35–42 1995.

Ron E, Modan B: Thyroid and other neoplasms following childhood scalp irradiations, in Boice JD, Fraumeni JF (eds): *Radiation Carcinogenesis: Epidemiology and Biological Significance*. New York: Raven Press, 1984, pp 139–151.

Rowland RE, Stehney AF, Lucas HF: Dose response relationships for female radium dial painters. *Radiat Res* 76:368–383, 1978.

Ruzer LS, Nero AV, Harley NH: Assessment of lung deposition and breathing rate of underground miners in Tadjikistan. *Radia Protect Dosimet* 261–268, 1995.

Samet JM: Radon and lung cancer. *JNCI* 81:745–757, 1989.

Samet JM, Stolwijk J, Rose SL: Summary: International workshop on residential radon epidemiology. *Health Phys* 60:223–227, 1991.

Schoenberg J, Klotz J: *A Case-Control Study of Radon and Lung Cancer Among New Jersey Women*. New Jersey State Department of Health Technical Report, Phase I. Trenton: NJDH, 1989.

Schoenberg JB, Klotz JB, Wilcox HB, Szmaciasz SF: A case-control study of radon and lung cancer among New Jersey women, in Cross FT (ed): 29th Hanford Symposium on Health and the Environment: *Indoor Radon and Lung Cancer: Reality or Myth*. Columbus, OH: Battelle Press, 1990 pp 905–922.

Schulz R, Albert RE: Dose to organs of the head from the X-ray treatment of tinea capitis. *Arch Environ Health* 17:935–950, 1963.

Sevc J, Kunz E, Tomasek L, et al: Cancer in man after exposure to Rn daughters. *Health Phys* 54:27–46, 1988.

Shimizu Y, Kato H, Schull WJ, et al: *Life Span Study Report 11, Part 1. Comparison of Risk Coefficients for Site-Specific Cancer Mortality Based on the DS86 and T65DR Shielded Kerma and Organ Doses. Technical Report TR 12-87*. Hiroshima, Japan: RERF, 1987a.

Shimizu Y, Kato H, Schull WJ: *Life Span Study Report 11, Part 2. Cancer Mortality in the Years 1950–85 Based on the Recently Revised Doses (DS86)*. RERF Report TR-5-88. Hiroshima, Japan: RERF, 1988.

Shore RE: Issues and epidemiological evidence regarding radiation-induced thyroid cancer. *Radiat Res* 131:98–111, 1992.

Shore RE, Albert RE, Pasternack BS: Follow-up of patients treated by x-ray epilation for tinea capitis. *Arch Environ Health* 31:21–28, 1976.

Shore RE, Albert RE, Reed M, et al: Skin cancer incidence among children irradiated for ringworm of the scalp. *Radiat Res* 100:192–204, 1984.

Sinclair WK, Abbatt HE, Farran HE, et al: A quantitative autoradiographic study of radioactive distribution and dosage in human thyroid glands. *Br J Radiol* 29:36–41, 1956.

Smith PG: Late effects of x-ray treatment of ankylosing spondylitis, in Boice JD, Fraumeni JF (eds): *Radiation Carcinogenesis: Epidemiology and Biological Significance*. New York: Raven Press, 1984.

Smith PG, Doll R: Mortality among patients with ankylosing spondylitis after a single treatment course with x-rays. *Br Med J* 1:449, 1982.

Smith WM, Doll R: Age and time dependent changes in the rates of radiation-induced cancers in patients with ankylosing spondylitis following a single course of x-ray treatment, in *Late Effects of Ionizing Radiation*. Vienna: IAEA, 1978, vol 1, p 205.

Spiess FW, Mays CW: Bone cancers induced by Ra-224 (ThX) in children and adults. *Health Physics* 19:713–729, 1970.

Spiess H, Mays CW: Protraction effect on bone sarcoma induction of Ra-224 in children and adults, in Sanders CL, Busch RH, Ballou JE, Mahlum DD (eds): *Radionuclide Carcinogenesis*. Springfield, VA: National Technical Information Service, 1973, pp 437–450.

Tirmarche M, Raphalen A, Allin F, et al: Mortality of a cohort of Rench uranium miners exposure to a relatively low radon exposure. *Br J Cancer* 67:1090–1097, 1993.

Tu KW, Knutson EO: Indoor radon progeny particle size distribution measurements made with two different methods. *Radiat Prot Dosimet* 24:251, 1988.

Turner JE: *Atoms, Radiation and Radiation Protection*. Elmsford, NY: Pergamon, 1986.

UNSCEAR: *Sources, Effects and Risks of Ionizing Radiation. Report of the United Nations Scientific Committee on the Effects of Atomic Radiation*. New York: United Nations, 1988.

UNSCEAR: *Sources and Effects of Ionizing Radiation*. United Nations Committee on the Effects of Atomic Radiation. New York: United Nations, 1993, pp 125–128.

UNSCEAR: *Sources and Effects of Ionizing Radiation*. New York: United Nations Scientific Committee on the Effects of Atomic Radiation, 1994, pp 60–63.

Weiss HA, Darby SC, Doll R: Cancer mortality following x-ray treatment for ankylosing spondylitis. *Int J Cancer* 59:327–338, 1994.

Whaling W: The energy loss of charged particles in matter, in Flugge S (ed): *Handbuch der Physik*. Berlin: Springer-Verlag, 1958, pp 193–217.

Wick RR, Chmelevsky D, Gossner W: 224Ra risk to bone and haematopoietic tissue in ankylosing spondylitis patients, in Gossner W, Gerber GB, Hagan U, Luz A (eds): *The Radiobiology of Radium and Thorotrast*. Munich: Urban and Schwarzenberg, 1986, pp 38–44.

Woodward A, Roder D, McMichael AJ, et al: Radon daughter exposures at the Radium Hill uranium mine and lung cancer rates among former workers 1952–1987. *Cancer Causes Control* 2:213–220, 1991.

Woodard HQ: *Radiation Carcinogenesis in Man: A Critical Review. Environmental Measurements Laboratory Report EML-380*. New York: U.S. Department of Energy, 1980.

Ziegler JF: *Helium Stopping Powers and Ranges in All Elemental Matter*. New York: Pergamon, 1977.

# CHAPTER 26

# TOXIC EFFECTS OF ANIMAL TOXINS

*Findlay E. Russell*

Venomous or poisonous animals are found in all the animal classes, including the birds. For the most part, they are widely distributed throughout the animal kingdom from the unicellular protistan *Alexandrium (Gonyaulax)* to certain chordates, including the platypus and the short-tailed shrew. Venomous marine animals are found in almost all seas and oceans. Although there are no exact figures on the numbers of such animals, there are approximately 1200 species of venomous or poisonous marine animals (Russell, 1984a), the number of venomous arthropods is countless, and there are about 400 species of snakes considered dangerous to humans.

The term "venomous animal" usually is applied to creatures that are capable of producing a poison in a highly developed secretory gland or group of cells and can deliver that toxin during a biting or stinging act. "Poisonous animals," by contrast, are generally regarded to be those whose tissues, either in part or in their entirety, are toxic. These animals have no mechanism or structure for the delivery of their poisons. Poisoning in these forms usually takes place through ingestion (Russell, 1965).

A venom may have one or several functions in an animal's armament. It may play a role in offense, as in the capture and digestion of food, or may contribute to the animal's defense, as in protection against predators or aggressors. It also may serve both functions. The principal biological property of the venom of a snake, however, is its food-securing potential. In this respect, venom is a superior modification to speed, size, strength, and better concealment as well as other characteristics seen in nonvenomous snakes. In addition, venom plays a role in the digestion of the prey. Finally, venom can play a role in a snake's defensive posture, as in spitting cobras and ringhals, and in kills or underkills in a defensive situation (Russell, 1984b).

The black widow spider and many other species of spiders use venom to paralyze their prey before extracting hemolymph and body fluids. It appears that the venom is not designed primarily to kill the prey, only to immobilize it. The venom apparatus of the stingray is used for defense. It is not employed in getting food, and for the most part its defensive use appears to have been spent eons ago. Lionfishes, stonefishes, and weeverfishes also use their venomous spines for defense. Scorpions, by contrast, can use their venom for both offense and defense.

Most venoms used in an offensive posture are associated with the oral pole of the animal, obviously the most functional place for their delivery. Defensively designed venoms usually are associated with the aboral pole, as in stingrays, or with dermal tissues, as in scorpionfishes and certain other fishes (Russell, 1965; Halstead, 1965).

In poisonous animals the poison or toxin may play a small role, if any, in the animal's offensive or defensive activities. The poison may be a product or by-product of metabolism or a product passed along in the food chain. In the case of Tetraodontidae, the responsible toxic organisms may be the Vibrionaceae and perhaps other bacteria. In ciguatera fish poisoning, the toxic organism, a dinoflagellate, is ingested by herbivores and then by carnivores. Ciguateric fishes in human poisonings have fed on smaller toxic fishes or other toxic marine animals, which in turn have ingested *Gambierdiscus* spp. or other toxic organisms. At each step in the feeding process, more toxin is accumulated; thus, while poisoning in humans may not result from eating the smaller toxic fishes or marine organisms, by the time a large grouper, barracuda, snapper, or other toxic fish that has fed on smaller toxic fishes is eaten, poisoning occurs. This sequence of events is known as the food-chain phenomenon, as described by Halstead (1965).

## PROPERTIES OF ANIMAL TOXINS

As one might expect from the various uses to which animals put their poisons, these toxins vary considerably in their chemistry and toxicology. Venoms, for instance, may be composed of proteins of both high and low molecular weight, including polypeptides and enzymes. They also may be amines, lipids, steroids, aminopolysaccharides, quinones, 5-hydroxytryptamine (5-HT), glycosides, or other substances. The biological properties of snake venoms have been reviewed by Zeller (1948), Russell (1967, 1983), Dowling and associates (1968), Minton and Minton (1969), Elliott (1978), Tu (1977), Lee (1979), and Habermehl (1981). With respect to the venoms of spiders, the text of Maretić and Lebez (1979) provides a fine description and ample references. Keegan's (1980) work on the scorpions is a basic text that provides a good overview of these arthropods. The toxins of marine animals have been thoroughly described by Halstead (1965, 1978) and Russell (1965, 1984a). The series of texts by Scheuer (1973, 1978) provides additional data on some marine animal toxins, as does the excellent work of Southcott (1979) and Sutherland (1983). Readers will find the book by Hashimoto (1979) a useful source of data on the biochemistry of marine toxins. Those specifically interested in ciguatera poisoning will find the recent contribution of the *Memoirs of the Queensland Museum* an excellent review.

One of the unfortunate facts in the study of the chemistry, pharmacology, and toxicology of venoms is that their structure and function are most easily researched by taking the venoms apart. This has two shortcomings: First, a destructive process is used in an attempt to understand an expedient and integrative one; second, the essential quality of the venom may be destroyed before a suitable acquaintance with it has been made. Often, the process of examination becomes so exacting that the end is lost sight of in the preoccupation with the means; in some cases the means may become a substitute for the end.

Another shortcoming in the study of venoms has been the naïve and oversimplified habit of classifying the whole poison or even its component parts as "neurotoxins," "cardiotoxins," "hemotoxins," "myotoxins," and other inexact synonyms. Most venoms probably exert their effects on almost all cells and tissues, and their pharmacological properties are determined by the amount of a specific biologically active component that accumulates at an activity site where it is capable of producing a change. That change probably has a common chemical basis in most tissues, specific not only to the component but also to the alteration in ion exchange it may cause at a cell or tissue site. Of course, most venoms have a more particular effect on one or several tissue sites, but recent experimental work has demonstrated the wide scope of the toxicological effects a venom or venom fraction can precipitate.

A clinician must never ignore any symptom or sign in a patient or minimize any manifestation on the naïve assumption that the venom has to be a "neurotoxin," "cardiotoxin," "hemotoxin," or "myotoxin" with its activity limited to one organ or system. While the patient may have respiratory distress from a "neurotoxic venom," he or she can also have changes in cardiac dynamics or vascular permeability, and these changes can become far more life-threatening, particularly if the physician centers his or her attention and therapy on the so-called neurotoxic activity of the venom (an effect that often can be treated adequately with simple positive-pressure respiration). The physician must guard his or her knowledge and experience zealously and be aware of the limits of application of pharmacological data that are based on animal experimentation.

Venoms may have important properties aside from the specific activities of their component parts. Important synergisms that are not obvious from the study of individual fractions may become apparent in studies of the activity of the whole venom. In addition, the whole venom may precipitate autopharmacological reactions that are not produced by individual fractions. Finally, the problem of the formation of metabolites in an envenomated organism has not been explored in a definitive manner, and this can be an important consideration in clinical cases.

The action of a venom or venom component is dependent on a number of variables, including its route of administration, absorption, distribution, passage across a succession of membranes, accumulation and action at a receptor site, and metabolism and excretion (Russell, 1980a). All these factors play a role in determining the action of the toxin. During the past two decades it has become increasingly clear that there are significant variations in the roles of these factors in different venoms and different species of animals. In some cases the variations in different animals are more important than the difference usually attributed solely to the weight of the animal. Studies carried out in pigs, opossums, certain species of rats, and other animals purport to show that these animals are more "immune" to a toxin than are mice. Such investigations do not take into account the dependent physiological variables involved in the availability and processing of a toxin in different kinds of animals, influences that are not related to any principle of immunity. It is a fallacious assumption to treat the $LD_{50}$ of mice and that of the opossum or another animal as direct products of the differences in their weights. In this respect, the toxicologist must always be concerned with the question of whether a particular difference between animals is caused by variables in the effectiveness of the toxin at the receptor site or in its absorption, distribution, metabolism, or excretion. The fate of a venom or venom fraction, as its activities are spent in the animal, has been discussed elsewhere (Russell, 1980a, 1980b, 1983).

## ANTIVENOMS (ANTIVENINS)

Because of their protein composition, many toxins produce an antibody response; this response is essential in producing antisera. An antivenom consists of venom-specific antiserum or antibodies concentrated from immune serum to the venom. Antisera contain neutralizing antibodies: one antigen (monovalent) or several antigens (polyvalent). Animals immunized with venom develop a variety of antibodies to the many antigens in the venom. The serum is harvested, partially or fully purified, and further processed before being administered to the patient. The antibodies bind to the venom molecules, rendering them ineffective. Antivenoms have been produced against most medically important snake, spider, scorpion, and marine toxins.

Antivenoms are available in several forms: intact IgG antibodies or fragments of IgG such as $F(ab)_2$ and Fab. They are prepared through $AmSO_4$ or $Na_2SO_4$ precipitation, pepsin or papain digestion, and other procedures, among which the elimination of the Fc, or complement-binding and complement-sensitizing fraction, is one of the most important. The molecular weight of the intact IgG is about 150,000, whereas that of Fab is approximately 50,000.

The molecular size of IgG prevents its renal excretion and produces a volume of distribution much smaller than that of Fab. The elimination half-life of IgG in the blood is approximately 50 h. Its ultimate fate is not known. Most IgG probably is taken up by the reticuloendothelial system and degraded with the antigen attached. Fab fragments have an elimination half-life of about 17 h and are small enough to permit renal excretion.

Since all antivenom products are produced through the immunization of animals, this increases the possibility of hypersensitivity. Type I (immediate) hypersensitivity reactions are caused by antigen cross-linking of endogenous IgE bound to mast cells and basophils. Binding of antigen by a mast cell may cause the release of histamine and other mediators, producing an anaphylactic reaction. Once initiated, anaphylaxis may continue despite discontinuation of antivenin administration. An additional concern is an *anaphylactoid* reaction. This is a term for a syndrome resembling an anaphylactic reaction; its etiology is unknown but appears to be associated with aggregated protein in the antiserum. Protein aggregates may activate the complement cascade, producing an anaphylactic-like syndrome. An important difference between anaphylactic and anaphylactoid reactions is that anaphylactoid reactions are dose-dependent and may be halted by removing the antigen. Type III hypersensitivity (serum sickness) may develop several days after antivenom administration. In these cases, antigen-antibody complexes are deposited in different areas of the body, often producing inflammatory responses in the skin, joints, kidneys, and other tissues. Fortunately, these reactions are rarely serious. The risks of anaphylaxis should always be considered when one is deciding whether to administer antivenom.

## REPTILES

From the beginnings of the human record, few subjects have stimulated the minds and imagination of humans more than the study of snakes and snake venoms. No animal has been more worshiped yet more cast out, more loved yet more despised, more collected yet more trampled on than the snake. The essence of the fascination for and fear of snakes lies in their venom. In times past, the consequences of the bites by venomous snakes often were attributed to forces beyond nature, sometimes to vengeful deities that were thought to be embodied in the serpents. To early peoples, the effects of snakebite were so surprising and so violent that snakes and their poisons were shrouded with myth and superstition.

Among the more than 3500 species of snakes, approximately 400 are considered sufficiently venomous to be dangerous to humans (Dowling et al., 1968; Minton and Minton, 1969; Harding and Welch, 1980; Russell, 1980b, 1983). Venomous species can be divided into the Elapidae: the cobras, kraits, mambas, and coral snakes; the Hydrophiidae: the true sea snakes; the Laticaudidae: the sea kraits; the Viperidae: the old world vipers and adders; the Crotalidae: the rattlesnakes, water moccasins, copperheads, fer-de-lances, and bushmaster of the Americas and some Asian species; and certain Colubridae, of which clinically the most important are the boomslang and bird snake of Africa and the rednecked keelback of Asia. However, several other colubrids must be viewed with concern (Minton and Minton, 1969; Minton, 1976; Mebs, 1977). There are no poisonous snakes in New Zealand, Hawaii, Ireland, and many other islands. The Gila monster, *Heloderma suspectum*, and the beaded lizard or escorpión, *H. horridum*, are the only venomous lizards and are confined to the southwestern United States and parts of Mexico.

Some medically important venomous snakes and their general distribution are shown in Table 26-1.

### Snake Venoms

The venoms of snakes are complex mixtures, chiefly proteins, a number of which have enzymatic activities. In some species, the most active component of the venom is a peptide or polypeptide. In addition, snake venoms contain inorganic substances such as sodium, calcium, potassium, magnesium, and small amounts of metals: zinc, iron, cobalt, manganese, and nickel. The importance of the metals in snake venoms is not known, although in the case of some elapid venoms zinc ions are necessary for anticholinesterase activity, and it has been suggested that calcium may play a role in the activation of phospholipase $A_2$ and the direct lytic factor. Some proteases appear to be metalloproteins. Some snake venoms also contain carbohydrates (glycoproteins), lipids, and biogenic amines, whereas others contain free amino acids (Russell, 1967, 1980b, 1983; Tu, 1977; Elliott, 1978; Lee, 1979; Habermehl, 1981).

**Enzymes.** The venoms of snakes contain at least 25 enzymes, although no single snake venom contains all of them. Enzymes are the proteins responsible for the catalysis of many specific biochemical reactions that occur in living matter. They are the agents on which cellular metabolism depends. Enzymes are universally accepted as proteins, although a few have crucial dependencies on certain nonprotein prosthetic groups, or cofactors. All living cells contain enzymes. Some of the more important snake venom enzymes are shown in Table 26-2.

Proteolytic enzymes catalyze the breakdown of tissue proteins and peptides. They are known as proteolytic enzymes, peptide hydrolases, proteases, endopeptidases, peptidases, and proteinases. There may be several proteolytic enzymes in a single venom. The proteolytic enzymes have molecular weights between 20,000 and 95,000. Some are inactivated by edetic acid (EDTA) and certain reducing agents (Lee, 1979). The role of metal ions in catalysis was demonstrated many years ago by Wagner and Prescott (1966). All crotalid venoms contain calcium. Metals appear to be intrinsically involved in the activity of certain venom proteases and phospholipases.

The crotalid venoms examined so far appear to be rich in proteolytic enzyme activity. Viperid venoms have lesser amounts, whereas elapid and sea snake venoms have no proteolytic activity or very little. Venoms that are rich in proteinase activity are associated with marked tissue destruction.

Arginine ester hydrolase is one of a number of noncholinesterases found in snake venoms. The substrate specificities are directed to the hydrolysis of the ester or peptide linkage to which an argine residue contributes the carboxyl group. This activity is found in many crotalid and viperid venoms and some sea snake venoms but is lacking in elapid venoms, with the possible exception of *Ophiophagus hannah*. It was first demonstrated by Deutsch and Diniz (1955) in 15 snake venoms and subsequently has been identified in many others. Some crotalid venoms contain at least three chromatographically separable arginine ester hydrolases. The bradykinin-releasing and perhaps bradykinin-clotting activities of some crotalid venoms may be related to esterase activity.

Thrombinlike enzymes are found in significant amounts in the venoms of the Crotalidae and Viperidae, whereas those of Elapidae and Hydrophiidae contain little or none. The mechanism of fibrinogen clot formation by snake venom thrombinlike enzymes invokes the preferential release of fibrinopeptide A (or B); thrombin releases fibrinopeptides A and B. Paradoxically, the thrombinlike enzymes have been shown to act as defibrinating anticoagulants in vivo, whereas in vitro they clot plasma, citrated or heparinized plasma, or purified fibrinogen. Because of the obvious clinical potential of these enzymes as defibrinating agents, more attention has been directed toward the characterization and study of the thrombinlike enzymes than toward those of the other venom procoagulant or anticoagulant enzymes (Lee, 1979; Russell, 1983). The proteolytic action of thrombin and thrombinlike snake venom enzymes is shown in Table 26-3.

Thrombinlike enzymes have been purified from the venoms of *Crotalus adamanteus* (Crotalase), *C. horridus horridus, Calloselasma (Agkistrodon) rhodostoma* (ancrod), *Agkistrodon contortrix contortrix, Deinagkistrodon (Agkistrodon) acutus, Bothrops atrox* (batroxobin), *B. marajoensis, B. moojeni, Trimeresurus gramineus, T. okinavensis,* and *Bitis gabonica.* Table 26-4 shows some of the physical and chemical properties of the thrombinlike enzymes. All these enzymes appear to be glycoproteins and, with the exception of two, appear to have molecular weights in the range of 29,000 to 35,000.

**Table 26–1**
**Some Medically Important Snakes of the World**

| SCIENTIFIC AND COMMON NAMES | DISTRIBUTION |
|---|---|
| Crotalids | |
| *Agkistrodon bilineatus*—cantil | Mexico south to Guatemala and Nicaragua |
| *Agkistrodon contortrix*—copperhead | New York south to Florida and west to Nebraska and Texas |
| *Agkistrodon halys*—mamushi | Caspian Sea to Japan |
| *Calloselasma (Agkistrodon) rhodostoma*—Malayan pit viper | Much of southeast Asia |
| *Bothrops asper* and/or *atrox*—fer-de-lance —barba amarillia —terciopelo | Southern Sonora to Peru and northern Brazil |
| *Bothrops jararaca*—jararaca | Brazil, Paraguay, and Argentina |
| *Bothrops jararacussu*—jararacussu | Brazil, Bolivia, Paraguay, and Argentina |
| *Bothrops neuwiedi*—jararaca pintada | Brazil, Bolivia, Paraguay, northern Argentina |
| *Crotalus adamanteus*—eastern diamondback rattlesnake | Southeastern United States |
| *Crotalus atrox*—western diamondback rattlesnake | Southwestern United States to central Mexico |
| *Crotalus basiliscus*—Mexican west-coast rattlesnake | Oaxaca and west coast of Mexico |
| *Trimeresurus flavoviridis*—habu | Amami and Okinawa islands |
| *Trimeresurus mucrosquamatus*—Chinese habu | Taiwan and southern China west through Vietnam and Laos to India |
| Viperids | |
| *Bitis arietans*—puff adder | Morocco and western Arabia through much of Africa |
| *Bitis caudalis*—horned adder | Angola south through Nambia into central and part of south Africa |
| *Causus* sp.—night adders | Most of Africa south of the Sahara |
| *Cerastes cerastes*—horned viper | Sahara, Arabian peninsula to Lebanon |
| *Cerastes vipera*—Sahara sand viper | Central Sahara to Lebanon |
| *Daboi (Vipera) russelli* | Indian subcontinent, southest China to Taiwan and parts of Indonesia |
| *Echis carinatus*—saw-scaled viper | Southern India to northern and tropical Africa |
| *Echis coloratus*—saw-scaled viper | Eastern Egypt, western Arabian peninsula north to Israel |
| *Vipera ammodytes*—long-nosed viper | Italy through southeast Europe, Turkey, Jordan to northwest Iran |
| *Vipera berus*—European viper | British Isles through Europe, to northern Asia |
| *Vipera lebetina*—Levantine viper | Cyprus through Middle East to Kashmir |
| *Vipera xanthina*—Near East viper | European Turkey and Asia Minor |
| Elapids | |
| Coral snakes (c.s.) | |
| *Calliophis* species—Oriental c.s. | Southeast Asia, Orient |
| *Micrurus alleni*—Allen's c.s. | Atlantic Nicaragua to Panama |
| *Micrurus corallinus*—c.s. | Southern Brazil to Uruguay, northern Argentina |
| *Micrurus frontalis*—southern c. s. | Southwestern Brazil, northern Argentina, Uruguay, Paraguay, and Bolivia |
| *Micrurus fulvius*—eastern c. s. | Southeastern, southern United States and north central Mexico |
| *Micrurus mipartitus*—black-ringed c.s. | Venezuela and Peru to Nicaragua |
| *Micrurus nigrocinctus*—black-banded c.s. | Southern Mexico to northwest Colombia |
| Cobras | |
| *Hemachatus haemachatus*—Ringhals cobra | Southeastern and southern Africa |
| *Naja haje*—Egyptian or brown cobra | Africa and part of Arabian peninsula |
| *Naja atra*—Chinese cobra | Thailand and South China to Taiwan |
| *Naja naja*—Indian cobra | Most of Indian subcontinent |
| *Naja nigricollis*—spitting cobra | West Africa and southern Egypt to near the Cape |
| *Naja oxiana*—Central Asian cobra | Northern Pakistan to Iran, southern Russia |
| *Naja philippinensis*—Philippine cobra | Philippines |
| *Naja sputatrix*—Malayan cobra | Malayan peninsula and Indonesia |

**Table 26–1**
**Some Medically Important Snakes of the World (*Continued*)**

| SCIENTIFIC AND COMMON NAMES | DISTRIBUTION |
|---|---|
| *Naja nivea*—Cape or yellow cobra | Nambia, Botswana south to the Cape |
| *Ophiophagus hannah*—king cobra | Indian subcontinent, China and Philippines |
| *Walterinnesia aegyptia*—desert blacksnake or desert cobra | Egypt to Iran |
| Kraits and mambas | |
| *Bungarus caeruleus*—Indian or blue krait | India, Pakistan, Sri Lanka, Bangladesh |
| *Bungarus candidus*—Malayan krait | Thailand, Malaysia, Indonesia |
| *Bungarus multicinctus*—many-banded krait | Southern China to Hainan, Taiwan |
| *Dendroaspis polylepis*—black mamba | Ethiopia and Somalia to Angola, Zambia, Nambia, southwest Africa |
| Australian elapids | |
| *Acanthophis antarcticus*—common death adder | Most of Australia, Moluccas, New Guinea |
| *Notechis scutatus*—tiger snake | Southeastern Australia |
| *Oxyuranus scutellatus*—Taipan | Northern coastal Australia, parts of New Guinea |
| *Pseudechis australis*—mulga | Most of Australia except southeast and southern coast, New Guinea |
| *Pseudonaja nuchalis*—western brown snake | Most of Australia except east and southeast coast |
| *Pseudonaja textilis*—eastern brown snake | Eastern Australia |

*Note*: The common names in this table are those generally employed as literature identifications for the snakes. However, these names may not be the ones used by people in the specific area where the snake abounds.

Thrombinlike enzymes have been used clinically and in animals for therapeutic and investigative studies. In experimentally induced venous thrombosis in dogs, treatment with ancrod before the formation of the thrombus prevented thrombosis and ensured vessel patency. However, ancrod had no thrombolytic effect when administered after thrombus formation. Trials of ancrod versus heparin and ancrod versus streptokinase in the treatment of deep venous thromboses of the lower leg have been conducted. It appears that neither heparin nor ancrod has a significant effect on thrombus resolution, whereas streptokinase produces more lysis of thrombi than does ancrod. Crotalase has been employed to evaluate the role of fibrin deposition in burns in animals (Bajwa and Markland, 1976). The role of fibrin deposition has been evaluated in tumor metastasis, in which fibrinogen is removed by treatment with ancrod or batroxobin. Ancrod also has been used to prevent the deposition of fibrin on prosthetic heart valves implanted in calves (Russell, 1980b, 1983).

Collagenase is a specific kind of proteinase that digests collagen. This activity has been demonstrated in the venoms of a number of species of crotalids and viperids. The venom of *Crotalus atrox* digests mesenteric collagen fibers but not protein. EDTA inhibits the collagenolytic effect but not the argine esterase effect.

**Table 26–2**
**Enzymes of Snake Venoms**

| | |
|---|---|
| Proteolytic enzymes | Phosphomonoesterase |
| Arginine ester hydrolase | Phosphodiesterase |
| Thrombinlike enzyme | Acetylcholinesterase |
| Collagenase | RNase |
| Hyaluronidase | DNase |
| Phospholipase $A_2$(A) | 5′-Nucleotidase |
| Phospholipase B | NAD-nucleotidase |
| Phospholipase C | L-Amino acid oxidase |
| Lactate dehydrogenase | |

SOURCE: Russell (1983).

Hyaluronidase catalyzes the cleavage of internal glycoside bonds in certain acid mucopolysaccharides. This results in a decrease in the viscosity of connective tissues. The breakdown in the hyaluronic barrier allows other fractions of venom to penetrate the tissues. The enzyme is thought to be related to the extent of edema produced by the whole venom, but the degree to which it contributes to clinical swelling and edema is not known. The enzyme also has been referred to as the "spreading factor."

Phospholipase enzymes are widely distributed throughout animals, plants, and bacteria. Snake venoms are the richest sources of phospholipase $A_2$ ($PLA_2$) enzymes. $PLA_2$ catalyzes the hydrolysis of the fatty acid ester at the 2-position of diacyl phosphatides, forming lysophosphatides and fatty acids, primarily unsaturated. The complete amino acid sequences of over 50 snake venom $PLA_2$ enzymes have been determined. The enzyme is widely distributed in the venoms of elapids, vipers, crotalids, sea snakes, and several colubrids. Although the sequences of these enzymes are homologous and their enzymatic active sites are identical, they differ widely in their lethal indexes and pharmacological properties. For example, taipoxin, a $PLA_2$ enzyme from the venom of the Australian elapid *Oxyuranus scutellatus* has an IV $LD_{50}$ in mice of 2 $\mu$g/kg, whereas the neutral $PLA_2$ from *Naja nigricollis* has an $LD_{50}$ of 10,200 $\mu$g/kg, even though *N. nigricollis* $PLA_2$ is enzymatically more active.

Recent studies have shown that $PLA_2$ enzymes can exert their pharmacological effects by different mechanisms: hydrolysis of membrane phospholipids, liberation of pharmacologically active products, and effects independent of enzymatic action. Similarly, snake venom $PLA_2$ enzymes can be

**Table 26–3**
**Proteolytic Action of Thrombin and Thrombinlike Snake Venom Enzymes**

| ENZYME | ACTION ON HUMAN FIBRINOGEN | | ACTIVATION OF FACTOR XIII | PROTHROMBIN FRAGMENT CLEAVAGE | PLATELET AGGREGATION AND RELEASE | ACTIVATION OF FACTOR VIII | ACTIVATION OF FACTOR V |
|---|---|---|---|---|---|---|---|
| | *Fibrinopeptides Released* | *Chain Degradation* | | | | | |
| Thrombin | A − B | $\alpha$(A) | Yes | Yes | Yes | Yes | Yes |
| Thrombinlike enzymes | A* | $\alpha$(A)† or $\beta$(B)‡ | No | Yes or no[§] | No | No | No |
| *Agkistrodon c. contortrix* venom | B | n.d.[#] | Incomplete | n.d. | No | n.d. | n.d. |
| *Bitis gabonica* venom | A + B | n.d. | Yes | n.d. | n.d. | n.d. | n.d. |

*Includes ancrod, batroxobin, crotalase, and the enzyme from *T. okinavensis*.
†Ancrod [batroxobin degrades $\alpha$(A) chain of bovine but not human fibrinogen].
‡Crotalase.
[§]Fragment I released by crotalase and *Agkistrodon contortrix* venom but not by ancrod or batroxobin.
[#]n. d. = not determined.
SOURCE: Russell (1983).

**Table 26–4**
**Comparison of Snake Venom Thrombinlike Enzymes**

| VENOM ENZYME | MOLECULAR WEIGHT | CARBOHYDRATE CONTENT % | $NH_2$-TERMINAL RESIDUE | ACTIVE SITE SERINE | ACTIVE SITE HISTIDINE |
|---|---|---|---|---|---|
| *Calloselasma rhodostoma* | 35,400 | 36.0 | Val | + | + |
| *Crotalus adamantus* | 33,700 | 5.4 | Val | + | + |
| *Bothrops marajoensis* | 31,400 | High | Val | + | n.d.* |
| *Bothrops moojeni* | 29,100 | 26.7 | Val | + | n.d. |
| *Crotalus horridus horridus* | 19,400 | Very low | n.d. | n.d. | n.d. |
| *Deinagkistrodon acutus* | 33,500 | 13.0 | n.d. | + | + |
| *Trimeresurus gramineus* | 29,500 | 25.0 | n.d. | + | n.d. |
| *Trimeresurus okinavensis* | 34,000 | 6.0 | n.d. | + | n.d. |
| *Agkistrodon contortrix contortrix* | 100,000 | n.d. | n.d. | + | n.d |
| *Bitis gabonica* | 32,500 | n.d. | n.d. | n.d. | n.d. |

*n.d. = not determined.
SOURCE: Russell (1983).

separated into three major groupings depending on their pharmacological activities: low-toxicity enzymes ($LD_{50} > 1$ mg/kg), high-toxicity enzymes (1 mg/kg $> LD_{50} >$ 0.1 mg/kg), and presynaptically acting toxins ($LD_{50} < 0.1$ mg/kg). Interested readers are referred to reviews by Rosenberg (1978, 1979, 1990).

Phosphomonoesterase (phosphatase) is widely distributed in the venoms of all families of snakes except the colubrids. It has the properties of an orthophosphoric monoester phosphohydrolase. There are two nonspecific phosphomonoesterases, and they have optimal pH at 5.0 and 8.5. Many venoms contain both acid and alkaline phosphatases, whereas others contain one or the other.

Phosphodiesterase has been found in the venoms of all five families of poisonous snakes. It is an orthophosphoric diester phosphohydrolase that releases 5-mononucleotide from the polynucleotide chain and thus acts as an exonucleotidase, attacking DNA and RNA. More recently, it has been found that it also attacks derivatives of arabinose.

Acetylcholinesterase was first demonstrated in cobra venom and is widely distributed throughout the elapid venoms. It is also found in sea snake venoms but is totally lacking in viperid and crotalid venoms. It catalyzes the hydrolysis of acetylcholine to choline and acetic acid. The role of the enzyme in snake venoms is not clear. Its so-called effect on ganglionic and neuromuscular transmission as a venom constituent is highly questionable.

RNase is present in some snake venoms in small amounts as the endopolynucleotidase RNase. It appears to have specificity toward pyrimidine-containing pyrimidyladenyl bonds in DNA. The optimum pH is 7 to 9 when ribosomal RNA is used as the substrate. This enzyme in *Naja oxiana* venom has a molecular weight of 15,900.

DNase acts on DNA and gives predominantly tri- or higher oligonucleotides that terminate in 3′ monoesterified phosphate. *Crotalus adamanteus* venom contains two DNases, with optimum pH at 5 and 9.

5′-Nucleotidase is a common constituent of all snake venoms, and in most instances it is the most active phosphatase in snake venoms. It specifically hydrolyzes phosphate monoesters, which link with a 5′ position of DNA and RNA. It is found in greater amounts in crotalid and viperid venoms than in elapid venoms. The molecular weight as determined from amino acid composition and gel filtration with *Naja naja atra* venom has been estimated at 10,000. The enzyme from *N. naja* venom is enhanced by $Mg^{2+}$, is inhibited by $Zn^{2+}$, is inactivated at 75°C at pH 7.0 or 8.4, and has an isoelectric point of about 8.6. That from *Agkistrodon halys blomhoffi* shows a pH optimum of 6.8 to 6.9, with activity being enhanced by $Mg^{2+}$ and $Mn^{2+}$ and inhibited by $Zn^{2+}$. The enzyme has a low order of lethality, and its pharmacological role in the venom is not understood (Russell, 1980b, 1983).

NAD nucleotidase has been found in a number of snake venoms. This enzyme catalyzes the hydrolysis of the nicotinamide *N*-ribosidic linkage of NAD, yielding nicotinamide and adenosine diphosphate riboside. Its optimum pH is 6.5 to 8.5; it is heat-labile, losing activity at 60°C. Its toxicological contribution to snake venoms is not understood.

L-Amino acid oxidase has been found in all snake venoms examined so far. It gives a yellow color to the venom. This enzyme catalyzes the oxidation of L-$\alpha$-amino and $\alpha$-hydroxy acids. This activity results from a group of homologous enzymes with molecular weights ranging from 85,000 to 150,000. It has a high content of acidic amino acids. We found that the mouse intravenous $LD_{50}$ of the enzyme from *Crotalus adamanteus* venom was 9.13 mg/kg body weight, approximately 4 times greater than the lethal value of the crude venom, and that this enzyme had no effect on nerve, muscle, or neuromuscular transmission (Russell, 1980b, 1983).

Lactate dehydrogenase reversibly catalyzes the conversion of lactic acid to pyruvic acid; it was found in nine elapid venoms but was not found in three others.

**Polypeptides.** Snake venom polypeptides are low-molecular-weight proteins that do not have enzymatic activity. Unfortunately, they are often logged under "neurotoxins," and this practice is not likely to change.

In 1938, Slotta and Fraenkel-Conrat isolated a crystalline protein from the venom of the tropical rattlesnake *Crotalus durissus terrificus*. The protein exhibited most of the toxic properties of the crude venom and was named crotoxin. In addition to the toxic nonenzymatic protein portion, it was found to contain the enzymes hyaluronidase and phospholipase and possibly several others. It did not appear to have proteolytic or coagulant properties or 5′-nucleotidase activity, but it had neurotoxic, indirect hemolytic, and smooth muscle–stimulating properties. After removal of phospholipase A, crotoxin was further separated into a general toxic principle known as crotactin, which was found to have a greater lethal index than that of crotoxin, and a second component that may have been crotamine. The word "crotoxin" has been retained in one form or another in the literature as an identification for 17 different separations of the venom of *Crotalus durissus terrificus* over the past 50 years. This has resulted in considerable confusion and disputes on research techniques which could be more easily resolved on the basis of a frank statement about the method of isolation. For a thorough review of crotoxin, see Haberman and Breithaupt (1978).

During the past 20 years, a number of peptides of snake venoms have been characterized. In 1965, the first paper on the amino acid composition of a snake venom peptide was published (Yang, 1965), and at the First International Symposium on Animal Toxins in 1966, Tamiya presented a paper on the chromatography, crystallization, electrophoresis, ultracentrifugation, and amino acid composition of the venom of the sea snake *Laticauda semifasciata*. Most of the lethal activity of the poison was recovered as two toxins, erabutoxin a and b, using carboxymethylcellulose chromatography; 30 percent of the proteins were erabutoxins. The homogeneity of the crystalline toxins was demonstrated by rechromatography, disk electrophoresis, and ultracentrifugation (Tamiya et al., 1967). At the same meeting, Su and colleagues (1967) reported the isolation of a cobra "neurotoxin." The toxin was separated by repeated fractionation with ammonium sulfate. The final product was a polypeptide and was approximately 7 times more lethal than the crude venom. Since 1966, more than 80 polypeptides with pharmacological activity have been isolated from snake venoms. Interested readers will find definitive reviews on these peptides in the works of Elliott (1978), Tu (1977), Rosenberg (1978), Lee (1979), Eaker and Wadström (1980), and Gopalakrishnakone and Tan (1992).

## Toxicology

It is not within the scope of this chapter to discuss all the pharmacological activities of snake venoms. Interested readers are referred to Russell (1967, 1983) and Mebs (1978) and to articles in the compendiums of the *International Society on Toxinology* for a more thorough consideration of the specific toxicological effects of these poisons and their components. However, some remarks will be made about the venoms of the North American crotalids, particularly the rattlesnakes. The $LD_{50}$'s of some North American snake venoms are shown in Table 26-5.

In general, the venoms of rattlesnakes and other new world crotalids produce alterations in the resistances (and often the integrity) of blood vessels, changes in blood cells and blood coagulation mechanisms, direct or indirect changes in cardiac and pulmonary dynamics, alterations in the nervous system, and changes in respiration. In humans, the course of the poisoning is determined by the kind and amount of venom injected; the site where it is deposited; the general health, size, and age of the patient; and the kind of treatment. Clinical experience indicates that death in humans occurs in less than 1 h to several days, with most deaths occurring between 18 and 32 h. Hypotension or shock is the major therapeutic problem. In some cases the hypotension is associated with acute blood loss secondary to bleeding and/or hemolysis, but in most patients shock is associated with a decrease in circulating fluid volume, with varying degrees of blood cell loss. It is not surprising therefore to find that numerous studies have been directed at determining the mechanisms responsible for snake venom poisoning, hypotension, and shock. These studies have been reviewed elsewhere (Russell, 1983).

Experimentally, it was found that an intravenous bolus injection of *Crotalus* venom caused an immediate fall in blood pressure and varying degrees of shock, which were associated with an initial hemoconcentration followed by a decrease in hematocrit values. There was increased blood volume in the lungs, an increase in pulmonary artery pressure with a concomitant decrease in pulmonary artery flow, and a relatively stable heart stroke volume (Russell et al., 1962). Other workers, using a 30-min perfusion of *Crotalus* venom, concluded that the hypotension was related to the formation of pulmonary thromboemboli in the pulmonary vascular bed (Halmagyi et al., 1965). Multiple pulmonary emboli may be found

**Table 26–5**
**$LD_{50}$ by Different Routes of Injection**

| VENOM | INTRAVENOUS | INTRAPERITONEAL | SUBCUTANEOUS |
|---|---|---|---|
| *Crotalus viridis helleri* | 1.29 | 1.60 | 3.65 |
| *Crotalus adamanteus* | 1.68 | 1.90 | 13.73 |
| *Crotalus atrox* | 2.18 | 3.71 | 17.75 |
| *Crotalus scutulatus* | 0.21 | 0.23 | 0.31 |
| *Agkistrodon piscivorus* | 4.17 | 5.10 | 25.10 |
| *Agkistrodon contortrix* | 10.92 | 10.50 | 26.10 |
| *Sistrurus miliarius* | 2.91 | 6.89 | 25.10 |

*Note*: All determinations were made in 20-g female mice of the same group. All mice were injected within a 1-h period and were observed for 48 h.

SOURCE: Russell (1983).

in animals that have received a fatal rattlesnake bite; however, the production of thromboembolism within 1 min after the administration of a bolus injection or even after a 30-min infusion of the venom might be a problematic explanation for the rapid onset of pulmonary hypotension and the precipitous fall in systemic arterial pressure. Clumping of blood cells in the lungs, thrombosis, or even multiple pulmonary emboli might conceivably cause pulmonary hypotension within this short period, but it seems unlikely that thromboembolism is responsible for the immediate circulatory failure. In postmortem reports on human victims who survived less than 3 h after a rattlesnake bite, there is no evidence of pulmonary thromboembolism (Russell, 1983).

*Crotalus* venom appears to produce a pooling of blood in the hepatosplanchnic bed in the dog (Vick et al., 1967). However, the hepatosplanchnic bed in the cat and the human is known to be a lesser target area in most shock states than it is in the dog, and it seems unlikely that this explanation for the hypotension is consistent with snake venom poisoning in humans. Again, postmortem examinations in humans have not shown a remarkable involvement of the hepatosplanchnic bed. Carlson and colleagues (1975) observed that when *Crotalus* venom is given intravenously and slowly over a 30-min period, there is hypovolemia secondary to an increase in capillary permeability to protein and red blood cells. The laboratory findings showed initial hemoconcentration, lactacidemia, and hypoproteinemia. In cats, the same findings are seen, followed by a fall in hematocrit and in some cases hemolysis that is related to the dose of venom. During this period the cat may be in shock or at near-shock levels, depending on the amount of venom injected or perfused. Respirations become labored, and if the period is prolonged, the animal becomes oliguric, rales develop, and the animal dies.

There appears to be no doubt that the shock or hypotension is caused by a decrease in circulating blood volume secondary to an increase in capillary permeability that leads to the loss of fluid, protein, and to some extent erythrocytes. The severity of the hypotension is dose-related, and restoration of circulating fluid volume can be achieved with intravenous fluids. In patients with venom hypovolemic shock, steroids are of no value, but the use of isoproterenol hydrochloride may be indicated. Antivenin in itself may not reverse a deep shock state, but a combination of parenteral fluids or plasma expanders, isoproterenol hydrochloride, and antivenin is definitely of value.

Evidence to the present time indicates that the fraction of the venom that most probably is responsible for the circulatory failure is a peptide. In 1970, Dubnoff and Russell reported the presence of two biologically active peptides in the venom of the rattlesnake *Crotalus viridis helleri*. Ion-exchange chromatography on carboxymethylcellulose and on IRC-50 indicated molecular weights of approximately 6000 each. The peptides moved as cations on cellulose acetate at pH 8.6. Peptide I was identified as the major peak. Subsequently, Bonilla and Fiero isolated highly basic proteins from the venoms of three subspecies of rattlesnakes: *Crotalus viridis viridis*, *C. horridus horridus*, and *C. h. atricaudatus*. The proteins were separated by recycling adsorption chromatography using Bio-Gel P-2 and by ion-exchange chromatography on carboxymethylcellulose. These fractions were of low molecular weight, had isoelectric points above pH 6.8 (Bonilla and Fiero, 1971), and showed pharmacological properties similar to those of *C. v. helleri* isolated by Dubnoff and Russell (1970).

Toxicological studies have been carried out on the various fractions of *C. v. helleri* venom. One peptide, *C. v. helleri* Peptide I, which moved as a cation on strip and gel electrophoresis and on ion-exchange chromatography, was resolved into three lethal peaks. The major fraction (*C. v. h.* Peptide Ic) was a basic polypeptide containing 43 amino acid residues with six half-cystine and had a molecular weight of 4490 as calculated from its sequence. Analysis showed that the peptide contained almost 20 percent lysine (Maeda et al., 1978). The peptide was found to be responsible for the hypotension or shock produced by the crude venom. When injected into rats, this peptide produced shock characterized by hypotension, lactacidemia, hemoconcentration, hypoproteinemia, and metabolic acidosis. Death occurred in some rats, and respiratory distress was observed just before death. Hemolysis did not occur, but hemolysis and hematuria were observed in rats given the non-peptide fractions (Schaeffer et al., 1978).

The primary action of the peptide on the cardiovascular system involves its ability to produce a transient increase in vascular permeability to plasma protein; this eventually, with certain other proteins, causes the loss of red blood cells. The peptide appears to alter the endothelial cells of the vascular wall, giving rise to the escape of plasma protein and some red blood cells. This finding for rattlesnake venom appears to differ from that presented for elapid venoms in that *C. viridis helleri* Peptide I is capable of producing rapid endothelial changes without enzyme involvement. Other protein components of the venom, some of which are enzymes, appear to have little effect on the vascular membrane but instead induce red blood cell changes or lysis. There may be some synergistic action, but for the most part the vascular properties are rather distinct.

## Lizard Venoms

The Gila monster, *Heloderma suspectum*, and the beaded lizard, *H. horridum*, are divided into five subspecies. These large, corpulent, relatively slow moving, and largely nocturnal reptiles have few enemies other than humans. They are far less dangerous than is generally believed. Their venom is transferred from venom glands in the lower jaw through ducts that discharge their contents near the base of the larger teeth of the lower jaw. The venom is then drawn up along grooves in the teeth by capillary action. The venom of this lizard has serotonin, amine oxidase, phospholipase A, proteolytic, and hyaluronidase activities but lacks phosphomonoesterase and phosphodiesterase, acetylcholinesterase, nucleotidase, ATPase, DNase, RNase, amino acid oxidase, and fibrinogenocoagulase activities. The high hyaluronidase content seems to be consistent with the tissue edema seen in many clinical cases, and the low proteolytic activity is also consistent with the minimal tissue breakdown seen in clinical cases. The injection of large doses of *Heloderma* venom produces a fall in systemic arterial pressure with a decrease in circulating blood volume, tachycardia, and respiratory distress; in lethal doses, there is a loss of ventricular contractility (Russell and Bogert, 1981). An excellent review on the biology of the Gila monster has been published by Brown and Carmony (1991).

## Clinical Problem

Snake venom poisoning is a medical emergency that requires immediate attention and the exercise of considerable judgment. Delayed or inadequate treatment may result in tragic consequences. However, before any treatment is instituted, it is essential that a working diagnosis be established. In making a diagnosis, it must be remembered that being bitten by a venomous snake does not necessarily mean being envenomated by that snake. A venomous snake may bite a person and not inject venom. Also, in treating snake venom poisoning, the physician should keep in mind that this is a case of multiple and complex poisoning. There is no single therapeutic measure other than antivenom that can effectively neutralize all the physiopharmacological activities of the venom.

The symptoms and signs of pit viper envenomation may include the presence of fang marks; swelling; pain; ecchymosis; weakness; various paresthesias; nausea and vomiting; alterations in temperature, pulse, and blood pressure; fasciculations; urinary changes; early hemoconcentration followed by a decreased hematocrit; decreased platelets; alterations in the clotting profile; petechial hemorrhages; and shock. The most diagnostic sign of crotalid envenomation is rapid, progressive swelling. In most patients, when venom has been injected, there is some swelling around the bite area within 5 to 10 min, and sometimes the swelling involves the entire finger, hand, toe, or foot within several hours. A common symptom after bites by some species of rattlesnakes is paresthesia about the mouth, sometimes the forehead and scalp, and less frequently the fingers and toes. This is usually present after the bites of the eastern diamondback rattlesnake (*Crotalus adamanteus*), the Pacific rattlesnakes (*C. viridis helleri* and *C. viridis oreganus*), and certain other species. The venom of some rattlesnake species, however, does not produce this complaint.

The degree of poisoning must always be determined on admission and as it progresses. A bite may appear minor at 1 h but prove serious or even fatal at 3 h. Most of the suggested grading systems for crotalid bites are precarious, for they usually depend on a few selected symptoms or signs that often are stipulated for a specific time, for instance, 12 h; this is beyond the effective time of antivenom administration.

It is far more simple and practical to grade envenomations as minimal, moderate, or severe on the basis of all clinical findings, including the laboratory data. One must remember that grading may need to be changed as the course of the poisoning or treatment progresses. This should always be noted on the patient's chart.

A determination should be made as to whether antivenom is necessary. It need not be given in trivial bites. The antivenom generally should be put in 250 to 1000 ml of an appropriate vehicle. It is compatible with commonly used dextrose and electrolyte solutions. The best results are obtained when it is administered during the first 4 h after the bite, but its efficacy, particularly in reversing clotting deficits, is apparent for at least 24 h after the bite and perhaps even longer. In most cases, antivenom is not needed for copperhead bites, but it may be indicated in water moccasin bites. A skin test should always be administered before the administration of antivenin. The patient should be slightly sedated if that is not contraindicated and put to bed, with the injured part lightly immobilized in a functional position slightly below heart level. Medication for tetanus, pain, sleep, and anxiety may be needed. In moderate or severe envenomations, laboratory work should be done on admission and at least twice a day thereafter. Food should be avoided during the first 24 h. Detailed clinical reports on bites by American species can be found in Russell (1977, 1983), Van Mierop (1976), Watt (1978), Parrish (1980), Dart and Russell (1992), and Gold and Wingert (1994).

# AMPHIBIA

The class Amphibia contains approximately 2600 species and is divided into the Anura (toads and frogs), and the Urodela (salamanders and newts). Although a number of amphibians are known to be poisonous, very few are dangerous to humans. The most important toxic Anura are toads of the family Bufonidae; frogs of the families Atelopodidae, Dendrobatidae, Discoglossidae, Hylidae, Phyllomedusae, Pipidae, and Ranidae; newts of the genera *Taricha* and *Triturus*; and certain salamanders of the genus *Salamandra* (Kaiser and Michl, 1958; Habermehl, 1981; Daly et al., 1993).

## Amphibian Toxins

The poisons of amphibians are produced in certain highly developed cutaneous secretory glands. These secretions generally are excreted in a steady state, although there may be increased elaboration under duress or other conditions. Although it is commonly believed that their only function is related to a deterrent posture, that is, defense against predators, it has been shown that in some amphibians an additional function is their role in protecting the host against microorganisms in the environment. When the skin is freed of the secretions of these particular glands, infection occurs and death may result. The secretions have been shown to inhibit the growth of bacteria and fungi in concentrations as low as $10^{-3}$ to $10^{-5}$ mol/liter (Habermehl, 1981; Bevins and Zasloff, 1990). There are nearly 300 known amphibian steroidal alkaloids, which generally are divided into two classes, batrachotoxins and Samandarines (Daly et al., 1993). Daly and associates (1991) have provided an excellent review of amphibian alkaloids.

The chemical composition of amphibian secretions is highly diversified. In toads, biogenic amines, including adrenaline, noradrenaline, dopamine, and epinine, are sometimes found, whereas among the indoalkylamines, the bases bufotenin, bufotenidin, and bufoviridin have been noted.

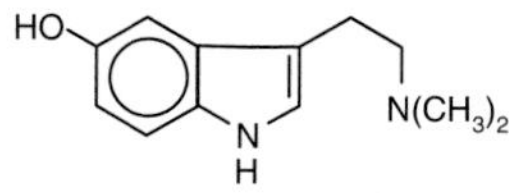

HO– … $N(CH_3)_2$

Bufotenin

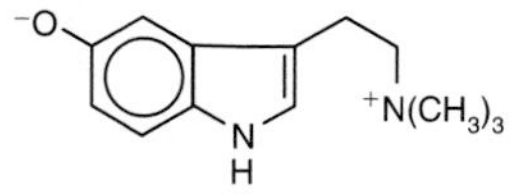

$^{-}O$– … $^{+}N(CH_3)_3$

Bufotenidin

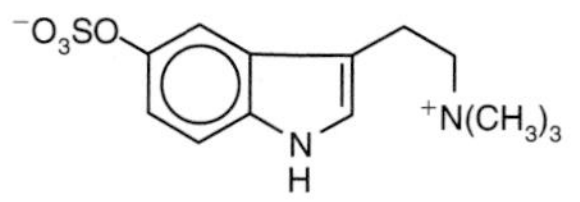

$^{-}O_3SO$– … $^{+}N(CH_3)_3$

Bufoviridin

These substances have been described as causing vasoconstriction, hypotension, and hallucinations. A second group of toxic secretions in toads consists of the bufogenines, of which bufotalin is representative. These toxins appear to have a marked effect on smooth muscle, including the heart (Meyer, 1949).

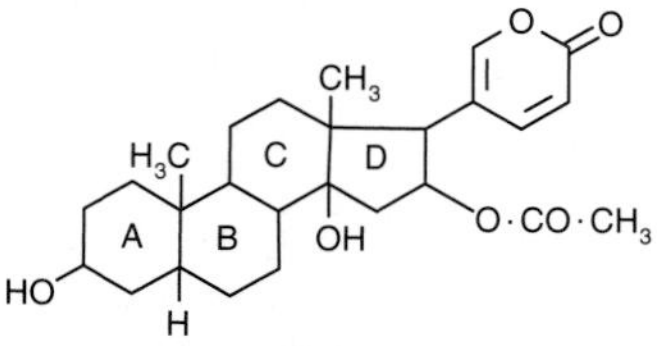

Bufotalin

Frog toxins are even more diversified chemically than are toad poisons. These toxins have been studied extensively by Daly and colleagues at the National Institutes of Health (NIH) (Daly et al., 1987, 1992). Contrary to popular opinion, only three extraordinarily toxic species of *Phyllobatis* have been used for poisonous blowgun darts, not arrows (Myers and Daly, 1993).

In the Atelopodidae, *Atelopus* species, there are a group of toxins known as zetekitoxins. The subcutaneous "lethal dose" in mice for zetekitoxin AB is 11 $\mu$g/kg; for zetekitoxin C, it is 80 $\mu$g/kg body weight. Tetrodotoxin has been isolated from the skin and egg clusters of *A. varius*, whereas both tetrodotoxin and chiriquitoxin have been found in the skin and eggs of *A. chiriquensis*. The bicyclic alkaloids are in several classes: pumiliotoxin-A, decahydroquinolines, and histrionicotoxins. Among the other steroid alkaloids are batrachotoxin, batrachotoxin A, homobatrachotoxin, dihydrobatrachotoxin, and 3-*O*-methylbatrachotoxin, all of which are found in certain *Phyllobates* species. Some representative structures are shown here (Daly et al., 1992):

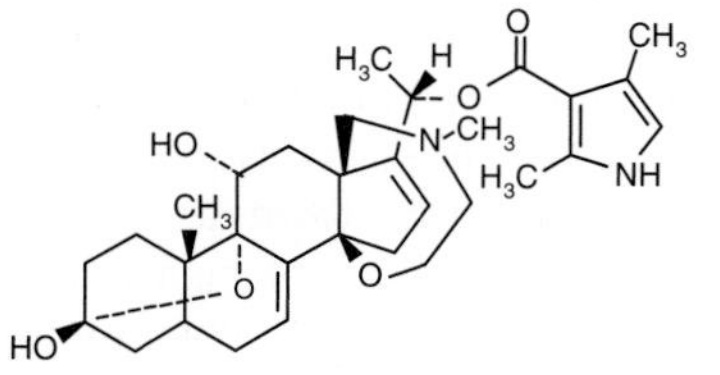

Batrachotoxin

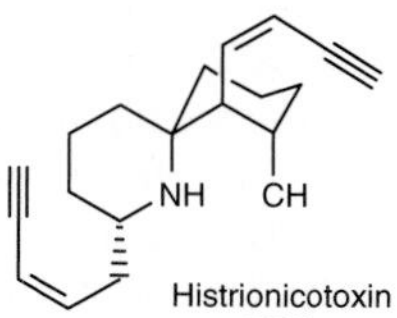

Histrionicotoxin
283A

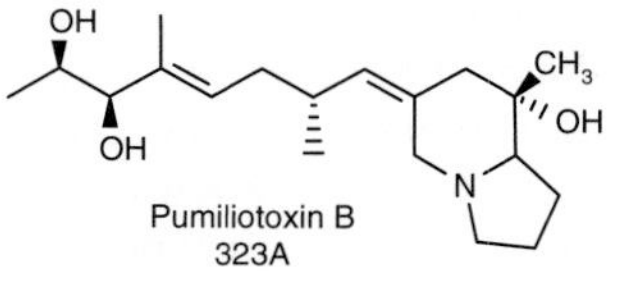

Pumiliotoxin B
323A

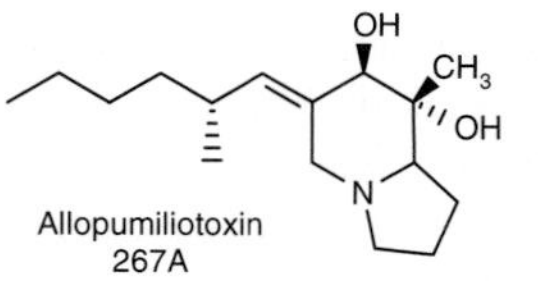

Allopumiliotoxin
267A

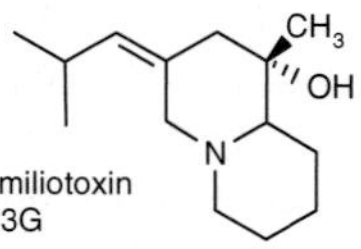

Homopumiliotoxin
223G

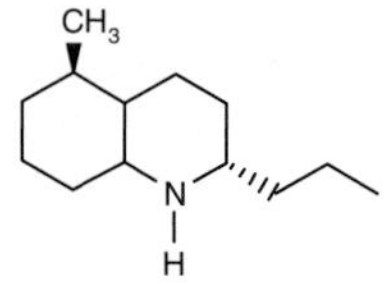

Decahydroquinoline
cis-195A

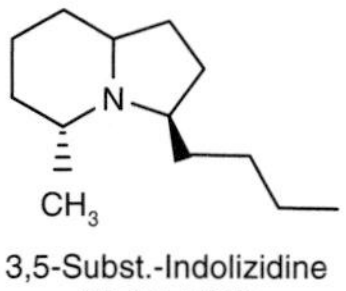

3,5-Subst.-Indolizidine
5E,9E-195B

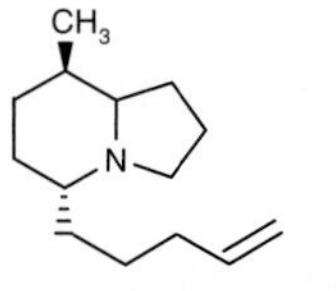

5,8-Subst.-Indolizidine
207A

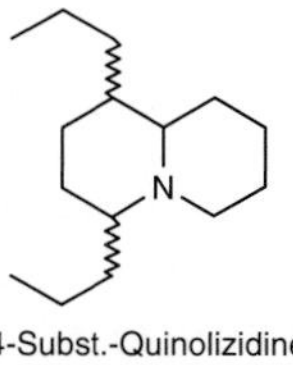

1.4-Subst.-Quinolizidine
223A

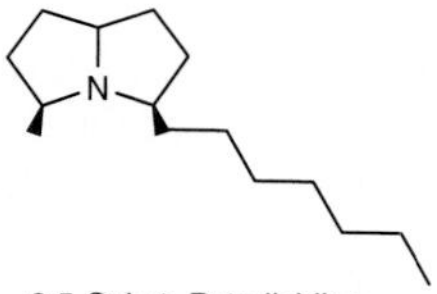

3,5-Subst.-Pytrolizidine
223H

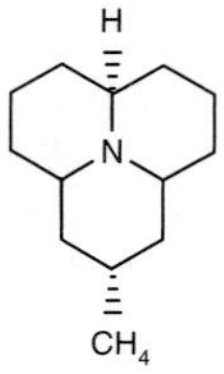

Tricyclic
193
precoccinoline

Batrachotoxin is one of the most toxic substances known, with the subcutaneous lethal dose in mice being 100 ng; the estimated lethal dose for humans is less than 200 $\mu$g. Although generally classified as a "neurotoxin," this alkaloid has a marked effect on the heart that is evident first as arrhythmias and then by changes leading to cardiac arrest. It has a direct effect on the peripheral nervous system, producing membrane depolarization, probably as a result of an increase in cell membrane permeability by sodium without related changes in potassium or calcium ions. Batrachotoxin also causes a massive release of acetylcholine in nerve muscle preparations. The ultrastructural changes in nerve and muscle precipitated by this toxin are thought to be caused by osmotic alterations produced by the massive influx of sodium ions (Daly, 1982).

From the skin secretions of *Dendrobates pumilio* and *D. auratus*, three alkaloids have been isolated: pumiliotoxins A ($C_{19}H_{33}NO_2$), B ($C_{19}H_{33}NO_3$), and C ($C_{13}H_{25}N$). Skin secretions from *D. auratus* have also yielded other alkaloids, whereas spiropiperidine alkaloids have been identified in the skin secretions of *D. histrionicus*. The subcutaneous "minimal lethal dose" in mice for pumiliotoxin A is 2.5 mg/kg body weight; for pumiliotoxin B, it is 1.5 mg/kg; and for pumiliotoxin C, it is 20 mg/kg. These doses produce ataxia, "clonic convulsions," and death within 20 min. Pumiliotoxin B potentiates both directly and indirectly evoked contractions of striated muscle. It does not appear to have an effect on sodium, potassium, or chloride conductances or on the resting membrane potential (Albuquerque et al., 1981). The skin secretions of *Bombina bombina* yield large amounts of serotonin, free amino acids, and basic peptides. In *B. variegata*, 12 $\alpha$-amino acids, gamma-aminobutyric acid, and serotonin, two nonpeptides, and a hemolytic polypeptide of 87,000 daltons have been demonstrated (Habermehl, 1981).

The poisons of newts and salamanders have undergone considerable study. Tarichatoxin has been isolated from three species of newts: *Taricha torosa*, *T. rivularis*, and *T. granulosa*. It is, of course, the same toxin found in the pufferfish *Sphaeroides* species and known as tetrodotoxin. Tarichatoxin, or tetrodotoxin, is also found in some species of frogs and at least one octopus as well as a number of other fishes besides the puffers. Among the steroid alkaloids found in the salamanders are samanine, samandenone, cycloneosamandaridine, cycloneosamandoine, samandarine, and samandaridine. Samandarines are very potent toxins that are said to act on the central nervous system and also have hypertensive and anesthetic properties.

## MARINE ANIMALS

Like snakes, venomous and poisonous marine animals have a fascinating history, including sea serpents that crawled ashore and copulated with vipers, others that sprayed their venom onto unsuspecting seamen on sailing ships and paralyzed them on the spot, and stingrays that stung and killed trees. Interested readers should consult the compendium of Halstead (1965, 1978) and the works of Kaiser and Michl (1958), Russell (1965, 1971, 1984a), Baslow (1969), Martin and Padilla (1973), Scheuer (1973, 1978), and Southcott (1979) for historical accounts of venomous marine animals.

Approximately 1200 species of marine organisms are known to be venomous or poisonous (Russell, 1983). For the most part, these animals are widely distributed throughout the marine fauna from the unicellular protistan *Alexandrium* (*Gonyaulax*) to certain of the chordates. In most areas, they do not constitute a medical or socioeconomic problem. However, in a few scattered regions, such as the South Pacific and the Caribbean, where ciguatera poisoning sometimes gives rise to serious public health and economic problems, and in the case of paralytic shellfish poisoning, poisonous marine animals have presented a threat to our health and economy.

### Marine Toxins

While the marine toxins as a whole are far more varied in their chemical composition than are those from terrestrial animals, there is some degree of component consistency within a particular genus or species in each group. Some organisms, such as clams and mussels, may be toxic only during a particular period or in one place but not elsewhere, while the toxicity in tetraodons varies with the species of fish, the organs studied, and other factors. Toxicity in ciguateric fishes is at the present time and for all practical purposes almost unpredictable with respect to species involved, location, and time of year.

Some marine toxins are proteins of low molecular weight, whereas others are of high molecular weight. Some marine venoms or poisons are composed of lipids, amines, quinones, quaternary ammonium compounds, alkaloids, guanidine bases, phenols, steroids, mucopolysaccharides, or halogenated compounds. Most fish venoms are unstable. In some marine organisms there are several toxins present, and in some instances two organisms are needed to produce one toxin. Finally, it is known that the venom of one species or genus in one phylum may be similar or even identical to that found in an animal in an entirely different phylum. The newt poison, tarichatoxin, and the pufferfish poison, tetrodotoxin, are one and the same.

As would be expected, the pharmacological and toxicological activities of marine toxins vary as remarkably as do their chemical properties. Some marine toxins provoke rather simple effects such as transient vasoconstriction or dilatation, pain, and localized erythema, whereas others produce more complex responses such as parasympathetic dysfunction and multiple concomitant changes in cardiovascular or blood dynamics. There is no doubt that in the evolution of marine toxins, as in snake and other terrestrial venoms (Russell, 1980a), synergistic and possibly antagonistic reactions may occur as a result of interactions between individual venom components. The release of autopharmacological substances by the action of marine poisons must also be taken into consideration in clinical cases of poisoning.

### Protista

Among the protistans are the various protozoans, algae, diatoms, bacteria, yeasts, and fungi. The marine Protista are widely distributed throughout neritic waters and in the high seas from the polar oceans to the tropics. At least 80 species are known to be toxic to humans and other animals. A listing of these species can be found in Russell (1984a). Most of the toxic organisms are of the order Dinoflagellata, of which there are more than 1200 species. Protistans have been shown to contain or release a toxin that (1) gives rise to paralytic shellfish poisoning through the food chain, (2) produces respiratory or gastrointestinal (GI) distress or dermatitis in humans, (3) causes mass mortality of marine animals, or (4) has been implicated in laboratory experiments as being toxic. Blooms of protistans sometimes occur and result in the phenomenon frequently referred to as "red tide," or "red water." However, the bloom may appear yellowish, brownish, greenish, bluish, or even milky in color, depending on the organism involved and other factors. Such blooms usually become visible when 20,000 or more of the organisms are present in 1 ml of water. However, some blooms may contain 50,000 or more organisms. The color of red tides probably is due to peridinin, a xanthophyll.

Paralytic shellfish poison (PSP), variously known as saxitoxin, *Gonyaulax* toxin, dinoflagellate poison, mussel or clam poison, or mytilotoxin, is a toxin or group of toxins found in certain mollusks, arthropods, echinoderms, and some other marine animals that have ingested toxic protistans and have become "poisonous." PSP through the food chain is well known in both domestic animals and humans.

The amount of poison in the shellfish or other organism is dependent on the number of toxic protistans filtered by the host animal. Off California, mussels become dangerous for human consumption when 200/ml protistans or more are found in the coastal waters. As the count rises, the mussels become more toxic. Within a week or two, in the absence of the toxic protistans, the mussels become relatively free of the poison. The toxin has been studied by extractions from shellfish, from dinoflagellates secured from natural blooms, and more recently from laboratory cultures. PSP can be obtained from all three sources in a similar form. Burke and associates (1960), Schantz and colleagues (1966), and Proctor and coworkers (1975) have grown *Alexandrium (Gonyaulax) catenella* in axenic cultures in cell densities equal to those occurring during natural blooms, and Schantz (1960) showed that the chromatographic properties of the toxin from the cultured organisms appear identical to those of the toxin found in natural blooms and mussels. It was not until 1975 that Schantz and associates presented the absolute configuration:

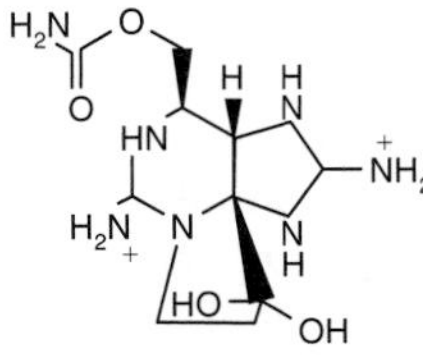

There is some question about how many toxins exist in the complex of PSP. In earlier works it was considered a single poison, but it must now be thought of as a complex of toxins. In the dinoflagellate *Alexandrium (Gonyaulax) tamarensis* there are several other toxins in addition to saxitoxin, and they differ from saxitoxin only in their weak binding ability on carboxylate resins. Further studies on organisms obtained from red tides along the New England coast have resulted in the isolation of two other toxins: gonyautoxin II ($GTX_2$) and gonyautoxin III ($GTX_3$) (Shimizu, 1978). Another toxin—neosaxitoxin—has also been isolated from *A. tamarensis*.

While a number of pharmacological and toxicological studies on shellfish poisons were carried out before the turn of this century, it was not until the reports of Meyer and associates (1928), Prinzmetal and colleagues (1932), and Sommer and Meyer (1937) that the more definitive work was reported. Prinzmetal and colleagues (1932) showed that the poison from the mussel *Mytilus californianus* was slowly absorbed from the GI tract and rapidly excreted by the kidneys. It was said to depress respiration, the cardioinhibitory and vasomotor centers, and conduction in the myocardium. Subsequent studies showed that saxitoxin had a marked effect on peripheral nerve and skeletal muscle in the frog. The "curarelike" action was attributed to a mechanism that prevented the muscle from responding to acetylcholine. The toxin produced progressive diminution in the amplitude of the endplate potential in the frog nerve-muscle preparation. It also depressed mammalian phrenic nerve potentials, suppressed indirectly elicited contractions of the diaphragm, and often reduced the directly stimulated contractions. With respect to the cardiovascular system, the toxin was shown to have a direct effect on the heart and its conduction system. It produced changes that ranged from a slight decrease in heart rate and contractile force with simple PR interval prolongation or ST segment changes to severe bradycardia and bundle branch block or complete cardiac failure. The poison provoked a prompt but reversible depression in the contractility of isolated cat papillary muscle (see Russell, 1984a, for references).

In 1967, Kao demonstrated that this toxin blocks action potentials in nerves and muscles by preventing, in a very specific manner, an increase in the ionic permeability that is normally associated with the inward flow of sodium. It appeared to do this without altering potassium or chloride conductances. Evans (1967) showed that in cats, mussel poison blocked transmission between the peripheral nerves and the spinal roots. The large myelinated sensory fibers were blocked by intravenous doses of 4.5 to 13 $\mu$g/kg, whereas the large motor fibers were not blocked until this dose was increased by 30 to 40 percent. Evans suggested that one of the layers in the connective tissue sheath of peripheral nerve is impermeable to saxitoxin, whereas the leptomeninges covering the spinal roots are either deficient in or lack this layer.

Sommer and Meyer (1937) found that 3000 *Gonyaulax* weighed 100 $\mu$g (wet weight) and that this number yielded 15 $\mu$g of the dry extract, which in turn gave 1 $\mu$g of pure poison, or 1 mouse unit. A mouse unit, or average lethal dose, was defined as the amount of toxin that would kill a 20-g mouse in 15 min (Prinzmetal et al., 1932; Sommer and Meyer, 1937). Thus, the amount of toxin contained in a single *Gonyaulax* was taken as 1/3000 of a mouse unit. McFarren and associates (1956) found the oral $LD_{50}$'s per kg body weight to vary considerably with the animal used and with its strain and weight. Their figures indicate that the human is twice as susceptible to the poison as is the dog and approximately 4 times more susceptible than is the mouse.

During the 1950s the Canadian–United States Conference on Shellfish Toxicology adopted a bioassay based on the use of the purified toxin isolated by Schantz and colleagues (1958). The intraperitoneal minimal lethal dose of the toxin for the mouse was approximately 9.0 $\mu$g/kg body weight. The intravenous minimal lethal dose for the rabbit was 3.0 to 4.0 $\mu$g/kg body weight, whereas the minimal lethal oral dose for humans was thought to be between 1.0 and 4.0 mg. Wiberg and

Stephenson (1960) demonstrated that the $LD_{50}$ of the then purified toxin in mice was

Oral route: 263 (251–267) $\mu$g/kg
Intravenous route: 3.4 (3.2–3.6) $\mu$g/kg
Intraperitoneal route: 10.0 (9.7–10.5) $\mu$/kg

More recently, various figures on the toxic and lethal doses for humans have been presented by various workers. The figures presented by Prakash and coworkers (1971) seem to be consistent with our calculations; that is, a mild case of poisoning can be caused by ingesting 1 mg of toxin, which might be the amount found in one to five poisonous mussels or clams weighing about 150 g each. A moderate case of poisoning could be caused by ingesting 2 mg of the poison, whereas a serious poisoning would be caused by 3 mg. One would expect that 4 mg of the toxin could be lethal to humans if vigorous treatment were not instituted.

The latest standards for toxicity are those set by the Association of Official Analytical Chemists (AOAC) (1975). However, these standards, like others, have several shortcomings. A number of assays have been proposed to circumvent these deficiencies. For example, an immunochemical technique has been suggested, whereas another method employs an analysis based on the oxidation of saxitoxin to a fluorescent derivative. Spectrophotometric analysis has been proposed, and a unique cockroach bioassay has been described. One of the most promising assays incorporates flow cytometric analysis of cellular saxitoxin, dependent on mithramycin fluorescent staining (see Russell, 1984a, for references). With the advent of the enzyme-linked immunosorbent assay (ELISA) and radioimmunology, new and improved techniques for determining toxicities have appeared.

## Porifera (Sponges)

Sponges are highly organized colonies of unicellular nomads composed of loosely integrated cells covered by a skin and, with few exceptions, supported internally by a skeleton of silica, calcite, or spongin. There are more than 5000 species, and they are found in almost every sea from midtide levels to the deepest parts of the oceans. Some sponges release a toxic substance into their environment. De Laubenfels (1932) observed that when *Tedania toxicalis* was placed in a bucket with fishes, crabs, mollusks, and worms, in an hour or perhaps less those animals would be found dead. Although the phenomenon has usually been considered a purely defensive reaction initiated when the sponge becomes endangered, Green (1977) suggested that the toxic material may be released as a continuous product into the surrounding water and thus serve as a warning or deterrent to an approaching predator.

The marine sponges of greater biological importance are described elsewhere (Russell, 1984a). Interested readers should also consult Halstead (1965), Jakowska and Nigrelli (1970), Stempien and associates (1970), Green (1977), and Bakus and Thun (1979) for more detailed data on the toxicity of these animals. It should be noted that some sponges of the same genus as those found to be toxic to fishes have been found to be nontoxic. The family Haliclonidae appears to have the most consistently toxic species.

Perhaps the most extensive studies on the toxic effects of sponges have been those by Bakus and colleagues. Essentially, their shipboard method for a preliminary toxicity assay involves grinding 5 g of the sponge in 10 ml of seawater, centrifuging, pouring the supernatant into a bowl with 300 ml of seawater, and then placing a 1.5- to 5-g sergeant major (*Abudefduf saxatilis*) into the water and observing the fish's behavior over a designated period. Toxicity is determined on the basis of the fish swallowing air, blowing bubbles, and being bitten by normal fish as well as equilibrium loss, erratic swimming behavior, slow swimming movements, escape responses, thrashing behavior, extreme lethargy or stupor, failure to recover when put in fresh water, and death (Bakus and Thun, 1979).

In 1906, Richet precipitated a substance from extracts of the siliceous sponge *Suberites domunculus*, which when injected into the dog produced vomiting, diarrhea, and dyspnea and caused hemorrhages in the gastric and intestinal mucosa, peritoneum, and endocardium. The lethal dose in dogs was 10 mg/kg, and the toxic substance was found to be nontoxic when administered orally. The poison was called "suberitine" (Richet, 1906; Lassablière, 1906). Arndt (1928) demonstrated that extracts from certain freshwater sponges produced diarrhea, dyspnea, prostration, and death when injected into homiothermic animals. The same extracts had some hemolytic effects on sheep and pig erythrocytes and blocked cardiac function in the isolated frog heart preparation. The extracts were heat-stable and produced no deleterious effects when taken orally. Das and colleagues (1971) found that extracts of *S. inconstans* produced a histaminelike effect on the guinea pig intestine and attributed this effect to histamine, which they found in the sponge. On paper chromatography, they detected five other amines, three with phenolic groups. Algelasine from *Agelas dispar* has activities of a saponin. A unique sesquiterpene, 9-isocyanopupukeanane, has been isolated from the nudibranch *Phyllidia varicosa* and has been found to be present in the sponge *Hymeniacidon* sp., on which the nudibranch feeds (Burreson et al., 1975).

Cariello and associates (1980) isolated and characterized Richet's suberitine. The toxin, which had an approximate molecular weight of 28,000, produced a marked hemolytic effect on human erythrocytes and showed some ATPase activity. Studies on the giant axon of the abdominal nerve of the crayfish indicated that in a concentration of 4.4 mg/ml there was depolarization followed by an irreversible block in the indirectly stimulated action potential. Wang and colleagues (1973) demonstrated that a preparation of an extract of *Haliclona rubens* exerted a depolarizing action on the end-plate membrane of the frog skeletal muscle and that a lesser depolarization occurred in the membrane in an area other than the end plate.

**Clinical Problem.** With respect to humans, poisoning probably occurs through deposition of the toxin or toxins in the superficial abrasions produced by the fine, sharp spicules of the sponge. It is known that traumatic injury to the human skin can be produced by spicules, particularly those of the hexactinellids, and it is believed that in many cases of poisoning this occurs before the deposition of the poison on the skin. Certainly, an abraded skin is more likely to absorb a toxin than is an uninjured one. The most frequently offending sponges are

*Tedania nigrescens, T. inconstans*, and *Neofibularia nolitangere*. The symptoms and signs consist of a burning or irritating sensation over the hands or other part contacted by the sponge, subsequent mild pain sometimes confined to the joints of the involved hand, pruritus (often severe), and malaise. The contact areas are warm to touch, and there may be mild edema. Systemic manifestations and infections are rare. Treatment consists of thoroughly washing the hands with soapy water and applying such as Itch Balm Plus (hydrocortisone, tetracaine, and diphenhydramine hydrochloride) four times a day.

## Cnidaria (Coelenterates)

The phylum Cnidaria (hydroids, jellyfish, sea anemones, and corals) are simple metazoans that possess the two basic tissues found in all higher animals, a layer of jellylike material with supporting elastic fibers between the ectoderm and endoderm known as "mesoglea," a gastrovascular cavity that opens only through the mouth, radial symmetry, and tentacles bearing abundant nematocysts. In the Portuguese man-of-war, *Physalia*, and in many other cnidarians, the tentacles contain long muscle strands that can be contracted to bring the animal's prey to the feeding polyps below the umbrella. The polyps engulf the prey and digest it. Venomous forms are found in all three classes of living cnidarians: Hydrozoa, or hydroids, hydromedusae, and fire corals; Scyphozoa, or true jellyfish; and Anthozoa, or sea anemones, sea feathers, and alcyonarion corals. The Hydrozoa are branched or simple polyps, some with budded medusae. The order Siphonophora includes the Portuguese man-of-war, *Physalia*. The Scyphozoa, true medusae or jellyfishes, are typified by a body, umbrella, or bell, which is usually convex above and concave below. The Cubomedusae, or sea wasps, are the most dangerous of all the cnidarians, particularly *Chironex fleckeri* and *Chiropsalmus quadrigatus*. The anemones are sedentary, flowerlike structures. The alcyonarians include the stony, soft, horny, and black corals as well as colonial sea pens and sea pansies. The cnidarians are of particular importance because of their stinging of humans and their unusual toxicological properties, which are noted elsewhere (Russell, 1984a).

The stinging unit of the cnidarians is the nematocyst. It might be an overstatement to say that all 9000 species of cnidarians have nematocysts. Nematocysts have been classified on the basis of their structure, function, and taxonomy. Weill (1934) described 17 categories of nematocyst, and while these categories have been qualified with the passing of time, in general this system still offers a basis for common communication. The nematocyst, which is a capsulated, ovoid cell varying in size from 4 to 225 $\mu$m, contains an operculum, a long coiled tube or hollow thread, a matrix, and venom. The nematocyst is formed as "metaplasmic organelle" within an interstitial cell, the cnidoblast. These cnidoblasts are distributed throughout the epidermis, except on the basal disk. The coiled tubule in the undischarged nematocyst varies in length from 50 $\mu$m to over 1 mm, depending on the species of cnidarian. When it is discharged, the operculum is released and the everted tubule explodes, remaining attached at the original site of the operculum. The nature of nematocyst discharge and the localized fashion in which these cells respond to stimuli, whether chemical, mechanical, or electrical, have been objects of extensive study (see Russell, 1984a, for references).

As in many of the earlier studies on marine venoms, the chemical and toxicological properties of the cnidarian toxins were investigated with crude saline or water extracts prepared from the whole animal or from one or several of its parts. It is apparent that some early workers were studying normal constituents of the animal's tissues. Substances such as thalassin, congestin, and the *Cyanea* principle probably were derived from tentacular tissues rather than from venom-bearing nematocysts.

The modern period of fire coral toxicology began with the work of Wittle and associates (1971) and Middlebrook and colleagues (1971). These investigators studied nematocyst toxin from *Millepora alcicornis*. They obtained a product with a molecular weight of approximately 100,000 and an intravenous mouse $LD_{50}$ of 0.04 mg/kg body weight. The sea whip, *Lophogorgia rigida*, contains a toxin known as lophotoxin; its formula is $C_{22}H_{24}O_8$. The toxin has a subcutaneous $LD_{50}$ in mice of 8.9 mg/kg body weight and was found to block the indirectly elicited contractions in a mammalian nerve-muscle preparation while not affecting the directly elicited contractions. It was concluded that lophotoxin produces an irreversible postsynaptic block, although the possibility of a presynaptic function could not be excluded (Culver and Jacobs, 1981).

While techniques for separating nematocysts are not new, the initial studies on a nematocyst preparation from *Physalia physalis* were performed by Lane and Dodge (1958). These authors found their nematocyst preparation to be a highly labile protein complex, rich in glutamic acid and having an approximate intraperitoneal lethal dose in mice of 0.037 ml/kg body weight of a preparation containing 0.02 percent total nitrogen. The toxin produced paralysis in fish, frogs, and mice. Animals killed after stingings by *Physalia* exhibited marked pulmonary edema and right-sided cardiac dilatation, with venous congestion of the larger vessels of the chest and portal circulations. Since the original work of Lane and Dodge, a number of advances in the preparation of nematocyst toxins from *P. physalis* have been made. These and the toxicological studies have been reviewed elsewhere (Russell, 1984a). Various investigations of crabs, rats, dogs, and a nerve-muscle preparation of the frog indicated that the toxin produced changes in the Na-K pump, resulting in depolarization of the cell membranes. In the rat, where the $LD_{50}$ was approximately 100 $\mu$g/kg body weight, low doses of the toxin caused an increase in the QT interval, a decrease in the PR interval, and P-wave inversion. Large doses produced marked electrocardiographic (ECG) changes leading to cardiac failure. Subsequent studies showed that the ability of skeletal muscle sarcoplasmic reticulum to bind ionic calcium and nuclear alterations and dissolution of intercellular collagen in cultured hamster ovary K-1 cells are important properties of the toxin (Calton and associates, 1973; Néeman and colleagues, 1981).

Tamkun and Hessinger (1981) obtained a hemolytic protein from *P. physalis*. This protein, physalitoxin, was also lethal to mice at the 0.20 mg protein/kg body weight level, whereas the $LD_{50}$ for the crude venom was 0.14 mg/kg. A molecular weight of 212,000 was calculated. These authors suggested that the toxin was composed of three subunits of unequal size, each of which is glycolated. Physalitoxin accounted for about 28 percent of the total nematocyst venom protein. Its carbohydrate content was 10.6 percent and represented the major glycoprotein of the crude venom. This hemolytic and lethal toxin was inactivated by concanavalin A.

Initial studies of extracts of the frozen tentacles of the sea wasp, *Chironex fleckeri*, indicated that the extracts had lethal, necrotizing, and hemolytic properties (Southcott and Kingston, 1959). Barnes (1967) isolated a *Chironex* nematocyst crude toxin by employing human amnion membrane and electrically stimulating the tentacles. In his initial study, Barnes (1960) found that the undiluted toxin was lethal to mice at the 0.005 ml/kg body weight level, but it was not known what this might be in dry weight, milligrams of protein, or protein nitrogen. Endean and coworkers (1969) found proteins, carbohydrates, cystine-containing compounds, and 3-indolyl derivatives in the nematocysts of the tentacles of *C. fleckeri*. Saline extracts of the contents of the nematocysts were highly toxic to prawns and fish and were lethal to mice and rats. In mice the intravenous $LD_{50}$ was between 20,000 and 25,000 nematocysts, whereas in rats the $LD_{50}$ was approximately 150,000 nematocysts. Using partially purified extracts of the tentacles, Freeman and Turner (1969) found that extracts produced respiratory arrest, which they attributed to a central origin. They also implicated deleterious cardiac changes leading to an atrioventricular block. Blood pressure and chemistry changes were consistent with a reduced circulating blood volume and hypoxia. The toxins had a nonspecific lytic effect on cells and had no particular differential effect on the guinea pig diaphragm preparation. It was found that 0.1 ml of a 5000-fold dilution of the tentacle extract would kill a 20-g mouse in less than 2 min, and that the toxin was hemolytic. The fraction was nondialyzable, and a molecular weight of 8000 was suggested.

Crone and Keen (1969) obtained two toxic proteins using tentacle extracts. The hemolytic activity was related to a protein component with a molecular weight of approximately 70,000. The second toxin had a molecular weight of about 150,000, and while both components had cardiotoxic activity, the larger fraction had considerably more than did the smaller fraction. Two *Chironex* tentacle extracts were studied by Freeman (1971), who found that both fractions produced an initial increase in systemic arterial pressure that was followed by a fall in pressure, bradycardia, and cardiac arrythmia. In the perfused guinea pig heart, both toxins caused a reduction in rate, amplitude of contraction, and coronary flow. The author concluded that the cardiovascular effects were due to "direct vasoconstriction, cardiotoxicity, a baroreceptor stimulation and possible depression of the vasomotor center."

It appears that the toxin or toxins derived from tentacles is quite different from that obtained from discharged or undischarged nematocysts. An attempt to resolve these discrepancies was made by Endean and Noble (1971). Using methods previously described by their group, they separated material within the nematocysts from the residual tentacular material. The two products were studied by injection into mice and rats, on the barnacle muscle preparation, the rat phrenic nerve–diaphragm preparation, the toad sciatic nerve–gastrocnemius and sciatic nerve conduction preparations, rat ilea and heart preparations, and several other isolated tissue preparations. It was found that after removal of the nematocysts from the tentacles, the remaining product possessed biological activities quite different from those extracted from the nematocysts. Although the work of Endean and Noble indicates certain differences, it is difficult to define them accurately in the absence of a standard tissue weight or solution. In addition, some of the differences demonstrated by the various investigators of *Chironex* toxins as well as several other cnidarian toxins might be due to dose relationships rather than the toxins employed. This is particularly true for the rat or guinea pig diaphragm–phrenic nerve preparation. Changes in the dose of toxins cause not only quantitative changes but qualitative ones. Furthermore, when the muscle of a mammalian nerve-muscle preparation is shortened, it is difficult to determine the effect on the indirectly elicited contraction. In fact, in a shortened muscle, it is even difficult to determine the significance of the direct effect. Obviously, a substance that is highly irritating to an entire muscle membrane presents a problem when one hopes to define its action on the nerve or even on the activity of a single muscle fiber.

Baxter and colleagues at the Commonwealth Serum Laboratories in Australia, using saline extracts of nematocysts obtained after the method of Barnes (1967) or as described by Endean and associates (1969), demonstrated that the biologically active fractions causing lethal, hemolytic, and dermonecrotizing reactions had molecular weights ranging from 10,000 to 30,000. In rabbits, a lethal intravenous dose of the venom caused labored and deep respirations, followed within several minutes by prostration, hyperextension of the head, "spasms," and respiratory and cardiac arrest. Similar manifestations were seen in sheep and primates. Postmortem examination revealed marked congestion of the vessels of the lungs and pulmonary edema; the right ventricle was engorged, the kidneys and liver were congested, and the vessels of the meninges of the cerebrum were engorged (Baxter et al., 1972).

Considerable study has been done on the nematocyst toxin of the sea nettle *Chrysaora quinquecirrha* by Burnett and his group at the University of Maryland School of Medicine (see Russell, 1984a, for references). Blanquet (1972) found that the toxin was contained within the nematocyst and that the discharged nematocyst capsules and threads were free of toxin. Further studies showed that the toxic material was associated with a protein fraction with a molecular weight above 100,000, which could be separated into two major fractions. The more toxic of these two proteins was found to be rich in aspartic and glumatic acids, which constituted approximately 27 percent of the total detectable amino acid content. Burnett and Calton (1977) reviewed the cardiotoxic, dermonecrotic, musculotoxic, and neurotoxic properties of the venom. Subsequently, it has been demonstrated that the toxin produced striking cytological changes, including nuclear alterations and dissolution of intercellular collagen. The lethal property is thought to exert its effect by altering the transport of calcium across the conduction system of the heart. From experiments on rat and frog nerve and muscle and on the neurons of *Aplysia californica*, it was concluded that the toxin appears to induce a nonspecific membrane depolarization through a sodium-dependent tetrodotoxin-insensitive mechanism that secondarily increases Ca influx.

The collagenase from *C. quinquecirrha* has been isolated and purified 237-fold. A monoclonal antibody to the lethal factor of the venom has also been prepared. Ascites fluid from a cloned hybridoma-breeding mouse showed an ELISA titer of 12,800 and neutralized an intravenous 2 × $LD_{50}$ injection of the crude venom.

Among the sea anemones, *Anemonia sulcata* is of particular interest because it is of considerable medical importance in the Adriatic Sea, where it inflicts numerous stings on bathers (Maretić and Russell, 1983). In 1973, a partially purified, toxic basic polypeptide from *A. sulcata* was isolated. Its molecular weight was estimated to be 6000, and its $LD_{100}$ in rats was 6 mg/kg body weight. In 1975, three toxic polypeptides were isolated. Toxin I contained 45 amino acid residues; toxin II, 44; and toxin III, 24. Toxins I and II had similar toxicological properties. When injected into a crustacean, fish, or mammal, these toxins produced paralysis and cardiovascular changes. When injected into crabs, the toxins caused convulsions and paralysis and were lethal at 2.0 mg/kg. They also caused paralysis and death in fishes. Toxin III caused neurotransmitter release from rat synaptosomes. Toxin II was far more toxic than was toxin I and produced a positive inotropic effect on isolated electrically driven atria of the guinea pig. At high concentrations it caused contracture and arrhythmia. On the Langendorff heart preparation, low concentrations enhanced the contractile force of the atrium and ventricle, whereas high concentrations caused contracture and arrhythmia, which appeared to be limited to the atrium. Ferlan and Lebez (1974) isolated a highly basic protein toxin, equinatoxin, from the sea anemone *Actinia equina*. It had a molecular weight of 20,000, with an isoelectric point of 12.5, and 147 amino acid residues. In rats, equinatoxin had an intravenous $LD_{50}$ of 33 $\mu$g/kg body weight and was found to have hemolytic, antigenic, cardiotropic, and certain other activities. Subsequently, it was found that equinatoxin, in vitro, exhibited strong lytic action on erythrocytes and did not have phospholipase activity. A cytolytic toxin, metridiolysin, from the anemone *Metridium senile* showed similar hemolytic activity. As with equinatoxin, the hemolytic activity was restricted to a relatively narrow pH range (see Russell, 1984a, for references).

Shapiro and Lilleheil (1969) at Harvard carried out a series of chemical and pharmacological studies on a stable acetone powder from tentacle homogenates of the large Caribbean anemone *Condylactis gigantea*. A toxin was obtained that acted as a basic protein and had an approximate molecular weight of 10,000 to 15,000. Assays on crayfish caused a paralysis characterized by an initial or spastic phase, followed by a flaccid phase. The immobilization dose was about 1 $\mu$g/kg body weight, and the yield from a 70-g anemone with 23 g of tentacles was 1 g of the acetone powder, or an amount sufficient to paralyze approximately 2100-kg of crayfish. Further studies on a crayfish preparation showed that the toxin had a direct effect on the crustacean nerve but not on the muscle membrane. No evidence for a truly synaptic effect was found. Using the lobster giant axon and crayfish slow-adapting preparations, it was found that the toxin transformed action potentials into prolonged plateau potentials of up to several seconds' duration and that the eventual conduction block was not due solely to depolarization (Shapiro and Lilleheil, 1969).

A central nervous system stimulant in the form of a basic polypeptide has been isolated from homogenized tissues of the anemone *Stoichactis kenti*. The stimulation was described as "fighting episodes." A partially purified toxin from *S. helianthus*, with a mouse intraperitoneal $LD_{50}$ of 0.25 mg/kg and hemolytic properties inhibited by sphingomyelin, has been reported (Bernheimer and Avigad, 1976). A cytotoxic poison from the anemone *S. helianthus* acts on black lipid membranes and liposomes through channel formation and detergent action. This mechanism is also suspected in the hemolytic activity of some of the other sea anemone "cytolytic" toxins. Hessinger and Lenhoff (1976) demonstrated that the toxin of *Aiptasia pallida* caused lysis through the action of phospholipase A on membrane phospholipids, while other workers suspect ionic or nonenzymatic roles. Several other Actiniidae species have been shown to contain toxins. A polypeptide termed anthopleurin A from *Anthopleura xanthogrammica* that closely resembles toxin II from *Anemonia sulcata* in its amino acid sequence has been described. In mice, anthopleurin A had an $LD_{50}$ of 0.3 to 0.4 mg/kg body weight and was said to stimulate cardiac activity. A second polypeptide toxin, anthopleurin B, has been identified in the same anemone (see Russell, 1984a, for references).

In 1967, Hashimoto and colleagues collected specimens of the file fish, *Alutera scripta*, from the Ryukyu Islands after a report that several pigs had died after eating the viscera of this fish. On examining the gut contents of the fish, the investigators found polyps of the zoanthid *Palythoa tuberculosa*. At about the same time, Scheuer and his group were investigating the toxin from *Palythoa toxica*, which is found at Hana off the island of Maui and is called *lima-make-O-Hana* (death seaweed of Hana). *Palythoa* toxin, palytoxin, was found to be a potent poison, having a mouse intravenous $LD_{50}$ of 0.15 $\mu$g/kg body weight. It has an approximate molecular weight of 3000.

**Clinical Problem.** As was pointed out by Halstead (1965), it has long been known that the nematocysts of certain cnidarians can penetrate the human skin. In 1984, approximately 78 of the 9000 species of cnidarians were noted to have been involved in injuries to humans (Russell, 1984a). While most nematocysts are capable of piercing only the thin membranes of the mouth or conjunctiva, some possess sufficient force to pierce the skin of the inner sides of the arms, legs, and more tender areas of the body. Still others can penetrate the thicker skin of the hands, arms, and feet (Russell, 1965). Swallowing the tentacles or even the umbrella can cause epigastric pain and discomfort (Maretić and Russell, 1983).

The cutaneous lesions, as well as other clinical manifestations produced by the cnidarians, vary considerably, depending on the species involved and the number of fired nematocysts. Contrary to common belief, the stings of many cnidarians produce little or no immediate pain. Sometimes itching is the first complaint that calls the victim's attention to the injured area, and this may not occur for hours after the initial contact. In the author's experience, stings by hydroids usually do not produce pain, although there may be subsequent localized discomfort. In most cases, the lesions produced by hydroids are minimal. The fire or stinging corals, *Millepora*, produce small reddened, somewhat papular eruptions, which appear 1 to 10 h after contact and usually subside within 24 to 96 h. In severe cases, the papules may proceed to pustular lesions and subsequent desquamation. The stinging usually is associated with some localized prickinglike pain that is generally of short duration and with some subsequent pruritus and minimal swelling.

Contact with the Portuguese man-of-war, *Physalia*, causes immediate pain, sometimes severe, and the early appearance of small reddened, linear papular eruptions. At first the papules are surrounded by an erythematous zone, but as their size increases, the area takes on the appearance of an inflammatory reaction with small periodic, demarcated hemorrhagic papules. In some cases, the papules are very close together, indicating multiple discharges of nematocysts as the tentacle passed over the injured part. The papules develop rapidly and often increase in size during the first hour. The affected area becomes painful, and severe pruritus is not uncommon. Pain may spread to the larger muscle masses in the involved extremity or even to the whole body. Pain sometimes involves the regional lymph nodes. In some cases, the papules proceed to vesiculation, pustulation, and desquamation. I have seen several cases in which hyperpigmentation of the lesions was obvious for years after a stinging (Russell, 1966). General systemic manifestations also may develop after *Physalia physalis* envenomation. Weakness, nausea, anxiety, headache, spasms in the large muscle masses of the abdomen and back, vascular spasms, lacrimation, nasal discharge, increased perspiration, vertigo, hemolysis, difficulty and pain on respiration described as being unable to "catch one's breath," cyanosis, renal failure, and shock have all been reported. Several deaths have been reported after *Physalia* stings.

Contact with most of the true jellyfishes gives rise in less severe cases to manifestations similar to those noted above for *Physalia*, with the symptoms sometimes disappearing within 10 h. In more severe cases, there is immediate, intense, burning pain, with contact areas appearing as swollen wheals that are sometimes purplish and often bear hemorrhagic papules. The areas may proceed to vesiculation and necrosis. Localized edema is common, and in more severe cases muscle mass pain, difficulty with respiration, and severe spasms of the back and abdomen with vomiting have been reported. Vertigo, mental confusion, changes in heart rate, and shock are sometimes seen, and death has occurred (Barnes, 1960; Halstead, 1965; Russell, 1965, 1984a).

The sea wasps, *Chironex fleckeri, Chiropsalmus quadrigatus*, and certain other related species, are extremely dangerous. The Cubomedusae have been responsible for a number of deaths, particularly in Indo-Pacific waters. Although systemic effects usually develop within 5 to 150 min after envenomation, some deaths have occurred in less than 5 min. Stings by these Cubomedusae cause a sharp prickling or burning sensation with the appearance of a wheal, which at first appears like a "rounded area of gooseflesh." An erythematous wheal soon develops and may become considerably larger than the area of contact. At first the lesion may not show a pattern that suggests whether the stinging had been by tentacles or by the animal's umbrella. The wheals may disappear when the stinging is minimal, or after an hour or so they may become enlarged. The nematocyst punctures become more apparent and appear as very small hemorrhagic vesicles surrounded by inflammation. A stinging pain develops and may persist for 1 to 3 h. In linear lesions the nematocyst injuries may be no more than 5 mm wide but may extend for 10 cm or more. Vesiculation and pustular formation may occur, and full-thickness skin necrosis is not uncommon. Edema about the area may persist for 10 days or more.

Stingings by anemones are usually of lesser consequence than those inflicted by jellyfishes, and they rarely are painful or disabling. The lesion area takes on a reddened and slightly raised appearance, bearing irregularly scattered pinhead-sized vesicles or hemorrhagic blebs. The area becomes painful, particularly to touch or heat. In stings by *Anemonia sulcata* seen by the author, there has been some diffuse edema around the injured site. Residual hyperpigmentation or hypopigmentation is unusual after anemone stings. Stings by the stony corals *(Acropora)* give rise to some minor pain often followed by itching and the development of small diffuse wheals which may progress to vesiculation but rarely necrosis. Small spicules of coral that sometimes break off and become embedded in the skin are troublesome, occasionally giving rise to infection.

Treatment consists of removing the tentacles, preferably with gloves, washing the affected area with seawater, immersing the part in vinegar for 20 to 30 min, applying a dry powder or shaving soap and scraping the area with a sharp knife to remove any nematocysts embedded in the skin, washing the area thoroughly with soapy water, and then applying a corticosteroid-analgesic-antihistamine ointment (Itch Balm Plus). Systemic manifestations are best treated symptomatically.

Chills and fever have been reported after the grinding of dried specimens of *Palythoa caribaeorum* that were being studied for the presence of wax esters. Toxic zoanthids have also been found in various parts of the Pacific. Accidental contact with the mucus of *Palythoa* through the abraded skin is said to produce weakness and malaise as well as localized irritation.

On some Pacific islands and elsewhere in the world, sea anemones are eaten after cooking, but some are apparently poisonous whether uncooked or cooked. *Rhodactis howesi* and *Physobrachia douglasi* are poisonous when eaten raw but are said to be safe when cooked. *Radianthus paumotensis* and another *Radianthus* species are said to be poisonous whether raw or cooked. Intoxication is typified by nausea, vomiting, abdominal pain, and hypoactive reflexes. In severe cases, marked weakness, malaise, cyanosis, stupor, and death have occurred.

## Echinodermata

In most cases, echinoderms are characterized by radial or meridional symmetry, a calcareous exoskeleton made up of separate plates or ossicles that often bear external spines, a well-developed coelom, a water-vascular system, and a nervous system but no special excretory system. Approximately 85 of the 6000 species in the four classes (Asteroidea, Ophiuroidea, Echinoidea, Holothuroidea) are known to be venomous or poisonous. Some of the more important toxic sea stars, sea urchins, and sea cucumbers have been described elsewhere (Russell, 1984a). Asteroids, sea stars, and starfishes have a central disk and five or more tapering rays or arms. On the upper surface there are many thorny spines of calcium carbonate in the form of calcite intermingled with organic materials. The calcite spines are covered by a thin integument composed of an epidermis and a dermis. Within the epidermis is an acidophilic cell that is thought to release a toxin. The toxin is discharged into the water or, as in the case of humans, directly onto the skin. In addition, sea stars have pedicellariae which contain poison glands in the concave cavity of their valves. Some sea stars produce poisoning after ingestion.

The regular sea urchins have rounded radially symmetric bodies, which are enclosed in a hard calcite shell from which calcareous spines and the venomous pedicellariae arise. The spines may be straight and pointed, curved, flat-topped, club-shaped, oar-shaped, umbrella-shaped, thorny, fan-shaped, or hooked. They may vary in length from less than 1 mm to over 30 cm. The spines serve in locomotion, protection, digging, feeding, and producing currents; certain primary and secondary spines bear poison glands.

The principal venom apparatus in the sea urchin, heart urchin, and sand dollar is the pedicellaria. In essence, pedicellariae are modified spines with flexible heads. There are four primary kinds, and some urchins possess all four. Pedicellariae function in food getting, grooming, and self-defense. The glandular, gemmiform, or globiferous type of pedicellaria serves as a venom organ. In most echinoids, the so-called head of the pedicellaria is composed of three calcareous jaws or valves, each with a rounded toothlike fang. The jaws are usually invested in a globose, fleshy, and somewhat muscular sac which has a single or double gland over each valve. A second trilobed gland system, anatomically and histologically distinct from the head gland, is present in several urchins. The primary and secondary spines of some urchins have specialized organs containing a gland, which is said to empty its contents through the hollow spine tip under certain conditions. The author's group found a toxin in the secondary spines of *Echinothrix calamaris* and *E. diadema* but not in the primary spines. The secondary spines of *Asthenosoma varium* and *Araesoma thetidis* contain a venom. According to Halstead (1978), the spine venom glands are best developed in the secondary aboral spines of *A. varium*.

The sea cucumbers, Holothuroidea, are soft-bodied animals covered by a leathery skin that contains only microscopic calcareous plates. According to Nigrelli and Jakowska (1960), at least 30 species belonging to four of the five orders are toxic. Some members have special defense organs known as Cuvierian tubules. When these animals are irritated, they emit these organs through the anus. The tubules become elongated by hydrostatic pressure so that once they pass through the anus, they become extremely sticky threads in which the attacking animal becomes ensnared. The process of elongation may split the outer layer of covering cells, releasing a proteinaceous material that forms an amorphous mass with strong adhesive properties. In some sea cucumbers, however, as in *Actinopyga agassizi*, the tubules do not become sticky or elongate but are expelled in a somewhat similar manner and discharge a toxin from certain highly developed structures filled with granules. The toxin is capable of killing fishes and other animals. In *Holothuria atra*, which does not have Cuvierian tubules, the toxin may be discharged through the body wall. In Guam, natives cut up common black sea cucumbers and squeeze the contents into crevices and pools to deactivate fish.

Many echinoderms secrete a mucus or liquid from their integument that appears to play a role in their defensive armament. The viscous discharge from the massive multicellular integumentary glands of the brittle star, *Ophiocomina nigra*, is characterized as a highly sulfated acid mucopolysaccharide containing amino sugars, sulfate esters, and other substances complexed to proteins. The pH of this discharge is approximately 1, and this probably makes it very offensive to other marine animals that might seek to prey on it. Among other substances isolated from the echinoderms is a quaternary ammonium base ($C_7H_7NO_2$, picolinic acid methyl betaine) known as homarine, several phosphagens (phosphoarginine and phosphocreatine), sterols, saponins, and other compounds (Hashimoto, 1979).

When the pedicellariae of *Toxopneustes pileolus* were allowed to sting the shaved abdomen of a mouse, the animal developed respiratory distress and exhibited a decrease in body temperature. The injection of thermostable extracts from the macerated pedicellariae of *Sphaerechinus granularis* and certain other species has been found to be lethal to isopods, crabs, octopods, sea stars, lizards, and rabbits. While the presence of a dialyzable, acetylcholinelike substance in the pedicellariae of *Lytechinus variegatus* has been reported, it was not until 1965 that the protein nature of pedicellarial toxin was first described. This protein had an intravenous $LD_{50}$ in mice, based on the quantity of precipitable protein nitrogen, of $1.59 \times 10^{-2}$ mg/kg body weight for the crude material and $1.16 \times 10^{-2}$ mg/kg for the protein (Alender and Russell, 1966). It possessed hemolytic activity against human type A and B, rabbit, guinea pig, beef, sheep, and fish erythrocytes. Intravenously, it produced a dose-related hypotension that was responsive to adrenaline. It had a deleterious effect on the isolated heart and guinea pig ileum. In both preparations, the toxin caused the release of histamine and serotonin. It seems to have little effect on isolated toad nerve. However, Parnas and Russell (1967), using the deep-extension abdominal muscle of the crayfish, showed that the toxin produced a rapid block in the response of the indirectly stimulated muscle. Even with low concentrations, there was an irreversible block in the muscle's response to intracellular stimulation. The compound action potential of the crayfish limb nerve was also blocked by the toxin, but this potential reappeared on washing. The toxin caused considerable damage to the muscle fibers. These findings seem to indicate that pedicellarial toxin blocks the response from both nerve and muscle and is cytolytic.

Subsequently, it was observed that pedicellarial toxin from *Tripneustes gratilla* elicited prolonged contractions of isolated guinea pig ileum. Chemical evidence was obtained for the release of histamine from ileal, cardiac, and pulmonary tissues as well as from the colonic and pulmonary tissues of the rat. The histamine release was quantitatively dependent on the concentration of the toxin acting on the tissue. The active material obtained from the reaction between crude sea urchin toxin and heated plasma was a mixture of pharmacologically active peptides, one of which was bradykinin (see Russell, 1984a, for references). Fleming and Howden (1974) obtained a partially purified toxin from the pedicellariae of *T. gratilla*. The toxin, as established by intraperitoneal injection in mice, was at the 5.0 to 5.1 isoelectric point. When this fraction was chromatographed, a molecular weight of $78{,}000 \pm 8000$ was found. This seems consistent with the sediment coefficient of 4.7 (67,000) that was previously reported.

It has been known since 1880 that the discharged tenacious filaments of sea cucumbers can produce lesions in humans and that eating the sea cucumber *Stichopus variegatus* can cause death. The initial studies of the poisonousness of sea cucumbers were carried out by Yamanouchi (1942), who observed that when fishes were placed in an aquarium to which aqueous extracts of *Holothuria vagabunda* were added, they subsequently died. Yamanouchi also obtained a toxic crystalline product termed holothurin and found it present in 24 of 27 species of sea cucumbers examined. Bakus and Green (1974) found that the more tropical the locality, the greater the probability that the sea cucumber will be toxic to fishes. The toxic substance (holothurin) extracted from the Bahamian sea cucumber *Actinopyga agassizi* was found to be composed of 60 percent glycosides and pigments; 30 percent salts, polypeptides, and free amino acids; 5 to 10 percent insoluble protein; and 1 percent cholesterol. The cholesterol-precipitated fraction, known as holothurin A, represented 60 percent of the crude holothurin and was given the empirical formula $C_{50\text{-}52}H_{81}O_{25\text{-}26}SNa$. Its provisional structure (Freiss et al., 1967) is

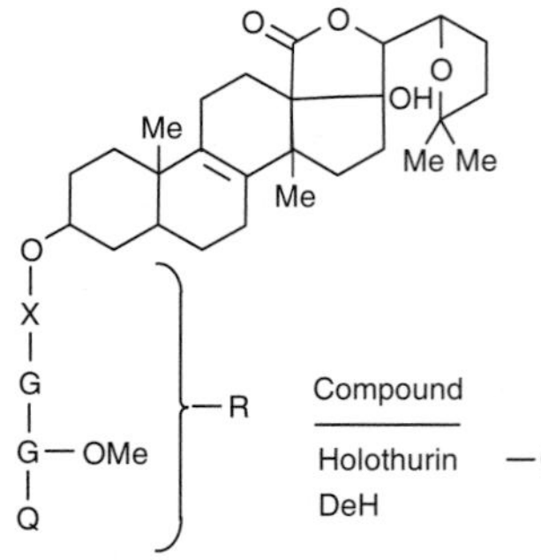

| Compound | R |
|---|---|
| Holothurin | $-OSO_3^-Na^-$ |
| DeH | $-H$ |

| SUGAR | SYMBOL |
|---|---|
| D-GLUCOSE | G |
| D-XYLOSE | X |
| D-QUINOVOSE | Q |
| 3-*O*-METHYLGLUCOSE | G—OMe |

In 10 ppm, holothurin was found to be lethal to *Hydra*, the mollusk *Planorbis*, and the annelid *Tubifex tubifex*. In the mammalian phrenic nerve–diaphragm preparation, holothurin A produced contracture of the muscle followed by some relaxation and a gradual decrease in the recorded amplitude of both the directly and the indirectly elicited contractions, with the latter decreasing at a slightly greater rate than the former. The intravenous $LD_{50}$ in mice was approximately 9 mg/kg body weight. In frogs, holothurin A produced an irreversible block and destruction of excitability on the single node of Ranvier in the sciatic nerve. The toxin does not produce any observable damage to the axonal walls or sheath (see Russell, 1984a, for references).

A major aglycone from the holothurin A of *H. vagabunda* was named holothurigenin ($C_{30}H_{44}O_5$). It contains three hydroxyls, a five-membered lactone, and a heteroannular diene. The toxins from the Cuvierian organ and body wall of a number of species have been described by Habermehl and Volkwein (1971). According to these authors, these compounds are glycosides of tetracyclic triterpenes which are derivatives of lanosterol and were the first glycoside triterpenes derived from animals. Holothurin has been shown to have hemolytic and cytolytic properties. It is considered one of the most potent saponin hemolysins known. In some concentrations it is lethal to animals and plants. The effects of various preparations of holothurin on the peripheral nervous system were the object of a number of studies by Friess and his group (Freiss et al., 1970). Holothurin in concentrations of $9.8 \times 10^{-3}$ *M* caused a decrease in the height of the propagated potential without reduction of the conduction velocity in the desheathed sciatic nerve of the frog. This change is concentration-dependent, independent of pH and is completely irreversible. A similar change was produced in the single fiber–single node of Ranvier preparation. In concentrations of $2.5 \times 10^{-5}$ to $1.0 \times 10^{-3}$ *M*, the toxin produced a diminution of the action current with a concomitant rise in the stimulation threshold. However, in approximately 80 percent of the preparations studied, the loss of nodal excitation caused by the same concentration was accompanied by a loss in basophilic macromolecular material from the exoplasm in and near the node of Ranvier.

**Clinical Problem.** In 1965, a student working with *Acanthaster planci*, who had inadvertently slipped and fallen, landing forcibly with his left hand impaled on the sea star, was treated at the Scripps Institute of Oceanography. Twenty minutes after the injury the patient had intense pain over the palm of the left hand, "shooting pains" up the volar aspect of the forearm, weakness, nausea, vertigo, and tingling in the fingertips. There were at least 10 puncture wounds over the hand, and some of them bled freely. I suggested that the patient put his hand in cold vinegar and water and be admitted to the hospital emergency room. When he arrived there 15 min later, the pain was less intense and the nausea had subsided somewhat. Unfortunately, the patient was given 100 mg meperidine hydrochloride and 5 min later was vomiting. The vomiting probably was due to the medication, and most of the other symptoms were due to hyperventilation. The patient was placed on cold vinegar and water and occasional aluminum acetate soaks over the next 2 days, and all symptoms and signs, including the mild edema, slowly resolved. Several broken spines were removed from the puncture wounds. Four days after the accident, the patient complained of burning and itching over the left palm. Examination revealed a scaly, erythematous dermatitis. Topical corticosteriods were used, but 2 days later the patient had to be placed on systemic corticosteroid therapy for the dermatitis, which cleared in 6 days.

A second episode involving *A. planci* was related by Dr. W. L. Orris in 1974 (personal correspondence). The patient had immediate, severe burning pain and localized edema. These symptoms responded to aluminum acetate soaks and corticosteroids. According to Endean (1964), the puncture wounds produced by *Asthenosoma periculosum* give rise to immediate and sometimes acute pain but few other symptoms or signs. The discharge from *Marthasterias glacialis* is said to cause edema of the lips. It is known that allergic dermatitis can occur after extensive contact with these animals.

Stings by the pedicellariae of certain sea urchins are well documented (Cleland and Southcott, 1965; Halstead, 1965; Russell, 1965, 1984a; Fisher, 1978). A biologist experienced severe pain; syncope; respiratory distress; partial paralysis of the lips, tongue, and eyelids; and weakness of the muscles of phonation and the extremities after a stinging by seven or eight pedicellariae from *Toxopneustes pileolus*. Another biologist experienced severe pain of several hours' duration at the site of a stinging by *Tripneustes gratilla*. The sting of a single globiferous pedicellaria from *T. gratilla* was found to be equal in pain severity to that experienced after a bee sting. Swelling appeared around the puncture wounds within minutes of the stinging, and a red wheal 1 cm in diameter soon developed. Subsequent stingings during the following 2-year period resulted in a more severe reaction. In one instance, the wheal was 12 cm in diameter and persisted for 8 h. In none of these experiences were there any systemic manifestations (Alender and Russell, 1966; Russell, 1971). It might be concluded that pedicellarial stings give rise to immediate pain, localized swelling and redness, and an aching sensation in the involved part. Other findings might include those reviewed by Halstead (1965).

As was previously noted, the secondary spines of *Echinothrix calamaris, E. diadema, Asthenosoma varium, Araesome thetidis* and the primary oral spines of *Phormosoma bursarium* are said to have a venom gland and are capable of envenomation (Alender and Russell, 1966). However, case reports on verified stingings are almost nonexistent, and in the several known to the author it is not possible to decide whether the pain, "dizziness," and minimal localized swelling were due to a venom or to the effects of a simple puncture wound complicated by hyperventilation.

The primary spines of almost 50 species of sea urchins have been implicated in injuries to humans. Urchins of the family Diadematidae are particularly troublesome because of their long length and fragility. When these spines break off in a puncture wound, they can be difficult to find and remove. I have attended injuries in which more than a dozen broken spine tips had to be surgically removed. With some species, there is no telltale dark color around the puncture wound and finding the broken spines is not easy. Although the fragments of some spines dissolve in tissue and cause no difficulties, others can give rise to granulomatous reactions, and some of these fragments may need to be removed. Still others may migrate through the foot or hand without causing complications. Occasionally, spines will lodge against a nerve or bone and cause complications requiring surgical intervention. Secondary infections from spine injuries are relatively rare.

It has long been known that the ovaries of sea urchins are toxic and perhaps lethal. Halstead (1980) noted that the gonads of *Paracentrotus lividus, Tripneustes ventricosus*, and *Centrechinus antillarium* are poisonous. Poisonings after the ingestion of certain sea cucumbers are not uncommon and have occurred frequently in the South Pacific, the Philippines, Japan, China, and southeast Asia. The most frequently implicated holothurian species are *Holothuria atra, H. axiologa, Stichopus variegatus*, and *Thelenota ananas*. The symptoms and signs are usually of short duration and without serious sequelae. Pruritus with mild swelling and redness of the hands has been reported after the handling of some sea cucumbers. Acute conjunctivitis has been observed in persons who have swum in waters polluted with the tissue discharge of sea cucumber Cuvierian organs.

## Mollusca

Mollusks are unsegmented invertebrates that have a mantle that often secretes a calcareous shell, a ventral muscular foot used for locomotion, a reduced coelom, an open circulatory system, and a radula or tonguelike organ (absent only in the bivalves). Jaws are present in some species. There are approximately 80,000 species of mollusks, of which about 85 have been implicated in poisonings of humans or are known to be toxic under certain conditions. The majority of the venomous or poisonous species are found in three of the five classes of mollusks, Gastropoda, Pelecypoda, and Cephalopoda. In the class Gastropoda, the univalve snails and slugs, the most dangerous members are in the genus *Conus*, in which there are perhaps 400 species. Cone shells are confined almost exclusively to tropical and subtropical seas and oceans and usually are found in shallow waters along reefs, although some of the more dangerous species are found on sandy bottoms. They range in length up to approximately 25 cm. The venom apparatus of *Conus* serves as an offensive weapon for the gaining of food and to a much lesser extent as a defensive weapon against predators. It consists of a muscular bulb, a long coiled venom duct, the radula (the radula sheath), and the radular teeth. The venom is thought to be secreted in the venom duct and to be forced under pressure exerted by the duct and the venom bulb into the radula and thus into the lumen of the radular teeth. The radular teeth are passed from the radula into the pharynx and then into the proboscis. They then are thrust by the proboscis into the prey during the stinging act. The radular teeth are needlelike, from 1 to 10 mm in length, and almost transparent. The reader is referred elsewhere for a more complete review of the structure of the venom apparatus of *Conus* (Halstead, 1965; Russell, 1984a).

The various species of Conidae have been divided into those that are vermivorous, molluscivorous, and piscivorous. Endean and coworkers (1967) demonstrated that in 37 species studied, the paralytic effects of the venoms were indeed directly related to the prey being hunted. They concluded that only the piscivorous Conidae were capable of causing serious injuries to humans.

Initial studies indicated that the venom was white, gray, yellow, or black, depending on the species involved; was viscous; and had a pH range of 7.6 to 8.2. The active principle was nondialyzable, and its toxicity was reduced by heating or incubation with trypsin. The lethal fraction was thought to be a protein or bound to a protein. It was found that the amount of venom in the ducts of *C. striatus* is sufficient to immobilize the small fish on which it preys but not large enough to cause serious injury to a human. A toxin with a molecular weight of over 10,000 and a low lethal index compared with other *Conus* species caused ataxia; depressed respirations, leading to apnea and cardiac arrest in mammals; precipitated a block in the compound action potential of the isolated toad sciatic nerve; blocked the directly and the indirectly elicited contractions of a mammalian nerve-muscle preparation; and markedly depressed the amplitude of intracellular recorded action potentials in the rat diaphragm. Various authors have reported that the active fraction is a protein, a poison with a molecular weight of about 10,000, or a peptide (see Russell, 1984a, for references).

Some abalones, such as *Haliotis*, are toxic when eaten. The toxin is concentrated in the digestive gland or liver and can be distinguished by its blue-green pigment. It is thought that the pigment pyropheophorbide *a* originates from chlorophyll in the seaweed on which the abalone feeds. Hashimoto (1979) noted that ingestion of the viscera of *Haliotis* caused dermatitis in cats and humans. On the basis of this observation, he carried out experiments demonstrating the importance of photosensitization in the development of the dermatitis and suggested an assay method. He also suggested that the use of fluorescent pigments in foods should be prohibited and that care should be taken to ensure that drugs are not transformed into fluorescent substances in the body. In the hypobranchial gland of *Murex*, there is a secretion that at first is colorless or yellow but on exposure to sunlight becomes brilliant violet and gives off a strong fetid odor. This gland also produces a toxic secretion. Subsequent studies indicated that two pharmacologically active substances were present: enteramine (5-hydroxytryptamine) and murexine ($C_{11}H_{18}O_3N_3$). Further investigations showed that murexine has the structure of $\beta$[imidazolyl-(4)]-acrylcholine; it was thus called urocanylcholine. Murexine also has been found in the midgut of the sea hare *Aplysia californica*. Senecioylcholine has been identified in the hypobranchial gland of *Thais floridana*, and acrylcholine in *Buccinum undatum*. The amount of these cholinesters in the hypobranchial gland was approximately 1 to 5 mg/g tissue. They exhibited muscarinelike and nicotinelike activity and caused cardiovascular changes with hypotension, increased respirations, gastric motility and secretions, and some contraction of the frog rectus muscle and guinea pig ileum. The intravenous $LD_{50}$ of murexine in mice was 8.1 to 8.7 mg/kg. Dihydromurexine has been isolated from the hypobranchial gland of *Thais haemastoma*, and the muricacean gastropod *Acanthina spirata* produces a paralytic substance with a high acetylcholine content in its hypobranchial and salivary–accessory gland complex. The toxin is thought to be a carboxylic ester of choline (see Russell, 1984a, for references).

A vasodilator and hypotensive agent from the salivary gland extract of the gastropod *Thais haemastoma* has been described. The extract produced behavioral changes in mice, followed by lethargy. When lethal doses were given, respirations first increased, then decreased, and then became shallow; death ensued. The toxin produced bradycardia and a fall in blood pressure, which was partly blocked by atropine. In the isolated rabbit heart, the extract produced a decrease in rate and contraction with a fall in heart output. It also produced contractions of the isolated guinea pig ileum and rabbit duodenum. The salivary poison of the gastropod *Neptunea arthritica* is thought to be tetramine ($C_4H_{12}N$). It has been suggested that histamine, choline, and choline ester, which are also found in the salivary glands of this mollusk, act synergistically with the tetramine in producing the poisoning. In *N. antiqua* the tetramine is probably responsible for almost all the biological activity of the salivary gland extract. In the viscera of the ivory shell, *Babylonia japonica*, a water-soluble toxin has been found that is slightly methanol- and ethanol-soluble, heat-labile, dialyzable, ninhydrin-positive, and Dragendorff- and biuret-negative. It has a potent mydriatic activity. The toxin is said to be a complex bromo compound with the formula $C_{25}H_{26}N_5O_{13}Br \cdot 7H_2O$ and a molecular weight of 810.53. It has been named surugatoxin (SGTX) after Suruga Bay, where the mollusks were taken (see Hashimoto, 1979, for references).

In the sea hare, *Aplysia californica*, acetone extracts of the digestive glands had an intraperitoneal $LD_{50}$ of approximately 30 mg sea hare tissue/kg mouse body weight. Signs in mammals included increased respiration, blanching and drooping of the ears, increased salivation, muscle fasciculations, agonal signs, ataxia, prostration, and death. The extract was found to be lethal when given orally at approximately 12 times the intraperitoneal dose. A partially purified toxin called aplysin had an immediate but transient hypotensive effect in the dog. There was some initial arrhythmia followed by a slower but regular rate. In the isolated heart of the frog, aplysin caused cardiac standstill. The anterior cervical sympathetic ganglion of the cat was stimulated initially and then was reversibly blocked by the toxin. The frog rectus abdominis muscle responded by contracture, and in the rat diaphragm–phrenic nerve preparation the neuromuscular junction was blocked. In another sea hare, two bromine-containing sesquiterpenes were isolated and were named aplysin and aplysinol. A debromo derivative, debromoaplysin, and subsequently a third bromo compound, diterpene aplysin-20, also have been isolated. Observation of a sea hare feeding on the alga *Laurencia nipponica* led to several experiments that indicated that steam distillates of the alga are toxic to worms and carp. Based on this observation, Irie and associates (1969) extracted aplysin, debromoaplysin, and aplysinol from the red alga *Laurencia okamurai*, whereas Waraszkiewicz and Erickson (1974) obtained aplysin from *L. nidifica*. From these observations, it was suggested that the bromo toxins originate in algae. Two lethal extracts, one ether-soluble and the other water-soluble, have been separated from the digestive glands of the Hawaiian sea hares *Dolabella auriculasia, Aplysia pulmonica, Stytocheilus longicauda*, and *Dolabrifera dolabriefa*. In mice, the ether-soluble toxin caused irritability, viciousness, and severe flaccid paralysis. The water-soluble toxin, in contrast, caused "convulsions" and respiratory distress. Sublethal doses of the ether-soluble residue produced hypertension when injected intravenously into rats, whereas the crude water-soluble residue produced transient hypotension, bradycardia, and apnea. The hypertension produced by the ether-soluble toxin was resistant to both alpha- and beta-adrenergic blocking agents. The hypotensive effect of the water-soluble extract was not abolished by vagotomy or pretreatment with either atropine or diphenhydramine. It was concluded that both extracts may have direct effects on the contractility of vascular smooth muscle that are not mediated by alpha-adrenergic or cholinergic mechanisms. Choline esters were found in the aqueous fraction of the digestive gland of *A. californica*. Both acetylcholine and urocanylcholine were identified. The urocanylcholine accounted for the cholinesterase-resistant cholinomimetic activity of extracts of the gland. An "antifeedant" has been observed in *A. brasiliana*; it is the aromatic bromoallene panacene. It has been suggested that the panacene is biosynthesized from a $C_{15}$ algal precursor (see Russell, 1984a, for references).

In the cephalopods—the cuttlefishes, squids, nautiluses, and octopods—there are venomous octopods and possibly several venomous and poisonous squid. The venom apparatus of the octopus is an integral part of the animal's digestive system. The secretions serve a digestive function in some ways similar to that of the venoms of snakes. The apparatus consists of paired posterior salivary glands, two short (salivary) ducts that join them with the common salivary duct, paired anterior salivary glands and their ducts, the buccal mass, and the mandibles, or beak. An impressive number of substances have been isolated from or identified in the salivary glands of various cephalopods. Many of these substances have been shown to have biological activity, although these activities were not always apparent in the physiopharmacological effect of the whole toxin, while some of these substances do not have a significant biological activity or the state of knowledge does not indicate which activity is present. It now appears that many of the substances reported in the literature are normal constituents of the tissues of the salivary glands of cephalopods and not necessarily venom constituents. Some of the substances found in the salivary glands are tyramine, octopine, agmatine, adrenaline, noradrenaline,

5-hydroxytryptamine, L-*p*-hydroxyphenylethanolamine, histamine, dopamine, tryptophan, and certain 11-hydroxysteroids, polyphenols, phenolamines, indoleamines, and guanidine bases.

The posterior salivary glands of *Octopus apollyon* and *O. bimaculatus* have been shown to contain decarboxylate L-3,4-dihydroxyphenalalanine (DOPA), DL-5-hydroxytryptophan, DL-*erythro*-3,4-dihydroxyphenylserine, and DL-*erythro*-*p*-hydroxyphenylserine as well as DL-*m*-tyrosine, DL-*erythro*-*m*-hydroxyphenylserine, histidine, L-histidine, DL-*erythro*-phenylserine, 3,4-dihydroxyphenylserine, tyrosine, and *m*-tyrosine. In general, the salivary glands of cephalopods contain little or no proteolytic enzymes, amylases, or lipases. A protein, cephalotoxin, from the posterior salivary glands of *Sepia officinalis* has been suggested as the biologically active component in the animal's toxin. The toxin contained no cholinesterase or aminoxidase activity. Analysis of cephalotoxin from the posterior salivary gland of *Octopus vulgaris* showed protein, 74.05 percent (N determination) or 64.25 percent (biuret reaction); carbohydrates, 4.17 percent; and hexosamines, 5.80 percent.

The posterior salivary glands of *Eledone moschata* and *E. aldrovandi* contain a substance that when injected into mammals causes marked vasodilatation and produces hypotension and stimulation of certain extravascular smooth muscles. The substance was first called moschatin but was later renamed eledoisin. It is an endecapeptide. Eledoisin is 50 times more potent than is acetylcholine, histamine, or bradykinin in its ability to provoke hypotension in the dog.

Reports of envenomation by Australian octopuses, some of which were fatal, stimulated renewed interest in the venom of cephalopods. A saline extract of homogenized glands of *Hapalochlaena maculosa* was found to be a dialyzable, heat-stable product that resisted mild acid hydrolysis. When it was studied in a number of pharmacological preparations, it was concluded that animals died of respiratory failure caused by a phrenic nerve block and/or deleterious changes at the neuromuscular junction. The product also produced bradycardia and hypotension without remarkable changes in the ECG. It was found that within 4 min of the placing of a live *H. maculosa* on the back of a rabbit, a small bleeding puncture wound surrounded by a blanched area could be seen, the rabbit became restless, and there was some exophthalmos and "one slight convulsion" with cessation of all muscular activity other than cardiac. Cyanosis developed, and death followed at 19 min. It was concluded that a young octopus has sufficient venom in its posterior salivary glands to cause paralysis in 750-g rabbits, that the gland extracts have a high concentration of hyaluronidase, and that neostigmine does not reverse or reduce the toxic effects of the venom.

Further investigations yielded an extract of gland tissue partially purified by filtration that was given the name maculotoxin. On the basis of lethality determinations, there appeared to be a close similarity between the toxin and tetrodotoxin, and it was concluded that maculotoxin appeared to resemble tetrodotoxin more closely than it did saxitoxin. Saline and water extracts of the homogenized whole glands of *H. maculosa* produced paralysis and death at the 1-mg-gland/2-kg-rabbit level. Antibodies were produced to a nontoxic high-molecular-weight component but not to the toxic low-molecular-weight component. It was suggested that the molecular weight below 540 accounted for the lack of antigenicity. Maculotoxin was found to block neuromuscular transmission in the isolated sciatic sartorius nerve–muscle preparation of the toad by inhibiting the action potential in the motor nerve terminals, and it had no postsynaptic effect. It was suggested that the toxin may block action potentials by displacing sodium ions from negatively charged sites in the membrane. In 1978, previous observations on the likeness of maculotoxin to tetrodotoxin were confirmed. Direct spectral and chromatographic comparisons showed these two toxins to be indistinguishable. This is of particular interest because this is a poison (tetrodotoxin) that is also a venom (maculotoxin). In tetrodotoxin, the presence of the poison is thought to be a product of metabolism, whereas in maculotoxin, the venom is used to immobilize and perhaps kill the prey (see Russell, 1984a, for references).

The Pelecypoda—scallops, oysters, clams, and mussels—are the principal transvectors of paralytic shellfish poisoning. The genera most often involved with PSP are *Mya, Mytilus, Modiolus, Protothaca, Spisula*, and *Saxidomus*, according to Halstead (1978). The eating of the ovaries of the Japanese callista, *Callista brevisiphonata*, has resulted in numerous cases of illness. The ovaries contain large amounts of choline but no histamine. Cats fed the shellfish showed few signs other than hypoactivity and some loss of coordination. Three of nine human volunteers who ate the ovaries developed urticaria and very mild symptoms. Venerupin poisoning is caused by the ingestion of the oyster *Crassostrea gigas*. In one series of 81 poisoned persons, 54 died (Halstead, 1965). In a second outbreak in 1941 involving six patients, five died, and from 1942 to 1950 there were 455 additional cases involving the eating of oysters and the short-necked clam *Tapes japonica* (Hashimoto, 1979). The toxin causes hemorrhage in the heart, lungs, and viscera, with diffuse hemorrhage, necrosis, and fatty degeneration of the liver.

**Clinical Problem.** A number of cones have been implicated in injuries to humans, including *Conus geographus, C. aulicus, C. gloria-maris, C. marmoreus, C. textile, C. tulipa, C. striatus, C. omaria, C. catus, C. obscurus, C. imperialis, C. pulicarius, C. quercinus, C. litteratus, C. lividus*, and *C. sponsalis*. The first would seem to be the most dangerous, because it is said to have the most highly developed venom apparatus (Halstead, 1978).

The sting often gives rise to immediate and sometimes intense localized pain at the site of the injury. Within 5 min the victim usually notes some numbness and ischemia around the wound, although in a case seen by the author the affected area was red and tender rather than ischemic. A tingling or numbing sensation may develop around the mouth, lips, and tongue and over the peripheral parts of the extremities. Other symptoms and signs during the first 30 min after the injury include hypertonicity, tremor, muscle fasciculations, nausea and vomiting, dizziness, increased lacrimation and salivation, weakness, and pain in the chest, which increases with deep inspiration. The numbness around the wound may spread to involve a good part of the extremity or injured part. In more severe cases, respiratory distress with chest pain, difficulties in swallowing and phonation, marked dizziness, blurring of vision and inability to focus, ataxia, and generalized pruritus have been reported. In fatal cases, "respiratory paralysis" precedes death (Russell, 1965).

Poisoning after the ingestion of the whelk, *Neptunea arthritica*, is characterized by dizziness, nausea, vomiting, weakness, ataxia, photophobia, external ocular weakness, dryness of the mouth, and occasionally urticaria. Ingestion of the toxic abalone produces erythema, swelling, and pain over the face and neck and sometimes the extremities and, in more severe cases, a fulminating dermatitis. Latin and medieval writers from the time of Pliny considered the sea hare *Aplysia* to be very poisonous. Halstead (1965) noted that extracts of *Aplysia* were "frequently employed to dispatch political enemies"; however, there are no recent reports of death from eating sea hares. Tasting them produces a burning sensation in the mouth and slight irritation of the oral mucosa. Handling the animals is not likely to be dangerous, but the author suspects that it would not be safe to rub one's eyes afterward. A number of poisonings occurred in Hokkaido, Japan, after the ingestion of *Callista brevisiphonata* in the early 1950s. These poisonings necessitated prohibiting the sale of the shellfish in the marketplace. The illness has a rapid onset, often occurring while the patient is still dining. It has been characterized as an "allergiclike" reaction which is thought to be due to the presence of excessive choline in the ovaries. The most common findings are flushing, urticaria, wheezing, and GI upset. It is self-limiting (Russell, 1971).

Hashimoto (1979) noted a total of 542 cases of venerupin poisoning in Japan with 185 deaths. Fortunately, there have been no reported cases since 1950. The poisoning was observed after the eating of the oyster *Crassostrea gigas* or the asari *Tapes japonica*. It is characterized by a long incubation period (24 to 48 h, and sometimes longer), anorexia, halitosis, nausea, vomiting, gastric pain, constipation, headache, and malaise. These findings may be followed by increased nervousness, hematemesis, and bleeding from the mucous membranes of the nose, mouth, and gums. In serious cases, jaundice may be present, and petechial hemorrhages and ecchymosis may appear over the chest, neck, and arms. Leukocytosis, anemia, and a prolonged blood-clotting time are sometimes observed. The liver is usually enlarged. In fatal poisonings, extreme excitation, delirium, and coma may occur.

The more common types of shellfish poisoning are recognized as GI, allergic, and paralytic. GI shellfish poisoning is characterized by nausea, vomiting, abdominal pain, weakness, and diarrhea. The onset of symptoms generally occurs 8 to 12 h after ingestion of the offending mollusk. This type of intoxication is caused by bacterial pathogens and usually is limited to GI signs and symptoms. It rarely persists for more than 48 h.

Allergic or erythematous shellfish poisoning is characterized by an allergic response that may vary between individuals. The onset of symptoms and signs occurs 30 min to 6 h after ingestion of the mollusk to which the individual is sensitive. The usual presenting signs and symptoms are diffuse erythema, swelling, urticaria, and pruritus involving the head and neck and then spreading to the body. Headache, flushing, epigastric distress, and nausea are occasional complaints. In more severe cases, generalized edema, severe pruritus, swelling of the tongue and throat, respiratory distress, and vomiting sometimes occur. Death is rare, but persons with a known sensitivity to shellfish should avoid eating all mollusks. The sensitizing material appears to be more capable of provoking a serious autopharmacological response than are most known sensitizing proteins.

Paralytic shellfish poisoning is known variously as gonyaulax poisoning, paresthetic shellfish poisoning, mussel poisoning, and mytilointoxication. Pathognomonic symptoms develop within the first 30 min after ingestion of the offending mollusk. Paresthesia, described as tingling, burning, or numbness, is noted first around the mouth, lips, and tongue; it then spreads over the face, scalp, and neck and to the fingertips and toes. Sensory perception and proprioception are affected to the point where the individual moves incoordinately and in a manner similar to that seen in another, more common form of intoxication. Ataxia, incoherent speech, and/or aphonia are prominent signs in severe poisonings. The patient complains of dizziness, tightness of the throat and chest, and some pain on deep inspiration. Weakness, malaise, headache, increased salivation and perspiration, thirst, and nausea and vomiting may be present. The pulse is usually thready and rapid; superficial reflexes are often absent, and deep reflexes may be hypoactive. If muscular weakness and respiratory distress grow progressively more severe during the first 8 h, death may ensue. If the victim survives the first 10 to 12 h, the prognosis is good. Death is usually attributed to "respiratory paralysis" (Russell, 1965, 1984a; Halstead, 1965).

Among the cephalopods that have been implicated in bites of humans are *Hapalochlaena (Octopus) maculosa, Octopus australis, O. lunulatus, O. doefleini, O. vulgaris, O. apollyon, O. bimaculatus, O. macropus, O. rubescens, O. fitchi, O. flindersi, Ommastrephes sloani pacificus, Eledone moschata, E. aldrovandi*, and *Sepia officinalis*. The bite of most octopods results in a small puncture wound; it appears to bleed more freely than one would expect from a similar nonenvenomated traumatic wound. Pain is minimal, and in the two cases seen by the author it was described as no greater than the pain produced by a sharp pin. The area around the wound is blanched but then becomes erythematous and in severe envenomations may become hemorrhagic. Tingling and numbness around the wound site are not uncommon complaints. Swelling is usually minimal immediately after the injury but may develop 6 to 12 h later. Muscle fasciculations have been noted after *H. maculosa* bites (Sutherland and Lane, 1969). Localized pruritus sometimes occurs over the edematous area. "Light-headedness" of several hours' duration and weakness were reported in both cases observed by this author; there were no other systemic symptoms or signs. The wounds healed without complications (Russell, 1965). In the case reported by Flecker and Cotton (1955), the patient was bitten by *H. maculosa* and complained of dryness in the mouth and difficulty in breathing but had no localized or generalized pain. Subsequently, breathing became more labored, swallowing became difficult, and the patient began to vomit. Severe respiratory distress and cyanosis developed, and the victim expired. The findings at autopsy were negative. Subsequently, Cleland and Southcott (1965) reviewed the literature on cephalopod bites and also noted several unreported bites in humans.

## Fishes

**Poisonous Fishes.** Approximately 700 species of marine fishes are known to be toxic or may on ingestion be poisonous to humans. This number does not include fishes that have caused a poisoning traceable to bacterial pathogens. Most, but by no means all, of these species are found in the coral reef belt. As a whole their distribution is spotty, even in a particular part of the ocean or around an island. They tend to occur in greater numbers around islands than along continental shores. Most species are nonmigratory. They may be either herbivores or carnivores. Some poisonous species have tissues that are toxic at all times, other species are poisonous only at certain periods or in certain areas, and still others have only specific organs that are toxic, and the toxicity of these tissues may vary with time and location.

Fish poisoning is synonymous with ichthyotoxism. Halstead (1964) divided the ichthyotoxic fishes into three subdivisions: (1) ichthyosarcotoxic, or fishes that contain a toxin within their musculature, viscera, or skin which when ingested produces deleterious effects, (2) ichthyootoxic, or fishes that produce a toxin that is related to gonadal activity; most members of this subdivision are freshwater species, and this group includes fishes whose roe is poisonous, and (3) icthyohemotoxic, or fishes that have a toxin in their blood. Some freshwater eels and several marine fishes make up this group. The word "ichthyocrinotoxic" is sometimes used for fishes that produce a poison through glandular secretions not associated with a venom apparatus. This word might be used for the soapfishes, certain gobies, some cyclostomes, boxfishes, toadfishes, lampreys, and hagfishes, which may release toxic skin secretions into the water, perhaps under stressful conditions, or as repellents or in defense.

**Ichthyosarcotoxism.** This type of poisoning is generally identified with the particular kind of fish involved: elasmobranch, chimaeroid, clupeoid, ciguatera, tetraodon, scombroid, and so on. It also includes hallucinatory fish poisoning.

***Ciguatera.*** The word "ciguatera" was perhaps first applied to a poisoning caused by the ingestion of the marine snail *Livona pica* ("cigua"), a staple seafood throughout the Caribbean. The word is now commonly used to indicate a type of fish poisoning characterized by certain gastrointestinal-neurological and sometimes cardiovascular manifestations. It may occur after the ingestion of certain tropical reef and semipelagic marine species, such as the barracudas, groupers, sea basses, snappers, surgeonfishes, parrotfishes, jacks, wrasses, and eels, as well as certain gastropods. A listing of the ciguateric fishes has been provided by Russell (1965), Halstead (1957), and Bagnis and colleagues (1970, 1979). Bagnis and colleagues (1970, 1979) noted approximately 400 species as ciguateric. Because almost all these fishes are normally edible and some are valuable food fishes in some parts of the world, ciguatera poisoning is not only the most common but also the most treacherous form of ichthyotoxism.

This form of fish poisoning is associated with the food chain or food web (Russell, 1952, 1965; Dawson et al., 1955; Randall, 1958; Halstead, 1965; Banner, 1976; Southcott, 1979). It has been shown to exist in both the South Pacific and the Caribbean. The responsible organism is a photosynthetic benthic dinoflagellate, *Gambierdiscus toxicus*, but the poison found in most ciguateric fishes is a combination of several toxins, the principal one being ciguatoxin and, in some cases, lesser ones such as maitotoxin and scaritoxin. The chemical structure of all the ciguatoxins has not been elucidated. The crude toxin is a colorless, heat-stable, hydroxylated lipid molecule with a molecular weight of about 1100, and it shows little olefinic character and no observable proton signals below 6. The toxin increases membrane permeability to sodium, causing depolarization, and in different doses produces changes in the rate and force of contraction of the heart. Large doses precipitate more severe cardiac changes. This toxin has been found to be antagonized by physostigmine.

The signs of poisoning in animals include increased salivation and lacrimation, lethargy, respiratory difficulties, cyanosis, decreased body temperature, ataxia and loss of reflexes, and prostration. In humans, the symptoms and signs include perioral parasthesia often with a feeling of loose teeth in the lower jaw, nausea and vomiting, abdominal pain, changes in sensory perception, pruritus, diarrhea, hypoactive reflexes, and bradycardia. The patient often complains of dizziness, marked weakness, and on occasion some myalgia and joint pain. Paresis, particularly of the legs, is a common finding in severe poisonings. The presence of the toxin can be demonstrated by ELISA and radioimmunoassay (RIA).

Tetrodotoxin, or puffer or fugu poison, is found in certain puffers, ocean sunfishes, and porcupinefishes. Tetrodotoxin (tarichatoxin) also is found in certain amphibian species of the family Salamandridae and the blue-ringed octopus among the animals. The puffers or pufferlike fishes appear to be the only fishes universally regarded as poisonous. Among the approximately 100 species of these fishes, over 50 have been involved in poisonings to humans or are known to be toxic under certain conditions. Some of the more important of the toxic species have been noted by Russell (1965), Kao (1966), Halstead (1965), and Hashimoto (1979). Table 26-6 shows the concentration of tetrodotoxin in various tissues of Tetraodontidae species and in the amphibian *Taricha torosa*. It can be seen that in most cases the toxin is concentrated in the ovaries and liver, with lesser amounts in the intestines and skin and very small amounts in the body musculature and blood. The appearance and amount of toxin in the fish appear to be related to the reproductive cycle and appear to be greatest just before spawning, which varies with the species involved and the locale. The chemistry of tetrodotoxin up until 1970 has been reviewed elsewhere (Russell, 1971). Its structure is

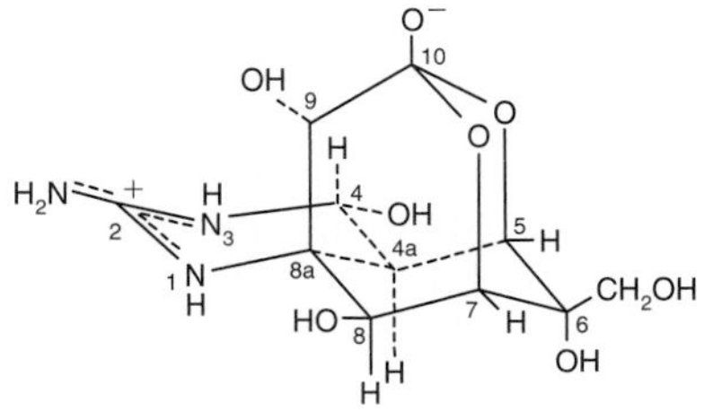

The lethal dose-response curve of tetrodotoxin is characteristically steep. The intraperitoneal minimal lethal dose in mice is 8 $\mu$g/kg, whereas the $LD_{99}$ is 12 $\mu$g/kg and the intraperitoneal $LD_{50}$ is approximately 10 $\mu$g/kg (Kao and Fuhrman, 1963). The oral $LD_{50}$ in mice is 322 $\mu$g/kg, whereas that in cats is in excess of 0.20 mg/kg. The toxin prevents the increase in the early transient ionic permeability of the nerve that normally is associated with the inward movement of sodium during excitation. This can be seen in the classic nerve preparations as a conduction block and in the voltage-clamp axon preparations as a decrease in the peak current of the inward

**Table 26–6**
**Concentrations of Tetrodotoxin in Tetraodontidae Fishes and a Newt**

| SPECIES | OVARY | LIVER | SKIN | INTESTINES | MUSCLE | BLOOD |
|---|---|---|---|---|---|---|
| *Sphaeroides niphobles* | 400 | 1000 | 40 | 400 | 4 | 1 |
| *Sphaeroides alboplumbeus* | 200 | 1000 | 20 | 40 | 4 | |
| *Sphaeroides pardalis* | 200 | 1000 | 100 | 40 | 1 | 1 |
| *Sphaeroides vermicularis* | 400 | 200 | 100 | 40 | 4 | |
| *Sphaeroides porphyreus* | 400 | 200 | 20 | 40 | 1 | |
| *Sphaeroides oscellatus* | 1000 | 40 | 20 | 40 | <0.2 | |
| *Sphaeroides basilewskianus* | 100 | 40 | 4 | 40 | <0.2 | |
| *Sphaeroides chrysops* | 40 | 40 | 20 | 4 | <0.2 | <0.2 |
| *Sphaeroides pseudommus* | 100 | 10 | 4 | 2 | <0.2 | |
| *Sphaeroides rubripes* | 100 | 100 | 1 | 2 | <0.2 | <0.2 |
| *Sphaeroides xanthopterus* | 100 | 40 | 1 | 4 | <0.2 | |
| *Sphaeroides stictonotus* | 20 | <0.2 | 2 | 1 | <0.2 | |
| *Lagocephalus inermis* | 0.4 | 1 | <0.2 | 0.4 | 0.4 | |
| *Canthigaster rivulatus* | <2 | 2 | 40 | 4 | <0.2 | |
| *Taricha torosa* ♀ | 25 | <0.1 | 25 | (0.1)* | 2 | 1 |
| *Taricha torosa* ♂ | <0.1† | <0.1 | 80 | (0. 5)* | 8 | 21 |

*Note*: Amounts expressed in μg toxin/g fresh tissue of female specimens.
*Visceral organ.
†Testis.
SOURCE: Kao (1966), © by Williams & Wilkins, 1966.

sodium. The subsequent outward movement of potassium is unaffected by the toxin.

To a lesser extent, tetrodotoxin blocks the skeletal muscle membrane. It has no direct effect on the junction exclusive of its effect on the nerve ending and the muscle membrane. It provokes hypotension and has a deleterious effect on respiration. It has some effects on the central nervous system but few effects on the autonomic nervous system. Tetrodotoxin has pharmacological and toxicological properties similar in many ways to those of saxitoxin, but the two are chemically distinct. Studies have shown that binding of tetrodotoxin, like that of saxitoxin, is a function separate from that of cation selectivity, which has been the basis of the cork-in-a-bottle model (Kao, 1981).

While fewer than 75 people now die from tetraodon poisoning in Japan each year, many people use the poison for suicide, with additional deaths reported from elsewhere in Asia and the Pacific. The total number of deaths worldwide is probably less than 125 annually. At one time the mortality rate was 80 percent, but through the years it has been reduced, part because of the fine work of Hashimoto and colleagues in licensing fugu restaurants in Japan. At the present time about 40 percent of those developing significant symptoms and signs subsequently die. The clinical case is characterized by the rapid onset (5 to 30 min) of weakness, dizziness, pallor, and paresthesia around the lips, tongue, and throat. The paresthesia usually is described as "tingling or pricking sensations" and often is noted in the limbs, particularly the fingers and toes, as the illness develops. Weakness is a common complaint. Increased salivation and diaphoresis are often present, and the patient may become hypotensive. Changes in heart rate are common. There may be vomiting, sometimes severe and frequent. Bradycardia, dyspnea, cyanosis, and shock may develop, and generalized flaccidity may ensue. Treatment consists of oxygen, intravenous fluids, atropine, and, if appropriate, activated charcoal, saline catharses, and nasoepigastric suctioning. Calcium, naloxone, and sedatives are contraindicated. The poison can be detected from autopsy material by gas chromatography.

Until recently, the basic source of tetrodotoxin through the food chain was a matter of speculation. With the work of Yasumoto and associates (1986), Simidu and colleagues (1987) and Simidu and coworkers (1990), it has been shown that certain bacteria are capable of producing the toxin and may be the source of the poison. The bacteria have been isolated from both red algae and pufferfish. Two strains are members of the genus *Listonella (Vibrio)*, while two others strains are from the genera *Alteromonas* and *Shewanella* (Simidu et al., 1990).

***Scombroid Poisoning.*** Certain mackerellike fishes (tunas, skipjacks, and bonitos) are occasionally involved in human poisonings. The clinical manifestations of such poisonings are quite different from those provoked by ciguatera toxin, although some of the same fishes may be implicated in ciguatera poisoning. Although more than 100 papers on this subject have been written during the past decade, they have added little to the report by Halstead (1965). A notable exception is the review by Arnold and Brown (1978). If scombroids are inadequately preserved, a toxic substance is formed in the body musculature. This substance was once thought to be histamine formed by the action of enzymes and bacteria or released by bacterial action after the death of the fish. However, more recent evidence seems to indicate that the toxic component is not histamine alone, although histamine is involved in the reaction. The toxic factor has been given the name "saurine" by some investigators. After ingestion of the offending fish, the victim usually complains of nausea, vomiting, and diarrhea; epigastric distress; and flushing of the face, headache, and burning of the throat, sometimes followed by numbness, thirst, and generalized urticaria. These signs and symptoms usually appear within 2 h of the meal and subside within 16 h. In more severe cases, there may be some muscular weakness. The poisoning is rarely serious. The offending fish is often said to have a "peppery taste" (Russell, 1971).

***Cyclostome Poisoning.*** The slime and flesh of certain lampreys and hagfishes appear to contain a toxin that may produce GI signs and symptoms.

***Elasmobranch Poisoning.*** Consumption of the musculature of the Greenland shark, *Somniosus microcephalus*, has caused poisonings in both humans and dogs, whereas the livers of several species of tropical sharks have caused severe poisonings and even deaths. Species reported to be poisonous at times include *Carcharhinus melanopterus, Heptranchias perlo, Hexanchus grisseus, Carcharodon carcharias*, and *Sphyrna zygaena*. In some cases, the poisoning appears to be ciguateric in nature. The eating of shark livers has been known to cause another kind of poisoning which appears to be due to hypervitaminosis A. Hypervitaminosis A is well known after the consumption of the livers of some polar bears, seals, and halibut (Russell, 1967; Halstead, 1965).

***Hallucinatory Fish Poisoning.*** Hallucinatory fish poisoning is characterized by central nervous system signs and symptoms and by a lack of GI manifestations. It has occurred after the ingestion of certain mullet and surmullet (goatfish). Among the species reported to have caused this poisoning are *Mugil cephalus, Neomyxus chaptalli, Paraupeneus chryserydros*, and *Upeneus arge*. Reports of poisoning have been filed in the tropical Pacific and Hawaii. The findings in human cases seem to indicate that the offending substance is different from that responsible for ciguatera poisoning. The onset of manifestations occurs 10 to 90 min after ingestion of the toxic fish. The victim complains of light-headedness or dizziness, weakness, muscular incoordination, and sometimes ataxia, hallucinations, and depression. In severe cases, there may be paresthesia around the mouth and some muscular paralysis and dyspnea. The agonal period is usually of short duration, 1 to 24 h, and few cases are serious enough to send the victim to a doctor. If the victim goes to sleep immediately after the poisoning, he or she is said to have violent nightmares. This complaint accounts for the term "nightmare weke" being given to the causative fish, *U. arge* (Helfrich and Banner, 1960).

**Ichthyootoxic Fishes.** A number of freshwater fishes and a few marine species produce a toxin that appears to be restricted to their gonads. In these fishes the body musculature and even the GI organs are edible. Poisoning occurs after ingestion of the roe or the gonads and roe. The eggs of the perchlike fish *Scorpaenichthys marmoratus* appear to be avoided by fish-eating and fish-scavenging birds as well as by the mink and raccoon. The roe of the alligator gar is also known to produce cardiovascular changes. An excellent review of this problem can be found in Fuhrman (1974). The poisoning is characterized by the rapid onset of nausea, vomiting, and epigastric distress. Diarrhea, dryness in the mouth, thirst, tinnitus, and malaise sometimes occur. In more severe cases, syncope, respiratory distress, chest pain, convulsions, and coma may ensue. Complete recovery usually occurs within a few days.

**Ichthyohemotoxic Fishes.** A toxic substance has been found in the blood of many species of fishes, although the principal contributions to our knowledge of the toxin have come from studies of the blood of the eels *Anguilla* and *Muraena*. Poisonings from the ingestion of fresh blood are extremely rare. The few cases reported have occurred in persons who of their own volition drank quantities sufficient to cause symptoms; most of these cases have occurred after the ingestion of blood from European freshwater eels or *M. helena*.

**Crinotoxic Fishes.** Halstead (1970) recorded approximately 50 teleost species as being crinotoxic. Hashimoto noted a few others, and with the studies of Cameron and associates (1981) and others, the total number now approaches 65. These fishes are known to release a toxic substance from the skin that is capable of repelling or killing other fishes and marine animals. This toxin appears to be part of the animal's defensive armament and probably is released as an alarm substance to deter predators. Cameron and associates (1981) suggested that in the case of the stonefish, the toxin liberated from the tubercle glands may be antibiotic in nature, protecting the fish against the plethora of potentially harmful organisms that occur in the immediate environment of the virtually scaleless integument of the fish.

A toxic factor has been separated from the skin secretions of the boxfish, or trunkfish, *Ostracion lentiginosis*. The toxin is heat-stable, nondialyzable, and soluble in water, methanol, ethanol, acetone, and chloroform but insoluble in diethyl ether and benzene. Repeated extractions of residues obtained from drying the skin secretions with acetone or chloroform and diethyl ether give a particulate substance that forms stable foams in aqueous solutions and is toxic to fish at concentrations of 1:1,000,000. Approximately 50 to 100 mg of the crude dried toxin can be obtained at one time from a single adult boxfish. The toxin was called ostracitoxin. Further studies showed that when a crude solution was extracted into 1-butanol, a 20-fold purification of the toxin was obtained. The product was called pahutoxin. Spectroscopic data, hydrolytic degradations, and synthesis gave the formula $C_{23}H_{46}NO_4Cl$ and the structure

$$CH_3-(CH_2)_{12}-\underset{\substack{|\\ OCOCH_3}}{\overset{\substack{H\\ |}}{C}}-CH_2-CO_2-(CH_2)_2-\overset{+}{N}(CH_3)_3Cl^-$$

Pahutoxin is thus the choline chloride ester of 3-acetoxyhexadecanoic acid. It and its $C_{14}$ and $C_{12}$ homologues have been synthesized as the racemates. When ostracitoxin was added to an aquarium containing other reef fishes, they exhibited "irritability," gasping, a decrease in opercular movements, loss of equilibrium and locomotion, and finally sporadic convulsions and death. When the skin mucus was injected into the boxfish, the fish immediately lost its balance, and death occurred within a few minutes. When injected into mice, ostracitoxin produced ataxia, labored respirations, coma, and death. The maximum lethal dose (MLD) was 200 mg/kg body weight. Ostracitoxin caused hemolysis of vertebrate erythrocytes in vitro. Pahutoxin was quantified for its hemolytic property, which correlated with its lethal property. The minimum lethal concentration for fish was found to be 0.176 $\mu$g/ml when death was measured at 1 h (see Russell, 1971, for references).

The Red Sea flatfish, *Pardachirus marmoratus*, has 212 to 235 secretory glands along its dorsal and anal fins. Its secretions are toxic to fishes, and the toxic factor, pardaxin, is a protein with a molecular weight of approximately 15,000, with a single chain and four disulfide bridges. The toxin has an intraperitoneal $LD_{50}$ in mice of 24.6 mg/kg and inhibits [$Na^+$, $K^+$] ATPase but enhances esterase activity. It causes hemolysis in dog red blood cells, which lack [$Na^+$, $K^+$] ATPase, but the toxin-induced hemolysis is not caused by inhibition. It was suggested that the different responses to the poison with respect to esterase and ATPase could be due to differences in the way those enzymes are anchored in the plasma membrane (Primor and Lazarovici, 1981).

## Venomous Fishes

More than 200 species of marine fishes, including stingrays, scorpionfishes, zebrafishes, stonefishes, weevers, toadfishes, stargazers, and certain sharks, ratfishes, catfishes, surgeonfishes, and a blenny, are known or thought to be venomous. The great majority of venomous piscines are nonmigratory and slow-swimming. They tend to live in protected habitats or around rocks, corals, or kelp beds. Stingrays spend much of their time buried in sand. Most species use their venom apparatus as a defensive weapon. The toxins of the venomous fishes differ markedly in their chemical, pharmacological, and toxicological properties from the toxins of the poisonous fishes as well as the toxins of other venomous animals. A common characteristic of the toxins of venomous fishes is their relative instability. Few of them are stable at room temperatures, and toxicity appears to be lost or markedly reduced on lyophilization of even freshly prepared crude extracts. The reader is referred to the works of Russell (1965, 1969, 1971, 1984a) and Halstead (1965, 1978) for a review of the toxins of venomous fishes.

**Stingrays.** The stingrays include the families Dasyatidae, the whiprays; Urolophidae, the round stingrays; Myliobatoidae, the bat-rays or eagle-rays; Gymnuridae, the butterfly rays; and Potamotrygonidae, or river rays. These elasmobranchs range in size from several inches in diameter to over 14 feet in length. For the most part, they are nonmigratory shallow-water fishes. The venom apparatus of the stingray consists of bilaterally serrated, dentinal caudal spines on the dorsum of the animal's tail. The spine is encased in an integumentary sheath. The venom is contained in certain highly specialized secretory cells in this sheath. Unlike many venomous marine animals, the stingray has no true venom gland. The venom is contained in the secretory cells in the grooves of the caudal spine, and these cells and their supporting tissues must be ruptured to release the toxin, as occurs during the traumatic act of stinging (Russell, 1965; Halstead, 1965; Smith et al., 1978).

Stingray venom is known to exert a deleterious effect on the mammalian cardiovascular system. Low concentrations of the venom give rise to either vasodilatation or vasoconstriction, with mild bradycardia and an increase in the PR interval. Cats receiving larger amounts of the venom show, in addition to the PR interval change, almost immediate ST, T-wave change indicative of ischemia and in some animals true heart muscle injury. High concentrations cause vasoconstriction and produce marked changes in heart rate and the amplitude of systole and often cause complete, irreversible cardiac standstill (Russell and van Harreveld, 1954). While small doses of the venom may cause some increase in the respiratory rate, large doses depress respiration. Part of this depression is secondary to the cardiovascular changes, but the venom may provoke changes in behavior. The venom has little or no effect on neuromuscular transmission. The $LD_{99}$ in mice has been calculated as 28.0 mg/kg for crude extracts of the tissue from the ventrolateral grooves of the spine. However, the author has found that the peak II portion of a Sephadex G-200 fraction has an intravenous $LD_{50}$ in mice of approximately 2.9 mg protein/kg body weight (see Russell, 1971, for references).

**Scorpionfishes.** The family Scorpanenidae, the scorpionfishes or rockfishes, contains approximately 80 species that have been implicated in poisonings to humans or whose venom has been studied by chemists and toxicologists. Included in this group are the sculpins, zebrafishes, stonefishes, bullrout, and waspfish. They are widely distributed throughout tropical and more temperate seas. A few are found in Arctic waters. In most, the venom apparatus consists of a number of dorsal, several anal, and two pelvic spines. The spines differ considerably in size and structure. The enveloping integumentary sheath and the glandular complex lying within the anterolateral grooves make up the remaining components of the venom apparatus. The venom apparatuses of these fishes have been divided into three types. More thorough reviews of the variations in the venom gland structures, the chemistry, and the toxicology of the venom have been provided by Halstead (1970) and Russell (1971). The pharmacological properties are summarized in Table 26-7.

**Weeverfishes.** The weevers, members of the family Trachinidae, are small marine fishes confined to the eastern Atlantic and Mediterranean coasts. The name "weever" is probably derived from a corruption of the Angle-Saxon "wivre," meaning viper. These fish are found in large numbers in the shallow waters of certain offshore sandy grounds along the British coast, in the continental southern North Sea, and along the coasts of the English Channel and the Mediterranean and Adriatic seas. The venom apparatus of weeverfishes consists of two opercular spines, five to eight dorsal spines, and the tissues contained in the integumentary sheaths surrounding the spines. The five to eight dorsal spines are enclosed in individual integumentary sheaths connected by their interspinous membranes. The venom is contained in the various grooves of the spines. These spines and the venom have been described elsewhere (Russell and Emery, 1960; Russell, 1971, 1984a; Halstead, 1978).

***Clinical Problem.*** Stings by venomous marine fishes are common in many areas of the world. Approximately 750 people have reported stings by stingrays along the North American coasts in a single year. Fortunately, deaths from the effects of the venom are very rare. Stings by *Scorpaena* are very common. Approximately 300 persons in the United States are stung by *S. guttata* or related species each year (see Russell, 1971, for references). Envenomations by lionfishes and zebrafishes were once rare, but with the importation of lionfishes for tropical sea aquariums, more than 50 cases of stings by

**Table 26–7**
**Some Properties of Scorpaenidae Venoms**

| | PTEROIS | SYNANCEJA | SCORPAENA |
|---|---|---|---|
| Small dose | Decreased arterial pressure<br>Minimal ECG changes<br>Increased respiratory rate<br>Muscular weakness in mice | Decreased arterial pressure<br>Minimal ECG changes<br>Increased respiratory rate<br>Tremor | Slight decrease in arterial pressure<br>Increased, then decreased venous pressure<br>Minimal ECG changes<br>Increased respiratory rate with decreased respiratory excursions |
| Medium dose | Marked fall in arterial pressure<br>Myocardial ischemia, injury or conduction defects<br>Increased respiratory rate<br>Partial paralysis of legs in mice | Marked fall in arterial pressure<br>Myocardial ischemia, injury or conduction defects<br>Increased respiratory rate<br>Muscular weakness in mice<br>Tremor | Fall in arterial pressure<br>Myocardial ischemia, injury or conduction defects<br>Changes in venous and CSF pressures<br>Increased respiratory rate with decreased respiratory excursions |
| Lethal dose | Precipitous, irreversible fall in systemic arterial pressure<br>Extensive ECG changes<br>Markedly decreased respiratory rate → cessation<br>Complete paralysis of legs in mice<br>Intravenous $LD_{50}$ mice, 1.1 mg protein/kg body weight | Precipitous, irreversible fall in systemic arterial pressure<br>Extensive ECG changes<br>Markedly decreased respiratory rate → cessation<br>Some paralysis of legs in mice<br>Possible neuromuscular junction changes<br>Produces tremors, convulsions, marked muscular weakness, coma: myotoxic<br>Intravenous $LD_{50}$ mice, 200 $\mu g$ protein/kg body weight | Precipitous, irreversible fall in arterial pressure<br>Extensive ECG changes<br>Markedly decreased respiratory rate → cessation<br>Some paralysis of legs in mice<br>Intravenous $LD_{50}$ mice, in excess 2.0 mg protein/kg body weight |

SOURCE: Russell (1971).

these fish were reported in 1978–1979. Injuries inflicted by weeverfishes are also common in certain coastal areas of Europe. However, no deaths attributable to the stings of these fishes have been reported in recent years.

Of 1097 stingray injuries reported over an 8-year period in North America from 1952 to 1959, 232 patients were seen by a physician at some time during the course of their recovery. That is not true today. Only about 5 percent are now seen by physicians because of the effective first aid provided by lifeguard services. Unlike the injuries inflicted by many venomous animals, wounds produced by the stingray may be large and severely lacerated, requiring extensive debridement and surgical closure. A spine no wider than 5 mm may produce a wound 3.5 cm long, and larger stings may produce wounds 17.5 cm long. The sting itself is rarely broken off in the wound, but that may happen. The stinging is followed by the immediate onset of intense pain out of proportion to that which might be produced by a similar nonvenomous injury. While the onset of pain is usually limited to the area of injury, it spreads rapidly, though it gradually diminishes in severity over 6 to 48 h.

For the most part, the symptoms and signs of the poisoning are limited to the injured area. However, syncope, weakness, nausea, and anxiety are common complaints and may be attributed in part to peripheral vasodilatation and in part to the reflex phenomenon precipitated by the severe pain. Vomiting, diarrhea, sweating, fasciculations in the muscles of the affected extremity, generalized cramps, inguinal or axillary pain, and respiratory distress are infrequently reported. True paralysis is extremely rare, if it occurs at all. Examination reveals either a puncture or a lacerated wound, usually the latter, jagged, bleeding freely, and often contaminated with parts of the sting's integumentary sheath. The edges of the wound may be discolored. However, within 2 h the discoloration may extend several centimeters from the wound. Subsequent necrosis of this area occasionally occurs in untreated cases.

To be successful, treatment must be instituted early. The standard procedure for the treatment of fish stings is well established. Injuries to an extremity should be irrigated with the salt water at hand. An attempt should be made to remove the integumentary sheath if it is present in the wound. The extremity should then be submerged in water at as high a temperature as the patient can tolerate without injury for 30 to 90 min. The addition of sodium chloride or magnesium sulfate to the hot water is optional. The wound should then be further cleaned, debrided, and sutured if necessary. The appropriate antitetanus agent should be administered. Infections of these wounds are rare in properly treated cases. Elevation of the injured extremity for several days is advised.

Envenomation by *Scorpaena* such as the California sculpin, *S. guttata*, is followed almost immediately by intense, sometimes pulsating pain in the area of the injury. Almost all stings are inflicted on the hands of fishers while they are attempting to dislodge the fish from their hooks. The area around the wound may appear ischemic at first, but in time the injured part becomes red and swollen. The pain may extend up the forearm and into the axilla within 15 min of the injury. Nausea, vomiting, weakness, pallor, syncope, and urgency to urinate are frequent complaints. Increased perspiration, headache, conjunctivitis, and diarrhea sometimes are reported. Paresthesia around the injured part and even up the forearm may occur. Swelling and tenderness of the axillary nodes occurred in at least 20 percent of one series of untreated cases. The pain subsides in 3 to 8 h, although the swelling and tenderness may persist for several days. In severe stingings the pain may be excruciating. Primary shock may occur, and in several cases seen by the author the patients were brought to the hospital under oxygen. Respirations may become labored and painful. Pulmonary edema has been reported, and abnormal ECG has been demonstrated. In one case known to the author, the patient had a pulmonary embolism and was hospitalized for 24 days. The standard first-aid treatment for *S. guttata* stings has consisted of soaking the injured part in hot water for 30 min. In many cases, fishers add household ammonia.

Envenomation by the lionfish gives rise to immediate intense, sometimes burning pain, which often radiates within minutes from the wound area. The tissues around the wound may appear blanched, and the victim may complain of numbness, weakness, and paresthesia around the injury or even over the entire affected part. Weakness, dizziness, and shock may ensue but are not common. In cases of shock, there is bradycardia, hypothermia, and respiratory distress. The wound site is sometimes discolored, edematous, and tender. Necrosis may occur around the wound. The pain often persists for 8 to 12 h, and the injured part may be sore and edematous for several weeks. First-aid treatment is the same as for stingray injuries. Meperidine hydrochloride may be needed to control pain. Intravenous calcium gluconate has been said to afford some relief. Cardiovascular tone should be maintained with intravenous fluids and vasopressor agents.

Stingings by the stonefishes, *Synanceja horrida* and *S. trachynis*, are usually more serious than those inflicted by any other venomous fishes. The clinical course after poisoning by a stonefish is similar to, although considerably more severe than, that previously described for stingrays and lionfishes. Necrosis of tissues at the site of the injury and the subsequent sloughing of these tissues are more common after stings by *Synanceja* than after injuries by other venomous fishes. Treatment of wounds produced by stonefishes must be instituted immediately after envenomation. Immersion of the injured part in hot water, as described for stingray wounds, should be tried. Injection of emetine hydrochloride directly into the wound has been tried with indifferent results. In one case seen by the author, a soap solution was injected directly into the wound area 15 min after the hot water treatment had been initiated. There were no untoward effects, and no local tissue changes developed. An antivenin is now prepared by the Commonwealth Serum Laboratories of Australia and should be used when the seriousness of the poisoning warrants.

The weeverfishes, *Trachinus*, may inflict either a single or a multiple puncture-type wound. Persons stung by these fishes reported having received a sharp, immediately painful stab. It increased in severity during the first 20 to 50 min and persisted for 16 to 24 h if treatment was not instituted. As was noted by Halstead (1957), the pain can be so severe that a victim stung by one of these fishes while in the water may experience difficulty reaching the shore. The author has received similar reports from bathers along the Devon and Cornwall coasts of Great Britain. It seems likely that it is the excruciating pain rather than true muscular paralysis that is responsible for the victim's motor incapacity. The degree of swelling around the wound varies, although some swelling appears to be a constant finding. The tissues adjacent to the wound often appear discolored, and the surrounding area may be somewhat blanched. Localized necrosis at the wound site may occur, and sloughing of these tissues has been reported. It is possible that repeated stings, the effects of the venom, and low-grade infection are contributing factors in cases of arthritis seen among trawler fishers in the North Sea (see Russell, 1971, for references).

In severe cases of envenomation by weevers, there may be weakness, dizziness, nausea, primary shock, and respiratory distress. Fishers at Ijmuiden, Holland, told the author that there was often an urgency to urinate and that in severe stings there was axillary and chest pain as well as changes in pulse and respirations.

A few thoughts on the treatment of weeverfish stings are indicated, along with an additional reflection on the therapeutics of the injuries produced by venomous fishes in general. After having seen and treated a good many such injuries during the past four decades, the author has been impressed by the differences between the advice found in medical texts and that suggested and used by fishers and lifeguards or even persons familiar with envenomations by fishes. In most cases the nonmedical advice has proved not only more effective but more rational. Much of the advice given in texts devoted to tropical and wilderness medicine, in which the problem of venomous animal injury is most often discussed, stems from the false and antiquated idea that all venoms are related chemically and thus all respond to similar therapeutic measures. For instance, from early studies on snake venoms, a number of remedies found their way into the therapeutics for venomous fish injuries. Among these were acetic acid, alcohol, formaldehyde, urine, potassium permanganate, ink, gold salts, carbolic acid, cassava bread, and cauterization. While all these measures have been found to be ineffective, some are still advised in medical texts. The more recent therapeutic fads for corticosteroids, fig juice, and ice water as "shotgun" therapeutic methods are slowly waning, fortunately for the patient.

A review of the literature during the past few decades reveals a highly effective method of treatment that is based on substantial clinical trials. When the author suggested (Russell and Emery, 1960) that the use of hot water in weeverfish stings might be effective, it was on the basis of its very effective use in stingray and scorpionfish injuries and a limited number of case histories and observations on weeverfish stings that the author studied in Great Britain, France, and Holland in 1958 (Russell, 1963). Subsequently, the author reviewed the extensive earlier literature on this problem and found a great number of statements concerning the effectiveness of heat in the treatment of weeverfish poisonings (Russell, 1965). In a controlled experiment in humans, we found that the methods suggested for the treatment of stingray, scorpionfish, and catfish injuries are equally effective in alleviating the severe pain and other symptoms provoked by the venom of the weeverfishes. Maretić (1957) successfully used intravenous calcium gluconate to relieve the pain of this injury. Local injections of procaine may be of some value in less severe poisonings, and intramuscular or intravenous meperidine is of definite value in cases in which there is severe pain after the first hour following the injury. An antivenin has been developed at the Institute of Immunology in Zagreb and has been shown to be effective in a limited number of clinical tests (Maretić, personal communication, 1981). However, its use probably should be limited to more serious stings with significant manifestations.

## Venomous Arthropods

Only a relatively small number of arthropods are sufficiently venomous to be potentially dangerous to humans. Nevertheless, arthropods are implicated in far more poisonings in humans than are all the other phyla combined. Almost all the 30,000 species of spiders are venomous, but luckily for humans, only a relatively small number have fangs long and strong enough to penetrate the human skin (Gertsch, 1979). There are some 500 species of scorpions, and all are venomous, although again, only a small number are sufficiently dangerous to be a problem for humans. In the order Hymenoptera—the bees, wasps, yellow jackets, and ants—there are numerous species of medical importance, particularly because of the anaphylactic problems they may precipitate. Among the ticks, caterpillars, kissing bugs, water bugs, moths, butterflies, grasshoppers, centipedes, and millipedes are additional arthropods of medical importance. The venoms of arthropods are highly diversified, and if the spider venoms so far studied are any indication, these poisons may prove to be more complex than was originally suspected. Like snake venoms, arthropod poisons exert their deleterious effects at the cellular level. Arthropod venoms have been reviewed in detail by Bettini (1978).

The number of deaths from arthropod stings and bites is not known, and most countries do not keep records of the incidence of such injuries. In Mexico, parts of Central and South America, north Africa, and India, deaths from scorpion stings may exceed several thousand a year. Spider bites probably do not account for more than 200 deaths a year worldwide. The number of deaths from arthropod bites or stings in the temperate countries is far greater than the number of deaths from snakebite. However, most of these deaths are anaphylactic in nature. In the underdeveloped countries of the tropics, a far greater number of deaths from arthropods are due to the direct effects of the venom.

A common problem in suspected arthropod bites or stings relates to the differential diagnosis. Of approximately 600 suspected spider bites seen in one series of cases, 80 percent were found to be caused by arthropods other than spiders or by other disease states (Russell and Gertsch, 1983). The arthropods most frequently involved in the misdiagnoses were ticks (including their embedded mouth parts), mites, bedbugs, fleas (infected flea bites), lepidopterous insects, flies, vesicating beetles, water bugs, and various stinging Hymenoptera. Among the disease states that have been confused with spider bites or arthropod bites or stings are erythema chronicum migrans, Stevens-Johnson syndrome, toxic epidermal necrolysis, erythema nodosum, herpes simplex, purpura fulminans, diabetic ulcer, poison oak, and gonococcal arthritic dermatitis. As with a snake, a spider or another arthropod may bite or sting and not eject venom, but this must be a rare event.

Anaphylactic reactions and anaphylaxis are sometimes encountered after arthropod injuries and may become medical emergencies. More common are other autopharmacological reactions which may mistakenly be attributed to the direct action of the venom. The author has seen many unusual responses, varying from mild agitation to a vesicle-pustule-ulcer-eschar lesion after the sting of a bee. Also, the development of a lesion or lesions at a previous sting may follow a new sting elsewhere and present difficulties in differential diagnosis unless a careful history is taken. Finally, some arthropod venom poisonings give rise to the symptoms and signs of a previously undiagnosed subclinical disease. The problem of diverse disease states after the bites or stings of various venomous animals has been recognized (Russell, 1979), and when a case of venom poisoning persists or develops into a new syndrome, the patient should be reexamined for the possible presence of an undiagnosed disease. In some cases, stings or bites may induce stress reactions and the patient may present with a more complex and distressing problem.

**Spiders.** At least 200 species of spiders have been implicated in significant bites of humans. Some of the more important of these spiders are noted in Table 26-8. A more complete review of spider bites can be found in the excellent work of Maretić and Lebez (1979) and the lesser contributions of Southcott (1976) and Russell and Gertsch (1983).

**Latrodectus *Species (Widow Spiders).*** These spiders are commonly known as the black widow, brown widow, or red-legged spider in the United States. They have many other common names in English: hourglass, poison lady, deadly spider, red-bottom spider, T-spider, gray lady spider, and shoe-button spider. Widow spiders are found almost circumglobally in all continents with temperate or tropical climates. In the United States, there are four species of widow spiders, with the possibility of a fifth species from the Pacific northwest. Although both male and female widow spiders are venomous, only the female has fangs large and strong enough to penetrate the human skin. Mature females range in body length from 10 to 18 mm, whereas males range from 3 to 5 mm. These spiders have a globose abdomen varying in color from gray to brown to black, depending on the species. In the black widow, the abdomen is shiny black with a red hourglass or red spots and sometimes white ones on the venter.

The chemistry of the venom has been reviewed by Bettini and Maroli (1978) and Maretić and Lebez (1979). The difficulties with many of the biochemical and toxicological studies of this spider's venom relate to the nature of the starting material. Most studies have been done on extracts of homogenized glands rather than on the venom itself. Thus, the chemical nature of the venom cannot be separated or determined from the normal constituents of the venom gland. The pharmacological properties reported in the literature often also reflect the activities of the whole gland, and because some of the reported properties carried out on definitive preparations are not consistent with human experiences, their clinical application is open to question.

Most workers have isolated five or six active proteins from the venom or venom glands (see Bettini and Maroli, 1978, for references). The so-called neurotoxin appears to have a high content of isoleucine and leucine and a low content of

**Table 26–8**
**Genera of Spiders for Which Significant Bites on Humans Are Known**

| GENUS | FAMILY | COMMON NAME | DISTRIBUTION |
|---|---|---|---|
| *Aganippe* species | Ctenizidae | Trap-door spider | Australia |
| *Aphonopelma* species | Theraphosidiae | Tarantula | North America |
| *Araneus* species | Araneidae | Orbweaver | Worldwide |
| *Arbanitis* species | Ctenizidae | Trap-door spider | Australia, East Indies |
| *Argiope* species | Araneidae | Argiope | Worldwide |
| *Atrax* species | Macrothelinae | Funnel-web spider | Australia |
| *Bothriocyrtum* species | Ctenizidae | Trap-door spider | California |
| *Chiracanthium* species | Clubionidae | Running spider | Europe, north Africa, Orient, North America |
| *Cupiennius* species | Ctenidae | Banana spider | Central America |
| *Drassodes* species | Gnaphosidae | Running spider | Worldwide |
| *Dyarcyops* species | Ctenizidae | Trap-door spider | Australia |
| *Dysdera* species | Dysderidae | Dysderid | Eastern hemisphere, Americas |
| *Elassoctenus* species | Ctenidae | Ctenid | Australia |
| *Filistata* species | Filistatidae | Hackled-band spider | Temperate and tropical worldwide |
| *Harpactirella* species | Barychelidae | Trap-door spider | South Africa |
| *Heteropoda* species | Heterodidae | Giant crab spider | East Indies, tropical Asia, south Florida |
| *Isopoda* species | Sparassidae | Giant crab spider | Australia, East Indies |
| *Ixeuticus* species | Amaurobiidae | Amaurobiid | New Zealand, southern California |
| *Lampona* species | Gnaphosidae | Running spider | Australia, New Zealand |
| *Latrodectus* species | Theridiidae | Widow spider | Temperate and tropical regions worldwide |
| *Liocranoides* species | Clubionidae | Running spider | Appalachia and California |
| *Litkvphantes* species (*Steatoda* species) | Theridiidae | Sheet-web weaver | Worldwide |
| *Loxosceles* species | Loxoscelidae | Brown or violin spider | Americas, Africa, Europe, eastern Asia, Pacific Islands |
| *Lycosa* species | Lycosoidae | Wolf spider | Worldwide |
| *Missulena* species | Actinopodidae | Trap-door spider | Australia |
| *Misumenoides* species | Thomisidae | Crab spider | North and South America |
| *Miturga* species | Theraphosidae | Running spider | Australia |
| *Mopsus* species | Salticidae | Jumping spider | Australia |
| *Neoscona* species | Araneidae | Orbweaver | Worldwide |
| *Olios* species | Sparassidae | Giant crab spider | North and South America |
| *Pamphobeteus* species | Theraphosidae | Tarantula | South America |
| *Peucetia* species | Oxyopidae | Green lynx spider | Worldwide |
| *Phidippus* species | Salticidae | Jumping spider | North and South America |
| *Phoneutria* species | Ctenidae | Hunting spider | Central and South America |
| *Selenocosmia* species | Theraphosidae | Tarantula | East Indies, India, Australia, tropical Africa |
| *Steatoda* species | Theridiidae | False black widow | Worldwide |
| *Thiodina* species | Salticidae | Jumping spider | North and South America |
| *Trechona* species | Dipluridae | Funnel-web spider | West Indies, South America |
| *Ummidia* species | Ctenidae | Trap-door spider | North and South America |

tyrosine. The fraction has a suspected molecular weight of 130,000. It affects the frog neuromuscular junction and is active on rat brain synaptosomes. Lipoproteins are also present. A proteolytic enzyme was absent from extracts of the venom glands, whereas venom taken from the fangs possessed that activity. The presence of hyaluronidase is also dependent on the original material. The average amount of venom from each spider was 0.22 mg, and the intravenous $LD_{50}$ in mice was 0.55 mg/kg body weight (Russell and Buess, 1970).

***Clinical Problems.*** In most patients there is a history of having received a sharp, pinpricklike bite, but in some cases the bite is so minor that it goes unnoticed. The initial pain sometimes is followed by a dull, occasionally numbing pain in the affected extremity and by pain and cramps in one or several of the large muscle masses. Rarely is there any local skin reaction, but piloerection in the bite area is sometimes seen. Muscle fasciculations frequently can be seen within 30 min of the bite. Sweating is common, and the patient may complain of weakness and pain in the regional lymph nodes, which are often tender on palpation and occasionally are enlarged; lymphadenitis is frequently observed. Pain in the low back, thighs, or abdomen is a common complaint, and rigidity of the abdominal muscles is seen in most cases in which envenomation has been severe. Severe paroxysmal muscle cramps may occur, and arthralgia has been reported. "Facies latrodectismica" is uncommon in bites by American species.

In bites on the upper extremities and sometimes on the lower extremities, there is rigidity of the muscles of the shoulders and back, sometimes accompanied by pain on inspiration and varying degrees of headache, dizziness, and ptosis. Edema of the eyelids, conjunctivitis, skin rash, hyperemia, and pruritus sometimes are observed. The patient may become very restless and have difficulty sitting or standing still. Reflexes are usually accentuated. There may be a fine body tremor, and nausea and vomiting are not uncommon. The patient sometimes gropes along slowly when attempting to walk. Hypertension is a common finding, particularly in the elderly, after moderate to severe envenomations. Blood studies are usually normal.

There is no effective first-aid treatment. In most cases, intravenous calcium gluconate 10 ml of 10 percent will relieve muscle pain, but this may need to be repeated at 4- to 6-h intervals for optimum effect. Muscle relaxants such as methocarbamol 10 ml by slow push as directed or diazepam 5 to 10 mg tid can be used. Meperidine hydrochloride 50 to 100 mg has been used when respiratory deficits have not been a problem. Acute hypertensive crises may require intravenous nitroprusside, 3 $\mu$g/kg/min. The use of antivenin (antivenin, *Latrodectus mactans*) should be restricted to more severe cases and when other measures have proved unsuccessful. One ampoule intravenously is usually sufficient. In patients who are under 16 or over 60 years or have any history of hypertension or hypertensive heart disease and who show significant symptoms and signs, the use of antivenin seems warranted; it also is appropriate in cases involving pregnancy (Russell et al., 1979).

**Loxosceles** ***Species (Brown or Violin Spiders).*** These primitive spiders are variously known in North America as the fiddle-back or violin spider or the brown recluse. There are over 100 species of *Loxosceles*. Twenty of these species range from temperate South Africa northward through the tropics into the Mediterranean region and southern Europe. Another 84 species are known from North, Central, and South America and the West Indies. The most widely distributed is *L. rufescens*, the so-called cosmopolitan species. It is found in the Mediterranean area, southern Russia, most of north Africa including the Azores, Madagascar, the Near East, Asia from India to southern China and Japan, parts of Malaysia and Australia, some islands of the Pacific, and North America. *Loxosceles laeta* is mostly South American, but it has been introduced into Central America; small areas in Cambridge, Massachusetts; Sierra Madre and Alhambra, California; and the zoology building of the University of Helsinki. The abdomen of these spiders varies in color from grayish through orange and reddish-brown to dark brown. The "violin" on the carapace is brown to blackish and is distinct from the pale yellow to reddish-brown background of the cephalothorax. This spider has six eyes grouped in three dyads, forming a recurved row. Females average 8 to 12 mm in body length, whereas males average 6 to 10 mm. Both males and females are venomous. The most important species in the United States are *L. reclusa* (brown recluse spider), *L. deserta* (desert violin spider), and *L. arizonica* (Arizona violin spider).

The chemistry and toxicology of *Loxosceles* venom were reviewed by Schenone and Suarez (1978). Early work indicated that the venom was composed of approximately 26 percent protein and that the average amount of venom protein per spider in *L. reclusa* was about 68 $\mu$g. On fractionation of the venom, two major components were separated. The high-molecular-weight fraction was lethal to mice, whereas the low-molecular-weight fraction was nonlethal. The venom contained a considerable number of enzymes. Injection of the venom in mammals produced, in addition to the local tissue reaction, varying degrees of thrombocytopenia, some intravascular hemolysis, and hemolytic anemia. More recently, *Loxosceles* sp. venom has been found to contain sphingomyelinase D (perhaps the most important component), phospholipase, protease, esterase, collagenase, hyaluronidase, deoxyribonuclease, ribonuclease, dipeptides, dermanecrosis factor 33, and dermanecrosis factor 37. This venom has coagulation and vasoconstriction properties. It causes selective damage to the vascular endothelium; there are adhesions of neutrophils to the capillary wall with sequestration and activation of passing neutrophils by the perturbed endothelial cells (Patel and associates, 1994).

***Clinical Manifestations.*** The bite of this spider produces about the same degree of pain as does the sting of an ant, but sometimes the patient may be unaware of the bite. In most cases, a local burning sensation develops around the injury that may last for 30 to 60 min. Pruritus over the area often occurs, and the area becomes red with a small blanched area surrounding the reddened bite site. Skin temperature usually is elevated over the lesion area. The reddened area enlarges and becomes purplish during the subsequent 1 to 8 h. It often becomes irregular in shape, and as time passes, hemorrhages may develop throughout the area. A small bleb or vesicle forms at the bite site and increases in size. It subsequently ruptures, and a pustule forms. The red hemorrhagic area continues to enlarge, as does the pustule. The whole area may become swollen and painful, and lymphadenopathy is common. During the early stages the lesion often takes on a bull's-eye appearance, with a central white vesicle surrounded by the reddened area, ringed by a whitish or bluish border. The central pustule ruptures, and necrosis to various depths can be visualized.

In serious bites the lesion can measure 8 by 10 cm with severe necrosis invading muscle tissue. On the face, large lesions resulting in extensive tissue destruction and requiring subsequent plastic surgery sometimes are seen after bites by *L. laeta* in South America. Systemic symptoms and signs include fever, malaise, stomach cramps, nausea and vomiting, jaundice, spleen enlargement, hemolysis, hematuria, and thrombocytopenia. Fatal cases, while rare, usually are preceded by intravascular hemolysis, hemolytic anemia, thrombocytopenia, hemoglobinuria, and renal failure. There have been no deaths in the United States from the bites of this spider, contrary to reports in the media.

There are no first-aid measures of value. In fact, all first-aid procedures should be avoided, as the natural appearance of the lesion is most important in determining the diagnosis. A cube of ice may be placed on the wound. At one time, excision of the bite area with ample margins was advised when this could be done within an hour or so of the bite and when *Loxosceles* was definitely implicated. The value of steroids has been questioned. This writer, however, has had seemingly good results after placing the patient on a corticosteroid, such as intramuscular dexamethasone, 4 mg every 6 h during the acute phase. If the poisoning is severe, hydrocortisone should be given intravenously, 300 to 500 mg in divided doses daily, until the patient begins to improve. Subsequent doses should be determined by clinical judgment, followed by decremental doses over a 4-day period. Antihistamines are of questionable value. The use of dapsone was suggested by King and Rees (1983). The results have been encouraging, but care must be exercised with this drug. Oxygen delivered to the wound through an improvised plastic bag is helpful. If skin grafting becomes necessary, the procedure is best deferred for 4 to 6 weeks after the injury. Systemic manifestations should be treated symptomatically (Russell, 1982). Antivenom is not commercially available but has been used in Tennessee (King, personal correspondence, 1990).

**Steatoda *Species (Cobweb Spiders).*** These small spiders, variously called the false black widow, combfooted, or cupboard spiders, are abundant in the old world and reached the Americas through trading sources. According to Gertsch (personal correspondence, 1983), they are gaining such a wide range that they deserve to be called cosmopolitan. These spiders often are mistaken for black widow spiders, and indeed, the first clinical case of *Steatoda grossa* envenomation directed to the author in 1961 was thought to be caused by *L. mactans*, owing to misidentification of the spider. The female of *S. grossa* differs from *L. mactans* and *L. hesperus* in having a purplish-brown abdomen rather than a black one; it is less shiny, and its abdomen is more oval than round. It may have pale yellow or whitish markings on the dorsum of the abdomen and no markings on the venter. The abdomen of some species is orange, brown, or chestnut in color and often bears a light band across the front dorsum.

According to Maretić and Lebez (1979), *S. paykulliana* gives rise to "strong motor unrest, clonic cramps, exhaustion, ataxia and then paralysis in guinea pigs." This writer, however, has never seen such a syndrome after the bites of *S. grossa* or *S. fulva* in the United States. Instead, bites have been followed by local pain, induration, pruritus, and the occasional breakdown of tissue at the bite site. The wound should be debrided and covered with a sterile dressing. Signs should be treated symptomatically.

**Phidippus *Species (Jumping Spiders).*** These spiders, variously known as crab spiders and eyebrow spiders, are large-eyed jumping spiders usually less than 20 mm in length and have a somewhat elevated, rectangular cephalothorax that tends to blunt anteriorly. The abdomen is often oval or elongated. There is a great deal of variation in the color of these spiders. In the female, the cephalothorax may be black, brown, red, orange, or yellowish-orange and the abdomen tends to be slightly lighter in color. In most species there are various white, yellow, orange, or red spots or markings on the dorsum of the abdomen. The bite of this spider produces a sharp pinprick pain, and the area immediately around the wound may become painful and tender. The pain usually lasts 5 to 10 min. An erythematous wheal slowly develops. In cases seen by the author, the wheal measured 2 to 5 cm in diameter. A dull, sometimes throbbing pain may subsequently develop over the injured part, but it rarely requires attention. A small vesicle may form at the bite site. Around this is an irregular, slightly hyperemic area, which in turn may be surrounded by a blanched region that is tender to touch and pressure. Generally, there is only mild lymphadenitis. Swelling of the part may be diffuse and is often accompanied by pruritus. The symptoms and signs usually abate within 48 h. There is no specific treatment for the bite of this spider.

**Chiracanthium *Species (Running Spiders).*** The 160 species of this genus have an almost circumglobal distribution, although only four or five species have been implicated in bites of humans. Maretić and Lebez (1979) named *C. punctorium, C. inclusum, C. mildei*, and *C. diversum* as the spiders most often implicated in envenomations. The abdomen is convex and egg-shaped and varies in color from yellow, green, or greenish-white to reddish-brown, and the cephalothorax is usually slightly darker than the abdomen. The chelicerae are strong, and the legs are long, hairy, and delicate. The spider ranges in length from 7 to 16 mm. Like *Phidippus*, but even more so, *Chiracanthium* tends to be tenacious and sometimes must be removed from the bite area. For that reason, there is a high degree of identification of these spiders. The author's experiences with 10 bites by *C. inclusum* have been very similar, and the following description is based on those experiences. The patient usually describes the bite as sharp and painful, with the pain increasing during the first 30 to 45 min. The patient complains of some restlessness and dull pain over the injured part. A reddened wheal with a hyperemic border develops. Small petechiae may appear near the center of the wheal. Skin temperature over the lesion is often elevated, but body temperature is usually normal. Lymphadenitis and lymphadenopathy may develop (see Russell, 1984b, for references).

**Scorpions.** Approximately 75 of the 800 species of scorpions can be considered of sufficient importance to warrant medical attention. Some of the more important of these species are noted in Table 26-9. In addition, members of the genera *Pandinus, Hadrurus, Vejovis, Nebo*, and some of the others are

**Table 26–9**
**Medically Important Scorpions**

| GENUS | DISTRIBUTION |
|---|---|
| *Androctonus* species | North Africa, Middle East, Turkey |
| *Buthus* species | France and Spain to Middle East and north Africa, Mongolia, China |
| *Buthotus* species | Africa, Middle East, central Asia |
| *Centruroides* species | North, Central, South America |
| *Heterometrus* species | Central and southeast Asia |
| *Leiurus* species | North Africa, Middle East, Turkey |
| *Mesobuthus* species | Turkey, India |
| *Parabuthus* species | Southern Africa |
| *Tityus* species | Central and South America |

capable of inflicting a painful and often erythematous lesion. The problem of scorpion stings has been reviewed by Keegan (1980).

**Centruroides *Species.*** There are approximately 30 species of this genus confined to the new world. Of these, about seven species are of considerable medical importance, and most of them are found in Mexico. In the United States, they are commonly referred to as "bark scorpions" because of their preference for hiding under the loose bark of trees or in dead trees or logs. They often frequent human dwellings. Their general color is straw to yellowish-brown or reddish-brown, and they are often easily distinguishable from other scorpions in the same habitat by their long, thin telson, or tail, and the thin pedipalps, or pincerlike claws. Adults of this genus show a considerable difference in length. *C. exlicauda (sculpturatus)* in the southwestern United States and adjacent Mexico reaches a length of approximately 5.5 cm, while *C. vittatus* of the Gulf states and adjacent Mexico is generally slightly larger. *C. suffusus*, a particularly dangerous Mexican species, may attain a length of 9 cm, but *C. noxious*, another important species, seldom exceeds 5 cm in length. In Mexico between 1940 and 1949 and 1950 to 1957 there were 20,352 deaths from scorpion envenomation. Most of these deaths occurred in children less than 3 years of age. Various estimates of the total number of stings per year in Mexico range from 20,000 to 70,000. Working in Mexico in 1953, this writer estimated that there were over 40,000 stings that year, of which 10,000 were treated or reported. The total number of deaths, usually in infants, appeared to be slightly less than 1500. As with other scorpions, envenomation by this genus appears to vary with the species.

In children, a sting by *C. exilicauda* produces initial pain, although it rarely is severe. However, some children do not complain of pain and are unaware of the injury. The area becomes sensitive to touch, and merely pressing lightly over the injury will elicit immediate retraction. Usually there is little or no local swelling or erythema. The child becomes tense and restless and shows abnormal and random head and neck movements. Often the child will display roving eye movements. In their review of *C. sculpturatus* stings, Rimsza and coworkers (1980) noted visual signs, including roving eye movements, nystagmus, and oculogyric movements, in 12 of their 24 patients stung by this scorpion. Loud noises, such as banging the examination table behind the child's back, often cause the patient to jump. Tachycardia is usually evident within 45 min, and hypertension, although it is not seen in children as early and is not as severe as in adults, often is present 1 h after the sting. Respiratory and heart rates are increased, and by 90 min after the bite the child may appear quite ill. Fasciculations may be seen over the face or large muscle masses, and the child may complain of generalized weakness and display some ataxia or motor weakness. The respiratory distress may proceed to respiratory paralysis. Excessive salivation is often present and may further embarrass respiratory function. Slurring of speech may be present, and convulsions may occur. If death does not occur, the child usually becomes asymptomatic within 36 to 48 h.

In adults the clinical picture is somewhat similar, but there are some differences. Almost all adults complain of immediate pain after the sting, regardless of the *Centruroides* species involved. Adults do not show the restlessness seen in children. Instead, they are tense and anxious. They develop tachycardia and hypertension, and respirations are increased. They may complain of difficulties in focusing and swallowing, as may children. In some cases, there is some general weakness and pain on moving the injured extremity. Convulsions are very rare, but ataxia and muscle incoordination may occur. Most adults are asymptomatic within 12 h but may complain of generalized weakness for 24 h or more.

A review of the therapy for scorpion stings will provide the reader with a fascinating mixture of mythology, folklore, hunches (educated and otherwise), and a listing of all sorts of therapeutic devices from electroshock to mechanical compression bandages. The list of drugs that have been tried includes atropine, barium, digitalis, epinephrine, heparin, hyoscine, iodine, procaine, morphine, physostigmine, reserpine, steroids, vitamin C, and snake, spider, and scorpion antivenins, to mention only a few. Other than scorpion antivenom, there is no evidence that any of these drugs are of value. There are no first-aid measures of value. In any severe scorpion envenomation by one of the known dangerous species or in infants and children, the specific or suggested polyvalent scorpion antivenom should be considered. The author generally gives twice the recommended dose intravenously unless otherwise indicated. The antivenom should be diluted with 100 to 200 ml of 5% dextrose in water or physiological saline and should be given over 30 to 90 min. Mild sedation is often indicated. If convulsions occur, intravenous phenobarbital is suggested, but great care must be used with respect to the dose. Diazepam may be of value. Assisted ventilation is sometimes necessary, particularly in children. Hypertension that does not respond to antivenom may have to be treated with the appropriate antihypertensive drugs. Inderal has been used for tachycardia. In patients who decompensate, digitalis and diuretics may be of value. Stings by species of *Vejovis* and *Hadrurus*, though far more common in the United States than those of *Centruroides*, rarely require anything more than treatment for the local pain. However, it is wise to put any person stung by a scorpion, particularly a child, on bed rest for 4 h after the accident.

## Centipedes and Millipedes

Some of the larger centipedes of the genus *Scolopendra* can inflict a painful bite with some localized swelling and erythema. Lymphangitis and lymphadenitis are not uncommon. Necrosis is rare, and infection is almost unknown. The symptoms and signs seldom persist for more than 48 h. Millipedes do not bite but when handled may discharge a toxic secretion that can cause local skin irritation and in severe cases local tissue changes and necrosis. Some species not found in the United States can spray a highly irritating repugnant secretion that may cause conjunctival reactions. In centipede bites, an ice cube over the area usually controls the pain. Corticosteroids have been used as anti-inflammatory agents. The toxic secretions of millipedes should be washed from the skin with copious amounts of soap and water. Cleansing with alcohol should be avoided. A corticosteroid lotion or cream should be applied if a skin reaction develops. Eye injuries require immediate irrigation and the application of a corticosteroid-analgesic ointment.

## Hymenoptera (Ants, Bees, Wasps, and Hornets)

The stings of Hymenoptera are responsible for more deaths in the United States than are the bites and stings of all other venomous creatures. This is due to sensitization to the venom from previous stings, resulting in anaphylactic reactions, including acute anaphylaxis. In most cases, those not sensitive to bee venom may tolerate up to 100 simultaneous stings, but any number over this can be fatal. The venom of these insects contains peptides, nonenzymatic proteins such as apamin and melittin or kinins, enzymes such as phospholipase A and B and hyaluronidase, and amines such as histamine and 5-hydroxytryptamine. The sting of a Hymenoptera may remain in the skin and should be removed by teasing or scraping rather than pulling. An ice cube placed over the sting area will reduce pain; an analgesic-corticosteroid lotion is often useful. Persons with known hypersensitivity to such stings should carry a kit containing an antihistamine and epinephrine when in endemic areas. Desensitization can be carried out using insect whole-body antigen or, preferably, whole-venom antigens (Russell, 1982). The medical problem of Africanized bee stings has been reviewed by Franca and associates (1994).

## Ticks and Mites

Ticks are vectors of many diseases. In addition to these disorders, ticks can be involved in venom poisonings. In North America, some species of *Dermacentor* and *Amblyomma* cause tick paralysis. Symptoms and signs include anorexia, lethargy, muscle weakness, incoordination, nystagmus, and ascending flaccid paralysis. Bulbar or respiratory paralysis may develop. The bites of some *Ornithodorus* ticks ("pajaroello") in Mexico and the southwestern United States cause local vesiculation and pustulation, which may lead to rupture, ulceration, and eschar, with varying degrees of local swelling and pain. Ticks are best removed by applying gasoline or by slowly withdrawing the arthropod in a rotating motion with flat-tip forceps. Care should be taken not to leave the capitulum in the wound, as it may induce chronic inflammation or migrate into deeper tissues and give rise to a granuloma. Infections are not uncommon during the ulcer stage but rarely require more than local antiseptic measures.

# REFERENCES


Albuquerque EX, Warnick JE, Maleque MA, et al: The pharmacology of pumiliotoxin-B: I. Interaction with calcium sites in the sarcoplasmic reticulum of skeletal muscle. *Mol Pharmacol* 19:411, 1981.

Alender CB, Russell FE: Pharmacology, in Boolootin RA (ed): *Physiology of Echinodermata*. New York: Interscience, 1966, p 529.

Arndt W: Die Spongern als kryptotoxische Tiere. *Zoo Jahrb* 45:343, 1928.

Arnold SH, Brown WD: Histamine toxicity from fish products. *Adv Food Res* 24:113, 1978.

Association of Official Analytical Chemists: Paralytic shellfish poison biological method, in *Official Methods of Analysis*, 12th ed. Washington, DC: Association of Official Analytical Chemists, 1975, p 319.

Bagnis RA, Berglund F, Elias PS, et al: Problems of toxicants in marine food products. *Bull WHO* 42:69, 1970.

Bagnis RA, Kuberski T, Langier S: Clinical observations on 3,009 cases of ciguatera (fish poisoning) in the South Pacific. *Am J Trop Med Hyg* 28:1067, 1979.

Bajwa SS, Markland FS: Defibrinogenation studies with crotalase: Possible clinical applications. *Proc West Pharmacol Soc* 21:461, 1978.

Bakus GJ, Green G: Toxicity in sponges and holothurians: A geographic pattern. *Science* 185:951, 1974.

Bakus GJ, Thun M: Bioassays on the toxicity of Caribbean sponges. *Biol Spongiaries* 291:417, 1979.

Banner AH: Ciguatera: A disease from coral reef fish, in Jones OE, Endean R (eds): *Biology and Geology of Coral Reefs*. New York: Academic Press, 1976, vol III, p 177.

Barnes JH: Observations of jellyfish stingings in North Queensland. *Med J Aust* 2:993, 1960.

Barnes JH: Extraction of cnidarian venom from living tentacle, in Russell FE, Saunders PR (eds): *Animal Toxins*. Oxford: Pergamon Press, 1967, p 115; see also *Toxicon* 4:292, 1967.

Baslow MH: *Marine Pharmacology*. Baltimore: Williams & Wilkins, 1969.

Baxter EH, Walden NB, Marr AG: Fatal intoxication of rabbits, sheep and monkeys by the venom of the sea wasp *(Chironex fleckeri)*. *Toxicon* 10:653, 1972.

Bernheimer AW, Avigad LS: Properties of a toxin from the sea anemone *Stoichactis helianthus*, including specific binding to sphingomyelin. *Proc Natl Acad Sci USA* 73:467, 1976.

Bettini S: *Arthropod Venoms*. New York: Springer-Verlag, 1978.

Bettini S, Maroli M: Venoms of Theridiidae, genus *Latrodectus*, in Bettini S (ed): *Arthropod Venoms*. New York: Springer-Verlag, 1978, p 149.

Bevins CL, Zasloff, M: Peptides from frog skin. *Am Rev Biochem* 59:395, 1990.

Blanquet RS: A toxic protein from the nematocysts of the scyphozoan medusa *Chrysaora quinquecirrha*. *Toxicon* 10:103, 1972.

Bonilla CA, Fiero MK: Comparative biochemistry and pharmacology of salivary gland secretions: II. Chromatographic separation of the basic proteins from North American rattlesnake venoms. *J Chromatogr* 56:253, 1971.

Brown DE, Carmony NB: *Gila Monster*. Silver City, N.M.: High Lonesome Books, 1991.

Burke JM, Marichisotto J, McLaughlin JJ, et al: Analysis of the toxin produced by *Gonyaulax catenella* in axenic culture. *Ann NY Acad Sci* 90:837, 1960.

Burnett JW, Calton HJ: The chemistry and toxicology of some venomous pelagic coelenterates. *Toxicon* 15:177, 1977.

Burreson BJ, Christophersen C, Scheuer PJ: Cooccurrence of a terpenoid isocyanideformamide pair in the marine sponge *Halichondria* sp. *Am Chem Soc* 97:201, 1975.

Calton GJ, Burnett JW, Rubenstein H, et al: The effect of two jellyfish toxins on calcium ion transport. *Toxicon* 11:357, 1973.

Cameron AM, Surridge J, Stablum W, et al: A crinotoxin from the skin tubercle glands of a stonefish (*Synanceia trachynis*). *Toxicon* 19:159, 1981.

Cariello L, Zanetti L, Rathmayer W: Isolation, purification and some properties of suberitine, the toxic protein from the marine sponge, *Suberites domuncula*, in Eaker D, Wadström T (eds): *Natural Toxins*. Oxford: Pergamon Press, 1980, p 631.

Carlson RW, Schaeffer RC, Russell FE, et al: A comparison of corticosteroid and fluid treatment after rattlesnake venom shock in rats. *Physiologist* 18:160, 1975.

Cleland JB, Southcott RV: *Injuries to Man from Marine Invertebrates in the Australian Region*. Canberra, Australia: 1965, p 195.

Crone HD, Keen TEB: Chromatographic properties of the hemolysin from the cnidarian *Chironex fleckeri*. *Toxicon* 7:79, 1969.

Culver P, Jacobs RS: Lophotoxin: A neuromuscular acting toxin from the sea whip (*Lophogorgia rigida*). *Toxicon* 19:825, 1981.

Daly JW: Biologically active alkaloids from poison frogs (*Dendrobatidae*). *Toxin Rev* 1:33, 1982.

Daly JW, Garraffo HM, Spande TF: Amphibian alkaloids. *Alkaloids* 43:186, 1993.

Daly JW, McNeal ET, Gusovsky F, et al: Cardiotoxic activities of pumiliotoxin $B_1$ pyrethroids and a phorbol ester and their relationships with phosphatidylinositol turnover. *Biochem Biophys Acta* 930: 470, 1987.

Daly JW, Myers CW, Whittaker N: Further classification of skin alkaloids from neotropical poisonous frog toxic/noxious substances in amphibia. *Toxicon* 25:1023, 1991.

Daly JW, Secunda SI, Gaáraffo HM, et al: Variability in alkaloid profiles in neotropical poison frogs (*Dendrobatidae*): Genetic versus environmental determinants. *Toxicon* 30:887, 1992.

Dart RC, Russell FE: Animal poisoning, in Hall JB, Schmidt GA, Wood LD (eds): *Principles of Critical Care*. New York: McGraw-Hill, 1992, p 2163.

Das NP, Lim HS, Teh YF: Histamine and histamine-like substances in the marine sponge *Suberites inconstans*. *Comp Gen Pharmacol* 2:473, 1971.

Dawson EY, Aleem AA, Halstead BW: Marine algae from Palmyra Island with special reference to the feeding habits and toxicology of reef fishes. *Occ Pap Allan Hancock Fdn* 17:1, 1955.

De Laubenfels MW: The marine and freshwater sponges of California. *Proc US Nat Mus* 81:1, 1932 (Publ. 2927).

Deutsch HF, Diniz CR: Some proteolytic activities of snake venoms. *J Biol Chem* 216:17, 1955.

Dowling HG, Minton SA, Russell FE: *Poisonous Snakes of the World*. Washington, D.C.: U.S. Government Printing Office, 1968.

Dubnoff JW, Russell FE: Isolation of lethal protein and peptide from *Crotalus viridis helleri* venom. *Proc West Pharmacol Soc* 13:98, 1970.

Eaker D, Wadström T (eds): *Natural Toxins*. Elmsford, N.Y.: Pergamon Press, 1980.

Elliott WB: Chemistry and immunology of reptilian venoms, in Gans C (ed): *Biology of the Reptilia*. London: Academic Press, 1978, vol 8, p 163.

Endean R: A new species of venomous echinoid from Queensland waters. *Mem Queensland Mus* 14:95, 1964.

Endean R, Duchemin C, McColm D, et al: A study of the biological activity of toxic material derived from nematocysts of the cubomedusan *Chironex fleckeri*. *Toxicon* 6:179, 1969.

Endean R, Izatt J, McColm D: The venom of the piscivorous gastropod *Conus striatus*, in Russell FE, Saunders PR (eds): *Animal Toxins*. Oxford: Pergamon Press, 1967, p 137.

Endean R, Noble M: Toxic material from the tentacles of the cubomedusan *Chironex fleckeri*. *Toxicon* 9:255, 1971.

Evans MH: Block of sensory nerve conduction in the cat by mussel poison and tetrodotoxin, in Russell FE, Saunders PR (eds): *Animal Toxins*. Oxford: Pergamon Press, 1967, p 97; see also *Toxicon* 5:289, 1967.

Ferlan I, Lebez D: Equinatoxin, a lethal protein from *Actinia equina*: I. Purification and characterization. *Toxicon* 12:57, 1974.

Fisher AA: *Atlas of Aquatic Dermatology*. New York: Grune & Stratton, 1978.

Flecker H, Cotton BC: Fatal bites from octopus. *Med J Aust* (2):329, 1955.

Fleming WJ, Howden MEH: Partial purification and characterization of steroid glycosides from the starfish *Acanthaster planci*. *Comp Biochem Physiol* 53b:267, 1974.

Franca FOS, Benevenuti LA, Fan HW, et al: Severe and fatal mass attacks by "killer" bees (Africanized honey bees—*Apis mellifera scutellata*) in Brazil: Clinicopathological studies with measurement of serum venom concentrations. *Q J Med* 87:269, 1994.

Freeman SE: Cardiovascular effects of toxins isolated from the cnidarian *Chironex fleckeri* Southcott. *Br J Pharmacol* 41:154, 1971.

Freeman SE, Turner RJ: A pharmacological study of the toxin of a cnidarian *Chironex fleckeri* Southcott. *Br J Pharmacol* 35:510, 1969.

Friess SL, Chanley JD, Hudak WV, et al: Interactions of the echinoderm toxin holothurin A and its desulfated derivative with the cat superior cervical ganglion preparation. *Toxicon* 8:211, 1970.

Friess SL, Durant RC, Chanley JD, et al: Role of the sulphate charge center in irreversible interactions of holothurin A with chemoreceptors. *Biochem Pharmacol* 16:1617, 1967.

Fuhrman FA: Fish eggs, in Liener IE (ed): *Toxic Constituents of Animal Foodstuffs*. New York: Academic Press, 1974, p 73.

Gertsch WJ: *American Spiders*, 2d ed. New York: Van Nostrand Reinhold, 1979.

Gold BS, Wingert WA: Snake venom poisoning in the United States. *South Med J* 87:579, 1994.

Gopalakrishnakone P, Tan CK (eds): *Recent Advances in Toxinology Research*. Singapore: National University of Singapore, 1992.

Green G: Ecology of toxicity in marine sponges. *Mar Biol* 40:207, 1977.

Habermann E, Breithaupt H: The crotoxin complex: An example of biochemical and pharmacological protein complementation. *Toxicon* 16:19, 1978.

Habermehl GG: *Venomous Animals and Their Toxins*. Berlin: Springer-Verlag, 1981.

Habermehl GG, Volkwein G: Aglycones of the toxins from the cuvierian organs of *Holothuria forskåli* and a new nomenclature for the aglycones from Holothurioideae. *Toxicon* 9:319, 1971.

Halmagyi DFJ, Starzecki B, Horner GJ: Mechanism and pharmacology of shock due to rattlesnake venom in sheep. *J Appl Physiol* 20:709, 1965.

Halstead BW: Weever stings and their medical management. *US Armed Forces Med J* 8:1441, 1957.

Halstead BW: Fish poisonings: their diagnosis, pharmacology and treatment. *Clin Pharmacol Ther* 5:615, 1964.

Halstead BW: *Poisonous and Venomous Marine Animals of the World*. Washington, DC: U.S. Government Printing Office, vol I, 1965; vol II, 1967; vol III, 1970.

Halstead BW: *Poisonous and Venomous Marine Animals of the World*, rev ed. Princeton, NJ: Darwin Press, 1978.

Halstead BW: *Dangerous Marine Animals*, 2d ed. Centreville, MD: Cornell Maritime Press, 1980, p 77.

Harding KA, Welch KRG: *Venomous Snakes of the World: A Checklist*. Elmsford, NY: Pergamon Press, 1980.

Hashimoto Y: *Marine Toxins and Other Bioactive Metabolites*. Tokyo: Japan Scientific Society, 1979.

Hashimoto Y, Konosu S, Yasumoto T, et al: Occurrence of toxic crabs in Ryukyu and Amami Islands. *Toxicon* 5:85, 1967.

Helfrich P, Banner AH: Hallucinatory mullet poisoning. *J Trop Med Hyg* 63:86, 1960.

Hessinger DA, Lenhoff HM: Membrane structure and function: Mechanism of hemolysis induced by nematocyst venom: Roles of phospholipase and direct lytic factor. *Arch Biochem Biophys* 173:603, 1976.

Irie T, Suzuki M, Hayakawa Y: Isolation of aplysin, debromoaplysin and aplysinol from *Laurencia okamurai* Yamada. *Bull Chem Soc Jpn* 42:843, 1969.

Jakowska S, Nigrelli RF: Antimicrobial substances from sponges. *Ann NY Acad Sci* 90:913, 1970.

Kaiser E, Michl H: *Die Biochemie der Tierischen Gifte*. Wien: Franz Deuticke, 1958.

Kao CY: Tetrodotoxin, saxitoxin and their significance in the study of the excitation phenomena. *Pharmacol Rev* 18:997, 1966.

Kao CY: Comparison of the biological actions of tetrodotoxin and saxitoxin, in Russell FE, Saunders PR (eds): *Animal Toxins*. Oxford: Pergamon Press, 1967 p 109.

Kao CY: New perspectives on the tetrodotoxin and saxitoxin receptors, in Singer TP, Ondarza PN (eds): *Molecular Basis of Drug Action*. New York: Elsevier/North-Holland, 1981.

Kao CY, Fuhrman FA: Pharmacological studies on tarichatoxin, a potent neurotoxin. *J Pharmacol Exp Ther* 140:31, 1963.

Keegan HL: *Scorpions of Medical Importance*. Jackson: University Press of Mississippi, 1980.

King LE, Rees RS: Dapsone treatment of a brown recluse bite. *JAMA* 250:648, 1983.

Lane CE, Dodge E: The toxicity of Physalia nematocysts. *Biol Bull* 115:219, 1958.

Lassablière MP: Influences des injections intraveineuses de subéritine sur la résistance globulaire. *C R Seances Soc Biol* 61:600, 1906.

Lee C-Y (ed): *Snake Venoms*. New York: Springer-Verlag, 1979.

Lewis RJ, Jell PA: *Memoirs of the Queensland Museum* 343:193, 1994.

Maeda N, Tamiya N, Pattabhiraman TK, et al: Some chemical properties of the venom of the rattlesnake *Crotalus viridis helleri*. *Toxicon* 16:431, 1978.

Maretić Z: Erfahrungen mit Stichen von Giftfischen. *Acta Trop (Basel)* 14:157, 1957.

Maretić Z, Lebez D: *Araneism*. Belgrade, Yugoslavia: Nolit Belgrade, 1979.

Maretić Z, Russell FE: Stings by the sea anemone *Anemonia sulcata* in the Adriatic Sea. *Am J Trop Med Hyg* 32:891, 1983.

Marki F, Witkop B: The venom of the Colombian arrow poison frog *Phyllobates bicolor*. *Experientia* 19:329, 1963.

Martin DF, Padilla GM (eds): *Marine Pharmacognosy*. New York: Academic Press, 1973.

McFarren EF, Schafer ML, Campbell JF, et al: Public health significance of paralytic shellfish poison: A review of literature and unpublished research. *Proc Natl Shellfish Assoc* 47:114, 1956.

Mebs D: Bissverletzungen durch "ungiftige" Schlangen. *Dtsch Med Wochenschr* 102:1429, 1977.

Mebs D: Pharmacology of reptilian venoms, in Gans C (ed): *Biology of the Reptilia*. London: Academic Press, 1978, vol 8, p 437.

Meyer K: Über herzaktive Krötengifte. *Pharm Acta Helv* 24:222, 1949.

Meyer KF, Sommer H, Schoenholz P: Mussel poisoning. *J Prev Med* 2:365, 1928.

Middlebrook RE, Wittle LW, Scura ED, et al: Isolation and purification of a toxin from *Millepora dichotoma*. *Toxicon* 9:333, 1971.

Minton SA Jr: A list of colubrid envenomations. *Kentucky Herp* 7:4, 1976.

Minton SA Jr, Minton MG: *Venomous Reptiles*. New York: Scribner, 1969.

Myers CW, Daly JW: Tropical poison frogs. *Science* 262:1193, 1993.

Néeman I, Calton GJ, Burnett JW: Purification of an endonuclease present in *Chrysaora quinquecirrha* venom. *Proc Soc Exp Biol Med* 166:374, 1981.

Nigrelli RF, Jakowska S: Effects of holothurin, a steroid saponin from the Bahamian sea cucumber (*Actinopyga agassizi*), on various biological systems. *Ann NY Acad Sci* 90:884, 1960.

Parnas I, Russell FE: Effects of venoms on nerve muscle and neuromuscular junction, in Russell FE, Saunders PR (eds): *Animal Toxins*. Oxford: Pergamon Press, 1967, p 401.

Parrish HM: *Poisonous Snakebites in the United States*. New York: Vantage Press, 1980.

Patel KA, Modur V, Zimmerman GA: The necrotic venom of the brown recluse spider induces dysregulated endothelial cell-dependent neutrophil activation. *Am Soc Clin Invest* 94:631, 1994.

Phillips C, Brady WH: *Sea Pests: Poisonous or Harmful Sea Life of Florida and the West Indies*. Miami: University of Miami Press, 1953.

Prakash A, Medcof JC, Tennant AD: Paralytic shellfish poisoning in eastern Canada. *Bull Fish Res Bd Can* 177:1, 1971.

Primor N, Lazarovici P: *Pardachirus marmoratus* (Red Sea flatfish) secretion and its isolated toxic fraction *pardaxin*: The relationship between hemolysis and ATPase inhibition. *Toxicon* 19:573, 1981.

Prinzmetal M, Sommer H, Leake CD: The pharmacological action of "mussel poison." *J Pharmacol Exp Ther* 46:63, 1932.

Proctor NH, Chan SL, Taylor AJ: Production of saxitoxin by cultures of *Gonyaulax catenella*. *Toxicon* 13:1, 1975.

Randall JE: A review of ciguatera tropical fish poisoning with a tentative explanation of its cause. *Bull Mar Sci Gulf Carib* 8:236, 1958.

Richet C: De la variabilité de la dose toxique de subéritine. *C R Soc Biol* 61:686, 1906.

Rimsza ME, Zimmerman DR, Bergeson PS: Scorpion envenomation. *Pediatrics* 66:298, 1980.

Rosenberg P: Pharmacology of phospholipase $A_2$ from snake venoms, in Lee C-Y (ed): *Snake Venoms: Handbook of Experimental Pharmacology*. Berlin: Springer-Verlag, 1979, vol 52, p 403.

Rosenberg P: Phospholipases, in Shier WT, Mebs D (eds): *Handbook of Toxinology*. New York: Marcel Dekker, 1990, p 67.

Rosenberg P (ed): *Toxins: Animal, Plant, and Microbial*. Elmsford, NY: Pergamon Press, 1978.

Russell FE: Poisonous fishes. *Eng Sci* 15:11, 1952.

Russell FE: Venomous animals and their toxins. *London Times Sci Rev* 49:10, 1963.

Russell FE: Marine toxins and venomous and poisonous marine animals, in Russell FS (ed): *Advances in Marine Biology*. London: Academic Press, 1965, vol III, p 255.

Russell FE: *Physalia* stings: A report of two cases. *Toxicon* 4:65, 1966.

Russell FE: Comparative pharmacology of some animal toxins. *Fed Proc* 26:1206, 1967.

Russell FE: Poisons and venoms, in Hoar WS, Randall DJ (eds): *Fish Physiology*. New York: Academic Press, 1969, vol III, p 401.

Russell FE: Pharmacology of toxins of marine origin, in Raskova H (ed): *International Encyclopedia of Pharmacology and Therapeutics*. Oxford: Pergamon Press, 1971, sec 71, vol 2, p 3.

Russell FE: Envenomation and diverse disease states (letter). *JAMA* 238:581, 1977.

Russell FE, Marcus P, Strong JA: Black widow spider envenomation during pregnancy: Report of a case. *Toxicon* 17:188, 1979.

Russell FE: Pharmacology of venoms, in Eaker D, Wadström T (eds): *Natural Toxins*. Elmsford, NY: Pergamon Press, 1980a, p 13.

Russell FE: Venomous bites and stings, in Berkow R (ed): *The Merck Manual*, 14th ed. Rahway, NJ: Merck Sharp & Dohme, 1982, p 2451.

Russell FE: *Snake Venom Poisoning*. Philadelphia: Lippincott, 1980b; Great Neck, NY: Scholium International, 1983.

Russell FE: Marine toxins and venomous and poisonous marine animals, in Blaxter JHS, Russell FS, Yonge CM (eds): *Advances in Marine Biology*. London: Academic Press, 1984a, p 60.

Russell FE: Snake venoms, in Ferguson MWJ (ed): *The Structure, Development and Evolution of Reptiles* (Symposia of the Zoological Society of London). London: Academic Press, 1984b, p 469.

Russell FE, Bogert CM: Gila monster, its biology, venom and bite: A review. *Toxicon* 19:341, 1981.

Russell FE, Buess FW: Gel electrophoresis: A tool in systematics studies with *Latrodectus mactans* venom. *Toxicon* 8:81, 1970.

Russell FE, Buess FW, Strassburg J: Cardiovascular response to Crotalus venom. *Toxicon* 1:5, 1962.

Russell FE, Carlson RW, Wainschel J, et al: Snake venom poisoning in the United States: Experiences with 550 cases. *JAMA* 233:341, 1975.

Russell FE, Emery JA: Venom of the weevers *Trachinus draco* and *Trachinus vipera. Ann NY Acad Sci* 90:805, 1960.

Russell FE, Gertsch WJ: Letter to the editor (arthropod bites). *Toxicon* 21:337, 1983.

Russell FE, van Harreveld A: Cardiovascular effects of the venom of the round stingray, *Urobatis halleri. Arch Intern Physiol* 62:322, 1954.

Schaeffer RC Jr, Carlson RW, Whigham H, et al: Acute hemodynamic effects of rattlesnake *Crotalus viridis helleri* venom, in Rosenberg P (ed): *Toxins: Animal, Plant, and Microbial.* Oxford: Pergamon Press, 1978, p 383.

Schantz EJ: Biochemical studies on paralytic shellfish poisons. *Ann NY Acad Sci* 90:843, 1960.

Schantz EJ, Ghazarossian VE, Schnoes HK, et al: The structure of saxitoxin. *J Am Chem Soc* 97:1238, 1975.

Schantz EJ, Lynch JM, Vayvada G, et al: The purification and characterization of the poison produced by *Gonyaulax catenella* in axenic culture. *Biochemistry* 5:1191, 1966.

Schantz EJ, McFarren EF, Schaffer ML, et al: Purified shellfish poison for bioassay standardization. *J Assoc Off Agric Chem* 41:160, 1958.

Schenone H, Suarez G: Venoms of Scytodidae Genus *Loxosceles*, in Bettini S (ed): *Arthropod Venoms.* New York: Springer-Verlag, 1978, p 247.

Scheuer PJ: *Chemistry of Marine Natural Products.* New York: Academic Press, 1973.

Scheuer PJ (ed): *Marine Natural Products: Chemical and Biological Perspectives.* New York: Academic Press, vols 1 and 2, 1978; vol 3, 1980; vol 4, 1981.

Shapiro BI, Lilleheil G: The action of anemone toxin on crustacean neurons. *Comp Biochem Physiol* 28:1225, 1969.

Shimizu Y: Dinoflagellate toxins, in Scheuer PJ (ed): *Marine Natural Products: Chemical and Biological Perspectives.* New York: Academic Press, 1978, vol I, p 1.

Simidu U, Noguchi T, Kon T, et al: Marine bacteria that produce tetrodotoxin. *Appl Environ Microbiol* 53:1714, 1987.

Simidu U, Kita-Tsukamoto K, Yashumoto T, et al: Taxonomy of four marine bacterial strains that produce tetrodotoxin. *Int J Syst Bactiol* 40:331, 1990.

Slotta K, Fraenkel-Conrat H: Two active proteins from rattlesnake venom. *Nature* 142:213, 1938.

Smith DS, Cayer ML, Russell FE, et al: Fine structure of stingray spine epidermis with special reference to a unique microtubular component of venom secreting cells, in Rosenberg P (ed): *Toxins:Animal, Plant, and Microbial.* Oxford: Pergamon Press, 1978, p 565.

Sommer A, Meyer KF: Paralytic shellfish poisoning. *Arch Pathol* 24:560, 1937.

Southcott RV: Arachnidism and allied syndromes in the Australian region. *Rec Adelaide Children's Hosp* 1:97, 1976.

Southcott RV: Marine toxins, in Cohen NH, Klawans HL (eds): *Handbook of Clinical Neurology.* Amsterdam: Elsevier/North-Holland, 1979, vol 37, p 27.

Southcott RV, Kingston CW: Lethal jellyfish stings: A study in sea-wasps. *Med J Aust* 1:443, 1959.

Stempien MF, Ruggieri GD, Nigrelli RF, et al: Physiologically active substances from extracts of marine sponges, in Youngken HW (ed): *Food-Drugs from the Sea Conference.* Washington, DC: Marine Technical Society, 1970, p 295.

Su C, Chang C, Lee C-Y: Pharmacological properties of the neurotoxin of cobra venom, in Russell FE, Saunders PR (eds): *Animal Toxins.* Oxford: Pergamon Press, 1967, p 259.

Sutherland SK: *Australian Animal Toxins.* Melbourne: Oxford University Press, 1983.

Sutherland SK, Lane WR: Toxins and mode of envenomation of the common ringed or blue-banded octopus. *Med J Aust* 1:893, 1969.

Tamiya N, Arai H, Sato S: Studies on sea snake venoms: Crystallization of "erabutoxins" a and b from *Laticauda semifasciata* venom and of "laticotoxin" a from *Laticauda laticaudata* venom, in Russell FE, Saunders PR (eds): *Animal Toxins.* Oxford: Pergamon Press, 1967, p 249.

Tamkun MM, Hessinger DA: Isolation and partial characterization of a hemolytic and toxic protein from the nematocyst venom of the Portuguese man-of-war *Physalia physalis. Biochem Biophys Acta* 667:87, 1981; see also *Fed Proc* 38:824, 1979 (abstract).

Torda AE, Norton RS: Proton NMR realization study of the dynamics of anthopleurin-A in solution. *Biopolymers* 28:703, 1989.

Tu A: *Chemistry and Molecular Biology.* New York: Wiley, 1977.

Van Mierop LHS: Poisonous snakebite: A review. *J Fla Med Assoc* 63:191, 1976.

Vick JA, Ciuchta HP, Manthei JH: Pathophysiological studies on ten snake venoms, in Russell FE, Saunders PR (eds): *Animal Toxins.* Oxford: Pergamon Press, 1967, p 269.

Wagner FW, Spiekerman AM, Prescott JM: *Leucostoma* peptidase A: Isolation and physical properties. *J Biol Chem* 243:4486, 1968.

Wang CM, Narahashi R, Mendi TJ: Depolarizing action of *Haliclona* toxin on end-plate and muscle membranes. *Toxicon* 11:499, 1973.

Waraszkiewicz SM, Erickson KL: Halogenated sesquiterpenoids from the Hawaiian marine alga *Laurencia nidifica*: Nidificene and nidifidiene. *Tetrahedron Lett* 23:2003, 1974.

Watt CH Jr: Poisonous snakebite treatment in the United States. *JAMA* 240:654, 1978.

Weill R: *Contributions a l'étude des Cnidaires et de leur Nématocystes.* Paris: *Trav Stat Zool Wimiereux*, 1934.

Wiberg GS, Stephenson NR: Toxicologic studies on paralytic shellfish poison. *Toxicol Appl Pharmacol* 2:607, 1960.

Wittle LW, Middlebrook RE, Lane CE: Isolation and partial purification of a toxin from *Millepora alcicornis. Toxicon* 9:327, 1971.

Yamanouchi T: Study of poisons contained in holothurians, in Japanese. *Teikoku Gakush Hokoku* 17:73, 1942.

Yang CC: Crystallization and properties of cobrotoxin and their relationship to lethality. *Biochem Biophys Acta* 133:346, 1965.

Yasumoto T, Yamazaki Y, Meguro, et al: Production of tetrodotoxin and its derivatives by *Pseudomonas* sp. isolated from the skin of a pufferfish. *Toxicon* 25:225, 1986.

Zeller EA: Enzymes of snake venoms and their biological significance, in Nord FF (ed): *Advances in Enzymology.* New York: Interscience, 1948, vol 8, p 459.

# CHAPTER 27

# TOXIC EFFECTS OF PLANTS

*Stata Norton*

In its broadest aspect, plant toxicology includes more than the signs, symptoms, and treatment of humans and livestock poisoned by exposure to plants containing various types of chemicals. Also included is extensive research into the mechanism of action of toxic substances in the body. Some chemicals that plants manufacture have medical and environmental importance because they have lethal effects, for example, on cancer cells, or can be used in the environment to control some species of animals, especially invertebrates.

Until the twentieth century, when there was a dramatic shift in medicine toward the use of pure chemicals as drugs, unintentional poisoning from plants was common. Plants altered only by drying and grinding had been a major part of the materia medica since the first medicines were administered to the first ailing humans. Historical records document the use of plants as poisons at least from the period of Mithridates Eupator, King of Pontus on the Black Sea, who lived from 135 to 65 B.C. As the story goes, Mithridates made himself immune to poisons—a common method for removing kings—by eating small quantities of various poisons and gradually increasing the doses to build up his tolerance. Although that was hardly a successful method for developing protection against most toxic chemicals, the story speaks for early recognition of dose response. Throughout the Middle Ages toxicology was the province of professional poisoners, and the skill of the practitioners was such that different degrees and kinds of outcomes could be had for hire. Poisoning was used to produce sickness or incapacitation as well as death. Taylor (1875) described a case in which a thief poisoned some individuals at a meal with *Datura stramonium* (jimsonweed) until they were too mentally deranged to stop the robbery. Unfortunately for the thief, he partook too generously of the food and after departing with his booty succumbed, like his victims, to the belladonna alkaloids in the plant and was caught. Perhaps the thief lacked accuracy in the dose of the plant because the plant he used contained more belladonna alkaloids than he expected. Variability in the production of toxic chemicals by plants under different growing conditions and in different strains of the same species has been known for a long time. One of the most serious problems faced by physicians before the advent of pure chemicals as drugs was the variability in the concentration of the active principle manufactured and stored by medicinal plants. Variability in concentration still is a source of uncertainty in cases of poisoning resulting from the ingestion of plants. This variability has several causes:

1. Different portions of the plant (root, stem, leaves, seeds) often contain different concentrations of chemicals. For example, taxol, an antineoplastic drug from species of *Taxus* (yew), is present in various parts of *Taxus cuspidata*. A recent report has listed, in order of descending concentration of taxol, the needles → bark → wood → mature male cones (Fett-Netto and Di Cosmo, 1992).
2. The age of the plant contributes to variability. Young plants may contain more or less of some constituents than do mature plants.
3. Climatic and soil differences alter the synthesis of some chemicals.
4. Genetic differences within a species may alter the ability of that species to synthesize some chemicals.

The ability of plants to synthesize related toxic chemicals often occurs in taxonomically related species, as a characteristic of a genus, and sometimes as a familial characteristic. For example, various species of *Ranunculus* (buttercup) produce an acrid juice that releases the irritating chemical anemonin. Some other genera of the same plant family (Ranunculaceae) also release anemonin. Many genera in the mint family (Labiatiae) are rich in essential oils that are pleasing to humans but toxic to insects. In fact, some aspects of the unique biochemistry of plants are being used to establish taxonomic relationships, adding to the traditional role of morphology.

## TOXIC EFFECTS BY ORGAN

### Gastrointestinal System

The most common outcome of ingestion of a toxic plant is gastrointestinal disturbance—nausea, vomiting, and diarrhea—from irritation of the mucous membranes. Many different kinds of chemicals are responsible for this. Some have found a place in medicine as mild purgatives, such as cascara sagrada. The name "cascara sagrada" means "sacred bark" from its use by Native Americans. Cascara is obtained from the bark of *Rhamnus purshiana* (California buckthorn). The active ingredient in the plant is emodin.

*Wisteria floribunda* (Fam. Leguminosae) is a common ornamental climbing vine or small tree with lilac-colored flowers from which pods containing several seeds develop in the fall. The plant is of interest as a research tool because the seeds contain a lectin with affinity for *N*-acetylgalactosamine. Lectins are a heterogeneous group of glycoproteins classified by their ability to bind specific carbohydrate ligands and by the number of protein chains linked by disulfide bonds in a lectin. The seeds of wisteria cause severe gastroenteritis when ingested. A few seeds can result in headache, nausea, and diarrhea within hours, followed by dizziness, confusion, and hematemesis (Rondeau, 1993).

*Ricinus communis* (castor bean) is a member of the Family Euphorbiaceae, which contains several genera that produce toxic chemicals. The castor bean is an ornamental plant introduced from India and grown in temperate regions as an annual. The seeds are large and attractively mottled. If the seeds are eaten, children and adults experience no marked symptoms of poisoning for several days. In this interval there is some loss of appetite with nausea, vomiting, and diarrhea gradually developing. After that, gastroenteritis becomes severe with persistent vomiting, bloody diarrhea, dehydration, and icterus in fatal cases. Death occurs in 6 to 8 days. The fatal dose for a child can be 5 to 6 seeds; it is about 20 seeds for an adult. Postmortem examination shows foci of necrosis in the liver, spleen, lymph glands, intestine, and stomach. Fatality is low in individuals who eat these seeds—less than 10 percent when a "fatal dose" is consumed—because the toxic protein is largely destroyed in the intestine. Death from the ingestion of castor beans is caused by two lectins in the beans: ricin I and ricin II. The more toxic is ricin II. Ricin II consists of two chains of amino acids. The A chain (molecular weight 30,000), which inactivates the 60s ribosomal subunit of cells and blocks protein synthesis, is endocytosed into the cell cytosol after the B chain (molecular weight 33,000) binds to a terminal galactose residue on the cell membrane. The two chains are linked by a disulfide bond. Similar toxic lectins are found in the seeds of *Abrus precatorius* (jequirity bean), attractive scarlet and black beans that have been made into necklaces. Abrin-a, one of four isoabrins from the plant, has the highest inhibitory effect on protein synthesis and consists of an A chain of 250 amino acids and a B chain of 267 amino acids (Tahirov et al., 1994). The $LD_{50}$ of abrin injected in mice is less than 0.1 $\mu$g/kg, making abrin one of the most toxic substances known.

Ricin-type lectins with both A and B chains are potentially deadly if they pass, even in small quantities, through the gastrointestinal (GI) tract, as their potency when injected clearly demonstrates. Plants that produce only A chains without the B chains offer much less risk when ingested. Young shoots of pokeweed (*Phytolacca americana*) are sometimes used in the spring as a salad green. Mature leaves and berries may cause GI irritation with nausea and diarrhea. The plant contains a lectin that can inhibit protein synthesis in cells by inactivating rRNA. The lectin is a single-chain protein with a molecular weight of about 30,000. Single-chain ribosome-inhibiting proteins do not enter intact cells, but if the cell wall has been breached by a virus, they may enter the cell and block viral replication by inhibiting protein synthesis (Monzingo et al., 1993). Lectins that bind strongly to and are endocytosed by the cells lining the small intestine may be "nutritionally toxic" if they are consumed over a long period. Experimentally, reduction in weight gain has been the major finding from the presence of high quantities of some lectins in the diet. A correlation between strength of binding to the brush border of the jejunum and effectiveness as an antinutrient has been reported recently (Pusztai et al., 1993).

*Aesculus hippocastanum* (horse chestnut) and *Aesculus glabra* (Ohio buckeye) are common trees with attractive panicles of flowers in spring. The nuts of both trees contain a glucoside called esculin. When it is eaten by humans, the main effect is gastroenteritis, which may be severe if several nuts are consumed. Esculin is poorly absorbed from the GI tract in humans, and its systemic effects are limited. In cattle the glucoside may be hydrolyzed in the rumen, releasing the aglycone to cause systemic effects. Cattle develop signs of nervous system stimulation: a stiff-legged gait and, in severe poisoning, tonic seizures with opisthotonos (Casteel et al., 1992). While the most common poisoning of cattle occurs from ingestion of nuts, they also may be poisoned in a spring pasture by eating new leaves and buds.

Colchicine is best known in western medicine for its antimitotic effect, which is particularly useful in attacks of gout. Colchicine is the major alkaloid in the bulbs of *Colchicum autumnale* (autumn crocus, Fam. Liliaceae), which is native to Asia Minor and blossoms in fall. Severe gastroenteritis (nausea, vomiting, diarrhea, and dehydration) follows ingestion of the bulbs. Systemic effects may develop, including confusion, delirium, hematuria, neuropathy, and renal failure. Bone marrow aplasia results from block of mitosis in bone marrow by colchicine. The antimitotic effect is caused by a block of the formation of microtubules from tubulin and subsequent failure of the mitotic spindle. In southern Europe, hay for cattle may contain the wild autumn crocus and deaths occur if contamination is heavy. In other countries similar poisoning has been found after human ingestion of tubers of *Gloriosa superba* (glory flower, Fam. Liliaceae), an ornamental plant that contains colchicine. The plant grows wild in Sri Lanka, and poisoning by Gloriosa tubers has been reported as the most common plant poisoning in that country. Poisoning has also been reported in India (Mendis, 1989).

## Skin

The genus Euphorbia (Fam. Euphorbiaceae, spurge family) contains hundreds of species dispersed over most temperate and tropical regions. Characteristically, the stems and leaves exude milky latex when damaged. The latex is irritating to the skin and contains diterpene esters (Gundidza et al., 1992). One of the major esters, resiniferatoxin, is found in the latex of *E. resinifera* and several other species of *Euphorbia*. It is a potent irritant and mimics the action of capsaicin, exciting and then desensitizing primary afferent nerve fibers (Maggi et al., 1990). This property has been used in medicine to relieve pain through topical application, presumably by causing degeneration of the fine C-fiber sensory neurons (Szallasi and Blumberg, 1989).

*E. marginata* (snow-on-the-mountain) is a common plant in the United States, growing wild from Minnesota to Texas and cultivated for its attractive foliage. Individuals using the plant in flower arrangements may come in contact with the latex and develop skin irritation (Urushibata and Kase, 1991). Serious eye irritation also has been reported (Frohn et al., 1993). The latex from *E. marginata* has been shown to be mutagenic to human lymphocytes (Stirpe et al., 1993). Another species, *E. tirucalli,* grows in the "lymphoma belt" of Africa, an area in which Burkitt's lymphoma, a childhood tumor, is found with unusual frequency. It has been hypothesized that the diterpene ester in the latex may activate the Epstein-Barr virus and in this way be related to the development of lymphoma (van den Bosch et al., 1993). The latex of *E. bougheii*, another African species, experimentally promotes the formation of skin tumors (Gundidza and Kufa, 1993).

*Philodendron* (Fam. Araceae, arum family) and *Toxicodendron* (Fam. Anacardiaceae, cashew family) are not closely related plants, but species of both genera cause contact dermatitis as an allergic reaction. *Philodendron scandens* is a common houseplant, while *Toxicodendron radicans* (poison ivy) is native to large sections of North America. The active ingredients in *P. scandens* are resorcinols, especially 5-*n*-heptadecatrienyl resorcinol (Knight, 1991). In *T. radicans* the allergenic component is a mixture of catechols called urushiol. The most active chemical in urushiol is 3-*n*-pentadecadienyl catechol, representing approximately 60 percent of urushiol (Johnson et al., 1972). The chemicals most likely to cause allergic dermatitis after contact with these plants have in common partly unsaturated straight side chains. As in allergies in general, there is no response to the initial exposure. Individuals show marked variation in the severity of response to subsequent exposures. The allergic dermatitis resulting from urushiol has been investigated extensively, in part because the allergen will sensitize about 70 percent of the persons exposed, making it a powerful allergen that is responsible for the most common form of allergic contact dermatitis in the United States. Urushiol is fat-soluble, penetrates the stratum corneum, and binds to Langerhans cells in the epidermis. These haptenated cells then migrate to lymph nodes where T cells are activated and return to the skin, where they are involved in the dermatitis (Kalish and Johnson, 1990).

Flower growers and other individuals who handle bulbs and cut flowers of narcissus, hyacinths, daffodils, and tulips sometimes develop dermatitis from contact with the sap. These conditions occur frequently enough to have achieved common names: "lily rash," "hyacinth itch," "daffodil itch," and "tulip fingers." Most of the skin rashes are due to irritation from alkaloids (masonin, lycorin, and several related alkaloids) (Fig. 27-1) or to needlelike crystals of calcium oxalate in the bulbs (Gude et al., 1988). Most of these alkaloids do not act as allergens, but one, tulipalin-A, which causes "tulip fingers" from sorting and peeling tulip bulbs, has allergenic properties.

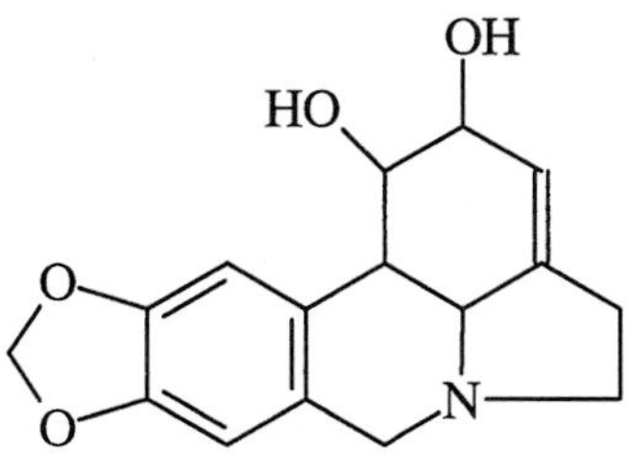

**LYCORIN**

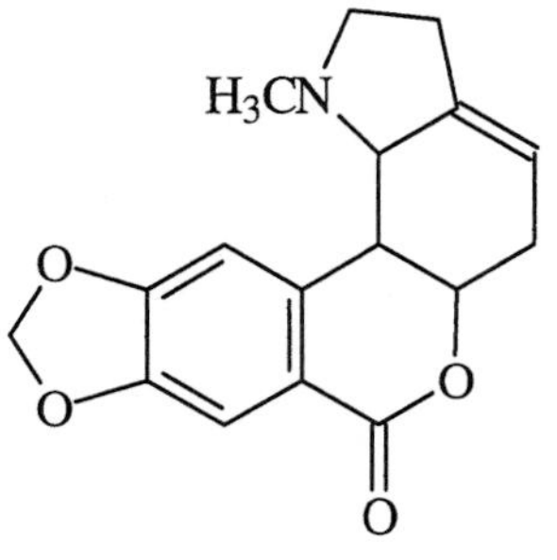

**MASONIN**

***Figure 27–1. Alkaloids causing skin irritation.***

Tulipalin-A, alpha-methylene-gamma-butyrolactone, is present in some cultivars in a concentration as high as 2%. A safe threshold for this allergen is considered to be a concentration of 0.01% (Hausen et al., 1983).

The two most common exposures to toxic substances in plants reported to poison control centers in the United States come from the houseplants *Philodendron* and *Dieffenbachia*. Children and workers in plant nurseries are the usual patients. Both plants belong to the Arum family, but their toxicities are different. *Dieffenbachia* does not cause allergic dermatitis. When the leaves or stems of *Dieffenbachia* (dumb cane) are broken, the juice is immediately irritating to mucous membranes. Children may chew leaves of the plant, and workers in greenhouses cut the plant in the course of their work. Contact with the juice to the eye or tongue results in pain and the rapid development of edema and inflammation, which may take days or weeks to subside. The toxicity is due to a combination of factors. The leaves contain irritating calcium oxalate crystals and a trypsinlike inflammatory protein. The release of a histaminelike or serotoninlike chemical may be involved in the immediate pain (Pamies et al., 1992). The needlelike crystals of calcium oxalate, which are called raphides, are located in ampoule-shaped ejector cells throughout the surface of the leaf. Slight pressure on these cells causes expulsion of the raphides. The raphides are coated with the trypsinlike enzyme, which increases the irritation from the crystals (McIntire et al. 1990).

Acute dermatitis is caused by some of the small hairs (called trichomes) on many plants. One of the most common skin contacts in the United States is with species of *Urtica* (nettles). Even gentle contact with the hairs causes pain and erythema. The trichomes readily penetrate skin. In the stinging nettles, *U. urens* and *U. dioica* (Fam. Urticaceae), the trichomes covering the leaves and stems consist of fine tubes with bulbs at the tips. On contact with skin, the hairs puncture the skin and the bulbs break off and release fluid containing histamine, acetylcholine, and serotonin, causing the acute response (Oliver et al., 1991). Exposure to a related species, *U. ferox* (poisonous tree nettle), that is widespread in areas of New Zealand has caused death in humans and animals. A defense against ingestion by animals similar to that of nettles has been developed by *Mucuna pruriens* (cowhage), a legume, whose pods are covered with barbed trichomes that cause pain, itching, erythema, and vesication on the skin. The trichomes of *M. pruriens* contain mucunain, a proteinase that is considered to be responsible for the pruritis (Southcott and Haegi, 1992).

Several species of *Ranunculus* (buttercup) cause contact dermatitis. These plants contain ranunculin, which releases the toxic principle, protoanemonin, which also is present in *Anemone*, another genus of the buttercup family. Protoanemonin is readily converted to anemonin, which has marked irritant properties. For many years the juice of *Ranunculus bulbosus* (bulbous buttercup) was used in medicine as a vesicant when blistering of the skin was a common practice in several remedial procedures. Ingestion of plants containing protoanemonin may result in severe irritation of the GI tract (Kelch et al., 1992).

Not all cases of dermatitis from plants are due to skin contact. Poisoning of livestock from *Hypericum perforatum* (Saint-John's-wort) has been reported in New Zealand, Australia, North Africa, Iraq, Europe, and the United States. The poisonous principle is hypericin (hexahydroxydimethylnaphthodianthrone), which is present throughout the plant. Sheep are the most commonly affected animal, ingesting the plant in pasturage. Hypericin is lost upon drying of the plant. The effect in sheep is development of edematous lesions of the skin, especially in areas not well covered with hair, including the ears, nose, and eyes. Hypericin causes photosensitization, and lesions appear after exposure to sunlight (Sako et al., 1993).

## Cardiovascular System

*Veratrum viride* (American hellebore), a member of the lily family native to eastern North America, produces several toxic alkaloids that are distributed in all parts of the plant. European hellebore (*V. album*) and *V. californicum* of western North America have similar properties. *V. album* and later *V. viride* were part of the "vegetable materia medica" for centuries. They were employed to "slow and soften the pulse," particularly in eclampsia (Underhill, 1924). These species of *Veratrum* contain a mixture of alkaloids including protoveratrine, veratramine, and jervine (Fig. 27-2). After ingestion of the plant, the alkaloids cause nausea, emesis, hypotension, bradycardia, and sometimes muscle spasm. The primary effect of the veratrum alkaloids on the heart is repetitive response to a single stimulus resulting from prolongation of the sodium current (Jaffe et al., 1990).

*Taxus baccata* (European yew) is a common ornamental evergreen shrub in the United States; it is native to Europe, North Africa, and western Asia. With its wide geographic distribution, it is not surprising that the poisonous qualities of the needles and berries of yew have been known since antiquity.

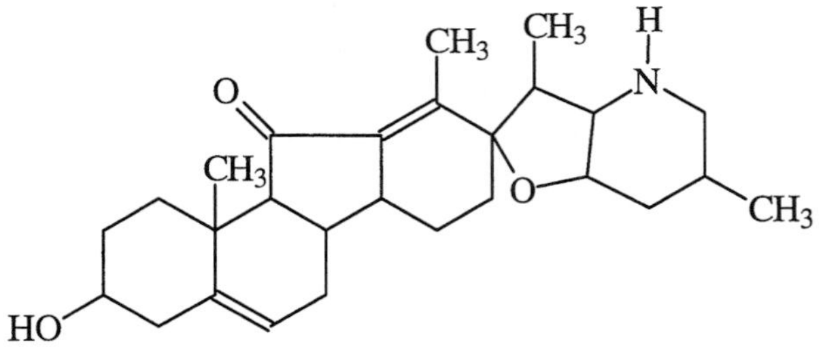

**JERVINE**

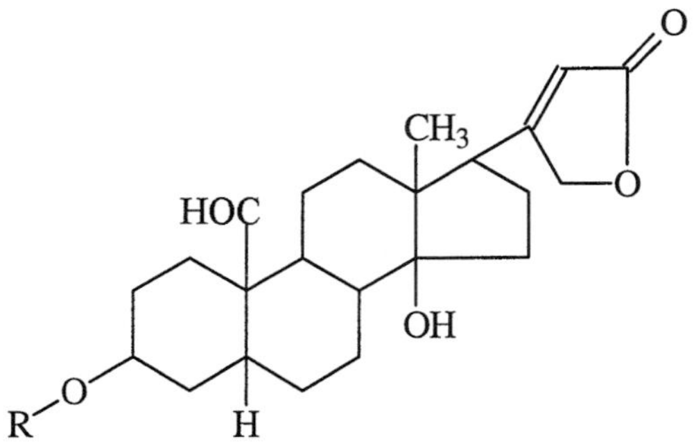

**THEVETIN A**
**(R = thevetose-gentiobiose)**

***Figure 27–2. Plant chemicals affecting the cardiovascular system.***

Human poisoning is relatively rare because of the large amount needed to produce serious effects. Nevertheless, deaths have occurred from ingestion of the leaves (Musshoff et al., 1993). Death results from cardiac or respiratory failure. Cattle, which ingest large amounts, show similar acute effects. Several alkaloids known as taxines have been isolated from European yew. The most poisonous is taxine A. The mechanism of action on the heart has been proposed to be inhibition of calcium ion currents (Panter et al., 1993). A different alkaloid from the Pacific yew (*Taxus brevifolia*), taxol, is of interest as a chemotherapeutic agent. The action of taxol is not like that of the taxines but is related to the ability of taxol to prevent dissociation of microtubules into tubulin in dividing cells.

Several disparate families of plants contain species with cardioactive glycosides, the best known of which is *Digitalis purpurea* (foxglove, Fam. Scrophulariaceae). In the lily family, squill (*Scilla maritima*) contains scillaren and *Convallaria majalis* (lily-of-the-valley) contains convallatoxin in the bulbs, both of which have actions resembling the effects of digitalis. Poisoning has occurred from their improper use for cardiac effects.

Two plants in the Family Apocyanceae contain cardioactive glycosides. *Nereum oleander* (bay laurel) is native to the Mediterranean area but is grown ornamentally in many regions. The major glycosides, oleandrum and neroside, may be present in concentrations as high as 0.5 mg/g plant material. Animals and humans have been poisoned by eating the leaves or seeds. The effect is identical to digitalis toxicity: nausea, vomiting, cardiac arrhythmias, and hyperkalemia (Clark et al., 1991). A related plant, *Thevetia peruviana* (yellow oleander), is a common ornamental in the United States and other parts of the world. Human poisoning has been reported in Australia, Melanesia, Thailand, and India. The seeds are the major source of the cardiac glycosides, the most active of which are thevetin A and B (Fig. 27-2). The fatal dose to an adult is 8 to 10 seeds (Prabhasankar et al., 1993).

*Aconitum* species have been used in western and eastern medicine for centuries. The European plant *Aconitum napellus* (monkshood) is a perennial grown in gardens for its ornamental blue flowers. The roots of *A. kusnezoffii* (chuanwu) and *A. carmichaeli* (caowu) are in the Chinese materia medica. Poisoning may occur from intentional or accidental ingestion, and the concentration of the toxic alkaloids—aconitine, mesaconitine, and hypoaconitine—varies depending on species, place of origin, time of harvest, and processing procedure (Chan et al., 1994). In addition to cardiac arrhythmias and hypotension, the alkaloids cause GI upset and neurological symptoms, especially numbness of the mouth and paresthesia in the extremities. Aconitine has been used experimentally in the study of cardiac arrhythmias. The alkaloid causes a prolonged sodium current in cardiac muscle with slowed repolarization (Peper and Trautwein, 1967). The neurological effects are due to a similar action on voltage-sensitive sodium currents in nerve fibers (Murai et al.,1990).

In Greece almost 2500 years ago, Xenophon described a serious condition that developed in his soldiers after they consumed honey. The condition has been called "mad honey poisoning" and consists of marked bradycardia, hypotension, oral paresthesias, weakness, and GI upset, resembling aconitine poisoning. In severe poisoning there is respiratory depression and loss of consciousness. The condition is caused by eating honey contaminated with grayanotoxins. Much of the action of grayanotoxins appears to be central. Grayanotoxin I (andromedotoxin) slows both the opening and the closing of sodium channels in nerves (Narahashi, 1986). Honey poisoning has been reported in Turkey, Japan, Nepal, Brazil, Europe, and some parts of North America. Grayanotoxins are produced exclusively by several genera of Ericaceae (heath family). They have been isolated from *Rhododendron ponticum* (Onat et al., 1991) and *Kalmia angustifolia* (Burke and Daskotch, 1990). The toxin gets into honey from nectar collected by bees from the flowers. The grayanotoxins are present throughout the plants, including the leaves, flowers, pollen, and nectar. Livestock have been poisoned by eating leaves of the plants. Toxicity also has been reported in goats and sheep eating leaves of *Rhododendron macrophyllum* (Casteel and Wagstaff, 1989).

A strange case of alternative medical uses of plants took place in eighteenth-century New England. A native plant, *Lobelia inflata* (Indian tobacco, bluebell family), was used to excess as a cure-all by Samuel Thomson, a self-trained "medical botanist." Thomson was charged with causing the death of some of his patients by administering the plant in repeated doses. The active alkaloid in *L. inflata*, lobeline (Fig. 27-3), has a high affinity for nicotinic acetylcholine receptors (Libri et al., 1992) and produces effects almost identical to those of nicotine. In toxic doses both cause emesis, and they cause cardiovascular effects through actions on the autonomic nervous system. Lobeline is found throughout the plant, including the seeds.

Mistletoe is a parasitic plant on trees that has over the centuries been considered both holy and demonic. In Norse mythology the plant that killed Balder, the god of summer, was mistletoe. In 1597 John Gerarde in his herbal described a case of poisoning from mistletoe berries in which the tongue was inflamed and swollen, the mind distraught, and strength of heart and wits enfeebled. The plant causing the condition was identified when the individual vomited mistletoe seeds. Shakespeare, writing at about the same time, referred to the "baleful mistletoe." The mistletoe that appears in shops at Christmastime in the United States is *Phoradendron tomentosum*, a member of the same family as European mistletoe (*Viscum album*) and also a parasitic plant on trees. The American mistletoe contains phoratoxin, a polypeptide with a molecular weight of about 13,000. Experimentally, phoratoxin produces effects in animals that resemble the effects of viscotoxins: hypotension, bradycardia, negative inotropic effects on heart muscle, and vasoconstriction of the vessels of skin and skeletal muscle. Phoratoxin is only one-fifth as active as are viscotoxins (Rosell and Samuelsson, 1966). Viscotoxins are basic polypeptides (molecular weight about 5000). Poisoning from European mistletoe is rare but resembles that from American mistletoe, including GI distress and hypotension. Several lectins have been isolated from European mistletoe in addition to the viscotoxins, the best known of which is viscumin (ML-I), a cytotoxic lectin with A and B chains. Recently, extracts of *V. album* have been used widely in alternative medicine in Europe as anticancer drugs, and controversy has arisen over the effectiveness of these extracts. The evidence has been reviewed (Franz, 1986). It has even been proposed that alkaloids from the host plants are absorbed by the parasitic mistletoe and may have additive effects with chemicals produced by the mistletoe.

Of the various fungi that produce toxic principles, some are parasitic or symbiotic on grasses used as food by humans and livestock. *Claviceps purpurea* (ergot) is a fungus parasitic on grains of rye. This fungus has caused outbreaks of strange poisonings in several European countries since the Middle Ages. At that time the disease was called "St. Anthony's fire" from the blackened appearance of the limbs of some sufferers. The main symptom caused by ergot alkaloids is vasoconstriction of blood vessels, primarily in the extremities, followed by gangrene. Abortion in pregnant women is also common after ingestion of contaminated rye. Ergot alkaloids are derivatives of lysergic acid. Some of the alkaloids have been used in therapeutics, especially ergotamine and ergonovine. Although the ergot alkaloids have been studied extensively over the years, treatment of vasospasm is still being investigated (McKiernan et al., 1994). Another fungus, *Acremonium coenophialum*, grows symbiotically on the forage grass tall fescue (*Festuca*

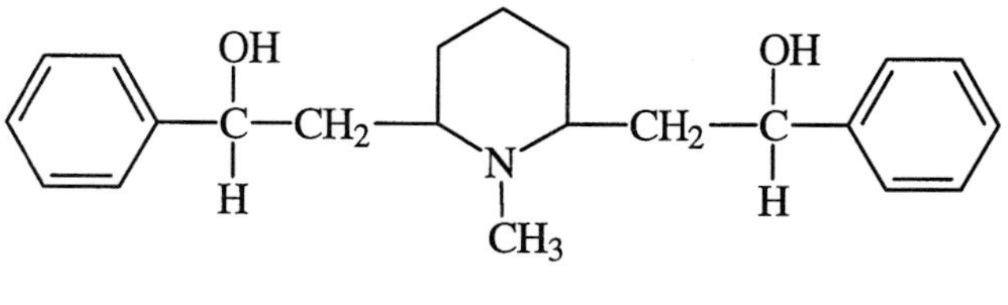

OH OH
C—CH2 N CH2—C
H CH3 H

**LOBELINE**

N CH3 =N
HOOC—C(H)(NH2) O NH O
H2C(NH2) O NH O

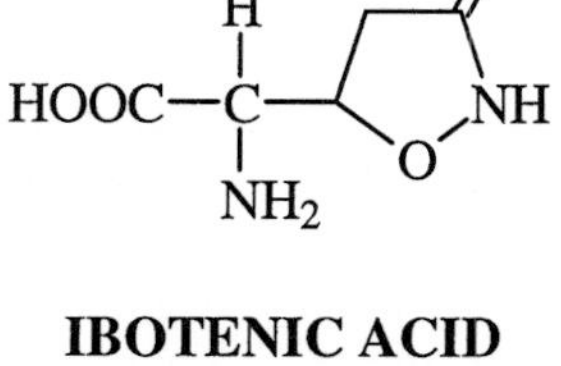

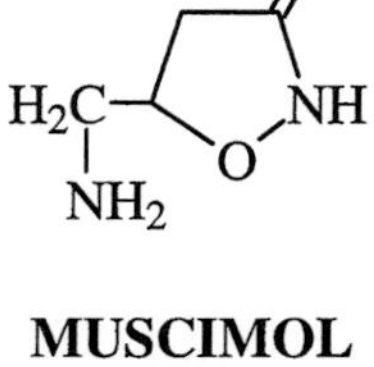

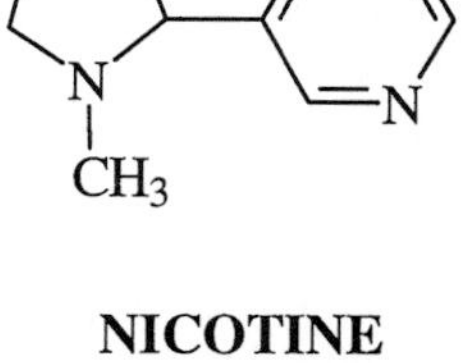

**NICOTINE** **IBOTENIC ACID** **MUSCIMOL**

***Figure 27–3. Plant chemicals affecting the nervous system.***

*arundinacea*) and produces some ergot alkaloids and other lysergic acid derivatives. The fungus causes "fescue toxicosis" in cattle that graze on infected plants (Hill et al., 1994). The condition in cattle includes decreased weight gain, decreased reproductive performance, and peripheral vasoconstriction. In the southwestern United States, *Stirpa robusta* (sleepy grass) is infected with an *Acremonium* fungus. Horses grazing in areas where the perennial grass grows become somnolent, presumably as a result of ingestion of lysergic acid amide, ergonovine, and related alkaloids produced by the fungus (Petroski et al., 1992).

## Nervous System

Curare, the South American arrow poison, is a potent neuromuscular blocking agent in skeletal muscle and kills by stopping respiration. Curare is obtained from tropical species of *Strychnos* and *Chondrodendron*. However, not all plants producing neuromuscular blocking agents are of tropical origin. In warm weather in temperate climates, blooms of blue-green algae are not uncommon in farm ponds, particularly those enriched with fertilizer. Under these conditions, one species of alga, *Anabena flos-aquae*, produces a neurotoxin, anatoxin A, which blocks acetylcholine receptors, both nicotinic and muscarinic, causing death in animals that drink the pond water. The lethal effects develop rapidly, with death in minutes to hours from respiratory arrest caused by neuromuscular block (Short and Edwards, 1990). Anatoxin A is 2-acetyl-9-azabicyclo [4.2.1] non-2-ene (Hyde and Carmichael, 1991).

Methyllycaconitine is an alkaloid present in *Delphinium barbeyi* (tall larkspur) and some related species. The plant contaminates western pastures in this country and causes the death of livestock. Poisoned cattle show muscle tremors, ataxia, and prostration and die from respiratory failure. The alkaloid has a high affinity for the cholinergic receptor and causes death by blocking the action of acetylcholine at the neuromuscular junction, much as curare does. Physostigmine has been used successfully as an antagonist in some cases of methyllycaconitine poisoning (Pfister et al., 1994). Methyllycaconitine is being used experimentally as a selective probe for discriminating different acetylcholine-binding sites in the brain (Alkodon et al., 1992).

Swainsonine is an indolizidine alkaloid found in *Swainsona canescens*, an Australian plant, and in *Astragalus lentiginosus* (spotted locoweed) and *Oxytropis sericea* (locoweed) in the western United States. Cattle consume these plants in pastures. The common name comes from the most obvious consequences of ingestion of the locoweeds: abberrant behavior with hyperexcitability and locomotor difficulty. In animals dying from locoweed poisoning there is cytoplasmic foamy vacuolation of cerebellar cells. The toxic chemical swainsonine causes marked inhibition of liver lysosomal and cytosomal alpha-D-mannosidase and Golgi mannosidase II. Inhibition of the Golgi enzyme results in abnormal brain glycoproteins and accumulation of mannose-rich oligosaccharides (Tulsiani et al., 1988). The pathology is not limited to the nervous system, and the effects of swainsonine poisoning are present in several tissues, especially the liver.

Excitatory amino acids (EAAs) are produced by widely divergent species of plants. These amino acids mimic in varying degrees the actions of the natural transmitters glutamic acid and aspartic acid on neurons in the central nervous system with specialized receptors for amino acids. However, these EAAs can cause the death of neurons from excessive stimulation. Several human and livestock diseases have been tied to EAAs. Some of the simplest plants structurally are the algae; nevertheless, they produce some of the most effective EAAs. The best known EAA is kainic acid (2-carboxy-4-(1-methylenelyl)-3-pyrrolidine acetic acid), which is present in the red alga *Digenea simplex*. Domoic acid is a constituent of a green alga, *Chondria armata*, growing in northern oceans and also is found in some marine protozoa, such as the diatom *Nitchia pungens*. Under some conditions the alga reproduces rapidly. Filter-feeding mussels accumulate domoic acid by ingesting the alga, and humans can be poisoned by eating the mussels. In 1987 there was a serious outbreak of poisoning in Canada among individuals eating Atlantic mussels. The acute symptoms were GI distress, headache, hemiparesis, confusion, and seizures. There were some prolonged neurological symptoms, including severe memory deficits and sensorimotor neuronopathy (Teitelbaum et al., 1990). The prolonged pathology has been linked to selective death of neurons sensitive to EAAs.

A little farther up the evolutionary ladder from the algae are the fungi. One fungus, *Amanita muscaria* (fly agaric), got its name from its poisonous qualities to flies. The toxic ingredient is the EAA ibotenic acid. Poisoning from two common woodland mushrooms, *A. muscaria* and *A. pantherina* (panther amanita, common in the western United States), is due to the content of ibotenic acid (and possibly to its derivative, muscimol) (Fig. 27-3). The effects are somewhat variable: central nervous system depression, ataxia, hysteria, and hallucinations. Myoclonic twitching and seizures may develop (Benjamin, 1992). The content of ibotenic acid varies with the time of year; more has been reported in mushrooms in spring than in fall.

The occurrence of EAAs extends to the complex vascular plants. The pea family contains several species which produce EAAs in the seeds. Willardiine [1-(2-amino-2-carboxyethyl) pyrimidine-2,4-dione] has been isolated from *Acacia Willardiana*, *A. lemmoni*, *A. millefolia,* and *Mimosa asperata* (Gmelin, 1961). Willardiine acts as an agonist on the kainate receptor (Patneau et al., 1992). Other important EAAs are present in species of *Lathyrus*. *Lathyrus sylvestris* (flat pea) is a perennial pea indigenous to Europe and central Asia and naturalized in Canada and the northern United States. The plant is eaten by livestock in areas where it is common. The seeds contain DABA (2,4-diaminobutyric acid) and lower quantities of BOAA (beta-*N*-oxalylamino-l-alanine). Both DABA and BOAA are excitatory neurotoxins. Seeds of *L. sativus* (chickling pea) contain more BOAA than DABA, and seeds of this plant are used as food by humans in parts of Africa. Lathyrism is a condition developing in humans who consume large quantities of *L. sativus* seeds over periods of months or longer. BOAA is an excitotoxic analogue of l-glutamate and is thought to be the cause of upper motor neuron degeneration in lathyrism. Affected individuals have severe spastic muscle weakness and atrophy with little sensory involvement (Spencer et al., 1986). *L. sylvestris* has caused an acute neurological condition in sheep that begins with weakness and progresses to tremors and prostration, sometimes with clonic movements and seizures. DABA may be responsible for the effects in sheep (Rasmussen et al., 1993).

*Karwinskia humboldtiana*, family Rhamnaceae, is a shrub of the southwestern United States, Mexico, and Central America. Common names are buckthorn, coyotillo, and tullidora. Anthracenones are found in the seeds, and there is marked variation in the content of the anthracenones. Green fruit may be more toxic than ripe fruit (Bermudez et al., 1986). Both human and livestock poisonings occur, occasionally in epidemic proportions. The clinical syndrome that develops after a latency of several days is symmetrical polyneuropathy beginning in the lower legs and progressing to the upper limbs and in fatal cases leading to bulbar paralysis. The neuropathology includes peripheral segmental demyelination of large motor axons with sparing of sensory fibers (Hernandez-Cruz and Munoz-Martinez, 1984). In addition to neurotoxicity, the anthracenones in *Karwinskia*, especially T-514 and T-544, cause atelectasis and emphysema in lungs and massive liver necrosis. T-514 [3,3′-dimethyl-3,3′,8,8′,9,9′-hexahydroxy-3,3′,4,4′-tetrahydro-(7,10 bianthracene)-1,1′(2H,2′H)-dione] is markedly toxic to hepatocytes both in vivo and in vitro (Garza-Ocanas et al., 1992).

The belladonna alkaloids, which are present in several genera of plants, are among the best known plant alkaloids. The plants are widely distributed and have had a place in the materia medica of many cultures. The alkaloids are l-hyoscyamine, atropine (d,l-hyoscyamine), and scopolamine. *Datura stramonium* (jimsonweed) is native to India and contains primarily scopolamine; *Hyoscyamine niger* (henbane) is native to Europe and contains mostly l-hyoscyamine; *Atropa belladonna* (deadly nightshade), which also is native to Europe, contains atropine; and *Duboisia myoporoides* (pituri) in Australia contains l-hyoscyamine. Of the two active alkaloids, l-hyoscyamine and scopolamine, the latter has the greater action on the central nervous system, while l-hyoscyamine acts primarily to block muscarinic receptors of the parasympathetic nervous system. The effects of modest doses of l-hyoscyamine or atropine are referable to muscarinic block: dry mouth, dilated pupils, and decreased GI motility. Large doses of either or scopolamine affect the central nervous system. Confusion, bizarre behavior, hallucinations, and subsequent amnesia are characteristic of toxic doses. Deaths are rare, although recovery may take several days. Poisoning from belladonna alkaloids results from accidental or intentional ingestion of the leaves, seeds, or roots of the plants. "Datura tea," a water extract of the leaves, has been used as a domestic remedy and has been responsible for poisoning. Other species of *Datura* also contain belladonna alkaloids. *Datura (Brugmansia) suaveolens* (angel's trumpet) is used as an ornamental houseplant and contains significant quantities of atropine and scopolamine (Smith et al., 1991). The plant is grown in pots, and when it is cut back, the juice of the plant may contact the eye, resulting in marked asymmetrical mydriasis that may be mistaken for a neurological disorder (Wilhelm et al., 1991). Seeds of the weed *Datura ferox* are contaminants in animal feed in some parts of Europe, and these seeds contain the belladonna alkaloids. In some areas where seeds for human consumption are not carefully sorted before milling and where *D. stramonium* and *D. metel* are common weeds, millet, wheat, rye, corn, and beans sometimes are contaminated with the seeds. The amount needed to poison an adult is about 20 seeds. The symptoms made from eating bread made from contaminated flour are typical of poisoning from belladonna alkaloids (van Meurs et al., 1992).

The postsynaptic receptors at terminations of parasympathetic nerve fibers are called "muscarinic" after the selective stimulation of these receptors by muscarine, which first was extracted from the mushroom *Amanita muscaria*. However, this mushroom contains only trace amounts of muscarine, and poisoning from it is due to its content of ibotenic acid. Some mushrooms of the genera *Inocybe* and *Clitocybe* (for example, *I. sororia* and *C. dealbata*) contain significant amounts of muscarine, and the consumption of these mushrooms may cause diarrhea, sweating, salivation, and lacrimation, all referable to stimulation of parasympathetic receptors (Stollard and Edes, 1989).

## Liver

In 1884 cases of "hepatitis" in cattle in Iowa were discovered to have been caused by the ingestion of species of *Senecio* (ragwort or groundsel). *Senecio* (Fam. Compositae) is a large genus of plants with worldwide distribution. Species that contain significant concentrations of some pyrrolizidine alkaloids are responsible for the liver damage, a form of hepatic veno-occlusive disease. Species in three other genera, *Crotalaria, Helotropium,* and *Symphytum*, also contain the pyrrolizidine alkaloids. *Crotalaria* (rattle box) is a legume, and *Helotropium* (heliotrope) and *Symphytum* (comfrey) are in the borage family. Species of all four genera are known to cause similar hepatic damage. Human deaths have been reported in several countries, including South Africa, Jamaica, and Barbados. In Afghanistan there was an epidemic of hepatic veno-occlusive disease from consumption of a wheat crop contaminated with seeds of a species of *Heliotropium* (Tandon et al., 1978). The clinical signs associated with the liver damage resemble those of cirrhosis and some hepatic tumors and may be mistaken for those conditions (McDermott and Ridker, 1990). The clinical condition has been described as a form of the Budd-Chiari syndrome with portal hypertension and obliteration of small hepatic veins (Ridker et al., 1985). Damage to hepatocytes has been proposed to be due to the formation of pyrrole metabolites from pyrrolidizine alkaloids by liver microsomal oxidation, with cross-linking of DNA strands by the pyrrole metabolites (Carballo et al., 1992).

*Symphytum* and *Senecio* have been included in some herbal preparations of domestic medicines. The ingestion of "comfrey tea" or "groundsel tea" has resulted in poisoning in children and adults. Hepatitis in cattle grazing on these plants, most commonly *Senecio*, has been reported in Africa and Asia as well as the United States. Cows and horses are seriously affected. The condition is progressive, and death occurs after weeks or months of grazing in contaminated pastures. The toxic alkaloid in *Senecio vulgaris* (common groundsel) is retrorsine; it is jacobine in *Senecio jacobaea* (stinking willie) and monocrotaline in *Crotalaria spectabilis* (showy rattlebox) (Fig. 27-4).

Many of the nonedible mushrooms may cause GI effects, but most of those effects are not life-threatening. Most deaths from mushroom poisoning worldwide are due to the consumption of *Amanita phalloides*, appropriately called "death cap." *A. ocreata* (death angel) is equally dangerous. *A. phalloides* contains two different types of toxic chemicals: phalloidin and amatoxins. Phalloidin is a cyclic heptapeptide that

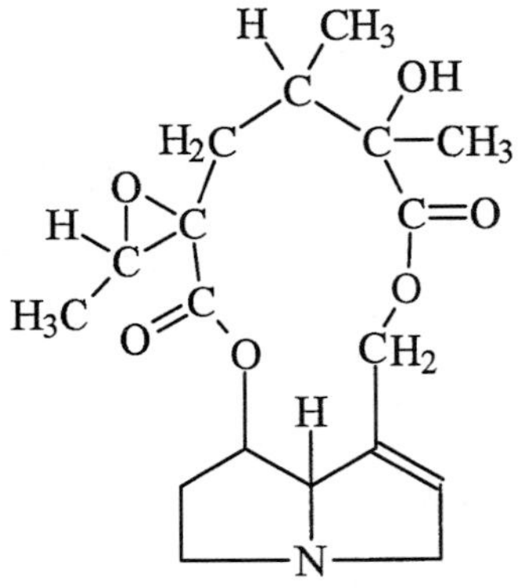

JACOBINE

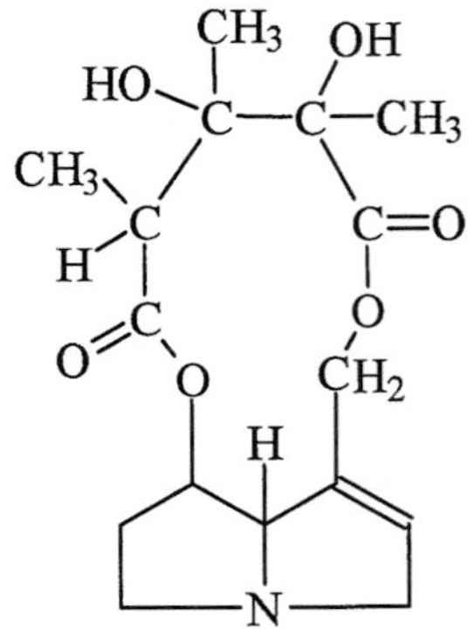

MONOCROTALINE

*Figure 27–4. Pyrrolizidine alkaloids affecting the liver.*

may be responsible for some of the diarrhea that develops 10 to 12 h after the ingestion of *A. phalloides*. Phalloidin combines with actin in muscle cells to interfere with the function of those cells but is not absorbed (Cappell and Hassan, 1992). The amatoxins are bicyclic peptides (molecular weight 900) and are absorbed. The most toxic, alpha-amanitin, has a strong affinity for hepatocytes and binds to RNA polymerase II, thus inhibiting protein synthesis (Jaeger et al., 1993). Serious clinical signs of liver effects develop slowly, beginning on about the third day after ingestion. Treatment in a severe case may require a liver transplant; there is no other specific treatment. Renal lesions also are found in cases of serious poisoning, with damage most prominent in proximal tubules. In addition to *A. phalloides* and *A. ocreata*, several species of Lepiota (parasol mushrooms) produce amatoxins, notably *Lepiota helveola* and *L. bruneo-incarnata*. A novel treatment to disrupt the enterohepatic circulation of amatoxin has been proposed in cases of ingestion of the poisonous mushrooms: administration of silymarin, the active principle of the thistle *Silybum marianum,* in the form of its soluble hemisuccinate. It has been shown in the rat that silymarin can suppress the uptake of amanitin into liver cells if therapy is started in time (Wieland and Faulstich, 1991).

Fumonisins are toxins produced by the fungus *Fusarium*, primarily by *F. moniliforme* growing on corn. Ingestion by horses of corn contaminated with *F. moniliforme* has been shown to be the cause of "moldy corn poisoning," or equine leukoencephalomalacia. The signs in affected horses are lethargy, ataxia, convulsions, and death (Norred, 1993). In other animals there are different target organs, but the liver is a primary target in every species: in horses, it is liver and brain; in pigs, liver and lung; in rats, liver and kidney; and in chickens, liver (Riley et al., 1994). In humans an association with esophageal cancer has been suggested (Yoshizawa et al., 1994). The structure of fumonisins is similar to that of sphingosine, and their toxicity has been proposed to be related to block of enzymes in sphingolipid biosynthesis (Norred, 1993).

*Cestrum laevigatum* (Fam. Solanaceae) is occasionally a contaminant of hay in Europe. Ingestion of the dried plant material by cattle can result in moderate to severe hepatic damage characterized by centrilobular to midzonal hemorrhagic necrosis (van der Lugt et al., 1991). Sheep develop a similar liver necrosis. The signs in poisoned animals include nervous system changes, ataxia, and tremors. *C. laevigatum* is known to have calcinogenic effects in chickens, just as *Solanum malacoxylon* does (Mello and Habermehl, 1992), as described in "Bone," below.

Ingestion of locoweeds (species of *Astragalus* and *Oxytropis*) by livestock results in marked nervous system signs (see "Nervous System," above). However, the general inhibition of mannosidase in cells by swansonine, the toxic chemical in locoweeds, causes many tissue alterations. A major effect is congestive heart failure, especially in animals grazing at high altitudes. This condition is sufficiently specific to have been given the name "high mountain disease" (James et al., 1991). Affected animals also have centrilobular lesions in the liver.

*Lantana camara* has been described as one of the 10 most noxious weeds in the world (Sharma et al., 1988). It is an attractive flowering shrub that is native to Jamaica and is cultivated in greenhouses in many parts of the world. *L. camara* thrives outdoors in hot, dry climates. An unusual property of the plant is that it inhibits the growth of neighboring plants. In India livestock poisoning from *L. camara* is a serious problem. Cattle grazing on the plant develop cholestasis and hyperbilirubinemia. The leaves also are toxic to nonruminants, including rabbits and guinea pigs. Several triterpenoids have been isolated from the plant. One that has been shown to induce hepatotoxicity is lantanene A (22-beta-angeloyloxy-3-oxo-olean-12-en-28-oic acid) (Sharma et al., 1991).

## Skeletal Muscle

Ataxia and generalized muscle weakness can develop from various causes. However, direct damage to skeletal muscle fibers has been demonstrated in some plant poisonings.

Species of *Thermopsis* (Fam. Leguminosae) grow commonly in the foothills and plains of the Rocky Mountains. Mature seeds of these plants are formed in pods, as in many legumes. Seeds of the poisonous species of *Thermopsis* contain quinolizidine alkaloids, principally anagyrine (see Fig. 27-7) and thermopsine. Human poisoning from eating the seeds is rare, but cases have been reported in young children (Spoerke et al., 1988). The symptoms in children are abdominal cramps, nausea, vomiting, and headache lasting up to 24 h. Serious poisoning has occurred in livestock grazing on *Thermopsis montana* (false lupine). The animals develop depression, prolonged recumbency, and microscopic areas of necrosis in skeletal muscle (Keeler and Baker, 1990).

Among the common contaminants of animal feeds are seeds of *Cassia obtusifolia* (sicklepod, Fam. Leguminosae). Another species, *C. acutifolia* (senna), is used as a laxative. Senna contains emodin, an anthraquinone that increases peristalsis in the human lower GI tract. Consumption of the seeds of *C. obtusifolia* causes illness in cattle, swine, and chicken. The toxic effect is a degenerative myopathy of cardiac and skeletal muscle. It has been shown that extracts of *C. obtusifolia* inhibit NADH-oxidoreductase activity in bovine and porcine heart mitochondria in vitro (Lewis and Shibamoto, 1989), possibly related to the anthraquinone content of *C. obtusifolia*.

## Blood

Cyanogens are constituents of several different kinds of plants. One that is present in the kernels of apples, cherries, peaches, and related genera in the Rosaceae (rose family) is called amygdalin and is found in the highest amounts in the seeds of the bitter almond, *Prunus amygdalus,* var. *amara*. In the 1960s amygdalin (Fig. 27-5) achieved some popular use as a cancer cure under the name Laetrile, although its value was never demonstrated. Amygdalin is not present in the seeds of the sweet almond, the nuts used as food. The amount of cyanogen in peach kernels is enough to cause poisoning in small children if several kernels are eaten. The small seeds of apples do not contain enough cyanogen to present a problem. Taylor (1875), when asked his professional opinion regarding a case of cyanide poisoning presumed to result from eating apples and swallowing the seeds, estimated that the required amount would involve the consumption at one time of the seeds from 160 apples, an unlikely event even for a dedicated apple lover. However, bitter almonds contain enough amygdalin to cause serious poisoning. In the stomach, amygdalin releases hydrocyanic acid, which combines with ferric ion in cytochrome oxidase or methemoglobin. The result of the ingestion of several bitter almond seeds is classic cyanide poisoning with death as in asphyxia.

Cassava is a staple food starch from *Manihot esculenta*, which is grown extensively in some parts of Africa as a major food source. The untreated root contains linamarin, a cyanogenic glucoside (Fig. 27-5). During processing of the root for human consumption, the cyanogen is removed. However, local processing may be inadequate. Chronic ingestion of linamarin in cassava has been proposed as the cause of epidemics of konzo, a form of tropical myelopathy with a sudden onset of spastic paralysis (Tylleskar et al., 1992). Another plant containing linamarin is flax, *Linum usitatissumum*, the seed of which is the source of linseed oil. In some European countries, as a domestic remedy, linseeds are soaked overnight and the extract is used as a laxative, exposing these individuals to cyanide from the content of linamarin (Rosling, 1993).

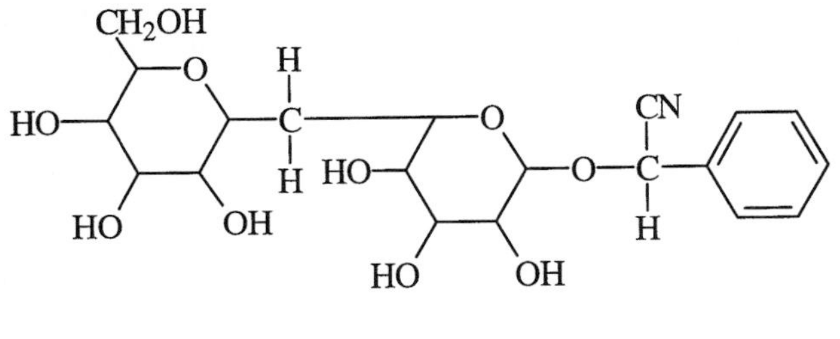

## Bone

In 1967, Worker and Carrillo proposed that a decrease of calcification and wasting in grazing cattle along the eastern coastal plains of South America was due to the consumption of *Solanum malacoxylon* (nightshade family, Solanaceae). They recognized the association of the presence of the plant in the fields with the condition. The disease, known in Argentina as "*enteque seco*," is characterized by calcification of the entire vascular system, especially the heart and aorta. Lungs, joint cartilage, and kidney are affected in the worst cases. The general picture resembles vitamin D intoxication. A water-soluble vitamin D–like substance, a glycoside of 1,25-dihydroxycholecalciferol [1,25-(OH)2-$D_3$], has been isolated from the leaves of the plant. Sheep and cows are both affected by ingestion of the plant. In experiments, rats that received doses of the vitamin $D_3$ derivative purified from the plant showed hyperosteoidosis followed by mineralization of the excessive osteoid after the cessation of dosing (Woodard et al., 1993).

*Cestrum diurnum* (day-blooming jasmine) is a calcinogenic plant that causes hypercalcemia and extensive soft tissue calcification in grazing animals in Florida, resembling the action of *S. malacoxylon*. A dihydroxyvitamin $D_3$ glycoside in the leaves has been proposed as the toxic agent (Hughes et al., 1977).

## Lung

Pyrrolidizine alkaloids are well known for causing a form of hepatitis in humans and livestock. Monocrotaline from seeds of *Crotalaria spectabilis* is one of these alkaloids (Fig. 27-4). In the laboratory, mice and guinea pigs are resistant while rats are highly susceptible. At doses below those causing severe hepatic venous endophlebitis, rats develop pulmonary disease. The condition in rats has been used to study the pathogenesis of pulmonary hypertension. In the rat monocrotaline is converted in the liver into an active pyrrolic metabolite that is responsible for the cardiopulmonary lesions (Schultze et al.,

AMYGDALIN

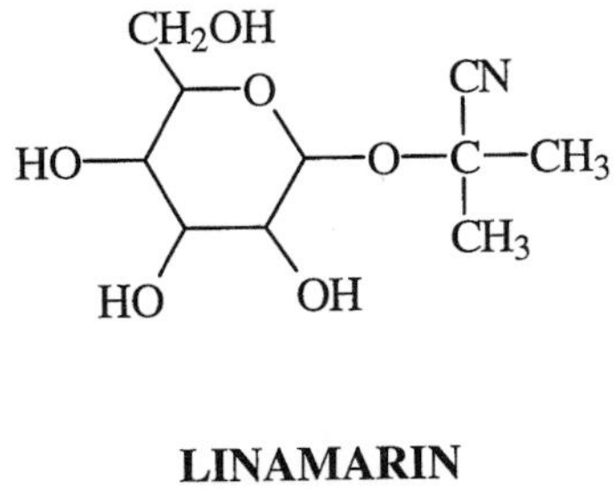

LINAMARIN

***Figure 27–5. Plant cyanogens.***

1991). The transport of pyrrole metabolites to lung from liver is augmented by red blood cells (Pan et al., 1991).

It has been found that workers who handle certain peppers, *Capsicum annum* (cayenne pepper) and *C. frutescens* (chili pepper), have a significantly increased incidence of cough during the day. The irritant ingredient in *Capsicum* is capsaicin (Fig. 27-6). Capsaicin-sensitive nerves in the airway are involved in the irritation and cough (Blanc et al., 1991). Sensory endings of C fibers are part of the cough reflex, and the principal neurotransmitter for these fibers is the neuropeptide substance P. Pure capsaicin depletes substance P stores and blocks further synthesis. The initial release of the transmitter causes pain and irritation, followed by reversible local anesthesia from depletion of substance P. This property of capsaicin has been used in skin creams prescribed for pain. High concentrations of capsaicin can be very irritating. Individuals handling the peppers may experience severe skin irritation and vesication.

## Reproductive System and Teratogenesis

Embryonic loss and teratogenesis in herbivores caused by the ingestion of some plants constitute a serious factor in livestock production worldwide. The types of plants and the abortifacient or teratogenic chemicals they contain are diverse.

*Veratrum californicum* is native to the mountains of western North America where sheep are grazed. An incidence of teratogenesis as high as 25 percent has been reported in pregnant sheep in these areas, along with an incidence of early embryonic death as high as 75 percent (Keeler, 1990). The teratogenic manifestations are dependent on the developmental stage at the time of ingestion, as with many teratogens. The malformations in the offspring involve cyclopia, exencephaly, and microphthalmia. During the fourth and fifth weeks of gestation, limb defects are common; by gestational day 31 to 33, the result of ingestion is stenosis of the trachea (Omnell et al., 1990). The alkaloids in *Veratrum* that are responsible for the defects are jervine (Fig. 27-2), 11-deoxojervine, and 3-*O*-glucosyl-11-deoxojervine. Although there is species difference in sensitivity, birth defects occur in cows and goats grazing on *V. californicum* and can be produced experimentally in chickens, rabbits, rats and mice (Omnell et al., 1990), hamsters (Gaffield and Keeler, 1993), and rainbow trout embryos (Crawford and Kocan, 1993). It has been hypothesized that the *Veratrum* alkaloids are teratogenic by virtue of competing with cytosolic receptors for steroid hormones (Omnell et al., 1990).

A cluster of fetal malformations characterized by deformation of limbs and the spinal cord is found after the ingestion of several related alkaloids during a sensitive gestational period (Fig. 27-7). This syndrome has been found in cattle grazing on *Lupinus caudatus* and *L. formosus* (lupines), *Conium maculatum* (water hemlock), and *Nicotiana glauca* (tree tobacco) (Panter et al., 1990). The active alkaloids in these plants have been identified as anagyrine (*L. caudatus*), ammodendrine (*L. formosus*), anabasine (*N. glauca*), and coniine (*C. maculatum*). It has been proposed that these alkaloids depress fetal movements during susceptible gestational periods and in this way cause bone malformations (Keeler and Panter, 1989).

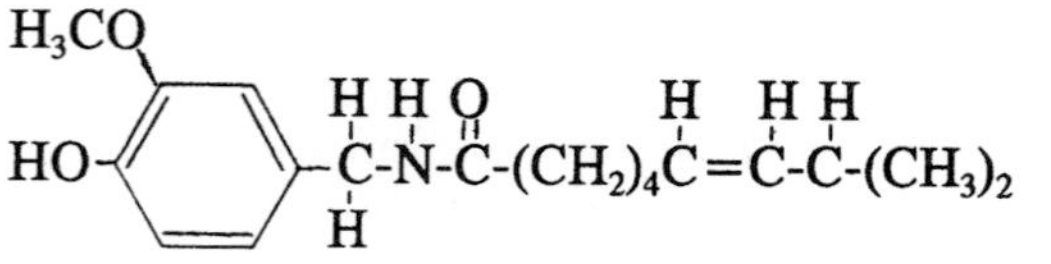

$H_3CO$ / HO / H H O H H H / $-C-N-C-(CH_2)_4C=C-C-(CH_3)_2$ / H

CAPSAICIN

*Figure 27–6. Plant chemical affecting the lung.*

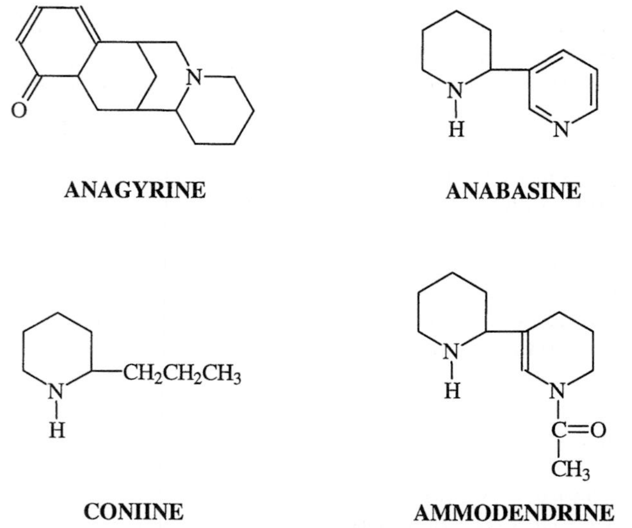

ANAGYRINE ANABASINE

$CH_2CH_2CH_3$ / N–H / $C=O$ / $CH_3$

CONIINE AMMODENDRINE

*Figure 27–7. Plant chemicals causing teratogenesis.*

Two genera from the legume family, *Astragalus* and *Oxytropis*, are both known as locoweed. The active alkaloid is swansonine, the action of which has been described above in the section on the nervous system. Ingestion by pregnant livestock of plants containing swansonine frequently causes abortion (Bunch et al., 1992).

# USES OF TOXIC CHEMICALS FROM PLANTS

Some of the best known toxic chemicals are from plants and have achieved fame as drugs but originally were used for other reasons. One is from a woody climber native to the Malabar coast of India and other mountainous forests of southeastern Asia. In these areas the dark red fruits of the plant *Anamirta cocculus* have been used by throwing the fruit into small ponds to stupefy fish and make them easy to catch. The fruit contains picrotoxin, a powerful convulsant. In the same family of plants to which *Anamirta* belongs, the Menispermaceae, is a plant that produces an equally potent but paralyzing chemical known as curare. The plant is called *Chondrodendron tomentosum* and is found in the jungles of South America, where an extract from it has been used to kill game.

Many plant chemicals are toxic to invertebrates, notably to insects that must consume annually far more plants than do all the large mammalian herbivores. Insecticides abound in plants. The original pyrethrum came from *Pyrethrum roseum* and was known in the nineteenth century as "Persian Powder."

There are many examples of efforts to control populations of invertebrates with plant toxins. One example is the current attempt to control schistosomiasis. Schistomiasis is a widespread parasitic disease of humans in tropical and subtropical regions. The intermediate hosts are species of snails, and the distribution of schistosomiasis is governed by the presence of suitable snails. The latex of *Euphorbia splendens*, a plant native to Brazil, where schistomiasis is endemic, has marked molluscicidal activity at low concentrations and has been proposed for use in controlling snail populations (Schall et al., 1991). Its mechanism of lethality to snails has not been described, but the latex of *E. splendens*, like that of many other species of *Euphorbia*, is irritating to tissues (Freitas et al., 1991).

A saponin with high molluscicidal activity is found in *Phytolacca dodecandra* (Ethiopian soapberry). Saponins are present in concentrations as high as 25 percent of the weight of dried seeds (Parkhurst et al., 1989). The aim is to find a substance toxic to mollusks at concentrations that do not severely alter the ecological balance of other species.

## SUMMARY

Worldwide, there are thousands of plants poisonous to animals in various ways. In the United States alone, Kingsbury (1980) has estimated the number causing serious toxicity to be about 700. Of this number, it is possible to review only a few here. The plants included have been chosen because they are representative of the types of toxic effects caused by plants or because exposure to the plant is of high frequency or importance. Plant toxins are being used as scientific tools as never before, and investigation into the uses of and risks of exposure to toxic plants is correspondingly expanding.

The focus of this review has not been on the treatment of plant poisonings. In the fourth edition of this book, Lampe (1990) covered the treatment of poisoning in detail. Various other reference sources on the treatment of human poisonings are available (*AMA Handbook*, 1985; *Medical Toxicology*, 1988).

# REFERENCES

Alkodon M, Periera EFR, Wonnacott S, Albuquerque EX: Blockade of nicotinic currents in hippocampal neurons defines methyllycaconitine as a potent and specific receptor antagonist. *Mol Pharmacol* 41:802–808, 1992.

*AMA Handbook of Poisonous and Injurious Plants*. Chicago: American Medical Association, 1985.

Benjamin DR: Mushroom poisoning in infants and children. *J Toxicol Clin Toxicol* 30:13–22, 1992.

Bermudez MV, Gonzalez-Spencer D, Guerrero M, et al: Experimental intoxication with fruit and purified toxins of buckthorn (*Karwinskia humboldtiana*). *Toxicon* 24:1091–1097, 1986.

Blanc P, Liu D, Juarez C, Boushey HA: Cough in hot pepper workers. *Chest* 99:27–32, 1991.

Bunch TD, Panter KD, James LK: Ultrasound studies of the effects of certain poisonous plants on uterine function and fetal development in livestock. *J Anim Sci* 70:1639–1643, 1992.

Burke JW, Doskotch RW: High field 1 H- and 13 C-NMR assignments of grayanotoxins I, IV and XIV isolated from *Kalmia angustifolia*. *J Nat Prod* 53:131–137, 1990.

Cappell MS, Hassan T: Gastrointestinal and hepatic effects of *Amanita phalloides* ingestion. *J Clin Gastroenterol* 15:225–228, 1992.

Carballo M, Mudry MD, Larripa IB, et al: Genotoxic action of an aqueous extract of *Heliotropium curassavicum* var. *argentinum*. *Mutat Res* 279:245–253, 1992.

Casteel SW, Johnson GC, Wagstaff DJ: *Aesculus glabra* intoxication in cattle. *Vet Hum Toxicol* 34:55, 1992.

Casteel SW, Wagstaff J: *Rhododendron macrophyllum* poisoning in a group of sheep and goats. *Vet Hum Toxicol* 31:176–177, 1989.

Chan TYF, Tomlinson B, Critchley JAJH, Cockram CS: Herb-induced aconitine poisoning presenting as tetraplegia. *Vet Hum Toxicol* 36:133–134, 1994.

Clark RF, Selden BS, Curry SC: Digoxin-specific Fab fragments in the treatment of Oleander toxicity in a canine model. *Ann Emerg Med* 20:1073–1077, 1991.

Crawford L, Kocan RM: Steroidal alkaloid toxicity to fish embryos. *Toxicol Lett* 66:175–181, 1993.

Fett-Netto AG, DiCosmo F: Distribution and amounts of taxol in different shoot parts of *Taxus cuspidata*. *Planta Med* 58:464–466, 1992.

Franz H (ed): Mistletoe: Pharmacologically relevant components of *Viscum album* L. *Oncology* 43(Suppl 1):1–70, 1986.

Freitas JC, Presgrave OA, Fingola FF, et al: Toxicological study of the molluscicidal latex of *Euphorbia splendens*: Irritant action on skin and eye. *Mem Inst Oswaldo Cruz* 86(Suppl 2):87–88, 1991.

Frohn A, Frohn C, Steuhl KP, Thiel H: Wolfsmilchverätzung. *Ophthalmology* 90:58–61, 1993.

Gaffield W, Keeler RF: Implications of C-5, C-6 unsaturation as a key structural factor in steroidal alkaloid-induced mammalian teratogenesis. *Experientia* 49:922–924, 1993.

Garza-Ocanas L, Hsieh GC, Acosta D, et al: Toxicity assessment of toxins T-514 and T-544 of buckthorn (*Karwinskia humboldtiana*) in primary skin and liver cell cultures. *Toxicology* 73:191–201, 1992.

Gmelin R: Isolierung von Willardiin (3-(1-uracyl)-L-alanin) aus den samen von *Acacia millefolia*, *Acacia lemmoni* and *Mimosa asperata*. *Acta Chem Scand* 15:1188–1189, 1961.

Gude M, Hausen MD, Heitsch H, Konig WA: An investigation of the irritant and allergenic properties of daffodils (*Narcissus pseudonarcissus* L., Amaryllidaceae): A review of daffodil dermatitis. *Contact Dermatitis* 19:1–10, 1988.

Gundidza M, Kufa A: Skin irritant and tumour promoting extract from the latex of *Euphorbia bougheii*. *Cent Afr J Med* 39:56–60, 1993.

Gundidza M, Sorg B, Hecker E: A skin irritant phorbol ester from *Euphorbia cooperi* N E Br. *Cent Afr J Med* 38:444–447, 1992.

Hausen BM, Prater E, Schubert H: The sensitizing capacity of Alstroemeria cultivars in man and guinea pig. *Contact Dermatitis* 9:46–54, 1983.

Hernandez-Cruz A, Munoz-Martinez EJ: Tullidora (*Karwinskia humboldtiana*) toxin mainly affects fast conducting axons. *Neuropathol Appl Neurobiol* 10:11–24, 1984.

Hill NS, Thompson FN, Dawe DL, Stuedemann JA: Antibody binding by circulating ergot alkaloids in cattle grazing tall fescue. *Am J Vet Res* 55:419–424, 1994.

Hughes MR, McCain TA, Chang SY, et al: Presence of 1,25-dihydroxyvitamin $D_3$-glycoside in the calcinogenic plant *Cestrum diurnum*. *Nature* 268:347–348, 1977.

Hyde EG, Carmichael WW: Anatoxin-a(s), a naturally occurring organophosphate, is an irreversible active site-directed inhibitor of acetylcholinesterase (E.C.3.1.1.7). *J Biochem Toxicol* 6:195–201, 1991.

Jaeger A, Jehl F, Flesch F, et al: Kinetics of amatoxins in human poisoning: Therapeutic implications. *Clin Toxicol* 31:63–80, 1993.

Jaffe AM, Gephardt D, Courtemanche L: Poisoning due to ingestion of *Veratrum viride* (false hellebore). *J Emerg Med* 8:161–167, 1990.

James LF, Panter KE, Broquist HP, Hartley WJ: Swainsonine-induced high mountain disease in calves. *Vet Hum Toxicol* 33:217–219, 1991.

Johnson RA, Baer H, Kirkpatrick CH, et al: Comparison of the contact allergenicity of the four pentadecylcatchols derived from poison ivy urushiol in human subjects. *J Allergy Clin Dermatol* 49:27–35, 1972.

Kalish RS, Johnson KL: Enrichment and function of urushiol (Poison Ivy)-specific T lymphocytes in lesions of allergic contact dermatitis to urushiol. *J Immunol* 145:3706–3713, 1990.

Keeler RF: Early embryonic death in lambs induced by *Veratrum californicum*. *Cornell Vet* 80:203–207, 1990.

Keeler RF, Baker DC: Myopathy in cattle induced by alkaloid extracts from *Thermopsis montana*, *Laburnum anagyroides* and a Lupinus sp. *J Comp Pathol* 103:169–182, 1990.

Keeler RF, Panter KE: Piperidine alkaloid composition and relation to crooked calf disease-inducing potential of *Lupinus formosus*. *Teratology* 40:423–432, 1989.

Kelch WJ, Kerr LA, Adair HS, Boyd GD: Suspected buttercup (*Ranunculus bulbosus*) toxicosis with secondary photosensitization in a Charolais heifer. *Vet Hum Toxicol* 34:238–239, 1992.

Kingsbury JM: Phytotoxicology, in Doull J, Klaassen CD, Amdur M (eds): *Casarett and Doull's Toxicology*, 2d ed. New York: Macmillan, 1980, pp 578–590.

Knight TE: Philodendron-induced dermatitis: Report of cases and review of the literature. *Cutis* 48:375–378, 1991.

Lampe KF: Toxic effects of plant toxins, in Amdur MO, Doull J, Klaassen CD (eds): *Casarett and Doull's Toxicology*, 4th ed. New York, Macmillan, 1990, pp 804–815.

Lewis DC, Shibamoto T: Effects of *Cassia obtusifolia* (sicklepod) extracts and anthraquinones on muscle mitochondrial function. *Toxicon* 27:519–529, 1989.

Libri V, Das B, Constanti A: Ganglionic nicotinic receptor agonists exhibit anti-muscarinic effects in guinea-pig olfactory cortical brain slices. *Eur J Pharmacol* 212:253–258, 1992.

Maggi CA, Palacchini R, Tramontana M, et al: Similarities and differences in the action of resiniferatoxin and capsaicin on central and peripheral endings of primary sensory neurons. *Neuroscience* 37:531–539, 1990.

McDermott WV, Ridker PM: The Budd-Chiari syndrome and hepatic veno-occlusive disease. *Arch Surg* 125:525–527, 1990.

McIntire MS, Guest JR, Porterfield JF: Philodendron—an infant death. *J Toxicol Clin Toxicol* 28:177–183, 1990.

McKiernan TL, Bock K, Leya F, et al: Ergot induced peripheral vascular insufficiency, noninterventional treatment. *Cathet Cardiovasc Diagn* 31:211–214, 1994.

*Medical Toxicology: Diagnosis and Treatment of Human Poisoning*. New York: Elsevier, 1988.

Mello JR, Habermehl: Calcinogenic plants and the incubation effect of rumen fluid. *DTW Dtsch Tierarztl Wochenschr* 99:371–376, 1992.

Mendis S: Colchicine cardiotoxicity following ingestion of *Gloriosa superba* tubers. *Postgrad Med J* 65:752–755, 1989.

Monzingo AF, Collins EJ, Ernst SR, et al: The 2.5 Å structure of pokeweed antiviral protein. *J Mol Biol* 233:705–715, 1993.

Murai M, Kimura I, Kimura M: Blocking effects of hypaconitine and aconitine on nerve action potentials in phrenic nerve-diaphragm muscles of mice. *Neuropharmacology* 29:567–572, 1990.

Musshoff F, Jacob B, Fowinkel C, Daldrup T: Suicidal yew leaves ingestion—phloroglucindimethylether (3,5-dimethylphenyl) as a marker for poisoning from *Taxus baccata*. *Int J Legal Med* 106:45–50, 1993.

Narahashi T: Modulators acting on sodium and calcium channels: Patch-clamp analysis. *Adv Neurol* 44:211–224, 1986.

Norred WP: Fumonisins—mycotoxins produced by *Fusarium moniliforme*. *J Toxicol Environ Health* 38:309–328, 1993.

Oliver F, Amon EU, Breathnach A, et al: Contact urticaria due to the common stinging nettle (*Urtica dioica*)—histological, ultrastructural and pharmacological studies. *Clin Exp Dermatol* 16:1–7, 1991.

Omnell ML, Sun FRP, Keeler RF, et al: Expression of Veratrum alkaloid teratogenicity in the mouse. *Teratology* 42:105–119, 1990.

Onat FY, Yegen BC, Lawrence R, et al: Mad honey poisoning in man and rat. *Rev Environ Health* 9:3–9, 1991.

Pamies RJ, Powell R, Herold AH, Martinez J: The Dieffenbachia plant: Case history. *J Fla Med Assoc* 79:760-761, 1992.

Pan LC, Lame MW, Morin D, et al: Red blood cells augment transport of reactive metabolites of monocrotaline from liver to lung in isolated and tandem liver and lung preparations. *Toxicol Appl Pharmacol* 110:336–346, 1991.

Panter KE, Bunch TD, Keeler RF, et al: Multiple congenital contractures (MCC) and cleft palate induced in goats by ingestion of piperidine alkaloid-containing plants: Reduction in fetal movement as the probable cause. *J Toxicol Clin Toxicol* 28:69–83, 1990.

Panter KE, Molyneux RJ, Smart RA, et al: English yew poisoning in 43 cattle. *J Am Vet Assoc* 202:1476–1477, 1993.

Parkhurst RM, Mthupha BM, Liang Y-S, et al: The molluscicidal activity of *Phytolacca dodecandra*: I. Location of the activating esterase. *Biochem Biophys Res Commun* 158:436–439, 1989.

Patneau DK, Mayer ML, Jane DE, Watkins JC: Activation and desensitization of AMPA/kainate receptors by novel derivatives of Willardiine. *J Neurosci* 12:595–606, 1992.

Peper K, Trautwein W: The effect of aconitine on the membrane current in cardiac muscle. *Pflugers Arch* 296:328–336, 1967.

Petroski RJ, Powell RG, Clay K: Alkaloids of *Stipa robusta* (sleepygrass) infected with an Acremonium endophyte. *Nat Toxins* 1:84–88, 1992.

Pfister JA, Panter KE, Manners GD: Effective dose in cattle of toxic alkaloids from tall larkspur (*Delphinium barbeyi*). *Vet Hum Toxicol* 36:10-11, 1994.

Prabhasankar P, Raguputhi G, Sundaravadivel B, et al: Enzyme-linked immunosorbent assay for the phytotoxin thevetin. *J Immunoassay* 14:279–296, 1993.

Pusztai A, Ewen SWB, Grant G, et al: Antinutritive effects of wheatgerm agglutinin and other *N*-acetylglucosamine-specific lectins. *Br J Nutr* 70:313–321, 1993.

Rasmussen MA, Allison MJ, Foster JG: Flatpea intoxication in sheep and indications of ruminal adaptation. *Vet Hum Toxicol* 35:123–127, 1993.

Ridker PM, Ohkuma S, McDermott WV, et al: Hepatic venocclusive disease associated with the consumption of pyrrolizidine-containing dietary supplements. *Gastroenterology* 88:1050-1054, 1985.

Riley RT, Hinton DM, Chamterlain WJ, et al: Dietary fumonisin $B_1$ induces disruption of sphingolipid metabolism in Sprague-Dawley rat: A new mechanism of nephrotoxicity. *J Nutr* 124:594–603, 1994.

Rondeau ES: Wisteria toxicity. *J Toxicol* 31:107–112, 1993.

Rosell S, Samuelsson G: Effect of mistletoe viscotoxin and phoratoxin on blood circulation. *Toxicon* 26:975–987, 1988.

Rosling R: Cyanide exposure from linseed. *Lancet* 341:177, 1993.

Sako MDN, Al-Sultan II, Saleem AN: Studies on sheep experimentally poisoned with *Hypericum perforatum*. *Vet Hum Toxicol* 35:298–300, 1993.

Schall VT, Vasconcellos MA, Valent GU, et al: Evaluation of the genotoxic activity and acute toxicity of *Euphorbia splendens* latex, a molluscicide for the control of schistosomiasis. *Braz J Med Biol Res* 24:573–582, 1991.

Schultze AE, Wagner JG, White SM, Roth RA: Early indications of monocrotaline pyrrole-induced lung injury in rats. *Toxicol Appl Pharmacol* 109:41–50, 1991.

Sharma OP, Dawra RK, Pattabhi V: Molecular structure, polymorphism, and toxicity of lantadene A, the pentacyclictriterpenoid from the hepatotoxic plant *Lantana camara*. *J Biochem Toxicol* 6:57–63, 1991.

Sharma OP, Makkar AP, Dawra RK: A review of the noxious plant *Lantana camara*. *Toxicon* 26:975–987, 1988.

Short SO, Edwards WC: Blue green algae toxicosis in Oklahoma. *Vet Hum Toxicol* 32:558–560, 1990.

Smith EA, Meloan CE, Pickell JA, et al: Scopolamine poisoning from homemade "Moon Flower" wine. *J Anal Toxicol* 15:216–219, 1991.

Southcott RV, Haegi LAR: Plant hair dermatitis. *Med J Aust* 156:623–628, 1992.

Spencer PS, Roy DN, Ludolph A, et al: Lathyrism: Evidence for the role of the neuroexcitatory amino acid, BOAA. *Lancet* 2:1066–1067, 1986.

Spoerke DG, Murphy MM, Wruck KM, Rumack BH: Five cases of Thermopsis poisoning. *J Toxicol Clin Toxicol* 26:397–406, 1988.

Stirpe F, Licastro F, Morini MC, et al: Purification and partial characterization of a mitogenic lectin from the latex of *Euphorbia marginata*. *Biochem Biophys Acta* 1158:33–39, 1993.

Stollard D, Edes TE: Muscarinic poisoning from medications and mushrooms. *Postgrad Med* 85(1):341–345, 1989.

Szallasi A, Blumberg PM: Resiniferatoxin, a phorbol-related diterpene, acts as an ultrapotent analog of capsaicin, the irritant constituent in red pepper. *Neuroscience* 30:515–520, 1989.

Tahirov THO, Lu T-H, Liaw Y-C, et al: A new crystal form of abrin-a from the seeds of *Abrus precatorius*. *J Mol Biol* 235:1152–1153, 1994.

Tandon HD, Tandon BN, Mattocks AR: An epidemic of veno-occlusive disease of the liver in Afghanistan. *Am J Gastroenterol* 70:607–613, 1978.

Taylor AS: *On Poisons*. Philadelphia: Henry C. Lea, 1875.

Teitelbaum JS, Zatorre RJ, Carpenter S, et al: Neurologic sequelae of domoic acid intoxication due to the ingestion of contaminated mussels. *N Engl J Med* 322:1781–1787, 1990.

Tulsiani DR, Broquest HP, James LF, Touster O: Production of hybrid glycoproteins and accumulation of oligosaccharides in the brain of sheep and pigs administered swansonine or locoweed. *Arch Biochem Biophys* 264:607–617, 1988.

Tylleskar T, Banea M, Bikongi N, et al: Cassava cyanogens and konzo, an upper motoneuron disease found in Africa. *Lancet* 339:208–211, 1992.

Underhill FP: *Toxicology*. Philadelphia: P. Blakiston's, 1924.

Urushibata O, Kase K: Irritant contact dermatitis from *Euphorbia marginata*. *Contact Dermatitis* 24:155–157, 1991.

Van den Bosch C, Griffin BE, Kazembe P, et al: Are plant factors a missing link in the evolution of endemic Burkitt's lymphoma? *Br J Cancer* 68:1232–1235, 1993.

van der Lugt JJ, Nel PW, Kitching JP: The pathology of *Cestrum laevigatum* (Schlechtd.) poisoning in cattle. *Onderstepoort J Vet Res* 58:211–221, 1991.

Van Meurs A, Cohen A, Edelbroek P: Atropine poisoning after eating chapattis contaminated with *Datura stramonium* (thorn apple). *Trans R Soc Trop Med Hyg* 86:221, 1992.

Wieland T, Faulstich H: Fifty years of amanitin. *Experientia* 47:1186–1193, 1991.

Wilhelm H, Wilhelm B, Schiefer U: Mydriasis caused by plant contact. *Fortschr Ophthalmol* 88:588–591, 1991.

Woodard JC, Berra G, Ruksan B, et al: Toxic effects of *Solanum malacoxylon* on sheep bone. *Bone* 14:787–797, 1993.

Worker NA, Carrillo BJ: "Enteque seco," calcification and wasting in grazing animals in the Argentine. *Nature* 215:72–74, 1967.

Yoshizawa T, Yamashita A, Luo Y: Fumonisin occurrence in corn from high- and low-risk areas for human esophageal cancer in China. *Appl Environ Microbiol* 60:1626–1629, 1994.

# UNIT 6

# ENVIRONMENTAL TOXICOLOGY

CHAPTER 28

# AIR POLLUTION

*Daniel L. Costa and Mary O. Amdur*

## AIR POLLUTION IN PERSPECTIVE

Despite early recognition and centuries of concern, pollution of the atmosphere remains a major public health issue. The fires of early cave dwellers polluted the indoor air of their homes and, when eventually vented outdoors, affected the air around their villages. With time and urbanization, energy demands led to the ambient release of sulfurous, sooty smoke from the burning of coal. The poor quality of urban air did not go unnoticed by early writers such as Seneca, the Roman philosopher, who in A.D 61 wrote: "As soon as I had gotten out of the heavy air of Rome, and from the stink of the chimneys thereof, which being stirred, poured forth whatever pestilential vapors and soot they had enclosed in them, I felt an alteration to my disposition" (Miller and Miller, 1993).

The regulation of air pollution evolved more slowly. Beginning in the thirteenth century, periodic community-based efforts were made, such as the banning of domestic burning of "sea coal" in London by Edward I. However, people had largely resigned themselves to accepting polluted air as part of urban life. Later, the industrial revolution, which was powered by the burning of mined coal, added a second dimension to pollution of the atmosphere. Power plants were built to provide energy for factories and to light homes. Steel mills grew up along riverbanks and lakeshores, oil refineries rose in port cities and near oil fields, and smelters roasted and refined metals in areas near large mineral deposits.

By 1925 air pollution was common to all industrialized nations, and many people found it intolerable. Public surveys were initiated—Salt Lake City in 1926, New York City in 1937, Leicester, Great Britain, in 1939—to bring attention to the problem and promote the need for controls (Miller and Miller, 1993). However, it was the great air pollution disasters in the Meuse Valley, Belgium, in 1930 and Donora, Pennsylvania, in 1948 and the great London fog of 1952 that fully indicted air pollution as a health problem. In the United States, California led the way with passage of the Air Pollution Control Act of 1947 to regulate the discharge of opaque smoke. Visibility problems in Pittsburgh during the 1940s prompted efforts to control smoke from local industries. It was the initiative of President Truman in the late 1940s that led to federal efforts to deal with air pollution that culminated in congressional passage of a series of acts starting with the Air Pollution Control Act of 1955.

Postwar America viewed belching smokestacks as a symbol of prosperity and economic status. In the 1950s, suburban communities sprawled around industrial centers and cities as the public sought healthier and cleaner lifestyles. It was the adoption of the commuting automobile that brought the third and perhaps most chemically complex dimension to air pollution. The term "smog," though originally coined to describe the mixture of smoke and fog that hung over large cities such as London, was curiously adopted to refer to the eye-irritating photochemical reaction products of auto exhaust that blanketed cities such as Los Angeles and Denver. Early federal legislation addressing stationary sources was soon expanded to include automobile-derived pollutants (the Clean Air Act of 1963, amended in 1967, and the Motor Vehicle Air Pollution Control Act of 1965). The Clean Air Act amendment of 1970 established the U.S. Environmental Protection Agency (EPA) and charged it with the responsibility to protect the public from the hazards of polluted outdoor air.

The latest chapter in the air pollution story concerns the fugitive release of specific chemicals or combustion products as a result of accidents or inadequate facility emission controls. Without doubt, no accidental release has had the political impact or personal devastation of the December 3, 1984, industrial release of 30 tons of methyl isocyanate vapor into the air over the shanty community in Bhopal, India. An estimated 3000 people died, and 200,000 were injured and/or permanently impaired. However, accidental releases or spills of toxic chemicals in the United States are surprisingly common, with 4375 cases recorded between 1980 and 1987, inflicting 11,341 injuries and 309 deaths (Waxman, 1994). Other chemicals, such as phosgene, benzene, butadiene, and dioxin, also occur in the air near populated industrial centers and draw concern regarding their chronic health effects. The slow progress of regulatory decisions (only eight between 1970 and 1990) on hazardous air pollutants led to mandated acceleration of the process under the amendments to the Clean Air Act of 1990. Section 112(b) listed 189 chemicals and substances for which special standards and risk assessments were required by the end of the decade. The chemicals listed were those of greatest concern on the basis of toxicity (including cancer) and estimated release volumes.

Internationally, the magnitude and control of air pollution vary considerably, especially among developing nations, which often forgo concerns for health and welfare because of cost and the desire to achieve prosperity. Figure 28-1 illustrates some of the variation among international megacities in regard to three major urban pollutants: total suspended particulate matter (TSP), sulfur oxides ($SO_x$), and ozone ($O_3$). Most recently, the political upheaval in eastern Europe has revealed that for decades that area has suffered considerably from uncontrolled industrial pollution. Clearly, the problems of air pollution remain significant even as we enter the twenty-first century. In all probability, "international pollution" will emerge as a major issue involving concerns such as the long-range transport of polluted air masses from one country to another. Such an issue can polarize neighboring nations, as has occurred with Canada and the United States as a result of the transport of midwestern industrial sulfates into southeastern Ontario. Organizations such as the World Health Organization

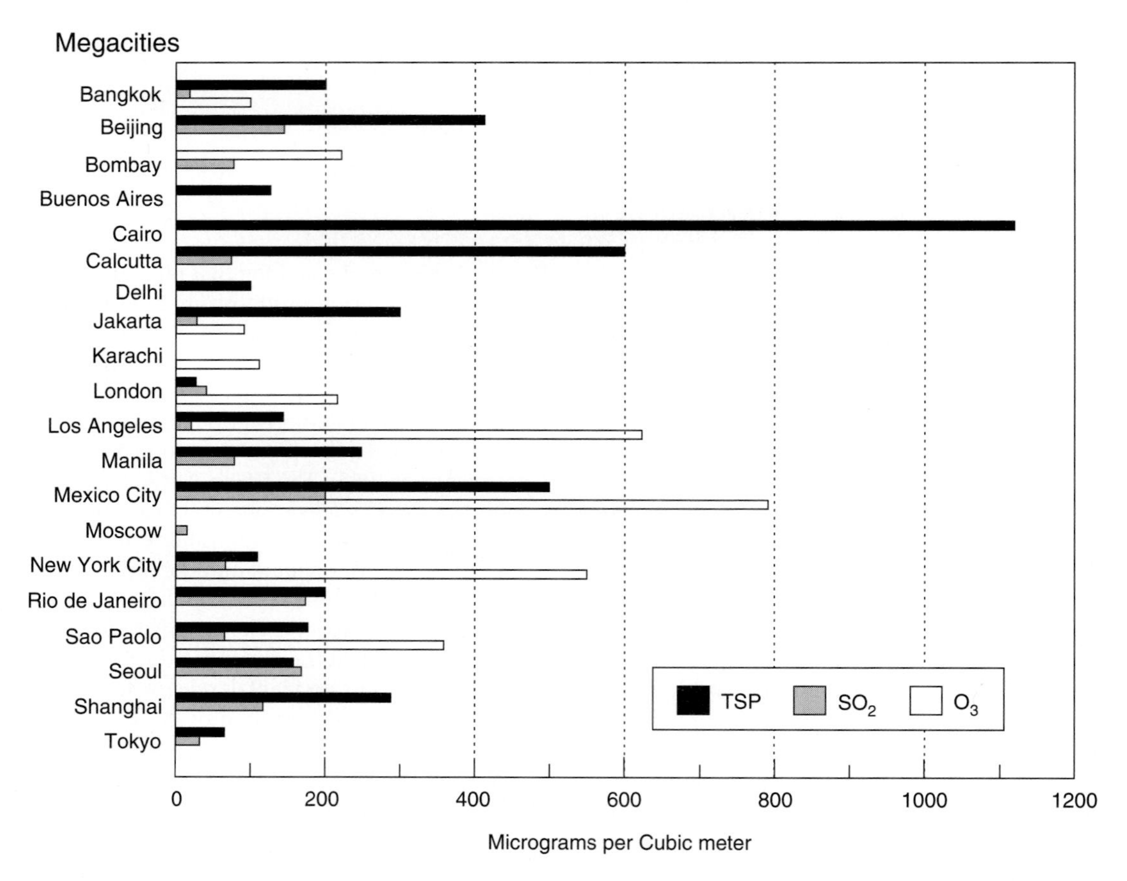


***Figure 28–1.** Comparison of ambient levels of 1-h maximum ozone, annual average of total suspended particulate matter, and sulfur dioxide in selected cities from around the world to illustrate the variation in these levels from country to country with respect to the United States. [Reproduced from the National Air Quality and Emission Trends Report (1992), with permission.]*

(WHO) are attempting to derive air quality standards as a rational basis for directing control measures within Europe, but to date such international recommendations are not binding (Lipfert, 1994).

## HEALTH RESEARCH IN AIR POLLUTION

The health database used to evaluate the hazards of specific air pollutants has been derived from animal toxicology, controlled human studies, and epidemiology. Because each of these research approaches has inherent strengths and limitations, an appropriate assessment of an air pollutant requires the careful integration and interpretation of data from all three methodologies. Thus, one should be aware of the attributes of each to assure the best possible assessment.

Animal toxicology is used to predict effects in humans and elucidate pathogenic mechanisms that may aid in extrapolation. Toxicology studies can involve methods that are not practical in human studies, including diversity of exposure concentrations and durations and an array of invasive biological endpoints. The minimization of uncontrolled variables (e.g., genetic variability and exposure) is perhaps the greatest strength of animal bioassays. However, the clear limitation of this approach lies in the extrapolation of the findings from animals to humans. Ideally, the animal is selected with the knowledge that it responds in a manner similar to the human response (*homology*). Qualitative extrapolation of homologous effects is frequently possible, but quantitative extrapolation is typically clouded by the uncertainties of the relative *sensitivity* of the animal or specific target tissue to the pollutant compared with that of humans as well as uncertainties about the target tissue dose (see below). With respect to the target tissue dose, in recent years animal toxicologists have attempted to keep exposure concentrations at fivefold to 10-fold that of the anticipated human exposure until appropriate dosimetric data are generated. Nevertheless, animal studies provide the largest database on a wide range of air toxicants and have proven utility in predicting human adverse responses to chemicals.

Studies that involve controlled human exposures have been used extensively in studying the most common air pollutants, notably several "Criteria Air Pollutants" regulated by the U.S. Environmental Protection Agency (EPA). For each of these pollutants there exists a Criteria Document, which is a detailed summary of the available database on a pollutant that is then integrated into a staff paper for use by the EPA administrator to set a National Ambient Air Quality Standard (NAAQS). These Criteria Pollutants (Table 28-1), with the exception of lead, which has irreversible effects, are pollutants to which most people are exposed frequently in their daily lives

**Table 28–1**
**U.S. National (Primary) Ambient Air Quality Standards**

| POLLUTANT | UNIT | AVERAGING TIME | CONCENTRATION | STATISTIC |
|---|---|---|---|---|
| Sulfur dioxide | $\mu g/m^3$ | Annual | 80 | Annual mean |
| | | 24 h | 365 | Maximum* |
| Carbon monoxide | $mg/m^3$ | 8 h | 10 | Maximum |
| | | 1 h | 40 | Maximum |
| Ozone | $\mu g/m^3$ | 1 h | 235 | Maximum† |
| Nitrogen dioxide | $\mu g/m^3$ | Annual | 100 | Annual mean |
| Inhalable particulate ($PM_{10}$) | $\mu g/m^3$ | Annual | 50 | Annual mean |
| | | 24 h | 150 | Maximum |
| Lead | $\mu g/m^3$ | 3 months | 1.5 | Quarterly average |

*Maximum values may be exceeded once per year.
†Not to be exceeded more than three times in 3 years.

and thus to which human volunteers can be justifiably exposed in a controlled environment to ascertain reversible responses. Such studies have the obvious advantage of being in the species of concern, eliminating this aspect of the extrapolation paradigm. Additionally, defined "sensitive" groups can be studied to better understand the breadth of response by the exposed public. However, clinical studies have limitations. Ethical issues are involved in every aspect of a clinical test; potentially irreversible effects and carcinogenicity are always of concern, along with the hyperresponsiveness of the so-called sensitive groups. There are obviously restrictions on the biological endpoints that can be studied, though sophistication in medical technology has made possible a greater array of study biomarkers than ever before (e.g., bronchoalveolar lavage fluids and biopsied cells). Also, the variety of toxicants which can be studied is limited, particularly if there is a lack of toxicity data to allay concerns about exposing human subjects. Finally, the cost of such studies, the limited numbers of subjects that usually can be evaluated, and the inability to address chronic exposure issues are also constraints on human testing.

Epidemiological studies have the advantage of revealing associations between exposure to a pollutant or pollutants and the health effect or effects in the *community* or *population* of interest. Because data are garnered directly under real exposure conditions and involve large numbers of humans, the data should be of direct utility to the regulatory community. Moreover, the data frequently are based on long-term exposures and theoretically can account for irreversible effects as well as responses even in population subsets (i.e., sensitive groups). Why, then, is this approach to the study of air pollution not the overwhelming choice of regulators? The difficulty here is that it is often difficult to control independent variables because of the diversity of the study population, its motility, or a lack of personal exposure (dose) data. Also, it is difficult to segregate an individual pollutant from copollutants and meteorological confounders. Thus, at best, associations can be drawn only between the exposure and the effect; rarely is a causal relationship discernible even with strong statistical significance. Recently, however, advances in exposure estimation and study design and analysis (e.g., time series) have allowed epidemiologists to examine relationships with greater confidence and specificity. This type of advance is clearly evident in the study of particulate matter (see below).

Health scientists must be experienced with these approaches if an appropriate estimation of toxic risk or potential hazard is to be determined. However, other scientific disciplines also are integral to the full assessment of the impact of air pollution on society. Chemical and engineering methodologies are used together to detect and control pollutants in the atmosphere and develop empirical test systems to gather information used to evaluate individual toxicity and/or physiochemical interactions. Meteorology relates to the real world by yielding information on the dispersion of pollutants from their sources and the conditions leading to the stagnation of air masses and the accumulation of pollutants. The study of plant pathology reveals the effects of pollutants on commercial and native vegetation. When this is considered along with the impact of pollution on human health and the deterioration of materials and edifices, the economist elucidates to regulators and the public at large the cumulative adversity of pollution and its effects on our standard of living. Plants can also act as sensitive "sentinels," warning us of the impact of pollution.

## EXTRAPOLATION ISSUES AND OTHER MITIGATING FACTORS

Extrapolation is the process of relating empirical study findings to real-world scenarios. Studies in animals are the most dependent on this process. Thus, the selection of an animal species as a toxicological model should involve more than a consideration of cost and convenience. Whenever possible, effects which are homologous between the study species and humans should guide selection of the test species. For example, if irritant responses to an upper airway irritant (sulfur dioxide or formaldehyde) are of interest, the guinea pig with its labile and reactive bronchoconstrictive reflex should be selected over the rat, which is not particularly responsive. By contrast, certain strains of rats exhibit a clear neutrophilic response to deep lung irritants such as ozone that resembles the human response. Other inherent differences between species, often biochemically based, may affect the sensitivity of a species to a particular toxicant (Slade et al., 1985). For that reason, any response revealed in an animal study builds greater confidence when it is replicated in another species. With the advent of new transgenic and knockout strains of mice, specially engineered animals provide toxicologists with a new instrument for the study of air pollutants.

An essential part of the species response is the relative dosimetry of the pollutant along the respiratory tree. Significant advances in studies of the distribution of gaseous and particulate pollutants have been made through the use of sophisticated mathematical models which incorporate parameters of respiratory anatomy and physiology, aerodynamics, and physical chemistry into predictions of deposition and retention. Empirical models combined with theoretical models aid in relating animal toxicity data to humans and help refine the study of injury mechanisms with better estimates of the target dose. Figure 28-2A, B illustrates the application of such an approach to the reactive gas ozone and insoluble 0.6-$\mu$m spherical particles, respectively, as each is distributed along the respiratory tract of humans and rats. Anatomic differences between the species clearly affect the deposition of both gases and particles, but the qualitative and to a large extent quantitative similarities in deposition profiles are noteworthy. This is not surprising if one argues teleologically that each species evolved with similar functional demands (i.e., $O_2$-$CO_2$ exchange) and environmental stresses on the pulmonary system. The extent to which this explanation holds is uncertain, but the utility of animal models for the study of air pollutants, when carefully applied, is evident.

Susceptible subpopulations that may hyperrespond to exposure to a pollutant deserve special mention in discussions of the toxicology of air pollution. Although federal statutes such as the Clean Air Act of 1970 specifically mandate that sensitive populations be protected in the development of NAAQS, little is known about these populations. There are some definable subgroups which are assumed to be susceptible, such as children, the elderly, and those with a preexisting disease (e.g., asthmatics), but the data to substantiate these assumptions are largely deficient. The reasons for this may lie in the difficulty in ethically conducting studies in those who are potentially at higher risk and the general lack of appropriate animal models of those groups. Inroads into this issue have been made, however, in part because of more precise definitions of potential risk factors as researchers design studies and the development of genetically defined animal models. Hence, studies in both animals and human subjects are being devised specifically to investigate the roles of diet (e.g., antioxidant content), exercise (as it relates to dosimetry), and age, gender, and race. In addition, studies in human subjects with mild asthma or heart-lung disease have been conducted to address the degree of sensitivity these compromised groups exhibit. Analogously, animal models with imposed cardiopulmonary impairments are being used more and more to address the same basic questions.

## AIR POLLUTION: SOURCES AND PERSONAL EXPOSURE

In terms of tons of anthropogenic material emitted annually (as of 1992), five major air pollutants account for 98 percent of pollution (Fig. 28-3): carbon monoxide (52 percent), sulfur oxides (14 percent), volatile organic compounds (14 percent), particulate matter (4 percent), and nitrogen oxides (14 percent). The remainder consists of lead, which is down 90 percent since 1983, when it was banned from gasoline, and a myriad of other compounds considered under the category of hazardous air pollutants. For any individual locality, this emission picture can vary widely. In the vicinity of a smelter, for example, sulfur oxides, metals, and/or particulate matter dominate the pollutant profile, while in suburban areas where the automobile is the main source of pollution, carbon monoxide, volatile organic compounds, and nitrogen oxides predominate.

Air pollution initially was distinguished on the basis of the oxidant nature of the atmosphere. The pollution classically referred to by Dickens as "London's particular," in which sulfur dioxide and smoke from incomplete combustion of coal accumulated under fog and in cool temperatures, was termed "reducing-type" air pollution. This reducing-type atmosphere, by the nature of its contaminants, was most often associated with large industrial centers such as New York and London. In contrast, Los Angeles had characteristic "oxidant-type" pollution consisting of hydrocarbons, oxides of nitrogen, and secondary photochemical oxidants such as ozone. In photochemical air pollution, atmospheric reaction products of automobile exhaust and sunlight are concentrated within a meteorologic inversion layer. This condition is today colloquially referred to as "smog."

Each type of air pollution is implicitly seasonal in nature by virtue of the time of year when oil and coal are burned to meet heating and industrial demands versus the time of year when sunlight is most intense and catalyzes reactions among the constituents of auto exhaust. Today, however, this distinction is academic, since modern industrial centers have experienced a considerable reduction in smoky, sulfurous emissions while the proliferation of automobiles contributes tons of oxidant precursors. Thus, major metropolitan areas, notably those in the northeastern United States, have atmospheres with both reducing and oxidant air pollutants. Los Angeles nevertheless remains the prototypical center of photochemical air pollution in this country. However, other megacities, such as Mexico City and Tokyo, have smog levels (not to mention reducing pollutants) that greatly surpass those of any U.S. city.

### Indoor versus Outdoor

People in the United States spend more than 70 percent of their time indoors at work, at school, and at home. This is particularly true of adults, who have relatively less time to participate in outdoor activities, especially at midday, when many pollutants are at the highest levels. Children and outdoor workers, by contrast, are much more likely to encounter outdoor air pollution at its worst, and in fact, because of the relatively high activity levels of these subgroups compared with inactive office workers, their lungs may incur a considerably larger dose. Thus, while it is important to characterize and track pollution levels in outdoor air, the most appropriate measure for exposure should involve a paradigm that addresses the total personal exposure of the individual or group of concern.

The indoor environment has only recently been appreciated in terms of its contribution to total personal exposure. Therefore, there is growing interest in defining exposure from myriad indoor sources. Even obvious sources such as unvented space heaters and poorly vented fireplaces and wood stoves have been poorly characterized until recently. Attention now is being directed toward less apparent and varied sources of indoor contaminants: certain soils and construction masonry

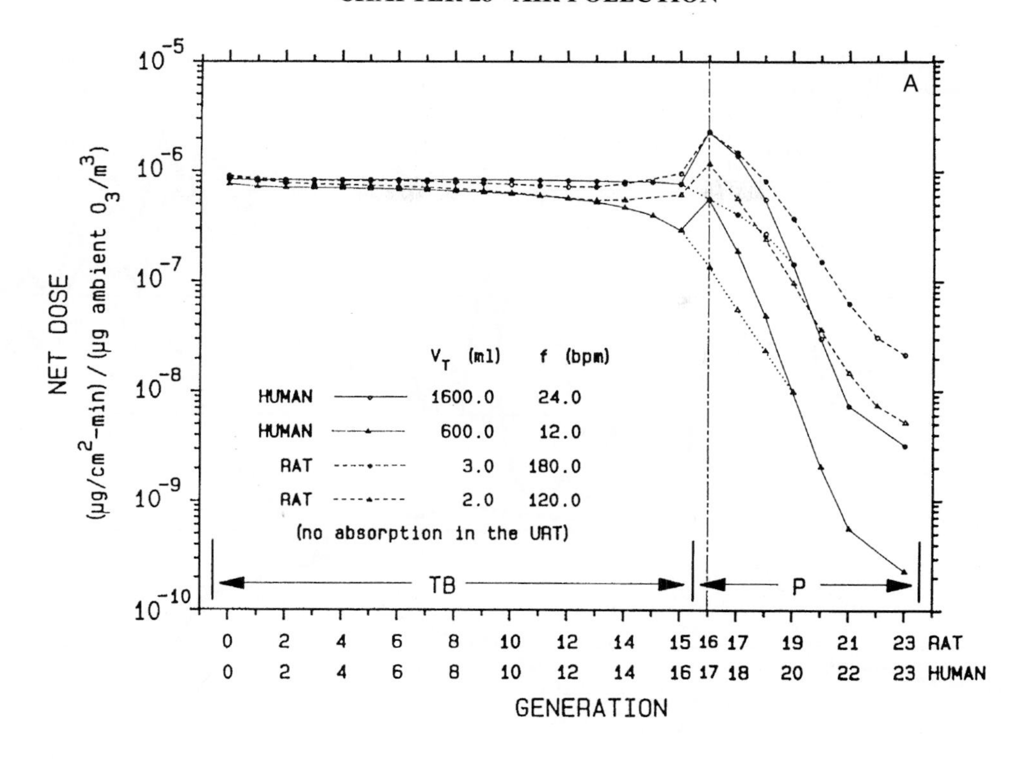


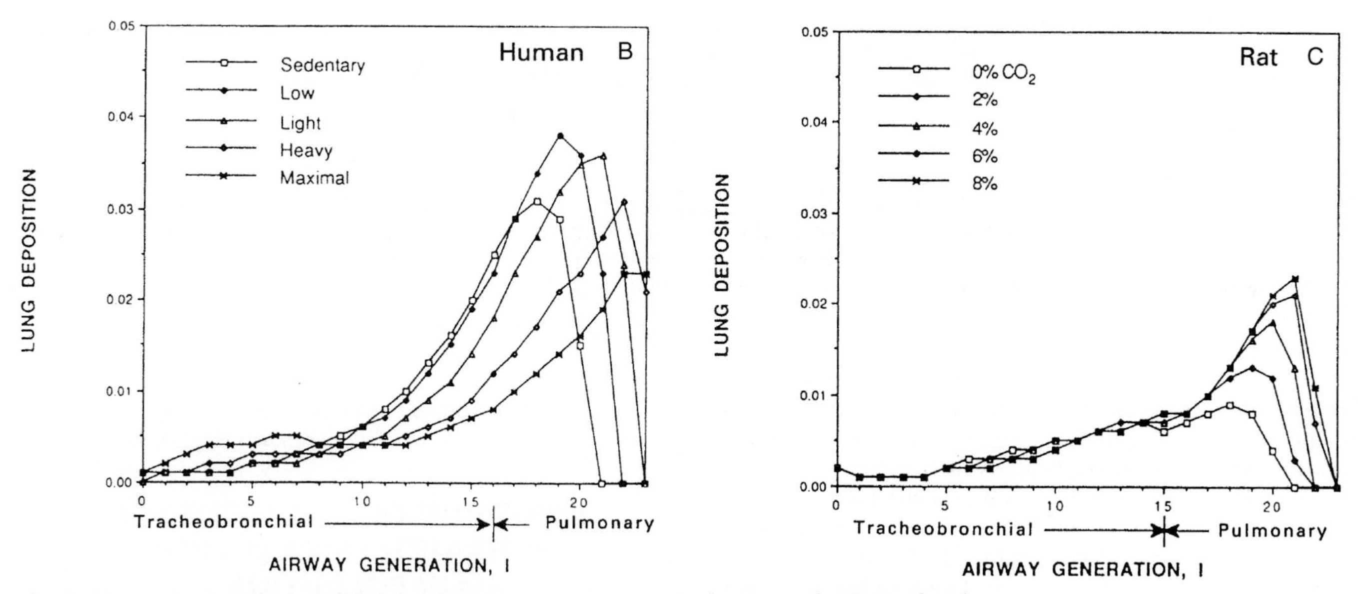


***Figure 28–2.** Theoretical normalized (to the concentration in inspired air) uptake curves for the reactive gas ozone in a resting/exercising human and a rat (A). Likewise, the percent deposition in the airways of a 0.6 µm insoluble particle in the respiratory tracts of a resting/exercising human (B) and rat (C). $CO_2$ in the rat augments ventilation up to threefold at 8 percent in the inspired air.*

Airway generation refers to that airway branch numbered from the trachea (0). [Panel A is from Overton and Miller (1987) and panels B and C are from Martonen et al. (1992). Reproduced with permission.]

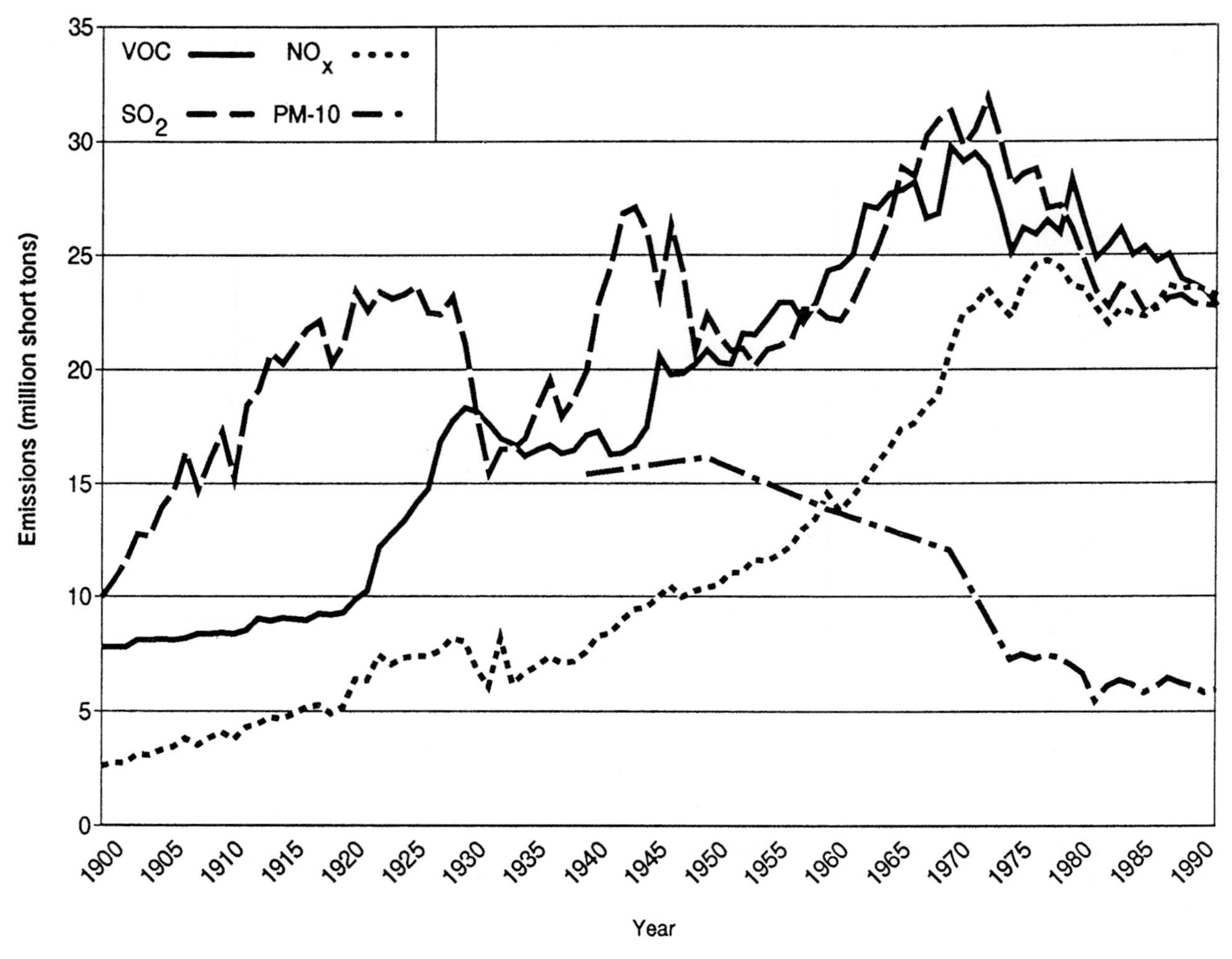


***Figure 28–3. Emission trend for volatile organic compounds (VOC), nitrogen oxides ($NO_x$), sulfur dioxide ($SO_2$), and particluate matter (<10 μm) from 1900 (or when records began) to 1990.***

Note that since the passage of the Clean Air Act of 1970 most emissions have decreased or, in the case of nitrogen oxides, leveled off. [Reproduced from *National Air Pollution Emission Trend, 1900–1992*, with permission.]

(radon), gas cooking appliances (nitrogen oxides), sidestream tobacco smoke (particulate matter, carbon monoxide, and a host of carcinogenic polyaromatics), and carpets, furnishings, dry-cleaned clothes, and household cleaning products [passively emitted volatile organic compounds (VOCs)]. As a result of these multiple sources, indoor air is chemically more complex in some respects than is outdoor air and often exhibits higher ambient concentrations of many of the compounds that had been thought to be limited to outdoor environments (e.g., nitrogen dioxide). Outdoor infiltration into indoor air is another more diffuse source of contamination but one that is poorly defined because of the many variables which determine indoor infiltration of outdoor air. The current evidence suggests that the average insulated home has about one air change per hour, resulting in indoor concentrations of about 30 to 80 percent of that outdoors (e.g., the indoor/outdoor ratio of ozone would be lower because of the reactivity of ozone; the ratio for fine particulate matter (<2.5 μm) would be higher since it can easily penetrate through cracks and open spaces). Clearly, to understand the nature of air pollution and its potential effects on humans, it is necessary to appreciate the complexity of the total exposure scenario (Fig. 28-4).

## EPIDEMIOLOGICAL EVIDENCE OF HEALTH EFFECTS FROM AIR POLLUTION

### Outdoor Air Pollution

**Acute and Episodic Exposures.** There have been a number of documented incidents in which the level of air pollution has risen to concentrations that are definitely hazardous to human health. On occasion, when a single chemical has been accidentally released (e.g., methyl isocyanate in Bhopal, India), establishing the relationship between cause and ill effect is straightforward. However, most air pollution situations involve relatively complex atmospheres, and establishing a specific cause other than the air pollution incident itself can be difficult. Three acute episodes of community air pollution have

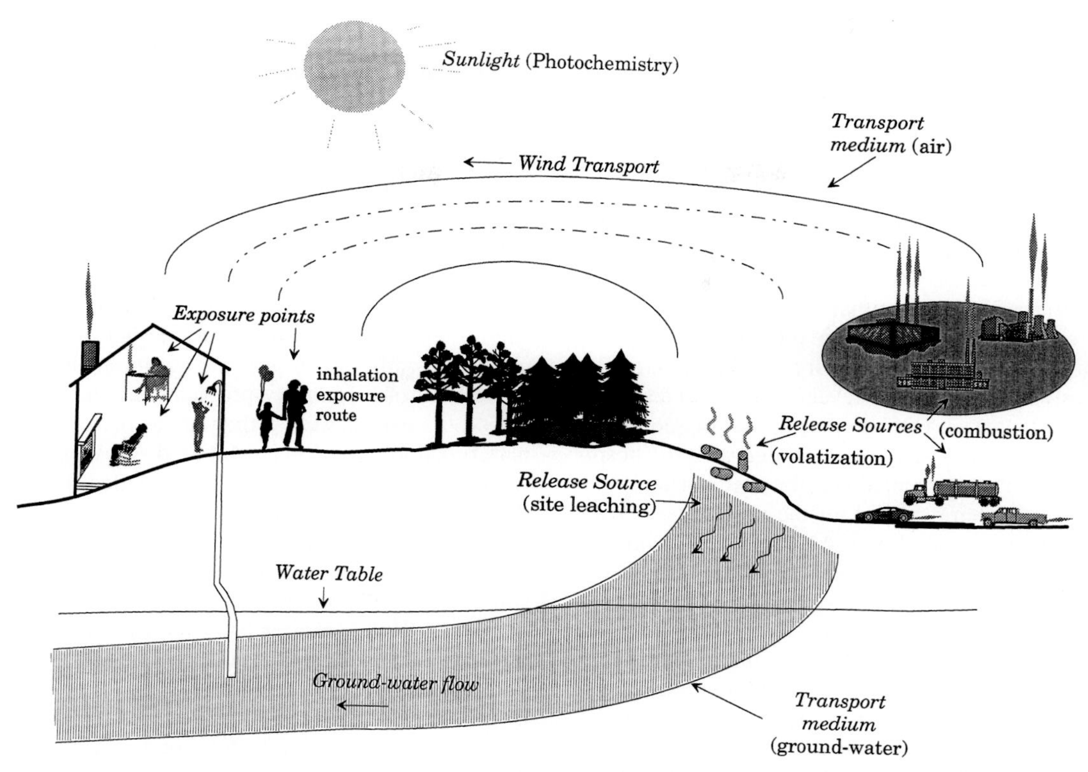


***Figure 28–4. Illustration of contributors to the total personal exposure paradigm showing how these indoor and outdoor factors interact.***

come to be considered classic in the history of air pollution. In each event, community members were clearly affected adversely, with a concomitant elevation in mortality. Although no single contaminant could be fully blamed, the air pollution was the "reducing type" in which coal-derived sulfurous gas and industrial particulate matter (including many metals) accumulated within a blanket of cool moist air (Meuse Valley, Donora, and London). In each case, a meteorologic inversion (cold air capped by warm air with little or no vertical mixing) prevailed for 3 or 4 days, during which time the concentration of pollutants rose well above the normal levels for these already heavily polluted areas. No actual measurements of pollution were made in the Meuse Valley and Donora, but crude measurements of the London fog recorded daily averages of smoke and sulfur dioxide, with the worst day having concentrations of 4.5 mg/m$^3$ and 1.34 ppm, respectively. Brief (on the order of hours) peak concentrations probably reached even higher levels. In the Meuse Valley 65 people died, while in Donora the number was 20. These deaths were considered "excess" deaths compared with normal death rates for that time of year.

The famous "London smog" of 1952 is estimated to have resulted in 4000 excess deaths. Hospital admissions increased dramatically, mainly among the elderly and those with preexisting cardiac and/or respiratory disease. Even otherwise healthy pedestrians, their visibility limited to as little as 3 ft, covered their noses and mouths in an attempt to minimize their exposure to the "choking " air. Those with preexisting health problems who died were unable to cope adequately or had their conditions worsened by the added stress imposed by breathing heavily polluted air. In light of the severity of this incident, it is ironic that 16 years earlier the prediction had been made that if an incident like that in the Meuse Valley occurred in London, some 3200 deaths would result. Historians and epidemiologists have since recounted that there were indeed many earlier incidents in London, though probably none as grave, in which pollution adversely affected the populace. Although the 1952 incident brought the issue of air pollution to consciousness, additional episodes occurred later, with 1956 and 1962 being among the most notable.

The mortality data from the 1952 London incident have been revisited, along with mortality and morbidity data from a host of other cities where particulate matter is a pollutant of relative prominence (Schwartz and Marcus, 1990). These studies have utilized novel time-series analyses to better discriminate the effects of particulate matter from the effects of other pollutants and potential confounders. The collective conclusion from more than 16 urban areas is that particulate matter, including its associated sulfates (see below), has effects on human health even at the level that is considered safe [50 $\mu$g/m$^3$, annual mean particulate matter of diameter $\leq$10 $\mu$m ($PM_{10}$) NAAQS]. Day-to-day fluctuations in the concentration of airborne particulate matter are associated with mortality trends, and for every 100 $\mu$g/m$^3$, there occurs an increase of about 6 percent (excess) mortality (Dockery and Pope, 1994). Moreover, morbidity in terms of hospital visits, inhaler use by asthmatics, and school absenteeism also is associated with ambient particulate levels; temperature, humidity, ozone, and sulfur dioxide per se do not explain the observed effects. Although effects are seen mostly in those already compromised by cardiopulmonary diseases, there is no accepted mechanism to account for these findings (Schwartz, 1994). These measurable effects are considerably below those previously thought to be of concern on the basis of diary studies in lung patients, which had suggested 24-h mean low effect levels for smoke and sulfur dioxide of 250 $\mu g/m^3$ and 0.19 ppm, respectively. As analytic approaches to the study of population responses continue to improve, other disturbing evidence of the adversity of air pollution may be detected.

Recently, a series of studies have shown acute effects of ambient levels of pollution that occur during the summer in areas of northeastern North America. These peaks of pollution are typified by increases in ozone and sulfate. The increase in sulfate reflects both acidic and atmospherically neutralized forms of sulfuric acid. In a southern Ontario–based study, there was a consistent association in the summer between hospital admissions for acute respiratory problems, especially among child asthmatics, and daily levels of ozone and sulfate. Interestingly, the apparent combined temporal or sequential patterns of ozone and sulfate were associated with the hospitalizations, not either constituent alone (Bates and Sizto, 1989). Similar results have been reported for the upstate New York area as well (Thurston et al., 1992). Acidity as $[H^+]$, which is common in summer haze, is thought to play a significant role in these responses. However, studies of children at summer camps where they are active outdoors most of the day have reported decrements in daily measured pulmonary function on days when both ozone and acidity levels were elevated but still below those which would be predicted to have a measurable effect (Lippmann, 1989). Animal toxicology and clinical studies in adolescent asthmatics lend further support to the belief that $H^+$ can affect airway function, particularly in the presence of ozone. Studies in the south and southwest similarly have found effects in young asthmatics, but these effects appear to relate more specifically to ozone. This finding is in agreement with earlier data from the Los Angeles area that showed a high degree of correlation between diminished performance of high school cross-country track runners and increased oxidant levels.

**Long-Term Exposures.** Epidemiological studies of the chronic effects of air pollution are difficult to conduct because of the nature of the goal: outcomes associated with long-term exposures. Retrospective and cross-sectional studies are frequently affected by confounding variables and poor historical exposure data. For example, there appears to be little question that there is a relationship between chronic bronchitis and emphysema and cigarette smoking. Air pollution also appears to be correlated with these respiratory diseases, but the effect of smoking is likely to be the greater contributing factor. Thus, the effect of smoking must be controlled in studies of human populations. Prospective studies have the advantage of more precise control of such confounding factors, but they are very expensive and require substantial time and dedication. They also can be plagued by subjects dropping out.

Despite these deficiencies, a number of air pollution studies of both types have been conducted and generally have suggested a positive association between urban pollution and progressive pulmonary impairment. Cross-sectional studies in the Los Angeles Air Basin have found more rapid "aginglike" loss of lung function in people living for extended periods in regions of dirty air where oxidant pollution builds up compared with areas where sea air circulates and lowers the overall pollutant concentration (Detels et al., 1991). Analogously, a prospective Dutch study has shown gradual impairment of lung function with chronic exposure to sulfur dioxide and particulate matter over 12 years (Van De Lende et al., 1981). Even rural areas can be affected, as demonstrated by a questionnaire-based study which indicated an association between respiratory symptoms and reducing-type pollutants transported into western Pennsylvania from midwestern industrialized areas (Schenker et al., 1983).

Among the most detailed epidemiological studies of the chronic health effects of current levels of air pollution has been the so-called Harvard Six Cities Study. The cities were chosen because of varying levels of pollution and access to routine air-monitoring data. The design of these studies includes the gathering of parental questionnaire data about the prevalence of respiratory problems in schoolchildren over a period of years as well as the regular performance of pulmonary function tests. When compared across cities, $[H^+]$ (measured in four of the six cities) was correlated (Fig. 28-5A) better than was sulfate with the prevalence of bronchitis in children age 10 to 12 (Speizer, 1989). However, as seen in Fig. 28-5B through D, the role of $[H^+]$ in excess acute mortality is less convincing; the excess mortality relates better to sulfate level or fine particulate matter (sulfates coassociate with fine particulates in the atmosphere) (Dockery et al., 1993). Additional findings from this study indicate that the life spans of people living in Steubenville, Ohio, an area of industrial reducing-type pollution, are significantly shortened in association with fine particulate exposure.

The role of air pollution in human lung cancer is difficult to assess because the vast majority of respiratory cancers result from cigarette smoking. Many compounds known to occur as urban air pollutants also are known to have carcinogenic potency. Indeed only about 10 percent of the more than 2800 compounds that have been identified in the air have been assayed for carcinogenic potency. Figure 28-6 gives estimates of the relative contributions of various chemicals to the noncigarette lung cancer rate, which for outdoor air is estimated to be about 2000 cases per year (Lewtas, 1993). This compares with about 2000 cases per year for passive environmental tobacco smoke and about 100,000 cases per year for smokers. Volatile organic compounds and nitrogen-containing and halogenated organics account for most of the compounds that have been studied with animal and genetic bioassays. Most of these compounds are derived from combustion sources ranging from tobacco to power plants to incinerator emissions. Other potential carcinogens also arise from mobile sources as products of incomplete combustion and their atmospheric transformation products as well as fugitive or accidental chemical releases. This contrasts with indoor air, where the sources are thought to derive largely from environmental tobacco smoke and radon, with some contribution from the offgassed organics.

By and large, the carcinogenic potency of air pollution resides in the particulate fraction. Polycyclic organic chemicals along with a group of lower-boiling organics sometimes referred to as "semivolatiles" (including nitroaromatics) are associated with the particulate fraction and could have a prolonged residence time at sensitive sites in the respiratory tract when inhaled. Genetic bioassays have demonstrated potent mutagenicity and presumably carcinogenic potential of various chemical fractions of ambient aerosols (Lewtas, 1993). Copollutants such as irritant gases which initiate inflammation may promote carcinogenic activity. There is experimental evi-

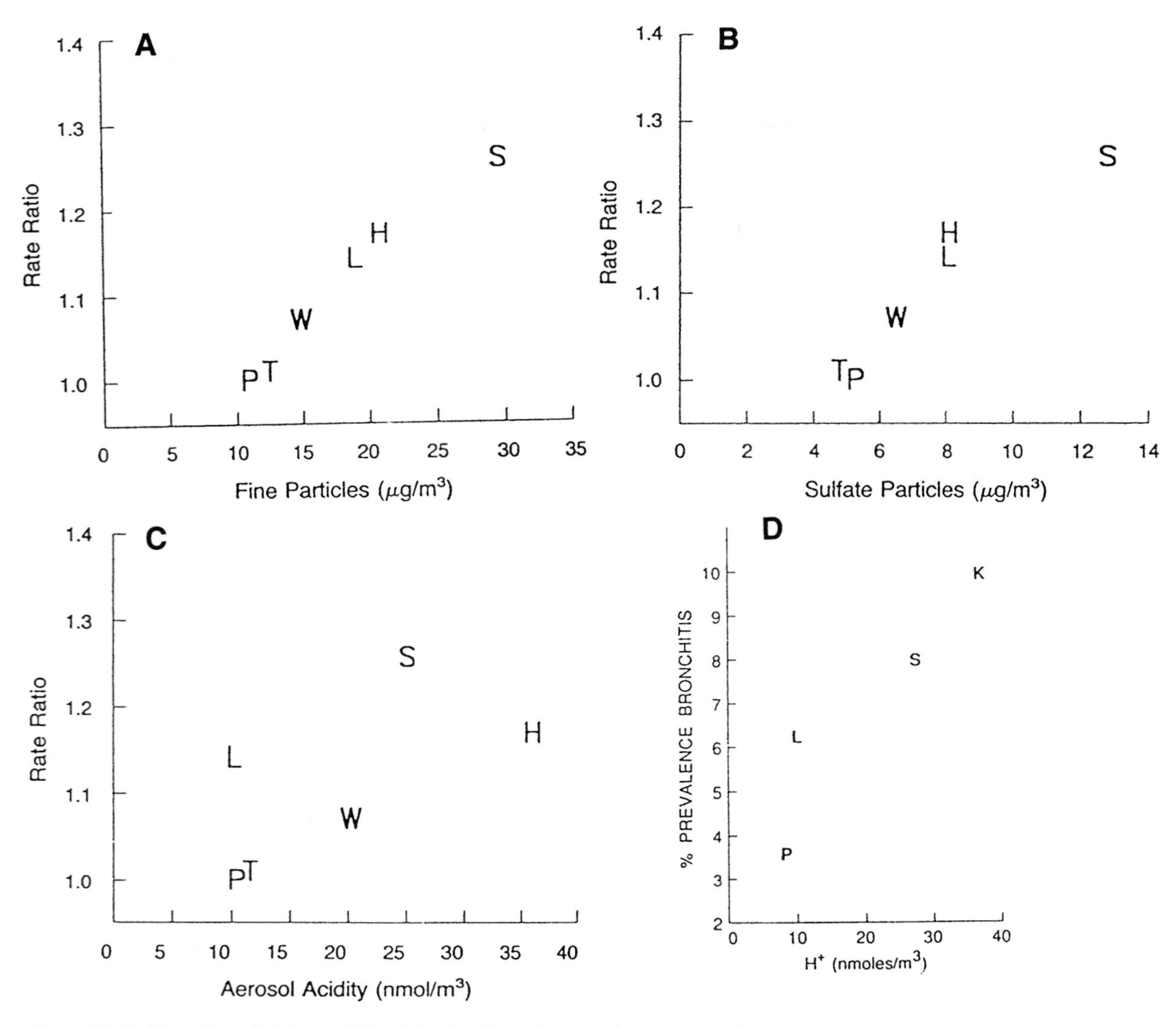


*Figure 28–5. Data from the Harvard Six Cities Studies indicating the superior relationship of $PM_{10}$ and sulfate to mortality rates (A–C) in contrast to acidity (D), which correlates better with the prevalence of bronchitis in children. [Reproduced from Speizer (1989) (D) and Dockery et al. (1993) (A–C), with permission.]*

dence that benzopyrene inhaled by rats whose respiratory tracts have been chronically irritated by sulfur dioxide inhalation results in bronchogenic carcinoma. Experimental evidence also indicates that when ozonized gasoline was inhaled by mice that had been infected with influenza virus, epidermoid carcinomas were produced. There is clearly an urban-rural gradient in the incidence of lung cancer that is verifiable when corrected for the effects of cigarette smoking, supporting the early notion of Kotin and Falk (1963): "Chemical, physical and biological data unite to form a constellation that strongly implicates the atmosphere as one dominant factor in the pathogenesis of lung cancer."

## Indoor Air Pollution

As outdoor air quality has improved over the last 20 to 30 years, an awareness of the potential effects of indoor air pollution on health has begun to emerge. Concerns about indoor air which at first brought skepticism are gaining respectability as various attributes of the indoor environment and its effect on health and well-being are being investigated. However, the issue remains controversial because many of the health problems associated with indoor air pollution have nonspecific symptomology and a wide range of potential toxicants and sources (Molhave et al., 1986). The response to indoor air pollution also may be affected by ambient comfort factors such as temperature and humidity. Two broadly defined illnesses are discussed below which are largely unique to the indoor environment (Brooks and Davis, 1992).

**Sick-Building Syndromes.** This collection of ailments, which is defined by a set of persistent symptoms (Table 28-2) occurring in at least 20 percent of those exposed, typically is of unknown specific etiology but is relieved sometime after an

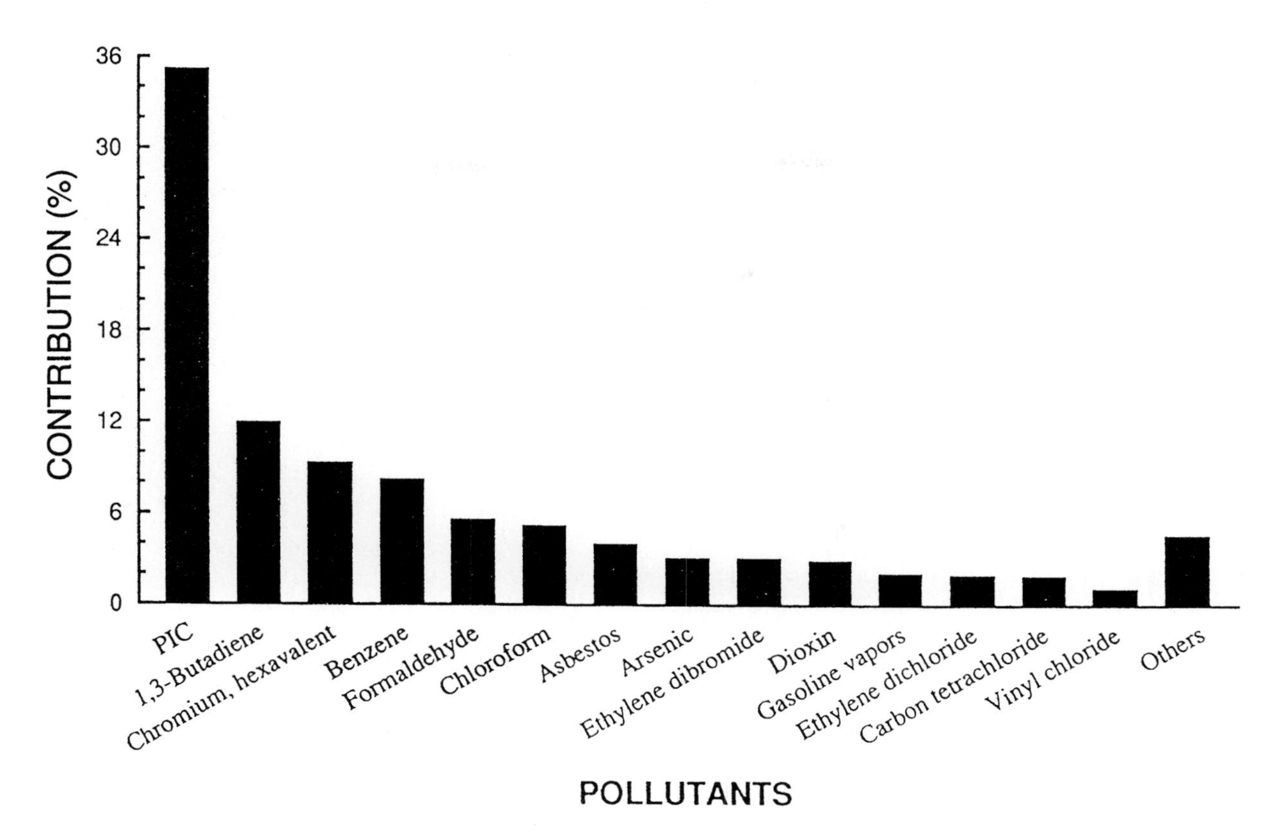


***Figure 28–6. Relative contribution of individual airborne hazardous pollutants to lung cancer rates after removal of tobacco smoke cancer.***

The total number of cancers from non-tobacco-smoke sources is estimated to be about 2000 per year. [Reproduced from Lewtas (1993), with permission.]

affected individual leaves the building. Frequently, but not always, this syndrome occurs in new, poorly ventilated, or recently refurbished office buildings. The suspected causes include combustion products, household chemicals, biological materials and vapors, and emissions from furnishings and are exacerbated by the effect of poor ventilation on comfort factors. The perception of irritancy to the eyes, nose, and throat ranks among the predominant symptoms which can become intolerable with repeated exposures. Controlled clinical studies have shown a concentration- and duration-dependent worsening of irritant discomfort after exposure to a complex mixture of 22 volatile organic compounds commonly found in the indoor environment (Molhave et al., 1986). The many factors contributing to such responses are poorly understood and warrant more attention.

**Table 28–2**
**Symptoms Commonly Associated with the Sick-Building Syndrome**

| Symptoms |
|---|
| Eyes, nose, and throat irritation |
| Headaches |
| Fatigue |
| Reduced attention span |
| Irritability |
| Nasal congestion |
| Difficulty breathing |
| Nosebleeds |
| Dry skin |
| Nausea |

SOURCE: Modified from Brooks and Davis (1992) with permission.

**Building-Related Illnesses.** This group of illnesses, in contrast to the sick-building syndrome, consists of well-documented conditions with defined diagnostic criteria and generally recognizable causes. These illnesses typically call for a conventional treatment regime since the symptoms are not readily reversed simply by exiting the building where the illness was contracted. Several of the biologically related illnesses (e.g., Legionnaires' disease, hypersensitivity pneumonitis, humidifier fever) fall into this group, as do allergies to animal danders, dust mites, and cockroaches. Some toxic inhalants might be classified in this group, such as carbon monoxide poisoning. In general, when the concentrations of carbon monoxide, nitrogen dioxide, and most volatile organic compounds result in less discernable or definable conditions, the responses would probably be considered among the sick-building syndromes. It should be noted, however, that many inhalants, such as nitrogen dioxide and trichloroethylene (a VOC common to the indoor air arising from chlorinated water or dry-cleaned clothes), have been shown in animal toxicology studies to suppress host defenses and allow opportunistic

pathogens to proliferate in the lung. Thus, complex indoor environments of chemicals and biologicals could have unexpected outcomes as a result of interactions.

## POLLUTANTS OF OUTDOOR AMBIENT AIR

### Classical Reducing-Type Air Pollution

Acute air pollution episodes made it clear that under certain meteorologic conditions reducing-type pollution characterized by sulfur dioxide and smoke is capable of producing disastrous effects. Studies in human subjects and animals have long stressed the toxicology of sulfur dioxide for its role in these incidents, while the potential for interactions among copollutants in the smoky, sulfurous mix has not been appreciated. The burning of fossil fuels and the smelting of metals emit a variety of particles in addition to sulfur dioxide into the atmosphere. These particles may have associated solubilized or surface-adducted metals that can promote the conversion of sulfur dioxide to the more irritating sulfuric acid. Particles of submicrometer size are of particular importance because they have a large surface area on which to foster interaction with the gas and are small enough to penetrate deep into the lung.

Summer haze, which consists of ozone and sulfate-associated particles, is not included in the classical reducing-type classification but is more typical of the modern-day complex oxidant atmosphere of large metropolitan areas and their suburban and rural neighbors downwind. These sulfates are formed by photochemical mechanisms, and as in the reducing-type atmosphere, they may exist as sulfuric acid or, more likely, as the partially or fully neutralized forms, ammonium bisulfate and ammonium sulfate. Fine sulfate aerosols may be transported long distances in the atmosphere and, in addition to posing a direct hazard to health, may contribute to acid rain (Fig. 28-7).

**Sulfur Dioxide.** ***General Toxicology.*** Sulfur dioxide is a water-soluble irritant gas. As such, it is predominantly an upper airway irritant which can stimulate bronchoconstriction and mucus secretion in a number of species, including humans. Sulfur dioxide has received more study over the years than has virtually any other air pollutant. Early studies showed airway injury and subsequent proliferation of goblet (mucus-secreting) cells, and this has led to the use of sulfur dioxide to produce laboratory animal models of bronchitis. The measurable presence of sulfur dioxide in the air in heavily industrialized areas ($\sim \frac{1}{1000}$ that used to produce animal models of bronchitis) has been associated with bronchitis among the residents of those areas. However, because sulfur dioxide is a precursor to the acid sulfates, which are typically more toxic, recent attention has been directed toward these descendant products.

Nevertheless, toxicology studies have shown that sulfur dioxide is itself capable of impairing macrophage-dependent host defenses in murine models. Exposed mice have a greater frequency and severity of infection. Analogously, rats exposed for 70 to 170 h to 0.1, 1.0, and 20 ppm exhibited reduced clearance of inert particles, while dogs exposed to 1 ppm for a year had slowed tracheal mucus transport. The fact that the low concentration exposures showed marked effects when extended over longer periods is consistent with the epidemiological associations with bronchitis. However, no evidence of pulmonary pathology was detected after the continuous exposure of guinea pigs or monkeys for a year or more to concentrations of 0.1 to 5 ppm (Alarie et al., 1970, 1972).

The penetration of sulfur dioxide to the lungs is greater during mouth breathing than it is during nose breathing. An

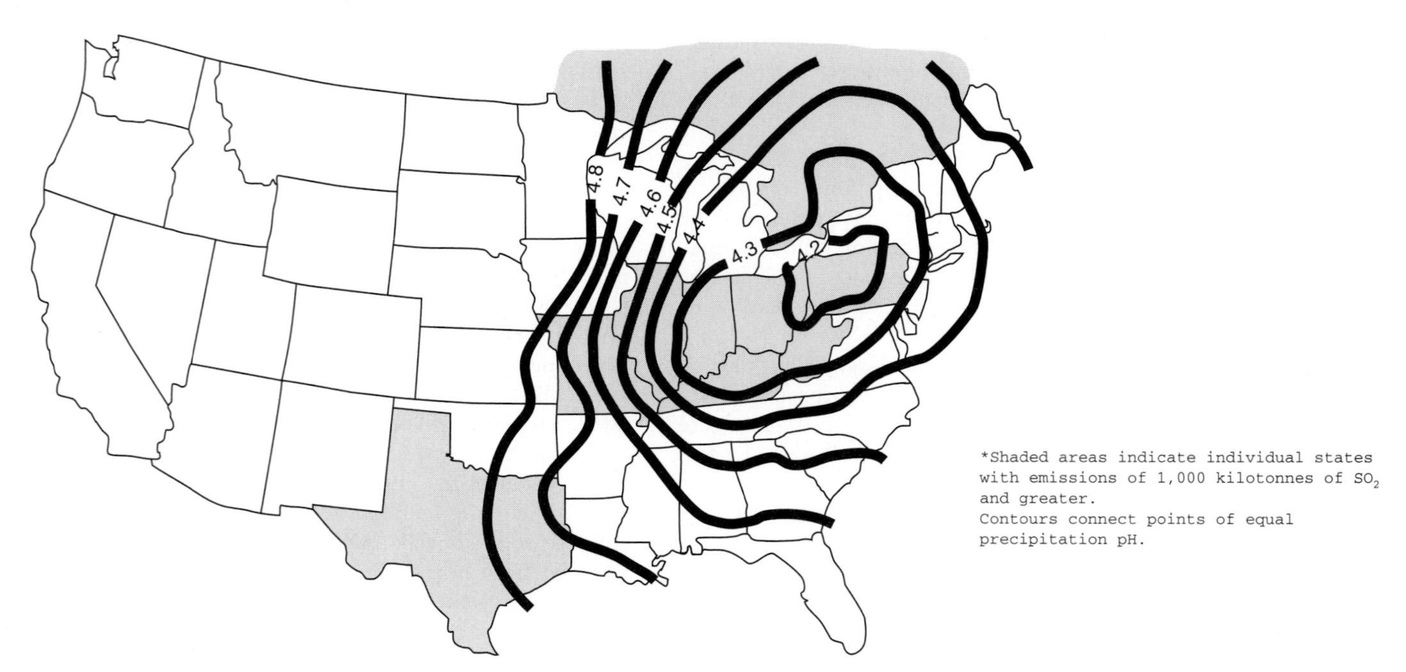


***Figure 28–7. Areas where precipitation in the east falls below pH 5: acid rain.***

The acidity of the air in the east is thought to result from air mass transport of fine sulfated particulate matter from the industrial centers of the midwest. (Reproduced from EPA-230-07-88-033 with permission.)

increase in the airflow rate also markedly increases penetration to the deeper lung. As a result, persons exercising in an area contaminated with sulfur dioxide (e.g., under a downdrafted plumb of a smokestack) can experience exacerbated acute responses to the irritant (see below). Once deposited, sulfur dioxide dissolves in airway and lung fluids as sulfite or bisulfite and is readily distributed throughout the body. Labeled $^{35}$sulfur dioxide studies indicate, however, that some residual sulfur dioxide (presumably as protein reaction products) persists in the respiratory system for a week or more after exposure (Yokoyama et al., 1971). In both rabbits and human subjects, the sulfite which reaches the plasma has been shown to form S-sulfonate products by reacting with the disulfide bonds of proteins (Gunnison and Palmes, 1974). It has not been determined whether S-sulfonate proteins lead to biochemical alterations in systemic organs or tissues.

***Pulmonary Function Effects.*** The basic physiological response to the inhalation of sulfur dioxide is a mild degree of bronchoconstriction, which is reflected as a measurable increase in airflow resistance. This concentration-related increase in resistance has been demonstrated in guinea pigs, dogs, cats, and human subjects. Airflow resistance in anesthetized dogs that were administered sulfur dioxide increased more when it was introduced through a tracheal cannula than when it was introduced through the nose, consistent with the bypassed scrubbing of the nose. Isolated nasal exposure increased resistance in that pathway, apparently as a result of mucosal swelling. When only a segment of the trachea was exposed, overall lung resistance was observed to increase, though not to the extent seen with whole-lung exposure, consistent with the extent of receptor stimulation (Frank and Speizer, 1965). Early study of bronchoconstrictive mechanisms of sulfur dioxide conducted in ventilated, tracheostomized cats (Nadel et al., 1965) indicated that pulmonary resistance increased during the first breath but reversed rapidly. Intravenous injection of atropine (parasympathetic receptor blocker) or cooling of the cervical vagosympathetic nerves abolishes bronchoconstriction; rewarming of the nerve reestablishes the response. The rapidity of the response and its reversal emphasizes the parasympathetically mediated tonal change in smooth muscle. Studies in human subjects have confirmed the predominance of parasympathetic mediation, but histamine from inflammatory cells may play a secondary role in the bronchoconstrictive responses of asthmatics (Sheppard et al., 1981).

Human subjects exposed to 1, 5, or 13 ppm sulfur dioxide for just 10 min also exhibited a rapid bronchoconstrictive response. Individuals with higher initial flow resistance were somewhat more responsive, especially at the lowest (1 ppm) concentration; this qualitatively parallels the responsiveness of asthmatics, who typically have higher base resistance values (Frank et al., 1962). Studies by other investigators have largely confirmed that the majority of subjects respond to concentrations of 5 ppm or higher, whereas only an occasional sensitive individual responds to 1 ppm. With exercise during exposure or mouth breathing, a concentration in the range of 1 to 3 ppm can increase airway resistance in normal individuals.

Concentrations of 3 ppm are unlikely as daily or hourly averages, though they could be encountered briefly as a downdrafted smoke plume. The fact that just a few deep breaths can produce increased airway resistance may be of significance to individuals with asthma and those who are otherwise hyperresponsive. Even stable concentrations of sulfur dioxide below the level usually of concern to normals (0.25 to 1 ppm) induce bronchoconstriction in adult and adolescent subjects with clinically defined mild asthma. These responses are most apparent with exposures through mouth breathing or exercise and are proportional to the severity of the subject's asthma (Sheppard et al., 1981; Koenig et al., 1981). Findings such as these (responses $<0.5$ ppm) have raised new concerns about potential adverse effects in this sensitive subpopulation when it is exposed to peaks of sulfur dioxide that are known to occur near point sources.

***Chronic Effects.*** Few long-term studies have been conducted with sulfur dioxide at levels approaching those likely to be in ambient air. Alarie and associates (1970) exposed guinea pigs to 0.13, 1.01, or 5.72 ppm sulfur dioxide continuously for a year without adverse impact on lung mechanics. Similarly, monkeys exhibited no alteration in pulmonary function when exposed continuously for 78 weeks to 0.14, 0.64, and 1.28 ppm sulfur dioxide (Alarie et al., 1972). Even in the presence of 0.1 mg/m$^3$ sulfuric acid, dogs exposed 16 h a day for 18 months to 0.5 ppm sulfur dioxide showed no impairment in pulmonary function (Vaughan et al., 1969). Only higher levels of sulfur dioxide for protracted periods of time [dogs to 5 ppm for 225 days (Lewis et al., 1969); rats to 350 ppm for 30 days (Reid, 1963)] have been shown to alter airway mucus secretion, goblet cell topography, or lung function, but these results are of little relevance to typical sulfur dioxide levels in ambient air.

**Sulfuric Acid and Related Sulfates.** Sulfur dioxide readily oxidizes to sulfate in the atmosphere when catalyzed by transition metals such as iron, manganese, and vanadium in dispersing smokestack plumes or via photochemical processes. During the smelting of metals or the combustion of fossil fuels, sulfuric acid can sorb on ultrafine metal oxide particles and occur as a primary emission. In some coals, for example, as much as 9 percent of the resident sulfur may be emitted in this form, sorbed on ultrafine ($<0.1$ $\mu$m) ash. Most of the oxidation of sulfur dioxide, however, occurs in the atmosphere. Sulfuric acid and its neutralization products ammonium bisulfate and ammonium sulfate exist typically as fine particulate matter ($<2.5$ $\mu$m) associated with metals in water droplets or on the surface of ash. As such, they may undergo long-range transport to areas distant from the emission source. Because acid sulfates are stronger irritants than sulfur dioxide is and are likely to be encountered in the atmosphere of industrial societies, considerable attention has been directed toward their impact on the pulmonary airways, where they are likely to be deposited upon inhalation. Sulfuric acid is the strongest of the atmospheric acids, including nitric acid (derived from nitrogen dioxide), which is more common in areas in the southwest. The limited database on nitric acid suggests that it may be mildly bronchoconstrictive in adolescent asthmatics (Koenig et al., 1989).

***General Toxicology.*** Sulfuric acid imparts irritation to respiratory tissues through its acidity (i.e., the availability of its $H^+$ to protonate receptor ligands and other biomolecules). Am-

monia, which exists in free air at about 25 ppb and in a much higher concentration in the mammalian nasopharynx/oropharynx, is capable of neutralizing the irritant potential of sulfates. The efficiency of this process is dependent on temperature, relative humidity, air mixing, and several other factors and thus is a likely source of variability in apparent biological responses. This is particularly true in animal studies involving standard whole-body exposure-chamber operation, in which excreta and bacteria may interact, giving rise to chamber ammonia concentrations up to 1100 ppb, more than enough to fully neutralize sulfuric acid up to several mg/m$^3$ (Higuchi and Davies, 1993). Similarly, endogenous ammonia such as that which exists in the mouth has been shown to inhibit responses up to 350 $\mu$g/m$^3$ sulfuric acid in exercising asthmatics (Utell et al., 1989).

Interestingly, there is also considerable species variability in sensitivity to sulfuric acid, with guinea pigs being quite reactive to acid sulfates, in contrast to rats, which are highly resistant. While the reasons for this difference between guinea pigs and rats are not fully understood, the sensitivity of healthy humans appears to fall somewhere in between, with asthmatic humans best modeled by the guinea pig. Overall, however, the collective data involving animals and humans are remarkably coherent, as reviewed in an article by Amdur (1989). To illustrate this point, Table 28-3 compares the acute toxicity of sulfur dioxide and sulfuric acid in animals and human subjects, using indexes that will be detailed below, airway resistance, and bronchial clearance. To allow direct comparisons, the concentrations are presented as $\mu$mol of the two compounds.

***Pulmonary Function Effects.*** Sulfuric acid produces an increase in flow resistance in guinea pigs, the magnitude of which is related to both concentration and particle size (Amdur, 1958; Amdur et al., 1978). Early studies indicated that as particle size was reduced from 7 $\mu$m to the submicron range, the concentration of sulfuric acid necessary to induce a response and the time to the onset of the response fell significantly. With the large particles, even the sensitive guinea pig was able to withstand an exceedingly high (30 mg/m$^3$) challenge with little change in pulmonary resistance, in contrast to the $<1$ mg/m$^3$ challenge needed with the 0.3-$\mu$m particles (Amdur et al., 1978). Human asthmatics exposed to 2 mg/m$^3$ of acid fog (10 $\mu$m) for 1 h, a very high concentration for an asthmatic, experienced variable respiratory symptoms suggesting irritancy but did not exhibit changes in spirometry (Hackney et al., 1989). The apparent reason for this size-based differential response is the scrubbing of large particles in the nose while the small particles are able to penetrate deep into the lung, reaching receptors that stimulate bronchoconstriction and mucus secretion. The thicker mucus blanket of the nose may blunt (by dilution or neutralization by mucus buffers) much of the irritancy of the deposited acid, limiting its effect to mucus secretion and some increase in nasal flow resistance which has little impact on overall pulmonary resistance. In contrast, the less shielded distal airway tissues with their higher receptor density would be expected to be more sensitive to the acid, as reflected by their responsiveness to the small particles which reach that area. This regional sensitivity and the longer residence time of a deposited particle relative to a gas probably were reflected in the relatively protracted recovery times in acid-exposed guinea pigs compared with those animals exposed to sulfur dioxide alone.

As with sulfur dioxide, asthmatic subjects appear to be more sensitive to the bronchoconstrictive effects of sulfuric acid than are healthy individuals, but for unknown reasons, this hypersensitivity is somewhat less consistent (both in occurrence and in time to expression) with the acid than with sulfur dioxide (Koenig et al., 1989; Utell et al., 1984). Some evidence suggests that the responsiveness of an asthmatic to nonspecific (e.g, carbachol, histamine, exercise) stimulation of bronchoconstriction may serve as a biomarker of the responsiveness of that individual to sulfuric acid bronchoconstriction (Hanley et al., 1992).

Airway hyperreactivity also has been observed as an acute response in guinea pigs 2 h after a 1-h exposure to 200 $\mu$g/m$^3$ sulfuric acid. In rabbits, increased airway reactivity appears to be associated with disturbances in arachidonate metabolism in a way that involves more than an infiltration of inflammatory cells. As can be seen in Table 28-3, the guinea pig appears to respond at levels of sulfuric acid in the range of responsive human asthmatics, suggesting that it might serve as a model of this sensitive subpopulation for further study of the

**Table 28–3**
**Comparative Toxicity of $SO_2$ and $H_2SO_4$ in Acute Studies**

| | $\mu$mol | | |
|---|---|---|---|
| | $SO_2$ | $H_2SO_4$ | REFERENCE |
| Guinea pigs: 1 h; 10% ↑ airway resistance | 6 | 1 | Amdur, 1974 |
| Donkeys: 30 min; 1-h altered bronchial clearance | 8875 | 2 | Spiegelman et al., 1968; Schlesinger et al., 1978 |
| Normal subjects: 7 min; 1-h altered bronchial clearance | 520 | 1 | Lippmann and Altshuler, 1976; Leikauf et al., 1981 |
| Normal subjects: 10 min; 5% ↓ tidal volume | 29 | 1.25 | Amdur, 1954 |
| Adolescent asthmatics: 40 min; equal ↑ airway resistance | 20 | 1 | Koenig et al., 1989 |

relationship between nonspecific responsiveness and sulfuric acid responsiveness.

***Effects on Mucociliary Clearance and Macrophage Function.*** Sulfuric acid alters the clearance of particles from the lung, interfering with a major defense mechanism. With insoluble, radioactively labeled ferric oxide particles, effects have been observed after as little as a single 1-h exposure in donkeys, rabbits, and human subjects. The effect on mucus clearance appears to vary directly with the acidity of the acid sulfate, with sulfuric acid having the greatest effect and ammonium sulfate the smallest (Schlesinger, 1984). There appears to be a biphasic response to the acid concentration as well as to its duration. In general, brief, single exposures of <250 $\mu g/m^3$ accelerate clearance, while high concentrations of >1000 $\mu g/m^3$ clearly depress clearance. Over several days, however, there appears to be a cumulative depression of clearance (concentration × time). Longer-term, low-level acid exposures of rabbits ultimately slow clearance in apparent concert with hyperplasia of airway mucosecretory cells (Gearhart and Schlesinger, 1989). Acidification of mucus by $H^+$ (i.e., a fall in pH) even locally is hypothesized to have potential effects on mucus rheology and viscosity (Holma, 1989); this is not unreasonable in light of the drop in macrophage intracellular pH reported in some acid studies (Qu et al., 1993).

Studies of bronchial clearance in rabbits and airway resistance in normal and asthmatic human subjects show that the irritant potency is sulfuric acid > ammonium bisulfate > ammonium sulfate. The irritant potency is thus related to relative acidity, as is bronchoconstriction. More recent studies (Schlesinger et al., 1990) examined the effect of in vivo exposure of rabbits to sulfuric acid and ammonium bisulfate on the phagocytic activity of alveolar macrophages harvested by pulmonary lavage. Phagocytosis was altered by a single exposure to sulfuric acid at a concentration of 500 $\mu g/m^3$ and by exposure to ammonium bisulfate at a concentration of 2000 $\mu g/m^3$. Identical levels of $H^+$ in the exposure-chamber atmosphere produced a lesser response with ammonium bisulfate than with sulfuric acid, although in vitro studies of incubated macrophages showed identical response at a given pH no matter which compound had been added to reach the level of acidity. These results suggest that speciation of acidic aerosols in the atmosphere may be an important cofactor and that a simple measurement of atmospheric acidity may not be sufficient to assess the potential effects on health.

***Chronic Effects.*** Sulfuric acid would be expected to induce the same qualitative effects along the airways that are found with sulfur dioxide at high concentrations. Because it is an aerosol, sulfuric acid would deposit deeper along the respiratory tree, and its high specific acidity would impart more damage or effect along its path of deposition. Thus, the primary concern in regard to acidic aerosols is the potential to cause bronchitis, since this has been a problem in industries troubled by employee exposures to sulfuric acid mists (e.g., battery plants). Early studies in the donkey that later were expanded in a rabbit model have provided fundamental data on this issue. Because brief acute exposures to sulfuric acid similarly depressed mucociliary clearance in donkeys and humans, the profound depression of clearance found in donkeys exposed repeatedly (100 $\mu g/m^3$ 1 h per day for 6 months) promoted the hypothesis that a similar response (i.e., chronic bronchitis) is a likely outcome in humans. This argument was strengthened by the similar bronchitogenic responses of the two species when chronically exposed to cigarette smoke.

Many studies conducted since that time in the rabbit are in general agreement with the findings of the donkey studies with sulfuric acid (Schlesinger et al., 1979; Schlesinger 1984). These studies have expanded our knowledge of the biological response and its exposure-based relationship. The initial stimulation of clearance with subsequent depression has been shown to occur over 12 months with as little as 2 h per day at 125 $\mu g/m^3$ sulfuric acid (Schlesinger et al., 1992). Related studies also have demonstrated that the airways of exposed animals became progressively more sensitive to challenge with acetylcholine, showed a progressive decrease in diameter, and experienced an increase in the number of secretory cells, especially in the smaller airways (Gearhart and Schlesinger, 1989).

Unlike other irritants, such as ozone (see below), sulfuric acid does not appear to stimulate a classic neutrophilic inflammation after exposure. However, eicosonoid homeostasis appears to be disturbed, and macrophage function as a critical element in host defense shows evidence of being altered, perhaps in part mediated by a decrease in intracellular pH. Long-term disease attributable to connective tissue disturbances induced by sulfuric acid seems to be of lesser concern than is the impact on mucocilliary function and the potential impact on ventilation and arterial oxygenation (Alarie et al., 1972, 1975). Therefore, it seems reasonable that chronic daily exposure of humans to sulfuric acid at levels of 100 $\mu g/m^3$ or above leads to impaired clearance and chronic bronchitis.

**Particulate Matter.** Particulate matter in the atmosphere is a melange of organic and inorganic materials whose relative compositional distribution can vary significantly, depending on point sources within a particular air shed. Long-range transport also can be a factor, particularly for fine (<2.5 $\mu m$) particles. The health effects of particulate matter revealed by epidemiology studies suggest significant short- and long-term toxicity at current ambient (near NAAQS) levels. These effects appear to be less affected by gross particle composition (inorganic versus organic) and nominal size (<10 $\mu m$) than by gravimetric estimates of ambient exposure. This perception appears to contradict the tenets of conventional air pollution toxicology, which are based on chemical-specific toxicity and the critical role of size in particle potency. However, at this time so little is understood about these epidemiological findings that the relatively crude ($PM_{10}$) mass-based correlation with the biological effects may be only a surrogate for the actual or proximal toxicant. Unfortunately, there is not a large database of animal toxicology in regard to this issue.

It is known that several metals and silicate-derived constituents of the inorganic phase of particulate matter can be cytotoxic to lung cells and that organic constituents theoretically can induce toxicity directly or via metabolism to genotoxic agents. Also, recent studies focusing on very small, ultrafine (<0.1 $\mu m$) particles suggest that though low in mass, these particles are high in number and thus can be very toxic with little or no impact on the apparent mass-based measure of exposure. Finally, our knowledge of the ability of particles to interact with coexistent gases is quite limited, derived largely from studies with soluble metals and sulfur dioxide.

***Metals.*** There have been many inhalation studies with specific metal compounds. The general toxicology of metal compounds is presented in detail elsewhere in this text, though their effect when delivered by inhalation may differ from their effect after systemic administration. Virtually all metals are found in some concentration in atmospheric particles, but the most common are metals released with oil and coal combustion (e.g., transition and heavy metals), metals common to the earth's crust (e.g., iron, sodium, and magnesium), and the anti-knock gasoline metal lead (much reduced since its ban in 1983). Fine ($<2.5\ \mu m$) particles usually are associated with anthropogenic metals, while coarse (2.5 to 10 $\mu m$) particles contain more of the crustal metals (e.g., $Fe_2O_3$) as part of their matrix.

Metal compounds generally fall into two classes: those that are essentially water-insoluble (e.g., metal oxides such as those that might be released from high-temperature combustion sources) and those that are soluble or partially soluble in water (often chlorides or sulfates such as those that might associate under acidic conditions in a smoke plume or leach from hydrated silicate particles in the atmosphere). Solubility appears to play a role in the toxicity of many inhaled metals by enhancing bioavailability (e.g., nickel chloride versus nickel oxide) or increasing pulmonary residence time (e.g., cadmium oxide versus cadmium chloride). There appears to be no hard and fast rule governing this relationship. Some metals, either in their soluble forms or coordinated to the surface of silicate materials (e.g., silicon dioxide and asbestos), can promote electron transfer to enhance the formation of reactive oxidants during inflammation (Ghio et al., 1992). It is likely that a number of mechanisms are involved in the action of inhaled metal-associated particles.

***Gas-Particulate Phase Interactions.*** The coexistence of pollutant gases and particles raises the concern that these phases may interact chemically or physiologically to result in enhanced effects. Many studies have shown that this generic process is feasible as a mechanism for altering the toxicity of either the particle or the gas. The guinea pig bronchoconstriction model used for many years by Amdur and associates has clearly shown that sulfur dioxide can interact with metal salts to potentiate its irritant effects. The mechanism or mechanisms behind this interaction involve the solubility of sulfur dioxide in a liquefied aerosol as well as the ability of the metal to catalyze the oxidation of the dissolved gas to sulfate. In the case of sodium chloride aerosol, potentiation appeared to be governed primarily by the solubility of sulfur dioxide in that salt droplet and its enhanced respiratory deposition, while metal salts such as manganese, iron, and vanadium functioned through the formation of the stronger irritant sulfate (Amdur and Underhill, 1968). The response of the mixture was dictated by the aerosol itself, indicating that it was the proximate irritant. Studies in humans have been less revealing about such interactions, perhaps in part as a result of differences in methodology.

Sulfuric acid sorbed on ultrafine (0.1 $\mu m$) metal oxide particles can be emitted by the smelting of metals or the combustion of coal. Analogous particles can be furnace-generated in the laboratory and diluted in cool clean air to expose animals (Amdur et al., 1986). These ultrafine particles are distributed widely and deeply in the lung and thus enhance the irritant potency beyond that predicted on the basis of sulfuric acid concentration alone. A concentration of 30 $\mu g/m^3$ sulfuric acid on the surface of ultrafine zinc oxide particles produces the same reduction in carbon monoxide–diffusing capacity ($DL_{CO}$) in guinea pigs as does a similar exposure to 300 $\mu g/m^3$ of conventionally generated sulfuric acid of the same size (Amdur, 1989). A single 3-h exposure of guinea pigs to 30 to 60 $\mu g/m^3$ sulfuric acid sorbed on ultrafine zinc oxide produced dose-dependent decreases in $DL_{CO}$, total lung capacity, and vital capacity and increases in cells, protein, and a variety of enzymes in lavage fluid that were not completely resolved 96 h after exposure. Though a single 20 $\mu g/m^3$ dose did not result in effects, repeated exposures appeared to be cumulative (Amdur, 1989). Some coals, such as Illinois No. 6, have a layer of sulfuric acid sorbed on the surface of the ultrafine ash, whereas other, more alkaline coals, such as Montana lignite, produce sorbed neutral sulfate. The acid-layered ash from Illinois No. 6 produced a greater response, even though the amount of sulfate was greater in the Montana lignite (Chen et al., 1990).

Gaseous pollutants may influence the clearance or metabolism of inhaled particulate material. Many years ago it was demonstrated that sulfur dioxide can enhance the carcinogenicity of benzo(*a*)pyrene, though the mechanism was never revealed. Rats exposed to ozone using an urban profile peaking at 0.25 ppm for 6 weeks and then exposed once for 5 h to asbestos were found to retain (not clear) 3 times as many fibers as did the controls 30 days later. Thus, realistic exposure scenarios of gaseous and particulate pollutants raise the prospect of interactions through physiological mechanisms which could enhance the risks associated with potentially carcinogenic particles.

***Organic and Carbonaceous Matter.*** Organic and carbonaceous matter can be found at the core or layered on the surface of urban particulates. Estimates of the carbonaceous content vary considerably but are nominally considered to be about 50 to 60 percent of the total mass of fine particulate material. The sources are varied and include natural smoke (e.g., forest fires), stationary-source combustion products (fly ash), and diesel exhaust particulate matter. The diesel particle itself is largely carbon with small amounts of various combustion-derived complex nitroaromatics but is not particularly toxic when administered acutely, even by intratracheal instillation. The limited acute studies with coal fly ash, which typically has a considerable organic fraction (in contrast to oil fly ash), have shown that it can induce some inflammation, but much of the response appears to be related to the metal content of the dust. The same appears to be true for samples of urban dust (Düsseldorf and Bochum, Germany), which when instilled into the lungs of rodents suppress host defenses against bacterial challenge (Hatch et al., 1985).

***Chronic Effects and Cancer.*** Chronic exposure studies have been conducted with a number of particles ranging from titanium dioxide and carbon to diesel exhaust and coal fly ash aerosol. Of these substances, diesel exhaust has been the most extensively studied, as reviewed by McClellan (1986). The diesel particle is of interest because it can constitute a significant portion of an urban particulate load and in many ways is representative of a class of relatively "inert" particles which have effects on the lung under some exposure conditions.

The evidence implicating diesel exhaust as a carcinogen in humans is not strong and has been suggested primarily by studies of railway yard and bus workers. The bulk of the evidence for potential carcinogenicity derives from chronic exposure studies in animals and in vitro data that indicate mutagenicity to *Salmonella* bacteria and enhanced sister chromatid exchange rates in Chinese hamster ovary cells. (These genotoxic effects are believed to be due to the nitroarenes associated with the diesel particles.) In vivo, chronic exposure studies show a pattern of tumorigenesis which appears to be an effect of the bulk loading of particulate material in the lungs of experimental animals. At higher concentrations of diesel particulate (3.5 and 7 mg/m$^3$), the normal mucociliary clearance mechanisms are gradually overwhelmed, resulting in a progressive buildup of particles in the lungs. By 12 months (and especially upon approaching 18 to 24 months), clearance essentially ceases and there is evidence of epithelial hyperplasia and fibrogenic activity around agglomerates of particles and phagocytic cells in the distal areas of the lung. The patchy inflammation at sites of accumulation is thought to be related to the mild fibrogenesis observed in the animals and perhaps to the adenosarcomas and squamous cell carcinomas that are observed.

The initiating events for these lesions are not well understood but are thought to be related to a phenomenon called lung "overload," a condition that could not occur in the ambient environment. Because "inert" particles of titanium dioxide and carbon black follow much the same course of toxicity that applies to diesel particulates, it is believed that these long-term effects, including the cancers, are due in part to chronic inflammation and other nonspecific events. The exact link and/or role of genotoxicity in the observed tumorigenesis has not been determined. Recent findings indicate that ultrafine carbon and titanium dioxide ($<0.1\mu m$) show greater inflammation, fibrogenesis, and tumorigenesis than do their larger-particle counterparts. This would support the hypothesis of a mechanistic role for inflammation linked to surface area–dependent toxicity. A small mass of ultrafines would provide many more particles to a given mass-based dose and thus could function as the proximal toxicant under the $PM_{10}$ measure.

**Photochemical Air Pollution.** Photochemical air pollution arises from a series of complex atmospheric reactions which result in a mixture of ozone, oxides of nitrogen, aldehydes, peroxyacetyl nitrates, and reactive hydrocarbons. If sulfur dioxide is present, sulfuric acid also may be formed, as nitric acid vapor can be formed from nitrogen dioxide. From the point of view of the toxicology of photochemical air pollutants, the hydrocarbons as such are of less concern, though they may fall into the hazardous pollutant category (perhaps associated with cancer). The concentrations of these substances in ambient air generally do not reach levels high enough to produce other toxic effects. They are important, however, because they enter into the chemical reactions that lead to the formation of photochemical smog.

The oxidant of critical importance in the photochemical atmosphere is ozone ($O_3$). Several miles above the earth's surface there is sufficient short-wave ultraviolet (UV) light to directly split molecular $O_2$ to atomic O· to combine with $O_2$ to form $O_3$. These UV wavelengths do not reach the earth's surface. In the troposphere, nitrogen dioxide efficiently absorbs longer-wavelength UV light, which leads to the following simplified series of reactions:

$$NO_2 + h\nu \rightarrow O\cdot + NO \quad (1)$$
$$O\cdot + O_2 \rightarrow O_3 \quad (2)$$
$$O_3 + NO\cdot \rightarrow NO_2 \quad (3)$$

This process is cyclic, with $NO_2$ regenerated by the reaction of the NO and $O_3$ formed. In the absence of hydrocarbons, this series of reactions would approach a steady state with no excess or buildup of $O_3$. The hydrocarbons, especially olefins and substituted aromatics, are attacked by the free atomic O·, resulting in oxidized compounds and free radicals that react with NO to produce more $NO_2$. Thus, the balance of the reactions shown in equations 1 to 3 is upset so that $O_3$ levels build up, particularly when the sun's intensity is greatest at midday, utilizing the $NO_2$ provided by morning commuters. These reactions are very complex and involve the formation of unstable intermediate free radicals that undergo a series of changes. Aldehydes are major products in these reactions. Formaldehyde and acrolein account for about 50 percent and 5 percent, respectively, of the total aldehyde in urban atmospheres. Peroxyacetyl nitrate ($CH_3COONO_2$), often referred to as PAN, and its homologues also arise in urban air, most likely from the reaction of the peroxyacyl radicals with $NO_2$.

**Smog Exposures and Vehicle Exhaust.** ***Short-Term Exposures to Smog.*** The complexity of photochemical air pollution challenged toxicologists early on to ascertain its potential to affect human health adversely. Although ozone was quickly suspected as a primary toxicant because of its reactivity and abundance, a number of studies were undertaken with actual (outdoor-derived) or synthetic (photolyzed laboratory-prepared atmospheres) smog in an attempt to assess the potency of a more realistic pollution mix. When human subjects were exposed to actual photochemical air pollution (Los Angeles ambient air pumped into a laboratory exposure chamber), they experienced changes in lung function similar to those described in controlled clinical studies of ozone (i.e., reduction in spirometric lung volumes; see below), thus supporting the notion that ozone is of primary concern.

Acute animal studies utilized more easily controlled synthetic atmospheres (usually irradiated auto exhaust) where the ozone target levels could be made to mimic high air pollution levels: $\sim <0.5$ ppm. Again, very much like ozone alone, just a few hours of exposure to irradiated exhaust resulted in deep lung damage, primarily within the alveolar or small airway epithelium. In some of these studies, early evidence of edema appeared in the interstitium, particularly in older animals. Additionally, similarly exposed mice were found to be more susceptible to bacterial challenge and lung pneumonias. With time after the termination of exposure, the end-airway lesions recovered and the susceptibility to infection waned, though some of the pathology in the distal lung persisted for more than 24 h. While ozone appeared to be the prime toxicant in these studies, that was not always the case. When guinea pigs were exposed to irradiated auto exhaust, airway resistance increased, indicating that a more soluble irritant probably was active, presumably reactive aldehydes. Thus, the array of effects of a complex atmosphere may be more diverse than would be predicted if it were assumed that ozone alone was responsible.

***Chronic Exposures to Smog.*** Studies of both humans and animals exposed to smog have attempted to link chronic lung effects with photochemical air pollution. Cross-sectional and prospective field studies have suggested an accelerated loss of lung function in people living in areas of high pollution relative to low pollution, but most of these studies have been imprecise because of confounding factors (meteorological factors, exposure imprecision, population variables). Recently, there has been a rejuvenation of interest in what are sometimes called "sentinel" studies, which allow a detailed study of animals exposed to the same highly polluted urban air to which people are exposed. This approach has had a troubled past, but newer studies have attempted to minimize or at least control for the problems of infection, animal care, and lack of control of the exposure atmosphere. In a study conducted in rats exposed for 6 months to the air of São Paulo, Brazil, considerable airway damage, lung function alteration, and altered mucus rheology were demonstrated (Saldiva et al., 1992). This collage of effects is not unlike a composite of injury one might suspect would result from an atmosphere of oxidants and acid particulates on the basis of controlled animal studies in the laboratory. At this time it is difficult to determine whether the effects exceed what would be predicted given the basic differences in the underlying study design and artifacts. The concentrations of ozone and particulate matter in the air of São Paulo frequently exceed daily maximum values (in the summer months of February and March) of 0.3 ppm and 75 $\mu g/m^3$, respectively.

Synthetic smog studies in animals were undertaken to eliminate some of the concerns about ambient smog exposures. The most extensive effort to evaluate the potential long-term health effects of synthetic smog was undertaken at the Cincinnati EPA laboratory in the mid-1960s. Beagle dogs were exposed to synthetic atmospheres on a daily basis (16 h) for 68 months, followed by a clean air recovery period of about 3 years (Lewis et al., 1974). After the exposure, a series of physiological measurements were made on the dogs, and they were moved to the College of Veterinary Medicine at the University of California at Davis after their 3-year recovery. The lungs of the dogs then underwent extensive morphological examination to correlate physiological and morphological observations. Seven exposure groups of 12 dogs were studied: (1) nonirradiated auto exhaust, (2) irradiated auto exhaust, (3) sulfur dioxide plus sulfuric acid, (4) and (5) the two types of exhaust plus the sulfur mixture, and (6) and (7) a high and a low level of nitrogen oxides. There was a control group of 20 dogs. The irradiated exhaust contained oxidant (measured as ozone) at about 0.2 ppm and nitrogen dioxide at about 0.9 ppm. The raw exhaust contained minimal concentrations of these materials and about 1.5 ppm nitric oxide. Both forms of exhaust contained about 100 ppm carbon monoxide. While the controls did not show time-related lung function changes, all the exposure groups had abnormalities, most of which persisted or worsened over the 3-year recovery period in clean air. Enlargement of air spaces and loss of interalveolar septa in proximal acinar regions were most severe in dogs that were exposed to oxides of nitrogen, oxides of sulfur, or oxides of sulfur with irradiated exhaust (Hyde et al., 1978). Oxidants such as ozone arising from the irradiated exhaust would be expected to act on the distal lung. These studies elucidated a morphological lesion that was degenerative and progressive in nature, not unlike that of chronic obstructive pulmonary disease (COPD), the condition most often noted in the epidemiological studies.

**Ozone.** ***General Toxicology.*** Ozone is the primary oxidant of concern in photochemical smog because of its inherent bioreactivity and concentration. Depending on the meteorologic pattern of a given year, 60 million to 135 million Americans live in areas not in compliance with the 1-h NAAQS of 0.12 ppm. Los Angeles frequently attains and occasionally exceeds levels of 0.2 to 0.3 ppm. Unlike sulfur dioxide and the reducing-type pollution profile discussed above, current mitigation strategies for ozone have been unsuccessful despite significant reductions in automobile emissions. These reductions have been offset by population growth, which brings with it additional vehicles. With the spread of suburbanization and the wind transport of air masses from populated areas to rural environments, the geographic distribution of those exposed has spread, as has the temporal profile of potential exposure. In other words, ozone exposures are no longer stereotyped as brief 1- to 2-h peaks. Instead, they are prolonged periods of exposure of 6 h or more at or near the NAAQS level and may occur either downtown or in the formerly cleaner suburban or rural areas downwind. This recently noted shift has given rise to concerns that *cumulative* damage from such prolonged exposures may be more significant than brief pulselike exposures and that many more people are being exposed than was previously thought. A thorough review of ozone toxicity in humans and animals, as well as an argument for a revised NAAQS of longer duration, was presented by Lippmann (1989).

Ozone has been the subject of considerable toxicological interest because it induces a variety of effects in humans and experimental animals at concentrations that occur in many urban areas. These effects include morphological, functional, immunologic, and biochemical alterations. Because of its poor water solubility, a substantial portion of inhaled ozone penetrates deep into the lung, but its reactivity is such that about 17 percent and 40 percent are scrubbed by the nasopharynx of resting rats and humans, respectively (Hatch et al, 1994; Gerrity et al., 1988). The reason for the higher degree of scrubbing in humans is unclear, but it is a reproducible finding and surprisingly does not differ from mouth scrubbing. On a surface area basis, the region of the lung that is predicted to have the greatest ozone deposition is the acinar region from the terminal bronchioles to the alveolar ducts, sometimes referred to as the proximal alveolar ductal region (Overton and Miller, 1988). This pattern parallels the profile of lung pathology (see below).

Because ozone penetration increases with increased tidal volume and flow rate, exercise increases the dose to the target area. Using $^{18}O_3$ (a nonradioactive isotope of oxygen), Hatch and coworkers have shown that the dose to the distal lung and the degree of damage to the lung as determined by extravasated protein into the alveolar space (as collected by bronchoalveolar lavage) in exercising human subjects exposed to 0.4 ppm for 2 h with intermittent periods of 15 min of exercise (threefold normal ventilation on average) are similar to those in resting rats exposed for the same length of time to

2.0 ppm. Thus, it is important to (1) consider the role of exercise in a study of ozone before making cross-study comparisons and (2) realize that the rat may not be very different from the human in actual distal lung dose with similar exposure conditions even though fractional uptake studies suggest about a twofold greater removal of ozone from the airstream by humans. With our many years of study of ozone, it is surprising that only now are we beginning to understand the nature of species differences with this toxicant.

Animal studies indicate that the acute morphological response to ozone involves epithelial cell injury along the entire respiratory tract, resulting in cell loss and replacement. Along the respiratory tree, ciliated cells appear to be most sensitive, while Clara cells and mucus-secreting cells are the least sensitive. In the distal lung, the type 1 epithelium is very sensitive to ozone, in contrast to the type 2 cell, which serves as the stem cell for the replacement of type 1 cells. Ultrastructural damage can be observed in rats after a few hours at 0.2 ppm, but sloughing of cells generally requires concentrations above 0.8 ppm. This acute injury is marked by an alteration in the permeability of the blood-air barrier of the lung as one of the first indications of an inflammatory response (see below). This injury is reversed within a couple days, and there appears to be no residual pathology. Hence, a single exposure to ozone is not likely to cause permanent damage. In fact, when a bronchoscope is used to peer down the bronchus of a human after ozone exposure, the airways appear "sunburned" but soon return to their original state.

***Pulmonary Function Effects.*** In exercising human subjects, ozone at ≥0.12 ppm produces reversible concentration-related decrements in forced exhaled volumes [forced vital capacity and forced expiratory volume in 1 s ($FEV_1$)] after 2 to 3 h of exposure (McDonnell et al., 1983). With the recent concern that prolonged periods of exposure (6 to 8 h) may lead to cumulative effects, similar protocols with lower exercise levels were extended up to 6.6 h. In these studies, exposures of 0.12, 0.10, and 0.08 ppm induced progressive lung function impairment during the course of the exposure (Horstman et al., 1989). The pattern of response was linearly cumulative as a function of exposure time so that changes not detectable at 1 or 2 h reached significance by 4 to 6 h. Decrements in $FEV_1$ after 6.6 h at 0.12 ppm averaged 13.6 percent and were comparable to effects after a 2-h exposure to 0.22 ppm with much heavier exercise. Another functional response to ozone is an increase in nonspecific airway reactivity. Unlike sulfuric acid and sulfur dioxide, which manifest clear airway effects such as bronchoconstriction and a clearly demonstrable enhancement of airway reactivity, ozone acts less on the airways, with only minor bronchconstriction and a modest influence on airway responsiveness, perhaps because of differences in deposition sites. Airway hyperreactivity caused by ozone has been observed after the typical 2-h high-level exposures as well as with the prolonged 6.6-h protocol in which sub-NAAQS exposures to 0.08, 0.10, and 0.12 ppm increased the response to methacholine by 56, 86, and 121 percent, respectively. This increased airway sensitivity could increase the response to other pollutants such as sulfuric acid or to aeroallergens that produce bronchoconstriction.

Compared to field studies, it appears that chamber exposures may underestimate the response for a given exposure to ozone. Greater decrements in pulmonary function per ppm ozone were found in children studied at summer camps than were found in a variety of studies of children after chamber exposures even though the exercise levels in the children at camp were lower than those observed in the chamber studies (Lippmann, 1989). This finding could relate to greater cumulative exposure in the children at camp. The relation between ozone levels the previous day and the pulmonary function of schoolchildren in the Kingston-Harriman area of Tennessee was similar to that observed in the summer camp studies even though the activity levels were lower (Kinney et al., 1988). Again, the role of simultaneous high levels of acid aerosol (which are common in summer haze) is not clear.

Animal studies are consistent with the fact that both duration and concentration are important in assessing the response to ozone exposure (Costa et al., 1989). Pulmonary function decrements increased with C × T (concentration × time) in rats exposed for 2, 4, or 8 h to ozone at 0.2, 0.4, and 0.8 ppm. Rats exposed for 7 h to 0.5 ppm with 8% $CO_2$ added to stimulate respiration showed functional decrements similar to those observed in human chamber studies of 6.6 h at 0.12 ppm when ventilation-adjusted C × T products were computed. This would imply that the rats and humans were responding with about the same sensitivity. It should be cautioned, however, that $CO_2$-stimulated breathing in the rat may have other attributes that contribute to the response beyond mere incrementing of the dose. In related studies without stimulated breathing, the 24-h postexposure response of the bronchoalveolar lavage fluid protein was also nearly linearly cumulative but appeared to have exaggerated responses at the higher concentrations, suggesting an exponential pattern (Highfill et al., 1992). These studies argue that the rat provides a good test model for the response of human subjects.

***Inflammation of the Lung and Host Defense.*** The mechanism by which ozone produces decrements in pulmonary function is not well understood. In contrast to sulfuric acid and sulfur dioxide, functional responses to ozone do not correlate with responsiveness to bronchoconstrictor challenge and are not enhanced in asthmatic subjects as is the case with the sulfated pollutants. Because the contribution of vagal mechanisms in the acute functional response to ozone appears to be minimal, attention has turned to the role of lung inflammation. Koren and colleagues (1989) found an eightfold increase in polymorphonuclear leukocytes (PMN) in lavage fluid 18 h after a 2-h exposure to 0.40 ppm. There was also evidence of increased epithelial permeability (a twofold increase in serum proteins and albumin). However, the inflammatory markers did not correlate well with functional impairment among the individuals tested. Arachidonate metabolism products, including the prostaglandins $PGE_2$ and $PGF_{2a}$ and the leukotriene thromboxane $B_2$, have also been seen to increase in human bronchoalveolar lavage fluid after 0.4 ppm ozone for 2 h (Seltzer et al., 1986). Pretreatment with the anti-inflammatory agents indomethacin and ibuprofen (cyclooxygenase inhibitors) decreased the pulmonary function deficit and $PGE_2$, but other indicators of injury in lavage fluid (PMNs, extravasated protein, and lactate dehydrogenase) were not attenuated after exposure to a similar ozone challenge (Hazucha et al., in press). Because $PGE_2$ can have either pro- or anti-inflammatory functions under certain conditions as well as bronchodilatory action on constricted airways, it remains to be seen whether there is any causal relationship between arachidonate metabolites and functional responses.

The potential for ozone to influence allergic sensitization or responses has received limited investigation in humans and animals. In general, animal studies have shown the ability to enhance the sensitization process under certain conditions (Osebold et al.,1980), but evidence of this in humans is lacking. Controlled studies of heightened responsiveness after sensitization are only suggestive, with enhancement of allergic rhinitis at 0.5 ppm for 4 h providing the only credible data to date. However, diary studies of asthmatics (in spite of their lack of exaggerated sensitivity to ozone) report worsened allergies and symptoms during periods of high ozone (Schwartz, 1989).

Exposure to ozone before a challenge with aerosols of infectious agents produces a higher incidence of infection than is seen in control animals (Coffin and Blommer, 1967). A recent study has demonstrated that this effect in a mouse model using an aerosol of *Streptococcus* (group C) bacteria is a direct result of altered phagocytosis by macrophages in the ozone-exposed animals (Gilmour et al., 1993), allowing the bacteria to develop a thickened capsule which reduces their attractiveness to phagocytes and enhances their virulence. This host resistance model has shown responsiveness to an exposure as low as 0.08 ppm for 3 h. The susceptibility of mice and hamsters to *Klebsiella pneumoniae* aerosol is also increased by prior exposure to ozone. In the rat, altered killing ability may relate to membrane damage in macrophages, thus impairing the production of bactericidal superoxide anion radicals.

***Chronic Effects.*** Morphometric studies of the acinar region of rats exposed for 12 h per day for 6 weeks to 0.12 or 0.25 ppm ozone showed hyperplasia of type I alveolar cells and major alterations in ciliated and Clara cells in small airways (Barry et al., 1988). To simulate the pattern of atmospheric exposure, rats were exposed daily for 13 h at 0.06 ppm plus a 9-h ramped peak 5 days per week to 0.25 ppm for up to 18 months. Hyperplasia of type I cells in the proximal alveoli occurred by 3 to 12 weeks and was linearly cumulative to the ozone $C \times T$ (Chang et al., 1991, 1992). This suggests that there is no threshold for cumulative lung damage over a period approximating an ozone season. Although many of these effects regressed with recovery in clean air, it is unclear whether repeated exposure in rats separated by a seasonal equivalent would in any way respond differently than is the case in the naive animal. Studies in rats and monkeys using an exposure pattern of alternating months of ozone (0.25 ppm) for 18 months resulted in end-airway lesions and interstitial thickening of about the same degree (even more in the monkey) regardless of the twofold difference in the cumulative exposure dose (Tyler et al., 1988, 1991). This would imply that a pattern of exposure resembling seasonal ozone patterns may result in greater lesions than does continuous ozone. Hence, the concept of more dose, more effect may not hold in chronic experiments as it appears to do in acute studies.

Lung function tests in humans chronically exposed to smog were discussed above. Pure ozone studies have never been possible. Studies in animals have been conducted but have provided mixed results. Generally, the effect is one of restriction or stiffened lungs, particularly at higher concentrations. The use of a realistic urban exposure profile for 18 months showed a similar but less dramatic restrictive effect (Costa et al., 1995) which was essentially found in recent National Toxicology Program (NTP) toxicity studies after 20 months at 0.5 ppm given 6 h per day. Interestingly, the cumulative $C \times T$ doses for the urban profile study and the NTP study were similar, but the fibrotic effect was more distinct (yet small) in the profile study, suggesting a possible influence of exposure pattern (known to be important with nitrogen dioxide; see below). Evidence of fibrosis in both studies was marginal histomorphometrically but indistinct biochemically (Last et al., 1994). Monkey and rat studies at higher concentrations have shown some biochemical evidence of fibrosis. This pattern of response appears to clash with the Cincinnati beagle study, which used a synthetic smog atmosphere and showed degenerative disease; unfortunately, the reasons for these differences are not apparent.

One aspect of ozone that is important in its long-term toxicity is its ability to induce tolerance to itself. This tolerance takes the form of protection in animals which received a low initial challenge 7 days before testing with a lethal ozone concentration as well as adaptation to nearly ambient levels, which begins after a single ozone exposure and progresses to completion in at most several days. This adaptive phenomenon has been reported a number of times for humans with regard to lung function tests and recently with inflammatory endpoints (Devlin et al., 1993). Lactate dehydrogenase and elastase markers associated with injury and lung tissue damage did not appear to adapt in humans. In rodents, adaptation of various functional and biochemical endpoints takes place, but the linkages between acute, adaptive, and long-term process are unclear, given that chronic morphological and functional effects do develop. The reduced sensitivity to ozone appears in part to be related to the induction of endogenous antioxidants such as ascorbic acid in the lung. The significance of this finding in humans is uncertain because ascorbic acid is not endogenously synthesized as it is in the rat. It suggests, however, a potential role of self-administration of ascorbate to provide protection from ozone, but no confirmatory data for this point exist.

***Ozone Interactions with Copollutants.*** An approach simplifying that of the synthetic smog studies yet addressing the issue of pollutant interactions involves the exposure of animals or humans to binary or tertiary mixtures of pollutants known to occur together in ambient air. Such studies have had a number of permutations, but most have attempted to address the interactions of ozone and nitrogen dioxide or those of ozone and sulfuric acid. These studies have found both potentiative and antagonistic effects on lung function, lung pathology, or indexes of injury as well as antioxidant or metabolic functions and occasionally have noted species differences overlaid on those responses, making a general interpretation difficult.

In a series of studies, concurrent ozone and nitrogen dioxide from a premixed retention chamber elicited damage in bronchoalveolar lavage endpoints in rats exceeding that of either toxicant alone or in temporal sequence (Gelzleichter et al., 1992). Fibrogenic potential also was increased (Last et al., 1994). Studies in rabbits at more realistic concentrations of 0.3 ppm ozone and 3.0 ppm nitrogen dioxide revealed only additivity on inflammatory eicosinoid metabolites in bronchoalveolar lavage (Schlesinger et al., 1991).

Interaction studies with acid also have shown both potentiative and antagonistic reactions. The diversity in study design and in the variables considered in the many investigations that have been conducted make it difficult to judge the relevance of the findings. Also, dependency on concentrations of each component, which often are relatively high compared with ambient levels, brings into question whether these interactions are likely to be encountered in the real world. However, field studies of children in camps and asthma admissions in the northeast and in Canada, as was noted above, have found an apparent interdependence of acid and ozone as part of the response to summer haze. In a long-term study, rabbits exhibited enhanced or antagonized secretory cell responses with combined ozone (0.1 ppm) and sulfuric acid (125 $\mu g/m^3$) at different points in the 1-year exposure (Schlesinger et al., 1992). Studies of even more complex atmospheres involving acid, ozone, nitrogen dioxide, and road dust at relevant levels show some evidence of interaction regarding macrophage toxicity. One difficulty with multicomponent studies is the statistical separation of the interacting responses from the individual or additive responses given the design demands of such studies. Nevertheless, it is the complex mixture to which people are exposed that we wish to evaluate for potential harm. Creative approaches to understanding mixture responses are a likely part of the new agenda that toxicologists will need to address in the next decade.

**Nitrogen Dioxide.** ***General Toxicology.*** Nitrogen dioxide, like ozone, is a deep lung irritant that can produce pulmonary edema if it is inhaled at high concentrations. This is a practical problem for farmers, as sufficient amounts can be liberated from ensilage to produce the symptoms of pulmonary damage known as silo filler's disease. Nitrogen dioxide is also an important indoor pollutant, especially in homes with unventilated gas stoves or kerosene heaters (Spengler and Sexton, 1983). Under such circumstances, children, who are especially sensitive, may show decrements in pulmonary function. The fact that nitrogen dioxide can cause effects similar to those produced by ozone is not surprising, but $NO_2$ is by far a much less potent irritant. The levels needed to produce effects are in general far above the levels that occur in ambient air. More recently, protocols that simulate an urban (rush hour) or household (cooking) pattern of two daily peaks superimposed on a low continuous background concentration have produced effects in experimental animals when continuous exposure to nitrogen dioxide did not.

Although the distal lung lesions produced by acute nitrogen dioxide are similar among species, there are considerable differences in species sensitivity. Where a direct comparison is possible, guinea pigs, hamsters, and monkeys are more sensitive than are rats, although comparative dosimetry information might explain some of this difference. Dosimetry studies indicate that nitrogen dioxide is deposited along the length of the respiratory tree, with its preferential site of deposition being the distal lung. Hence, the pattern of damage reflects this profile. In accordance with the dosimetry estimates, damage is most apparent in the terminal bronchioles, just a bit more proximal in the airway than is seen with ozone. At high concentrations, the alveolar ducts and alveoli are also affected, with type I cells again showing their sensitivity to oxidant challenge. In the airways of these animals there is also damage to epithelial cells in the bronchioles, notably with loss of ciliated cells, as well as a loss of secretory granules in Clara cells. The pattern of injury of nitrogen dioxide is quite similar to that of ozone, but the potency is about an order of magnitude lower.

***Pulmonary Function Effects.*** Exposure of normal human subjects to concentrations of nitrogen dioxide of 4 ppm or less for periods up to 3 h produced no consistent effects on spirometry. However, a study has shown slightly enhanced airway reactivity with 1.5 to 2.0 ppm. Interestingly, ascorbic acid pretreatment of the human subjects appeared to protect them from this hyperreactivity (Mohsenin, 1987). Whether asthmatics have a particular sensitivity to nitrogen dioxide is a controversial issue. A number of factors appear to be involved (e.g., exercise, inherent sensitivity of the asthmatic subject, exposure method). Some studies have reported effects in some individuals at 0.2 ppm, which would be the level of a household with an unvented gas stove. Very high concentrations (10 ppm) are required for guinea pigs to show deep irritant tachypnea relative to the levels a person probably would encounter in everyday life.

***Inflammation of the Lung and Host Defense.*** Unlike ozone, nitrogen dioxide does not induce significant neutrophilic inflammation in humans at acute exposure concentrations approximating those in the ambient outdoor environment. There is some evidence for bronchial inflammation after 4 to 6 h at 2.0 ppm, which approximates the highest transient peak indoor concentrations of this oxidant. Exposures at these higher levels (2.0 to 5.0 ppm) also have been shown to affect T lymphocytes, particularly CD8+ cells and natural killer cells, which function in host defenses against viruses. Epidemiological studies show an effect of nitrogen dioxide, especially in indoor environments, on respiratory infection rates in children, though not all studies have found positive associations. Animal models, by contrast, have for years shown associations between nitrogen dioxide and both viral and bacterial infection. The bacterial infectivity data in mice have been reviewed by Gardner (1984). Several different strains of bacteria have been used to demonstrate these effects, which appear to be governed more by the peak exposure concentration than by long, low-level exposures at similar $C \times T$s. These effects are ascribed to suppression of macrophage function and clearance from the lung. Altered function in the form of killing and/or motility was apparent in macrophages from rabbits exposed to 0.3 ppm for 3 days (Schlesinger, 1987) and from humans exposed to 0.10 ppm for 6.6 h (Devlin et al., 1991).

Studies with viruses are suggestive of enhanced infectivity. Squirrel monkeys infected with nonlethal levels of A/PR-8 influenza virus and then exposed continuously to 5 or 10 ppm nitrogen dioxide suffered mortality: six of six monkeys exposed to 10 ppm within 3 days and one of three exposed to 5 ppm (Henry et al., 1970). Other experiments suggested that the exposure of squirrel monkeys for 5 months to 5 ppm nitrogen dioxide depressed the formation of a protective antibody against this influenza virus. Controlled clinical studies in humans have been inconclusive, generally because of low subject numbers. One study showed decreased virus inactivation by macrophages in four of nine subjects when cultured in vitro after 3.5 h of 0.6 ppm nitrogen dioxide. These same macrophages also produced interleukin-1, which is a known cytokine modulator of immune cell function (Frampton et al., 1989). Thus, the issue of enhanced infection associated with nitrogen dioxide exposure remains controversial, particularly at the concentrations to which one is likely to be exposed.

***Chronic Effects.*** Concern about the chronic effects of nitrogen dioxide stem from observations that 30-ppm exposures for 30 days produce emphysema in hamsters. Whether this has a bearing on human exposures at 100-fold lower exposure concentrations is questionable. An 18-month study in rats exposed to an urban pattern of nitrogen dioxide in which a background of 0.5 ppm for 23 h per day peaked at 1.5 ppm for 4 h each day showed little ultrastructural damage to the distal lung (Chang et al., 1988). Other studies utilizing peak-base patterns of exposure have found some effect at nearly environmental levels of nitrogen dioxide using other biological endpoints. Mice exposed for a year to a base level of 0.2 ppm nitrogen dioxide with a 1-h spike of 0.8 ppm twice a day 5 days per week (Miller et al., 1987) yielded effects that differed between base-only and peak exposure groups. The base level produced no effects, while the spiked group experienced slight functional impairment and augmented susceptibility to bacterial infection. Early studies (Ehrlich and Henry, 1968) showed that clearance of bacteria from the lungs is suppressed with 0.5 ppm through 12 months of exposure. These and similar studies utilizing peak plus baseline versus baseline or peak alone exposures indicate that for nitrogen dioxide, the exposure profile may act as a determinant in the elicitation of a toxic effect.

**Other Oxidants.** While a number of reactive oxidants have been identified in photochemical smog, most are short-lived because of their reaction with available volatile organic compounds (VOCs), nitric oxides, and other reducing equivalents which have the effect of scrubbing them from the air before they can be breathed. One reactive, irritating constituent of the oxidant atmosphere is PAN, which is thought to be responsible for much of the eye-stinging activity of smog. It is more soluble and reactive than ozone is and hence dissipates in mucous membranes before it can get down into the lungs. The eyes have many irritant receptors and respond readily, while the PAN absorbed into the thicker mucous fluids of the proximal nose and mouth presumably never reaches its target. A few studies with high levels of PAN have shown that it can cause lung damage and have mutagenic activity in bacteria, but it is not likely that this is relevant to air pollution.

**Aldehydes.** Various aldehydes in polluted air are formed as reaction products in the photooxidation of hydrocarbons. The two aldehydes of major interest are formaldehyde (HCHO) and acrolein ($H_2C{=}CHCHO$). These materials contribute to the odor and eye irritation of photochemical smog. Formaldehyde accounts for about 50 percent of the estimated total aldehydes in polluted air, while acrolein, the more irritating of the two, may account for about 5 percent of the total aldehyde. Acetaldehyde and many other longer-chain aldehydes make up the remainder, but they are not as irritating because of their low concentration and lesser solubility in airway fluids. Both formaldehyde and acrolein are found in tobacco smoke, particularly acrolein (~90 ppm per drag), and are likely to be found in sidestream smoke as well. Empirical studies have shown that formaldehyde and acrolein compete for similar irritant receptors in the airway and thus can act as competitive agonists. Thus, irritation may be related not to "total aldehyde" but to specific concentrations of acrolein and formaldehyde. Their relative difference in solubility, with formaldehyde being somewhat more soluble and thus having more nasopharyngeal uptake, may distort this relationship under certain exposure conditions (e.g., exercise).

***Formaldehyde.*** Formaldehyde is a primary irritant. Because it is very soluble in water, it irritates mucous membranes in the nose, upper respiratory tract, and eyes. Concentrations of 0.5 to 1 ppm are detectable by odor, those of 2 to 3 ppm produce mild irritation, and those of 4 to 5 ppm are intolerable to most people. In guinea pigs, a 1-h exposure to ≥0.3 ppm formaldehyde produced an increase in pulmonary flow resistance accompanied by a lesser decrease in compliance (Amdur, 1960). The respiratory frequency and minute volume decreased, but changes in these factors did not become statistically significant until concentrations of 10 ppm and above were used. The overall pattern of respiratory response to formaldehyde is similar to that produced by sulfur dioxide.

A concentration of 0.05 ppm caused no alterations in any of the respiratory criteria used. Below concentrations of 50 ppm, the alterations were reversible within an hour after the exposure. The response to a given concentration of formaldehyde was greater when the gas was inhaled through a tracheal cannula, which bypassed the scrubbing effect of the upper respiratory tract and permitted a greater concentration of the irritant to reach the lungs. The response in these animals was readily reversible, and the flow resistance values returned to preexposure levels by 1 h after the end of exposure. When formaldehyde was inhaled simultaneously with submicron sodium chloride aerosol, irritancy was potentiated in proportion to the aerosol concentration. This response was greater than what could be accounted for by a simple carrying effect. Moreover, reversal of bronchoconstriction was slowed. It appeared that the aerosol itself constituted a new irritant species. Both the water-soluble particles and the carbon-based particles which exist in these atmospheres have shown the ability to interact with formaldehyde and hence could theoretically potentiate the relatively low concentration of ambient formaldehyde.

Two aspects of formaldehyde toxicology have brought it from relative obscurity to the forefront of the news. One is its presence in indoor atmospheres as an off-gassed product of construction materials such as plywood or improperly installed urea-formaldehyde foam insulation. This aspect is discussed at length in a review article (Spengler and Sexton, 1983). Complaints of formaldehyde irritation in industry have been reported at 50 ppb (Horvath et al., 1988). In studies relating household formaldehyde to chronic effects, children were found to have significantly lower peak expiratory flow rates (~22 percent in homes with 60 ppb) than did unexposed children or adults regardless of the household. Asthmatic children were affected below 50 ppb. Thus, this irritant vapor has the potential to cause respiratory effects at commonly experienced exposure levels (Krzyzanowski et al., 1990), and this may relate to evidence that formaldehyde is a weak sensitizer and is capable of initiating allergic responses.

Nasal cancer has been induced empirically with formaldehyde vapor in rodents. In a 2-year study, rats were exposed to 2, 6, or 14 ppm formaldehyde 6 h per day 5 days per week. The occurrence of nasal squamous cell carcinomas was zero in the control and 2-ppm groups, 1 percent in the 6-ppm group, and 44 percent in the 14-ppm group. An exposure-related induction of squamous metaplasia occurred in the respiratory epithelium of the anterior nasal passages in all exposed groups. Rats exposed 6 h per day for 5 days to 14 ppm had a greater than 20-fold increase in cell proliferation in the nasal epithelium. Mice were much less sensitive; only one carcinoma was seen at 14 ppm. The likely reasons for this species difference and the implications of these findings to the development of the observed carcinomas were reviewed by Starr and Gibson (1985). The detection of DNA adducts in the two species paralleled the difference in the incidence of tumors. With this collection of data, formaldehyde has been designated as a probable human carcinogen. Recent epidemiology studies, however, have failed to find an increased incidence of nasal cancer in exposed workers.

***Acrolein.*** Because it is an unsaturated aldehyde, acrolein is more irritating than formaldehyde. Concentrations below 1 ppm cause irritation of the eyes and the mucous membranes of the respiratory tract. Exposure of guinea pigs to >0.6 ppm reversibly increased pulmonary flow resistance and tidal volume but decreased respiratory frequency (Murphy et al., 1963). With irritants of this type, flow resistance is increased by concentrations below those which cause a decrease in frequency. This suggests that increases in flow resistance would be produced by far lower concentrations of acrolein than were tested. The mechanism of increased resistance appears to be mediated through a cholinergic reflex. Atropine (muscarinic blocker) and aminophylline, isoproterenol, and epinephrine (sympathetic agonists) partially or completely reversed the changes. The antihistamines pyrilamine and tripelennamine had no effect.

Exposures of rats to 0.4, 1.4, or 4.0 ppm for 6 h per day 5 days per week for 13 weeks resulted in apparently paradoxical effects on lung function (Costa et al., 1986). The lowest concentration resulted in hyperinflation of the lung with an apparent reduction in small airway flow resistance, while the highest concentration resulted in airway injury and peribronchial inflammation and fibrosis. The intermediate concentration was functionally not different from the control but did show some airway pathology. It appears that the high-concentration response reflected the cumulative irritant injury of repeated acrolein, while the low-concentration group was thought to have had slightly stiffened airways with little overt damage, perhaps a result of the protein cross-linking action of acrolein. The pathology in these animals contrasts with formaldehyde studies of similar duration in that there was much more airway involvement. Ambient exposure to acrolein probably would be about fivefold to tenfold lower than the low concentration used in the subchronic study discussed above.

**Carbon Monoxide.** Carbon monoxide is classed toxicologically as a chemical asphyxiant because its toxic action stems from its formation of carboxyhemoglobin, preventing oxygenation of the blood for systemic transport. The fundamental toxicology of carbon monoxide and the physiological factors that determine the level of carboxyhemoglobin attained in the blood at various atmospheric concentrations of carbon monoxide are detailed in Chapter 11.

The normal concentration of carboxyhemoglobin (COHb) in the blood of nonsmokers is about 0.5 percent. This is attributed to endogenous production of CO from heme catabolism. Uptake of exogenous CO increases blood COHb as a function of the concentration in air as well as the length of exposure and the ventilation rate of the individual. Uptake is said to be ventilation-limited, implying that virtually all the carbon monoxide inspired in a breath is absorbed and bound to the available hemoglobin. Continuous exposure of human subjects to 30 ppm CO leads to an equilibrium value of 5 percent COHb. About 80 percent of this value is approached in 4 h, and the remaining 20 percent is approached slowly over the next 8 h. It can be calculated (Haldane equation) that continuous exposure to 20 ppm CO gives an equilibrium COHb value of about 3.7 percent and that exposure to 10 ppm CO gives an equilibrium COHb value of 2 percent. The equilibrium values generally are reached after 8 h or more of exposure. The time required to reach equilibrium can be shortened by physical activity.

Analysis of data from air-monitoring programs in California indicates that 8-h average values, which may be exceeded 0.1 percent of the time, ranged from 10 to 40 ppm CO. Depending on the location in a community, CO concentrations can vary widely. Concentrations predicted inside the passenger compartments of motor vehicles in downtown traffic were almost 3 times those for central urban areas and 5 times those expected in residential areas. Occupants of vehicles traveling on expressways had CO exposures somewhere between those in central urban areas and those in downtown traffic. Concentrations above 87 ppm have been measured in underground garages, tunnels, and buildings over highways.

No overt human health effects have been demonstrated for COHb levels below 2 percent. At COHb levels of 2.5 percent resulting from about 90-min exposure to about 50 ppm CO, there is an impairment of time-interval discrimination; at approximately 5 percent COHb, there is an impairment of other psychomotor faculties. At levels as low as 5 percent COHb in nonsmokers (the median COHb value for smokers is about 5 percent), however, maximal exercise duration and maximal oxygen consumption are reduced (Aronow, 1981). Cardiovascular changes also may be produced by exposure sufficient to yield COHb in excess of 5 percent. These include increased cardiac output, arteriovenous oxygen difference, and coronary blood flow in patients without coronary disease. Decreased coronary sinus blood $P_{O_2}$ occurs in patients with coronary heart disease, and this would impair oxidative metabolism of the myocardium. Over the last several years a series of studies in subjects with cardiovascular disease were conducted to determine the potential for angina pectoris when they exercised moderately with COHb levels in the range of 2 to 6 percent (Allred et al., 1989). The results of these studies indicate that premature angina can result under these conditions but that the potential for the induction of ventricular arrhythmias remains uncertain. Thus, the reduction in ambient carbon monoxide brought about by newer controls should reduce the risk of myocardial infarct in predisposed persons.

**Hazardous Air Pollutants.** Hazardous air pollutants (so-called air toxics) represent an inclusive classification for pollutants in the air that are of anthropogenic origin, are of measurable quantity, and are not covered in the Criteria Pollutant list. The inclusive nature of this group of pollutants complicates a discussion of their toxicology because the group includes various classes of organic chemicals (by structure, e.g., acrolein, benzene), minerals (e.g., asbestos), polycyclic hydrocarbon particulate material [e.g., benzo(*a*)pyrene], and various metals and metal compounds (e.g., mercury, beryllium compounds) and pesticides (e.g., carbaryl, parathion). Section 112 b(1) of the 1990 Clean Air Act designates a priority list of 189 chemicals in the official list of hazardous air pollutants. The point of this discussion is not to discuss the regulatory aspects of these pollutants but to note the diversity and complexity of ambient air and the need for a better understanding of its potential health impact.

Most toxic air pollutants are of concern because of their potential carcinogenicity as shown in chronic bioassays, mutagenicity tests in bacterial systems, structure-activity relationships, or in a few special cases (e.g., benzene, asbestos) their known carcinogenicity in humans. Noncancer issues generally relate to direct lung toxicants which upon accidental release or as fugitive emissions over time might induce lung damage or lead to chronic lung disease. The assessment of risk of the non-cancer-attributed air toxics is based on the computation of long-term risk reference exposure concentrations (RfCs) to which individuals may be exposed over a lifetime without adverse, irreversible injury. This approach to hazardous air pollutant assessment is discussed in detail by Jarabek and Segal (1994). A short-term RfC method for brief or accidental exposures is being developed.

***Accidental versus "Fence-Line" Exposures.*** The relationship between the effects associated with an accidental release of a large quantity of a volatile chemical into the air from a point source such as a chemical plant and the effects associated with a chronic low-level exposure over many years or a lifetime is not clear. With regard to cancer, which for the present assumes a linearized model of dose and effect, the issue is fairly straightforward. Any exposure must be minimized, if not eliminated, if cancer risk is to be kept as close to zero as possible. With noncancer risks, the roles of nonspecific or specific host defenses, thresholds of response, and repair and recovery after exposure complicate the assessment of risk. In large part the issue here relates to C × T. Can we better relate disease or injury to *cumulative dose* or *peak* concentration for protracted exposures? Is there an exposure peak beyond which a cumulative approach fails (i.e., the effect is concentration-driven), or is concentration always the dominant determinant? Many of these questions have yet to be answered, not to mention their specificity with regard to individual compounds.

Methyl isocyanate provides a contrast between the effects of a large accidental release versus a small release of fugitive vapor such that it is detectable in ambient air but at very low levels. The reactive nature of methyl isocyanate with aqueous environments is of such magnitude that upon inspiration, almost immediate severe irritancy can be perceived by an exposed individual. The vapor undergoes hydrolysis within the mucous lining of the airways to generate hydrocyanic acid, which destroys the airway epithelium and causes acute bronchoconstriction and edema. The damage is almost immediately life-threatening at concentrations above 50 ppm and is damaging in minutes at 10 ppm. These concentrations are in the range of the dense vapor cloud that for several hours enshrouded the village of Bhopal bordering the Union Carbide pesticide plant.

Studies in guinea pigs showed the immediate irritancy of this isocyanate, which in just a few minutes also resulted in significant pathology (Alarie et al., 1987). Rats exposed to 10 or 30 ppm for 2 h also showed severe airway and parenchymal damage, which in surviving rats did not resolve; transient effects were seen at 3 ppm. Even 6 months after exposure, the airway and lung damage remained, having evolved into patchy, mostly peribronchial fibrosis with associated functional impairments (Stevens et al., 1987). There was also cardiac involvement secondary to the damage to the pulmonary parenchyma and arterial bed. As a result, there was pulmonary hypertension and right-sided heart hypertrophy. This same collection of biological signs appeared in the surviving exposed residents of Bhopal and is in large part associated with their above-average death rate.

In the United States, methyl isocyanate has been measured in Katawba Valley, Texas, as a result of small but virtually continual fugitive releases of the vapor into the community air ("fence-line") from an adjoining region with several chemical plants. While these levels of methyl isocyanate are not sufficient to cause the damage seen in Bhopal, there is concern that low-level exposure over many years may have more diffuse, chronic effects. Residents complain of odors and a higher frequency of respiratory disorders, but clear evidence of injury or disease is lacking.

Phosgene is best known for its use as a war gas, but it is also one of the most common intermediate reactants used in the chemical industry, particularly in pesticide formulation. It is also a constituent of photochemical smog. Because of its direct pulmonary reactivity, it lends itself to use as a model pulmonary toxicant for studies addressing C × T relationships. These studies suggest that there may be a threshold below which compensatory and other bodily defenses (e.g., antioxidants) may be able to cope with long-term low-level exposure (tolerance). For phosgene this appears to be at or below the current threshold limit value of 0.1 ppm for 8 h. At higher concentrations, however, concentration appears to be the primary determinant of injury or disease regardless of duration. Thus, even though there is some adaptation with time, there continues to be a concentration-driven response which exceeds that predicted by C × T. This relationship appears to be different from that of ozone at ambient levels, which can be approximated acutely by the C × T paradigm.

## CONCLUSIONS

Because this chapter was written for a textbook of toxicology, it has attempted to relate experimental studies to what we know in humans through epidemiological or controlled clinical study of specific pollutants identified in urban air. Data of this kind are among the factors considered in practical deliberations on the development of air quality criteria and standards as mandated by the Clean Air Act of 1970 and its most recent amendment in 1990. The initial step in this process is the preparation of an air quality criteria document that sets forth the state of knowledge in regard to the effects of a substance on animals, humans, plants, and materials. It is in this step that the availability of pertinent toxicological data is of prime importance. This has been and should continue to be an incentive to toxicologists to develop sensitive methods of assaying the response to low concentrations of materials that occur as air pollutants and to develop paradigms of exposure and species sensitivity to relate empirical toxicological data to real life.

# REFERENCES


Alarie Y, Ferguson JS, Stock MF, et al: Sensory and pulmonary irritation of methyl isocyanate in mice and pulmonary irritation and possible cyanidelike effects of methyl isocyanate in guinea pigs. *Environ Health Perspect* 72:159–168, 1987.

Alarie YC, Krumm AA, Busey WM, et al: Long-term exposure to sulfur dioxide, sulfuric acid mist, fly ash, and their mixtures: Results of studies in monkeys and guinea pigs. *Arch Environ Health* 30:254–262, 1975.

Alarie YC, Ulrich CE, Busey WM, et al: Long-term continuous exposure of guinea pigs to sulfur dioxide. *Arch Environ Health* 21:769–777, 1970.

Alarie YC, Ulrich CE, Busey WM, et al: Long-term continuous exposure to sulfur dioxide in cynomolgus monkeys. *Arch Environ Health* 24:115–128, 1972.

Allred EN, Bleeker ER, Chaitman BR, et al: Short-term effects of carbon monoxide exposure on individuals with coronary heart disease. *N Engl J Med* 321:1426–1432, 1989.

Altshuler B: Regional deposition of aerosols, in Aharonson FF et al (eds): *Air Pollution and the Lung*. New York:Wiley, 1976.

Amdur MO: Toxicological studies of air pollutants. *US Public Health Reports* 69:724–726, 1954.

Amdur MO: The respiratory response of guinea pigs to sulfuric acid mist. *AMA Arch Ind Health* 18:407–414, 1958.

Amdur MO: The response of guinea pigs to inhalation of formaldehyde and formic acid alone and with a sodium chloride aerosol. *Int J Air Pollut* 3:201–220, 1960.

Amdur MO: 1974 Cummings memorial lecture: The long road from Donora. *Am Ind Hyg Assoc J* 35:589–597, 1974.

Amdur MO: Sulfuric acid: The animals tried to tell us: 1989 Herbert E. Stokinger Lecture. *Appl Ind Hyg Assoc J* 4:189–197, 1989.

Amdur MO, Dubriel M, Creasia DA: Respiratory response of guinea pigs to low levels of sulfuric acid. *Environ Res* 15:418–423, 1978.

Amdur MO, Sarofim AF, Neville M, et al: Coal combustion aerosols and $SO_2$: An interdisciplinary analysis. *Environ Sci Tech* 20:139–145, 1986.

Amdur MO, Underhill DW: The effect of various aerosols on the response of guinea pigs to sulfur dioxide. *Arch Environ Health* 16:460–468, 1968.

Aronow WS: Aggravation of angina pectoris by two percent carboxyhemoglobin. *Am Heart J* 101:154–157, 1981.

Barry BE, Mercer RR, Miller FJ, Crapo JD: Effects of inhalation of 0.25 ppm ozone on the terminal bronchioles of juvenile and adult rats. *Exp Lung Res* 14:225–245, 1988.

Bates DV, Sizto R: The Ontario air pollution study: Identification of the causative agent. *Environ Health Perspect* 79:69–72, 1989.

Brooks BO, Davis WF: *Understanding Indoor Air Quality*. Boca Raton, FL: CRC Press, 1992.

Chang L, Huang Y, Stockstill BL, et al: Epithelial injury and interstitial fibrosis in the proximal alveolar regions of rats chronically exposed to a simulated pattern of urban ambient ozone. *Toxicol Appl Pharmacol* 115:241–252, 1992.

Chang L, Miller FJ, Ultman J, et al: Alveolar epithelial cell injuries by subacute exposure to low concentrations of ozone correlate with cumulative exposure. *Toxicol Appl Pharmacol* 109:219–234, 1991.

Chang LY, Mercer RR, Stockstill BL, et al: Effects of low levels of $NO_2$ on terminal bronchiolar cells and its relative toxicity compared to $O_3$. *Toxicol Appl Pharmacol* 96:451–464, 1988.

Chen LC, Lam HF, Kim EJ, et al: Pulmonary effects of ultrafine coal fly ash inhaled by guinea pigs. *J Toxicol Environ Health* 29:169–184, 1990.

Coffin DL, Blommer EJ: Acute toxicity of irradiated auto exhaust: Its indication by enhancement of mortality from streptococcal pneumonia. *Arch Environ Health* 15:36–38, 1967.

Costa DL, Hatch GE, Highfill J, et al: Pulmonary function studies in the rat addressing concentration vs. time relationships for ozone, in Schneider T, Lee SD, Wolters GJR, Grant LD (eds): *Atmospheric Ozone Research and Its Policy Implications*. Amsterdam: Elsevier, 1989, pp 733–743.

Costa DL, Kutzman RS, Lehmann JR, Drew RT: Altered lung function and structure in the rat after subchronic exposure to acrolein. *Am Rev Resp Dis* 133:286–291, 1986.

Costa DL, Tepper JS, Stevens MA, et al: Restrictive lung disease in rats chronically exposed to an urban profile of ozone. *Am J Resp Crit Care Med* 151:1512–1518, 1995.

Detels R, Tashkin DP, Sayre JW, et al: The UCLA population studies of CORD: X. A cohort study of changes in respiratory function associated with chronic exposure to $SO_X$, $NO_X$, and hydrocarbons. *Am J Public Health* 81:350–359, 1991.

Devlin RB, Folinsbee LJ, Biscardi F, et al: Attenuation of cellular and biochemical changes in the lungs of humans exposed to ozone for five consecutive days. *Am Rev Respir Dis* 147:A71, 1993.

Devlin RB, McDonnell WF, Mann R, et al: Exposure of humans to ambient levels of ozone for 6.6 hours causes cellular and biochemical changes in the lung. *Am J Respir Cell Mol Biol* 4:72–81, 1991.

Dockery DW, Pope CA: Acute respiratory effects of particulate air pollution. *Rev Public Health* 15:107–132, 1994

Dockery DW, Pope CA, Xu X, et al: An association between air pollution and mortality in six U.S. cities. *N Engl J Med* 329(24): 1753–1759, 1993.

Ehrlich R, Henry MC: Chronic toxicity of nitrogen dioxide: I. Effect on resistance to bacterial pneumonia. *Arch Environ Health* 17:860–865, 1968.

*Environmental Progress and Challenges: EPA's Update.* U.S. EPA, Office of Policy Planning and Evaluation (PM-219), EPA-230-07-88-033, 1988, p 29, Washington, DC.

Frampton MW, Smeglin AM, Roberts NJJ, et al: Nitrogen dioxide exposure *in vivo* and human macrophage inactivation of influenza virus *in vitro*. *Environ Res* 48:179–192, 1989.

Frank NR, Amdur MO, Worchester J, Whittenberger JL: Effects of acute controlled exposure to $SO_2$ on respiratory mechanics in healthy male adults. *J Appl Physiol* 17:252–258, 1962.

Frank NR, Speizer FE: $SO_2$ effects on the respiratory system in dogs: Changes in mechanical behavior at different levels of the respiratory system during acute exposure to the gas. *Arch Environ Health* 11:624–634, 1965.

Gardner DE: Oxidant induced enhanced sensitivity to infection in animal models and their extrapolation to man. *J Toxicol Environ Health* 13:423–439, 1984.

Gearhart JM, Schlesinger RB: Sulfuric acid-induced changes in the physiology and structure of the tracheobronchial airways. *Environ Health Perspect* 79:127–136, 1989.

Gelzleichter TR, Witschi H, Last JA: Synergistic interaction of nitrogen dioxide and ozone on rat lungs: Acute responses. *Toxicol Appl Pharmacol* 116:1–9, 1992.

Gerrity TR, Weaver RA, Bernsten J, et al: Extrathoracic and intrathoracic removal of ozone in tidal breathing humans. *J Appl Physiol* 65:393–400, 1988.

Ghio AJ, Kennedy TP, Whorton AR, et al: Role of surface complexed iron in oxidant generation and lung inflammation induced by silicates. *Am J Physiol* 263(*Lung Cell Mol Physiol* 7):L511–L518, 1992.

Gilmour MI, Park P, Doerfler D, Selgrade MK: Ozone-enhanced pulmonary infection with Streptococcus zooepidemicus in mice: The role of alveolar macrophage function and capsular virulence factors. *Am Rev Respir Dis* 147:753–760, 1993.

Gunnison AF, Palmes ED: S-Sulfonates in human plasma following inhalation of sulfur dioxide. *Am Ind Hyg Assoc J* 35:288–291, 1974.

Hackney JD, Linn WS, Avol EL: Acid fog: Effects on respiratory function and symptoms in healthy asthmatic volunteers. *Environ Health Perspect* 79:159–162, 1989.

Hanley QS, Koenig JQ, Larson TV, et al: Response of young asthmatic patients to inhaled sulfuric acid. *Am Rev Respir Dis* 145:326–331, 1992.

Hatch GE, Boykin E, Graham JA, et al: Inhalable particles and pulmonary host defense: *In vivo* and *in vitro* effects of ambient air and combustion particles. *Environ Res* 36:67–80, 1985.

Hatch GE, Slade R, Harris LP, et al: Ozone dose and effect in humans and rats: A comparison using oxygen-18 labeling and bronchoalveolar lavage. *Am J Respir Crit Care Med* 150:676–683, 1994.

Hazucha M, Madden M, Pape G, et al: Effect of cycloxygenase inhibition on ozone induced respiratory inflammation and lung function changes. *Environ J Appl Physiol Occup Health* (in press).

Henry MC, Findlay J, Spengler J, Ehrlich R: Chronic toxicity of $NO_2$ in squirrel monkeys: III. Effect on resistance to bacterial and viral infection. *Am Ind Hyg Assoc J* 20:566–570, 1970.

Highfill JH, Hatch GE, Slade R, et al: Concentration time models for the effects of ozone on bronchoalveolar lavage fluid protein in rats and guinea pigs. *Inhal Toxicol* 4:1–16, 1992.

Higuchi MA, Davies DW: An ammonia abatement system for whole-body animal inhalation exposures to acid aerosols. *Inhal Toxicol* 5:323–333, 1993.

Holma B: Effects of inhaled acids on airway mucus and its consequences for health. *Environ Health Perspect* 79:109–114, 1989.

Horstman DH, Folinsbee LJ, Ives PJ, et al: Ozone concentration and pulmonary response relationships for 6.6 hours with five hours of moderate exercise to 0.08, 0.10, and 0.12 ppm. *Am Rev Respir Dis* 142:1158–1162, 1989.

Horvath E, Anderson H, Pierce W, et al: Effects of formaldehyde on mucous membranes and lungs: A study of an industrial population. *JAMA* 259:701–707, 1988.

Hyde D, Orthoefer J, Dungworth D, et al: Morphometric and morphologic pulmonary lesions in beagle dogs chronically exposed to high ambient levels of air pollutants. *Lab Invest* 38(4):455–469, 1978.

Jarabek AM, Segal SA: Noncancer toxicity of inhaled toxic air pollutants: Available approaches for risk assessment and risk management, in Patrick DR (ed): *Toxic Air Pollution Handbook*. New York: Van Nostrand Reinhold, 1994, pp 100–132.

Kinney PJ, Ware JH, Spengler JD: A critical evaluation of acute epidemiology results. *Arch Environ Health* 43:168–173, 1988.

Koenig JQ, Covert DS, Pierson WE: Effects of inhalation of acidic compounds on pulmonary function in allergic adolescent subjects. *Environ Health Perspect* 79:127–137, 173–178, 1989.

Koenig JQ, Pierson WE, Horike M, Frank R: Effects of $SO_2$ plus NaCl aerosol combined with moderate exercise on pulmonary function in asthmatic adolescents. *Environ Res* 25:340–348, 1981.

Koren HS, Devlin RB, Graham DE, et al: Ozone-induced inflammation in the lower airways of human subjects. *Am Rev Respir Dis* 139:407–415, 1989.

Kotin P, Falk HF: Atmospheric factors in pathogenesis of lung cancer. *Cancer Res* 7:475–514, 1963.

Krzyzanowski M, Quackenboss JJ, Lebowitz MD: Chronic respiratory effects of indoor formaldehyde exposure. *Environ Res* 52:117–125, 1990.

Last JA, Gelzleichter TR, Harkema J, Hawk S: *Consequences of Prolonged Inhalation of Ozone on Fischer-344/N Rats: Collaborative Studies*. Part I: *Content and Cross-Linking of Lung Collagen*. Health Effects Institute: Res. Report No. 65, Cambridge, MA, April 1994.

Leikauf G. Yeates DB, Wales KA, et al: Effects of sulfuric acid aerosol on respiratory mechanics and mucociliary particle clearance in healthy nonsmoking adults. *Am Ind Hyg Assoc J* 42:273–282, 1981.

Lewis TR, Campbell KI, Vaughan TR Jr: Effects on canine pulmonary function: Via induced $NO_2$ impairment, particulate interaction, and subsequent $SO_X$. *Arch Environ Health* 18:596–601, 1969.

Lewis TR, Moorman WJ, Yang YY, Stara JF: Long-term exposure to auto exhaust and other pollutant mixtures. *Arch Environ Health* 21:102–106, 1974.

Lewtas J: Airborne carcinogens. *Pharmacol Toxicol* 72(Suppl 1):S55–S63, 1993.

Lipfert FW: *Air Pollution and Community Health: A Critical Review and Data Sourcebook*. New York: Van Nostrand Reinhold, 1994, pp 10–57.

Lippmann M: Health effects of ozone: A critical review. *J Air Pollut Control Assoc* 39:67–96, 1989.

Martonen TB, Zhang Z, Yang Y: Interspecies modeling of inhaled particle deposition patterns. *J Aerosol Sci* 23(4): 389–406, 1992.

McClellan RO: Health effects of diesel exhaust: A case study in risk assessment. *Am Ind Hyg Assoc J* 47:1–13, 1986.

McDonnell WF, Horstman DH, Hazucha MJ, et al: Pulmonary effects of ozone exposure during exercise: Dose-response characteristics. *J Appl Physiol* 5:1345–1352, 1983.

Miller FJ, Graham JA, Raub JA, et al: Evaluating the toxicity of urban patterns of oxidant gases: II. Effects in mice from chronic exposure to nitrogen dioxide. *J Toxicol Environ Health* 21:99–112, 1987.

Miller FW, Miller RM: *Environmental Hazards: Air Pollution—A Reference Handbook*. Contemporary World Issues. Santa Barbara, Ca.: ABC-CLIO, 1993, pp 1–18.

Mohsenin V: Effect of vitamin C on $NO_2$-induced airway hyperresponsiveness in normal subjects. *Am Rev Respir Dis* 136:1408–1411, 1987.

Molhave LB, Bach B, Pederson O: Human reactions to low concentrations of volatile organic compounds. *Environ Int* 12:165–167, 1986.

Murphy SD, Klingshirn DA, Ulrich CE: Respiratory response of guinea pigs during acrolein inhalation and its modification by drugs. *J Pharmacol Exp Ther* 141:79–83, 1963.

Nadel JA, Salem H, Tamplin B, Tokiwa Y: Mechanism of bronchoconstriction during inhalation of sulfur dioxide. *J Appl Physiol* 20:164–167, 1965.

*National Air Pollutant Emission Trends 1990–1992*. U.S. EPA, Office of Air Quality Planning and Standards, EPA-454/R-93-032, 1993, p E5–6, Research Triangle Park, NC.

National Air Quality and Emissions Trends Report, 1992. U.S. EPA: Office of Air Quality Planning and Standards. Research Triangle Park, NC. EPA 454 R-93-031, October 1993.

Osebold JW, Gershwin LJ, Zee YC: Studies on the enhancement of allergic lung sensitization by inhalation of ozone and sulfuric acid aerosol. *J Environ Pathol Toxicol* 3:221–234, 1980.

Overton JH, Miller FJ: Modeling ozone absorption in the respiratory tract. 80th Annual Meeting of the Air Pollution Control Association, paper no. 87-99.4, 1987.

Qu QS, Chen LC, Gordon T, et al: Alteration of pulmonary macrophage pH regulation by sulfuric acid aerosol exposures. *Toxicol Appl Pharmacol* 121(1):138–143, 1993.

Reid L: An experimental study of hypersecretion of mucus in the bronchial tree. *Br J Exp Pathol* 44:437–440, 1963.

Saldiva PHN, King M, Delmonte VLC, et al: Respiratory alterations due to urban air pollution: An experimental study in rats. *Environ Res* 57:19–33, 1992.

Schenker MB, Samet JM, Speizer FE, et al: Health effects of air pollution due to coal combustion in the Chestnut Ridge region of Pennsylvania: Results of cross-sectional analysis in adults. *Arch Environ Health* 38:325–330, 1983.

Schlesinger RB: Comparative irritant potency of inhaled sulfate aerosol: Effects on bronchial mucociliary clearance. *Environ Res* 34:268–279, 1984

Schlesinger RB: Intermittent inhalation of nitrogen dioxide: Effects on rabbit alveolar macrophages. *J Toxicol Environ Health* 21:127–139, 1987.

Schlesinger RB, Chen LC, Finkelstein I, Zelikoff JT: Comparative potency of inhaled acidic sulfates: Speciation and the role of hydrogen ion. *Environ Res* 52:210–224, 1990.

Schlesinger RB, Gorczynski JE, Dennison J, et al: Long-term intermittent exposure to sulfuric acid aerosol, ozone, and their combination: Alterations in tracheobronchial mucociliary clearance and epithelial secretory cells. *Exp Lung Res* 18:505–534, 1992.

Schlesinger RB, Halpern M, Albert RE, Lippmann M: Effects of chronic inhalation of sulfuric acid mist upon mucociliary clearance from the lungs of donkeys. *J Environ Pathol Toxicol* 2:1351–1367, 1979.

Schlesinger RB, Lippmann M, Albert RE: Effects of short-term exposures to sulfuric acid and ammonium sulfate aerosols upon bronchial airway function in the donkey. *Am Ind Hyg Assoc J* 39:275–286, 1978.

Schlesinger RB, Weidman PA, Zelikoff JT: Effects of repeated exposures to ozone and nitrogen dioxide on respiratory tract prostanoids. *Inhal Toxicol* 3:27–36, 1991.

Schwartz J: Lung function and chronic exposure to air pollution: A cross-sectional analysis of NHANES II. *Environ Res* 50:309–321, 1989.

Schwartz J: Air pollution and daily mortality: A review and meta analysis. *Environ Res* 64:36–52, 1994.

Schwartz J, Marcus A: Mortality and air pollution in London. *Am J Epidemiol* 131:185–194, 1990.

Seltzer J, Bigby BG, Stulbarg M, et al: $O_3$-induced change in bronchial reactivity to methacholine and airway inflammation in humans. *J Appl Physiol* 60:1321–1326, 1986.

Sheppard DA, Saisho A, Nadel JA, Boushey HA: Exercise increases sulfur dioxide induced bronchoconstriction in asthmatic subjects. *Am Rev Respir Dis* 123:486–491, 1981.

Slade R, Stead AG, Graham JA, Hatch GE: Comparison of lung antioxidant levels in humans and laboratory animals. *Am Rev Respir Dis* 131:742–746, 1985.

Speigelman JR, Hanson GD, Lazurus A, et al: Effect of acute sulfur dioxide exposure on bronchial clearance in the donkey. *Arch Environ Health* 17:321, 1968.

Speizer FE: Studies of acid aerosols in six cities and in a new multi-city investigation: Design issues. *Environ Health Perspect* 79:61–68, 1989.

Spengler JD, Sexton K: Indoor air pollution: A public health perspective. *Science* 221:9–17, 1983.

Starr TB, Gibson JE: The mechanistic toxicology of formaldehyde and its implications for quantitative risk assessment. *Annu Rev Pharmacol Toxicol* 25:745–767, 1985.

Stevens MA, Fitzgerald S, Menache MG, et al: Functional evidence of persistent airway obstruction in rats following a two-hour inhalation exposure to methyl isocyanate. *Environ Health Perspect* 72:89–94, 1987.

Thurston GD, Ito K, Kinney PL, Lippmann M: A multi-year study of air pollution and respiratory hospital admissions in three New York state metropolitan areas: Results for 1988 and 1989 summers. *J Expos Anal Environ Epidemiol* 2:429–450, 1992.

Tyler WS, Tyler NK, Hinds D, et al: Influence of exposure regimen on effects of experimental ozone studies: Effects of daily and episodic and seasonal cycles of exposure and post-exposure. Presented at the 84th annual meeting of the Air and Waste Management Assoc., Vancouver, BC, Canada. Paper No. 91-141.5, 1991.

Tyler WS, Tyler NK, Last JA, et al: Comparison of daily and seasonal exposures of young monkeys to ozone. *Toxicology* 50:131–144, 1988.

Utell MJ, Mariglio JA, Morrow PE, et al: Effects of inhaled acid aerosols on respiratory function: The role of endogenous ammonia. *J Aerosol Med* 2:141–147, 1989.

Utell MJ, Morrow PE, Hyde RW: Airway reactivity to sulfate and sulfuric acid aerosols in normal and asthmatic subjects. *J Air Pollut Control Assoc* 34:931–935, 1984.

Van De Lende R, Kok TJ, Reig RP, et al: Decreases in VC and $FEV_1$ with time: Indicators for effects of smoking and air pollution. *Bull Eur Physiopathol Respir* 17:775–792, 1981.

Vaughan TR Jr, Jennelle LF, Lewis TR: Long-term exposure to low levels of air pollutants: Effects on pulmonary function in the beagle. *Arch Environ Health* 19:45–50, 1969.

Waxman HA: Title III of the 1990 Clean Air Act Amendments, in Patrick DR (ed): *Toxic Air Pollution Handbook*. New York: Van Nostrand Reinhold, 1994, pp 25–32.

Yokoyama E, Toder RE, Frank NR: Distribution of $^{35}SO_2$ in the blood and its excretion in dogs exposed to $^{35}SO_2$. *Arch Environ Health* 22:389–395, 1971.

# CHAPTER 29

# AQUATIC AND TERRESTRIAL ECOTOXICOLOGY

*The Faculty of The Department of Environmental Toxicology and The Institute of Wildlife and Environmental Toxicology (ENTOX/TIWET), Clemson University**

## PRINCIPLES OF ECOTOXICOLOGY

Ecotoxicology is a rapidly developing discipline of environmental science (Connell and Miller, 1984; Duffus, 1980; Guthie and Perry, 1980; Hoffman et al., 1995; Moriarty, 1988; Truhaut, 1977). The term ecotoxicology was introduced by Truhaut in 1969 (Truhaut, 1977), and is a natural extension of toxicology. Ecotoxicology is best defined as the study of the fate and effects of toxic substances on an ecosystem and is based on scientific research employing both laboratory and field methods (Kendall, 1982; Kendall, 1992). The science itself requires an understanding of ecological principles, ecological theory, and of how chemicals potentially impact individuals, populations, communities, and ecosystems (Kendall and Lacher, 1994). Measurements are accomplished using either species-specific responses to toxicants (Smith, 1987) or impacts at higher levels of organization. Ecotoxicology builds on the science of toxicology and the principles of toxicological testing, though its emphasis is more at the level of populations, communities, and ecosystems (Moriarty, 1988). The ability to measure chemical transport and fate and exposure of organisms in ecotoxicological testing is critical to the ultimate development of an ecological risk assessment (USEPA, 1992; Suter, 1993; Maughan, 1993).

Descriptions of ecotoxicological testing methods and procedures have been offered by Cairns (1980) and colleagues (1978), and more recently by Hoffman and coworkers (1995). Unlike standard toxicological tests, which seek to define the cause-effect relationship with certain concentrations of toxicant exposure at a sensitive receptor site, ecotoxicological testing attempts to evaluate cause and effect at higher levels of organization, particularly on populations (National Academy of Sciences, 1975). To a large extent, the early tests (e.g., evaluating the effects of pesticides in fish and wildlife populations) generally employed species-specific tests in the laboratory (Smith, 1987). Tested species included aquatic species such as *Daphnia magna*, fathead minnows (*Pimephales promelas*), the top minnow (*Gambusia affinis*); and among wildlife, the northern bobwhite (*Colinus virginianus*) and mallard duck (*Anas platyrhynchos*) (Lamb and Kenaga, 1981). Arguments have continued over the last decade concerning the relevance of these few test organisms to the larger ecosystem at risk. Methods for laboratory bioassays to measure the impact of chemical and nonchemical stressors on aquatic and terrestrial plants and animals continue to evolve. In addition, extrapolation of the results of these assays to field conditions and their utility in ecological risk assessment are active areas of research.

A critical component in ecotoxicological testing is the integration of laboratory and field research (Kendall and Akerman, 1992). Laboratory toxicity bioassays define toxicant impact on individual organisms and on their biochemistry and physiology. Knowledge acquired in the laboratory is integrated with what is occurring under field conditions is critical to understanding the complex set of parameters with which an organism must deal in order to reproduce or survive under toxicant exposures. Laboratory testing often limits the complexity of stress parameters, except perhaps for isolating the toxicant. It is therefore difficult to interpret potential ecotoxicological effects resulting from laboratory studies without data from pertinent field investigations. For these reasons, integrating laboratory and field research ensures that ecotoxicological testing methods produce relevant data (Kendall and Lacher, 1994).

Demands on ecotoxicological testing methodologies will continue to increase as concern for environmental protection from chemical impacts increases. Scientific journals continue to publish increasing numbers of manuscripts on ecotoxicological studies. This chapter outlines some test methodologies for evaluating the effects of toxicants on invertebrates, vertebrates, and plants in aquatic and terrestrial ecosystems. The complexity and testing strategy in the aquatic versus terrestrial environment can be quite different. For this reason, this chapter is entitled "Aquatic and Terrestrial Ecotoxicology," to reflect the often different parameters involved with evaluating chemical impacts in aquatic versus terrestrial habitats.

## ENVIRONMENTAL CHEMISTRY AND CHEMODYNAMICS

### Role of Environmental Chemistry in Ecotoxicology

The study of the behavior of xenobiotic chemicals in the environment is no trivial matter (Tinsley, 1979). To characterize chemical behavior, it is necessary to measure the chemical in different environmental compartments (e.g., soil, water, and biological systems) and to understand the movement and transportation of the chemical within and among these compartments. During the past half-century, intensive effort has been directed toward developing analytical techniques to detect and quantify minute concentrations of chemicals in environmental

*Ronald J. Kendall, Catherine M. Bens, George P. Cobb III, Richard L. Dickerson, Kenneth R. Dixon, Stephen J. Klaine, Thomas E. Lacher, Jr., Thomas W. La Point, Scott T. McMurry, Raymond Noblet, and Ernest E. Smith.

matrices (Murray, 1993; Blaser et al., 1995). One needs only to look at the myriad of publications discussing parts per quadrillion (ppq) of 2,3,7,8-tetrachlorodibenzo-*p*-dioxin (TCDD) to realize that environmental analytical chemistry has progressed substantially to complement the ever-increasing sensitivity inherent in sublethal toxicological endpoints. Consider, for illustrative purposes, the fact that 1 ppq is 1 billion times smaller than a part per million (ppm). One ppq is approximately equal to 1 oz of salt in 31,250,000 tons of sugar. Nevertheless, it is well-documented that environmental concentrations less than 1 ppm of certain chemicals can have deleterious effects on different components of the ecosystem. A few examples include: 1 ppm phenol in water is lethal to some species of fish; 1 ppq of hydrogen fluoride gas in the atmosphere can injure peach trees; and, the acute oral $LC_{50}$ of TCDD to laboratory animals (e.g., guinea pigs) is $1 \mu g/kg$ (Rand and Petrocelli, 1985; Poland and Knutson, 1982).

Understanding chemical movement in the environment is necessary to ultimately characterize chemical concentrations and speciation in different environmental compartments. Understanding the environmental fate of the chemicals lays the foundation for ecological risk assessment. Exposure assessment relies on understanding chemical concentrations and speciation in different environmental compartments. Chemical transport (chemodynamics) occurs within compartments (intraphase) and between compartments (interphase) (Thibodeaux, 1979; MacKay, 1991). Chemodynamics is critical to understanding and interpreting environmental toxicology data. A likely scenario for a chemical released into the environment is as follows: a chemical is released into one environmental compartment; it is partitioned among environmental compartments; it is involved in movement and reactions within each compartment; it is partitioned between each compartment and the biota that reside in that compartment; it reaches an active site in an organism at a high enough concentration for long enough to induce an effect. Chemodynamics is, in essence, the study of all these steps.

Interphase transport is often predicted assuming thermodynamic equilibrium. While this assumption often does not hold, the approach is relatively straightforward and easy to apply. Although intraphase chemical transport is most easily approximated assuming thermodynamic equilibrium, better accuracy is possible using a steady-state model (MacKay, 1991). Abiotic and biotic reactions, which occur within a phase, result in significant changes in the physical and chemical properties of the compound, such as the oxidation state, lipophilicity, and volatility.

Combining these approaches facilitates prediction of the chemical concentration within the immediate vicinity of a particular organism. Chemodynamics also deals with chemical movement into organisms. This process, also known as bioavailability, is dependent on both interphase and intraphase chemical transport and is principally responsible for the potential toxicological action of the chemical. Detoxification mechanisms, such as partitioning into adipose tissue, metabolism, and accelerated excretion, can significantly reduce, eliminate, or in some cases increase the toxic action of the chemical. Thus, an appreciation of chemodynamics aids in the prediction of chemical concentrations in compartments and serves as a resource for designing toxicological experiments using the appropriate concentrations and form of the chemical in question.

## Single Phase Chemical Behavior

Chemical transport in and among environmental matrices, and the persistence of chemicals in the environment, are complex interdisciplinary subjects requiring chemistry, physics, systems analysis, modeling, engineering, and biology (Thibodeaux, 1979). Once a man-made chemical enters the environment, it is acted upon primarily by natural forces. Models are used to predict the effect of natural forces on the movement of chemicals in the environment. This requires the incorporation of abiotic variables into valid models. These variables include temperature, wind and water flow directions and velocities, incident solar radiation, atmospheric pressure and humidity, and the concentration of the chemical in one of four matrices. These matrices are those that have mobile phases—atmosphere (air) and hydrosphere (water)—and those that contain stationary phases—lithosphere (soil) and biosphere organisms. Chemical transport in the environment is thus divided into intraphase and interphase movement. Intraphase movement will be discussed first and consists of intraphase mass transfer, diffusion, or dispersion (Atkins, 1982). Concentration gradients result in movement within the medium. Contaminant persistence is a function of the stability of that chemical in a phase and its transport within that phase. Stability is a function of the physicochemical properties of a particular chemical and the kinetics of its degradation in the phase; these vary widely in and between classes of chemicals (Howard et al., 1991). Stability issues are difficult to predict and are often better handled by observation rather than modeling. Transport of chemicals in the environment, in contrast, is more predictable and will be discussed in detail below.

**Air.** The primary routes of entry of contaminants into the atmosphere are through evaporation and stack emissions. Significant amounts of contaminants enter the atmosphere through transport from other matrices. Contaminant transport in air is similar to that in the hydrosphere but generally occurs much more rapidly, as air has lower viscosity. Contaminant transport in air occurs primarily by diffusional processes or advection. Diffusion dominates in the very thin boundary layer between air and the other phases. The thickness of this boundary layer is thinner than that for the water-soil interface. The diffusion rate for a contaminant in air is approximately $10^6$-fold faster than for the same contaminant in water and is a function of the phase viscosity and existing concentration gradient. The contaminant diffusivity in air depends on its molecular weight compared to air, air temperature, the molecular separation at collision, the energy of molecular interaction, and Boltzmann's constant (Atkins, 1982). Wind currents transport airborne contaminants much more rapidly than does diffusion (Wark and Warner, 1981).The atmospheric stability affects the amount of turbulence and thus the degree of vertical mixing in the atmosphere. The stability of the atmosphere is considered neutral when the actual vertical temperature gradient is equal to the adiabatic lapse rate (Thibodeaux, 1979). Vertical mixing is at a maximum when the actual lapse rate is greater than the adiabatic lapse rate and it is at a minimum during inversion conditions. It is the latter condition that can trap higher concentrations of contaminants near the earth's surface.

**Water.** Contaminants enter the hydrosphere by direct application, spills, wet and dry deposition, and interphase movement. In addition, chemicals enter the hydrosphere by direct dissolution of lighter-than-water spills in the form of slicks or from pools on the bottom of channels, rivers, or other waterways. Chemical movement in the hydrosphere occurs through diffusion, dispersion, and bulk flow of the water. It is worthwhile to reintroduce the basic concepts of fluid flow at this point. In any flow, a stagnant boundary layer exists at the interface between phases or artificial boundaries. Overlying this layer is a section in which flow is laminar. Finally, above the laminar flow, the fluid is in turbulent flow. Contaminant movement in a mobile phase is dominated by the turbulence of the mobile phase, in this case, water. If the water is stagnant, (e.g., in close proximity to a stationary phase such as soil or an artificial boundary), the chemical moves by molecular diffusion. As described for the other fluid envirnomental compartment, air, the diffusion rate depends on fixed characteristics such as the molecular weight of the contaminant (solute), the molecular weight of the water (solvent), water temperature, viscosity, and the association factor for water and dynamic characteristics such as the magnitude of the concentration gradient of the contaminant. These characteristics are referred to as the diffusivity of the contaminant-water mixture. Diffusional processes in water are several orders of magnitude faster than in soil.

Away from the boundaries of other media (i.e, air and soil), transport in water is dominated by turbulence. Even in seemingly still water, water is constantly moving in vertical and horizontal eddies. These eddies are small pockets of water that form and subside and, during the process, carry the contaminant with them. This mode of transport is defined as *eddy diffusion*. In addition, the contaminant can be rapidly transported by bulk flow (also referred to as advection) in the cases of streams and rivers. In advection, the rate of transport is proportional to stream velocity.

**Soil.** Chemicals enter the lithosphere by processes similar to those for the hydrosphere. Soils have varying porosities, but pores are invariably filled with either gas or fluids. Chemical movement in the soil occurs by diffusion in these fluids or by the movement of water through the voids between soil particles. Fluid-borne contaminants partition with the solid fraction of soil by processes closely resembling chromatography (Willard et al., 1988), in that chemical solubility in porewater, adsorption to soil particles, and porewater velocity affect the rate of transport. The direction of diffusion will be from areas of high to areas of low concentration. The chemical diffusion rate in soil depends on molecular weight, soil temperature, the length of the path, and the magnitude of the concentration gradient (Shonnard et al., 1993), among other issues. Contaminants leave the soil by interphase transport or decomposition.

## Chemical Transport Between Phases

A chemical, once released, can enter any of the four matrices: the atmosphere by evaporation, the lithosphere by adsorption, the hydrosphere by dissolution, or the biosphere by absorption, inhalation or ingestion (depending on the species). Once in a matrix, the contaminant can enter another matrix by interphase transport. Absorption by biota is considered in the section on "Chemical Behavior and Bioavailability," below.

**Air:Water.** A chemical can leave the water by volatilization. Conversely, an airborne contaminant can move into an aqueous phase by adsorption. At equilibrium, the net rates of volatilization and adsorption are equal and the total mass transfer of the contaminant is zero. In nonequilibrium conditions, the rate of net movement of a chemical from one phase to another depends on how far the system is away from equilibrium as well as the magnitude of the overall mass transfer coefficient (MacKay, 1991). In turn, this mass transfer coefficient depends on the physical properties of the solute and the magnitude of the bulk flow of both the air and the water. For example, ammonia desorbs most quickly from shallow, rapidly flowing streams with a brisk crosswind.

**Soil:Water.** A contaminant can leave the soil and enter the water through the process of desorption. Water-borne contaminants can also adsorb on soil particles. Again, the rate of mass transfer depends on the contaminant-specific overall mass transfer coefficient and the bulk flow velocity of the water over the water-soil interface.

**Soil:Air.** A contaminant may leave the soil and be transported into the overlying air through the process of volatilization. This process is dependent on the vapor pressure of the chemical and its affinity for the soil. For example, more contaminant will be released from contaminated soil at higher temperatures and more contaminant will be released from sandy versus highly organic soil.

## Chemical Behavior and Bioavailability

Chemical bioavailability in various environmental compartments ultimately dictates toxicity. For example, in the aquatic environment it is important to understand that total mercury concentration in the sediment does not necessarily correlate with the chemical concentration in midge larvae of genus *Chironomus*. Important considerations in the case of mercury include the mercury species (e.g., the oxidation state, whether organic or inorganic) as well as physical and chemical characteristics of the sediment matrix (e.g., acid volatile sulfide concentration, pH, pE) (Tinsley, 1979). It also should be noted that in most cases mercury will not exist as a single species but will be distributed among several stable forms. Hence, a simple analytical result of total mercury content does not sufficiently describe the hazard associated with the presence of the metal in the sediment. Understanding the influence of soil, sediment, air, and water quality on the bioavailability of environmental chemicals are important research areas.

Chemical bioavailability in the water column has been studied for years, yet many questions are still unanswered. The behavior of dissolved metals, for example, has been studied for over two decades. In the early seventies, much research concerned the influence of pH and water hardness on metal toxicity to algae and other aquatic organisms. This work led to the development of a model to predict metal toxicity based on pH and water hardness (U.S. EPA, 1986a). This model, in turn, was used in the regulatory arena to generate water quality criteria to guide point-source discharge permits under the National Pollutant Discharge Elimination System (NPDES) (Macek, 1985) in the United States. Most of this work was based on total metal concentrations. More recently, the importance of

differentiating between total and dissolved metal concentrations was demonstrated and proposed to be incorporated into the NPDES permits.

A contaminant's organic chemical behavior and bioavailability in the water column has been shown to relate directly to its water solubility. However, the presence of certain constituents in water may affect the apparent water solubility of toxicants. Johnson-Logan and coworkers (1992) demonstrated the apparent solubility of the organochlorine insecticide, Chlordane (1,2,4,5,6,7,8,8-octachloro-2,3,3a,4,7,7a hexahydro-4,7-methanoindane), to be enhanced almost 500% in ground water containing 34 mg/L total organic carbon (TOC). This enhanced solubility resulted directly from partitioning of this hydrophobic insecticide into the dissolved organic carbon (DOC) fraction within the water column. The apparent increase in water solubility did not necessarily indicate an increase in pesticide bioavailability. DOC may increase transport and mobility of organic contaminants in the water column but may reduce their bioavailability.

The behavior and bioavailability of sediment-incorporated xenobiotics is a complex phenomenon studied only recently. The awareness that many aquatic contaminants settle into sediments has prompted studies of metals and organics to characterize their fate and disposition within the complex sediment matrix. Deposition is a combination of physical, chemical, and biological processes that may ultimately change the form of the xenobiotic. Many metals, for example, are abiotically or biotically reduced as they are incorporated into sediments. Mercury is methylated through microbial reactions in the sediment. Methylmercury is much more bioavailable and toxic than inorganic mercury.

Characterization of processes that control metal bioavailability in sediments would facilitate the development of models to predict toxic threshold concentrations of metals in different sediments. Much work with sediment-incorporated metals has emphasized divalent cations in anaerobic environments. Under these conditions, a growing body of evidence suggests that acid volatile sulfides (AVS) preferentially bind divalent cations. Initial work with AVS focused on cadmium (DiToro et al., 1990), which can react with the solid phase AVS to displace iron and form a cadmium sulfide precipitate:

$$Cd^{2+} + FeS_{(s)} \leftrightarrows CdS_{(s)} + Fe^{2+}$$

If the AVS quantity in sediment exceeds the quantity of added cadmium, the cadmium concentration in the interstitial water is not detectable and the cadmium is not bioavailable, hence it is not toxic. This process can be extended to other cations including nickel, zinc, lead, copper, mercury, and perhaps chromium, arsenic, and silver (Ankley et al., 1991). Furthermore, there is thermodynamic evidence that the presence of one divalent cation, copper for example, may displace a previously bound divalent cation with weaker binding strength such as cadmium. This results in a greater concentration of bioavailable cadmium while sulfide-bound copper is less bioavailable. Thus, the bioavailable fraction of metals in sediments can be predicted by measuring AVS and the simultaneously extracted metals (SEM) that result during AVS extraction. If the molar ratio of SEM to AVS is $<1$, little or no toxicity should be expected; if the molar ratio of SEM to AVS is $>1$, the mortality of sensitive species can be expected (DiToro et al., 1992). This approach is not without controversy and, while many scientists believe that AVS plays a significant role in the bioavailability of divalent cations in anaerobic sediments, most would agree that AVS alone does not predict metal bioavailability. Other sediment factors including oxide and hydroxide layers undoubtedly play a role in metal bioavailability. In addition, the ability of sediment-dwelling organisms to oxidize their surrounding environment, thus breaking metal-sulfide bonds, should be further studied.

Organic chemicals residing in the sediment matrix undergo a variety of abiotic and biotic transformations and may be incorporated into a variety of different phases. Predicting the intraphase movement of organics in sediments is extremely difficult and the processes, in general, that control such movement are poorly understood. For nonionic, nonmetabolized, nonpolar organics, however, equilibrium partitioning theory has been proposed as the basis for developing sediment quality criteria. This theory suggests that, in the sediment matrix, certain chemicals partition between interstitial water and the organic carbon fraction of the solids. At equilibrium, this partitioning can be predicted using laboratory-generated partitioning coefficients, $K_{oc}$s. The resulting interstitial water concentration should induce the same exposure as a water-only exposure. Thus, the toxicity of chemicals in interstitial water can be predicted using the results of water column bioassays with the chemical. One assumption of this theory is that, for these chemicals, exposure of sediment-dwelling organisms occurs through interstitial water only and that chemicals partitioned onto solids are not bioavailable. A good review of this theory and supporting data can be found in the 1991 report of DiToro and colleagues.

## THE USE OF BIOMARKERS IN ASSESSING THE IMPACT OF ENVIRONMENTAL CONTAMINANTS

A fundamental problem in ecological risk assessment is relating the release of a chemical into the environment with a valid prediction of ensuing risk to potential biological receptors. Adverse health effects to biological receptors begin with the release of a contaminant into the environment; air, water, soil, or food. Subsequent exposure of wildlife by contact to contaminated environmental media is defined as an external dose, whereas internalization of the contaminated media, via inhalation, ingestion, or dermal absorption, results in an internal dose. The amount of this internal dose necessary to elicit a response or health effect is referred to as the *biologically effective dose*.

Traditionally, environmental risk has been assessed by chemical residue determination in samples of the environmental media from affected sites. This approach, although it yielded useful information, has several limitations. First, the determination of chemical residues in environmental matrices is not simple and may require extensive sample cleanup (U.S. EPA, 1986b). Moreover, the cost per sample may be high for certain classes of chemicals. Secondly, the availability of the chemicals from the environmental matrix to the biological receptor (bioavailability) cannot be quantified by this approach. Depending upon the chemical, the receptor, and the environmental matrix, bioavailability may range from 100 percent to a fraction of a percent. To overcome this problem

chemical residue analysis of tissues from the biological receptor may be performed (ATSDR, 1994). However, this approach is often more difficult and more expensive than the cost of the analysis of environmental matrices. In addition, the toxicokinetics and toxicodynamics of a contaminant in a particular species determines whether an exposure is capable of an adverse response. A biomarker-based approach resolves many of these difficulties by providing a direct measure of toxicant effects in the affected species (Dickerson et al., 1994).

## What Are Biomarkers?

The National Academy of Sciences defines a *biomarker* or *biological marker* as a xenobiotically induced alteration in cellular or biochemical components or processes, structures, or functions that is measurable in a biological system or sample. Therefore, biomarkers can be broadly categorized as markers of exposure and effects (ATSDR, 1994). Toxicologists have recently developed a strong interest in biomarkers to evaluate exposure, effects, and susceptibility in animal studies, and they are currently pursuing development of new biomarkers in animal systems (Henderson et al., 1989). The selection of appropriate biomarkers to be used for risk assessment is based on the mechanism of a chemically induced disease state.

Dosing with an adequate concentration of a toxicant produces a continuum of events beginning with exposure and possibly resulting in the development of a disease. These events begin with external exposure, followed by the establishment of an internal dose leading to delivery of a contaminant to a critical site. This is followed either by reversible or irreversible adverse alterations to the critical site, resulting in the development of recognizable disease states. A clearer understanding of a chemically induced disease state in a species leads to an increase in the number of specific and useful biomarkers that may be extrapolated to other species. It is readily apparent that the earlier these effects can be measured at a critical site, the more sensitive the evaluation of risk. However, in many cases the exact mechanism of injury is not well understood.

## Biomarkers of Exposure

The presence of a xenobiotic substance or its metabolite(s) or the product of an interaction between a xenobiotic agent and some target molecule or cell that is measured within a compartment of an organism can be classified as a biomarker of exposure (ATSDR, 1994). In general, biomarkers of exposure are used to predict the dose received by an individual, which can then be related to changes resulting in a disease state. In many cases, biomarkers of exposure are among the most convenient to determine because the contaminant or its metabolites can be quantitated from nonlethal samples of urine, feces, blood, or breast milk, as well as tissues obtained through biopsy or necropsy. The former sources are the most desirable because they can be used for multiple determinations over time; thus making the marker more useful by providing more information and reducing variability.

The utility of biomarkers of exposure is readily apparent when comparing the indices of exposure and the biomarkers of exposure in personnel exposed to TCDD either occupationally in Viet Nam or accidentally in Missouri (i.e., Times Beach). An exposure index comparison of over 600 Operation Ranch Hand personnel showed an inverse correlation of estimated exposure to actual serum TCDD levels (Michalek, 1992).

Some very useful biomarkers of cancer involve detecting the ability of chemical carcinogens to form adducts with cellular macromolecules such as DNA or protein. Most chemical carcinogens are either strong electrophiles or are converted to an electrophilically active substance through metabolic activation (Miller and Miller, 1981). These carcinogens react with nucleophilic biomacromolecules to form adducts. If the biomacromolecule is sufficiently stable, the adducts can then be detected by a variety of means and then used to detect exposure to electrophiles. Stable biomacromolecules can also provide measurement of the dose of a chemical carcinogen received by animals and humans. Adduct detection can be accomplished by total hydrolysis of the protein to alkylated amino acids (histidine, cysteine adducts), mild hydrolysis to release adducts (adducts that form esters to carboxyl groups or sulfonamides), immunodetection, or modified Edman degradation (adducts to N-terminal valines on Hb). These techniques have been used to identify adducts formed by simple alkylating agents and their metabolites, aromatic amines, nitrosamines, and polynuclear aromatic hydrocarbons. One major advantage to this method of cancer risk determination is that blood samples are easily obtained and multiple samples can be obtained to determine patterns of exposure.

## Biomarkers of Effect

Biomarkers of effect are defined as any measurable biochemical, physiological, or other alteration within an organism that, depending on the magnitude, can be recognized as an established or potential health impairment or disease (ATSDR, 1994). One classification of biomarkers of effect is by the degree of validation required of the test and the specificity of the test. These are referred to as Gold, Silver, or Bronze Standard tests (Peakall, 1994). A Gold Standard test must be able to stand alone. As such, it does not need chemical analysis or additional biological tests for confirmation. These tests are highly specific for individual chemicals and thus have a fairly limited application. Examples of Gold Standard tests include inhibition of cholinesterase, inhibition of aminolevulinic acid, and eggshell thinning.

Silver Standard tests are also well-validated but they have wider applications and tend to respond to classes of chemicals. Examples of Silver Standard tests are the induction of mixed function oxidases, the formation of DNA adducts, other DNA alterations such as sister chromatid exchange and strand breakage, and immunological changes.

Finally, there is a list of tests referred to as Bronze Standard tests. These tests have been used with varying degrees of success as biomarkers but require further validation before they can be used in risk assessment. Thyroid function, retinol levels, porphyrin levels, and stress proteins fall into this classification. For example, the induction of cytochrome P4501A1 (CYP1A) enzymes in fish liver is generally recognized as a useful biomarker of the exposure of fish to anthropogenic contaminants (Collier et al., 1995), but these results are not compound-specific.

Biomarkers can be used to characterize the effects caused by environmental contaminants. For example, because the

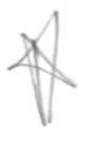

liver and kidney are target organs in both humans and animals, pentachlorophenol elevated serum glutamate oxaloacetate transaminase (SGOT) and serum glutamate pyruvate transaminase (SGPT) (Armstrong et al., 1969; Bergner et al., 1965; Gordon, 1956; Klemmer, 1972; ATSDR, 1994). Pentachlorophenol also increased enzyme levels and levels of blood urea nitrogen and accelerated the loss of proximal tubular alkaline phosphatase activity in the kidney (Greichus et al., 1979; Kimbrough and Linder, 1978; Nishimura et al., 1980); in this manner they can be used to assess the clinical manifestations of the effects of pentachlorophenol. Indices of changes in hepatic oxidative phosphorylation may also be useful as biomarkers for pentachlorophenol-induced liver changes (ATSDR, 1994). These effects are not specific for exposure to pentachlorophenol. They have been associated with other compounds such as some mycotoxins and chlorinated hydrocarbons. Target organs of 1,1,1-trichloro-2,2-*bis*(ρ-chlorophenyl)ethane (DDT), 1,1-dichloro-2-2-*bis*(ρ-chlorophenyl)ethylene (DDE) and 1,1-dichloro-2,2-*bis*(ρ-chlorophenyl)ethane (DDD) toxicity include the nervous system, the reproductive system, and the liver. In addition to the induction of hepatic microsomal enzymes in both humans and animals, serotonin and norepinephrine in the brain decrease, while the metabolites increase following DDT exposure. Increased levels of excitatory amino acids in the brain—for example, aspartate and glutamate—have also been reported (Hudson et al., 1985; ATSDR, 1994).

In another example, stress proteins as biomarkers are important tools which enable toxicologists to predict reliably and to detect exposures to xenobiotics and the resultant cell injury. Cellular stress response is involved in protecting organisms from damage due to exposure to a wide variety of stressors, including elevated temperatures, ultraviolet light, heavy metals, and xenobiotics (Sanders, 1993). This stress response entails the rapid synthesis of a suite of proteins upon exposure to adverse environmental conditions. A number of studies have demonstrated that stress proteins or their messages are induced and accumulate in organisms under realistic environmental conditions. Because the de novo synthesis of stress proteins can be detected at an early stage of exposure to some agents, analysis of toxicant-induced changes in gene expression, that is, alterations in patterns of protein synthesis, may be useful in developing biomarkers of exposure and toxicity (Goering et al., 1993). Furthermore, because the stress response is involved in protecting tissues from environmental damage, its potential to integrate stressor-induced damage may provide a direct measure of the physiological state of target tissues. As a quantitative response, it has the added benefit of providing a measure of the extent to which an organism is stressed (Sanders, 1993).

Biomarkers of reproductive and developmental toxicants are useful in detecting effects generated by endocrine-disrupting xenobiotics and teratogens. Estrogenic and antiestrogenic effects are well-characterized and provide useful biomarkers for the indication of toxicity. These effects include alterations in uterine wet weight, changes in vaginal cornification, induction of estrogen-induced protein synthesis, changes in estrogen metabolism, and alteration in phenotypic sex ratios. These biomarkers also are useful in detecting exposure to xenobiotics such as DDT, dioxins, certain mycotoxins, and phytoestrogens (Travis, 1993). In particular, changes in sexual phenotype show great promise in detecting the effects of estrogenic pesticides on aquatic reptiles (Guillette et al., 1994).

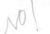

## AQUATIC TOXICOLOGY

The impact of chemicals and other anthropogenic materials on aquatic ecosystems can be evaluated at several levels. These range from laboratory bioassays that provide toxicological information under standardized regimes to whole-ecosystem bioassays with limited control over the myriad of variables that may influence toxicological information. Each approach has limitations and benefits. In both, however, it is critical to understand temporal and spatial changes in water quality and toxicant concentration, and how these influence the toxicological endpoint(s) measured.

There is evidence that direct measures of toxicity taken in the laboratory are protective of the environment (Cairns and Mount, 1990). In Mayer and Ellersieck (1986), the results of nearly 5000 tests on 66 species exposed to 410 chemicals indicated that for 88 percent of the tests, three species (*Daphnia sp., Gammarus fasciatus*, and *Salmo gairdneri*) provided the lowest indication of toxicity. Hence, if these species and tests were to be used to establish the lower limits of chemical effects, one could make the argument that the system would be protected. By how much is still problematic. Yet, laboratory tests provide information useful for regulatory purposes: the physiological or biochemical mode of action of the chemical can be established; the tests provide an objective assessment of the chemical effect in clean water, that is to say maximizing exposure and bioavailability of the chemical; and a concentration-response function can be established, within which certain concentrations raise a red flag. The reason ecotoxicological testing is undertaken is to assess the response of individuals and populations under actual exposure conditions, to assess the potential for indirect, sublethal effects, and to determine whether threshold levels for effect, measured in the laboratory, have validity for ecosystems (Cairns and Mount, 1990; Cairns, 1992). Assessing ecotoxicity experimentally or via biomonitoring programs requires integrating chemical, physical, and biological methods. Such complex ecosystem-level problems may only be understood or mitigated when multiple scientific disciplines are linked for such studies. Such multidisciplinary approaches have been given a great impetus through the development of ecological risk characterization and assessment (NAS, 1986; NRC, 1981; U.S. EPA, 1992a). The goals of such assessments are broader than the evaluation of a single-chemical cause and effect; rather, they seek to quantify the effects of human activities on entire biotic communities.

In the simplest sense, the chief reason for incorporating field tests is that field testing involves direct measures of contaminants' fate (as the net result of the myriad physical, chemical, and biological interactions involved) and subsequently links them to models (Neely and Mackay, 1982; Landrum et al., 1992). Macek (1988) states that the shift from laboratory toxicity studies to field testing concerns the "real variable" in hazard and exposure assessment. A great number of chemical and physical factors (e.g., hardness, pH, incident radiation, temperature, nutrient levels, etc.) influence chemical hydrolysis, photodegradation, and biodegradation (Rijstenbil and Poortvliet, 1992). Hence, field tests and monitoring programs serve to verify fate models and estimates of biological hazard developed from laboratory toxicity tests (Bergman and Meyer, 1982).

The rationale for using aquatic biota as indicators of ecotoxicity has been described previously (La Point and Fairchild, 1992). Briefly, indigenous aquatic organisms (e.g., algae, fish, macroinvertebrates) complete all or most of their life cycles in water and can serve as monitors of water quality. Because water quality may fluctuate widely with respect to the generation time of a given species, the use of numerous taxa has a benefit. Organisms with short life spans and high reproductive capacity may serve as early warning indicators. For bioaccumulable chemicals, longer-lived organisms may serve as sentinel species (Muir and Yarechewski, 1988). Field assessment of natural populations directly measures damage; extrapolations for interspecies sensitivity, water quality differences, or chemical interaction (additivity, antagonism, or synergism) are not necessary. Also, results of the assessment of indigenous populations are more biologically interpretable, which should quantify damage in a manner easily understood by resource managers, regulators, and the general public. Finally, understanding how ecosystems respond to contaminants allows us to use surrogate species to evaluate their effectiveness protecting aquatic communities.

Regulatory requirements for using ecosystem testing can lead to better insight into how interacting populations within a community respond to contaminant exposure. The key to isolating contaminant effects from natural variation in biotic community structure and function is to incorporate the use of reference stations, streams, or watersheds and to follow seasonal variation in physical, chemical, and biological parameters. Furthermore, the large variations typically associated with biological responses measured in the field begs the question of the ecological significance of population responses occurring at levels below our ability to detect them. There needs to be much more emphasis on determining the statistical differences in community responses that have ecological relevance and yet possess coefficients of variation greater than 30 to 50 percent. Presently, such interrelationships among community parameters have been quantified using multivariate analytic approaches (Corkum, 1991).

## Requirements for Ecotoxicological Measures in the Aquatic Environment

Biomonitoring programs must include the ancillary, independent variables that influence the abundance and distribution of invertebrates and fish. Such information is often necessary for understanding the factors affecting natural variation in population distribution. A sound experimental design is critical to an assessment of ecological damage (Westman, 1985). Prior to deciding the nature of the sampling program, a rationale for and an approach to the study needs to be given careful thought. The design requires understanding the complexity of the aquatic ecosystem such that confounding factors (e.g., depth, light penetration, substrate size, organic matter, nutrients, etc.) are controlled or accounted for in sample site comparisons (Platts et al., 1983). Habitats to be sampled and sites within the habitats need to be chosen to minimize differences among each of these with respect to physical and chemical parameters. Kerans and coworkers (1992) stress the requirement for sampling habitats in proportion to their abundance in the system of interest.

Westman (1985) details several questions and concerns to be considered prior to beginning a survey. Careful attention needs to be given to the boundaries of potential impact, to the major ecological components affected, and to which variables affect baseline conditions. Herricks and Cairns (1982) recommend close coupling of prediction and monitoring and the incorporation of appropriate toxicological testing in biomonitoring programs. Criteria for "biological test systems" have been established (Cairns and Mount, 1990; Hammons, 1981). Certain of these apply to field monitoring programs to assess damage to an aquatic ecosystem (Kapustka et al., 1989):

1. The method should be as simple as possible, yet unambiguously indicate the response of the aquatic community to the perturbation. Also, the method should be accepted among the scientific community, well-documented, and, if possible, standardized.
2. The method must be economical, although the expense of its use must be viewed in relation to the cost of potential resource damage if no action were taken.
3. The procedure used must have a generality in that it predicts population and community responses to a wide range of organic and inorganic chemicals.
4. Data generated from application of the method should be appropriate for inclusion into mathematical and statistical models of contaminant fate and effect.

In any given effects study, careful consideration must be given to the comparability of samples collected among stations. Not only must the type of sampler chosen be appropriate for the situation, but the sampler type and sampling effort must be uniform among different stations (Green, 1979). In any case, the experimental design must be developed prior to initiation of the study; mistakes in study design cannot be statistically corrected after the sampling is concluded. Standardized methods (ASTM, 1986; APHA, 1989) provide helpful directions when sampling periphyton, macrophyton, and macroinvertebrates. The use of standard techniques aids the comparability of samples among sites and investigators. The degree of success in using spatial distributions to assess ecological damage depends upon statistical considerations of sufficient sample number (Chutter, 1972; Morin, 1985) and upon the ability to characterize water quality characteristics that influence species distributions independent of contaminant influences (La Point et al., 1984; Wiederholm, 1984; Kuwabara, 1992).

Experimental ecosystems (mesocosms and microcosms) have been used to validate exposure models and to determine the potential hazard of exposure to aqueous and sediment-bound chemicals (Touart and Slimak, 1989). Pond mesocosms are valuable for determining the ecotoxicity of pesticides, as mesocosms simulate ponds, lakes, and riverine backwater habitats (AEDG, 1992; Crossland and La Point, 1992). However, successful extrapolation of results collected from experimental ecosystems to surface waters depends, in part, on how biological responses within the mesocosms are interpreted. This remains a serious research and regulatory problem.

Although most published ecotoxicological studies have included indicators from a series ranging from individual toxicity bioassays through community- or ecosystem-level tests, linkages across landscapes remain less studied. Toxic responses measured at the community level, as the initial response or the subsequent "recovery," are typically measures of species richness and composition within the community's structure, and relative abundances (the number of individuals in any given species, relative to the total number of individuals in the community) of periphytic, planktonic, benthic, or fish communities. These tests present a formidable problem in the regulation of pesticides because changes in relative abundance or species richness have not yielded readily interpretable information. The difficulties have stemmed as much from a lack of a theoretical basis on which to base the results observed as from a lack of understanding of the secondary effects (i.e., food web relationships). Johnson and colleagues (1991) had difficulties in accurately measuring chemical fate within aquatic ecosystems.

The desirable aspects of system comparability are perhaps best provided by experimental ecosystems in which individual units are constructed as replicate systems and dosed in a concentration gradient. In such ecotoxicity testing, *primary* toxic responses (defined as the responses of the taxa that are expected to be affected immediately by the chemical) are compared to population variation in control units. The concentration-response series of measures are quantified using statistical techniques (Graney et al., 1989; Liber et al., 1992). However, indirect effects and underlying causes leading to reductions in a population or trophic guild (or some deviation from "stability") are not handled well using analysis of variance or regression techniques. Dewey and deNoyelles (1994) and others have used path analysis to measure the rate at which the so-called stable state changes in experimental ecosystems. They acknowledge the difficulty of measuring population or community stability at all. However, for experimental and biomonitoring purposes, concepts of population and community descriptors, such as species composition, trophic structures, and stability, have to be operationally defined and made relative to control (undosed) ecosystems (Suter, 1993; Levin, 1992).

However, too many biomonitoring or mesocosm studies have resulted in collections of data without sufficient forethought given to how the data will be used. Often, the focus of ecological effects studies is determined by the individual strengths (or biases) of the principal investigators, the nature of their expertise, the availability of sampling sites, and the biota that are familiar to the investigators. Very often, this type of program has not worked well in assigning cause and effect because the correct questions were not asked prior to the study. Separate studies on the same watershed may give rise to conflicting conclusions, resulting simply from methodological differences in approach and data gathering, rather than from true differences in species' distributions. As a result, information generated in these biomonitoring programs can be of limited utility to other scientists or to the public. To overcome this criticism, criteria for selecting indicators of ecosystem effect and recovery have been proposed by Kelly and Harwell (1990). These authors present a rationale for choosing indicators, not necessarily mutually exclusive, which include (1) intrinsic importance, such as endangered or economically important species; (2) early warning indicators, when a rapid response to a stress is desired; (3) sensitive indicators, known to predictably respond to the stress; and (4) process indicators, when a community function (e.g., primary production) is known to respond to a stress.

Relative abundance is a measure of how the number of individuals in a community are distributed among the species present. Historically, the use of this measure has given rise to derived measures: indices of dominance, evenness, and diversity (Ford, 1989). The idea of how well a species tracks changes in an aquatic habitat has been useful in monitoring responses of the communities to contaminant perturbations. Green (1979) and others (Sokal and Rohlf, 1981) discuss the drawbacks of using derived measures. Such measures include most diversity measures, ratios, indices of eutrophication, and other indices. The drawbacks to their use stem from the lack of coherence in the variances of the numerator and denominator components of a derived variable. Information attached to the original variables is lost.

When the appropriate limitations are addressed, the utility of such indices may be improved. However, it should be kept in mind that indices lose the variances and quantitative information about the variables used to derive the ratio. Hence, the use of derived indices must be carefully couched in terms of the original variables used to calculate the derived variable. Furthermore, derived indices must be discussed relative to the presence and abundance of the organisms of interest.

Early on, the concept of indicator species was shown to be important in studies of eutrophication (Kolkwitz and Marsson, 1908). This concept continues to have a use in the development of the mussel watch program and in other projects, such as monitoring the abundance of amphibians. Also, in communities dominated by critical keystone species, the theory of contaminant effects on such important species is germane, as the influences of a chemical on a keystone species may affect the remainder of the biotic community, even if the resident species are not sensitive to the chemical (Giesy and Allred, 1985). More recently, examples of this approach have employed groups of macroinvertebrate taxa (Hilsenhoff, 1988; Bergman and Meyer, 1982), specifically, the numbers of Ephemeroptera, Plecoptera, and Trichoptera, to assess community disturbance.

The question arises concerning the overall ramifications of contaminants in the environment and their effects on organisms that are part of the aquatic food chain. For instance, amphibians have been shown to be sensitive to certain synthetic pyrethroids (Materna, 1991). Species of mammals such as mink (*Mustela vison*) and raccoons (*Procyon lotor*) rely on aquatic invertebrates for food. Bioaccumulation of lipophilic compounds may affect population abundance and the survival of organisms not resident in the aquatic systems, yet which are completely dependent upon it for sustenance. For regulatory purposes, there is an increasing emphasis on the movement of contaminants from the aqueous to the terrestrial environments. These studies present formidable sampling difficulties, yet, with thoughtful approaches, they may truly integrate studies of chemical fate and effect at the ecosystem or watershed level.

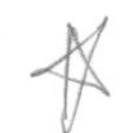

## TERRESTRIAL TOXICOLOGY

Terrestrial toxicology is the science of the exposure to and effects of toxic compounds in terrestrial ecosystems. Investigations in terrestrial toxicology are often complex endeavors because of a number of intrinsic and extrinsic factors associ-

ated with terrestrial systems. All organisms function at several levels, from the individual level to the level of the ecosystem, interacting with others within the constraints of social ranking, food webs, and niches. Many terrestrial species are very mobile, covering significant areas while defending territories, foraging, migrating, and dispersing. Terrestrial toxicology includes all aspects of the terrestrial system while attempting to elucidate the effects on the biota following contaminant exposure. Exploring exposures to and the effects of environmental contaminants in terrestrial systems is a recent endeavor relative to work that has been conducted historically in aquatic systems. Like aquatic toxicology, however, terrestrial toxicology relies heavily on interdisciplinary scientific exploration.

The early 1900s witnessed the realization that chemicals used in the environment could impact nontarget organisms. Studies were conducted on the exposures to and effects of arsenicals, pyrethrums, mercurials, and others on terrestrial organisms (Peterle, 1991). In later years, synthetic pesticides became increasingly important in controlling pest species in agricultural crops, although little was known about their effects on nontarget organisms. As pesticide use continued, however, reports of wildlife mortalities and declining avian populations spawned concern among biologists in several countries. Studies demonstrated residues of DDT and DDT metabolites, other chlorinated hydrocarbon insecticides, and industrial chemicals, including polychlorinated biphenyls (PCBs). Although reduced nesting success was apparent in some avian species (e.g., osprey, bald eagles, Bermuda petrels, herring gulls, and brown pelicans) (Ames, 1966; Peterle, 1991; Wurster and Wingate, 1968; Keith, 1966; Schreiber and DeLong, 1969), the underlying mechanism was not completely understood.

Studies of the toxic effects of chemicals on terrestrial organisms witnessed its most dramatic growth in the 1980s (Kendall and Akerman, 1992). Requirements for detailed and accurate information on the effects of pesticides on terrestrial wildlife species played a large part in the development of terrestrial toxicology methodologies. Persistent pesticides such as DDT and Mirex [1,1a,2,2,3,3a,4,5,5,5a,5b,6-dodecachloro-octahydro-1,3,4-metheno-1H-cyclobuta(cd)pentalene] were shown to accumulate in wildlife species. Development of new insecticides, such as organophosphates, lessened the problem of persistence although toxicity was still a concern. An obvious need existed by which scientifically sound investigations could be conducted to explore the direct and indirect effects of chemicals on terrestrial wildlife populations.

Work on the effects of chemicals on avian populations was the primary focus for many years. This problem became more apparent as the link was established between DDT contamination and declining bird populations. The classic case of eggshell thinning in raptor eggs was established by Ratcliffe (1967) in studies on declining sparrow hawk (*Accipiter nisus*) and peregrine falcon (*Falco peregrinus*) populations in the United Kingdom. Other studies soon followed and it became apparent that many avian species suffered reduced productivity resulting from eggshell thinning and decreased hatching success. Other studies have demonstrated a plethora of adverse pesticide effects on avian as well as other terrestrial species. For example, acute exposure of domestic sheep to dieldrin (1,2,3,4,10,10-hexachloro-6,7-epoxy-1,4,4a,5,6,7,8,8a-octahydro-endo,exo-1,4:5,8-dimethanonaphthalene) resulted in a 21 to 76 percent decline in vigilance behavior (Sandler et al., 1969).

Interactions between toxicants and natural environmental stressors have been demonstrated experimentally. American kestrels (*Falco sparverius*) died following exposure to methyl parathion [phosphorothioic acid O,O-di-methyl O-(4-nitrophenyl ester)] and cold stress compared to nonlethal responses with the chemical alone (Rattner and Franson, 1984). Sublethal effects of pesticide exposure also have been shown. Northern bobwhite (*Colinus virginianus*) exposed to methyl parathion showed a dose-dependent susceptibility to predation (Galindo et al., 1985; Buerger et al., 1991). These studies represent but a few examples of the numerous intricacies involved with the mechanisms and responses of species exposed to contaminants. As such, they exemplify the complexity involved in adequately designing strategies for monitoring the exposure to and effect of environmental contaminants in terrestrial ecosystems.

## Acute and Chronic Toxicity Testing

Acute and chronic toxicity tests are designed to determine the short- and long-term effects of chemical exposure on a variety of endpoints, including survival, reproduction, and physiological and biochemical responses. Toxicity testing of terrestrial animal and plant species serves a number of purposes in terrestrial toxicology. Understanding the effects of a single compound provides a foundation for assessing the effects of complex contaminant mixtures. Methods for measuring endpoints include the $LD_{50}$ and $LC_{50}$, the $ED_{50}$ and $EC_{50}$, and reproductive tests (e.g., fertility, egg hatchability, neonate survival), among others. These can be used to assess toxicity in a variety of terrestrial animals including earthworms (*Eisenia foetida*), honey bees (*Apis mellifera*), northern bobwhite, mallards (*Anas platyrhynchos*), mink, and European ferrets (*Mustela purofius furo*) (Menzer et al., 1994). Likewise, specialized tests for determining toxicity in plants are used to assess lethal and nonlethal response to contaminants. Standardized tests for toxicity in plants include germination assays for lettuce seeds (*Latuca sativa*), root elongation in seedlings, and analysis of whole plants such as soybean (*Glycine max*) and barley (*Hordeum vulgare*) (Wang, 1985; Greene et al., 1989; Pfleeger et al., 1991; Ratsch, 1983). Other plant and animal species, including domestic and wild types, can be used in standardized testing systems as dictated by specific site requirements (Lower and Kendall, 1990).

Results derived from acute and chronic tests can be used to determine the pathological effects of contaminants, to provide data necessary for analyzing the effects discovered in field tests, to identify the potential effects to be aware of under field conditions, and to provide dose response data for comparison to exposure levels in the field. Initial laboratory tests performed under United States Environmental Protection Agency (U.S. EPA) guidelines include acute oral $LD_{50}$s and dietary $LC_{50}$s on northern bobwhite quail and mallard ducks. Also, mammalian toxicity tests include acute oral $LD_{50}$s on rats (Rattus) using estimated environmental concentrations of the chemical in question. Avian and mammalian reproductive toxicity testing may be required under certain circumstances, depending on such factors as food tolerance, indications of repeated or continued exposure, the persistence of chemicals in the environment, and chemical storage or accumulation in plant or animal tissues (U.S. EPA, 1982).

Contaminants may exist singly or as complex mixtures, and they may be found as the parent compound or as one or more breakdown products. Because of the complex possibilities under typical field conditions, acute and chronic toxicity testing provides a critical foundation for evaluating the exposures and effects encountered in the field and for linking cause and effect to specific chemicals. For example, brain and plasma cholinesterase (ChE) inhibition has proven to be an excellent tool for monitoring exposure and in some cases for diagnosing the effect in animals exposed to organophosphate and carbamate pesticides (Mineau, 1991). Advances in terrestrial toxicology have resulted in an expanding search for new sentinel plant and animal species for assessing contaminant exposure and effects. In turn, new sentinel prospects require testing to determine their sensitivity and the precision of their responses. Acute and chronic toxicity testing represent that initial step toward validating new species as useful sentinels of environmental contamination.

## Field Testing

Field studies in terrestrial ecosystems are designed to address potential hazards suggested by laboratory studies. As the effects of environmental contaminants on wild populations of animals have become more apparent (Kendall and Akerman, 1992), the need and usefulness of field testing strategies has needed improvement. Whether the U.S. EPA requires field testing depends both on laboratory testing results and professional judgement. Chemical properties of the compound, intended use patterns (e.g., pesticides), difference between the estimated environmental concentration (EEC) and the lowest observed effect level (LOEL), and dose-response relationships are considered in combination when exploring the need for conducting field studies.

Under the guidelines of the U.S. EPA, there are two categories of field tests; screening studies and definitive studies (Fite et al., 1988). Screening studies are designed primarily to demonstrate that a hazard suggested by lower-tier laboratory studies does not exist under actual field use conditions (i.e., to rebut the presumption of risk). Typically, results from screening tests are limited to an effect-or-no-effect interpretation and address acute toxic effects on wildlife survival and behavior. Definitive studies, in contrast, rely on a detailed approach designed to quantify the magnitude of the impacts identified in a screening study, mortality incidents, or from other information. The basic objectives in a definitive study are to quantify the effects of a chemical application on the magnitude of acute mortality, the existence and extent of impaired reproduction in nontarget species, and the extent to which survival is influenced.

Field studies are conducted in complex ecological systems where plants and animals are affected by numerous natural stressors (e.g., nutrient restriction, disease, predation) that might possibly confound the measurement of contaminant exposure and effects. In addition, life history characteristics vary dramatically among species. Issues of habitat use, home range size, foraging characteristics, and other factors must be considered when designing a field study. Field study design must be robust to noncontaminant influences, and some important considerations include censusing techniques, sampling units, site replication, scale, ecological similarity among sites, and choice of study organisms. Grue and Shipley (1981) concluded in their study that conventional censusing techniques and population estimators may be inadequate for assessing changes in bird populations due to the confounding effects of pesticide exposure on bird behavior.

Traditional methods used by biologists and wildlife ecologists have been used successfully in terrestrial toxicology field studies, and resources are available that describe the various techniques for trapping, remote sensing, and sampling terrestrial biota (Bookhout, 1994; Menzer et al., 1994). Ligature techniques used for birds have improved the process of collecting food from nestlings raised on contaminated sites, allowing researchers to better determine the composition of the diet and to ascertain the contaminant loads in foodstuffs (Mellott and Woods, 1993). The published results of field studies have provided information on the impacts of contaminants on wildlife abundance and survival (Rowley et al., 1983), acute mortality (Babcock and Flickinger, 1977; Kendall et al., 1992), food chain relationships (Korschgen, 1970), reproduction (Clark and Lamont, 1976; Hooper et al., 1990), and behavior (Grue et al., 1982). Basic laboratory techniques are often integrated with field methods to determine the ecological significance and mechanisms of exposure and effects on populations (Kendall, 1992).

The U.S. EPA has recommended field methods for examining the effects of pesticides and hazardous waste on wildlife (Fite et al., 1988; Warren-Hicks et al., 1989). Approaches include a protocol for assessing the reproductive effects of contaminant exposure on European starlings (*Sturnus vulgaris*), which provides a model for assessing other cavity-nesting passerines with similar life history traits (Kendall et al., 1989). Starlings are cavity nesting birds that readily occupy artificial nest cavities and will colonize study sites when provided with nest boxes. Colony behavior promotes large numbers of adults and nestlings, from which information on reproductive success, behavioral response, exposure routes, and physiological and biochemical perturbations can be obtained during the breeding season.

## Enclosure Studies

Enclosure studies incorporate a variety of outdoor, open-air facilities to enclose test organisms during toxicological testing. The purpose of using enclosures is to simulate natural field conditions while maintaining a level of control over experimental conditions (e.g., exposure period, nutritional condition, test organism, sex ratios, age, genetic similarity, habitat type). In essence, enclosure-based experiments can be used to bridge the gap between laboratory and field investigations. Study organisms are more readily accessible when housed in enclosures, making it easier to take multiple samples from and administer treatments to individuals and to monitor behavior and reproduction. The flexibility afforded under these conditions makes it possible to explore a number of questions regarding the potential interactions between the contaminant and natural stressors in the environment. Enclosure studies may be required by the U.S. EPA under the Federal Insecticide, Fungicide and Rodenticide Act (FIFRA) guidelines for pesticide registration, if they can potentially yield useful information about pesticide impacts on wildlife.

Enclosure studies have been used successfully with birds and mammals to explore the effects of pesticides and chemical contaminants on abundance, reproduction, immune function, and biochemical response (Barrett, 1968; Pomeroy and Barrett, 1975; Barrett, 1988; Dickerson et al., 1994; Gebauer and Weseloh, 1993; Weseloh et al., 1994; Hooper and La Point, 1994). Basic approaches to using enclosures to study the impacts of chemicals on terrestrial organisms vary widely. There is considerable variation in enclosure size; they range from less than 1 meter square to more than a hectare. Small stainless steel enclosures, approximately 0.5 × 1.5 m, have been used to house laboratory raised deer mice (*Peromyscus maniculatus*) for the assessment of contaminant uptake and biomarker response in mice on sites contaminated with polynuclear aromatic hydrocarbons (Dickerson et al., 1994). Larger enclosures can be used to monitor population-level responses and community interactions. Barrett (1988) and Pomeroy and Barrett (1975) used enclosures constructed of galvanized sheet metal to assess population and community responses of several rodent species to controlled applications of Sevin insecticide (1-naphthyl-N-methylcarbamate). Studies incorporating pinioned ducks on contaminated waste ponds provide an equivalent method for avian species (Gebauer and Weseloh, 1993; Weseloh, 1994).

Although large enclosures offer the advantage of addressing population- and community-level issues of toxicant effects, they can be restrictive in cost and space. Smaller pens can be very beneficial for site-specific evaluations and are more affordable. They can be easily moved among locations, making them an excellent strategy for short-term testing and determining the efficacy of site remediation. However, the choice of enclosure depends on the goals of the study.

## Trophic Level Transfer of Contaminants

Although contaminant exposure may occur through inhalation, dermal contact, or ingestion from preening or grooming behavior, significant exposure also occurs through food chain transport. Depending on specific properties, contaminants may accumulate in either soft or hard tissues of prey species. Species that normally do not directly contact contaminated media may be exposed through ingestion of contaminated prey, promoting biomagnification of contaminants in higher trophic levels. Earthworms in soils contaminated with organochlorines and heavy metals can accumulate quantities of contaminants known to be deleterious to sensitive species (Beyer and Gish, 1980; Beyer and Cromartie, 1987). The use of pesticides to control plant pests often coincides with the reproductive periods of many wildlife species, enhancing exposure potential in juveniles that often rely on invertebrates as a primary food source (Korschgen, 1970).

The foraging habits of individual species dictate the potential for contaminant exposure through food chain transport. In a field study in Canada, Daury and coworkers (1993) found a higher percentage of ring-necked ducks (*Aythya collaris*) with elevated blood lead concentrations compared to American black ducks (*Anas rubripes*). The difference was attributed primarily to foraging habits, as ring-neck ducks are divers and may consume up to 30 percent invertebrates in their diet, compared with American black ducks who forage on the surface of the water. Even when contaminated prey is ingested, exposure may be minimal in certain species. American kestrels fed pine voles (*Microtus pinetorum*) with mean body burdens of 48 $\mu$g/g DDE, 1.2 $\mu$g/g dieldrin, and 38 $\mu$g/g lead accumulated approximately 1 $\mu$g/g lead in bone and liver tissue but 232 $\mu$g/g DDE and 5.9 $\mu$g/g dieldrin in carcasses after 60 days. Mean lead concentration in regurgitated pellets from kestrels was 130 $\mu$g/g, demonstrating a lack of lead accumulation from contaminated prey (Stendell et al., 1989). Secondary poisoning from food chain transfer has also been implicated in the mortality of endangered species. Lead poisoning was apparently responsible for the deaths of several California condors (*Gymnogyps californianus*) found in California. The probable source of the lead was considered to be bullet fragments consumed by condors feeding on hunter killed deer (Wiemeyer et al., 1988).

The potential exposure of predatory species may be enhanced due to the altered behavior of contaminant-exposed prey. Affected prey may be easier to catch, leading predators to concentrate their foraging efforts on contaminated sites, thus increasing their direct exposure and the trophic level transfer of toxicants (Bracher and Bider, 1982; Mendelssohn and Paz, 1977). As contaminants move through food chains they may be translocated from their source. Migrating individuals may transport contaminants considerable distances, resulting in potential exposure and effects in organisms that otherwise would not be in contact with contaminated sites (Braestrup et al., 1974).

## Sublethal Effects

Mortality represents an important nonreversible endpoint of interest in terrestrial toxicology. However, documenting die-offs can be challenging, as success is affected by search efficiency and rapid disappearance of carcasses (Rosene and Lay, 1963). Also, many contaminants exist in smaller, nonlethal amounts or exist in relatively unavailable forms, such that acute mortality is unlikely. Thus, understanding and monitoring the sublethal effects of contaminant exposure in terrestrial systems is of great interest.

The existence of sublethal effects in exposed organisms has been used as an advantage in monitoring strategies. Many biochemical and physiological measurement endpoints have been developed or adapted from other sources and, in turn, used with various plant and animal sentinels to assess exposure and effect in terrestrial species (Lower and Kendall, 1990; Kendall et al., 1990). Inhibition of ChE's has proven an excellent marker that is both sensitive and diagnostic for organophosphate and carbamate insecticide exposure (Mineau, 1991). Induction of enzyme systems, such as the mixed-function oxygenases, are also useful as sublethal biomarkers of exposure to many types of environmental pollutants (Elangbam et al., 1989; Rattner et al., 1989). Other strategies for monitoring sublethal effects include monitoring immune function (McMurry et al., 1995), genotoxicity (McBee et al., 1987), and reproductive endpoints (Kendall et al., 1990).

Sublethal effects of contaminant exposure reach beyond the intrinsic physiological and biochemical responses to many behavioral traits of the individual. Decreased predator avoidance may expose individuals to increased susceptibility to pre-

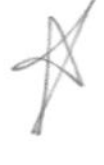

dation (Bildstein and Forsyth, 1979). Foraging behavior may be altered by chemicals, such that foraging efficiency is diminished (Peterle and Bentley, 1989). Migration and homing (Snyder, 1974) also may be affected, decreasing the general fitness of the individual. Altered breeding behavior may decrease fecundity through impaired nest building and courtship behavior, territory defense, and parental care of the young (McEwen and Brown, 1966).

## Chemical Interactions and Natural Stressors

As more information is becoming available on chemical effects in terrestrial organisms, there is increasing interest in understanding the interactive effects of exposure to multiple contaminants as well as the interactions between contaminants and inherent stressors (e.g., nutritional stress, disease, predation, climate). This area of terrestrial toxicology is one of the least understood because of the a priori need to understand the more direct exposure and effects scenarios. Nevertheless, it represents an interesting part of toxicology and is generating interest in the research community.

Perhaps the greatest inherent stressors faced by many species of wildlife are nutritional restriction and seasonal shifts in climatic extremes. Daily food restriction of as little as 10 percent below normal intake has been shown to enhance the overall decline in courtship behavior, egg laying and hatching, and number of young fledged by ringed turtle doves (*Streptopelia risoria*) exposed to DDE (Keith and Mitchell, 1993). Antagonistic relationships also exist. Methionine supplementation effectively negated the detrimental effects of selenium toxicity on mortality in mallard ducklings (Hoffman et al., 1992). Effects also have been found for the interaction between temperature stress and chemical exposure. Cold stress has been shown to augment the effects of pesticide exposure, resulting in increased mortality of several wildlife species (Fleming et al., 1985; Rattner and Franson, 1984; Montz and Kirkpatrick, 1985). However, more subtle interactive effects on energy acquisition and allocation were less conclusive in deer mice exposed to aldicarb 2-methyl-2-(methylthio)propanal O-[(methylamino)carbonyl]oxime and cold stress (French and Porter, 1994). Other areas of interest include interactions between chemical exposure and social stress (Brown et al., 1986) and interactions between different chemicals (Stanley et al., 1994).

# MODELING AND GEOGRAPHIC INFORMATION SYSTEMS

The role of modeling in ecotoxicology is to predict the effects of toxic compounds on the environment. The environment can be characterized by various ecosystems. Terrestrial ecosystems include forests, grasslands, and agricultural areas, whereas aquatic ecosystems include lakes, rivers, and wetlands. Each of these systems is a collection of interconnected components, or subsystems, that functions as a complete entity. Because the dynamics of real systems are quite complex, understanding the impacts of toxicants on a system can be enhanced by modeling the system.

The components or compartments of a system are represented by state variables that define the system. Once we have defined a system, it is possible to identify stimuli or disturbances from exogenous toxic substances, called inputs, from outside the system. These inputs operate on the system to produce a response called the output. The adverse effects of many toxic inputs are directly related to their ability to interfere with the normal functioning of both physiological and environmental systems. For example, emissions of heavy metals from a lead ore processing complex caused perturbations to the litter-arthropod food chain in a forest ecosystem (Watson et al., 1976). Elevated concentrations of lead, zinc, copper, and cadmium caused reduced arthropod density and microbial activity, resulting in a lowered rate of decomposition and a disturbance of forest nutrient dynamics.

In applying modeling to ecotoxicology, we are interested in studying a real-world system and the effects of various toxicants on that system. A model is a necessary abstraction of the real system. The level of abstraction, however, is determined by the objectives of the model. Our objective is to simulate the behavior of a system perturbed by a toxicant. This requires a mechanistic approach to modeling.

The modeling process involves three steps: (1) identification of system components and boundaries, (2) identification of component interactions, and (3) characterization of those interactions using quantitative abstractions of mechanistic processes. Once the model has been defined, it is implemented on a computer. Measurements obtained from the real system are compared to the model projections in a process of model validation. Several iterations of comparing model behavior to that of the real system are usually required to obtain a satisfactory or "valid" model.

## Types of Models

Models can be described in a variety of ways. In ecotoxicology modeling, the primary classifications are (1) Individual-based vs. aggregated models, (2) stochastic vs. deterministic models, and (3) spatially distributed vs. lumped models.

**Individual-Based Models versus Aggregated Models.** Models that simulate all individuals simultaneously are referred to as individual-based models. Each individual in the simulation has a unique set of characteristics: age, size, condition, social status, location in the landscape, as well as its own history of daily foraging, reproduction, and mortality.

Several individual-based models have been described by Huston and coworkers (1988) and by DeAngelis and Gross (1992), among others. This approach has several advantages. It enables the modeler to include complex behavior and decision-making by individual organisms in the model. But importantly, it allows one to model populations in complex landscapes, where different individuals may be exposed to very different levels of toxicant concentration (DeAngelis, 1994).

There are two general ways in which models of individuals can be extended to a population as a whole. First, one can simulate not just one individual, but all individuals that make up the population of interest. Second, one can aggregate various population members into classes, such as age classes. The model then follows not individual organisms but variables representing the numbers of individuals per age class. In simulating a complex environmental system, both individual-based and aggregated models will be needed. Usually, individual-based models are used to represent top-level predators and large herbivores while aggregated models are used to represent organisms at lower classification levels.

**Stochastic vs. Deterministic Models.** Model coefficients not only can be functions of other variables, they can be functions of random variables and thus can be random variables themselves. In this way of classifying models, those with random (stochastic) variables are called stochastic models and those without are called deterministic models. Random variables are used to represent the random variation or unexplained variation in the state variables. Stochastic models can include random variables expressed either as random inputs or as parameters with a random error term.

In a stochastic model, random variables representing state variables or model parameters (or both) take on values according to some statistical distribution. In other words, there will be a probability associated with the value of the parameter or state variable.

Monte Carlo is a numerical technique of finding a solution to a stochastic model. For those random features of the model, values are chosen from a probability distribution. Repeated runs of the model then will result in different outcomes. A probability distribution can be calculated for a state variable in the model along with its mean and variance. Suppose the model has random variables for parameters $p_1$, $p_2$, $p_3$, . . . $p_n$; the state variable will be a function of the $n$ parameters. A value for each parameter is calculated by sampling from its individual distribution function. A value for the state variable $X$ then is obtained by running a simulation of the model. We repeat the process until we have $N$ values of the state variable $X$. Finally we determine the mean $\mu$ and variance $\sigma^2$ for $X$.

**Spatially Distributed vs. Lumped Models.** Lumped models spatially integrate the entire area being modeled (Moore et al., 1993). Parameters for lumped models are averaged over the same spatial area. Spatially distributed models are based upon identifiable geographic units within the area being modeled. These subunits can represent physiographic areas, such as hydrologic or atmospheric basins that can be identified using a geographic information system (GIS). A GIS can be used to further identify homogeneous polygons or grid cells based upon soil and terrain features. Model parameters for each subunit can be geographically referenced and stored in the GIS database. The distributed model then can be used to simulate the response to a spatially distributed toxicant by replicating the model for each geographic subunit. Responses to toxicants are likely to be spatially nonlinear. Therefore, a lumped model using mean parameter values will not yield the expected value of the combined results of a distributed model. Modeling in ecotoxicology then usually will involve individual-based, stochastic, spatially distributed models.

## Modeling Exposure

Exposure of organisms to toxicants requires contact between the organism and the toxicant of concern. Modeling exposure requires a model to predict the spatial and temporal distributions of the toxicant and a model to predict the organism's geographical position relative to the toxicant concentration. Transport and fate models are used to predict the spatial distribution of toxicants. Atmospheric transport models (e.g., SCREEN and ISC2; U.S. EPA, 1992b,c, respectively) predict groundlevel concentrations of toxicants from stack emissions. Dixon and Murphy (1979) used these models to predict exposure concentrations as a series of *plume events* at any point on the ground. Exposure can occur from inhalation, immersion, ingestion, or a combination of these routes. Some vegetation models, such as CERES (Dixon et al., 1978a,b; Luxmoore et al., 1978) and PLANTX (Trapp et al., 1994), can predict uptake of atmospheric and soil concentrations of toxicants. Surface hydrologic models, such as HSPF (Donigian et al., 1983) and GLEAMS (Leonard et al., 1987), predict the runoff of toxicants from the land surface. Lake and stream models obtain input from surface runoff models and predict the change in toxicant concentration within the body of water.

Most vertebrates are mobile enough to move from an area of high toxicant concentration to an area of low toxicant concentration (or vice versa). The actual exposure of an individual will depend upon the concentration levels at the geographic locations visited by that animal at a given time. An integrated time- and space-averaged exposure $E_i$ can be calculated using the model (Henriques and Dixon, 1996; Ott et al., 1986):

$$E_i = \sum_{j=1}^{J} c_j t_{ij} \tag{1}$$

where $c_j$ = exposure concentration in microenvironment $j$;
$t_{ij}$ = time spent by animal $i$ in microenvironment $j$; and
$J$ = total number of microenvironments occupied by animal $i$.

The prediction of real-time exposure requires linking models of contaminant transport with behavioral models of animal movement. Models of animal movement can be based upon matching spatial patterns of observed behavior (Siniff and Jessen, 1969), rules based upon mechanisms governing the response of an individual to its environment (Wolff, 1994), or theoretical constructs such as random walk models (Holgate, 1971; Tyler and Rose, 1994).

## Modeling Effects

The effect of a toxicant on an organism depends upon the dose (the concentration reaching the target organ) and the physiological response to the dose. The dose depends upon the concentration of the chemical at the exposure site and the duration of the exposure. To predict the concentration reaching the target organ, we need to know how much of the chemical is taken up and absorbed by the organism. We also need to know where the chemical is distributed among the organism's tissues and organs and the rate at which the chemical is excreted from the same tissues and organs.

The dynamics of the disposition of a toxicant in the body of an organism is the subject of toxicokinetics. The dynamics involve the changes, over time, of the concentration of a toxicant in various tissues and the rate processes that control the movement from one part of the organism to another (Fig. 7-5).

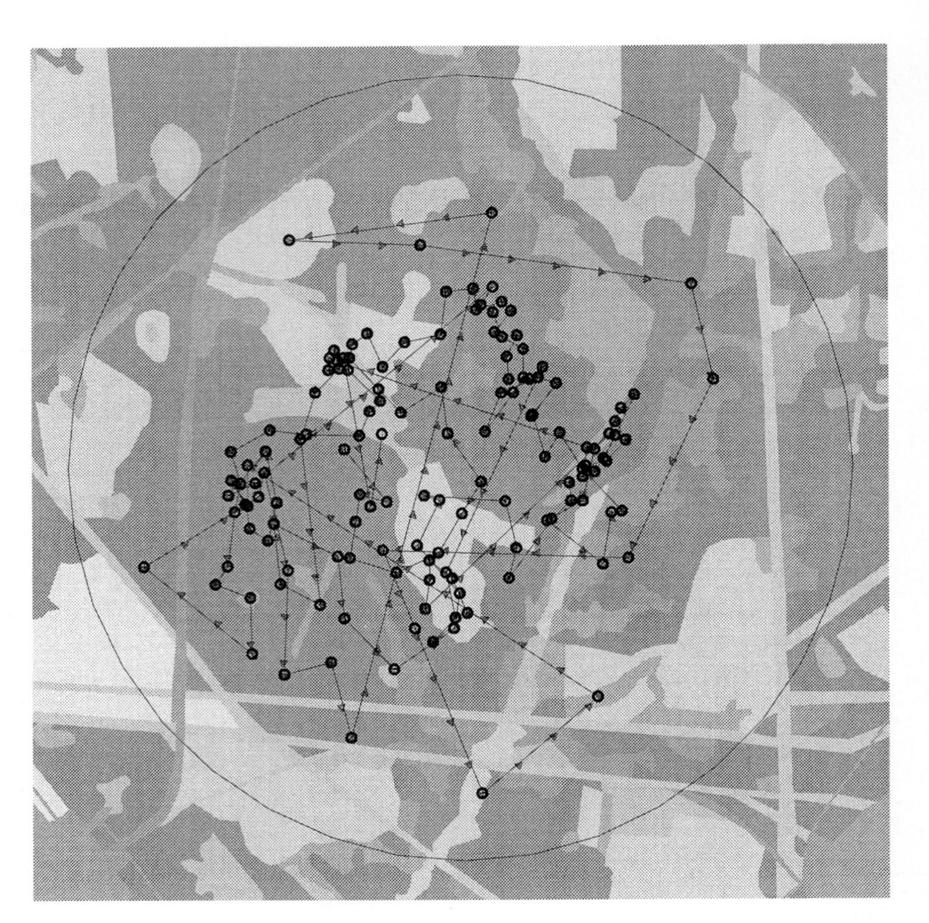

A

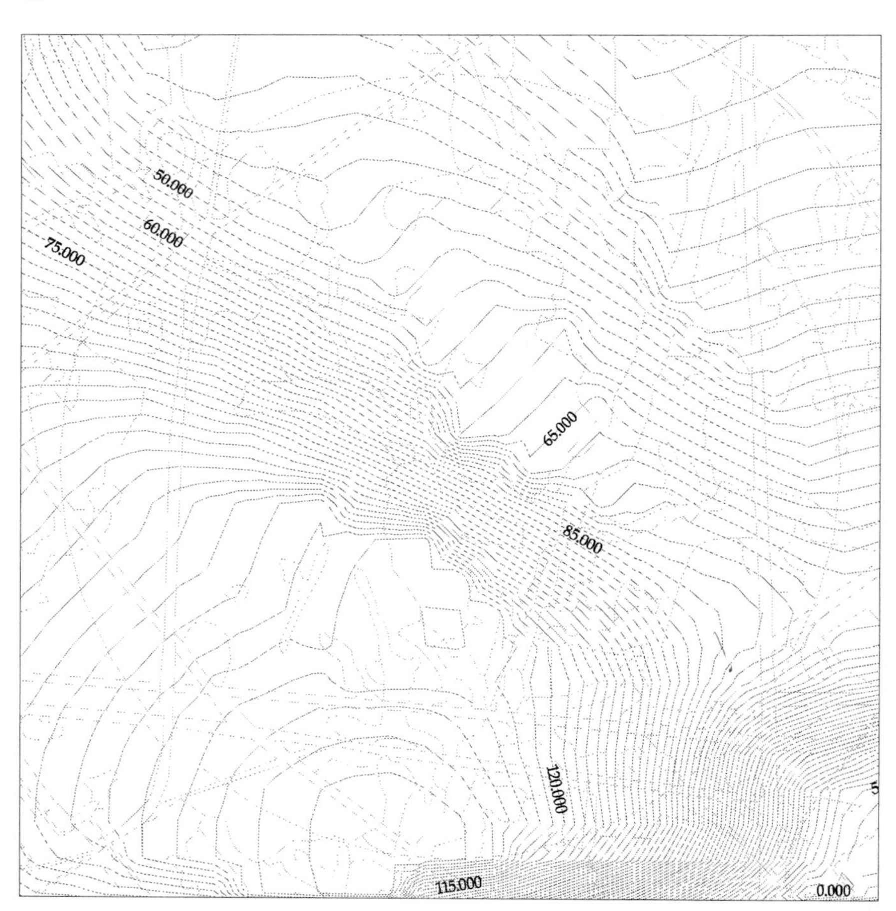


B

***Figure 29–1. Example of an animal's movement predicted by a spatial behavior model (A). Example of static ambient ground-level concentrations of a toxicant predicted by Gaussian plume model (B). Isopleths show lines of equal concentration. Units are in $\mu g/m^3$.***

DATA SOURCE: Henriques and Dixon, 1996.

The dynamics of a toxic gas or vapor in the lungs, $dC_l/dt$ ($\mu$g/h), can be simulated with the model:

$$\frac{dC}{dt} = 10^{-9}\, Y \cdot V_T \cdot f - k \cdot C \qquad (2)$$

where: $Y$ = exposure concentration ($\mu$g/m$^3$),
$V_T$ = tidal volume (ml/breath), and
$f$ = breathing frequency (breaths/h)
$k$ = transfer rate from lungs to bloodstream (1/h).

A solution to equation 2, with the input from the discrete-event exposure model, can be obtained by integrating over a defined time period with a given initial concentration.

## Linking Models to Geographic Information Systems

The GIS can be used to map the observed and predicted concentrations of toxic substances, as well as the resulting effects of exposure to these concentrations. By linking models with GIS, the ability to explicitly model the spatial dynamics of toxicant concentrations is greatly enhanced. There are different levels of integration of models with a GIS. First, a set of utility programs, external to both the model and the GIS, can be used to transfer data between the model and the GIS. Secondly, routines and macros can be written in the GIS language to run the models and analyze the results. Thirdly, the GIS computer code can be modified to run the models and display the results of the simulations as part of the GIS procedures.

## Mapping Exposure and Effects

Results from simulation models with spatially referenced output can be mapped as static or dynamic data in a GIS. Static data are spatially explicit but are expressed as a point (snapshot), as an average, or as a summed response over time. Dynamic data consider responses of state variables at points in space or a sum of the responses for an area. These data can be graphed as a function of time, or time series.

In our lung model example, static exposure can be mapped using the spatial behavior model (Fig. 29-1*A*) and the discrete-event Gaussian plume model (Fig. 29-1*B*). The resulting effect (lung dose) also can be mapped spatially (Fig. 29-2). The results from the discrete-event plume model and the lung concentra-

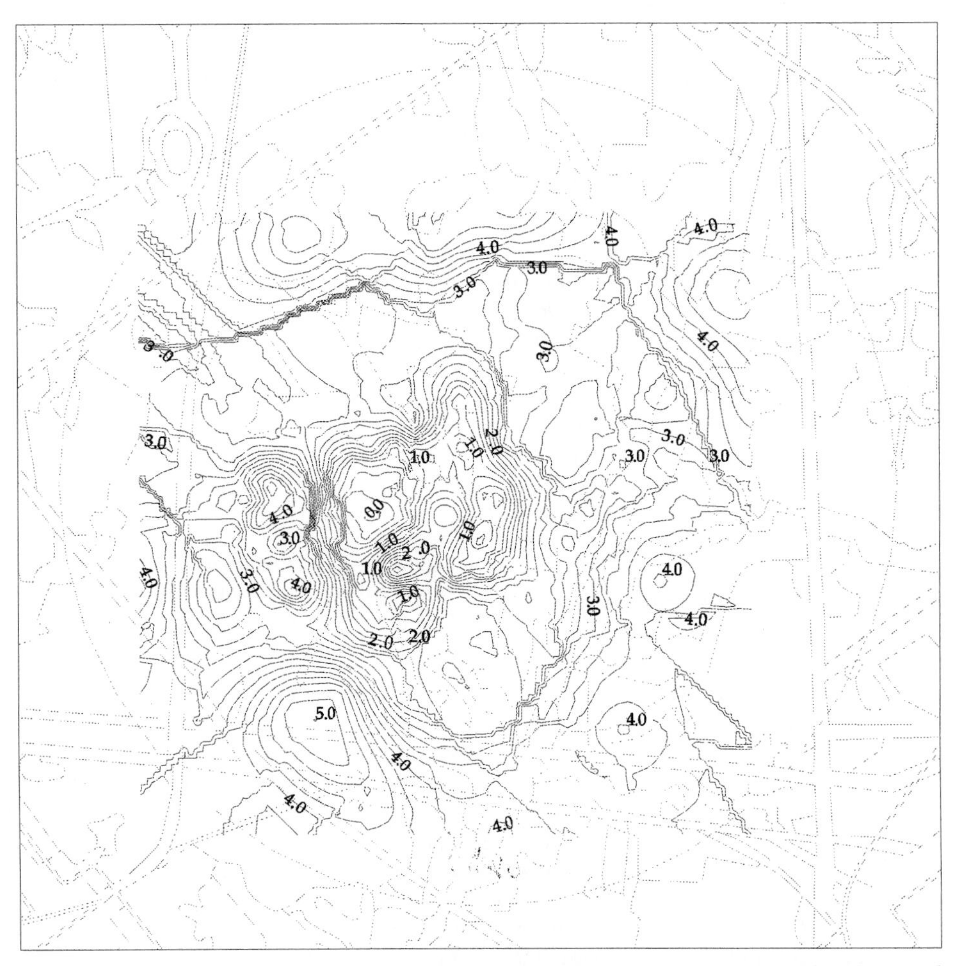


***Figure 29–2. Predicted dose to the lungs from exposure to ambient toxicant concentration as the animal moves according to the pattern in Fig. 29-1A.***

Dose depends upon the exposure concentration (Fig. 29-1B) and the time the animal spends at each location in Fig. 29-1A. Isopleths are lines of equal lung dose in units of $\mu$g.

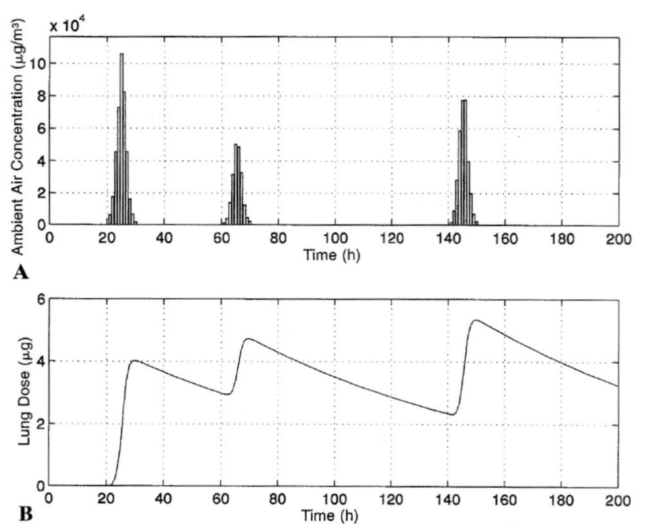


***Figure 29–3. A. Ambient air concentrations of toxicant predicted by discrete-event Gaussian plume model over time. Each pulse represents the ground level concentration at a given location. The shape of the pulse depends upon wind direction, wind speed, and atmospheric stability. B. Lung dose of toxicant predicted from lung model (equation 2) with input from plume model.***

Dose increases as plume passes over animal's location. Dose decreases as plume changes direction and concentration in lung decreases by diffusion to blood stream.

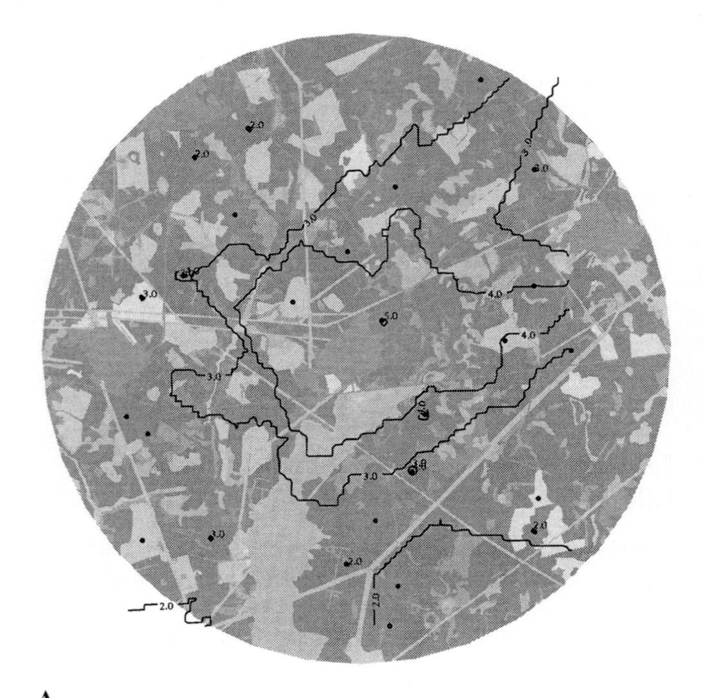


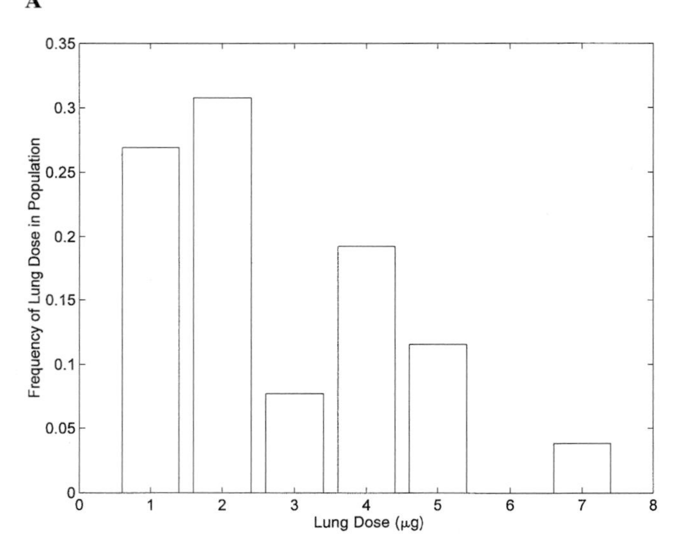


***Figure 29–4. A. Predicted static population lung dose for 26 individual animals. B. Frequency of occurrence of lung dose in population mapped in A.***

tion model can be graphed as a time series (Fig. 29-3*A,B*). This response is a result of the animal moving in space and time and the different concentrations of toxicant to which it is exposed at those places and times. A population response can be predicted by repeating the procedure for all the individuals in the exposed population. A spatial map of the steady-state lung concentrations in the population (Fig. 29-4*A*) shows a static response. The population response also can be expressed as a probability distribution (Fig. 29-4*B*) to show the variability in the population that results from the different individual responses.

Displaying both spatial and temporal responses simultaneously is more difficult, although developments in the area of computer visualization make this possible. Dynamic shifts in spatial maps of animal behavior (home range) and ambient concentrations can be illustrated in a "movie" sequence of maps. It is also possible to use visualization methods to show real-time movements of an animal in space and simultaneously display the time-series graph of lung dose. These techniques can enhance our understanding of the effects of toxicants in the environment and provide for more realistic estimates of the risk attached to those toxicants.

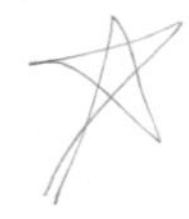

## ECOLOGICAL RISK ASSESSMENT

With the growth of the field of environmental toxicology comes the need to appropriately assess the impact of toxic chemicals on organisms, their populations, and communities in ecosystems. Earlier techniques to conduct risk assessments utilizing human health approaches were not appropriate for ecological systems. For this reason, the U.S. EPA has recently issued a new paradigm for conducting ecological risk assessment (Fig. 29-5). This new paradigm allows for the assessment of the impact of toxic chemicals, as well as other stressors, on ecological systems (U.S. EPA, 1992a). A basic overview of the ecological risk assessment paradigm is appropriate and applicable to the topics of this chapter.

The risk of toxic chemicals to wildlife or other biota within the ecosystem requires a knowledge of the environmental fate or exposure of the toxic substance in question in addition to hazard data (Table 29-1). Hazard data for species of concern at either the individual or population level also is needed (Kendall and Akerman, 1992). The evolution of the ecological risk assessment process is so new that currently there are relatively few examples. However, it is imperative in the problem formulation phase that an appropriate overview be considered for the ecotoxicological issue of concern, to

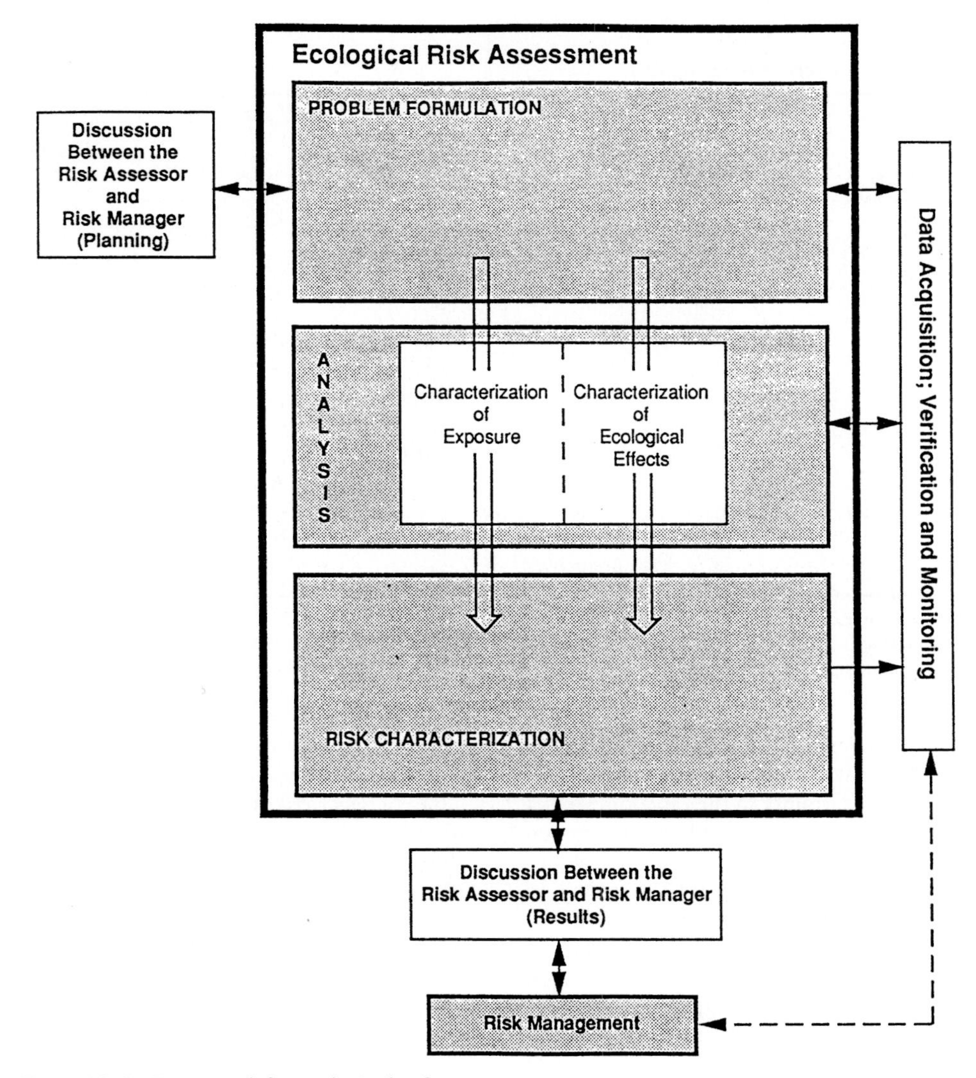


*Figure 29–5. Framework for ecological risk assessment.*

answer the question of what toxic substance and/or other stressors might have an impact on important species and/or their populations.

Subsequent to a full evaluation and the development of the problem formulation phase of ecological risk assessment, it is important that a conceptual model be identified before proceeding to the analysis phase to assess effects and exposure.

In an ecological risk assessment, effects may be registered at the individual or population levels (Kendall and Lacher, 1994) through a tiered framework for testing (Table 29-2). Under FIFRA testing requirements, for instance, laboratory bioassay data is often used to generate hazard information as part of the risk assessment. These laboratory bioassays, discussed above, in "The Use of Biomarkers in Assessing the Impact of Environmental Contaminants," include assays to measure the effects of chemicals on northern bobwhite and mallard ducks raised in a laboratory. These important dose-response data sets provide a better understanding of the potential biological effects and endpoints of concern. These endpoints include lethality, reproductive impairment, or health impacts such as those involving biochemical processes or physiological functions (Kendall, 1982).

One recent example involving the assessment of the ecological risk to wildlife of exposure to the insecticide carbofuran (a carbamate) has been published by the U.S. EPA (Houseknecht, 1993). Ecological risk assessment revealed widespread and repeated mortality events, particularly in locations where birds ingested carbofuran granules in agricultural ecosystems. According to legislation promulgated by FIFRA and extended to the international sphere by the Migratory Bird Treaty Act, environmental regulations do not permit the killing of migratory songbirds or waterfowl with a pesticide. Under FIFRA, through a Special Review, the U.S. EPA took regulatory action against carbofuran use in a large number of agroecosystems in which such use was associated with wildlife mortality.

The quotient method of assessing risk is often utilized in ecological risk assessment (Bascietto et al., 1990). The quotient method employs the formula of the expected environmental concentration divided by the toxic impact of concern (e.g., $LC_{50}$ or $EC_{50}$). If the quotient exceeds 1, then a significant risk may be indicated. Indeed, granular carbofuran products utilized in a broad range of agricultural uses resulted in quotients exceeding 1, and, as mentioned earlier, wildlife mortality has been identified (Houseknecht, 1993).

**Table 29–1**
**Ecotoxicological Assessment Criteria for Pesticides***

| PRESUMPTION OF MINIMUM HAZARD | HAZARD THAT MAY BE MITIGATED BY RESTRICTED USE | LEVEL OF CONCERN (LOC) |
|---|---|---|
| Mammals and Birds | Granular Formulations | |
| $LD_{50}$/sq. ft. < $\frac{1}{5}$ $LD_{50}$ | $\frac{1}{5} \leq LD_{50}$/sq. ft. < $\frac{1}{2}$ $LD_{50}$<br>$LD_{50} \geq 50$ mg/kg | $LD_{50}$/sq. ft. > $\frac{1}{2}$ $LD_{50}$ |
| | Acute Toxicity | |
| EEC* < $\frac{1}{5}$ $LC_{50}$<br>mg/kg/day < $\frac{1}{5}$ $LD_{50}$ | $\frac{1}{5}$ $LC_{50} \leq$ EEC < $\frac{1}{2}$ $LC_{50}$<br>$\frac{1}{5}$ $LD_{50} \leq$ mg/kg/day < $\frac{1}{2}$ $LD_{50}$ | EEC $\geq \frac{1}{2}$ $LC_{50}$<br>mg/kg/day $\geq \frac{1}{2}$ $LD_{50}$ |
| Aquatic Organisms<br>EEC < $\frac{1}{10}$ $LC_{50}$ | $\frac{1}{10}$ $LC_{50} \leq$ EEC < $\frac{1}{2}$ $LC_{50}$ | EEC $\geq \frac{1}{2}$ $LC_{50}$ |
| Mammals, Birds, and Aquatics | Chronic Toxicity | |
| EEC < Chronic<br>No effect level | N/A | EEC ≥ effect level<br>(including reproductive) |

Current EPA guidelines provided by Edward Fite, Office of Pesticide Programs, Ecological Effects Branch, EPA Headquarters, Washington, DC. From: *Wildlife Toxicology and Populations Modeling: Integrated Studies of Agroecosystem*. Boca Raton, FL: CRC/Lewis, 1994, with permission.

* Estimated environmental concentration. This is typically calculated using a series of simple nomographs to complex exposure models.

In the U.S. EPA Risk Assessment Paradigm, risk characterization offers the opportunity to put the ecological risk in perspective and to identify uncertainty in the development of the risk assessment. Although carbofuran could not be proven to cause significant adverse effects on bird populations, extensive mortality was evident and regulatory action was taken (Houseknecht, 1993; U.S. EPA, 1989). Evidence of carbofuran killing bald eagles (*Haliaeetus leucocephalus*) was also reported. Under the auspices of the Endangered Species Act, endangered species in the United States require special consideration because of their limited numbers and possible susceptibility to extinction.

Ecological risk assessment continues to evolve as a science (Suter, 1993). Much work still needs to be done to further refine risk assessments so that they reflect actual risk in the environment. The key to understanding ecological risk assessment in ecotoxicology is considering more than just chemical toxicity. We must consider ecological risk assessment in the context of exposure and other issues such as sublethal effects or ecosystem impacts. Indeed, we now know that predator-

**Table 29–2**
**Tiered Framework for Pesticide Toxicity Testing in Birds under FIFRA.**

Tier I
- Laboratory testing (acute)
  - $LD_{50}$—Adult mallard and northern bobwhite (single oral dose)
  - $LC_{50}$—2-week-old mallard and northern bobwhite (concentration in feed)
  - Songbirds may be included for comparative toxicology.

Tier II
- Laboratory testing (subchronic-chronic)
  - Reproductive toxicity where pairs of northern bobwhite and mallards are exposed in their food during breeding period; available data includes egg production, embryo survival, hatchability, and survival of hatched young to 2 weeks of age.

Tier III
- Field—pen testing
- Field testing (acute-subacute)
- Field pens are used to confirm wildlife exposure to pesticides in certain treatment areas; data acquired includes mortality.

Tier IV
- Field—full-scale testing (acute-subacute-subchronic-chronic)
  - Field testing using level I or II designs; level I design or "screening study" generally focuses on assessment of pesticide residues plus mortality and bird use data of agricultural fields; level II design seeks to quantify responses of wildlife populations exposed to pesticides through radiotelemetry, nest box techniques, blood/fecal sampling, and extensive residue chemistry.

From: *Wildlife Toxicology and Population Modeling: Integrated Studies of Agroecosystems*. Boca Raton, FL: CRC/Lewis, 1994, with permission.

prey relationships can be affected by chemical exposure in prey (Galindo et al., 1985). In addition, sublethal effects assessment or "biomarkers" offers new technology to assess sublethal impacts of chemicals on fish and wildlife populations (Dickerson et al., 1994). The availability of data from laboratory and field ecotoxicological experiments generated under Good Laboratory Practices (GLP), discussed below, will improve the quality and ultimate value of ecological risk assessments. GLP data may offer new opportunities to integrate validated information into ecological effect or exposure models for use in risk assessment (Kendall and Lacher, 1994). The contribution of ecological models in the ecological risk assessment process is in its infancy and offers significant opportunities for the extrapolation of data from laboratory and field experiments to a broader range of applications for the protection of the environment and its fish, wildlife, and other biotic resources.

## GOOD LABORATORY PRACTICE IN ECOTOXICOLOGY TESTING

Good scientific practices which result in high quality data are of paramount importance in the field of toxicology. There is a great public demand for personal and environmental safety, which is supported by environmental requirements under FIFRA, the Toxic Substances Control Act (TSCA), the Food and Drug Act (FDA) and the Occupational Safety and Health Administration (OSHA). With regulatory agencies increasingly being held accountable for environmental standards, there is a strong demand for formal and legal assurance that the toxicological data generated are accurate and that sufficient documentation exists to support the study conclusions. Requirements are designed to ensure that the studies are conducted under high ethical and scientific standards. Thus it is critical in today's regulated environment that toxicological data are produced and reported in a manner that ensures the study is reconstructible and that there are sufficient assurances of the quality and integrity of the data.

The principles and practices of quality assurance and quality control are perhaps best exemplified by the GLPs. The GLPs are regulations that define conditions under which a toxicology study should be planned, conducted, monitored, reported, and archived, and they have been adopted by many national and international governments and agencies. The GLPs outline study management procedures and documentation practices, which, if followed, will limit the influence of extraneous factors on study results. GLPs include provisions for such factors as personnel management and training, facilities support and operation, equipment design, maintenance and calibration, independent quality assurance monitoring, handling of test systems and materials, documentation of study conduct, written standard operation procedures and study protocols, reporting study results, and retention of records and samples.

In 1983, the U.S. EPA implemented GLP regulations under the mandate of FIFRA (40 CFR Part 160) and TSCA (40 CFR Part 792) for pesticide and toxic chemical registration and use. By 1989, these regulations were amended to cover field studies as well as laboratory studies.

# REFERENCES


Agency for Toxic Substances and Disease Registry (ATSDR): *Toxicological Profile for 4,4′DDT,4,4′-DDE,4,4′-DDD.* U.S. Dept. of Health and Human Services, TP-93/05, Atlanta, Ga., 1994.

Agency for Toxic Substances and Disease Registry (ATSDR): *Toxicology Profile for Pentachlorophenol.* Atlanta, GA: U.S. Dept of Health and Human Services, TP 93/13, 1994.

American Public Health Association (APHA): *Standard Methods for the Examination of Water and Wastewater*, 17th ed. Washington, DC: American Water Works Association, Water Pollution Control Federation, 1989.

American Society for Testing and Materials (ASTM): *Annual Book of Standards*, Philadelphia: American Society for Testing and Materials, 1986, vol 11.04.

Ames PL: DDT residues in the eggs of the osprey in the northeastern United States and their relation to nesting success. *J Appl Ecol (Suppl)* 3:87–97, 1966.

Ankley GT, Phipps GL, Leonard EN, et al: Acid volatile sulfide as a factor mediating cadmium and nickel bioavailability in contaminated sediments. *Environ Toxicol Chem* 10(10):1299–1307, 1991.

Aquatic Effects Dialogue Group (AEDG), World Wildlife Fund: *Improving Aquatic Risk Assessment under FIFRA: Report of the Aquatic Effects Dialogue Group.* Washington, DC: RESOLVE, 1992.

Armstrong RW, Eichner ER, Klein DE: Pentachlorophenol poisoning in a nursery for newborn infants: II. Epidemiologic and toxicologic studies. *J Pediatr* 75:317–325, 1969.

Atkins PW: *Physical Chemistry*, 2d ed. San Francisco: Freeman, 1982.

Babcock KM, Flickinger EL: Dieldrin mortality of lesser snow geese in Missouri. *J Wildl Manage* 41:100–103, 1977.

Barrett GW: The effects of an acute insecticide stress on a semi-enclosed grassland ecosystem. *Ecology* 49:1019–1035, 1968.

Barrett GW: Effects of sevin on small-mammal populations in agricultural and old-field ecosystems. *J Mammal* 69:731–739, 1988.

Bascietto J, Hinckley D, Platkin J, Slimak M: Ecotoxicity and ecological risk assessment. *Environ Sci Technol* 24:10–15, 1990.

Bergman HL, Meyer JS: Complex effluent fate modeling, in Dickson KL, Maki AW, Cairns J Jr (eds): *Modeling the Fate of Chemicals in the Aquatic Environment.* Ann Arbor, MI: Ann Arbor Science, 1982, pp 247–267.

Bergner H, Constantinidis P, Martin JH: Industrial pentachlorophenol poisoning in Winnipeg. *Can Med Assoc J* 92:448–451, 1965.

Beyer WN, Gish CD: Persistence in earthworms and potential hazards to birds of soil applied DDT, dieldrin and heptachlor. *J Appl Ecol* 17:295–307, 1980.

Beyer WN, Cromartie EJ: A survey of Pb, Cu, Zn, Cd, Cr, As, and Se in earthworms and soil from diverse sites. *Environ Monitor Assess* 8:27–36, 1987.

Bildstein KL, Forsyth DJ: Effects of dietary dieldrin on behavior of white-footed mice (*Peromyscus leucopus*) toward an avian predator. *Bull Environ Contam Toxicol* 21:93–97, 1979.

Blaser WW, Bredeweg RA, Harner RS, et al: Process Analytical Chemistry, in *Application Reviews.* Washington, DC: American Chemical Society, 1995, pp 47R–70R.

Bookhout TA: *Research and Management Techniques for Wildlife and Habitats.* Bethesda: The Wildlife Society, 1994.

Bracher GA, Bider JR: Changes in terrestrial animal activity of a forest community after an application of aminocarb (Metacil). *Can J Zool* 60:1981–1997, 1982.

Braestrup L, Clausen J, Berg O: DDE, PCB and aldrin levels in arctic birds of Greenland. *Bull Environ Contam Toxicol* 11:326–332, 1974.

Brown C, Gross WB, Ehrich M: Effects of social stress on the toxicity of malathion in young chickens. *Avian Diseases* 30:679–682, 1986.

Buerger TT, Kendal RJ, Mueller BS, DeVos T, Williams BA: Effects of methyl parathion on northern bobwhite survivability. *Environ Toxicol Chem* 10:527–532, 1991.

Cairns J Jr, Dickson KL, Maki AW (eds): *Estimating the Hazard of Chemical Substances to Aquatic Life*. Philadelphia: American Society for Testing and Materials, Special Technical Publication 657, 1978.

Cairns J Jr, Dickson KL, Maki AW: Scenarios on alternative futures for biological monitoring, 1978–1985, in Worf DL (ed): *Biological Monitoring for Environmental Effects*. Lexington, MA: Heath, 1980, pp 11–21.

Cairns J Jr, Mount DI: Aquatic toxicology. *Environ Sci Technol* 24:154–159, 1990.

Cairns J Jr, Mount DI: The threshold problem in ecotoxicology. *Ecotoxicology* 1:3–16, 1992.

Chutter M: A reappraisal of Needham and Usinger's data on the variability of a stream fauna when sampled with a Surber sampler. *Limnol Oceanogr* 17:139–141, 1972.

Clark DR, Lamont TG: Organochlorine residues and reproduction in the big brown bat. *J Wildl Manage* 40:249–254, 1976.

Collier TK, Anulacion BF, Stein JE, et al: A field evaluation of Cytochrome P4501A as a biomarker of contaminant exposure in three species of flatfish. *Environ Toxicol Chem* 14(1):143–152, 1995.

Connell DW, Miller GJ: *Chemistry and Ecotoxicology of Pollution*. New York: Wiley, 1984.

Corkum LD: Spatial patterns of macroinvertebrate distributions along rivers in eastern deciduous forest and grassland biomes. *J NABS* 10:358–371, 1991.

Crossland NO, La Point TW: The design of mesocosm experiments. *Environ Toxicol Chem* 11:1–4, 1992.

Daury RW, Schwab RE, Bateman MC: Blood lead concentrations of waterfowl from unhunted and heavily hunted marshes of Nova Scotia and Prince Edward Island, Canada. *J Wildl Dis* 29:577–581, 1993.

DeAngelis DL, Gross LJ (eds): *Individual-Based Models and Approaches in Ecology*. New York: Chapman and Hall, 1992.

DeAngelis DL: What food web analysis can contribute to wildlife toxicology, in Kendall RJ, Lacher TE Jr (eds): *Wildlife Toxicology and Population Modeling: Integrated Studies of Agroecosystems*. Boca Raton, FL: Lewis/CRC, 1994, pp 365–382.

Dewey SL, deNoyelles F Jr: On the use of ecosystem stability measurements in ecological effects testing, in Graney RL, Kennedy JH, Rodger JH Jr (eds): *Aquatic Mesocosm Studies in Ecological Risk Assessment*. Boca Raton, FL: Lewis/CRC, 1994, pp 605–625.

Dickerson RL, Hooper MJ, Gard NW, et al: Toxicological foundations of ecological risk assessment: Biomarker development and interpretation based on laboratory and wildlife species. *Environ Hlth Perspect* 102(12):65–69, 1994.

DiToro DM, Mahony JD, Hansen DJ, et al: Toxicity of cadmium in sediments: the role of acid volatile sulfides. *Environ Toxicol Chem* 9(12):1487–1502, 1990.

DiToro DM, Mahony JD, Hansen DJ, et al: Acid volatile sulfide predicts the acute toxicity of cadmium and nickel in sediments. *Environ Sci Technol* 26:96–101, 1992.

DiToro DM, Zarba CS, Hansen DL, et al: Technical basis for establishing sediment quality criteria for nonionic organic chemicals by using equilibrium partitioning. *Environ Toxicol Chem* 10(12):1541–1583, 1991.

Dixon KR, Luxmoore RJ, Begovich CL: CERES—A model of forest stand biomass dynamics for predicting trace contaminant, nutrient, and water effects. I. Model description. *Ecol Modelling* 5:17–38, 1978a.

Dixon KR, Luxmoore RJ, Begovich CL: CERES—A model of forest stand biomass dynamics for predicting trace contaminant, nutrient, and water effects. II. Model application. *Ecol Modelling* 5:93–114, 1978b.

Dixon KR, Murphy BD: A discrete event approach to predicting the effects of atmospheric pollutants on wildlife populations using C-14 exposure in meadow voles (*Microtus pennsylvanicus*) as a model, in *Animals as Monitors of Environmental Pollutants*. Washington, DC: National Academy of Sciences, ISBN 0-309-02871-X, 1979, pp 15–20.

Donigian AS Jr, Imhoff JC, Bichnell BR: Predicting water quality resulting from agricultural nonpoint source pollution via simulation—HSPF, in Schaller FW, Bailey GW (eds): *Agricultural Management and Water Quality*. Ames, IA: State Univ. Press, 1983, pp 200–249.

Duffus JH: *Environmental Toxicology*. New York: Wiley, 1980.

Elangbam CS, Qualls CW Jr, Lochmiller RL, Novak J: Development of the cotton rat (*Sigmodon hispidus*) as a biomonitor of environmental contamination with emphasis on hepatic cytochrome P-450 induction and population characteristics. *Bull Environ Contam Toxicol* 42:482–488, 1989.

Fite EC, Turner LW, Cook JJ, et al: *Guidance Document for Conducting Terrestrial Field Studies*. Technical Report 540/09-88-109, Washington, DC: Environmental Protection Agency, 1988.

Fleming WJ, Heinz GH, Franson JC, Rattner BA: Toxicity of ABATE® 4E (Temephos) in mallard ducklings and the influence of cold. *Environ Toxicol Chem* 4:193–199, 1985.

Ford J: The effects of chemical stress on aquatic species composition and community structure, in Levin SA, Harwell MA, Kelly JR, Kimball KD (eds): *Ecotoxicology: Problems and Approaches*. New York: Springer-Verlag, 1989, pp 99–144.

French JB Jr, Porter WP: Energy acquisition and allocation in *Peromyscus maniculatus* exposed to aldicarb and cool temperatures. *Environ Toxicol Chem* 13:927–933, 1994.

Galindo JC, Kendall RJ, Driver CJ, Lacher TE: The effect of methyl parathion on susceptibility of bobwhite quail (*Colinus virginianus*) to domestic cat predation. *Behav Neural Biol* 43:21–36, 1985.

Gebauer MB, Weseloh DV: Accumulation of organic contaminants in sentinel mallards utilizing confined disposal facilities at Hamilton Harbour, Lake Ontario, Canada. *Arch Environ Contam Toxicol* 25:234–243, 1993.

Giesy JP Jr, Allred PM: Replicability of aquatic multispecies test systems, in Cairns J Jr (ed): *Multispecies Toxicity Testing*. Elmsford, NY: Pergamon, 1985, pp 187–247.

Goering PL, Kish CL, Fisher BR: Stress protein synthesis induced by cadmium cysteine in rat kidney. *Toxicology* 85:25–39, 1993.

Gordon D: How dangerous is pentachlorophenol? *Med J Australia* 43:485–488, 1956.

Graney RL, Giesy JP, DiToro D: Mesocosm experimental design strategies: advantages and disadvantages in ecological risk assessment, in Voshell JR Jr (ed): *Using Mesocosms to Assess the Aquatic Ecological Risk of Pesticides: Theory and Practice*. Lanham, MD: Entomological Society of America, 1989, No. 75, pp 74–88.

Green RH: *Sampling Design and Statistical Methods for Environmental Biologists*. New York: Wiley, 1979.

Greene JC, Bartels CL, Warren-Hicks WJ, et al: *Protocols for Short Term Toxicity Screening of Hazardous Waste Sites*. EPA/600/3-88/029. Washington, DC: Environmental Protection Agency, 1989.

Greichus YA, Libal GW, Johnson DD: Diagnosis and physilogic effects of pentachlorophenols on young pigs: Part 1. Effects of purified pentachlorophenol. *Bull Environ Contam Toxicol* 23:418–422, 1979.

Grue CE, Shipley BK: Interpreting population estimates of birds following pesticide applications-behavior of male starlings exposed to an organophosphate pesticide. *Studies in Avian Biology* 6:292–296, 1981.

Grue CE, Powell GVN, McChesney MJ: Care of nestlings by wild female starlings exposed to an organophosphate pesticide. *J Appl Ecol* 19:327–335, 1982.

Guillette LJ Jr, Gross TS, Masson GR, et al: Developmental Abnormalities of the gonad and abnormal sex hormone concentrations in juvenile alligators from contaminated and control lakes in Florida. *Environ Hlth Perspect* 102(8):680–688, 1994.

Guthie FE, Perry JJ (eds): *Introduction to Environmental Toxicology*. New York: Elsevier, 1980.

Hammons AS: *Methods for Ecological Toxicology*. Ann Arbor, MI: Ann Arbor Science, 1981.

Henderson RF, Bechtold WE, Bond JA, Sun JD: The use of biological markers in toxicology. *Crit Rev Toxicol* 20:65–82, 1989.

Henriques WD, Dixon KR: Estimating spatial distribution of exposure by integrating radiotelemetry, computer simulation, and GIS. *Human and Ecological Risk Assessment* (invited paper, in press), 1996.

Herricks EE, Cairns J Jr: Biological monitoring, Part III: Receiving system methodology based on community structure. *Water Res* 16:141–153, 1982.

Hilsenhoff WL: Rapid field assessment of organic pollution with a family level biotic index. *J NABS* 7:65–68, 1988.

Hoffman DJ, Rattner BA, Burton GA Jr, Cairns J Jr: *Handbook of Ecotoxicology*. Boca Raton, FL: Lewis/CRC, 1995.

Hoffman DJ, Sanderson CJ, LeCaptain LJ, et al: Interactive effects of selenium, methionine, and dietary protein on survival, growth, and physiology in mallard ducklings. *Arch Environ Contam Toxicol* 23:163–171, 1992.

Holgate P: Random walk models for animal behavior, in Patil GP, Pielou EC, Waters WC (eds): *Statistical Ecology*. University Park, PA: State Univ. Press, 1971, vol 2, pp 1–12.

Hooper MJ, Brewer LW, Cobb GP, Kendall RJ: An integrated laboratory and field approach for assessing hazards of pesticide exposure to wildlife, in Somerville L, Walker CH (eds): *Pesticide Effects on Terrestrial Wildlife*. London: Taylor and Francis, 1990, pp 271–283.

Hooper MJ, La Point TW: Contaminant effects in the environment: their use in waste site assessment. *Centr Eur J Pub Hlth* 2(Suppl):65–69, 1994.

Houseknecht CR: Ecological risk assessment case study: Special review of the granular formulations of carbofuran based on adverse effects on birds, in: *A Review of Ecological Assessment Case Studies from a Risk Assessment Perspective*. Environmental Protection Agency Risk Assessment Forum. EPA/630/R-92-005, Washington, DC: Environmental Protection Agency, 1993, 3:1–25.

Howard PH, Boethling RS, Jarvis WF, et al: *Handbook of Environmental Degradation Rates*. Chelsea, MI: Lewis Publ., 1991.

Hudson P, Chen P, Tilson H: Effects of $\rho,\rho'$-DDT on the rat brain concentrations of biogenic amine and amino acid neurotransmitters and their association with $\rho,\rho'$-DDT-induced tremor and hyperthermia. *J Neurochem* 45:1349–1355, 1985.

Huston MA, DeAngelis DL, Post WM: New computer models unify ecological theory. *Bioscience* 38:682–691, 1988.

Johnson ML, Huggins DG, deNoyelles F Jr: Ecosystem modeling with LISREL: A new approach for measuring direct and indirect effects. *Ecol Appl* 1:383–398, 1991.

Johnson-Logan LR, Broshears RE, Klaine SJ: Partitioning behavior and the mobility of chlordane in groundwater. *Environ Sci Technol* 26(11):2234–2239, 1992.

Kapustka LA, La Point TW, Fairchild JF, et al: *Field Assessments: Ecological Assessment of Hazardous Waste Sites*. U.S. Environmental Protection Agency, EPA/600/3-89/013, Corvallis, Or., 1989.

Keith JA: Reproduction in a population of herring gulls (*Larus argentatus*) contaminated by DDT. *J Appl Ecol* 3(Suppl):57–70, 1966.

Keith JO, Mitchell CA: Effects of DDE and food stress on reproduction and body condition of ringed turtle doves. *Arch Environ Contam Toxicol* 25:192–203, 1993.

Kelly JR, Harwell MA: Indicators of ecosystem recovery. *Environ Manage* 14:527–545, 1990.

Kendall RJ: Wildlife Toxicology. *Environ Sci Technol* 16(8):448A–453A, 1982.

Kendall RJ: Farming with agrochemicals: the response of wildlife. *Environ Sci Technol* 26(2):238–245, 1992.

Kendall RJ, Akerman J: Terrestrial wildlife exposed to agrochemicals: An ecological risk assessment perspective. *Environ Toxicol Chem* 11(12):1727–1749, 1992.

Kendall RJ, Brewer LW, Hitchcock RR, Mayer JR: American wigeon mortality associated with turf application of diazinon AG500. *J Wildl Dis* 28:263–267, 1992.

Kendall RJ, Brewer LW, Lacher TE, et al: *The Use of Starling Nest Boxes for Field Reproductive Studies: Provisional Guidance Document and Technical Support Document*. EPA/600/8—89/056. Washington, DC: Environmental Protection Agency, 1989.

Kendall RJ, Funsch JM, Bens CM: Use of wildlife for on-site evaluation of bioavailability and ecotoxicology of toxic substances in hazardous waste sites, in Sandhu SS, Lower WR, deSerres FJ, et al (eds): *In Situ Evaluations of Biological Hazards of Environmental Pollutants*. New York: Plenum, 1990, pp 241–255.

Kendall RJ, Lacher TE Jr (eds): *Wildlife Toxicology and Population Modeling: Integrated Studies of Agroecosystems*. Chelsea, MI: Lewis, 1994.

Kerans BL, Karr JR, Ahlstedt SA: Aquatic invertebrate assemblages: Spatial and temporal differences among sampling protocols. *J NABS* 11:377–390, 1992.

Kimbrough RF, Linder RE: The effect of technical and purified pentachlorophenol on the rat liver. *Toxicol Appl Pharmacol* 46:151–162, 1978.

Klemmer HW: Human health and pesticides: Community pesticide studies. *Res Rev* 41:55–63, 1972.

Kolkwitz R, Marsson M: Oekologie der pflanzlichen saprobien. *Berlin Deutsche Botanische Ges* 26:505–519, 1908.

Korschgen LJ: Soil-food-chain-pesticide wildlife relationships in aldrin-treated sites. *J Wildl Mange* 34:186–199, 1970.

Kuwabara JS: Associations between benthic flora and diel changes in dissolved arsenic, phosphorus, and related physico-chemical parameters. *J NABS* 11:218–228, 1992.

Lamb DW, Kenaga EE (eds): *Avian and Mammalian Wildlife Toxicology: Second Conference*. Philadelphia: American Society for Testing and Materials, 1981.

Landrum PF, Lee H II, Lydy MJ: Toxicokinetics in aquatic systems: model comparisons and use in hazard assessment. *Environ Toxicol Chem* 11:1709–1725, 1992.

La Point TW, Fairchild JF: Evaluation of sediment contaminant toxicity: The use of freshwater community structure, in Burton GA Jr (ed): *Sediment Toxicity Assessment*. Ann Arbor, MI: Lewis, 1992, p 110.

La Point TW, Melancon SM, Morris MK: Relationships among observed metal concentrations, criteria values, and benthic community structural responses in 15 streams. *J Water Pll Control Red* 56:1030–1038, 1984.

Leonard RA, Knisel WG, Still DA: GLEAMS: Groundwater loading effects of agricultural management systems. *Trans ASAE* 30:1403–1418, 1987.

Levin SA: The problem of pattern and scale in ecology. *Ecology* 73:1943–1967, 1992.

Liber K, Kaushik NK, Solomon KR, Carey JH: Experimental designs for aquatic mesocosm studies: A comparison of the "ANOVA" and "regression" design for assessing the impact of tetrachlorophenol on zooplankton populations in limnocorrals. *Environ Toxicol Chem* 11:61–77, 1992.

Lower WR, Kendall RJ: Sentinel species and sentinel bioassay, in

McCarthy JF, Shugart LR (eds): *Biomarkers of Environmental Contamination*. Boca Raton, FL: Lewis/CRC, 1990, pp 309–331.

Luxmoore RJ, Begovich CL, Dixon KR: Modelling solute uptake and incorporation into vegetation and litter. *Ecol Modelling* 5:137–171, 1978.

Macek KJ: Aquatic toxicology: ten years in review and a look at the future, in Adams WJ, Chapman GA, Landis WG (eds): *Aquatic Toxicology and Hazard Assessment*. Philadelphia: American Society for Testing and Materials, 1988, vol 10, pp 18.

Macek KJ: Effluent evaluation, in Rand GM, Petrocelli SR (eds): *Fundamentals of Aquatic Toxicology: Methods and Applications*. Bristol, PA: Taylor and Francis, 1985, pp 636–649.

MacKay D: *Multimedia Environmental Models: The Fugacity Approach*. Chelsea, MI: Lewis, 1991.

Materna EJ: Effects of the synthetic pyrethroid insecticide, esfenvalerate, on larval amphibians. M.S. Thesis, University of Missouri-Columbia, Missouri, 1991.

Maughan JT: *Ecological Assessment of Hazardous Waste Sites*. New York: Van Nostrand Reinhold, 1993.

Mayer FL Jr, Ellersieck MR: *Manual of Acute Toxicity: Interpretation and Data Base of 410 Chemicals and 66 Species of Freshwater Animals*. Washington, DC: U.S. Dept of the Interior, Fish and Wildlife Service Resource Publication 160, 1986.

McBee K, Bickham JW, Brown KW, Donnelly KC: Chromosomal aberrations in native small mammals (*Peromyscus leucopus* and *Sigmodon hispidus*) at a petrochemical waste disposal site. 1. Standard karyology. *Arch Environ Contam Toxicol* 16:681–688, 1987.

McEwen LC, Brown LC: Acute toxicity of dieldrin and malathion to wild sharp-tailed grouse. *J Wildl Manage* 30:604–611, 1966.

McMurry ST, Lochmiller RL, Chandra SAM, Qualls CW Jr: Sensitivity of selected immunological, hematological, and reproductive parameters in the cotton rat (*Sigmodon hispidus*) to subchronic lead exposure. *J Wildl Dis* 31:193–204, 1995,.

Mellott RS, Woods PE: An improved ligature technique for dietary sampling in nestling birds. *J Field Ornithol* 64:205–210, 1993.

Mendelssohn H: Mass mortality of birds of prey caused by azodrin, an organophosphorus insecticide. *Biol Conserv* 11:163–170, 1977.

Menzer RE, Lewis MA, Fairbrother A: Methods in environmental toxicology, in Hayes AW (ed): *Principles and Methods of Toxicology*, 3d ed. New York: Raven, 1994.

Michalek JE, Tripathi RC, Caudill SP, Pirkle JL: Investigation of TCDD half-life heterogeneity in veterans of operation Ranch Hand. *J Tox Env Health* 35:29–38, 1992.

Miller EC, Miller JA: Mechanisms of chemical carcinogenesis. *Cancer* 47:1055–1064, 1981.

Mineau P (ed): *Cholinesterase Inhibiting Insecticides: Their Impact on Wildlife and the Environment*. New York: Elsevier, 1991.

Montz WE Jr, Kirkpatrick RL: Effects of cold temperatures on acute mortality of *Peromyscus leucopus* dosed with parathion. *Bull Environ Contam Toxicol* 35:375–379, 1985.

Moore ID, Turner AK, Wilson JP, et al: GIS and land-surface-subsurface process modeling, in Goodchild MR, Parks BO, Steyaert LT (eds): *Environmental Modeling with GIS*. New York: Oxford, 1993, pp 198–230.

Moriarty F: *Ecotoxicology: The Study of Pollutants in Ecosystems*. 2d ed. New York: Academic, 1988.

Morin A: Variation of density estimates and the organization of sampling programs for stream benthos. *Can J Fish Aquat Sci* 42:1530–1534, 1985.

Muir DCG, Yarechewski AL: Dietary accumulation of four chlorinated dioxincongeners by rainbow trout and fathead minnows. *Environ Toxicol Chem* 7:227–236, 1988.

Murray RW (ed): Application reviews. *J Anal Chem* 1991 and 1993.

National Academy of Sciences (NAS): *Principles for Evaluating Chemicals in the Environment*. Washington, DC: National Academy Press, 1975.

National Academy of Sciences (NAS): *Ecological Knowledge and Environmental Problem Solving: Concepts and Case Studies*. Washington, DC: National Academy Press, 1986.

National Research Council (NRC): *Testing for Effects of Chemicals on Ecosystems*. Washington, DC: National Academy Press, 1981.

Neely WB, Mackay D: Evaluative model for estimating environmental fate, in Dickson KL, Maki AW, Cairns J Jr (eds): *Modeling the Fate of Chemicals in the Aquatic Environment*. Ann Arbor, MI: Ann Arbor Science, 1982, pp 143–172.

Nishimura H, Nishimura N, Oshima H: Experimental studies on the toxicity of pentachlorophenol. *J Aichi Med Unib Assoc* 8:203–209, 1980.

Ott W, Wallace L, Mage D, et al: The Environmental Protection Agency's research program on total human exposure. *Environ Int* 12:475–494, 1986.

Peakall DB: Biomarkers: the way forward in environmental assessment. *TEN* 1(2):55–60, 1994.

Peterle TJ: *Wildlife Toxicology*. New York: Van Nostrand Reinhold, 1991.

Peterle TJ, Bentley R: Effects of a low OP dose on seed/bead discrimination in the kangaroo rat, *Diopodomys. Bull Environ Contam Toxicol* 43:95–100, 1989.

Pfleeger T, McFarlane JC, Sherman R, Volk G: A short-term bioassay for whole plant toxicity, in Gorsuch JW, Lower WR, Lewis MA, Wang W (eds): *Plants for Toxicity Assessment*. Philadelphia: American Society for Testing and Materials, Publ. 04-011150-16, 1991, vol 2, pp 355–364.

Platts WS, Megahan WF, Minshall GW: *Methods for Evaluating Stream, Riparian, and Benthic Conditions*. U.S. Dept of Agriculture, Forest Service Technical Report INT-138, Ogden, Ut., 1983.

Poland A, Knutson JC: 2,3,7,8-Tetrachlorodibenzo-p-dioxin and related halogenated aromatic hydrocarbons: examination of the mechanism of toxicity. *Ann Rev Pharmacol Toxicol* 22:517–554, 1982.

Pomeroy SE, Barrett GW: Dynamics of enclosed small mammal populations in relation to an experimental pesticide application. *Am Midl Natur* 93:91–106, 1975.

Rand GM, Petrocelli SR (eds): *Fundamentals of Aquatic Toxicology: Methods and Applications*. Washington, DC: Hemisphere, 1985.

Ratcliffe DA: Decrease in eggshell weight in certain birds of prey. *Nature* 215(5097):208–210, 1967.

Ratsch H: *Interlaboratory Root Elongation Testing of Toxic Substances on Selected Plant Species*. NTIS, PB 83-226. Washington, DC: Environmental Protection Agency, 1983.

Rattner BA, Franson JC: Methyl parathion and fenvalerate toxicity in American kestrels: Acute physiological responses and effects of cold. *Can J Physiol Pharmacol* 62:787–792, 1984.

Rattner BA, Hoffman DJ, Marn CM: Use of mixed-function oxygenases to monitor contaminant exposure in wildlife. *Environ Contam Toxicol* 8:1093–1102, 1989.

Rijstenbil JW, Poortvliet TCW: Copper and zinc in estuarine water: chemical speciation in relation to bioavailability to the marine planktonic diatom *Ditylum brightwellii. Environ Toxicol Chem* 11:1615–1625, 1992.

Rosene W Jr, Lay DW: Disappearance and visibility of quail remains. *J Wildl Manage* 27:139–142, 1963.

Rowley MH, Christian JJ, Basu DK, et al: Use of small mammals (voles) to assess a hazardous waste site at Love Canal, Niagara Falls, New York. *Arch Environ Contam Toxicol* 12:383–397, 1983.

Sanders BM: Stress proteins in aquatic organisms: an environmental perspective. *Crit Rev Toxicol* 23:49–75, 1993.

Sandler BE, Van Gelder GA, Elsberry DD, et al: Dieldrinexposure and vigilance behavior in sheep. *Psychon Sci* 15:261–262, 1969.

Schreiber RW, DeLong RL: Brown pelican status in California. *Aud Field Notes* 23:57–59, 1969.

Shonnard DR, Bell RL, Jackman AP: Effects of nonlinear sorption on the diffusion of benzene and dichloromethane from two air-dry soils. *Environ Sci Technol* 27(3):457–465, 1993.

Siniff DB, Jessen CR: A simulation model of animal movement patterns. *Adv in Ecol Res* 6:185–219, 1969.

Smith GJ: *Pesticide Use and Toxicology in Relation to Wildlife: Organophosphorus and Carbamate Compounds*. Washington, DC: U.S. Dept of the Interior, Fish and Wildlife Service Resource Publ. 170, 1987.

Snyder RL: Effects of dieldrin on homing and orientation in deer mice. *J Wildl Manage* 38:362–364, 1974.

Sokal RR, Rohlf FJ: *Biometry*. San Francisco: W.H. Freeman, 1981.

Stanley TR Jr, Spann JW, Smith GJ, Rosscoe R: Main and interactive effects of arsenic and selenium on mallard reproduction and duckling growth and survival. *Arch Environ Contam Toxicol* 26:444–451, 1994.

Stendell RC, Beyer WN, Stehn RH: Accumulation of lead and organochlorine residues in captive American kestrels fed pine voles from apple orchards. *J Wildl Dis* 25:388–391, 1989.

Suter GW II: *Ecological Risk Assessment*. Chelsea, MI: Lewis, 1993.

Thibodeaux LJ: *Chemodynamics: Environmental Movement of Chemicals in Air, Water, and Soil*. New York: Wiley, 1979.

Tinsley IJ: *Chemical Concepts in Pollutant Behavior*. New York: Wiley, 1979.

Touart LW, Slimak MW: Mesocosm approach for assessing the ecological risk of pesticides, in Voshell JR Jr (ed): *Using Mesocosms to Assess the Aquatic Ecological Risk of Pesticides: Theory and Practice*. Lanham, MD: Entomological Society of America, No. 75, 1989, pp 33–40.

Trapp S, McFarlane C, Matthies M: Model for uptake of xenobiotics into plants: Validation with bromacil experiments. *Environ Toxicol Chem* 13:413–422, 1994.

Travis CC: *Use of Biomarkers in Assessing Health and Environmental Impacts of Chemical Pollutants*. New York: Plenum, 1993.

Truhaut R: Ecotoxicology: objectives, principles and perspectives. *Ecotoxicol Environ Safety* 1:151–173, 1977.

Tyler JA, Rose KA: Individual variability and spatial heterogeneity in fish population models. *Reviews in Fish Biology and Fisheries* 4:91–123, 1994.

United States Environmental Protection Agency (U.S. EPA): *Final Report: Pesticide Assessment Guidelines, Subdivision E-Hazard Evaluation: Wildlife and Aquatic Organisms*. EPA/540/9-82/024, Washington, DC, 1982.

U.S. EPA: *Quality Criteria for Water*. Appendix A. USEPA Office of Water Regulation and Standards. EPA 440/5-86-0001, Washington, DC, 1986a.

U.S. EPA: *Test Methods for Evaluating Solid Waste*. 3d Ed. vol 1C: Laboratory Manual Physical/Chemical Methods. SW846, Washington, DC, 1986b.

U.S. EPA: *Carbofuran Special Review Technical Support Document*. 540/09-89/027, Washington, DC, 1989.

U.S. EPA: *Risk Assessment Forum: Framework for Ecological Risk Assessment*. EPA/630/R-92/001, Washington, DC, 1992a.

U.S. EPA: *Screening Procedures for Estimating the Air Quality Impact of Stationary Sources*. Revised. EPA-454/R-92-019, Washington, DC, 1992b.

U.S. EPA: *User's Guide for the Industrial Source Complex (ISC2) Dispersion Models—User Instructions*. EPA-450/4-92-008a, Washington, DC, 1992c, vol 1.

Wang W: The use of plant seeds in toxicity tests of phenolic compounds. *Environ Internat* 11:49–55, 1985.

Wark K, Warner C: *Air Polution: Its Origin and Control*. New York: Harper and Row, 1981, pp 69–73.

Warren-Hicks W, Parkhurst BR, Baker SS: *Ecological Assessments of Hazardous Waste Sites: A Field and Laboratory Reference Document*. EPA/600/3-89/01, Washington, DC: Environmental Protection Agency, 1989.

Watson AP, Van Hook RI, Jackson DR, Reichle DE: Impact of a lead mining-smelting complex on a forest-floor litter arthropod fauna in the new lead belt region of southeast Missouri. Oak Ridge National Laboratory, ORNL/NSF/EATC-30, Oak Ridge, TN, 1976.

Weseloh DV, Struger J, Hebert C: White pekin ducks (*Anas platyrhynchos*) as monitors of organochlorine and metal contamination in the Great Lakes. *J Great Lakes Res* 20:277–288, 1994.

Westman WE: Summarizing and evaluating impacts, in *Ecology, Impact Assessment and Environmental Planning*. New York: Wiley, 1985, pp 131–197.

Wiederholm T: Responses of aquatic insects to environmental pollution, in Resh VH, Rosenberg DM (eds): *The Ecology of Aquatic Insects*. New York: Praeger, 1984, pp 508–557.

Wiemeyer SN, Scott JM, Anderson MP, et al: Environmental contaminants in California condors. *J Wildl Manage* 52:238–247, 1988.

Willard WW, Merritt LL, Dean JA, Settle FA: *Instrumental Methods of Analysis*, 7th ed. Belmont, CA: Wadsworth, 1988.

Wolff WF: An individual-oriented model of a wading bird nesting colony. *Ecol Modelling* 72:75–114, 1994.

Wurster CF, Wingate DB: DDT residues and declining reproduction in the Bermuda petrel. *Science* 159(3818):979–981, 1968.

# UNIT 7

# APPLICATIONS OF TOXICOLOGY

## CHAPTER 30

# FOOD TOXICOLOGY

*Frank N. Kotsonis, George A. Burdock,*
*and W. Gary Flamm*

Food toxicology is different from other subspecialties in toxicology, largely because of the nature and chemical complexity of food. This chapter describes the general principles of food toxicology and explains how those principles have been shaped by existing food laws and applied to the safety assessment of foods, food ingredients, and food contaminants. The necessity for practical and workable approaches to the assessment of food safety is addressed throughout the chapter.

In addition to macronutrients and micronutrients, the typical western diet contains hundreds of thousands of substances which are naturally present in food and many more which form in situ when food is cooked or prepared. These substances may be *organoleptic*, i.e., conferring flavor, texture, color, or aroma to food, and there is a wide range of other substances which do not affect the organoleptic characteristics of food. An understanding of the meaning of food safety cannot ignore the fact that naturally present in food are hundreds of thousands of organic substances which, for example, make an apple look, taste, and smell like an apple. The Federal Food, Drug and Cosmetic (FD&C) Act gives the federal government the authority to ensure that all food involved in interstate commerce is safe within the meaning of the act. Congress, in writing the FD&C Act, understood that safety cannot be proved absolutely and indicated instead that the safety standard for substances added to food can be no more than a reasonable certainty that no harm will occur. As will be pointed out in other sections of this chapter, the language of the FD&C Act effectively provides for practical and workable approaches to the assessment of safety for food, food ingredients, and food contaminants. Because food is highly complex, the legal framework provided by Congress in the FD&C Act for the regulation of food and substances in food was kept simple so that it would work. The basic element of the framework is that food, which is defined as articles or components of articles used for food or drink for humans or animals [section 201(f) of FD&C Act], bears the presumption of safety [section 402(a)(1) of the FD&C Act]. This means that a steak or a potato is presumed to be safe unless it contains a poisonous or deleterious substance *in an amount* which is shown to make it *ordinarily injurious* to health [section 402(a)(1) of the FD&C Act]. In essence, this presumption of safety was born of necessity. If the hundreds of thousands of substances that are naturally present in food were subject to the same strictures and limitations that apply to added substances, food shortages and chaos affecting food availability could easily result. To avoid such crises, Congress, recognizing the innate complexity of food, developed a safety standard which would not force regulatory authorities to ban common, traditional foods.

In cases where the substance is not naturally present in food but is a contaminant or added ingredient, the safety standard established by the FD&C Act is quite different. This standard states that a food is adulterated if it contains any poisonous or deleterious substance which *may render* the food injurious to health [section 402(a)(1) of the FD&C Act]. Therefore, the presence of a substance which is not a *natural* component of a food involves a far higher standard of safety. The mere possibility that such a substance *may render* the food injurious to health suffices to ban the food containing that substance. Thus, for additives and contaminants, Congress recognized that these substances are not as complex as food and hence can reasonably meet a higher standard of safety.

An understanding of the term "safe" within the meaning of the FD&C Act is necessary in deciding how many studies and what types of studies must be conducted to determine that an added substance is safe. Wisely, the act does not give explicit instructions about how safety should be assessed or determined and does not explicitly define safety. Because neither the law nor Food and Drug Administration (FDA) and U.S. Department of Agriculture (USDA) regulations explicitly define the term "safety" for substances added to food, scientists—toxicologists, pathologists, chemists, and statisticians—and their legal and regulatory counterparts have worked out operational definitions for the safety of food ingredients. The one principle on which there has been unanimous agreement is that safety concerns in regard to an added substance should focus on both the nature of the substance and its intended conditions of use. It is recognized that substances are not inherently unsafe; it is only the level at which they are presented in the diet which makes them unsafe. The level present in the diet is determined by the intended conditions of use and limitations of use of the substance.

As with food, practical and workable solutions must be found for the constituents of additives, because all substances contain a myriad of impurities at trace and even undetectable levels. Decisions concerning the safety of impurities and the development of appropriate specifications for food and color additives to assure that they are of suitable purity must similarly constitute a workable approach. In this case, the workable approach involves setting specification limits on contaminants that are intended to exclude the possibility that the level of contaminants present in an additive *may render* the food to which the substance is added *unsafe*. As a practical matter and because of time and cost considerations, established specifications must be relatively simple and straightforward and must provide reasonable assurance that an ingredient is of suitable purity for its intended conditions of use. However, it generally is not necessary or practical to require extensive analysis and identification of all individual impurities to establish the fact that a substance is of "food grade purity." It should be emphasized that specifications can serve their purpose of assuring suitable purity only if the manufacturing processes used are adequately controlled to assure consistency in the quality and purity of the product. It should be understood that the philosophy by which specifications are established for substances added to food embodies the belief that not all risks are worthy of regulatory concern and control. Implicit in this philosophy is the concept of *threshold of regulation*, which is an important unifying concept in food safety assessment (Flamm et al., 1994).

To understand the meaning in the FD&C Act of the term "safe for intended conditions of use" for a substance added to food, it is important to recognize that such a determination must rest on a general understanding of the risks posed by food itself. The requirement that substances added to food be safe to a reasonable degree of certainty demands consideration of the far higher theoretical risk posed by food itself. Food, as was stated earlier, contains hundreds of thousands of substances, most of which have not been fully characterized or tested. The presumption that a food is safe is based on a history of common use as food and the understanding that the consumption of food is essential to life and that the consumption of certain specific foods is deeply rooted in tradition. While an individual substance added to food can be studied with every available toxicological test, such total scrutiny is not required to meet the standard of a "reasonable certainty of no harm." When the uncertainty about the risk of the added substance is small compared with the uncertainties attending food itself, the standard of "reasonable certainty of no harm" has been satisfied.

From the perspective of food safety, substances added to food (i.e., additives) generally can be divided into two major categories on the basis of the level of consumption and similarity to food itself. The first category contains additives which are virtually indistinguishable from food, such as fats, oils, fatty acids, modified fats, starches, modified starches, cellulose, modified cellulose, sugars and sugar alcohols, proteins, hydrolyzed proteins, and amino acids. Such substances are regulated (approved for specific or general use in food provided that specified limitations are met) in the Code of Federal Regulations (CFR) by the FDA as either direct food additives (21 CFR 172) or as generally recognized as safe (GRAS) substances (21 CFR 182 and 184). These substances may be added in relatively substantial amounts to food, in some instances at levels representing more than 1 percent of dietary intake. The second category consists of substances typically added in much smaller amounts (i.e., far below 1 percent and in many cases far below 1 ppm). Included in this category are indirect food additives, which are substances that may migrate into food from packaging or other food contact surfaces and are typically present in the total diet at concentrations below 0.05 ppm. Generally, indirect food additives and other members of this group, including processing aids and flavor substances, are present at concentrations far less than 1 percent in the total diet.

As a broad generalization, these two categories of additives carry with them separate but equally compelling presumptions that support the demonstration of their safety under their intended conditions of use in food. For the first category of foodlike substances, the presumption is that the substance resembles food, is digested and metabolized as food, and consequently raises fewer toxicological and safety-related questions than do non-food-like substances. For the second category of substances, which are added either directly or indirectly in only very small or trace amounts, the low levels of exposure and the large margins of safety [difference in exposure between the no observable effect level (NOEL) in test animals and anticipated human exposure] aid in demonstrating that the intended conditions of use of these substances are safe. These conclusions do not suggest that the presumptions of safety are sufficiently dispositive for substances added to food, as is the case, under the FD&C Act, for food itself. Instead, comprehensive testing of added substances is required by the FDA, but the requirements for testing are and should be tempered by considerations of (1) the basic nature of the substance, (2) the level to which consumers will be exposed as a result of the intended conditions of use of the substance, and (3) the inherent nature of food.

For substances that are similar to food and digestion products of food that are used at levels resulting in dietary exposures that do not exceed 0.05 ppm, minimal testing is required (acute oral toxicity and in vitro mutagenicity). However, for substances whose use results in dietary concentrations above 0.05 ppm but below 1 ppm, extensive testing involving subchronic toxicity studies in rats and dogs and reproductive and teratology studies in one rodent species and one nonrodent species are recommended. For substances whose use results in dietary concentrations in excess of 1 ppm, the full battery of toxicological tests, including chronic/carcinogenicity studies in two rodent species (in addition to all the tests listed above), is often required. It should be recognized, however, that for many foodlike substances derived from food under current good manufacturing practice (CGMP), using methods employed for producing GRAS substances, these requirements are excessive in that they probably exceed what is required to demonstrate safety under the standards of "reasonable certainty of no harm."

Over the past 5 years, new concepts about food and its components have been presented to the public and to regulators. These "designer foods," "functional foods," and "nutraceuticals" have been presented as the next generation of food, providing specific physiological, health-promoting, and even disease-preventing benefits (Mackey and Hill, 1994). Thus, consumer demands for better, safer, and healthier food with less cholesterol, less saturated fat, less salt, fewer calories, more fiber, and greater nutrition and wholesomeness have started a revolution in the food industry. However, it is not easy to reconcile the innovations demanded by the public with the framework used to assess safety by regulatory bodies because the latter is a scheme designed principally to assess the safety of exogenous synthetic organic chemicals added to food as opposed to the safety assessment of novel foods.

Finally, it should be recognized that in most of the world, microbiological contamination of food represents by far the greatest food-borne risk facing consumers. Thus, while vigilance in assuring the safety of substances added to food under their intended conditions of use is appropriate, we should not lose sight of the major concern of food safety.

## UNIQUENESS OF FOOD TOXICOLOGY

### Uniqueness of Food and Nutritional Considerations

The nature of food is responsible for the uniqueness of food toxicology. Food not only is essential to all life but also is a major contributor to the quality of life. Food and drink are enjoyed for their appearance, aroma, flavor, and texture. They are significant factors in defining cultures and societies. For example, ethnic foods and gourmet foods have a status which far exceeds their nutritional benefits, but any proposal to ban an ethnic food because new data have raised questions about its safety would be met with strong resistance.

As food occupies a position of central importance in virtually all cultures and because most food cannot be commercially produced in a definable environment under strict quality controls, food generally cannot meet the rigorous standards of chemical identity, purity, and good manufacturing practice met by most consumer products. The fact that food is harvested from the soil, the sea, or inland waters or is derived from land animals, which are subject to the unpredictable forces of nature, makes the consistency of raw food unreliable. Food in general is more complex and variable in composition than are all the other substances to which humans are exposed. However, there is nothing to which humans have greater exposure despite the uncertainty about its chemical identity, consistency, and purity.

Experience has supported the safety of commonly consumed foods, and the good agricultural practices under which food is grown or produced address the need for quality controls. Nevertheless, it is clear that food is held to a different standard as a practical matter dictated by necessity.

Food also acquires uniqueness from its essential nutrients, which, like vitamin A, may be toxic at levels only 10-fold above those required to prevent deficiencies. The evaluation of food ingredient substances (i.e., food additives, GRAS substances) often must rely on reasoning unique to food science in the sense that such substances may be normal constituents of food or modified constituents of food as opposed to the types of substances ordinarily addressed in the fields of occupational, environmental, and medical toxicology. Assessing the safety of these types of substances, which are added to food for their technical effects, often focuses on digestion and metabolism occurring in the gastrointestinal (GI) tract. The reason for this focus is that in many cases an ingested substance is not absorbed through the GI tract; only products of its digestion are absorbed, and these products may be identical to those derived from natural food. In these cases, it is only the ingested substance that differs from natural food; digestion products and absorbed substances are identical to those from natural food.

## Nature and Complexity of Food and Human Consumption of Food

**Nutrient and Anutrient Substances.** Food is an exceedingly complex mixture of nutrient and anutrient substances whether it is consumed in the "natural" (unprocessed) form or as a highly processed ready-to-eat microwaveable meal (Table 30-1). Among the "nutrient" substances, the western diet consists of items of caloric and noncaloric value; that is, carbohydrates supply 47 percent of caloric intake, fats supply 37 percent, and protein supplies 16 percent ("macronutrients") (Technical Assessment Systems, Inc., 1992) whereas minerals and vitamins, the so-called micronutrients, obviously have no caloric value but are no less essential for life.

**Table 30–1**
**Food as a Complex Mixture**

| NUTRIENTS | ANUTRIENTS |
|---|---|
| Carbohydrates | Naturally occurring substances |
| Proteins | Food additives |
| Lipids | Contaminants |
| Minerals | Products of food processing |
| Vitamins | |

SOURCE: Smith (1991). Used with permission.

**Anutrient Substances.** Anutrient substances are often characterized in the popular literature as being contributed by food processing, but nature provides the vast majority of anutrient constituents. For instance, in Table 30-2 one can see that even among "natural" (or minimally processed) foods, there are far more anutrient than nutrient constituents. Nature did not develop these foods for consumption by humans as the final goal. Many of these anutrient substances are vital for the growth and survival of the plant, including hormones and naturally occurring pesticides (estimated at approximately 10,000 by Gold et al., 1992). Some of these substances may be antinutrient (e.g., goiterogens in *Brassica*, trypsin and/or chymotrypsin inhibitors in soybeans, and antithiamines in fish and plants) or even toxic (e.g., tomatine, cycasin) to humans. An idea of the large number of substances present in food is given in the series edited by Maarse and associates (1993), in which approximately 5500 volatile substances are noted as occurring in one or more of 246 different foods. However, this is only the tip of the iceberg, as the number of unidentified natural chemicals in food vastly exceeds the number that has been identified (Miller, 1991).

Anutrient substances are added as a result of processing, and in fact, 21 CFR 170.3(o) lists 32 categories of direct additives, in which there are about 3000 individual substances. Approximately 1800 are flavor ingredients, most of which already occur naturally in food. Of the 1800 flavoring ingredients that may be added to food, approximately one-third are used at concentrations below 10 ppm (Hall and Oser, 1968), about the same concentration as is found naturally.

**Table 30–2**
**Anutrient Substances in Food**

| FOOD | NUMBER OF IDENTIFIED ANUTRIENT CHEMICALS |
|---|---|
| Cheddar cheese | 160 |
| Orange juice | 250 |
| Banana | 325 |
| Tomato | 350 |
| Wine | 475 |
| Coffee | 625 |
| Beef (cooked) | 625 |

SOURCE: Smith (1991). Used with permission.

## Importance of the Gastrointestinal Tract in Food Toxicology

Food toxicology deals with ingested substances taken as food or as components of food and begins and often ends in the GI tract. Many food ingredients are modified proteins, carbohydrates, fats, or components of such substances. Understanding the changes these substances undergo in the GI tract, their possible effect on the GI tract, and whether they are absorbed or affect the absorption of other substances is critical to an understanding of food toxicology and safety assessment.

It is essential to appreciate the fact that the gut is a large, complex, and dynamic organ with several layers of organization and a vast absorptive surface that has been estimated to be from 200 to 4500 $m^2$ (Concon, 1988). The GI transit time provides for adequate exposure of ingesta to a variety of environmental conditions (i.e., variable pH), digestive acids and enzymes (trypsin, chymotrypsin, etc., from the pancreas and carbohydrases, lipases, and proteases from the enterocytes), saponification agents (in bile), and a luxuriant bacterial flora presenting an extensive system of metabolism-possessing capabilities not shared by the host (e.g., fermentation of "nondigestible" sugars such as xylitol and sorbitol; this may also be important in the activation of carcinogens) (Drasar and Hill, 1974). The enterocytes (intestinal epithelium) possess an extensive capacity for the metabolism of xenobiotics which may be second only to the liver, with a full complement of phase (type) I and phase (type) II reactions present. The enteric monooxygenase system is analogous to the liver, as both systems are located in the endoplasmic reticulum of cells, require NADPH and $O_2$ for maximum activity, are inhibited by SKF-525A and carbon monoxide, and are qualitatively identical in their response to enzyme induction (Hassing et al., 1989). Induction of xenobiotic metabolism by the enteric monooxygenase system has been demonstrated in a number of substances, including commonly eaten foods and their constituents (Table 30-3). Dietary factors also may decrease metabolic activity. For example, in one study iron restriction and selenium deficiency decreased cytochrome P450 values, but a vitamin A–rich diet had the same effect (Kaminsky and Fasco, 1991).

The constituents of food and other ingesta (e.g., drugs, contaminants, inhaled pollutants dissolved in saliva and swallowed) are a physicochemically heterogeneous lot, and because the intestine has evolved into a relatively impermeable membrane, mechanisms of absorption have developed that allow substances to gain access to the body from the intestinal lumen. The four primary mechanisms for absorption are passive or simple diffusion, active transport, facilitated diffusion, and pinocytosis. Each of these mechanisms characteristically transfers a defined group of constituents from the lumen into the body (Table 30-4). As is noted in the table, xenobiotics and other nutrients may compete for passage into the body.

Aiding this absorption is the rich vascularization of the intestine, with a normal rate of blood flow in the portal vein of approximately 1.2 L/h/kg. However, after a meal, there is a 30

**Table 30–3**
**Induction of Xenobiotic Metabolism in the Rat Intestine**

| INDUCER | SUBSTRATE OR ENZYME | REFERENCE |
|---|---|---|
| Butylated hydroxyanisole, benzo[*a*]pyrene | UDP-glucuronic acid | Goon and Klaassen, 1992 |
| Benzo[*a*]pyrene, cigarette smoke, charcoal-broiled ground beef (vs. ground beef cooked on foil), Purina Rat Chow (vs. semisynthetic diet), chlorpromazine, chlorcyclizine | Phenacetin | Pantuck et al., 1974, 1975 |
| Cabbage or brussels sprouts | Phenacetin, 7-ethoxycoumarin, hexobarbital | Pantuck et al., 1976 |
| Ethanol | Benzo[*a*]pyrene | Van de Wiel et al., 1992 |
| Indole-3-carbinol (present in brussels sprouts) | Pentoxy- and ethoxyresorufin, testosterone | Wortelboer et al., 1992b |
| Fried meat, dietary fat | 7-ethoxyresorufin *O*-deethylase | Kaminsky and Fasco, 1991 |
| Brussels sprouts | Aryl hydrocarbon hydroxylase, 7-ehtoxyresorufin *O*-deethylase | Kaminsky and Fasco, 1991 |
| Brussels sprouts | Ethoxyresorufin deethylastion, glutathione-S-transferase, DT-diaphorase | Wortelboer et al., 1992 |

**Table 30–4**
**Systems Transporting Enteric Constituents**

| SYSTEM | ENTERIC CONSTITUENT |
|---|---|
| Passive diffusion | Sugars (e.g., fructose, mannose, xylose, which may also be transported by facilitated diffusion), lipid-soluble compounds, water |
| Facilitated diffusion | D-xylose, 6-deoxy-1,5-anhydro-D-glucitol, glutamic acid, aspartic acids, short-chain fatty acids, xenobiotics with carboxy groups, sulfates, glucuronide esters, lead, cadmium, zinc |
| Active transport | Cations, anions, sugars, vitamins, nucleosides (pyrimidines, uracil, and thymine, which may be in competition with 5-fluorouracil and 5-bromouracil), cobalt, manganese (which compete for the iron transportation system) |
| Pinocytosis | Long-chain lipids, vitamin $B_{12}$ complex, azo dyes, maternal antibodies, botulinum toxin, hemagglutinins, phalloidins, *E. coli* endotoxins, virus particles. |

percent increase in blood flow through the splanchnic area (Concon, 1988). It follows, then, that substances which affect blood flow also tend to affect the absorption of compounds; an example is alcohol, which tends to increase blood flow to the stomach and thus enhances its own absorption. Few stimuli tend to decrease flow to this area, with the possible exception of energetic muscular activity and hypovolemic shock.

Lymph circulation is important in the transfer of fats, large molecules (such as botulinum toxin), benzo[*a*]pyrene, 3-methylcholanthrene, and *cis*-dimethylaminostilbene (Chhabra and Eastin, 1984). Lymph has a flow rate of about 1 to 2 ml/h/kg in humans, and few factors are known to influence its flow, with the exception of tripalmitin, which has been shown to double the flow and therefore double the absorption of *p*-aminosalicylic acid and tetracycline (Chhabra and Eastin, 1984). Another factor that lends importance to lymph is the fact that the lymph empties via the thoracic duct into the point of junction of the left internal jugular and subclavian veins, preventing "first-pass" metabolism by the liver, unlike substances transported by the blood.

Some of the factors which may affect GI absorption and the rate of absorption are listed in Table 30-5.

## SAFETY STANDARD FOR FOODS, ADDITIVES AND CONTAMINANTS

### The FD&C Act Provides for a Practicable Approach

As was discussed above, the FD&C Act presumes that traditionally consumed foods are safe if they are free of contaminants. For the FDA to ban such foods, it must have clear evidence that death or illness traced to consumption of a food has occurred. The fact that foods contain many natural substances, some of which are toxic at a high concentration, is in itself an insufficient basis under the FD&C Act for declaring a food as being unfit for human consumption.

**The Pragmatic Use of Tolerances.** If a food contains an unavoidable contaminant (unavoidable by CGMP), it may be declared unfit as food if the contaminant has the potential to render that food injurious to health. Thus, for a food to be declared unfit, it must be ordinarily injurious, while an unavoidable contaminant in food need only pose the risk of harm

**Table 30–5**
**Factors Affecting Intestinal Absorption and Rate of Absorption**

| FACTOR | EXAMPLE |
|---|---|
| Gastric emptying rate | Increased fat content |
| Gastric pH | Antacids, stress, $H_2$-receptor blockers |
| Intestinal motility | Diarrhea due to intercurrent disease, laxatives, dietary fiber, disaccharide intolerance, amaranth |
| Food content | Lectins of *Phaseolus vulgaris* (inhibition of glucose absorption and transport) |
| Surface area of small intestine | Short-bowel syndrome |
| Intestinal blood flow | Alcohol |
| Intestinal lymph flow | Tripalmitin |
| Enterohepatic circulation | Chlordecone (prevented by cholestyramine) |
| Permeability of mucosa | Inflammatory bowel disease, celiac disease |
| Inhibition of digestive processes | Catechins of tea which inhibit sucrase and therefore glucose absorption |
| Concomitant drug therapy | Iron salts/tetracycline |

SOURCE: Modified from Hoensch and Schwenk (1984). Used with permission.

**Table 30–6**
**FDA Action Levels for Aflatoxins (Compliance Policy Guides 7120.26, 7106.10, and 7126.33)**

| COMMODITY | LEVEl, ng/g |
|---|---|
| All products, except milk, designated for humans | 20 |
| Milk | 0.5 |
| Corn for immature animals and dairy cattle | 20 |
| Corn for breeding beef cattle, swine, and mature poultry | 100 |
| Corn for finishing swine | 200 |
| Corn for finishing beef cattle | 300 |
| Cottonseed meal (as a feed ingredient) | 300 |
| All feedstuffs other than corn | 20 |

for that food to be found unfit and subject to FDA action. The reason for the dichotomy is practicability. Congress recognized that if authority were granted to ban traditional foods for reasons that go beyond clear evidence of harm to health, the agency would be subject to pressure to ban certain foods.

Foods containing unavoidable contaminants are not automatically banned because such foods are subject to the provisions of section 406 of the FD&C Act, which states that the quantity of unavoidable contaminants in food may be limited by regulation for the protection of public health and that any quantity of a contaminant which exceeds the fixed limit shall be deemed unsafe. This authority has been used by the FDA to set limits on the quantity of unavoidable contaminants in food by regulation (tolerances) and by informal action levels which do not have the force of law. Such action levels have been set for aflatoxin in peanuts, grain, and milk (Table 30-6). Action levels have the advantage of offering greater flexibility than is provided by tolerances established by regulation. Whether tolerances or action levels are applied to unavoidable contaminants of food, the FDA attempts to balance the health risk posed by unavoidable contaminants against the loss of a portion of the food supply. Recognition by Congress of the premier status of food mandates a thoughtful approach to regulation.

In contrast, contaminants in food that are *avoidable* by CGMP are deemed to be unsafe under section 406 if they are considered poisonous or deleterious. Under such circumstances, the food is typically declared *adulterated* and unfit for human consumption. The extent to which consumers who are already in possession of such food must be alerted depends on the health risk posed by the contaminated food. If there is a reasonable probability that the use of or exposure to such a food will cause serious adverse health consequences or death, the FDA will seek a Class I recall which provides the maximum public warning, the greatest depth of recall, and the most follow-up. Classes II and III represent progressively less health risk and require less public warning, less depth of recall, and less follow-up (21 CFR 7.3).

**The Pragmatic Application of Experience: GRAS.** The FD&C Act permits the addition of substances to food to accomplish a specific technical effect if the substance is determined to be GRAS by experts qualified by scientific training and experience to evaluate food safety. The FD&C Act does not require that this determination be made by the FDA, though it does not exclude the agency from making such decisions. The act instead requires that scientific experts base a GRAS determination on the adequacy of safety, as shown through scientific procedures or through experience based on common use in food before January 1, 1958, under the intended conditions of use of the substance [FD&C Act, section 201(s)].

In addition to allowing GRAS substances to be added to food, the act provides for a class of substances that are regulated food additives, which are defined as "any substances the intended use of which results in its becoming a component . . . of any food . . . if such substance is not generally recognized . . . to be safe." Hence, a legal distinction is drawn between regulated food additives and GRAS substances. Regulated food additives must be approved and regulated for their intended conditions of use by the FDA under 21 CFR 172–179 before they can be marketed. Under section 409 of the act, the requirements for data to support the safe use of a food additive are described in general terms. The exact requirements or recommended methods for establishing safe conditions of use for an additive are available in the form of a guideline issued by FDA (*Toxicological Principles for the Safety Assessment of Direct Food Additives and Color Additives Used in Food*). These guidelines, referred to as the Redbook, provide substance and definition to the safety standard applicable to regulated food additives: "reasonable certainty of no harm under conditions of intended use."

## Methods Used to Evaluate the Safety of Foods, Additives, and Contaminants

**Safety Evaluation of Food and Color Additives.** The FDA has stated its safety assessment strategy in the form of four precepts: (1) The agency "should possess at least some toxicologic or other biologic safety data for each additive," (2) the extent of toxicological evaluation is set by the agency's "concern about potential public health consequences," which in turn is related to exposure, (3) a level of concern* can be determined as a function of the level of exposure and the

*Level of concern [concern level (CL)] is the term used by FDA to determine the extent of toxicity testing required. The CL results from an algorithm based on exposure and structure-activity relationships. The procedure is described in detail in the Redbook (USFDA, 1982).

correlation of molecular structure activity with other substances of known toxicity, and (4) the results from preliminary toxicological studies can lead to a substance's being placed in a higher CL. Thus, toxicity and exposure from the intended conditions of use are the driving force in safety evaluation.

**Exposure and Dose: The Estimated Daily Intake.** Before 1958, the FDA employed the philosophy that additives (and contaminants) should be harmless per se; that is, an additive should not be harmful at *any* level. The impractical nature of this philosophy is illustrated by two examples: A reasonable person would assume that pure, distilled water is harmless, but if enough is ingested to cause electrolyte imbalance, death may result; similarly, sulfuric acid in its concentrated form can dissolve steel, but when used to control pH during the processing of alcoholic beverages or cheeses, it is considered GRAS by the FDA (*Principles*, 1991). Clearly, exposure should be the driving engine of safety evaluation. This philosophy is reflected in the FDA's *Toxicological Principles for the Safety Assessment of Direct Food Additives and Color Additives Used in Food* (the Redbook) (USFDA, 1982),* in which exposure is a key factor in an algorithm used to determine which types of testing should be carried out on a substance.

Exposure is most often referred to as an estimated daily intake (EDI) and is based on two factors: the daily intake (I) of the food in which the substance will be used and the concentration (C) of the substance in that food:

$$EDI = C \times I$$

In most cases, an additive is used in several different food categories, but for the sake of simplicity, we can assume that the additive is used only in baked goods. If the additive is used at a level that does not exceed 10 ppm and the mean daily intake of baked goods is 137 g/person/day, the EDI for this substance is 1370 $\mu$g/person/day.

Because most additives are used in more than one food, the total exposure (dose) is the sum of the exposures from each of the food categories. The formula for exposure to substance XYZ is

$$EDI_{xyz} = (C_{xyz}f \times I_f) + (C_{xyz}g \times I_g) + (C_{xyz}h \times I_h) + (C\ldots)$$

where $C_{xyz}f$ and $C_{xyz}g$ are the concentration of XYZ in food category f and the concentration of XYZ in food category g, respectively. $I_f$ and $I_g$ are the daily intake of food category f, food category g, and so on. Therefore, the EDI is the sum of the individual contributions of XYZ in each of the food categories.

Many of the same principles can be applied to an estimation of the consumption of residue from enzyme preparations [total organic solids (TOS)], residue from secondary direct additives (substances not intended to remain in a food after the technical effect has been accomplished; this includes but is not limited to mold release agents, solvents, defoaming agents, and chemicals used in washing fruits), and contaminants.

These concepts give rise to two questions: (1) How does one determine how much is added to each of the food categories? and (2) What are the food categories, and how are they determined? First, the agency will use as the basis for its calculations the highest end of the range of use level for the new substance, but what ensures that these food group maximums will not be exceeded by a food manufacturer? This is also covered by a regulation—CGMPs (21 CFR 110)—in which a manufacturer is bound not to add more of an additive than is reasonably required to achieve its specific technical effect. That is, if the desired red color of strawberry ice cream is achieved with the addition of 1 ppm of red dye and additional

*At the time of this writing Redbook II, dated 1993, remains in draft form and may undergo significant revision before finalization. For this reason, the 1982 version is used in this chapter except where noted.

**Table 30–7**
**Food Categories**

| NUMBER | DESIGNATION | DESCRIPTION | EXAMPLES |
|---|---|---|---|
| 170.3(n) | | | |
| (1) | Baked goods and baking mixes | Includes all ready-to-eat and ready-to-bake products, flours, and mixes requiring preparation before serving | Doughnuts, bread, croissants, cake mix, cookie dough |
| (2) | Beverages, alcoholic | Includes malt beverages, wines, distilled liquors, and cocktail mix | Beer, malt liquor, whiskey, liqueurs, wine coolers |
| (3) | Beverages and beverage bases, nonalcoholic | Includes only special or spiced teas, soft drinks, coffee substitutes, and fruit- and vegetable-flavored gelatin drinks | Herbal tea (non-tea-containing "teas"), soda pop, chicory |
| (4) | Breakfast cereals | Includes ready-to-eat and instant and regular hot cereals | Oatmeal (both regular and instant), farina, corn flakes, wheat flakes |

**Table 30–8**
**Databases for Estimating Food Intake**

| |
|---|
| The Nationwide Food Consumption Survey, USDA, 1987–1988* |
| Foods Commonly Consumed by Individuals, USDA (Pay et al., 1984) |
| Continuing Survey of Food Intakes by Individuals, USDA, 1985, 1986, 1989*, 1990, 1991 |
| The 1977 Survey of Industry on the Use of Food Additives by the NRC/NAS, Volume III. |
| Estimates of Daily Intake (NRC/NAS, 1979) (Abrams, 1992) |
| USDA Economic Research Service Reports |
| The FDA Total Diet Study (Pennington and Gunderson, 1987) |

*Indicates current use by FDA.
SOURCE: Information kindly provided by Technical Assessment Systems, Inc., Washington, D.C.

dye does not increase the color or the intensity of the color, it is in violation of CGMPs to add an amount greater than 1 ppm. (A discussion of CGMPs may be found in the *Food Chemicals Codex*, 3d ed., 1981.)

In regard to the second question on food categories, one set of 43 food categories is listed in 21 CFR 170.3(n), which grew out of a survey of food additives conducted by the National Academy of Sciences/National Research Council and published in 1972. A sample of those categories is shown in Table 30-7. This survey pioneered the use of food categorization, but changing lifestyles of the population and shifts in food preferences have necessitated the generation of additional, more timely data.

The newer food consumption surveys provide more contemporary data on food intake (Table 30-8). All these databases (and others) have characteristics that serve a particular purpose. For example, one database may be only a 3-day "snapshot" of consumption, another may cover average consumption over 14 days, while yet another provides a detailed breakout of particular subpopulations (e.g., teenagers, the elderly, Hispanics). The majority of these databases are available to the public but may not be particularly "user-friendly," and private industry has made some of them available on a fee basis.

In its estimates of consumption and/or exposure, the agency also considers other sources of consumption for the proposed intended use of the additive if it already is used in food for another purpose, occurs naturally in foods, or is used in nonfood sources (e.g., drugs, toothpaste, lipstick).

Thus, to estimate human consumption of a particular food substance, it is necessary to know (1) the levels of the substance in food, (2) the daily intake of each food containing the substance, (3) the distribution of intakes within the population, and (4) the potential consumption of or exposure to the substance from nonfood sources. (A discussion of chemical intake is covered in Rees and Tennant, 1994.)

***Structure-Activity Relationships.*** Structure-activity (SA) relationships are now the basis for developing many therapeutic drugs, pesticides, and food additives. These relationships are put to good use in the Redbook (USFDA, 1982), which describes a qualitative "decision tree" that assigns categories to substances on the basis of the structural and functional groups in the molecule. Additives with functional groups with a high order of toxicity are assigned to category C, those of indeterminant or intermediate toxicity are assigned to category B, and those with a low potential for toxicity are assigned to category A. For example, a simple saturated hydrocarbon alcohol such as pentanol would be assigned to category A. Similarly, a substance containing an $\alpha,\beta$-unsaturated carbonyl function, epoxide, thiazole, or imidazole group would be assigned to category C.

***Assignment of Concern Level.*** According to the algorithm, the CLs are assigned as shown in Table 30-9. Thus, a substance in Structure Category B added to food at a level of 0.03 ppm would be assigned the concern level II.

***Tests for Concern Levels.*** Once the CL is established, a specific test battery is prescribed, as shown in Table 30-10. The

**Table 30–9**
**Assignment of Concern Level**

| STRUCTURE CATEGORY A | STRUCTURE CATEGORY B | STRUCTURE CATEGORY C | CONCERN LEVEL |
|---|---|---|---|
| <0.05 ppm in the total diet (<0.0012 mg/kg/day) | <0.025 ppm in the total diet (<0.0063 mg/kg/day) | <0.0125 ppm in the total diet (<0.00031 mg/kg/day) | I |
| or | or | or | |
| ≥0.05 ppm in the total diet (≥0.0012 mg/kg/day) | ≥0.025 ppm in the total diet (≥0.00063 mg/kg/day) | ≥0.0125 ppm in the total diet (≥0.00031 mg/kg/day) | II |
| or | or | or | |
| ≥1 ppm in the total diet (≥0.25 mg/kg/day) | ≥0.5 ppm in the total diet (≥0.0125 mg/kg/day) | ≥0.25 ppm in total diet (≥0.0063 mg/kg/day) | III |

**Table 30–10**
**Tests for Each Concern Level**

| CONCERN LEVEL | TESTS REQUIRED |
|---|---|
| I | Short-term feeding study (at least 28 days in duration) |
| | Short-term tests for carcinogenic potential that can be used for determining priority for conduction of lifetime carcinogenicity bioassays and may assist in the evaluation of results from such bioassays, if conducted |
| II | Subchronic feeding study (at least 90 days in duration) in a rodent species |
| | Subchronic feeding study (at least 90 days in duration) in a nonrodent species |
| | Multigeneration reproduction study (minimum of two generations with a teratology phase) in a rodent species |
| | Short-term tests for carcinogenic potential |
| III | Carcinogenicity studies in two rodent species |
| | A chronic feeding study at least 1 year in duration in a rodent species (may be combined with a carcinogenicity study) |
| | Long-term (at least 1 year in duration) feeding study in a nonrodent species |
| | Multigenerational reproduction study (minimum of two generations) with a teratology phase in a rodent species |
| | Short-term tests for carcinogenic potential |

tests for CL III are the most demanding and provide the greatest breadth for the determination of adverse biological effects, including effects on reproduction. The tests are comprehensive enough to detect nearly all types of observable toxicity, including malignant and benign tumors, preneoplastic lesions, and other forms of chronic toxicity. The tests for CL II are of intermediate breadth. These tests are designed to detect the most toxic phenomena other than late-developing histopathological changes. The short-term (genotoxicity) tests are intended to identify substances for which chronic testing becomes critical. The CL I test battery is the least broad, as is appropriate for the level of hazard which substances in this category may pose. However, if untoward effects are noted, additional assessment becomes necessary. The Redbook (USFDA, 1982) is careful to note that although not specifically required for any CL, studies of the absorption, distribution, metabolism, and elimination characteristics of a test substance are recommended before the initiation of toxicity studies longer than 90 days' duration. Of particular importance for many proposed food ingredients is data on their processing and metabolism in the GI tract.

Unique to food additive carcinogenicity testing is the controversial use of protocols that include an *in utero* phase. Under such protocols, parents of test animals are exposed to the test subtances for 4 weeks before mating and throughout mating, gestation, and lactation. Most countries and international bodies do not subscribe to the combining of an *in utero* phase with a rat carcinogenicity study, as this presents a series of logistical and operational problems and substantially increases the cost of conducting a rat carcinogenicity study. The FDA began requesting *in utero* studies of the food industry in the early 1970s, when it was discovered from lifetime feeding studies that the artificial sweetener saccharin produced bladder tumors in male rats when *in utero* exposure was introduced. Subsequently, the FDA required the food, drug, and cosmetic color industries to conduct lifetime carcinogenicity feeding studies of 18 color additives in rats using an *in utero* exposure phase. This testing has provided the largest database available to date on the performance of *in utero* testing.

Special note should also be made of genetic toxicity testing. Genetic toxicity tests are performed for two reasons: (1) to test chemicals for potential carcinogenicity and (2) to assess whether a chemical may induce heritable genetic damage. Currently, genetic toxicity assays can be divided into three major groups: (1) forward and reverse mutation assays (e.g., point mutations, deletions), (2) clastogenicity assays detecting structural and numerical changes in chromosomes (e.g., chromosome aberrations, micronuclei), and (3) assays that identify DNA damage (e.g., DNA strand breaks, unscheduled DNA synthesis).

Because the correlation between carcinogens and mutagens has proved to be less than desirable, as has been demonstrated by false-positive and false-negative findings when carcinogens and noncarcinogens have been examined in genetic toxicity tests, the FDA has recommended that several tests be selected from a battery of tests. A list of some of the tests and their endpoint descriptions is given in the Redbook. It should be kept in mind that as the number of tests used increases, the possibility of false-negative results increases as well. Consequently, the National Toxicology Program (NTP) has advised that only a single gene mutational assay be used (*Salmonella typhimurium*) to optimize the prediction of carcinogenicity (Tennant and Zeiger, 1993).

**Safety Determination of Indirect Food Additives.** Indirect food additives are substances that are defined as food additives under the FD&C Act [section 201(s)] and that are not added directly to food but enter food by migrating from surfaces that contact food. These surfaces may be from packaging material (cans, paper, plastic) or the coating of packaging materials or surfaces used in processing, holding, or transporting food.

Essential to demonstrating the safety of an indirect additive are extraction studies with food-simulating solvents. The FDA recommends the use of three food-simulating solvents—8% ethanol, 50% ethanol, and corn oil or a synthetic triglyceride—for aqueous, alcoholic, and fatty foods, respectively (FDA, 1988). The conditions of extraction depend in

**Table 30–11**
**Exposure Estimate Calculations (Package Type)**

| | | FOOD-TYPE DISTRIBUTION ($f_T$) | | | |
|---|---|---|---|---|---|
| PACKAGE CATEGORY | CF* | AQUEOUS | ACIDIC | ALCOHOLIC | FATTY |
| Glass | 0.08 | 0.08 | 0.36 | 0.47 | 0.09 |
| Metal, polymer-coated | 0.17 | 0.16 | 0.35 | 0.40 | 0.69 |
| Metal, uncoated | 0.03 | 0.54 | 0.25 | 0.01† | 0.20 |
| Paper, polymer-coated | 0.21 | 0.55 | 0.04 | 0.01† | 0.40 |
| Paper, uncoated | 0.10 | 0.57 | 0.01† | 0.01† | 0.41 |
| Polymer | 0.41 | 0.49 | 0.16 | 0.01 | 0.34 |

*As discussed in the text, a minimum CF of 0.05 is used initially for all exposure estimates.
†1% or less.

part on the intended conditions of use. If the package material is intended to be retorted, the petitioner must conduct extractions for at least 2 h at 275°F. For all conditions of use, high-temperature extraction (conducted at 275°, 250°, or 212°F) is followed by a minimum of 238 h at 120°F except for refrigerated foods (in which 70°F is used) and frozen food (in which only 120 h of extraction is required).

Extraction studies are used to assess the level or quantity of a substance which might migrate and become a component of food, leading to consumer exposure. The prescribed extraction tests are believed to overestimate the amount of an indirect additive that is likely to migrate to food and thus are unlikely to underestimate consumer exposure.

To convert extraction data from packaging material into anticipated consumer exposure, the FDA has determined the fraction of the U.S. diet which comes into contact with different classes of material: glass, metal-coated, metal-uncoated, paper-uncoated, paper-coated, and polymers. For each class, FDA has assigned a "consumption factor" (CF), which is the fraction of the total diet that comes into contact with an individual class of material (Table 30-11).

The fraction of individual food types (aqueous, acidic, alcoholic, fatty) for which such packaging material is used is referred to as the food-type-distribution factor ($f_T$). To calculate consumer exposure (EDI), the following equation is used:

$$\text{EDI} = \text{C.F.} \times [f_T \text{ aqueous} \times \text{ppm in } 8\% \text{ ethanol} + f_T \text{ acidic} \times \text{ppm in } 8\% \text{ ethanol} + f_T \text{ alcohol} \times \text{ppm in } 50\% \text{ ethanol} + f_T \text{ fatty} \times \text{ppm in corn oil}] \times 3 \text{ kg} = \text{mg/person/day*}$$

For additives with virtually no migration in which the EDIs correspond to less than 0.05 ppm exposure, acute toxicology data are considered sufficient to provide an assurance of safety for the intended conditions of use of the additive. Migration levels, as determined by extraction studies, that are greater than 0.05 ppm to 1 ppm exposure generally require subchronic (90-day) feeding studies in rodent and nonrodent (usually the dog) species.

Other studies may be indicated by the data or information available on the substance, for example, the possible need for a teratology or reproduction study or short-term tests for carcinogenicity potential. Judgment is required, however, to determine the extent of testing needed after each food additive situation is considered on the basis of its own merits and to determine whatever ancillary data and information may be available that bear on the question of safety.

Where there is significant migration—that is, more than around 1 ppm exposure—long-term toxicological data involving carcinogenicity/chronic toxicity testing in rodents, at least 1 year in a nonrodent, and multigeneration reproduction testing to a minimum of two generations and with a teratology phase in a rodent, are recommended by the FDA. Other testing may be suggested or indicated by the data or information obtained.

**Safety Requirements for GRAS Substances.** While the courts have ruled that GRAS substances must be supported by the same quantity and quality of safety data that support food additives, this ruling should not be interpreted to mean that the supporting data must be identical in nature and character to those supporting a food additive. For uses of substances to be eligible for classification as GRAS, there must be common knowledge throughout the scientific community about the safety of substances directly or indirectly added to food (21 CFR 170.30).

The studies relied on for concluding that a given use of a substance is GRAS ordinarily are based on generally available data and information published in the scientific literature. Such data are unlikely to be conducted in accordance with FDA-recommended protocols, as these studies often are conducted for reasons unrelated to FDA approval.

GRAS status also can be based on experience with common use in food before January 1, 1958, which further distinguishes GRAS data requirements from those demanded of food additives. Such experience need not be limited to the United States, but if it comes from outside the United States, it must be documented by published or other information which is corroborated by information from an independent source.

**Transgenic Plant (and New Plant Varieties) Policy.** The safety of new plant varieties (transgenic plants, genetically modified plants) is regulated primarily under the FDA's postmarket authority [section 402(a)(1) of the FD&C Act]. This section had previously been applied to occurrences of unsafe levels of

*The 3 kg is FDA's value for daily food consumption which, when multiplied by mg/kg (ppm) and the weighting factors, reduces to milligrams of the additive per day.

toxicants in food. Now it is applied to new plant varieties whose composition has been altered by an added substance. The new policy has been applied to plants containing substances that are GRAS [*Federal Register* 57(104): 22984–23005]. This *Federal Register* notice (May 29, 1992) states that "[i]n most cases, the substances expected to become components of food as a result of genetic modification of a plant will be the same as or substantially similar to substances commonly found in food, such as proteins, fats and oils, and carbohydrates." Although the notice acknowledges the responsibility of the FDA to exercise the premarket review process when the "objective characteristics of the substance raise questions of safety," the policy recognizes the validity of GRAS status for new plant varieties.

In regard to substances within the new variety that are not similar to substances commonly found in food, a food additive petition may have to be filed. For example, if a food derived from a new plant variety contains a novel chemical as a result of the genetic modification of the plant, that chemical probably will require the submission of a food additive petition and approval by the FDA before marketing.

Further, the *Federal Register* notice offers points of consideration for the safety assessment of new plant varieties (Table 30-12). Accompanying these points of consideration are a decision flowchart and advice that the FDA be consulted on certain findings, for example, transference of allergens from one plant to another, a change in the concentration or bioavailability of nutrients, and the introduction of a new macroingredient.

### Assessment of Carcinogens

***Carcinogenicity as a Special Problem.*** As was discussed above, Congress provided the FDA with wide latitude in assessing safety and assuring a safe food supply with one exception. That exception is a provision of the FD&C Act known as the Delaney clause, which prohibits the approval of regulated food additives "found to induce cancer when ingested by man or animals" [section 409(c)(3)(A)]. The Delaney clause is found in two other sections of the act. The three clauses—sections 409(c)(3)(A), 706(b)(5)(B), and 512(d)(1)(H)—constitute the Delaney clause.

It needs to be emphasized that the Delaney proscription applies only to the approval of food additives, color additives, and animal drugs; it does not apply to unavoidable contaminants or GRAS substances or ingredients sanctioned by the FDA or USDA before 1958. The clause also does not apply to carcinogenic constituents that are present in food or color additives or animal drugs as nonfunctional contaminants, provided that the level of such contaminants can be demonstrated to be safe and the whole additive, including its contaminants (permitted by specification and regulations), is not found to induce cancer in humans or animals. This interpretation of the Delaney clause was set forth by the FDA in its so-called constituent policy published on April 2, 1982, as an Advanced Notice of Proposed Rulemaking (ANPR). The policy mandates the development and use of animal carcinogenicity data and probabilistic risk assessment to establish a safe level for the contaminant in the additive under its intended conditions of use.

**Table 30–12**
**Points of Consideration in the Safety Assessment of New Plant Varieties**

| |
|---|
| Toxicants known to be characteristic of the host and donor species |
| The potential that food allergens will be transferred from one food source to another |
| The concentration and bioavailability of important nutrients for which a food crop is ordinarily consumed |
| The safety and nutritional value of newly introduced proteins |
| The identity, composition and nutritional value of modified carbohydrates or fats and oils |

The constituent policy and, as will be discussed later, the implementation of the so-called DES (diethylstilbestrol) proviso for animal drugs under the Delaney clause have forced the FDA to develop a means for establishing safe levels for carcinogenic substances. The DES proviso allows the addition of carcinogenic animal drugs to animal feed if they leave no residue in edible tissue as determined by an approved analytic procedure. To do this, the FDA has turned to the use of probabilistic risk assessment in which tumor data in animals are mathematically extrapolated to an upperbound risk in humans exposed to particular use levels of the additive. The FDA takes the position that considering the many conservative assumptions inherent in the procedure, an upperbound lifetime risk of one cancer in a million individuals is the biological equivalent of zero.

Much controversy surrounds the use of risk assessment procedures, in part because estimates of risk are highly dependent on the many assumptions which must be made. The tendency is to be "risk-averse" and favor assumptions which exaggerate risk. As these exaggerations are multiplicative, the total overestimation of risk can be several orders of magnitude. Table 30-13 provides some rough estimates of potential ranges of uncertainty which might lead to large overestimates (Flamm and Lorentzen, 1988).

The common practice of testing at a maximum tolerated dose (MTD) (Williams and Weisburger, 1991) raises the question of appropriateness to human exposure. Do high test doses cause physiological changes unlike those from human exposure? The basic assumption in quantitative risk assessment (QRA) that the dose-response curve is linear beneath the lowest observable effect may result in the calculation of relatively high risks even at doses that are much lower than the lowest dose that produces cancer in experimental animals (Flamm and Lorentzen, 1988). QRA is more a process than a science; many steps in the process are based on assumptions, not proven scientific facts. If only the most conservative assumptions are made throughout the process, many will represent overestimates of human risk by 10- or 100-fold, leading to a combined overestimate of perhaps a millionfold or more.

Risk assessment cannot be used for either food additives or color additives because of the Delaney clause. If these additives are found to induce cancer, they cannot be approved for foods or colors no matter how small the estimated risk is. Because of the harsh consequences of finding a food additive to be a carcinogen, the FDA has interpreted this clause as

**Table 30–13**
**Uncertainty Parameters and Their Associated Range of Risk Factors**

| UNCERTAINTY PARAMETERS | ESTIMATED RANGE (FACTOR) |
|---|---|
| Extrapolation model | 1–10,000 |
| Total dose vs. dose rate | 30–45 |
| Most sensitive sex/strain vs. average sensitivity | 1–100 |
| Sensitivity of human vs. test animal | 1–1000 |
| Potential synergism or antagonism with other carcinogens or promoters | 1–1000? |
| Total population vs. target population, potential vs. actual market penetration | 1–1000 |
| Absorptive rate (gut, skin, lung) for animals at high dose vs. humans at low dose | 1–10 |
| Dose scaling: mg/kg body weight, ppm (diet, water, feed) surface area | 1–15 |
| Upper confidence on users or exposed | 1–10 |
| Specifics or tolerances | 1–10 |
| Limits of detection vs. actual levels | 1–1000 |
| Additivity vs. nonadditivity of multiple sites | 1–3 |
| Survival or interim sacrifice adjustments | 1–2 |
| Knowledge of only high-end plateau dose response | 1–10 |
| Error or variation in detection methods | 1–10 |
| Adjustments for less than lifetime bioassays | 1–100 |
| Adjustment for intermittent and less than lifetime human exposure | 1–100 |
| Use vs. nonuse of historical data | 1–2 |
| Upper confidence and lower confidence limits vs. expected values in extrapolation level of acceptable risk | 1–1000 |
| Level of acceptable risk | 1–1000 |
| Adding or not adding theoretical risks from many substances | 1–100 |

SOURCE: Flamm and Lorentzen (1988).

requiring an affirmative finding of a clear and unequivocal demonstration of carcinogenicity upon ingestion. Historically, the FDA has employed a high threshold for establishing that a food or color additive has been found to induce cancer when ingested by humans or animals. Very few substances have been disapproved or banned because of the Delaney clause. Two indirect food additives (Flectol H and mercaptoimidazoline) that migrate from packaging material were banned. Among direct additives, safrole, cinnamyl anthranilate, thiourea, and diethylpyrocarbonate were banned because of the Delaney clause, diethylpyrocarbonate because it forms urethane.

A number of substances [e.g., butylated hydroxyanisole (BHA), xylitol, methylene chloride, sorbitol, trichloroethylene, nitrilotriacetic acid (NTA), diethylhexyl phthalate, melamine, formaldehyde, bentonite] listed in the Code of Federal Regulation as regulated food additives are also listed as carcinogens by National Toxicology Program (NTP), the International Agency for Research on Cancer (IARC), or the state of California (under the Safe Drinking Water and Toxic Enforcement Act of 1986, also known as Proposition 65). How is this possible, and on what basis do these food additive listings continue?

Despite the fact that tests and conditions exist under which each of these substances will produce cancer in animals, the FDA has found it possible to continue listing these substances as food additives. The reasoning applied in almost every case is based on secondary carcinogenesis. The one exception is formaldehyde; formaldehyde is carcinogenic only on inhalation, and there are compelling reasons to believe that inhalation is not an appropriate test in this case (Flamm and Frankos, 1985). Therefore, formaldehyde is not treated as a "Delaneyable" carcinogen.

For BHA, which induces forestomach cancer, the concept has been advanced that its carcinogenicity is attributable primarily to irritation, restorative hyperplasia, and so on (Clayson et al., 1986). For xylitol, a sugar alcohol, an increase in bladder tumors and adrenal pheochromocytomas is considered secondary to calcium imbalance resulting from the indigestibility of sugar alcohols and their fermentation in the lower GI tract. Sorbitol, another sugar alcohol, behaves in a similar manner. For NTA, the argument is secondary carcinogenesis, and although specific explanations vary, the mechanism involving zinc imbalance has considerable scientific support. The review of diethylhexyl phthalate is ongoing, but the possibility that peroxisome proliferation is involved has been offered, as has the possibility that hepatocellular proliferation is primary to the subsequent development of tumors.

Thus, the FDA has generally interpreted the phrase "found to induce cancer when ingested by man or animals" as excluding cancers that arise through many secondary means. Therefore, to be a "Delaneyable" carcinogen, a food or color additive must be demonstrated to induce cancer by primary means when ingested by humans or animals or to induce cancer by other routes of administration that are found to be appropriate. This is interpreted to mean that the findings of cancer must be clearly reproducible and that the cancers found are not secondary to nutritional, hormonal, or physiological imbalances. This position allows the agency to argue that changing the level of protein or fat in the diet does not induce cancer but simply modulates tumor incidence (Kritschevsky, 1994). Given the many modulating factors and influences connected with food and diet, the FDA has to be careful about what it declares to be a carcinogen under the Delaney clause.

Thus, the FDA has always had to look at the mechanistic question and has been doing that for more than 30 years.

***Biological versus Statistical Significance.*** Much can be learned about the proper means of assessing carcinogenicity data by studying large databases for substances that have been tested for carcinogenicity many times. The artificial sweetener cyclamate is an example. The existence of more than a dozen studies on cyclamate and the testing of multiple hypotheses at dozens of different organ and tissue sites in all these studies led to the awareness that the overall false-positive error rate (i.e., higher cancer incidence at a specific organ site in treated subjects versus controls as a result of chance) could be inflated if individual findings were viewed out of context (FDA, 1984). Therefore, very careful attention must be paid to the totality of the evidence.

The possibility of false-negative error is always of concern because of the need to protect public health. However, it should be recognized that any attempt to prove absolutely that a substance is not carcinogenic is futile. Therefore, an unrelenting effort to minimize false-negative errors can produce an unacceptably high probability of a false positive. Further, demanding certainty (i.e., a zero or implicitly an extremely low probability of false-negative error) has negative consequences for an accurate decision-making process. This is the case because it severely limits the ability to discriminate between carcinogens and noncarcinogens on the basis of bioassays (FDA, 1984).

In addition to the false-positive/false-negative trap, which is a statistical matter, there are many potential biological traps. The appearance of a higher incidence of tumors at a specific organ site in treated animals may not demonstrate by itself a carcinogenic action of the substance employed in the treatment. This is the case because the incidence of tumors at specific organ sites can be influenced and controlled by many biological processes which may affect tumor incidence.

The test substance, typically administered at high MTDs, may affect one or more of the many biological processes known to modulate tumor incidence at a specific organ site without causing an induction of tumors at that or any other site. Nutritional imbalances such as choline deficiency are known to lead to a high incidence of liver cancer in rats and mice. Simple milk sugar (lactose) is known to increase the incidence of Leydig's cell tumors in rats. Caloric intake has been shown to be a significant modifying factor in carcinogenesis. Impairment of immune surveillance by a specific or nonspecific means (stress) affecting immune responsiveness and hormonal imbalance can result in higher incidences of tumors at specific organ sites. Hormonal imbalance, which can be caused by hormonally active agents (e.g., estradiol) or by other substances that act indirectly, such as vitamin D, may result in an increased tumor incidence. Chronic cell injury and restorative hyperplasia resulting from treatment with lemon flavor (*d*-limonene) probably are responsible for renal tumor development in male rats by mechanisms that are of questionable relevance to humans (Flamm and Lehman-McKeeman, 1991).

In these examples, the increases in tumor incidence at specific organ sites probably are secondary to significant changes in normal physiological balance and homeostasis. Moreover, the increases in tumor incidence, and hence the increases in the risk of cancer, probably would not occur except at toxic doses.

To preserve the ability of a bioassay to discriminate, the possibility of false-positive or false-negative results and the possibility of secondary effects must be considered. To be meaningful, evaluations must be based on the weight of evidence, which must be reviewed as carefully as possible. Particular attention must be given to the many factors that are used in deciding whether tumor incidences are biologically as well as statistically significant. These factors include (1) the historical rate of the tumor in question (is it a rare tumor, or does it occur frequently in the controls?), (2) the survival histories of dosed and test animals (did dosed animals survive long enough to be considered "at risk"? What effect did chemical toxicity and reduced survival have in the interpretation of the data?), (3) the patterns of tumor incidence (was the response dose-related?), (4) the biological meaningfulness of the effect (was it experimentally consistent with the evidence from related studies? Did it occur in a target organ?), (5) the reproducibility of the effect with other doses, sexes, or species, (6) evidence of hyperplasia, metaplasia, or other signs of an ongoing carcinogenic process (is the effect supported by a pattern of related nonneoplastic lesions, particularly at lower doses?), (7) evidence of tumor multiplicity or progression, and (8) the strength of the evidence of an increased tumor incidence (what is the magnitude of the *p* value? for pairwise comparison? for trend?).

A good discussion of the use of these factors by scientists in deciding whether a substance induces cancer in animals is contained in the notice of a final rule permanently listing FD&C Yellow No. 6 (51 FR 41765–41783, 1988). An elevation of tumor incidence in rats was identified at two organ and/or tissue sites: (1) medullary tumors of the adrenal glands in female rats only and (2) renal cortical tumors in female rats only.

Scientists at the FDA concluded that the increase in medullary tumors of the adrenal glands in female rats did not suffice to establish that FD&C Yellow No. 6 is a carcinogen. The basis for the decision was (1) a lack of dose response, (2) the likelihood of false positives, (3) the lack of precancerous lesions, (4) morphological similarity of adrenal medullary lesions in treated and control rats, (5) an unaffected latency period, (6) a lack of effect in male rats, and (7) a comparison with other studies in which there was an association between exposure to FD&C Yellow No. 6 and the occurrence of adrenal medullary tumors.

A similar judgment was made with respect to the cortical renal lesions in female rats, which were not found to provide a basis for concluding that FD&C Yellow No. 6 can induce cancer of the kidneys. The main reasons leading to this conclusion were (1) the relatively common occurrence of proliferative renal lesions in aged male control rats (28 months or older), (2) the lack of renal tumors in treated males despite their usually greater sensitivity to renal carcinogens, (3) the lack of malignant tumors indicating no progression of adenomas to a malignant state, (4) the lack of a decreased latency period compared with controls, (5) the coincidence of renal proliferative lesions and chronic renal disease, (6) the lack of genotoxicity, and (7) a lack of corroborative evidence from other studies that suggests a treatment-related carcinogenic effect of FD&C Yellow No. 6 on the kidney. In both these cases, FDA scientists emphasize the importance of considering all the evidence in attempting to decide the significance of any subset of data.

***Carcinogenic Contaminants.*** The Delaney clause, which prohibits the addition of carcinogens to food, may, if interpreted strictly, ban all food additives and color additives if it includes carcinogenic contaminants of additives within its definition. Clearly, this was not Congress's intent, and just as clearly, the FDA needed to develop a commonsense policy for addressing the problem that all substances, including food and color additives, may contain carcinogenic contaminants at some trace level.

Toward this end, the agency argued in its 1982 ANPR (FDA, 1982) that banning food and color additives simply because they have been found or are known to contain a trace level of a known carcinogen does not make sense because all substances may contain carcinogenic contaminants. The agency asserted that the mere fact that an additive contains a contaminant known to be carcinogenic should not automatically lead the agency to ban that food additive under the Delaney clause but should instead cause the agency to consider the health risks it poses based on its level of contamination and the conditions of its use. In the ANPR, the agency stated that by using highly conservative scientific assumptions and a highly conservative methodology for extrapolating cancer risk from high dose to low and from animals to humans, the agency could estimate such risks in a manner that would assure that the actual risks posed to humans would not be underestimated. This reaffirmed the agency's position taken in the proposal on the addition of carcinogens to the feed of food-producing animals (FDA, 1977).

## FUNCTIONALITY OF FOOD INGREDIENTS

### Direct Food Additives

An additive is identified as a substance with a specific technical function (functionality). The FDA recognizes 32 such functionalities (Table 30-14).

### Color Additives

The term "color additive" refers to a material which is a dye, pigment, or other substance made by a process of synthesis or extracted and isolated from a vegetable, animal, or mineral source [FD&C Act 201(t)]. Blacks, whites, and intermediate grays also are included in this definition. When such additives are added or applied to a food, drug, or cosmetic or to the human body, they are capable of imparting color. Color additives are not eligible for GRAS status.

There are two distinct types of color additives that have been approved for food use: those requiring certification by FDA chemists and those exempt from certification. Certification, which is based on chemical analysis, is required for each batch of most organic synthesized colors because they may contain impurities that may vary from batch to batch.

Most certified colors approved for food use bear the prefix FD&C. They include FD&C Blue No. 1, FD&C Blue No. 2, FD&C Green No. 3, FD&C Red No. 3, FD&C Red No. 40, FD&C Yellow No. 5, and FD&C Yellow No. 6. Orange B and Citrus Red No. 2 are the only certified food colors which lack the FD&C designation (21 CFR 74 Subpart A).

The basis for the certification of these color additives is the finding that each batch is of suitable purity and can be safely used as prescribed by regulation (FD&C Act, section 721). Certification involves in-depth chemical analysis of major and trace components of each individual batch of color additives by FDA chemists and is required before any batch can be released for commercial use. Such color additives consist of aromatic amines or aromatic azo structures (FD&C Blue No. 1, FD&C Blue No. 2, FD&C Green No. 3, FD&C Red No. 40, FD&C Yellow No. 5, and FD&C Yellow No. 6) which cannot be synthesized without a variety of impurities.

Despite the fact that aromatic amines are generally considered relatively toxic substances, the FD&C colors are notably nontoxic. Table 30-15, which is adopted from a publication of the National Academy of Sciences (NAS) (Committee on Food Protection, 1971), shows that certified food colors have a low order of acute toxicity. The principal reason involves sulfonation of the aromatic amine or azo compound that constitutes a color additive. Such sulfonic acid groups are highly polar, which, combined with their high molecular weight, prevents them from being absorbed by the GI tract or entering cells. All the FD&C food colors have been extensively tested in all CL III tests and have been found to be remarkably nontoxic.

Food colors that are exempt from certification typically have not been subjected to such extensive testing requirements. The exempt food colors are derived primarily from natural sources. While synthetic food colors have received the majority of public, scientific, and regulatory attention, natural color agents are also an important class. Currently, 25 color additives have been given exemption from certification in 21 CFR 73. These agents consist of a variety of natural compounds generally obtained by various extraction and treatment technologies. Included in this group of colors are preparations such as dried algae meal, beet powder, grape skin extract, fruit juice, paprika, caramel, carrot oil, cochineal extract, ferrous gluconate, and iron oxide. A problem encountered in attempts to regulate these additives is the lack of a precise chemical definition of many of these preparations. With a few exceptions, such as caramel, which is the most widely used color, the natural colors have not been heavily used. In part, this may be due to economic reasons, but these colors generally do not have the uniformity and intensity characteristic of the synthetic colors, therefore necessitating higher concentrations to obtain a specific color intensity. They also lack the chemical and color stability of the synthetic colors and have a tendency to fade with time.

Intake of color additives varies among individuals. The maximal intake of food colors is estimated to be approximately 53.5 mg/day, whereas the average intake per day is approximately 15 mg (Committee on Food Protection, 1971). Only about 10 percent of the food consumed in the United States contains food colors. The foods that utilize food colors in order of the quantity of color utilized are (1) beverages, (2) candy and confections, (3) dessert powders, (4) bakery goods, (5) sausages (casing only), (6) cereals, (7) ice cream, (8) snack foods, and (9) gravies, jams, jellies, and so forth (Committee on Food Protection, 1971).

**Table 30–14**
**Direct Food Additives by Functionality**

| NUMBER | DESIGNATION | DESCRIPTION | EXAMPLES |
| --- | --- | --- | --- |
| 170.3(o) (1) | Anticaking agents and free-flow agents | Substances added to finely powdered or crystalline food products to prevent caking, lumping, or agglomeration | Glucitol, sodium ferrocyanide, silicon dioxide |
| (2) | Antimicrobial agents | Substances used to preserve food by preventing growth of microorganisms and subsequent spoilage, including fungistats, mold, and rope inhibitors and the effects listed by the NAS/NRC under "preservatives" | Nisin; methyl-, ethyl-, propyl-, or butyl- ester of *p*-hydroxybenozoic acid; sodium benzoate; sorbic acid and its salts |
| (3) | Antioxidants | Subtances used to preserve food by retarding deterioration, rancidity, or discoloration due to oxidation | Butylated hydroxyanisole (BHA), butylated hydroxytoluene (BHT), propyl gallate |
| (4) | Colors and coloring adjuncts | Substances used to impart, preserve, or enhance the color or shading of a food, including color stabilizers, color fixatives, color-retention agents | FD&C Yellow No. 5 (tartrazine), FD&C Red No. 4, $\beta$-carotene, annatto, turmeric |
| (5) | Curing and pickling agents | Substances imparting a unique flavor and/or color to a food, usually producing an increase in shelf life | Calcium chloride, glucitol |
| (6) | Dough strengtheners | Substances used to modify starch and gluten, producing a more stable dough, including the applicable effects listed by the NAS/NRC under "dough conditioners" | Calcium bromate, baker's yeast extract, calcium carbonate |
| (7) | Drying agents | Substances with moisture-absorbing ability used to maintain an environment of low moisture | Calcium stearate, cobalt caprylate, cobalt tallate |
| (8) | Emulsifiers and emulsifier salts | Substances that modify surface tension in the component phase of an emulsion to establish a uniform dispersion or emulsion | Phosphate esters of mono- and diglycerides, acetylated monoglycerides, calcium stearate |
| (9) | Enzymes | Enxymes used to improve food processing and the quality of the finished food | Papain, rennet, pepsin |
| (10) | Firming agents | Substances added to precipitate residual pectin, strengthening the supporting tissue and preventing its collapse during processing | Calcium acetate, calcium carbonate |
| (11) | Flavor enhancers | Substances added to supplement, enhance, or modify the original taste and/or aroma of a food without imparting a characteristic taste or aroma of their own | Monosodium glutamate, inositol |
| (12) | Flavor agents and adjuvants | Substances added to impart or help impart a taste or aroma in food | Cinnamon, citral, *p*-cresol, thymol, zingerone |

**Table 30–14**
**Direct Food Additives by Functionality (*Continued*)**

| NUMBER | DESIGNATION | DESCRIPTION | EXAMPLES |
|---|---|---|---|
| (13) | Flour-treating agents | Substances added to milled flour at the mill to improve its color and/or baking qualities, including bleaching and maturing agents | Calcium bromate |
| (14) | Formulation aids | Substances used to promote or produce a desired physical state or texture in food, including carriers, binders, fillers, plasticizers, film formers, and tableting aids | Palm kernel oil, tallow |
| (15) | Fumigants | Volatile substances used for controlling insects or pests | Aluminum phosphide, potassium bromide |
| (16) | Humectants | Hygroscopic substances incorporated in food to promote retention of moisture, including moisture-retention agents and antidusting agents | Arabic gum, calcium chloride |
| (17) | Leavening agents | Substances used to produce or stimulate production of carbon dioxide in baked goods to impart a light texture, including yeast, yeast foods, and calcium salts listed by the NAS/NRC under "dough conditioners" | Carbon dioxide, adipic acid |
| (18) | Lubricants and release agents | Substances added to food contact surfaces to prevent ingredients and finished products from sticking to them | Mineral oil, acetylated monoglycerides |
| (19) | Nonnutritive sweeteners | Substances having less than 2 percent of the caloric value of sucrose per equivalent unit of sweetening capacity | Acesulfame, aspartame, saccharin |
| (20) | Nutrient supplements | Substances that are necessary for the body's nutritional and metabolic processes | Calcium carbonate |
| (21) | Nutritive sweeteners | Substances that have greater than 2 percent of the caloric value of sucrose per equivalent unit of sweetening capacity | Lactitol, hydrogenated starch hydrolysate |
| (22) | Oxidizing and reducing agents | Substances that chemically oxidize or reduce another food ingredient, producing a more stable product, including the applicable effects listed by the NAS/NRC under "dough conditioners" | Calcium peroxide, chloride, hydrogen peroxide |
| (23) | pH control agents | Substances added to change or maintain active acidity or basicity, including buffers, acids, alkalis, and neutralizing agents | Acetic acid, propionic acid, calcium acetate, calcium carbonate, carbon dioxide |
| (24) | Processing aids | Substances used as manufacturing aids to enhance the appeal or utility of a food or food component, including clarifying agents, clouding agents, catalysts, flocculents, filler aids, and crystallization inhibitors | Carbon dioxide, ammonium carbonate, ammonium sulfate, potassium bromide |

**Table 30–14**
**Direct Food Additives by Functionality (*Continued*)**

| NUMBER | DESIGNATION | DESCRIPTION | EXAMPLES |
|---|---|---|---|
| (25) | Propellants, aerating agents, and gases | Gases used to supply force to expel a product or reduce the amount of oxygen in contact with the food in packaging | Carbon dioxide, nitrous oxide |
| (26) | Sequestrants | Substances that combine with polyvalent metal ions to form a soluble metal complex to improve the quality and stability of products | Acetate salts, citrate salts, gluconate salt, metaphosphate, edetic acid, calcium acetate |
| (27) | Solvents and vehicles | Substances used to extract or dissolve another substance | Acetic acid, acetylated monoglycerides |
| (28) | Stabilizers and thickeners | Substances used to produce viscous solutions or dispersions, to impart body, improve consistency, or stabilize emulsions, including suspending and bodying agents, setting agents, jellying agents, and bulking agents | Calcium acetate, calcium carbonate |
| (29) | Surface-active agents | Substances used to modify suface properties of liquid food components for a variety of effects other than emulsifiers but including solubilizing agents, dispersants, detergents, wetting agents, rehydration enhancers, whipping agents, foaming agents, and defoaming agents | Sorbitan monostearate, mono- and diglycerides, polysorbate 60, acetostearin |
| (30) | Surface-finishing agents | Substances used to increase palatability, preserve gloss, and inhibit discoloration of foods, including glazes, polishes, waxes, and protective coatings | Ammonium hydroxide, arabic gum |
| (31) | Synergists | Substances used to act or react with another food ingredient to produce a total effect different from or greater than the sum of the effects produced by the individual ingredients | Acetic acid, propionic acid |
| (32) | Texturizers | Substances that affect the appearance or feel of food | Calcium acetate |

## GRAS Substances

In spite of the fact that the FD&C Act and the regulations (21 CFR 170.3, etc.) scrupulously avoid defining food except in a functional sense—"food means articles used for food or drink for man or other animals . . . [and includes] chewing gum, and . . . articles used for components of any such article"—it regards foods as GRAS when they are added to other food, for example, green beans in vegetable soup (Kokoski et al., 1990). It also regards a number of food ingredients as GRAS, and these ingredients are listed under 21 CFR 182, 184, and 186. However, it is important to note that not all substances regarded by the FDA as GRAS are listed as such. The language used in 21 CFR 182.1(a) acknowledges that there are substances the FDA regards as GRAS which are not listed in the CFR. This accomplishes two things: (1) It leaves the door open for additional nonlisted substances to be affirmed as GRAS by the agency and (2) reinforces the concept that substances can be deemed GRAS whether or not they are listed by the FDA or on a publicly available list. A list of examples of substances regarded as GRAS is given in Table 30-16. It is important to note that GRAS substances, though *used* like food additives, are *not* food additives, because the act states in section 201(s): "The term 'food additive' means any substance the intended use of which results . . . in its becoming a component . . . of any food . . . , if such substance is not generally recognized . . . to be safe." Therefore, to be GRAS is not to be a regulated food additive. Although the distinction may seem to

**Table 30–15**
**Data on Certified Food Colors Permanently Listed in the United States**

| COLOR | NO ADVERSE EFFECT DIETARY LEVELS AND ANIMAL STUDIES | SAFE LEVEL FOR HUMANS mg/day | ESTIMATED MAXIMUM INGESTION, mg/day/person |
|---|---|---|---|
| FD&C Blue No. 1 | 5.0% rats<br>2.0% dogs | 363 | 1.23 |
| FD&C Blue No. 2 | 1.0% rats, dogs | 181 | 0.29 |
| FD&C Green No. 3 | 5.0% rats<br>1.0% dogs<br>2.0% mice | 181 | 0.07 |
| Orange B | 5.0% rats<br>1.0% dogs<br>5.0% mice | 181 | 0.31 |
| Citrus Red No. 2 | 0.1% rats | 18 | Not applicable |
| FD&C Red No. 3 | 0.5% rats<br>2.0% dogs<br>2.0% mice | 91 | 1.88 |
| FD&C Yellow No. 5 | 2.0% rats<br>2.0% dogs | 363 | 16.3 |
| FD&C Yellow No. 6 | 2.0% rats<br>2.0% dogs<br>2.0% mice | 363 | 15.5 |

SOURCE: Committee on Food Protection (1971).

be one of semantics, it allows GRAS substances to be exempt from the premarket clearance restrictions enforced by the FDA and exempt from the Delaney clause, because that clause pertains only to food additives.

## Importance of the GRAS Concept to the Production of Healthier Foods

The importance of the GRAS provision is obvious from its many applications. Many substances, for example, that are used in food processing have never received formal FDA approval. The use of these substances in the manufacture of food products is considered appropriate under CGMPs, while the substance itself is considered GRAS for such purposes. Similarly, certain substances are permitted as optional ingredients in standardized foods [foods with standards of identity specified by regulation (21 CFR 130-169)] even though they are not approved food additives and are not on any of the GRAS lists.

The GRAS concept as traditionally applied in the United States also has applicability to certain novel foods which may differ only slightly from traditional foods or which, after careful consideration, can be regarded as raising no issues or questions of safety beyond that raised by the traditional foods they

**Table 30–16**
**Examples of GRAS Substances and Their Functionality**

| CFR NUMBER | SUBSTANCE | FUNCTIONALITY |
|---|---|---|
| | Substances Generally Recognized as Safe<br>21 CFR 182 | |
| 182.2122 | Aluminum calcium silicate | Anticaking agent |
| 182.5065 | Linoleic acid | Dietary supplement |
| | Direct Food Substances Affirmed as Generally Recognized as Safe<br>21 CFR 184 | |
| 184.1005 | Acetic acid | Several |
| 184.1355 | Helium | Processing aid |
| | Indirect Food Substances Affirmed as Generally Recognized as Safe<br>21 CFR 186 | |
| 186.1025 | Caprylic acid | Antimicrobial |
| 186.1374 | Iron oxides | Ingredient of paper and paperboard |

are intended to replace. The GRAS approach may therefore permit the introduction of novel foods that contain less saturated fat and/or cholesterol or more fiber or are in other ways viewed as healthier foods.

In a recent policy announcement, the FDA indicated its intention to consider qualifying new foods derived from new plant varieties as GRAS (54 FR 22984–23005, 1992). This policy includes transgenic plants such as the transgenic tomato. For example, in discussing the inserted DNA of transgenic foods, the FDA stated: "Nucleic acids are present in the cells of every living organism, including every plant and animal used for food by humans . . . and do not raise a safety concern. . . . In regulatory terms, such material is presumed to be GRAS."

**Methods for Establishing Safe Conditions of Use for Novel Foods.** Novel foods, including those derived from new plant varieties and macroingredient substitutes, present new challenges and require new methods of determining safety. For example, with each new additive, it has been traditional (and rooted in a regulation such as 21 CFR 170.22) to establish an acceptable daily intake (ADI), which is usually based on 1/100 of the NOEL established in animal testing. This works well for additives projected to be consumed at a level of 1.5 g/day or less (which is equal to or less than 25 mg/kg), for this extrapolates at a 100-fold safety factor to consumption by a rat at a level of 2500 mg/kg/day (about 5 percent of the rat's diet). The problem arises when a new food or macroingredient substitute becomes a substantive part of the diet (estimated to constitute as much as 15 to 20 percent) (Borzelleca, 1992a). For example, a macroingredient substitute or food projected to be consumed at a level of just 5 percent of the diet (150 g/day) would require the test animal (rat) to consume 250 g/kg/day, or slightly more than the rat's body weight. This is an untenable test requirement, for at those levels, the investigator would establish an effect level only for malnutrition, not for the toxicity of the macroingredient. The converse is true for some essential nutrients, such as vitamins A and D and iron, which at doses 100 times the nutritional use level would be toxic (Kokoski et al., 1990).

This situation leaves the investigator with two problems: (1) how to describe the toxicity of the compound in a way which does not allow for dosing at the traditional multiples of the estimated intake and (2) because of the ingested volume of this substance, the other (secondary) effects that might be considered. For example, at these high dose levels for a nonabsorbable fat substitute or nonabsorbable carbohydrate, there may be no toxicity as a direct effect of the substance; instead, toxicity may result from the secondary effects. The answer therefore lies in careful interpretation of toxicological data and the conduction, where appropriate, of special studies to assess drug interactions, nutrient interactions (e.g., what effects consumption might have on micronutrient status, such as selenium in certain grains), changes in gut flora, changes in gut activity, and the like (Borzelleca, 1992a, 1992b; Munro, 1990). Also, it may be appropriate to consider what effect, if any, macroingredients may have on individuals with compromised digestive tracts, those dependent on laxatives, and those on high-fiber diets.

The combination of traditional toxicity studies, special studies, and possibly postmarketing surveillance will ensure the safety of consumers and satisfy the requirement of section 170.22 that evidence has been submitted to satisfy a safety factor different from 100. (For a thorough discussion of postmarketing surveillance, refer to Butchko et al., 1994).

## SAFETY OF FOOD

### Food Intolerance

In a survey of Americans, 30 percent indicated that they or someone in their immediate families had a food sensitivity. Although this number is likely too high, as much as 7.5 percent of the population may be allergic to some food or component thereof (Taylor et al., 1989). Lactose intolerance (a deficiency of the disaccharide enzyme lactase) is very high among some groups; for example, there is an incidence of 27 percent in black children age 12 to 24 months, which may increase to 33 percent by age 6 years (Juambeltz et al., 1993). The percentage of young (northern European) children allegedly intolerant to food additives ranges from 0.03 to 0.23 percent (Wuthrich, 1993) to 1 to 2 percent (Fuglsang et al., 1993). Further, there are certain drug-food incompatibilities about which physicians and pharmacists are obligated to warn patients, such as taking monoamine oxidase (MAO) inhibitors and tyramine in cheese. People who are prescribed tetracycline also must be alerted not to take milk with this antibiotic. By any standard, there are large numbers of real and perceived adverse reactions to or incompatibilities with food. The first step in understanding these reactions is to define the nomenclature, a task undertaken by the American Academy of Allergy and Immunology (Committee on Adverse Reactions to Foods) and the National Institute of Allergy and Infectious Diseases (Anderson and Sogn, 1984). A modification of their attempt at definitions and classification is represented in Table 30-17.

In the table, the definitions proceed from general to most specific. Obviously, there is little to distinguish the terms "adverse reaction" and "sensitivity" to a food or a food "intolerance," except perhaps in the lexicon of the individual, colored by his or her own experience. That is, an "adverse reaction" may indicate something as simple as an unpleasing esthetic or hedonic quality such as an unpleasant taste, which may in fact have a genetic basis as in the ability to taste phenylthiocarbamide (Guyton, 1971), or may indicate a fatal outcome resulting from an immune or toxic reaction.

Clinical descriptions of adverse reactions to food are not new. Hippocrates (460–370 B.C.) first recorded adverse reactions to cow's milk which caused gastric upset and urticaria, and Galen (A.D. 131–210) described allergic symptoms to goat milk. However, the immunologic basis of many adverse reactions to food was not established until the passive transfer of sensitivity to fish was described in the early 1960s (Frankland, 1987; Taylor et al., 1989). This test, which evolved into the (skin) prick test and later the Radioallergosorbent (RAST) test, allowed a distinction to be made between immunologically based adverse reactions (true allergies) and adverse reactions with other causation.

#### Food Allergy

***Description.*** Food hypersensitivity (allergy) refers to a reaction involving an immune-mediated response. Such a response

**Table 30–17**
**Adverse Reactions to Food: Definition of Terms**

| TERM | DEFINITION | CHARACTERISTICS/EXAMPLES |
|---|---|---|
| Adverse reaction (sensitivity) to a food | General term that can be applied to a clinically abnormal response attributed to an ingested food or food additive | Any untoward pathological reaction resulting from ingestion of a food or food additive. May be immune-mediated |
| Food hypersensitivity (allergy) | An immunologic reaction resulting from the ingestion of a food or food additive. This reaction occurs only in some patients, may occur after only a small amount of the substance is ingested, and is unrelated to any physiological effect of the food or food additive | Immune-mediated (cellular or humoral response), requires prior exposure to antigen or cross-reacting antigen. First exposure may have been asymptomatic |
| Food anaphylaxis | A classic allergic hypersensitivity reaction to food or food additives | A humoral immune response most often involving IgE antibody and release of chemical mediators. Mortality may result |
| Food intolerance | A general term describing an abnormal physiological response to an ingested food or food additive; this reaction may be an immunologic, idiosyncratic, metabolic, pharmacological, or toxic response | Any untoward pathological reaction resulting from ingestion of a food or food additive. May be immune-mediated. Celiac disease (intolerance to wheat, rye, barley, oats) |
| Food toxicity (poisoning) | A term used to imply an adverse effect caused by the direct action of a food or food additive on the host recipient without the involvement of immune mechanisms. This type of reaction may involve nonimmune release of chemical mediators. Toxins may be contained within food or released by microorganisms or parasites contaminating food products | Not immune-mediated. May be caused by bacterial endo- or exotoxin (e.g., hemorrhagic *E. coli*), fungal toxin (e.g., aflatoxin), tetrodotoxin from pufferfish, domoic acid from mollusks, histamine poisoning from fish (scombroid poisoning), nitrate poisoning (i.e., methemoglobinuria) |
| Food idiosyncrasy | A quantitatively abnormal response to a food substance or additive; this reaction differs from its physiological or pharmacological effect and resembles hypersensitivity but does not involve immune mechanisms. Food idiosyncratic reactions include those which occur in specific groups of individuals who may be genetically predisposed | Not immune-mediated. Favism (hemolytic anemia related to deficiency of erythrocytic glucose-6-phosphate dehydrogenase) fish odor syndrome, beetanuria, lactose intolerance, fructose intolerance, asparagus urine, red wine intolerance |
| Anaphylactoid reaction to a food | An anaphylaxislike reaction to a food or food additive as a result of nonimmune release of chemical mediators. This reaction mimics the symptoms of food hypersensitivity (allergy) | Not immune-mediated. Scombroid poisoning, sulfite poisoning, red wine sensitivity |
| Pharmacological food reaction | An adverse reaction to a food or food additive as a result of a naturally derived or added chemical that produces a druglike or pharmacological effect in the host | Not immune-mediated. Tyramine in patients treated with MAO inhibitors, fermented (alcohol-containing) foods in disulfiram-treated patients. |
| Metabolic food reaction | Toxic effects of a food when eaten in excess or improperly prepared | Cycasin, vitamin A toxicity, goiterogens |

SOURCE: Adapted from Anderson and Sogn (1984).

is generally (immunoglobulin) IgE-mediated, although (immunoglobulin) $IgG_4$- and cell-mediated immunity also may play a role in some instances (Fukutomi et al., 1994). What generally distinguishes food allergy from other reactions is the involvement of immunoglobulins, basophils, or mast cells (the latter being a source of mediating substances including histamine and bradykinin for immediate reactions and prostaglandins and leukotrienes for slower-developing reactions) and a need for a prior exposure to the allergen or a cross-reactive allergen. An allergic reaction may be manifested by one or more of the symptoms listed in Table 30-18. The list of foods known to provoke allergies is long and is probably limited only by what people are willing to eat. Although cutaneous reactions and anaphylaxis are the most common symptoms associated with food allergy, the body is replete with a repertoire of responses which are rarely confined to only a few foods.

A curious type of food allergy, the so-called exercise-induced food allergy, is apparently provoked by exercise which has been immediately preceded or followed by the ingestion of certain foods (Kivity et al., 1994), including shellfish, peach, wheat, celery, and "solid" food (Taylor et al., 1989). The exact mechanism is unknown, but it may involve enhanced mast cell responsiveness to physical stimuli and/or diminished metabolism of histamine similar to red wine allergy (Taylor et al., 1989). On the other hand, food intolerance in patients with chronic fatigue may have less to do with allergic response and has been shown to be a somatization trait of patients with depressive symptoms and anxiety disorders (Manu et al., 1993).

***Chemistry of Food Allergens.*** Most allergens (antigens) in food are protein in nature, and although almost all foods contain one or more proteins, a few foods are associated more with allergic reactions than are others. For example, anaphylaxis to peanuts is more common than is anaphylaxis to other legumes (e.g., peas, soybeans). Similarly, although allergies may occur from bony fishes, there is no basis for cross-reactivity to other types of seafood (e.g., mollusks and crustaceans), although dual (and independent) sensitivities may exist (Anderson and Sogn, 1984). Interestingly, patients who are allergic to milk usually can tolerate beef and inhaled cattle dander, and patients who are allergic to eggs usually can tolerate ingestion of chicken and feather-derived particles (Anderson and Sogn, 1984), although in the "bird-egg" syndrome patients can be allergic to bird feathers, egg yolk, egg white, or any combination of the three (deBlay et al., 1994; Szepfalusi et al., 1994).

**Table 30–18**
**Symptoms of IgE-Mediated Food Allergies**

| | |
|---|---|
| Cutaneous | Urticaria (hives), eczema, dermatitis, pruritus, rash |
| Gastrointestinal | Nausea, vomiting, diarrhea, abdominal cramps |
| Respiratory | Asthma, wheezing, rhinitis, bronchospasm |
| Other | Anaphylactic shock, hypotension, palatal itching, swelling including tongue and larynx, methemoglobinemia* |

*An unusual manifestation of allergy reported to occur in response to soy or cow milk protein intolerance in infants (Murray and Christie, 1993).

SOURCE: Adapted from Taylor et al (1989). Used with permission.

Some of the allergenic components of common food allergens are listed in Table 30-19.

Although food avoidance is usually the best means of protection, it is not always possible because (1) the content of some prepared foods may be unknown (e.g., the presence of eggs or cottonseed oil), (2) there is the possibility of contamination of food from unsuspected sources [e.g., *Penicillium* in cheeses or meat, *Candida albicans* (Dayan, 1993; Dorion et al., 1994), and cow's milk antigens in the breast milk of mothers who have consumed cow's milk (Halken, et al., 1993)], and (3) there is a lack of knowledge about the phylogenetic relationships between food sources [legumes include peas, soybeans, and peanuts; some Americans are not aware that ham is a pork product (personal communication, 1994)].

**Table 30–19**
**Known Allergenic Food Proteins**

| FOOD | ALLERGENIC PROTEINS |
|---|---|
| Cows' milk | Casein (Dorion et al., 1994; Stoger and Wuthrich, 1993) |
| | $\beta$-Lactoglobulin (Piastra et al., 1994; Stoger and Wuthrich, 1993) |
| | $\alpha$-Lactalbumin (Bernaola et al., 1994; Stoger and Wuthrich, 1993) |
| Egg whites | Ovomucoid (Bernhiesel-Broadbent et al., 1994) |
| | Ovalbumin (Fukotomi et al., 1994, Bernhiesel-Broadbent et al., 1994) |
| Egg yolks | Livetin (de Blay et al., 1994; Szepfalusi et al., 1994) |
| Peanuts | Ara h II (Dorion et al., 1994) |
| | Peanut I (Sachs et al., 1981) |
| Soybeans | $\beta$-Conglycinin (7S fraction) (Rumsey et al., 1994) |
| | Glycinin (11S fraction) (Rumsey et al., 1994) |
| | Gly mIA (Gonzalez et al., 1992) |
| | Gly mIB (Gonzalez et al., 1992) |
| | Kunitz trypsin inhibitor (Brandon et al., 1986) |
| Codfish | Gad cI (O'Neil et al., 1993) |
| Shrimp | Antigen II (Taylor et al., 1989) |
| Green peas | Albumin fraction (Taylor et al., 1989) |
| Rice | Glutelin fraction (Taylor et al., 1989) |
| | Globulin fraction (Taylor et al., 1989) |
| Cottonseed | Glycoprotein fraction (Taylor et al., 1989) |
| Peach, guava, banana, mandarin, strawberry | 30-kD protein (Wadee et al., 1990) |
| Tomato | Several glycoproteins (Taylor et al., 1989) |
| Wheat | Gluten (Stewart-Tull and Jones, 1992) |
| | Gliadin (O'Hallaren, 1992) |
| | Globulin (O'Hallaren, 1992) |
| | Albumin (O'Hallaren, 1992) |
| Okra | Fraction I (Manda et al., 1992) |

SOURCE: Modified from Taylor et al (1989). Used with permission.

***Demographics of Food Allergy.*** Although children appear to be the most susceptible to food allergy, with adverse reactions occurring in 4 to 6 percent of infants, the incidence appears to taper off with maturation of the digestive tract, with only 1 to 2 percent of young children (4 to 15 years) being susceptible (Fuglsang et al., 1993). The increase in the number of adults exhibiting food allergy may be due in part to an expanded food universe, that is, an increased willingness to try different foods. In one study, allergies among young children were most commonly to milk and eggs, while allergies that developed later in life tended to be to fruit and vegetables (Kivity et al., 1994).

Familial relationships also play a role. Schrander and colleagues (1993) noted that among infants with cow's milk protein intolerance, 65 percent had a positive family history (first- or second-degree relatives) for atopy compared with 35 percent of healthy controls.

**Food Toxicity (Poisoning).** See "Substances for Which Tolerances May Not Be Set."

**Food Idiosyncrasy.** Food idiosyncrasies are generally defined as *quantitatively* abnormal responses to a food substance or additive; this reaction differs from the physiological effect, and although it may resemble hypersensitivity, it does not involve immune mechanisms. Food idiosyncratic reactions include those which occur in specific groups of individuals who may be genetically predisposed. Examples of such reactions and the foods that probably are responsible are given in Table 30-20.

Probably the most common idiosyncratic reaction is lactose intolerance, a deficiency of the lactase needed for the metabolism of the lactose in cow's milk. A lack of this enzyme results in fermentation of lactose to lactic acid and an osmotic effect in the bowel, with resultant symptoms of malabsorption and diarrhea. Lactose intolerance is lowest in northern Europe at 3 to 8 percent of the population; it reaches 70 percent in southern Italy and Turkey and nearly 100 percent in southeast Asia (Gudmand-Hoyer, 1994; Anderson and Sogn, 1984).

**Anaphylactoid Reactions.** Anaphylactoid reactions are historically thought of as reactions mimicking anaphylaxis

**Table 30–20**
**Idiosyncratic Reactions to Foods**

| FOOD | REACTION | MECHANISM | REFERENCE |
|---|---|---|---|
| Fava beans | Hemolysis, sometimes accompanied by jaundice and hemoglobinuria; also, pallor, fatigue, nausea, dyspnea, fever and chills, abdominal and dorsal pain | Pyrimidine aglycones in fava bean cause irreversible oxidation of GSH in G-6-PD-deficient erythrocytes by blocking NADPH supply, resulting in oxidative stress of the erythrocyte and eventual hemolysis | Chevion et al., 1985 |
| Chocolate | Migraine headache | Phenylethylamine-related (?) | Gibb et al., 1991; Settipane, 1987 |
| Beets | Beetanuria: passage of red urine (often mistaken for hematuria) | Excretion of beetanin in urine after consumption of beets | Smith, 1991 |
| Asparagus | Odorous, sulfurous-smelling urine | Autosomal dominant inability to metabolize methanthiol of asparagus and consequent passage of methanthiol in urine | Smith, 1991 |
| Red wine | Sneezing, flush, headache, diarrhea, skin itch, shortness of breath | Diminished histamine degradation; deficiency of diamine oxidase (?) Histamines present in wine | Wantke et al., 1994 |
| Choline- and carnitine-containing foods | Fish odor syndrome: foul odor of body secretions | Choline and carnitine metabolized to trimethylamine in gut by bacteria, followed by absorption but inability to metabolize to odorless trimethylamine *N*-oxide | Ayesh et al., 1993 |
| Lactose intolerance | Abdominal pain, bloating, diarrhea | Lactase deficiency | Mallinson, 1987 |
| Fructose-containing foods | Abdominal pain, vomiting, diarrhea, hypoglycemia | Reduced activity of hepatic aldolase B toward fructose-1-phosphate | Frankland, 1987; Catto-Smith and Adams, 1993 |

through direct application of the primary mediator of anaphylactic reactions: histamine. Ingestion of scombroid fish (e.g., tuna, mackerel, bonito) as well as nonscombroid fish (mahimahi and bluefish) that have been acted upon by microorganisms to produce histamine may result in an anaphylactoid reaction (Table 30-21). The condition was reported to be mimicked by the direct ingestion of 90 mg of histamine in unspoiled fish (van Geldern et al., 1992), but according to Taylor (1986), the effect of simply ingesting histamine does not produce the equivalent effect. Instead, Taylor stated that histamine ingested with spoiled fish appears to be much more toxic than is histamine ingested in an aqueous solution as a result of the presence of histamine potentiators in fish flesh. These potentiators included putrefactive amines (putrescine and cadaverine) and pharmacological potentiators such as aminoguanidine and isoniazid. The mechanism of potentiation involves the inhibition of intestinal histamine-metabolizing enzymes (diamine oxidase), which causes increased histamine uptake. However, Ijomah and coworkers (1991) claimed that dietary histamine is not a major determinant of scombrotoxicosis, since potency is not positively correlated with the dose and volunteers tend to fall into susceptible and nonsusceptible subgroups. Ijomah and coworkers (1991) suggested that endogenous histamine released by mast cells plays a significant role in the etiology of scombrotoxicosis, whereas the role of dietary histamine is minor. An exception to this endogenous histamine theory was described by Morrow and colleagues (1991), who found the expected increase in urinary histamine in scombroid-poisoned individuals but did not find an increase in urinary 9$\alpha$,11$\beta$-dhydroxy-15-oxo-2,3,18,19-tetranorprost-5-ene-1,20-dioic acid, the principal metabolite of prostaglandin $D_2$, a mast cell secretory product; thus, no mast cell involvement was indicated. Obviously, additional research is needed on this subject.

Smith (1991) described sulfite-induced bronchospasm (sometimes leading to asthma), which was first noticed as an acute sensitivity to metabisulfites sprayed on restaurant salads (and salad bars) and in wine. Sulfite normally is detoxicated rapidly to inorganic sulfate by the enzyme sulfite oxidase. In sensitive individuals, there is apparently a deficiency in this enzyme, making them supersensitive to sulfites. (The FDA has taken the position that the addition of sulfite to food is safe only when properly disclosed on the food label.)

**Pharmacological Food Reactions.** Also referred to as "false food allergies" (Moneret-Vautrin, 1987), these adverse reactions are characterized by exaggerated responses to pharmacological agents in food (Table 30-22). These reactions are distinguished from other classifications because they are not associated with a specific anomaly of metabolism (e.g., lactose intolerance or favism) but may be a receptor anomaly instead. These, then, are common pharmacological agents acting in a very predictable manner, but at exceptionally low levels.

**Metabolic Food Reactions.** Metabolic food reactions are distinct from other categories of adverse reactions in that the foods are more or less commonly eaten and demonstrate toxic effects only when eaten to excess or improperly processed

**Table 30–21**
**Anaphylactoid Reactions to Food**

| FOOD | REACTION | MECHANISM | REFERENCE |
|---|---|---|---|
| Western Australian salmon (*Arripis truttaceus*) | Erythema and urticaria of the skin, facial flushing and sweating, palpitations, hot flushes of the body, headache, nausea, vomiting, and dizziness | Scombroid poisoning; high histamine levels demonstrated in the fish | Smart, 1992 |
| Fish (spiked with histamine) | Facial flushing, headache | Histamine poisoning; histamine concentration in plasma correlated closely with histamine dose ingested | Van Gelderen et al., 1992 |
| Cape yellow tail (fish) (*Seriola lalandii*) | Skin rash, diarrhea, palpitations, headache, nausea and abdominal cramps, paraesthesia, unusual taste sensation, and breathing difficulties | Scombroid poisoning, treated with antihistamines | Muller et al., 1992 |
| Sulfite sensitivity | Bronchospasm, asthma | Sulfite oxidase deficiency to metabisulfites in foods and wine | Smith, 1991 |
| Tuna, albacore, mackerel, bonito, mahimahi, and bluefish | Reaction resembling an acute allergic reaction | Scombroid poisoning treated with antihistamines and cimetidine | Lange, 1988 |
| Cheese | Symptoms resembling acute allergic reaction | Responds to antihistamines; histamine poisoning? | Taylor, 1986 |

**Table 30–22**
**Pharmacological Reactions to Food**

| FOOD | REACTION | MECHANISM | REFERENCE |
|---|---|---|---|
| Cheese, red wine | Severe headache, hypertension | Tyramine from endogenous or ingested tyrosine | Settipane, 1987 |
| Nutmeg | Hallucinations | Myristicin | Anderson and Sogn, 1984 |
| Coffee, tea | Headache, hypertension | Methylxanthine (caffeine) acting as a noradrenergic stimulant | Anderson and Sogn, 1984 |
| Chocolate | Headache, hypertension | Methylxanthine (theophylline) acting as a noradrenergic stimulant | Anderson and Sogn, 1984 |

(Table 30-23). The susceptible population exists as a result of its own behavior, that is, the "voluntary" consumption of food as a result of a limited food supply or an abnormal craving for a specific food. Such an abnormal craving was reported by Bannister and associates (1977), who noted hypokalemia leading to cardiac arrest in a 58-year-old woman who had been eating about 1.8 kg of licorice per week. In "glycyrrhizism," or licorice intoxication, glycyrrhizic acid is the active component, with an effect resembling that of aldosterone, which suppresses the renin-angiotensin-aldosterone axis, resulting in the loss of potassium. Clinically, hypokalemia with alkalosis, cardiac arrhythmias, muscular symptoms together with sodium retention and edema, and severe hypertension are observed. The syndrome may develop at a level of 100 g licorice per day but gradually abates upon withdrawal of the licorice (Tonnesen, 1979).

This category also includes the ingestion of improperly prepared food such as cassava or cycad, which if prepared properly will result in a toxin-free food. For example, cycad (*Cacaos circinalis*) is a particularly hardy tree in tropical to subtropical habitats around the world. Cycads often survive when other crops have been destroyed (e.g., a natural disaster such as a typhoon or drought) and therefore may serve as an alternative source of food. Among people who have used cycads for food, the method of detoxification is remarkably similar despite the wide range of this plant: The seeds and stems are cut into small pieces and soaked in water for several days and then are dried and ground into flour. The effectiveness of leaching the toxin (cycasin) from the bits of flesh is most directly dependent on the size of the pieces, the duration of soaking, and the number of water changes. Shortcuts in processing may have grave consequences (Matsumoto, 1985).

## Importance of Labeling

The FDA has held that the populace reads labels and knows which raw or processed food may contain harmful constituents and thus avoids them. Labeling is perceived as a remedy for processed foods when potentially susceptible individuals have no other means of knowing about the potentially harmful contents. Thus, food labeling is seen as a critical component of establishing safe conditions of use for a food ingredient.

# TOLERANCE SETTING FOR FOODS

## Pesticide Residues

A pesticide is defined under the FD&C Act as any substance which is used as a pesticide, within the meaning of the Federal Insecticide, Fungicide and Rodenticide Act (FIFRA), in the production, storage, or transportation of raw agricultural commodities (food in its raw or natural state) [Section 201(q)]. The Pesticide amendments of 1956 to the FD&C Act (section 408) were the first congressional action requiring premarket clearance evaluations of the safety of chemicals added to food. Currently, the U.S. Environmental Protection Agency (EPA) is responsible for evaluating the safety of pesticides before issuing tolerances.

The regulation of pesticides and their safety is accomplished under both FIFRA and the FD&C Act. FIFRA governs the registration of pesticides. Registration addresses specific uses of a pesticide, and without such registration a pesticide cannot be lawfully sold for such use in the United States. A major part of the registration process involves tolerance setting. Pesticides intended for use on food crops must be granted tolerances or exempted from tolerances under the FD&C Act. There are two types of tolerances: one permitting the presence of pesticide residues in or on raw agricultural commodities and the other permitting such residues in processed foods. The EPA cannot register the use of a pesticide on food crops unless tolerances have first been granted to cover residues that are expected to remain in or on food.

Tolerances for raw food are granted by the EPA under 40 CFR 180 on a commodity-by-commodity basis. An example of such tolerances is shown in Table 30-24 for the pesticide dodine under 40 CFR 180.172.

Two sections of the FD&C Act apply to the setting of tolerances. Section 408 governs tolerances for pesticide residues in or on raw agricultural commodities, and section 409 governs tolerances for pesticide residues that are concentrated in processed foods. Under section 408, tolerances are to be set at levels deemed necessary to protect public health, and as there is no Delaney anticancer provision in this section, tolerances for carcinogenic pesticides can be established. Residues of a pesticide on a raw agricultural commodity that exceed a section 408 tolerance or of a pesticide for which no tolerance has been established are as a matter of law unsafe within the meaning of

**Table 30–23**
**Metabolic Food Reactions**

| FOOD | REACTION | MECHANISM | REFERENCE |
|---|---|---|---|
| Lima beans, cassava roots, millet (sorghum) sprouts, bitter almonds, apricot and peach pits | Cyanosis | Cyanogenic glycosides releasing hydrogen cyanide on contact with stomach acid | Anderson and Sogn, 1984 |
| Cabbage family, turnips, soybeans, radishes, rapeseed, and mustard | Goiter (enlarged thyroid) | Isothiocyanates, goitrin, or *S*-5-vinyl-thiooxazolidone interferes with utilization of iodine | Anderson and Sogn, 1984; vanEtten and Tookey, 1985 |
| Unripe fruit of the tropical tree *Blighia sapida*, common in the Caribbean and Nigeria | Severe vomiting, coma, and acute hypoglycemia sometimes resulting in death, especially among the malnourished | Hypoglycin A, isolated from the fruit, may interfere with oxidation of fatty acids, so that glycogen stores have to be metabolized for energy, with depletion of carbohydrates, resulting in hypoglycemia | Evans, 1985 |
| *Leguminosae, Cruciferae* | Lathyritic symptoms: neurological symptoms of weakness, leg paralysis, and sometimes death | L-2,4-Diaminobutyric acid inhibition of ornithine transcarbamylase of the urea cycle, inducing ammonia toxicity | Evans, 1985 |
| Licorice (glycyrrhizic acid) | Hypertension, cardiac enlargement, sodium retention | Glycyrrhizic acid mimicking mineralocorticoids | Farese et al., 1991 |
| Polar bear and chicken liver | Irritability, vomiting, increased intracranial pressure, death | Vitamin A toxicity | Bryan, 1984 |
| Cycads (cycad flour) | Amyotrophic lateral sclerosis (humans), hepatocarcinogenicity (rats and nonhuman primates) | Cycasin (methylazoxymethanol); primary action is methylation, resulting in a broad range of effects from membrane destruction to inactivation of enzyme systems | Matsumoto, 1985; Sieber et al., 1980 |

section 402 of the FD&C Act, and commodities bearing these residues are considered adulterated and subject to seizure.

However, as was discussed above, section 409 of the FD&C Act provides broad authority to regulate substances that are added to food. Nevertheless, the definition expressly excludes pesticide residues in or on raw agricultural commodities, presumably because they are covered by section 408. By implication, however, pesticide residues in processed foods are "food additives" and thus are subject to the requirements of section 409, which include the Delaney clause prohibition against the approval of carcinogenic food additives.

Although the FDA has the primary responsibility for implementing section 409, the EPA has the responsibility for evaluating the safety of pesticide residues and, under section 409, the safety of pesticide residues that are food additives as well as for setting tolerances. These food additive tolerances are listed under 40 CFR 185. As with section 408–based tolerances, food additive tolerances are granted on a food-by-food basis.

To deny a petition requesting the establishment of a tolerance under section 409 or to withdraw such a tolerance, the responsible agency must find specifically that the data in support of the additive fail to establish that the proposed use would be "safe." Such a safety question can hinge on the applicability of the Delaney clause if the EPA finds that the additive "induces cancer" in humans or laboratory animals.

Many important pesticides require food additive tolerances for certain of their uses. Some, such as benomyl, captan, ethylene oxide, trifluralin, mancozeb, oxyfluorfen, propargite, and simazine, have been implicated as possibly carcinogenic (59 FR 33941–33946, 1994). Before 1992, the EPA considered it lawful to grant food additive tolerance for carcinogenic pesticides on the grounds that the risk was "negligible" (less than a lifetime risk of one cancer in a million individuals). A court

**Table 30–24**
**Section 180.172: Dodine: Tolerances for Residues**

(a) Tolerances are established for residues of the fungicide dodine (*n*-do-decylguanidine acetate) in or on the following raw agricultural commodities

| COMMODITIES | ppm |
|---|---|
| Apples | 5.0 |
| Cherries, sour | 5.0 |
| Cherries, sweet | 0 |
| Meat | 0 |
| Milk | 5.0 |
| Peaches | 5.0 |
| Pears | 0.3 |
| Strawberries | 5.0 |
| Walnuts | 0.3 |

decision in 1992 (*Les v. Reily*) struck down the EPA's negligible risk policy, forcing the agency to conform to the strict language of the Delaney clause.

## Drugs Used in Food-Producing Animals

An animal drug "means any drug intended for use for animals other than man" [section 201(w) of the FD&C Act]. Animal drugs, which typically are used for growth promotion and increased food production, present a complex problem in the safety assessment of animal drug residues in human food. Determination of the potential human health hazards associated with animal drug residues is complicated by the metabolism of an animal drug, which results in residues of many potential metabolites. The sensitivity of modern analytic methodologies designed to quantitate small quantities of drugs and their various metabolites has made the evaluation problem more complex.

The primary factors which must be considered in the evaluation of animal drugs are (1) consumption and absorption by the target animal, (2) metabolism of the drug by the target food animal, (3) excretion and tissue distribution of the drug and its metabolites in food animal products and tissues, (4) consumption of food animal products and tissues by humans, (5) potential absorption of the drug and its metabolites by humans, (6) potential metabolism of the drug and its metabolites by humans, and (7) potential excretion and tissue distribution in humans of the drug, its metabolites, and the secondary human metabolites derived from the drug and its metabolites. Thus, the pharmacokinetic and biotransformation characteristics of both the animal and the human must be considered in an assessment of the potential human health hazard of an animal drug.

When an animal drug is considered GRAS, the safety assessment of the drug is handled as described under the section on GRAS. With respect to new animal drugs, safety assessment is concerned primarily with residues that occur in animal food products (milk, cheese, etc.) and edible tissues (muscle, liver, etc.). Toxicity studies in the target species (chicken, cow, pig, etc.) should provide data on metabolism and the nature of metabolites, along with data on the drug's pharmacokinetics. If this information is not available, these studies must be performed using the animal species that is likely to be exposed to the drug. During this phase, the parent drug and its metabolites are evaluated both qualitatively and quantitatively in the animal products of concern (eggs, milk, meat, etc.). This may involve the development of sophisticated analytic methodologies. Once these data are obtained, it is necessary to undertake an assessment to determine potential human exposure to these compounds from the diet and other sources. If adequate toxicity data are available, it is possible to undertake a safety assessment pursuant to the establishment of a tolerance.

To comply with the congressional intent regarding the use of animal drugs in food-producing animals as required in the no residue provision of the Delaney clause, the FDA began to build a system for conducting risk assessment of carcinogens in the early 1970s (FDA, 1977). In the course of developing a policy and/or regulatory definition for "no residue," the FDA was compelled to address the issue of residues of metabolites of animal drugs known to induce cancer in humans or animals. As the number of metabolites may range into the hundreds, it became apparent that as a practical matter, not every metabolite could be tested with the same thoroughness as the parent animal drug. This forced the FDA to consider threshold assessment for the first time. Threshold assessment combines information on the structure and in vitro biological activity of a metabolite for the purpose of determining whether carcinogenicity testing is necessary (Flamm et al., 1994). If testing is necessary and if the substance is found to induce cancer, the FDA's definition of no residue under current regulations is applicable. That definition states that a lifetime risk of one in a million as determined by a specified methodology is equivalent to the meaning of "no residue" as intended by Congress.

## Unavoidable Contaminants

**Heavy Metal Contaminants.** There are 92 natural elements; approximately 22 are known to be essential nutrients of the mammalian body and are referred to as micronutrients (Concon, 1988). Among the micronutrients are iron, zinc, copper, manganese, molybdenum, selenium, iodine, cobalt, and even aluminum and arsenic. However, among the 92 elements, lead, mercury, and cadmium are familiar as contaminants or at least have more specifications setting their limits in food ingredients (e.g., Food Chemicals Codex, 1981). The prevalence of these elements as contaminants is due to their ubiquitousness in nature but also to their use by humans.

***Lead.*** Although the toxicity of lead is well known, lead may be an essential trace mineral. A lead deficiency induced by feeding rats ≤50 ppb (versus 1000 ppb in controls) over one or more generations produced effects on the hematopoietic system, decreased iron stores in the liver and spleen, and caused decreased growth (Kirchgessner and Reichmayer-Lais, 1981), but apparently not as a result of an effect on iron absorption (Reichmayer-Lais and Kirchgessner, 1985). Although the toxic effects of lead are discussed elsewhere in this text, it is important to note that the effects are profound (especially in children) and appear to be long-lasting, since mechanisms for excretion appear to be inadequate in comparison to those for uptake (Linder, 1991).

Over the years, recognition of the serious nature of lead poisoning in children has caused the World Health Organization (WHO) and FDA to adjust the recommended tolerable total lead intake from all sources of not more than 100 $\mu$g/day for infants up to 6 months old and not more than 150 $\mu$g/day for children from 6 months to 2 years of age to the considerably lower range of 6 to 18 $\mu$g/day as a provisional tolerable range for lead intake in a 10-kg child.

Initiatives to reduce the level of lead in foods, such as the move to eliminate lead-soldered seams in soldered food cans that was begun in the 1970s, and efforts to eliminate leachable lead from ceramic ware glazes, have resulted in a steady decline in dietary lead intake. Although food and water still contribute lead to the diet, data from the FDA's Total Diet Study indicated a reduction in mean dietary lead intake for adult males from 95 $\mu$g/day in 1978 to 9 $\mu$g/day in the period 1986–1988 (Shank and Carson, 1992).

Some lead sources are difficult to curtail as lead often survives food processing; for example, lead in wheat remains in the finished flour (Linder, 1991). Therefore, reducing the contribution from dietary sources remains a challenge, but elimination of lead-soldered cans, lead-soldered plumbing, and especially the use of tetraethyl lead as a gasoline additive has produced substantial reductions in lead ingestion. What is needed now is continued vigilance of largely imported lead-based ceramic ware, lead-containing calcium supplements, and lead leaching into groundwater (Shank and Carson, 1992).

***Arsenic.*** Arsenic is a ubiquitous element in the environment; it ranks twentieth in relative abundance among the elements of the earth's crust and twelfth in the human body (Concon, 1988). (Since arsenic is discussed in detail elsewhere in this text, the discussion here is limited to its relationship to foods.) There is some competition for arsenic absorption with selenium, which is known to reduce arsenic toxicity; arsenic is also known to antagonize iodine metabolism and inhibit various metabolic processes, as a result affecting a number of organ systems. There are a number of sources of arsenic, including drinking water, air, and pesticides (Newberne, 1987), but arsenic consumed via food is largely in proportion to the amount of seafood eaten (74 percent of the arsenic in a market basket survey came from the meat-poultry-fish group, of which seafood has the consistently highest concentration) (Johnson et al., 1981). Although arsenic is used as an animal feed additive, this source does not contribute much to the body burden, as 0.1% arsanilic acid or docecylamine-*p*-cholorophenylarsonate fed to turkeys resulted in tissue residues of only 0.31 and 0.24 ppm in fresh muscle (Underwood, 1973).

Acute poisoning with arsenic often results from mistaking arsenic for sugar, baking powder, and soda and adding it to food. The time between exposure and symptoms is 10 min to several days, and the symptoms include burning of the mouth or throat, a metallic taste, vomiting, diarrhea (watery and bloody), borborigmi (rumbling of the bowels caused by movement of gas in the GI tract), painful tenesmus (spasm of the anal or vesical sphincter), hematuria, dehydration, jaundice, oliguria, collapse, and shock. Headache, vertigo, muscle spasm, stupor, and delirium may occur (Bryan, 1984).

***Cadmium.*** Cadmium is a relatively rare commodity in nature and usually is associated with shales and sedimentary deposits. It is often found in association with zinc ores and in lesser amounts in fossil fuel. Although rare in nature, it is a nearly ubiquitous element in American society because of its industrial uses in plating, paint pigments, plastics, and textiles. Exposure to humans often occurs through secondary routes as a result of dumping at smelters and refining plants, disintegration of automobile tires (which contain rubber-laden cadmium), subsequent seepage into the soil and groundwater, and inhalation of combustion of cadmium-containing materials. The estimated yearly release of cadmium from automobile tires ranges from 5.2 to 6.0 metric tons (Davis, 1970; Lagerwerff and Specht, 1971).

Although, like mercury, cadmium can form alkyl compounds, unlike mercury, the alkyl derivatives are relatively unstable and consumption almost always involves the inorganic salt. Of two historical incidents of cadmium poisoning, one involved the use of cadmium-plated containers to hold acidic fruit slushes before freezing. Up to 13 to 15 ppm cadmium was found in the frozen confection, 300 ppm in lemonade, and 450 in raspberry gelatin. Several deaths resulted. A more recent incident of a chronic poisoning involved the dumping of mining wastes into rice paddies in Japan. Middle-aged women who were deficient in calcium and had had multiple pregnancies seemed to be the most susceptible. Symptoms included hypercalciuria; extreme bone pain from osteomalacia; lumbago; pain in the back, shoulders, and joints; a waddling gait; frequent fractures; proteinuria; and glycosuria. The disease was called *itai itai* (ouch-ouch disease) as a result of the pain with walking. The victims had a reported intake of 1000 $\mu$g/day, approximately 200 times the normal intake in unexposed populations (Yamagata and Shigematsu, 1970). Cadmium exposure also has been associated with cancer of the breast, lung, large intestine, and urinary bladder (Newberne, 1987).

**Chlorinated Organics as Food Contaminants.** Chlorinated organics have been with us for some time, and given their stability in water and resistance to oxidation, ultraviolet light, microbial degradation, and other sources of natural destruction, chlorinated organics will continue to reside in the environment for some time to come, albeit in minute amounts. However, with the introduction of chlorinated hydrocarbons as pesticides in the 1930s, diseases associated with an insect vector such as malaria were nearly eliminated. In the industrialized world, chlorinated organics brought the promise of nearly universal solvents, and their extraordinary resistance to degradation made them suitable for use as heat transfer agents, carbonless copy paper, and fire retardants (Table 30-25).

As persistent as these substances are in the environment and despite the degree of toxicity that might be implied, the possible hazard from chlorinated substances is relatively low. Ames and associates (1987) described a method for interpreting the differing potencies of carcinogens and human exposures: the percentage HERP (*h*uman *e*xposure dose/*r*odent *p*otency dose). Using this method, Ames and associates (1987) demonstrated that the hazard from trichloroethylene-contaminated water in Silicon Valley or Woburn, Massachusetts, or the daily dietary intake from DDT (or its product, DDE) at a HERP of 0.0003 to 0.004 percent is considerably less than the hazard presented by the consumption of symphytine in a single cup of comfrey herb tea (0.03 percent) or the hazard presented by aflatoxin in a peanut butter sandwich (0.03 percent). The FDA's authority to set tolerances has been used only once in establishing levels for polychlorinated biphenyls (21 CFR 109.15 and 109.30).

The literature reveals a case of mass poisoning—*yusho*, or rice oil disease—from rice oil contamination by polychlorinated biphenyls (PCBs). The most vulnerable individuals were newborn infants of poisoned mothers. The liver and skin were the most severely affected. Symptoms included dark brown pigmentation of nails; acnelike eruptions; increased eye discharge; visual disturbances; pigmentation of the skin, lips, and gingiva; swelling of the upper eyelids; hyperemia of the conjunctiva; enlargement and elevation of hair follicles; itching; increased sweating of the palms; hyperkeratotic plaques on the soles and palms; and generalized malaise. Recovery requires several years (Anderson and Sogn, 1984).

**Nitrosamines, Nitrosamides, and *N*-Nitroso Substances.** Nitrogenous compounds such as amines, amides, guanidines, and ureas can react with oxides of nitrogen ($NO_x$) to form *N*-nitroso compounds (NOCs) (Hotchkiss et al., 1992). The NOCs may be divided into two classes: the nitrosamines, which are *N*-nitroso derivatives of secondary amines, and nitrosamides, which are *N*-nitroso derivatives of substituted ureas, amides, carbamates, guanidines, and similar compounds (Mirvish, 1975).

Nitrosamines are stable compounds, while many nitrosamides have half-lives on the order of minutes, particularly at pH > 6.5. Both classes are potent carcinogens, but by different mechanisms. In general, the biological activity of an NOC is thought to be related to alkylation of genetic macromolecules. *N*-nitrosamines are metabolically activated by hydroxylation at an $\alpha$-carbon. The resulting hydroxyalkyl moiety is eliminated as an aldehyde, and an unstable primary nitrosamine is formed. The nitrosamine tautomerizes to a diazonium hydroxide and ultimately to a carbonium ion. Nitrosamides spontaneously decompose to a carbonium ion at physiological pH by a similar mechanism (Hotchkiss et al., 1992). This is consistent with in vitro laboratory findings because nitrosamines require S9 for activity and nitrosamides are mutagenic de novo.

NOCs originate from two sources: environmental formation and endogenous formation (Table 30-26). Environmental sources have declined over the last several years but still include foods (e.g., nitrate-cured meats) and beverages (e.g., malt beverages), cosmetics, occupational exposure, and rubber products (Hotchkiss, 1989). NOCs formed in vivo may actually constitute the greatest exposure and are formed from nitrosation of amines and amides in several areas, including the stomach, where the most favorable conditions exist (pH 2 to 4), although consumption of $H_2$-receptor blockers or antacids decreases the formation of NOCs.

Environmentally, nitrite is formed from nitrate or ammonium ions by certain microorganisms in soil, water, and sewage. In vivo, nitrite is formed from nitrate by microorganisms in the mouth and stomach, followed by nitrosation of secondary amines and amides in the diet. Sources of nitrate and nitrite in the diet are given in Table 30-27. Many sources of nitrate are also sources of vitamin C. Another possibly significant source of nitrate is well water; although the levels are generally in the range of 21 $\mu M$, average levels of 1600 $\mu M$ (100 mg/liter) have been reported (Hotchkiss et al., 1992). However, on the average, western diets contain 1 to 2 mmol nitrate/person/day (Hotchkiss et al., 1992).

Nitrosation reactions can be inhibited by preferential, competitive neutralization of nitrite with naturally occurring and synthetic materials such as vitamin C, vitamin E, sulfamate, and antioxidants such as BHT, BHA, gallic acid, and even amino acids or proteins (Hotchkiss, 1989; Hotchkiss et al., 1992).

**Food-Borne Molds and Mycotoxins.** Molds have served humans for centuries in the production of foods (e.g., ripening cheese) and have provided various fungal metabolites with

**Table 30–25**
**Examples of Levels of Chlorinated Hydrocarbons in British Food**

| | CHLORINATED HYDROCARBONS, $\mu$g/kg | | | | | | | | |
|---|---|---|---|---|---|---|---|---|---|
| FOOD | $CHCl_3$ | $CCl_4$ | TCE | TCEY | TTCE | PCE | HCB | HCBD | PerCE |
| Milk | 5.0 | 0.2 | | 0.3 | — | — | 1.0 | 0.08 | 0.3 |
| Cheese | 33.0 | 5.0 | | 3.0 | 0.0 | 0.0 | 0.0 | 0.0 | 2.0 |
| Butter | 22.0 | 14.0 | | 10.0 | — | — | — | 2.0 | 13.0 |
| Chicken eggs | 1.4 | 0.5 | | 0.6 | 0.0 | 0.0 | 0.0 | 0.0 | 0.0 |
| Beef steak | 4.0 | 7.0 | 3.0 | 16.0 | 0.0 | 0.0 | 0.0 | 0.0 | 0.9 |
| Beef fat | 3.0 | 8.0 | 6.0 | 12.0 | | | | | 1.0 |
| Pork liver | 1.0 | 9.0 | 4.0 | 22.0 | 0.5 | 0.4 | | | 5.0 |
| Margarine | 3.0 | 6.0 | — | | 0.8 | | | | 7.0 |
| Tomatoes | 2.0 | 4.5 | — | 1.7 | 1.0 | | 70.1 | 0.8 | 1.2 |
| Bread (fresh) | 2.0 | 5.0 | 2.0 | 7.0 | — | — | — | — | 1.0 |
| Fruit drink (canned) | 2.0 | 0.5 | — | 5.0 | | 0.8 | | | 2.0 |

$CHCl_3$ = chloroform; $CCl_4$ = carbon tetrachloride; TCE = trichloroethane; TCEY = trichloroethylene; TTCE = tetrachloroethane; PCE = pentachloroethane; HCB = hexachlorobenzene; HCBD = hexachlorobutadiene; Per CE = perchloroethylene.

SOURCE: Modified from McConnell et al. (1975), with kind permission from Elsevier Science Ltd, The Boulevard, Langford Lane, Kidlington OX5 1GB, UK.

**Table 30–26**
**Sources of Dietary NOCs**

The use of nitrate and/or nitrite as intentional food additives, both of which are added to fix the color of meats, inhibit oxidation, and prevent toxigenesis
Drying processes in which the drying air is heated by an open flame source. $NO_x$ is generated in small amounts through the oxidation of $N_2$, which nitrosates amines in the foods. This is the mechanism for contamination of malted barley products
NOCs can migrate from food contact materials such as rubber bottle nipples
NOCs can inhabit spices which may be added to food
Cooking over open flames (e.g., natural gas flame) can result in NOC formation in foods by the same mechanism as drying

SOURCE: Hotchkiss et al (1992). Used with permission.

important medicinal uses; they also may produce metabolites with the potential to produce severe adverse health effects. Mycotoxins represent a diverse group of chemicals that can occur in a variety of plant foods. They also can occur in animal products derived from animals that consume contaminated feeds. The current interest in mycotoxicoses was generated by a series of reports in 1960–1963 that associated the death of turkeys in England (so-called turkey X disease) and ducklings in Uganda with the consumption of peanut meal feeds containing mold products produced by *Aspergillus flavus* (Stoloff, 1977). The additional discovery of aflatoxin metabolites (for example, aflatoxin $m_1$) led to more intensive studies of mycotoxins and to the identification of a variety of these compounds associated with adverse human health effects, both retrospectively and prospectively. Moldy foods are consumed throughout the world during times of famine, as a matter of taste, and through ignorance of their adverse health effects. Epidemiological studies designed to ascertain the acute or chronic effects of such consumption are few. Data from animal studies indicate that the consumption of food contaminated with mycotoxins has a high potential to produce a variety of human diseases (Miller, 1991).

With some exceptions, molds can be divided into two main groups: "field fungi" and "storage fungi." The former group contains species that proliferate in and under field conditions and do not multiply once grain is in storage. Field fungi are in fact superseded and overrun by storage fungi if conditions of moisture and oxygen allow. Thus, for instance, *Fusarium* spp., a field fungus commonly found on crops, is seldom found after about 6 weeks of storage, its place being taken by *Aspergilli* and *Penicillia*, both of which represent several species of storage fungi (Harrison, 1971). However, the presence of mold does not guarantee the presence of mycotoxin, which is elaborated only under certain conditions. Further, more than one mold can produce the same mycotoxin (e.g., both *Aspergillus* and *Penicillium* may produce the mycotoxin cyclopiazonic acid) (Truckness et al., 1987; El-Banna et al., 1987). Also, more than one mycotoxin may be present in an intoxication; that is, as in the outbreak of turkey X disease, there is evidence that aflatoxin and cyclopiazonic acid both exerted an effect, but the profound effects of aflatoxin overshadowed those of cyclopiazonic acid (Miller, 1989). Although there are many different mycotoxins and subgroups (Table 30-28), this discussion will be confined largely to two of the more toxicologically and economically important: aflatoxins and trichothecenes.

**Table 30–27**
**Nitrate and Nitrite Content of Food**

| VEGETABLES | NITRATE, PPM | NITRITE, PPM | MEAT | NITRATE, PPM | NITRITE, PPM |
|---|---|---|---|---|---|
| Artichoke | 12 | 0.4 | Unsmoked side bacon | 134 | 12 |
| Asparagus | 44 | 0.6 | Unsmoked back bacon | 160 | 8 |
| Green beans | 340 | 0.6 | Peameal bacon | 16 | 21 |
| Lima beans | 54 | 1.1 | Smoked bacon | 52 | 7 |
| Beets | 2400 | 4 | Corned beef | 141 | 19 |
| Broccoli | 740 | 1 | Cured corned beef | 852 | 9 |
| Brussels sprouts | 120 | 1 | Corned beef brisket | 90 | 3 |
| Cabbage | 520 | 0.5 | Pickled beef | 70 | 23 |
| Carrots | 200 | 0.8 | Canned corn beef | 77 | 24 |
| Cauliflower | 480 | 1.1 | Ham | 105 | 17 |
| Celery | 2300 | 0.5 | Smoked ham | 138 | 50 |
| Corn | 45 | 2 | Cured ham | 767 | 35 |
| Radish | 1900 | 0.2 | Belitalia (garlic) | 247 | 5 |
| Rhubarb | 2100 | NR | Pepperoni (beef) | 149 | 23 |
| Spinach | 1800 | 2.5 | Summer sausage | 135 | 7 |
| Tomatoes | 58 | NR | Ukranian sausage (Polish) | 77 | 15 |
| Turnip | 390 | NR | German sausage | 71 | 17 |
| Turnip greens | 6600 | 2.3 | | | |

NR = not reported.
SOURCE: Hotchkiss et al (1992). Used with permission.

***Aflatoxins.*** Among the various mycotoxins, the aflatoxins have been the subject of the most intensive research because of the extremely potent hepatocarcinogenicity and toxicity of aflatoxin $B_1$ in rats. Epidemiological studies conducted in Africa and Asia suggest that it is a human hepatocarcinogen, and various other reports have implicated the aflatoxins in incidences of human toxicity (Krishnamachari et al., 1975; Peers et al., 1976).

Generally, aflatoxins occur in susceptible crops as mixtures of aflatoxins $B_1$, $B_2$, $G_1$, and $G_2$, with only aflatoxins $B_1$ and $G_1$ demonstrating carcinogenicity. A carcinogenic hydroxylated metabolite of aflatoxin $B_1$ (termed aflatoxin $M_1$) can occur in the milk from dairy cows that consume contaminated feed. Aflatoxins may occur in a number of susceptible commodities and products derived from them, including edible nuts (peanuts, pistachios, almonds, walnuts, pecans, Brazil nuts), oil seeds (cottonseed, copra), and grains (corn, grain sorghum, millet) (Stoloff, 1977). In tropical regions, aflatoxin can be produced in unrefrigerated prepared foods. The two major sources of aflatoxin contamination of commodities are field contamination, especially during times of drought and other stresses which allow insect damage that opens the plant to mold attack, and inadequate storage conditions. Since the discovery of their potential threat to human health, progress has been made in decreasing the level of aflatoxin in specific commodities. Control measures include ensuring adequate storage conditions and careful monitoring of susceptible commodities for aflatoxin level and the banning of lots that exceed the action level for aflatoxin $B_1$.

Aflatoxin $B_1$ is acutely toxic in all species studied, with an $LD_{50}$ ranging from 0.5 mg/kg for the duckling to 60 mg/kg for the mouse (Wogan, 1973). Death typically results from hepatotoxicity. This aflatoxin is also highly mutagenic, hepatocarcinogenic, and possibly teratogenic. A problem in extrapolating animal data to humans is the extremely wide range of species susceptibility to aflatoxin $B_1$. For instance, whereas aflatoxin $B_1$ appears to be the most hepatocarcinogenic compound known for the rat, the adult mouse is essentially totally resistant to its hepatocarcinogenicity.

Aflatoxin $B_1$ is an extremely biologically reactive compound, altering a number of biochemical systems. The hepatocarcinogenicity of aflatoxin $B_1$ is associated with its biotransformation to a highly reactive electrophilic epoxide which forms covalent adducts with DNA, RNA, and protein. Damage to DNA is thought to be the initial biochemical lesion resulting in the expression of the pathological tumor growth (Miller, 1978). Species differences in the response to aflatoxin may be due in part to differences in biotransformation and susceptibility to the initial biochemical lesion (Campbell and Hayes, 1976; Monroe and Eaton, 1987).

Although the aflatoxins have received the greatest attention among the various mycotoxins because of their hepatocarcinogenicity in certain species, there is no compelling evidence that they have the greatest potential to produce adverse human health effects.

***Trichothecenes.*** Trichothecenes represent a group of toxic substances in which it is likely that several forms may be consumed concomitantly. They represent over 40 different chemical entities, all containing the trichothecene nucleus, and are produced by a number of commonly occurring molds, including *Fusarium, Myrothecium, Trichoderma*, and *Cephalosporium*. The trichothecenes were first discovered during attempts to isolate antibiotics, and although some show antibiotic activity, their toxicity has precluded their pharmacological use. Trichothecenes most often occur in moldy cereal grains. There have been many reported cases of trichothecene toxicity in farm animals and a few in humans. One of the more famous cases of presumed human toxicity associated with the consumption of trichothecenes occurred in Russia during 1944 around Orenburg, Siberia. Disruption of agriculture caused by World War II resulted in millet, wheat, and barley being overwintered in the field. Consumption of these commodities resulted in vomiting, skin inflammation, diarrhea, and multiple hemorrhages, among other symptoms. This exposure was fatal to over 10 percent of the individuals who consumed the moldy grain (Ueno, 1977). The extent of toxicity associated with the trichothecenes in humans and farm animals is currently unknown owing to the number of entities in this group and the difficulty of assaying for these compounds. The acute $LD_{50}$'s of the trichothecenes range from 0.5 to 70 mg/kg, and though there have been reports of possible chronic toxicity associated with certain members of this group, more research will be needed before the magnitude of their potential to produce adverse human health effects is understood (Sato and Ueno, 1977).

Another mycotoxin produced by *Fusarium* is zearalenone. It was first discovered during attempts to isolate an agent from feeds that produced a hyperestrogenic syndrome in swine that was characterized by a swollen and edematous vulva and actual vaginal prolapse in severe cases (Stob et al., 1962). Zearalenone can occur in corn, barley, wheat, hay, and oats as well as other agricultural commodities (Mirocha et al., 1977). Zearalenone consumption can decrease the reproductive potential of farm animals, especially swine.

## SUBSTANCES FOR WHICH TOLERANCES MAY NOT BE SET

### Seafood Toxins in Fish, Shellfish, and Turtles

There are a number of seafood toxins (to be distinguished from marine venoms), many of which are not confined to a single species (over 400 species have been incriminated in ciguatera toxicity) and are therefore most likely to be influenced by the environment. However, some seafood toxins are specific to a single species or genus. A complicating factor in the study of seafood toxins is the infrequency and nonpredictability of the presence of the toxin.

Seafood toxins generally can be classified according to the location of the poison. For example, (1) ichthyosarcotoxin is concentrated in the muscles, skin, liver, or intestines or is otherwise not associated with the reproductive system or circulatory system, (2) ichthyootoxin is associated with reproductive tissue, (3) ichthyohemotoxin is confined to the circulatory system, and (4) ichthyohepatotoxin is confined to the liver. In general, seafood toxins under FDA policy have a zero tolerance, with any detectable level being considered a cause for regulatory action.

**Table 30-28**
**Selected Mycotoxins Produced by Various Molds**

| MYCOTOXIN | SOURCE | EFFECT | COMMODITIES CONTAMINATED |
|---|---|---|---|
| Aflatoxins $B_1$, $B_2$, $G_1$, $G_2$ | *Aspergillus flavus, parasiticus* | Acute aflatoxicosis, carcinogenesis | Corn, peanuts, and others |
| Aflatoxin $M_1$ | Metabolite of $AFB_1$ | Hepatotoxicity | Milk |
| Fumonisins $B_1$, $B_2$, $B_3$, $B_4$, $A_1$, $A_2$ | *Fusarium moniliforme* | Carcinogenesis | Corn |
| Trichothecenes | *Fusarium, Myrothecium* | Hematopoietic toxicity, meningeal hemorrhage of brain, "nervous" disorder, necrosis of skin, hemorrhage in mucosal epithelia of stomach and intestine | Cereal grains, corn |
| T-2 toxin | *Trichoderma* | | Corn, barley, sorghum |
| Trichodermin | *Cephalosporium* | | |
| Zearalenones | *Fusarium* | Estrogenic effect | Corn, grain |
| Cyclopiazonic acid | *Aspergillus, Penicillium* | Muscle, liver, and splenic toxicity | Cheese, grains, peanuts |
| Kojic acid | *Aspergillus* | Hepatotoxic? | Grain, animal feed |
| 3-Nitropropionic acid | *Arthrinium sacchari, saccharicola, phaeospermum* | Central nervous system impairment | Sugarcane |
| Citreoviridin | *Penicillium citreoviride, toxicarium* | Cardiac beriberi | Rice |
| Cytochalasins E, B, F, H | *Aspergillus* and *Penicillium* | Cytotoxicity | Corn, cereal grain |
| Sterigmatocystin | *Aspergillus versiolar* | Carcinogenesis | Corn |
| Penicillinic acid | *Penicillium cyclopium* | Nephrotoxicity, abortifacient | Corn, dried beans, grains |
| Rubratoxins A, B | *Penicillium rubrum* | Hepatotoxicity, teratogenic | Corn |
| Patulin | *Penicillium patulatum* | Carcinogenesis, liver damage | Apple and apple products |
| Ochratoxin | *A. ochraceus, P. viridicatum* | Balkan nephropathy, carcinogenesis | Grains, peanuts, green coffee |
| Ergot alkaloids | *Cladosporium purpurea* | Ergotism | Grains |

**Dinoflagellate Poisoning (Paralytic Shellfish Poisoning).** The etiologic agent in this type of poisoning is saxitoxin or related compounds and is found in mussels, cockles, clams, soft shell clams, butter clams, scallops, and shellfish broth. Bivalve mussels are the most common vehicles. Saxitoxin is a neurotoxin that blocks neural transmission at the neuromuscular junction. The toxin produces neuromuscular weakness without hypotension and lacks the emetic and hypothermic action of tetrodotoxin. Eighty $\mu$g of purified toxin per 100 g of tissue may be lethal. The toxin is an alkaloid and is relatively heat stable. The toxin is produced by at least two genera of plankton (*Gonyaulax catenella, G. acatenella*, and *G. tamarensis* and *Pyrodinium phoneus*), and during red tides blooms may reach 20 million to 40 million per milliliter. Toxic materials are stored in various parts of the body of shellfish. Digestive organs, liver, gills, and siphons contain the greatest concentrations of poison during the warmer months.

Symptoms including tingling or burning numbness around

lips and fingertips, ataxia, giddiness, staggering, drowsiness, dryness and gripping in the throat, incoherent speech, aphasia, rash, fever, and respiratory paralysis. Patients often report a feeling of lightness, as if floating in the air (Bryan, 1984).

**Ciguatera Poisoning.** Ciguatoxin is an ichthyosarcotoxic neurotoxin (anticholinesterase) and is found in 11 orders, 57 families, and over 400 species of fish as well as in oysters and clams. Given this distribution within the animal kingdom, it is reasonable to assume that these species are merely transvectors to a toxin that some day may be classified with algal toxins. The toxin appears to pass through the food chain unabated in its toxicity and without harm to the vector. The asymptomatic period is 3 to 5 h after consumption but may last up to 24 h. The onset is sudden, and symptoms may include abdominal pain, nausea, vomiting, and watery diarrhea; muscular aches; tingling and numbness of the lips, tongue, and throat; a metallic taste; temporary blindness; and paralysis. Deaths have occurred. Recovery usually occurs within 24 h, but tingling may continue for a week or more (Bryan, 1984).

**Puffer Fish Poisoning.** Tetrodon or puffer fish poisoning may be caused by the improper preparation and consumption of any of about 90 species of puffer fish (fugu, blowfish, globefish, porcupine fish, molas, burrfish, balloonfish, toadfish, etc.). The toxin (tetrodotoxin) is located in nearly all the tissues, but the ovaries, roe, liver, intestines, and skin are the most toxic. Toxicity is highest during the spawning period, although a species may be toxic in one location but not in another.

Tetrodotoxin is a neurotoxin and causes paralysis of the central nervous system and peripheral nerves by blocking the movement of all monovalent cations. The toxin is water-soluble and is stable to boiling except in an alkaline solution. The victim is asymptomatic for 10 to 45 min but may have a reprieve for as long as 3 or more h. Toxicity is manifested as a tingling or prickly sensation of the fingers and toes; malaise; dizziness; pallor; numbness of the lips, tongue, and extremities; ataxia; nausea, vomiting, and diarrhea; epigastric pain; dryness of the skin; subcutaneous hemorrhage and desquamation; respiratory distress; muscular twitching, tremor, incoordination, and muscular paralysis; and intense cyanosis. Fatality rates are high (Bryan, 1984).

### Other Types of Seafood Poisoning

***Moray Eel Poisoning.*** This involves an ichthyohemotoxin and is destroyed when heated to 60 to 65°C. Drying does not affect the toxicity. The toxin is found in the blood or serum of raw moray, conger, and anguillid eels, although the flesh is not toxic. Symptoms require 30 min to 24 h to develop and consist of diarrhea, bloody stools, nausea, vomiting, frothing at the mouth, skin eruptions, cyanosis, weakness, paralysis, and respiratory distress. Topical application of the toxin results in burning, redness of mucosa, and hypersalivation (Bryan, 1984).

***Fish Liver Poisoning.*** This type of poisoning involves an ichthyohepatotoxin and may be related to or cause hypervitaminosis A. It occurs after the consumption of the liver of sawara (Japanese mackerel) and ishingai (sea bass, sandfish, and porgy). After an asymptomatic period of 30 min to 12 h, the victim experiences nausea, vomiting, fever, headache, mild diarrhea, rash, loss of hair, dermatitis, desquamation, bleeding from the lips, and joint pain (Bryan, 1984).

***Fish Roe Poisoning.*** This type of poisoning involves a group of ichthyootoxins found in the roe and ovaries of carp, barbel, pike, sturgeons, gar, catfish, tench, bream, minnows, salmon, whitefish, trout, blenny, cabezon, and other freshwater and saltwater fish. Poisonings have been reported in Europe, Asia, and North America. Within this group of ichthyootoxins are heat-stable toxins and lipoprotein toxins. The asymptomatic period is 1 to 6 h, followed by a bitter taste, dryness of the mouth, intense thirst, headache, fever, vertigo, nausea, vomiting, abdominal cramps, diarrhea, dizziness, cold sweats, chills, and cyanosis. Paralysis, convulsions, and death may occur in severe cases (Bryan, 1984; Furman, 1974).

***Abalone Poisoning.*** Abalone poisoning is caused by abalone viscera poison (located in the liver and digestive gland) and is unusual in that it causes photosensitization. The toxin is stable to boiling, freezing, and salting. It is found in Japanese abalone, *Haliotis discus* and *H. sieboldi*. The development of symptoms is contingent on exposure to sunlight. The symptoms are of sudden onset and include a burning and stinging sensation over the entire body, a prickling sensation, itching, erythema, edema, and skin ulceration on parts of the body exposed to sunlight (Bryan, 1984).

***Sea Urchin Poisoning.*** The etiologic agent here is unknown but apparently forms during the reproductive season and is confined to the gonads. The sea urchins involved include *Paracentrotus lividus, Tripneustes ventricosus*, and *Centrechinus antillarum*. The symptoms include abdominal pain, nausea, vomiting, diarrhea, and migrainelike attacks (Bryan, 1984).

***Sea Turtle Poisoning.*** The etiologic agent here is chelonitoxin, which is found in the liver (greatest concentration) but also in the flesh, fat, viscera, and blood. Toxicity is sporadic, and the poison may be derived from toxic marine algae. Most outbreaks occur in the Indo-Pacific region. The turtles involved include the green sea turtle and the hawksbill and leatherback turtles. The symptoms appear over a few hours to several days and include vomiting; diarrhea; sore lips, tongue, and throat; foul breath, difficulty in swallowing; a white coating on the tongue, which may become covered with pin-sized, pustular papules; tightness of the chest; coma; and death. Fatality occurs in approximately one-fourth of the victims (Bryan, 1984).

## Microbiological Agents

Despite the fact that the United States has as safe a food supply as any country in the world, most food-related illness in the United States results from microbial contamination. If all the food-borne health concerns could be divided into two large categories—poisonings and infections—the former would include *chemical poisonings* (e.g., contaminants such as chlorinated hydrocarbons) and *intoxications*, which may have a plant, animal, or microbial origin. Toxins of microbial origin may be further subdivided into algal toxins, mycotoxins, and bacterial toxins that have contaminated food and gain access to vulnerable tissues upon ingestion.

In the infections category, food acts as a vector for organisms which exhibit their pathogenicity once they have multiplied inside the body. Infections include the two subcategories enterotoxigenic infections (with the release of toxins following colonization of the GI tract) and invasive infections in which the GI tract is penetrated and the body is invaded by organisms (bacteria, protozoans, viruses, or rickettsiae).

Food-borne disease outbreaks are tracked by the Centers for Disease Control and Prevention (CDC) in Atlanta, Georgia. The CDC reports that there are approximately 400 outbreaks of food-borne disease per year involving 10,000 to 20,000 people. However, the actual frequency may be as much as 10 to 200 times as high because (1) an outbreak is classified as such only when the source can be identified as affecting two or more people and (2) most home poisonings are mild or have a long incubation time and are therefore not connected to the ingested food and go unreported. Naturally, because of differences in virulence and opportunity, some species are more likely than others to cause outbreaks. The microorganisms with the greatest propensity for food-borne illness are listed in Table 30-29 (Johnson and Pariza, 1989), although *Escherichia coli* (O157:H7) and *Listeria monocytogenes* may be added to the list soon because of their newly recognized presence, virulence, and ability to grow at low temperatures (psychrotrophism) (Kraft, 1992).

**Table 30–29**
**Etiologic Agents Most Often Associated with Food-Borne Intoxication**

| |
|---|
| *Salmonella* spp. |
| *Staphylococcus aureus* |
| *Clostridium perfringens* |

**Food-Borne Bacterial Disease.** Bacteria are not created equal in terms of the numbers required to produce symptoms; for example, only several hundred *Shigella* or less than 100 *E. coli* (O157:H7) versus $10^9$ organisms for some enterotoxigenic *E. coli* are required to produce the symptomatology characteristically associated with each of these organisms (Banwell, 1984). This variability is referred to as virulence or pathogenicity, an expression of a phenotype unrelated (directly) to viability or other characteristics. The virulence of an organism derives from two components: toxins, and surface agents which may include phagocytosis-resistant capsules, flagella for motility, adherence mechanisms, and so on. These virulence factors may not always be exhibited from one strain to another, but the presence in some organisms is associated with certain growth phases or nutrient conditions. Because of the difference in virulence, the amount required for an infectious dose is quantitated and is referred to as an $ID_{50}$.

Most of the etiologic agents relevant to this discussion can be grouped into some well-defined taxonomic groups, as seen in Table 30-30. It is important to note that a number of these organisms are psychrotrophs; that is, they can grow at temperatures of 5°C or less, although optimum growth- and toxin-producing temperatures may be higher. Other pathogens may not fit the accepted definition of psychrotrophs but grow at low temperatures (above 5°C) and survive in refrigerated or frozen foods (Kraft, 1992).

The number of food-borne agents present as a result of improper preparation, handling, and storage is considerable and represents a persistent hazard to the consuming public. In fact, the overwhelming concern for food safety in the United States and elsewhere remains directed toward preserving the microbiological integrity of food (Shank and Carson, 1992; Lechowich, 1992; Pariza, 1989).

The following agents are most popularly associated with food "poisoning" or infection and may cause a range of effects from localized GI discomfort, malaise, and fever to profound systemic distress and/or death.

**Table 30–30**
**Food-Borne Bacterial Pathogens**

| PATHOGEN | ORGANISM | GRAM STAINING | $O_2$ REQUIREMENTS | GROWTH TEMPERATURE, °C |
|---|---|---|---|---|
| Enterobacteriaceae | *Escherichia coli* | – | Facultatively | <5 |
| | *Salmonella* | – | anaerobic | >5 |
| | *Shigella* | – | | <5 |
| | *Yersinia* | – | | <5 |
| Vibrionaceae | *Vibrio* | – | Facultatively anaerobic | <5 |
| | *Campylobacter* | – | Microaerophilic | <5 |
| Others | *Mycobacterium* | – | Aerobic | |
| | *Brucella* | – | Aerobic | <5 |
| | *Bacillus cereus* | + | Anaerobic | >5 |
| Spore formers | *Clostridium botulinum* | + | Anaerobic | >5 |
| | *Clostridium perfringens* | + | Anaerobic | >5 |
| Cocci | *Staphylococcus* | + | Aerobic | >5 |
| | *Streptococcus* | + | Aerobic | <5 |
| Others | *Listeria* | + | Aerobic | <5 |

**Salmonella *spp.*** Salmonellosis may be caused by *Salmonella choleraesuis* and *S. enteritidis* serotypes Heidelberg, Derby, Java, Infantis, and others. There are over 1600 serotypes known, but only about 50 commonly occur. Usually more than $10^5$ organisms are required to cause illness. The foods involved include meat, poultry, and eggs and their products. Other incriminated foods include coconut, yeast, cottonseed protein, smoked fish, dry milk, and chocolate candy (Bryan, 1979, 1984; Eickhoff, 1978; Hubbert et al., 1975; Dupont and Pickering, 1980; Committee on *Salmonella* 1969; Edwards and Ewing, 1972; Kauffman, 1972; Rubin and Weinstein, 1977; Van Oye, 1964).

*Salmonella typhi* is the agent responsible for typhoid fever. Foods associated with typhoid fever include high-protein foods, milk, shellfish and cooked foods that have been handled and then eaten without further heat treatment (Bryan, 1979, 1984; Budd, 1977; Rubin and Weinstein, 1977; Van Oye, 1964).

**Escherichia coli.** There are both enterotoxigenic and invasive strains of *E. coli* which produce both heat-stable and heat-labile enterotoxins. The much publicized O157:H7 strain produces an enterohemorrhagic type of toxin and is one of the most virulent food-borne pathogens known. The symptomatology of the invasive type is characterized by fever, chills, headache, myalgia, abdominal cramps, and profuse watery diarrhea similar to shigellosis. The enterotoxigenic type is characterized by diarrhea (rice water stools), vomiting, dehydration, and shock, similar to cholera. This organism is probably important in travelers' diarrhea. Documented food sources include cheese, coffee substitutes, and salmon. (Eickhoff, 1978; DuPont and Pickering, 1980; Bryan, 1979, 1984; Sack, 1975).

**Yersinia *spp.*** The etiologic agents responsible for yersiniosis are *Y. enterocolitica* and *Y. pseudotuberculosis. Yersinia* is psychrotrophic, and about $10^9$ organisms can cause illness in volunteers. Foods associated with yersiniosis include pork and other meats, raw milk, and chocolate milk (Eickhoff, 1978; Bottone, 1981; Bryan, 1979; Morris and Feeley, 1976; Noah et al., 1980).

**Campylobacter.** *Campylobacter jejuni* causes campylobacteriosis (*Campylobacter jejuni* enteritis). *C. jejuni* is of moderate virulence, with $10^6$ organisms causing illness in a volunteer. Reservoirs of organisms and sources of infection include the intestine, liver, and gallbladder of cattle, sheep, pigs, poultry, and other animals. Contact with infected animals or their tissues can transmit the organism, and water-borne infections have been documented. The foods involved include raw milk, raw beef liver, meat, poultry, and water (Blazer et al., 1979; Bryan, 1979, 1984; Butzler and Skirrow, 1979; Smibert, 1978).

**Listeria monocytogenes.** *Listeria* grow well in 10% NaCl media and survive in 20%. The beta-hemolytic type grows well at 39°F and survives 176°F for 5 min. The incubation period is probably 4 days to 3 weeks. The sources of this organism include tissues, urine, and milk of infected animals. Foods associated with outbreaks include milk, milk products (cream, sour milk, cottage cheese, other cheeses), eggs, meat, and poultry.

**Clostridium botulinum.** Botulism is a product of the various toxins A, B, E, and F of *C. botulinum*; toxins C and D cause botulism in animals. Type G has not caused any human cases. The toxin is elaborated in foods, wounds, and infant gut and is neurotoxic, interfering with acetylcholine at peripheral nerve endings. Although the spores are among the most heat-resistant, the toxins are heat-labile. The symptoms may include respiratory distress and respiratory paralysis which may persist for 6 to 8 months. The case fatality rate is 35 to 65 percent, and the poison is fatal in 3 to 10 days. Sources and reservoirs include soil, mud, water, and the intestinal tracts of animals. Foods associated with botulinum toxin include improperly canned low-acid foods (green beans, corn, beets, asparagus, chili peppers, mushrooms, spinach, figs, olives, and tuna). The toxin also may occur in smoked fish, fermented food (seal flippers, salmon eggs), and improperly home-cured hams (Bryan, 1984; Hobbs, 1976; Meyer and Eddie, 1965; Public Health Laboratory Service, 1976; Smith, 1977; U.S. Department of Health, Education and Welfare, Public Health Service, 1979).

**Staphylococcus aureus.** Staphylococcal intoxication includes staphlyloenterotoxicosis and staphylococcus food poisoning. The toxin is a protein (18 amino acids) which is heat-stable. Less than 1 $\mu$g can cause illness. Sources include nose and throat discharges, hands and skin, infected cuts, wounds, burns, boils, pimples, acne, and feces. The anterior nares of humans are the primary reservoirs. Other reservoirs include mastitic udders of cows and ewes and arthritic and bruised tissues of poultry. Foods usually are contaminated after cooking by persons cutting, slicing, chopping, or otherwise handling them and then keeping them at room temperature for several hours or storing them in large containers. Foods associated with staphylococcal poisoning include cooked ham; meat products, including poultry and dressing; sauces and gravy; cream-filled pastry; potatoes; ham; poultry; fish salads; milk; cheese; bread pudding; and generally high protein leftover foods (Bryan, 1976, 1984; Bergdoll, 1979; Cohen, 1972; Minor and Marth, 1976).

**Clostridium perfringens.** *Clostridium perfringens (welchii)* type A is responsible for certain types of gastroenteritis. Large numbers ($10^6$) of vegetative cells must be ingested. The enterotoxin, a protein, is released during sporulation in the gut. Strains form either heat-resistant (some survive boiling for 1 to 5 h) or heat-sensitive spores. Heating encourages spores to germinate. The symptoms are of short duration: 1 day or less. Sources include the feces of infected persons and animals, soil, dust, and sewage. Both raw and cooked foods are frequently contaminated with *C. perfringens*. Foods associated with *C. perfringens* poisoning include cooked meat or poultry, gravy, stew, and meat pies (Bryan, 1984; Duncan, 1976; Hauschild, 1971; Hobbs, 1979; Hobbs et al., 1953; Walker, 1975).

**Bacillus cereus.** *Bacillus cereus* is a causative agent of emetic or diarrheagenic exo- and enterotoxins elaborated in food. It produces a diarrheagenic thermolabile toxin (133°F for 20 min) and an emetic thermostable toxin (surviving 259°F for 90 min). Reservoirs are soil and dust. Foods associated with this organism and its toxic properties include boiled and fried rice, custards, cereal products, puddings, sauces, vegetable dishes, soups, and meat loaf (Bryan, 1984; Gilbert, 1979; Goepfert et al., 1972).

**Shigella** ***spp.*** Shigellosis, or bacillary dysentery, may be caused by *Shigella sonnei, S. flexneri, S. dysenteriae*, or *S. boudii*. There are more than 30 serotypes. This is a very virulent organism, with as few as 10 *S. dysenteriae* and 100 *S. flexneri* having caused illness in human volunteers. Foods associated with dysentery include moist mixed food such as potato, tuna, shrimp, turkey, and macaroni salads; milk, beans, apple cider, and poi also have been reported (Bryan, 1979, 1984; Dupont and Pickering, 1980; Edwards and Ewing, 1972; Weissman et al., 1974).

**Bovine Spongiform Encephalopathy.** Bovine spongiform encephalopathy (BSE) was first identified in Great Britain in 1986. Since that time over 100,000 cattle have died or been destroyed in Great Britain as a result of BSE infection (59 FR 44591–44594, 1994). BSE is a neurological disease classified as a transmissible spongiform encephalopathy (TSE) and is similar to TSEs such as scrapie in sheep and Creutzfeldt-Jakob disease (CJD) in humans. Epidemiological evidence suggests that BSE results from feeding cattle protein derived from sheep infected with scrapie.

The cause of TSE diseases is unknown, and it is not known whether BSE is transmissible to humans. As a precautionary measure, regulatory agencies throughout the world have moved to reduce exposure to products from infected cows. The European Commission (EC) has issued new rules (Decision 474/94) requiring that beef which comes from farms with one or more cases of BSE in the previous 6 years be trimmed to remove possibly contaminated tissue (e.g., nervous, lymphatic, and fat tissue).

The etiologic agent in BSE has not been identified. Research on other TSEs indicates that the agent is smaller than the smallest known virus and is resistant to proteases, nucleases, and many other substances and treatments that would inactivate most conventional viruses. Also, there is no clear immune response to infection with TSE agents. Numerous hypotheses have been advanced concerning the biochemical nature of the pathogen or pathogens that cause TSEs, including speculation that it is an infectious carbohydrate or lipid. Scrapie has served as a primary focus of TSE research, as it has been known for decades.

Currently, three hypotheses about the nature of the scrapie agent are under active investigation: (1) a virus which has eluded detection by conventional techniques, (2) a "virino," which is hypothesized to be composed of foreign nucleic acid complexed with normal host components, and (3) a "prion," which is operationally defined as a proteinaceous infectious particle that may be devoid of nucleic acid (Prusiner, 1991). No compelling evidence has been produced to refute or confirm any of these hypotheses.

## Substances Produced by Cooking

Tolerances cannot be set for contaminants which are produced as a result of an action taken by the consumer. An example of this type of contaminant is heterocyclic amines, which are generated during cooking. Heterocyclic amines were discovered serendipitously by Japanese investigators who, while examining the mutagenicity of smoke generated by charred foods, found that the extracts of the charred surfaces of the meat and fish were quantitatively more mutagenic than could be accounted for by the presence of polycyclic aromatic hydrocarbons (Sugimura et al., 1989). Collectively, these substances are called heterocyclic amines (HCAs) and are formed as a result of high-temperature cooking of proteins (especially those containing high levels of creatinine) and carbohydrates. Normally, as a result of such heating, desirable flavor components are formed, for example, pyrazines, pyridines, and thiazoles. Intermediates in the formation of these substances are dihydropyrizines and dihydropyridines, which in the presence of oxygen form the flavor components; however, in the presence of creatinine, HCAs are formed (Munro et al., 1993) (Table 30-31).

There are at least 21 heterocyclic amines, the most prominent of which are 2-amino-3-methylimidazo[4,5-*f*]quinoline (IQ), 2-amino-3,4-dimethyl-3H-imidazo[4,5-*f*]quinoline (MeIQ), 2-amino-3,8-dimethylimidazo[4,5-*f*]quinoxaline (MeIQx), 2-amino-3,4,8 (or 3,7,8)-trimethylimidazo[4,5-*f*]quinoxaline (diMeIQx), 2-amino-*N*-methyl-5-phenylimidazopyridine (PhIP), 3-amino-1,4-dimethyl-5H-pyrido[4,3-*b*]indole (Trp-P-1), 3-amino-1-methyl-5H-pyrido[4,3-*b*]indole (Trp-P-2), 2-amino-6-methyldipyrido[1,2-*a*:3′,2′-*d*]imidazole (Glu-P-1), and 2-aminodipyrido[1,2-*a*:3′,2′-*d*]imidazole (Glu-P-2). These substances are rapidly absorbed by the GI tract, are distributed to all organs, and decline to undetectable levels within 72 h.

HCAs behave as do electrophilic carcinogens (Table 30-32). They are activated through *N*-hydroxylation by cytochrome P-450 or P-448, depending on the specific HCA. The *N*-hydroxy forms require further activation by *O*-acetylation

**Table 30–31**
**Amounts of Heterocyclic Amines in Cooked Foods**

| | AMOUNT, ng/g IN COOKED FOOD | | | | |
|---|---|---|---|---|---|
| SAMPLE | IQ | MeIQx | 4,8-DiMeIQx | Trp-P-1 | Trp-P-2 |
| Broiled beef | 0.19 | 2.11 | | 0.21 | 0.25 |
| Fried ground beef | 0.70 | 0.64 | 0.12 | 0.19 | 0.21 |
| Broiled chicken | | 2.33 | 0.81 | 0.12 | 0.18 |
| Broiled mutton | | 1.01 | 0.67 | | 0.15 |
| Food-grade beef extract | | 3.10 | | | |

SOURCE: Sugimura et al (1989). Used with permission. Adamson, 1990.

or *O*-sulfonation to react with DNA. DNA adducts are formed with guanosine in various organs, including the liver, heart, kidney, colon, small intestine, forestomach, pancreas, and lung. Unreacted substances are subject to phase II detoxication reactions and are excreted via the urine and feces (Munro et al., 1993). In vitro, HCAs require metabolic activation, with some requiring *O*-acetyltransferase and others not requiring it. Although much of the mutagenicity testing has been carried out in TA98 and TA100, these substances are mutagenic in mammalian cells both in vitro and in vivo, *Drosophila*, and other strains of *Salmonella*.

## Miscellaneous Contaminants in Food

Sometimes the items under the miscellaneous heading are the most interesting. For example, Rodricks and Pohland (1981) pointed out an interesting historical case of the possible transfer of a toxic botanic chemical from an animal to humans which was first identified by Hall (1979). It is found in the Bible, Book of Numbers, 11:31–33, which describes hungry Israelites inundated with quail blown in from the sea; those who ate the quail quickly died. Hall speculated that the quail had consumed various poisonous berries, including hemlock, while they overwintered in Africa. The hemlock berry contains coniine, a neurotoxic alkaloid to which quail are resistant and which can accumulate in their tissue. Humans are not resistant to coniine, and consumption of large quantities of quail tissue containing the neurotoxin could result in death as described in the biblical text.

Mountain laurel, rhododendron, and azaleas all possess andromedotoxin in their shoots, leaves, twigs, and flowers. Honey made from flowers of these plants is toxic to humans, and after an asymptomatic period of 4 to 6 h, salivation, malaise, vomiting, diarrhea, tingling of the skin, muscular weakness, headache, visual difficulties, coma, and convulsions occur. Needless to say, beekeepers maintain apiaries well away from these species of plants. A similar poisoning occurs with oleander (*Nerium oleander* and *N. indicum*), where honey made from the flowers, meat roasted on oleander sticks, or milk from a cow that eats the foliage can produce prostrating symptoms. The oleander toxin consists of a series of cardiac glycosides: thevetin, convallarin, steroidal, helleborein, ouabain, and digitoxin. Sympathetic nerves are paralyzed; the cardiotoxin stimulates the heart muscles similar to the action of digitalis, and gastric distress ensues (Anderson and Sogn, 1984).

Other contaminations include contamination of milk with pyrrolizidine and other alkaloids after a cow has fed on tansy ragwort (*S. jacobaea*) and tremetol contamination of milk from white snakeroot (*Eupatorium rugusum*).

# CONCLUSIONS

Food toxicology differs in many respects from other subspecialties of toxicology largely because of the nature and chemical complexity of food. Food consists of hundreds of thousands of chemical substances in addition to the macro- and micronutrients that are essential to life. The federal law defining food safety in the United States, the FD&C Act, provides a workable scheme for establishing the safety of foods, food ingredients, and contaminants. While the act does not specify how the safety of food and its components and ingredients is to be

**Table 30-32**
**Mutagenicity and Carcinogenicity of Heterocyclic Amines**

| HCA | NUMBER OF REVERTANTS/μg (STRAIN TA98) | CARCINOGENICITY | |
|---|---|---|---|
| | | SPECIES | STATISTICALLY SIGNIFICANT TUMORS |
| MeIQ | 47,000,000 | Mouse | Liver, forestomach |
| | | Rat | Zymbal gland, oral cavity, colon, skin, mammary gland |
| IQ | 898,000 | Mouse | Liver, forestomach, lung |
| | | Rat | Liver, mammary gland, Zymbal gland |
| | | Monkey | Liver, metastasis to lungs |
| MeIQx | 417,000 | Mouse | Liver, lung, lymphoma, leukemia |
| | | Rat | Liver, Zymbal gland, clitoral gland, skin |
| Glu-P-1 | 183,000 | Mouse | Liver, blood vessels |
| | | Rat | Liver, small and large intestine, brain, clitoral gland, Zymbal gland |
| DiMeIQx | 126,000 | No data | |
| Trp-P-2 | 92,700 | Mouse | Liver, lung |
| | | Rat | Liver, clitoral gland |
| Trp-P-1 | 8,990 | Mouse | Liver |
| | | Rat | Liver, metastasis to lungs |
| PhIP | 1,800 | Mouse | Liver, lung, lymphoma |
| | | Rat | Colon, mammary gland |
| Glu-P-2 | 930 | Mouse | Liver, blood vessels |
| | | Rat | Liver, small and large intestine, Zymbal gland, brain, clitoral gland |

SOURCE: Adapted from Sugimura et al (1989). Used with permission.

demonstrated, it emphasizes the need for reasonable approaches in both the application of tests and their interpretation. The specific examples of reasonable approaches and interpretations of safety data discussed in this chapter illustrate both the means and the necessity for reasonableness. New policies that are consistent with the safety provisions of the act are being devised to demonstrate the safety of novel foods which may be derived from new plant varieties or genetically engineered foods.

Contaminants found in food may be divided into two large classes: those that are unavoidable by current good manufacturing practice and those that are not. The former class is represented by substances such as certain chlorinated organic compounds, heavy metals, and mycotoxins which have been determined to be unavoidable by current food-manufacturing practice and for which tolerances or action levels may be established. Additionally, pesticide residues and residues of drugs used in food-producing animals may have tolerances established when necessary to protect public health. In the case of the latter class of contaminants, tolerances cannot be set either because the law requires zero tolerance or because contamination occurs in the home (e.g., during cooking).

It is important to emphasize that the vast majority of food-borne illnesses in developed countries is attributable to microbiological contamination of food arising from the pathogenicity and/or toxigenicity of the contaminating organism. Thus, the overwhelming concern for food safety in the United States remains directed toward preserving the micorbiological integrity of food.

# REFERENCES


Abrams IJ: Using the menu census survey to estimate dietary intake—Post-market surveillance of aspartame, in Finley JW, Robinson SF, Armstrong DJ (eds): *Food Safety Assessment*. Washington DC: American Chemical Society, 1992, pp 201–213.

Adamson RH: Mutagens and carcinogens formed during cooking of foods and methods to minimize their formation. *Cancer Prev* 1–7, 1990.

Ames BN, Magaw R, Gold LS: Ranking possible carcinogenic hazards. *Science* 236:271, 1987.

Anderson JA, Sogn DD (eds): *Adverse Reactions to Foods*. Washington, DC: U.S. Department of Health and Human Services, 1984.

Ayesh R, Mitchell SC, Zhang A, Smith RL: The fish odour syndrome: Biochemical, familial and clinical aspects. *Br Med J* 307:655, 1993.

Bannister B, Gibsburg G, Shneerson T: Cardiac arrest due to licorice induced hypokalemia. *Br Med J* 2:738, 1977.

Banwell JG: Environmental contaminant effects on human intestinal function, in Schiller CM (ed): *Intestinal Toxicology*. New York: Raven Press, 1984, pp 193–208.

Bernhisel-Broadbent J, Dintzis HM, Dintzis RZ, Sampson HA: Allergenicity and antigenicity of chicken egg ovomucoid (Gal d III) compared with ovalbumin (Gal d I) in children with egg allergy and in mice. *J Allergy Clin Immunol* 93:1047, 1994.

Bergdoll MS: Staphylococcal intoxication, in Reimann H, Bryan FL (eds): *Foodborne Infections and Intoxications*, 2d ed. New York: Academic Press, 1979, pp 59–73.

Bernaola G, Echechipia S, Urrutia I, et al: Occupational asthma and rhinoconjunctivitis from inhalation of dried cow's milk caused by sensitization to alpha-lactalbumin. *Allergy* 49:189, 1994.

Blazer MJ, Berkowitz ID, LaForce M, et al: *Campylobacter* enteritis: Clinical and epidemiologic features. *Ann Intern Med* 91:179, 1979.

Borzelleca JF: Macronutrient substitutes: Safety evaluation. *Regul Toxicol Pharmacol* 16:253, 1992a.

Borzelleca JF: The safety evaluation of macronutrient substitutes. *Crit Rev Food Sci Nutr* 32:127, 1992b.

Bottone EJ (ed): *Yersinia enterocolitica*. Boca Raton, FL: CRC Press, 1981.

Brandon DL, Haque S, Friedman M: Antigenicity of native and modified Kunitz soybean trypsin inhibitors. *Adv Exp Med Biol* 199:449, 1986.

Bryan FL: *Staphylococcus aureus*, in Defigueiredo MP, Splittstoesser DF (eds): *Food Microbiology: Public Health and Spoilage Aspects*. Westport, CT: AVI, 1976.

Bryan FL: Infections and intoxications due to other bacteria, in Reimann H, Bryan FL (eds): *Food-Borne Infections and Intoxications*, 2d ed. New York: Academic Press, 1979, pp 95–105.

Bryan FL: Diseases transmitted by foods—a classification and summary, in Anderson JA, Sogn DN (eds): *Adverse Reactions to Foods*. Washington, DC: US Department of Health and Human Services, 1984, Appendix, pp 1–101.

Budd W: *Typhoid: Its Nature, Mode of Spreading and Prevention*. New York: Arno Press, 1977.

Butchko HH, Tschanz C, Kotsonis FN: Postmarketing surveillance of food additives. *Regul Toxicol Pharmacol* 20:105, 1994.

Butzler JP, Skirrow MB: *Campylobacter* enteritis. *Clin Gastroenterol* 8:737, 1979.

Campbell TC, Hayes JR: The role of aflatoxin metabolism in its toxic lesion. *Toxicol Appl Pharmacol* 35:199, 1976.

Catto-Smith AG, Adams A: A possible case of transient hereditary fructose intolerance. *J Inherit Metab Dis* 16:73, 1993.

Chevion M, Mager J, Glaser G: Naturally occurring food toxicants: Favism-producing agents, in Rechcigl M Jr (ed): *CRC Handbook of Naturally Occurring Food Toxicants*. Boca Raton, FL: CRC Press, 1985, pp 63–79.

Chhabra RS, Eastin WC Jr: Intestinal absorption and metabolism of xenobiotics in laboratory animals, in Schiller CM (ed): *Intestinal Toxicology*. New York: Raven Press, 1984, pp 145–160.

Clayson DB, Iverson F, Nera F, et al: Histopathological and radioautographical studies on the forestomach of F344 rats treated with butylated hydroxyanisole and related chemicals. *Food Chem Toxicol* 24:1171, 1986.

Cohen JO (ed): *The Staphylococci*. New York: Wiley-Interscience, 1972.

Committee on Food Protection: *Food Colors*. Washington, DC: National Academy of Sciences, 1971.

Committee on *Salmonella*, National Research Council: *An Evaluation of the Salmonella Problem*. Washington, DC: National Academy of Sciences, 1969.

Concon J: *Food Toxicology*. New York: Marcel Dekker, 1988.

Davis WE: *National Inventory of Sources and Emissions of Cadmium, Nickel, and Asbestos. Cadmium*, section 1. Report PB 192250, Springfield, VA: National Technical Information Service, 1970.

Dayan AD: Allergy to antimicrobial residues in food: Assessment of the risk to man. *Vet Microbiol* 35:213, 1993.

DeBlay F, Hoyet C, Candolfi E, et al: Identification of alpha livetin as a cross reacting allergen in bird-egg syndrome. *Allergy Proc* 15:77, 1994.

Dorion BJ, Burks AW, Harbeck R, et al: The production of interferon-gamma in response to a major peanut allergy, Arh h II, correlates with serum levels of IgE anti-Ara h II. *J Allergy Clin Immunol* 93:93, 1994.

Drasar BS, Hill MJ: *Human Intestinal Flora*. New York: Academic Press, 1974.

Duncan C: *Clostridium perfringens*, in Defigueiredo MP, Splittstoesser DF (eds): *Food Microbiology: Public Health and Spoilage Aspects*. Westport, CT: AVI, 1976.

DuPont HL, Pickering LK: *Infections of the Gastrointestinal Tract*. New York: Plenum Press, 1980.

Edwards PR, Ewing WH: *Identification of Enterobacteriaceae*, 3d ed. Minneapolis: Burgess, 1972.

Eickhoff TC (ed): Vol III: *Bacterial Diseases, Rickettsial Infections*; Vol IV: *Virus Infections, Parasitic Infections*, in *Practice of Medicine*. Hagerstown, MD: Harper & Row, 1978.

El-Banna AA, Pitt JI, Leistner L: Production of mycotoxins by Penicillium species. *Systematic Appl Microbiol* 10(1):42–46, 1987.

Evans CS: Naturally occurring food toxicants: Toxic amino acids, in Rechcigl M Jr (ed): *CRC Handbook of Naturally Occurring Food Toxicants*. Boca Raton, FL: CRC Press, 1985, pp 3–14.

Farese, RV, Biglieri EG, Shackleton CHL, et al: Licorice-induced hypermineralocorticoidism. *N Engl J Med* 325:1223, 1991.

Food Chemicals Codex. Washington, DC: National Academy Press, 1981.

FDA: Food producing animals: Criteria and procedures for evaluating assays for carcinogenic residues. *Fed Reg* 42: 1977.

FDA: Policy for regulating carcinogenic chemicals in food and color additives. *Fed Reg* 47:14464, 1982.

FDA: Scientific review of the long-term carcinogen bioassays performed on the artificial sweetener, cyclamate. Report of the Cancer Assessment Committee for Food Safety and Applied Nutrition. Washington, DC: Food and Drug Administration, 1984.

FDA: Recommendations for chemistry data for indirect food additive petitions. Chemistry Review Branch. Washington, DC: Food and Drug Administration, 1988.

Flamm WG, Frankos V: Nitrates: Laboratory evidence, in Walk NJ, Doll R (eds): *Interpretation of Negative Epidemiological Evidence for Carcinogenicity*. Lyons, France: IARC Scientific Publications No 65, 1985, pp 85–90.

Flamm WG, Kotsonis FN, Hjelle JJ: Threshold of regulation: A unifying concept in food safety assessment, in Kotsonis F, Mackey M, Hjelle J (eds): *Nutritional Toxicology*. New York: Raven Press, 1994, pp 223–234.

Flamm WG, Lehman-McKeeman LD: The human relevance of the renal tumor-inducing potential of d-limonene in male rats: Implications for risk assessment. *Regul Toxicol Pharmacol* 13:70, 1991.

Flamm WG, Lorentzen RL: Quantitative risk assessment (QRA): A special problem in approval of new products, in Mehlman M (ed): *Risk Assessment and Risk Management*. Princeton, NJ: Princeton Scientific Publishing, 1988, pp 91–108.

Frankland AW: Anaphylaxis in relation to food allergy, in Brostoff J, Challacombe SJ (eds): *Food Allergy and Intolerance*. Philadelphia: Bailliere and Tindall, 1987, pp 456–466.

Fuglsang G, Madsen C, Saval P, Osterballe O: Prevalence of intolerance to food additives among Danish school children. *Pediatr Allergy Immunol* 4(3):123, 1993.

Fukutomi O, Kondo N, Agata H, et al: Timing of onset of allergic symptoms as a response to a double-blind, placebo-controlled food challenge in patients with food allergy combined with a radioallergosorbent test and the evaluation of proliferative lymphocyte responses. *Int Arch Allergy Immunol* 104(4):352, 1994.

Furman FA: Fish eggs, in Lienec IE (ed): *Toxic Constituents of Animal Feedstuffs*. New York: Academic Press, 1974, pp 16–28.

Gibb CM, Davies PT, Glover V, et al: Chocolate is a migraine-provoking agent. *Cephalalgia* 11(2):93, 1991.

Gilbert R: *Bacillus cereus* gastroenteritis, in Reimann H, Bryan FL (eds): *Food-Borne Infections and Intoxications*, 2d ed. New York: Academic Press, 1979.

Goepfert JM, Spira WM, Kim HU: *Bacillus* cereus: Food poisoning organism: A review. *J Milk Food Technol* 35:213, 1972.

Gold LS, Slone TH, Stern BR, et al: Rodent carcinogens: Setting priorities. *Science* 258:261, 1992.

Gonzalez R, Polo F, Zapatero L, et al: Purification and characterization of major inhalant allergens from soybean hulls. *Clin Exp Allergy* 22(8):748, 1992.

Goon D, Klaassen CD: Effects of microsomal enzyme inducers upon UDP-glucuronic acid concentration and UDP-glucuronosyltransferase activity in the rat intestine and liver. *Toxicol Appl Pharmacol* 115(2):253, 1992.

Gudmand-Hoyer E: The clinical significance of disaccharide maldigestion. *Am J Clin Nutr* 59(Suppl 3):735S, 1994.

Guyton AC: The chemical senses—taste and smell, in *Textbook of Medical Physiology*, 4th ed. Philadelphia: Saunders, 1971, pp 639–646.

Halken S, Host A, Hansen LG, Osterballe O: Preventive effect of feeding high-risk infants a casein hydrolysate formula or an ultrafiltrated whey hydrolysate formula. A prospective, randomized, comparative clinical study. *Pediatr Allergy Immunol* 4(4):173, 1993.

Hall R, Oser B: The safety of flavoring substances. *Residue Rev* 24:1, 1968.

Hall RL: *Proceedings of Marabou Symposium on Foods and Cancer*. Stockholm: Caslan Press, 1979.

Harrison J: Food moulds and their toxicity. *Trop Sci* 13:57, 1971.

Hassing JM, Al-Turk WA, Stohs SJ: Induction of intestinal microsomal enzymes by polycyclic aromatic hydrocarbons. *Gen Pharmacol* 20(5):695, 1989.

Hauschild AHW: *Clostridium perfringens* enterotoxin. *J Milk Food Technol* 34:596, 1971.

Hobbs BC: *Clostridium perfringens* infection, in Reimann H, Bryan FL (eds): *Food-Borne Infections and Intoxications*, 2d ed. New York: Academic Press, 1979, pp 35–58.

Hobbs BC, Smith ME, Oakley CL, Warrack GH: *Clostridium welchii* food poisoning. *J Hyg* 51:75, 1953.

Hobbs G: *Clostridium botulinum* and its importance in fishery products. *Adv Food Res* 22:135, 1976.

Hoensch HP, Schwenk M: Intestinal absorption and metabolism of xenobiotics in humans, in Schiller CM (ed): *Intestinal Toxicology*. New York: Raven Press, 1984, pp 169–192.

Hotchkiss JH: Relative exposure to nitrite, nitrate, and N-nitroso compounds from endogenous and exogenous sources, in Taylor SL, Scanlan RA (eds): *Food Toxicology: A Perspective on the Relative Risks*. New York: Marcel Dekker, 1989, pp 57–100.

Hotchkiss JH, Helser MA, Maragos CM, Weng Y-M: Nitrate, nitrite, and *N*-nitroso compounds: Food safety and biological implications, in Finley JW, Robinson SF, Armstrong DJ (eds): *Food Safety Assessment*. Washington, DC: American Chemical Society, 1992, pp 400–418.

Hubbert WT, McCulloch WF, Schnurrenberger PR (eds): *Disease Transmitted from Animals to Man*, 6th ed. Springfield, IL: Charles C Thomas, 1975.

Ijomah P, Clifford MN, Walker R, et al: The importance of endogenous histamine relative to dietary histamine in the aetiology of scombrotoxicosis. *Food Addit Contam* 8(4):531, 1991.

Johnson EA, Pariza MA: Microbiological principles for the safety of foods, in Middlekauff RD, Shubik P (eds): *International Food Regulation Handbook*. New York: Marcel Dekker, 1989, pp 135–174.

Johnson RD, Manske DD, New DH, Podrebarac DS: Food and feed pesticides, heavy metal and other chemical residues in infant and toddler total diet samples. *Pest Monitor J* 15:39, 1981.

Juambeltz JC, Kula K, Perman J: Nursing caries and lactose intolerance. *ASDC J Dent Child* 60(4):377, 1993.

Kaminsky LS, Fasco MJ: Small intestinal cytochromes P450. *Crit Rev Toxicol* 21(6):407, 1991.

Kauffman F: *Serological Diagnosis of Salmonella Species*. Baltimore: Williams & Wilkins, 1972.

Kirchgessner M, Reichlmayer-Lais AM: *Trace Element Metabolism in Man and Animals (TEMA-4)*. Canberra: Australian Academy of Science, 1981.

Kivity S, Sunner K, Marian Y: The pattern of food hypersensitivity in patients with onset after 10 years of age. *Clin Exp Allergy* 24:1, 1994.

Kokoski CJ, Henry SH, Lin CS, Ekelman KB: Methods used in safety evaluation, in Branen AL, Davidson PM, Salminen S (eds): *Food Additives*. New York: Marcel Dekker, 1989.

Kraft AA: *Psychrotrophic Bacteria in Foods—Disease and Spoilage*. Boca Raton, FL: CRC Press, 1992.

Krishnamachari KAVR, Bhat RV, Nagarajan V, Tilak TBG: Hepatitis due to aflatoxicosis. *Lancet* 1(7915):1061–1063, 1975.

Kritschevsky D: The role of fat, calories and fiber in disease, in Kotsonis F, Mackey M, Hjelle J (eds): *Nutritional Toxicology*. New York: Raven Press, 1994, pp 67–93.

Lagerwerff JV, Sprecht AW: Occurrence of environmental cadmium and zinc and their uptake by plants, in Hemphill DD (ed): *Proceedings of the University of Missouri 4th Annual Conference on Trace Substances in Environmental Health*. Columbia: University of Missouri, 1971, pp 85–93.

Lange WR: Scombroid poisoning. *Am Fam Physician* 37:163, 1988.

Lechowich RV: Current concerns in food safety, in Finley JW, Robinson SF, Armstrong DJ (eds): *Food Safety Assessment*. Washington, DC: American Chemical Society, 1992, pp 232–242.

Linder MC: *Nutritional Biochemistry and Metabolism*, 2d ed. Norwalk, CT: Appleton and Lange, 1991.

Maarse H, Visscher CA, Willemsens LC, Boelens MH: *Volatile Compounds in Food: Qualitative and Quantitative Data*. Supplement 4: *TNO Nutrition and Food Research*. Zeist, Netherlands: TNO Nutrition and Food Research, 1993, pp 622.

Mackey MA, Hill BA: Health claims regulations and new food concepts, in Kotsonis F, Mackey M (eds): *Nutrition in the 90's*. New York: Marcel Dekker, 1994, vol 2, pp 143–164.

Mallinson CN: Basic functions of the gut, in Brostoff J, Challacombe SJ (eds): *Food Allergy and Intolerance*. Philadelphia: Bailliere and Tindall, 1987, pp 27–53.

Manda F, Tadera K, Aoyama K: Skin lesions due to Okra (*Hibiscus esculentus* L.): Proteolytic activity and allergenicity of okra. *Contact Dermatitis* 26(2):95, 1992.

Manu P, Matthews DA, Lane TJ: Food intolerance in patients with chronic fatigue. *Int J Eat Disorder* 13:203, 1993.

Matsumoto H: Cycasin, in Rechcigl M Jr (ed): *CRC Handbook of Naturally Occurring Food Toxicants*. Boca Raton, FL: CRC Press, 1985, pp 43–61.

McConnell G, Ferguson DM, Pearson CR: Chlorinated hydrocarbons and the environment. *Endeavour* 34:13, 1975.

Meyer KF, Eddie B: *Sixty-five Years of Human Botulism in the United States and Canada*. San Francisco: Hooper Foundation, University of California, 1965.

Miller CD: Selected toxicological studies of the mycotoxin cyclopiazonic acid in turkeys. (dissertation). Ann Arbor, MI: University of Michigan Dissertation Services, 1989.

Miller EC: Some current perspectives on chemical carcinogenesis in humans and experimental animals: presidential address. *Cancer Res* 38:1479, 1978.

Miller SA: Food additives and contaminants, in Amdur MO, Doull J, Klaassen CD (eds): *Toxicology: The Basic Science of Poisons*. New York: Raven Press, 1991, pp 819–853.

Minor TE, Marth EH: *Staphylococci and their Significance in Foods*. Amsterdam: Elsevier, 1976.

Mirocha CJ, Pathre SV, Christensen CM: Zearalenone, in Rodericks JV, Hesseltine CW, Mehlman MA (eds): *Mycotoxins in Human and Animal Health*. Park Forest South, IL: Pathtox, 1977, pp 345–364.

Mirvish SS: Formation of N-nitroso compounds: Chemistry kinetics, and *in vivo* occurrence. *Toxicol Appl Pharmacol* 31:325, 1975.

Moneret-Vautrin DA: Food intolerance masquerading as food allergy: False food allergy, in Brostoff J, Challacombe SJ (eds): *Food Allergy and Intolerance*. Philadelphia: Balliere Tindall, 1987, pp 836–849.

Monroe DH, Eaton DL: Comparative effects of butylated hydroxyanisole on hepatic *in vivo* DNA binding and *in vitro* biotransformation of aflatoxin $B_1$ in the rat and mouse. *Toxicol Appl Pharmacol* 90:401–409, 1987.

Morris GK, Feeley JC: *Yersinia enterocolitica*: A review of its role in food hygiene. *Bull WHO* 54:179, 1976.

Morrow JD, Margiolies GR, Rowland J, Roberts LJ II: Evidence that histamine is the causative toxin of scombroid-fish poisoning. *N Engl J Med* 324(11):716, 1991.

Muller GJ, Lamprecht JH, Barnes JM, et al: Scombroid poisoning: Case series of 10 incidents involving 22 patients. *S African Med J* 81(8):427, 1992.

Munro IC: Issues to be considered in the safety evaluation of fat substitutes. *Food Chem Toxicol* 28:751, 1990.

Munro IC, Kennepohl E, Erickson RE, et al: Safety assessment of ingested heterocyclic amines: Initial report. *Regul Toxicol Pharmacol* 17:S1, 1993.

Murray KF, Christie DL: Dietary protein intolerance in infants with transient methemoglobinemia and diarrhea. *J Pediatr* 122:90, 1993.

Newberne PM: Mechanisms of interaction and modulation of response, in Vouk VB, Butler GC, Upton AC, et al (eds): *Methods for Assessing the Effects of Mixtures of Chemicals*. New York: Wiley, 1987, pp 555–588.

NRC/NAS (National Research Council/National Academy of Science): *The 1977 Survey of Industry on the Use of Food Additives by the NRC/NAS*. October 1979, U.S. Department of Commerce, NTIS PB 80-113418. Volume III: *Estimates of Daily Intake*. Committee on GRAS list survey—Phase III Food and Nutrition Committee, National Research Council, 1979.

Noah ND, Bender AE, Raidi GB, Gilbert RJ: Food poisoning from red kidney beans. *Br Med J* 281:236, 1980.

O'Hollaren MT: Bakers' asthma and reactions secondary to soybean and grain dust, in Bardana EJ Jr, Montanaro A, O'Hallaren MT (eds): *Occupational Asthma*. Philadelphia: Hanley and Belfus, 1992, pp 107–116.

O'Neil C, Helbling AA, Lehrer SB: Allergic reactions to fish. *Clin Rev Allergy* 11(2):183, 1993.

Pantuck EJ, Hsiao K-C, Kuntzman R, Conney AH: Intestinal metabolism of phenacetin in the rat: Effect of charcoal-broiled beef and rat chow. *Science* 187:744, 1975.

Pantuck EJ, Hsiao K-C, Maggio A, et al: Effect of cigarette smoking on phenacetin metabolism. *Clin Pharmacol Ther* 15:9, 1974.

Pantuck EJ, Kuntzman R, Conney AH: Intestinal drug metabolism and the bioavailability of drugs, in Mehlman MA, Shapiro RE, Blumenthal H (eds): *New Concepts in Safety Evaluation*. Washington DC: Hemisphere, 1976, pp 345–368.

Pariza MW: A perspective on diet and cancer, in Taylor SL, Scanlan RA (eds): *Food Toxicology A Perspective on the Relative Risks*. New York: Marcel Dekker, 1989, pp 1–10.

Pay EM, Fleming KH, Guenther PM, Mickle SJ: *Foods Commonly Eaten by Individuals: Amount per Day and per Eating Occasion*. Washington, DC: USDA (HERR No. 44), 1984.

Peers FG, Gilman GA, Linsell CA: Dietary aflatoxins and human liver cancer: A study in Swaziland. *Int J Cancer* 17:167, 1976.

Pennington JAP, Gunderson EL: History of the Food Drug Administration total diet study—1961–1987. *J Assoc Off Anal Chem* 70:772, 1987.

Personal communication: Telephone conversation between author

Burdock and Ms. Robin Cline of the National Pork Council, 1994.

Piastra M, Stabile A, Fioravanti G, et al: Cord blood mononuclear cell responsiveness to beta-lactoglobulin: T-cell activity in "atopy-prone" and "non-atopy-prone" newborns. *Int Arch Allergy Immunol* 104:358, 1994.

*Principles for Estimating Exposure to Substances Found in or Added to the Diet*. Division of Food Chemistry and Technology, Regulatory Feed Chemistry Branch. Food and Color Additives Review Section. Washington, DC: Food and Drug Administration, 1991.

Prusiner SB: Prion diseases of animals and humans. Washington, DC: Toxicology Forum, 1991, pp 203–234.

Public Health Laboratory Service: Unusual outbreak of food poisoning. *Br Med J* 2:1268, 1976.

Rees N, Tennant D: Estimation of food chemical intake, in Kotsonis FN, Mackey M, Hjelle J (eds): *Nutritional Toxicology*. New York: Raven Press, 1994 pp 199–221.

Reichlmayer-Lais MM, Kirchgessner M: *Trace Elements in Man and Animals 6*. New York: Plenum, 1985.

Rodricks JV, Pohland AE: Food hazards of animal origin, in Roberts HR (ed): *Food Safety*. New York: Wiley, 1981, pp 181–237.

Rubin RH, Weinstein L: *Salmonellosis: Microbiologic, Pathologic and Clinical Features*. New York: Stratton Intercontinental, 1977.

Rumsey GL, Siwicki AK, Anderson DP, Bowser PR: Effect of soybean protein on serological response, non-specific defense mechanisms, growth, and protein utilization in rainbow trout. *Vet Immunol Immunopathol* 41:323, 1994.

Sachs MI, Jones RT, Yunginger JW: Isolation and partial characterization of a major peanut allergen. *J Allergy Clin Immunol* 67:27, 1981.

Sack B: Human diarrheal disease caused by enterotoxigenic *Escherichia coli*. *Annu Rev Microbiol* 29:333, 1975.

Sato N, Ueno Y: Comparative toxicities of trichothecenes, in Rodericks JV, Hesseltine CW, Mehlman MA (eds): *Mycotoxins in Human and Animal Health*. Park Forest South, IL: Pathtox Publishers, 1977, pp 295–307.

Schrander JJ, van den Bogart JP, Forget PP, et al: Cow's milk protein intolerance in infants under 1 year of age: A prospective epidemiological study. *Eur J Pediatr* 52(8):640, 1993.

Settipane GA: The restaurant syndromes. *N Engl Reg Allergy Proc* 8:39, 1987.

Shank FR, Carson KL: What is safe food? in Finley JW, Robinson SF, Armstrong DJ (eds): *Food Safety Assessment*. Washington, DC: American Chemical Society, 1992, pp 26–35.

Sieber SM, Correa P, Dalgard DW, et al: Carcinogenicity and hepatotoxicity of cycasin and its aglycone methylazoxymethanol acetate in nonhuman primates. *JNCI* 65:177, 1980.

Smart DR: Scombroid poisoning: A report of seven cases involving the Western Australian salmon, *Arripis truttaceus*. *Med J Aust* 157:748, 1992.

Smibert RM: The genus *Campylobacter*. *Annu Rev Microbiol* 32:673, 1978.

Smith LDS: *Botulism: The Organism, Its Toxins, the Disease*. Springfield, IL: Charles C Thomas, 1977.

Smith RL: Does one man's meat become another man's poison? *Trans Med Soc Lond* Nov. 11, 1991, pp 6–17.

Stewart-Tull DE, Jones AC: Adjuvanted oral vaccines should not induce allergic responses to dietary antigens. *FEMS Microbiol Lett* 79:489, 1992.

Stob M, Baldwin RS, Tuite J, et al: Isolation of an anabolic, uterotropic compound from corn infected with *Gibberella zeae*. *Nature* 196:1318, 1962.

Stoger P, Wuthrich B: Type I allergy to cow milk proteins in adults: A retrospective study of 34 adult milk- and cheese-allergic patients. *Int Arch Allergy Immunol* 102:399, 1993.

Stoloff L: Aflatoxins—an overview, in Rodericks JV, Hesseltine CW, Mehlman MA (eds): *Mycotoxins in Human and Animal Health*. Park Forest South, IL: Pathtox, 1977.

Sugimura T, Wakahayashi K, Nagao M, Ohgaki H: Heterocyclic amines in cooked food, in Taylor SL, Scanlan RA (eds): *Food Toxicology A Perspective on the Relative Risks*. New York: Marcel Dekker, 1989, pp 31–55.

Szepfalusi Z, Ebner C, Pandjaitan R, et al: Egg yolk alpha-livetin (chicken serum albumin) is a cross-reactive allergen in the bird-egg syndrome. *J Allergy Clin Immunol* 93:932, 1994.

Taylor SL: Histamine food poisoning: Toxicology and clinical aspects. *Crit Rev Toxicol* 17(2):91, 1986.

Taylor SL, Nordlee JA, Rupnow JH: Food allergies and sensitivities, in Taylor SL, Scanlan RA (eds): *Food Toxicology: A Perspective on the Relative Risks*. New York: Marcel Dekker, 1989, pp 255–295.

Technical Assessment Systems: *Evaluation of the Current Dietary Status of the U.S. Population using the USDA Nationwide Food Consumption Survey Results*. Washington, DC, 1992.

Tennant R, Zeiger E: Genetic toxicology: Current status of methods of carcinogen identification. *Environ Health Perspect* 100:307, 1993.

Tonnesen P: Licorice poisoning. *Ugeskr Laeger* 141:513, 1979.

Truckness MW, Mislivec PB, Young K, et al: Cyclopiazonic acid production by cultures of aspergillus and penicillium species isolated from dried beans, corn meal, macaroni, and pecans. *J Assoc Off Anal Chem* 70:123, 1987.

Ueno Y: Trichothecenes: Overview address, in Rodericks JV, Hesseltine CW, Mehlman MA (eds): *Mycotoxins in Human and Animal Health*. Park Forest South, IL: Pathtox, 1977, pp 189–208.

Underwood JE: Trace elements, in *Toxicants Occurring Naturally in Foods*, 2d ed. Washington, DC: National Academy of Sciences, 1973, pp 178–213.

U.S. Department of Health, Education, and Welfare, Public Health Service: *Botulism in the United States, 1899–1977*. Atlanta: Centers for Disease Control, 1979.

USFDA: *Toxicological Principles for the Safety Assessment of Direct Food Additives and Color Additives Used in Food*. Washington, DC: U.S. Food and Drug Administration, Bureau of Foods, 1982.

Van de Wiel JA, Meuwissen M, Kooy H, et al: Influence of long-term ethanol treatment on in vitro biotransformation of benzo(a)pyrene in microsomes of the liver, lung and small intestine from male and female rats. *Biochem Pharmacol* 44:1977, 1992.

VanEtten CH, Tookey HL: Glucosinolates, in Rechcigl J Jr (ed): *CRC Handbook of Naturally Occurring Food Toxicants*. Boca Raton, FL: CRC Press, 1985, pp 15.

Van Gelderen CE, Savelkoul TJ, van Ginkel LA, van Dokkum W: The effects of histamine administered in fish samples to healthy volunteers. *J Toxicol Clin Toxicol* 30(4):585, 1992.

Van Oye E (ed): *The World Problem of Salmonellosis*. The Hague, Netherlands: W. Junk, 1964.

Wadee AA, Boting L2DA, Rabson AR: Fruit allergy: Demonstration of IgE antibodies to a 302Dkd protein present in several fruits. *J Allergy Clin Immunol* 85:801, 1990.

Walker HW: Foodborne illness from *Clostridium perfringens*. *CRC Crit Rev Food Sci Nutr* 7:71, 1975.

Wantke F, Gotz M, Jarisch R: The red wine provocation test: Intolerance to histamine as a model for food intolerance. *Allergy Proc* 15(1):27, 1994.

Weissman JB, Gangarosa EJ, Barker WH Jr: Shigellosis, in Eickhoff TC (ed): *Practice of Medicine*, Vol III: *Bacterial Diseases, Rickettsial Infections*. Hagerstown, MD: Harper & Row, 1974.

Williams GM, Weisburger JH: Chemical carcinogenesis, in Amdur MO, Doull J, Klaassen CD (eds): *Toxicology: The Basic Science of Poisons*. New York: Raven Press, 1991, pp 127–200.

Wogan GN: Aflatoxin carcinogenesis, in Busch H (ed): *Methods in Cancer Research*. New York: Academic Press, 1973, pp 309–344.

Wòrtelboer HM, de Kruif CA, van Iersel AA, et al: Effects of cooked brussels sprouts on cytochrome P-450 profile and phase II enzymes in liver and small intestinal mucosa of the rat. *Food Chem Toxicol* 30:17, 1992a.

Wortelboer HM, van der Linden EC, de Kruif CA, et al: Effects of indole-3-carbinol on biotransformation enzymes in the rat: *In vivo* changes in liver and small intestinal mucosa in comparison with primary hepatocyte cultures. *Food Chem Toxicol* 30:589, 1992b.

Wuthrich B: Adverse reactions to food additives. *Ann Allergy* 71(4):379, 1993.

Yamagata N, Shigematsu I: Cadmium pollution in perspective. *Inst Public Health Tokyo Bull* 19:1, 1970.

# CHAPTER 31

# ANALYTIC/FORENSIC TOXICOLOGY

*Alphonse Poklis*

It is impossible to consider the topic of forensic toxicology without discussing analytic toxicology in detail. However, analytic toxicology has its roots in forensic applications. Therefore, it is logical to discuss these mutually dependent areas together.

Analytic toxicology involves the application of the tools of analytic chemistry to the qualitative and/or quantitative estimation of chemicals which may exert adverse effects on living organisms. Generally, the chemical that is to be measured (the analyte) is a xenobiotic which may have been altered or transformed by metabolic actions of the organism. Frequently, the specimen that is to be analyzed presents a matrix consisting of body fluids or solid tissues from the organism. Both the identity of the analyte and the nature of the matrix present formidable problems to an analytic toxicologist.

Forensic toxicology involves the use of toxicology for the purposes of the law (Cravey and Baselt, 1981). Although this broad definition includes a wide range of applications, such as regulatory toxicology and urine testing to detect drug use, by far the most common application is to identify any chemical which may serve as a causative agent in inflicting death or injury on humans or in causing damage to property. Frequently, as a result of such unfortunate incidents, charges of liability or criminal intent are brought which must be resolved by the judicial system. At times, indirect or circumstantial evidence is presented in an attempt to prove cause and effect. However, there is no substitute for an unequivocal identification of a specific chemical substance that is demonstrated to be present in tissues from the victim at a sufficient concentration to explain the injury with a reasonable degree of scientific probability or certainty. For this reason, forensic toxicology and analytic toxicology have long shared a mutually supportive partnership.

Some forensic toxicological activities have been deemed so important by society that a great effort is expended to initiate and implement analytic procedures in a forensically credible manner as an aid in deciding whether adverse effects have been produced by certain chemicals. Attempts to control drivers whose driving ability may be impaired by ethanol or certain drugs are evidenced by laws prescribing punishment to individuals who are so impaired. The measurement of ethanol in blood or breath at specific concentrations is generally required to prove impairment by this agent (Fisher et al., 1968). Similarly, the decade of the 1980s saw a growing response by society to the threat of drug abuse. Attempts to identify drug users by testing urine for the presence of drugs or their metabolites, using methods and safeguards developed by forensic toxicologists, have become required by law (Department of Health and Human Services, 1988).

The diagnosis and treatment of health problems induced by chemical substances (Blanke and Decker, 1986) and the closely allied field of therapeutic drug monitoring (Moyer et al., 1986) also rely greatly on analytic toxicology. Although the analytes are present in matrices similar to those seen in forensic toxicology, the results must be reported rapidly to be of use to clinicians in treating patients. This requirement of a rapid turnaround time limits the number of chemicals which can be measured because methods, equipment, and personnel must all be available for an instant response to toxicological emergencies.

Occupational toxicology (Chap. 33) and regulatory toxicology (Chap. 34) require analytic procedures for their implementation or monitoring. In occupational toxicology, the analytic methods used to monitor threshold limit values (TLVs) and other means of estimating the exposure of workers to toxic hazards may utilize simple, nonspecific, but economical screening devices. However, to determine the actual exposure of a worker, it is necessary to analyze blood, urine, breath, or another specimen by employing methods similar to those used in clinical or forensic toxicology. For regulatory purposes, a variety of matrices (food, water, air, etc.) must be examined for extremely small quantities of analytes. Frequently, this requires the use of sophisticated methodology with extreme sensitivity. Both of these applications of analytic toxicology impinge on forensic toxicology because an injury or occupational disease in a worker can result in a legal proceeding, just as a violation of a regulatory law may.

Other applications of analytic toxicology occur frequently during the course of experimental studies. Confirmation of the concentration of dosing solutions and monitoring of their stability often can be accomplished with the use of simple analytic techniques. The bioavailability of a dose may vary with the route of administration and the vehicle used. Blood concentrations can be monitored as a means of establishing this important parameter. In addition, an important feature in the study of any toxic substance is the characterization of its metabolites as well as the distribution of the parent drug, together with its metabolites, to various tissues. This requires sensitive, specific, and valid analytic procedures. Similar analytic studies can be conducted within a temporal framework to gain an understanding the dynamics of the absorption, distribution, metabolism, and excretion of toxic chemicals.

It is evident that analytic toxicology is intimately involved in many aspects of experimental and applied toxicology. Because toxic substances include all chemical types and because the measurement of toxic chemicals may require the examination of biological or nonbiological matrices, the scope of analytic toxicology is broad. Nevertheless, a systematic approach and a reliance on the practical experience of generations of forensic toxicologists can be used in conjunction with the sophisticated tools of analytic chemistry to provide the data needed to understand the hazards of toxic substances more completely. These concepts will be described in detail in the rest of this chapter.

## ANALYTIC TOXICOLOGY

In light of the statement by Paracelsus five centuries ago, "All substances are poisons: there is none which is not a poison" (Klaassen et al., 1986), analytic toxicology potentially encompasses all chemical substances. Forensic toxicologists learned long ago that when the nature of a suspected poison is unknown, a systematic, standardized approach must be used to identify the presence of most common toxic substances. An approach which has stood the test of time was first suggested by Chapuis in 1873 in *Elements de Toxicologie*. It is based on the origin or nature of the toxic agent (Peterson et al., 1923). Such a system can be characterized as follows:

1. Gases
2. Volatile substances
3. Corrosive agents
4. Metals
5. Anions and nonmetals
6. Nonvolatile organic substances
7. Miscellaneous

Closely related to this descriptive classification is the method for separating a toxic agent from the matrix in which it is embedded. The matrix is generally a biological specimen such as a body fluid or a solid tissue. The agent of interest may exist in the matrix in a simple solution or may be bound to protein and other cellular constituents. The challenge is to separate the toxic agent in sufficient purity and quantity to permit it to be characterized and quantified. At times, the parent compound is no longer present in large enough amounts to be separated. In this case, known metabolites may indirectly provide a measure of the parent substance (Hawks and Chiang, 1986). With other substances, interaction of the poison with tissue components may require the isolation or characterization of a protein adduct (SanGeorge and Hoberman, 1986). Methods for separation have long provided a great challenge to analytic toxicologists. Only recently have methods become available which permit direct measurement of some analytes without prior separation from the matrix.

*Gases* are most simply measured by means of gas chromatography. Some gases are extremely labile, and the specimen must be collected and preserved at temperatures as low as that of liquid nitrogen. Generally, the gas is carefully liberated by incubating the specimen at a predetermined temperature in a closed container. The gas, freed from the matrix, collects over the specimen's "headspace," where it can be sampled and injected into the gas chromatograph. Other gases, such as carbon monoxide, interact with proteins. These gases can be carefully released from the protein, or the adduct can be measured independently, as in the case of carboxyhemoglobin.

*Volatile substances* are generally liquids of a variety of chemical types. The temperature at which they boil is sufficiently low that older methods of separation utilized microdistillation or diffusion techniques. Gas-liquid chromatography is the simplest approach for simultaneous separation and quantitation in favorable cases. The simple alcohols can be measured by injecting a diluted body fluid directly onto the column of the chromatograph. A more common approach is to use the headspace technique, as is done for gases, after incubating the specimen at an elevated temperature.

*Corrosives* include mineral acids and bases. Many corrosives consist of ions which are normal tissue constituents. Clinical chemical techniques can be applied to detect these ions when they are in great excess over normal concentrations. Because these ions are normal constituents, the corrosive effects at the site of contact of the chemical, together with other changes in blood chemistry values, can confirm the ingestion of a corrosive substance.

*Metals* are encountered frequently as occupational and environmental hazards. Elegant analytic methods are available for most metals even when they are present at extremely low concentrations. Classical separation procedures involve destruction of the organic matrix by chemical or thermal oxidation. This leaves the metal to be identified and quantified in the inorganic residue. Unfortunately, this prevents a determination of the metal in the oxidation state or in combination with other elements, as it existed when the metal compound was absorbed. For example, the toxic effects of metallic mercury, mercurous ion, mercuric ion, and dimethylmercury are all different. Analytic methods must be selected which determine the relative amount of each form present to yield optimal analytic results. The analytic difficulty in doing this has lent support to the unfortunate practice of discussing the toxicity of metals as if each metal existed as a single entity.

*Toxic anions and nonmetals* are a difficult group for analysis. Some anions can be trapped in combination with a stable cation, after which the organic matrix can be destroyed, as with metals. Others can be separated from the bulk of the matrix by dialysis, after which they are detected by colorimetric or chromatographic procedures. Still others are detected and measured by ion-specific electrodes. There are no standard approaches for this group, and other than phosphorus, they are rarely encountered in an uncombined form.

The *nonvolatile organic substances* constitute the largest group of substances which must be considered by analytic toxicologists. This group includes drugs, both prescribed and illegal, pesticides, natural products, pollutants, and industrial compounds. These substances are solids or liquids with high boiling points. Thus, separation procedures generally rely on differential extractions, either liquid-liquid or solid-liquid in nature (Fig. 31-1). These extractions often are not efficient, and recovery of the toxic substance from the matrix may be poor. When the nature of the toxic substance is known, immunoassay procedures are useful because they allow a toxicologist to avoid using separation procedures.

These compounds can be classified as

Organic strong acids
Organic weak acids
Organic bases
Organic neutral compounds
Organic amphoteric compounds

Separation generally is achieved by adjusting the acidity of the aqueous matrix and extracting with a water-immiscible solvent or a solid-phase absorbent material (Fig. 31-2).

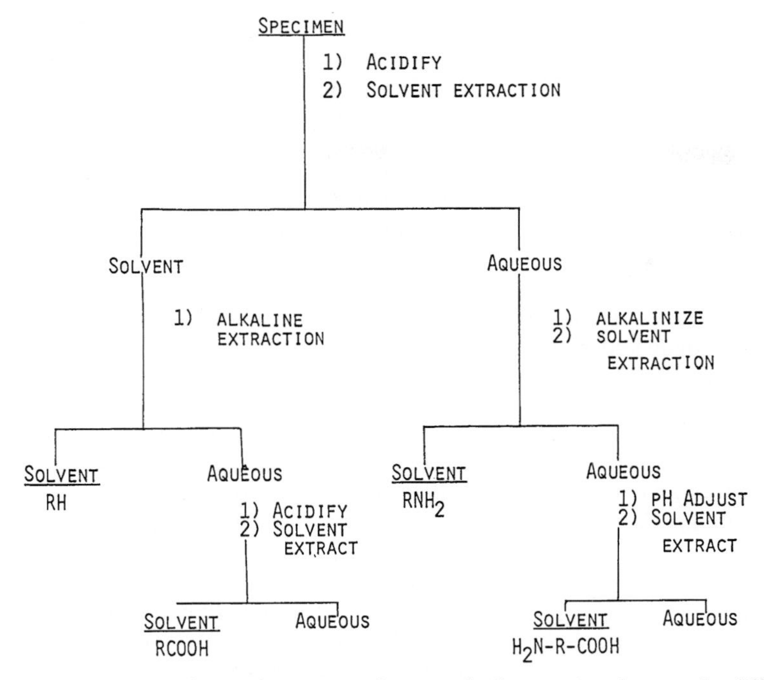


*Figure 31–1. A scheme of separation for nonvolatile organic substances by differential solvent extraction.*

Finally, a *miscellaneous* category must be included to cover the large number of toxic agents which cannot be detected by the routine application of the methods described above. Venoms and other toxic mixtures of proteins or uncharacterized constituents fall into this class. Frequently, if antibodies can be grown against the active constituent, immunoassay may be the most practical means of detecting and measuring these highly potent and difficult to isolate substances. Unfortunately, unless highly specific monoclonal antibodies are used, the analytic procedure may not be acceptable for forensic purposes. Most frequently, specific analytic procedures must be developed for each analyte of this type. At times, biological endpoints are utilized to semiquantify the concentration of the isolated product.

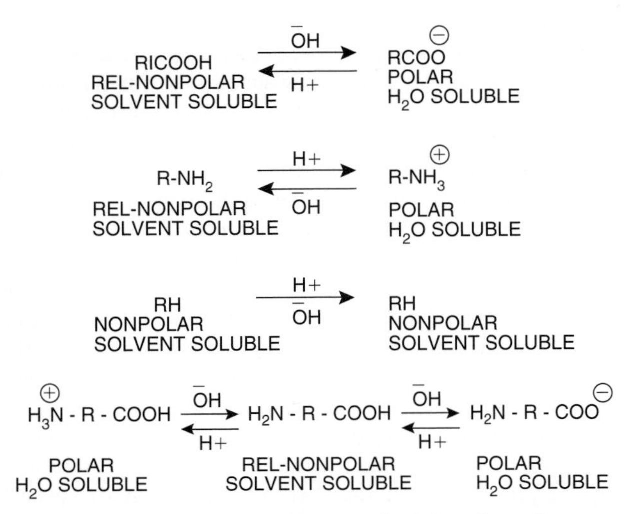


*Figure 31–2. Effects of manipulating pH of the solvent for separation of nonvolatile organic substances by solvent extractions.*

After this brief description of the scope of analytic toxicology, we shall now show how it is applied to a variety of aspects of toxicology.

## ANALYTIC ROLE IN GENERAL TOXICOLOGY

In almost all experimental studies in toxicology, an agent, generally a single chemical substance, is administered in known amounts to an organism. It is universally acknowledged that the chemical under study must be pure or the nature of any contaminants must be known to interpret the experimental results with validity. However, it is common practice to proceed with the experimental study without verifying the purity of the compound. Not only does this practice lead to errors in establishing an accurate dose, but, depending on the nature of the study, other erroneous conclusions may be drawn. For example, the presence of related compounds in the dosage form of a tricyclic antidepressant led to erroneous conclusions about the metabolic products of the drug when it was administered together with the unidentified contaminants (Saady et al., 1981).

An even greater error may result when a small amount of a contaminant may be supertoxic. A well-publicized example of this error involved the presence of dioxin in mixtures of the defoliants 2,4-D and 2,4,5-T (Panel on Herbicides, 1971) used during the Vietnam war as Agent Orange. Some of the adverse effects of Agent Orange may have been due to the low concentration of dioxin in those mixtures. Other researchers have reported that the toxicity of mixtures of polybrominated biphenyls may be due to the high toxicity of specific components, while other brominated biphenyls are relatively nontoxic (Mills et al., 1985).

A related application of analytic toxicology is in monitoring dosage forms or solutions for stability throughout the course of an experimental study. Chemicals may degrade in contact with air, by exposure to ultraviolet or other radiation, by interaction with constituents of the vehicle or dosing solution, and by other means. Developing an analytic procedure by which these changes can be recognized and corrected is essential in achieving consistent results throughout a study (Blanke, 1989).

Finally, analytic methods are important in establishing the bioavailability of a compound that is under study. Some substances with low water solubility are difficult to introduce into an animal, and a variety of vehicles may be tried. However, measuring blood concentrations of the compound under study provides a simple means of comparing the effectiveness of vehicles. Introducing a compound to the stomach in an oil vehicle may not be the most effective means of enhancing the absorption of that compound (Granger et al., 1987). Rather than observing dose-effect relationships, it may be more accurate to describe blood (plasma) concentration–effect relationships.

## ANALYTIC ROLE IN FORENSIC TOXICOLOGY

The duties of a forensic toxicologist in postmortem investigations include the qualitative and quantitative analysis of drugs or poisons in biological specimens collected at autopsy and the interpretation of the analytic findings in regard to the physiological and behavioral effects of the detected chemicals on the deceased at the time of death.

The complete investigation of the cause or causes of sudden death is an important civic responsibility. Establishing the cause of death rests with the medical examiner, coroner, or pathologist, but success in arriving at the correct conclusion often depends on the combined efforts of the pathologist and the toxicologist. The cause of death in cases of poisoning cannot be proved beyond contention without a toxicological analysis which establishes the presence of the toxicant in the tissues and body fluids of the deceased.

Many drugs or poisons do not produce characteristic pathological lesions, and their presence in the body can be demonstrated only by chemical methods of isolation and identification. If toxicological analyses are avoided, deaths resulting from poisoning may be erroneously ascribed to an entirely different cause or poisoning may be designated as the cause of death without definite proof. Such erroneous diagnoses may have significant legal and social consequences.

Additionally, a toxicologist can furnish valuable evidence concerning the circumstances surrounding a death. Such cases commonly involve demonstrating the presence of intoxicating concentrations of ethanol in victims of automotive or industrial accidents or such concentrations of carbon monoxide in fire victims. The degree of carbon monoxide saturation of the blood may indicate whether the deceased died as a result of the fire or was dead before the fire started. Arson is commonly used to conceal homicide. Also, licit or illicit psychoactive drugs often play a significant role in the circumstances associated with sudden or violet death. The behavioral toxicity of many illicit drugs may explain the bizarre or "risk-taking" behavior of the deceased that led to his or her demise. At times, a negative toxicological finding is of particular importance in assessing the cause of death. For example, toxicology studies may demonstrate that a person with a seizure disorder was not taking the prescribed medication and that this contributed to the fatal event.

Additionally, the results of postmortem toxicological testing provide valuable epidemiological and statistical data. Forensic toxicologists are often among the first to alert the medical community to new epidemics of substance abuse (Poklis, 1982) and the dangers of abusing over-the-counter drugs (Garriott et al., 1985). Similarly, they often determine the chemical identity and toxicity of novel analogues of psychoactive agents that are subject to abuse, including "designer drugs" such as "china white" (methylfentanyl) (Henderson, 1988) and "ecstasy" (methylenedioxymethamphetamine) (Dowling et al., 1987).

Today there are numerous specialized areas of study in the field of toxicology; however, it is the forensic toxicologist who is obliged to assist in the determination of the cause of death for a court of law who has been historically recognized by the title "toxicologist."

Until the nineteenth century, physicians, lawyers, and law enforcement officials harbored extremely faulty notions about the signs and symptoms of poisoning (Thorwald, 1965). It was traditionally believed that if a body was black, blue, or spotted in places or "smelled bad," the decedent had died from poison. Other mistaken ideas were that the heart of a poisoned person could not be destroyed by fire and that the body of a person killed by arsenic poisoning would not decay. Unless a poisoner was literally caught in the act, there was no way to establish the fact that the victim died from poison. In the early eighteenth century, a Dutch physician, Hermann Boerhoave, theorized that various poisons in a hot, vaporous condition yield characteristic odors. He placed substances suspected of containing poisons on hot coals and tested their smells. While Boerhoave was not successful in applying his method, he was the first to suggest a chemical method for proving the presence of poison.

During the Middle Ages, professional poisoners sold their services to royalty and the common populace. The most common poisons were substances from plants (hemlock, aconite, belladonna) and toxic metals (arsenic and mercury salts). During the French and Italian Renaissance, political assassination by poisoning was raised to an art by Pope Alexander VI and Cesare Borgia.

The murderous use of white arsenic (arsenic trioxide) became so widespread that arsenic acquired the name "inheritance powder." Given this popularity, it is not surprising that the first milestones in the chemical isolation and identification of a poison in body tissues and fluids centered on arsenic. In 1775, Karl Wilhelm Scheele, a Swedish chemist, discovered that white arsenic is converted to arsenous acid by chlorine water. The addition of metallic zinc reduced the arsenous acid to poisonous arsine gas. If gently heated, the evolving gas would deposit metallic arsenic on the surface of a cold vessel. In 1821, Serullas utilized the decomposition of arsine for the detection of small quantities of arsenic in stomach contents and urine in poisoning cases. In 1836, James M. Marsh, a chemist at the Royal British Arsenal in Woolwich, applied Serullas's observations in developing the first reliable method to determine the presence of an absorbed poison in body tissues and fluids such as liver, kidney, and blood. After acid digestion of the tissues, Marsh generated arsine gas, which was drawn through a heated capillary tube. The arsine decomposed, leaving a dark deposit of metallic arsenic. Quantitation was performed by comparing the length of the deposit from known concentrations of arsenic with those of the test specimens.

The 1800s witnessed the development of forensic toxicology as a scientific discipline. In 1814, Mathieiv J. B. Orfila (1787–1853), the "father of toxicology," published *Traité des Poisons*, the first systematic approach to the study of the chemical and physiological nature of poisons (Gettler, 1977). Orfila's role as an expert witness in many famous murder trails, particularly his application of the Marsh test for arsenic in the trial of the poisoner Marie Lafarge, aroused both popular and scholarly interest in the new science. As dean of the medical faculty at the University of Paris, Orfila trained numerous students in forensic toxicology.

The first successful isolation of an alkaloidal poison was done in 1850 by Jean Servials Stas, a Belgian chemist, using a solution of acetic acid in ethyl alcohol to extract nicotine from the tissues of the murdered Gustave Fougnie. As modified by the German chemist Fredrick Otto, the Stas-Otto method was quickly applied to the isolation of numerous alkaloidal poisons, including colchicine, coniine, morphine, narcotine, and strychnine. In the latter half of the nineteenth century, European toxicologists were in the forefront of the development and application of forensic sciences, providing valuable evidence against many poisoners. A number of these trials became "causes celèbres," and the testimony of forensic toxicologists captured the imagination of the public and increased awareness of the development and application of toxicology. Murderers could no longer poison with impunity.

In the United States, Rudolph A. Witthaus, professor of chemistry at Cornell University Medical School, made many contributions to toxicology and called attention to the new science by performing analyses for the city of New York in several famous morphine poisoning cases, including the murder of Helen Potts by Carlyle Harris and that of Annie Sutherland by Dr. Robert W. Buchanan. In 1911, Witthaus and Tracy C. Becker edited a four-volume work on medical jurisprudence, forensic medicine, and toxicology, the first standard forensic textbook published in the United States. In 1918, the city of New York established a medical examiner's system, and the appointment of Dr. Alexander O. Gettler as toxicologist marked the beginning of modern forensic toxicology in this country. Although Dr. Gettler made numerous contributions to the science, perhaps his greatest was the training and direction he gave to future leaders in forensic toxicology. Many of his associates went on to direct laboratories within coroners' and medical examiners' systems in major urban centers throughout the country.

In 1949, the American Academy of Forensic Sciences was established to support and further the practice of all phases of legal medicine in the United States. The members of the toxicology section represent the vast majority of forensic toxicologists working in coroners' or medical examiners' offices. Several other international, national, and local forensic science organizations, such as the Society of Forensic Toxicologists and the California Association of Toxicologists, offer a forum for the exchange of scientific data pertaining to analytic techniques and case reports involving new or infrequently used drugs and poisons. The International Association of Forensic Toxicologists, founded in 1963, with over 750 members in 45 countries, permits worldwide cooperation in resolving the technical problems confronting toxicology.

In 1975, the American Board of Forensic Toxicology was created to examine and certify forensic toxicologists. One of the stated objectives of the board is "to make available to the judicial system, and other publics, a practical and equitable system for readily identifying those persons professing to be specialists in forensic toxicology who possess the requisite qualifications and competence." Those certified as Diplomates of the board must have a doctor of philosophy or doctor of science degree, have at least 3 years of full-time professional experience, and pass a written examination. In 1993, the board began certifying "forensic toxicology specialists." Specialists must have a master's degree and 6 years of full-time professional experience and must pass a written examination. At present, there are approximately 200 diplomates and 15 specialists certified by the board.

## TOXICOLOGICAL INVESTIGATION OF A POISON DEATH

The toxicological investigation of a poison death may be divided into three steps: (1) obtaining the case history and suitable specimens, (2) the toxicological analyses, and (3) the interpretation of the analytic findings.

### Case History and Specimens

Today, there are readily available to the public thousands of compounds which are lethal if ingested, injected, or inhaled. Only a limited amount of material on which to perform analyses is available; therefore, it is imperative that before the analyses are initiated, as much information as possible concerning the facts of the case be collected. The age, sex, weight, medical history, and occupation of the decedent as well as any treatment administered before death, the gross autopsy findings, the drugs available to the decedent, and the interval between the onset of symptoms and death should be noted. In a typical year, a postmortem toxicology laboratory will perform analyses for such diverse poisons as prescription drugs (analgesics, antidepressants, hypnotics, tranquilizers), drugs of abuse (hallucinogens, narcotics, stimulants), commercial products (antifreeze, aerosol products, insecticides, rodenticides, rubbing compound, weed killers), and gases (carbon monoxide, cyanide). Obviously, an identification of the poison before analysis can be helpful.

The collection of postmortem specimens for analysis is usually performed by the pathologist at autopsy. Specimens of many different body fluids and organs are necessary, as drugs and poisons display varying affinities for body tissues. A large quantity of each specimen is needed for thorough toxicological analysis because a procedure which extracts and identifies one compound or class of compounds may be ineffective in extracting and identifying others (Table 31-1).

In collecting the specimens, the pathologist labels each container with the date and time of autopsy, the name of the decedent, the identity of the sample, an appropriate case identification number, and his or her signature or initials. It is paramount that the handling of all specimens, their analysis,

**Table 31–1**
**Suggested List of Specimens and Amounts to Be Collected at Autopsy**

| SPECIMEN | QUANTITY |
|---|---|
| Brain | 100 g |
| Liver | 100 g |
| Kidney | 50 g |
| Heart blood | 25 g |
| Peripheral blood | 10 g |
| Vitreous humor | All available |
| Bile | All available |
| Urine | All available |
| Gastric contents | All available |

SOURCE: From Appendix, Report of the Laboratory Guidelines Committee, Society of Forensic Toxicologist and Toxicology Section, American Academy of Forensic Sciences. *J Anal Toxicol* 14:18A, 1990.

and the resultant reports be authenticated and documented. A form developed at the collection site which identifies each specimen is submitted to the laboratory with the specimens. The form is signed and dated by the pathologist and subsequently by any individual handling, transferring, or transporting the specimens from one individual or place to another. In legal terms, this form constitutes a "chain of custody" of specimens, documenting by time, date, name, and signature all persons transferring or receiving the specimens. The chain of custody enables a toxicologist to introduce his or her results into legal proceedings, having established that the specimens analyzed came from the decedent.

Specimens should be collected before embalming, as this process may destroy or dilute the poisons present, rendering their detection impossible. Conversely, methyl or ethyl alcohol may be a constituent of embalming fluid, giving a false indication of the decedent's drinking before death.

On occasion, toxicological analysis is requested for cases of burned, exhumed, and skeletal remains. In such instances, it is necessary to analyze unusual specimens such as bone marrow, hair, skeletal muscle, vitreous humor, and even maggots (Inoue, 1992). Numerous drugs have been successfully identified in bone marrow and bone washings from skeletal remains even after decomposition and burial (Benko, 1985). Similarly, the vitreous humor of the eye is isolated and sequestered from putrefaction, charring, and trauma; thus, it is a useful specimen for the detection of most drugs, anions, and even volatile poisons such as alcohols, ketones, and glycols (Coe, 1993). Hair analysis is a rapidly growing technique in forensic toxicology. Recently, numerous therapeutic agents, such as antibiotics and antipsychotic drugs, as well as drugs subject to abuse (morphine, phencyclidine, and cocaine), have been identified in hair (Tagliro, 1993). Limited data are available to support a direct correlation between hair values and drug doses or between physiological and behavioral effects. At present, the interpretation of quantitative hair data is debatable (Poklis, 1994); however, qualitative results have been accepted as indicators of drug use. In severely decomposed bodies, the absence of blood and/or the scarcity of solid tissues suitable for analysis have led to the collection and testing of maggots (fly larvae) feeding on the body (Pounder, 1991). The fundamental premise underlying maggot analysis is that if drugs or intoxicants are detected, they could only have originated from tissues on which the larvae were feeding: those of the decedent. Surprisingly, analysis of maggots is rather straightforward, requiring no special methodology beyond that routinely applied in toxicology laboratories. Case reports have documented the detection of numerous drugs and intoxicants in maggots on decomposed bodies. The compounds detected include barbiturates, benzodiazepines, phenothiazines, morphine, and malathion. Controlled studies in which maggots were allowed to feed on tissues to which drugs had been added have demonstrated the accumulation of propoxphene and amitriptyline in the larvae (Goff et al., 1993).

## Toxicological Analysis

Before the analysis begins, several factors must be considered: the amount of specimen available, the nature of the poison sought, and the possible biotransformation of the poison. In cases involving oral administration of the poison, the gastrointestinal (GI) contents are analyzed first, because large amounts of residual unabsorbed poison may be present. The urine may be analyzed next, as the kidney is the major organ of excretion for most poisons and as high concentrations of toxicants and/or their metabolites often are present in urine. After absorption from the GI tract, drugs or poisons are carried to the liver before entering the general systemic circulation; therefore, the first analysis of an internal organ is conducted on the liver. If a specific poison is suspected or known to be involved in a death, the toxicologist first analyzes the tissues and fluids in which the poison concentrates.

A knowledge of drug biotransformation is often essential before an analysis is performed. The parent compound and any major physiologically active metabolites should be isolated and identified. In some instances, the metabolites provide the only evidence that a drug or poison has been administered. Many screening tests, such as immunoassays, are specifically designed to detect not the parent drug but its major urinary metabolite. An example of the relationship of pharmacokinetic and analytic factors is provided by cocaine. The major metabolites of cocaine biotransformation are benzoylecgonine and ecgonine methylester (Fig. 31-3). The ingestion of alcohol combined with the administration of cocaine results in the hepatic transesterification of cocaine to form cocaethylene (Hime et al., 1991) (Fig. 31-3). The disposition of these compounds in various body fluids and hair is shown in Fig. 31-4. Thus, the initial testing of urine to determine cocaine use is performed with immunoassays specifically designed to detect the presence of benzoylecgonine, the major urinary metabolite. If saliva or hair is tested, parent cocaine is the analyte sought. To determine a cocaine profile of each compound present in a specimen, chromatographic procedures such as gas chromatography/mass spectrometry (GC/MS), which allows the simultaneous separation and quantification of each compound, are used.

The analysis may be complicated by the normal chemical changes that occur during the decomposition of a cadaver. The autopsy and toxicological analysis should be started as soon after death as possible. The natural enzymatic and nonenzymatic processes of decomposition and microbial metabolism may destroy a poison that was present at death or produce

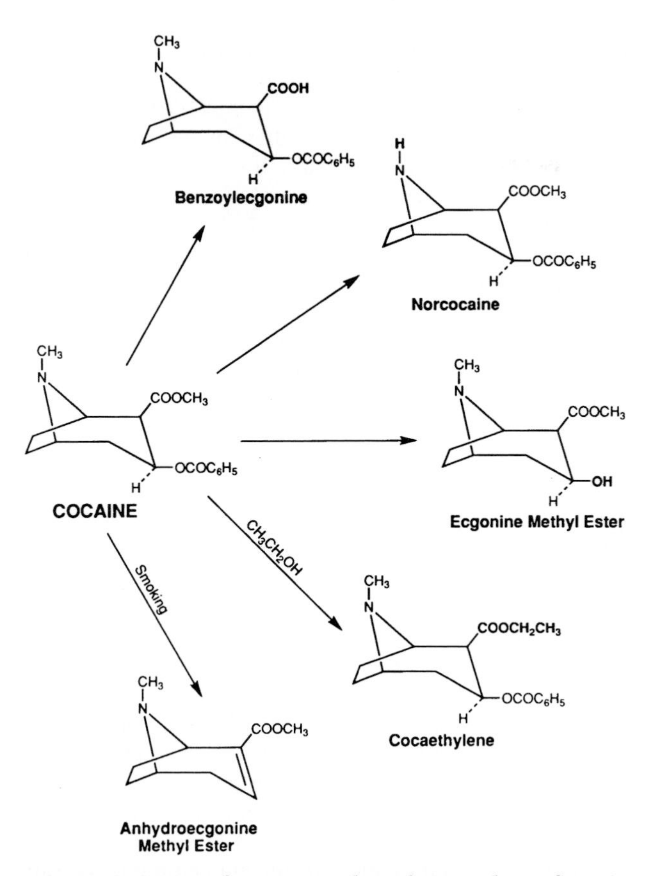


*Figure 31–3. Biotransformation and pyrolysis products of cocaine.*

substances or compounds with chemical and physical properties similar to those of commonly encountered poisons. As early as the 1870s, so-called cadaveric alkaloids isolated from the organs of putrefied bodies were known to produce color test reactions similar to those produced by morphine and other drugs. These cadaveric alkaloids resulted from the bacterial decarboxylation of the amino acids ornithine and lysine, producing putrescine and cadaverine, respectively (Evans, 1963). Similarly, during decomposition, phenylalanine is converted to phenylethylamine, which has chemical and physical properties very similar to those of amphetamine. The hydrolysis, oxidation, or reduction of proteins, nucleic acids, and lipids may generate numerous compounds, such as hydroxylated aliphatic and aromatic carboxylic acids, pyridine and piperidine derivatives, and aromatic heterocyclics such as tryptamine and norharmone (Kaempe, 1969). All these substances may interfere with the isolation and identification of the toxicants being sought. The concentration of cyanide and ethyl alcohol and the carbon monoxide saturation of the blood may be decreased or increased, depending on the degree of putrefaction and microbial activity. However, many poisons, such as arsenic, barbiturates, mercury, and strychnine, are extremely stable and may be detectable many years after death.

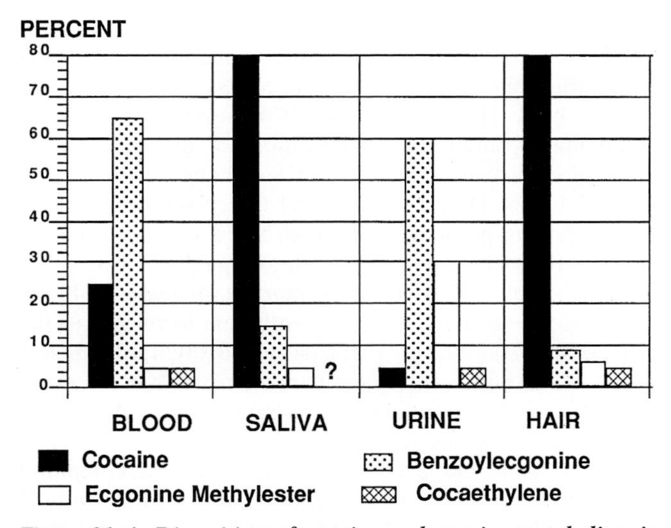


*Figure 31–4. Disposition of cocaine and cocaine metabolites in human fluids and hair. (Data redrawn form Spiehler V: Society of Forensic Toxicologist Conference on Drug Testing in Hair, Tampa, FL, October 29, 1994.)*

Before analysis, the purity of all chemicals should be established. The primary reference material used to prepare calibrators and controls should be checked for purity, and the salt form or degree of hydration should be determined (Blanke, 1989). All reagents and solvents should be of the highest grade possible and should be free of contaminants which may interfere with or distort analytic findings. For example, the chloroform contaminants phosgene and ethyl chloroformate may react with primary or secondary amine drugs to form carbamyl chloride and ethyl carbamate derivatives (Cone et al., 1982). Specimen containers, lids, and stoppers should be free of contaminants such as plasticizers, which often interfere with chromatographic or GC/MS determinations. Care should be exercised to ensure a clean laboratory environment. This is a particular concern in the analysis of metals, as aluminum, arsenic, lead, and mercury are ubiquitous environmental and reagent contaminants.

Forensic toxicology laboratories analyze specimens by using a variety of analytic procedures. Initially, nonspecific tests designed to determine the presence or absence of a class or group of analytes may be performed directly on the specimens. Examples of tests used to rapidly screen urine are the FPN (*f*erric chloride, *p*erchloric, and *n*itric acid) color test for phenothiazine drugs and immunoassays for the detection of barbiturates, benzodiazepines, and opiate derivatives. Positive results obtained with these tests must be confirmed by a second analytic procedure which identifies the particular drug. The detection limit of the confirmatory test should be lower than that of the initial nonspecific test.

Some analytic procedures identify specific compounds. Even in such instances, a second test should be performed to identify the analyte. The second test should be based on a chemical or physical principle different from that of the first test. Such additional testing is performed to establish an unequivocal identification of the drugs or poisons present. Whenever possible, the most specific test for the compound of interest should be performed. Today, GC/MS is generally accepted as unequivocal identification for most drugs. However, even GC/MS has limitations in drug identification.

The limit of detection, the smallest concentration of analyte reliably identified by the assay, and the specificity of all qualitative methods should be well documented. The laboratory must demonstrate that the assay response to blank or negative calibrators does not overlap with the response of the lowest positive calibrator.

In certain instances, qualitative identification of a poison or drug is sufficient to resolve forensic toxicology issues. However, most cases require reliable estimates of poison concentrations for forensic interpretation. For quantitative analysis, the linearity, precision, and specificity of the procedure must be established. Linearity should be determined by using at least three calibrators whose concentrations bracket the anticipated concentrations in the specimen. Precision, which statistically demonstrates the variance in the value obtained, is determined by multiple analyses of a specimen of a known concentration. For a variety of reasons, a quantitative result occasionally will deviate spuriously from the true value. Therefore, replicate quantitative determinations should be performed on all specimens, at least in duplicate (Blanke, 1987).

When unusual samples such as bone marrow, hair, and maggots are analyzed, the extraction efficiency of a procedure may vary greatly, depending on the nature of the specimens. Therefore, all calibrators and controls should be prepared in the same matrix as the specimens and analyzed concurrently with the specimens. Often the matrix is "unique" or impossible to match, such as decomposed or embalmed tissue. In these instances, the method of "standard additions" may be used. Known amounts of the poison of interest are added to specimen aliquots, and quantitation is performed by comparing the proportional response of the "poison added" specimens to that of the test specimens.

## Interpretation of Analytic Results

Once the analysis of the specimens is complete, a toxicologist must interpret his or her findings in regard to the physiological or behavioral effects of the toxicants on the decedent at the concentrations found. Specific questions must be answered, such as the route of administration, the dose administered, and whether the concentration of the toxicant present was sufficient to cause death or alter the decedent's actions enough to cause his or her death. Assessing the physiological meanings of analytic results is often the most difficult problem faced by a forensic toxicologist.

In determining the route of administration, a toxicologist notes the results of the analysis of the various specimens. As a general rule, the highest concentrations of a poison are found at the site of administration. Therefore, the presence of large amounts of drugs and/or poisons in the GI tract and liver indicates oral ingestion, higher concentrations in the lungs than in other visceral organs can indicate inhalation, and detection of a drug in the tissue surrounding an injection site generally indicates a fresh intramuscular or intravenous injection. Smoking is a popular route of administration for abusers of controlled substances such as cocaine, heroin, and phencyclidine. Pyrolysis of these drugs leads to the inhalation of not only the parent drug but also characteristic breakdown products of combustion. For example, a major pyrolysis product of "crack" cocaine smoking is anhydroecgonine methylester (Martin et al., 1989) (Fig. 31-3). Thus, identification of relatively high concentrations of this compound along with cocaine in urine or other body fluids or tissues indicates smoking as the route of cocaine administration (Jacob et al., 1990).

The presence of a toxic material in the GI tract, regardless of the quantity, does not provide sufficient evidence to establish that agent as the cause of death. It is necessary to demonstrate that absorption of the toxicant has occurred and that it has been transported by the general circulation to the organs where it has exerted a fatal effect. This is established by blood and tissue analysis. An exception to the rule is provided by strong corrosive chemicals such as sulfuric acid, lye, and phenol, which exert their deleterious effects by directly digesting tissue, causing hemorrhage and shock.

The results of urine analysis are often of little benefit in determining the physiological effects of a toxic agent. Urine results establish only that some time before death the poison was present in the body. Correlation of urine values with physiological effects is poor as a result of various factors that influence the rate of excretion of specific compounds and the urine volume.

The physiological effects of most drugs and poisons are correlated with their concentrations in blood or blood fractions such as plasma and serum. Indeed, in living persons, this association is the basis of therapeutic drug monitoring. However, postmortem blood has been described as a fluid obtained from the vasculature after death which resembles blood. Therefore, interpretation of postmortem blood results requires careful consideration of the case history, the site of collection, and postmortem changes. The survival time between the administration of a poison and death may be sufficiently long to permit biotransformation and excretion of the agent. Blood values may appear to be nontoxic or consistent with therapeutic administration. Death from hepatic failure after an acetaminophen overdose usually occurs at least 3 to 4 days after ingestion. Postmortem acetaminophen concentrations in blood may be consistent with the ingestion of therapeutic doses (Fig. 31-5). Emergency medical treatment such as the administration of fluids, plasma extenders, diuretics, and blood transfusions may dilute or remove toxic agents. Similarly, prolonged survival on a mechanical respirator, hemodialysis, or hemoperfusion may significantly reduce initially lethal blood concentrations of poisons.

Until recently, it was generally assumed that postmortem blood drug concentrations are more or less uniform throughout the body. However, in the 1970s, several investigators noted that postmortem concentrations of digoxin in heart blood greatly exceeded those in simultaneously collected femoral blood. They also observed that postmortem blood concentrations, particularly in heart blood, exceeded the expected values at the time of death (Vorpahl and Coe, 1978; Aderjan et al., 1979). This postmortem increase in blood digoxin concentrations was apparently due to release of the drug from tissue stores, particularly the myocardium. Recently, other researchers have demonstrated that for many drugs, blood concentrations in the same body vary greatly depending on the site from which the specimen is collected: subclavian vein, thoracic aorta, inferior vena cava, femoral vein, and so forth. For example, in a case of fatal multiple drug ingestion, analysis of postmortem blood collected from 10 different sites demonstrated imipramine concentrations that differed by as much as 760 percent (2.1 to 16.0 mg/liter) (Jones and Pounder, 1987). In an extensive investigation,

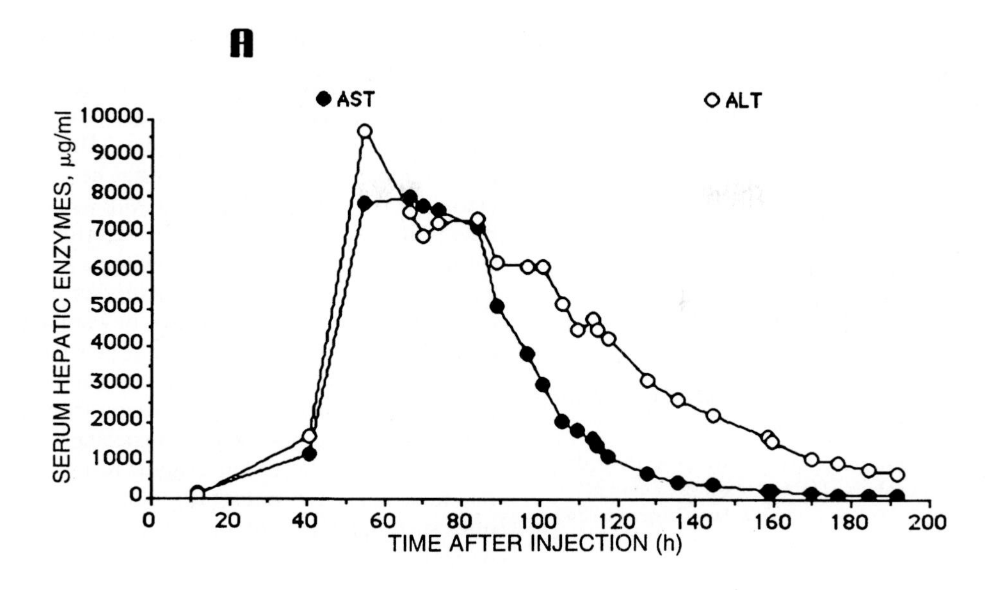


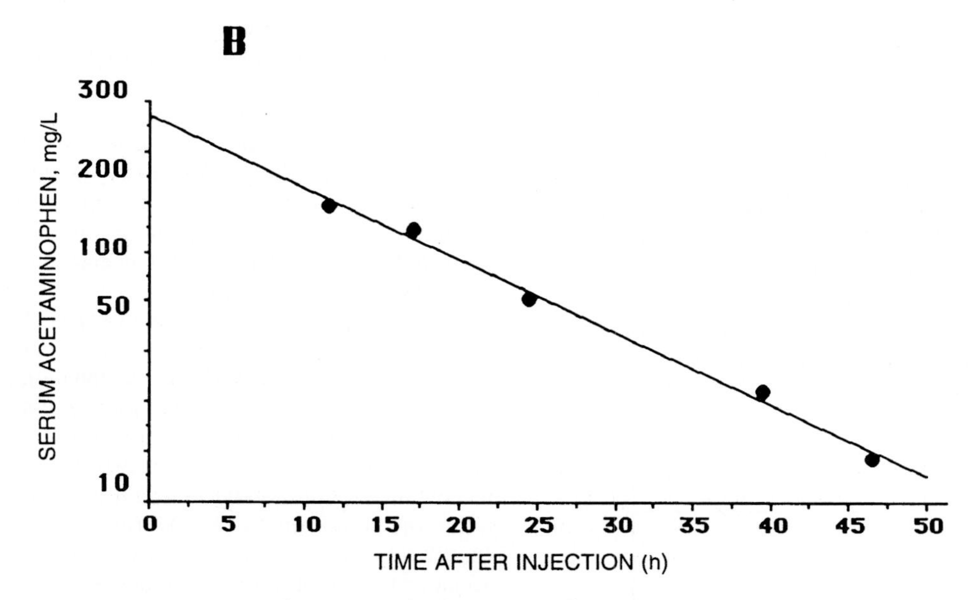


***Figure 31–5. Laboratory findings in a fatal acetaminophen poisoning.***

(*A*) Hepatotoxicity demonstrated by elevation and exhaustion of hepatic enzymes: alanine aminotransferase (ALT) and aspartate aminotransferase (AST). (*B*) Serum acetaminophen concentrations decline to those consistent with therapeutic values within 2 days after ingestion. (Data redrawn from Price LM, Poklis A, Johnson DE: Fatal acetaminophen poisoning with evidence of subendocardial necrosis of the heart. *J Forensic Sci* 36:930–935, 1991.)

Prouty and Anderson (1990) demonstrated that postmortem blood drug concentrations not only were site-dependent but increased greatly over the interval between death and specimen collection, particularly in heart blood. This increase over the postmortem interval was most pronounced for basic drugs with large apparent volumes of distribution, such as tricyclic antidepressants.

In an overt drug overdose, postmortem blood concentrations are elevated sufficiently to render an unmistakable interpretation of fatal intoxication. However, in many cases, the postmortem redistribution of drugs may significantly affect the interpretation of analytic findings. For drugs whose volume of distribution, plasma half-life, and renal clearance vary widely from person to person or undergo postmortem redistribution, tissue concentrations readily distinguish therapeutic administration from drug overdose (Apple, 1989) (Fig. 31-6). Therefore, to provide a foundation of reasonable medical certainty in regard to the role of a drug in the death of an individual, it is recommended that in addition to heart blood, a peripheral blood specimen and tissues be analyzed.

Postmortem toxicology results often are used to corroborate investigative findings. For example, the analysis of sequential sections of hair provides a reliable correlation with the pattern of arsenic exposure. Significant increases in the arsenic content of the root and the first 5 mm of the hair occur within hours after the ingestion of arsenic (Smith, 1964). The germinal cells are in relativity close equilibrium with circulating arsenic; thus, as arsenic concentrations in

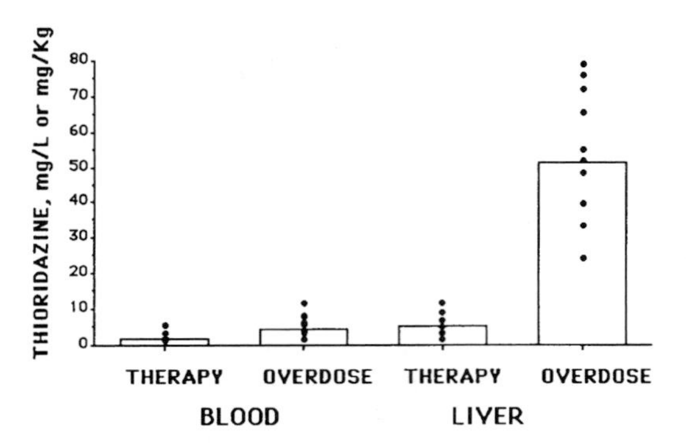


***Figure 31–6. Comparison of thioridazine blood and liver concentration after therapeutic and overdose ingestion.***

Liver concentrations clearly differentiate drug overdose from drug therapy. Bars represent mean values. (Data taken from Baselt RC et al: *J Anal Toxicol* 2:41–43, 1978; Poklis A et al: *J Anal Toxicol* 6:2250–2252, 1982.)

blood rise or fall, so does arsenic deposition in growing hair. Normal arsenic content in hair varies with nutritional, environmental, and physiological factors; however, the maximum upper limit of normal with a 99 percent confidence limit in persons not exposed to arsenic is 5 mg/kg (Shapiro, 1967). Hair grows at a rate of approximately 12.5 mm (½ in.) per month. Therefore, analysis of 1.0-cm segments provides a monthly pattern of exposure (Fig. 31-7). Such analyses often are performed in cases of homicidal poisoning to demonstrate that increases in arsenic deposition in the victim's hair correlate with times when a poisoner had an opportunity to administer the poison. Continuously elevated hair arsenic values indicate chronic rather than acute poisoning as the cause of death.

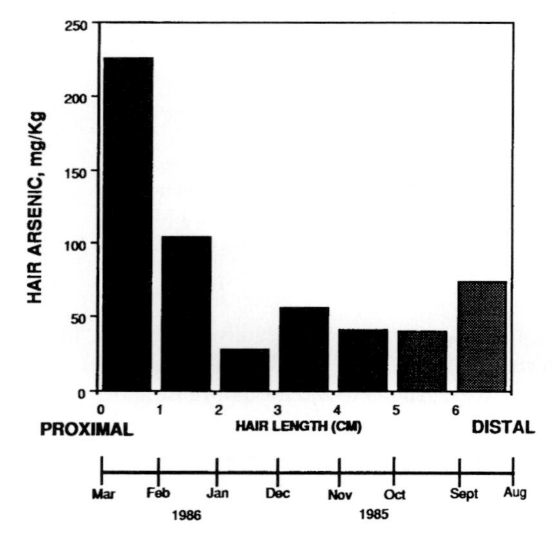


***Figure 31–7. Results of neutron activation analysis for arsenic in sequential sections of hair, demonstrating chronic arsenic poisoning. Increased exposure in the first two sections is consistent with fatal events. Lower values in section 3 are consistent with 2 weeks of hospitalization. (Data redrawn from Poklis A, Saady JJ: Arsenic poisoning: Acute or chronic? Suicide or murder?* **Am J Forensic Med Pathol** *11:226–232, 1990.)*

## COURTROOM TESTIMONY

A forensic toxicologist often is called to testify in legal proceedings. As a general rule of evidence, a witness may testify only to facts known to him or her. The witness may offer opinions solely on the basis of what he or she has observed (Moenssens et al., 1973). Such a witness is called a "lay witness." However, a toxicologist is referred to as an "expert witness." A court recognizes a witness as an expert if that witness possesses knowledge or experience in a subject which is beyond the range of ordinary or common knowledge or observation. An expert witness may provide two types of testimony: objective and "opinion." Objective testimony by a toxicologist usually involves a description of his or her analytic methods and findings. When a toxicologist testifies as to the interpretation of his or her analytic results or those of others, that toxicologist is offering an "opinion." Lay witnesses cannot offer such opinion testimony, as it exceeds their ordinary experience.

Before a court permits opinion testimony, the witness must be "qualified" as an expert in his or her particular field. In qualifying someone as an expert witness, the court considers the witness's education, on-the-job training, work experience, teaching or academic appointments, and professional memberships and publications as well as the acceptance of the witness as an expert by other courts. Qualification of a witness takes place in front of the jury members, who consider the expert's qualifications in determining how much weight to give his or her opinions during their deliberations.

Whether a toxicologist appears in criminal or civil court, worker's compensation or parole hearings, the procedure for testifying is the same: direct examination, cross-examination, and redirect examination. Direct examination is conducted by the attorney who has summoned the witness to testify. Testimony is presented in a question-and-answer format. The witness is asked a series of questions which allow him or her to present all facts or opinions relevant to the successful presentation of the attorney's case. During direct examination, an expert witness has the opportunity to explain to the jury the scientific bases of his or her opinions. Regardless of which side has called the toxicologist to court, the toxicologist should testify with scientific objectivity. Bias toward his or her client and prejudgments should be avoided. An expert witness is called to provide informed assistance to the jury. The guilt or innocence of the defendant is determined by the jury, not by the expert witness.

After direct testimony, the expert is questioned by the opposing attorney. During this cross-examination, the witness is challenged as to his or her findings and/or opinions. The toxicologist will be asked to defend his or her analytic methods, results, and opinions. The opposing attorney may imply that the expert's testimony is biased because of financial compensation, association with an agency involved in the litigation, or personal feelings regarding the case. The best way to prepare for such challenges before testimony is to anticipate the questions the opposing attorney may ask.

After cross-examination, the attorney who called the witness may ask additional questions to clarify any issues raised during cross-examination. This allows the expert to explain apparent discrepancies in his or her testimony raised by the opposing attorney.

Often an expert witness is asked to answer a special type of question, the "hypothetical question." A hypothetical question contains only facts that have been presented in evidence. The expert is then asked for his or her conclusion or opinion, based solely on this hypothetical situation. This type of question serves as a means by which appropriate facts leading to the expert's opinion are identified. Often these questions are extremely long and convoluted. The witness should be sure he or she understands all the facts and implications in the question. Like all questions, this type should be answered as objectively as possible.

## FORENSIC URINE DRUG TESTING

Concerns about the potentially adverse consequences of substance abuse both to the individual and to society have led to widespread urine analysis for the detection of controlled or illicit drugs (Gust and Walsh, 1989). Currently, such testing is conducted routinely by the military services, regulated transportation and nuclear industries, many federal and state agencies, public utilities, federal and state criminal justice systems, and numerous private businesses and industries. Significant ethical and legal ramifications are associated with such testing. Those having positive test results may not receive employment, be dismissed from a job, be court-martialed, or suffer a loss of reputation.

To assure the integrity of urine testing, two certification programs currently accredit forensic urine-testing laboratories. Laboratories conducting testing of federal employees are required to be certified under the Department of Health and Human Services Mandatory Guidelines for Workplace Drug Testing as published in the April 11, 1988, *Federal Register* (Department of Health and Human Services, 1988). The College of American Pathologists (CAP) also conducts a certification program for urine-testing laboratories. The federal program regulates a specific program from specimen collection through testing to the reporting of results, whereas the CAP program allows flexibility in the construction of programs servicing a broad range of clients. Both programs involve periodic on-site inspection of laboratories and proficiency testing.

Forensic urine drug testing (FUDT) differs from other areas of forensic toxicology in that urine is the only specimen analyzed and testing is performed for a limited number of drugs. At present, under the federal certification program, analyses are performed for only five drug classes or drugs of abuse (Table 31-2). While FUDT laboratories typically analyze 100 to 1000 urine specimens daily, only a relatively small number of those specimens are positive for drugs. To handle this large workload, initial testing is performed by immunoassays on high-speed, large-throughput analyzers. A confirmation analysis in FUDT certified laboratories is performed by GC/MS.

Proper FUDT is a challenge to good laboratory management. As with all forensic activities, every aspect of the laboratory operation must be thoroughly documented: specimen collection, chain of custody, quality control, procedures, testing, qualifications of personnel, and the reporting of the results. The facility must be constructed and operated to assure total security of specimens and documents. Confidentiality of all testing results is paramount; only specifically authorized persons should receive the results.

The presence of a controlled or illicit drug in a single random urine specimen is generally accepted as proof of recent or past substance abuse. However, positive urine drug findings are only evidence that at some time before the collection of the sample the individual was administered, self-administered, or was exposed to the drug. Positive urine tests do not prove impairment from the drug or abuse or addiction.

FUDT results are reported only as positive or negative for the drugs sought. Cutoff values are established for both the initial and confirmation assays (Table 31-2). The cutoff value is a concentration at or above which the assay is considered positive. Below the cutoff value, the assay is negative. Obviously, drugs may be present below the cutoff concentration. However, the use of cutoff values allows uniformity in testing and reporting results. All test reports indicate the drug tested and its cutoff value.

**Table 31–2**
**Forensic Urine Drug-Testing Analytes and Cutoff Concentrations**

| | CONCENTRATION, ng/ml | |
|---|---|---|
| | INITIAL TEST | CONFIRMATORY TEST |
| Marijuana metabolite(s) | 50 | 15† |
| Cocaine metabolite(s) | 300 | 150‡ |
| Opiate(s) | 300* | — |
| Morphine | — | 300 |
| Codeine | — | 300 |
| Phencyclidine | 25 | 25 |
| Amphetamines | 1000 | — |
| Amphetamine | — | 500 |
| Methamphetamine | — | 500 |

* 25 ng/ml if immunoassay specific for free morphine.
† Δ-9-tetrahydrocannabinol-9-carboxylic acid.
‡ Benzoylecognine.
SOURCE: Department of Health and Human Services, *Mandatory Guidelines for Federal Workplace Drug Testing Programs, Federal Register*, April 11, 1988, p 11983; revised: *Federal Register*, January 25, 1993, p 6063.

FUDT laboratories must be thoroughly familiar with all regulatory and analytic issues related to urine testing and devise strategies to resolve uncertainties. Many individuals who are subject to regulated urine testing have devised techniques to mask their drug use either by physiological means such as the ingestion of diuretics or by attempts to directly adulterate the specimen with bleach, vinegar, or other products which interfere with the initial immunoassay tests (Warren, 1989). In fact a miniindustry has developed to sell various products which are alleged to "fool drug testers." Thus, specimens are tested for adulteration by checking urinary pH, creatinine, and specific gravity and noting an unusual color or smell. Additionally, there may be valid reasons other than substance abuse that account for positive drug findings, such as therapeutic use of controlled substances, inadvertent intake of drugs via food, and passive inhalation. For example, the seed of *Papaver somniferum*, poppy seed, is a common ingredient in many pastries and breads. Depending on their botanical source, poppy seeds may contain significant amounts of morphine. Several studies have demonstrated that the ingestion of certain poppy seed foods results in the urinary excretion of readily detectable concentrations of morphine (ElSohly and Jones, 1989). Morphine is a major urinary metabolite of heroin. Therefore, to readily differentiate heroin abuse from poppy seed ingestion, analysis may be performed for 6-acetylmorphine, a unique heroin metabolite (Fehn and Megges, 1985).

Even over-the-counter medications may present potential problems for laboratories conducting urine drug testing. Methamphetamine may occur as a racemic mixture of *d* and *l* optical isomers. *d*-Methamphetamine, a Schedule II controlled substance, is a potent central nervous system stimulant subject to illicit drug abuse, while *l*-methamphetamine (*l*-desoxyephedrine) is an alpha-adenergic stimulant available in over-the-counter Vicks inhalers as a nasal decongestant. Cross-reactivity of *l*-desoxyephedrine with the initial immunoassay screening test may occur after excessive use of Vicks inhalers (Poklis and Moore, 1995). Additionally, the most popular confirmational GC/MS products for amphetamines are achiral. Therefore, if such analyses are performed, a "false-positive" result for *d*-methamphetamine may be reported. This dilemma is easily resolved if confirmational testing is done with a *chiral* GC/MS procedure which can readily resolve the stereoisomers of methamphetamine (Fitzgerald et al., 1988).

## HUMAN PERFORMANCE TESTING

Forensic toxicology activities also include the determination of the presence of ethanol and other drugs and chemicals in blood, breath, or other specimens and the evaluation of their role in modifying human performance and behavior. The most common application of human performance testing is to determine driving under the influence of ethanol (DUI) or drugs (DUID). Over the past half century, an enormous amount of data has been developed correlating blood ethanol concentrations with intellectual and physiological impairment, particularly of the skills associated with the proper operation of motor vehicles (Table 31-3). Numerous studies have demonstrated a direct relationship between an increased blood ethanol concentration (BAC) in drivers and an increased risk of involvement in road accidents (Council on Scientific Affairs, 1986). Alcohol-impaired drivers are responsible for 25 to 35 percent of all crashes causing serious injury. The threshold BAC for diminished driving performance is 0.05 g/dl, although the statutory definition of DUI in most states in the United States is 0.10 g/dl. In single-vehicle accidents, 55 to 65 percent of fatally injured drivers have BACs of 0.10 g/dl or greater.

During the past decade, there has been growing concern about the deleterious effects on driving performance of drugs other than ethanol. Several studies have demonstrated a relatively high occurrence of drugs in impaired or fatally injured drivers (White et al., 1981; Mason and McBay, 1984). These studies tend to report the highest drug use incidence rates which are associated with illicit or controlled drugs such as cocaine, benzodiazepines, marijuana, and phencyclidine. However, most studies test only for a few drugs or drug classes, and the repeated reporting of the same drugs may be a function of limited testing. Before DUID testing is as readily accepted by the courts as ethanol testing is, many legal and scientific problems concerning drug concentrations and driving impairment must be resolved (Consensus Report, 1985). The ability of analytic methodology to routinely measure minute concentrations of drug in blood must be established. Also, drug-induced driving impairment at specific blood concentrations in controlled tests and/or actual highway experience must be demonstrated.

## ANALYTIC ROLE IN CLINICAL TOXICOLOGY

Analytic toxicology in a clinical setting plays a role very similar to its role in forensic toxicology. As an aid in the diagnosis and treatment of toxic incidents, as well as in monitoring the effectiveness of treatment regimens, it is useful to clearly identify the nature of the toxic exposure and measure the amount of the toxic substance which has been absorbed. Frequently, this information, together with the clinical state of the patient, permits a clinician to relate the signs and symptoms observed to the anticipated effects of the toxic agent. This may permit a clinical judgment as to whether the treatment must be vigorous and aggressive or whether simple observation and symptomatic treatment of the patient are sufficient.

A cardinal rule in the treatment of poisoning cases is to remove any unabsorbed material, limit the absorption of additional poison, and hasten its elimination. The clinical toxicology laboratory serves an additional purpose in this phase of the treatment by monitoring the amount of the toxic agent remaining in circulation or measuring what is excreted. In addition, the laboratory can provide the data needed to permit estimations of the total dosage or the effectiveness of treatment by changes in known pharmacokinetic parameters of the drug or agent ingested. Some examples from our laboratory serve as illustrations of these aspects.

Ethylene glycol is a toxic solvent commonly used as an antifreeze in a number of commercial products found around the home. Upon ingestion, it is metabolized, in part by alcohol dehydrogenase, to a series of mixed aldehydes and carboxylic acids and eventually to oxalic acid (Mundy et al., 1974). Some of these metabolites are toxic to the kidney and can result in renal shutdown (Berman et al., 1957). Derivatives of ethylene glycol such as mono- and diesters produce similar toxic effects, as do diethylene glycol and its ether and ester derivatives.

**Table 31–3**
**Stages of Acute Alcoholic Influence/Intoxication**

| BLOOD-ALCOHOL CONCENTRATION (g/100 ml) | STAGE OF ALCOHOLIC INFLUENCE | CLINICAL SIGNS/SYMPTOMS |
|---|---|---|
| 0.01–0.05 | Subclinical | No apparent influence<br>Behavior nearly normal by ordinary observation<br>Slight changes detectable by special tests |
| 0.03–0.12 | Euphoria | Mild euphoria, sociability, talkativeness<br>Increased self-confidence; decreased inhibitions<br>Diminution of attention, judgment, and control<br>Beginning sensorimotor impairment<br>Slowed information processing<br>Loss of efficiency in finer performance tests |
| 0.09–0.25 | Excitement | Emotional instability; loss of critical judgment<br>Impairment of perception, memory, and comprehension<br>Decreased sensitory response; increased reaction time<br>Reduced visual acuity, peripheral vision, and glare recovery<br>Sensorimotor incoordination; impaired balance |
| 0.18–0.30 | Confusion | Disorientation, mental confusion; dizziness<br>Exaggerated emotional states (fear, rage, sorrow, etc.)<br>Disturbances of vision (diplopia, etc.) and of perception of color, form, motion, dimensions<br>Increased pain threshold<br>Increased muscular incoordination; staggering gait; slurred speech<br>Apathy, lethargy |
| 0.25–0.40 | Stupor | General inertia; approaching loss of motor functions<br>Markedly decreased response to stimuli<br>Marked muscular incoordination; inability to stand or walk<br>Vomiting; incontinence of urine and feces<br>Impaired consciousness; sleep or stupor |
| 0.35–0.50 | Coma | Complete unconsciousness; coma; anesthesia<br>Depressed or abolished reflexes<br>Subnormal temperature<br>Incontinence of urine and feces<br>Impairment of circulation and respiration<br>Possible death |
| 0.45+ | Death | Death from respiratory arrest |

SOURCE: Copyright © by Kurt M. Dubowski, Ph.D, DABFT, and reprinted with his permission.

Propylene glycol, by contrast, is relatively nontoxic, as are other polyethylene glycols. Labels for commercial products may not specify the type of glycol present. If ethylene glycol is not found to be present, the patient may still be at risk. However, if propylene glycol is present, aggressive therapy may not be indicated. It is important that the testing procedure discriminate between various glycols and other related substances. A chromatographic method such as gas chromatography is useful in such situations (Edinboro et al., 1993).

Treatment of ethylene glycol poisoning may involve the administration of ethanol, the preferred substrate for alcohol dehydrogenase, thus saturating the enzyme and permitting the excretion of ethylene glycol without metabolism to the toxic aldehydes and acids (Wacker et al., 1965). By monitoring the patient continuously for serum ethanol and ethylene glycol concentrations, a clinical toxicology laboratory can make sure that the appropriate concentration of ethanol is maintained and follow the excretion of ethylene glycol in order to determine when it is safe to discontinue the ethanol therapy.

Overdoses of drugs and toxic chemicals may lead to a variety of other changes in a patient which can be monitored by a clinical toxicology laboratory. The common analgesic acetaminophen, which is available for sale without a prescription, may be ingested excessively or accidentally by children. A portion of this drug is metabolized by the cytochrome P-450 mixed-function oxidase system to a toxic metabolite which is bound by glutathione and is excreted as a nontoxic conjugate. If enough drug is ingested to produce more of the metabolite than can be detoxified, hepatic necrosis can occur. A clinical toxicology laboratory can aid in the assessment of these patients by measuring the serum acetaminophen concentration at timed intervals. A significant increase in the half-life of the drug may indicate that hepatic injury has occurred, and aggressive therapy then may be initiated (Chap. 32).

It is evident that the utilization of the analytic capabilities of a clinical toxicology laboratory has increased enormously in recent years. Not only can toxic agents be ruled into consideration in a diagnosis, the absence of a toxic agent also may be of use to the clinician. Other uses of this laboratory service may include the assessment of ethanol or drugs in terms of behavior modification. It can be important to include this parameter in trauma cases, particularly when the patient is unable to communicate and surgery with the administration of anesthetic agents or analgesic agents is indicated. Psychiatrists need to know the effects of any self-administered drugs before performing psychiatric or neurological examinations.

While the instrumentation and the methodology used in a clinical toxicology laboratory are similar to those utilized by a forensic toxicologist, a major difference between these two applications is responsiveness. In the clinical setting, test results must be communicated to the clinician within hours for the results to be meaningful for therapy. A forensic toxicologist may carefully choose the best method for a particular test and conduct replicate procedures to assure maximum accuracy. A clinical laboratory cannot afford this luxury and frequently sacrifices accuracy for a rapid turnaround time. In addition, because it is impossible to predict when toxicological emergencies will occur, a clinical laboratory must be staffed and operated constantly. The necessity for staffing three shifts each day with trained analysts makes this type of clinical laboratory activity costly.

To partially offset these costs, it is frequently effective to apply the same trained analysts and special facilities to the measurement of drugs in patients receiving drugs for therapeutic purposes. Monitoring the serum concentration of drugs in patients undergoing a routine regimen of dosing generally is not an emergency procedure. The required assays can be planned to conform to a predetermined work schedule. This permits a more efficient utilization of staff and equipment than is the case when they are applied solely to clinical toxicology.

## ANALYTIC ROLE IN THERAPEUTIC MONITORING

Historically, the administration of drugs for long-term therapy was based largely on experience. A dosage amount was selected and administered at appropriate intervals, based on what the clinician had learned was generally tolerated by most patients. If the drug seemed ineffective, the dose was increased; if toxicity developed, the concentration was decreased or the frequency of dosing was altered. At times, a different dosage form might be substituted. Establishing an effective dosage regimen was particularly difficult in children and the elderly.

The factors responsible for individual variability in responses to drug therapy have been studied extensively. The important factors are summarized in Fig. 31-8 (Blaschke et al., 1985). In a given patient, when the various factors are assumed to be constant, the administration of the same dose of a drug at regular intervals eventually produces a steady-state condition (Fig. 31-9) (Moyer et al., 1986). When a steady state is established, the average plasma concentration of the drug remains relatively constant and is proportional to the fractional bioavailability of the dose and inversely related to the clear-

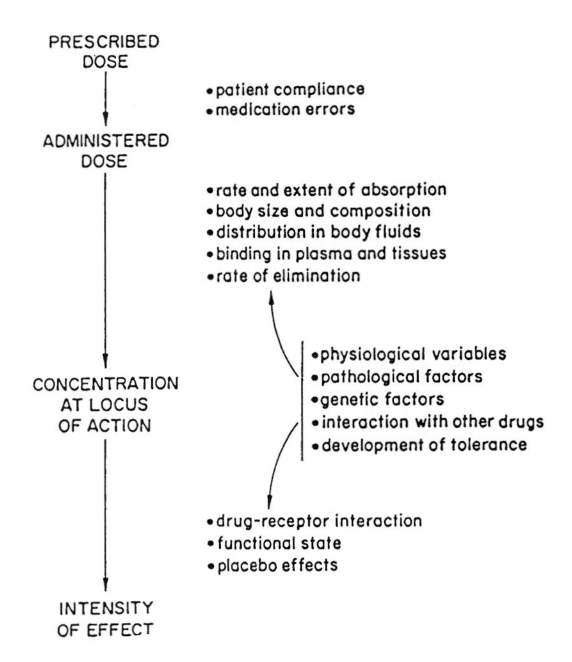


***Figure 31–8. Factors that determine the relationship between prescribed drug dosage and drug effect. (Modified from Koch-Weser J: Serum drug concentrations as therapeutic guides.* N Engl J Med *287:227–231, 1972.)***

ance of the drug from the plasma and the time interval of dosing:

$$C_{ss} = \frac{F \cdot \text{dose}}{Cl \cdot T}$$

Monitoring the plasma concentration at regular intervals will detect deviations from the average plasma concentration, which in turn may suggest that one or more of the variables

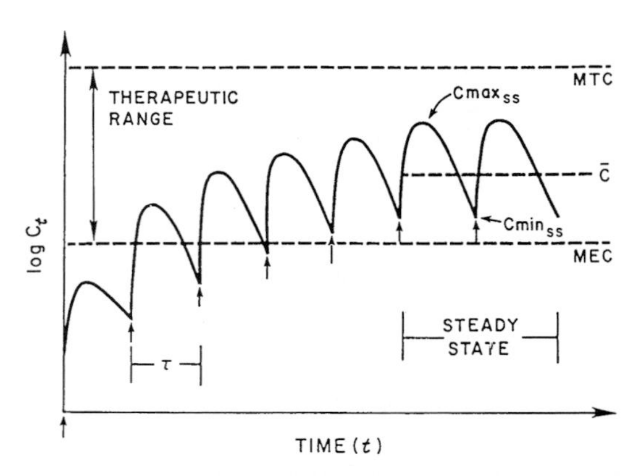


***Figure 31–9. Sequence of drug concentration changes with multiple identical doses.***

Note that at steady state peak and trough concentrations lie within the therapeutic range (or therapeutic window) and that five to seven half-lives are required to reach steady state. $C_{max}$ and $C_{min}$ = maximum and minimum steady-state concentrations; C = average steady state concentration; T = dosing interval; π = dose; MTC = minimum toxic concentration; MEC = minimum effective concentration. [Modified from Gilman AG, Goodman L, Gilman A (eds): *The Pharmacological Basis of Therapeutics*, 6th ed. New York: Macmillan, 1980, p 24.]

which cause deviations from the average plasma concentration need to be identified and corrected (Fig. 31-8).

Because the drug being administered is known, qualitative characterization of the analyte generally is not required. Quantitative accuracy is required, however. Frequently, the methodology applied is important, particularly in regard to its selectivity. For example, methods which measure both the parent drug and one of the metabolites are not ideal unless the individual analytes can be quantified separately. Depending on the drug, metabolites may not be active or may be active to a different degree than is the parent drug. The cardiac antiarrythmic drug procainamide is acetylated during metabolism to form *N*-acetylprocainamide (NAPA). This metabolite has antiarrythmic activity of almost equal potency to that of procainamide. There is bimodal genetic variation in the activity of the *N*-acetyltransferase for procainamide so that in "fast acetylators" the concentration of NAPA in the plasma may exceed that of the parent drug. For optimal patient management, information should be available about the concentrations of both procainamide and NAPA in plasma (Bigger and Hoffman, 1985).

Since absolute characterization of the analyte is not necessary for many drugs, immunoassay procedures are commonly used. This is particularly true of drugs with extremely low plasma concentrations, such as cardiac glycosides, and drugs which are difficult to extract because of a high degree of polarity, such as the aminoglycoside antibiotics. In these cases, plasma can be conveniently assayed directly by using commercially available kits for immunoassays.

The chromatographic methods, in which an appropriate internal standard is added, are favored when more than one analyte is to be measured or if metabolites with structures similar to those of the parent drugs must be distinguished. Since the nature of drugs is varied, many different analytic techniques may be applied, including atomic absorption spectrometry for measuring lithium used to treat manic disorders. Virtually all the tools of the analyst may be used for specific applications of analytic toxicology.

## ANALYTIC ROLE IN BIOLOGICAL MONITORING

In the workplace, good industrial hygiene practices require monitoring of the environment to which workers are exposed in order to identify potentially harmful amounts of hazardous chemicals. Despite these precautions, it has become apparent that monitoring a worker directly can be a better indicator of exposure because it can show what has actually been absorbed. This is biological monitoring, and it can take a variety of forms. Often environmental exposures are to a mixture of compounds and/or to compounds which are converted to physiologically important metabolites. Thus, analytic methods must be capable of separating a family of chemical agents and their major metabolites (Fig. 31-10). Additionally, methods most be sufficiently specific and sensitive to measure minute concentrations of the compounds in complex biological matrices.

An example of biological monitoring is presented in Table 31-4, which shows data relating to benzene exposure of chemists engaged in pesticide residue analysis in a state regulatory laboratory. Air-monitoring devices in this laboratory indicated

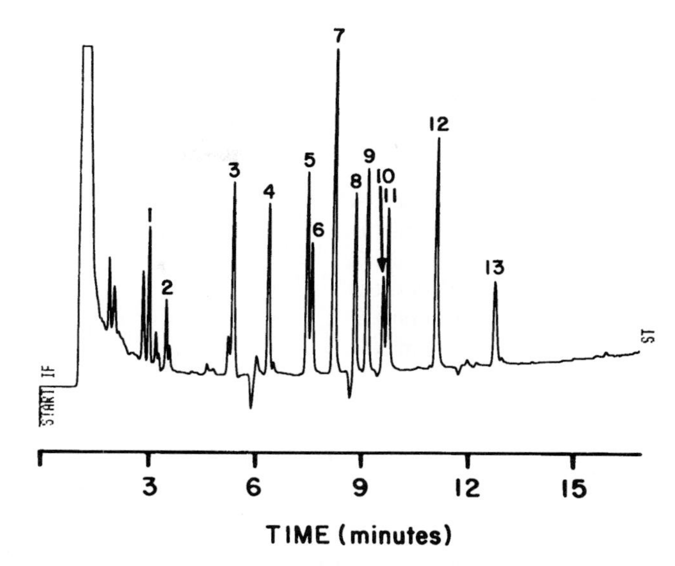


***Figure 31–10. Capillary gas chromatographic separation of chlorinated hydrocarbon pesticides added to human serum at concentrations ranging from 1 to 4 ng/ml.***

Peak number 1, $\alpha$-lindane; 2, $\gamma$-lindane; 3, heptachlor; 4, internal standard; 5, heptachlor epoxide; 6, oxychlordane; 7, $\gamma$-chlordane; 8, $\alpha$-chlordane; 9, trans-nonachlor; 10, dieldrin; 11, *p,p'*-DDE; 12, *p,p*-DDD; 13, *p,p'*-DDT. (Separation based on the method of Saady JJ, Poklis A: Determination of chlorinated hydrocarbon pesticides by solid phase extraction and capillary GC with electron capture detection. *J Anal Toxicol* 14:301–304, 1990.)

that the ambient benzene concentration never exceeded the time-weighted average (TWA) of 32 mg/m$^3$ (10 ppm). Monitoring of the breathing zone at different locations around the laboratory where benzene was in use showed other concentrations of this material. When expired air was monitored, one worker showed a significantly greater amount of benzene exposure than did others. Upon questioning, she recalled spilling some of the solvent on a laboratory bench, in the process saturating a portion of her laboratory coat. Presumably, her exposure by inhalation and skin absorption was considerably greater than was indicated by the air monitor.

In addition to the measurement of the chemical or its metabolites in the body fluids, hair, or breath of the worker, other, more indirect methods may be employed. Substances which interact with macromolecules may form adducts which persist for long periods. These adducts can be sampled periodically and potentially can serve as a means of integrating exposure to certain substances over long periods. For example, adducts of ethylene oxide with DNA or hemoglobin have been studied in workers. This technique also may be applicable in other situations that are not necessarily related to occupational hazards. Acetaldehyde, a metabolite of ethanol, forms adducts with hemoglobin. This marker may be of use in forensic cases (Stockham and Blanke, 1988).

Another approach that is useful in biological monitoring is to measure changes of normal metabolites induced by xenobiotics. The profile of glucuronic acid metabolites excreted in urine can be altered after exposure to substances which induce monooxygenase activity. Although monitoring the alteration of the urinary excretion of these metabolites may not indicate exposure to specific substances, this technique can be used in a generic fashion to flag a potentially harmful exposure to a

**Table 31–4**
**Benzene Exposure of Chemists Performing Pesticide Residue Analysis**

| SOURCE | BREATH BENZENE, ppm | AIR BENZENE, ppm |
|---|---|---|
| Chemist A | 0.45 | — |
| Chemist B | 0.13 | — |
| Chemist C | 0.41 | — |
| Chemist D | 0.48 | — |
| Chemist E | 0.34 | — |
| Chemist F | 0.37 | — |
| Chemist G | 2.50 | — |
| Chemist H | 0.56 | — |
| Fume hood breathing zone | — | 14.2 |
| Fume hood breathing zone | — | 51.2 |

hepatotoxic agent (Saady and Blanke, 1990). The early recognition of a toxicological problem may permit the protection of a worker before irreversible effects occur.

## SUMMARY

The analytic techniques initiated by forensic toxicologists have continued to expand in complexity and improve in reliability. Many new analytic tools have been applied to toxicological problems in almost all areas of the field, and the technology continues to open new areas of research. Forensic toxicologists continue to be concerned about conducting unequivocal identification of toxic substances in such a manner that the results can withstand a legal challenge. The problems of substance abuse, designer drugs, increased potency of therapeutic agents, and widespread concern about pollution and the safety and health of workers present challenges to the analyst's skills. As these challenges are met, analytic toxicologists continue to play a significant role in the expansion of the discipline of toxicology.

# REFERENCES


Aderjan R, Bahr H, Schmidt G: Investigation of cardiac glycoside levels in human postmortem blood and tissues determined by a special RIA procedure. *Arch Toxicol* 42:107–114, 1979.

Apple FS: Postmortem tricyclic antidepressant concentrations: Assessing cause of death using parent drug to metabolite ratio. *J Anal Toxicol* 13:197–198, 1989.

Benko A: Toxicological analysis of amobarbital and glutethimide from bone tissue. *J Forensic Sci* 30:708–714, 1985.

Berman LB, Schreiner GE, Feys J: The nephrotoxic lesion of ethylene glycol. *Ann Intern Med* 46:611–619, 1957.

Bigger JT Jr, Hoffman BF: Antiarrhythmic drugs, in Gilman AG, Goodman LS, Rall TW, Murad F (eds): *The Pharmacological Basis of Therapeutics*, 7th ed. New York: Macmillan, 1985, p 763.

Blanke RV: Quality assurance in drug-use testing. *Clin Chem* 33:41B–45B, 1987.

Blanke RV: *Validation of the Purity of Standards*. Irving, TX: Abbott Laboratories, Diagnostic Division, 1989.

Blanke RV, Decker WJ: Analysis of toxic substances, in Tietz NW (ed): *Textbook of Clinical Chemistry*. Philadelphia: Saunders, 1986, pp 1670–1744

Blaschke TF, Nies AS, Mamelock RD: Principles of therapeutics, in Gilman AG, Goodman LS, Rall TW, Murad F (eds): *The Pharmacological Basis of Therapeutics*, 7th ed. New York: Macmillan, 1985, p 52.

Chapuis: *Elements de toxicologie*, 1873, cited in Peterson F, Haines WS, Webster RW: *Legal Medicine and Toxicology*. 2d ed. Philadelphia: Saunders, 1923, vol 2.

Coe JI: Postmortem chemistry update: Emphasis on forensic applications. *Am J Forensic Med Pathol* 14:91–117, 1993.

Cone EJ, Buchwald WF, Darwin WD: Analytical controls in drug metabolism studies: 11. Artifact formation during chloroform extraction of drugs and metabolites with amine substitutes. *Drug Metab Dispos* 10:561–567, 1982.

Consensus Report: Drug Concentrations and Driving Impairment. *JAMA* 254:2618–2621, 1985.

Council on Scientific Affairs: Alcohol and the driver. *JAMA* 255:522–527, 1986.

Cravey RH, Baselt RC: The science of forensic toxicology, in Cravey RH, Baselt RC (eds): *Introduction to Forensic Toxicology*. Davis, CA: Biomedical Publications, 1981, pp 3–6.

Department of Health and Human Services, ADAMHA: Mandatory Guidelines for Federal Workplace Drug Testing: Final Guidelines: Notice. *Federal Register* 53(69):11970–11989, 1988.

DHHS, ADAMHA: Mandatory Guidelines for Federal Workplace Drug Testing Programs: Final Guidelines: Notice. *Federal Register* 53(69):11970–11989, 1988.

Dowling GP, McDonough ET, Bost RO: "Eve" and "Ecstasy": A report of five deaths associated with the use of MDEA and MDMA. *JAMA* 257:1615–1617, 1987.

Edinboro LE, Nanco CR, Soghoian DM, Poklis A: Determination of ethylene glycol in serum utilizing direct injection on a wide bore capillary column. *Ther Drug Monit* 15:220–223,1993

ElSohly MA, Jones AB: Morphine and codeine in biological fluids: Approaches to source differentiation. *Forensic Sci Rev* 1:13–22, 1989.

Evans WED: *The Chemistry of Death*. Springfield, IL: Charles C Thomas, 1963.

Fehn J, Megges G: Detection of O6-monoacetylmorphine in urine samples by GC/MS as evidence for heroin use. *J Anal Toxicol* 9:134–138, 1985.

Fisher RS, Hine CH, Stetler CJ (Committee on Medicolegal Problems): *Alcohol and the Impaired Driver: A Manual on the Medicolegal Aspects of Chemical Tests for Intoxication*. Chicago: American Medical Association, 1968.

Fitzgerald RL, Ramos JM, Bogema SC, Poklis A: Resolution of methamphetamine stereoisomers in urine drug testing: Urinary excretion of R(-)-methamphetamine following use of nasal inhalers. *J Anal Toxicol* 12: 255–259, 1988.

Garriott JS, Simmons LM, Poklis A, Mackell MS: Five cases of fatal overdose from caffeine-containing 'look-alike' drugs. *J Anal Toxicol* 9:141–143, 1985.

Gettler AD: Poisoning and toxicology, forensic aspects: Part 1. Historical aspects. *Inform* 9:3–7, 1977.

Goff ML, Brown WA, Omori AI, LaPointe DA: Preliminary observations of the effects of amitriptyline in decomposing tissue on the development of parasarcophaga ruficornis (Diptera: Sarcophagidae) and implications of this effect to estimation of postmortem interval. *J Forensic Sci* 38:316–322,1993.

Granger RH, Condie LW, Borzelleca JF: Effect of vehicle on the relative uptake of haloalkanes administered by gavage. *The Toxicologist* 40:1, 1987.

Gust SW, Walsh JM: *Drugs in the Workplace: Research and Evaluation Data*. NIDA Research Monograph 91. Washington, DC: U.S. Government Printing Office, 1989.

Hawks RL, Chiang CN: Examples of specific drug assays, in Hawks RL, Chiang CN (eds): *Urine Testing for Drugs of Abuse*. NIDA Research Monograph 73. Rockville, MD: U.S. Department Health and Human Services, PHS, ADAMHA, 1986, p 93.

Henderson GL: Designer drugs: Past history and future prospects. *J Forensic Sci* 33:569–575, 1988.

Hime GW, Hearn WL, Rose S, Cofino J: Analysis of cocaine and cocaethylene in blood and tissues by GC-NPD and GC-Ion Trap mass spectrometry. *J Anal Toxicol* 15:241, 1991.

Inoue T, Seta S: Analysis of drugs in unconventional samples. *Forensic Sci Rev* 4:89–107, 1992.

Jacob P, Lewis ER, Elias-Baker BA, Jones RT: A pyrolysis product, anhydroecgonine methyl ester (methylecgonidine), is in the urine of cocaine smokers. *J Anal Toxicol* 14:353, 1990.

Jones GR, Pounder DJ: Site-dependence of drug concentrations in postmortem blood—a case study. *J Anal Toxicol* 11:186–190, 1987.

Kaempe B: Interfering compounds and artifacts in the identification of drugs in autopsy material, in Stolman A (ed): *Progress in Chemical Toxicology*. New York: Academic Press, 1969, vol 4, pp 1–57.

Klaassen CD, Amdur MO, Doull J: *Casarett and Doull's Toxicology: The Basic Science of Poisons*, 3d ed. New York: Macmillan, 1986.

Martin BR, Lue LP, Boni JP: Pyrolysis and volatization of cocaine. *J Anal Toxicol* 13:158, 1989.

Mason AP, McBay AJ: Ethanol, marijuana, and other drug use in 600 drivers killed in single-vehicle crashes in North Carolina. *J Forensic Sci* 29:987–1026, 1984.

Mills RA, Millis CD, Dannan GA, et al: Studies on the structure-activity relationships for the metabolism of polybrominated biphenyls by rat liver microsomes. *Toxicol Appl Pharmacol* 78:96–104, 1985.

Moenssens AA, Moses RE, Inbau FE: *Scientific Evidence in Criminal Cases*. Mineola, NY: Foundation Press, 1973.

Moyer TP, Pippenger CE, Blanke RV: Therapeutic drug monitoring, in Tietz NW (ed): *Textbook of Clinical Chemistry*. Philadelphia: Saunders, 1986, pp 1615–1669.

Mundy RL, Hall LM, Teague RS: Pyrazole as an antidote for ethylene glycol poisoning. *Toxicol Applied Pharmacol* 28:320–322, 1974.

Panel on Herbicides: Report on 2,4,5-T, in *A Report of the Panel on Herbicides of the President's Science Advisory Committee*. Executive Office of the President, Office of Science and Technology, Washington, DC: U.S. Government Printing Office, 1971.

Petersen F, Haines WS, Webster RW: *Legal Medicine and Toxicology*, 2d ed. Philadelphia: Saunders, 1923, vol II.

Poklis A: Pentazocine/tripelennamine (T's and blues) abuse: A five year survey of St. Louis, Missouri. *Drug Alcohol Depend* 10:257–267, 1982.

Poklis A: Revised consensus opinion on applicability of hair analysis for drugs of abuse: Policy statement. Prepared by the SOFT advisory committee, October 15, 1992. *Forensic Sci Intern* 65:61–63, 1994.

Poklis A, Moore KA: Response of emit amphetamine immunoassays to urinary desoxyephedrine following Vicks inhaler use. *Ther Drug Monit* 17:89–94, 1995.

Pounder DJ: Forensic entomo-toxicology. *J Forensic Sci Soc* 31:469–472, 1991.

Prouty BS, Anderson WH: The forensic science implications of site and tempered influences on postmortem blood-drug concentrations. *J Forensic Sci* 35:243–270, 1990.

Saady JJ, Blanke RV: Measurement of glucuronic acid metabolites by high resolution gas chromatography. *J Chromatogr Sci* 28:282–287,1990.

Saady JJ, Narasimhachari N, Friedel RO: Unsuspected impurities in imipramine and desipramine standards and pharmaceutical formulations. *Clin Chem* 27:343–344, 1981.

SanGeorge RC, Hoberman RD: Reaction of acetaldehyde with hemoglobin. *J Biol Chem* 262:6811–6821, 1986.

Shapiro HA: Arsenic content of human hair and nails: Its interpretation. *J Forensic Med* 14:65–71, 1967.

Smith H: The interpretation of the arsenic content of human hair. *J Forensic Sci Soc* 4:192–199, 1964.

Stockham TL, Blanke RV: Investigation of an acetaldehyde-hemoglobin adduct in alcoholics: Alcoholism. *Clin Exp Res* 12:748–754, 1988.

Tagliro F (ed): *Hair Analysis as a Diagnostic Tool for Drugs of Abuse Investigation*. Proceeding of the 1st International Meeting, Genoa, Italy, December 10–11, 1992. Special Issue. *Forensic Sci Intern* 63:1–316,1993.

Thorwald J: *The Century of the Detective*. New York: Harcourt, 1965.

Vorpahl TE, Coe JI: Correlation of antemortem and postmortem digoxin levels. *J Forensic Sci* 23:329–334, 1978.

Wacker WEC, et al: Treatment of ethylene glycol poisoning with ethyl alcohol. *JAMA* 194:1231–1233, 1965.

Warren A: Interference of common household chemicals in immunoassay methods for drugs of abuse. *Clin Chem* 35:648–651,1989.

White JM, Clardy MS, Groves MH, et al: Testing for sedative-hypnotic drugs in the impaired driver: A survey of 72,000 arrests. *Clin Toxicol* 18:945–957, 1981.

# CHAPTER 32

# CLINICAL TOXICOLOGY

*Wayne R. Snodgrass*

Clinical toxicology is a rapidly expanding area that encompasses both acute and chronic exposure to drugs, chemicals, and naturally occurring toxins. Human toxicological exposures range from acute overdoses (accidental and deliberate) to chronic exposures (environmental and occupational). Treatment of a poisoned patient that is based on pharmacological principles promotes the use of rational methods that are beneficial to recovery. There is a great need for additional prospective, randomized, controlled, blinded clinical trials of treatment modalities in clinical toxicology. These are difficult studies to carry out in many instances. In the absence of such information, one must evaluate recommended therapies and procedures with appropriate skepticism and in the context of the best benefit-risk ratio for the individual patient.

This chapter reviews some of the principles of clinical management and current theory along with treatment of the more commonly encountered clinical toxicology events.

## TOXICOKINETICS

The application of pharmacokinetic principles to exposure to toxic substances may be useful in selected specific poisonings for the purpose of monitoring the severity and clinical course of the poisoning and for determining therapeutic maneuvers. Calculation of the body burden of a drug and its half-life and knowledge about its route or routes of excretion and other kinetic characteristics may be important in making decisions such as the use of activated charcoal, gastric lavage, whole-bowel irrigation, hemodialysis, and hemoperfusion. However, it is important to recognize that published drug and/or chemical human kinetic data often are based on therapeutic doses, not overdoses, in which the kinetics may be quite different. Thus, it is important for a physician to attempt to determine whether the data on which decisions are to be based are relevant to the overdose situation.

### $LD_{50}$ and MLD

$LD_{50}$ and MLD (median lethal dose) values generally are not of practical value for evaluating clinical toxicity. These parameters are determined in various animal species and are not directly or at times even proportionally extrapolatable to humans. The clinical history obtained in an overdose and/or exposure in an attempt to estimate the dose is known to be inaccurate in one-half or more of all cases. Thus, $LD_{50}$ and MLD often are disregarded; instead, careful monitoring, along with the clinical history, is done. A clinically useful estimate is MS (margin of safety), which may be defined as $LD_1/ED_{99}$, that is, the lethal dose (mg/kg) in 1 percent of a given human population divided by the therapeutically effective dose (mg/kg) in 99 percent of the population. This is a more conservative variation of the therapeutic index ($TI = LD_{50}/ED_{50}$). The $LD_1$ often may be approximated from the published case report literature on overdoses or exposures. The $ED_{99}$ in the case of drugs may be estimated from therapeutic clinical trial data on efficacy. A drug with a high MS ratio value generally requires a considerably higher dose relative to the therapeutic dose to cause toxicity in a patient. Overall, the adage "Treat the patient, not the poison" represents the most basic and important principle in clinical toxicology.

### Half-Life

The purpose of determining a drug or chemical half-life during a poisoning is to evaluate the rate at which a patient is getting rid of the excessive amount of drug in the body and to assess the effectiveness of a therapeutic procedure. The half-life is a measure of rate for the time required to eliminate one-half of a quantity of a chemical in the body. For drugs exhibiting first-order kinetics, the half-life can be calculated by the following equation, where *Kel* is the elimination rate constant:

$$t_{1/2} = \frac{0.693}{Kel}$$

A simple way to approximate the half-life in an individual patient is to estimate it graphically. In this process, one plots at least three plasma concentrations of the drug and/or chemical against time on semilogarithmic paper. Once at least three points have been plotted, if there is linear kinetics, a straight line should be evident. The amount of time it takes for the drug concentration to decrease by half from any point on the line can be estimated from the graph.

For some drugs, half-life values in the overdose situation are prolonged compared with values at therapeutic doses. Therefore, procedures to increase elimination in order to shorten a drug's half-life may be desirable.

### Kinetic Relationships

The volume of distribution is the apparent space in which an agent is distributed after absorption and subsequent distribution in the body. Salicylate is distributed in total body water, or about 60 percent of body mass. Digoxin, in contrast, has an enormous volume of distribution of 500 liters or more in a 70-kg human (approximately 7 liters/kg). Since this is impossible practically, the term "apparent" volume of distribution is utilized. While this is the apparent volume based on the measured value of the drug in the blood, the drug is concentrated or sequestered somewhere out of the blood, that is, in tissue compartments (Chaps. 5 and 7).

Some useful mathematic relationships are

$$Vd = \frac{D}{Cp} \qquad Cp = \frac{D}{Vd} \qquad D = Cp \cdot Vd$$

Where $Vd$ = volume of distribution
$D$ = dose administered
$Cp$ = plasma concentration (at zero time)

$$Cl = Kel \cdot Vd$$

Where $Cl$ = clearance of drug
$Kel$ = elimination rate constant

$$Kel = \frac{0.693}{t_{1/2}}$$

Thus, if the history is that of a 25-kg child who is estimated to have consumed 500 mg of phenobarbital and the $Vd$ for phenobarbital is approximately 60 percent body weight, the estimated blood level will be 33.3 $\mu$g/ml. This approximates phenobarbital's high therapeutic range.

Example calculations:

$$25 \text{ kg} \times 0.60 \text{ liter/kg} = 15 \text{ liters} = Vd$$

$$500 \text{ mg}/15 \text{ liters} = 33.3 \text{ mg/liter or } 33.3\ \mu\text{g/ml}$$

In this case, the decision will be made clinically that the maximum possible dose by history, assuming total absorption, can produce toxicity. Therefore, the child probably needs to be seen and observed by medical personnel.

## MEASURES TO ENHANCE ELIMINATION

Once a patient has been observed clinically to be in a seriously toxic state, it must be determined whether the agent can be eliminated more rapidly, thus shortening the duration of coma and lessening toxic manifestations. Procedures for enhancing elimination may be indicated in severely poisoned patients.

### Diuresis

The basic principle of diuresis is ion trapping. Urinary flow was increased to two to three times normal in the past, but this has been replaced with adjustment of urine pH and maintenance of normal urine flow. The ion-trapping phenomenon occurs when the $pK_a$ of the agent is such that after glomerular filtration in the renal tubules, alteration of the pH of the urine can ionize and "trap" the agent. Once the toxin is ionized, reabsorption from the renal tubules is impaired, and as a result, more of the drug is excreted in the urine. Salicylate and phenobarbital elimination is significantly enhanced by an alkaline diuresis. Because of problems with acid diuresis, this procedure is rarely used. Even though a drug's $pK_a$ may indicate that the drug might be successfully eliminated by this method, other factors, such as high lipid solubility and a large volume of distribution, may render this method ineffective (Table 32–1).

**Table 32–1**
**Toxicokinetic Data of Drugs and Toxins (Numbers Expressed as a Mean or as a Range)**

| AGENT | $pK_a$ | $Vd$ l/kg | THER. $t_{1/2}$ h | O.D. $t_{1/2}$ h | URINE ENHANCEMENT | DIALYSIS | SPECIFIC THERAPY |
|---|---|---|---|---|---|---|---|
| Acetaminophen | 9.5 | 0.75 | 2 | 4 | No | No | *N*-Acetylcysteine |
| Amitriptyline | 9.4 | 40+ | 36 | 72 | No | No | |
| Amobarbital | 7.9 | 2.4 | 16 | 36+ | No | No | |
| Amphetamine | 9.8 | 0.60 | 8–12 | 18–24 | Acid | Yes | Chlorpromazine |
| Bromide | — | 40+ | 300 | 300 | Yes | Yes | |
| Caffeine | 13 | 0.75 | 3.5 | 4–120 | No | No | |
| Chloral hydrate | — | 0.75 | 8 | 10–18 | No | No | |
| Chlorpromazine | 9.3 | 40+ | 16–24 | 24–36 | No | No | |
| Codeine | 8.2 | 3 | 2 | 2 | No | No | Naloxone |
| Coumadin | 5.7 | 0.1 | 36–48 | 36–48 | No | No | Vitamin K |
| Desipramine | 10.2 | 50+ | 18 | 72 | No | No | |
| Diazepam | 3.3 | 1–2 | 36–72 | 48–144 | No | No | |
| Digoxin | — | 7–10 | 36 | 13 | No | No | Fab antibodies |
| Diphenhydramine | 8.3 | — | 4–6 | 4–8 | No | No | |
| Ethanol | — | 0.6 | 2–4 | — | No | No | |
| Ethchlorvynol | 8.7 | 3–4 | 1–2 | 36–48 | No | No | |
| Glutethimide | 4.5 | 20–25 | 8–12 | 24+ | No | No | |
| Isoniazid | 3.5 | 0.60 | 2–4 | 6+ | No | Yes | Pyridoxine |
| Methadone | 8.3 | 6–10 | 12–18 | 12–18 | No | No | Naloxone |
| Methicillin | 2.8 | 0.60 | 2–4 | 2–4 | Yes | Yes | |
| Pentobarbital | 8.11 | 2.0 | 10–20 | 50+ | No | No | |
| Phencyclidine | 8.5 | — | — | 12–48 | Acid | Yes | |
| Phenobarbital | 7.4 | 0.75 | 36–48 | 72–120 | Alkaline | Yes | |
| Phenytoin | 8.3 | 0.60 | 24–30 | 36–72 | No | No | |
| Quinidine | 4.3, 8.4 | 3 | 7–8 | 10 | No | No | |
| Salicylate | 3.2 | 0.1–0.3 | 2–4 | 25–30 | Alkaline | Yes | |
| Tetracycline | 7.7 | 3 | 6–10 | 6–10 | No | No | |
| Theophylline | 0.7 | 0.46 | 4.5 | 6+ | No | Yes | |

In theory, for drugs whose renal elimination is flow-dependent, increasing urine output through the use of fluids or diuretics may enhance drug or toxin elimination. Few drugs are responsive solely to urine flow. The risks of fluid diuresis include pulmonary edema and cardiac arrhythmias or failure.

## Dialysis

The dialysis technique, either peritoneal dialysis or hemodialysis, relies on passage of the toxic agent through a semipermeable dialysis membrane so that it can equilibrate with the dialysate and subsequently be removed. This is in part dependent on the molecular weight of the compound. Some drugs, such as phenobarbital, can readily cross these membranes and go from a high concentration in plasma to a lower concentration in the dialysate. Because the volume of distribution of phenobarbital is 75 percent of body weight, there is a reasonable opportunity for enough drug to be removed from the total body burden to make the technique valuable in serious cases. Conversely, drugs with large volumes of distribution can be expected to be poorly dialyzable. Similarly, drugs that are highly serum protein bound are not expected to be well removed by dialysis (Watanabe, 1977) (Table 32–2).

# APPROACH TO THE POISONED PATIENT

Estimation of the severity of poisoning is an important initial step. A thorough history and details of exposure and/or poisoning should be obtained, and a physical examination should be performed.

Clinical evaluation includes the use of one of several available clinical scoring systems for coma, hyperactivity, and withdrawal. These scoring systems serve as useful monitoring parameters to follow in order to determine whether the patient's condition is improving or deteriorating. They also are useful to semiquantitate clinically the response to therapy. Table 32–3 identifies these scoring methods and criteria.

In the United States and most developed countries, there are now regional poison centers with expertise available for consultative toxicology services. These poison centers are available by telephone to physicians and toxicologists who seek information from their large toxicology databases (Rumack, 1994; Thompson et al., 1983).

## Emesis

Published clinical trials of patients with oral overdose ingestions do *not* show that induced emesis (usually with ipecac syrup; much less frequently used is apomorphine or a mild liquid detergent) improves patient outcome compared with the use of oral or gastrically instilled activated charcoal. Note that the more clinically relevant measure of efficacy is patient outcome, not the percentage of gastric contents removed. In fact, the data in the majority of published prospective clinical trials show that activated charcoal alone or activated charcoal preceded by gastric lavage is superior to ipecac. By contrast, some studies do show that induced emesis results in a greater risk of adverse effects, primarily aspiration pneumonitis resulting from aspiration of gastric contents into the trachea and lung. No published studies show that induced emesis results in

**Table 32–2**
**Drug Toxin Removal by Dialysis, Intensive Supportive Care, and Use of Activated Charcoal**

| *Well Adsorbed by Activated Charcoal* | |
|---|---|
| Amphetamines | Nicotine |
| Antimony | Opium |
| Antipyrene | Oxalates |
| Atropine | Parathion |
| Arsenic | Penicillin |
| Barbiturates | Phenol |
| Camphor | Phenolphthalein |
| Cantharides | Phenothiazine |
| Cocaine | Phosphorus |
| Digitalis | Potassium permanganate |
| Glutethimide | Quinine |
| Iodine | Salicylates |
| Ipecac | Selenium |
| Malathion | Silver |
| Mercuric chloride | Stramonium |
| Methylene blue | Strychnine |
| Morphine | Sulfonamides |
| Muscarine | |
| *Increased Clearance with Multiple Doses of Activated Charcoal* | |
| Carbamazepine | Nadolol |
| Dapsone | Phenobarbital |
| Digoxin | Salicylates |
| Digitoxin | Theophylline |
| *Dialysis Indicated on Basis of Condition of Patient* | |
| Amphetamines | Isoniazid |
| Anilines | Meprobamate (Equanil, Miltown) |
| Antibiotics | Paraldehyde |
| Boric acid | Phenobarbital |
| Bromide | Potassium |
| Calcium | Salicylates |
| Chloral hydrate | Strychnine |
| Fluorides | Thiocynates |
| Iodides | |
| *Dialysis Not Indicated Except for Support in the Following Poisons; Therapy Is Intensive Supportive Care* | |
| Antidepressants (tricyclic and MAO inhibitors also) | |
| Antihistamines | |
| Chlordiazepoxide (Librium) | |
| Digitalis and related | |
| Diphenoxylate (Lomotil) | |
| Ethchlorvynol (Placidyl) | |
| Glutethimide (Doriden) | |
| Hallucinogens | |
| Heroin and other opiates | |
| Methaqualone (Quaalude) | |
| Noludar (Methyprylon) | |
| Oxazepam (Serax) | |
| Phenothiazines | |
| Synthetic anticholinergics and belladonna compounds | |

**Table 32–3**
**Scoring Systems for Coma, Hyperactivity, and Withdrawal**

| | *Classification of Coma* |
|---|---|
| 0 | Asleep but can be aroused and can answer questions |
| 1 | Comatose; does withdraw from painful stimuli; reflexes intact |
| 2 | Comatose; does not withdraw from painful stimuli; most reflexes intact; no respiratory or circulatory depression |
| 3 | Comatose; most or all reflexes are absent but without depression of respiration or circulation |
| 4 | Comatose; reflexes absent; respiratory depression with cyanosis, circulatory failure, or shock |

| | *Classification of Hyperactivity* |
|---|---|
| 1+ | Restlessness, irritability, insomnia, tremor, hyperreflexia, sweating, mydriasis, flushing |
| 2+ | Confusion, hyperactivity, hypertension, tachypnea, tachycardia, extrasystoles, sweating, mydriasis, flushing, mild hyperpyrexia |
| 3+ | Delirium, mania, self-injury, marked hypertension, tachycardia, arrhythmias, hyperpyrexia |
| 4+ | Above plus convulsions, coma, circulatory collapse |

*Classification of Withdrawal*

Score the following findings on a 0-, 1-, 2-point basis:

| | | |
|---|---|---|
| Diarrhea | Hypertension | Restlessness |
| Dilated pupils | Insomnia | Tachycardia |
| Gooseflesh | Lacrimation | Yawning |
| Hyperactive bowel sounds | Muscle cramps | |

1–5, mild
6–10, moderate
11–15, severe

Seizures indicate severe withdrawal regardless of the rest of the score

fewer adverse effects compared with oral activated charcoal (Kulig et al., 1985; Albertson et al., 1989; Merigian et al., 1990; Rumack, 1985; Vale et al., 1986; Rodgers et al., 1986; Kornberg et al., 1991; Underhill et al., 1990; Saetta et al., 1991; Saetta and Quinton, 1991). Thus, the use of ipecac syrup typically should be limited to individual patients in whom it is likely to make a difference in outcome, in whom it appears to be the most effective method available in that particular set of circumstances, or in whom it is the only method available to achieve the goal of gastric emptying.

## Lavage

The efficacy with which gastric lavage removes gastric contents decreases with time after ingestion. Gastric lavage should be considered only if a patient has ingested a life-threatening amount of a toxic agent, usually within 1 h or a very few hours previously. Gastric lavage with a large-bore tube (36 to 40 French size) is a rapid way to remove some of the contents of the stomach; however, some contents may be pushed beyond the pylorus into the small intestine, increasing unwanted absorption of the drug and/or chemical. There is no strong clinical evidence to support the opinion that in general lavage later than 1 h or a few hours after a toxic ingestion will benefit patients; this includes ingested drugs with anticholinergic activity and/or drugs that delay gastric emptying, such as tricyclic antidepressants and aspirin. Nevertheless, uncommonly in individual patients, large amounts of gastric contents have been removed many hours after ingestion (Kulig et al., 1985; Albertson et al., 1989; Merigian et al., 1990; Underhill et al., 1990).

## Cathartics

The use of cathartics is no longer recommended routinely in the management of orally ingested poisons. There is no strong evidence to indicate that the use of cathartics improves patient outcome. Recent data suggest that cathartics may not alter patient outcome when adequate continuous intragastric activated charcoal is infused (e.g., 0.2 g/kg/h with bowel sounds present). When cathartics are used alone, the absorption of some drugs [area under the curve (AUC)] is increased (Picchioni et al., 1982; Al-Shareef et al., 1990). One must not repeatedly administer a cathartic to a patient with absence of bowel sounds. The uncommon pseudoobstruction of the intestine during the administration of multiple-dose activated charcoal may not be prevented with the cathartic sorbitol (Longdon et al., 1992). The reported adverse effects of cathartics include dehydration, hypernatremia, hypermagnesemia, hyperphosphatemia, hypokalemia, and hypocalcemia. For serious oral poisonings in which rapid clearing of the intestine beyond the pyloris is indicated, the use of whole-bowel irrigation utilizing Golytely or Colyte may offer greater efficacy with minimal evidence of fluid or electrolyte shifts. Typical cathartics include magnesium citrate and sorbitol. Oil-based cathartics almost never should be considered because of the risk of aspiration (Shannon et al., 1986; Sue et al., 1994; Farley, 1986; Krenzelok et al., 1985; Neuvonen et al., 1986).

## Whole-Bowel Irrigation

Whole-bowel irrigation (WBI) is not a routine procedure but may be used in selected patients with a reasonable expectation of good efficacy (when measured as reduction of bioavailability) and relatively less evidence of adverse effects. WBI involves the enteral administration of large volumes of an isosmotic electrolyte lavage solution containing polyethylene glycol (PEG-ELS) (e.g., Colyte or GoLytely) by orogastric or nasogastric tube at a rapid rate until the rectal effluent becomes clear. The purpose of this procedure is to irrigate out the contents of the gastrointestinal (GI) tract to prevent or decrease the absorption of toxic substances. The PEG-ELS is isosmotic and results in minimal or not measurable electrolyte and fluid changes in most patients. Published results typically show an approximately 65 to 75 percent reduction in the bioavailability of ingested drugs in volunteer studies. Adverse effects include vomiting from overly rapid infusion rates. Contraindications include ileus, GI hemmorrhage, GI obstruction, and GI perforation. Relative contraindications include compromised circulation and a compromised airway. Indications include excessive ingestions of iron, lithium, and sustained-release resin-form tablets/capsules and possibly acute ingestion of heavy metals [e.g., paint chips containing lead (Pb)]. WBI has been used to hasten rectal passage of packets of illicit drugs (e.g., swallowed condoms containing cocaine) ingested for the purpose of smuggling drugs. The WBI procedure consists of orogastric or nasogastric tube administration of PEG-ELS at about 25 to 40 ml/kg/h. The duration of infusion is determined by the goal of therapy, which is passage of a clear rectal effluent (Tenenbein et al., 1987; Kirshenbaum et al., 1989; Smith et al., 1991; Buckley et al., 1993).

## Activated Charcoal

Activated charcoal currently is the single most useful agent for the prevention of absorption of ingested drugs and chemicals. In many cases of acute oral overdose, it may be administered (typically 1.0 g/kg per orogastric tube or nasogastric tube of plain activated charcoal not containing sorbitol) without prior ipecac-induced emesis or gastric lavage. When the ingested agent is not adsorbed to charcoal or the situation warrants a different approach based on patient presentation and clinical judgment, other means of GI decontamination may be considered. Table 32–2 indicates agents for which charcoal and dialysis may be useful.

Prospective, randomized, controlled clinical trials in overdose patients have indicated that charcoal alone, compared with gastric emptying procedures with or without charcoal, results in at least similar patient outcomes with fewer complications (Kulig et al., 1985; Albertson et al., 1989; Merigian et al., 1990).

Table 32-4 lists substances not significantly adsorbed to activated charcoal and substances which sometimes are cited as not being adsorbed to activated charcoal but for which there is published evidence that significant adsorption occurs. There is a great need for additional published comprehensive and detailed in vivo laboratory animal data (AUC, repeat plasma drug and/or chemical concentration measurements, and degree of change/nonchange of $LD_{50}$ or $LD_{90}$) to determine the in vivo efficacy/nonefficacy of single-dose and multiple-dose activated charcoal for a variety of important clinically encountered drug/chemical oral, parenteral, or inhaled overdoses and/or exposures. Drugs and toxins for which there is a great need for in vivo laboratory animal data for activated charcoal efficacy/nonefficacy include but are not limited to verapamil, flecainide, clonidine, propranolol, procainamide, disopyramide, amiodarone, sotalol, flosequinan, glyburide, glypizide, chlorpropamide, cocaine, ephedrine, phenylpropanolamine, cyclosporin, azathioprine, methotrexate, vincristine, cyclophosphamide, doxorubicin, mercaptopurine, cisplatin, bleomycin, colchicine, podophyllin, etoposide, diazepam, baclofen, bupropion, buspirone, clozapine, risperidone, ethchlorvynol, pargyline, phenelzine, tranylcypromine, isocarboxazid, delta-9-tetrahydrocannabinol, terfenadine, diphenhydramine, methapyriline, etretinate, isotretinoin, acyclovir, amantadine, amphotericin, gentamicin, minoxidil, ibuprofen, ketorolac, mefenamic acid, ethylene glycol, camphor, toluene, benzene, paraquat, diazinon, chlorpyrifos, furniture polish, food poisoning toxins, alpha-amanitin (mushroom), rattlesnake venom, brown recluse spider venom, black widow spider venom, Pb, mercury/mercuric chloride/methylmercury/phenyl mercury, arsenic/organic arsenicals, strychnine, tetrachloroethylene, trichloroethylene, lindane, deet (Off), ricin (castor bean plant), solanine alkaloids (various plants), aconitine (various plants and herbal medicines), coniine (poison hemlock), cicutoxin (water hemlock), saxitoxin (paralytic shellfish poisoning), and ciguatera toxin.

**Table 32–4**

| *Substances Not Significantly* Adsorbed to Activated Charcoal as Demonstrated by Published Studies* |
|---|
| Iron |
| Lithium |
| Borates |
| Bromide |
| Potassium |
| Mineral acids and alkalis |
| Ethanol† |
| *Substances Sometimes Cited as Not Being Adsorbed to Activated Charcoal but for Which There Is Published Evidence That Significant* Adsorption Occurs* |
| Cyanide |
| Malathion |
| Diazinon |
| DDT |
| Carbamates |
| Mercuric chloride |
| Methanol |
| *N*-methyl carbamate |
| Ethylene glycol |
| Kerosene |
| Turpentine |
| Isopropyl alcohol |
| Tolbutamide |

* "Significant" in this context is arbitrarily defined when 50 g of activated charcoal could adsorb a toxic dose (significant symptoms expected) in adults based on an extrapolation of in vitro data or in vivo studies in which toxicity or morbidity was shown to be decreased by charcoal.

† Ethanol appears to be adsorbed in vitro but not in vivo, including in humans.

Multiple-dose activated charcoal (MDAC) involves the repeated administration (more than two doses) of oral or orogastric/nasogastric tube activated charcoal to enhance the elimination of drugs already absorbed into the body. Studies in animals and human volunteers have shown that MDAC increases drug elimination significantly, but few prospective randomized controlled clinical studies in poisoned patients have been published showing a reduction in morbidity or mortality. The early use of MDAC is an attractive alternative to more complex methods of enhancing toxin elimination, such as hemodialysis and hemoperfusion, although only in a relatively small subset of patients. Generally, patients with mild to moderate intoxications may benefit the most from MDAC. The decision to use MDAC depends on the physician's clinical judgment regarding the expected clinical outcome, the efficacy of MDAC for the specific condition of the patient, the presence of contraindications (e.g., intestinal obstruction) to the use of MDAC, and the effectiveness of alternative methods of therapy.

MDAC is thought to produce its beneficial effect by interrupting the enteroenteric-enterohepatic circulation of drugs and by binding any drug which diffuses from the circulation into the gut lumen. After absorption, a drug may reenter the gut lumen by passive diffusion if the intraluminal concentration is lower than that in blood. The rate of this passive diffusion depends on the concentration gradient and the intestinal surface area, permeability, and blood flow. Under these "sink" conditions, a concentration gradient is maintained and drug passes continuously into the gut lumen, where it is adsorbed to charcoal. Pharmacokinetic characteristics of drugs that favor enhanced elimination by MDAC include (1) significant enteroenteric-enterohepatic circulation, including the formation of active recirculating metabolites, (2) prolonged plasma half-life after an overdose, (3) small (<1.0 liter/kg) volume of distribution, (4) limited (<60 percent) plasma protein binding, (5) a $pK_a$ that maximizes transport of drug across cell membranes, (6) sustained-release/resin-form tablets and/or capsules, and (7) onset of organ failure (e.g., kidney) of a major route of elimination of drug that is no longer available so that MDAC may make a considerable contribution to total body clearance.

The technique for MDAC is to give via an orogastric tube or nasogastric tube a loading dose of 1.0 g/kg of plain activated charcoal (not the combination product that contains sorbitol) followed by a continuous infusion intragastrically of 0.2 g/kg/h. The duration of infusion depends on the clinical status of the patient and repeated monitoring of plasma drug levels where indicated (Ilkhanipour et al., 1992; Ohning et al., 1986; Chyka et al., 1993; Goulbourne et al., 1994; Mofenson et al., 1985; Park et al., 1983, 1986; Pollack et al., 1981; Van de Graaff et al., 1982).

### Hemoperfusion

Passing blood through a column of charcoal or adsorbent resin is an important technique for extracorporeal drug and/or toxin removal. While some agents are better removed by this technique because of the adsorptive capacity of the column, the volume of distribution of an agent may limit removal in a similar manner to hemodialysis. Theophylline is an example of an agent that is amenable to this technique. If the drug is highly tissue bound, such as in fat stores, and only a small proportion is presented via the blood compartment to a device, only the proportion that is in blood is available for removal. To date, few agents have been found that are able to significantly displace toxins from either fat stores or tissue binding sites. The application of digoxin Fab antibodies in digoxin overdose represents one clinically useful example (Smith, 1985).

### Laboratory

Measurement of plasma, urine, or gastric levels of drugs or toxins when done in appropriate relationship to time after ingestion and clinical status can have a significant impact in the clinical management of a poisoned patient. Qualitative screens on blood and urine are helpful in identifying ingested toxins, whereas quantitative analyses are useful in determining appropriate therapy with selected toxins (e.g., methanol, iron, acetaminophen). When a toxic screen is requested, the clinician must know which drugs are actually being examined. Too often the clinician interprets a negative toxic screen to mean that there are no toxic agents on board. Interpretation of a patient's levels should be related to the therapeutic levels from the same laboratory. Statements such as "lethal level" are not relevant because toxicologists assume that most patients who arrive alive in the emergency department will eventually recover. Where possible, specific relationships of blood levels will be presented with each drug discussed in the following sections of this chapter (Curry, 1974).

## ACETAMINOPHEN

Acetaminophen has been utilized as an analgesic and antipyretic since the mid-1950s and has become more prominently recognized as a potential hepatotoxin in the overdose situation since the original British reports in the late 1960s (Proudfoot and Wright, 1970). Work on the mechanisms of the liver toxicity of this drug has provided a theoretical basis for therapy (Mitchell et al., 1973).

Acetaminophen in normal individuals is inactivated by sulfation (approximately 52 percent) and glucuronide conjugation (42 percent). About 2 percent of the drug is excreted unchanged. The remaining 4 percent is biotransformed by the cytochrome P-450 mixed-function oxidase system. This P-450 metabolic process results in a potentially toxic metabolite that is detoxified by conjugation with glutathione and excreted as the mercapturate. Evidence extrapolated from animals indicates that when 70 percent of endogenous hepatic glutathione is consumed, the toxic metabolite becomes available for covalent binding to hepatic cellular components. The ensuing hepatic necrosis can be expected to take place after absorption of 15.8 g of acetaminophen, the amount needed to deplete glutathione in a normal 70-kg human. Other factors may alter this figure. Ingestion of 15.8 g may not produce toxicity if the dose is not entirely absorbed, if the history is inaccurate, if the patient has a biotransformation inhibitor on board such as piperonyl butoxide, or if the patient suffers from anorexia nervosa. However, patients on long-term biotransformation enhancers (microsomal enzyme inducers) such as phenobarbital may produce more than 4 percent of the toxic metabolite. The range of metabolic response and the difficulty of estimating accurately the amount ingested and absorbed preclude the possibility of making therapeutic decisions on a historical predictive basis alone (Peterson and Rumack, 1977).

The clinical presentation of these patients is also sufficiently confusing in some cases to make waiting for the appearance of symptoms inadequate for diagnosis.

Follow-up liver biopsy studies of patients who have recovered 3 months to a year after hepatotoxicity have demonstrated no long-term sequelae or chronic toxicity (Clark et al., 1973). A very small percentage (0.25 percent) of patients in the national multiclinic study conducted in Denver may progress to hepatic encephalopathy with subsequent death. The clinical nature of the overdose is one of a sharp peak of serum glutamic-oxalocaetic transaminase (SGOT) by day 3, with recovery to less than 100 IU/liter by day 7 or 8. Patients with SGOT levels as high as 20,000 IU/liter have shown complete recovery and no sequelae 1 week after ingestion (Arena et al., 1978).

Laboratory evaluation of a potentially poisoned patient is crucial in terms of both hepatic measures of toxicity and plasma levels of acetaminophen. Accurate estimation of acetaminophen in the plasma should be done on samples drawn 4 h after ingestion, when peak plasma levels can be expected.

Once an accurate plasma level has been obtained, it should be plotted on the Rumack-Matthew nomogram to determine whether therapy is indicated (Fig. 32-1). This nomogram is based on a series of patients with and without hepatotoxicity and their corresponding blood levels. While half-life was once considered an accurate way to determine potential acetaminophen hepatotoxicity, it is no longer considered adequate because the toxic metabolite constitutes about 4 percent of the total biotransformation. Similarly, back extrapolation of data to the zero-hour axis may not accurately reflect initial levels because the slope of the excretion curve does not necessarily reflect hepatic toxicity.

Treatment should be instituted in any patient with a plasma level in the potentially toxic range. Standard support with gastric lavage should be followed by oral administration of *N*-acetylcysteine (Mucomyst). A major national multiclinic open study has demonstrated a protective effect of *N*-acetylcysteine (NAC) in acetaminophen poisoning when contrasted with controls not receiving antidotal therapy (Rumack et al., 1981; Smilkstein et al., 1988). Because NAC is most effective if it is given prior to 16 h after ingestion, patients in whom blood levels cannot be obtained should have NAC treatment instituted and therapy terminated only if levels are nontoxic. The dosing regimen for NAC is a loading dose of 140 mg/kg orally,

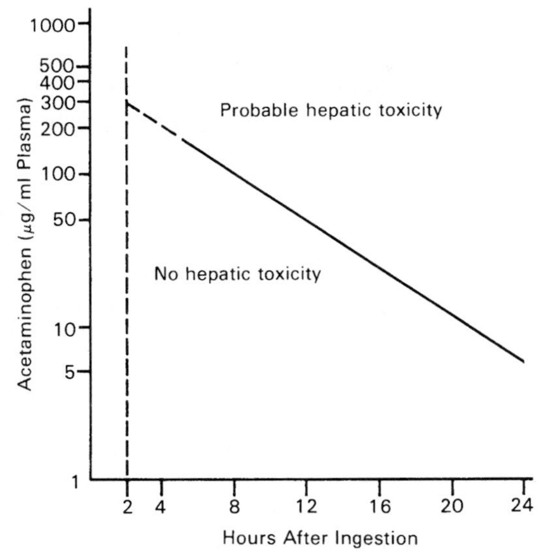


***Figure 32–1. Rumack-Matthew nomogram for acetaminophen poisoning.***

Cautions for use of chart: (1) The time coordinates refer to time of ingestion. (2) Serum levels drawn before 4 h may not represent peak levels. (3) The graph should be used only in relation to a single acute ingestion. (4) A half-life greater than 4 h indicates a high likelihood of significant hepatic injury. [From Rumack and Matthew (1975). Copyright American Academy of Pediatrics 1975.]

followed by 70 mg/kg orally for 17 additional doses (Peterson and Rumack, 1977).

Children less than 9 to 12 years of age have a lower incidence of hepatotoxicity after an overdose than do adults (Rumack, 1984).

Daily SGOT, serum glutamate pyruvate transaminase (SGPT), bilirubin, and prothrombin time should be monitored. Chronic ethanol ingestion is additive in its hepatotoxicity when acetaminophen poisoning is superimposed, whereas acute ethanol ingestion as a single ingestion concomitantly with acetaminophen is protective (Rumack et al., 1981). The same effect occurs in children (Rumack, 1984).

## ACIDS

Acids such as hydrochloric acid, nitric acid, sulfuric acid, and sodium bisulfate are commonly found around the home in products such as toilet bowl cleaners, automobile batteries, and swimming pool cleaning agents. Despite the fact that these agents have various degrees of toxicity, even a very small amount (milliliters) can result in serious sequelae that can occasionally progress to death, for example, if the caustic acid agent is aspirated. Clinically, the patient may present with irritation and crying in association with inability to swallow, pain on swallowing, mucous membrane burns, circumoral burns, hematemesis, abdominal pain, respiratory distress (secondary to epiglottal edema), shock, and renal failure. Once the patient has been treated through the initial stages of the ingestion, residual sequelae may occur with lesions of the esophagus and GI tract that may progress to scarring and strictures. Ingestion of concentrated acids has led to necrosis of esophageal tissue, with death occurring 1 to 5 days after ingestion.

The use of emetics and lavage is absolutely contraindicated (Penner, 1980; Friedman and Lovejoy, 1984). Dilution or therapy with water or milk *immediately* after ingestion represents the treatment of choice, as these substances do not result in an exothermic chemical reaction. Alkaline substances and carbonate preparations are contraindicated because when administered, they may produce increased amounts of heat and carbonates may form carbon dioxide gas, which presents an unacceptable risk of gastric perforation. Immediate irrigation with copious amounts of water should be instituted to the exposed areas of skin, mucous membranes, and other affected areas. Analgesics administered by the parenteral route may be indicated. The development of shock requires appropriate treatment with fluid therapy and pressor agents as indicated. Development of laryngoedema may require placement of an endotracheal tube, and esophagoscopy should be considered in all patients with significant symptoms that indicate extensive burn involvement. Acids are more likely to produce gastric burns than esophageal burns. Corticosteroid therapy for the prevention of stricture and scar formation with acid burns has not been proved to be of benefit.

## ALKALIES

Strong alkaline substances are found in products such as Drano, Liquid Plummer, and Clinitest Tablets, all of which contain compounds such as sodium hypochlorite, sodium hydroxide, and potassium hydroxide. Experience has shown that strongly basic substances such as these are likely to produce injuries more severe than those seen after acidic caustic ingestions. Chlorinated bleaches, which contain a 3 to 6 percent concentration of sodium hypochlorite, are not very toxic. After an ingestion of sodium hypochlorite, this compound interacts with the acidic milieu of the stomach, producing hypochlorous acid, which is an irritant to the mucous membranes and skin but does not cause stricture formation. More serious problems are presented after ingestions of compounds such as Drano, which can cause burns of the skin, mucous membranes, and eyes almost immediately on contact. However, the absence of evidence of burns, irritation, erythema, and other such signs in the oral or circumoral area does not necessarily indicate that esophageal injury does not exist (Gaudreault et al., 1983). There have been cases demonstrating the absence of oral involvement, with subsequent esophagoscopy proving esophageal burns. Edema of the epiglottis may result in respiratory distress, and inhalation of fumes may result in pulmonary edema or pneumonitis. Shock may occur. "Button" batteries, which contain concentrated solutions of sodium or potassium hydroxide, represent a serious risk for leakage, corrosion, and perforation when lodged in the esophagus (Litovitz, 1983).

Alkaline caustic exposures require immediate irrigation of the affected areas with large amounts of water. Exposures to the eyes require irrigation for a minimum of 20 to 30 min and may require instillation of a local anesthetic to treat the blepharospasm. Oral ingestions require immediate dilution therapy with water or milk. Vinegar and lemon juice are absolutely contraindicated (Lacouture et al., 1986). Ingestion of chlorinated bleaches does not necessarily require esophagoscopy unless a highly concentrated solution has been ingested or the patient is demonstrating symptoms or signs of esophageal burns. Dexamethasone has not been beneficial (Anderson et al., 1990). Bougienage (passage of a cannula) has been reported to be of some benefit for subsequent dilation of strictures of the esophagus. Antibiotic therapy should be instituted if mediastinitis occurs. Further information on the treatment of alkaline poisoning can be found in several publications (Haller, 1971; Burrington, 1974; Rumack and Temple, 1977; Howell, 1986).

## AMPHETAMINE AND RELATED DRUGS

Stimulant drugs such as amphetamine and methylphenidate can produce anxiety, hyperpyrexia, hypertension, and severe central nervous system (CNS) stimulation. A paranoid psychosis is not uncommon, especially as the patient begins to come off the "high." These tablets and capsules are used as "diet" pills even though they are clearly not effective as anorexic agents after 2 weeks of therapy. Street "speed," "crystal," or "crystal ice" may contain in addition to or in lieu of amphetamine compounds such as caffeine, strychnine, phencyclidine (PCP), or phenylpropanolamine (Pentel, 1984; Linden et al., 1985).

Therapy for a severely agitated patient should be directed toward tranquilization with chlorpromazine and acid diuresis to ion-trap and promote excretion (Espelin and Done, 1968; Linden et al., 1985). The dose of chlorpromazine should be 1 mg/kg in a pure amphetamine overdose and 0.5 mg/kg if the amphetamine has been mixed with a barbiturate. A major problem with this therapy is the interaction of chlorpromazine with several street drugs, such as STP, MDA, and DMT, which may produce dramatic hypotension. If the history is not definitive for amphetamine, diazepam at 0.1 to 0.3 mg/kg as a starting intravenous dose should be administered.

Acid diuresis may rarely be instituted in severe cases with sufficient intravenous fluids to produce a urine flow of 3 to 6 ml/kg/h. Ammonium chloride, at 75 mg/kg/dose administered intravenously four times per day, to a maximum of 6 g total dose per day, may be used. This will produce a urine with a pH range of 4.5 to 5.5. Rhabdomyolysis (myoglobinuria) seen with phencyclidine poisoning is a contraindication to acid diuresis.

## ANTICHOLINERGICS

A number of agents may produce anticholinergic toxicity after an acute overdose; these agents include drugs such as antihistamines (Benadryl, Dramamine, Chlor-Trimeton), atropine, homatropine, over-the-counter sleeping medications (which contain both antihistamines and belladonnalike agents), and certain plants (e.g., jimsonweed, deadly nightshade) (Rumack et al., 1974; Mikolich et al., 1975; Bryson et al., 1978). Antihistamines are readily available in many common nonprescription products as well as in prescription medications. Plants containing belladonna alkaloids, such as jimsonweed, are frequently used in folk medicine cures for the common cold or as hallucinogens by thrill seekers. Patients with anticholinergic toxicity may present with atropinic symptoms, including dry mouth; thirst; fixed, dilated pupils; flushed face; fever; hot, dry red skin; and tachycardia. Speech and swallowing may be impaired in association with blurred vision. In infants, particularly those ingesting antihistamines, paradoxic excitement may occur, followed by a more characteristic CNS depression. Severe overdoses can present with hallucinationlike delirium, tremors, convulsions, coma, respiratory failure, or cardiovascular collapse. Potentially fatal doses of most antihistamines have been estimated to be approximately 25 to 30 mg/kg.

Immediate treatment may include lavage followed by the administration of activated charcoal. Severe prolonged seizures may respond to the cautious use of physostigmine 0.5 to 2.0 mg IV repeated if needed every 15 to 30 min.

## CYANIDE

Cyanide is commonly found in certain rat and pest poisons, silver and metal polishes, photographic solutions, and fumigating products. Compounds such as potassium cyanide can be readily purchased from chemical stores. Cyanide is readily absorbed from all routes, including the skin and mucous membranes, and by inhalation, although the alkali salts of cyanide are toxic only when ingested. Death may result from the ingestion of even small amounts of sodium or potassium cyanide and can occur within minutes to several hours, depending on the route of exposure. Inhalation of toxic fumes represents a potentially rapidly fatal type of exposure. Sodium nitroprusside (Smith and Kruszyna, 1974) and apricot seeds (Sayre and Kaymakcalan, 1964) also have caused cyanide poisoning. A blood cyanide level greater than 0.2 $\mu$g/ml may be associated with toxic manifestations. Lethal cases usually have involved levels above 1 $\mu$g/ml. Clinically, cyanide poisoning is reported to produce a bitter, almond odor on the breath of the patient; however, approximately 20 percent of the population is genetically unable to discern this characteristic odor. Typically, cyanide has a bitter, burning taste, and after poisoning, symptoms of salivation, nausea without vomiting, anxiety, confusion, vertigo, giddiness, lower jaw stiffness, convulsions, opisthotonos, paralysis, coma, cardiac arrhythmias, and transient respiratory stimulation followed by respiratory failure may occur (Hall et al., 1987). Bradycardia is a common finding, but in most cases heartbeat outlasts respirations (Wexler et al., 1947). A prolonged expiratory phase is considered to be characteristic of cyanide poisoning.

Artificial respiration with 100% oxygen should be started immediately in patients with respiratory difficulty or apnea. Administration of 1 to 2 ampoules of amyl nitrite by inhalation to the patient for 15 to 30 s every minute should be instituted concurrently while sodium nitrite is prepared for intravenous administration (Chen and Rose, 1952; Graham et al., 1977). Amyl nitrite has the ability to induce methemoglobin, which has a higher affinity for cyanide than does hemoglobin; however, amyl nitrite alone can produce only a 5 percent methemoglobin level (Stewart, 1974). The Lilly cyanide kit (Lilly stock no. M76) contains ampoules of amyl nitrite, sodium nitrite, and sodium thiosulfate with appropriate instructions. Sodium nitrite, 300 mg intravenously, should be administered to adults to attain a desired methemoglobin level of approximately 25 percent. However, doses this high should not be administered to children, as potentially fatal methemoglobinemia may result (Berlin, 1970). Children weighing less than 25 kg must be dosed on the basis of their hemoglobin levels and weight. In the absence of immediate serum hemoglobin levels, a dose of 10 mg/kg is considered safe (Berlin, 1970). Once intravenous sodium nitrite is administered, sodium thiosulfate should be given immediately. Thiosulfate combines with available cyanide to form thiocyanate, which is readily excreted in the urine (Chen and Rose, 1952; Stewart, 1974; Graham et al., 1977). Oxygen also should be given, as it increases the effectiveness of the nitrites and the thiosulfate. Oxygen therapy should be maintained during and after thiosulfate therapy to ensure adequate oxygenation of the blood. A methemoglobin level greater than 50 percent is an indication for exchange transfusion or administration of blood. Since cyanide toxicity may recur, the patient should be observed for no less than 24 to 48 h, and recurrence is an indication for retreatment with sodium nitrite and sodium thiosulfate in one-half the recommended doses. Data indicate that the use of hydroxycobalamin may be of value in the treatment of cyanide poisoning (Bain and Knowles, 1967; Hillman et al., 1974; Posner et al., 1976). However, experience in the United States with this compound is limited owing to its lack of availability. Further clinical experience is required to evaluate the role of these agents in the treatment of cyanide poisoning.

## DIGITALIS GLYCOSIDES

Digitalis glycosides are available in prescription medications as digoxin (Lanoxin) and digitoxin as well as through a number of plant sources (oleander, foxglove). Many ingestions of digitalis occur in infants who inadvertently get into a grandparent's heart medication, although the drug has been used on occasion for suicide. Acute toxic manifestations of the digitalis glycosides represent extensions of the compound's vagal effects. The clinical manifestations seen in an acute overdose include nausea, vomiting, bradycardia, heart block, cardiac arrhythmia, and cardiac arrest. Younger individuals without significant heart disease tend to present with bradycardia and heart block, whereas other patients may present with ventricular arrhythmias, with or without heart block (Ekins and Watanabe, 1978). While hypokalemia is a frequent hallmark associated with chronic digitalis poisoning, in the acute overdose situation hyperkalemia is found more frequently. Serum digoxin levels in excess of 5 $\mu$g/liter (ng/ml) are often seen.

Emesis or lavage is indicated, followed by the administration of activated charcoal with saline cathartics. Potassium administration is contraindicated unless there is documented hypokalemia, as potassium administration with unsuspected concurrent digitalis-induced hyperkalemia in an overdose situation may result in heart block progressing to sinus arrest. Patients should be monitored by ECG, and antiarrhythmics should be instituted for the treatment of arrhythmias. Phenytoin (Dilantin) is considered to be the antiarrhythmic of choice for ventricular arrhythmia (Rumack et al., 1974), whereas atropine has been shown to be useful in the treatment of severe bradycardia. Pacemaker therapy may be required in refractory cases. The use of resin-binding agents such as cholestyramine (Cuemid, Questran) and colestipol has been recommended to minimize the absorption of cardiac glycosides as well as to interrupt the enterohepatic circulation of these compounds. A major advance in the treatment of digitalis poisoning is the use of Fab fragments for digoxin's specific antibodies (Lloyd and Smith, 1978). Clinical experience with this method is now available and has clearly shown its efficacy for digoxin and digitoxin overdose (Smith et al., 1982; Smith, 1985).

## ETHANOL

Excessive consumption of ethanol produces a depressed state that may be additive if depressants such as sedatives, hypnotics, and tranquilizers have also been consumed. The following tabulation (Lambecier and DuPan, 1968) summarizes clinical findings at various blood levels:

| BLOOD ETHANOL | |
|---|---|
| 50–150 mg/100 ml | Incoordination, slow reaction time, and blurred vision |
| 150–300 mg/100 ml | Visual impairment, staggering, and slurred speech; marked hypoglycemia, especially in children |
| 300–500 mg/100 ml | Marked incoordination, stupor, hypoglycemia, and convulsion |
| 500 mg and over/100 ml | Coma and death, except in tolerant individuals |

One patient who was reported to exhibit a peak level of 780 mg/100 ml was capable of holding a normal conversation at 520 mg/100 ml and related a history of chronic alcoholism (Hammond et al., 1973). Hypoglycemia occurring as ethanol levels are falling is a complication of ethanol poisoning in children.

Absorption of ethanol from the GI tract is rapid, particularly in the fasting state, with peak blood levels attained within 30 to 60 min after ingestion. Metabolism in adults eliminates 7 to 11 g of ethanol per hour, which is equivalent to 0.5 to 1 oz of 50-proof beverage per hour. A rule of thumb is that 1 ml of absolute ethanol per kilogram of body weight results in a level of 100 mg/100 ml in 1 h (Elbel and Schleyer, 1956). Although ethanol is considered to be biotransformed according to zero-order kinetics (Wilkinson, 1976), some patients with high levels have been found to have ethanol metabolism that demonstrates first-order kinetics (Hammond et al., 1973; David and Spyker, 1979).

Treatment of ethanol overdose consists of intensive supportive care. Attention must be directed toward hypoglycemia and acidosis. Chronic alcoholics may experience delirium tremens. During ethanol withdrawal, conservative management and benzodiazepines or other sedatives can adequately control these symptoms and prevent convulsions. Dialysis is rarely indicated unless the patient is unable to dispose of the ethanol because of hepatic or renal failure.

## HYDROCARBONS—PETROLEUM DISTILLATES

Hydrocarbons and petroleum distillates are available in a wide variety of forms, including motor oil, gasoline, kerosene, red seal oil, and furniture polish, and in combination with other chemicals as a vehicle or solvent. The toxicity of hydrocarbons generally is indirectly proportional to the agent's viscosity, with products having high viscosity (150 to 250), such as heavy greases and oils, being considered to have only limited toxicity. Products with viscosity in the range of 30 to 35 or lower present an extreme aspiration risk and include agents such as mineral seal oil, which is found in furniture polishes. It is important to realize that even small amounts of a low-viscosity material, once aspirated, can involve a significant portion of the lung and produce a chemical pneumonitis. Oral ingestion of hydrocarbons often is associated with symptoms of mucous membrane irritation, vomiting, and CNS depression. Cyanosis, tachycardia, and tachypnea may appear as a result of aspiration, with subsequent development of chemical pneumonitis. Other clinical findings include albuminuria, hematuria, hepatic enzyme derangement, and cardiac arrhythmias. Doses as low as 10 ml orally have been reported to be potentially fatal, whereas other patients have survived the ingestion of 60 ml of petroleum distillates (Baldochin et al., 1964; Rumack, 1977; Truempier et al., 1987). A history that presents with coughing or choking in association with vomiting strongly suggests aspiration and hydrocarbon pneumonia. Hydrocarbon pneumonia is an acute hemorrhagic necrotizing disease that can develop within 24 h after the ingestion. Pneumonia may require several weeks for complete resolution.

Activated charcoal and/or emesis may be indicated in some hydrocarbon ingestions in which absorption may produce systemic effects. Agents such as asphalt, tar, heavy lubricants, Vaseline, and mineral oil are considered relatively nontoxic and do not require removal. Chlorinated hydrocarbon solvents or any hydrocarbon or petroleum distillate with a potentially dangerous additive (camphor, pesticide, heavy metals) in some cases may be treated with activated charcoal or emesis. Petroleum naphtha derivatives, gasoline, kerosene, and mineral seal oil (or signal oil) as found in furniture polish and oil polishes produce severe and often prolonged chemical pneumonitis (Beaman et al., 1976; Rumack, 1977). These compounds are poorly absorbed from the stomach but are very damaging to the lung if inhaled. They should *not* be removed by emesis unless very large amounts are ingested (greater than 12 to 18 ml/kg) (Bratton and Haddow, 1974). Gastric lavage is not indicated for hydrocarbon ingestion because of the risk of aspiration if the patient vomits around the lavage tube (Ng et al., 1974). X-rays taken early in the course of ingestion may not demonstrate chemical pneumonia; even if it is demonstrated, the clinical severity does not correlate well with the degree of x-ray findings. However, x-rays should be repeated on follow-up to detect the development of pneumonitis or demonstrate pneumatoceles (Bergson, 1975; Subcommittee on Accidental Poisoning, 1976). Patients who arrive coughing probably already have aspirated and should be monitored closely for the development of pneumonitis. The decision for hospitalization should be based on clinical criteria (e.g., cyanosis, respiratory distress) rather than on x-ray findings alone (Anas et al., 1981). Steroid therapy may be harmful (Marks et al., 1972; Brown et al., 1974). Antibiotics, oxygen, and positive end-expiratory pressure should be instituted as indicated (Steele et al., 1972; Rumack, 1977).

## CHRONIC SOLVENT EXPOSURE AND CHRONIC ENVIRONMENTAL CHEMICAL EXPOSURE

Chronic solvent exposure, especially at high long-term dose levels in some occupational settings, now is increasingly recognized as a risk for the development of neurotoxicity in humans. In its more severe form, the term "solvent encephalopathy" has been used. Typically, there is about 12 to 14 or more years of work exposure to solvents, often to aromatic hydrocarbons but also to aliphatic hydrocarbons and halogenated hydrocarbons. Impairment may consist of decrements in memory functioning, cognitive functioning, and sometimes neuromotor function such as maintaining standing and/or walking balance and coordination (Hartman, 1988; Hogstedt et al., 1980; Gilli et al., 1990; Antoine et al., 1986; Axelson et al., 1988; Ekberg et al., 1988; Seppalainen, 1988; van Vliet et al., 1989).

Objective findings on physical examination may include increased risk for color vision and shades of gray impairment, abnormal neurophysiological testing (e.g., evoked potentials), and abnormal neuropsychological testing (e.g., Halstead-Reitan group of tests for intellectual functioning, memory, perceptual-motor speed and accuracy, and psychomotor abilities) (Mergler et al., 1987, 1990; Ghittori et al., 1987; Droz et al., 1989; Ledin et al., 1989; Kelsey et al., 1989; Bolla et al., 1990; Morrow et al., 1990; Odkvist et al., 1983; Hagstadius et al., 1989; NIOSH, 1987).

Chronic solvent exposure should not be confused with persons claiming so-called multiple chemical sensitivity the [preferred terminology is multiple environmental complaints (MEC)], which has been shown to be a psychological malfunction, often a somatization disorder, with no proven relationship to the toxicity of chemicals (Simon et al., 1993).

## INSECTICIDES

### Chlorinated Hydrocarbons

Chlorinated hydrocarbon insecticides are stable lipophilic chemicals and usually are contained in various organic solvents or as petroleum distillates. Often the petroleum distillates or organic solvents used as vehicles for the chemicals are as toxic as are the pesticides themselves, and in the event of a significant ingestion, the vehicle toxicity should be considered as well (i.e., hydrocarbon pneumonitis). Many chlorinated hydrocarbon insecticides are rapidly absorbed and produce CNS toxicity. Because of the halogenated nature of these organic compounds, hepatotoxicity, renal toxicity, and myocardial toxicity also may occur. Examples of chlorinated hydrocarbons include chlordane, DDT, dieldrin, chlordecone (Kepone), lindane, toxaphene, and *p*-dichlorobenzene. Clinical manifestations after ingestion include apprehension, agitation, vomiting, GI upset, abdominal pain, and CNS depression. Convulsions may occur at higher doses and may be preceded by symptoms of ataxia, muscle spasms, and fasciculations.

In cases of ingestion, activated charcoal often is indicated. Epinephrine is contraindicated because it may induce ventricular fibrillation as a result of sensitization of the myocardium by chlorinated hydrocarbons. Convulsions may be treated with lorazepam or diazepam in a dose of 0.1 mg/kg administered intravenously to a maximum of 10 mg. Methods to enhance elimination have not been successful other than as a supportive measure for hepatic and renal failure. Cholestyramine, which has been shown to bind chlordecone (Kepone) in the intestinal tract, may offer a means to treat chronic Kepone poisoning and, pending further study, may have application to other agents (Boylan et al., 1978).

### Organophosphates

Organophosphate insecticides such as diazinon, malathion, parathion, TEPP, and DFP are potent cholinesterase enzyme inhibitors that act by interfering with the metabolism of acetylcholine, resulting in the accumulation of acetylcholine at neuroreceptor transmission sites. Exposure produces a broad spectrum of clinical effects that are indicative of massive overstimulation of the chlorinergic system, including muscarinic effects (parasympathetic), nicotinic effects (sympathetic and motor), and CNS effects (Namba, 1971; Minton and Murray, 1988). These effects present clinically as feelings of headache, weakness, dizziness, blurred vision, psychosis, respiratory difficulty, paralysis, convulsions, and coma. Typical findings are given by the mnemonic SLUD (*s*alivation, *l*acrimation, *u*rination, and *d*efecation). A small percentage of patients may fail to demonstrate miosis, a classic diagnostic hallmark (Mann, 1967). The onset of the clinical manifestation of organophosphate poisoning usually occurs within 12 h of exposure. Measurement of red cell cholinesterase usually is diagnostic; when there is a reduction to 50 percent or less of control values, this indicates significant poisoning and is an indication for the institution of 2-PAM [pralidoxime (Protopam)], a cholinesterase-regenerating agent. Efforts must be made to ensure that the patient does not become reexposed through contaminated clothing or reexposure to the contaminated environment. Decontamination may be achieved by using soap washings followed by alcohol-soap washings with tincture of green soap. Rescuers and medical personnel should be protected from contamination by using rubber gloves and aprons.

Maintaining adequate respiratory function should be the first treatment measure taken. In cases of ingestion, activated charcoal is indicated. Atropine is the drug of first choice (especially in patients with respiratory problems) and should be administered until lung sounds of rales or rhonchi decrease or until signs of atropinism occur, such as dry mouth and tachycardia. In some cases, large doses (up to 2 g of atropine) may be required to reverse cholinergic excess. The presence of significant cholinesterase depression in red blood cells requires treatment with 2-PAM in conjunction with atropine. In an adult, a dose of 1 g intravenously should be given and repeated every 8 to 12 h, or a continuous infusion of approximately 3 mg/kg/h preceded by a single loading dose of 4 mg/kg will on average result in a plasma level of pralidoxime of about 4 $\mu$g/ml (Thompson et al., 1987). The pediatric dose consists of the same continuous infusion regimen or 250 mg/dose administered slowly by the intravenous route and repeated every 8 to 12 h.

## IRON

Iron is available in a wide variety of preparations, including iron supplement tablets (ferrous sulfate, ferrous gluconate, ferrous fumarate), multiple-vitamin preparations, and prenatal vitamin preparations. As described on the labels of these preparations, the amount of iron given may be calculated in terms of a milligram amount of the salt form (e.g., ferrous sulfate 300 mg or ferrous gluconate 320 mg) or by the actual amount of elemental iron. It is important to note that iron toxicity relates to the amount of *elemental* iron; therefore, for the salt forms, the actual elemental iron content must be calculated.

| SALT FORM | % ELEMENTAL IRON |
|---|---|
| Ferrous fumarate | 33 |
| Ferrous gluconate | 12 |
| Ferrous sulfate (exsiccated) | 30 |
| Ferrous sulfate | 20 |

Clinically, there are generally five phases of toxicity subsequent to the ingestion of iron (Jacobs et al., 1965). The *first phase* lasts from 30 min to 2 h after ingestion and may be characterized by symptoms of lethargy, restlessness, hematemesis, abdominal pain, and bloody diarrhea. Necrosis of the GI mucosa results from the direct corrosive effect of iron on tissue and may lead to severe hemorrhagic necrosis with the development of shock. Iron absorbed through intact mucosa also may cause shock. The *second phase* presents as an apparent recovery period, which then progresses into the third phase. The *third phase* occurs 2 to 12 h after the first phase and is characterized by the onset of shock, metabolic acidosis, cyanosis, and fever. Acidosis results from the release of hydrogen ion from the conversion of ferric ($Fe^{3+}$) to ferrous ($Fe^{2+}$) ion forms and the accumulation of lactic and citric acids. The *fourth phase* occurs 2 to 4 days after ingestion and sometimes is characterized by the development of hepatic necrosis, which is thought to be due to a direct toxic action of iron on mitochondria. The *fifth phase* occurs from 2 to 4 weeks after ingestion and is characterized by GI obstruction secondary to gastric or pyloric scarring and healed tissue. Oral ingestion of iron is a potentially fatal occurrence, and ingestions of over 30 mg/kg body weight may be considered for hospital admission for observation, depending on the clinical symptoms and findings (Stein et al., 1976). Qualitative methods for determining the ingestion of iron include (1) a consistent history and physical examination, (2) a positive abdominal x-ray for iron tablets, and (3) a semiquantitative color change that is demonstrable when gastric aspirate containing iron is mixed with deferoxamine (McGuigan et al., 1979). Quantitative methods used in iron overdose include (1) a white blood cell count greater than 15,000 or a blood sugar greater than 150 mg/dl obtained within 6 h of ingestion (Lacouture et al., 1981), (2) a positive urinary deferoxamine challenge (excretion of a vin rosé color), although this is not always reliable, and (3) an elevated serum iron level (Lacouture et al., 1981).

Emesis or lavage with a large-bore tube is indicated (Proudfoot et al., 1986). Whole-bowel irrigation may be indicated in some cases. Abdominal x-rays may reveal full tablets or tablet fragments in the GI tract, as these tablets are radiopaque. Sodium bicarbonate or Fleet phosphates given orally are no longer used because of a high incidence of adverse effects and unclear efficacy. The use of oral deferoxamine may be useful in severe poisonings, but this drug may induce hypotension after oral doses. When used, the dose is 2 to 10 g of deferoxamine dissolved in 25 ml of lavage fluid, followed by a second dose of 50 percent of the initial dose in 4 h and a similar third dose in 8 to 12 h. If free iron is present in serum, if the patient is exhibiting shock or coma, or if the serum iron is greater than 350 $\mu$g/ml, deferoxamine may be administered at a rate of 15 mg/kg/h for 8 h followed by additional chelation if needed (Stein et al., 1976; Robotham and Leitman, 1980; Lovejoy, 1982). Shock with dehydration should be treated with appropriate fluid therapy (Robertson, 1971).

## MERCURY

Mercury in its various forms is available widely as metallic mercury (thermometers, Miller-Abbot tubes), fungicides, hearing aid and watch batteries, paints, mercurial drugs, and antiquated cathartics and ointments. Poisoning may occur from either chronic or acute exposure to such agents or through the food chain (Eyl, 1971). The toxicity of mercury is related primarily to its form (Chap. 19), as metallic mercury is relatively nontoxic unless it is converted to an ionized form, such as occurs on exposure to acids or strong oxidants. In general, the mercuric salts are more soluble and produce more serious poisoning than do the mercurous salts (Goldwater, 1972). Inorganic forms of mercury are corrosive and produce symptoms of metallic taste, burning, irritation, salivation, vomiting, diarrhea, upper GI tract edema, abdominal pain, and hemorrhage. These effects are seen acutely and may subside with subsequent lower GI ulceration (Goldwater, 1972). Large ingestions of mercurial salts may produce kidney damage, which may present with nephrosis, oliguria, and anuria. Ingestion of organic mercurials such as ethylmercury may produce symptoms of nausea, vomiting, abdominal pain, and diarrhea, but in most cases the main toxicity is neurological involvement presenting with paresthesias, visual disturbances, mental disturbances, hallucinations, ataxia, hearing defects, stupor, coma, and death. The symptoms may occur for several weeks after exposure. Exposure and poisoning can occur after the ingestion of mercury-contaminated seafood or grains or the inhalation of vaporized organomercurials. Chronic inorganic mercury poisoning may occur after repeated environmental exposure and may present with a neurological syndrome often described as the "mad hatter syndrome."

Therapy should be initiated with activated charcoal with or without prior lavage. Blood and urine levels of mercury may be of value in determining the indication for the administration of chelating agents such as D-penicillamine and dimercaprol (BAL) (Kark, 1971). D-Penicillamine is administered in a dose of 250 mg orally four times a day in adults and 100 mg/kg/day in children, to a maximum recommended dose of 1 g per day for 3 to 10 days, with continuous monitoring of mercury urinary excretion. In patients who cannot tolerate penicillamine, BAL can be administered in a dose of 3 to 5 mg/kg/dose every 4 h by deep intramuscular injection for the first 2 days, followed by 2.5 to 3 mg/kg/dose intramuscularly every 6 h for 2 days and then 2.5 to 3 mg/kg/dose every 12 h intramuscularly for 1 week. Adverse reactions associated with BAL administration, such as urticaria, often can be controlled with antihistamines such as diphenhydramine. The development of renal failure contraindicates penicillamine therapy because the kidney is the main route of renal excretion for penicillamine. BAL therapy can be used cautiously in spite of renal failure because BAL is excreted in the bile; however, BAL toxicity, which consists of fever, rash, hypertension, and CNS stimulation, must be closely monitored. Dialysis does not remove either chelated or free mercury metal (Robillard et al., 1976).

## NARCOTIC OPIATES

Narcotic overdose may occur in a number of different situations, such as in a newborn infant, in addition to drug addiction. Accidental or intentional overdoses frequently involve Lomotil, Darvon, Talwin, morphine, and dextromethorphan. Acute overdoses of any narcotic drug may result in respiratory arrest and coma with an initial clinical presentation of pinpoint pupils, hypotension, bradycardia, respiratory depression, urinary retention, muscle spasm, and itching. Propoxyphene overdose has been associated with convulsions (Lovejoy et al., 1974). Other signs, such as leukocytosis, hyperpyrexia, and pulmonary edema, may occur, particularly in drug abusers who inject street drugs intravenously. Ingestions of methadone or propoxyphene may have a prolonged or protracted clinical course lasting 24 to 48 h or more (Lovejoy et al., 1974). Chronic narcotic use often is associated with skin abscesses, cellulitis, endocarditis, myoglobinuria, cardiac arrhythmias, tetanus, and thrombophlebitis. Lomotil ingestion is frequently complicated by the presence of atropine in the proprietary dosage forms, with a resultant mixed picture of narcotic and anticholinergic symptoms (Rumack and Temple, 1974).

Emesis or lavage should always be performed because delayed gastric emptying is common after narcotic ingestions (Rumack and Temple, 1974; Fuzltz and Senay, 1975; Lawson and Northridge, 1987). Emesis can be induced in an alert patient; however, if seizures and/or coma exist, intubation and gastric lavage with a large-bore (28 French or larger) Ewald tube should be carried out. Activated charcoal at 5 to 10 times the estimated weight of the ingested drug (minimum of 10 g) should be instilled after emesis or lavage. Other basic supportive measures should be provided as needed. Naloxone at a dose of 0.03 mg/kg in children and 1.2 mg/kg in adolescents and adults intravenously is the drug of choice for all narcotic ingestions, including pentazocine and propoxyphene as well as methadone, morphine, and codeine (Martin, 1976). In some cases, doses of naloxone as high as 0.1 mg/kg in a child or 2 to 4 mg in an adolescent or adult may be required for those who fail to respond to the initial dose, and there is little evidence that such doses of naloxone are associated with any ill effects (Moore et al., 1980). Owing to the short duration of action of naloxone (60 to 90 min) (Evans et al., 1974), repeated doses of naloxone may be necessary until the narcotic is biotransformed, particularly in the treatment of methadone overdoses (Aronow et al., 1972; Frand et al., 1972; Lovejoy et al., 1974). In some cases of narcotic overdose, up to 20 mg of naloxone may be required (Moore et al., 1980). Other narcotic antagonists, such as nalorphine (Nalline) and levallorphan (Lorfan), possess narcotic agonist effects, that is, respiratory depressant effects (Foldes et al., 1969), and are no longer recommended.

## PHENOTHIAZINES

The phenothiazine class of antipsychotic agents includes a broad group of drugs with similar therapeutic effects. Individual agents, depending on the class of phenothiazine (aliphatic, piperidine, or piperazine), differ primarily in their milligram potencies and their tendencies to produce extrapyramidal symptoms, sedation, and hypotension. Agents such as fluphenzine (Prolixin) and trifluoperazine (Stelazine) have a high tendency to produce extrapyramidal effects, whereas chlorpromazine (Thorazine) and thioridazine (Mellaril) have a lesser tendency to produce such effects but a greater tendency to produce sedation and hypotension. Two other classes of antipsychotic drugs that are non-phenothiazine-related include butyrophenones such as haloperidol (Haldol) and the thioxanthine class such as chlorprothixene (Taractane) and thiothixene (Navane). These non-phenothiazine-class drugs have a greater tendency to produce extrapyramidal symptoms rather than sedation and hypotension. These drugs have significant anticholinergic, alpha-adrenergic blocking, quinidinelike, and extrapyramidal effects. In addition, phenothiazines lower the seizure threshold (Logothetis, 1967). Overdose with these drugs may result in CNS depression, which can present initially with reduced activity, emotional quieting, and affective indifference, although these patients also may exhibit a period of agitation, hyperactivity, or convulsions before the depressed state (Barry et al., 1983). Hyperthermia or hypothermia may develop as a result of phenothiazine's effects on the temperature-regulating mechanisms in the hypothalamus. Tachycardia with hypotension as a result of anticholinergic and alpha-blocking effects may occur. In addition, widening of the QRS complex resulting from the "quinidinelike" effect of these drugs can occur and may result in ventricular tachycardia. Extrapyramidal symptoms presenting as torticollis, stiffening of the body, spasticity, impaired speech, and opisthotonos may occur (Gupta and Lovejoy, 1967). These symptoms may occur frequently in children who have been administered prochlorperazine (Compazine) for the treatment of nausea and vomiting.

Lavage is indicated, followed by the administration of activated charcoal. Phenothiazines are radiopaque, and unabsorbed drug in the form of full or partial tablets may be visualized in the GI tract by abdominal x-ray (Barry et al., 1973). The development of convulsions should be treated with intravenous diazepam in a dose of 0.1 to 0.3 mg/kg in pediatric patients and 5 to 10 mg in adults. Hypotension requires the use of a pure alpha agonist such as norepinephrine (levarterenol or Levophed) because the administration of epinephrine may cause hypotension (Benowitz et al., 1979). Dialysis is ineffective in removing phenothiazine because these drugs are highly tissue bound. Cardiac arrhythmias may respond to the use of phenytoin (Dilantin) or lidocaine; in patients with refractory arrhythmias, a cardiac pacemaker may be required. Extrapyramidal reactions are usually adequately treated with intravenous diphenhydramine (Benadryl) in a dose of 1 to 2 mg/kg (Gupta and Lovejoy, 1967; Davies, 1970). Hypothermia or hyperthermia should be treated appropriately. Drugs that can potentiate the depressant effect of phenothiazine, such as barbiturates, sedatives, alcohol, narcotics, and anesthetics, are best avoided.

## SALICYLATES

Accidental or intentional ingestion of salicylates by children and adults continues to represent a major poisoning problem, although the frequency has decreased. Salicylates have widespread availability, are found in numerous proprietary and nonproprietary products and preparations, and receive mass promotion through advertising media (McGuigan, 1987). Most salicylate poisonings involve the use of aspirin or acetylsalicylic acid, although other serious salicylate exposures may result from compounds such as oil of wintergreen (methylsalicylate). Generally, the ingestion of doses larger than 150 mg/kg (70 mg/lb) can produce toxic symptoms such as tinnitus, nausea, and vomiting. Serious toxicity can be seen with ingestions greater than 400 mg/kg (approximately 180 mg/lb), with severe vomiting, hyperventilation, hyperthermia, confusion, coma, convulsions, hyper- or hypoglycemia, and acid-base disturbances such as respiratory alkalosis and metabolic acidosis (Pierce, 1974; Gabow et al., 1978). In severe cases, the clinical course may progress to pulmonary edema, hemorrhage, acute renal failure, or death (Anderson et al., 1976). It is important to note that a salicylate overdose patient can progress to a more serious condition over time as additional drug is absorbed from the GI tract. Chronic salicylism presents clinically in a similar fashion to the acute situation, although it often is associated with higher morbidity and mortality as well as more pronounced hyperventilation, dehydration, coma, seizures, and acidosis (Gaudreault et al., 1982). Although acute overdoses may be associated with salicylate levels of 25 to 35 mg/100 ml or more, chronic salicylism can occur at lower salicylate levels, that is, as low as 10 to 15 mg/100 ml. It is important to remember that the kinetics of salicylates are dose-dependent, and at higher serum concentrations of salicylate the drug's half-life may be prolonged to 15 to 30 h. While the half-life typically should not be used for zero-order processes, this calculation will provide a useful clinical guide. The Done nomogram (Fig. 32-2) can be utilized as an aid in interpreting

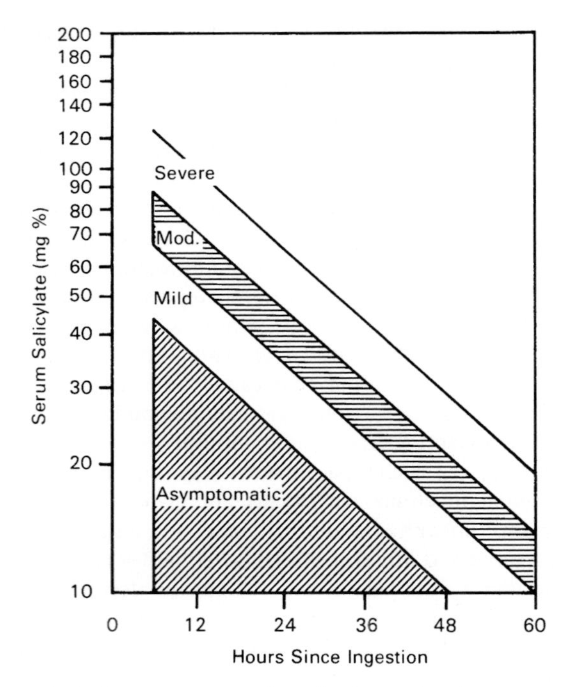


***Figure 32–2. Done nomogram for salicylate poisoning.***

Cautions for use of chart: (1) The patient has taken a single acute ingestion and is not suffering from chronic toxicity. (2) The blood level to be plotted on the nomogram was drawn 6 h after *ingestion*. (3) Levels in the toxic range drawn before 6 h should be treated. (4) Levels in the nontoxic range drawn before 6 h should be repeated to see if the level is increasing. [From Done (1960). Copyright American Academy of Pediatrics, 1960.]

a given salicylate level as long as the blood sample was not drawn prior to 6 h after ingestion. The Done nomogram is not useful in cases of chronic salicylism. Salicylates are sensitive to pH changes, with the resulting ionization changes having a pronounced effect on disposition in the body. Acidosis, which is a common finding in acute salicylate overdose, can result in a larger percentage of the drug being distributed into the CNS. Similarly, alkalinization of the urine results in ion trapping of salicylate in the kidney tubule, causing greater urinary excretion (Hill, 1973).

Orogastric intubation usually may be done to perform gastric lavage, using a large-bore tube such as a 36 French size. Subsequently, activated charcoal should be administered. Repetitive doses of activated charcoal enhance gut elimination of salicylates and shorten the half-life. Alkalinization of the urine can result in a 10-fold increase in salicylate excretion by increasing urinary pH to more than 8.0. Hypokalemia secondary to respiratory alkalosis induced by salicylate poisoning should be corrected because this condition may make alkalinization of urine difficult (Temple, 1981).

Acetazolamide (Diamox) is contraindicated for urine alkalization because this drug may contribute to metabolic acidosis. Hemodialysis, peritoneal dialysis, exchange transfusion, and hemoperfusion can be effective in removing salicylate from blood compartments but are indicated for only the most severe cases or when alkalinization of the urine is ineffective or contraindicated. Adequate fluid therapy should be instituted to prevent dehydration and correct electrolyte imbalances. Systemic acidosis should be corrected promptly with sodium bicarbonate. If hemorrhagic complications in association with a prolonged prothrombin time occur, vitamin $K_1$ or phytonadione is indicated. It is important to note that salicylates may cause coagulation defects as a result of platelet effects that are not responsive to vitamin K administration (Pierce, 1974). The patient's serum electrolytes, renal function, and cardiac status should be monitored. If hyperpyrexia occurs, appropriate treatment measures should be instituted (Hill, 1973).

## SEDATIVE-HYPNOTICS

Sedative-hypnotics include a wide range of pharmacological agents used in the treatment of anxiety, nervousness, and sleep disorders. The most widely known agents are the barbiturates (short-acting and long-acting), benzodiazopines, chloral hydrate, ethchlorvynol (Placidyl), meprobamate (Miltown), methyprylon (Noludar), glutethimide (Doriden), and methaqualone (Quaalude). After chronic overuse or abuse, these agents have a propensity to cause physical addiction, and the possibility of physical withdrawal symptoms should be considered in the treatment of patients overdosed on sedative-hypnotics. Patients presenting with a sedative-hypnotic overdose may manifest symptoms of confusion, poor coordination, ataxia, respiratory distress, apnea, and coma. Barbiturate overdose cases may present characteristically with "barb burns" or clear vesicular bullous skin lesions appearing on the hands and buttocks and between the knees (Groschel et al., 1970). Glutethimide may present with a clinical course characterized by an unusually prolonged coma or cyclic coma with periods of alternating unconsciousness and wakefulness (Decker, 1970). Much of the severity of this drug's toxicity is related to its biotransformation to and accumulation of a metabolite, 4-hydroxy-glutethimide, that has a long half-life and is twice as potent as the parent drug (Hansen et al., 1975). Gastric drug mass or drug bezoar formation has been reported, particularly in association with sedative-hypnotic agents that are poorly soluble in water (Schwartz, 1976). In some cases, gastrotomy has been required to surgically remove drug bezoars.

In the vast majority of sedative-hypnotic overdoses, conservative treatment represents the most successful approach to managing these patients (McCarron et al., 1982). If the patient is conscious, vomiting may be indicated, although in many cases gastric lavage followed by the administration of activated charcoal is required to terminate the exposure. Maintaining a patent airway, providing adequate ventilation and control of hypotension, and other supportive measures are the mainstays of therapy. In some cases, such as with phenobarbital, alkalinization of the urine has been shown to be of benefit in hastening the elimination of the drug. For lipid-soluble drugs such as glutethimide, methaqualone, and ethchlorvynol, dialysis procedures have not been shown to be effective. Some data suggest that meprobamate may be adequately treated in severe cases with the use of diuresis and/or dialysis, whereas chloral hydrate may be significantly removed by hemodialysis (Stalker et al., 1978). Analeptics and other stimulants (e.g., caffeine) have never been shown to be of any value and are therefore contraindicated. In sedative-hypnotic overdose, patients may develop pulmonary edema or shock that should be treated appropriately.

## TRICYCLIC ANTIDEPRESSANTS

The tricyclic antidepressants are available in a wide variety of brands, including amitriptyline (Elavil), doxepin (Sinequan), and imipramine (Tofranil), and in combination with phenothiazine drugs in Triavil and Etrafon. Tricyclic antidepressants have three primary pharmacological actions: anticholinergic effects, reuptake blockade of catecholamines at the adrenergic neuronal site, and quinidinelike (fast sodium channel) effects on cardiac tissue. The newer tricyclic antidepressants, such as amoxapine, have a significantly higher incidence of seizures and a lower incidence of cardiac arrhythmia than do the older tricyclic antidepressants. Tricyclic antidepressant overdose represents a life-threatening episode (Crome, 1986; Frommer et al., 1987). The initial symptoms seen are CNS depression with manifestations of lethargy, disorientation, ataxia, respiratory depression, hypothermia, and agitation. Severe toxicity may be associated with hallucinations, loss of deep tendon reflexes, muscle twitching, coma, and convulsions. The anticholinergic or atropinic effects of these drugs include dry mouth, hyperpyrexia, dilated pupils, urinary retention, tachycardia, and reduced GI motility, which may result in marked delay of the onset of symptoms. Life-threatening sequelae of the tricyclic antidepressants are the cardiovascular effects, resulting in cardiac arrhythmias such as supraventricular tachycardia, premature ventricular contractions, ventricular tachycardia, ventricular flutter, and ventricular fibrillation that progresses to hypotension and shock. ECG characteristically demonstrates a prolonged PR interval, widening of the QRS complex, QT prolongation, T-wave flattening or inversion, ST segment depression, and varying degrees of heart block progressing to cardiac standstill (Tobis and Das, 1976). Widening of the QRS complex has been reported to correlate well with the severity of the toxicity after acute overdose ingestions (Bigger, 1977b). Widening of the QRS complex past 100 ms or greater within the first 24 h is an indication of severe toxicity (Boehnert and Lovejoy, 1985).

Lavage may be indicated as appropriate, followed by the administration of activated charcoal. Patients admitted with tricyclic antidepressant overdose but without symptoms should be monitored for a minimum of 6 h to detect any possible delayed onset of symptoms. Vital signs and the ECG should be monitored in symptomatic patients, as fatal cardiac arrhythmias have occurred late in the course. Hypotension should be treated with fluids and a vasopressor such as norepinephrine (levarterenol or Levophed) administered as needed. Adjustment of blood pH with bicarbonate to pH greater than 7.45, coupled with appropriate antiarrhythmia drugs (lidocaine, phenytoin, etc.), is the primary approach to therapy for cardiac arrhythmias. Seizures are responsive to phenytoin, diazepam, and barbiturates (Bigger, 1977a).

# REFERENCES


Albertson TE et al: Superiority of activated charcoal alone compared with ipecac and activated charcoal in the treatment of acute toxic ingestions. *Ann Emerg Med* 18:56–59, 1989.

Al-Shareef AH et al: The efficacy of charcoal and sorbitol (alone and in combination) on plasma theophylline concentrations after sustained-release formulation ingestion. *Hum Exp Toxicol* 9:179–182, 1990.

Anas N, Namasonthi V, Ginsburg CM: Criteria for hospitalizing children who have ingested products containing hydrocarbons. *JAMA* 246:840–843, 1981.

Anderson KD, Rouse TM, Randolph JG: A controlled trial of corticosteroid in children with corrosive injury of the esophagus. *N Engl J Med* 323:637–640, 1990.

Anderson RJ, Potts DE, Gabow PA, et al: Unrecognized adult salicylate intoxication. *Ann Intern Med* 85:745–748, 1976.

Antoine SR et al: Environmentally significant volatile organic pollutants in human blood. *Bull Environ Contam Toxicol* 36:364–371, 1986.

Arena JM, Rourke MH, Sibrach CD: Acetaminophen: Report of an unusual poisoning. *Pediatrics* 61:68–72, 1978.

Aronow R, Shashi DP, Wooley PV: Childhood poisoning and unfortunate consequences of methadone availability. *JAMA* 219:321–324, 1972.

Axelson O et al: On the health effects of solvents, in Zenz C: *Occupational Medicine: Principles and Practical Applications*, 2d ed. Chicago: Year Book, 1988, pp 775–784.

Bain JTB, Knowles EL: Successful treatment of cyanide poisoning. *Br Med J* 2:763, 1967.

Baldochin BJ, Melmed RN: Clinical and therapeutic aspects of kerosene poisoning: A series of 200 cases. *Br Med J* 2:28–30, 1964.

Barry D, Meyskens FL Jr, Becker CE: Phenothiazine poisoning: A review of 48 cases. *Cal Med* 118:1, 1973.

Beaman R, Seigel C, Landers G: Hydrocarbon ingestion in children: A six year retrospective study. *J Am Coll Emerg Physicians* 5:771–775, 1976.

Benowitz NL, et al: Cardiopulmonary catastrophes in drug-overdosed patients. *Med Clin North Am* 63:267, 1979.

Bergson F: Pneumatocoeles following hydrocarbon ingestion. *Am J Dis Child* 129:49–54, 1975.

Berlin CM Jr: The treatment of cyanide poisoning in children. *Pediatrics* 46:793, 1970.

Bigger JT: Is physostigmine effective for cardiac toxicity of tricyclic antidepressant drugs? *JAMA* 273:1311, 1977a.

———: Tricyclic antidepressant overdose: Incidence of symptoms. *JAMA* 238:135–138, 1977b.

Boehnert MT, Lovejoy FH Jr: Value of QRS, duration versus the serum drug level in predicting seizures and ventricular arrhythmias after an acute overdose of tricyclic antidepressants. *N Engl J Med* 313:474–479, 1985.

Bolla KI et al: Subclinical neuropsychiatric effects of chronic low-level solvent exposure in US paint manufacturers. *J Occup Med* 32:671–677, 1990.

Boylan JL, Egle JL, Guzelian PD: Cholestyramine: Use as a new therapeutic approach for chlordecone (Kepone) poisoning. *Science* 199:893–895, 1978.

Bratton L, Haddow JE: Ingestion of charcoal lighter fluid. *J Pediatr* 84:396–401, 1974.

Brown J, Burke B, DaJanias C: Experimental kerosene pneumonia: Evaluation of some therapeutic regimens. *J Pediatr* 84:396–401, 1974.

Bryson PD, Watanabe AS, Rumack BH, Murphy RC: Burdock root tea poisoning: Case report involving a commercial preparation. *JAMA* 239:2157, 1978.

Buckley N et al: Slow-release verapamil poisoning: Use of polyethylene glycol whole bowel lavage and high-dose calcium. *Med J Aust* 158:202–204, 1993.

Burrington JP: Clinitest burns of the esophagus. *Ann Thorac Surg* 20:400, 1974.

Chen KK, Rose CL: Nitrite and thiosulfate therapy in cyanide poisoning. *JAMA* 149:113, 1952.

Chyka PA et al: Evaluation of a porcine model to study repeat-dose activated charcoal therapy. *Vet Hum Toxicol* 35:367, 1993.

Clark R, Borirakchanyavat V, Davidson AR, et al: Hepatic damage and death from overdose of paracetamal. *Lancet* 1:66, 1973.

Crome P: Poisoning due to tricyclic antidepressant overdose. *Med Toxicol* 1:261–285, 1986.

Curry AS: *The Poisoned Patient: The Role of the Laboratory*. Amsterdam: Elsevier, 1974.

David DJ, Spyker DA: The acute toxicity of ethanol: Dosage and kinetic nomograms. *Vet Hum Toxicol* 21:272, 1979.

Davies DM: Treatment of drug-induced dyskinesias. *Lancet* 1:567, 1970.

Decker WJ: Gluthethimide rebound. *Lancet* 1:778, 1970.

Done AK: Salicylate intoxication, Significance of measurements of salicylate in blood in cases of acute intoxication. *Pediatrics* 26:800–807, 1960.

Droz PO et al: Variability in biological monitoring of organic solvent exposure: II. Application of a population physiological model. *Br J Ind Med* 46:547–558, 1989.

Ekberg K et al: Psychologic effects of exposure to solvents and other neurotoxic agents in the work environment, in Zenz C: *Occupational Medicine: Principles and Practical Applications*, 2d ed. Chicago: Year Book, 1988, pp 785–795.

Ekins BR, Watanabe AS: Acute digoxin poisoning: Review of therapy. *Am J Hosp Pharm* 35:268–277, 1978.

Elbel H, Schleyer F: In *Blutalkatal: Die Wissenschaftlichen Grudlagen der Beruteilung von Blutalkoholbefunden bei Strassenverke-Msdelkien Stuttgart*. Heidelberg: Georg Thieme, 1956, p 226.

Espelin DE, Done AK: Amphetamine poisoning: Effectiveness of chlorpromazine. *N Engl J Med* 278:1361–1365, 1968.

Evans JM, Hogg MIJ, Lynn JN, Rosen M: Degree and duration of reversal by naloxone of effects of morphine in conscious subjects. *Br Med J* 2:589–591, 1974.

Eyl TB: Organic-mercury food poisoning. *N Engl J Med* 284:706, 1971.

Farley TA: Severe hypernatremic dehydration after use of an activated charcoal-sorbitol suspension. *J Pediatr* 109:719–721, 1986.

Fischer DS, Parkman R, Finch SC: Acute iron poisoning in children. *JAMA* 218:1179–1184, 1971.

Foldes FF, Duncalf D, Kuwabara S: The respiratory, circulatory, and narcotic antagonistic effects of nalorphine, levallorphan, and naloxone in anesthetized subjects. *Can Anaesth Soc J* 16:151–161, 1969.

Frand UI, Chang SS, Williams MH Jr: Methadone induced pulmonary edema. *Ann Intern Med* 76:975–979, 1972.

Friedman EM, Lovejoy FH Jr: The emergency management of caustic ingestions. *Emerg Med Clin North Am* 2:77–86, 1984.

Frommer DA, Kulig KW, Marx JA, Rumack B: Tricyclic antidepressant overdose: A review. *JAMA* 257:521–526, 1987.

Fuzltz JM, Senay EC: Guidelines for the management of hospitalized addicts. *Ann Intern Med* 82:815–818, 1975.

Gabow PA, Anderson RJ, Potts DE: Acid-based disturbances in the salicylate-intoxicated adult. *Arch Intern Med* 138:1481–1484, 1978.

Gaudreault P, Parent M, McGuigan MA, et al: Predictability of esophageal injury from signs and symptoms: A study of caustic ingestion in 378 children. *Pediatrics* 71:767–770, 1983.

Gaudreault P, Temple AR, Lovejoy FH Jr: The relative severity of acute versus chronic salicylate poisoning in children. *Pediatrics* 70:566–569, 1982.

Ghittori S et al: The urinary concentration of solvents as a biological indicator of exposure: Proposal for the biological equivalent exposure limit for nine solvents. *Am Ind Hyg Assoc J* 48:786–790, 1987.

Gilli G et al: Volatile halogenated hydrocarbons in urban atmosphere and in human blood. *Arch Environ Health* 45:101–106, 1990.

Goldwater LJ: *Mercury: A History of Quicksilver*. Baltimore: York Press, 1972.

Goulbourne KB et al: Small-bowel obstruction secondary to activated charcoal and adhesions. *Ann Emerg Med* 24:108–109, 1994.

Graham DL, Laman D, Theodore J: Acute cyanide poisoning complicated by lactic acidosis and pulmonary edema. *Arch Intern Med* 137:1051–1055, 1977.

Groschel, D, Gerstein AR, Rosenbaum JM: Skin lesions as a diagnostic aid in barbiturate poisoning. *N Engl J Med* 403:409–410, 1970.

Gupta JM, Lovejoy FH Jr: Acute phenothiazine toxicity in children. *Pediatrics* 71:890–894, 1967.

Hagstadius S et al: Regional cerebral blood flow at the time of diagnosis of chronic toxic encephalopathy induced by organic-solvent exposure and after the cessation of exposure. *Scand J Work Environ Health* 15:130–135, 1989.

Hall AH et al: Clinical toxicology of cyanide: North American clinical experiences, in Ballantyne B, Marrs TC (eds): *Clinical and Experimental Toxicology of Cyanides*. Bristol, UK: Butterworth (John Wright), 1987.

Haller JA Jr: Pathophysiology and management of acute corrosive burns of the esophagus. *J Pediatr Surg* 6:578, 1971.

Hammond RB, Rumack BH, Rodgerson DO: Blood ethanol: A report of unusually high levels in a living patient. *JAMA* 226:63–64, 1973.

Hansen AR, Kennedy KA, Ambre JJ, Fischer LJ: Glutethimide poisoning—a metabolite contributes to morbidity and mortality. *N Engl J Med* 292:250–252, 1975.

Hartman DE: *Neuropsychological Toxicology: Indentification and Assessment of Human Neurotoxic Syndromes*. New York: Pergamon Press, 1988.

Hill JB: Salicylate intoxication. *N Engl J Med* 2–8:1110, 1113, 1973.

Hillman B, Bardham KD, Bain JTB: The use of dicobalt edetate (Kelocyanor) in cyanide poisoning. *Postgrad Med J* 50:171–174, 1974.

Hogstedt C et al: Diagnostic and health care aspects of workers exposed to solvents, in Zenz C: *Developments in Occupational Medicine*. Chicago, Year Book, 1980, pp 249–258.

Howell JM: Alkaline ingestions. *Ann Emerg Med* 15:820–825, 1986.

Ilkhanipour K et al: The comparative efficacy of various multiple-dose activated charcoal regimens. *Am J Emerg Med* 10:298–300, 1992.

Jacobs J, Greene H, Gendel BR: Acute iron intoxication. *N Engl J Med* 273:1124–1127, 1965.

Kark RAP: Mercury poisoning and its treatment with *N*-acetyl-D,L-penicillamine. *N Engl J Med* 285:1, 1971.

Kelsey KT et al: Sister chromatid exchange in painters recently exposed to solvents. *Environ Res* 50:248–255, 1989.

Kirshenbaum LA et al: Whole bowel irrigation versus activated charcoal in sorbitol for the ingestion of modified release pharmaceuticals. *Clin Pharmacol Ther* 46:264–271, 1989.

Kornberg AE et al: Pediatric ingestion: Charcoal alone versus ipecac and charcoal. *Ann Emerg Med* 20:648–651, 1991.

Krenzelok EP et al: Gastrointestinal transit times of cathartics combined with charcoal. *Ann Emerg Med* 14:1152–1155, 1985.

Kulig KW, Bar-Or D, Cantrill SV, et al: Management of acutely poisoned patients without gastric emptying. *Ann Emerg Med* 14:562–567, 1985.

Lacouture PG, Gaudreault P, Lovejoy FH Jr: Clinitest tablet ingestion: An *in-vitro* investigation concerned with initial emergency management. *Ann Emerg Med* 15:143–146, 1986.

Lacouture PG, Wason S, Temple AR, et al: Emergency assessment of severity in iron overdose. *J Pediatr* 99:89–91, 1981.

Lambecier MR, DuPan RM: L'intoxication alcooligue aigue et les accidents d'automobile. *Schweiz Med Wochenschr* 76:395–398, 421–428, 1968.

Lawson AAH, Northridge DB: Dextropropoxyphene. *Med Toxicol* 2:430–444, 1987.

Ledin T et al: Posturography findings in workers exposed to industrial solvents. *Acta Otolaryngol (Stockh)* 107:357–361, 1989.

Linden CH, et al: Amphetamines. *Topics Emerg Med* 7:18–32, 1985.

Litovitz TL: Button battery ingestions. *JAMA* 249:2495, 1983.
Lloyd BL, Smith TW: Contrasting rates of reversal of digoxin toxicity by digoxin specific IgG and Fab fragments. *Circulation* 58:280–283, 1978.
Logothetis J: Spontaneous epileptic seizures and EEG changes in the course of phenothiazine therapy. *Neurology* 17:869–877, 1967.
Longdon P et al: Intestinal pseudo-obstruction following the use of enteral charcoal and sorbitol and mechanical ventilation with papaveretum sedation for theophylline poisoning. *Drug Safety* 7:74–77, 1992.
Lovejoy FH Jr: Chelation therapy in iron poisoning. *Clin Toxicol* 19:871–874, 1982.
Lovejoy FH Jr, Mitchel AA, Goldman P: Management of propoxyphene poisoning. *J Pediatr* 85:98–100, 1974.
Mann JB: Diagnostic aids in organophosphate poisoning. *Ann Intern Med* 67:905–906, 1967.
Marks MI, Chicoine L, Legere G: Adrenocorticosteroid treatment of hydrocarbon pneumonia in children—a cooperative study. *J Pediatr* 81:366–369, 1972.
Martin WR: Naloxone. *Ann Intern Med* 85:765, 1976.
McCarron MM, Schulze BW, Walberg CB, et al: Short-acting barbiturate overdosage: Correlation of intoxication score with serum barbiturate concentration. *JAMA* 248:55–61, 1982.
McGuigan MA: A two-year review of salicylate deaths in Ontario. *Arch Intern Med* 147:510–512, 1987.
McGuigan M, Lovejoy FH Jr, Marino S, et al: Qualitative deferoxamine test for iron ingestion. *J Pediatr* 94:940–942, 1979.
Mergler D et al: Assessing color vision loss among solvent-exposed workers. *Am J Ind Med* 12:195–203, 1987.
Mergler D et al: Color vision loss among disabled workers with neuropsychological impairment. *Neurotoxicol Teratol* 12:669–672, 1990.
Merigian KS et al: Prospective evaluation of gastric emptying in self-poisoned patients. *Am J Emerg Med* 8:479–483, 1990.
Mikolich JR, Paulson GW, Cross CJ: Acute anticholinergic syndromes due to jimson weed ingestion. *Ann Intern Med* 83:321, 1975.
Minton NA, Murray VSG: A review of organophosphate poisoning. *Med Toxicol* 3:350–375, 1988.
Mitchell JR, Jollow DJ, Potter WZ, et al: Acetaminophen induced hepatic necrosis. *J Pharmacol Exp Ther* 187:185, 1973.
Mofenson HC et al: Gastrointestinal dialysis with activated charcoal and cathartic in the treatment of adolescent intoxications. *Clin Pediatr (Phila)* 24:678–684, 1985.
Moore RA, Rumack BH, Conner CS, Peterson RG: Naloxone: Underdosage after narcotic poisoning. *Am J Dis Child* 134:156–158, 1980.
Morrow LA et al: Alterations in cognitive and psychological functioning after organic solvent exposure. *J Occup Med* 32:444–450, 1990.
Namba T: Poisoning due to organophosphate insecticides: Acute and chronic manifestations. *Am J Med* 50:475–492, 1971.
Neuvonen PJ et al: Effect of purgatives on antidotal efficacy of oral activated charcoal. *Hum Toxicol* 5:255–263, 1986.
Ng R, Darwich H, Stewart DA: Emergency treatment of petroleum distillate and turpentine ingestion. *CMA J* 111:538, 1974.
NIOSH: *Organic Solvent Neurotoxicity*. NIOSH Current Intelligence Bulletin 48, DHHS (NIOSH) publication no. 87–104, March 31, 1987.
Odkvist L et al: Vestibulo-oculomotor disturbances caused by industrial solvents. *Otolaryngol Head Neck Surg* 91:537–539, 1983.
Ohning BL et al: Continuous nasogastric administration of activated charcoal for the treatment of theophylline intoxication. *Pediatr Pharmacol* 5:241–245, 1986.
Park GD et al: Effects of size and frequency of oral doses of charcoal on theophylline clearance. *Clin Pharmacol Ther* 34:663–666, 1983.
Park GD, et al: Expanded role of charcoal in the poisoned and overdosed patient. *Arch Intern Med* 146:969–973, 1986.
Penner GE: Acid ingestion: Toxicology and treatment. *Ann Emerg Med* 9:374–379, 1980.
Pentel P: Toxicity of over-the-counter stimulants. *JAMA* 252:1898–1903, 1984.
Peterson RG, Rumack BH: Treatment of acute acetaminophen poisoning with acetylcysteine. *JAMA* 237:2406–2407, 1977.
Picchioni AL et al: Evaluation of activated charcoal-sorbitol suspension as an antidote. *J Toxicol Clin Toxicol* 19:433–444, 1982.
Pierce AW: Salicylate poisoning. *Pediatrics* 54:342–347, 1974.
Pollack MM et al: Aspiration of activated charcoal and gastric contents. *Ann Emerg Med* 10:528–529, 1981.
Posner MA, Tobey RE, McElroy H: Hydraoxocobalamine therapy of cyanide intoxication in guinea pigs. *Anesthesiology* 44:157, 1976.
Proudfoot AT, Wright N: Acute paracetamol poisoning. *Br Med J* 2:557, 1970.
Proudfoot AT, Simpson D, Dyson EH: Management of acute iron poisoning. *Med Toxicol* 1:83–100, 1986.
Robertson WO: Treatment of acute iron poisoning. *Mod Treat* 8:552–560, 1971.
Robillard JE, Rames LK, Jensen RL, Roberts RJ: Peritoneal dialysis in mercurialdiuretic intoxication. *J Pediatr* 88:79–81, 1976.
Robotham JL, Leitman PS: Acute iron poisoning—a review. *Am J Dis Child* 134:875–879, 1980.
Rodgers GC et al: Gastrointestinal decontamination for acute poisoning. *Pediatr Clin North Am* 33:261–285, 1986.
Rumack BH: Hydrocarbon ingestions in perspective. *JACEP* 6:4, 1977.
———: Acetaminophen overdose in young children: Treatment and effects of alcohol and other additional ingestants in 417 cases. *Am J Dis Child* 138:428–433, 1984.
———: Ipecac use at home. *Pediatrics* 75:1148, 1985.
———: *Poisindex*. Denver: Micromedex: 1994.
Rumack BH, Anderson RH, Wolfe R, et al: Ornade and anticholinergic toxicity: Hypertension, hallucination and arrhythmias. *Clin Toxicol* 7:573–581, 1974.
Rumack BH, Matthew H: Acetaminophen poisoning and toxicity. *Pediatrics* 55:871, 1975.
Rumack BH, Peterson RC, Koch GG, Amara IA: Acetaminophen overdose: 662 cases with evaluation of oral acetylcysteine treatment. *Arch Intern Med* 141:380–385, 1981.
Rumack BH, Temple AR: Lomotil poisoning. *Pediatrics* 53:495–500, 1974.
——— (eds): *Management of the Poisoned Patient*. Princeton, NJ: Science Press, 1977.
Rumack BH, Wolfe RR, Gilfrich H: Phenytoin treatment of massive digoxin overdose. *Br Heart J* 36:405–408, 1974.
Saetta JP et al: Gastric emptying procedures in self-poisoned patients: Are we forcing gastric contents beyond the pylorus? *J R Soc Med* 84:274–276, 1991.
Saetta JP, Quinton DN: Residual gastric content after gastric lavage and ipecac-induced emesis in self-poisoned patients: An endoscopic study. *J R Soc Med* 84:35–38, 1991.
Sayre JW, Kaymakcalan S: Cyanide poisoning from apricot seeds among children in central Turkey. *N Engl J Med* 270:1113, 1964.
Schwartz HS: Acute meprobamate poisoning with gastrostomy and removal of a drug contained mass. *N Engl J Med* 295:1177, 1976.
Seppalainen AM: Occupational neurology, in Zenz C: *Occupational Medicine: Principles and Practical Applications*, 2d ed. Chicago, Year Book, 1988, pp 796–805.
Shannon M et al: Cathartics and laxatives: Do they still have a place in management of the poisoned patient? *Med Toxicol* 1:247–252, 1986.
Simon GE et al: Immunologic, psychological, and neuropsychological factors in multiple chemical sensitivity: A controlled study. *Ann Intern Med* 119:97–103, 1993.
Smilkstein MJ, Knapp GL, Kulig KW, Rumack BH: Efficacy of oral *N*-acetylcysteine in the treatment of acetaminophen overdose. *N Engl J Med* 319:1557–1562, 1988.

Smith RP, Kruszyna H: Nitroprusside produces cyanide poisoning via a reaction with hemoglobin. *J Pediatr* 191:557, 1974.

Smith SW et al: Whole bowel irrigation as a treatment for acute lithium overdose. *Ann Emerg Med* 20:536–539, 1991.

Smith TW: New advances iin the assessment and treatment of digitalis toxicity. *J Clin Pharmacol* 25:522–528, 1985.

Smith TW, Butler VP, Haber E, et al: Treatment of life-threatening digitalis intoxication with digoxin-specific Fab antibody fragments. *N Engl J Med* 307:1357–1362, 1982.

Stalker NE, Gamertoglio JG, Fukumitsu CJ, et al: Acute massive chloral hydrate intoxication treated with hemodialysis: A clinical pharmacokinetic analysis. *J Clin Pharmacol* 18:136–142, 1978.

Steele RW, Conklin RH, March HM: Corticosteroids and antibiotics for the treatment of fulminant hydrocarbon aspiration. *JAMA* 219:1434–1437, 1972.

Stein M, Blayney D, Feit T, et al: Acute iron poisoning in children. *West J Med* 125:289–297, 1976.

Stewart R: Cyanide poisoning. *Clin Toxicol* 7:561, 1974.

Subcommittee on Accidental Poisoning: Kerosene and related petroleum distillates, in *Handbook of Common Poisonings in Children*. FDA-76-7004. Rockville, MD: U.S. Department of HEW, 1976, pp 1–87.

Sue YJ et al: Efficacy of magnesium citrate cathartic in pediatric toxic ingestions. *Ann Emerg Med* 24:709–712, 1994.

Temple AR: Acute and chronic effects of aspirin toxicity and their treatment. *Arch Intern Med* 141:364–369, 1981.

Tenenbein M et al: Whole bowel irrigation as a decontamination procedure after acute drug overdose. *Arch Intern Med* 147:905–907, 1987.

Thompson DF, Trammel HL, Robertson NJ, Reigart JR: Evaluation of regional and nonregional poison centers. *N Engl J Med* 308:191–194, 1983.

Tobis J, Das EN: Cardiac complications in amitriptyline poisoning—successful treatment with physostigmine. *JAMA* 234:1474–1476, 1976.

Truempier E, Reyes de la Rocha S, Atkinson SD: Clinical characteristics, pathophysiology and management of hydrocarbon ingestion: Case report and review of the literature. *Pediatr Emerg Care* 3:187–193, 1987.

Underhill TJ et al: A comparison of the efficacy of gastric lavage, ipecacuanha, and activated charcoal in the emergency management of acetaminophen overdose. *Arch Emerg Med* 7:148–154, 1990.

Vale JA et al: Syrup of ipecacuanha: Is it really useful? *Br Med J* 293:1321, 1986.

Van de Graaff WB et al: Adsorbent and cathartic inhibition of enteral drug absorption. *J Pharmacol Exp Ther* 221:656–663, 1982.

Van Vliet C et al: Exposure-outcome relationships between organic solvent exposure and neuropsychiatric disorders: Results from a Dutch case-control study. *Am J Ind Med* 16:707–718, 1989.

Watanabe AS: Pharmacokinetic aspects of the dialysis of drugs. *Drug Intell Clin Pharm* 11:407–416, 1977.

Wexler J, Whittenberger JL, Dumke PR: The effect of cyanide on the electrocardiogram of man. *Am Heart J* 34:163–173, 1947.

Wilkinson PK: Blood ethanol concentrations during and following constant rate IV infusion of alcohol. *Clin Pharmacol Ther* 19:213, 1976.

# CHAPTER 33

# OCCUPATIONAL TOXICOLOGY

*Robert R. Lauwerys*

The main objective of industrial toxicology is the prevention of health impairments in workers who handle or who are exposed to industrial chemicals. This objective can only be met if conditions of exposure or work practices are defined that do not entail an unacceptable health risk.

In practice this implies a definition for *permissible* levels of exposure to industrial chemicals. These levels can be expressed either in terms of allowable atmospheric concentrations [maximum allowable concentrations (MACs); threshold limit values (TLVs); time-weighted averages (TWAs); threshold limit value-ceiling (TLV-C); occupational exposure limits (OELs); short-term exposure limits (STELs)] or in terms of permissible biological levels for the chemical or its metabolites or the amount bound to the critical sites (biological TLV; biological exposure indices; biologically permissible values). It is important to stress that these atmospheric or biologically allowable concentrations do not correspond to exposure conditions devoid of any health risk. The concept of acceptable exposure level must be understood as the level of exposure below which the risk—that is, the probability of impairing the health of the exposed workers—is acceptable. To conclude that a risk is acceptable, one must identify and quantify it, which requires knowledge of the relationship between exposure intensity (dose) and the health effects and that between exposure intensity and the response (i.e., the prevalence of subjects exhibiting a defined adverse effect). One must first identify the nature of the biological effects likely to occur and their severity when exposure (intensity-duration) to a chemical agent(s) increases. One must then define which effect is acceptable. This choice may be the object of intense controversy. Between being in good health and being ill following exposure to chemicals, there is no strict barrier but a continuum of changes from simple asymptomatic biochemical and/or functional changes to clinical disease.

The health significance of all the identified changes resulting from chemical exposure must be assessed in order to decide which ones are adverse or nonadverse. Following this assessment, one must then take into account the interindividual variability in the susceptibility to chemicals. There is not one single dose-effect relationship but as many as there are exposed subjects. Therefore, to recommend an acceptable exposure level to an industrial chemical, one must also attempt to define the dose (exposure)-response (probability of occurrence of early adverse effects in populations at risk) relationship. Another choice must then be made, that is, the percentage of exposed subjects who may still develop an adverse effect at the proposed acceptable exposure level. This acceptable response of course will vary according to the type of potential adverse effects (e.g., inhibition of an enzyme without functional consequences, reversible local irritant effect, genotoxicity, etc.).

To evaluate with some degree of confidence the level of exposure at which the risk of health impairment is acceptable, a body of toxicological information is required that derives from two main sources: experimental investigations on animals and clinical surveillance of exposed workers (including retrospective studies on previously exposed workers). In some circumstances, limited investigations on volunteers can also be considered.

The large-scale use of any chemical in industry should be preceded by certain types of toxicological investigations on animals in order to establish a tentative acceptable exposure level. Other important information that may also be derived from these investigations concerns the relationships between the metabolic handling of the chemical and its interactions with target molecules (mechanism of action), identification of methods for biological monitoring of exposure and early health effects and of preexisting pathological states that may increase the susceptibility to the chemical. However, animal testing can provide only an estimate of the toxicity of a chemical for humans. Animals do not always respond to chemical exposure the same way humans do.

The comparative toxicity of 2,3,7,8-tetrachlorodibenzo-*p*-dioxin to animals and humans illustrates this point (Kimbrough, 1991). Dioxin is much less acutely toxic to humans than to several other species probably because the affinity with which dioxin binds to the cytoplasmic receptor Ah is lower in humans than in other species. Because of interspecies differences in their metabolism and/or mechanism of action, certain chemicals are more likely to induce cancer in rats than in humans (e.g., kidney cancer in male rats chronically exposed to unleaded gasoline may be related to the accumulation in proximal tubular cells of a rat specific protein, $\alpha_{2U}$-globulin) (Hard et al., 1993).

The opposite may occur, e.g., skin and internal cancers caused in humans by excessive oral exposure to inorganic arsenic have not been reproduced during classical carcinogenicity studies in animals (ATSDR, 1993). There is also a great risk of missing respiratory sensitization properties in testing new materials in animals because so far no predictive tests (e.g., mouse IgE test, guinea pig model) have been validated (Briatico-Vangosa et al., 1994). Thus, when the compound is actually handled in industry, monitoring of the workplace and careful clinical surveillance of the workers are essential. The design of these clinical surveys will to a large extent depend on the information collected during the first experimental phase of the investigations. The main objectives of the clinical work are (1) to test the validity of the provisional permissible level of exposure based on animal experiments; (2) to detect as early as possible hypersensitive reactions or other effects that are unpredictable from animal investigations; and (3) to confirm the usefulness of biological methods of monitoring workers (assessment of exposure and early detection of adverse effects). One must, however, recognize that for many chemicals, toxicological investigations on animals have not been performed before the chemicals' use in industry. In that case, clinical work (retrospective epidemiological studies; historical prospective studies; case-control studies; cross-sectional studies) is aimed at identifying the potential health risks and at defining the acceptable exposure level directly in humans.

In some circumstances exposure of volunteers can be considered when the information (e.g., threshold for upper respiratory tract irritation) is not easily obtainable by other means and when the experiments entail no risk for the volunteers (which means that extensive biological information should already be available before any experiments on volunteers are undertaken). Experimental investigations on animals and clinical studies on workers or volunteers are closely related, and the following discussion illustrates how collaboration between these disciplines or approaches helps accomplish more rapid progress in the field of industrial toxicology.

## PRELIMINARY TESTING ON ANIMALS

It is evident that certainty as to the complete safety of a chemical can never be obtained, whatever the extent of toxicological investigations performed on animals. Nevertheless, some basic requirements can be suggested to estimate with some degree of confidence the level of exposure at which the risk of health impairment is negligible and thus acceptable. We are excluding from the following considerations chemicals that have only very limited use, as in a research laboratory, and can be handled by a limited number of skilled persons in a way that prevents any exposure.

General guidelines for assessing experimentally the toxicological hazards of chemicals have been formulated by various national or international agencies. These tests include local and systemic acute toxicity tests, skin sensitization tests, toxicity following repeated exposure (including interference with the immune system), short-term tests for detecting potential mutagens and carcinogens, studies of effect on reproduction and of teratogenic activity, chronic studies to detect carcinogenesis and other long-term effects, investigations of metabolism and mechanism of action, and interaction studies that have been described extensively in previous chapters. The following discussion stresses a few points that are important or especially pertinent to the field of industrial toxicology.

The need for performing some (or all) of those investigations should be carefully evaluated for any industrial chemical to which workers will be exposed. In selecting the studies most appropriate for safety evaluation, the toxicologist is guided by an understanding of the physicochemical properties of the chemical (including speciation for inorganic compounds, which may have important consequences in their toxicokinetics and biological reactivity); the conditions of use and degree of exposure, including the possibility of generating toxic derivatives when the chemical is submitted to various chemical and physical factors (heat, pH change, etc.); the type of exposure, which may be continuous or accidental; and possibly toxicological information already available on other chemicals with similar chemical structure and reactive chemical groups. It should be stressed that conclusions drawn from any toxicological investigation are valid only if the exact composition (e.g., the nature and concentration of impurities or degradation products) of the tested preparation is known.

The assessment of the toxicity of the pesticides malathion and 2,4,5-T illustrates this point. Malathion, an organophosphorus insecticide normally devoid of significant human toxicity, was responsible for an episode of mass poisoning in Pakistan in 1976 because the technical preparation used contained various impurities (mainly isomalathion) capable of inhibiting tissue and plasma carboxyesterases (Baker et al., 1978; Aldridge et al., 1979). The teratogenic hazard of the herbicide 2,4,5-T is estimated differently, depending on the content of the highly toxic impurity 2,3,7,8-tetrachlorodibenzodioxin (TCDD) in the preparation tested (Courtney and Moore, 1971; Emerson et al., 1971). Accurate methods of analysis of the chemical in air and in biological material also should be available.

Flexibility of approach is essential in deciding the duration of tests necessary to establish a reasonable acceptable level for occupational exposure. This depends mainly on the type of toxic action that is suspected, but it is generally recognized that, for systematically acting chemicals, subacute and short-term toxicity studies are usually insufficient for proposing permissible exposure levels. Subacute and short-term toxicity tests are usually performed to find out whether the compound exhibits immunotoxic properties and cumulative characteristics and to select the doses for long-term exposure and the kind of tests that may be most informative when applied during long-term exposures. Several studies have drawn attention to the fact that the reproductive system may also be the target organ of industrial chemicals (e.g., some glycolethers, monochlorodibromopropane). Studies designed to evaluate reproductive performance and teratogenic action should therefore also be considered during routine toxicologic testing of industrial chemicals.

Information derived from exposure routes similar to those sustained by workers (e.g., skin, lung) is clearly most relevant. For airborne pollutants, inhalation exposure studies provide the basic data on which provisional permissible levels are based. Experimental methodology is certainly much more complicated for inhalation studies than for oral administration experiments. For example, in the case of exposure to an aerosol, particle size distribution should be estimated and the approximate degree of retention in the respiratory tract of the animal species selected should be known. Ideally, particle size should be selected according to the deposition pattern of solid or liquid aerosols in the particular animal species used. It also should be kept in mind that the concentration of the material in the air and the duration of exposure do not give a direct estimate of the dose, which is also dependent on the minute volume and percent retention. The measurement of pulmonary dust retention following a brief exposure to a radiolabeled test aerosol at various times during prechronic or chronic studies of insoluble inhaled dust has been recommended in order to assess whether the selected levels of exposure may overwhelm pulmonary clearance mechanisms (Lewis et al., 1989).

The appropriateness of studying the effects of other routes of administration (usually oral) in combination with limited data from tests by inhalation or skin application must be evaluated scientifically for each chemical (depending on its main site of action, metabolism, etc.). The morphological, physiological, and biological parameters that usually are evaluated, either at regular intervals in the course of the exposure period or at its termination, are described in Chaps. 11 through 21, in Unit 4 (Target Organ Toxicity). It is evident that investigations that can make use of specific physiological or biochemical tests, based on knowledge of the critical organ or function, produce highly valuable information and hence increase confidence in the atmospheric or biological TLV derived from them (see "Practical Applications," below).

In the field of industrial toxicology, knowledge of the disposition (absorption, distribution, biotransformation, and excretion) of the chemical and/or its mechanism of action is of major interest. Indeed, as indicated at the beginning of this chapter the main objective of occupational toxicology is to prevent the development of occupational diseases. In this respect, the biological monitoring of workers exposed to various industrial chemicals may play an important role, by detecting excessive exposures as early as possible, before the occurrence of significant biological disturbances or at least when they are still reversible or have not yet caused any health impairment. A rational biological monitoring of exposure and of early health effects is possible only when sufficient toxicological information has been gathered on the mechanism of action and/or the metabolism of xenobiotics to which workers may be exposed (see below, "Observations on Workers/Practical Applications"). These studies must be performed first on animals.

## OBSERVATIONS ON WORKERS

When a new chemical is being used on a large scale, the careful clinical survey of workers and monitoring of workplaces should be planned. In addition to determining the specific actions to be taken immediately if any adverse effect on the health of the workers is discovered, a clinical survey may have two main, general objectives: (1) to evaluate the validity of the acceptable exposure level derived from animal experiments and (2) to test the validity of a biological method of monitoring (in sum, the assessment of exposure and early detection of adverse effects).

### Evaluation of the Validity of Animal Experiments

Evaluation of the validity of the proposed permissible exposure level derived from animal experiments is certainly the prime objective since, as Barnes stated in 1963, "studies and observations on man will always be the final basis for deciding whether or not a MAC set originally on the basis of tests on animals is, in fact, truly acceptable as one that will not produce any signs of intoxication." This means that behavioral, clinical, biochemical, physiological, or morphological tests that are considered to be the most sensitive for detecting an adverse effect of the chemical should be made on the workers at the same time their overall exposure is evaluated. An important point with regard to the clinical studies (prospective or cross-sectional studies) is that, like the experimental studies (animal tests) mentioned above (this section), they should rely on sensitive biological effect parameters as much as possible. The diagnostic tools used in clinical medicine frequently reveal only advanced pathological states and, with a few exceptions, are not designed to detect early adverse effects at a stage when they are still reversible, if preventive actions are taken. To give an example, the measurement of serum creatinine is still the most widely used clinical test for assessing renal integrity; yet it is known that the filtration capacity of the kidney (its main function) must be reduced by more than 60 percent before serum creatinine significantly rises. What can be said for the kidney is true for most other organs or functions.

The main limitation of current permissible airborne concentrations or biological limit values is that they are usually based on limited experimental data or clinical studies in which only late effects have been looked for and correlated with past exposure. Furthermore, several biological TLVs are derived from the study of external-internal exposure relationships and not from that of internal dose-early adverse effects relationships (see below, this section). The validity of an acceptable exposure level is much stronger if it is based on the study of the dose-effects/dose-response relationships in which the dose is expressed in terms of the cumulative target dose and the monitored effect reflects a critical biological event. However, it should be noted that for some chemicals and/or adverse effects (e.g., induction of hypersensitivity state and possibly genotoxic effects) the frequency of peak exposure may be more important for health risk assessment than the integrated dose.

As illustrated in Fig. 33-1, the epidemiological studies designed to assess the dose-effect/dose-incidence relationships can be carried out by using different parameters for assessing the exposure and the resulting health changes. Exposure may be characterized qualitatively (e.g., by job classification or through a questionnaire) or quantitatively through ambient or personal monitoring or through measurement of the internal dose or the target dose. The adverse effects may be expressed in terms of increased death rate, clinical diseases, irreversible or reversible functional changes, or critical biological changes (i.e., changes that are predictive of health impairment if they are maintained or if they occur repeatedly). It is evident that the assessment of the health risk resulting from exposure (and the permissible exposure level derived therefrom) will have more validity if it results from dose-effects and dose-incidence studies in which both the target dose and the critical biological changes are monitored. Of course, the use of such parameters requires knowledge of the fate of the chemical in the organism and its mechanism of action.

Because the adverse effects under scrutiny for the early detection of health impairment are subtle and individual variations exist in the response to a chemical insult, results can only be evaluated on a statistical basis. This means that the dose-prevalence curves found for exposed workers should always be compared with those derived from observations of a group of unexposed workers matched for other variables such as age, sex, socioeconomic status, and smoking habits. The importance of selecting a control group that is well matched with the exposed group and that undergoes exactly the same standardized clinical, biological, or physiological evaluation at the same time as the exposed group must be emphasized. Because an employed population is a group selected to a

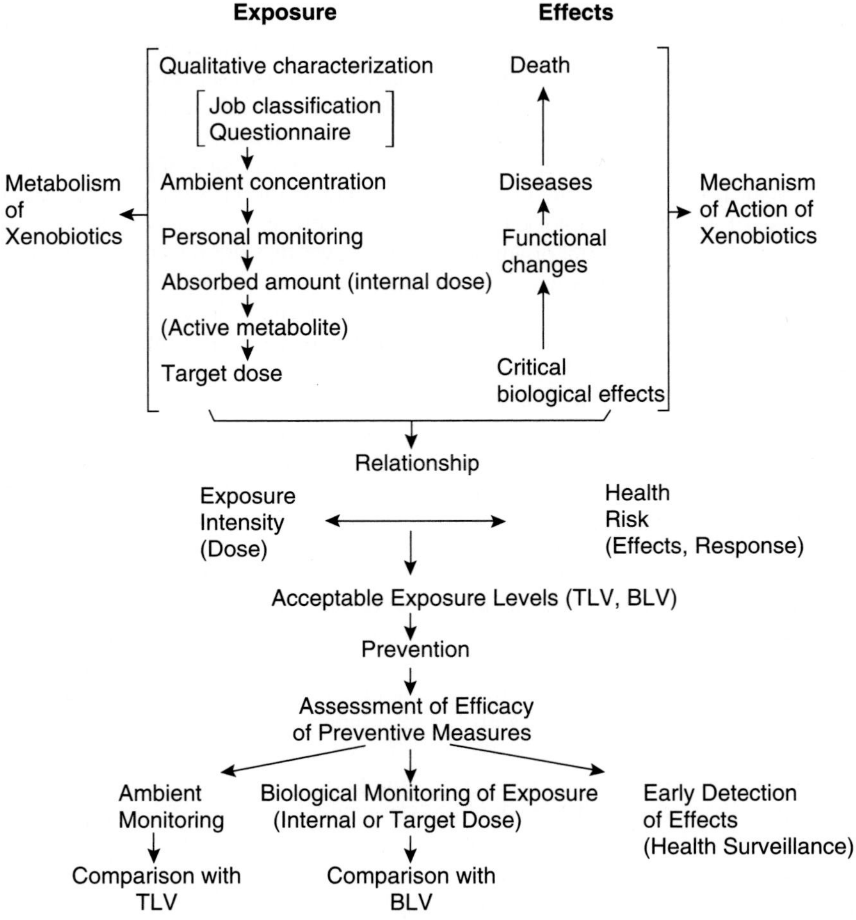


***Figure 33–1. Factors involved in the relationship of exposure and effects in the workplace.***

TLV, threshold limit value; BLV, biological limit value.

certain degree for health, comparison with the general population is not valid. Since such a survey may last for several years (prospective survey or observational cohort study or large-scale cross sectional study), the importance of good standardization of all methods of investigation, such as questionnaires related to subjective complaints, instrumentation, and analytical techniques, must be stressed before the start of the survey. If labor turnover is too high to allow a typical cohort study (i.e., regular examination of the same exposed and control workers), repeated cross sectional studies of exposed and matched controls should be undertaken but it should be kept in mind that such an approach may underestimate the risk, due to the loss of follow-up. If exposure is above the threshold level of effect it is expected that these studies may permit (1) establishment of the relationship between integrated exposure (intensity $\times$ time) and frequency of abnormal results and, consequently, (2) a redefinition of the permissible exposure level.

When a meaningful surveillance program has not been planned before the introduction of a new chemical, it is more difficult to obtain the desired information through investigations designed after the fact. Indeed, in this case evaluation depends on retrospective cohort studies or case-control studies or cross-sectional studies on workers who already may have sustained variable exposure conditions. Because the information regarding the past exposure of the workers is often incomplete and because only late effects are looked for usually in retrospective or case-control studies, a correct evaluation of the no-adverse-effect level is much more difficult. Provided that a satisfactory assessment of past exposure is possible, cross-sectional studies that rely on preclinical signs of toxicity may, to a certain extent, overcome these difficulties. Whether or not clinical investigations are planned from the introduction of a new chemical or process, it is essential to keep standardized records of workers' occupational histories and exposure. The need may arise for mortality or case history studies in order to answer an urgent question on a suspected risk. The evaluation of the acceptable exposure level of benzene in humans illustrates this point (Rinsky et al., 1987).

In addition to these clinical surveys, it is useful to report in case studies any particular observations resulting from exposure to the chemicals (e.g., accidental acute intoxications). Although such isolated observations are not helpful for determining the no-effect level in humans, they are still of interest mainly for new chemicals. They may indicate whether human symptomatology is similar to that found in animals and hence may suggest the functional or biological tests that might prove useful for routine monitoring of exposed workers.

### Testing the Validity of a Biological Method of Monitoring

Experimental work may suggest a biological method for the monitoring of exposure (e.g., evaluation of current exposure, internal load, or target dose). Clinical investigations must then be made to test the applicability of such methods in industrial situations. A brief review of the main biological monitoring methods presently available for evaluating exposure to some industrial toxicological hazards is presented at the end of this chapter.

Likewise, studies in animals may reveal biological effects that precede or are predictive of irreversible functional and/or morphological changes if exposure is prolonged. Epidemiological studies must then be designed to assess the relevance of these parameters for detecting workers at risk.

## EXPERIMENTAL STUDIES ON VOLUNTEERS

Experimental studies on volunteers are usually designed to answer very specific questions, for example, regarding the time course of metabolite excretion during and after exposure; evaluation of the threshold concentration for sensory responses (odor, irritation of the nasal mucosa, etc.); acute effect of solvent exposure on perception, vigilance, and the like. For evident ethical reasons, such studies can only be undertaken when the same results cannot be obtained through other means and under circumstances in which the risk for volunteers can reasonably be estimated as nonexistent. The experimentation should comply with the Declaration of Helsinki (1964), that is, it should be carried out under proper medical supervision on duly-informed volunteers.

## THE NEED FOR SHARING DATA BETWEEN ANIMAL STUDIES AND CLINICAL STUDIES OF WORKERS (OR VOLUNTEERS)

In the field of industrial toxicology, perhaps more than in other areas of toxicology, close cooperation between animal studies and clinical studies of workers plays an important role in explaining the potential risk linked with overexposure to chemicals and, hence, in suggesting preventive measures to protect the health of workers. A few examples will illustrate the complementarity of these disciplines in occupational toxicology.

Several occupational carcinogens have been identified clearly through combined epidemiological and experimental approaches (IARC, 1987). For example, the carcinogenicity of vinyl chloride was first demonstrated in rats (Viola et al., 1971), and a few years later, epidemiological studies confirmed the same carcinogenic risk for humans (Creech and Johnson, 1974; Monson et al., 1974). This observation stimulated several investigations on its metabolism in animals and on its mutagenic activity in various in vitro systems. Identification of vinyl chloride metabolites led to the conclusion that an epoxy derivative is first formed, which is suspected to be the proximate carcinogen. This report triggered a number of investigations on the biotransformation of structurally related halogenated ethylenes, such as vinylbromide, vinylidene chloride, 1,2-dichloroethene, trichloroethylene, perchloroethylene (Bonse et al., 1975; Uehleke et al., 1977; Dekant et al., 1987). All give rise to epoxy intermediates. Comparison of the oncogenic activity of haloethylenes in relation to their metabolism led to the formulation of the "optimum stability" theory of the epoxides. An optimum between the stability and reactivity in both reaching the DNA target and reacting with it after being formed at the monooxygenase site would determine their genotoxic risk (Bolt, 1984). According to this theory, trichloroethylene and perchloroethylene would not represent a significant genotoxic hazard. Clinical evidence, however, is still controversial (IARC, 1987). Furthermore, the possibility of conjugation with glutathione, leading to production of *S*-(1,2 dichlorovinyl)-L-cysteine which, under the action of a beta-lyase, may liberate a reactive thiol in the kidney, cannot be ignored (Dekant et al., 1986, 1987). Indeed it has been shown that in renal cells in culture, *S*-(1,2 dichlorovinyl)-L-cysteine can induce DNA breaks and some oncogene expression (Vamvakas and Köster, 1993). In addition, the finding of *N*-acetyl-*S*-dichlorovinylcysteine in urine of subjects exposed to technical trichloroethylene indicates that a glutathione metabolite can be formed in humans (Birner et al., 1993). Therefore, large-scale retrospective epidemiological studies on persons who have been occupationally exposed to these widely used solvents still are needed.

Dioxane is an industrial solvent with a variety of applications in industry. When it is administered at high doses, the principal toxic effects in rats are centrilobular hepatocellular, renal tubular epithelial degeneration and necrosis, and induction of hepatic and nasal carcinoma (Kociba et al., 1974). The major metabolite in rats was identified as either $\beta$-hydroxyethoxyacetic acid (HEAA) or *p*-dioxane-2-one, depending on the acidity and the alkalinity of the solution. It was found, however, that the biotransformation of dioxane to HEAA may be saturated by high doses of dioxane. This observation led Young to suggest that the toxicity of dioxane occurs when doses sufficient to saturate the metabolic pathway for detoxification are given (Young et al., 1976b). On the premise that the similarity between the metabolic pathway of dioxane in rats and humans would greatly facilitate the extrapolation of toxicological data from rats to humans, Young and coworkers (1976a) examined the urine of plant personnel exposed to dioxane vapor. In the urine of workers exposed to a TWA concentration of 1.6 ppm dioxane for 7.5 h, they found the same product (HEAA) as found previously in the rat. Furthermore, the high ratio of HEAA to dioxane, 118:1, suggests that at a low-concentration dioxane is rapidly metabolized to HEAA. The authors concluded that since metabolic saturation with dioxane in rats was correlated with toxicity, their results on humans supported the hypothesis that low levels of dioxane vapor in the workplace pose a negligible hazard. This conclusion is debatable, however, since dioxane is carcinogenic in rats and guinea pigs and the existence of a threshold level for such chemicals is controversial (Dinman, 1972; Claus et al., 1974; Henschler, 1974). Furthermore, Woo et al. (1977) have reported that *p*-dioxane-2-one is more toxic than dioxane, and its production in vivo may be related to dioxane toxicity and/or carcinogenicity, in view of the fact that a number of lactones with a similar structure are known to be carcinogenic. If it can be shown that *p*-dioxane-2-one is really a proximate carcinogen, workers found to excrete the metabolite will have to be considered at risk.

Dimethylformamide (DMF) is a hepatotoxic solvent extensively used in laboratories and in the production of acrylic resins. Exposure of workers occurs mainly by inhalation of vapor and through skin contact. DMF is rapidly metabolized in vivo. A negligible fraction of the absorbed dose is excreted unchanged in urine and in the gastrointestinal tract. It was initially believed that the biotransformation of DMF in vivo in the rat, dog, and human consisted of a direct demethylation mediated by the microsomal mixed-function oxidases to yield *N*-methylformamide (NMF) and formamide (F) (Kimmerle and Eben, 1975a,b; Maxfield et al., 1975; Krivanek et al., 1978; Lauwerys et al., 1980; Scailteur et al., 1981). It has now been demonstrated that the metabolite identified as NMF by gas chromatography (Barnes and Henry, 1974) is mainly *N*-hydroxymethyl-*N*-methylformamide (DMF-OH), a stable carbinolamine that breaks down in the injector of the gas chromatograph to give NMF (Scailteur and Lauwerys, 1984a,b; Scailteur et al., 1984).

By analogy, *N*-hydroxymethylformamide (NMF-OH) is considered to be the metabolite initially described as F. Only a very small percentage of the absorbed DMF, however, is transformed into NMF and F (probably less than 5%). NMF is more toxic than DMF, and the differences between DMF and NMF toxicity were difficult to explain when NMF was thought to represent the principal in vivo metabolite of DMF. The metabolic studies demonstrating that, following DMF administration, the main urinary metabolites are in fact DMF-OH and NMF-OH and not NMF (Mraz and Nohova, 1992) now offer a logical explanation for these apparent discrepancies, since DMF-OH has been shown to be less acutely toxic than NMF (Scailteur and Lauwerys, 1984b). However, it has been demonstrated that in humans *N*-acetyl-*S*-(*N*-methylcarbamoyl) cysteine (AMCC) is a common urinary metabolite of DMF and NMF (Mraz and Turecek, 1987), and it has been postulated that this biotransformation pathway is responsible for the hepatotoxicity of both solvents possibly because of the formation of methylisocyanate as a reactive intermediate.

It is also possible that in vivo AMCC may release methylisocyanate in different tissues (Slatter et al., 1991). The different amount of reactive intermediate produced from DMF and NMF also might explain the different hepatotoxicity of both compounds (Mraz et al., 1989). It also has been shown that DMF can transiently inhibit its own activation and this phenomenon is probably responsible for the delayed hepatotoxic effect after acute intoxication (Mraz et al., 1993). Observations of workers have clearly demonstrated that for a substance like DMF, which can enter the organism not only by inhalation but also through skin contact, DMF-OH + NMF analysis in urine (both detected as a single NMF peak by gas chromatography) currently appears to be the most pratical method for assessing exposure (Lauwerys, 1986). Further studies are required to assess whether the determination of AMCC in urine may be a more relevant indicator of the health risk (Gesher, 1993).

These examples (vinyl chloride, dioxane, dimethylformamide) demonstrate that the study of the metabolic handling of an industrial chemical in animals is very important because it may lead to the characterization of reactive intermediates, suggesting as yet unsuspected risks, or it may indicate new methods of biological monitoring, which first must be validated by a field study. Conversely, clinical observations on workers may stimulate the study of the metabolism or the mechanism of toxicity of an industrial chemical in animals. This may help in predicting the human response to structurally related compounds or in evaluating the health significance of a biological disturbance. In 1973, an outbreak of peripheral neuropathy occurred in workers exposed to the solvent methyl butyl ketone (MBK) (Billmaier et al., 1974; McDonough, 1974; Allen et al., 1975). The same lesion was reproduced in animals (Duckett et al., 1974; Mendell et al., 1974; Spencer et al., 1975). Biotransformation studies were then undertaken in rats and guinea pigs (Abdel-Rahman et al., 1976; DiVincenzo et al., 1976, 1977), and some MBK metabolites (2,5-hexanedione, 5-hydroxy-2-hexanone) were also found to possess neurotoxic activity (Spencer and Schaumburg, 1975; DiVincenzo et al., 1977). Similar oxidation products are formed from *n*-hexane, the neurotoxicity of which is probably due to the same active metabolite as that produced from MBK. According to DiVincenzo et al. (1977), the most probable active intermediate is 2,5-hexanedione. Since methyl isobutyl ketone and methyl ethyl ketone cannot give rise to 2,5-hexanedione (DiVincenzo et al., 1976), they should preferably replace MBK as solvents. *n*-Hexane derivatives that are oxidized to 2,5-hexanedione are probably also neurotoxic for humans (DiVincenzo et al., 1977).

Organic metabolites of arsenic—namely, monomethylarsonic (MMA) and dimethylarsinic (DMA) acids—have been identified in human urine after ingestion of inorganic arsenic in either the trivalent or pentavalent state (Buchet et al., 1980, 1981a,b). The methylation reaction can be regarded as a detoxification mechanism. In vivo studies on healthy human volunteers and patients suffering from liver diseases and observations on subjects acutely intoxicated with inorganic arsenic (Buchet et al., 1981b, 1984; Mahieu et al., 1981) have shown that the production of DMA is transiently inhibited when inorganic arsenic intake exceeds a certain level and that liver insufficiency significantly modifies the ratio of the methylated metabolites excreted in urine (decreased excretion of MMA and increased excretion of DMA). In vitro studies with rat tissues (Buchet and Lauwerys, 1985, 1988) and in vivo investigation in rats (Buchet and Lauwerys, 1987) have elucidated the mechanism of arsenic biotransformation and the factors influencing it. These studies have demonstrated that the liver cytosol is the main site of biotransformation of inorganic arsenic, which involves two different enzymatic activities for the monomethylated and dimethylated arsenical synthesis. Inorganic arsenic must be in the trivalent state to be methylated, and the process requires the presence of *S*-adenosylmethionine and reduced glutathione. The latter cofactor is only required for the first methylation reaction, which is rate limiting. An excess of substrate inhibits the dimethylation reaction, and this finding is in agreement with the human observations mentioned above. Laboratory studies also suggest that the changes in arsenic methylation observed in patients with liver insufficiency result from a depletion of liver GSH.

Hard metals are alloys of tungsten carbide in a matrix of cobalt metal. They are almost as hard as diamonds and are used for a number of industrial purposes, such as the manufacture of cutting and boring tools. Cases of parenchymal lung disease characterized by a subacute or chronic alveolitis which, in some instances, progresses to interstitial fibrosis (hard metal disease) have been reported among workers exposed to hard metal particles (Balmes, 1987).

Cobalt, which is present in small amounts in hard metals, frequently has been implicated as the causal agent mainly because tungsten carbide alone is considered an inert dust. However, in vitro studies on alveolar macrophage and in vivo studies on rats have clearly demonstrated that cobalt alone is not the only component responsible for the toxicity of hard metal particles on the lung parenchyma (Lison and Lauwerys, 1990, 1992, 1994; Lasfargues et al., 1992). An interaction between cobalt and tungsten carbide, possibly generating oxygen radical species, is responsible for the induction of alveolitis. This interaction explains that studies on workers only exposed to cobalt in cobalt producing plants never revealed any parenchymal impairment (Swennen et al., 1993).

These few examples illustrate the advantage of sharing of information between experimental and clinical studies in the area of industrial toxicology. More rapid achievement of the control of occupational hazards can be accomplished if close cooperation between disciplines is further stimulated.

## PRACTICAL APPLICATIONS

Three important applications of toxicological investigations are stressed here, that is, the proposal of permissible airborne concentrations of chemicals, the development of methods for the biological evaluation of the intensity of exposure to chemicals, and the recommendation of early markers of adverse effects (Fig. 33-1). The basis of these three applications is illustrated by Fig. 33-2, which summarizes the fate of a chemical exerting systemic biological effects from the environment to the target molecules in the organism (Lauwerys, 1984b).

### Permissible Levels of Exposure to Airborne Industrial Chemicals

It is a cliché to say that the best practice in occupational hygiene is to maintain concentrations of all atmospheric contaminants as low as is practical, but even this does not always preclude overexposure to toxic levels of chemicals. The industrial physician must have guidelines to judge the potential health hazards of industrial chemicals and to evaluate whether the general preventive methods in use in the factory are adequate or must be improved or must be complemented by the use of personal

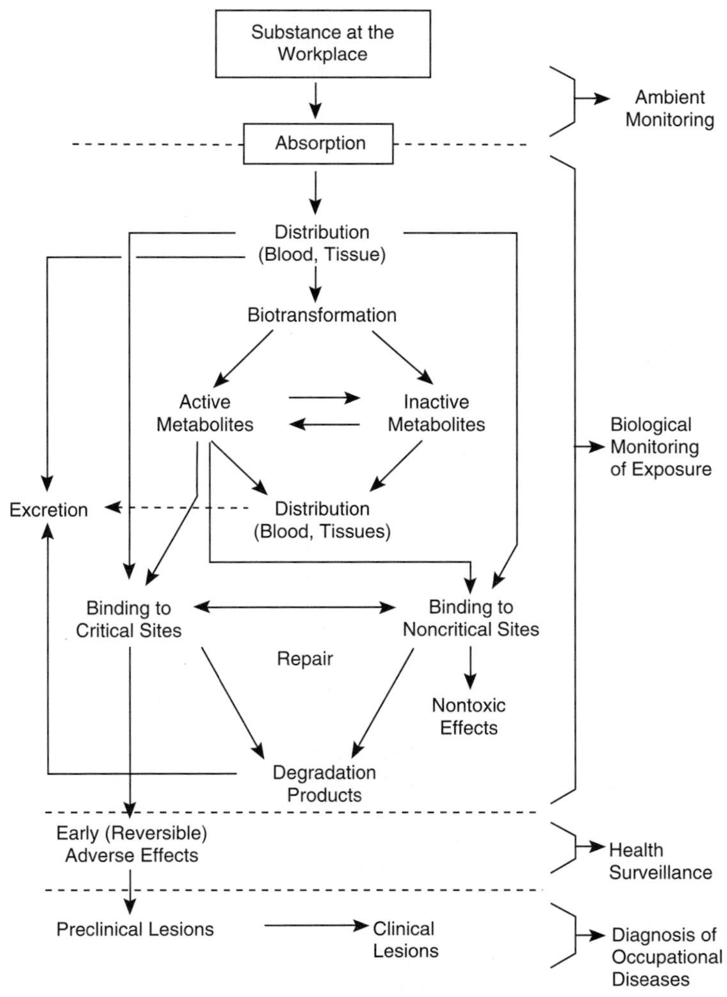


*Figure 33–2. Relationship of metabolic information to biological monitoring of workers.*

protective devices. As indicated above, an important objective of experimental and clinical investigations in industrial toxicology is the proposal of "safe" (i.e., acceptable) levels of exposure. Various private and official institutions regularly review the toxicological information on chemicals in order to propose permissible levels of exposure. ECETOC (1994) has prepared an overview of the work done by 21 organizations involved in reviewing or evaluating data pertaining to the possible hazards posed by more than 3000 industrial chemicals. The database is available in computerized format. Depending on the type of sampling system selected—stationary or personal—the estimate of the risk may be carried out on a group or individual basis. It is evident that with the accumulation of new information on the toxicity of industrial chemicals, the proposed permissible levels must be reevaluated at regular intervals. It should also be made clear that these levels are only guides and should not take the place of close medical surveillance of the workers.

## Biological Assessment of Exposure

Biological monitoring of exposure assesses the health risk through the evaluation of the internal dose. Depending on the chemical and the analyzed biological parameter, the term *internal dose* may cover different concepts (Bernard and Lauwerys, 1986, 1987). It may mean the amount of chemical absorbed recently. Hence, a biological parameter may reflect the amount of chemical absorbed either shortly before sampling (e.g., the concentration of a solvent in the alveolar air or in the blood during the workshift) or during the preceding day (e.g., the concentration of a solvent in alveolar air or in blood collected 16 h after the end of exposure) or during the last months when the chemical has a long biological half-life (e.g., the concentration of some metals in the blood). Internal dose also may mean the amount of chemical stored in one or in several body compartments or in the whole body (the *body burden*). This usually applies to cumulative toxic chemicals. For example, the concentration of polychlorinated biphenyls in the blood is a reflection of the amount accumulated in the main sites of deposition (i.e., fatty tissues). Finally, with ideal biological monitoring, the internal dose means the amount of active chemical species bound to the critical sites of action (the *target dose*). Such tests can be developed when the critical sites are easily accessible (e.g., hemoglobin in the case of exposure to carbon monoxide or to methemoglobin agents) or when the chemical interacts with a blood constituent in a similar way as with the critical target molecule.

When biological measurements are available to assess the internal dose, the approach offers important advantages over monitoring the air of the workplace (Lauwerys, 1984c). Its greatest advantage is the fact that the biological parameter of exposure is more directly related to the adverse health effects that one attempts to prevent than any environmental measurement. Therefore, it may offer a better estimate of the risk than ambient monitoring. Biological monitoring takes into consideration absorption by routes other than the lungs. Many industrial chemicals can enter the organism by absorption through the skin or the gastrointestinal tract. For example, it has been demonstrated that in an acrylic fiber factory, skin absorption of the solvent dimethylformamide, which is used for the dissolution of the polymer (see "The Need for Sharing Data between Animal Studies and Clinical Studies of Workers," above), is more likely to be absorbed by the cutaneous route than by inhalation (Lauwerys et al., 1980). In some industries, ingestion of lead- or cadmium-containing dust may significantly contribute to the overall intake of the metals (Adamsson et al., 1979; Roels et al., 1982).

Even if there exists a relationship between the airborne concentration, the overall dustiness of the workplace, and hence the amount of industrial pollutant entering the organism by any route, one cannot expect that a determination of the airborne concentration will allow for estimation of the total amount of the chemical absorbed by the exposed workers (Lauwerys, 1984a). First, personal hygiene habits (hand washing, smoking at the workplace, etc.) vary from one person to another. Second, it is well known that great individual variation exists in the absorption rate of a chemical through the lungs, the skin, or the gastrointestinal tract. Even if strict personal hygiene measures can be implemented so that the pollutant can enter the organism only by inhalation (in addition to the amount transported from the lungs by mucociliary clearance to the gastrointestinal tract), there is no reason to postulate the existence of a relationship between the airborne concentration and the amount absorbed. This has been demonstrated clearly for lead by King and associates (1979). Many physicochemical and biological factors (particle size distribution, ventilatory parameters, etc.) preclude the existence of such a correlation. For example, a physical load of 100 watts increases by a factor of 2 to 3 the respiratory uptake of trichloroethylene by comparison with the uptake at rest (Monster et al., 1976). The daily uptake of xylene by volunteers exposed to the same TWA concentration varies with the environmental conditions (constant or peak exposures) and the work load (Riihimaki et al., 1979). A biological parameter may take all these different toxicokinetic factors into consideration.

Because of its ability to encompass and evaluate the overall exposure (whatever the route of entry), biological monitoring also can be used to test the efficacy of various personal protective measures, such as gloves, masks, or barrier creams (Lauwerys et al., 1980).

Another advantage of biological monitoring is the fact that the nonoccupational background exposure (leisure activity, residency, dietary habits, smoking, etc.) also may be expressed in the biological level. The organism integrates the total external (environmental and industrial) exposure into one internal load (Zielhuis, 1979). So it is clear that for many industrial pollutants the control of any concentration in air may not necessarily prevent an undue intake by the exposed workers.

Despite this observation, the rational biological monitoring of exposure is possible when sufficient toxicological information has been gathered on the mechanism of action and/or the metabolism (absorption, biotransformation, distribution, excretion) of xenobiotics to which workers may be exposed (Fig. 33-2) (Lauwerys, 1986). When a biological exposure monitoring method is based on the determination of the chemical or its metabolite in biological media, it is essential to know how the substance is absorbed via the lung, the gastrointestinal tract, and the skin, to be distributed subsequently to the different compartments of the body, biotransformed, and finally eliminated. It is also important to know whether the chemical may accumulate in the body. These different kinetic aspects must be kept in mind when selecting the time of sampling.

Biological monitoring of exposure is of practical value only when certain relationships between external exposure, internal dose, and adverse effects are known. Normally, biological monitoring of exposure cannot be used for assessing exposure to substances that exhibit their toxic effects at the sites of first contact (e.g., primary lung irritants) and are poorly absorbed. In this situation, the only useful quantitative relationship is that between external exposure and the intensity of the local effects.

For the other chemicals that are significantly absorbed and/or exert a systemic toxic action, a biological monitoring test may provide different information, depending on our current knowledge of the relationships among external exposure, internal exposure, and the risk of adverse effects, as illustrated in Fig. 33-3 (Lauwerys and Bernard, 1985). If just the relationship between external exposure and the internal dose is known, this biological parameter can be used as an index of exposure, but it provides little information on the health risk (situation (a), Fig. 33-3). In other words, biological monitoring performed under these conditions is much more an assessment of the exposure intensity than of the potential health risk. But if a quantitative relationship has been established between internal dose and adverse effects (situation (c), Fig. 33-3), that is if the internal dose-effects and the internal dose-incidence relationships are known, biological monitoring allows for a direct health risk assessment and thus for an effective prevention of the adverse effects. It is indeed possible to derive a biologically permissible value from these dose-effects and dose-incidence relationships, which is essential to make biological exposure monitoring operational. Unfortunately, the majority of the published studies in this field have focused on the relationship between the internal dose and the external exposure rather than on that between the internal parameter reflecting the internal dose and the adverse effects. Consequently, for many chemicals, the latter relationship is insufficiently documented for a reliable estimation of the biological limit values. In other words, the biologically permissible values are often derived indirectly from the exposure limits in air, through relationships (a) and (b) as shown in Fig. 33-3, a method that is obviously much less reliable than one based on the knowledge of the internal dose-effects and the internal dose-response relationships.

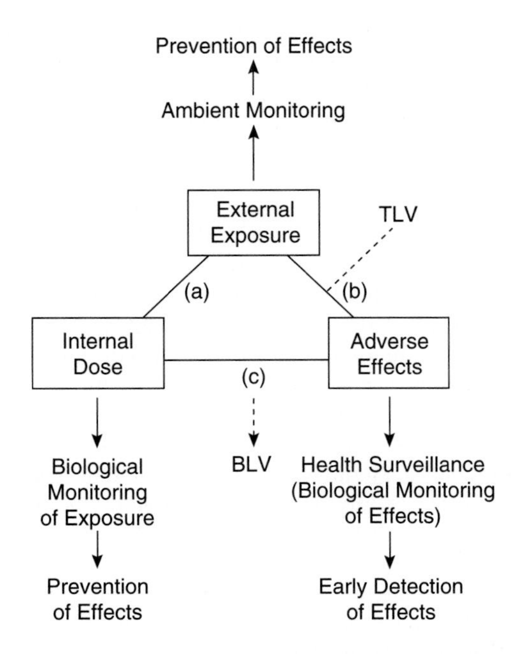


***Figure 33–3. Relationship of external exposure, internal exposure and adverse effects.***

TLV, threshold limit value; BLV, biological limit value.

It must also be kept in mind that the relationships described here may be modified by various factors that influence the fate of an industrial chemical in vivo. Metabolic interactions can be predicted when workers are exposed simultaneously to chemicals that are biotransformed through identical pathways. Exposure to industrial chemicals that modify the activity of the biotransformation enzymes (e.g., microsomal enzyme inducers or inhibitors) may also influence the fate of another compound. Furthermore, metabolic interferences may occur between industrial agents and alcohol, food additives, pesticide residues, drugs, or even tobacco. Changes in any of several biological variables (sex, weight, fatty mass, pregnancy, diseases, etc.) also may modify the metabolism of an industrial chemical. In summary, the relationship between total uptake of an industrial chemical, its concentration or that of its metabolites in biological media, and the risk of adverse effects may be modified by various environmental and biological factors. These may have to be taken into consideration when interpreting the results of biological exposure tests. Whatever the biological parameter measured (the substance itself, its metabolite[s], the target dose), the test must be sufficiently sensitive (not too many false-negative results) and specific to be of practical value (not too many false-positive results).

Other conditions should be fulfilled before attempting to implement biological exposure monitoring methods in industry. The ethical aspects must not be neglected; in particular, the collection of biological specimens cannot involve any health risk for the workers, and the individual results should be considered confidential (Zielhuis, 1978). The selected parameter should be sufficiently stable to allow storage of the biological sample for a certain period of time, and it should be amenable to a non-time-consuming analysis by a not-too-sophisticated technique. The sensitivity, precision, and accuracy of the analysis should be satisfactory. Several intercomparison programs for the analysis of industrial chemicals in biological media indeed have stressed the analytical difficulties sometimes associated with these measurements and the importance of implementing adequate internal and external quality control programs (Elinder et al., 1988). For many industrial chemicals, one or all of the preceding conditions are lacking, which limits the possibilities for biological monitoring of exposure.

It is therefore evident that environmental monitoring still has an important role to play for evaluating and hence for preventing excessive exposure to industrial pollutants. Moreover, as stressed above in this Chap., the prevention of acute toxic effects on the respiratory tract or the eye mucosa can only be achieved by keeping the airborne concentration of the irritant substance below a certain level. Local acute effects of industrial chemicals do not lend themselves to a biological surveillance program. Likewise, biological monitoring is usually not indicated for detecting peak exposure to dangerous chemicals (e.g., $AsH_3$, CO, HCN). Furthermore, identification of emission sources and the evaluation of the efficiency of engineering control measures are usually best performed by ambient air analysis.

In summary, environmental and biological monitoring programs should not be regarded as opposites but, on the contrary, as truly complementary. They should be integrated as much as possible to ensure low levels of contaminants for the optimal health of workers.

The results of a biological monitoring program can be interpreted either on an individual or group basis. Interpretation on an individual level, which is usually carried out by the occupational physician, is possible only if the intraindividual variability of the parameter is not too great and its specificity is sufficiently high. The results may also be interpreted on a group basis by considering their distribution. If all the observed values are below the biologically permissible value, the working conditions are satisfactory. If all or the majority of the results are above the biologically permissible value, the overall exposure conditions must certainly be corrected. A third situation also may occur, which is that the majority of the workers may have values below the biologically permissible level but a few of them have abnormally high values (the distribution is bimodal or polymodal). Two interpretations can be put forward: (1) either the subjects exhibiting the high values perform activities exposing them to higher levels of the pollutant, in which case the biological monitoring program has identified job categories for which work conditions need to be improved, or (2) these workers do not perform different activities and their higher internal dose must result from different hygiene habits or nonoccupational exposure.

Table 33-1 lists some industrial chemicals for which a biological determination may be useful for evaluating the internal dose (Lauwerys and Hoet, 1993). The interpretation of these data requires some comment. Some industrial chemicals have a long biological half-life in various body compartments, and the time of sampling (e.g., blood, urine) may not be critical. For other chemicals, the time of sampling is, on the contrary, critical because following exposure, the compounds and/or their metabolites may be rapidly eliminated from the organism. In these cases, the biological sample is usually collected during exposure, at the end of the exposure period, or sometimes just before the next work shift (16 h after the end of exposure) or even before resuming work after the weekend (i.e., 60 to 64 h after the last exposure).

When biological monitoring consists of sampling and analyzing urine, it is usually performed in "spot" specimens because routine collection of 24-h samples from workers is impractical (Elkins et al., 1974). It is usually advisable to correct the results for the dilution of the urine. Two methods of correction have been routinely used: (1) expression of the results per gram of creatinine or (2) adjustment to a constant specific gravity. Although there is no general superiority for creatinine adjustment over specific gravity, in general creatinine correction is better for concentrated and dilute samples (Elkins et al., 1974). Furthermore, in the case of glucosuria and probably proteinuria, the specific gravity adjustment may give erroneous results. Whatever the method of correction, analyses performed on very dilute urine samples (specific gravity less than 1.010, creatinine concentration less than 0.3 g/liter) are not reliable and should be repeated. In some circumstances, it may be feasible to report results in excretion rate (i.e., quantity/time unit) or one variant (standardization for a diuresis of 1 ml/min) (Araki et al., 1986). Since creatinine excretion depends to a certain extent on urinary flow, Greenberg and Levine (1989) have also proposed to correct creatinine concentration in "spot" urine for the effects of varying hydration. One must, however, recognize that these standardization procedures, which suppose the collection of urine during a known period of time, are usually too elaborate for the routine control of worker exposure. Furthermore, there are compounds for which the expression of urinary results in excretion rate does not improve the accuracy of the exposure estimate.

When the large interindividual variability and/ or the high "background" level of the biological parameter selected makes the interpretation of a single measurement difficult, it is sometimes useful to analyze biological material collected before and after the exposure period. The change in the biological parameter specifically due to exposure can sometimes be better assessed by this method.

When expired air is analyzed, it is preferable to collect end-exhaled samples, which represent alveolar air.

For each chemical agent listed in Table 33-1, the proposed biological parameters, their reference value, and, when data were available, the tentative maximum permissible values are indicated. The significance of the latter proposals must be kept clearly in mind. They are simply tentative guidelines based on the currently available scientific knowledge. Like the airborne TLVs, these guidelines should be subject to regular revision in the light of new scientific data.

## Early Detection of Adverse Effects (Health Surveillance)

A biological monitoring program designed to evaluate the intensity of exposure of workers to industrial chemicals must always be complemented by a health surveillance program (Fig. 33-2). The objective of the latter is to detect as early as possible any adverse biological and functional effects in exposed workers (e.g., release of hepatic enzymes into the plasma, bronchoconstriction, etc.), that is, effects that are likely to be reversible or that do not progress to significant functional impairments when exposure conditions are improved. As defined, health surveillance should not be simply assimilated with the diagnosis of occupational diseases, which, of course, is not any more a preventive activity. Such a program should be implemented even when the results of the environmental or biological monitoring program of exposure indicate that the latter is probably below the acceptable level. Indeed, this level may sometimes contain a large factor of uncertainty, and, this aside, an internal exposure considered safe according to the present state of knowledge may still cause some adverse effects in susceptible individuals.

The implementation of tests capable of detecting early adverse biological effects of industrial chemicals requires a knowledge of their main target organs and their mechanism of action. A review of the tests available for the early detection of adverse effects to various organs or functions following occupational exposure to chemicals is outside the scope of this

**Table 33–1**
**Proposed Methods for the Biological Monitoring of Exposure to Industrial Chemicals**

| CHEMICAL AGENT | BIOLOGICAL PARAMETER | BIOLOGICAL MATERIAL | REFERENCE VALUE | TENTATIVE MAXIMUM PERMISSIBLE CONCENTRATION | REMARKS |
|---|---|---|---|---|---|
| | | *A. Inorganic and Organometallic Substances* | | | |
| Aluminium | Aluminium | Serum | <1 µg/100 ml | | |
| | | Urine | <50 µg/g creat. | 150 µg/g creat. | |
| Antimony | Antimony | Urine | <1 µg/g creat. | 35 µg/g creat. | |
| Arsenic | Total arsenic | Urine | <40 µg/g creat. | | Influence of arsenic of marine origin |
| | | Blood | | | |
| | | Hair | <1 µg/g | | |
| | Sum of inorganic arsenic and methylated metabolites | Urine | <10 µg/g creat. | 50 µg/g creat. if TWA 30 µg/g creat. if TWA : 10 µg/m$^3$ | No interference of arsenic from marine origin |
| Barium | Barium | Urine | <15 µg/g creat. | | |
| | | Blood | <0.8 µg/100 ml | | |
| Beryllium | Beryllium | Urine | <2 µg/g creat. | | Nonsmokers |
| Cadmium | Cadmium | Urine | <2 µg/g creat. | 5 µg/g creat. | |
| | | Blood | <0.5 µg/100 ml | 0.5 µg/100 ml | |
| | Metallothionein | Urine | | | |
| Carbon disulfide | Iodine-azide test | Urine | | >6.5 (Vasak index) | To detect exposure >100 mg/m$^3$ |
| | 2-Thiothiazolidine-4-carboxylic acid (TTCA) | Urine | <1 mg/g creat. | 5 mg/g creat. | |
| Chromium VI (soluble compounds) | Chromium | Urine | <5 µg/g creat. | 30 µg/g creat. | |
| | | Red blood cells | | | |
| Cobalt | Cobalt | Urine | <2 µg/g creat. | 20 µg/g creat. | |
| | | Blood | <0.2 µg/100 ml | | |
| | | Serum | <0.05 µg/100 ml | | |
| Copper | Copper | Urine | <50 µg/g creat. | | |
| | | Serum | <0.14 mg/100 ml | | |
| Fluoride | Fluoride | Serum | | | |
| | | Urine | <0.5 mg/g creat. | 3-4 mg/g creat. | Postshift minus preshift value |
| Germanium | Germanium | Urine | <1 µg/g creat. | | |
| Lead | Lead | Blood | <25 µg/100 ml | 40 µg/100 ml | |
| | | Urine | <50 µg/g creat. | 50 µg/g creat. | |
| | (after 1 g EDTA IV or 2 g DMSA PO) | Urine | <600 µg/24 h | 600 µg/24 h | |

**Table 33–1**
**Proposed Methods for the Biological Monitoring of Exposure to Industrial Chemicals *(Continued)***

| CHEMICAL AGENT | BIOLOGICAL PARAMETER | BIOLOGICAL MATERIAL | REFERENCE VALUE | TENTATIVE MAXIMUM PERMISSIBLE CONCENTRATION | REMARKS |
|---|---|---|---|---|---|
| | Free porphyrin | Red blood cells | <75 $\mu$g/100 ml RBC | 80 $\mu$g/100 ml RBC | |
| | Zinc protoporphyrin | Blood | <40 $\mu$g/100 ml | 40 $\mu$g/100 ml | |
| | | | <2.5 $\mu$g/g Hb | 3 $\mu$g/g Hb | |
| | $\delta$-Aminolevulinic acid (ALA) | Urine | <4.5 mg/g creat. | 5 mg/g creat. | |
| | Coproporphyrins | Urine | <100 $\mu$g/g creat. | 100 $\mu$g/g creat. | |
| | ALA dehydratase | Red blood cells | | | |
| | Pyrimidine-5′-nucleotidase | Red blood cells | | | |
| Lead tetraethyl | Lead | Urine | <50 $\mu$g/g creat. | 100 $\mu$g/g creat. | |
| Manganese | Manganese | Urine | <3 $\mu$g/g creat. | | |
| | | Blood | <1 $\mu$g/100 ml | | |
| Mercury, inorganic | Mercury | Urine | <5 $\mu$g/g creat. | 50 $\mu$g/g creat. | |
| | | Blood | <1 $\mu$g/100 ml | 2 $\mu$g/100 ml | |
| | | Saliva | | | |
| Methylmercury | Mercury | Blood | <1 $\mu$g/100 ml | 10 $\mu$g/100 ml | |
| | | Hair | | | |
| Nickel (soluble compounds) | Nickel | Urine | <2 $\mu$g/g creat. | 30 $\mu$g/g creat. | |
| | | Plasma | <0.05 $\mu$g/100 ml | | |
| Nickel carbonyl | Nickel | Urine | | | |
| Nitrous oxide | $N_2O$ | Urine | | 60 $\mu$g/g creat. | |
| | $N_2O$ | Expired air | | | |
| Selenium | Selenium | Serum | <15 $\mu$g/100 ml | | |
| | | Urine | <25 $\mu$g/g creat. | | |
| Silver | Silver | Urine | <1 $\mu$g/g creat. | | |
| | | Serum | <0.5 $\mu$g/100 ml | | |
| Tellurium | Tellurium | Urine | <1 $\mu$g/g creat. | | |
| Thallium | Thallium | Urine | <1 $\mu$g/g creat. | 50 $\mu$g/g creat. | |
| | | Blood | <0.1 $\mu$g/100 ml | | |
| Uranium | Uranium | Urine | <0.1 $\mu$g/g creat. | | |
| | | Blood | <0.01 $\mu$g/100 ml | | |
| Vanadium | Vanadium | Urine | <1 $\mu$g/g creat. | 50 $\mu$g/g creat. | |
| | | Blood | <0.1 $\mu$g/100 ml | | |
| Zinc | Zinc | Urine | <0.9 mg/g creat. | | |
| | | Serum | <170 $\mu$g/100 ml | | |

| | | | | | |
|---|---|---|---|---|---|
| **1. Nonsubstituted Aliphatic and Alicyclic Hydrocarbons** | | | | | |
| *n*-Hexane | 2-Hexanol | Urine | | 0.2 mg/g creat. | |
| | 2,5-Hexanedione | Urine | | 2 mg/g creat. | End of first workday in week |
| | *n*-Hexane | Blood | | 15 μg/100 ml | During exposure |
| | | Expired air | | 50 ppm | During exposure |
| 2-Methylpentane | 2-Methyl-2-pentanol | Urine | | | |
| | 2-Methylpentane | Expired air | | 1500 μg/L | |
| | 2-Methylpentane | Blood | | 35 μg/100 ml | |
| 3-Methylpentane | 3-Methyl-2-pentanol | Urine | | | |
| | 3-Methylpentane | Expired air | | 1500 μg/L | |
| | 3-Methylpentane | Blood | | 35 μg/100 ml | |
| Cyclohexane | Cyclohexanol | Urine | 3.2 mg/g creat. | | |
| | 1,2-Cyclohexane diol | Urine | | | |
| | 1,4-Cyclohexane diol | Urine | | | |
| | Cyclohexane | Blood | | 45 μg/100 ml | Durng exposure |
| | | Expired air | | 220 ppm | During exposure |
| **2. Nonsubstituted Aromatic Hydrocarbons** | | | | | |
| Benzene | Phenol | Urine | <20 mg/g creat. | 45 mg/g creat. | If TWA : 10 ppm |
| | | | | <20 mg/g creat. | If TWA : 1 ppm |
| | Muconic acid | Urine | <0.5 mg/g creat. | 1.4 mg/g creat. | If TWA : 1 ppm |
| | Benzene | Expired air | | <0.022 ppm | If TWA : 1 ppm (during exposure) |
| | | Blood | | <5 μg/100 ml | If TWA : 1 ppm (during exposure) |
| Toluene | Hippuric acid | Urine | <1.5 g/g creat. | 2.5 g/g creat. | |
| | *o*-Cresol | Urine | <0.3 mg/g creat. | 1 mg/g creat. | |
| | Toluene | Expired air | | 20 ppm | During exposure |
| | | Blood | | 0.1 mg/100 ml | During exposure |
| Ethylbenzene | Mandelic acid | Urine | | 1 g/g creat. | |
| | Ethylbenzene | Blood | | 0.15 mg/100 ml | During exposure |
| | | Expired air | | | |
| Cumene (isopropylbenzene) | 2-Phenylpropanol | Urine | | 200 mg/g creat. | |
| | Cumene | Expired air | | | |
| | Cumene | Blood | | | |
| Trimethylbenzenes (mesitylene, pseudocumene) | Dimethylbenzoic acids | Urine | | | |
| Styrene | Mandelic acid | Urine | | 800 mg/g creat. | |
| | Phenylglyoxylic acid | Urine | | 250 mg/g creat. | |
| | Styrene | Blood | | 0.1 mg/100 ml | |
| | | | | 0.002 mg/100 ml | 16 h After end of exposure |
| | | Expired air | | 9 ppm | |
| | | Urine | | 50 μg/L | |

**Table 33–1**
**Proposed Methods for the Biological Monitoring of Exposure to Industrial Chemicals *(Continued)***

| CHEMICAL AGENT | BIOLOGICAL PARAMETER | BIOLOGICAL MATERIAL | REFERENCE VALUE | TENTATIVE MAXIMUM PERMISSIBLE CONCENTRATION | REMARKS |
|---|---|---|---|---|---|
| α-Methylstyrene | Atrolactic acid | Urine | | | |
| Xylene | Methylhippuric acid | Urine | | 1.5 g/g creat. | |
| | Xylene | Expired air | | | |
| | Xylene | Blood | | 0.3 mg/100 ml | During exposure |
| Biphenyl | 2,4-Hydroxy-biphenyl | Urine | | 1.5 mg/g creat. | |
| Polycyclic hydrocarbons | 1-Hydroxypyrene | Urine | <2 μg/g creat. | 2.7 μg/g creat. | |
| | Hemoglobin adducts | Red blood cells | | | |
| | DNA Adducts | Lymphocytes | | | |
| **3. Halogenated Hydrocarbons** | | | | | |
| Monochloromethane (methylchloride) | *S*-Methylcysteine | Urine | | | |
| Monobromomethane | *S*-Methylcysteine | Urine | | | |
| | Bromide | Blood | | | |
| | | Urine | <10 mg/L | | |
| Dichloromethane | HbCO | Blood | <1% | 2% | Nonsmokers |
| | Dichloromethane | Blood | | 0.05 mg/100 ml | |
| | | Expired air | | 15 ppm | |
| 1,2-Dibromoethane | *N*-acetyl-*S*-(2-hydroxyethyl) cysteine | Urine | | | |
| Vinyl chloride | Thiodiglycolic acid | Urine | <2 mg/g creat. | | |
| Trichlorethylene | Trichloroethanol | Urine | | 150 mg/g creat. | |
| | Trichloroacetic acid | Urine | | 75 mg/g creat. | |
| | Trichloroethanol | Plasma | | 0.25 mg/100 ml | After 5-day exposure |
| | Trichloroethylene | Expired air | | 0.5 ppm | 16 h After the end of exposure |
| | | | | 10 ppm | During exposure |
| | Trichloroacetic acid | Plasma | | 5 mg/100 ml | After 5-day exposure |
| | Trichloroethylene | Blood | | 0.06 mg/100 ml | During exposure |
| 1,1,1-Trichloroethane (methylchloroform) | Trichloroethanol + trichloro-acetic acid | Urine | | 40 mg/g creat. | End of workweek |
| | Trichloroacetic acid | Urine | | 10 mg/g creat. | End of workweek |
| | Trichloroethanol | Urine | | 30 mg/g creat. | |
| | Trichloroethanol | Blood | | 0.1 mg/100 ml | |

| | | | | | |
|---|---|---|---|---|---|
| | Trichloroethane | Blood | | 100 μg/100 ml | |
| | Trichloroethane | Urine | | 800 μg/g creat. | |
| | Trichloroethane | Expired air | | 30 pp | 16 h After the end of exposure |
| Tetrachloroethylene | Tetrachloroethylene | Expired air | | 60 ppm | During exposure |
| | | | | 8 ppm | 16 h After end of exposure |
| | | Blood | | 100 μg/100 ml | 16 h After end of exposure |
| | | Urine | | 70 μg/g creat. | 16 h After end of exposure |
| | Trichloroacetic acid | Urine | | 5 mg/g creat. | End of week |
| Hexachlorobutadiene | Hexachlorobutadiene | Blood | | | |
| Monochlorobenzene | 4-Chlorocatechol | Urine | | | |
| | 4-Chlorophenol | Urine | | | |
| *p*-Dichlorobenzene | *p*-Dichlorobenzene | Urine | | 250 μg/g creat. | |
| | 2,5-Dichlorophenol | Urine | | | |
| Halothane | Trifluoroacetic acid | Urine | | 10 mg/g creat. | After 5-day exposure If TWA : 5 ppm |
| | | Blood | | 0.25 mg/100 ml | After 5-day exposure If TWA : 5 ppm |
| | Halothane | Urine | | 90 μg/g creat. | If TWA : 50 ppm |
| | | | | 10 μg/g creat. | If TWA : 5 ppm |
| | | Expired air | | 0.5 ppm | If TWA : 5 ppm |
| Enflurane (Ethrane) | Enflurane | Urine | | 3.5 μg/L | |
| 2,3,7,8-Tetrachloro-dibenzo-*p*-dioxine (TCDD) | TCDD | Serum | | | |
| | | Blood | | | |
| Polychlorinated biphenyl | Polychlorinated biphenyl | Serum | | | |
| | | Adipose tissue | | | |
| | Trichlorobiphenyl | Blood | | | |
| Other volatile halogenated hydrocarbons (carbon tetrachloride, chloroform, halogenated anesthetics, etc.) | | | | | |
| | Other substances | Expired air | | | |
| | | Blood | | | |
| **4. Aminoderivatives and Nitroderivatives** | | | | | |
| Triethylamine (TEA) | TEA+triethylamine-*N*-oxide | Urine | | 60 mg/g creat. | If TWA : 2.5 ppm |
| Dimethylethylamine (DMEA) | DMEA+dimethylelamine-*N*-oxide | Urine | | 90 mg/g creat. | If TWA : 5 ppm |
| Aniline | Aniline | Urine | | | |
| | *p*-Aminophenol | Urine | | 30mg/g creat. | |
| | Methemoglobin | | <2% | 5% | |
| | Aniline released from hemoglobin adducts | Blood | | 10 μg/100 ml | |
| Nitroglycerine | Nitroglycerine | Blood | | | |
| Ethyleneglycol dinitrate | Ethyleneglycol dinitrate | Urine | | | |
| | | Blood | | | |

**Table 33–1**
**Proposed Methods for the Biological Monitoring of Exposure to Industrial Chemicals *(Continued)***

| CHEMICAL AGENT | BIOLOGICAL PARAMETER | BIOLOGICAL MATERIAL | REFERENCE VALUE | TENTATIVE MAXIMUM PERMISSIBLE CONCENTRATION | REMARKS |
|---|---|---|---|---|---|
| Isopropylnitrate | Isopropylnitrate | Blood | | | |
| | | Urine | | | |
| | | Expired air | | | |
| Several aromatic amino and nitro compounds | Methemoglobin | Blood | <2% | | |
| | Diazo-positive metabolite | Urine | | | |
| | Parent compounds, e.g., benzidine, *β*-naphtylamine | Urine | | | |
| | Hemoglobin adducts | Blood | | | |
| Nitrobenzene | *p*-Nitrophenol | Urine | | 5 mg/g creat. | |
| | Methemoglobin | Blood | <2% | 5% | |
| 4,4′-Methylene bis (2-chloroaniline) (MOCA) | MOCA | Urine | | | |
| Methylene dianiline (MDA) | MDA | Urine | | | |
| Benzidine-derived azo compounds | Benzidine | Urine | | | |
| Monoacetylbenzidine-derived azo compounds | Monoacetylbenzidine | Urine | | | |
| 2,4-Dinitrotoluene | 2,4-Dinitrobenzoic acid | Urine | | | |
| Trinitrotoluene | 2,4- and 2,6-Dinitroamino toluene | Urine | | | |
| **5. Alcohols** | | | | | |
| Methanol | Methanol | Urine | <2.5 mg/g creat. | 25 mg/g creat. | |
| | | Blood | | | |
| | Formic acid | Urine | <60 mg/g creat. | | |
| | | Blood | | | |
| Isopropanol | Acetone | Urine | <2 mg/g creat. | 30 mg/g creat. | |
| | Isopropanol | Expired air | | 500 mg/m$^3$ | |
| Furfuryl alcohol | Furoic acid | Urine | <65 mg/g creat. | | |
| **6. Glycols and Derivatives** | | | | | |
| Ethyleneglycol | Oxalic acid | Urine | <50 mg/g creat. | | |
| | Glycolic acid | Urine | | | |
| | Ethyleneglycol | Serum | | | |

| | | | | | |
|---|---|---|---|---|---|
| Ethyleneglycol monomethylether (methylcellosolve) | Methoxyacetic acid | Urine | | | |
| Ethyleneglycol monoethylether (ethylcellosolve or 2-ethoxyethanol) | Ethoxyacetic acid | Urine | | 150 mg/g creat. | If TWA : 5 ppm |
| Ethyleneglycol monoethylether acetate (2-ethoxy-ethanol acetate) | Ethoxyacetic acid | Urine | | 150 mg/g creat. | If TWA : 5 ppm |
| Ethyleneglycol monobutylether (butylcellosolve) | Butoxyacetic acid | Urine | | | |
| Ethyleneglycol phenylether (phenylcellosolve) | Phenoxyacetic acid | Urine | | | |
| Propyleneglycol monomethylether | Propyleneglycol | Urine | | | |
| $\gamma$-Isomer (1-methoxy-2-propanol) | Propyleneglycol monomethylether | Blood | | 4 mg/100 ml | |
| | | Urine | | 10 mg/g creat. | |
| Propyleneglycol-monomethylether $\beta$-isomer (2-methoxy-1-propanol) | Methoxypropionic acid | Urine | | | |
| Dioxane | $\beta$-Hydroxy-ethoxyacetic acid | Urine | | | |
| **7. Ketones** | | | | | |
| Acetone | Acetone | Urine | <2 mg/g creat. | 30 mg/g creat. | |
| | | Blood | <0.2 mg/100 ml | 5 mg/100 ml | |
| | | Expired air | | | |
| Cyclohexanone | Cyclohexanol | Urine | | 20 mg/g creat. | |
| | 1,2-Cyclohexane diol | Urine | | | |
| | 1,4-Cyclohexane diol | Urine | | | |
| Methylethylketone | Methylethylketone | Urine | | 2.5 mg/g creat. | |
| | | Blood | | | |
| | | Expired air | | | |
| | 3-Hydroxy-2-butanone | Urine | | | |
| Methyl-*n*-butylketone | 2,5-Hexanedione | Urine | | 4 mg/g creat. | End of workweek |
| Methylisobutylketone | Methylisobutylketone | Urine | | 0.5 mg/g creat. | |
| **8. Aldehydes** | | | | | |
| Furfural | Furoic acid | Urine | <65 mg/g creat. | 80 mg/g creat. | |

**Table 33–1**
**Proposed Methods for the Biological Monitoring of Exposure to Industrial Chemicals *(Continue)***

| CHEMICAL AGENT | BIOLOGICAL PARAMETER | BIOLOGICAL MATERIAL | REFERENCE VALUE | TENTATIVE MAXIMUM PERMISSIBLE CONCENTRATION | REMARKS |
|---|---|---|---|---|---|
| **9. Amides and Anhydrides** | | | | | |
| Dimethylformamide | *N*-Methylformamide† | Urine | | 30 mg/g creat. | |
| | Dimethylformamide | Blood | | 0.15 mg/100 ml | |
| | *N*-Methylformamide† | Blood | | 0.1 mg/100 ml | |
| | Dimethylformamide | Expired air | | 2.5 ppm | During exposure |
| | *N*-Acetyl-*S*-(*N*-methyl-carbamoyl) cysteine | Urine | | | |
| Dimethylacetamide | *N*-Methylacetamide | Urine | | | |
| Acrylamide | *S*-(2-Carboxyethyl cysteine) | Urine | | | |
| | Hemoglobin adducts | Red blood cells | | | |
| Maleic anhydride | Maleic acid | Urine | | | |
| Phtalic anhydride | Phtalic acid | Urine | | 8 mg/g creat. | If TWA : 1 ppm |
| Hexahydrophtalic anhydride | Hexahydrophtalic acid | Urine | | 8 mg/g creat. | If TWA : 0.1 ppm |
| **10. Phenols** | | | | | |
| Phenol | Phenol | Urine | <20 mg/g creat. | 250 mg/g creat. | |
| *p*-Tert-Butylphenol | *p*-Tert-butylphenol | Urine | | 2 mg/g creat. | |
| **11. Carbon Monoxide** | | | | | |
| Carbon monoxide | Carboxyhemoglobin | Blood | <1% | 3.5% | Nonsmokers |
| | Carbon monoxide | Blood | <0.15 ml/100 ml | 7 ml/100 ml | Nonsmokers |
| | | Expired air | <2 ppm | 12 ppm | Nonsmokers |
| **12. Cyanides and Nitriles** | | | | | |
| Cyanides and aliphatic nitriles | Thiocyanate | Urine | <2.5 mg/g creat. | 6 mg/g creat. | Nonsmokers |
| | | Plasma | <0.6 mg/100 ml | | Nonsmokers |
| | Cyanide | Blood | <10 μg/100 ml | | Nonsmokers |
| | | Blood | <50 μg/100 ml | | Smokers |
| | SCN (mg/g creat.) ÷ HbCO (%) | Urine + blood | | 3 | |
| Acrylonitrile | Acrylonitrile | Urine | | | |
| | Thiocyanate | Urine | <2.5 mg/g creat. | | Nonsmokers |
| Methemoglobin-forming agents except for specific compounds mentioned elsewhere | Methemoglobin | Blood | <2% | 5% | |
| **13. Isocyanates** | | | | | |
| Toluene diisocyanate | Toluenediamine | Urine | | | |

| | | | | | |
|---|---|---|---|---|---|
| **14. Cyanamides** | | | | | |
| Cyanamide | Acetylcyanamide | Urine | | | |
| **15. Pesticides** | | | | | |
| Organophosphorus | Cholinesterase | Red blood cells | | 30% Inhibition | |
| | | Plasma | | 50% Inhibition | |
| | | Whole blood | | 30% Inhibition | |
| | Dialkylphosphates | Urine | | | |
| Parathion | *p*-Nitrophenol | Urine | | 0.5 mg/g creat. | |
| Carbamates insecticides | Cholinesterase | Red blood cells | | 30% Inhibition | |
| | | Plasma | | 50% Inhibition | |
| | | Whole blood | | 30% Inhibition | |
| Carbaryl | 1-Naphtol | Urine | | 10 mg/g creat. | |
| Baygon | 2-Isopropoxyphenol | Urine | | | |
| DDT | DDT | Serum | | | |
| | DDT+DDE+DDD | Blood | <10 μg/100 ml | | |
| | DDA | Urine | | | |
| Dieldrin | Dieldrin | Blood | <1 μg/100 ml | 15 μg/100 ml | |
| | Dieldrin | Urine | | | |
| Lindane | Lindane | Blood | | 2 μg/100 ml | |
| Endrin | Endrin | Blood | | 5 μg/100 ml | |
| | Anti-12-hydroxy-endrin | Urine | <1 μg/g creat. | 0.13 mg/g creat. | |
| Hexachlorobenzene | Hexachlorobenzene | Blood | <0.3 μg/100 ml | 30 μg/100 ml | |
| | 2,4,5-Trichlorophenol | Urine | | | |
| | Pentachlorophenol | Urine | <30 μg/g creat. | | |
| Pentachlorophenol | Pentachlorophenol | Urine | <30 μg/g creat. | 1 mg/g creat. | |
| | | Plasma | | 0.05 mg/100 ml | |
| Chlorophenoxyacetic acid derivatives (2,4-D; 2,4,5-T; MCPA) | 2,4-D | Urine | | | |
| | 2,4,5-T | Urine | | | |
| | MCPA | Urine | | | |
| Synthetic pyrethroids | Cyclopropane Carboxylic acid | Urine | | | |
| Dinitroorthocresol | Dinitroorthocresol | Blood | | 1 mg/100 ml | |
| | Amino-4-nitro-orthocresol | Urine | | | |
| Ethylene oxide | Ethylene oxide | Expired air | | 0.5 mg/m$^3$ | During exposure |
| | Ethylene oxide | Blood | | 0.8 μg/100 ml | During exposure |
| | *N*-Acetyl-*S* (-2-hydroxyethyl)cysteine | Urine | | | |
| **16. Hormones** | | | | | |
| Diethylstilbestrol | Diethylstilbestrol | | | 30 mg/g creat. | 24-h Urine collection |

**Table 33–1**
**Proposed Methods for the Biological Monitoring of Exposure to Industrial Chemicals *(Continued)***

| CHEMICAL AGENT | BIOLOGICAL PARAMETER | BIOLOGICAL MATERIAL | REFERENCE VALUE | TENTATIVE MAXIMUM PERMISSIBLE CONCENTRATION | REMARKS |
|---|---|---|---|---|---|
| **17. Mutagenic and carcinogenic substances** | | | | | |
| | Mutagenic activity | Urine | | Comparison with a control group | |
| | Thioethers | Urine | | | |
| | Chromosome analysis | Lymphocytes | | | |
| | Spermatozoa analysis | Sperm | | | |
| | Protein adducts | Blood | | | |
| | DNA Adducts | Lymphocytes | | | |
| | Nucleic acid adducts | Urine | | | |
| | Oncogen proteins | Serum | | | |
| **18. Other substances** | | | | | |
| Cyclophosphamide | Cyclophosmadine | Urine | | | |
| Ethylene oxide | Ethylene oxide | Expired air | | 0.5 $mg/m^3$ | |
| | Ethylene oxide | Blood | | 0.8 $\mu g$/100 ml | |
| | *N*-Acetyl-S-(2-hydroxy-ethyl)cysteine | Urine | | | |
| Toluene di-isoyanate | Toluenediamine | Urine | | | |
| Hexamethylene di-isocyanate | Hexamethylenediamine | Urine | | | |

*Analyses performed on biological materials collected at the end of the workday unless otherwise indicated.
†The metabolite measured as *N*-methylformamide by gas chromatography is mainly *N*-hydroxymethyl-*N*-methylformamide

chapter. They are covered in previous chapters, and several publications also specifically deal with this biological monitoring activity (Lauwerys and Bernard, 1989; Rempel, 1990).

## CONCLUSION

The working environment will always present the risk of workers' overexposure to various chemicals. It is self-evident that the control of these risks cannot wait until epidemiological studies have defined the no-adverse-effect level directly in humans. However, extrapolation from animal data has its limitations. A combined experimental and clinical approach is certainly the most effective for evaluating the potential risks of industrial chemicals, hence, for recommending adequate preventive measures and for applying the most valid screening procedures on workers.

Thus the field of industrial toxicology provides many opportunities for scientists with different backgrounds (physicians, chemists, biologists, hygienists) who are convinced of the usefulness of working in close collaboration to understand and prevent the adverse effects of industrial chemicals on workers' health.

# REFERENCES


Abdel-Rahman MS, Hetland LB, Couri D: Toxicity and metabolism of methyl n-butylketone. *Am Ind Hyg Assoc J* 37:95–102, 1976.

Adamsson E, Piscator M, Nogawa K: Pulmonary and gastrointestinal exposure to cadmium oxide dust in a battery factory. *Environ Health Perspect* 28:219–222, 1979.

Aldridge WN, Miles JM, Mount DL, Verschoyle RD: The toxicological properties of impurities in malathion. *Arch Toxicol* 42:95–106, 1979.

Allen N, Mendell JR, Billmaier DJ, et al: Toxic polyneuropathy due to methyl n-butylketone. *Arch Neurol* 32:209–218, 1975.

Araki S, Aono H, Murata K: Adjustment of urinary concentration of urinary volume in relation to erythrocyte and plasma concentrations: An evaluation of urinary heavy metals and organic substances. *Arch Environ Health* 41:171–177, 1986.

ATSDR (Agency for Toxic Substances and Disease Registry): *Toxicological Profile for Arsenic*. Atlanta: U.S. Department of Health & Human Services, 1993.

Baker EL, Zack M, Miles JV, et al: Epidemic malathion poisoning in Pakistan malaria workers. *Lancet* i:31–33, 1978.

Balmes JR: Respiratory effects of hard metal dust exposure. *Occupational Medicine: State of the Art Reviews* 2:327–344, 1987.

Barnes JM: The basis for establishing and fixing maximum allowable concentrations. *Trans Assoc Ind Med Off* 13:74–76, 1963.

Barnes JR, Henry NW III: The determination of N-methylformamide and N-methylacetamide in urine. *Am Ind Hyg Assoc J* 35:84–87, 1974.

Bernard A, Lauwerys R: Present status and trends in biological monitoring of exposure to industrial chemicals. *J Occup Med* 28:559–562, 1986.

Bernard A, Lauwerys R: General principles for biological monitoring of exposure to chemicals, in Ho MH, Millon HK (eds): *Biological Monitoring of Exposure to Chemicals: Organic Compounds*. New York: Wiley, 1987, pp 1–16.

Billmaier D, Yee HT, Allen N, et al: Peripheral neuropathy in a coated fabrics plant. *J Occup Med* 16:665–671, 1974.

Birner G, Vamvakas S, Dekant W, Henschler D: Nephrotoxic and genotoxic N-acetyl-S-dichlorovinyl-L-cysteine is a urinary metabolite after occupational 1,1,2-trichloroethylene exposure in humans: Implications for the risk of trichloroethene exposure. *Environ Health Perspect* 99:281–284, 1993.

Bolt HN: Metabolism of genotoxic agents: Halogenated hydrocarbons, in Berlin A, Draper M, Hemminki K, Vainio H (eds): *Monitoring Human Exposure to Carcinogenic and Mutagenic Agents*. Lyons, France: IARC No. 59, 1984, pp 63–72.

Bonse G, Urban T, Reichert D, Henschler D: Chemical reactivity, metabolic oxirane formation and biological reactivity of chlorinated ethylenes in the isolated perfused rat liver preparation. *Biochem Pharmacol* 24:1829–1834, 1975.

Briatico-Vangosa G, Braun CLJ, Cookman G, et al: Respiratory allergy: Hazard identification and risk assessment. *Fund Appl Toxicol* 23:145–158, 1994.

Buchet JP, Geubel A, Pauwels S, et al: The influence of liver disease on the methylation of arsenic in humans. *Arch Toxicol* 55:151–154, 1984.

Buchet JP, Lauwerys R: Study of inorganic arsenic methylation by rat liver *in vitro*: relevance for the interpretation of observations in man. *Arch Toxicol* 57:125–129, 1985.

Buchet JP, Lauwerys R: Study of factors influencing the *in vivo* methylation of inorganic arsenic in rats. *Toxicol Appl Pharmacol* 91:65–74, 1987.

Buchet JP, Lauwerys R: Role of thiols in the *in vitro* methylation of inorganic arsenic by rat liver cytosol. *Biochem Pharmacol* 37:3149–3153, 1988.

Buchet JP, Lauwerys R, Roels H: Comparison of several methods for the determination of arsenic compounds in water and in urine. Their application for the study of arsenic metabolism and for the monitoring of workers exposed to arsenic. *Int Arch Occup Environ Health* 46:11–29, 1980.

Buchet JP, Lauwerys R, Roels H: Comparison of the urinary excretion of arsenic metabolites after a single oral dose of sodium arsenite, monomethylarsonate or dimethylarsinate in man. *Int Arch Occup Environ Health* 48:71–79, 1981a.

Buchet JP, Lauwerys R, Roels H: Urinary excretion of inorganic arsenic and its metabolites after repeated ingestion of sodium metaarsenite by volunteers. *Int Arch Occup Environ Health* 48:111–118, 1981b.

Claus G, Krisko I, Bolander K: Chemical carcinogens in the environment and in the human diet: can a threshold be established? *Food Cosmet Toxicol* 12:737–746, 1974.

Courtney KD, Moore JA: Teratology studies with 2,4,5-trichlorophenoxyacetic acid and 2,3,7,8-tetrachlorodibenzo-*p*-dioxin. *Toxicol Appl Pharmacol* 20:396–403, 1971.

Creech JL, Johnson HM: Angiosarcoma of the liver in the manufacture of polyvinylchloride. *J Occup Med* 16:150–151, 1974.

Dekant W, Martens G, Vamvakas S, et al: Bioactivation of tetrachloroethylene. *Drug Metab Dispos* 15:702–709, 1987.

Dekant W, Metzler M, Henschler D: Identification of S-1,2-dichlorovinyl-N-acetyl-cysteine as a urinary metabolite of trichloroethylene: A possible explanation for its nephrocarcinogenicity in male rats. *Biochem Pharmacol* 35:2455–2458, 1986.

Dinman BD: "Non-concept" of "no-threshold" chemicals in the environment. *Science* 175:495–497, 1972.

DiVincenzo GD, Kaplan CJ, Dedinas J: Characterization of the metabolites of methyl-n-butyl ketone, methyl iso-butyl ketone, and methyl ethyl ketone in guinea pig serum and their clearance. *Toxicol Appl Pharmacol* 36:511–522, 1976.

DiVincenzo GD, Hamilton ML, Kaplan CJ, Dedinas J: Metabolic fate and disposition of $^{14}$C-labeled methyl n-butyl ketone in the rat. *Toxicol Appl Pharmacol* 41:547–560, 1977.

Duckett S, Williams N, Francis S: Peripheral neuropathy associated with inhalation of methyl n-butyl ketone. *Experientia* 30(11):1283–1284, 1974.

ECETOC (European Centre for Ecotoxicology and Toxicology of Chemicals): Existing Chemicals: Literature reviews and evaluations. Technical Report No. 30(5). Brussels: ECETOC, 1994, pp 1–275.

Elinder CG, Gerhardsson L, Oberdoerster G: Biological monitoring of toxic metals—Overview, in Clarkson TW, Friberg L, Nordberg GF, Sager PL (eds): *Biological Monitoring of Toxic Metals*. New York: Plenum, 1988, pp 1–72.

Elkins HB, Pagnotto LD, Smith HL: Concentration adjustments in urine analysis. *Am Ind Hyg Assoc J* 35:559–565, 1974.

Emerson JL, Thompson DJ, Strebing RJ, et al: Teratogenic studies on 2,4,5-trichlorophenoxyacetic acid in the rat and rabbit. *Food Cosmet Toxicol* 9:395–404, 1971.

Gesher A: Metabolism of N,N-dimethylformamide: Key to the understanding of its toxicity. *Chem Res Toxicol* 6:245–251, 1993.

Greenberg G, Levine R: Urinary creatinine excretion is not stable: A new method for assessing urinary toxic substance concentrations. *J Occup Med* 31:832–838, 1989.

Hard GC, Rodgers IS, Baetcke KP, et al: Hazard evaluation of chemicals that cause accumulation of $\alpha_2\mu$-globulin, hyaline droplet nephropathy, and tubule neoplasia in the kidneys of male rats. *Environ Health Perspect* 99:313–349, 1993.

Henschler D: New approaches to a definition of threshold values for "irreversible" toxic effects? *Arch Toxicol* 32:63–67, 1974.

IARC (International Agency for Research on Cancer): *IARC Monographs on the Evaluation of Carcinogenic Risks to Humans*. Supplement 7, Lyons, France, 1987.

Kimbrough RD: Uncertainties in risk assessment. *Appl Occup Environ Hyg* 6:759–763, 1991.

Kimmerle G, Eben A: Metabolism studies of N,N-dimethylformamide. I. Studies in rats and dogs. *Int Arch Arbeitsmed* 34:109–126, 1975a.

Kimmerle G, Eben A: Metabolism studies of N-N-dimethylformamide. II. Studies in persons. *Int Arch Arbeitsmed* 14:127–136, 1975b.

King E, Conchie A, Hiett D, Milligan B: Industrial lead absorption. *Ann Occup Hyg* 22:213–239, 1979.

Kociba RJ, McCollister SB, Park C, et al: 1,4-Dioxane. I. Results of a 2-year ingestion study in rats. *Toxicol Appl Pharmacol* 30:275–286, 1974.

Krivanek ND, McLaughlin M, Fayerweather WE: Monomethylformamide levels in human urine after repetitive exposure to dimethylformamide vapor. *J Occup Med* 20:179–182, 1978.

Lasfargues G, Lison D, Maldague P, Lauwerys R: Comparative study of the acute lung toxicity of pure cobalt powder and cobalt-tungsten carbide mixture in the rat. *Toxicol Appl Pharmacol* 112:41–50, 1992.

Lauwerys R: Current use of ambient and biological monitoring: Reference workplace hazards. Inorganic toxic agents—cadmium, in Berlin A, Yodaiken RE, Henman BA (eds): *Assessment of Toxic Agents at the Workplace. Roles of Ambient and Biological Monitoring.* Boston: Martinus Nijhoff, 1984a, pp 109–119.

Lauwerys R: Basic concepts of human exposure monitoring, in Berlin A, Draper M, Hemminki K, Vainio H (eds): *Monitoring Human Exposure to Carcinogenic and Mutagenic Agents*. IARC Scientific Publication No. 59, Lyons, France: IARC, 1984b, pp 31–36.

Lauwerys R: Objectives of biological monitoring in occupational health practice, in Aitio A, Riihimaki V, Vainio H, et al (eds): *Biological Monitoring and Surveillance of Workers Exposed to Chemicals*. Washington, DC: Hemisphere, 1984c, pp 3–6.

Lauwerys R: Dimethylformamide, in Alessio L, Berlin A, Boni M, Roi R (eds): Biological Indicators for the Assessment of Human Exposure to Industrial Chemicals. Commission of the European Communities, EUR 10704 EN, Luxembourg, 1986.

Lauwerys R, Bernard A: La surveillance biologique de l'exposition aux toxiques industriels. Position actuelle et perspectives de développement. *Scand J Work Environ Health* 11:155–164, 1985.

Lauwerys R, Bernard A: Preclinical detection of nephrotoxicity: Description of the tests and appraisal of their health significance. *Toxicol Lett* 46:13–29, 1989.

Lauwerys R, Hoet P: *Industrial Chemical Exposure. Guidelines for Biological Monitoring*. 2d ed. Boca Raton, FL: Lewis, 1993, pp 210–305.

Lauwerys R, Kivits A, Lhoir M, et al: Biological surveillance of workers exposed to dimethylformamide and the influence of skin protection on its percutaneous absorption. *Int Arch Occup Environ Health* 45:189–203, 1980.

Lewis TR, Morrow PE, McClellan RO, et al: Establishing aerosol exposure concentrations for inhalation toxicity studies. *Toxicol Appl Pharmacol* 99:377–383, 1989.

Lison D, Lauwerys R: *In vitro* cytotoxic effects of cobalt-containing dusts on mouse peritoneal and rat alveolar macrophages. *Environ Res* 52:187–198, 1990.

Lison D, Lauwerys R: Study of the mechanism responsible for the elective toxicity of tungsten carbide–cobalt powder toward macrophages. *Toxicol Lett* 60:203–210, 1992.

Lison D, Lauwerys R: Cobalt bioavailability from hard metal particles. Further evidence that cobalt alone is not responsible for the toxicity of hard metal particles. *Arch Toxicol* 68:528–531, 1994.

Mahieu P, Buchet JP, Roels H, Lauwerys R: The metabolism of arsenic in humans acutely intoxicated by $As_2O_3$. Its significance for the duration of BAL therapy. *Clin Toxicol* 18:1067–1075, 1981.

Maxfield ME, Barnes JR, Azar A, Trochimowicz HT: Urinary excretion of metabolite following experimental human exposures to DMF or to DMAC. *J Occup Med* 17:506–511, 1975.

McDonough JR: Possible neuropathy from methyl n-butyl ketone. *N Engl J Med* 290:695, 1974.

Mendell JR, Saida K, Ganasia MF, et al: Toxic polyneuropathy produced by methyl-n-butyl ketone. *Science* 185:787–789, 1974.

Monson RR, Peters JM, Johnson MN: Proportional mortality among vinyl-chloride workers. *Lancet* 2(7877):397–398, 1974.

Monster AC, Boersma G, Duba WC: Pharmacokinetics of trichloroethylene in volunteers, influence of workload and exposure concentration. *Int Arch Occup Environ Health* 38:87–102, 1976.

Mraz J, Cross H, Gescher A, et al: Differences between rodents and humans in the metabolic toxification of N,N-dimethylformamide. *Toxicol Appl Pharmacol* 98:507–516, 1989.

Mraz J, Jheeta P, Gesher A, et al: Investigation of the mechanistic basis of N,N-dimethylformamide toxicity. Metabolism of N,N-dimethylformamide and its deuterated isotopomers by cytochrome P4502E1. *Chem Res Toxicol* 6:197–207, 1993.

Mraz J, Nohova H: Absorption, metabolism and elimination of N,N-dimethylformamide in humans. *Int Arch Occup Environ Health* 64:85–92, 1992.

Mraz J, Turecek F: Identification of N-acetyl-S-(N-methylcarbamoyl)cysteine, a human metabolite of N,N-dimethylformamide and N-methylformamide. *J Chromatogr* 414:399–404, 1987.

Rempel D (ed): *Medical Surveillance in the Workplace. Occupational Medicine. State of the Art Reviews*. Philadelphia: Hanley & Belfus, 1990, vol 5, pp 435–652.

Riihimaki V, Pfaffli P, Savolainen K: Kinetics of m-xylene in man. Influence of intermittent physical exercise and changing environmental concentrations on kinetics. *Scand J Work Environ Health* 5:232–248, 1979.

Rinsky RA, Smith AB, Hornuing R, et al: Benzene and leukemia. An epidemiologic risk assessment. *N Engl J Med* 316:1044–1049, 1987.

Roels H, Buchet JP, Truc J, et al: The possible role of direct ingestion on the overall absorption of cadmium or arsenic in workers exposed to CdO or $As_2O_3$ dust. *Am J Ind Med* 3:53–65, 1982.

Scailteur V, Buchet JP, Lauwerys R: The relationship between dimethylformamide metabolism and toxicity, in Brown SS, Davies DS (eds): *Organ-Directed Toxicity, Chemical Indices and Mechanisms*. Oxford, England: Pergamon, 1981, pp 169–74.

Scailteur V, de Hoffmann E, Buchet JP, Lauwerys R: Study on *in vivo* and *in vitro* metabolism of dimethylformamide in male and female rats. *Toxicology* 29:221–234, 1984.

Scailteur V, Lauwerys R: *In vivo* and *in vitro* oxidative biotransformation of dimethylformamide in rat. *Chem Biol Int* 50:327–337, 1984a.

Scailteur V, Lauwerys R: *In vivo* metabolism of dimethylformamide and relationship to toxicity in the male rat. *Arch Toxicol* 56:87–91, 1984b.

Slatter JG, Rashed MS, Pearson PG, et al: Biotransformation of methylisocyanate in the rat. Evidence for glutathione conjugation as a major pathway of metabolism and implications for isocyanate-mediated toxicities. *Chem Res Toxicol* 4:157–161, 1991.

Spencer PS, Schaumburg HH: Experimental neuropathy produced by 2,5-hexanedione—a major metabolite of the neurotoxic industrial solvent methyl n-butyl ketone. *J Neurol Neurosurg Psychiatry* 38:771–775, 1975.

Spencer PS, Schaumburg HH, Raleigh RL, Terhaar CJ: Nervous system degeneration produced by the industrial solvent methyl n-butyl ketone. *Arch Neurol* 32:219–222, 1975.

Swennen B, Buchet JP, Stanescu D, et al: Epidemiologic survey on workers exposed to cobalt oxides, cobalt salts and cobalt metal. *Br J Ind Med* 50:835–842, 1993.

Uehleke H, Tabarelli-Poplawski S, Bonse G, Henschler D: Spectral evidence for 2,2,3-trichloro-oxirane formation during microsomal trichloroethylene oxidation. *Arch Toxicol* 37:95–105, 1977.

Vamvakas S, Köster U: The nephrotoxin dichlorovinylcysteine induces expression of the protooncogenes C-FOS and C-MYC in LLC-PK1 cell. A comparative investigation with growth factors and 12-0-tetradeconoylphorbolacetate. *Cell Biol Toxicol* 9:1–13, 1993.

Viola PL, Bigotti A, Caputo A: Oncogenic response of rat skin, lungs, and bones to vinyl chloride. *Cancer Res* 31:516–522, 1971.

Woo YT, Arcos JC, Argus MF: Metabolism *in vivo* of dioxane: Identification of p-dioxane-2-one as the major urinary metabolite. *Biochem Pharmacol* 26:1535–1538, 1977.

Young JD, Braun WH, Gehring PJ, et al: 1,4-Dioxane and *B*/-hydroxyethoxyacetic acid excretion in urine of humans exposed to dioxane vapors. *Toxicol Appl Pharmacol* 38:643–46, 1976a.

Young JD, Braun WH, LeBeau JE, Gehring PJ: Saturated metabolism as the mechanism for the dose dependent fate of 1,4-dioxane in rats. *Toxicol Appl Pharmacol* 37:138, 1976b.

Zielhuis RL: Biological monitoring: Guest lecture given at the 26th Nordic Symposium on Industrial Hygiene, Helsinki, October 1977. *Scand J Work Environ Health* 4:1–18, 1978.

Zielhuis RL: General aspects of biological monitoring, in Berlin A, Wolff AH, Hasegawa Y (eds): The Use of Biological Specimens for the Assessment of Human Exposure to Environmental Pollutants. Proceedings of the International Workshop at Luxembourg, 18–22 April 1977. The Hague: Martinus Nijhoff, 1979, p 341.

# CHAPTER 34

# REGULATORY TOXICOLOGY

*Richard A. Merrill*

## THE ROLES OF SCIENCE AND REGULATION

This chapter deals with the use of the results of toxicological studies by governmental regulatory agencies and with the requirements these agencies impose for the conduct of such studies. It does not attempt to justify government agencies' handling of toxicology-related issues but rather seeks to explore the interaction of scientific and regulatory institutions in this field.

This explanation begins by recognizing a central difference between the goals of science and government: Science investigates and attempts to explain natural phenomena; it is cautious, incremental, and truth-seeking. Government, in its capacity as regulator, seeks to affect human behavior and settle human disputes; it is episodic and peremptory and pursues resolution rather than truth. It often happens that a regulator cannot withhold a decision or reserve judgment on a problem even when the facts appear to call for a delay, for even a pause to delay out of respect for "getting all the information" has real-world consequences. Because the field of toxicology continuously generates information about the effects of chemicals (though it less often provides information about the magnitude of their effects or the frequency of exposure associated with these effects), regulators invariably are forced to intervene (i.e., to decide) before knowledge is complete.

Scientists often are frustrated by another feature of American regulatory institutions. In the United States, government officials are accorded less discretion to make political or social judgments than in any other industrialized society. Government actions affecting private interests are constrained by the demand that they be authorized by the legislature and that they rest on a factual predicate that it specifies for such decisions. Furthermore, our legal system requires regulators to set forth the facts on which they rely and we allow the opponents of regulatory measures numerous opportunities to contest them. Participants in the regulatory process start from the assumption that the available evidence can be construed in the light most favorable to their position. Regulators, for their part, often overstate the evidence for their decisions, just as those who challenge them do, with the result that both sides frequently appear to distort the facts.

## THE RELATIONSHIP BETWEEN THE DISCIPLINE OF TOXICOLOGY AND REGULATORY INSTITUTIONS

The foregoing observations could apply to any scientific discipline whose investigations underpin governmental decision making. But over the past two decades regulation and toxicology have become intertwined in distinctive ways. The most obvious connection is that regulators whose job is to protect health rely heavily on toxicological principles and experimental data for their evaluation of problems that present the need for a decision. Whether the decision is to assign priorities among a group of compounds or to approve a new substance or restrict the use of an old one, the findings of toxicological investigations are likely to be influential, often decisive.

Regulators are not merely consumers of experimental results but also shape toxicological science in ways that may be unexpected. Regulatory demands have provided a major impetus for improvements in toxicological methods and they have stimulated a demand for major toxicological studies. Some programs, such as the Food and Drug Administration's (FDA) programs for licensing drugs and food additives and Environmental Protection Agency's (EPA) program for registering pesticides, explicitly demand toxicological studies of new, and in some cases marketed, compounds. Such studies constitute a major part of the discipline's research agenda. But even if no government agency were empowered to demand toxicological studies, concern for public health would lead marketers of new products to turn to toxicology to evaluate their possible health hazards.

Regulatory agencies also have exercised important influence over the design and conduct of toxicological studies. For example, the EPA is empowered by the Toxic Substances Control Act (TSCA) to promulgate standards for different types of toxicological (and other scientific) investigations. The FDA has long issued guidelines for laboratory studies submitted in support of food additives and drugs. Both agencies have adopted requirements governing laboratory operations and practice.

Communication between government officials and laboratory scientists flows in both directions. Government testing standards are influenced strongly by the prevailing consensus among toxicologists, many of whom work in regulatory agencies. The procedures for adopting these standards always permit if not encourage the expression of privately held views by members of the discipline.

The balance of this chapter focuses on two of these prominent linkages between toxicology and regulation. The next section outlines the legal and administrative contexts in which regulators rely on toxicological data in making critical decisions. In the final section the focus is on government as a regulator of toxicology, as the source of guidance for and limitations on the design and conduct of laboratory experiments. This chapter does not, however, provide a comprehensive treatment of the legal and regulatory requirements that impinge on toxicology, nor does it discuss every program that relies on toxicological data. It also omits such topics as the laws and regulations designed to protect laboratory personnel, legal restrictions on the handling of dangerous substances, and local requirements for the operation of laboratories.

# REGULATORY PROGRAMS THAT RELY ON TOXICOLOGY

## An Overview of Approaches to Toxic Chemical Regulation

This section surveys current federal programs for controlling human exposure to toxic chemicals. The discussion highlights the features of regulatory programs that influence both the quantity and the quality of data needed to support an agency's decisions.

One such regulatory feature, sometimes overlooked by nonlawyers, is the law's allocation of the "burden of proof," which is the responsibility for demonstrating whether a substance is safe or hazardous. The range of possible approaches can be observed by comparing laws such as the Food Additives Amendment, which requires users of new substances to prove lack of hazard *before* humans may be exposed, with laws such as the Occupational Safety and Health Act (1970), which requires regulators to show that a substance *is* hazardous *before* exposures can be restricted. The approach chosen by Congress largely determines an agency's ability to require comprehensive toxicological investigation of compounds and thus affects the quality of data on which decisions ultimately are based.

A parallel distinction, observable even in programs that mandate premarket testing of new products, is made between substances not yet on the market and those previously approved on the basis of studies that inevitably appear inadequate as investigatory methods improve.

**Typology of Regulatory Approaches.** At least two issues must be resolved to justify government action to regulate human exposure to a substance. First, it must be determined that the substance is capable of harming persons who may be exposed. Second, it must be determined that humans are likely to be exposed to the substance in ways that could be harmful. In the absence of affirmative answers to both questions, government intervention to control exposure would be difficult to justify. A few statutes require only these two findings. Most laws under which chemicals are regulated, however, mandate or permit consideration of other criteria as well, such as the *magnitude* of the risk posed by a substance and the *consequences* of regulating it.

**Agencies Involved.** At the federal level, four agencies are chiefly responsible for regulating human exposure to chemicals: the FDA, the EPA, the Occupational Safety and Health Administration (OSHA), and the Consumer Product Safety Commission (CPSC). Together they administer some two-dozen statutes whose primary goal is the protection of health. The statutes administered by these four agencies convey different levels of concern about risks to human health and about the weight to be given economic costs (OTA, 1981). This diversity has several explanations. The statutes were enacted in different eras. They originated with, and remain under the influence of, different political constituencies. Perhaps most significant, statutory standards often reflect differences in the technical capacity to control different types of exposures and they embody different congressional judgments about the economic benefits of limiting exposures.

**Summary of Current Approaches.** For at least two decades, federal regulatory agencies have distinguished between cancer and all other toxic effects. However, it is in their treatment of carcinogens that existing statutes appear to display the greatest diversity. For other (noncarcinogenic) chemicals, regulators have generally embraced a standard safety assessment formula, built around the concept of *acceptable daily intake* (ADI). The ADI for a chemical is derived by applying a safety factor—usually 100, but sometimes a larger number if the toxicological data are sparse or occasionally a smaller number if the data are very good—to the human equivalent of the lowest no-observed-effect level (NOEL) revealed in animal experiments. When estimated human exposure to a chemical falls below the ADI, it—or the quantity of it that results in that exposure—is adjudged "safe." It is only when exposure is likely to exceed the ADI that the regulator must turn to any other considerations made relevant by the applicable statute.

However, this traditional approach to conventional toxicants has not been considered appropriate for carcinogens. Regulators in the United States and many of their counterparts in other countries have operated on the premise that carcinogens as a class cannot be assumed to have "safe" or threshold doses. Furthermore, they have assumed that any chemical shown convincingly in animal studies to cause cancer should be considered a potential human carcinogen. Accordingly, for this group of compounds, which has grown to exceed 500 as more chemicals have been subjected to long-term testing, United States regulators have assumed that no finite level of human exposure can be considered risk-free. This set of assumptions has profoundly affected the way carcinogenic chemicals have been regulated in this country.

***No Risk.*** This approach is epitomized by the famous Delaney Clause, enacted in 1958 as part of the Food Additives Amendment. The amendment itself requires that any food additive be found safe before the FDA may approve its use (FD&C Act, 1958). The Delaney proviso stipulates that this finding may not be made for a food additive that has been shown to induce cancer in humans or in experimental animals. The Delaney Clause has been characterized as a categorical risk-benefit judgment by Congress that no food additive is likely to offer benefits sufficient to outweigh any risk of cancer (Turner, 1971).

***Negligible Risk.*** Because the risk posed even by a carcinogenic substance depends on the dose, as well as its potency, it may be possible to reduce human exposure to such low levels that any associated risk is small enough to ignore without considering any other criteria. No current health statute explicitly prescribes such a "negligible risk" approach, but the FDA has adopted it administratively for some classes of environmental carcinogens. For example, under a 1962 amendment to the Delaney Clause, the FDA may approve a carcinogenic drug for use in food-producing animals if no residue will be found in edible tissues of treated animals (FD&C Act, 1938). The FDA announced that it will calibrate its tests for residues so that they only register toxins with carcinogenic potency (FDA, 1985) and will approve a carcinogenic drug if the sponsor provides an analytic method capable of detecting residues in meat, milk, or eggs large enough to pose a lifetime dietary risk greater than 1 in 1 million, as determined by extrapolation from animal bioassays.

Any such "negligible risk" approach requires data depicting carcinogenic potency. This is not a major problem when an agency can require a product's sponsor to conduct the necessary tests, but programs in which regulation responds to already extant exposures often lack such leverage. The approach also requires the selection of a method for quantifying the risk associated with low doses of a carcinogen. As a practical matter, a negligible risk approach will not suffice when exposures to toxic substances cannot be reduced to very low levels without sacrificing other values.

***Trade-off Approaches.*** These embrace a variety of formulas that have one common feature: Each requires the regulatory agency to weigh factors in addition to the health risks posed by substances targeted for regulation. One version is illustrated by the Occupational Safety and Health Act, which directs OSHA, in setting workplace standards for toxic materials, to elect the standard "which most adequately assures, *to the extent feasible* . . . that no employee will suffer material impairment of health or functional capacity" (OSHA, 1970). OSHA has interpreted "feasibility" as requiring it to consider, in addition to the risk posed by a substance, the availability of technology for reducing exposure and the financial ability of the responsible industries to pay for the necessary controls. The agency need not, however, balance the health benefits of mandated exposure controls against the costs of achieving them (*American Textile Manufacturers Institute v. Donovan*, 1982).

A more expansive "trade-off" law is the Federal Insecticide, Fungicide, and Rodenticide Act (FIFRA), which requires the EPA to refuse or withdraw registration of a pesticide if its use is likely to result in "unreasonable adverse effects on health or the environment" (FIFRA, 1972). The EPA interprets this language as requiring that it weigh all the effects of a pesticide—its contribution to food production as well as its possible adverse effects on applicators, consumers, and the natural environment—in determining whether, or on what terms, to permit registration. The Toxic Substances Control Act (TSCA, 1976) uses more explicit language to mandate the balancing of risks and benefits.

## Programs for Regulating Chemical Hazards

**Food and Drug Administration.** The oldest of the major health regulation laws, the Food, Drug, and Cosmetic Act, was enacted in 1938 and covers food for humans and animals, human and veterinary drugs, medical devices, and cosmetics.

***Food.*** The original 1906 Food and Drugs Act contained two prohibitions addressed to foods containing hazardous constituents; both remain part of the current law. The first forbids the marketing of any food containing "any *added* poisonous or deleterious *substance which may render it injurious* to health," a provision that the FDA has interpreted as barring foods presenting any significant risk. The second forbids the marketing of foods containing *nonadded* toxicants that make them "*ordinarily injurious* to health," a standard that accords a preferred status to traditional components of the American diet (FD&C Act § 402(a)). Neither of these original provisions required premarket approval; the FDA had the burden of proving that a food was, in the legal vernacular, "adulterated."

Congress has since amended the Act several times to improve the FDA's ability to ensure the safety of foods. Each time, it identified a class of additives for which it prescribed a form of premarket approval, thus giving the FDA the authority not only to evaluate a substance's safety before humans are exposed but also to specify the kinds of studies necessary to obtain approval (FDA, 1994).

The most important of these amendments was the 1958 Food Additives Amendment. For food additives, the law requires safety to be demonstrated prior to marketing. The critical standard for approval is that the substance is "reasonably certain to be safe"; no inquiry into the benefits of an additive is undertaken or authorized (Cooper, 1978). But the amendment does not apply to all food ingredients. Congress excluded substances that are "generally recognized as safe" (GRAS) by qualified scientific experts. In effect, it instructed the FDA to pay less attention to ingredients that had been in use for many years without observable adverse effects. Congress also excepted ingredients sanctioned by either the FDA or the USDA prior to 1958. The practical significance of this exception is that a "prior-sanctioned" ingredient is not subject to the Delaney Clause because it is not technically a food additive.

Three classes of indirect food constituents—pesticide residues, animal drug residues, and food contact materials—are subject to distinct regulatory standards. Pesticide residues on raw agricultural commodities are regulated by the EPA under a 1954 amendment to the FD&C Act, which allows residues if they meet a tolerance established by the agency (FD&C Act § 348). In setting tolerances, the EPA may consider both the potential adverse health effects of residues and the value of pesticide uses. Pesticide residues that satisfy established tolerances are exempt from the food additive provisions of the FD&C Act, including the Delaney Clause. If the concentration of a pesticide in a processed food exceeds the established tolerance, however, and the pesticide is a carcinogen, the Delaney Clause prohibits its approval for that use (*Les v. Reilly*, 1992).

Any animal drug residue must be shown to be safe for humans under essentially the same standards that apply to food additives, with a notable exception. The FDA has interpreted the 1962 authorization for approval of carcinogenic compounds ("if . . . no residue of the additive will be found") as allowing residues that pose no more than a negligible risk.

A food contact substance requires approval as a food additive if, when used as intended, it "may reasonably be expected to become a component of food." This vague language presents two issues. First, the Delaney Clause appears to preclude approval if the material induces cancer, as some important food-packaging materials, such as acrylonitrile and polyvinylchloride, clearly do. Second, the scientific principle of diffusion supports the argument that all food contact substances are properly characterized as food additives. The FDA has attempted to cushion this potential collision between toxicological findings and advances in analytic chemistry. It has declined to apply the Delaney Clause to carcinogenic migrants whose extrapolated risk does not exceed 1 in 1 million because these migrants present only a minimal risk (FDA, 1984). And the FDA has proposed a rule that would exempt noncarcinogenic food-contact substances from the food additive requirements when the potential for migration is trivial. The proposal establishes a dietary concentration of 0.5 ppb as the "threshold of regulation" for food-contact substances (FDA, 1993).

Environmental contaminants constitute the final category of food constituents that is of concern to regulators. The FDA relies on a provision of the 1938 act authorizing the establishment of tolerances for "added poisonous or deleterious substances" that cannot be avoided through good manufacturing practice. In setting such tolerances, the FDA weighs three factors: (1) the health effects of the contaminant, usually estimated on the basis of animal data: (2) the ability to measure the contaminant; and (3) the effects of various tolerance levels on the price and availability of the food (Merrill and Schewel, 1980).

***Human Drugs.*** Preclinical studies play an important role in the FDA's evaluation of human drugs. The current law requires premarket approval, for both safety and efficacy, of all "new" drugs, a category that embraces virtually all prescription drug ingredients introduced since 1938 (Hutt and Merrill, 1991). Investigation of therapeutic agents in humans has long been accepted, and the primary evidence of safety accordingly comes from clinical and not laboratory studies. However, animal studies are the sole source of information about a substance's biological effects before human trials are begun, and their results influence not only the decision whether to expose human subjects but also the design of clinical protocols (FDA, 1994).

***Medical Devices.*** In 1976, Congress overhauled the FD&C Act's requirements for medical devices, according the FDA major new authority to regulate their testing, marketing, and use. The elaborate new scheme contemplates three tiers of control, the most restrictive of which is premarket approval similar to that required for new drugs. To obtain FDA approval of a so-called class III device, the sponsor must demonstrate safety and efficacy. The bulk of the data supporting such applications will be derived from clinical studies but also will include toxicological studies of any constituents likely to be absorbed by the patient.

***Cosmetics.*** The statutory provisions governing cosmetics do not require premarket approval of any product or demand that manufacturers test their products for safety, though most manufacturers routinely do so. The basic safety standard for cosmetics is similar to that for food ingredients; no product may be marketed if it contains "a poisonous or deleterious substance which may render it injurious to health" (FD&C Act § 601(a)). The case law establishes that this language, too, bars distribution of a product that poses any significant risk of more than transitory harm when used as intended, but it places on the FDA the burden of proving violations (Hutt and Merrill, 1991). The FDA has brought few cases under this standard, in part because acute toxic reactions are readily detected and immediately result in abandonment of the offending ingredient.

While the law does not require premarket proof of safety for most cosmetic ingredients generally, it does mandate safety testing for color additives. The scheme enacted by Congress in 1960 (FD&C Act § 706) resembles that for food additives, except that no colors are exempt; every color additive must be shown, with "reasonable certainty," to be safe. A separate version of the Delaney Clause precludes approval of any carcinogenic color additive, no matter how small a risk it presents (*Public Citizen v. Young*, 1987).

**Environmental Protection Agency.** Created in 1970, the EPA immediately became responsible for administering numerous existing laws protecting human health and the environment. Congress has since enacted almost a dozen additional statutes that provide the core of the EPA's current authority. A comprehensive review of the EPA's many programs is not possible here; the following summary focuses on those EPA activities in which toxicological evidence plays a central role: pesticide regulation, regulation of industrial chemicals, regulation of drinking water supplies, hazardous waste control, and regulation of toxic pollutants of water and of air.

***Pesticides.*** Under the Federal Insecticide, Fungicide, and Rodenticide Act (FIFRA), no pesticide may be marketed unless it has been registered by the EPA. The law specifies that a pesticide shall be registered if it is effective, bears proper labeling, and "when properly used . . . will not generally cause unreasonable adverse effects on the environment" (FIFRA § 136b). Congress defined this last criterion as "any unreasonable risk to man or the environment, taking into account the economic, social and environmental costs and benefits of the use of any pesticide." Most of the data supporting a product's initial registration—mainly toxicological studies—are provided by the sponsor.

In the early 1970s, the EPA engendered controversy by canceling registrations for a number of pesticides based primarily on studies suggesting they were carcinogenic in animals. Criticism of its "hair-trigger" approach to regulation, coupled with court rulings that the agency was obligated to initiate the process of cancellation whenever a pesticide's safety came into question, led to important changes in the law. Congress added procedural safeguards for pesticide manufacturers and created a panel of outside scientists to review contemplated actions against pesticides (FIFRA, 1972). The EPA itself established a procedure, now named "special review," for public ventilation of disputes over the risks and benefits of pesticides before the formal cancellation process is undertaken (EPA, 1980). A pesticide will be subjected to close scrutiny if the EPA concludes that it induces cancer in experimental mammalian species or in man. The agency has published general guidelines for assessing whether a pesticide or any other substance poses a cancer risk to humans (EPA, 1984). Even if a pesticide is convincingly shown to be a carcinogen, however, the law would allow it to be registered if the EPA concluded that its economic benefits outweighed the risk.

The EPA has for over a decade been engaged in a comprehensive review of previously registered pesticides and "reregistration" of those that meet contemporary standards for marketing. Under this program, many older pesticides have been subjected to comprehensive toxicological testing, including carcinogenicity testing, for the first time, and the results have required modification of the terms of approved use and, in some instances, cancellation for several agents. In 1988, Congress amended the law to require the EPA to accelerate this reregistration effort (FIFRA Amendments, 1988). The agency was specifically requested to increase the stringency of its requirements for neurotoxic and behavioral testing to include tests "related to chronic exposure, prenatal, and neonatal effects." The EPA has since published additional testing data requirements for 160 active pesticide ingredients and has issued decisions on reregistration eligibility for over 70 ingredients.

***Industrial Chemicals.*** The Toxic Substance Control Act (TSCA) (1976) represents Congress's most ambitious effort to control the hazards of chemicals in commercial production. The TSCA covers all chemical substances manufactured or processed in or imported into the United States, except for substances already regulated under other laws. A *chemical substance* is defined broadly as "any organic or inorganic substance of a particular molecular identity."

The TSCA gives the EPA three main powers. The agency is empowered to restrict, including banning the manufacture, processing, distribution, use, or disposal of, a chemical substance when there is a reasonable basis to conclude any such activity poses an "unreasonable risk of injury to health or environment." In determining whether a chemical substance presents an unreasonable risk, the agency is instructed (TSCA § 6) to consider

> the effects of such substance or mixture on the health and the magnitude of the exposure of human beings to such substance or mixture; the effects of such substance or mixture on the environment and the magnitude of the exposure of the environment to such substance or mixture; the benefits of such substance for various uses and the availability of substitutes; and the reasonably ascertainable economic consequences of the rule, after consideration of the effect on the national economy, small business, technological innovation, the environment and public health.

The EPA also must consider any rule's positive impact on the development and use of substitutes as well as its negative impact on manufacturers or processors of the chemical and weigh the economic savings to society resulting from reduction of the risk.

The TSCA's trade-off approach to regulation has proved a major challenge to the EPA. The agency has not often used its authority often under TSCA § 6. In 1989, it issued a comprehensive rule prohibiting the future manufacture, importation, processing, and distribution of almost all products containing asbestos. Despite the documented hazards of asbestos, a court overturned the rule; the ban failed to satisfy the statutory requirement that the EPA promulgate the "least burdensome" regulation required to protect the environment (*Corrosion Proof Fittings v. Environmental Protection Agency*, 1991). The ban continues to govern products that were not in manufacture as of mid-1989, but the EPA has not attempted to issue a new rule regulating existing asbestos-containing products.

If the EPA suspects that a chemical *may* pose an unreasonable risk but lacks sufficient data to take action, the TSCA empowers it to require testing to develop the necessary data. Similarly, it may order testing if the chemical will be produced in substantial quantities that may result in significant human exposure whose effects cannot be predicted on the basis of existing data. In either case, the EPA must consider the "relative costs of the various test protocols and methodologies" and the "reasonably foreseeable availability of the facilities and personnel" needed to perform the tests (TSCA § 4).

Finally, to enable the EPA to evaluate chemicals before humans are exposed, the TSCA requires the manufacturer of a new chemical substance to notify the agency 90 days prior to production or distribution (TSCA § 5(a)(1)). The manufacturer's or distributor's notice must include any health effects data it possesses. However, the EPA is not empowered to require that manufacturers routinely conduct testing of all new chemicals to permit an evaluation of their risks; Congress declined to confer that kind of premarket approval authority that the FDA exercises for drugs and food additives and EPA exercises for pesticides.

The system for regulating new and existing chemical substances in the European Union (E.U.) highlights both the advantages and disadvantages of the U.S. system under the TSCA. Since 1979, the E.U. has required manufacturers of new chemical substances to submit notification to a member state at least 45 days prior to *marketing* the substance. The notification for substances produced in excess of one ton per year must include a base set of data that assesses acute and subacute toxicity, mutagenicity, and carcinogenic screening. Additional tests may be required if the production level exceeds specified volumes or if the base set of data suggests a possible hazard. In 1992, the E.U. expanded its regulatory scheme by imposing health effects testing requirements on chemicals produced in amounts of less than one ton per year and by lengthening the waiting period from 45 to 60 days. In addition, member states that receive notification are now obligated to conduct risk assessments on new substances in accordance with guidelines adopted by the E.U.

The E.U. and U.S. systems for regulating new chemicals thus differ significantly. The E.U. scheme requires manufacturers to generate and submit a base set of data concerning the health risks of most new chemicals; the EPA is authorized to order testing only in limited situations. The TSCA, however, permits regulatory intervention at a much earlier stage than the E.U. by requiring notification prior to manufacturing. Perhaps most importantly, the E.U. system addresses only notification, labeling, and packaging, while member states retain their independent authority over the control of new substances.

In 1993, the E.U. adopted a scheme for regulating approximately 100,000 existing chemicals that are listed on the European Inventory of Existing Chemical Substances (EINECS). The E.U. system for regulating existing chemicals closely resembles the TSCA approach. Manufacturers of existing chemicals must submit existing data on the chemicals. Based on this data, E.U. regulators select priority chemicals each year and assign the responsibility for assessing these chemicals to member states. Manufacturers of priority chemicals must submit data for the assessments and perform new studies if necessary.

***Hazardous Wastes.*** Several statutes administered by the EPA regulate land disposal of hazardous materials. The principal law is the Resource Conservation and Recovery Act (RCRA), enacted in 1976. The RCRA established a comprehensive federal scheme for regulating hazardous waste. Directed to promulgate criteria for identifying hazardous wastes, the EPA has specified these as ignitability, corrosivity, reactivity, and toxicity. The agency has identified accepted protocols for determining these characteristics and established a list of substances whose presence will make waste hazardous.

The RCRA directs the EPA to regulate the activities of generators, transporters, and those who treat, store, or dispose of hazardous wastes. Standards applicable to generators, transporters, and handlers of hazardous wastes must "protect human health and the environment." The EPA's regulations applicable to generators and transporters establish a manifest system that is designed to create a paper trail for every shipment of waste, from generator to final destination, to ensure proper handling and accountability. The agency has the broadest authority over persons who own or operate hazardous waste treatment, storage, or disposal facilities. Pursuant to the RCRA, it issued regulations prescribing methods for treating, storing, and disposing of wastes; governing the location, design, and construction of facilities; mandating contingency plans to minimize negative impacts from such facilities; setting qualifications for ownership, training, and financial responsibility; and requiring permits for all such facilities (EPA, 1993).

***Toxic Water Pollutants.*** The EPA has had responsibility for regulating toxic water pollutants since 1972. As originally enacted, Section 307 of the Federal Water Pollution Control Act required the EPA to publish within 90 days and periodically add to a list of toxic pollutants for which effluent standards (discharge limits) would then be established.

Section 307(a)(4) of the Federal Water Pollution Control Act originally specified that in establishing standards for any listed pollutant the EPA was to provide an "*ample margin of safety*," a difficult criterion to meet for most toxic pollutants and arguably impossible for any known to be carcinogenic. The law also mandated both a rapid timetable and a complex procedure for standard-setting.

The EPA's slow implementation of these instructions precipitated a series of lawsuits. The agency eventually reached a court-sanctioned settlement that fundamentally altered federal policy toward toxic pollutants of the nation's waterways. The settlement allowed the EPA to act under other provisions of the act that allow consideration of economic costs and technological feasibility in setting limits. Congress incorporated the terms of this settlement in 1977 amendments to the statute.

In 1987, Congress again amended the Federal Water Pollution Control Act to toughen standards for toxic pollutants. Under the 1977 amendments, the EPA had developed health-based "water quality criteria" for 126 compounds it had identified as toxic. These criteria described *desirable* maximum contamination levels which, because the EPA's discharge limits were technology-based, generally were substantially lower than the levels actually achieved. The 1987 amendments gave these theretofore advisory criteria real bite by requiring that states incorporate them in their own mandatory standards for water quality and impose on operations discharging into below-standard waterways additional effluent limits (Heineck, 1989).

***Drinking Water.*** The 1974 Safe Drinking Water Act (SDWA) was enacted to ensure that public water supply systems "meet minimum national standards for the protection of public health." Under the SDWA, the EPA is required to regulate any contaminants "which may have an adverse effect on human health." The EPA was to establish national primary drinking water regulations for public water systems. For each contaminant of concern, the agency was to prescribe a maximum contaminant level (MCL) or a treatment technique for its control.

The 1974 act prescribed a two-stage process. The EPA first was required to promulgate interim national primary drinking water regulations, uniform minimum standards that would "protect health to the extent feasible . . . (taking costs into consideration)." These interim regulations were later supplanted by regulations formulated on the basis of a series of reports by the National Academy of Sciences (NAS). The charge to the NAS Safe Drinking Water Committee was to recommend the MCLs necessary to protect humans from any known or anticipated adverse health effects. In turn, the EPA was to specify MCLs as close as feasible to the levels recommended by the NAS. By 1986, the EPA had established MCLs for 23 contaminants but treatment techniques for none.

In that year Congress amended the Safe Drinking Water Act to cover more contaminants, to apply more pressure to states and localities to clean up their drinking water supplies, and to strengthen EPA's enforcement role. The EPA was required to adopt regulations for a total of 83 contaminants within 3 years (including all but one of those originally regulated). It was directed to prescribe regulations for two treatment techniques for public water systems—filtration and disinfection. In translating recommended MCLs (now maximum contaminant level goals) into feasible and enforceable regulations, the EPA was directed to assume installation of the best available technology (Gray, 1986).

Continuing criticism of the SDWA over the last decade has prompted yet another attempt at reform. Congress failed to pass amendments at the end of the 1994 session, but further revisions to the SDWA are expected in the near future. Congress will likely abandon the current requirement that the EPA issue standards for 25 additional contaminants every 3 years, in order to permit the EPA to choose contaminants for regulation based on scientific criteria. There is also support for a cost-benefit approach to standard-setting that would relax the current feasibility requirement for standards.

***Toxic Air Pollutants.*** Section 112 of the Clean Air Act (CAA) provides a list of 189 hazardous air pollutants, to which the EPA may add or delete pollutants. The EPA must establish national emissions standards for sources that emit any listed pollutant. The original 1970 version of section 112 required the standards to provide "an ample margin of safety to protect the public health from such hazardous air pollutants." The implication of this language, that standards were to be set without regard to the costs of emissions control, generated intense debate from the beginning and contributed to the EPA's glacial pace of implementation.

The EPA finally attempted to escape the strict interpretation of the CAA when it issued a standard for vinyl chloride in 1986. In this instance the agency claimed it could consider costs and declined to adopt a standard that would assure safety. A court set aside this standard because the EPA had improperly considered costs, but it did make clear that in determining what emissions level was safe, even for a carcinogen, the EPA need not eliminate exposure. Additionally, the decision said the EPA could consider costs in deciding what, if any, additional margin of protection to prescribe (*Natural Resources Defense Council, Inc. v. United States Environmental Protection Agency*, 1987).

The 1990 amendments to the CAA responded to the difficulties presented by the strict approach of Section 112. The Amendments replace the health-based standard with a two-tiered system of regulation. The EPA must first issue standards that are technology-based, designed to require the "maximum degree of emission reduction achievable" (MACT) (CAA § 112(d)(2)). If the MACT controls are insufficient to protect human health with an "ample margin of safety," the EPA must issue residual risk standards (CAA § 112(f)). The 1990 Amendments essentially define "ample margin of safety" for carcinogens by requiring the EPA to establish residual risk standards for any pollutant that poses a lifetime excess cancer risk of greater than one in one million.

**Occupational Safety and Health Administration.** The 1970 Occupational Safety and Health Act requires employers to provide employees safe working conditions and empowers OSHA to prescribe mandatory occupational safety and health standards (OSHA, 1970). OSHA's most controversial standards have been exposure limits for toxic chemicals.

While manufacturers of food additives, drugs, and pesticides must demonstrate the safety of their products prior to marketing, no employer need obtain advance approval of new processes or materials or conduct tests to ensure that its operations will not jeopardize worker health. OSHA must first discover that a material already in use threatens worker health before it may attempt to control exposure. Standards for toxic chemicals typically set maximum limits on employee exposure and prescribe changes in employer procedures or equipment to achieve this level.

The Act specifies that in regulating toxic chemicals OSHA shall adopt the standard "which most adequately assures, to the extent feasible, on the basis of the best available evidence, that no employee will suffer material impairment of health or physical capacity" [OSH Act § 6 (b)(5)]. The meaning of these contradictory phrases was for many years a source of controversy. Court decisions made clear that the "best available evidence" did not require proof of causation or even positive epidemiological studies; animal data alone could support regulation of a toxic substance. The debate focused on OSHA's obligation to weigh the economic costs of its standards. The agency acknowledged that it was required to consider technological achievability and viability for industry, but it denied that it was obliged to balance health benefits and economic costs.

Judicial challenges to OSHA standards have clarified OSHA's responsibilities. In 1980, the Supreme Court overturned OSHA's benzene standard because the agency had not shown that prevailing worker exposure levels posed a "significant" health risk (*Industrial Union Department, AFL-CIO v. American Petroleum Institute*, 1980). This prerequisite proved difficult when OSHA attempted to establish standards for 428 air contaminants in a single proceeding in 1989. Although it found that OSHA's generic approach to regulation was permissible in theory, a court vacated the standards because OSHA failed to show that each individual contaminant posed a "significant risk" at current levels (*American Federation of Labor v. OSHA*, 1992). However, the Supreme Court earlier upheld OSHA's cotton dust standard, rejecting arguments that the agency was obligated to weigh the costs of individual standards for concededly hazardous substances (*American Textile Manufacturers Institute v. Donovan*, 1982).

**Consumer Product Safety Commission.** Of the four agencies discussed here, the CPSC has played the least important role in federal efforts to control toxic chemicals. The commission was created in 1972 by the Consumer Product Safety Act (CPSA) with authority to regulate products that pose an unreasonable risk of injury or illness to consumers. The commission is empowered to promulgate safety standards "to prevent or reduce an unreasonable risk of injury" associated with a consumer product. If no feasible standard "would adequately protect the public from the unreasonable risk of injury" posed by a consumer product, the commission may ban the product (CPSA § 8). In assessing the need for a standard or ban, the agency must balance the likelihood that a product will cause harm, and the severity of harm it will likely cause, against the effects of reducing the risk on the product's utility, cost, and availability to consumers.

The CPSC also administers the older Federal Hazardous Substances Act (FHSA). The FHSA authorizes the CPSC to regulate, primarily through prescribed label warnings, products that are toxic, corrosive, combustible, or radioactive or that generate pressure. The FHSA is unusual among federal health laws because it contains detailed criteria for determining toxicity. It defines "highly toxic" in terms of a substance's acute effects in specified tests in rodents; substances capable of producing chronic effects thus fall within the "toxic" category. The FHSA contains another unique provision (FHSA § 2(h)(2)) specifically addressing the probative weight of animal and human data on acute toxicity:

> If the [commission] finds that available data on human experience with any substance indicates results different from those obtained on animals in the above-named dosages or concentrations, the human data shall take precedence.

The CPSC has prescribed labeling for products containing numerous substances that are acutely toxic. It has also acted to ban from consumer products several substances that pose a cancer risk, including asbestos, vinyl chloride as a propellant, benzene, TRIS, and formaldehyde (Merrill, 1981). Its ban of urea formaldehyde foam insulation was set aside by a reviewing court in an opinion that is remarkable for its detailed critical analysis of the agency's handling of toxicological data (*Gulf South Insulation v. CPSC*, 1983).

The CPSC's regulation of asbestos under the FHSA illustrates the overlap of regulatory jurisdictions of different agencies. In 1986, the CPSC issued an enforcement policy requiring accurate labeling of the hazards of asbestos for all asbestos-containing household products (CPSC, 1986). It characterized the labeling requirement as an "interim measure" because the EPA had proposed a ban of asbestos in household products under TSCA. However, as discussed earlier, a court overturned the EPA's asbestos ban (*Corrosion Proof Fittings v. Environmental Protection Agency*, 1991). Neither the EPA nor the CPSC has since attempted to restrict asbestos-containing products.

The Labeling of Hazardous Art Materials Act of 1988 (LHAMA) amended the FHSA. The LHAMA authorizes the CPSC to require labeling of art materials that have "the potential for producing chronic adverse health effects with customary or reasonably foreseeable use." The LHAMA also requires a producer or repackager of an art material to submit the material to a toxicologist for review. The toxicologist must determine whether the material presents a chronic health hazard and must recommend appropriate labeling.

The CPSC has issued guidelines, applicable to both the LHAMA and the FHSA, for determining whether a material presents a chronic health hazard (CPSC, 1992). Manufacturers are encouraged to use these guidelines in order to ensure appropriate labeling.

## REGULATORY CONTROLS OVER TOXICOLOGY

Previous sections of this chapter have surveyed contexts in which regulators draw on toxicological data to decide whether and how to control environmental chemicals. Modern toxicology has grown significantly in response to the information needs of contemporary regulation. But government impinges on the discipline in more direct ways as well. Regulatory agencies often prescribe the content and characteristics of studies that are conducted to meet regulatory requirements. In recent years, pressure to protect animals used in research has produced laws and regulations that govern toxicologists themselves.

### Different Ways Regulation Impinges on Toxicology

An agency's influence over the conduct of toxicological studies depends on its regulatory responsibilities. An agency such as the FDA or the EPA that must confirm the safety of new substances before marketing can dictate the kinds of tests that manufacturers must conduct to gain approval. By contrast, an agency that has no premarket approval function has less leverage.

Statutory terms often do not reveal an agency's real power. For example, the FD&C Act does not in so many words authorize the FDA to prescribe the kinds of preclinical tests a manufacturer of human drugs must conduct; it merely says that no new drug may be marketed until the manufacturer has satisfied the FDA, "by all methods reasonably applicable," that it is "safe" (FD&C Act § 505(c)). However, the agency's power to withhold approval when it has doubts about a drug's safety provides it the practical leverage necessary to demand whatever tests its reviewers believe necessary. Some laws, notably the TSCA, explicitly accord power to prescribe testing, but if an agency has the ability to prevent marketing until safety is proved, doubts about its legal authority to prescribe testing requirements are academic; the important issues are the procedures by which its requirements are adopted, their scope and scientific support, and their legal effect.

The last issue is important for laboratory scientists and test sponsors, as well as for lawyers. Two significant legal distinctions should be noted. The first is the distinction between the requirements that an agency imposes for testing of specific compounds and generic requirements prescribed for all compounds within a class (e.g., direct food additives). An agency such as the FDA could impose its views of appropriate toxicological testing without ever enunciating any general testing standards. When a compound's sponsor seeks approval, it could be told that the tests it had conducted were inadequate. Alternatively, an individual sponsor could solicit the agency's advice about what tests were necessary before it undertook testing. The first approach wastes resources, and the second—unless agency advice is broadly disseminated—fails to guide other potential sponsors and allows inconsistency in the treatment of similar compounds.

For these reasons, the FDA and the EPA have moved increasingly toward establishing generic test standards or guidelines. Both agencies have issued guidelines for the design and conduct of studies of the health effects of compounds submitted for agency approval (EPA, 1993; FDA, 1993). In addition, the EPA has established guidelines for several of the tests that it may mandate by rule or consent agreement for individual chemicals under TSCA § 4 (EPA, 1993). Multinational bodies like the Organization for Economic Cooperation and Development have sought to secure multilateral adherence to standardized test guidelines and minimum testing requirements for new chemicals (Page, 1982).

This trend has focused attention on a second legal distinction: the distinction between binding regulations and advisory guidelines. Any time a regulatory agency wants to provide guidance for private behavior, it confronts a choice between establishing standards that have the force of law and merely conveying its current best judgment of what conduct will satisfy the law. A regulation typically specifies what the law mandates; failure to comply (e.g., failure to perform a test or follow a specified protocol) constitutes a violation of law just as if the regulation had been enacted by Congress. A test guideline describes performance that will satisfy legal requirements; but failure to follow the guidelines is not forbidden. The agency may accept another approach that employs, for example, a different set of studies or studies conducted using different protocols, if it concludes that they meet the law's basic objectives.

Regulations ensure consistency and are more easily enforced than guidelines, but they are more rigid because they restrict the agency, and the procedures for their adoption are cumbersome. The design and conduct of toxicological studies, it is often argued, should take into account the characteristics of the test compound, the endpoints to be evaluated, the resources available, and perhaps even laboratory capabilities. Accordingly, both the FDA and the EPA have preferred to announce their standards as guidelines, permitting sponsors and scientists to consider alternative approaches.

It is increasingly common for U.S. agencies to specify the types of tests they require before they will consider the safety of a compound (e.g., tests for acute toxicity, subchronic effects, and chronic effects). Within each of these categories, an agency might set out more detailed requirements, essentially enumerating its "base set" data demands. As noted above, an agency may also describe methods for executing particular tests, for instance, a bioassay for carcinogenesis. It is these descriptions that in the U.S. usually take the form of guidelines.

Both the FDA and the EPA have adopted another set of requirements that specify laboratory procedures for conducting tests required or submitted for regulatory consideration. These good laboratory practice (GLP) regulations prescribe essential but often mundane features of sound laboratory science, such as animal husbandry standards and record-keeping practices (EPA, 1993; FDA, 1993). All of these types of requirements are intended to contribute to sound regulatory decision making by ensuring the quality and integrity of toxicological data submitted to support agency decisions. In addition, toxicologists have confronted another form of direct regulation in recent years whose goal is protection of the subjects of laboratory studies—experimental animals.

## FDA and EPA Testing Standards

It would serve little purpose here to detail existing agency requirements for the design and conduct of toxicological studies; they change frequently enough that any summary would soon be outdated. This chapter thus only attempts to acquaint the reader with the principal federal programs that specify standards for toxicity testing. The discussion focuses on the FDA and the EPA.

**Food and Drug Administration.** The FDA exercises premarketing approval authority over several classes of compounds of which the most important, for present purposes, are new human drugs and direct and indirect additives to food.

***Toxicological Testing Requirements for Human Drugs.*** In 1962, Congress expressly authorized the FDA to exempt investigational drugs from the premarket approval requirement so that they could be shipped for use in clinical testing, subject to conditions the agency believed appropriate to protect human subjects (FD&C Act § 505(i)). One condition that the FDA established was that an investigational drug first must have been evaluated in preclinical studies. This requirement appears in current regulations that amplify, in the text and in referenced guidelines, the types of tests that are to be performed and the design they should follow (FDA, 1994). Almost invariably, a drug's sponsor will consult agency personnel to get a precise understanding of what sorts of toxicological studies they expect. Preclinical studies of substances that are candidates for use as human drugs must meet the standards set by the FDA's GLP regulations (FDA, 1994). These regulations apply to all laboratories—university, independent, and manufacturer-owned—in which such studies are conducted.

The work of the International Conference on Harmonisation of Technical Requirements for Registration of Pharmaceuticals for Human Use (ICH) highlights the trend toward international agreement on test methods. In 1994 the ICH, comprised of the European Union, Japan, and the United States, issued six draft guidelines on various toxicology testing methods for human drugs. The testing requirements applicable in the U.S. surely will evolve as the international community reaches consensus on the appropriate methodology.

***Testing Requirements for Food Additives.*** The Food Additives Amendment and the Color Additive Amendments require premarket approval of new additives to human food. Both laws assume that laboratory studies in animals will provide the principal data for assessing safety. A petitioner must submit "full reports of investigations made with respect to the safety for use of such additives, including full information as to the methods and control used" (FD&C Act § 409(c)).

The FDA's regulations contain only general statements about the need for and features of toxicological studies. For many years, the agency maintained an advice-giving system in which it prescribed the type and design of tests to be performed. In 1982, the FDA first codified this "common law" in *Toxicological Principles for the Safety Assessment of Direct Food Additives and Color Additives Used in Food*, known thereafter as "the Red Book." The Red Book describes the types of tests the FDA believes necessary to evaluate an additive's safety. The agency's requirements, which are in the form of guidelines rather than regulations, are calibrated to the purposes for which the additive will be used, to estimated levels of human exposure, and to the results of sequential studies. The FDA recently issued a draft revision, "Redbook II," under the same title as the original. Tests of food color and additives must comply with the FDA's good laboratory practice regulations (FDA, 1993).

**Environmental Protection Agency.** The EPA's premarket approval authority over pesticides places it, like the FDA, in a position to dictate the design and conduct of studies on such compounds. The 1976 Toxic Substances Control Act gave the EPA authority to mandate testing of other chemicals in use or scheduled for introduction and to specify, by regulation, test standards.

***Toxicology Requirements for Pesticides.*** The FIFRA clearly contemplates the submission of toxicological studies, as well as other types of investigations, to support the EPA's evaluation of a pesticide (FIFRA § 136(b)). The statute also requires the EPA to "publish guidelines specifying the kinds of information which will be required to support the registration of a pesticide and to revise such guidelines from time to time."

The EPA's regulations state broadly that pesticide registration depends on evaluation of "all available, pertinent data," which must satisfy the minimum requirements set forth in registration guidelines (EPA, 1993). The agency has issued regulations outlining the procedures for submission of registration petitions and their basic content (EPA, 1978, 1993). Animal studies of pesticides must also comply with EPA's own good laboratory practice regulations, which were inspired by the same investigations that led the FDA to promulgate its standards for testing laboratories and impose similar requirements.

***Testing of Industrial Chemicals.*** The primary means by which the EPA can mandate health effects testing of new or existing industrial chemicals is Section 4(a) of the TSCA. That provision states that the administrator "shall by rule require that testing be conducted to develop data with respect to the health and environmental effects for which there is an insufficiency of data and experience" to permit assessment of whether a substance presents an unreasonable risk. This obligation to order testing is triggered by an administrative finding that a chemical presents a potential risk (based on the suspicion of toxicity) or that humans or the environment will be exposed to substantial quantities. The statute creates an Interagency Testing Committee (ITC) with members from EPA, OSHA, CEQ, NIOSH, NIEHS, NCI, NSF, and the Department of Commerce to recommend a list of chemicals that should be tested and in what order of priority. Once the ITC has recommended a chemical substance for testing, the EPA must either initiate testing or publish its reasons for not doing so, within 12 months.

This last requirement, coupled with the statute's formal procedures for adopting test rules, led the EPA initially to rely on negotiations with chemical producers to secure voluntary agreements for the conduct of tests it thought appropriate for chemicals identified by the ITC (GAO, 1982). The practice was challenged by public interest organizations, who were excluded from the negotiations, and ultimately it was declared unlawful (*Natural Resources Defense Council, Inc. v. United States Environmental Protection Agency*, 1984). The agency amended its regulations to recognize two forms of mandates for testing: test rules and enforceable testing consent agreements (EPA, 1993). By the end of 1993, the EPA had adopted test rules for approximately 33 commercial chemicals and 22 constituents of industrial waste and had entered into consent orders for the testing of 36 other chemicals (EPA, 1993).

TSCA test rules are subject to judicial challenge. Manufacturers challenged a 1988 test rule for cumene, arguing that the EPA had failed to support its finding that the substance enters the environment in substantial quantities with the potential for substantial human exposure. Although the court ultimately upheld the rule, it ordered the agency to articulate standards governing the definition of "substantial" (*Chemical Manufacturers Association v. EPA*, 1990). Another court challenge to a test rule requiring neurotoxicity studies of ten widely used and intensively marketed organic solvents resulted in a settlement with the EPA. The settlement required the EPA to enter into consent agreements with reduced testing requirements for seven chemicals, to eliminate testing requirements for two, and to postpone its decision on one.

Both test rules and testing consent agreements specify what types of tests are to be done. Their design is governed either by general "test methodology guidelines" that the EPA has issued for several types of tests or by the rule or the agreement itself. All toxicological studies required by the EPA under the TSCA must comply with its GLP regulations.

***Locating Testing Guidelines.*** The EPA usually publishes toxicology testing guidelines that apply to a specific regulatory program in the *Code of Federal Regulations* (*C.F.R.*). For example, the TSCA testing guidelines appear at 40 *C.F.R.* Part 798. The health effects testing guidelines applicable to the FIFRA appear in the *Federal Register* or may be obtained directly from the agency.

The EPA occasionally issues generic guidelines applicable to several of its regulatory programs. The agency is currently in the process of revising several of its generic guidelines, including cancer assessment guidelines that it first issued in 1986. The proposed guidelines offer a more flexible approach to the assessment of cancer risk. For example, they support the use of several types of data, including biological, pharmacokinetic, and tumor development data, for hazard identification. The EPA also proposes to abandon the assumption of a linear dose-response model and intends to replace its existing alphanumeric rankings of cancer risk with narrative descriptions (EPA, 1994).

## Interagency Testing Criteria and Programs

The foregoing summary of regulatory programs that mandate toxicological tests (see "FDA and EPA Testing Standards," above) suggests the possibility of inconsistencies in testing standards. In the late 1970s, the responsible regulatory agencies (OSHA and the CPSC as well as the FDA and the EPA) combined to form the Interagency Regulatory Liaison Group (IRLG) to secure agreement on the design of standard toxicological tests. Though the IRLG has long since collapsed, both the FDA and the EPA, along with the White House Office of Science and Technology Policy, have continued to work to achieve internal consistency.

The National Toxicology Program (NTP) was established in 1978 as an administrative umbrella for coordinating the numerous federal efforts to improve test methods and to coordinate toxicological studies then under way, primarily in the Department of Health and Human Services. NTP assumed responsibility for what had been the National Cancer Institute's (NCI's) bioassay program. An NTP committee that includes representatives of all four regulatory agencies is responsible for selecting chemicals to be tested at public expense. Attention continues to be focused on improving health risk assessment research techniques. In 1993 the congressional Office of Technology Assessment recommended the establishment of an independent risk assessment research agency to administer research funding (OTA, 1993).

## Animal Welfare Requirements

Researchers who conduct studies funded by federal agencies must comply with the Animal Welfare Act (AWA), and some may also be subject to restrictions imposed by the Public Health Service (PHS). Recipients of grants from the Department of Education, the Department of Health and Human Services, the Department of Agriculture, or the EPA are subject only to the AWA. Those funded by the Department of Energy or by the PHS must also comply with PHS policies. Restrictions on animal use also appear in the GLP regulations adopted by the FDA and the EPA (Reagan, 1986).

**Animal Welfare Act.** The AWA is administered by the Animal and Plant Health Inspection Service (APHIS), a part of the U.S. Department of Agriculture. The AWA, which protects only warm-blooded animals and excludes birds, rats, and mice, requires all covered research facilities to register with APHIS and agree to comply with applicable AWA standards. Each facility must file an annual report signed by a responsible official that shows that "professionally acceptable standards governing the care, treatment, and use of animals" were followed for the year in question. The report must include:

1. Assurances that alternatives to painful procedures were considered in the design of the studies conducted there.
2. A summary and brief explanation of all exceptions to the standards and regulations that were approved by the Institutional Animal Care and Use Committee, including the species and number of animals affected.
3. The common names and the numbers of animals used in three research categories: (1) research involving no pain,

distress, or use of pain-relieving drugs; (2) research involving pain and distress and for which pain-relieving drugs were used; and (3) research involving pain or distress, in which no pain-relieving drugs were used because of adverse effects on the procedures, results, or interpretation.

4. The common names and the numbers of animals bred, conditioned, or held for research purposes but not yet used.

Pursuant to the AWA, APHIS has established specific requirements for the humane handling, care, and transportation of dogs and cats, guinea pigs and hamsters, rabbits, nonhuman primates, marine mammals, and other warm-blooded animals. The regulations governing facilities address living space, heating, lighting, ventilation, and drainage. The health and husbandry provisions address feeding, watering, sanitation, veterinary care, grouping of animals, and the number and qualifications of caretakers (APHIS, 1994).

The APHIS has strengthened the content and broadened the scope of its regulations, which were amended in an attempt to achieve more consistency with those of the PHS, while favoring flexible guidelines rather than strict standards. The 1991 amendments to the specifications for the humane handling, care, and treatment of dogs and nonhuman primates require research facilities to develop plans to ensure appropriate exercise for dogs as well as an environment that promotes the psychological well-being of nonhuman primates (APHIS, 1991). Within the last 5 years the APHIS also has clarified the question of whether horses and other farm animals are subject to its regulations (APHIS, 1990).

Despite these initiatives, several animal welfare groups and individuals have sued the agency in an attempt to further strengthen the regulations. One lawsuit challenged the APHIS's exclusion of rats, mice, and birds from coverage under the AWA (*Animal Legal Defense Fund v. Madigan*, 1992). A second lawsuit challenged the regulations governing the exercise of dogs and the psychological well-being of nonhuman primates on the grounds that the discretionary standard failed to guarantee minimum requirements (*Animal Legal Defense Fund v. Secretary of Agriculture*, 1993). Both suits were dismissed on the ground that the petitioners, including researchers, members of institutional oversight committees, and animal welfare organizations, lacked standing to challenge the regulations.

The AWA requires each research facility to establish an Institutional Animal Care and Use Committee (IACUC), composed of three or more members, one of whom must be a veterinarian and one of whom must represent community interests and who may not be affiliated with the institution. In 1989, the APHIS expanded the responsibilities of the IACUC. At least one member of the IACUC must now review and approve the animal care and use components of all proposed research activities. Prerequisites to approval include the avoidance or minimization of discomfort, distress and pain; the use of pain-relieving drugs where appropriate; the consideration of pain-free alternatives; and euthanization when an animal would otherwise experience severe or chronic pain or distress that cannot be relieved.

The IACUC is also responsible for conducting semiannual inspections of the facility itself and of the program for humane care and use of animals. Committee reports are filed with the APHIS and with any federal agency funding the research.

**Public Health Service Policy.** The PHS Policy on Humane Care and Use of Laboratory Animals by Awardee Institutions applies to research using all vertebrates, and thus it has a broader reach than the AWA. The PHS policy requires each facility to submit an annual report, called an "Assurance," which is evaluated by the National Institutes of Health (NIH) Office for Protection from Research Risks (OPRR) to determine the sufficiency of animal care.

The PHS policy imposes two primary obligations on researchers: Each institution must adopt a Program for Animal Care and Use, and it must establish an IACUC. The IACUC must be comprised of at least five members including a veterinarian, an animal research scientist, a nonscientist, and a person who cares for or studies animals who is not affiliated with the facility. The IACUC must review all applications for research funding and review the institution's programs to ensure compliance with NIH standards.

The Health Research Extension Act of 1985 requires that PHS-funded institutions provide training on methods to reduce animal suffering similar to that mandated by the AWA for its personnel. It also requires that researchers' grant applications justify any proposed use of animals (NRC, 1988).

Research facilities subject to either the AWA or PHS may wish to consult a National Academy of Sciences report that details suggestions for developing institutional compliance programs (National Research Council, 1991). Scientists working with no federal funding who expect their research to be submitted to the FDA or the EPA are not subject to the AWA or PHS policies, but they must comply with the animal protection provisions of those agencies' GLP regulations. These regulations prescribe adequate living conditions, detail requirements for veterinary treatment, and impose specific record-keeping requirements (EPA, 1993; FDA, 1994).

# REFERENCES

## Cases

*American Federation of Labor v. OSHA*, 965 F.2d 962 (11th Cir. 1992).

*American Textile Manufacturers Institute v. Donovan*, 452 U.S. 490, 495 (1982).

*Animal Legal Defense Fund v. Madigan*, 781 F. Supp. 797 (D.D.C. 1992), *vacated and remanded sub nom. Animal Legal Defense Fund v. Espy*, 23 F.3d 496 (D.C. Cir. 1994).

*Animal Legal Defense Fund v. Secretary of Agriculture*, 813 F. Supp. 882 (D.D.C. 1993), *vacated and remanded sub nom. Animal Legal Defense Fund v. Espy*, 29 F.3d 720 (D.C. Cir. 1994).

*Chemical Manufacturers Association v. EPA*, 899 F.2d 344 (5th Cir. 1990).

*Corrosion Proof Fittings v. Environmental Protection Agency*, 947 F.2d 1201 (5th Cir. 1991).

*Environmental Defense Fund, Inc. v. Environmental Protection Agency*, 548 F.2d 998 (D.C. Cir. 1976).

*Environmental Defense Fund, Inc. v. Ruckelhaus*, 439 F.2d 584 (D.C. Cir. 1971).

*Environmental Defense Fund, Inc. and National Audubon Society v. Environmental Protection Agency*, 510 F.2d 1292 (D.C. Cir. 1975)

*Gulf South Insulation v. CPSC*, 701 F.2d 1137 (5th Cir. 1983).

*Industrial Union Department, AFL-CIO v. American Petroleum Institute*, 448 U.S. 607 (1980).

*Industrial Union Department, AFL-CIO v. Hodgson*, 499 F.2d 467 (D.C. Cir. 1974).

*Les v. Reilly*, 968 F.2d 985 (9th Cir. 1992).

*Monsanto v. Kennedy*, 613 F.2d 947 (D.C. Cir. 1979).

*Natural Resources Defense Council, Inc. v. United States Environmental Protection Agency*, 595 F. Supp. 1255 (S.D.N.Y. 1984).

*Natural Resources Defense Council, Inc. v. United States Environmental Protection Agency*, 824 F.2d 1146 (D.C. Cir. 1987)

*NRDC v. Train*, 8 E.R.C. 2120 (D.D.C. 1976).

*Public Citizen v. Young*, 831 F.2d 1108 (D.C. Cir. 1987).

*Society of the Plastics Industry, Inc. v. OSHA*, 509 F.2d 9301 (2d Cir. 1975).

SECONDARY SOURCES

Berger J, Riskin S: Economic and technological feasibility under the Occupational Safety and Health Act. *Ecology L Q* 7:285, 1978.

Bruser J, Harris R, Page T: Waterborne carcinogens: An economist's view, in *The Scientific Basis of Health and Safety Regulation*. Washington, DC: Brookings Institution, 1981.

Cooper R: The role of regulatory agencies in risk-benefit decision-making. *Food Drug Cosmet L J* 33:755–757, 1978.

Douglas I: Safe Drinking Water Act of 1975—history and critique. *Environ Affairs* 5:501, 1976.

EPA: *Draft Revisions to the Guidelines for Carcinogen Risk Assessment*. Report by the U.S. Environmental Protection Agency, 1994.

GAO: *EPA Implementation of Selected Aspects of the Toxic Substances Control Act*. Report by the U.S. General Accounting Office, Washington, DC, December 1982.

Gray K: The Safe Drinking Water Act Amendments of 1986: Now a tougher act to follow. *Environ L Rep* 16:10338, 1986.

Heineck D: New clean water act toxics control initiatives. *Nat Resources Environ* 1:10, 1989.

Hutt PB, Merrill R: *Food and Drug Law: Cases and Materials*. Mineola, NY: Foundation Press, 1991.

Merrill R: Regulating carcinogens in food: A legislator's guide to the food safety provisions of the federal Food, Drug, and Cosmetics Act. *Mich L Rev* 77:179–184, 1979.

Merrill R: CPSC regulation of cancer risks in consumer products: 1972–81. *Va L Rev* 67:1261, 1981. A

Merrill R, Schewel M: FDA regulation of environmental contaminants of food. *Va L Rev* 66:1357, 1980.

*National Institute of Health, Department of Health and Human Services: Guide for the Care and Use of Laboratory Animals*, Publ. No. 23. Guide for Grants and Contracts: Special ed. Laboratory Animal Welfare June, (Suppl.) 1985.

National Research Council: *A Guide for Developing Institutional Programs*. Washington, DC: National Academy, 1991.

National Research Council: *Use of Laboratory Animals in Biomedical and Behavioral Research*. Washington, DC: National Academy, 1988.

HHS: *National Toxicology Program Annual Plan for Fiscal Year 1988*. Report by the U.S. Department of Health and Human Services, January 1988.

Page NP: Testing for health and environmental effects: The OECD guidelines. *Toxic Substances J* 4:135, Autumn 1982.

Reagan K: Federal regulation of testing with laboratory animals: Future directions. *Pace Environ L Rev* 3:165, 1986.

Reed PD: The trial of hazardous air pollution regulation. *Environ L Register* 16:10066–10072, 1986.

OTA: *Researching Health Risks*. Report by the Office of Technology Assessment, Washington, DC: U.S. Government Printing Office, November 1993.

OTA: *Assessment of Technologies for Determining the Cancer Risks from the Environment*. Report by the Office of Technology Assessment. Washington, DC: US Government Printing Office, June 1981.

FDA: *Toxicological Principles for the Safety Assessment of Direct Food Additives and Color Additives Used in Food*. Report by the U.S. Food and Drug Administration, Washington, DC, 1982.

FDA: *Toxicological Principles for the Safety Assessment of Direct Food Additives and Color Additives Used in Food*. Draft Report by the U.S. Food and Drug Administration, Washington, DC, 1993.

Turner J: The Delaney anticancer clause: A model environmental protection law. *Vand L Rev* 24:889, 1971.

STATUTES AND REGULATIONS

Animal Welfare, 9 *CFR* Parts 2 & 3 (1994).

Animal Welfare Act (1988), 7 U.S.C. § 2131 et seq.

Animal Welfare; Standards. *Fed Reg* 56(32):6426, February 15, 1991.

APHIS: (part of USDA) Intent to Regulate Horses and Other Farm Animals Under the Animal Welfare Act; Technical Amendment and Definition. *Fed Reg* 55(66): 12630, April 5, 1990.

Applications for FDA Approval to Market a New Drug or an Antibiotic Drug, 21 C.F.R. Part 314 (1994).

Clean Air Act (1976), 42 U.S.C. § 7401 et seq.

Color Additive Amendments of 1960 to the Federal Food, Drug, and Cosmetic Act, 21 U.S.C. § 706.

Color Additive Petitions, 21 C.F.R. Part 71 (1994).

Consumer Product Safety Act (1972), 15 U.S.C. § 2051 et seq.

CPSC: Labeling of Asbestos-Containing Household Products; Enforcement Policy. *Fed Reg* 51(185):33910, September 24, 1986.

CPSC: Labeling of Hazardous Art Materials Act (1988), 15 U.S.C. § 1277.

CPSC: Labeling Requirements for Art Materials Presenting Chronic Hazards; Guidelines for Determining Chronic Toxicity of Products Subject to the FHSA; Supplementary Definition of "Toxic" Under the Federal Hazardous Substances Act. *Fed Reg* 57(197):46626, October 9, 1992.

Data Requirements for Registration, 40 C.F.R. Part 158 (1993).

Drug Amendments of 1962 to the Federal Food, Drug, and Cosmetic Act, 21 U.S.C. § 360(b).

Environmental Effects Testing Guidelines, 40 C.F.R. Part 797 (1993).

EPA: Good Laboratory Practice Standards for Health Effects: Environmental Protection Agency. *Fed Reg* 44(91):27362, May 9, 1979.

EPA: Hazardous Waste Management System: General, 40 C.F.R. Part 260 (1993).

EPA: Proposed Guidelines for Carcinogen Risk Assessment; Request for Comments. *Fed Reg* 49(227):46293–46301, November 23, 1984.

FDA: Food Additive Petitions, 21 C.F.R. Part 171 (1994).

FDA: Food Additives; Threshold of Regulation for Substances Used in Food-Contact Articles. *Fed Reg* 58(195): 52719, October 12, 1993.

FDA: Good Laboratory Practice for Nonclinical Laboratory Studies, 21 C.F.R. Part 58 (1994).

FDA: Indirect Food Additives: Polymers; Acrylonitrile/Styrene Copolymers. *Fed Reg* 49(183):36635–36644, September 19, 1984.

FDA: Policy for Regulating Carcinogenic Chemicals in Food and Color Additives: Advanced Notice of Proposed Rulemaking: Food and Drug Administration. *Fed Reg* 47(64):14464–14469, April 2, 1982.

FDA: *Sponsored Compounds in Food Producing Animals,* Fed Reg 50(284): 45530, October 31, 1995.

Federal Food, Drug, and Cosmetic Act (1938), 21 U.S.C. § 321 et seq.

Federal Hazardous Substances Act (1976), 15 U.S.C. § 1261 et seq.

Federal Insecticide, Fungicide, and Rodenticide Act (1972), 7 U.S.C. § 135 et seq.
Federal Insecticide, Fungicide, and Rodenticide Act Amendments of 1988, Pub. L. No. 100–532, 102 Stat. 2654.
Federal Water Pollution Control Act Amendments of 1972, 33 U.S.C. § 307.
Food Additive Amendments to the Federal Food, Drug, and Cosmetic Act (1958), 21 U.S.C. § 348 et seq.
Good Laboratory Practice Standards, 40 C.F.R. Part 160 (1993).
Good Laboratory Practice Standards, 40 C.F.R. Part 792 (1993).
Health Effects Testing Guidelines, 40 C.F.R. Part 798 (1993).
Identification of Specific Chemical Substance and Mixture Testing Requirements, 40 C.F.R. Part 799 (1993).
New Drugs, 21 C.F.R. Part 310 (1994).
Occupational Safety and Health Act (1970), 29 U.S.C. § 651 et seq.
OSHA: Identification, Classification and Regulation of Potential Occupational Carcinogens: Occupational Safety and Health Act. *Fed Reg* 45(15):5002, January 22, 1980.
OSHA: Identification, Classification and Regulation of Potential Occupational Carcinogens: Occupational Safety and Health Act. *Fed Reg* 47(2):187–190, January 5, 1982.
Pesticide Residue Amendments to the Federal Food, Drug, and Cosmetic Act (1954), 21 U.S.C. § 348 et seq.
Proposed Guidelines for Registering Pesticides in the United States: Environmental Protection Agency. *Fed Reg* 43(163):37336, August 22, 1978.
Proposed Health Effects Test Standards for Toxic Substances Control Act Test Rules: Environmental Protection Agency. *Fed Reg* 44(145):44054, July 26, 1979.
Proposed Interim Primary Drinking Water Regulations: Environmental Protection Agency. *Fed Reg* 43(130):29135–29137, July 6, 1978 (to be codified at 40 C.F.R. § 141).
Provisional Test Guidelines, 40 C.F.R. Part 795 (1993).
Rebuttable Presumption Against Registration (RPAR) Proceedings and Hearings Under Section 6 of the Federal Insecticide, Fungicide, and Rodenticide Act (FIFRA): Environmental Protection Agency. *Fed Reg* 45(154):52628–52674, August 7, 1980.
Resource Conservation and Recovery Act (1976), 42 U.S.C.A. § 6901.
Safe Drinking Water Act (1974), 42 U.S.C. §§ 300f to 300j-9.
Specific Chemical Test Rules, 40 C.F.R. Part 799 (1993).
Sponsored Compounds in Food Producing Animals: Proposed Rule and Notice. *Fed Reg* 50(211):45529–45556, October 31, 1985.
Testing Consent Orders, 40 C.F.R. § 799.5000 (1993).
Toxic Substances Control Act (1976), 15 U.S.C. § 2601.
Toxic Substances Control Act, § 4, 15 U.S.C. § 2603(b)(1) (1988).
Toxic Substances Control Act, § 6, 15 U.S.C. § 2605 (1988).

**APPENDIX**

# RECOMMENDED LIMITS FOR EXPOSURE TO CHEMICALS

*John Doull*

The occupational exposure levels in this listing were taken from the recommendations of the 1994–95 chemical substances threshold limit values (TLVs) from the American Conference of Governmental Industrial Hygienists (ACGIH) and the 1989 OSHA permissible exposure levels (PELs). The drinking water recommendations are from the 1994 National Primary Drinking Water Standards and Health Advisories of the Office of Water of the U.S. Environmental Protection Agency. Values in the occupational exposure listings include the time-weighted average (TWA) for a normal 8-h workday and, when appropriate, short-term exposure limits (STEL) or ceiling (C) recommendations. The information in this listing is intended to illustrate the type of chemicals for which recommendations have been made and the range and type of values recommended for the agents. This listing does not include all of the information provided in the source documents and since the values are reviewed and updated frequently, interested readers should contact the sponsoring organization to obtain the current information and supporting documentation for the values. This documentation also provides information on other adverse effects (fetotoxicity, carcinogenicity, etc.), recommendations for dealing with mixtures, and various other types of useful information.

Abbreviations used in the listing:

ppm, parts per million
m/M, milligrams per cubic meter
f/cc, fibers per cubic centimeter
A1, Confirmed human carcinogen
A2, Suspected human carcinogen
A3, Animal carcinogen
A4, Not classifiable
A5, Not suspected as a worker carcinogen
MCL, Maximum contaminant level (milligrams per liter)
MCLG, Maximum contaminant level goal (milligrams per liter)
RfD, Reference dose (milligrams per kilogram per day)

**1994–1995 Threshold Limit Values (TLV) and Permissible Exposure Limits (PEL)**

| | | ACGIH TLV | | OSHA PEL | |
|---|---|---|---|---|---|
| NAME | CAS NO. | TWA | STEL | TWA | STEL |
| Acetaldehyde | 000075-07-0 | | C25 ppm A3 | 100 ppm | 150 ppm |
| Acetic acid | 000064-19-7 | 10 ppm | 15 ppm | 10 ppm | |
| Acetic anhydride | 000108-24-7 | 5 ppm | | | C5 ppm |
| Acetone | 000067-64-1 | 750 ppm | 1000 ppm | 750 ppm | 1000 ppm |
| Acetone cyanohydrin, as CN | 000075-86-5 | | C4.7 ppm Skin | | |
| Acetonitrile | 000075-05-8 | 40 ppm | 60 ppm | 40 ppm | 60 ppm |
| Acetophenone | 000098-86-2 | 10 ppm | | | |
| Acetylene | 000074-86-2 | Asphyxiant | | | |
| Acetylene dichloride (1,2-dichloroethylene) | 000540-59-0 | 200 ppm | | 200 ppm | |
| Acetylene tetrabromide | 000079-27-6 | 1 ppm | | 1 ppm | |
| Acetylsalicylic acid (aspirin) | 000050-78-2 | 5 m/M | | 5 m/M | |
| Acrolein | 000107-02-8 | 0.1 ppm | 0.3 ppm | 0.1 ppm | 0.3 ppm |
| Acrylamide | 000079-06-1 | 0.03 m/M Skin A2 | | 0.03 m/M Skin | |
| Acrylic acid | 000079-10-7 | 2 ppm Skin | | 10 ppm Skin | |
| Acrylic acid, *n*-butyl ester (*n*-butyl acrylate) | 000141-32-2 | 10 ppm | | 10 ppm | |
| Acrylic acid, ethyl ester (ethyl acrylate) | 000140-88-5 | 5 ppm, A2 | 15 ppm, A2 | 5 ppm Skin | 25 ppm Skin |
| Acrylic acid, methyl ester (methyl acrylate) | 000096-33-3 | 10 ppm Skin | | 10 ppm Skin | |
| Acrylonitrile (vinyl cyanide) | 000107-13-1 | 2 ppm, A2 Skin | | 2 ppm Skin | C 10 ppm |
| Adipic acid | 000124-04-9 | 5 m/M | | | |

| NAME | CAS NO. | ACGIH TLV | | OSHA PEL | |
|---|---|---|---|---|---|
| | | TWA | STEL | TWA | STEL |
| Adiponitrile | 000111-69-3 | 2 ppm Skin | | | |
| Aldrin | 000309-00-2 | 0.25 m/M Skin | | 0.25 m/M Skin | |
| Allyl alcohol | 000107-18-6 | 2 ppm Skin | 4 ppm Skin | 2 ppm Skin | 4 ppm Skin |
| Allyl chloride | 000107-05-1 | 1 ppm | 2 ppm | 1 ppm | 2 ppm |
| Allyl glycidyl ether (AGE) | 000106-92-3 | 5 ppm | 10 ppm | 5 ppm | 10 ppm |
| Allyl propyl disulfide | 002179-59-1 | 2 ppm | 3 ppm | 2 ppm | 3 ppm |
| *a*-Alumina (aluminum oxide) | 001344-28-1 | 10 m/M | | | |
| Aluminum hydroxide | 021645-51-2 | | | | |
| Aluminum metal dust [7429-90-5] | | 10 m/M | | 15 m/M | |
| Aluminum, pyro powders, as Al | | 5 m/M | | 5 m/M | |
| Aluminum, welding fumes, as Al | | 5 m/M | | 5 m/M | |
| Aluminum, soluble salts, as Al | | 2 m/M | | 2 m/M | |
| Aluminum, alkyls, not otherwise classified as Al | | 2 m/M | | 2 m/M | |
| Aluminum oxide | | 10 m/M | | 10 m/M | |
| 2-Aminoethanol (ethanolamine) | 000141-43-5 | 3 ppm | 6 ppm | 3 ppm | 6 ppm |
| 2-Aminopyridine (2-nitro-4-aminophenol) | 000504-29-0 | 0.5 ppm | | 0.5 ppm | |
| 3-Amino-1,2,4-triazole (amitrole) | 000061-82-5 | 0.2 m/M | 0.2 m/M | | |
| Amitrole (3-amino-1,2,4-triazole) | 000061-82-5 | 0.2 m/M | | 0.2 m/M | |
| Ammonia | 007664-41-7 | 25 ppm | 35 ppm | 25 ppm | 35 ppm |
| Ammonium chloride fume | 012125-02-9 | 10 m/M | 20 m/M | 10 m/M | 20 m/M |
| Ammonium perfluoro-octanoate | 003825-26-1 | 0.01 m/M, A3 Skin | | | |
| Ammonium sulfamate | 007773-06-0 | 10 m/M | | 10 m/M | |
| Amosite (asbestos) | 012172-73-5 | 0.5 f/cc, A1 | | 0.2 f/cc | |
| *n*-Amyl acetate | 000628-63-7 | 100 ppm | | 100 ppm | |
| sec-Amyl acetate | 000626-38-0 | 125 ppm | | 125 ppm | |
| Aniline and homologues | 000062-53-3 | 2 ppm Skin | | 2 ppm Skin | |
| Anisidine (*o*-, *p*-isomers) | 029191-52-4 | 0.5 m/M Skin | | 0.5 m/M | |
| Antimony [7440-36-0] and compounds, as Sb | | 0.5 m/M | | 0.5 m/M | |
| Antimony trioxide, handling and use, as Sb | 001309-64-4 | 0.5 m/M | | | |
| ANTU (*a*-naphthylthiourea) | 000086-88-4 | 0.3 m/M | | 0.3 m/M | |
| Argon | 007440-37-1 | Asphyxiant | | | |
| Arsenic, elemental [7440-38-2] and inorganic compounds (except arsine), as As | | 0.01 m/M A1 | | 0.05 m/M | |
| Arsenous acid, arsenic acid and salts | | 0.01 m/M A1 | | | |
| Arsine | 007784-42-1 | 0.05 ppm | | 0.05 ppm | |
| Asbestos, amosite | 012172-73-5 | 0.5 f/cc A1 | | 0.2 f/cc | 1 f/cc |
| Asbestos, chrysotile | 012001-29-5 | 2 f/cc A1 | | 0.2 f/cc | 1 f/cc |
| Asbestos, crocidolite | 012001-28-4 | 0.2 f/cc A1 | | 0.2 f/cc | 1 f/cc |
| Asbestos, other forms | | 2 f/cc A1 | | 0.2 f/cc | 1 f/cc |
| Asphalt (petroleum) fumes | 008052-42-4 | 5 m/M | | | |
| Atrazine | 001912-24-9 | 5 m/M | | 5 m/M | |
| Azinphos-methyl (Guthion) | 000086-50-0 | 0.2 m/M Skin | | 0.2 m/M Skin | |

| NAME | CAS NO. | ACGIH TLV | | OSHA PEL | |
|---|---|---|---|---|---|
| | | TWA | STEL | TWA | STEL |
| Barium [7440-39-3] soluble compounds, as Ba | | 0.5 m/M | | 0.5 m/M | |
| Barium sulfate | 007727-43-7 | 10 m/M | | 10 m/M | |
| Beech wood dust | | 1 m/M | | 5 m/M | 10 m/M |
| Benomyl | 017804-35-2 | 0.84 ppm | | | |
| Benzene | 000071-43-2 | 10 ppm A2 | | 1 ppm | 5 ppm |
| *p*-Benzoquinone (quinone) | 000106-51-4 | 0.1 ppm | | 0.1 ppm | |
| Benzoyl peroxide | 000094-36-0 | 5 m/M | | 5 m/M | |
| Benzo[a]pyrene | 000050-32-8 | A2 | | 0.2 m/M | |
| Benzylchloride | 000100-44-7 | 1 ppm | | 1 ppm | |
| Beryllium [7440-41-7] and compounds, as Be | | 0.002 m/M A2 | | 0.002 m/M | C0.0005 m/M |
| Biphenyl (diphenyl) | 000092-52-4 | 0.2 ppm | | 0.2 ppm | |
| Bismuth telluride, undoped, as $Bi_2Te_3$ | 001304-82-1 | 10 m/M | | 15 m/M | |
| Bismuth telluride, Se-doped, as $Bi_2Te_3$ | 001304-82-1 | 5 m/M | | 5 m/M | |
| Bitumen | 008052-42-4 | 5 m/M | | | |
| Borates, tetra, sodium salts, anhydrous | 001303-96-4 | 1 m/M | | 10 m/M | |
| Borates, tetra, sodium salts, decahydrate | 001303-96-4 | 5 m/M | | 10 m/M | |
| Borates, tetra, sodium salts, pentahydrate | 001303-96-4 | 5 m/M | | 10 m/M | |
| Boron oxide | 001303-86-2 | 10 m/M | | 10 m/M | |
| Boron tribromide | 010294-33-4 | | C1 ppm | | C1 ppm |
| Boron trifluoride | 007637-07-2 | | C1 ppm | | C1 ppm |
| Bromacil | 000314-40-9 | 1 ppm | | 1 ppm | |
| Bromine | 007726-95-6 | 0.1 ppm | 0.2 ppm | 0.1 ppm | 0.3 ppm |
| Bromine pentafluoride | 007789-30-2 | 0.1 ppm | | 0.1 ppm | |
| Bromochloromethane (chlorobromomethane) | 000074-97-5 | 200 ppm | | | 200 ppm |
| Bromoethane (ethyl bromide) | 000074-96-4 | 5 ppm Skin A2 | | 200 ppm | 250 ppm |
| Bromoform (tribromomethane) | 000075-25-2 | 0.5 ppm Skin | | 0.5 ppm Skin | |
| 1,3-Butadiene | 000106-99-0 | 2 ppm A2 | | 1000 ppm | |
| Butane | 000106-97-8 | 800 ppm | | 800 ppm | |
| Butanethiol (butyl mercaptan) | 000109-79-5 | 0.5 ppm | | 0.5 ppm | |
| *n*-Butanol (*n*-butyl alcohol) | 000071-36-3 | | C50 ppm Skin | 100 ppm Skin | C50 ppm Skin |
| *sec*-Butanol (*sec*-butyl alcohol) | 000078-92-2 | 100 ppm | | 100 ppm | |
| *tert*-Butanol (*tert*-butyl alcohol) | 000075-65-0 | 100 ppm | | 100 ppm | 150 ppm |
| 2-Butanone (methyl ethyl ketone [MEK]) | 000078-93-3 | 200 ppm | 300 ppm | 200 ppm | 300 ppm |
| 2-Butoxyethanol (ethylene glycol monobutyl ether) | 000111-76-2 | 25 ppm Skin | | 25 ppm Skin | |
| 2-Butoxyethyl acetate (ethylene glycol monobutyl ether acetate) | 000112-07-2 | | | | |
| *n*-Butyl acetate | 000123-86-4 | 150 ppm | 200 ppm | 150 ppm | 200 ppm |
| *sec*-Butyl acetate | 000105-46-4 | 200 ppm | | 200 ppm | |
| *tert*-Butyl acetate | 000540-88-5 | 200 ppm | | 200 ppm | |
| *n*-Butyl acrylate (acrylic acid, n-butyl ester) | 000141-32-2 | 10 ppm | | 10 ppm | |
| *n*-Butylamine | 000109-73-9 | | C5 ppm Skin | | C5 ppm Skin |
| *tert*-Butyl chromate, as $CrO_3$ | 001189-85-1 | | C0.1 m/M Skin | | C0.1 m/M Skin |

| NAME | CAS NO. | ACGIH TLV | | OSHA PEL | |
|---|---|---|---|---|---|
| | | TWA | STEL | TWA | STEL |
| *n*-Butyl glycidyl ether (BGE) | 002426-08-6 | 25 ppm | | 25 ppm | |
| *n*-Butyl lactate | 000138-22-7 | 5 ppm | | 5 ppm Skin | |
| Butyl mercaptan (butanethiol) | 000109-79-5 | 0.5 ppm | | 0.5 ppm | |
| *o*-sec-Butylphenol | 000089-72-5 | 5 ppm Skin | | 5 ppm Skin | |
| *p*-tert Butyltoluene | 000098-51-1 | 1 ppm | | 10 ppm | 20 ppm |
| *n*-Butyronitrile | 000109-74-0 | | | | 8 ppm |
| Cadmium [7440-43-9] and compounds, as Cd | | 0.01 m/M | | 0.005 m/M | |
| Calcium carbonate (limestone; marble) | 001317-65-3 | 10 m/M | | 15 m/M | |
| Calcium chromate, as Cr | 013756-19-0 | 0.001 m/M A2 | | | |
| Calcium cyanamide | 000156-62-7 | 0.05 m/M | | 0.05 m/M | |
| Calcium hydroxide | 001305-62-0 | 5 m/M | | 5 m/M | |
| Calcium oxide | 001305-78-8 | 2 m/M | | 5 m/M | |
| Calcium silicate (synthetic) | 001344-95-2 | 10 m/M | | 15 m/M | |
| Calcium sulfate (gypsum; plaster of paris) | 007778-18-9 | 10 m/M | | 15 m/M | |
| Camphor, synthetic | 000076-22-2 | 2 ppm | 3 ppm | 2 m/M | |
| Caprolactam dust | 000105-60-2 | 1 m/M | 3 m/M | 1 m/M | 3 m/M |
| Caprolactam vapor | 000105-60-2 | 5 ppm | 10 ppm | 5 ppm | 10 ppm |
| Captafol | 002425-06-1 | 0.1 m/M Skin | | 0.1 m/M | |
| Captan | 000133-06-2 | 5 m/M | | 5 m/M | |
| Carbaryl (sevin) | 000063-25-2 | 5 m/M | | 5 m/M | |
| Carbofuran | 001563-66-2 | 0.1 m/M | | 0.1 m/M | |
| Carbon black | 001333-86-4 | 3.5 m/M | | 3.5 m/M | |
| Carbon dioxide | 000124-38-9 | 5000 ppm | 30,000 ppm | 10,000 ppm | 30,000 ppm |
| Carbon disulfide | 000075-15-0 | 10 ppm Skin | | 4 ppm Skin | 12 ppm Skin |
| Carbon monoxide | 000630-08-0 | 25 ppm | | 35 ppm | C200 ppm |
| Carbon tetrabromide | 000558-13-4 | 0.1 ppm | 0.3 ppm | 0.1 ppm | 0.3 ppm |
| Carbon tetrachloride (tetrachloromethane) | 000056-23-5 | 5 ppm A3 Skin | 10 ppm A3 Skin | 2 ppm | |
| Carbonyl chloride (phosgene) | 000075-44-5 | 0.1 ppm | | 0.1 ppm | |
| Carbonyl fluoride | 000353-50-4 | 2 ppm | 5 ppm | 2 ppm | 5 ppm |
| Catechol (pyrocatechol) | 000120-80-9 | 5 ppm Skin | | 5 ppm Skin | |
| Cellulose | 009004-34-6 | 10 m/M | | 15 m/M | |
| Cesium hydroxide | 021351-79-1 | 2 m/M | | 2 m/M | |
| Chlordane | 000057-74-9 | 0.5 m/M Skin | | 0.5 m/M Skin | |
| Chlorinated camphene (toxaphene) | 008001-35-2 | 0.5 m/M Skin | 1 m/M Skin | 0.5 m/M Skin | 1 m/M Skin |
| Chlorinated diphenyl oxide | 031242-93-0 | 0.5 m/M | | 0.5 m/M | |
| Chlorine | 007782-50-5 | 0.5 ppm | 1 ppm | 0.5 ppm | 1 ppm |
| Chlorine dioxide | 010049-04-4 | 0.1 ppm | 0.3 ppm | 0.1 ppm | 0.3 ppm |
| Chlorine trifluoride | 007790-91-2 | | C0.1 ppm | | C0.1 ppm |
| Chloroacetaldehyde | 000107-20-0 | | C1 ppm | | C1 ppm |
| Chloroacetone | 000078-95-5 | | C1 ppm Skin | | |
| *α*-Chloroacetophenone (phenacyl chloride) | 000532-27-4 | 0.05 ppm | | 0.05 ppm | |
| Chloroacetyl chloride | 000079-04-9 | 0.05 ppm Skin | 0.15 ppm Skin | 0.05 ppm | |
| Chlorobenzene (mono-chlorobenzene) | 000108-90-7 | 10 ppm | | 75 ppm | |
| *o*-Chlorobenzylidene malononitrile | 002698-41-1 | | C0.05 ppm Skin | | C0.05 ppm Skin |
| Chlorobromomethane (bromochloromethane) | 000074-97-5 | 200 ppm | | 200 ppm | |
| 2-Chloro-1,3-butadine (*β*-chloroprene) | 000126-99-8 | 10 ppm Skin | | 10 ppm Skin | |

| NAME | CAS NO. | ACGIH TLV | | OSHA PEL | |
|---|---|---|---|---|---|
| | | TWA | STEL | TWA | STEL |
| Chlorodifluoromethane | 000075-45-6 | 1000 ppm | | 1000 ppm | |
| Chlorodiphenyl (42% chlorine) | 053469-21-9 | 1 m/M Skin | | 1 m/M Skin | |
| Chlorodiphenyl (54% chlorine) | 011097-69-1 | 0.5 m/M Skin | | 0.5 m/M Skin | |
| 1-Chloro,2,3-epoxypropane (epichlorohydrin) | 000106-89-8 | 2 ppm Skin | | | |
| Chloroethane (ethyl chloride) | 000075-00-3 | 1000 ppm | | 1000 ppm | |
| 2-Chloroethanol (ethylene chlorohydrin) | 000107-07-3 | | 1 ppm Skin | | C1 ppm Skin |
| Chloroethylene (vinyl chloride) | 000075-01-4 | 5 ppm A1 | | 1 ppm | 5 ppm |
| Chloroform (trichloromethane) | 000067-66-3 | 10 ppm A2 | | 2 ppm | |
| *bis*(Chloromethyl) ether | 000542-88-1 | 0.001 ppm A1 | | | |
| 1-Chloro-1-nitropropane | 000600-25-9 | 2 ppm | | 2 ppm | |
| Chloropentafluorethane | 000076-15-3 | 1000 ppm | | 1000 ppm | |
| Chloropicrin (trichloronitromethane) | 000076-06-2 | 0.1 ppm | | 0.1 ppm | |
| *β*-Chloroprene | 000126-99-8 | 10 ppm Skin | | 10 ppm Skin | |
| 2-Chloropropionic acid | 000598-78-7 | 0.1 ppm Skin | | | |
| *o*-Chlorostyrene | 002039-87-4 | 50 ppm | 75 ppm | 50 ppm | 75 ppm |
| *o*-Chlorotoluene | 000095-49-8 | 50 ppm | | 50 ppm | |
| 2-Chloro-6-(trichloromethyl) pyridine (nitrapyrin) | 001929-82-4 | 10 m/M | 20 m/M | 15 m/M | |
| Chlorpyrifos | 002921-88-2 | 0.2 m/M Skin | | 0.2 m/M Skin | |
| Chromates, alkaline, as Cr | | 0.05 m/M A1 | | | C0.1 m/M |
| Chromic acid [1066-30-4] and chromates | | 0.05 m/M A1 | | | C0.1 m/M |
| Chromite ore processing (chromate), as Cr | | 0.05 m/M A1 | | | |
| Chromium (II) compounds, as Cr | | | | 0.5 m/M | |
| Chromium (III) compounds as Cr | | 0.5 m/M A4 | | 0.5 m/M | |
| Chromium (VI) compounds, as Cr, water soluble | | 0.05 m/M A1 | | | C0.1 m/M |
| Chromium (VI) compounds, as Cr, certain water insoluble | | 0.05 m/M A1 | | | |
| Chromium metal | 007440-47-3 | 0.5 m/M A4 | | 1 m/M | |
| Chromium trioxide, as Cr | 001333-82-0 | 0.05 m/M A1 | | | C0.1 m/M |
| Chromyl chloride | 014977-61-8 | 0.025 ppm | 0.005 m/M | | |
| Chrysene | 000218-01-9 | A2 | | | 0.2 m/M |
| Chrysotile (asbestos, chrysotile) | 012001-29-5 | 2 f/cc A1 | | 2 f/cc | |
| Clopidol | 002971-90-6 | 10 m/M | | 15 m/M | |
| Coal dust | | 2 m/M | | 2 m/M | |
| Coal tar pitch volatiles, as benzene solubles | 65996-93-20 | 0.2 m/M A1 | | 0.2 m/M | |
| Cobalt, elemental [7440-48-4], and inorganic compounds, as Co | | 0.02 m/M A3 | | 0.05 m/M | |
| Cobalt carbonyl, as Co | 010210-68-1 | 0.1 m/M | | 0.1 m/M | |
| Cobalt hydrocarbonyl, as Co | 016842-03-8 | 0.1 m/M | | 0.1 m/M | |
| Coke oven emissions | | | | 0.15 m/M | |
| Copper fume | 007440-50-8 | 0.2 m/M | | 0.1 m/M | |
| Copper [7440-50-8] dusts and mists, as Cu | | 1 m/M | | 1 m/M | |
| Cotton dust, raw | | 0.2 m/M | | 1 m/M | |
| Cotton dust | | | | 0.2 m/M | |
| Cotton dust, in textile slashing and weaving operations | | | | 0.75 m/M | |

| NAME | CAS NO. | ACGIH TLV | | OSHA PEL | |
|---|---|---|---|---|---|
| | | TWA | STEL | TWA | STEL |
| Cresol, all isomers | 001319-77-3 | 5 ppm Skin | | 5 ppm Skin | |
| Cristobalite (silica-crystalline) | 014464-46-1 | 0.05 m/M | | 0.05 m/M | |
| Crocidolite (asbestos, crocidolite) | 012001-28-4 | 0.2 f/cc A1 | | 0.2 f/cc | |
| Crotonaldehyde | 004170-30-3 | 2 ppm | | 2 ppm | |
| Crufomate | 000299-86-5 | 5 m/M | | 5 m/M | |
| Cumene | 000098-82-8 | 50 ppm Skin | | 50 ppm Skin | |
| Cyanamide | 000420-04-2 | 2 m/M | | 2 m/M | |
| Cyanide, calcium, as CN | 000592-01-8 | | C5 m/M Skin | 5 m/M | |
| Cyanide, potassium, as CN | 000151-50-8 | | C5 m/M | 5 m/M | |
| Cyanide, sodium, as CN | 000143-33-9 | | C5 m/M Skin | 5 m/M | |
| Cyanogen | 000460-19-5 | 10 ppm | | 10 ppm | |
| Cyanogen chloride | 000506-77-4 | | C0.3 ppm | | C0.3 ppm |
| Cyclohexane | 000110-82-7 | 300 ppm | | 300 ppm | |
| Cyclohexanol | 000108-93-0 | 50 ppm Skin | | 50 ppm Skin | |
| Cyclohexanone | 000108-94-1 | 25 ppm Skin | | 25 ppm Skin | |
| Cyclohexene | 000110-83-8 | 300 ppm | | 300 ppm | |
| Cyclohexylamine | 000108-91-8 | 10 ppm | | 10 ppm | |
| Cyclonite (RDX) | 000121-82-4 | 1.5 m/M Skin | | 1.5 m/M Skin | |
| Cyclopentadiene | 000542-92-7 | 75 ppm | | 75 ppm | |
| Cyclopentane | 000287-92-3 | 600 ppm | | 600 ppm | |
| Cyhexatin (tricyclohexyltin hydroxide) | 013121-70-5 | 5 m/M | | 5 m/M | |
| 2,4-D (2,4-dichlorophenoxyacetic acid) | 000094-75-7 | 10 m/M | | 10 m/M | |
| DDT (Dichlorodiphenyltrichloroethane) | 000050-29-3 | 1 m/M | | 1 m/M Skin | |
| Decaborane | 017702-41-9 | 0.05 ppm Skin | 0.15 ppm Skin | 0.05 ppm Skin | 0.15 ppm Skin |
| Demeton-methyl (methyl demeton) | 008022-00-2 | 0.5 m/M Skin | | 0.5 m/M Skin | |
| Demeton (Systox) | 008065-48-3 | 0.01 ppm Skin | | 0.1 m/M Skin | |
| Diacetone alcohol (4-hydroxy-4-methyl-2-pentanone) | 000123-42-2 | 50 ppm | | 50 ppm | |
| 1,2-Diaminoethane (ethylenediamine) | 000107-15-3 | 10 ppm | | 10 ppm | |
| Diatomaceous earth (silica-amorphous) | 061790-53-2 | 10 m/M | | 6 m/M | |
| Diazinon | 000333-41-5 | 0.1 m/M Skin | | 0.1 m/M Skin | |
| Diazomethane | 000334-88-3 | 0.2 ppm | | 0.2 ppm | |
| Diborane | 019287-45-7 | 0.1 ppm | | 0.1 ppm | |
| Dibrom (naled) | 000300-76-5 | 3 m/M Skin | | 3 m/M Skin | |
| 1,2-Dibromo-3-chloropropane (DBCP) | 000096-12-8 | | | 0.001 | |
| 1,2-Dibromoethane (ethylene dibromide) | 000106-93-4 | | | 20 ppm | C30 ppm |
| 2-N-Dibutylaminoethanol | 000102-81-8 | 0.5 ppm Skin | | 2 ppm | |
| Dibutyl phosphate | 000107-66-4 | 1 ppm | 2 ppm | 1 ppm | 2 ppm |
| Dibutyl phenyl phosphate | 002528-36-1 | 0.3 ppm Skin | | | |
| Dibutyl phthalate | 000084-74-2 | 5 m/M | | 5 m/M | |
| Dicholoroacetylene | 007572-29-4 | | C0.1 ppm | | C0.1 ppm |
| *o*-Dichlorobenzene (1,2-dichlorobenzene) | 000095-50-1 | 25 ppm Skin | 50 ppm Skin | | C50 ppm Skin |
| *p*-Dichlorobenzene (1,4-dichlorobenzene) | 000106-46-7 | 10 ppm A3 | | 75 ppm | 110 ppm |
| 1,4-Dichloro-2-butene | 000764-41-0 | 0.005 ppm Skin A2 | | | |

| NAME | CAS NO. | ACGIH TLV TWA | ACGIH TLV STEL | OSHA PEL TWA | OSHA PEL STEL |
|---|---|---|---|---|---|
| Dichlorodifluoromethane | 000075-71-8 | 1000 ppm | | 1000 ppm | |
| 1,3-Dichloro-5,5-dimethyl hydantoin | 000118-52-5 | 0.2 m/M | 0.4 m/M | 0.2 m/M | 0.4 m/M |
| Dichlorodiphenyltrichloroethane (DDT) | 000050-29-3 | 1 m/M | | 1 m/M Skin | |
| 1,1-Dichloroethane (ethylidene chloride) | 000075-34-3 | 100 ppm | | 100 ppm | |
| 1,2-Dichloroethane (ethylene dichloride) | 000107-06-2 | 10 ppm | | 1 ppm | 2 ppm |
| 1,1-Dichloroethylene (vinylidene chloride) | 000075-35-4 | 5 ppm | 20 ppm | 1 ppm | |
| 1,2-Dichloroethylene (acetylene dichloride) | 000540-59-0 | 200 ppm | | 200 ppm | |
| Dichloroethyl ether | 000111-44-4 | 5 ppm Skin | 10 ppm Skin | 5 ppm Skin | 10 ppm Skin |
| Dichlorofluoromethane (dichloromonofluoromethane) | 000075-43-4 | 10 ppm | | 10 ppm | |
| Dichloromethane (methylene chloride) | 000075-09-2 | 50 ppm A2 | | 500 ppm | C100 ppm |
| 1,1-Dichloro-1-nitroethane | 000594-72-9 | 2 ppm | | 2 ppm | C10 ppm |
| 2,4-Dichlorophenoxyacetic acid (2,4-D) | 000094-75-7 | 10 m/M | | 10 m/M | |
| 1,2-Dichloropropane (propylene dichloride) | 000078-87-5 | 75 ppm | 110 ppm | 75 ppm | 110 ppm |
| 1,3-Dichloropropene | 000542-75-6 | 1 ppm Skin | | 1 ppm Skin | |
| 2,2-Dichloropropionic acid | 000075-99-0 | 1 ppm | | 1 ppm | |
| Dichlorotetrafluoroethane | 000076-14-2 | 1000 ppm | | 1000 ppm | |
| Dichlorvos (DDVP) | 000062-73-7 | 0.1 ppm Skin | | 1 m/M Skin | |
| Dicrotophos | 000141-66-2 | 0.05 m/M Skin | | 0.25 m/M Skin | |
| Dicyclopentadiene | 000077-73-6 | 5 ppm | | 5 ppm | |
| Dicyclopentadienyl iron (ferrocene) | 000102-54-5 | 10 m/M | | 10 m/M | |
| Dieldrin | 000060-57-1 | 0.25 m/M Skin | | 0.25 m/M Skin | |
| Diethanolamine | 000111-42-2 | 0.46 ppm Skin | | 3 ppm | |
| Diethylamine | 000109-89-7 | 5 ppm A4 | 15 ppm A4 | 10 ppm | 25 ppm |
| 2-Diethylaminoethanol | 000100-37-8 | 2 ppm Skin | | 10 ppm Skin | |
| Diethylene glycol monobutyl ether | 000112-34-5 | | | | |
| Diethylene triamine | 000111-40-0 | 1 ppm Skin | | 1 ppm | |
| Diethyl ether (ethyl ether) | 000060-29-7 | 400 ppm | 500 ppm | 400 ppm | 500 ppm |
| Di(2-ethylhexyl)phthalate (DEHP; di-sec-octylphthalate | 000117-81-7 | 5 m/M | 10 m/M | 5 m/M | 10 m/M |
| Diethyl ketone | 000096-22-0 | 200 ppm | | 200 ppm | |
| Diethyl phthalate | 000084-66-2 | 5 m/M | | 5 m/M | |
| Difluorodibromomethane | 000075-61-6 | 100 ppm | | 100 ppm | |
| Diglycidyl ether (DGE) | 002238-07-5 | 0.1 ppm | | 0.1 ppm | C0.5 ppm |
| Dihydroxybenzene (hydroquinone) | 000123-31-9 | 2 m/M | | 2 m/M | |
| Diisobutyl ketone (2,6-dimethyl-4-heptanone) | 000108-83-8 | 25 ppm | | 25 ppm | |
| Diisopropylamine | 000108-18-9 | 5 ppm Skin | | 5 ppm Skin | |
| Dimethoxymethane (methylal) | 000109-87-5 | 1000 ppm | | 1000 ppm | |
| *N,N*-Dimethyl acetamide | 000127-19-5 | 10 ppm Skin | | 10 ppm Skin | |
| Dimethylamine | 000124-40-3 | 5 ppm | 15 ppm | 10 ppm | |

| NAME | CAS NO. | ACGIH TLV |  | OSHA PEL |  |
|---|---|---|---|---|---|
|  |  | TWA | STEL | TWA | STEL |
| Dimethylaminobenzene (xylidine) | 001300-73-8 | 0.5 ppm Skin A2 |  | 2 ppm Skin |  |
| Dimethylaniline (*N,N*-dimethylaniline) | 000121-69-7 | 5 ppm Skin | 10 ppm Skin | 5 ppm Skin | 10 ppm Skin |
| Dimethylbenzene (xylene) | 001330-20-7 | 100 ppm | 150 ppm | 100 ppm | 150 ppm |
| Dimethyl-1,2-dibromo-2, 2-dichloroethyl phosphate (dibrom; naled) | 000300-76-5 | 3 m/M Skin |  | 3 m/M Skin |  |
| Dimethylethoxysilane | 014857-34-2 |  | 1.5 ppm |  |  |
| Dimethylformamide | 000068-12-2 | 10 ppm Skin |  | 10 ppm Skin |  |
| 2,6-Dimethyl-4-heptanone (diisobutyl ketone) | 000108-83-8 | 25 ppm |  | 25 ppm |  |
| 1,1-Dimethylhydrazine | 000057-14-7 | 0.5 ppm Skin A2 |  | 0.5 ppm Skin |  |
| Dimethylphthalate | 000131-11-3 | 5 m/M |  | 5 m/M |  |
| Dimethyl sulfate | 000077-78-1 | 0.1 ppm Skin A2 |  | 0.1 ppm 1 Skin |  |
| Dinitolmide (3,5-dinitro-*o*-toluamide) | 000148-01-6 | 5 m/M |  | 5 m/M |  |
| Dinitrobenzene 528-29-0; 99-65-0; 100-25-4; 25154-54-5 |  | 0.15 ppm Skin |  | 1 m/M Skin |  |
| Dinitro-*o*-cresol | 000534-52-1 | 0.2 m/M Skin |  | 0.2 m/M Skin |  |
| 3,5-Dinitro-*o*-toluamide (dinitolmide) | 000148-01-6 | 5 m/M |  | 5 m/M |  |
| Dinitrotoluene | 025321-14-6 | 0.15 m/M A2 Skin |  | 1.5 m/M Skin |  |
| 1,4-Dioxane | 000123-91-1 | 25 ppm Skin |  | 25 ppm Skin |  |
| Dioxathion | 000078-34-2 | 0.2 m/M Skin |  | 0.2 m/M Skin |  |
| Diphenyl (biphenyl) | 000092-52-4 | 0.2 ppm |  | 0.2 ppm |  |
| Diphenylamine | 000122-39-4 | 10 m/M |  | 10 m/M |  |
| Diphenylmethane-4,4′-diisocyanate (methylene bisphenyl isocynate; MDI) | 000101-68-8 | 0.005 ppm |  |  | C0.02 ppm |
| Dipropylene glycol methyl-ether | 034590-94-8 | 100 ppm Skin | 150 ppm Skin | 100 ppm Skin | 150 ppm Skin |
| Dipropyl ketone | 000123-19-3 | 50 ppm |  | 50 ppm |  |
| Diquat | 02764-72-9 | 0.5 m/M |  | 0.5 m/M |  |
| Di-*sec*-octyl-phthalate [di(2-ethylhexyl) phthalate] (DEHP) | 000117-81-7 | 5 m/M | 10 m/M | 5 m/M | 10 m/M |
| Disulfiram | 000097-77-8 | 2 m/M |  | 2 m/M |  |
| Disulfoton | 000298-04-4 | 0.1 m/M Skin |  | 0.1 m/M Skin |  |
| 2,6-Di-*tert*-butyl-*p*-cresol | 000128-37-0 | 10 m/M |  | 10 m/M |  |
| Diuron | 000330-54-1 | 10 m/M |  | 10 m/M |  |
| Divinyl benzene | 001321-74-0 | 10 ppm |  | 10 ppm |  |
| Emery | 001302-74-5 | 10 m/M |  | 10 m/M |  |
| Endosulfan | 000115-29-7 | 0.1 m/M Skin |  | 0.1 m/M Skin |  |
| Endrin | 000072-20-8 | 0.1 m/M Skin |  | 0.1 m/M Skin |  |
| Enflurane | 013838-16-9 | 75 ppm |  |  |  |
| Enzymes, proteolytic (subtilisins) | 001395-21-7 |  | C0.00006 m/M |  | C0.00006 m/M |
| Epichlorohydrin (1-chloro-2,3-epoxypropane) | 000106-89-8 | 2 ppm Skin |  | 2 ppm Skin |  |
| EPN | 002104-64-5 | 0.1 m/M Skin |  | 0.5 m/M Skin |  |
| 1,2-Epoxypropane (propylene oxide) | 000075-56-9 | 20 ppm |  | 20 ppm |  |
| 2,3-Epoxy-1-propanol (glycidol) | 000556-52-5 | 25 ppm |  | 25 ppm |  |

| NAME | CAS NO. | ACGIH TLV TWA | ACGIH TLV STEL | OSHA PEL TWA | OSHA PEL STEL |
|---|---|---|---|---|---|
| Ethanethiol (ethyl mercaptan) | 000075-08-1 | 0.5 ppm | | 0.5 ppm | C10 ppm |
| Ethanol (ethyl alcohol) | 000064-17-5 | 1000 ppm | | 1000 ppm | |
| Ethanolamine (2-amino-ethanol) | 000141-43-5 | 3 ppm | 6 ppm | 3 ppm | 6 ppm |
| Ethion | 000563-12-2 | 0.4 m/M Skin | | 0.4 m/M Skin | |
| 2-Ethoxyethanol (ethylene glycol, monoethyl ether) | 000110-80-5 | 5 ppm Skin | | 200 ppm Skin | |
| 2-Ethoxyethyl acetate (ethylene glycol, mono-ethyl ether acetate | 000111-15-9 | 5 ppm Skin | | 100 ppm Skin | |
| Ethyl acetate | 000141-78-6 | 400 ppm | | 400 ppm | |
| Ethyl acrylate (acrylic acid, ethyl ester) | 000140-88-5 | 5 ppm A2 | 15 ppm A2 | 5 ppm Skin | 25 ppm Skin |
| Ethyl alcohol (ethanol) | 000064-17-5 | 1000 ppm | | 1000 ppm | |
| Ethylamine | 000075-04-7 | 5 ppm Skin | 15 ppm Skin | 10 ppm | |
| Ethyl amyl ketone (5-methyl-3-heptanone) | 000541-85-5 | 25 ppm | | 25 ppm | |
| Ethyl benzene | 000100-41-4 | 100 ppm | 125 ppm | 100 ppm | 125 ppm |
| Ethyl bromide (bromoethane) | 000074-96-4 | 5 ppm A2 | | 200 ppm | 250 ppm |
| Ethyl butyl ketone (3-heptanone) | 000106-35-4 | 50 ppm | | 50 ppm | |
| Ethyl chloride (chloroethane) | 000075-00-3 | 1000 ppm | | 1000 ppm | |
| Ethylene | 000074-85-1 | Asphyxiant | | | |
| Ethylene chlorohydrin (2-chloroethanol) | 000107-07-3 | | C1 ppm Skin | | C1 ppm Skin |
| Ethylenediamine (1,2-diaminoethane) | 000107-15-3 | 10 ppm | | 10 ppm | |
| Ethylene dibromide (1,2-dibromoethane) | 000106-93-4 | | | 20 ppm | C30 ppm |
| Ethylene dichloride (1,2-dichloroethane) | 000107-06-2 | 10 ppm | | 1 ppm | 2 ppm |
| Ethylene glycol | 000107-21-1 | | C50 ppm | | C50 ppm |
| Ethylene glycol dinitrate | 000628-96-6 | 0.05 ppm Skin | | | C0.2 ppm Skin |
| Ethylene glycol methyl ether acetate (2-methoxyethyl acetate) | 000110-49-6 | 5 ppm Skin | | 25 ppm Skin | |
| Ethylene glycol mono-butyl ether (2-butoxy-ethanol) | 000111-76-2 | 25 ppm Skin | | 25 ppm Skin | |
| Ethylene glycol mono-ethyl ether (2-ethoxyethanol) | 000110-80-5 | 5 ppm Skin | | 200 ppm | |
| Ethylene glycol mono-ethyl ether acetate (2-ethoxyethyl acetate) | 000111-15-9 | 5 ppm Skin | | 100 ppm Skin | |
| Ethylene glycol mono-methyl ether (2-methoxyethanol) | 000109-86-4 | 5 ppm Skin | | 25 ppm | |
| Ethylene glycol mono-methyl ether acetate (2-methoxyethyl acetate) | 000110-49-6 | 5 ppm Skin | | 25 ppm | |
| Ethylene oxide | 000075-21-8 | 1 ppm A2 | | 1 ppm | C5 ppm |
| Ethyleneimine | 000151-56-4 | 0.5 ppm Skin | | | |
| Ethyl ether (diethyl ether) | 000060-29-7 | 400 ppm | 500 ppm | 400 ppm | 500 ppm |
| Ethyl formate (formic acid, ethyl ester) | 000109-94-4 | 100 ppm | | 100 ppm | |

| NAME | CAS NO. | ACGIH TLV TWA | ACGIH TLV STEL | OSHA PEL TWA | OSHA PEL STEL |
|---|---|---|---|---|---|
| Ethylidene chloride (1,1-dichloroethane) | 000075-34-3 | 100 ppm | | 100 ppm | |
| Ethylidene norbornene | 016219-75-3 | | C5 ppm | | C5 ppm |
| *N*-Ethylmorpholine | 000100-74-3 | 5 ppm Skin | | 5 ppm Skin | |
| Ethyl mercaptan (ethanethiol) | 000075-08-1 | 0.5 ppm | | 0.5 ppm | C10 ppm |
| Ethyl silicate (silicic acid, tetraethyl ester) | 000078-10-4 | 10 ppm | | 10 ppm | |
| Fenamiphos | 022224-92-6 | 0.1 m/M Skin | | 0.1 m/M Skin | |
| Fensulfothion | 000115-90-2 | 0.1 m/M | | 0.1 m/M | |
| Fenthion | 000055-38-9 | 0.2 m/M | | 0.2 m/M | |
| Ferbam | 014484-64-1 | 10 m/M | | 10 m/M | |
| Ferrocene (dicyclopentadienyl iron) | 000102-54-5 | 10 m/M | | 10 m/M | |
| Ferrovanadium dust | 012604-58-9 | 1 m/M | 3 m/M | 1 m/M | 3 m/M |
| Fibrous glass dust (glass, fibrous or dust) | None | 10 m/M | | | |
| Fluorides as F | None | 2.5 m/M | | 2.5 m/M | |
| Fluorides and hydrogen fluoride (where both are simultaneously present) | None | | | | |
| Fluorine | 007782-41-4 | 1 ppm | 2 ppm | 0.1 ppm | |
| Fluorotrichloromethane (trichlorofluoromethane) | 000075-69-4 | | C1000 ppm | | C1000 ppm |
| Fluroxene | 000406-90-6 | | | | |
| Fonofos | 000944-22-9 | 0.1 m/M Skin | | | |
| Formaldehyde | 000050-00-0 | | C0.3 ppm A2 | 0.75 ppm | 2 ppm |
| Formamide | 000075-12-7 | 10 ppm Skin | | 20 ppm | 30 ppm |
| Formic acid | 000064-18-6 | 5 ppm | 10 ppm | 5 ppm | |
| Formic acid, ethyl ester (ethyl formate) | 000109-94-4 | 100 ppm | | 100 ppm | |
| Formic acid, methyl ester (methyl formate) | 000107-31-3 | 100 ppm | | 100 ppm | 150 ppm |
| Furfural | 000098-01-1 | 2 ppm Skin | | 2 ppm Skin | |
| Furfuryl alcohol | 000098-00-0 | 10 ppm Skin | 15 ppm Skin | 10 ppm Skin | 15 ppm Skin |
| Gasoline | 008006-61-9 | 300 ppm | 500 ppm | 300 ppm | 500 ppm |
| Germanium tetrahydride | 007782-65-2 | 0.2 ppm | | 0.2 ppm | |
| Glutaraldehyde | 000111-30-8 | | C0.2 ppm | | C0.2 ppm |
| Glycerin mist | 000056-81-5 | 10 ppm | | | 10 m/M |
| Glycidol (2,3-epoxy-1-propanol) | 000556-52-5 | 25 ppm | | 25 ppm | |
| Glycol monoethyl ether (2-ethoxyethanol) | 000110-80-5 | 5 ppm Skin | | 200 ppm Skin | |
| Grain dust (oat, wheat, barley) | | 4 m/M | | 10 m/M | |
| Graphite (natural) | 007782-42-5 | 2 m/M | | 2.5 m/M | |
| Graphite (synthetic) | | 2 m/M | | 10 m/M | |
| Guthion (azinphos-methyl) | 000086-50-0 | 0.2 m/M | | 0.2 m/M | |
| Gypsum (calcium sulfate) | 013397-24-5 | 10 m/M | | 15 m/M | |
| Hafnium | 007440-58-6 | 0.5 m/M | | 0.5 m/M | |
| Halothane | 000151-67-7 | 50 ppm | | | |
| Helium | 007440-59-7 | Asphyxiant | | | |
| Heptachlor and heptachlor epoxide | 000076-44-8 | 0.5 m/M | | 0.5 m/M | |
| Heptane (*n*-heptane) | 000142-82-5 | 400 ppm | 500 ppm | 400 ppm | 500 ppm |
| 2-Heptanone (methyl *n*-amyl ketone) | 000110-43-0 | 50 ppm | | 100 ppm | |
| 3-Heptanone (ethyl butyl ketone) | 000106-35-4 | 50 ppm | | 50 ppm | |

| | | ACGIH TLV | | OSHA PEL | |
|---|---|---|---|---|---|
| NAME | CAS NO. | TWA | STEL | TWA | STEL |
| Hexachlorobenzene (HCB) | 000118-74-1 | 0.025 m/M A3 Skin | | | |
| Hexachlorobutadiene | 000087-68-3 | 0.02 ppm Skin A2 | | 0.02 ppm | |
| γ-Hexachlorocyclohexane (lindane) | 000058-89-9 | 0.5 m/M Skin | | 0.5 m/M Skin | |
| Hexachlorocyclopentadiene | 000077-47-4 | 0.01 ppm | | 0.01 ppm | |
| Hexachloroethane | 000067-72-1 | 1 ppm Skin A2 | | 1 ppm Skin | |
| Hexachloronaphthalene | 001335-87-1 | 0.2 m/M Skin | | 0.2 m/M Skin | |
| Hexafluoroacetone | 000684-16-2 | 0.1 ppm Skin | | 0.1 ppm Skin | |
| Hexamethylene diisocyanate | 000822-06-0 | 0.005 ppm | | | |
| Hexane (*n*-hexane) | 000110-54-3 | 50 ppm | | 50 ppm | |
| Hexane, other isomers | | 500 ppm | 1000 ppm | 500 ppm | 1000 ppm |
| 1,6-Hexanediamine | 000124-09-4 | 0.5 ppm | | | |
| 2-Hexanone (methyl *n*-butyl ketone) | 000591-78-6 | 5 ppm Skin | | 5 ppm | |
| Hexone (methyl isobutyl ketone) | 000108-10-1 | 50 ppm | 75 ppm | 50 ppm | 75 ppm |
| *sec*-Hexyl acetate | 000108-84-9 | 50 ppm | | 50 ppm | |
| Hexylene glycol | 000107-41-5 | | C25 ppm | | C25 ppm |
| Hydrazine | 000302-01-2 | 0.1 ppm Skin A2 | | 0.1 ppm Skin | |
| Hydrogen | 001333-74-0 | Asphyxiant | | | |
| Hydrogenated terphenyls | 061788-32-7 | 0.5 ppm | | 0.5 ppm | |
| Hydrogen bromide | 010035-10-6 | | C3 ppm | | C3 ppm |
| Hydrogen chloride | 007647-01-0 | | C5 ppm | | C5 ppm |
| Hydrogen cyanide | 000074-90-8 | | C4.7 ppm Skin | 10 ppm Skin | 4.7 ppm Skin |
| Hydrogen fluoride, as F | 007664-39-3 | | C3 ppm | 3 ppm | 6 ppm |
| Hydrogen peroxide | 007722-84-1 | 1 ppm | | 1 ppm | |
| Hydrogen selenide, as Se | 007783-07-5 | 0.05 ppm | | 0.05 ppm | |
| Hydrogen sulfide | 007783-06-4 | 10 ppm | 15 ppm | 10 ppm | 15 ppm |
| Hydroquinone (dihydroxy benzene) | 000123-31-9 | 2 m/M | | 2 m/M | |
| 4-Hydroxy-4-methyl--2-pentanone (diacetone alcohol) | 000123-42-2 | 50 ppm | | 50 ppm | |
| 2-Hydroxypropyl acrylate | 000999-61-1 | 0.5 ppm Skin | | 0.5 ppm Skin | |
| Indene | 000095-13-6 | 10 ppm | | 10 ppm | |
| Indium [7440-74-6] and compounds, as In | | 0.1 m/M | | 0.1 m/M | |
| Iodine | 007553-56-2 | | C0.1 ppm | | C0.1 ppm |
| Iodoform | 000075-47-8 | 0.6 ppm | | 0.6 ppm | |
| Iron oxide dust and fume ($Fe_2O_3$), as Fe | | 5 m/M | | 10 m/M | |
| Iron pentacarbonyl as Fe | 013463-40-6 | 0.1 ppm | 0.2 ppm | 0.1 ppm | 0.2 ppm |
| Iron salts, soluble, as Fe | | 1 m/M | | 1 m/M | |
| Isoamyl acetate | 000123-92-2 | 100 ppm | | 100 ppm | |
| Isoamyl alcohol | 000123-51-3 | 100 ppm | 125 ppm | 100 ppm | 125 ppm |
| Isobutyl acetate | 000110-19-0 | 150 ppm | | 150 ppm | |
| Isobutyl alcohol | 000078-83-1 | 50 ppm | | 50 ppm | |
| Isooctyl alcohol | 026952-21-6 | 50 ppm Skin | | 50 ppm Skin | |
| Isophorone | 000078-59-1 | | C5 ppm | 4 ppm | |
| Isophorone diisocyanate | 004098-71-9 | 0.005 ppm | | 0.005 ppm Skin | 0.02 ppm Skin |
| Isopropoxyethanol | 000109-59-1 | 25 ppm Skin | | 25 ppm | |
| Isopropyl acetate | 000108-21-4 | 250 ppm | 310 ppm | 250 ppm | 310 ppm |
| Isopropyl alcohol | 000067-63-0 | 400 ppm | 500 ppm | 400 ppm | 500 ppm |
| Isopropylamine | 000075-31-0 | 5 ppm | 10 ppm | 5 ppm | 10 ppm |
| *N*-Isopropylaniline | 000768-52-5 | 2 ppm Skin | | 2 ppm Skin | |
| Isopropyl ether | 000108-20-3 | 250 ppm | 310 ppm | 500 ppm | |
| Isopropyl glycidyl ether (IGE) | 004016-14-2 | 50 ppm | 75 ppm | 50 ppm | 75 ppm |

| NAME | CAS NO. | ACGIH TLV | | OSHA PEL | |
|---|---|---|---|---|---|
| | | TWA | STEL | TWA | STEL |
| Kaolin | 001332-58-7 | 2 m/M | | 10 m/M | |
| Ketene | 000463-51-4 | 0.5 ppm | 1.5 ppm | 0.5 ppm | 1.5 ppm |
| Lead elemental [7439-92-1], and inorganic compounds, as Ph | | 0.15 m/M | | 0.05 m/M | |
| Lead arsenate, as $Pb(AsO_4)_2$ | 003687-31-8 | 0.15 | | 0.01 | |
| Lead chromate | 007758-97-6 | 0.05 m/M A2 | | | |
| Lead phosphate | 007446-27-7 | 0.15 m/M | | 0.05 m/M | |
| Limestone (calcium carbonate) | 001317-65-3 | 10 m/M | | 15 m/M | |
| Lindane ($\gamma$-hexachloro-cyclohexane) | 000058-89-9 | 0.5 m/M Skin | | 0.5 m/M Skin | |
| Lithium hydride | 007580-67-8 | 0.025 m/M | | 0.025 m/M | |
| LPG (liquified petroleum gas) | 068476-85-7 | 1000 ppm | | 1000 ppm | |
| Magnesite | 000546-93-0 | 10 m/M | | 15 m/M | |
| Magnesium oxide fume | 001309-48-4 | 10 m/M | | | |
| Malathion | 000121-75-5 | 10 m/M Skin | | 10 m/M Skin | |
| Maleic anhydride | 000108-31-6 | 0.25 ppm | | 0.25 ppm | |
| Manganese, elemental [7439-96-5], and inorganic compounds as Mn | | 5 m/M | | | C5 m/M |
| Manganese fume, as Mn | 007439-96-5 | 1 m/M | 3 m/M | 1 m/M | 3 m/M |
| Manganese cyclopentadienyl tricarbonyl, as Mn | 012079-65-1 | 0.1 m/M Skin | | 0.1 m/M Skin | |
| Manganese tetroxide, as Mn | 001317-35-7 | | | 1 m/M | |
| Marble (calcium carbonate) | 001317-65-3 | 10 m/M | | 15 m/M | |
| Mercury, alkyl compounds, as Hg | | 10 m/M | | 15 m/M | |
| Mercury, aryl compounds, as Hg | | 0.01 m/M Skin | 0.03 m/M Skin | 0.01 m/M Skin | 0.03 m/M Skin |
| Mercury, inorganic compounds, as Hg | | 0.025 m/M A4 Skin | | | C0.1 m/M Skin |
| Mercury, vapor, as Hg | | 0.025 A4 Skin | | 0.05 m/M | |
| Mesityl oxide | 000141-79-7 | 15 ppm | 25 ppm | 15 ppm | 25 ppm |
| Methacrylic acid | 000079-41-4 | 20 ppm | | 20 ppm Skin | |
| Methacrylic acid, methyl ester | 000080-62-6 | 100 ppm | | 100 ppm | |
| Methane | 000074-82-8 | Asphyxiant | | | |
| Methanethiol (methyl mercaptan) | 000074-93-1 | 0.5 ppm | | 0.5 ppm | C10 ppm |
| Methanol (methyl alcohol) | 000067-56-1 | 200 ppm Skin | 250 ppm Skin | 200 ppm Skin | 250 ppm Skin |
| Methomyl | 016752-77-5 | 2.5 m/M | | 2.5 m/M | |
| Methoxychlor | 000072-43-5 | 10 m/M | | 10 m/M | |
| 2-Methoxyethanol (ethylene glycol mono-methyl ether) | 000109-86-4 | 5 ppm Skin | | 25 ppm | |
| 2-Methoxyethyl acetate (ethylene glycol mono-methyl ether acetate) | 000110-49-6 | 5 ppm Skin | | 25 ppm Skin | |
| 4-Methoxyphenol | 000150-76-5 | 5 m/M | | 5 m/M | |
| Methyl acetate | 000079-20-9 | 200 ppm | 250 ppm | 200 ppm | 250 ppm |
| Methyl acetylene (propyne) | 000074-99-7 | 1000 ppm | | 1000 ppm | |
| Methyl acetylene-propadiene mixture (MAPP) | | 1000 ppm | 1250 ppm | 1000 ppm | 1250 ppm |
| Methyl acrylate (acrylic acid, methyl ester) | 000096-33-3 | 10 ppm Skin | | 10 ppm Skin | |
| Methylacrylonitrile | 00126-98-7 | 1 ppm Skin | | 1 ppm Skin | |
| Methylal (dimethoxymethane) | 00109-87-5 | 1000 ppm | | 1000 ppm | |
| Methyl alcohol (methanol) | 000067-56-1 | 200 ppm Skin | 250 ppm Skin | 200 ppm Skin | 250 ppm Skin |

| NAME | CAS NO. | ACGIH TLV | | OSHA PEL | |
|---|---|---|---|---|---|
| | | TWA | STEL | TWA | STEL |
| Methylamine | 000074-89-5 | 5 ppm | 15 ppm | 10 ppm | |
| Methyl amyl alcohol (methyl isobutyl carbinol; 4-methyl-2-pentanol) | 000108-11-2 | 25 ppm Skin | 40 ppm Skin | 25 ppm Skin | 40 ppm Skin |
| Methyl *n*-amyl ketone (2-hepatone) | 000110-43-0 | 50 ppm | | 100 ppm | |
| *N*-Methyl aniline (monomethyl aniline) | 000100-61-8 | 0.5 ppm Skin | | 0.5 ppm Skin | |
| 2-Methylaziridine (propylene imine) | 000075-55-8 | 2 ppm Skin A2 | | 2 ppm Skin | |
| Methyl bromide | 000074-83-9 | 5 ppm Skin | | 5 ppm Skin | C20 ppm Skin |
| Methyl-*tert*-butyl ether | 001634-04-4 | 40 ppm | | | |
| Methyl *n*-butyl ketone (2-hexanone) | 000591-78-6 | 5 ppm Skin | | 5 ppm | |
| Methyl cellosolve (2-methoxyethanol) | 000109-86-4 | 5 ppm Skin | | 25 ppm Skin | |
| Methyl cellosolve acetate (2-methoxyethyl acetate) | 000110-49-6 | 5 ppm Skin | | 25 ppm Skin | |
| Methyl chloride | 000074-87-3 | 50 ppm Skin | 100 ppm Skin | 50 ppm | 100 ppm |
| Methyl chloroform (1,1,1-trichloroethane) | 000071-55-6 | 350 ppm | 450 ppm | 350 ppm | 450 ppm |
| Methyl-2-cyanoacrylate | 000137-05-3 | 2 ppm | 4 ppm | 2 ppm | 4 ppm |
| Methylcyclohexane | 000108-87-2 | 400 ppm | | 400 ppm | |
| Methylcyclohexanol | 025639-42-3 | 50 ppm | | 50 ppm | |
| *o*-Methylcyclohexanone | 000583-60-8 | 50 ppm Skin | 75 ppm Skin | 50 ppm Skin | 75 ppm Skin |
| 2-Methylcyclopentadienyl manganese tricarbonyl, as Mn | 012108-13-3 | 0.2 m/M | | 0.2 m/M | |
| Methyl demeton (demeton-methyl) | 008022-00-2 | 0.5 m/M Skin | | 0.5 m/M Skin | |
| Methylene bisphenyl isocyanate (diphenylmethane-4,4′-diisocyanate; MDI) | 000101-68-8 | 0.005 ppm | | | C0.02 ppm |
| Methylene chloride (dichloromethane) | 000075-09-2 | 50,A2 ppm | | 500 ppm | C1000 ppm |
| 4,4′-Methylene bis (2-chloroaniline) (MBOCA) | 000101-14-4 | 0.01 ppm Skin A2 | | 0.02 ppm Skin | |
| Methylene bis(4-cyclohexylisocyanate) | 005124-30-1 | 0.005 ppm | | | C0.01 ppm |
| 4,4′-Methylene dianiline | 000101-77-9 | 0.1 ppm Skin A2 | | 0.01 ppm | 0.1 ppm |
| Methyl ethyl ketone (MEK; 2-butanone) | 000078-93-3 | 200 ppm | 300 ppm | 200 ppm | 300 ppm |
| Methyl ethyl ketone peroxide | 001338-23-4 | | C0.2 ppm | | C0.7 ppm |
| Methylformate (formic acid, methyl ester) | 000107-31-3 | 100 ppm | 150 ppm | 100 ppm | 150 ppm |
| 5-Methyl-3-heptanone (ethyl amyl ketone) | 000541-85-5 | 25 ppm | | 25 ppm | |
| Methylhydrazine | 000060-34-4 | C0.2 ppm Skin A2 | | | C0.2 ppm Skin |
| Methyliodide | 000074-88-4 | 2 ppm A2 | | 2 ppm Skin | |
| Methylisoamyl ketone | 000110-12-3 | 50 ppm | | 50 ppm | |
| Methylisobutyl carbinol (methyl amyl alcohol) | 000108-11-2 | 25 ppm Skin | 40 ppm Skin | 25 ppm Skin | 40 ppm Skin |
| Methylisobutyl ketone (hexone) | 000108-10-1 | 50 ppm | 75 ppm | 50 ppm | 75 ppm |
| Methylisocyanate | 000624-83-9 | 0.02 ppm Skin | | 0.02 ppm Skin | |
| Methylisopropyl ketone | 000563-80-4 | 200 ppm | | 200 ppm | |

| NAME | CAS NO. | ACGIH TLV TWA | ACGIH TLV STEL | OSHA PEL TWA | OSHA PEL STEL |
|---|---|---|---|---|---|
| Methylmercaptan (methanethiol) | 000074-93-1 | 0.5 ppm | | 0.5 ppm | |
| Methylmercury | 022967-92-6 | 0.01 m/M Skin | 0.03 m/M Skin | 0.01 m/M Skin | 0.03 m/M Skin |
| Methylmethacrylate | 000080-62-6 | 100 ppm | | 100 ppm | |
| Methylparathion | 000298-00-0 | 0.2 m/M Skin | | 0.2 m/M Skin | |
| 4-Methyl-2-pentanol (methyl amyl alcohol) | 000108-11-2 | 25 ppm Skin | 40 ppm Skin | 25 ppm Skin | 40 ppm Skin |
| Methylpropyl ketone (2-pentanone) | 000107-87-9 | 200 ppm | 250 ppm | 200 ppm | 250 ppm |
| Methylsilicate | 000681-84-5 | 1 ppm | | 1 ppm | |
| *a*-Methylstyrene | 000098-83-9 | 50 ppm | 100 ppm | 50 ppm | 100 ppm |
| Methyl styrene (all isomers) (vinyl toluene) | 025013-15-4 | 50 ppm | 100 ppm | 100 ppm | |
| Metribuzin | 021087-64-9 | 5 m/M | | 5 m/M | |
| Mevinphos (Phosdrin) | 007786-34-7 | 0.01 ppm Skin | 0.03 ppm Skin | 0.01 ppm Skin | 0.03 ppm Skin |
| Mica | 012001-26-2 | 3 m/M | | 3 m/M | |
| Mineral wool fiber | | 10 m/M | | | |
| Molybdenum [7439-98-7], soluble compounds, as Mo | | 5 m/M | | 5 m/M | |
| Molybdenum [7439-98-7], insoluble compounds, as Mo | | 10 m/M | | 10 m/M | |
| Monochlorobenzene (chlorobenzene) | 000108-90-7 | 10 ppm | | 75 ppm | |
| Monocrotophos | 006923-22-4 | 0.025 m/M Skin | | 0.025 m/M | |
| Morpholine | 000110-91-8 | 20 ppm Skin | | 20 ppm Skin | 30 ppm Skin |
| Naled (Dibrom) | 000300-76-5 | 3 m/M Skin | | 3 m/M Skin | |
| Naphtha (coal tar) (rubber solvent) | 008030-30-6 | 400 ppm | | 100 ppm | |
| Naphthalene | 000091-20-3 | 10 ppm | 15 ppm | 10 ppm | 15 ppm |
| *a*-Naphthylthiourea (ANTU) | 000086-88-4 | 0.3 m/M | | 0.3 m/M | |
| Neon | 007440-01-9 | Asphyxiant | | | |
| Nickel, elemental | [7440-02-0] | 1 m/M A1 | | 1 m/M | |
| Nickel, insoluble compounds, as Ni | | 1 m/M Skin A1 | | 1 m/M | |
| Nickel, soluble compounds, as Ni | | 0.1 m/M | | 0.1 m/M | |
| Nickel, carbonyl, as Ni | 013463-39-3 | 0.05 ppm | | 0.001 ppm | |
| Nickel sulfide roasting, fume and dust, as Ni | | 1 m/M A1 | | | |
| Nicotine | 000054-11-5 | 0.5 m/M Skin | | 0.5 m/M Skin | |
| Nitrapyrin (2-chloro-6-trichloromethyl pyridine) | 001929-82-4 | 10 m/M | 20 m/M | 15 m/M | |
| Nitric acid | 007697-37-2 | 2 ppm | 4 ppm | 2 ppm | 4 ppm |
| Nitric oxide | 010102-43-9 | 25 ppm | | 25 ppm | |
| *p*-Nitroaniline | 000100-01-6 | 3 m/M Skin | | 3 m/M Skin | |
| Nitrobenzene | 000098-95-3 | 1 ppm Skin | | 1 ppm Skin | |
| *p*-Nitrochlorobenzene | 000100-00-5 | 0.1 ppm Skin | | 1 m/M Skin | |
| Nitroethane | 000079-24-3 | 100 ppm | | 100 ppm | |
| Nitrogen | 007727-37-9 | Asphyxiant | | | |
| Nitrogen dioxide | 010102-44-0 | 3 ppm | 5 ppm | | 1 ppm |
| Nitrogen trifluoride | 007783-54-2 | 10 ppm | | 10 ppm | |
| Nitroglycerin (NG) | 000055-63-0 | 0.05 ppm Skin | | | C0.2 ppm Skin |
| Nitromethane | 000075-52-5 | 20 ppm | | 100 ppm | |
| 1-Nitropropane | 000108-03-2 | 25 ppm | | 25 ppm | |
| 2-Nitropropane | 000079-46-9 | 10 ppm A2 | | 10 ppm | |
| Nitrotoluene, *o*-isomer | 000088-72-2 | 2 ppm Skin | | 2 ppm Skin | |

| NAME | CAS NO. | ACGIH TLV TWA | ACGIH TLV STEL | OSHA PEL TWA | OSHA PEL STEL |
|---|---|---|---|---|---|
| Nitrotoluene, *m*-isomer | 00099-08-1 | 2 ppm Skin | | 2 ppm Skin | |
| Nitrotoluene, *p*-isomer | 000099-99-0 | 2 ppm Skin | | 2 ppm Skin | |
| Nitrotrichloromethane (chloropicrin) | 000076-06-2 | 0.1 ppm | | 0.1 ppm | |
| Nitrous oxide | 010024-97-2 | 50 ppm | | | |
| Nonane | 000111-84-2 | 200 ppm | | 200 ppm | |
| Nuisance particulates (particulates not otherwise classified [PNOC]) | | 10 m/M | | 15 m/M | |
| Octachloronaphthalene | 002234-13-1 | 0.1 m/M Skin | 0.3 m/M Skin | 0.1 m/M Skin | 0.3 m/M Skin |
| Octane | 000111-65-9 | 300 ppm | 375 ppm | 300 ppm | 375 ppm |
| *n*-Octylmercaptan | 000111-88-6 | | | | |
| Oil mist, mineral, severely refined | | 5 m/M | | 5 m/M | |
| Osmium tetroxide, as Os | 020816-12-0 | 0.0002 ppm | 0.0006 ppm | 0.0002 ppm | 0.0006 ppm |
| Oxalic acid | 000144-62-7 | 1 m/M | 2 m/M | 1 m/M | 2 m/M |
| Oxygen difluoride | 007783-41-7 | | C0.05 ppm | | C0.05 ppm |
| Ozone | 010028-15-6 | | C0.1 0.2 ppm | 0.1 ppm | 0.3 ppm |
| Paraffin wax fume | 008002-74-2 | 2 m/M | | 2 m/M | |
| Paraquat | 004685-14-7 | 0.5 m/M | | 0.1 m/M Skin | |
| Parathion | 000056-38-2 | 0.1 m/M Skin | | 0.1 m/M Skin | |
| Partic. polycycl. arom. hydrocarb. (PPAH; coal tar pitch volatiles) | | 0.2 m/M A2 | | 0.2 m/M | |
| Particulates not otherwise classified (PNOC) (nuisance particulates) | | 10 m/M | | 15 m/M | |
| Pentaborane | 019624-22-7 | 0.005 ppm | 0.015 ppm | 0.005 ppm | 0.015 ppm |
| Pentachloronaphthalene | 001321-64-8 | 0.5 m/M Skin | | 0.5 m/M Skin | |
| Pentachloronitrobenzene | 000082-68-8 | 0.5 m/M | | | |
| Pentachlorophenol | 000087-86-5 | 0.5 m/M Skin | | 0.5 m/M Skin | |
| Pentaerythritol | 000115-77-5 | 10 m/M | | 10 m/M | |
| Pentane | 000109-66-0 | 600 ppm | 750 ppm | 600 ppm | 750 ppm |
| 2-Pentanone (methyl propyl ketone) | 000107-87-9 | 200 ppm | 250 ppm | 200 ppm | 250 ppm |
| Perchloroethylene (tetrachloroethylene) | 000127-18-4 | 25 ppm A3 | 100 ppm A3 | 25 ppm | |
| Perchloromethyl mercaptan | 000594-42-3 | 0.1 ppm | | 0.1 ppm | |
| Perchloryl fluoride | 007616-94-6 | 3 ppm | 6 ppm | 3 ppm | 6 ppm |
| Perfluoroisobutylene | 000382-21-8 | | C0.01 ppm | | |
| Perlite | 093763-70-3 | 10 m/M | | 15 m/M | |
| Petroleum distillates (gasoline; Stoddard solvent; VM&P naphtha) | | | | 400 ppm | |
| Phenacyl chloride (α-Chloroacetophenone) | 000532-27-4 | 0.05 ppm | | 0.05 ppm | |
| Phenol | 000108-95-2 | 5 ppm Skin | | 5 ppm Skin | |
| Phenothiazine | 000092-84-2 | 5 m/M Skin | | 5 m/M Skin | |
| *o*-Phenylenediamine | 000095-54-5 | 0.1 m/M A2 | | | |
| *m*-Phenylenediamine | 000108-45-2 | 0.1 m/M | | | |
| *p*-Phenylenediamine | 000106-50-3 | 0.1 m/M Skin | | 0.1 m/M Skin | |
| Phenyl ether, vapor | 000101-84-8 | 1 ppm | 2 ppm | 1 ppm | |
| Phenyl ether-biphenyl mixture, vapor | | | | 1 ppm | |
| Phenylethylene (Styrene, monomer) | 000100-42-5 | 50 ppm Skin | 100 ppm | 50 ppm | 100 ppm |

| NAME | CAS NO. | ACGIH TLV TWA | ACGIH TLV STEL | OSHA PEL TWA | OSHA PEL STEL |
|---|---|---|---|---|---|
| Phenyl glycidyl ether (PGE) | 000122-60-1 | 0.1 ppm Skin | | 1 ppm | |
| Phenylhydrazine | 000100-63-0 | 0.1 ppm Skin A3 | | 5 ppm Skin | 10 ppm Skin |
| Phenyl mercaptan | 000108-98-5 | 0.5 ppm | | 0.5 ppm | C0.1 |
| Phenylphosphine | 000638-21-1 | | C0.05 ppm | | C0.05 ppm |
| Phorate | 000298-02-2 | 0.05 m/M Skin | 0.2 m/M Skin | 0.05 m/M Skin | 0.2 m/M Skin |
| Phosdrin (mevinphos) | 007786-34-7 | 0.01 ppm Skin | 0.03 ppm Skin | 0.01 ppm Skin | 0.03 ppm Skin |
| Phosgene (carbonyl chloride) | 000075-44-5 | 0.1 ppm | | 0.1 ppm | |
| Phosphine | 007803-51-2 | 0.3 ppm | 1 ppm | 0.3 ppm | 1 ppm |
| Phosphoric acid | 007664-38-2 | 1 m/M | 3 m/M | 1 m/M | 3 m/M |
| Phosphorus (yellow) | 007723-14-0 | 0.02 ppm | | 0.1 m/M | 0.1 m/M |
| Phosphorus oxychloride | 010025-87-3 | 0.1 ppm | | 0.1 ppm | |
| Phosphorus pentachloride | 010026-13-8 | 0.1 ppm | | 1 m/M | |
| Phosphorus pentasulfide | 001314-80-3 | 1 m/M | 3 m/M | 1 m/M | 3 m/M |
| Phosphorus trichloride | 007719-12-2 | 0.2 ppm | 0.5 ppm | 0.2 ppm | 0.5 ppm |
| Phthalic anhydride | 000085-44-9 | 1 ppm | | 1 ppm | |
| *m*-Phthalodinitrile | 000626-17-5 | 5 m/M | | 5 m/M | |
| Picloram | 001918-02-1 | 10 m/M | | 10 m/M | |
| Picric acid (2,4,6-trinitrophenol) | 000088-89-1 | 0.1 m/M | | 0.1 m/M Skin | |
| Pindone (2-pivalyl-1, 3-indandione) | 000083-26-1 | 0.1 m/M | | 0.1 m/M | |
| Piperazine dihydrochloride | 000142-64-3 | 5 m/M | | 5 m/M | |
| 2-Pivalyl-1, 3-indandione (pindone) | 000083-26-1 | 0.1 m/M | | 0.1 m/M | |
| Plaster of paris (calcium sulfate) | 026499-65-0 | 10 m/M | | 15 m/M | |
| Platinum, metal | 007440-06-4 | 1 m/M | | 1 m/M | |
| Platinum, soluble salts, as Pt | 007440-06-4 | 0.002 m/M | | 0.002 m/M | |
| Portland cement | 065997-15-1 | 10 m/M | | 10 m/M | |
| Potassium hydroxide | 001310-58-3 | | C2 m/M | | C2 m/M |
| Precipitated silica (silica–amorphous) | 112926-00-8 | 10 m/M | | 6 m/M | |
| Propane | 000074-98-6 | | | 1000 ppm | |
| Propargyl alcohol | 000107-19-7 | 1 ppm Skin | | 1 ppm Skin | |
| *β*-Propiolactone | 000057-57-8 | 0.5 ppm A2 | | | |
| Propionic acid | 000079-09-4 | 10 ppm | | 10 ppm | |
| Propoxur | 000114-26-1 | 0.5 m/M | | 0.5 m/M | |
| *n*-Propyl acetate | 000109-60-4 | 200 ppm | 250 ppm | 200 ppm | 250 ppm |
| *n*-Propyl alcohol | 000071-23-8 | 200 ppm Skin | 250 ppm Skin | 200 ppm | 250 ppm |
| Propylene | 000115-07-1 | Asphyxiant | | | |
| Propylene dichloride (1,2-dichloropropane) | 000078-87-5 | 75 ppm | 110 ppm | 75 ppm | 110 ppm |
| Propylene glycol dinitrate | 006423-43-4 | 0.05 ppm Skin | | 0.05 ppm | |
| Propylene glycol monomethyl ether | 000107-98-2 | 100 ppm | 150 ppm | 100 ppm | 150 ppm |
| Propylene imine (2-methylaziridine) | 000075-55-8 | 2 ppm Skin A2 | | 2 ppm Skin | |
| Propylene oxide (1,2-epoxypropane) | 000075-56-9 | 20 ppm | | 20 ppm | |
| *n*-Propylnitrate | 000627-13-4 | 25 ppm | 40 ppm | 25 ppm | 40 ppm |
| Propyne (methylacetylene) | 000074-99-7 | 1000 ppm | | 1000 ppm | |
| Pyrethrum | 008003-34-7 | 5 m/M | | 5 m/M | |
| Pyridine | 000110-86-1 | 5 ppm | | 5 ppm | |
| Pyrocatechol (catechol) | 000120-80-9 | 5 ppm | | 5 ppm Skin | |
| Quartz (silica-crystalline) | 014808-60-7 | 0.1 m/M | | 0.1 m/M | |
| Quinone | 000106-51-4 | 0.1 ppm | | 0.1 ppm | |

| NAME | CAS NO. | ACGIH TLV TWA | ACGIH TLV STEL | OSHA PEL TWA | OSHA PEL STEL |
|---|---|---|---|---|---|
| RDX (cyclonite) | 000121-82-4 | 1.5 m/M Skin | | 1.5 m/M Skin | |
| Resorcinol | 000108-46-3 | 10 ppm | 20 ppm | 10 ppm | 20 ppm |
| Rhodium, metal | 007440-16-6 | 1 m/M | | 0.1 m/M | |
| Rhodium, insoluble compounds, as Rh | | 1 m/M | | 0.1 m/M | |
| Rhodium, soluble compounds, as Rh | | 0.1 m/M | | 0.001 m/M | |
| Ronnel | 000299-84-3 | 10 m/M | | 10 m/M | |
| Rosin core solder pyrolysis products as formaldehyde | | | | 0.1 m/M | |
| Rotenone (commercial) | 000083-79-4 | 5 m/M | | 5 m/M | |
| Rouge | | 10 m/M | | 10 m/M | |
| Rubber solvent (Naphtha) | 008030-30-6 | 400 ppm | | 100 ppm | |
| Selenium [7782-49-2] and compounds, as Se | | 0.2 m/M | | 0.2 m/M | |
| Selenium hexafluoride, as Se | 007783-79-1 | 0.05 ppm | | 0.05 ppm | |
| Sesone (sodium-2,4-dichlorophenoxyethyl sulfate) | 000136-78-7 | 10 m/M | | 10 m/M | |
| Silane (silicon tetrahydride) | 007803-62-5 | 5 ppm | | 5 ppm | |
| Silica—amorphous diatomaceous earth (uncalcined) | 061790-53-2 | 10 m/M | | 6 m/M | |
| Silica—amorphous precipitated silica | 112926-00-8 | 10 m/M | | 6 m/M | |
| Silica—amorphous silica fume | 069012-64-2 | 2 m/M | | | |
| Silica—amorphous silica, fused | 060676-86-0 | 0.1 m/M | | 0.1 m/M | |
| Silica—amorphous silica gel | 112926-00-8 | 10 m/M | | 6 m/M | |
| Silica—crystalline cristobalite | 014464-46-1 | 0.05 m/M | | 0.05 m/M | |
| Silica—crystalline quartz | 014808-60-7 | 0.1 m/M | | 0.1 m/M | |
| Silica—crystalline tridymite | 015468-32-3 | 0.05 m/M | | 0.05 m/M | |
| Silica—crystalline tripoli | 001317-95-9 | 0.1 m/M | | 0.1 m/M | |
| Silica fume (silica—amorphous) | 069012-64-2 | 2 m/M | | | |
| Silica, fused (silica—amorphous) | 060676-86-0 | 0.1 m/M | | 0.1 m/M | |
| Silica gel (silica—amorphous) | 112926-00-8 | 10 m/M | | 6 m/M | |
| Silica, precipitated (silica—amorphous) | 112926-00-8 | 10 m/M | | 6 m/M | |
| Silicic acid, tetraethyl ester (ethyl silicate) | 000078-10-4 | 10 ppm | | 10 ppm | |
| Silicon | 007440-21-3 | 10 m/M | | 10 m/M | |
| Silicon carbide | 000409-21-2 | 10 m/M | | 10 m/M | |
| Silicon tetrahydride (silane) | 007803-62-5 | 5 ppm | | 5 ppm | |
| Silver, metal | 007440-22-4 | 0.1 m/M | | 0.01 m/M | |
| Silver, soluble compounds, as Ag | | 0.01 m/M | | 0.01 m/M | |
| Soapstone | | 6 m/M | | 6 m/M | |
| Sodium azide | 026628-22-8 | | C0.11 ppm | | C0.1 ppm |
| Sodium bisulfite | 007631-90-5 | 5 m/M | | 5 m/M | |
| Sodium-2,4-dichlorophenoxyethyl sulfate (sesone) | 000136-78-7 | 10 m/M | | 10 m/M | |
| Sodium fluoroacetate | 000062-74-8 | 0.05 m/M Skin | | 0.05 m/M Skin | 0.15 m/M Skin |
| Sodium hydroxide | 001310-73-2 | | C2 m/M | | C2 m/M |
| Sodium metabisulfite | 007681-57-4 | 5 m/M | | 5 m/M | |
| Starch | 009005-25-8 | 10 m/M | | 15 m/M | |

| NAME | CAS NO. | ACGIH TLV | | OSHA PEL | |
|---|---|---|---|---|---|
| | | TWA | STEL | TWA | STEL |
| Stearates | | 10 m/M | | | |
| Stibine | 007803-52-3 | 0.1 ppm | | 0.1 ppm | |
| Stoddard solvent | 008052-41-3 | 100 ppm | | 100 ppm | |
| Strontium chromate, as Cr | 007789-06-2 | 0.005 m/M A2 | | | C0.1 m/M |
| Strychnine | 000057-24-9 | 0.15 m/M | | 0.15 m/M | |
| Styrene, monomer (phenylethylene; vinyl benzene) | 000100-42-5 | 50 ppm Skin | 100 ppm Skin | 50 ppm | 100 ppm |
| Subtilisins (proteolytic enzymes as 100% pure ... | 001395-21-7 | | C0.00006 m/M | | 0.00006 m/M |
| Sucrose | 000057-50-1 | 10 m/M | | 15 m/M | |
| Sulfometuron methyl | 074222-97-2 | 5 m/M A4 | | | |
| Sulfotep (TEDP) | 003689-24-5 | 0.2 m/M Skin | | 0.2 m/M Skin | |
| Sulfur dioxide | 007446-09-5 | 2 ppm | 5 ppm | 2 ppm | 5 ppm |
| Sulfur hexafluoride | 002551-62-4 | 1000 ppm | | 1000 ppm | |
| Sulfuric acid | 007664-93-9 | 1 m/M | 3 m/M | 1 m/M | |
| Sulfur monochloride | 010025-67-9 | | C1 ppm | | C1 ppm |
| Sulfur pentafluoride | 005714-22-7 | | C0.01 ppm | | C0.01 ppm |
| Sulfur tetrafluoride | 007783-60-0 | | C0.1 ppm | | C0.1 ppm |
| Sulfuryl fluoride | 002699-79-8 | 5 ppm | 10 ppm | 5 ppm | 10 ppm |
| Sulprofos | 035400-43-2 | 1 m/M | | 1 m/M | |
| Systox (demeton) | 008065-48-3 | 0.01 ppm Skin | | 0.1 ppm Skin | |
| 2,4,5-T (2,4,5-Trichloro-phenoxyacetic acid) | 000093-76-5 | 10 m/M | | 10 m/M | |
| Talc (containing no asbestos fibers) | 014807-96-6 | 2 m/M | | 2 m/M | |
| Tantalum metal | 007440-25-7 | 5 m/M | | 5 m/M | |
| Tantalum, oxide dusts | 001314-61-0 | 5 m/M | | 5 m/M | |
| TEDP (sulfotep) | 003689-24-5 | 0.2 m/M Skin | | 0.2 m/M Skin | |
| Tellurium (13494-80-9) and compounds, as Te | | 0.1 m/M | | 0.1 m/M | |
| Tellurium hexafluoride, as Te | 007783-80-4 | 0.02 ppm | | 0.02 ppm | |
| Temephos | 003383-96-8 | 10 m/M | | 10 m/M | |
| TEPP (tetraethyl pyrophosphate) | 000107-49-3 | 0.004 ppm Skin | | 0.05 m/M Skin | |
| Terephthalic acid | 000100-21-0 | 10 m/M | | | |
| Terphenyls | 026140-60-3 | | C0.53 ppm | | C0.5 ppm |
| 1,1,2,2-Tetrabromoethane | 79-27-6 | | | | |
| 1,1,1,2-Tetrachloro-2,2-difluoroethane | 000076-11-9 | 500 ppm | | 500 ppm | |
| 1,1,2,2-Tetrachloro-1,2-difluoroethane | 000076-12-0 | 500 ppm | | 500 ppm | |
| 1,1,2,2-tetrachloroethane | 630-20-6 | 1 ppm Skin | | 1 ppm Skin | |
| Tetrachloroethylene (perchloroethylene) | 000127-18-4 | 25 ppm A3 | 100 ppm A3 | 25 ppm | |
| Tetrachloromethane (carbon tetrachloride) | 000056-23-5 | 5 ppm Skin A3 | 10 ppm Skin A3 | 2 ppm | |
| Tetrachloronaphthalene | 001335-88-2 | 2 m/M | | 2 m/M Skin | |
| Tetraethyl lead, as Pb | 000078-00-2 | 0.1 m/M Skin | | 0.075 m/M Skin | |
| Tetraethyl pyrophosphate (TEPP) | 000107-49-3 | 0.004 ppm Skin | | 0,05 m/M Skin | |
| Tetrahydrofuran | 000109-99-9 | 200 ppm | 250 ppm | 200 ppm | 250 ppm |
| Tetramethyl lead, as Pb | 000075-74-1 | 0.15 m/M Skin | | 0.075 m/M Skin | |
| Tetramethyl succinonitrile | 003333-52-6 | 0.5 ppm Skin | | 0.5 ppm Skin | |
| Tetranitromethane | 000509-14-8 | 0.005 ppm A2 | | 1 ppm | |
| Tetrasodium pyrophosphate | 007722-88-5 | 5 m/M | | 5 m/M | |

| NAME | CAS NO. | ACGIH TLV TWA | ACGIH TLV STEL | OSHA PEL TWA | OSHA PEL STEL |
|---|---|---|---|---|---|
| Tetryl (2,4,6-Trinitrophenylmethylnitramine) | 000479-45-8 | 1.5 m/M | | 1.5 m/M Skin | |
| Thallium, soluble compounds, as TI | | 0.1 m/M Skin | | 0.1 m/M Skin | |
| 4,4′-Thiobis (6-tert-butyl-*m*-cresol) | 000096-69-5 | 10 m/M | | 10 m/M | |
| Thioglycolic acid | 000068-11-1 | 1 ppm Skin | | 1 ppm Skin | |
| Thionyl chloride | 007719-09-7 | | C1 ppm | | C1 ppm |
| Thiram | 000137-26-8 | 1 m/M | | 5 m/M | |
| Tin, metal | 007440-31-5 | 2 m/M | | 2 m/M | |
| Tin, oxide and inorganic compounds, except $SnH_4$ as Sn | | 2 m/M | | 2 m/M | |
| Tin, organic compounds, as Sn | | 0.1 m/M Skin | 0.2 m/M Skin | 0.1 m/M Skin | |
| Tin oxide, as Sn | 021651-19-4 | 1 m/M | | 2 m/M | |
| Titanium dioxide | 013463-67-7 | 10 m/M | | 10 m/M | |
| Toluene (toluol) | 000108-88-3 | 50 ppm Skin | | 100 ppm | 150 ppm |
| Toluene-2,4-diisocyanate (TDI) | 000584-84-9 | 0.005 ppm | 0.02 ppm | 0.005 ppm | 0.02 ppm |
| *o*-Toluidine | 000095-53-4 | 2 ppm A2 Skin | | 5 ppm Skin | |
| *m*-Toluidine | 000108-44-1 | 2 ppm Skin | | 2 ppm Skin | |
| *p*-Toluidine | 000106-49-0 | 2 ppm Skin A2 | | 2 ppm Skin | |
| Toluol (toluene) | 000108-88-3 | 50 ppm Skin | | 100 ppm | 150 ppm |
| Toxaphene (chlorinated camphene) | 008001-35-2 | 0.5 m/M Skin | 1 m/M Skin | 0.5 m/M Skin | 1 m/M Skin |
| Tremolite | 001332-21-4 | 2 f/cc A1 | | 0.2 f/cc | 1 fcc |
| Tribromomethane (bromoform) | 000075-25-2 | 0.5 ppm Skin | | 0.5 ppm Skin | |
| Tributyl phosphate | 000126-73-8 | 0.2 ppm | | 0.2 ppm | |
| Trichloroacetic acid | 000076-03-9 | 1 ppm | | 1 ppm | |
| 1,2,4-Trichlorobenzene | 000120-82-1 | | C5 ppm | | C5 ppm |
| 1,1,1-Trichloroethane (methyl chloroform) | 000071-55-6 | 350 ppm | 450 ppm | 350 ppm | 450 ppm |
| 1,1,2-Trichloroethane | 000079-00-5 | 10 ppm Skin | | 10 ppm Skin | |
| Trichloroethylene | 000079-01-6 | 50 ppm A5 | 100 ppm A5 | 50 ppm | 200 ppm |
| Trichlorofluoromethane (fluorotrichloromethane) | 000075-69-4 | | C1000 ppm | | C1000 ppm |
| Trichloromethane (chloroform) | 000067-66-3 | 10 ppm A2 | | 2 ppm | |
| Trichloronaphthalene | 001321-65-9 | 5 m/M Skin | | 5 m/M Skin | |
| Trichloronitromethane (chloropicrin) | 000076-06-2 | 0.1 ppm | | 0.1 ppm | |
| 2,4,5-Trichlorophenoxyacetic acid (2,4,5-T) | 000093-76-5 | 10 m/M | | 10 m/M | |
| 1,2,3-Trichloropropane | 000096-18-4 | 10 ppm Skin | | 10 ppm | |
| 1,1,2-Trichloro-1,2,2-trifluoroethane | 000076-13-1 | 1000 ppm | 1250 ppm | 1000 ppm | 1250 ppm |
| Tricyclohexyltin hydroxide (cyhexatin) | 013121-70-5 | 5 m/M | | 5 m/M | |
| Tridymite (silica-crystalline) | 015468-32-3 | 0.05 m/M | | 0.05 m/M | |
| Triethanolamine | 000102-71-6 | 5 m/M | | | |
| Triethylamine | 000121-44-8 | 1 ppm Skin A4 | 3 ppm Skin A4 | 10 ppm | 15 ppm |
| Trifluorobromomethane | 000075-63-8 | 1000 ppm | | 1000 ppm | |
| Trimellitic anhydride | 000552-30-7 | | C0.04 m/M | 0.005 ppm | |
| Trimethylamine | 75-50-3 | 5 ppm | 15 ppm | 10 ppm | 15 ppm |
| Trimethyl benzene | 025551-13-7 | 25 ppm | | 25 ppm | |
| Trimethyl phosphite | 000121-45-9 | 2 ppm | | 2 ppm | |

| NAME | CAS NO. | ACGIH TLV | | OSHA PEL | |
|---|---|---|---|---|---|
| | | TWA | STEL | TWA | STEL |
| 2,4,6-Trinitrophenol (picric acid) | 000088-89-1 | 0.1 m/M Skin | | 0.1 m/M Skin | |
| 2,4,6-Trinitrophenylmethylnitramine (tetryl) | 000479-45-8 | 15 m/M | | 15 m/M Skin | |
| 2,4,6-Trinitrotoluene (TNT) | 000118-96-7 | 0.5 m/M Skin | | 0.5 m/M Skin | |
| Triorthocresyl phosphate | 000078-30-8 | 0.1 m/M Skin | | 0.1 m/M Skin | |
| Triphenyl amine | 000603-34-9 | 5 m/M | | 5 m/M | |
| Triphenyl phosphate | 000115-86-6 | 3 m/M | | 3 m/M | |
| Tripoli (silica—crystalline) | 001317-95-9 | 0.1 m/M | | 0.1 m/M | |
| Tungsten [7440-33-7] and insoluble compounds, as W | | 5 m/M | 10 m/M | 5 m/M | 10 m/M |
| Tungsten, soluble compounds, as W | | 1 m/M | 3 m/M | 1 m/M | 3 m/M |
| Turpentine | 008006-64-2 | 100 ppm | | 100 ppm | |
| 1-Undecanethiol | 005332-52-5 | | | | |
| Uranium (natural [7440-61-1], soluble and insolube compounds), as U | | 0.2 m/M | 0.5 m/M | 0.05 m/M | 0.6 m/M |
| *n*-Valeraldehyde | 000110-62-3 | 50 ppm | | 50 ppm | |
| Vanadium pentoxide, as $V_2O_5$, respirable dust or fume | 001314-62-1 | | 0.05 m/M | | 0.05 m/M |
| Vegetable oil mists | | 10 m/M | | 15 m/M | |
| Vinyl acetate | 000108-05-4 | 10 ppm A3 | 15 ppm A3 | 10 ppm | 20 ppm |
| Vinyl benzene (styrene, monomer) | 000100-42-5 | 50 ppm Skin | 100 ppm Skin | 50 ppm | 100 ppm |
| Vinyl bromide | 000593-60-2 | 5 ppm A2 | | 5 ppm | |
| Vinyl chloride (chloroethylene) | 000075-01-4 | 5 ppm A1 | | 1 ppm | 5 ppm |
| Vinyl cyanide (acrylonitrile) | 000107-13-1 | 2 ppm Skin A2 | | 2 ppm | C10 ppm |
| Vinyl cyclohexene | 000100-40-3 | 0.1 ppm A2 | | | |
| Vinyl cyclohexene dioxide | 000106-87-6 | 10 ppm Skin A2 | | 10 ppm Skin | |
| Vinyl fluoride | 000072-02-5 | | | | |
| Vinylidene chloride (1,1-dichloroethylene) | 000075-35-4 | 5 ppm | 20 ppm | 1 ppm | |
| Vinylidene fluoride monomer (1,1-difluoroethylene) | 000075-38-7 | | | | |
| Vinyl toluene (methyl styrene, all isomers) | 025013-15-4 | 50 ppm | 100 ppm | 100 ppm | |
| VM & P Naphtha | 008032-32-4 | 300 ppm | | 300 ppm | 400 ppm |
| Warfarin | 000081-81-2 | 0.1 m/M | | 0.1 m/M | |
| Welding fumes (NOC)* (*not otherwise classified) | | 5 m/M | | 5 m/M | |
| Wood dust (certain hard woods as beech and oak) | | 1 m/M | | 5 m/M | 10 m/M |
| Wood dust, soft wood | | 5 m/M | 10 m/M | 5 m/M | 10 m/M |
| Wood dust, western red cedar | | | | 2.5 m/M | |
| Xylene (*o*-, *m*-, *p*-isomers) 1330-20-7; 95-47-6; 108-38-3; 106-42-3 | | 100 ppm | 150 ppm | 100 ppm | 150 ppm |
| *m*-Xylene *a*,*a*′-diamine | 001477-55-0 | | C0.1 m/M | | C0.1 m/M |
| Xylidine (mixed isomers) | 001300-73-8 | 0.5 ppm A2 Skin | | 2 ppm Skin | |
| 2,4-Xylidine | 000095-68-1 | | | | |
| Yttrium [7440-65-5] metal and compounds, as Y | | 1 m/M | | 1 m/M | |
| Zinc beryllium silicate, as Be | 039413-47-3 | 0.0002 m/M A2 | | 0.0002 m/M | C0.0005 m/M |
| Zinc chloride fume | 007646-85-7 | 1 m/M | 2 m/M | 1 m/M | 2 m/M |

| NAME | CAS NO. | ACGIH TLV | | OSHA PEL | |
|---|---|---|---|---|---|
| | | TWA | STEL | TWA | STEL |
| Zinc chromates, as Cr 13530-65-9; 11103-86-9; 37300-23-5 | | 0.02 m/M A1 | | | C0.1 m/M |
| Zinc oxide, dust | 001314-13-2 | 10 m/M | | 10 m/M | |
| Zinc oxide, fume | 001314-13-2 | 5 m/M | 10 m/M | 5 m/M | 10 m/M |
| Zinc stearate | 000557-05-1 | 10 m/M | | 10 m/M | |
| Zirconium (7440-67-7) compounds, as Zr | | 5 m/M | 10 m/M | 5 m/M | 10 m/M |

**1994 EPA Drinking Water Standards and Health Advisories**

| | STANDARDS | | HEALTH ADVISORIES |
|---|---|---|---|
| CHEMICALS | MCLG (mg/L) | MCL (mg/L) | RfD (mg/kg/day) |
| Acenaphthene | — | — | 0.06 |
| Acifluorfen | Zero | — | 0.013 |
| Acrylamide | Zero | TT | 0.002 |
| Acrylonitrile | Zero | — | — |
| Adipate (diethylhexyl) | 0.4 | 0.4 | 0.6 |
| Alachlor | Zero | 0.002 | 0.01 |
| Aldicarb | 0.007 | 0.007 | 0.001 |
| Aldicarb sulfone | 0.007 | 0.007 | 0.001 |
| Aldicarb sulfoxide | 0.007 | 0.007 | 0.001 |
| Aldrin | — | — | 0.00003 |
| Ametryn | — | — | 0.009 |
| Ammonium sulfamate | — | — | 0.28 |
| Anthracene (PAH) | — | — | 0.3 |
| Atrazine | 0.003 | 0.003 | 0.035 |
| Baygon | — | — | 0.004 |
| Bentazon | 0.02 | — | 0.0025 |
| Benz(a)anthracene (PAH) | Zero | 0.0001 | — |
| Benzene | Zero | 0.005 | — |
| Benzo(a)pyrene (PAH) | Zero | 0.0002 | — |
| Benzo(b)fluoranthene (PAH) | Zero | 0.0002 | — |
| Benzo(k)fluoranthene (PAH) | Zero | 0.0002 | — |
| *bis*-2-Chloroisopropyl ether | — | — | 0.04 |
| Bromacil | — | — | 0.13 |
| Bromochloromethane | — | — | 0.013 |
| Bromodichloromethane (THM) | Zero | 0.1/0.08 | 0.02 |
| Bromoform (THM) | Zero | 0.1/0.08 | 0.02 |
| Bromomethane | — | — | 0.001 |
| Butyl benzyl phthalate (PAE) | Zero | 0.1 | 0.2 |
| Butylate | — | — | 0.05 |
| Carbaryl | — | — | 0.1 |
| Carbofuran | 0.04 | 0.04 | 0.005 |
| Carbon tetrachloride | Zero | 0.005 | 0.0007 |
| Carboxin | — | — | 0.1 |
| Chloral hydrate | 0.04 | 0.06 | 0.0002 |
| Chloramben | — | — | 0.015 |
| Chlordane | Zero | 0.002 | 0.00006 |
| Chlorodibromomethane (THM) | 0.06 | 0.1/0.08 | 0.02 |
| Chloroform (THM) | Zero | 0.1/0.08 | 0.01 |
| Chloromethane | — | — | 0.004 |
| Chlorophenol (2-) | — | — | 0.005 |
| Chlorothalonil | — | — | 0.015 |
| *o*-Chlorotoluene | — | — | 0.02 |
| *p*-Chlorotoluene | — | — | 0.02 |
| Chlorpyrifos | — | — | 0.003 |
| Chrysene (PAH) | Zero | 0.0002 | — |
| Cyanazine | 0.001 | — | 0.002 |
| *p*-Cymene | — | — | — |
| 2,4-D | 0.07 | 0.07 | 0.01 |
| DCPA (dacthal) | — | — | 0.5 |
| Dalapon | 0.2 | 0.2 | 0.026 |
| Di[2-ethylhexyl]adipate | 0.4 | 0.4 | 0.6 |
| Diazinon | — | — | 0.00009 |
| Dibenz(a,h)anthracene (PAH) | Zero | 0.0003 | — |
| Dibromoacetonitrile | — | — | 0.02 |
| Dibromochloropropane (DBCP) | Zero | 0.0002 | — |

| CHEMICALS | STANDARDS MCLG (mg/L) | STANDARDS MCL (mg/L) | HEALTH ADVISORIES RfD (mg/kg/day) |
|---|---|---|---|
| Dibutyl phthalate (PAE) | — | — | 0.1 |
| Dicamba | — | — | 0.03 |
| Dichloroacetic acid | Zero | 0.06 | 0.004 |
| Dichloroacetonitrile | — | — | 0.008 |
| *o*-Dichlorobenzene | 0.6 | 0.6 | 0.09 |
| *m*-Dichlorobenzene | 0.6 | 0.6 | 0.09 |
| *p*-Dichlorobenzene | 0.075 | 0.075 | 0.1 |
| Dichlorodifluoromethane | — | — | 0.2 |
| 1,2-Dichloroethane | Zero | 0.005 | — |
| 1,1-Dichloroethylene | 0.007 | 0.007 | 0.009 |
| *cis*-1,2-Dichloroethylene | 0.07 | 0.07 | 0.01 |
| *trans*-1,2-Dichloroethylene | 0.1 | 0.1 | 0.02 |
| Dichloromethane | Zero | 0.005 | 0.06 |
| 2,4-Dichlorophenol | — | — | 0.003 |
| 1,2-Dichloropropane | Zero | 0.005 | — |
| 1,3-Dichloropropene | Zero | — | 0.0003 |
| Dieldrin | — | — | 0.00005 |
| Diethyl phthalate (PAE) | — | — | 0.8 |
| Diethylhexyl phthalate (PAE) | Zero | 0.006 | 0.02 |
| Diisopropyl methylphosphonate | — | — | 0.08 |
| Dimethrin | — | — | 0.3 |
| Dimethyl methylphosphonate | — | — | 0.2 |
| 1,3-Dinitrobenzene | — | — | 0.0001 |
| 2,4-Dinitrotoluene | — | — | 0.002 |
| 2,6-Dinitrotoluene | — | — | 0.001 |
| Dinoseb | 0.007 | 0.007 | 0.001 |
| Diphenamid | — | — | 0.03 |
| Diphenylamine | — | — | 0.03 |
| Diquat | 0.02 | 0.02 | 0.0022 |
| Disulfoton | — | — | 0.00004 |
| 1,4-Dithiane | — | — | 0.01 |
| Diuron | — | — | 0.002 |
| Endothall | 0.1 | 0.1 | 0.02 |
| Endrin | 0.002 | 0.002 | 0.0003 |
| Epichlorohydrin | Zero | TT | 0.002 |
| Ethylbenzene | 0.7 | 0.7 | 0.1 |
| Ethylene dibromide (EDB) | Zero | 0.00005 | — |
| Ethylene glycol | — | — | 0.00008 |
| ETU | — | — | 0.00025 |
| Fenamiphos | — | — | 0.00025 |
| Fluometron | — | — | 0.013 |
| Fluorene (PAH) | — | — | 0.04 |
| Fluorotrichloromethane | — | — | 0.3 |
| Fonofos | — | — | 0.002 |
| Formaldehyde | — | — | 0.15 |
| Glyphosate | 0.7 | 0.7 | 0.1 |
| Heptachlor | Zero | 0.0004 | 0.0005 |
| Heptachlor epoxide | Zero | 0.0002 | 1E-5 |
| Hexachlorobenzene | Zero | 0.001 | 0.0008 |
| Hexachlorobutadiene | 0.001 | — | 0.002 |
| Hexachlorocyclopentadiene | 0.05 | 0.05 | 0.007 |
| Hexachloroethane | — | — | 0.001 |
| Hexazinone | — | — | 0.033 |
| HMX | — | — | 0.05 |
| Indeno(1,2,3,-c,d)pyrene (PAH) | Zero | 0.0004 | — |
| Isophorone | — | — | 0.2 |
| Isopropyl methylphosphonate | — | — | 0.1 |

| CHEMICALS | STANDARDS | | HEALTH ADVISORIES |
|---|---|---|---|
| | MCLG (mg/L) | MCL (mg/L) | RfD (mg/kg/day) |
| Lindane | 0.0002 | 0.0002 | 0.0003 |
| Malathion | — | — | 0.02 |
| Maleic hydrazide | — | — | 0.5 |
| MCPA | — | — | 0.0015 |
| Methomyl | — | — | 0.025 |
| Methoxychlor | 0.04 | 0.04 | 0.005 |
| Methyl parathion | — | — | 0.00025 |
| Methyl tert butyl ether | — | — | 0.005 |
| Metolachlor | — | — | 0.1 |
| Metribuzin | — | — | 0.025 |
| Monochlorobenzene | 0.1 | 0.1 | 0.02 |
| Naphthalene | — | — | 0.004 |
| Nitroguanidine | — | — | 0.1 |
| *p*-Nitrophenol | — | — | 0.008 |
| Oxamyl (vydate) | 0.2 | 0.2 | 0.025 |
| Paraquat | — | — | 0.0045 |
| Pentachlorophenol | Zero | 0.001 | 0.03 |
| Phenol | — | — | 0.6 |
| Picloram | 0.5 | 0.5 | 0.07 |
| Polychlorinated biphenyls (PCBs) | Zero | 0.0005 | — |
| Prometon | — | — | 0.015 |
| Pronamide | — | — | 0.075 |
| Propachlor | — | — | 0.013 |
| Propazine | — | — | 0.02 |
| Propham | — | — | 0.02 |
| Pyrene (PAH) | — | — | 0.03 |
| RDX | — | — | 0.003 |
| Simazine | 0.004 | 0.004 | 0.005 |
| Styrene | 0.1 | 0.1 | 0.2 |
| 2,4,5-T | — | — | 0.01 |
| 2,3,7,8-TCDD (dioxin) | Zero | 3E-08 | 1E-09 |
| Tebuthiuron | — | — | 0.07 |
| Terbacil | — | — | 0.013 |
| Terbufos | — | — | 0.00013 |
| 1,1,1,2-Tetrachloroethane | — | — | 0.03 |
| Tetrachloroethylene | Zero | 0.005 | 0.01 |
| Toluene | 1 | 1 | 0.2 |
| Toxaphene | Zero | 0.003 | 0.1 |
| 2,4,5-TP | 0.05 | 0.05 | 0.0075 |
| Trichloroacetic acid | 0.3 | 0.06 | 0.1 |
| 1,2,4-Trichlorobenzene | 0.07 | 0.07 | 0.01 |
| 1,3,5-Trichlorobenzene | — | — | 0.006 |
| 1,1,1-Trichloroethane | 0.2 | 0.2 | 0.035 |
| 1,1,2-Trichloroethane | 0.003 | 0.005 | 0.004 |
| Trichloroethylene | Zero | 0.005 | — |
| 1,2,3-Trichloropropane | — | — | 0.006 |
| Trifluralin | — | — | 0.0075 |
| Trinitrotoluene | — | — | 0.0005 |
| Vinyl chloride | Zero | 0.002 | 0.0005 |
| Xylenes | 10 | 10 | 2 |
| Antimony | 0.006 | 0.006 | 0.0004 |
| Arsenic | — | 0.05 | — |
| Asbestos (fibers/L>10 mm length) | 7 MFL | 7 MFL | — |
| Barium | 2 | 2 | 0.07 |
| Beryllium | 0.004 | 0.004 | 0.005 |
| Boron | — | — | 0.09 |
| Bromate | Zero | 0.01 | — |

| CHEMICALS | STANDARDS | | HEALTH ADVISORIES |
|---|---|---|---|
| | MCLG (mg/L) | MCL (mg/L) | RfD (mg/kg/day) |
| Cadmium | 0.005 | 0.005 | 0.0005 |
| Chloramine | 4 | 4 | 0.1 |
| Chlorine | 4 | 4 | 0.1 |
| Chlorine dioxide | 0.3 | 0.8 | 0.01 |
| Chlorite | 0.08 | 1 | 0.003 |
| Chromium (total) | 0.1 | 0.1 | — |
| Copper | 1.3 | TT | — |
| Cyanide | 0.2 | 0.2 | 0.022 |
| Fluoride | 4 | 4 | 0.12 |
| Hypochlorite | 4[1] | — | — |
| Hypochlorous acid | 4[1] | — | — |
| Lead (at tap) | Zero | TT | — |
| Manganese | — | — | 0.14[2], 0.005[3] |
| Mercury (inorganic) | 0.002 | 0.002 | 0.0003 |
| Molybdenum | — | — | 0.005 |
| Nickel | 0.1 | 0.1 | 0.02 |
| Nitrate (as N) | 10 | 10 | 1.6 |
| Nitrite (as N) | 1 | 1 | 0.16 |
| Nitrate + nitrite (both as N) | 10 | 10 | — |
| Selenium | 0.05 | 0.05 | 0.005 |
| Silver | — | — | 0.005 |
| Strontium | — | — | 0.6 |
| Thallium | 0.0005 | 0.002 | 0.00007 |
| White phosphorous | — | — | 0.00002 |
| Zinc | — | — | 0.3 |
| Zinc chloride (measured as zinc) | — | — | 0.3 |

TT, under review.

[1]Regulated as chlorine.

[2]In food.

[3]In water.

# INDEX

## D

## H

**J**

## Q



## R

## T

## U



## V

**W**

ISBN 0-07-105476-6